DELMAR'S
Comprehensive
Medical
Assisting

Administrative and Clinical Competencies

Wilburta Q. Lindh, CMA (AAMA)

Marilyn S. Pooler, RN, MEd, RMA (AMT)

Carol D. Tamparo, CMA (AAMA), PhD

Barbara M. Dahl, CMA (AAMA), CPC

Julie A. Morris, RN, BSN, CBCS, CCMA, CMAA

Angela P. Rein, RMA (AMT), AS, BSHM, CPC MAHS, CPC-H

FIFTH EDITION

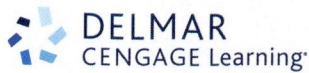

DELMAR
CENGAGE Learning®

Australia • Brazil • Japan • Korea • Mexico • Singapore • Spain • United Kingdom • United States

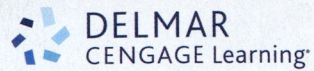

DELMAR
CENGAGE Learning®

Delmar's Comprehensive Medical Assisting: Administrative and Clinical Competencies, Fifth Edition

Wilburta Q. Lindh, Marilyn S. Pooler, Carol D. Tamparo, Barbara M. Dahl, Julie A. Morris

Vice President, Careers & Computing: Dave Garza

Publisher: Stephen Helba

Executive Editor: Rhonda Dearborn

Director, Development-Career and Computing: Marah Bellegarde

Product Development Manager: Juliet Steiner

Product Manager: Lauren Whalen

Editorial Assistant: Courtney Cozzy

Executive Brand Manager: Wendy Mapstone

Senior Market Development Manager: Nancy Bradshaw

Senior Production Director: Wendy Troeger

Production Manager: Andrew Crouth

Content Project Manager: Brooke Greenhouse

Senior Art Director: Jack Pendleton

Technology Project Manager: Brian Davis

Media Editor: William Overocker

Cover image(s): www.Shutterstock.com

© 2014, 2010, 2006, 2002, 1997 Delmar, Cengage Learning

ALL RIGHTS RESERVED. No part of this work covered by the copyright herein may be reproduced, transmitted, stored, or used in any form or by any means graphic, electronic, or mechanical, including but not limited to photocopying, recording, scanning, digitizing, taping, Web distribution, information networks, or information storage and retrieval systems, except as permitted under Section 107 or 108 of the 1976 United States Copyright Act, without the prior written permission of the publisher.

For product information and technology assistance, contact us at
Cengage Learning Customer & Sales Support, 1-800-354-9706

For permission to use material from this text or product,
submit all requests online at **www.cengage.com/permissions**
Further permissions questions can be e-mailed to
permissionrequest@cengage.com

Library of Congress Control Number: 2013933619

Book Only ISBN-13: 978-1-1336-0283-5

Package ISBN-13: 978-1-1336-0286-6

Delmar
5 Maxwell Drive
Clifton Park, NY 12065-2919
USA

Cengage Learning is a leading provider of customized learning solutions with office locations around the globe, including Singapore, the United Kingdom, Australia, Mexico, Brazil, and Japan. Locate your local office at: **international.cengage.com/region**

Cengage Learning products are represented in Canada by Nelson Education, Ltd.

To learn more about Delmar, visit **www.cengage.com/delmar**

Purchase any of our products at your local college store or at our preferred online store **www.cengagebrain.com**

Notice to the Reader

Publisher does not warrant or guarantee any of the products described herein or perform any independent analysis in connection with any of the product information contained herein. Publisher does not assume, and expressly disclaims, any obligation to obtain and include information other than that provided to it by the manufacturer. The reader is expressly warned to consider and adopt all safety precautions that might be indicated by the activities described herein and to avoid all potential hazards. By following the instructions contained herein, the reader willingly assumes all risks in connection with such instructions. The publisher makes no representations or warranties of any kind, including but not limited to, the warranties of fitness for particular purpose or merchantability, nor are any such representations implied with respect to the material set forth herein, and the publisher takes no responsibility with respect to such material. The publisher shall not be liable for any special, consequential, or exemplary damages resulting, in whole or part, from the readers' use of, or reliance upon, this material.

Printed in the United States of America
1 2 3 4 5 6 7 17 16 15 14 13

Table of Contents

List of Procedures xiii
How to Use the Book xvi
Preface xx
About the Authors xxvi
Acknowledgments xxviii
Contributors xxx
Reviewers xxxi

SECTION I: GENERAL PROCEDURES   1

Unit I: Introduction to Medical Assisting and Health Professions   3

Chapter 1: The Medical Assisting Profession   4

Historical Perspective of the
Profession 6
Career Opportunities 7
Education of the Medical Assistant 7
Courses in a Medical Assisting Program 8
Practicum 8
Associate and Bachelor Degrees 8
Accreditation of Medical Assisting
Programs 9
CAAHEP 9
ABHES 9
Attributes of a Medical Assistant
Professional 9
Communication 12
Presentation 12
Competency 14
Initiative 14
Integrity 15
American Association of Medical
Assistants 15
Certification 16
Continuing Education 16
American Medical Technologists 16
Registered Medical Assistant 17
Certified Medical Administrative
Specialist 17
Continuing Education 17
Other Certification 17
National Healthcareer Association 17
National Center for Competency
Testing (NCCT) 17
Regulation of Health Care Providers 18
Scope of Practice 18

Chapter 2: Health Care Settings and the Health Care Team   22

Ambulatory Health Care Settings 24
Individual and Group Medical
Practices 24
Urgent Care Centers 26
Managed Care Operations 26
"Boutique" or "Concierge"
Medical Practices 26
The Health Care Team 27
The Title "Doctor" 27
Health Care Professionals and
Their Roles 27
Integrative Medicine and
Alternative Health Care Practitioners 28
Future of Integrative Medicine 31
Allied Health Professionals
and Their Roles 32
The Role of the Medical Assistant 32
Health Unit Coordinator 33
Medical Laboratory Technologist 33
Registered Dietitian 33
Pharmacist 35
Pharmacy Technician 35
Phlebotomist 35
Physical Therapist 35
Physical Therapy Assistant 35
Nurse 35
Physician Assistant 36
The Value of the Medical
Assistant to the Health Care Team 36

Chapter 3: History of Medicine   40

Cultural Heritage in Medicine 42
Medical Specialists in History 43
History of Medical Education 43
History of Attitudes
Toward Illness 44
Historical Medical Treatments 44
The Scourge of Epidemics 46
Other Threats to Health 47
Significant Contributions
to Medicine 48
Women in Medicine 48
Frontiers in Medicine 48

Unit II: The Therapeutic Approach   55

Chapter 4: Coping Skills for the Medical Assistant   56

What Is Stress? 58
The Body's Response to Stress 59

Factors Causing Stress 59
Stress in the Work Environment 60
Effect of Prolonged Stress—Burnout 61
Persons Most Vulnerable to Burnout 62
General Stress Management
Techniques 62
Goal Setting as a Stress Reliever 63

Chapter 5: Therapeutic Communication Skills   68

Importance of Communication 70
The Communication Cycle 70
The Sender 70
The Message 71
The Receiver 71
Feedback 71
Listening Skills 72
Types of Communication 72
Verbal Communication 72
Nonverbal Communication 73
Congruency in Communication 76
Factors Affecting Therapeutic
Communication 76
Age Barriers 76
Economic Barriers 76
Education and Life Experience
Barriers 76
Bias and Prejudice Barriers 78
Verbal Roadblocks to Therapeutic
Communication 78
Defense Mechanisms as Barriers 78
Barriers Caused by Cultural
and Religious Diversity 80
Human Needs as Barriers
to Therapeutic Communication 82
Maslow's Hierarchy of Needs 82
Patients with Special Needs 83
Environmental Factors 83
Time Factors 84
Establishing Multicultural
Communication 84
Cultural Brokering 84
Therapeutic Communication in Action ... 85
Interview Techniques 85
Point of Care Techniques 86
Community Resources 87

Chapter 6: The Therapeutic Approach to the Patient with a Life-Threatening Illness   92

Life-Threatening Illness 94
Cultural Perspective on
Life-Threatening Illness 94
Choices in Life-Threatening Illness 95

iv   Contents

The Range of Psychological Suffering 97
The Therapeutic Response to the
Patient with HIV/AIDS 98
The Therapeutic Response to the
Patient with Cancer 98
The Therapeutic Response to the
Patient with End-Stage Renal Disease 99
The Stages of Grief 99
Denial 99
Anger 99
Bargaining 100
Depression 100
Acceptance 100
The Challenge for the Medical
Assistant 100

Unit III: Responsible
Medical Practice   105

Chapter 7: Legal Considerations   106
Sources of Law 108
Statutory Law 109
Common Law 109
Criminal Law 109
Civil Law 110
Administrative Law 110
Title VII of the Civil Rights Act 110
Equal Pay Act of 1963 111
Federal Age Discrimination Act 111
Americans with Disabilities Act 111
Family and Medical Leave Act 111
Health Insurance Portability and
Accountability Act 112
Occupational Safety and Health Act 112
Controlled Substances Act 112
Uniform Anatomical Gift Act 113
Regulation Z of the Consumer
Protection Act 113
Medical Practice Acts 114
Contract Law 114
Termination of Contracts 115
Tort Law 115
Standard of Care and Scope of Practice . . . 115
Classification of Torts 117
Common Torts 117
Informed Consent 118
Implied Consent 120
Consent and Legal Incompetence 120
Risk Management 120
Professional Liability Coverage 121
Civil Litigation Process 121
Subpoenas 121
Discovery 122
Pretrial Conference 122
Trial 122
Statute of Limitations 123
Public Duties 124
Reportable Diseases/Injuries 124
Abuse 124
Good Samaritan Laws 125
Advance Directives 125
Living Wills/Advance Directives 129

Durable Power of Attorney for
Health Care 129
Patient Self-Determination Act 129

Chapter 8: Ethical Considerations   136
Ethics 138
Principle-Centered Leadership 140
Five Ps of Ethical Power 141
Ethics Check Questions 141
Keys to the AAMA Code of Ethics 142
Ethical Guidelines for Health
Care Providers 142
Advertising 143
Confidentiality 143
HIPAA 143
Medical Records 143
Professional Fees and Charges 143
Professional Rights and
Responsibilities 144
Disaster Response and Emergency
Preparedness 144
Treatment for a Culturally Diverse
Clientele 144
Care of the Poor 144
Abuse 144
Bioethics 146
Allocation of Scarce Medical Resources . . 146
Health Care: A Right or a Privilege? 148
HIV and AIDS 148
Reproductive Issues 148
Abortion and Fetal Tissue
Research 149
Genetic Engineering/Manipulation 150
Dying and Death 151
Hospice 151

Chapter 9: Emergency Procedures
and First Aid   156
Recognizing an Emergency 158
Responding to an Emergency 159
Primary Survey 160
Using the 911 or Emergency
Medical Services System 161
Good Samaritan Laws 161
Blood, Body Fluids, and Disease
Transmission 162
Preparing for an Emergency 162
The Medical Crash Tray
or Cart 162
Common Emergencies 164
Shock 164
Wounds 165
Burns 168
Musculoskeletal Injuries 171
Heat- and Cold-Related Illnesses 173
Poisoning 174
Sudden Illness 175
Cerebral Vascular Accident 178
Heart Attack 178
Breathing Emergencies
and Cardiac Arrest 178
Rescue Breathing 179

Cardiopulmonary Resuscitation 179
Safety and Emergency Practices 181

**SECTION II:
ADMINISTRATIVE
PROCEDURES   187**

Unit IV: Integrated
Administrative Procedures   189

Chapter 10: Creating the Facility
Environment   190
Creating a Welcoming
Environment 193
The Reception Area 193
The Receptionist 194
Cultural Considerations 195
When Children Are Patients 195
Education in the Reception Area 195
Clinic Design and Environment 196
Ventilation and Infection
Control 196
Lighting 196
Nature, Music, Water,
and Color 197
Noise Reduction 198
Legal Compliance in the Facility 198
HIPAA 198
Americans with Disabilities Act 198
Safety 199
Creating a Safe Environment 199
Evacuation Procedures 199
Fire Safety 200
Response to Natural Disaster
or Emergency 200
The Medical Assistant's Response
to Disaster Preparedness 202
Opening the Facility 202
Closing the Facility 202
The Future Environment
for Ambulatory Care 203

Chapter 11: Computers in the
Ambulatory Care Setting   210
The Computer System 212
Basic System 212
Types of Computer Systems 212
Components of a Computer
System 214
Hardware 215
Software 216
Documentation 217
Hardware and Software
Compatibility 217
Computer Networks 217
Systems Security 218
Cloud Computing 221
Computer Maintenance
by Clinic Personnel 221

Use of Computers in the Medical Clinic **222**
General Clinic Procedures 222
Electronic Health Records 222
Clinical and Laboratory Applications 223
Portable Computers in the Medical Clinic 223
Design Considerations for a Computerized Medical Clinic **223**
Software Selection 225
Hardware Selection 225
Scheduling the Changeover 226
Ergonomics **226**
Eyestrain 226
Cumulative Trauma Disorder 226
Posture 226
Patient Confidentiality in the Computerized Medical Clinic **227**
HIPAA Standards for Safeguarding Protected Health Information (PHI) **228**
Professionalism in the Computerized Medical Clinic **229**

Chapter 12: Telecommunications   **238**
Telecommunications in the Electronic Health Record Environment **240**
Basic Telephone Techniques **241**
Telephone Personality 241
Professional Telephone Etiquette 242
Answering Incoming Calls 242
Routing Calls in the Medical Clinic **245**
Types of Calls the Medical Assistant Can Take 246
Types of Calls Referred to the Provider . . 247
Special Consideration Calls 248
Telephone Documentation **250**
Using Telephone Directories **250**
Placing Outgoing Calls **251**
Placing Long-Distance Calls **251**
Legal and Ethical Considerations **252**
HIPAA Guidelines for Telephone Communications **253**
Americans with Disabilities Act (ADA) . . . **254**
Telephone Technology **254**
Automated Routing Units 254
Answering Services and Machines 255
Voice over Internet Protocol (VoIP) Telecommunications 255
Facsimile (Fax) Machines 256
Electronic Mail (Email) 257
Clinical Email 259
Interactive Videoconferencing 260
Cellular Service 261
Professionalism in Telecommunications . **261**

Chapter 13: Patient Scheduling   **270**
Tailoring the Scheduling System **272**
Scheduling Styles **273**
Open Hours 273
Double Booking 273
Clustering 275

Wave Scheduling 275
Modified Wave Scheduling 275
Stream Scheduling 275
Practice-Based Scheduling 276
Analyzing Patient Flow **276**
Waiting Time 277
Legal Issues **277**
Interpersonal Skills **277**
Guidelines for Scheduling Appointments **278**
Screening Calls 278
Referral Appointments 278
Recording Information 278
Appointment Matrix 279
Telephone Appointments 279
Patient Check-In 280
Patient Cancellation and Appointment Changes 280
Reminder Systems 281
Scheduling Pharmaceutical Representatives 282
Scheduling Software and Materials **282**
Appointment Schedule 282
Computer Scheduling Software 283
Inpatient and Outpatient Admissions Procedures **283**

Chapter 14: Medical Records Management   **294**
The Purpose of Medical Records **296**
Ownership of Medical Records **296**
Authorization to Release Information **297**
Manual or Electronic Medical Records . . . **297**
The Importance of Accurate Medical Records **299**
Creating Paper and Electronic Charts 299
Correcting Medical Records 299
Types of Medical Records **300**
Problem-Oriented Medical Record 300
Source-Oriented Medical Record 301
Strict Chronological Arrangement 301
Equipment and Supplies **301**
Vertical Files 301
Open-Shelf Lateral Files 301
Movable File Units 302
File Folders 302
Identification Labels 302
Guides and Positions 302
Out Guides 303
Basic Rules for Filing **303**
Indexing Units 303
Filing Patient Charts 304
Filing Identical Names 305
Steps for Filing Medical Documentation in Patient Files **305**
Inspect 305
Index 305
Code 305
Sort 305
File 306

Filing Techniques and Common Filing Systems **306**
Color Coding 306
Alphabetic Filing 308
Numeric Filing 308
Subject Filing 309
Choosing a Filing System 310
Filing Procedures **311**
Cross-Referencing 311
Tickler Files 312
Release Marks 312
Checkout System 313
Locating Missing Files or Data 313
Filing Chart Data 313
Retention and Purging 314
Correspondence **315**
Filing Procedures for Correspondence . . . 315
Electronic Medical Records **316**
Archival Storage 317
Transfer of Data 317
Confidentiality 317

Chapter 15: Written Communications   **324**
Composing Correspondence **326**
Writing Tips 326
Spelling 327
Proofreading 327
Proofreading in the Cloud 327
Components of a Business Letter **328**
Date Line 328
Inside Address 328
Salutation 329
Subject Line 329
Body of Letter 329
Complimentary Closing 331
Keyed Signature 331
Reference Initials 331
Enclosure Notation 331
Copy Notation 332
Postscripts 332
Continuation Page Heading 332
Letter Styles **332**
Full Block 333
Modified Block 333
Simplified 334
Supplies for Written Communication **334**
Letterhead 335
Second Sheets 335
Printing Multipage Business Letters 335
Envelopes 336
Mail Merge 337
Other Types of Correspondence **337**
Memoranda 337
Meeting Agendas 337
Meeting Minutes 338
Processing Incoming and Outgoing Mail **338**
Incoming Mail and Shipments 338
Outgoing Mail and Shipments 339

Postal Classes 340
Formats for Efficient Mail
Processing. 340
International Mail 341
Legal and Ethical Issues 341

Chapter 16: Medical Documents   352

**The Changing Role of Medical
Transcription. 354**
Electronic Medical Records 354
Outsourcing 355
Voice Recognition Software 356
Medical Transcriptionist as Editor 356
Authentication 357
Confidentiality and Legal Issues. 358
Health Insurance Portability and
Accountability Act Regulations 358
Protocols. 358
Types of Medical Documents 359
Chart Notes and Progress Notes 360
History and Physical Examination
Reports 360
Radiology and Imaging Reports 360
Operative Reports 361
Pathology Reports 362
Consultation. 363
Discharge Summaries 363
Autopsy Reports. 363
Correspondence. 363
Turnaround Time and Productivity 365
Medical Transcription as a Career 366
Professionalism Related to
Medical Transcription 368

**Unit V: Managing Facility
Finances   373**

Chapter 17: Medical Insurance   374

**Understanding the Role of Health
Insurance. 376**
Medical Insurance Terminology 377
Terminology Specific to Insurance
Policies 377
Terminology Specific to Billing
Insurance Carriers 380
**Types of Medical Insurance
Coverage 380**
Traditional Insurance 380
Managed Care Insurance 382
Medicare. 384
Medicare Supplemental Insurance. 386
Medicaid Insurance 386
TRICARE 387
Civilian Health and Medical Program
of the Veterans Administration. 387
Workers' Compensation Insurance 387
Self-Insurance. 388
Medical Tourism Insurance. 388
Screening for Insurance 388
Referrals and Authorizations 389
Determining Fee Schedules 390
Usual, Customary, and Reasonable Fees. . . 390
Resource-Based Relative Value Scale
(RBRVS) 390

Diagnosis-Related Groups 391
Hospital Inpatient Prospective
Payment System 391
Hospital Outpatient Prospective
Payment System 391
Capitation. 392
Legal and Ethical Issues 392
Insurance Fraud and Abuse 392
Professional Careers in Insurance 393

**Chapter 18: Medical Insurance
Coding   400**

Insurance Coding Systems Overview 402
ICD-10-CM and ICD-10-PCS 402
Coding of Medical Procedures. 403
CPT Manual Organization and Use 404
Modifiers. 406
**Healthcare Common Procedure
Coding System (HCPCS) 406**
Coding of Medical Diagnoses 406
ICD-9-CM Manual Organization
and Use. 406
External Cause Codes (E Codes) 407
Supplementary Health Factor
Codes (V Codes) 407
Morphology Codes (M Codes) 408
Code References 408
Coding Accuracy 408
Coding the Claim Form 409
Third-Party Guidelines 412
Completing the CMS-1500 (08-05) 412
Uniform Bill 04 Form 415
Using the Computer to Complete
Forms 415
Common Errors in Completing
Claim Forms. 417
**Benefits of Submitting Claims
Electronically. 417**
Managing the Claims Process 417
Documentation of Referrals 417
Point-of-Service Device 417
Maintaining a Claims Registry. 418
Following Up on Claims 418
The Insurance Carrier's Role 419
Explanation of Benefits. 419
Legal and Ethical Issues 419
Compliance Programs. 419

**Chapter 19: Daily Financial
Practices   430**

Patient Fees. 432
Helping Patients Who
Cannot Pay 432
Determining Patient Fees 432
Discussion of Fees 433
Adjustment of Fees 433
Credit Arrangements. 434
Payment Planning 434
The Bookkeeping Function. 434
Managing Patient Accounts. 434
Recording Patient Transactions 436
Encounter Form. 436
Patient Account or Ledger 437
Day Sheet 439

Receipts 439
Month-End Activities 439
Computerized Patient Accounts. 440
Banking Procedures 440
Online Banking 440
Types of Accounts 441
Types of Checks 443
Depositing Checks 443
Cash on Hand 443
Accepting Checks. 444
Lost or Stolen Checks 445
Writing and Recording Checks. 445
Reconciling a Bank Statement 445
**Purchasing Supplies
and Equipment 446**
Preparing a Purchase Order 446
Verifying Goods Received 448
Petty Cash 448
Establishing a Petty Cash Fund 448
Tracking, Balancing, and
Replenishing Petty Cash 448

**Chapter 20: Billing and
Collections   462**

Billing Procedures. 464
Credit and Collection Policies 465
Payment at Time of Service 465
Truth-In-Lending Act. 466
**Components of a Complete
Statement 466**
Computerized Statements. 467
Monthly and Cycle Billing. 468
Monthly Billing 468
Cycle Billing 469
Past-Due Accounts. 469
Collection Process. 469
Collection Ratio 469
Accounts Receivable Ratio 470
Aging Accounts 470
Computerized Aging 470
Collection Techniques 470
Billing Insurance Carriers 471
Telephone Collections. 472
Collection Letters. 472
**Use of an Outside Collection
Agency. 472**
Use of Small Claims Court 474
Special Collection Situations 475
Bankruptcy. 475
Estates. 475
Tracing "Skips". 475
Statute of Limitations 475
Maintain a Professional Attitude. 476

**Chapter 21: Accounting
Practices   484**

**Bookkeeping and
Accounting Systems. 486**
Single-Entry System 486
Pegboard System 487
Double-Entry System 487
Total Practice Management System 487
Computer and Billing Service
Bureaus. 488
Day-End Summary. 489

Tips for Finding Errors 489
Accounts Receivable Trial Balance 489
Accounts Payable **490**
Disbursement Records. 490
The Accounting Function **490**
Cost Analysis **491**
Fixed Costs 491
Variable Costs. 491
Financial Records **491**
Income Statement 491
Balance Sheet. 491
Useful Financial Data **491**
Accounts Receivable Ratio 494
Collection Ratio. 494
Cost Ratio 494
Legal and Ethical Guidelines **494**
Bonding 495
Payroll. 495

SECTION III: CLINICAL PROCEDURES   499

Unit VI: Integrated Clinical Procedures   501

Chapter 22: Infection Control and Medical Asepsis   502

Impact of Infectious Diseases. 505
The Process of Infection **505**
Growth Requirements for
Microorganisms 506
Infection Cycle **506**
Infectious Agents 506
Reservoir. 511
Portal of Exit 511
Modes of Transmission 513
Portal of Entry 514
Susceptible Host. 514
The Body's Defense Mechanisms
for Fighting Infection and Disease 515
The Body's Natural Barriers 515
Inflammatory Response. 516
The Immune System and Immunity. 516
Stages of Infectious Diseases **518**
Incubation Stage 518
Prodromal Stage 519
Acute Stage. 519
Acme. 519
Declining Stage 519
Convalescent Stage 519
Sequelae 519
Disease Transmission **519**
Human Immunodeficiency
Virus and Hepatitis B and C **526**
HIV and AIDS 526
Acute Viral Hepatitis Diseases. 526
Reporting Infectious Disease **529**
Standard Precautions **529**
Transmission-Based Precautions. 531
Blood and Body Fluids. 533
Personal Protective Equipment. 536
Needlestick. 536
Disposal of Infectious Waste 537

Federal Organizations and
Infection Control. 538
OSHA Regulations **539**
The Bloodborne Pathogen Standard 539
OSHA Regulations and Students **546**
Avoiding Exposure to Bloodborne
Pathogens 546
Principles of Infection Control. 547
Medical Asepsis. 547
Hand Washing 548
Sanitization. 548
Disinfection 550
Sterilization 551
Bioterrorism **551**

Chapter 23: The Patient History and Documentation   564

The Purpose of the Medical History **566**
Preparing for the Patient **567**
A Cross-Cultural Model. 567
Patient Information Forms **568**
Demographic Data Form. 568
Financial Information Form 568
Privacy Information Form 568
Release of Information Form 568
Medical History Form 568
Computerized Health History **571**
The Patient Intake Interview **571**
Interacting with the Patient 571
Displaying Cultural Awareness 572
Being Sensitive to Patient Needs. 573
Approaching Sensitive Topics 573
Communication across the Life Span 574
The Medical Health History **574**
SOAP/SOAPER and CHEDDAR 574
Chief Complaint. 575
History of Present Illness. 576
Medical History 576
Family History 577
Social History 577
Review of Systems (ROS) 577
The Patient Record and
its Importance **579**
HIPAA Compliance 580
Contents of Medical Records 580
Continuity of Care Record 580
Methods of Charting/Documentation . . . 581
Source-Oriented Medical Records 581
Problem-Oriented Medical Records. 581
Electronic Medical Records (EMR) **583**
Rules of Charting **583**
Abbreviations Used in Charting 585
Chart Organization 587

Chapter 24: Vital Signs and Measurements   592

The Importance of Accuracy **594**
Temperature **594**
Terms Used to Describe Body
Temperature. 595
Phaseout of Mercury Thermometers
and Other Mercury-Containing
Equipment 597
Types of Thermometers. 597

Measuring Temperature 599
Recording Temperature 600
Cleaning and Storage of
Thermometers 601
Pulse **601**
Pulse Sites 601
Measuring and Evaluating a Pulse 602
Normal Pulse Rates 602
Pulse Abnormalities. 602
Recording Pulse Rates 603
Respiration **603**
Respiration Rate. 603
Abnormalities. 603
Blood Pressure **604**
Equipment for Measuring Blood
Pressure 605
Measuring Blood Pressure. 608
Recording Blood Pressure
Measurement 609
Normal Blood Pressure Readings 609
Blood Pressure Abnormalities. 609
Height and Weight. 611
Height. 611
Weight. 611
Significance of Weight. 613
Measuring Chest Circumference **613**

Chapter 25: The Physical Examination   628

Methods of Examination. 630
Observation or Inspection. 630
Palpation. 631
Percussion. 631
Auscultation 632
Mensuration 632
Manipulation 633
Positioning and Draping **633**
Examination Positions. 633
Equipment and Supplies for
the Physical Examination **636**
Basic Components of a Physical
Examination **636**
Patient Appearance 638
Gait 638
Stature. 638
Posture. 638
Body Movements 638
Speech 638
Breath Odors 638
Weight. 639
Skin and Appendages 639
The Physical Examination Sequence **639**
Head 639
Eyes 642
Ears 642
Nose 642
Mouth and Throat. 643
Neck 643
Chest. 643
Breast 643
Abdomen 643
Genitals. 643
Rectum 644
Reflexes 644
After the Examination. 644

Unit VII: Assisting with Specialty Examinations and Procedures   651

Chapter 26: Obstetrics and Gynecology   652

Obstetrics **655**
Initial Prenatal Visit 655
Subsequent or Return Prenatal Visits 659
Disorders of Pregnancy 662
Parturition 667
Postpartum Period 668
Contraception 668
Gynecology **673**
The Gynecologic Examination 674
Gynecologic Diseases and Conditions . . 684
Other Diagnostic Tests and Treatments
for Reproductive System Diseases 686
Complementary Therapy in
Obstetrics and Gynecology 693

Chapter 27: Pediatrics   706

What Is Pediatrics? **708**
Preparation of Vaccines for
Administration 709
Recommended Vaccination
Schedule 717
Considerations for Vaccine
Administration 718
Giving Injections to Pediatric
Patients 720
Theories of Growth and
Development **723**
Newborns 723
Infants 723
Toddlers 725
Preschoolers 725
School-Aged Children 726
Adolescents 726
Growth Patterns **727**
Length and Weight Measurements 727
Infant Holds and Positions 727
Height and Weight Measuring
Devices 730
Measuring Head Circumference 731
Measuring Chest Circumference 732
Infant/Child Failure to Thrive 733
Pediatric Vital Signs **733**
Temperature 733
Pulse 733
Respirations 734
Blood Pressure 734
Collecting a Urine Specimen from
an Infant **734**
Screening Infants for Hearing
Impairment **735**
Screening Infant and Child
Visual Acuity **735**
Common Disorders and Diseases **736**
Otitis Media 736
The Common Cold 737
Tonsillitis 737
Pediculosis 737
Asthma 737

Croup 738
Pertussis (Whooping Cough) 738
Respiratory Syncytial Virus 738
Attention Deficit Hyperactivity
Disorder 738
Child Abuse 738
Male Circumcision **739**

Chapter 28: Male Reproductive System   752

Anatomy of Male Reproductive
System **754**
External Anatomy 754
Internal Anatomy 756
Disorders of the Penis **757**
Priapism 757
Erectile Dysfunction 757
Penile Cancer 757
Other Disorders of the Penis 758
Disorders of the Testes **758**
Testicular Trauma 758
Testicular Torsion 758
Testicular Cancer 759
Epididymitis 760
Hypogonadism 760
Disorders of the Prostate **760**
Prostatitis 760
Benign Prostatic Hyperplasia 761
Prostate Cancer 762
Other Disorders of the Male
Reproductive System **762**
Sexually Transmitted Diseases 762
Infertility 763
Assisting with the Male Reproductive
Examination **763**

Chapter 29: Gerontology   768

Societal Bias **770**
Facts about Aging **770**
Physiologic Changes **771**
Senses 771
Integumentary System 772
Nervous System 773
Musculoskeletal System 773
Respiratory System 774
Cardiovascular System 774
Gastrointestinal System 774
Urinary System 775
Reproductive System 775
Prevention of Complications **775**
Psychological Changes **776**
The Medical Assistant and
the Geriatric Patient **776**
Memory-Impaired Older Adults 776
Visually Impaired Older Adults 777
Hearing-Impaired Older Adults 777
Elder Abuse 777
Healthy and Successful Aging **779**

Chapter 30: Examinations and Procedures of Body Systems   784

Integumentary System **786**
Allergy Skin Testing 787
Neurologic System **792**

Components of a Neurologic
Screening 792
Sensory System **798**
The Eye **798**
The Ear 805
The Nose 808
Respiratory System **809**
Signs and Symptoms of Respiratory
Conditions and Disorders 809
Diagnostic Tests 813
Spirometry 813
Peak Expiratory Flow Rates 814
Pulse Oximetry 814
Inhalers 815
Circulatory System **815**
Blood and Lymph System **818**
Musculoskeletal System **820**
Fractures, Casting, and Cast
Removal 821
Digestive System **827**
Signs and Symptoms of Digestive
Conditions and Disorders 827
Diagnostic Tests 827
Bariatrics 841
Urinary System **844**
Signs and Symptoms of Urinary
Conditions and Disorders 844
Diagnostic Tests 844
Urinary Catheterization 848

Unit VIII: Advanced Techniques and Procedures   885

Chapter 31: Assisting with Office/ Ambulatory Surgery   886

Surgical Asepsis and Sterilization **888**
Hand Cleansing (Hand Hygiene)
for Medical and Surgical Asepsis 890
Sterile Principles **890**
Methods of Sterilization **891**
Gas Sterilization 891
Dry Heat Sterilization 891
Chemical ("Cold") Sterilization 891
Steam Sterilization (Autoclave) 892
Common Surgical Procedures
Performed in Providers'
Offices and Clinics **896**
Additional Surgical Methods **896**
Electrosurgery 896
Cryosurgery 897
Laser Surgery 897
Suture Materials and Supplies **898**
Suture/Ligature 898
Suture Needles 899
Staples 899
Staple Removal 899
Instruments **900**
Structural Features 900
Categories and Uses 900
Care of Instruments 907
Supplies and Equipment **910**
Drapes 911
Sponges and Wicks 911
Solutions/Creams/Ointments 911

Dressings and Bandages 912
Anesthetics 912
Patient Care and Preparation 915
Patient Preparation and Education 915
Informed Consent 915
Medical Assisting Considerations 915
Postoperative Instructions 916
Wounds, Wound Care, and the
Healing Process 916
Basic Surgery Setup 918
Basic Rules and Concepts for
Setup of Surgical Trays 918
Surgery Process. 918
Preparation for Surgery 920
Using Dry Sterile Transfer Forceps 921

Chapter 32: Diagnostic Imaging   954

Radiation Safety 956
Radiography Equipment 957
Contrast Media 958
Patient Preparation 958
Positioning the Patient 961
Fluoroscopy. 962
Bone Densitometry 962
Diagnostic Imaging 963
Positron Emission Tomography
(PET) 963
Computerized Tomography (CT) 964
Magnetic Resonance Imaging (MRI) 964
X-Rays (Flat Plates) 965
Ultrasonography 966
Mammography 967
Filing Films and Reports 967
Radiation Therapy 967
Nuclear Medicine 968

**Chapter 33: Rehabilitation
and Therapeutic Modalities   972**

**The Role of the Medical Assistant
in Rehabilitation 974**
Principles of Body Mechanics. 975
Posture 975
**Using the Body Safely and
Effectively 976**
Lifting Techniques 976
Transferring Patients 976
Assisting Patients to Ambulate 978
Assistive Devices 978
Walkers 980
Crutches 980
Canes 984
Wheelchairs 984
Therapeutic Exercises. 985
Range of Motion 985
Muscle Testing 987
Types of Therapeutic Exercise 987
Electromyography 988
Electrostimulation of Muscle 988
Therapeutic Modalities. 988
Heat and Cold 988
Moist and Dry Heat 989
Moist and Dry Cold 991
Ultrasound 991
Massage Therapy 992

**Chapter 34: Nutrition in Health
and Disease   1006**

Nutrition and Digestion 1008
Types of Nutrients 1009
Energy Nutrients (Organic) 1010
Other Nutrients (Inorganic) 1014
Reading Food Labels 1023
Items on the Nutrition Label 1023
Comparing Labels 1024
**Nutrition at Various Stages
of Life 1025**
Pregnancy and Lactation. 1025
Breast-Feeding 1026
Infancy 1026
Childhood 1026
Adolescence 1027
Older Adults 1027
Therapeutic Diets 1028
Weight Control. 1028
Diabetes Mellitus 1029
Cardiovascular Disease 1030
Cancer. 1031
Diet and Culture 1032

**Chapter 35: Basic
Pharmacology   1040**

Uses of Medications 1042
Research and Development 1043
Drug Names 1043
History and Sources of Drugs. 1044
Plant Sources 1044
Animal Sources 1044
Mineral Sources 1044
Herbal Supplements 1044
Synthetic Drugs 1046
Genetically Engineered
Pharmaceuticals. 1046
**Drug Regulations and Legal
Classifications of Drugs 1046**
Controlled Substance Act
of 1970 1046
Prescription Drugs. 1049
Nonprescription Drugs 1050
Proper Disposal of Drugs. 1050
Administer, Prescribe, Dispense 1052
Drug References and Standards 1052
How to Use the PDR 1053
Other Reference Sources 1054
Classification of Drugs 1054
Principal Actions of Drugs 1054
Factors That Affect Drug Action 1054
Undesirable Actions of Drugs 1063
Drug Routes 1063
Forms of Drugs. 1064
Liquid Preparations 1064
Solid and Semisolid
Preparations 1064
Other Drug Delivery Systems 1064
**Storage and Handling of
Medications. 1065**
**Emergency Medications and
Supplies. 1066**
Bioterrorism 1066
Drug Abuse 1066

**Chapter 36: Calculation of
Medication Dosage and
Medication Administration   1078**

**Legal and Ethical Implications
of Medication Administration 1080**
Ethical Considerations. 1081
The Medication Order 1081
The Prescription 1081
Drug Dosage 1084
Age 1084
Weight. 1085
Sex. 1085
Other Factors 1085
Pediatric Considerations 1085
The Medication Label. 1085
Calculation of Drug Dosages 1086
Understanding Ratio 1087
Understanding Proportion 1087
Weights and Measures 1088
Medications Measured in Units 1090
How to Calculate Unit Dosages. 1091
Insulin. 1091
Diabetes 1091
Calculating Adult Dosages 1093
The Proportional Method 1094
Understanding the Formula
Method 1094
Calculating Children's Dosages. 1096
Body Surface Area 1096
Kilogram of Body Weight 1096
Administration of Medications 1098
The "Six Rights" of Proper Drug
Administration 1099
Medication Errors 1101
Patient Assessment. 1101
**Administration of Oral
Medications. 1102**
Equipment and Supplies for Oral
Medications 1102
**Administration of Parenteral
Medications. 1102**
Hazards Associated with Parenteral
Medications 1103
Reasons for Parenteral Route
Selection 1103
Parenteral Equipment and Supplies. . . . 1103
Principles of Intravenous Therapy 1108
Site Selection and Injection Angle 1110
Marking the Correct Site for
Intramuscular Injection. 1111
**Basic Guidelines for Administration
of Injections 1114**
**Z-Track Method of Intramuscular
Injection 1115**
**Administration of Allergenic
Extracts 1115**
**Administration of Inhaled
Medications. 1116**
Implications for Patient Care 1116
Administration of Oxygen. 1116

Chapter 37: Electrocardiography   1140

Anatomy of the Heart 1142
**Electrical Conduction System
of the Heart. 1143**

The Cardiac Cycle and the
ECG Cycle........................... 1145
Calculation of Heart Rate
on ECG Graph Paper................. 1146
Types of Electrocardiographs......... 1146
Single-Channel Electrocardiograph.... 1146
Multichannel Electrocardiograph..... 1146
Automatic Electrocardiograph
Machines.......................... 1146
Electrocardiograph Telephone
Transmissions...................... 1148
Facsimile Electrocardiograph......... 1148
Interpretive Electrocardiograph....... 1148
ECG Equipment 1149
Electrocardiograph Paper............. 1149
Electrolyte.......................... 1149
Sensors or Electrodes................ 1149
Lead Wires......................... 1149
Electrocardiograph Machine 1149
Care of Equipment 1149
Lead Coding 1150
The Electrocardiograph and
Sensor Placement 1150
Standard Limb or Bipolar Leads...... 1150
Augmented Leads 1150
Chest Leads or Precordial Leads 1151
Standardization and Adjustment
of the Electrocardiograph........... 1153
Standard Resting Electrocardiography.. 1153
Mounting the ECG Tracing.......... 1154
Interference or Artifacts............. 1154
Somatic Tremor Artifacts............ 1154
AC Interference 1154
Wandering Baseline Artifacts 1155
Interrupted Baseline Artifacts........ 1155
Patients with Unique Problems....... 1155
Myocardial Infarctions (Heart
Attacks) 1156
Cardiac Arrhythmias............... 1156
Atrial Arrhythmias 1156
Ventricular Arrhythmias 1157
Defibrillation..................... 1159
Other Cardiac Diagnostic Tests 1160
Holter Monitor (Portable
Ambulatory Electrocardiograph) 1160
Loop ECG.......................... 1162
Treadmill Stress Test or Exercise
Tolerance ECG..................... 1162
Thallium Stress Test................. 1163
Echocardiography/
Ultrasonography 1163
Coronary MRI and CT Imaging 1164
Cardiac Procedures................. 1164
Procedures for Heart Disease 1164
Procedures for Arrhythmias 1164

Unit IX: Laboratory
Procedures   1173

Chapter 38: Regulatory Guidelines
in the Medical Laboratory   1174

Clinical Laboratory Improvement
Amendments of 1988 1177
The Intention of CLIA '88 1178
General Program Description........ 1178

Categories of Testing 1179
Contents of the Law................. 1179
Criteria for PPMP................... 1181
Criteria for CLIA Waived Tests 1182
CLIA '88 Regulation for Quality
Control in Automated Hematology 1182
Aftermath of CLIA '88.............. 1182
Impact of CLIA on Medical Assistants .. 1183
Where to Find More Information
Regarding CLIA '88................ 1184
OSHA Regulations 1184
The Standard for Occupational
Exposure to Hazardous Chemicals
in the Laboratory.................. 1184
Chemical Hygiene Plan.............. 1184
OSHA Regulations and Students 1190
Avoiding Exposure to Chemicals 1190
Ergonomics and Cumulative
Trauma Disorders 1191

Chapter 39: Introduction
to the Medical Laboratory   1194

The Laboratory.................... 1196
Purposes of Laboratory Testing 1197
Types of Laboratories................ 1198
Laboratory Personnel 1199
Laboratory Departments 1199
Panels of Laboratory Tests........... 1203
Billing for Laboratory Services....... 1203
Quality Controls/Assurances in the
Laboratory 1205
Control Tests 1205
Proficiency Testing................. 1205
Preventive Maintenance 1205
Instrument Validations 1205
The Medical Assistant's Role......... 1205
Laboratory Requisitions
and Reports..................... 1205
The Specimen 1209
Proper Procurement, Storage,
and Handling..................... 1209
Processing and Sending Specimens
to a Laboratory.................... 1210
Microscopes 1211
Types of Microscopes............... 1211
How to Use a Microscope 1212
How to Care for a Microscope 1213

Chapter 40: Phlebotomy: Venipuncture
and Capillary Puncture   1218

Why Collect Blood?................. 1220
The Medical Assistant's Role
in Phlebotomy.................... 1220
Anatomy and Physiology
of the Circulatory System 1221
Blood Collection.................. 1223
Plasma and Whole-Blood Collection ... 1223
Collection of Blood Specimens....... 1223
Venipuncture Equipment 1224
Syringes and Needles 1225
Safety Needles and Blood
Collection Systems................. 1227
Vacuum Tubes and Adapters/
Holders.......................... 1228

Anticoagulants, Additives, and Gels 1228
Order of Draw 1231
Tourniquets 1231
Specimen Collection Trays 1232
Venipuncture Technique........... 1232
Approaching the Patient............. 1232
Preparing Supplies and Greeting
the Patient 1233
Patient and Specimen Identification ... 1233
Positioning the Patient 1234
Selecting the Appropriate
Venipuncture Site.................. 1234
Applying the Tourniquet 1235
Performing a Safe Venipuncture 1236
Specimen Collection............... 1237
The Syringe Technique 1237
Vacuum Tube Specimen Collection 1239
Butterfly Needle Collection System 1239
Blood Cultures.................... 1240
Patient Reactions 1240
The Unsuccessful Venipuncture....... 1240
Criteria for Rejection of a Specimen ... 1241
Factors Affecting Laboratory Values.... 1241
Capillary Puncture 1244
Composition of Capillary Blood 1244
Capillary Puncture Sites 1244
Preparing the Capillary Puncture Site ... 1244
Performing the Puncture 1244
Collecting the Blood Sample 1245

Chapter 41: Hematology   1266

Hematologic Tests................. 1268
Hemoglobin and Hematocrit Tests..... 1271
Hemoglobin....................... 1271
Hematocrit........................ 1272
White and Red Blood Cell Counts 1273
White Blood Cells and Differential..... 1273
Red Blood Cells 1275
Platelets......................... 1276
Erythrocyte Indices............... 1277
Understanding RBC Indices 1278
Using Erythrocyte Indices
to Diagnose....................... 1278
Erythrocyte Sedimentation
Rates (ESR or Sed Rate)........... 1278
Wintrobe Method 1279
Westergren Method................. 1279
Using the ESR to Screen 1280
C-Reactive Proteins............... 1280
Coagulation Studies 1281
Automated Hematology 1281

Chapter 42: Urinalysis   1292

Urine Formation.................. 1294
Filtration......................... 1294
Reabsorption 1295
Secretion......................... 1295
Urine Composition 1296
Safety............................ 1296
Quality Control................... 1296
Clinical Laboratory Improvement
Amendments of 1988 (CLIA '88) 1297
Urine Containers.................. 1297
Urine Collection.................. 1298
Urine Specimen Types.............. 1298

Collection Methods 1299
Culture and Sensitivity of Urine **1299**
Examination of Urine **1299**
Physical Examination of Urine 1301
Chemical Examination of Urine 1303
Microscopic Examination
of Urine Sediment 1307
Urinalysis Report 1310
Drug Screening **1311**

Chapter 43: Basic Microbiology   1326

**The Medical Assistant's Role in the
Microbiology Laboratory** **1328**
Microbiology **1329**
Classification 1329
Nomenclature 1329
Cell Structure 1330
Equipment **1331**
Autoclave 1331
Microscope 1331
Safety Hood 1331
Incubator 1332
Anaerobic Equipment 1332
Inoculating Equipment 1332
Incinerator 1333
Media 1333
Refrigerator 1333
**Safety when Handling Microbiology
Specimens** **1333**
Personal Protective Equipment 1334
Work Area 1334
Specimen Handling 1334
Disposal of Waste and Spills 1334
Quality Control **1334**
Collection Procedures **1335**
Specific Collection Requirements
for Cultures 1335
Foodborne Illnesses **1337**
**Microscopic Examination
of Bacteria** **1338**
Bacterial Shapes 1338
Dyes (Stains) 1339
Simple Stain 1340
Differential Stain 1340
Acid-Fast Stain 1341
Special Techniques 1341
Potassium Hydroxide
Preparation 1341
Culture Media **1341**
Media Classification 1342
Microbiology Culture **1343**
Inoculating the Media 1343
Other Types of Streaking 1343
Primary Culture 1344
Subculture 1345
**Rapid Identification
Systems** **1345**
Streptococcus Screening
(Rapid Strep Testing) 1345
Sensitivity Testing **1346**
Parasitology **1347**
Examination Methods 1348
Specimen Collection 1348
Common Parasites 1348
Mycology **1350**

Chapter 44: Specialty
Laboratory Tests   1358

Urine Pregnancy Tests **1360**
**Commercial/Home Urine
Pregnancy Tests** **1360**
**False/Positive Pregnancy
Test Results** **1361**
Infectious Mononucleosis **1361**
Transmission of EBV 1361
Symptoms of IM 1361
Treatment of IM 1362
Diagnosis of IM 1362
CLIA Waived IM Tests 1362
Prothrombin Time **1362**
Blood Typing **1362**
ABO Blood Typing 1362
Rh Blood Typing 1363
Semen Analysis **1364**
Semen Composition 1365
Altering Factors in Semen Analysis . . . 1365
Phenylketonuria Test **1366**
Blood Testing for PKU 1366
Tuberculosis **1366**
Cause of TB 1367
Resistance in Mycobacteria 1367
Transmission of Infectious TB 1367
Diagnosis of TB 1367
Screening for TB: Skin Testing 1368
The Mantoux Test 1368
Blood Glucose **1369**
Fasting Blood Glucose 1370
Two-Hour Postprandial Blood
Glucose 1370
Glucose Tolerance Test 1371
Automated Methods of Glucose
Analysis 1372
Testing Panels 1373
Glycosylated Hemoglobin 1373
**Cholesterol, Lipids and Systemic
Inflammation** **1373**
The Chemistry of Cholesterol 1375
Functions of Cholesterol 1375
Lipoproteins and Cholesterol
Transport 1376
Triglyceride 1376
Inflammation 1377
Blood Chemistry Tests **1377**
Alanine Aminotransferase (ALT) 1377
Albumin 1378
Alkaline Phosphatase (ALP) 1378
Aspartate Aminotransferase (AST) 1378
Bilirubin, Total and Direct 1378
Blood Urea Nitrogen Test 1378
Calcium 1378
Chloride 1379
Carbon Dioxide (CO_2) 1379
Creatinine 1379
Gamma Glutamyltransferase (GGT) . . . 1379
Lactate Dehydrogenase (LDH) 1379
Phosphorus (Phosphate) 1379
Potassium (K) 1379
Sodium 1379
Total Protein 1379
Uric Acid 1379

SECTION IV:
PROFESSIONAL
PROCEDURES   1391

Unit X: Clinic
and Human Resources
Management   1393

Chapter 45: The Medical
Assistant as Clinic Manager   1394

**The Medical Assistant as Clinic
Manager** **1396**
Qualities of a Manager **1397**
Clinic Manager Attitude 1398
Professionalism 1398
Management Styles **1399**
Authoritarian Style 1399
Participatory Style 1399
Management by Walking Around 1399
Risk Management **1400**
Importance of Teamwork **1400**
Getting the Team Started 1401
Using a Team to Solve a Problem 1401
Planning and Implementing
a Solution 1401
Recognition 1401
Supervising Personnel **1401**
Staff and Team Meetings 1402
Conflict Resolution 1402
Harassment in the Workplace **1403**
Assimilating New Personnel 1403
Employees with Chemical
Dependencies or Emotional
Problems 1405
Evaluating Employees and
Planning Salary Review 1405
Dismissing Employees 1409
Procedure Manual **1409**
Organization of the Procedure
Manual 1409
Updating and Reviewing
the Procedure Manual 1410
HIPAA Implications **1410**
Travel Arrangements **1410**
Itinerary 1411
Time Management **1411**
Marketing Functions **1413**
Seminars 1413
Brochures 1413
Newsletters 1415
Press Releases 1415
Special Events 1415
Social Media in the Medical Clinic **1416**
**Records and Financial
Management** **1417**
Electronic Health Records
and the Clinic Manager 1417
Records and Financial Management . . . 1417
Payroll Processing 1417
Facility and Equipment Management . . . **1421**
Administrative and Clinical
Inventory of Supplies and Equipment . . 1422

Administrative and Clinical
Equipment Calibration and
Maintenance........................ 1422
Liability Coverage and Bonding **1423**
Legal Issues....................... **1423**

Chapter 46: The Medical
Assistant as Human
Resources Manager   1434
**Tasks Performed by the Human
Resources Manager**................. **1436**
The Clinic Policy Manual **1437**
**Recruiting and Hiring Clinic
Personnel** **1438**
Job Descriptions.................... 1438
Recruiting......................... 1439
Preparing to Interview Applicants 1439
The Employment Interview........... 1440
Selecting the Finalists 1441
Orienting New Personnel **1442**
Dismissing Employees............... **1443**
Exit Interview 1443
Maintaining Personnel Records **1443**
Complying with Personnel Laws....... **1444**
Special Policy Considerations........ **1444**
Temporary Employees................ 1444
Smoking Policy..................... 1445
Discrimination 1445
**Providing/Planning Employee
Instruction and Education** **1445**

Unit XI: Entry into
the Profession   1451

Chapter 47: Preparing for Medical
Assisting Credentials   1452
Purpose of Certification **1454**
Certification Agencies 1455
**Preparing for Certification
Examinations**..................... **1455**
**American Association of Medical
Assistants (AAMA)**................. **1456**
Certified Medical Assistant (AAMA)
Examination Format and Content 1457
Certified Medical Assistant (AAMA)
Application Process 1457
Certified Medical Assistant (AAMA)
Examination Scheduling
and Administration 1457

Certified Medical Assistant (AAMA)
Recertification 1458
**American Medical Technologists
(AMT)** **1459**
Registered Medical Assistant (AMT)
Examination Format and Content 1459
Registered Medical Assistant (AMT)
Application Process 1459
Registered Medical Assistant (AMT)
Examination Scheduling
and Administration 1460
Registered Medical Assistant (AMT)
Recertification 1460
**National Healthcareer
Association (NHA)** **1460**
Certified Clinical Medical
Assistant and Certified Medical
Administrative Assistant
Examination Format and Content 1461
Certified Clinical Medical Assistant
and Certified Medical Administrative
Assistant Application Process 1461
Certified Clinical Medical Assistant
and Certified Medical Administrative
Assistant Examination Scheduling and
Administration..................... 1461
Certified Clinical Medical Assistant
and Certified Medical Administrative
Assistant Recertification 1461
Professional Organizations........... **1462**
American Association of Medical
Assistants (AAMA) 1462
American Medical Technologists
(AMT)........................... 1462
National Healthcareer
Association (NHA)................. 1463

Chapter 48: Employment
Strategies   1466
Developing a Strategy **1468**
Attitude and Mindset............... 1468
Self-Assessment.................... 1469
Job Search Analysis and Research...... **1470**
Social Media in Your Job Search....... **1471**
Résumé Preparation **1472**
Résumé Specifications............... 1472
Clear and Concise Résumés 1472
Accomplishments................... 1472
References 1472
Accuracy.......................... 1474

Résumé Styles...................... 1474
Vital Résumé Information............ 1480
Application/Cover Letters **1480**
Completing the Application Form **1481**
The Interview Process............... **1483**
The Look of Success 1483
Preparing for the Interview.......... 1484
The Actual Interview 1484
Interviewing the Employer 1485
Closing the Interview............... 1486
Interview Follow-Up **1486**
Follow-Up Letter 1486
Follow-Up by Telephone 1487
After You Are Employed **1487**
Dealing with Difficult People 1488
Getting a Raise 1488
Professionalism.................... **1488**

Appendix A: Common
Medical Abbreviations
and Symbols   1491

Appendix B: Top 200
Brand-Name Drugs in the
U.S. Market by Dispensed
Prescriptions, 2010   1498

Appendix C: AAMA 2007–2008
Occupational Analysis of the
CMA (AAMA)   1501

Appendix D: Medical
Assisting Task List   1504

Appendix E: Software Support: The
Critical Thinking Challenge and
Medical Office Simulation
Software   1507

Glossary of Terms   1517

Glosario de términos   1539

Index   1564

List of Procedures

5-1   Identifying Community Resources

9-1   Control of Bleeding

9-2   Applying an Arm Splint

10-1   Develop a Personal and/or Employee Safety Plan in Case of a Disaster

10-2   Demonstrate Proper Use of a Fire Extinguisher

11-1   Instructions for Performing Routine Maintenance of Clinic Computers and Ancillary Equipment with Documentation

11-2   Software Installation

11-3   Hardware Installation

12-1   Answering and Screening Incoming Calls

12-2   Taking a Telephone Message

12-3   Calling a Pharmacy to Refill an Authorized Prescription

12-4   Handling Problem Calls

12-5   Preparing, Sending, and Receiving a Fax

13-1   Establishing the Appointment Matrix in a Paper System

13-2   Establishing the Appointment Matrix Using Medical Office Simulation Software (MOSS)

13-3   Making an Appointment Using Paper Scheduling

13-4   Making an Appointment Using Medical Office Simulation Software (MOSS)

13-5   Checking in Patients in a Paper System

13-6   Checking in Patients Using Medical Office Simulation Software (MOSS)

13-7   Cancelling and Rescheduling Procedures Using Paper Scheduling

13-8   Cancelling a Patient Appointment Using MOSS

13-9   Rescheduling a Patient Appointment Using MOSS

13-10   Scheduling Inpatient and Outpatient Admissions and Procedures

14-1   Establishing a Paper Medical Chart for a New Patient

14-2   Registering a New Patient Using Medical Office Simulation Software (MOSS)

14-3   Correcting a Paper Medical Record

14-4   Updating Patient Registration Information Using Medical Office Simulation Software (MOSS)

14-5   Steps for Manual Filing with an Alphabetic System

14-6   Steps for Manual Filing with a Numeric System

14-7   Steps for Manual Filing with a Subject Filing System

15-1   Preparing and Composing Business Correspondence Using All Components (Computerized Approach)

15-2   Addressing Envelopes According to United States Postal Regulations

15-3   Folding Letters for Standard Envelopes

15-4   Creating a Mass Mailing Using Mail Merge

15-5   Preparing Outgoing Mail According to United States Postal Regulations

16-1   Transcribe Medical Referral Letters Using Medical Office Simulation Software (MOSS)

17-1   Applying Managed Care Policies and Procedures

17-2   Screening for Insurance

17-3   Verifying Insurance Eligibility Using Medical Office Simulation Software (MOSS)

17-4   Obtaining Referrals and Authorizations

17-5   Computing the Medicare Fee Schedule

18-1   Current Procedural Terminology Coding

18-2   International Classification of Diseases, 9th Revision, Clinical Modification Coding

18-3   Applying Third-Party Guidelines

18-4   Completing a Medicare CMS-1500 (08-05) Claim Form

19-1   Recording/Posting Patient Charges, Payments, and Adjustments in a Manual System

19-2   Balancing Day Sheets in a Manual System

19-3   Posting Procedure Charges and Payments Using Medical Office Simulation Software (MOSS)

19-4   Insurance Billing Using Medical Office Simulation Software (MOSS)

19-5   Posting Insurance Payments and Adjustments Using Medical Office Simulation Software (MOSS)

19-6   Processing Credit Balances and Refunds Using Medical Office Simulation Software (MOSS)

19-7   Preparing a Deposit

19-8   Recording a Nonsufficient Funds Check in a Manual System

19-9   Writing a Check

19-10   Reconciling a Bank Statement

19-11 Establishing and Maintaining a Petty Cash Fund

20-1   Explaining Fees in the First Telephone Interview

20-2   Prepare Itemized Patient Accounts for Billing in a Manual System

20-3   Identifying Accounts Receivable Using Medical Office Simulation Software (MOSS)

20-4   Preparing Itemized Patient Statements Using Medical Office Simulation Software (MOSS)

20-5   Preparing Collection Letters Using Medical Office Simulation Software (MOSS)

20-6   Posting Non-Sufficient Fund (NSF) Checks Using Medical Office Simulation Software (MOSS)

20-7   Post/Record Collection Agency Adjustments in a Manual System

20-8   Post/Record Collection Agency Adjustments Using Medical Office Simulation Software (MOSS)

21-1   Preparing Accounts Receivable Trial Balance in a Manual System

21-2   Preparing Accounts Receivable Trial Balance Using Medical Office Simulation Software (MOSS)

22-1   Medical Asepsis Hand Wash (Hand Hygiene)

22-2   Correct Use of Alcohol-Based Hand Rubs (ABHR)

22-3   Removing Contaminated Gloves

22-4   Transmission-Based Precautions: Donning a Gown, Mask, Gloves, and Cap (Isolation Technique)

22-5   Sanitization of Instruments

23-1   Taking a Medical History for a Paper Medical Record

24-1   Measuring an Oral Temperature Using an Electronic Thermometer

24-2   Measuring an Aural Temperature Using a Tympanic Thermometer

24-3   Measuring a Temperature Using a Temporal Artery (TA) Thermometer

24-4   Measuring a Rectal Temperature Using a Digital Thermometer

24-5   Measuring an Axillary Temperature

24-6   Measuring an Oral Temperature Using a Disposable Oral Strip Thermometer

24-7   Measuring a Radial Pulse

24-8   Taking an Apical Pulse

24-9   Measuring the Respiration Rate

24-10 Measuring Blood Pressure

24-11 Measuring Height

24-12 Measuring Adult Weight

25-1   Assisting with a Complete Physical Examination

26-1   Assisting with Routine Prenatal Visits

26-2   Assisting with Pelvic Examination and Pap Test (Conventional and ThinPrep® Methods)

26-3   Assisting with Insertion of an Intrauterine Device (IUD)

26-4   Assisting with Insertion of a Hormonal Contraceptive (Implanon®)

26-5   Wet Prep/Wet Mount and Potassium Hydroxide (KOH) Prep

26-6   Amplified DNA ProbeTec Test for Chlamydia and Gonorrhea

27-1   Administration of a Vaccine

27-2   Maintaining Immunization Records

27-3   Measuring the Infant: Weight, Length, Head and Chest Circumference

27-4   Taking an Infant's Rectal Temperature with a Digital Thermometer

27-5   Taking an Apical Pulse on an Infant

27-6   Measuring Infant's Respiratory Rate

27-7   Obtaining a Urine Specimen from an Infant or Young Child

28-1   Instructing Patient in Testicular Self-Examination

30-1   Assisting the Provider during a Lumbar Puncture or Cerebrospinal Fluid Aspiration

30-2   Assisting the Provider with a Neurologic Screening Examination

30-3   Performing Visual Acuity Testing Using a Snellen Chart

30-4   Measuring Near Visual Acuity

30-5   Testing Color Vision Using the Ishihara Plates

30-6   Performing Eye Instillation

30-7   Performing Eye Patch Dressing Application

30-8   Performing Eye Irrigation

30-9   Performing Ear Irrigation

30-10 Assisting with Audiometry

30-11 Performing Ear Instillation

30-12 Assisting with Nasal Examination

30-13 Cautery Treatment of Epistaxis

30-14 Performing Nasal Instillation

30-15 Administer Oxygen by Nasal Cannula for Minor Respiratory Distress

30-16 Instructing Patient in the Use of a Metered Dose Inhaler with and Without a Spacer

30-17 Spirometry

30-18 Pulse Oximetry

30-19 Assisting with Plaster Cast Application

30-20 Assisting with Cast Removal

30-21 Fecal Occult Blood Test

30-22 Urinary Catheterization of a Male Patient

30-23 Urinary Catheterization of a Female Patient

31-1   Applying Sterile Gloves

31-2   Chemical "Cold" Sterilization of Endoscopes

31-3   Preparing Instruments for Sterilization in Autoclave

31-4   Sterilization of Instruments (Autoclave)

31-5   Setting Up and Covering a Sterile Field

31-6   Opening Sterile Packages of Instruments and Supplies and Applying Them to a Sterile Field

31-7   Pouring a Sterile Solution into a Cup on a Sterile Field

31-8   Assisting with Clinic/ Ambulatory Surgery

31-9   Dressing Change

31-10   Wound Irrigation

31-11   Preparation of Patient's Skin before Surgery

31-12   Suturing of Laceration or Incision Repair

31-13   Sebaceous Cyst Excision

31-14   Incision and Drainage of Localized Infection

31-15   Aspiration of Joint Fluid

31-16   Hemorrhoid Thrombectomy

31-17   Suture/Staple Removal

31-18   Application of Sterile Adhesive Skin Closure Strips

33-1   Transferring Patient from Wheelchair to Examination Table

33-2   Transferring Patient from Examination Table to Wheelchair

33-3   Assisting the Patient to Stand and Walk

33-4   Care of the Falling Patient

33-5   Assisting a Patient to Ambulate with a Walker

33-6   Teaching the Patient to Ambulate with Crutches

33-7   Assisting a Patient to Ambulate with a Cane

34-1   Provide Instruction for Health Maintenance and Disease Prevention

35-1   Proper Disposal of Drugs

36-1   Administration of Oral Medications

36-2   Withdrawing Medication from a Vial

36-3   Withdrawing Medication from an Ampule

36-4   Administration of Subcutaneous, Intramuscular, and Intradermal Injections

36-5   Administering a Subcutaneous Injection

36-6   Administering an Intramuscular Injection

36-7   Administering an Intradermal Injection of Purified Protein Derivative (PPD)

36-8   Reconstituting a Powder Medication for Administration

36-9   Z-Track Intramuscular Injection Technique

37-1   Perform Single-Channel or Multichannel Electrocardiogram

37-2   Holter Monitor Application (Cassette and Digital)

39-1   Using the Microscope

40-1   Palpating a Vein and Preparing a Patient for Venipuncture

40-2   Venipuncture by Syringe

40-3   Venipuncture by Vacuum Tube System

40-4   Venipuncture by Butterfly Needle System

40-5   Capillary Puncture

40-6   Obtaining a Capillary Specimen for Transport Using a Microtainer Transport Unit

40-7   Obtaining Blood for Blood Culture

41-1   Hemoglobin Determination Using a CLIA Waived Hemoglobin Analyzer

41-2   Microhematocrit Determination

41-3   Erythrocyte Sedimentation Rate

41-4   Prothrombin Time (Using CLIA Waived ProTime Analyzer)

42-1   Assessing Urine Volume, Color, and Clarity (Physical Urinalysis)

42-2   Using the Refractometer to Measure Specific Gravity Urinalysis (Physical Urinalysis, Continued)

42-3   Performing a Chemical Urinalysis

42-4   Preparing Slide for Microscopic Examination of Urine Sediment

42-5   Performing a Complete Urinalysis

42-6   Utilizing a Urine Transport System for C&S

42-7   Instructing a Patient in the Collection of a Clean-Catch, Midstream Urine Specimen

43-1   Obtaining a Throat Specimen for Culture

43-2   Wet-Mount and Hanging Drop Slide Preparations

43-3   Performing Strep Throat Testing

43-4   Instructing a Patient on Obtaining a Fecal Specimen

44-1   Pregnancy Test

44-2   Performing Infectious Mononucleosis Test

44-3   Obtaining Blood Specimen for Phenylketonuria (PKU) Test

44-4   Measurement of Blood Glucose Using an Automated Analyzer

44-5   Cholesterol Testing

45-1   Completing a Medical Incident Report

45-2   Preparing a Meeting Agenda

45-3   Supervising a Student Practicum

45-4   Developing and Maintaining a Procedure Manual

45-5   Making Travel Arrangements with a Travel Agent

45-6   Making Travel Arrangements via the Internet

45-7   Processing Employee Payroll

45-8   Perform an Inventory of Equipment and Supplies

45-9   Perform Routine Maintenance and Calibration of Clinical Equipment

46-1   Develop and Maintain a Policy Manual

46-2   Prepare a Job Description

46-3   Conduct Interviews

46-4   Orient Personnel

HOW TO USE THE BOOK

Chapter Openers

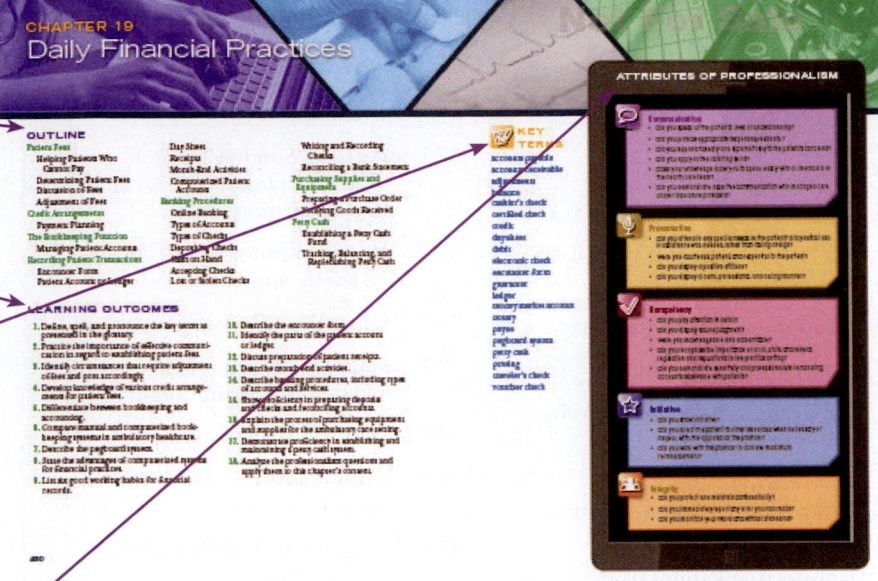

Outline

The **Outline** provides a road map for each chapter.

Learning Outcomes

The **Learning Outcomes** state chapter goals and outcomes.

Key Terms

Key Terms identify important vocabulary for the chapter. Each term appears in bold-face color the first time it is used in the chapter, and also appears in the glossary with a definition.

Attributes of Professionalism

The **Attributes of Professionalism** feature lists questions pertaining to five categories of professional behavior: communication, presentation, competency, initiative, and integrity. As you read each chapter, you are encouraged to keep these questions in mind, and apply them to your own interactions with patients and fellow medical staff. Refer to page 10 in Chapter 1 for a comprehensive list of the Attributes of Professionalism questions.

Total Practice Management Figures

Total Practice Management Figures are special figures that illustrate how specific content fits in to the overall total practice management data flow. Refer to page 224 in Chapter 11 for the entire figure showing the TPMS data flow.

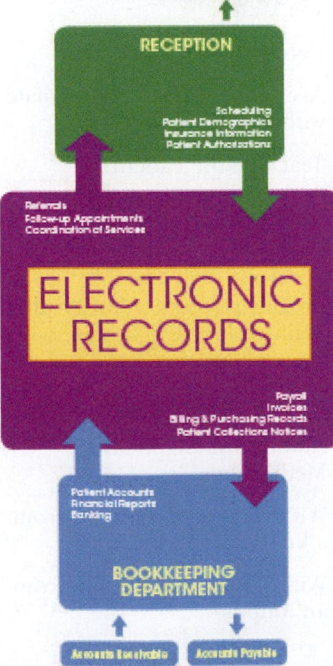

Figure 19-2 Total practice management system diagram illustrating the connection between daily financial practices, patients' electronic medical records, and reception/scheduling activities.

Icons

Icons appear throughout the book to highlight chapter material on topics important to today's medical assistant:

 Key Terms

 Cultural Diversity

 Electronic Health Records (EHR)

 HIPAA Compliance

 Legal Issues

 Safety and Security

 Procedures

To enhance the Attributes of Professionalism feature, five professionalism icons also appear throughout the text:

 Communication

 Presentation

 Competency

 Initiative

 Integrity

SCENARIO

At the clinic of Drs. Lewis and King, many different types of patients are seen. Most have some kind of insurance, either a traditional plan or an HMO plan; some are on Medicare; a few are on Medicaid; and occasionally a patient does not have any insurance or any financial resources to pay for treatment. Whoever schedules the first patient appointment also opens a courteous discussion with the patient about provider fees and the patient's anticipated method of payment. Initiating this discussion of fees at the beginning of the provider–patient relationship keeps patients informed of their responsibility for payment and helps the medical assistants at Drs. Lewis and King's practice make any necessary credit arrangements with the patient before treatment begins.

Scenario

A **Scenario** box appears at the beginning of each chapter, describing a real-world situation applicable to that chapter's content.

Spotlight on Certification

The **Spotlight on Certification** feature maps the chapter material to the content outlines for the RMA (AMT), CMA (AAMA), and CMAS exams to help you prepare to obtain medical assistant credentials.

SPOTLIGHT ON CERTIFICATION

RMA (AMT) Content Outline
- Financial and bookkeeping

CMA (AAMA) Content Outline
- Equipment and supply inventory
- Bookkeeping systems
- Accounting and banking procedures

CMAS Content Outline
- Managing practice finances
- Bookkeeping systems
- Banking procedures

Patient Education

Patient Education boxes present important issues to discuss with patients before and during tests and examinations.

PATIENT EDUCATION

One way to easily provide information to patients regarding fees is to include in the clinic brochure policies regarding fees, insurance, co-payments, and how third-party payments are handled. If credit and debit cards are allowed, include that information as well.

Critical Thinking

Critical Thinking boxes help you think about and deal with issues you may face on the job.

CRITICAL THINKING

Discuss with another student the advantages and disadvantages of adopting a computer system that allows the practice to start with one component and add more components at a later time.

Step-by-Step Procedures

Step-by-step procedures, grouped together at the end of most chapters, give instruction on all important administrative, clinical, and general competencies. They feature graphical illustration of the steps to be performed as well as rationales and correct documentation. Affective (behavior) steps are called out with bold, italicized text, and the professionalism icons indicate which affective skills are emphasized.

PROCEDURE 10-1

Develop a Personal and/or Employee Safety Plan in Case of a Disaster

PURPOSE:
To develop a plan of action in case of a disaster that promotes personal safety and can also be applied to both employees and patients in ambulatory care.

EQUIPMENT/SUPPLIES:
Computer
Clear plastic protector envelope for plan

PROCEDURE STEPS:

1. *Be proactive* by reviewing state and local recommendations for emergency preparedness. *Pay attention to detail.* RATIONALE: Some areas of the country are prone to particular natural disasters such as floods, tornados, or hurricanes. Your plan should be pertinent to your geographical area.

2. *Show initiative* by gathering family members or other employees together to discuss a disaster plan. RATIONALE: When those close to you are involved in the process, they are more likely to participate in the activity and understand the importance of the actions to be taken.

3. List supplies necessary for your supply kit. Be certain to include any special needs required in your supplies. Allow each person 1 personal item for the kit. Plan your needs for a minimum of 48 hours. RATIONALE: A detailed list of the supply kit items reminds you of what you will need to purchase, when items will expire or lose their usefulness, and what one item is most important to each individual.

4. Plan for evacuation. Where are the exits? Identify the safest route for exit. List the steps to take prior to evacuation. RATIONALE: Planning ahead makes it easier to function in the time of great stress. Who will be responsible for picking up the supply kit? A first aid kit? Who will turn off electricity, gas, water?

5. Determine a communication or contact plan to follow should you be separated from others during the disaster. Where will you meet? Name a "neutral" person or friend in another location who can be a telephone contact. RATIONALE: Following any disaster, the first concern is always for the well-being of your loved ones and those closest to you. Knowing how to reach one another will reduce this stress.

6. Schedule updates to the personal safety plan at least every quarter, *developing strategic plans to achieve your goals.* RATIONALE: This time frame allows for changes that may be necessary in the supply kit, reinforcing the safety protocol you have devised, and the ability to make any other changes necessary.

7. Make certain everyone has a copy of the plan. Post a copy of your plan in a prominent place where it is noticed regularly. RATIONALE: Unless everyone has a copy of the plan and it is posted where everyone is continually reminded, the plan loses its effectiveness.

Case Studies

The **Case Studies** provide you with real-world scenarios, and ask you how you would handle such situations in your own career.

CASE STUDY 19-2

Joann Crier has completed her 3-month probation period with Drs. Lewis and King. She is doing quite well and has demonstrated skill in accurate financial documentation. She has been asked to take over reconciling the monthly bank statements and managing all the accounts payable, including getting the checks ready for the provider's signature. She has difficulty, however, completing these tasks until after hours when the clinic is closed and quiet. Marilyn Johnson has told her that it must be done within normal working hours unless special permission is granted.

CASE STUDY REVIEW

1. What suggestions can you make to Joann to allow her to complete these tasks during normal working hours?

2. What impact does the time of day, day(s) of the month, or place where the tasks are completed have on your suggestions?

3. Are there any circumstances you can identify when overtime might be warranted to allow Joann to complete the tasks after hours?

Chapter Summaries

The **Chapter Summaries** provide an overview and summation of the main learning outcomes within the chapter.

SUMMARY

In this chapter, we discussed the daily financial duties in an ambulatory care setting: patient bookkeeping, working with the checkbook, purchasing supplies and equipment, and petty cash. By becoming proficient in these functions, you will be prepared to handle the day-to-day financial aspects of any ambulatory care setting.

Patient bookkeeping involves not only a responsibility to your employer (you are keeping track of income) but also to the patient, to be certain that charges for services rendered are correct and that payments are properly credited. The pegboard system is a comprehensive manual system for posting and tracking these data. Computerized bookkeeping offers many advantages of speed, high accuracy, and elimination of some routine tasks while providing the same important financial data.

STUDY FOR SUCCESS

To reinforce your knowledge and skills of information presented in this chapter:

- Review the *Key Terms*.
- Role-play with other students to apply attributes of professionalism pertinent to this chapter.
- Consider the *Case Studies* and discuss your conclusions.
- Answer the questions in the *Certification Review*.
- Apply your knowledge by completing the *Activities* in the *Study Guide* and the *Games and Quizzes* in the StudyWARE software on the *Premium Website*.
- Perform the *Procedures* using the *Competency Assessment Checklists* in the *Competency Manual*.
- Practice your problem-solving skills with the *Critical Thinking Challenge 3.0* on the *Premium Website*.

Additional resources for this chapter include:

- Module 10 of the *Medical Assisting Learning Lab*
- *CourseMate for Delmar's Comprehensive Medical Assisting*
- *WebTutor for Delmar's Comprehensive Medical Assisting*

Study for Success

The **Study for Success** boxes at the end of each chapter reinforce your understanding of the concepts covered through activities in the Study Guide, Competency Manual, Premium Website, Learning Lab, CourseMate, and WebTutor. Use this element as a study plan and checklist to get the most out of the entire learning package.

CERTIFICATION REVIEW

1. The debit column of a ledger is:
   a. the column to the right of the balance column
   b. the column on the left; used to enter charges, procedure codes, and description of services
   c. the column at the far right that records the difference between the debit and credit columns
   d. the column that indicates the patient's debt to the practice
2. The use of debit/credit cards by patients to pay for services in ambulatory care settings is:
   a. never done
   b. unethical
   c. sure to compromise the integrity of the clinic
   d. a financial arrangement increasingly being used

Certification Review

The **Certification Review** solidifies your understanding of the chapter through certification-style review questions.

Preface

The world of health care continues to change rapidly, and, as medical assistants, you will be called on to do more and respond to an increasing number of clinical and administrative responsibilities. Now is the time to equip yourself with the skills you will need to excel in the field to maximize your potential, expand your base of knowledge, and dedicate yourself to becoming the best multifaceted, multiskilled medical assistant that you can be.

The new edition of *Delmar's Comprehensive Medical Assisting: Administrative and Clinical Competencies* will guide you on this journey. The word *comprehensive* is not used lightly here, for this text is part of a dynamic learning system that includes software, study guide, and online materials. Together, this learning package includes coverage of the entry-level competencies identified by the Accrediting Bureau of Health Education Schools (ABHES) and the Commission on Accreditation of Allied Health Education Programs (CAAHEP). It will also help you prepare for certification examinations from the American Association of Medical Assistants (AAMA), the American Medical Technologists (AMT), and the National Healthcareer Association (NHA).

You will find this edition continues to provide you with opportunities to use your critical thinking skills through case studies, critical thinking boxes, Patient Education boxes, and scenarios. You will also see that the text addresses topics that will make you workplace-ready, including electronic health records (EHR), Total Practice Management System (TPMS) software, professionalism, and confidentiality and privacy issues.

Some of the special new features and updates to this edition include:

- Continued emphasis on EHR and TPMS software; where appropriate, each chapter includes a figure illustrating how the chapter content relates to TPMS
- Refreshed learning outcomes that map to CAAHEP and ABHES competencies
- A new *Attributes of Professionalism* figure in each chapter opener that emphasizes behavioral skills
- More than 50 new photos and illustrations portraying a greater number of procedures and showing the latest equipment
- Updated procedures that include language emphasizing professionalism skills; the text also includes several new procedures further utilizing Medical Office Simulation Software (MOSS) 2.0
- Updated end of chapter-content, including an expanded Certification Review section with multiple choice questions that mimic the medical assisting certification examinations
- Updated certification and examination information for AAMA, AMT, and NHA
- Additional Critical Thinking boxes throughout the text

- In most instances, the term *clinic* has replaced the term *office*. In today's medical environment very few single physician practices are left to compete with large corporate or non-profit medical facilities and specialty clinics. The change in terms was made to reflect this alteration in the delivery of medical services.

HOW THE TEXT IS ORGANIZED

Section I, General Procedures (Chapters 1 through 9), provides the groundwork for understanding the role and responsibilities of the medical assistant. Topics include the medical assisting profession, the health care team, the history of medicine, communication skills, legal and ethical issues, and emergency and first aid procedures.

New material in this section includes:

- Introduction to the Attributes of Professionalism figure
- Five medical specialties added to Table 2-1
- The order of Chapters 4 and 5 has been switched, to create a better flow of information
- Information on the Equal Pay Act and the Federal Age Discrimination Act
- Scope of Practice for both providers and medical assistants
- Expanded coverage of reproductive issues
- Patient Bill of Rights appropriate for ambulatory care
- Patient Protection and Affordable Care Act of 2010
- A table identifying Erikson's stages of human growth and development
- New topics in Section I: Retail stores entering into ambulatory and urgent care; use of silence as a therapeutic communication technique; patients with physical limitations and ADA accommodations; choices individuals can make when facing a life-threatening illness; professional liability coverage; health care—a right or a privilege?

Section II, Administrative Procedures (Chapters 10 through 21), provides up-to-date information on all administrative competencies required of medical assistants. Topics include the facility environment, using computers and technology, clinic communications, scheduling, creating and managing medical records, insurance and coding, and financial practices.

New material in this section includes:

- Several new procedures, including procedures that utilize additional functionality in Medical Office Simulation Software (MOSS) 2.0—to give exposure to both paper-based and electronic administrative procedures
- Expanded information on emergency preparedness, including two new procedures on creating a disaster plan and safely operating a fire extinguisher
- Legal compliance in the facility, including HIPAA and ADA
- Performing routine maintenance of clinic computers and ancillary equipment
- The transition from paper to EHR documents
- Discussion of the American Reinvestment and Recovery Act (ARRA), including criteria for Meaningful Use
- Implementation of ICD-10-CM and ICD-10-PCS
- New topics in Section II: Education in the reception area; cloud computing; using a smartphone; encryption of email; job outlook for the medical transcriptionist

Section III, Clinical Procedures (Chapters 22 through 44), gives you a thorough understanding of the clinical, diagnostic, and laboratory procedures you will be performing and assisting with in the medical clinic. Topics include asepsis, patient history, vital signs, body system examinations, specialty examinations, minor surgery, diagnostic imaging, nutrition, ECG, pharmacology, dosage calculation, venipuncture, urinalysis, and laboratory tests.

New material in this section includes:

- Chapters 28 and 30 have been internally reorganized to improve the flow of content
- All laboratory procedures have been updated to reflect the latest equipment technology and processes
- 2010 CPR Guidelines
- Updated immunization guidelines
- Point of Care Testing has been updated
- Information on CLIA Waived Tests qualifications has been revised
- Comparison of blood collection methods
- Anticoagulant medications and studies
- New topics in Section III: 2011 MyPlate program; rapid ESR test; C-Reactive Protein test

Section IV, Professional Procedures (Chapters 45 through 48), examines the role of the medical assistant as clinic manager and human resources manager and provides tools and techniques to use when preparing for practicums, medical assistant credentials, and employment.

New material in this section includes:

- Updated certification and examination information
- Using social media in the job search
- Online résumés and e-applications
- Critical thinking activities directed toward the student seeking employment
- Updated discussion on the recommended length of a resume
- New topics in Section IV: Social media in the medical clinic; what potential employees might expect from a human resources manager

THE COMPLETE LEARNING PACKAGE: STUDENT SUPPLEMENTS

Premium Website (www.cengagebrain.com)

This robust, password-protected website is designed to maximize learning by providing a multimedia approach to learning the concepts presented in this text. Follow the directions on the printed access card to log on at (www.cengagebrain.com). In the student resources:

- Download the **Work Documentation** forms needed to complete the Competency Checklists. The forms can be completed electronically and saved or printed and completed manually.
- Practice chapter concepts with the **StudyWARE™ Software** (described later in this section).
- Practice your pronunciation and recognition of medical terms by using the **Audio Library**; you may search for terms by word or body system.
- Complete the popular **Critical Thinking Challenge 3.0**, **Competency Challenge 2.0**, and **Virtual Administrative Skills for the Medical Assistant** programs (described later in this section).

Critical Thinking Challenge 3.0

The Critical Thinking Challenge 3.0 software simulates a 3-month practicum in a medical clinic. You will be confronted with a series of situations

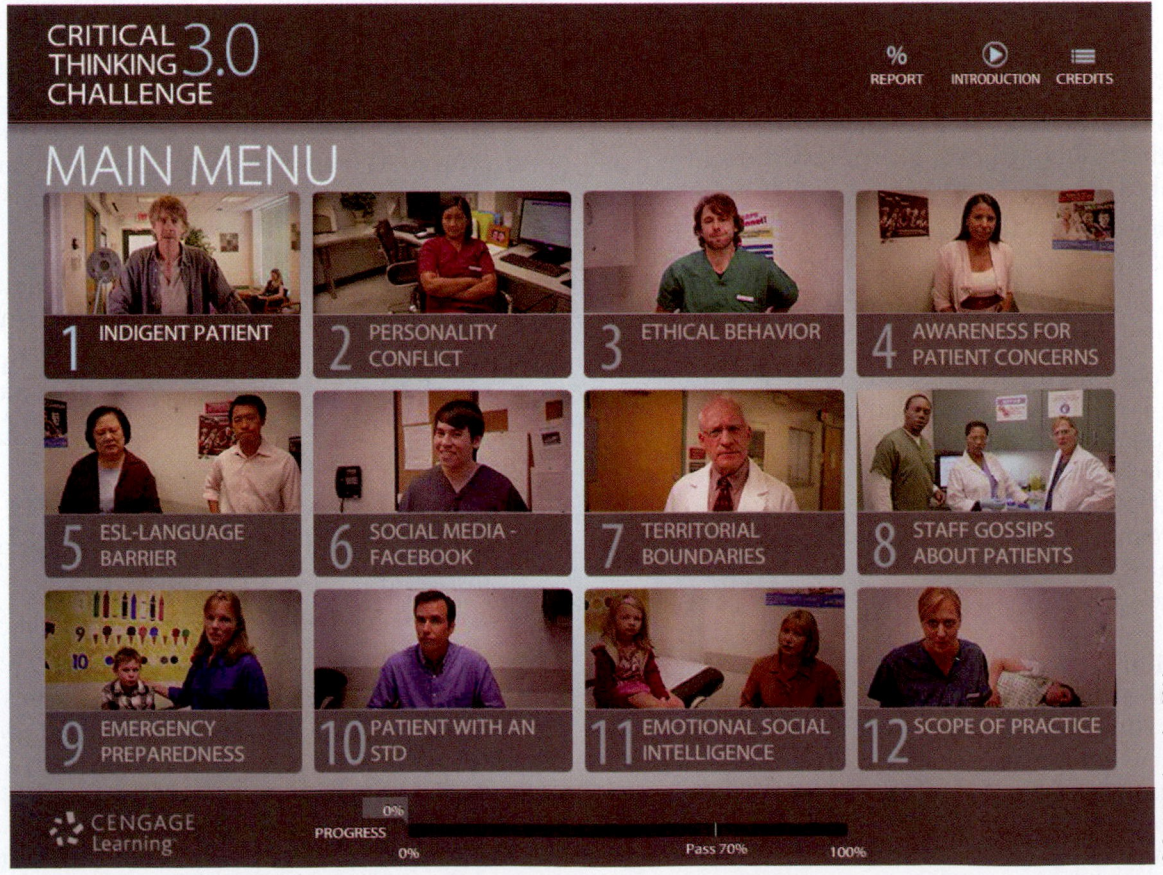

in which you must use your critical thinking skills to choose the most appropriate action in response to the situation. Your decisions will be evaluated in three categories: how your decisions affect the practice, the patient, and your career. The 3.0 version includes 12 all-new video-based scenarios with more branching options. After successfully completing the program, print out a Certification of Completion. *See Appendix E for more information about the Critical Thinking Challenge 3.0.*

Competency Challenge 2.0

The Competency Challenge 2.0 features interactive activities, better assessment, and a new concluding capstone element. To help practice the competencies necessary to become a medical assistant, you are "virtually" externing at a local medical clinic.

- Days 1 through 4 focus on 26 video-based case studies with interactive exercises.
- Day 5 is a "day in the life" capstone event that applies the competencies practiced to a realistic patient case study. In the case study, you will follow a new patient through a clinic visit for a physical exam.
- Features printable quiz scoring and competency checklists.

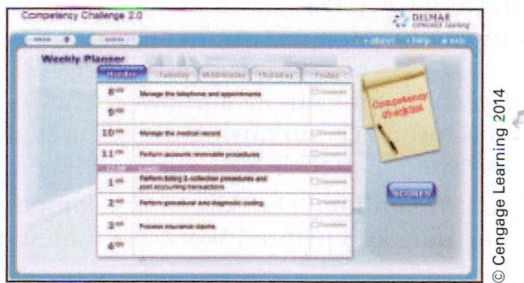

© Cengage Learning 2014

Virtual Administrative Skills for the Medical Assistant

This exciting new digital learning simulation focuses on key administrative tasks performed in the medical clinic. Each task requires you to demonstrate your professionalism and knowledge to complete a variety of customer service, financial, and clinic maintenance activities. Resources, feedback, and reporting guide and assess you throughout as you gain proficiency in performing these tasks. The program provides flexibility to complete tasks

in any order, and includes a printable performance review with scores to assess your work. Through successful completion of the simulation, you can feel more confident in your ability and skills to begin a career as an administrative medical assistant.

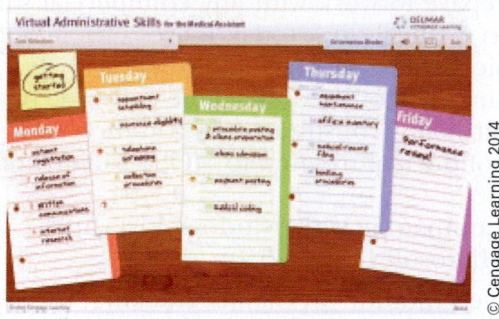

© Cengage Learning 2014

StudyWARE™ Software

StudyWARE™ is interactive software consisting of two programs:

1. **StudyWARE™** is interactive software with learning activities and quizzes to help study key concepts and test your comprehension. The activity and quiz content corresponds with each chapter in the text book:
   - Multiple choice, true/false, and fill-in-the-blank quizzes
   - Flash cards, concentration, hangman, case studies
   - Championship game
   - Visual instrument flash cards
   - Visual instrument concentration
   - Animations library

2. **Audio Library:** Practice pronouncing and recognizing medical terminology using the Audio Library. Search for terms by word or body system. Once a word is selected, it is pronounced correctly and defined on the screen.

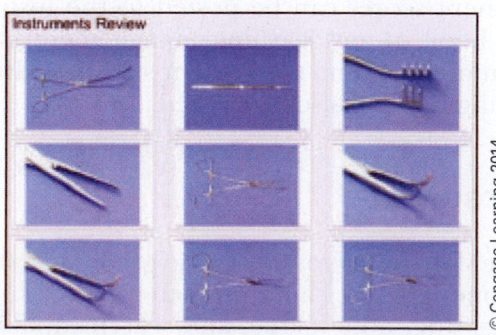

© Cengage Learning 2014

Medical Office Simulation Software (MOSS) 2.0

MOSS 2.0 (*CD-ROM in the front of the book*) is generic software built for educational purposes, to help users prepare to work with any commercial software used in medical clinic today. It uses a friendly, highly graphical interface that allows users to learn the fundamentals of medical clinic software packages without being constrained by a difficult interface. Some of the features new to MOSS 2.0 include:

- Compatible with Windows Vista and Microsoft Office 2010
- New module on Claims Tracking, to simulate receiving electronic explanations of benefits from individual carriers
- CMS-1500 (08-05) forms populate based on insurance type selected to meet the needs of medical billing programs
- Prebilling report added prior to generating claims
- Each insurance type has a fee schedule
- New financial reports added: Aging patient balance report, individual patient balance report
- Patient ledger report to track payment history

See Appendix E for more information about Medical Office Simulation Software 2.0.

Learning Lab

Learning Lab maps to learning objectives and includes interactive activities and case scenarios to build students' critical thinking skills and help retain the more difficult concepts. This simulated, immersive environment engages users with its real-life approach. Each Learning Lab has a pre-assessment, three to five learning activities, and a post-assessment organized around the units in this text. The post-assessment scores can be posted to the instructor grade book in any learning management system. The amount of time the student spends within the Learning Lab can also be tracked.

CourseMate

CourseMate helps you make the grade with several components: (1) an interactive eBook, with highlighting, note taking, and search capabilities; (2) interactive learning tools, including quizzes, flashcards, videos, games, and presentations; and

(3) Engagement Tracker, a first-of-its-kind tool that monitors student engagement in the course. Go to (www.cengagebrain.com) to access these resources and look for this icon, which 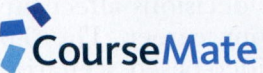 denotes a resource available within CourseMate.

Study Guide

The Study Guide has been fully revised to map closely to the book. Designed to reinforce and apply concepts and develop critical thinking, the Study Guide helps strengthen the knowledge and skills presented in the book.

The Assignment Sheets:

- Incorporate a mix of review exercises and application activities in the chapter assignment sheets
- Feature more hands-on application activities, case studies, forms to practice and certification exam practice

Competency Manual

The Competency Manual contains competency assessment checklists for each procedure that track all of the entry-level competencies designated by ABHES and CAAHEP.

Competency Assessment Checklists:

- Contain new source materials, scenarios, and forms accompanying the competency assessment checklists
- Are streamlined checklists, with competency mapping and printed Work Documentation forms

THE COMPLETE LEARNING PACKAGE: INSTRUCTOR SUPPLEMENTS

Instructor's Manual

The Instructor's Manual has been revised to be one comprehensive tool for instructors. Features include:

- Instructor Tips and Strategies for teaching, lesson planning, and evaluation
- Chapter Overviews, Outlines, and Activities

- Answers to Critical Thinking Boxes and Certification Reviews in the text
- Answers to all Study Guide activities

Instructor Resources

The Instructor Resources CD-ROM is a tool to help prepare for class, deliver effective presentations, and monitor student progress throughout the course. Create a total lesson plan, that includes visual examples, computer-generated tests, and more. Tools include:

- A Computerized Test Bank in ExamView with more than 1,200 questions and answers, organized by chapter
- Instructor slides created in PowerPoint for each chapter, which cover key concepts presented in the text and includes graphics, animations, and video clips
- An Image Library of more than 700 images from the text
- Complete, customizable Instructor's Manual files

Instructor Companion Site
(Access at www.cengage.com/login)

The Instructor Companion Site offers extra content for instructors. Log on to (www.cengage.com/login) to get these resources and more:

- CourseForward curriculum and curriculum mapping tools
- Customizable Competency Assessment Checklists
- Crossover and conversion guides
- Support documentation for software programs
- All resources found on the Instructor Resources CD-ROM
- All content found on the student Premium Website

CourseForward Curriculum

CourseForward is a modular curriculum solution that breaks down content into topics for ease of learning and serves as a road map for course material. CourseForward is designed for instructors to spend less time planning and more time teaching. Some of the features of CourseForward include:

- Equipment lists
- Homework assignments
- In-class discussion topics and suggested responses, individual and group activities
- Key Concepts table mapped to activities and assignments

WebTutor™ Advantage on Blackboard or Angel Platforms

WebTutor™ Advantage is an online classroom management tool that takes your course beyond the classroom wall. WebTutor™ provides rich communication and course management tools, including a course calendar, chat, email, threaded discussions, Web links, and a whiteboard. It also contains additional content to reinforce and enhance learning and test student learning, including:

- Learning Links explore health care topics through research on the Internet
- Critical thinking questions and case studies with video clips
- Discussion questions and quizzes for each chapter
- Quizzes by chapter, unit, and section
- A comprehensive terminal examination
- PowerPoint presentations that include animations and video clips

WebTutor™ Toolbox on Blackboard or Angel Platforms

WebTutor™ Toolbox is an online classroom management tool that takes your course beyond the classroom wall. WebTutor™ provides rich communication and course management tools, including a course calendar, chat, email, threaded discussions, Web links, and a whiteboard. Preloaded content includes objectives, advance preparation, and FAQs.

About the Authors

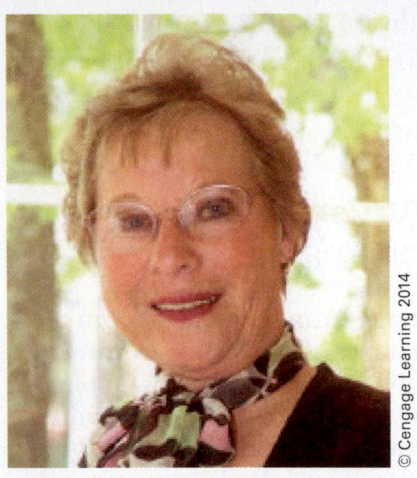

Wilburta (Billie) Q. Lindh, CMA, (AAMA), holds professor emeritus status at Highline Community College, Des Moines, Washington, where she was the former medical assisting program director and educator. Lindh was the honored recipient of the Outstanding Faculty Member of the Year award during her tenure. She participated in the original forum leading to the development and publication of Delmar's *Comprehensive Medical Assisting Administrative and Clinical Competencies* textbook. She is co-author of *Therapeutic Communications for Health Care* published by Delmar Cengage Learning, and she co-authored *The Radiology Word Book* and *The Ophthalmology Word Book*, texts frequently used by transcriptionists and other medical professions. She also authored the medical assistant chapter for *Guide to Careers in the Health Professions*. Ms. Lindh is a member of the SeaTac Chapter of the American Association of Medical Assistants (AAMA) and has lectured at AAMA seminars on the local, state, and national levels. She resides in Federal Way, Washington, with her husband DeVere.

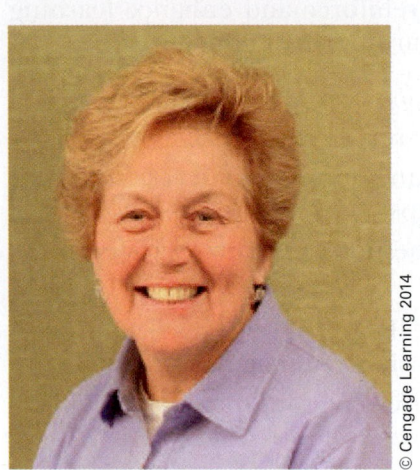

Marilyn S. Pooler, RN, MEd, RMA (AMT), served as a professor in medical assisting and taught for more than 25 years at Springfield Technical Community College in Springfield, Massachusetts, where she served as the medical assisting department chairperson for several years. Marilyn also served on the Certifying Board of the AAMA Task Force for test construction and was a site surveyor for the AAMA for many years. Ms. Pooler is a member of the Hampden District chapter of the American Association of Medical Assistants (AAMA), and she has been a speaker at local and state medical assisting meetings and seminars, emphasizing the importance of education, certification, and recertification of medical assistants. For a number of years, she was a member of the Executive Board of the Northeast Association of Allied Health Educators. Presently, she works at Baystate Medical Center in Springfield, Massachusetts, in their ambulatory/clinic areas, and for the Center of Business and Technology at Springfield Technical Community College, where she teaches review courses to medical assistants.

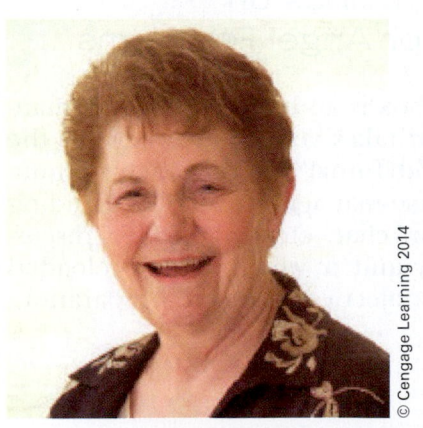

Carol D. Tamparo, CMA (AAMA), PhD, served as a medical assistant instructor for 24 years and as program director for medical assisting for 15 years at Highline Community College, Des Moines, Washington. She was the Dean of Business and Allied Health programs at Lake Washington Technical College in Kirkland, Washington, for 4 years. She is the co-author of *Therapeutic Communications for Health Care; Medical Law, Ethics, & Bioethics for Ambulatory Care;* and *Diseases of the Human Body*. She is a member of the SeaTac Chapter of AAMA and is a frequent speaker for medical assistants in the Northwest. You can find Ms. Tamparo on Facebook.

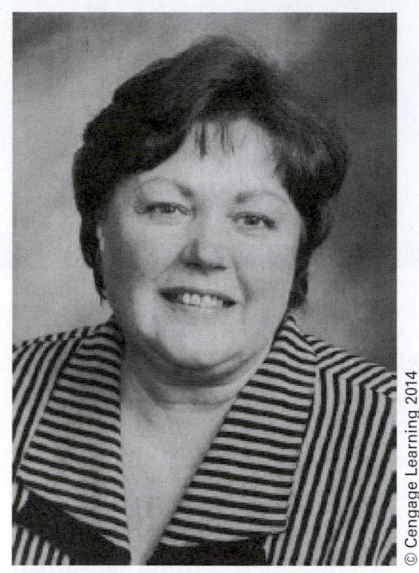

© Cengage Learning 2014

Barbara M. Dahl, CMA (AAMA), CPC, has dedicated her professional life to the recognition, education, and advancement of medical assistants through quality education, increased public awareness, legislative compliance, and positive professional development. She retired in 2010 from Whatcom Community College in Bellingham where she served as the Medical Assisting Program Coordinator and tenured faculty member for over 20 years. She is an active member of the Whatcom County Chapter of Medical Assistants, Washington State Society of Medical Assistants (WSSMA), the AAMA, and the Washington State Medical Assisting Educators. She is a former WSSMA state president and has served on and chaired many committees on the chapter, state, and national levels including state legislative committee and the Coalition for the Medical Assisting Scope of Practice for the state of Washington. She was instrumental in developing and designing the AAMA Excel Award–winning WSSMA website and continues to serve as the state co-webmaster. As a Certified Professional Coder she was a member of the AAPC for many years. She is a frequent speaker for many medical assisting conferences and seminars on both the local and state levels in clinical, administrative, legal, and leadership topics and has been a guest speaker at the Washington State Podiatric Medical Association for the past three years.

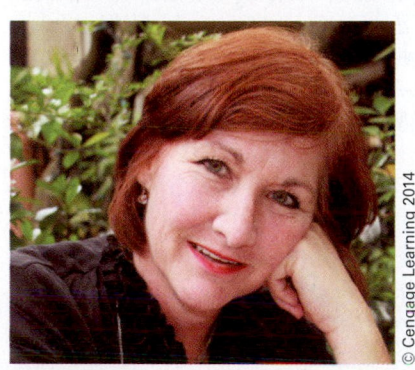

© Cengage Learning 2014

Julie A. Morris, RN, BSN, CBCS, CCMA, CMAA entered the field of medicine as a phlebotomist at the age of 16. She obtained a Bachelor of Science degree in nursing from Jacksonville State University. In her three-plus decades in health care she has experienced multiple facets of the profession including intensive care, cardiac catheterization lab, surgical nursing, and owning a home infusion company. She entered the education field in 2009 and served as an allied health program director for a large student population. Teaching has always been her passion. She has taught adult learners in critical care, medical assisting, and medical billing and coding. Ms. Morris is also a Subject Matter Expert, as well as a co-author, for Delmar, Cengage Learning. She is currently the Director of Career Services for Medtech College, placing allied health professionals in Atlanta, Georgia.

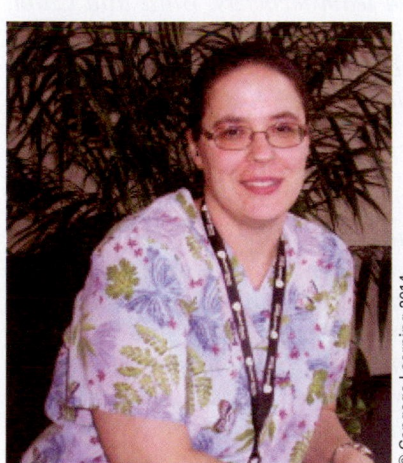

© Cengage Learning 2014

Angela P. Rein, RMA (AMT), AS, BSHM, CPC, MAHS, CPC-H has been in the medical field since 1994, when she graduated from Sanford-Brown College with a diploma in Medical Administrative Assistance. She earned the credential of Registered Medical Assistant from the AMT in 1996. After working in the field for many years, she continued her education and obtained three separate college degrees. In 2004, she completed her Associate of Science in Medical Assisting from High-Tech Institute. Ms. Rein completed her Bachelor of Science in Health Management from Anthem College in 2007. Finally, in 2008, she obtained her Master of Arts in Human Service from Liberty University, with a specialization in Health and Wellness. She has been a member of the AAPC since 2007 and holds the credentials of both the CPC and the CPC-H. She has been an officer a total of three times in the local AAPC Chapter of Maryville, Illinois, having served as the vice president (2009), president (2010), and member development officer (2011). She has taught in the post-secondary proprietary environment for over ten years, and is now the Medical Program Director for Vatterott College-Online Division in St. Louis, Missouri. She has done fund raising and coordinated her past students to do volunteer work at the Illinois Center for Autism. Ms. Rein resides in Collinsville, Illinois, with her husband and two sons.

Acknowledgments

A special thank you to my husband, DeVere, who continually supports, encourages, and assists me in so many ways. Thank you to my family and friends, who understood when I was not available for activities, but continually accepted and encouraged my commitment to excellence. Collaborating with the author team and those at Delmar, Cengage Learning encouraged forward thinking and a 5th edition that is progressive and current with technology to ensure that medical assisting students are well prepared for tomorrow's challenges.

Billie Q. Lindh

Many thanks are expressed to my husband, Tom, who assumed many household chores and took us out to dinner at just the right time. Writing a textbook, even the revision of a textbook, requires the input and dedication of many individuals, especially in the field of health care where changes occur almost daily. Collaborating with the other authors on this edition has ensured that the most recent information is included in this text. Thank you Lauren Whalen and Sarah Prime for your vision and guidance.

Carol D. Tamparo

First I would like to thank my husband, Ed, for his continued support and encouragement during this 5th edition revision. It has been an exciting experience; making sure our textbook is the best and most current representation of what today's medical assistant student needs to know to enter the profession, covering the cognitive, psychomotor, and affective domains, as well as using the most current technology and new clinical diagnostics and equipment. I appreciate the opportunity to continue working with my diversely talented team members, Billie and Carol, and I welcome the fresh perspective of our new team members, Julie and Angela. I also have a great deal of appreciation for the expertise and patience from Lauren Whalen and our Delmar/Cengage Learning team and S4Carlisle Publishing in updating this nationally respected resource.

Barbara M. Dahl

So many great moments have happened around me as I have worked on this text. I want to thank my children, Sam Huckaby and Casey Mountjoy for their understanding and love. From the bottom of my heart, I want to thank the love of my life, Phillip Rutledge, for his patience and forbearance as I have focused on this project. Every interaction with Cengage Learning has been one in which I have gained in experience and knowledge. Thank you Sarah Prime, Lauren Whalen, Rhonda Dearborn, et. al! I want to thank all the talented professionals that I have worked with during my career in health care. Everything I know, I learned from someone. I am grateful and sincerely hope that their influence is faithfully represented in this text, especially in the focus on the attributes of professionalism.

Julie A. Morris

Many special thanks to Lauren Whalen and Sarah Prime for all of your continuous guidance and support throughout this project. I wish to also thank everyone on the author team for their continuous feedback and strong desire for student success: Barb, Billie, Carol, and Julie. To my husband Eric for always being there for me and for taking care of our boys when I was so busy writing and working. Finally, to my mother Cathy Rombach—who always told me to reach for my dreams and to never give up.

Angela Rein

Contributors

Michelle Blesi, MBA, CMA (AAMA)
Program Director, Medical Assisting
Century College – East Campus
White Bear Lake, MN
Subject Matter Expert for the Critical Thinking Challenge 3.0

Cindy Correa
Former Educational Coordinator and Curricula Developer, Allied
    Health Program
City University of New York at Queens College
Flushing, NY
Administrative Procedures for Medical Office Simulation Software 2.0

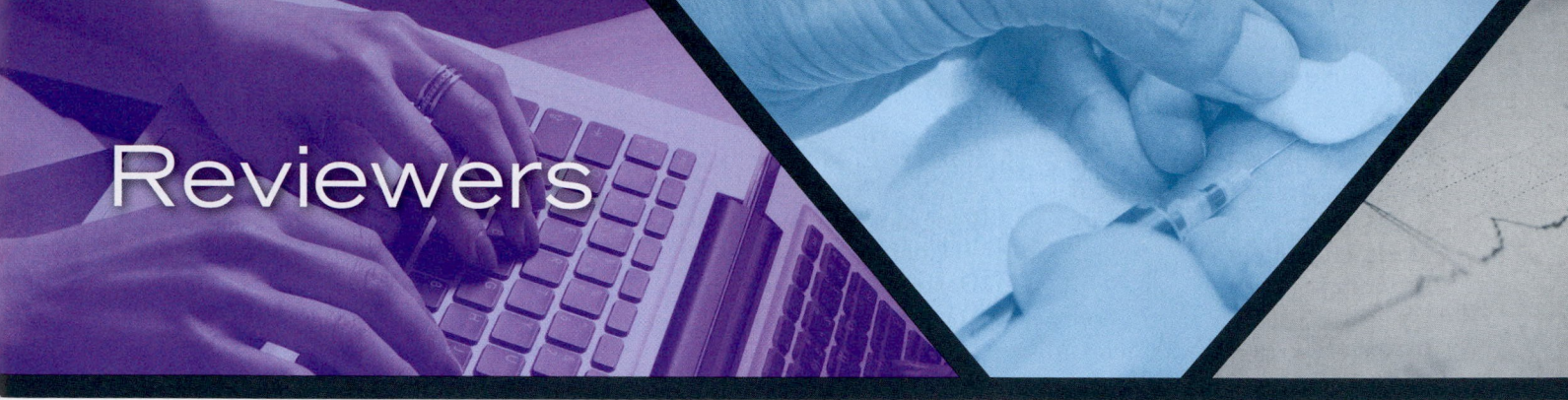

Reviewers

Rose T. Allain, RN, BSN, CCM
St. Vincent Hospital
Worcester, MA

Anthony Avenido, M.D.
Allied Health Department Chair
Brown Mackie College
Cincinnati, OH

Diane Roche Benson, CMA
(AAMA), MSA, BSHCA, CPC
Professor
Wake Technical Community
College, JCC/University of
Phoenix
Raleigh, NC

Cindy Brazell, B.S., M.A.
Program Director, Office
Administration
Salter College
West Boylston, MA

Deborah Bryant, BSHS, CMA
(AAMA)
Program Director/Teacher
Chattahoochee Technical
College
Acworth, GA

Tracy Carter, BS, RMA
Medical Assistant Instructor
Ross Medical Education Center
Portage, MI

Barbara Cerna, CMA (AAMA)
Instructor and Program Director
of Health Care Professions and
currently Business Division Chair
Highline Community College
Des Moines, WA

Lynn Cherry, RN, MSN
Director of Medical Programs
Dorsey Schools
Madison Heights, MI

Courtney Conrad, CMA, MBA,
MPH
Professor
Robert Morris University
Peoria, IL

Dana Curry, CMA (AAMA)
Program Director, Medical
Assisting AAMA
Boise, ID

Rhonda Epps, CMA (AAAMA),
RMA (AMT), BS
Director of Healthcare Education
National College
Knoxville, TN

Ekbal S. Fakhoury, MD,
DTM&H, MS
Director of Healthcare Programs
Heald College
Concord, CA

Jennifer Fendinger, MS eEd, MT
(ASCP), CET (NHA), CPT
(NHA)
Medical Assisting/Phlebotomy/
EKG Practicum Coordinator
Bryant & Stratton College –
Southtowns Campus
Orchard Park, NY

Angela K. Fulford, CMA
(AAMA), AAS
Administrative Instructor
Ross Medical Education Center
Fort Wayne, IN

Judee L. Gorczynski, M.Ed., BBS,
AAS, NR-CMA
Allied Health Department Chair
Fortis College
Cuyahoga, Falls, OH

Victoria Gottschalk, RMA, AHI
Medical Assistant Instructor,
Regional Trainer, Curriculum
Development
Ross Medical Education Centers
Brighton, MI

Kimberly Hockaday, NCMA,
NCET, NCICS, AS, BLS
Director of Medical Assisting
Carrington College
Reno, NV

Brina Hollis, PhD, MHHS, CST,
NCICS
Allied Health Programs Director
Bryant & Stratton College
Parma, OH

Cynthia Greiner Holmes, M.A.M.
Faculty
Prospect Education/Charter
College, LLC
Reno, NV

Cheryl D. Jerzak, BSHA, CMA
(AAMA)
Director of Medical Assistant
Program
Four-D College
Colton, CA

Faith Kallert
Medical Assistant Program
Supervisor
Lincoln Technical Institute
Mahwah, NJ

Linda A. Lee, RMA, RPT, EMT-P,
EECP-T, CCT, CRAT
Director of Healthcare Education
National College
Cleveland, OH

Penny Lee, CMA, CAHI
Program Director of Medical
   Assisting
Medtech College
Indianapolis, IN

Lynnae Lockett, RN, MSN, CMRS
Subject Area Coordinator
Bryant & Stratton College
Parma, OH

Wanda MacLeod, A.H.I.
Instructor
Ross Medical Education Center
Roosevelt Park, MI

Sheila Malahowski, CCA, MBA
Associate Professor, HIM
   Coordinator
Luzerne County Community
   College
Nanticoke, PA

Tammy Martin-Griffin, CMA,
   BS-HSM
Assistant Professor
Springfield Technical
   Community College
Springfield, MA

Michelle McClatchey, BS, CMRS
Program Chair
Westwood College-CHR
Calumet City, IL

Joann Monks, RN, BSN-BC, MBA,
   RMA
Salter College
West Boylston, MA

Tamara E. Mottler, B.A., CMA
   (AAMA)
Program Manager/Assistant
   Chair
Daytona State College
Daytona Beach, FL

Sherry Pearsall, RN, MSN, CAS
Medical Program Coordinator
Bryant & Stratton College
Syracuse, NY

Connie Pettengill, R.N., M.Ed.
Department Chairperson
Springfield Technical
   Community College
Springfield, MA

Blasé Romence, D.C., CMA
   (AAMA)
Professor, MA Curriculum Chair,
   Program Director (Central
   Region)
Robert Morris University
Springfield, IL

Margaret J. Roslasky, RN
Instructor
Lincoln Technical Institute
Mahwah, NJ

Stephanie Ross, PBT, CMA
   (AAMA), AAS, MA
Instructor
Chattahoochee Technical
   College
Georgia

Lori Starnes, AAS, CMA (AAMA)
Program Director, Medical
   Assisting
South Piedmont Community
   College
Polkton, NC

Arleen E. Stern, CMA-C (AAMA),
   PBT (ASCP)
Medical Instructor
Lincoln Technical Institute
Mahwah, NJ

Traci L. SuSong, MBA/HCM,
   CMA (AAMA), CMRS, CCS-P
Business Manager
Summa Health Systems
Akron, OH

Lottie Thompson, BSN, M. Ed.
Allied Health Director
Fortis College
Mobile, AL

Joy Williams, RMA
MA Program Director
Vatterott College
Quincy, IL

Shantreese Young, RMA, CRC
Allied Health Instructor
Fortis College
Mobile, AL

Patti Zint, CMA-NHA
Program Director, MA/HCA
Carrington College
Phoenix, AZ

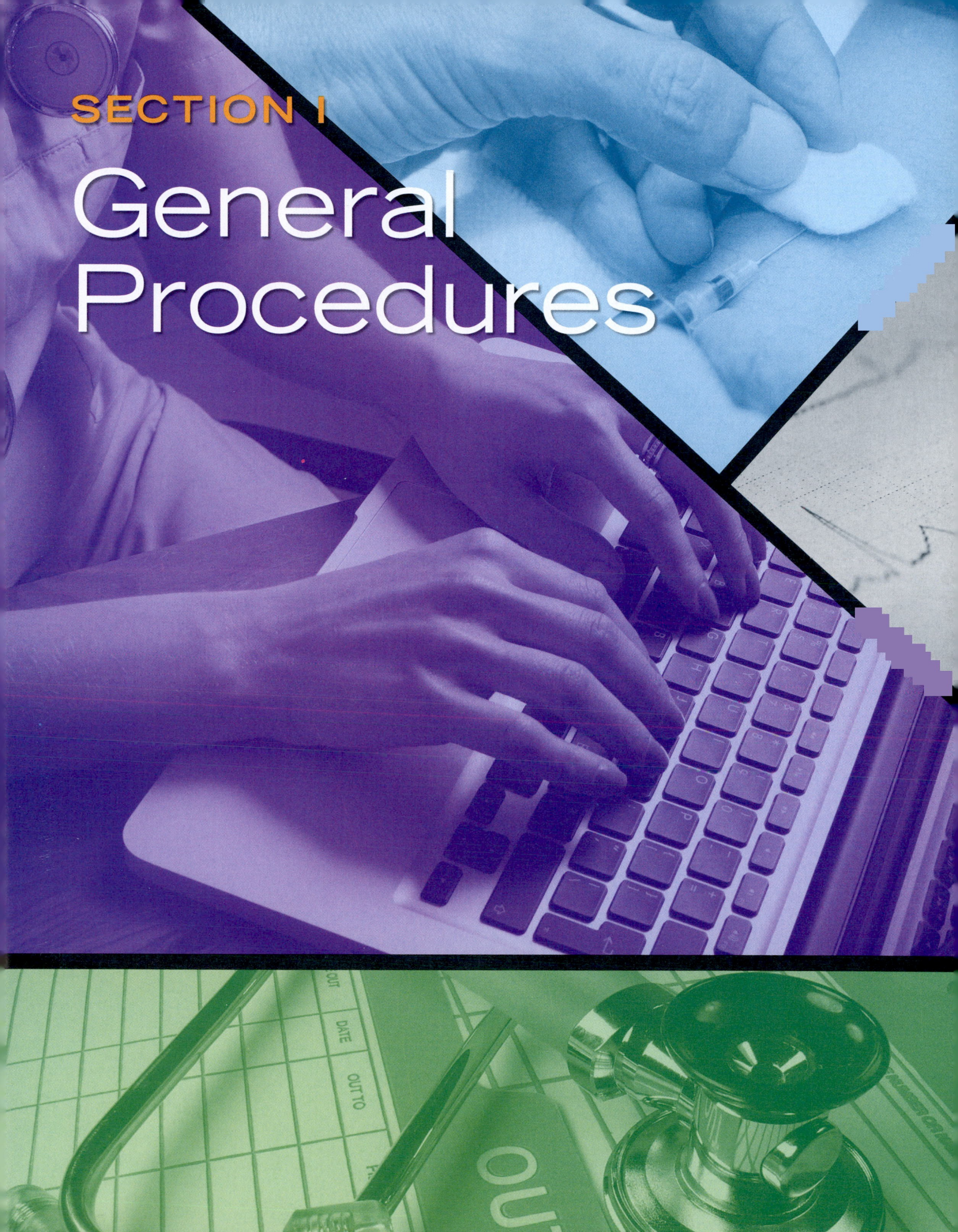

SECTION I

General Procedures

General
Procedures

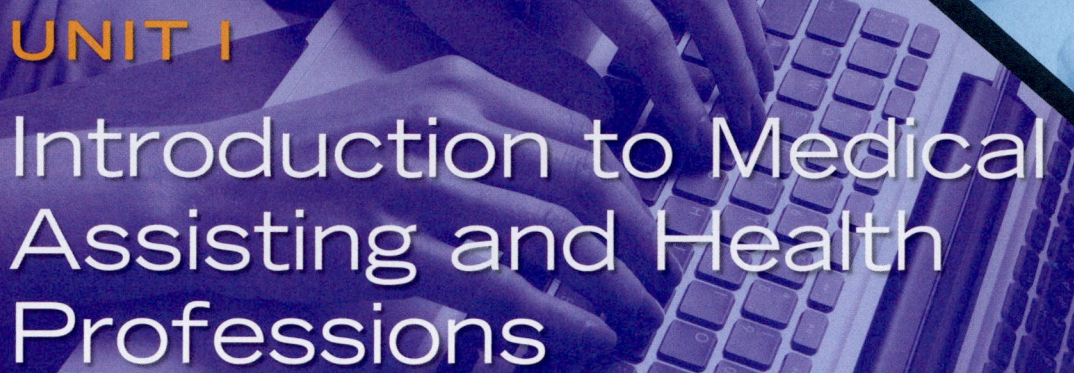

UNIT I
Introduction to Medical Assisting and Health Professions

CHAPTER 1
The Medical Assisting Profession 4

CHAPTER 2
Health Care Settings and the Health Care Team 22

CHAPTER 3
History of Medicine 40

The Medical Assisting Profession

OUTLINE

Historical Perspective of the Profession

Career Opportunities

Education of the Medical Assistant
  Courses in a Medical Assisting Program
  Practicum
  Associate and Bachelor Degrees

Accreditation of Medical Assisting Programs
  CAAHEP
  ABHES

Attributes of a Medical Assistant Professional
  Communication
  Presentation
  Competency
  Initiative
  Integrity

American Association of Medical Assistants
  Certification
  Continuing Education

American Medical Technologists
  Registered Medical Assistant

Certified Medical Administrative Specialist

Continuing Education

Other Certification
  National Healthcareer Association
  National Center for Competency Testing (NCCT)

Regulation of Health Care Providers
  Scope of Practice

LEARNING OUTCOMES

1. Define, spell, and pronounce the key terms as presented in the glossary.
2. Discuss the history of medical assisting.
3. Describe the practicum experience.
4. Recall two criteria for the selection of practicum sites.
5. List three benefits of the practicum to the student and the site.
6. Describe the profession of medical assisting and analyze its career opportunities in relationship to your interests.
7. Identify and discuss five attributes that are essential to a professional medical assistant's career.
8. Describe the American Association of Medical Assistants and discuss its major functions.
9. Discuss the role of the American Medical Technologists in the credentialing of medical assistants.
10. Explain the purpose of the National Healthcareer Association.
11. Explain accreditation, certification, and continuing education as they pertain to the professional medical assistant.
12. Differentiate the requirements for certification and recertification for each of the credentialing bodies.
13. Identify the importance of the accreditation process to an educational institution.
14. Recall at least two methods available to obtain recertification.
15. List five means of obtaining continuing education units.
16. Differentiate among certification, licensure, and registration.
17. State the importance of understanding the scope of practice for the medical assistant.
18. Analyze the professionalism questions and apply them to this chapter's content.

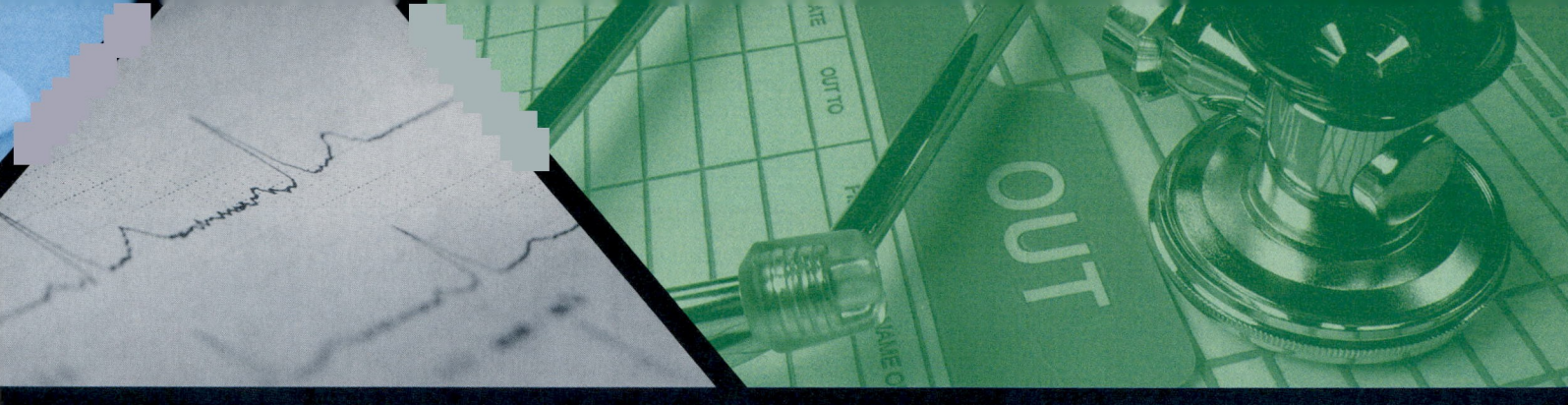

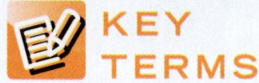 KEY TERMS

accreditation

ambulatory care setting

associate's degree

attribute

bachelor's degree

certification

Certified Clinical
Medical Assistant
(CCMA [AMT])

Certified Medical
Administrative
Assistant (CCMA)

Certified Medical
Assistant (CMA
[AAMA])

competency

compliance

credentialed

dexterity

diploma

disposition

empathy

externship

facilitate

improvise

internship

license

licensure

practicum

professionalism

proprietary

Registered
Medical Assistant
(RMA [AMT])

scope of practice

SCENARIO

A group of high school freshmen have come to tour the medical assisting class and laboratory areas. The Program Director of Medical Assisting is showing the students around the department. The Program Director then takes them into the medical assisting laboratory, where the senior medical assistant students are practicing their clinical skills. Each senior student pairs up with a high school freshman, and each pair talks about medical assisting, with the medical assistant students answering questions the others may have. The medical assistant students are in uniform as part of their preparation to go into various health care agencies to do their externship or practicum. The medical assistant students look professional, clean,

fresh, and motivated. They tell the high school students about medical assisting and describe the personal and physical attributes desirable for those who want to become medical assistants. They explain the importance of these attributes, as well as what duties a professional medical assistant performs and what education is needed to pursue a career in medical assisting.

Throughout the question and answer discussions, the senior medical assistant students and the program director stress the importance of ethics, empathy, attitude, dependability, and teamwork as favorable attributes. Individuals seeking a career in medical assisting should develop and maintain these characteristics.

INTRODUCTION

There are many fascinating aspects of the medical assisting profession. When a person pursues formal education to enter the world of medicine as a professional medical assistant, he or she may take on a new role in his or her family and community. In this new role, the medical assisting student can have a major, positive influence on the community-wide knowledge of health and the process for seeking medical care. This influence is just the beginning of the many highly rewarding aspects of becoming a medical assistant.

The medical assistant is defined by the American Association of Medical Assistants (AAMA) Board of Trustees as "A multi-skilled member of the health care team who performs administrative and clinical procedures under the supervision of licensed healthcare providers." The majority of medical assistants, about 62 percent, are employed by provider practices, though there are many career opportunities in many settings. The list of licensed health care providers that can supervise medical assistants has expanded to include Nurse Practitioners, Physician's Assistants, Podiatrists, Chiropractors, and Optometrists.

Medical assistants come from a variety of backgrounds and educational experiences. Today there are only a very few medical assistants trained on the job. Due to the sophistication of the health care consumer and the complexity of delivering health care, employers are seeking medical assistants who have already been educated and are credentialed for employment in their practices.

There is an entire body of knowledge—such as anatomy and physiology, medical terminology, and practical clinical skills—that must be acquired in your studies to become a professional medical assistant. An equally important aspect of a medical assistant's career is **professionalism**. *Professionalism combines your acquired knowledge and skills with the types of behavior that demonstrate your moral, ethical, and respectful attributes when interacting with patients and colleagues.*

HISTORICAL PERSPECTIVE OF THE PROFESSION

There is a rich history of medical assisting and the medical assistants who enjoy the profession. Historically, medicine has included the role of the handmaiden. This person served to assist the provider in his daily tasks caring for an ill population. This role was essential, but undefined. The first recognition of this important aspect of health care was nursing. As time progressed, another vital role emerged—that of the medical assistant.

The last 100 years have brought an acceleration of medical technology that has impacted both the diagnosis and treatment of many disease processes as well as the maintenance of wellness. With advancing technology, the provider has increased the demands on the staff of the practice. Nursing has held a traditional role of management, training, and assisting the provider in clinical procedures. As the availability of testing and treatment has moved from a more acute-care setting to the

SPOTLIGHT ON CERTIFICATION

RMA Content Outline
- Medical law
- Medical ethics
- Human relations

CMA (AAMA) Content Outline
- Professionalism
- Communication
- Medicolegal concepts and guidelines

CMAS Content Outline
- Legal and ethical considerations
- Professionalism

provider's clinic, there has been an expanding role for the medical assistant in the delivery of care. The medical assistant must possess a wide array of skills including excellent communication skills, clinical skills that relate to patient care, and administrative skills that are required to manage the facility and the practice finances. These skills are all part of the requirements for a professional medical assistant in today's market.

In 1978, the profession of medical assisting was formally recognized by the United States Department of Education. In 1991, the board of trustees of the American Association of Medical Assistants (AAMA) approved the current definition of medical assisting:

> Medical Assisting is an allied health profession whose practitioners function as members of the health care delivery team and perform administrative and clinical procedures.

Medical assisting has become well respected among the professions in allied health care.

CAREER OPPORTUNITIES

Medical assistants have been described as health care's most versatile, multifaceted professionals.

That medical assistants possess a broad scope of knowledge and skills makes them ideal professionals for any **ambulatory care setting**. Indeed, because of such versatility, medical assistants find employment in a variety of settings: clinics, medical laboratories, insurance companies, government agencies, pharmaceutical companies, educational institutions, surgical centers, urgent-care facilities, and electrocardiography (ECG or EKG) departments in hospitals. Other career opportunities are available to the medical assistant. Some medical assistants work as phlebotomists, coding specialists, medical laboratory assistants, and medical administrative specialists. The broad application of the skills of a medical assistant is relevant to many aspects of a medical practice. This ensures the continued growth of responsibilities and opportunities for medical assisting.

Currently, there are approximately half a million medical assistants in the workforce, with projections of more than 650,000 job opportunities by 2018, according to the United States Department of Labor. The job market for medical assistants is projected to grow much faster than average. Increased employment opportunities for medical assistants will result from the increased medical needs of an aging population, growth in the number of health care providers and their desire to hire the most qualified person for the task, increased diagnostic testing, greater volume and complexity of paperwork and computer information, managed care's emphasis on ambulatory care, and the insurance-mandated shorter stay of patients in hospitals.

EDUCATION OF THE MEDICAL ASSISTANT

Formal education of medical assistants takes place in community and junior colleges, as well as in **proprietary** schools. Educational requirements are based on current entry-level responsibilities that medical assistants perform in the medical clinic. These requirements were previously known as the Developing A CUrriculuM (DACUM) Analysis. In 1997, in coordination with the National Board of Medical Examiners, educators, and practicing **Certified Medical Assistants (CMAs)**, the AAMA developed the Medical Assistant Role Delineation Chart, now known as the Occupational Analysis of the CMA (AAMA) (see Appendix C to review this chart). Entry-level competencies must be mastered by students in academic programs.

Classroom instruction takes place in community colleges, proprietary schools, and junior colleges that offer courses in medical assisting. The lecture portion of classes takes place in a classroom setting. The skills portion takes place in a laboratory setting in which supplies and equipment similar to those in the medical clinic/ambulatory care setting are available for practice.

An important new mode of education is online education. Some schools offer medical assistant courses online, and, if the school is accredited, many students who cannot or desire not to take traditional classroom courses can work toward becoming certified or registered through this method. On graduation, the student will receive a **diploma** or certificate of completion. If a student decides to pursue additional courses, it could take another year to complete an **associate's degree** (a total of 2 years) or longer for a **bachelor's degree**.

Courses in a Medical Assisting Program

Some of the administrative, general, and clinical courses are listed in Table 1-1. Another aspect of an educational medical assisting program is the **practicum**, a period when students participate in an on-the-job training program. This provides an excellent opportunity to apply theory to practices.

Practicum

Practicum, **externship**, and **internship** are all terms used to define the transition period between the classroom and actual employment. A practicum is planned and supervised by a coordinator from the medical assisting program and the health care facility that agrees to become a partner in the education and employability of the student.

Practicum Sites.   Sites for practicums are chosen carefully to ensure that a variety of experiences are available for the student. The sites should provide the student with adequate administrative, clinical, and general experiences. The staff at the various sites must be willing to make a commitment to the medical assistant's education by spending appropriate time observing and instructing the student (see Chapter 45 for more information on supervising student practicums).

(see Chapter 45 for more information on supervising student practicums)

CRITICAL THINKING

Patients and providers prefer to have working for them professional medical assistants who have had the benefit of a formal education. Discuss the impact of this education on patients and employers. Why is it important to both groups?

Table 1-1   Some Typical Administrative, General, and Clinical Courses in an Accredited Medical Assisting Program

Administrative Courses	Electronic medical records (EMRs) and electronic health records (EHRs)
	Word processing
	Appointments and scheduling
	Insurance claims/coding
	Billing, collections, and patients' accounts
General Courses	Anatomy and physiology
	Medical terminology
	Diseases
	Law and ethics
	Patient education
Clinical Courses	Infection control
	Disease prevention
	Medical prevention
	Pharmacology
	Temperature, pulse, respirations, and blood pressure
	Assisting the provider with physical exams
	Assisting the provider with minor surgery
	Drawing blood samples
	Urine and blood testing in the laboratory
	CPR (provider-level certification), first aid

© Cengage Learning 2014

Benefits of Practicum.   The practicum experience is mutually beneficial to the student and staff at the health care facility that is providing the educational experiences. Students are able to apply classroom knowledge and skill in a real-world medical setting, while using the practicum experience to build a resume and begin to establish a network of support through colleagues. The staff at the health care facility are given the opportunity to educate and impart knowledge to the student.

Associate and Bachelor Degrees

The expanding role and applicable job openings for medical assistants has allowed a new focus on degrees in medical assisting. Both proprietary schools and more traditional educational institutions have added both associate's and bachelor's degrees in medical assisting to their curriculum.

The primary benefit of these degrees is positioning in the job market. With an expanded curriculum, the medical assistant is prepared with college-level classes that include college math, English, and psychology as well as more in-depth classes related to medical assisting. Employers are eager to hire candidates with a demonstrated commitment to education and to their profession. Movement up the career ladder in health care is assisted by educational credentials as well as job experience.

With the increase of allied health education programs in the United States ranging from the certificate level to degree levels, a new opportunity has been created for tenured medical assistants: that of instructor. Required credentials for instructors in each medical assisting program are outlined by the credentialing bodies of each educational organization.

ACCREDITATION OF MEDICAL ASSISTING PROGRAMS

Educational institutions seeking **accreditation** for a medical assisting program must develop the curricula to meet the *Standards and Guidelines* set by the Commission on Accreditation for Allied Health Education Programs (CAAHEP), or the standards set by the Accrediting Bureau of Health Education Schools (ABHES) to ensure the highest quality medical assistant education and employment preparedness.

CAAHEP

The Commission on Accreditation for Allied Health Education Programs (CAAHEP) is an accrediting body for medical assisting programs in private and public postsecondary institutions and programs that prepare individuals for entry into the profession.

A medical assisting program that is accredited by CAAHEP meets the standards as outlined in the *Standards and Guidelines for an Accredited Education Program for the Medical Assistant*. Standards are the minimum standards of quality used in accrediting programs that prepare individuals to enter the medical assisting profession.

On-site review teams evaluate the program's **compliance** with, or adherence to, the standards. All aspects of programs seeking accreditation status undergo scrutiny to ascertain the program's quality and to ensure continued compliance with the standards.

For more information, see the CAAHEP Web site at http://www.caahep.org.

ABHES

The Accrediting Bureau of Health Education Schools (ABHES) is the agency that also grants accreditation to medical assisting programs. ABHES is recognized by the United States Department of Education (USDE) as an accrediting agency of public and private schools and colleges that primarily offer health education. This includes medical assisting, medical laboratory technology, and surgical technology programs. Besides being recognized by the USDE, recognition for ABHES comes from the AAMA, American Medical Technologists (AMT), National League for Nursing Accrediting (NLNA), and National Board of Surgical Technology and Surgical Assisting (NBSTSA).

More information about ABHES can be obtained through the ABHES Web site at http://www.abhes.org.

ATTRIBUTES OF A MEDICAL ASSISTANT PROFESSIONAL

Medical assistants should strive to cultivate certain characteristics or personal qualities. These are the **attributes** that identify a true professional; when caring for patients, these qualities should be sincere. They will enable the patient to trust you, the caregiver. Figure 1-1 lists some of the important attributes of professionalism. As you interact with patients and colleagues, the questions listed in the figure will serve as guidelines for the type of professional behavior that is expected from medical assistants. It is difficult to list all of the requirements for presenting the demeanor of a competent professional. Many of the aspects of professionalism are those that cannot be measured. Communication and competency can be monitored and evaluated to improve performance, but other aspects—such as presentation, initiative, and integrity—are harder to quantify. Being a professional incorporates all of these attributes. You should continue to reflect on these important aspects of professionalism as you increase your knowledge of anatomy and physiology, medical terminology, procedures, and other concrete aspects of the profession.

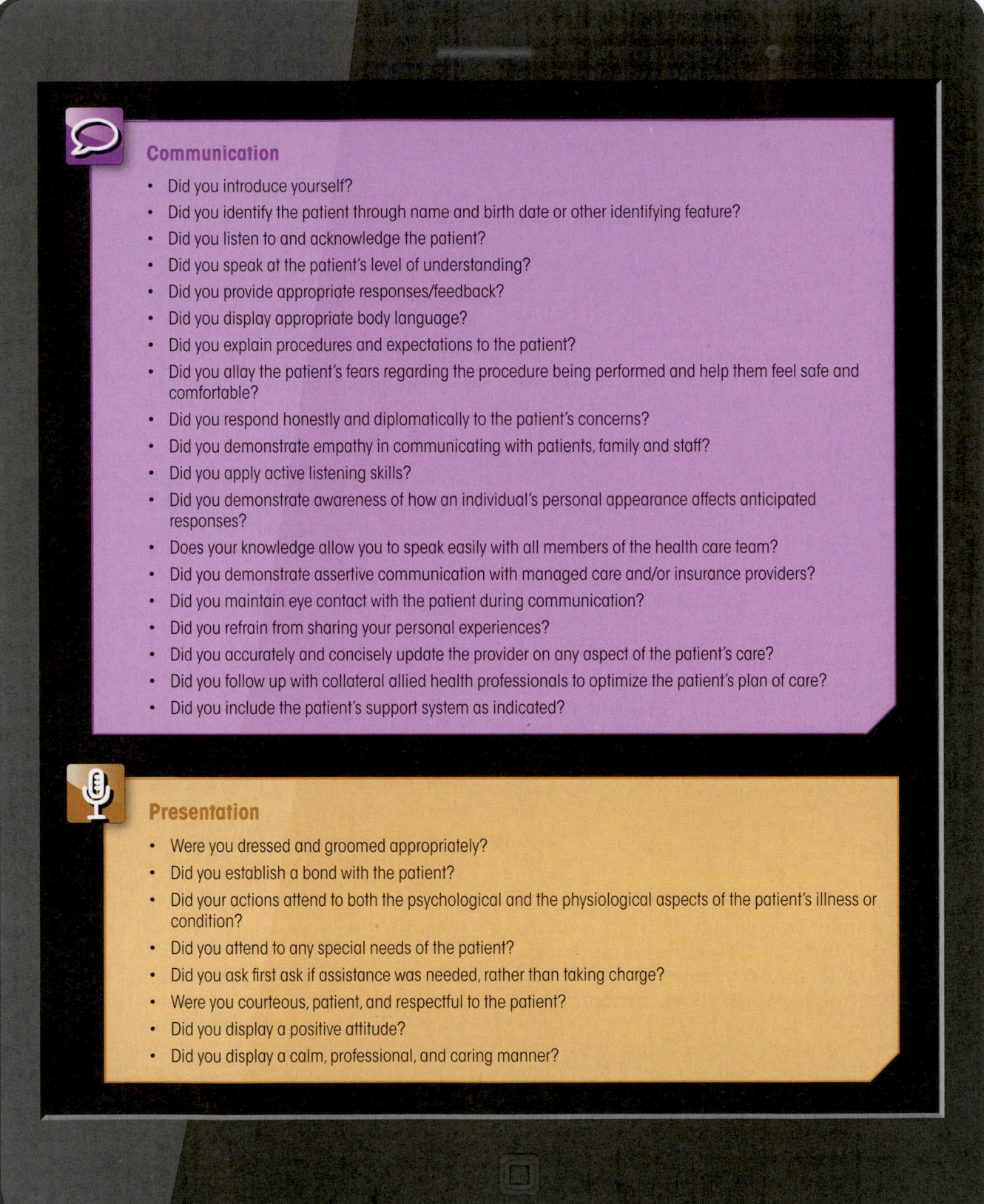

Communication

- Did you introduce yourself?
- Did you identify the patient through name and birth date or other identifying feature?
- Did you listen to and acknowledge the patient?
- Did you speak at the patient's level of understanding?
- Did you provide appropriate responses/feedback?
- Did you display appropriate body language?
- Did you explain procedures and expectations to the patient?
- Did you allay the patient's fears regarding the procedure being performed and help them feel safe and comfortable?
- Did you respond honestly and diplomatically to the patient's concerns?
- Did you demonstrate empathy in communicating with patients, family and staff?
- Did you apply active listening skills?
- Did you demonstrate awareness of how an individual's personal appearance affects anticipated responses?
- Does your knowledge allow you to speak easily with all members of the health care team?
- Did you demonstrate assertive communication with managed care and/or insurance providers?
- Did you maintain eye contact with the patient during communication?
- Did you refrain from sharing your personal experiences?
- Did you accurately and concisely update the provider on any aspect of the patient's care?
- Did you follow up with collateral allied health professionals to optimize the patient's plan of care?
- Did you include the patient's support system as indicated?

Presentation

- Were you dressed and groomed appropriately?
- Did you establish a bond with the patient?
- Did your actions attend to both the psychological and the physiological aspects of the patient's illness or condition?
- Did you attend to any special needs of the patient?
- Did you ask first ask if assistance was needed, rather than taking charge?
- Were you courteous, patient, and respectful to the patient?
- Did you display a positive attitude?
- Did you display a calm, professional, and caring manner?

Figure 1-1 Medical assistants should reflect on these questions to ensure that they are embodying the characteristics and qualities of a true medical professional.

Competency

- Did you pay attention to detail?
- Did you ask questions if you were out of your comfort zone or did not have the experience to carry out tasks?
- Did you display sound judgment?
- Did you remain calm in a crisis?
- Were you knowledgeable and accountable?
- Did you apply critical thinking skills in performing patient assessment and care?
- Did you recognize the importance of local, state, and federal legislation and regulations in the practice setting?
- Did you demonstrate sensitivity and professionalism in handling accounts receivable activities with patients?
- Do you recognize the effect of stress on all persons involved in emergency situations?
- Did you demonstrate self-awareness in responding to emergency situations?

Initiative

- Did you show initiative?
- Did develop a strategic plan to achieve your goals? Was your plan realistic?
- Did you seek out opportunities to expand your knowledge base?
- Were you flexible and dependable?
- Did you direct the patient to other resources when necessary or helpful, with the approval of the provider?
- Did you implement time management principles to maintain effective office function?
- Did you consider needs and limitations in establishment of a filing system?
- Did you work with provider to achieve the maximum reimbursement?
- Did you assist co-workers when appropriate?
- Did you seek ways to improve the morale of your work place?

Integrity

- Did you work within your scope of practice?
- Did you acknowledge the scope of practice of other health care professionals?
- Did you demonstrate sensitivity to patient's rights?
- Did you protect personal boundaries?
- Were you respectful of others?
- Did you demonstrate respect for individual diversity?
- Did you demonstrate an appreciation for the patient's attitude toward illness or condition?
- Did you protect and maintain confidentiality?
- Did you immediately report any error you had made?
- Did you report situations which were harmful or illegal?
- Did you maintain your moral and ethical standards?
- Did you do the 'right thing' even when no one was observing?

Figure 1-1 *(continued)*

Communication

It is important that medical assistants learn to develop the ability to communicate well both verbally and nonverbally with patients, staff, and other professionals (see Chapter 5). Written communications must be clear and concise and reflect on the practice's professional reputation. Letters and other professional communications must utilize correct grammar, punctuation, and medical terminology.

Compliance with the provider's treatment plan is important for a positive outcome of patients' illnesses (Figure 1-2). Also, patients will feel more comfortable and less threatened in a medical clinic or ambulatory center that encourages staff to keep them informed. Consistent kindness and concern help patients develop trust in you.

Presentation

Presentation is the style or manner in which something is displayed. The professional medical assistant is required to present professionalism even when there is no conversation going on, no procedure being performed, and no documentation being recorded. Medical assistants should always be groomed and dressed appropriately in order to project a professional image. In addition to maintaining a professional appearance, medical assistants must also be able to communicate and interact with patients, family, and staff in an effective and constructive manner. Treating others with care and respect, while displaying a positive attitude, are equally important aspects of presenting a professional image.

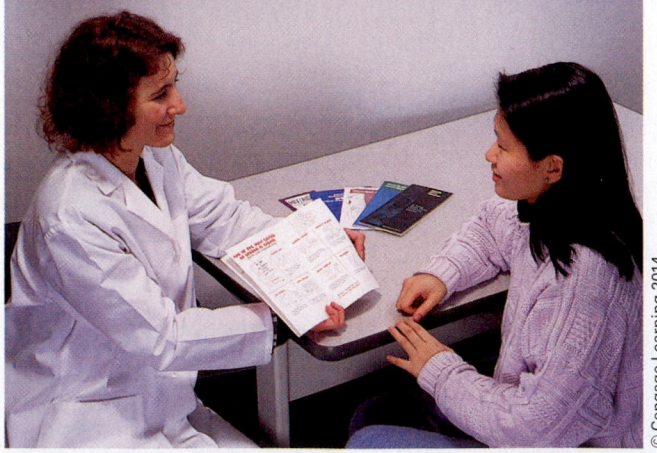

Figure 1-2 Patient education requires skill in communicating instructions to patients in language appropriate to their needs.

Physical Attributes. Appearance is important in patients' perceptions of the delivery of their care. Imparting the look of a professional requires an appearance that is clean, fresh, and wholesome—in general, an appearance that reflects good health habits (Figure 1-3). Good personal hygiene practices (daily shower, deodorant), weight control, and healthy-looking skin, hair, teeth, and nails all contribute to a professional appearance. Rest, good nutrition, scheduled dental care, regular exercise, and recreation all promote good health. A smile can help alleviate some of the anxiety a patient may be experiencing. Your smile gives a pleasant and encouraging appearance to the patient.

Female medical assistants should wear only appropriate light daytime makeup. For the safety of both the professional and the patient, no necklaces or dangling earrings should be worn. The only jewelry worn should be single earposts or wedding rings. Hair should be neat. Fingernails should be short and manicured. Male medical assistants should be clean-shaven and have short hair. Colognes, perfumes, and aftershave should not be worn at work. Body piercings and tattoos should not be visible. There are a variety of cosmetic products manufactured specifically for the covering of visible tattoos. These cosmetics come in a

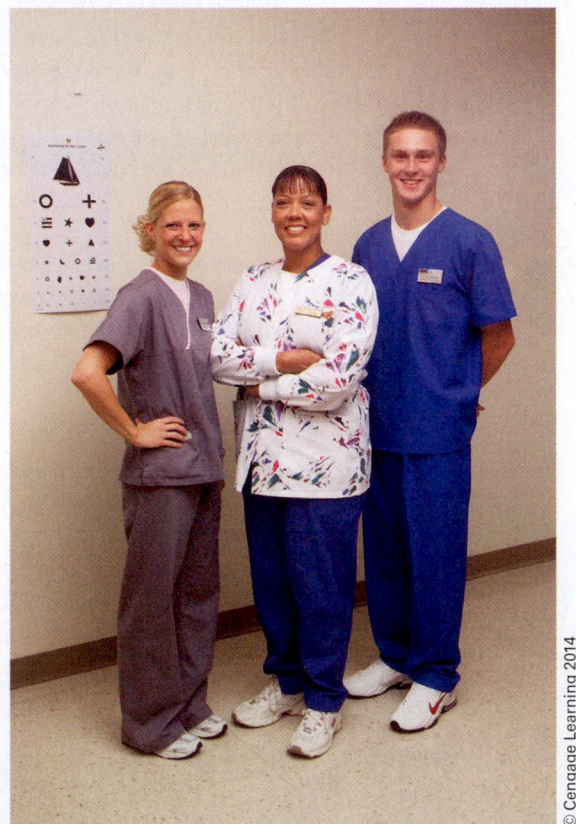

Figure 1-3 Medical assistants should always look very professional. Uniforms should always be crisp and clean.

variety of colors to match skin tone and are waterproof. Proper appearance has a positive effect on the patient.

It is important to know and follow the appropriate dress code for your facility. The Centers for Disease Control and Prevention (CDC) recommends that artificial nails and nail extenders not be worn when caring for "high-risk" (intensive care, surgery, or dialysis) patients. Many ambulatory facilities have more stringent rules about artificial nails and extenders.

Patient care can place physical demands on medical assistants. Lifting and moving patients are often required, and the use of correct body mechanics will help minimize injuries to the back. Although every reasonable accommodation is made for medical assistants with physical challenges, it is important to be mobile without assistance because medical assistants move about throughout the day while performing tasks and procedures. It is frequently necessary to bend, stoop, kneel, and crouch, especially when filing and retrieving patients' records, as well as for other tasks. Most procedures require that medical assistants have the ability to hear and see well for the accurate completion of tasks (Figure 1-4). Listening to blood pressures, taking a medical history, observing patients, performing phlebotomy, and identifying microorganisms under a microscope are some of the routine tasks and procedures performed daily in a medical facility.

Manual **dexterity** is also needed for manipulating certain instruments and for entering data using a computer.

Empathy. To have **empathy** means to consider the patient's welfare and to be kind. It means

stepping into the patient's place, discovering what the patient is experiencing, and then recognizing and identifying with those feelings.

Medical assistants should treat patients as they themselves would want to be treated. A visit to the providers' clinic is often a time of fear and anxiety. Patients can feel vulnerable. Apprehension can be allayed tremendously when patients realize that their caregiver understands their feelings and desires to make their lives more pleasant and comfortable (Figure 1-5).

It is important to realize that patients' health problems can have a profound effect on you, the medical assistant. By maintaining a balanced outlook, medical assistants can safeguard themselves from becoming too emotionally involved with patients' problems. Empathy is extremely important in the health care profession; however, emotionalism can cloud one's judgment.

Attitude. A friendly, warm **disposition** and a sense of humor will help patients feel more at ease. A sincere affection for people can be conveyed by actions that **facilitate** open and honest communication. Your attitude should radiate genuine interest. Be sure that all contact with patients is positive.

An essential aspect of a good attitude is respect. Every person that enters the presence of a professional medical assistant must be treated with esteemed reverence. Patients, peers, co-workers, and other clients of the practice must be held in regard. A medical professional's willingness to show appreciation and consideration is an attitude that facilitates a positive experience for all involved. Seeking health care is a very personal experience. On the part of the medical assistant, it necessitates a respect for the patient's

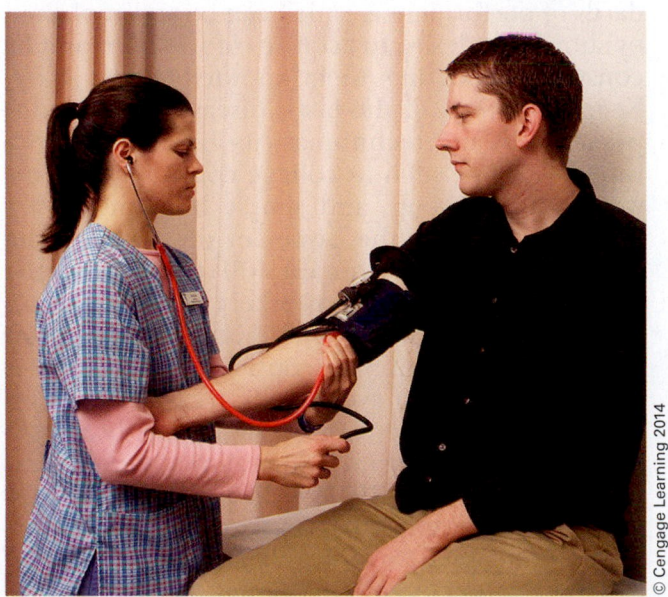

Figure 1-4 Measuring blood pressure is a task that requires the medical assistant to see and hear well.

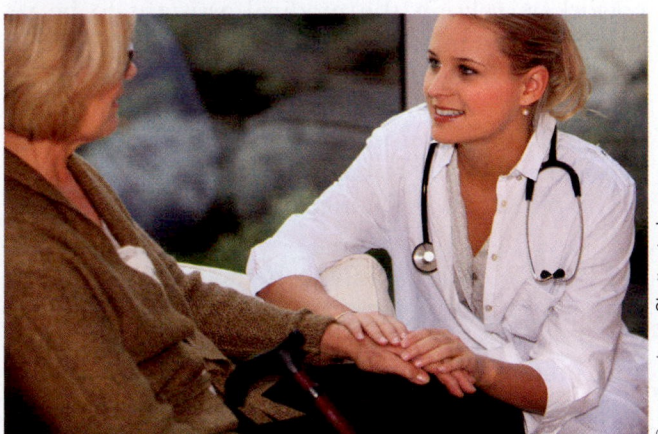

Figure 1-5 The medical assistant should have a friendly disposition and communicate empathy for the patient.

information, the resulting care, and the documentation of this care.

On occasion, difficult patients can test the tolerance level of the most experienced medical assistant because they seldom seem to be content with the care or services received. But no matter what the circumstances, patients should never be treated with disinterest or in an unfriendly manner. The medical assistant should always be pleasant and courteous.

 Patients should be treated equally, with no reservations about their disease, race, religion, economic status, or sexual orientation.

 As a member of the health care delivery team, the medical assistant needs to be cooperative and supportive of all other members, working with the team in an honest, open manner while keeping in mind the patient's right to privacy and confidentiality.

Competency

 Competency is the ability to perform a set of skills on a reproducible basis. Competent medical assistants have knowledge of the reason, the methods, and the expected outcomes of the tasks they perform, and are able to execute them consistently. Competency is not just doing your job well. It is a commitment to keeping skills sharp and presentation professional.

Dependability. When providing for a patient's well-being, it is important to focus attention on activities in the office or clinic environment that will demonstrate that you are well organized, accurate, and responsive to patients' needs.

Being dependable means that employer and coworkers rely on the medical assistant to be respectful of them, of patients, and of equipment and materials. Other members of the health care team will expect you to be accountable for the duties and responsibilities you undertake. A dependable person interacts with coworkers in a supportive manner, is punctual, and limits absences from work.

Flexibility. The ability to be adaptable is a trait that serves all professionals well. When caring for ill people, unexpected situations arise daily, and medical assistants must be able to respond to a variety of situations (many of them emergencies and unanticipated) without losing a sense of equilibrium. Finding solutions to problems and developing alternative action plans demonstrates flexibility. To **improvise**, or solve problems that

arise either routinely or spontaneously, is a characteristic worth nurturing. Willingness to help with various aspects of the clinic offers opportunities to adjust to various situations. It shows your adaptability and willingness to respond to new circumstances.

Initiative

 The willingness and ability to work independently shows initiative. A person with initiative is observant, notices work that needs to be done, and then takes action to complete those tasks without being told to do them. Employers and coworkers must be able to count on one another to anticipate patients' needs and be attentive to work that needs to be accomplished. The successful medical assistant will be ready to pitch in and recognize when others need assistance. Teamwork and a positive work ethic are valuable characteristics.

By asking appropriate questions and seeking information that will improve performance, medical assistants will demonstrate that they have the foresight and the "get up and go" needed to complete the numerous and varied tasks of the ambulatory care environment.

Desire to Learn. A willingness to continually learn and grow is the mark of a true professional. With the growing use of technology in medicine, there is an ongoing necessity for constant learning. Medical assistants must be dedicated to high standards of performance, which can be accomplished by showing a desire to acquire information and by constantly updating their knowledge and skills. Keeping abreast of the latest diseases, treatments, procedures, and techniques can be achieved in a variety of ways, such as college courses, seminars, workshops, reading, and simply by being observant. The sharper the power of observation, the more the medical assistant will learn from the provider-employer and coworkers.

The gaining and maintaining of **competency** through participation in continuing education is the responsibility of every medical assistant. Active involvement and membership in the medical assistant professional organizations allows students and CMAs (AAMA) and RMAs (AMT) to participate in meetings and events that can increase professional skills. This benefits medical assistant skills as well as future careers. Students can attend medical assisting meetings (usually free of charge), enjoy student discounts, and network at the meetings.

Integrity

Another crucial attribute of professionalism is integrity. Being honest is just one of the hallmarks of integrity. Adherence to moral and ethical principles also describes those who have integrity. The application of integrity is one of the professional characteristics that is in high demand in the profession of medical assisting. Integrity applies to every aspect of patient care, beginning with the first encounter with a patient and continuing through the end of the patient's episode of care. Integrity is not a learned trait, but rather a core personal attribute that can be nurtured and honed to become the cornerstone of one's reputation in the medical field.

Accountability.   Accountability is the willingness to accept responsibility. If you reflect upon the numerous aspects of the role of an allied health care provider, you will discover that responsibility plays a key role. The medical assistant is responsible for collecting data, maintaining accurate documentation, interacting with the financial record, planning, and patient teaching, just to name a few tasks. Being accountable means demonstrating the highest level of integrity when accepting the responsibility for a patient's care and management of his or her confidential information.

Ethical Behavior.   No discussion about personal attributes is complete without the mention of ethics. Ethics is a system of values each individual has that determines perceptions of right and wrong. Our life experiences mold this set of values, which is considered a personal code of ethics.

Medical ethics govern medical conduct or that behavior practiced as health care providers. These ethics involve relationships with patients, their families, fellow professionals, and society in general. Ethical behavior will have a positive impact on the profession of medical assisting and on the medical community as well.

By adhering to the medical assistants' Code of Ethics, we endeavor to elevate the profession to a position of dignity and respect. Medical assistants interact on a daily basis with patients and are entrusted with information about their medical and personal histories. Such information must, by law, be kept confidential. (A more in-depth discussion of ethics and the Code of Ethics can be found in Chapter 8.)

The personal qualities of empathy, professional attitude, dependability, initiative, integrity, accountability, flexibility, the desire to learn, a

wholesome physical presence, the ability to communicate well, and ethical behavior are some of the characteristics that most professionals have and that medical assistants should strive to develop. When entering into the profession of medical assisting, it is important to learn more about these and other qualities and to begin to use and refine them. Skills and knowledge alone do not guarantee success. There are personal characteristics that must go along with them.

Professional attitudes, attributes, and values are important for beginning medical assistant students to understand. Students' behaviors can impact the public's opinion of both the provider and the medical assistant profession.

The public has a right to expect that the medical assistant will be competent to practice medical assisting in accordance with the medical assistants' Code of Ethics (see Chapter 8) and with the standards and guidelines set by their professional organizations (AMT, AAMA).

AMERICAN ASSOCIATION OF MEDICAL ASSISTANTS

In the mid-fifties, there was a movement to form a national organization for medical assistants. The Kansas Medical Assistants Society met in Kansas City, Kansas, and accepted by vote the name "American Association of Medical Assistants" (AAMA) (see Figure 1-6). In 1956, this organization was supported

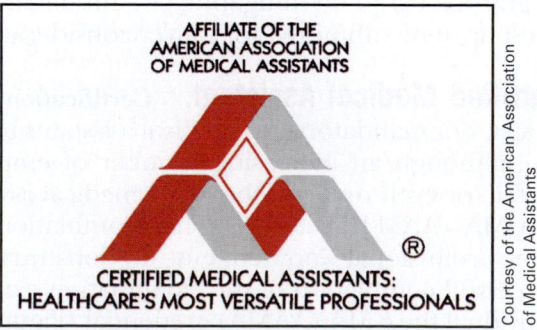

Figure 1-6   Logo of the AAMA, a professional organization founded in 1956.

by the American Medical Association by the passage of a resolution commending the objectives of the AAMA. By 1962, the AAMA had developed a sample certification exam, and in 1963 it offered the first certification. In order to continue to promote and gain recognition for this special set of medical assisting skills, with the collaboration of the American Medical Association, the AAMA began in 1966 to have influence over curriculum and accreditation of post-secondary levels of education. (See Chapter 47 for more information about credentialing for medical assisting).

Certification

As the profession grew and developed, some states came to require special licensure or certification to perform certain tasks; in other states, other health professionals were challenged by the skill and broad spectrum of the medical assistant's abilities. To defend medical assistants whose right to practice clinical procedures was being challenged, the AAMA responded at their 1995 convention with the following policy:

> that any candidate for the AAMA Certification Examination be a graduate of a CAAHEP-accredited medical assisting program or a graduate of an ABHES-accredited program with one year of documented work experience. Anticipated benefits of the recommendation are to: (1) safeguard the quality of care to the consumer; (2) ensure the CMA's role in the rapidly evolving health care delivery system; and (3) continue to promote the identity and stature of the profession.

In order to sit for the CMA exam, a medical assistant must have not only completed an accredited program, they must also have a clean legal record. If a candidate for the exam has pled guilty to or been convicted of a felony, they generally are not permitted to take the CMA exam. There is a waiver that may be granted based on mitigating circumstances. A request must be submitted for waiver consideration.

Certified Medical Assistant.   Certification is voluntary, not mandatory, for medical assistants to practice, although an increasing number of employers prefer (or even require) that their medical assistants be CMA (AAMA) certified. The examination measures professional knowledge at the job-entry level. Successful completion of the examination earns the individual the CMA (AAMA) credential (Figure 1-7). (For information on recertification, please see Chapter 47). The initials follow the individual's name. Conferring of the CMA (AAMA) status is referred to

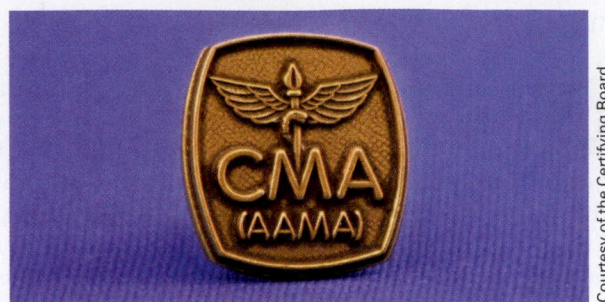

Figure 1-7   Certified medical assistant (CMA) pin awarded by the American Association of Medical Assistants on successful completion of the national certification examination.

as being **credentialed**. The Certification Program of the Certifying Board of the American Association of Medical Assistants is accredited by the National Commission for Certifying Agencies (NCCA) as a result of demonstrating compliance with the *NCCA Standards for the Accreditation of Certification Programs.*

Continuing Education

The AAMA vigorously encourages continuing education for all medical assistants. This can be accomplished through various means such as educational meetings, seminars, workshops, conventions, and the AAMA's self-study publications, a series of study courses for continuing education credit.

Membership in the AAMA is trilevel: local, state, and national. Educational meetings are held regularly at local and state meetings and conventions. The annual AAMA national convention provides an excellent forum for attaining knowledge through its educational offerings and for networking with other medical assistants.

Continuing an education is a lifelong process and serves as testimony to a commitment to professionalism (see the AAMA Web site at http://www.aama-ntl.org).

AMERICAN MEDICAL TECHNOLOGISTS

Founded in 1939, the American Medical Technologists (AMT) is a national certification and professional membership association that represents 60,000 allied health care individuals. Its purpose is to certify and credential medical assistants, clinical laboratory personnel, allied health instructors, dental assistants, medical administrative specialists, and others. The AMT has its own bylaws, conventions, committees, state chapters, officers, and registration and certification examinations.

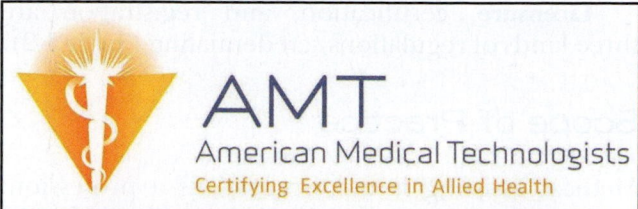

Figure 1-8A   AMT Logo.
Courtesy of the American Medical Technologists

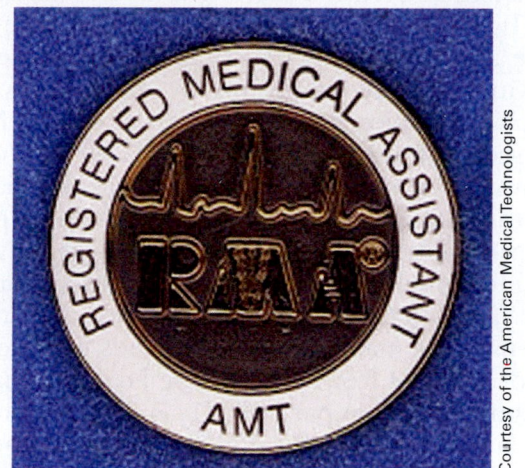

Figure 1-8B   Registered Medical Assistant (RMA) pin.

Registered Medical Assistant

In 1972, the AMT established the certification examination for medical assistants. The designation of **registered medical assistant (RMA)** is conferred on those individuals who successfully pass the examination (Figure 1-8).

The RMA certification examination includes general medical assisting topics, medical terminology, clinical medical assisting, medical law and ethics, human relations, administrative medical assisting, pharmacology, therapeutic modalities, laboratory procedures, electrocardiography, and first aid.

RMAs have been active in legislation to protect medical assistants, ensuring improvement in medical assistant education. American Medical Technologists advocate education and the evolution of professionalism in medical assisting.

Certified Medical Administrative Specialist

Another profession that the AMT certifies is the Medical Administrative Specialist (CMAS). Individuals who successfully pass the AMT certification examination are conferred with the credential of Certified Medical Administrative Specialist (CMAS). The CMAS exam is given in both computerized and paper and pencil formats.

The CMAS serves an important role in the hospital, clinic, or medical office. The CMAS is competent in a multitude of skills such as medical records management, coding and billing for insurance, practice finance management, information processing, and fundamental management practices. The CMAS also is familiar with the clinical and administrative concepts that are required to coordinate office functions in the health care setting.

Continuing Education

AMT encourages and promotes continuing education. The Certification Continuation Program (CCP) requires members to document activities that attest to their continued effort to carry the competencies needed to maintain certification. Proof of compliance is required every three years.

OTHER CERTIFICATION

National Healthcareer Association

The National Healthcareer Association (NHA) is a certifying body for health care professionals (Figure 1-9). Its main goals are to certify and to offer continuing education course development, membership services for professionals, and a registry for certified professionals. The NHA offers certification for many allied health professions, including the **Certified Clinical Medical Assistant (CCMA)** and the **Certified Medical Administrative Assistant (CMAA)**.

National Center for Competency Testing (NCCT)

The National Center for Competency Testing (NCCT) (Figure 1-10) is an independent certifying body for many allied health professions, including Medical Assistant, Medical Office Assistant, and Phlebotomy Technician. There are two routes to qualify to sit for a certification exam with NCCT.

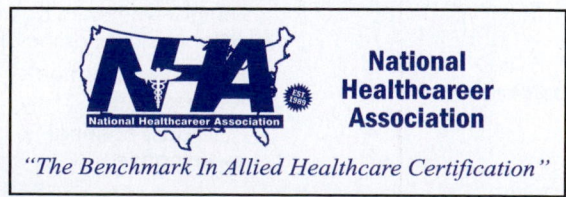

Figure 1-9   Logo of the National Healthcareer Association.
Courtesy of the National Healthcareer Association, www.nhanow.com

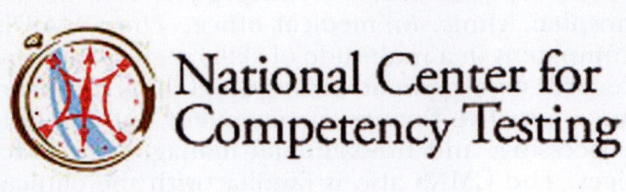

Figure 1-10 NCCT Logo.
Courtesy of the National Center for Competency Testing

These two routes are graduation from an approved educational program or qualifying work experience with the goal of validating competency.

National Certified Medical Assistant (NCMA).

The NCMA certification exam is offered by the NCCT. It measures job knowledge, skills and abilities in the front and back office, general medical clinic management duties, medical procedures, and pharmacology. To assure proficiency, this exam also tests knowledge of anatomy and physiology as well as medical terminology.

REGULATION OF HEALTH CARE PROVIDERS

One way health care providers can be regulated is through the process of credentialing. Credentialing recognizes health care providers who are professionally and technically competent. Recognition comes from professional associations, certifying agencies, and the state or federal government. Regulation ensures:

- The competence of health care providers
- A minimum standard of knowledge, training, and skill
- The limiting of the performance of certain procedures to a specific occupation

Licensure, certification, and registration are three kinds of regulations/credentialing (Table 1-2).

Scope of Practice

Medical assisting is not licensed as a profession; however, some states require that medical assistants be graduates of an accredited medical assisting program and be certified to work as medical assistants.

Two examples of licensed professions are medicine and nursing. A licensing body regulates the activities of these professions by enacting laws that specify educational requirements and by defining the **scope of practice**. A **license** is conferred on an individual who successfully completes specialized educational requirements and successfully passes an examination administered by the state in which the individual resides. The state grants a license to that individual to practice medicine or nursing. Licensure is mandatory and forbids anyone who is not licensed from performing activities that are designated by that particular license. For example, the law states that the medical license allows diagnosing and prescribing treatment. If someone were to diagnose or prescribe without a medical license, that individual would be committing an illegal act and would be practicing medicine without a license, which is considered a felony.

There are state laws that govern the practice of medicine and nursing (medical practice acts, nursing practice acts), and many states have acts that give providers the right to delegate certain clinical procedures to qualified allied health professionals. Because medical assistants are not required to be licensed, they can become certified voluntarily. They are allowed to perform clinical procedures only under the supervision of the provider or other licensed health care professional who is granted that right and who delegates the specific clinical procedures to the medical assistants.

Table 1-2 Comparison of Requirements for Certification, Licensure, and Registration

Practice Requirement	Voluntary	Mandatory	Voluntary
Conferred by	Nongovernmental agency or professional association If qualified and meets requirements Must pass national examination	Legislated by each state If qualified and meets requirements Must pass state examination	Professional association If qualified and meets requirements Listed on an official roster Passing examination not always required
How restrictive	Used by most professionals	Most restrictive	Least restrictive

© Cengage Learning 2014

In some states, including California, Washington, and others, unlicensed health care providers are required to have authorization from the state to perform allergy testing and venipuncture and to give injections. A registration fee and mandatory training are required. In such circumstances, medical assistants or other health care providers would be breaking the law if they performed these procedures without registration and training.

In some states, authorization is required for unlicensed health care providers to expose patients to X-rays.

On March 30, 2007 a bill called the CARE bill (Consistency, Accuracy, Responsibility and Excellence in Medical Imaging and Radiation Therapy) was introduced before the U.S. Senate. Had it passed, it would have required all persons who perform medical imaging (including X-rays) and radiation therapy (excluding ultrasound) procedures to meet specific federal education and credentialing standards in order to participate in Medicare and Medicaid. However, the bill did not receive the support it needed to be passed into law. In June 2012, a new version of the law was again introduced in the senate. Establishing a federal standard for education and certification will allow for a more uniform quality of care with some anticipated cost savings for Medicare. It is noted that the American Society of Radiologic Technologists (ASRT) have educated their congressional representatives on the importance of education and certification in this aspect of a patient's care. Presently, the law in some states requires only voluntary basic training standards. This situation allows individuals without formal education to perform imaging procedures.

The AAMA supports the legislation that would require specific educational and certification standards for individuals performing medical imaging. Medical assistants do not perform procedures for which they have not been educated and in which they are not proficient. The AAMA's Occupational Analysis for the CMA (AAMA) in Appendix C and the AMT's Medical Assisting Task List in Appendix D are excellent reference sources that identify the clinical, administrative, and general procedures medical assistants are educated to perform. However, because of the variability of state statutes, the medical assistant would be wise to check with the AAMA or AMT if in doubt about the legality of certain clinical procedures.

The AMT and the AAMA (the two leading organizations that certify medical assistants) agreed on a model state law outlining the medical assistant's scope of practice. Both the AMT and AAMA took from existing state laws regarding medical assistants' right to practice the most important aspects of these and developed the model. Both organizations agreed to require a medical assistant to graduate from an accredited medical assistant program and to obtain certification from AMT, AAMA, or other approved agencies that certify. A nonexclusive list of functions that a supervised medical assistant may perform was developed. The purpose of the Model State Legislation is to protect the medical assistant's right to practice. A copy of the model legislation is available at state medical assistant societies.

As the scope of medical assisting practice expands and diversifies, there are many questions regarding state-by-state legislation. Resources to answer these questions are available at www.aama-ntl.org.

CRITICAL THINKING

A medical assistant relates to a patient on the telephone that her symptoms are "probably the flu" and to "take over-the-counter cough syrup" for her cough. Is this an appropriate or inappropriate action for the medical assistant to take? Discuss your answer and explain why you came to your decision.

CASE STUDY 1-1

Refer to the scenario at the beginning of the chapter.

CASE STUDY REVIEW

1. If you were a freshman in high school and interested in medical assisting, would you like to have an opportunity to visit a program and tour the classroom and laboratories? Why or why not?

2. List three or four questions you might ask of the senior medical assistant students while you are touring the medical assisting department that would help to clarify what the profession is, the course requirements, etc.

SUMMARY

Progress has been made in the advancement of the profession of medical assisting since the first group of medical assistants gathered to become organized and formed the AAMA and the AMT. For example, the number of certified medical assistants has exceeded 65,000 and continues to grow since certification began in 1963. The total number of medical assistants in the work force is over 500,000, and employment opportunities continue to grow. Educational requirements have become increasingly important. The AAMA, the AMT, and the NHA continue to promote standards of excellence for its members, encouraging continuing education and awarding continuing education credits to members of AAMA, AMT, and the NHA via various means.

All of these factors are evidence of a strong professional perspective and should offer encouragement and support to any student or graduate of medical assisting education programs.

Becoming a professional is a gradual process and cannot be learned in its entirety from a textbook. The challenge of becoming a professional medical assistant will require open-mindedness and a desire for continued learning and education, certification and recertification of the CMA (AAMA) or RMA credential, and professional involvement through organizational participation.

As the scope of work done by medical assistants broadens and medical assistants seek and require formal education, the professional medical assistant will gain additional respect and be in even greater demand. Medical assistants must continuously pursue excellence, which is the hallmark of all professional behavior.

STUDY FOR SUCCESS

To reinforce your knowledge and skills of information presented in this chapter:

- Review the *Key Terms*
- Role-play with other students to apply attributes of professionalism pertinent to this chapter.
- Consider the *Case Study* and discuss your conclusions
- Answer the questions in the *Certification Review*
- Apply your knowledge by completing the *Activities* in the *Study Guide* and the *Games and Quizzes* in the StudyWARE (StudyWARE) software on the *Premium Website*
- Practice your problem-solving skills with the *Critical Thinking Challenge 3.0* on the *Premium Website*

Additional resources for this chapter include:

- Module 1 of the *Medical Assisting Learning Lab*
- *CourseMate for Delmar's Comprehensive Medical Assisting*
- *WebTutor for Delmar's Comprehensive Medical Assisting*

CERTIFICATION REVIEW

1. The designation "CMAS" is awarded by the:
   a. AAMA
   b. ABHES
   c. AMA
   d. AMT

2. Increased employment opportunities for medical assistants result from:
   a. regulation of diagnostic testing
   b. the volume of paperwork
   c. managed care's emphasis on ambulatory care
   d. "baby boomers" beginning to retire
   e. all of the above

3. Ethics is:
   a. a system of values each individual has that determines perceptions of right and wrong
   b. a code established by an agency that has nothing to do with the medical assistant's belief in right or wrong
   c. making patients more comfortable
   d. willingness to work as a team member
4. Accreditation means:
   a. meeting appropriate standards
   b. obtaining the CMA (AAMA) or RMA credential
   c. being listed on an official roster
   d. having a curriculum with courses that are unrestricted
5. Licensure is:
   a. voluntary and up to the individual practitioner
   b. unrestrictive in scope
   c. conferred on an individual through a nongovernment agency
   d. mandatory and legislated by states
6. Medical assistants have a skill set that is appropriate in the following settings:
   a. provider's clinics
   b. urgent care clinics
   c. insurance companies
   d. all of the above

7. Benefits of a medical assistant practicum or externship include:
   a. receiving a paycheck for experience gained
   b. obtaining references for future employment
   c. improving performance and knowledge
   d. both b and c
8. Which of the following statements are true?
   a. Medical assisting is a licensed profession.
   b. Medical assistants must obtain an associate's degree.
   c. Medical assistants are governed by state laws.
   d. Medical assistants have mandatory certification.
9. Which are the functions of the American Association of Medical Assistants (AAMA)?
   a. Provides certification for Registered Medical Assistant (RMA)
   b. Was the first national organization for medical assisting
   c. Defined the occupation of medical assisting
   d. Both b and c
10. Which of the following are attributes of the professional medical assistant?
    a. Communication skills
    b. Integrity
    c. Empathy
    d. All of the above

REFERENCES/BIBLIOGRAPHY

American Association of Medical Assistants, Executive Office, 20 N. Wacker Dr., Suite 1575, Chicago, IL 60606.

American Medical Technologists, Allied Health Professions, 10700 West Higgins Rd., Suite 150, Rosemont, IL 60018.

Balasa, D. (2000). Securing the future for medical assistants to practice. *Professional medical assistant,* January/February 2000, 6–7.

Balasa, D. (2003). Vigilance is key to protecting practice rights. *CMA Today, 36*(4). Retrieved April 15, 2007, from http://www.aama-ntl.org/cmatoday/archives

Balasa, D. (2004). Model legislation designed to protect practice rights. *CMA Today, 37*(2). Retrieved April 15, 2007, from http://www.aama-ntl.org/cmatoday/archives

Balasa, D. (2005). CARE bill gains momentum in Congress. *CMA Today, 38*(4). Retrieved April 15, 2007, from http://www.aama-ntl.org/cmatoday/archives

Balasa, D. (2012). Frequent questions about medical assistant's scope of practice. *CMA Today. 45*(2). Retrieved March 4, 2012 from http://www.aama-ntl.org/CMAToday/archives/publicaffairs/details.aspx?ArticleID=886

Carli, L. L., LaFleur, S. J., Loeber, C. C., Connell, F., & Geiser, R. (1995). Nonverbal behavior, gender, and influence. *Journal of Personality and Social Psychology, 68*(6), 1030–1041.

McCarty, M. (2003). The lawful scope of a medical assistant's practice. *AMT Events,* March 2003. Retrieved from http://hws.hrsa.gov/default.aspx?category=Auxiliary+Health&occu=Medical+Assistants http://www.bls.gov/oco/ocos164.htm

National Healthcareer Association, 7 Ridgedale Ave., Suite 203, Cedar Knolls, NJ 07927.

CHAPTER 2

Health Care Settings and the Health Care Team

OUTLINE

Ambulatory Health Care Settings

Individual and Group Medical Practices

Urgent Care Centers

Managed Care Operations

"Boutique" or "Concierge" Medical Practices

The Health Care Team

The Title "Doctor"

Health Care Professionals and Their Roles

Integrative Medicine and Alternative Health Care Practitioners

Future of Integrative Medicine

Allied Health Professionals and Their Roles

The Role of the Medical Assistant

Health Unit Coordinator

Medical Laboratory Technologist

Registered Dietitian

Pharmacist

Pharmacy Technician

Phlebotomist

Physical Therapist

Physical Therapy Assistant

Nurse

Physician Assistant

The Value of the Medical Assistant to the Health Care Team

LEARNING OUTCOMES

1. Define, spell, and pronounce the key terms as presented in the glossary.
2. Critique the three primary medical management models.
3. Analyze the benefits and limitations of working in the different ambulatory health care settings.
4. Assess the role of managed care in the health care environment.
5. Describe the function of the health care team.
6. List and describe a minimum of 12 health care providers.
7. Research a minimum of three alternative health care specialists.
8. Compare a minimum of 12 allied health professionals.
9. Discuss the role of the medical assistant in ambulatory health care.
10. Critique alternative therapies and discuss their role in today's health care setting.
11. Comment on the value of the medical assistant to the health care team.
12. Analyze the professionalism questions and apply them to this chapter's content.

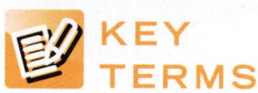

KEY TERMS

acupuncture

ambulatory care
  setting

fringe benefits

health maintenance
  organization (HMO)

homeopathy

independent provider
  association (IPA)

integrative medicine

managed care
  operation

preferred provider
  organization (PPO)

ATTRIBUTES OF PROFESSIONALISM

Communication
- Does your knowledge allow you to speak easily with all members of the health care team?

Presentation
- Were you courteous, patient, and respectful to the patient?
- Did you display a positive attitude?

Competency
- Did you display sound judgment?
- Did you remain calm in a crisis?
- Were you knowledgeable and accountable?

Initiative
- Did you assist coworkers when appropriate?

Integrity
- Did you work within the scope of your practice?
- Did you acknowledge the scope of practice of other health care professionals?

SCENARIO

You always had thought you wanted to be a medical assistant and work in a clinic where you would see a variety of patients. But after discussing this chapter in class, you are really intrigued with becoming a physical therapy assistant and want to investigate the profession further. What kind of research can you do to make certain you have chosen the right path? Consider working hours, rate of pay, patient contact, required schooling, and job availability.

INTRODUCTION

There are few professions in our society as rich and complex as the health care profession. Particularly in recent years, the health care environment has been very much in flux as the profession seeks ways to provide quality care while containing costs. This effort to curtail costs has resulted in the rise of managed care, which, in turn, has spawned a number of medical models such as **health maintenance organizations (HMOs)** *and* **preferred provider organizations (PPOs)**, *two well-known managed care entities.*

Many other types of networks and alliances are also being established as providers merge to give patients the best of care while controlling their costs. **Ambulatory care settings**, *where services are provided on an outpatient basis, have become increasingly pivotal to consumer health care as insurers direct dollars away from hospital inpatient care and toward ambulatory outpatient care. Hospitals are more frequently providing outpatient care as it has become more common for patients to appear at the emergency room (ER) for routine ailments when they have nowhere else to go. Large retail stores such as Walmart, Target, and CVS have also entered the field of outpatient care. These retail sites, commonly staffed by nurse practitioners, provide routine medical services for a set fee.*

Just as the medical setting continues to evolve to meet new societal needs, health care technology is ever changing. Health care is a dynamic, stimulating industry that requires the medical assistant and other professionals to constantly develop new skills if they are to contribute to the team effort. The range of skills within the health care team is astonishing and includes providers in more than 25 specialties, an increasing number of nontraditional alternative practitioners licensed to practice, and more than 20 kinds of allied health professionals.

AMBULATORY HEALTH CARE SETTINGS

Although medical assistants work in a number of different environments, including laboratories and hospitals, most are employed in an ambulatory

SPOTLIGHT ON CERTIFICATION

RMA Content Outline
- Knowledge of allied health professions
- Medical assistant general responsibilities
- Medical assistant scope of practice

CMA (AAMA) Content Outline
- Medical assistant scope of practice

CMAS Content Outline
- Medical assistant scope of practice

care setting such as a medical clinic (either a solo provider or group practice), an urgent or primary care center, or a managed care organization where they give outpatient care.

Often, the medical assistant chooses to work in one setting rather than another based on interests, personality, and work preferences. For instance, the individual practice may provide medical assistants with the opportunity to use their full array of skills, whereas in urgent care centers, the work of the medical assistant is often more specialized in nature.

It is helpful if medical assistants recognize the three major forms of medical practice management and how they affect salary, benefits, and liability issues (Figure 2-1).

Individual and Group Medical Practices

For years, the most common form of ambulatory health care was the individual provider or group practice. This model competes with a variety of other models such as urgent and managed care

FORMS OF MEDICAL PRACTICE MANAGEMENT

Medical assistants employed in ambulatory care settings or medical offices and clinics are likely to see three major forms of medical practice management: sole proprietorships, partnerships, and corporations.

Whatever form of management is chosen by providers, they are responsible for the employees that serve with them. (Refer to the discussion of *respondeat superior* in Chapter 7.) Employers and their medical assistants must have the kind of healthy working relationship where mutual trust and respect are apparent. The provider must understand the skill level of the medical assistant, and the medical assistant must feel secure enough to ask any necessary questions or admit any errors. Critical errors are often made when this trust does not exist between employer and employee. This causes a breakdown in the delivery of the best health care for patients.

Sole Proprietorships

In the past, many providers preferred a solo practice. A solo practice entitles the sole proprietor to hold exclusive right to all aspects of the medical practice or sole proprietorship, including profits and debts. If the business fails, the sole proprietor's personal property may also be attached.

A sole proprietorship may employ other providers to participate in the practice. The employed provider(s) is entitled to any employee **fringe benefits** such as health insurance and paid vacation, but the solo practitioner is not so entitled.

Partnerships

When two or more providers join together under a legal agreement to share in the total business operations of the practice, a partnership is formed. Several providers who share a facility and practice medicine are often referred to as a group. Partners share income, expenses, debt, equipment, records, and personnel according to a predetermined agreement. Partners are liable for only their own actions but may be liable for the whole amount of the partnership debts.

Corporations

Providers may form a corporation, usually referred to as a professional service corporation. The shareholders are considered employees of the corporation. A corporation allows income and tax advantages to all employees. A variety of fringe benefits can be offered to the employees, which may include pension; profit-sharing plans; medical expense reimbursement; and life, health, and disability insurance. These benefits are separate from salary. Another advantage is that professional employees of a corporation are liable only for their own acts, and personal property cannot be attached in litigation. A sole proprietor may incorporate if the practice is large enough.

The health maintenance organization (HMO) is one type of corporation in which providers often practice. Basically, providers are employees of the HMO and are paid by various methods; providers in the HMO usually serve as the primary care provider (PCP). In this situation, a referral from the PCP may be necessary before a patient can see a specialist or allied health professional.

© Cengage Learning 2014

Figure 2-1 Different forms of medical practice management.

centers, but many medical assistants find the individual or group practice the most challenging place of employment.

Individual Practices. In the individual practice, also called the solo practice, one primary provider sees and treats all patients. Although this type of arrangement is limited in the number of people it can serve, many patients feel secure in this kind of health care setting because they come to know and trust their provider. Because they always see the same provider, they feel their health care is being managed in a personal way. The solo-provider practice, however, can be an expensive arrangement,

because one provider must undertake the costs of clinic space, equipment, and personnel. Today, the majority of solo providers are found in many of the nontraditional alternative or integrative medical practices.

Group Practices. Group practices are attractive arrangements where two or more providers can share the costs of space, equipment, and personnel. The advantages of a group practice, however, are not solely economic; providers learn from and consult one another, and patients receive the benefit of this exchange of information and knowledge. Often, a group practice has more than one clinic, and some employees are asked to travel between sites to cut overhead. Group practices may be formed to offer specialized care, such as oncology or women's health care. Most medical practices are still groups of three or four providers.

In most group practices, patients may request that they see the same provider for all appointments, although sometimes patients are assigned to the next available provider. For emergencies, group practices have the staff and flexibility to ensure that there is always a provider on call.

Many providers in small groups allowed large practice management firms to acquire their assets and manage the business side of their practice. In some cases, these practice management firms were sold to even larger practice management companies that eventually went bankrupt, forcing them to shed all their practices. This dilemma left providers with no recourse except to start over. Therefore, a number of providers are returning to the preferred provider organization (PPO), where providers network to offer discounts to employers and other purchasers of health insurance as well as agree to discounted fees for services.

Urgent Care Centers

Urgent care centers are usually private, for-profit centers that provide services for primary care, routine injuries and illnesses, and minor surgery. Sometimes laboratory services and a radiology department are located on the premises. Providers and other health care professionals in the center are often salaried employees, not owners who share in the profits, and they may also be associated with other medical facilities.

The pace in many urgent care centers is brisk, and typically a number of providers are working at one time. Patients are usually encouraged to make appointments, but drop-ins are accepted, especially for emergencies. As mentioned earlier, certain retail chain stores, including Walmart, Target, and CVS, have entered into this market. All over the country, there are walk-in urgent care chains such as MDNow and Patient First entering into the field. According to the Urgent Care Association of America, an estimated 3 million patients visit these centers each week. About 25% of patients who patronize these locations have a primary care provider, but feel they can be seen quicker in this environment. It is also estimated that close to 25% of urgent care patients are uninsured and expect to pay cash for their services.

Because these centers often see a higher volume of patients during expanded hours (often 10 AM to 10 PM, 365 days of the year), usually for a lower cost than a hospital emergency room, experts predict that urgent care centers will continue to grow in popularity.

Managed Care Operations

Health maintenance organizations, or HMOs, have become the most familiar **managed care operation**. Originally, HMOs were designed to provide a full range of health care services under one roof. More recently, the "HMO without walls" has become common and typically consists of a network of participating providers within a defined geographic area.

Originally, the HMO with walls was conceived to provide patients with comprehensive health care services at one facility. Today, as managed care and managed competition sweep through the health care industry, other arrangements include the preferred provider organization (PPO), where providers network to offer discounts to employers and other purchasers of health insurance, and the **independent provider association (IPA)**, the members of which agree to treat patients for an agreed-upon fee.

"Boutique" or "Concierge" Medical Practices

According to the American Academy of Family Physicians, there are now more than 5,000 "boutique" or "concierge" practices in the United States that are growing in popularity with both patients and providers. Providers who are discouraged by their shrinking insurance reimbursements and by managed care plans dictating what procedures and tests will be performed have turned to another avenue for providing health care. Patients who are disappointed in the quality of care received and frustrated by being bounced from one insurer to another as employers seek a cost reduction in their health care benefits are increasingly willing to pay the extra amount for the "concierge" care.

Concierge care generally offers patients the following services:

- Immediate access to their provider by phone 24 hours a day, 7 days a week
- Convenient and unhurried same-day appointments

CRITICAL THINKING

What is your opinion of the concierge type of medical practice? Would you feel comfortable working in such an environment? Why or why not?

- Unlimited email, fax, or phone consultation with their provider
- Home or work visits as needed
- Coordination of specialist referrals
- Friendly staff who understand a patient's unique health needs
- Free parking

Patients who choose this type of service pay a set fee per year from $2,000 to $3,000 for one individual, and up to $5,000 to include a spouse or $6,000 to include children. Patients are expected to carry a major medical plan to cover referrals to specialists, hospitalization, and emergency care.

Ethical concerns have been raised regarding concierge services. Some say the "extra" services should be available to everyone; others believe the extra fees make the service very exclusive. Some providers follow a "retainer" model for concierge services, where patients pay a monthly fee for priority access to their provider, unlimited clinic visits, annual physicals, preventive care, and wellness screenings.

Providers practicing in a concierge service report a greater satisfaction with their chosen profession, enjoy really getting to know their patients, and serve a few hundred patients rather than a few thousand in a traditional practice. Patients report satisfaction in receiving more time and personal care from a provider who determines the best options for maintaining their health.

THE HEALTH CARE TEAM

In every kind of health care setting, the team concept is critical to the quality of patient care. A primary care provider is most likely the main source of health care for patients. From time to time, however, a specialist is sought or recommended. A number of different allied health professionals, including the medical assistant, supply additional health care as ordered by the provider. Increasingly, patients are looking outside traditional medicine for portions of their health care. The Centers for Disease Control and Prevention's (CDC)

2008 National Health Interview Survey revealed that 38% of adults in the United States use some form of complementary and/or alternative medical (CAM) care. The number is closer to 47% for those persons 50 years and older. The survey also indicated greater use of CAM among women and individuals with higher education. In 2007, the World Health Organization (WHO) estimated that between 65% and 80% of the world's population relied on alternative medicine as their primary health care source. One third of all medical schools in the United States now have courses in alternative medicine, and many people in the United States seem to desire a more "natural" approach to health care whenever possible. Although alternative care is not always covered by medical insurance, traditional and nontraditional health care practices are nonetheless blending in many areas.

In whatever manner health care is sought, all members of the health care team must communicate with one another, sometimes in person and sometimes just through the medical history and record, to ensure quality patient care. The Patient Education box on page 30 discusses the role of another major member of the health care team.

The Title "Doctor"

The public is often confused by the title *doctor*. The term implies an earned academic degree of the highest level in a particular area of study. Physicians have earned the MD, or Doctor of Medicine, degree. Other medical degrees include the Doctor of Osteopathy (DO), Doctor of Dentistry (DDS), Doctor of Optometry (OD), Doctor of Podiatric Medicine (DPM), Doctor of Chiropracty (DC), and Doctor of Naturopathy (ND). In the medical field, the abbreviation *Dr.* is used and the title *Doctor* is used to address these individuals qualified by education, training, and licensure to practice medicine.

In nonmedical disciplines, persons who have achieved a doctorate conferred by a college or university include the Doctor of Education (EdD), the Doctor of Philosophy (PhD), and the Doctor of Psychology (PSYD). All three have several areas of specialty and are referred to as *doctor*.

Health Care Professionals and Their Roles

Doctor of Medicine. A doctorate degree in medicine and a license to practice allows a person to diagnose and treat medical conditions. The doctor of medicine candidate attends four years of medical school after receiving a bachelor's degree. Newly graduated MDs enter into a residency program that consists of three to seven years of additional training and education depending on the specialty chosen. This residency comes under the direct supervision of senior medical doctor educators. Family practice, internal medicine, and pediatrics each require a three-year residency; general surgery requires a five-year residency. Some refer to the first year of residency as an internship; however, the American Medical Association (AMA) no longer uses this term. At this point, many medical doctors choose to be board certified, which is optional and voluntary. Certification assures the public that the doctor's knowledge, experience, and skills in a particular specialty area have been tested and deemed qualified to provide care in that specialty. Doctors of medicine can be certified through 24 specialty medical boards and in 88 subspecialty fields. Table 2-1 gives a partial listing of these fields.

Medical doctors must still obtain a license to practice medicine from the state or jurisdiction of the United States in which they are planning to practice. They apply for the permanent license after completing a series of examinations and completing a minimum number of years of graduate medical education. Medical doctors must continue to receive a certain number of continuing medical education (CME) requirements each year to ensure that their knowledge and skills are current. CME requirements vary by state, professional organizations, and hospital staff organizations. Medical assistants are often required to maintain their employer's CME records for easier reporting at the time of license renewal.

Doctor of Osteopathy. Osteopaths are generally recognized as equal to medical doctors in all respects. The Doctor of Osteopathy, or DO, is a fully qualified provider licensed to perform surgery and prescribe medication. The training and education are quite similar to that of the MD. Osteopathic medicine was established in 1874 by Dr. Andrew Taylor Still, who was one of the first practitioners to study the attributes of good health to better understand the process of disease. He identified the musculoskeletal system as a key element of health and encouraged preventive medicine, eating properly, and keeping fit. The education of an osteopath includes a four-year undergraduate degree plus four years of medical school. After graduation from medical school, a DO can choose to practice in any of the 18 American Osteopathic Association specialty areas, requiring from two to six years of additional

training. Approximately 65% of all osteopaths practice in primary care areas such as family practice, pediatrics, obstetrics/gynecology, and internal medicine. DOs must pass a state licensure examination and maintain currency in their education. Most patients find little difference between an MD and a DO. However, doctors of osteopathy can incorporate osteopathic manipulative treatment (OMT) in their treatment of patients as deemed helpful.

Integrative Medicine and Alternative Health Care Practitioners

Many **integrative medicine** and alternative health care practitioners also carry the title *Doctor,* but they have a different training regimen than required for the MD or DO. The training is highly specialized and specific; when licensed, these professionals are allowed to diagnose and treat medical conditions.

As mentioned earlier, alternative therapies are increasingly being perceived as complements to traditional health care in a form of integrative medicine. In this text, three broad alternative therapy disciplines are identified: chiropractic, naturopathy, and Oriental medicine/acupuncture.

Doctor of Chiropractic. Chiropractic is a branch of the healing arts that gives special attention to the physiological and biochemical aspects of the body's structure and it includes procedures for the adjustment and manipulation of the bones, joints, and adjacent tissues of the human body, particularly of the spinal column. Chiropractic is a nonsurgical science that does not include pharmaceuticals or surgery.

The roots of chiropractic care can be traced back to the beginning of recorded time. Writings from China and Greece written in 2700 BC and 1500 BC, respectively, mention spinal manipulation and maneuvering of the lower extremities to ease lower back pain. Daniel David Palmer founded the chiropractic profession in the United States in 1895. Throughout the twentieth century, doctors of chiropractic gained legal recognition and licensure in all 50 states.

Doctors of chiropractic (DC) complete four to five years of study at an accredited chiropractic college. The curriculum includes a minimum of 4,200 hours of classroom, laboratory, and clinical experience. About 555 hours are devoted to adjustive techniques and spinal analysis. This specialized education must be preceded by a minimum of 90 hours of undergraduate courses focusing on science. On successful completion of their education

Table 2-1   Selected Medical and Surgical Specialties

Specialties	Title of Doctor	Description
Anesthesiology	Anesthesiologist	Evaluates sleep and pain control.
Allergy and Immunology	Allergist and Immunologist	Evaluates diseases/disorders of the immune system and problems related to asthma and allergy.
Cardiology	Cardiologist	Evaluates and treats medical conditions of the heart.
Dermatology	Dermatologist	Evaluates disorders/diseases of skin, hair, nails, and related tissues.
Emergency Medicine	Emergency Medical Doctor	Evaluates and treats medical conditions that result from trauma or sudden illness; manages the emergency department.
Family Practice	Family Practitioner	Treats the whole family from infancy to death.
Internal Medicine	Internist	Provides comprehensive care, practices preventive care, and treats long-term and chronic conditions.
Medical Genetics	Geneticist	Provides information in medical and genetic pathology.
Nuclear Medicine	Doctor of Nuclear Medicine	Evaluates molecular and metabolic conditions using radiopharmaceuticals.
Obstetrics and Gynecology	Obstetrician and Gynecologist	Provides care to pregnant women, delivers babies, and treats disorders/diseases of the female reproductive system.
Ophthalmology	Ophthalmologist	Provides comprehensive care of the eye and its structures and offers vision services.
Orthopedic Surgeon	Orthopedist	Examines, diagnoses, and treats diseases and injuries of the musculoskeletal system.
Otolaryngology	Otolaryngologist	Treats diseases/disorders of the ears, nose, and throat.
Pathology	Pathologist	Evaluates body tissues.
Pediatrics	Pediatrician	Treats diseases/disorders of children and adolescents; monitors growth and development of children.
Physical Medicine and Rehabilitation	Doctor of Physical Medicine and Rehabilitation	Evaluates pain, orders rehabilitation, and practices sports medicine.
Preventative Medicine	Doctor	Encourages healthy living.
Psychiatry and Neurology	Psychiatrist and Neurologist	Diagnoses and treats patients with mental, emotional, or behavioral disorders as well as disorders of the brain and central nervous system.
General Surgery	Surgeon	Operates to repair or remove diseased or injured parts of the body.
Colon and Rectal Surgery	Colorectal Surgeon	Operates to remove or repair diseased colon and rectal areas of the body.
Neurological Surgery	Neurosurgeon	Treats conditions of the nervous systems, often through surgery.
Plastic Surgery	Plastic Surgeon	Repairs and reconstructs physical defects; provides cosmetic enhancements.
Thoracic Surgery	Thoracic Surgeon	Performs surgery on the respiratory system, chest, heart, and cardiovascular system.

continues

Table 2-1 Selected Medical and Surgical Specialties (Continued)

Specialties	Title of Doctor	Description
Radiology	Radiologist	Interprets diagnostic images, performs special procedures, and manages radiological services.
Urology	Urologist	Treats diseases/disorders of the urinary tract.

© Cengage Learning 2014

PATIENT EDUCATION

Continually remind your patients of the important role they play in their own health care. *Only your patients* know exactly what happens to their bodies and minds in any particular illness. *Only your patients* know if their pain is too much to bear. *Only your patients* know whether they will remain on any treatment regimen established. *Only your patients* know if they are already embracing some alternative form of treatment. *Only your patients* know how much financial burden they can handle for health care. In initial interviews and pre-provider preparations, ask your patients questions that encourage them to tell you what is happening, whether they are coping, and how their particular problem affects their daily lives. Listen to them carefully. Do not rush or second-guess their responses. Be mindful of the special needs of elderly patients and individuals for whom English is their second language. They are likely to be unfamiliar with taking a major role in their own health care. Always remember to be therapeutic and observe nonverbal cues. Empower your patients to be a member of their own health care team.

CRITICAL THINKING

Discuss with a peer what action might be taken when patients refuse all opportunities to be a member of their own health care team. How might you encourage patients to take even a small part in their own health care? How would major decisions be made?

and training, doctors of chiropractic must also pass the national board examination and all examinations or licensure requirements identified by the particular state in which the individual wishes to practice.

Doctors of chiropractic frequently treat patients with neuromusculoskeletal conditions such as headaches, joint pain, neck pain, lower back pain, and sciatica. Chiropractors also treat patients with osteoarthritis, spinal disk conditions, carpal tunnel syndrome, tendonitis, sprains, and strains. Chiropractors also may treat a variety of other conditions such as allergies, asthma, and digestive disorders. There are obstacles to chiropractors in some areas, however, because states vary in what they authorize chiropractors to practice and may limit their ability to practice **homeopathy** or **acupuncture** or to dispense or sell dietary supplements.

Doctor of Naturopathy. Naturopathy, often referred to as "natural medicine," is based on the belief that the cause of disease is violation of nature's laws. The goal of the naturopath is to remove the underlying causes of disease and to stimulate the body's natural healing processes. Naturopathic treatments may include fasting; adhering to natural food diets; taking vitamins and herbs; tissue minerals; counseling; homeopathic remedies; manipulation of the spine and extremities; massage; exercise; naturopathic hygienic remedies; acupuncture; and applications of water, heat, cold, air, sunlight, and electricity. Most of these treatment methods are used to detoxify the body and strengthen the immune system.

In the United States, a Doctor of Naturopathy (ND) or Doctor of Naturopathic Medicine (NMD) receives education, training, and credentials from a full-time naturopathy college. Full-time education includes two years of science courses and two years of clinical work. Naturopaths are currently licensed to practice in 15 states, four Canadian provinces, and Puerto Rico and the Virgin Islands. The number of states licensing NDs is expected to increase. In many states, naturopaths practice independently and unlicensed, or they practice under the direction of a physician.

Oriental Medicine and Acupuncture.

Oriental medicine is a comprehensive system of health care with a history of more than 3,000 years. Oriental medicine includes acupuncture, Chinese herbology and bodywork, dietary therapy, and exercise based on traditional Oriental medicine principles. This form of health care is used extensively in Asia and is rapidly growing in popularity in the West.

Oriental medicine is based on an energetic model rather than the biochemical model of Western medicine. The ancient Chinese recognized a vital energy behind all life-forms and processes called *qi* (pronounced "chee"). Oriental healing practitioners believe that energy flows along specific pathways called *meridians*. Each pathway is associated with a particular physiological system and internal organ. Disease is the result of deficiency or imbalance of energy in the meridians and their associated physiological systems. Acupuncture points are specific sites along the meridians. Each point has a predictable effect on the vital energy passing through it. Modern science has measured the electrical charge at these points, corroborating the locations of the meridians. Traditional Oriental medicine uses an intricate system of pulse and tongue diagnosis, palpation of points and meridians, medical history, and other signs and symptoms to create a composite diagnosis. A treatment plan then is formulated to induce the body to a balanced state of health.

The WHO recognizes acupuncture and traditional Oriental medicine's ability to treat many common disorders, including the following:

- *Gastrointestinal disorders.* Food allergies, peptic ulcer, chronic diarrhea, constipation, indigestion, anorexia, gastritis
- *Urogenital disorders.* Stress incontinence, urinary tract infections, sexual dysfunction
- *Gynecological disorders.* Irregular, heavy, or painful menstruation; premenstrual syndrome (PMS); infertility
- *Respiratory disorders.* Emphysema, sinusitis, asthma, allergies, bronchitis
- *Neuromusculoskeletal disorders.* Arthritis; migraine headaches; neuralgia; insomnia; dizziness; low back, neck, and shoulder pain
- *Circulatory disorders.* Hypertension, angina pectoris, arteriosclerosis, anemia
- *Eye, ear, nose, and throat disorders.* Otitis media, sinusitis, sore throats
- *Emotional and psychological disorders.* Depression; anxiety; addictions to alcohol, nicotine, and drugs
- *Pain.* Elimination or control of pain for chronic and painful debilitating disorders

In the hands of a comprehensively trained acupuncturist, patients do not find acupuncture painful. Sterile, very fine, flexible needles about the diameter of a human hair are used in treatment. Practitioners may also recommend herbs, dietary changes, and exercise, together with lifestyle changes.

Training for acupuncture and Oriental medicine can be obtained in schools and colleges accredited by the Accreditation Commission for Acupuncture and Oriental Medicine. A minimum of two years of undergraduate study is required, and some colleges prefer applicants to have a bachelor's degree. Most of these specialized programs are three years, and on completion graduates are conferred with a Master's Degree in Acupuncture and Oriental Medicine (MAOM) or a Master's Degree in Acupuncture (MA) degree. Nearly all states regulate the practice of acupuncture and Oriental medicine, either through licensure or a ruling by the Board of Medical Examiners. It is likely that passing a national certification examination or other testing procedure is required before licensure. Many doctors (MDs, DOs, DCs, and NDs) have become qualified to perform acupuncture and to use Oriental medicine in their practices through additional education and training.

Future of Integrative Medicine

There was a time when osteopaths and chiropractors were not accepted by the medical establishment and had difficulty with licensure. Naturopaths, acupuncturists, and Oriental medicine practitioners face similar challenges, and states vary greatly in their regulations of any form of alternative medicine.

The road may be bumpy for alternative practitioners, but their numbers are increasing rapidly.

By 2010, the number of chiropractors, naturopaths, and Oriental medicine practitioners had increased by 88% over previous numbers. Managed care health plans are offering increased access to alternative medicine practitioners, mostly because of the ability to expand patient choices at a lower cost. It is expected that states will broaden their licensure to increased numbers of well-educated and trained alternative practitioners.

Neither the growth in the number of alternative medicine practitioners nor the laws and insurance practices that facilitate their access by patients likely would have occurred without broad public acceptance of alternative and complementary medicine. Americans seem quite willing to pay out-of-pocket expenses for alternative forms of treatment, such as massage therapy, aromatherapy, biofeedback, guided imagery, hydrotherapy, hypnotherapy, and homeopathy. Furthermore, many patients are seeking the more integrated form of medicine that occurs when primary care providers are willing to refer to an alternative practitioner and vice versa. Table 2-2 gives a brief description of a few alternative modalities that integrate fairly easily with traditional medical practices.

ALLIED HEALTH PROFESSIONALS AND THEIR ROLES

In the health care team, allied health professionals bring specific educational backgrounds and a broad array of skills to the medical environment. Medical assistants are allied health professionals with a very specific set of skills for ambulatory care.

The Role of the Medical Assistant

 In the ambulatory care setting, a critical and most beneficial allied health professional is the medical assistant. The medical assistant, performing both administrative and clinical

Table 2-2 Selected Alternative Medicine Modalities

Acupressure	A massage technique that applies pressure to specific acupuncture-like points on the body; pressure encourages the flow of vital energy (*qi*) along the meridian pathways. It is used to control chronic pain, migraine headaches, and backaches.
Aromatherapy	The inhalation and bodily application of essential oils from aromatic plants to relax, balance, rejuvenate, restore, or enhance the body's mind and spirit. It strengthens the self-healing process by indirect stimulation of the immune system.
Biofeedback	Biofeedback machines gauge internal bodily functions and help patients tune in to these functions and identify the triggers that evoke symptoms. Relaxation can be taught to relieve the symptoms.
Guided Imagery	Uses images or symbols to train the mind to create a definitive physiological or psychological effect; relieves stress and anxiety and reduces pain.
Homeopathy	Healing that claims highly diluted doses of certain substances can leave an energy imprint in the body and bring about a cure. Homeopathic remedies are made from naturally occurring plant, animal, or mineral substances and are manufactured by pharmaceutical companies under strict guidelines.
Hydrotherapy	Hydrotherapy uses the buoyancy, warmth, and effects of water and its turbulence to speed recovery after surgery and to reduce pain and stress, spasm and discomfort. It is especially beneficial for work- or sports-related injuries and arthritis.
Hypnotherapy	Hypnotherapy facilitates communication between the right and left sides of the brain with the patient in a state of focused relaxation when the subconscious mind is open to suggestions. It is currently used to help people lose weight; stop smoking; reduce stress; and relieve pain, anxiety, and phobias.
Massage	Massage reduces stress, manages chronic pain, promotes relaxation, and increases circulation of the blood and lymph. Hand stroking on the body helps patients become more familiar with their pain.

tasks under the direction of the provider, is an important link between patient and provider. The medical assistant serves in many capacities—receptionist, secretary, office manager, bookkeeper, insurance coder and biller, sometimes transcriptionist, patient educator, and clinical assistant. The latter requires the medical assistant to be able to administer injections, perform venipuncture, prepare patients for examinations, assist with examinations and special procedures, and perform electrocardiography and various laboratory tests. Medical assistants screen and assess patient needs when scheduling appointments and tests. However, although medical assistants have a broad range of responsibilities, it is critical that they perform only within the scope of their training, education, and personal capabilities and always function within ethical and legal boundaries and state statutes. To perform outside the scope of training is both illegal and unethical.

Because medical assistants are often the patient's first contact with the facility and its providers, a positive attitude is important (see Chapter 1). They must be excellent communicators, both verbally and nonverbally, and project a professional image of themselves and their employer. Medical assistants who believe in their work, who are proud of their career, and who convey compassion and caring provide a positive experience for patients who are ill or in a great deal of discomfort.

Table 2-3 lists some of the allied health professionals recognized by the Commission on Accreditation of Allied Health Education Programs (CAAHEP) and the Accrediting Bureau of Health Education Schools (ABHES).

As a medical assistant, you may not work directly with all the identified allied health care professionals, but you likely will have contact with many of them by telephone and written or electronic communication. Knowledge of the roles these health professionals play enables you to interact more intelligently with all members of the health care team.

In addition to the professionals listed in Table 2-3, you may encounter some or all of the following health care professionals in daily patient care.

Health Unit Coordinator

Health unit coordinators (HUCs) perform non-clinical patient care tasks for the nursing unit of a hospital. HUCs maintain patients' charts, schedule tests, order supplies, screen new patients, and give directions to visitors. This profession requires a self-motivated, mature individual who can handle the stress and hectic pace of coordinating personnel and their duties at the nurses' station. Also called unit secretary, administrative specialist, ward clerk, or ward secretary, a health unit coordinator receives on-the-job training or completes a six-month to one-year certificate program.

Medical Laboratory Technologist

Medical laboratory technologists (MLTs) physically and chemically analyze, as well as culture, urine, blood, and other body fluids and tissues. They work closely with specialists such as oncologists, pathologists, and hematologists. Knowledge of specimen collection, anatomy and physiology, biochemistry, laboratory equipment, asepsis, and quality control is essential. The American Society of Clinical Pathology (ASCP) is a professional organization that oversees credentialing and education in the medical laboratory professions (Figure 2-2).

Registered Dietitian

Registered dietitians (RDs) have specialized training in the nutritional care of groups and individuals and have successfully completed an examination conducted by the Commission on Dietetic Registration. Dietitians assist patients in regulating their diets. Although they are typically employed in hospitals and clinics, they can also be found working

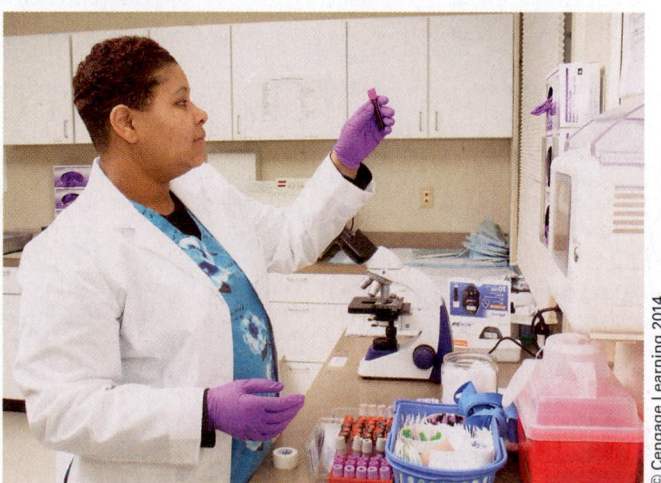

Figure 2-2   Medical laboratory personnel performing blood analysis.

© Cengage Learning 2014

Table 2-3 Selected Allied Health Professions

Occupation	Abbreviations	Job Description
Anesthesiologist Assistant	AA	Performs preoperative tasks; performs airway management and drug administration for induction and maintenance of anesthesia during surgery under direction of a licensed and qualified anesthesiologist
Athletic Trainer	AT	Provides a variety of services including injury prevention, recognition, immediate care, treatment, and rehabilitation after athletic trauma
Clinical Laboratory Technician *Associate Degree*	CLT	Performs all routine tests in a medical laboratory and is able to discriminate and recognize factors that directly affect procedures and results. Works under direction of pathologist, provider medical technologist, or scientist
Diagnostic Medical Sonographer	DMS	Provides patient services using medical ultrasound under the supervision of a provider
Electroneurodiagnostic Technologist	EEG-T	Possesses the knowledge, attributes, and skills to obtain interpretable recordings of a patient's nervous system functions
Emergency Medical Technician— Paramedic	EMT-P	Recognizes, assesses, and manages medical emergencies of acutely ill or injured patients in prehospital care settings, working under the direction of a provider (often through radio communication)
Medical Assistant	MA	Functions under the supervision of licensed medical professionals and is competent in both administrative/office and clinical/laboratory procedures
Medical Illustrator	MI	Creates visual material designed to facilitate the recording and dissemination of medical, biological, and related knowledge through communication media
Occupational Therapist	OT	Educates and trains individuals in the application of purposeful, goal-oriented activity in the evaluation, diagnosis, and treatment of loss of ability to cope with the tasks of daily living and impairment caused by physical injury, illness, or emotional disorder; congenital or developmental disability; or the aging process
Ophthalmic Medical Technician or Technologist	OMT	Assists ophthalmologists to perform diagnostic and therapeutic procedures
Personal Fitness Trainer	PFT	Develops activity plan for each individual that integrates a complete approach to fitness and wellness through exercise, strength training, and proper diet
Radiographer	RT(R)	Provides patient services using imaging modalities, as directed by providers qualified to order and perform radiologic procedures
Registered Health Information Administrator	RHIA	Manages health information systems consistent with the medical, administrative, ethical, and legal requirements of the health care delivery system
Registered Health Information Technician	RHIT	Possesses the technical knowledge and skills necessary to process, maintain, compile, and report patient data
Respiratory Therapist	RRT	Applies scientific knowledge and theory to practical clinical problems of respiratory care
Surgical Technologist	ST	Works as an integral member of the surgical team, which includes surgeons, anesthesiologists, registered nurses, and other surgical personnel delivering patient care and assuming appropriate responsibilities before, during, and after surgery

with the public in personal nutritional counseling. Education includes a bachelor's degree with a major in dietetics, food and nutrition, or food service systems management, in addition to completion of an approved internship.

Pharmacist

Pharmacists (RPh) are licensed by each state to prepare and dispense all types of medications as well as medical supplies related to medication administration. They can practice in hospitals, medical centers, and pharmacies. The minimum training for a pharmacist is a five-year bachelor's degree; some pharmacists pursue a Doctor of Pharmacy degree (PharmD), which is offered by major universities in the United States.

Pharmacy Technician

Pharmacy technicians assist the pharmacist with preparation and administration of medications; they also perform receptionist and billing duties. In hospitals, nursing homes, and assisted living facilities, their responsibilities may include reading patient charts and preparing and delivering medications to patients. Pharmacists must check all orders before delivery. The technician can copy the information about the prescribed medication onto the patient's profile. Professional certification of pharmacy technicians varies from state to state and is administered by state pharmacy associations (Figure 2-3).

Phlebotomist

Phlebotomists are trained in the art of drawing blood for diagnostic laboratory testing. Phlebotomists are also referred to as laboratory liaison technicians. Phlebotomists may be nationally certified and are employed in medical clinics, hospitals, and laboratories. Training consists of one to two semesters in a community college program or on-the-job training.

Physical Therapist

Physical therapists (PTs) are licensed professionals who assist in the examination, testing, and treatment of physically disabled or challenged people. They also assist in physical rehabilitation of patients after an accident, injury, or serious illness, using special exercises, application of heat or cold, ultrasound therapy, and other techniques. Educational requirements for a PT are a minimum of a four-year bachelor's degree (Bachelor of Science) or a special certificate course after obtaining the Bachelor of Science in a related field. PTs must also successfully complete a state licensure examination (Figure 2-4).

Physical Therapy Assistant

Physical therapy assistants (PTAs) are trained to use and apply physical therapy procedures, such as exercise, and physical agents under the supervision of a physical therapist. The PTA has earned an Associate of Science degree from an accredited program and must pass a licensure or registry examination in selected states.

Nurse

Neither ABHES nor CAAHEP is responsible for nurse education or accreditation, but they are listed here as a major participant in health care. Nurses are licensed by the state in which they practice. Although nurses' education and training are oriented to bedside care, some may be employed in medical clinics as clinical assistants, especially in clinics where surgery is performed. Nurses play a number of roles on the health care team.

Registered Nurse. In the United States, registered nurses (RNs) are professionals who have completed, at a minimum, a two-year course of study at a state-approved school of nursing and have passed the National Council Licensure Examination (NCLEX-RN). Employment settings most often include hospitals, convalescent homes, clinics, and home health care.

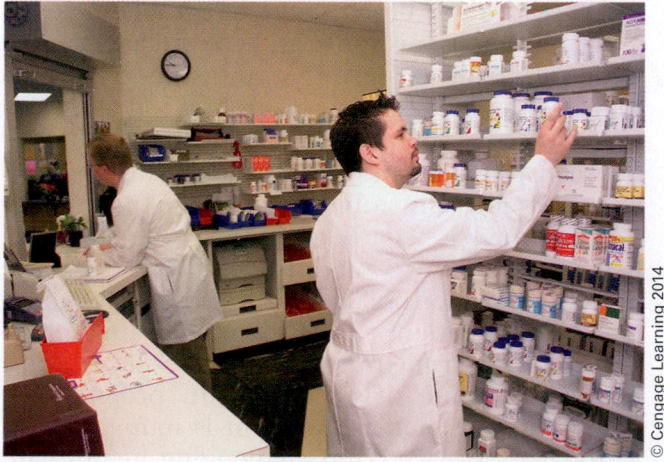

© Cengage Learning 2014

Figure 2-3 Pharmacy technician working with pharmacist preparing medications.

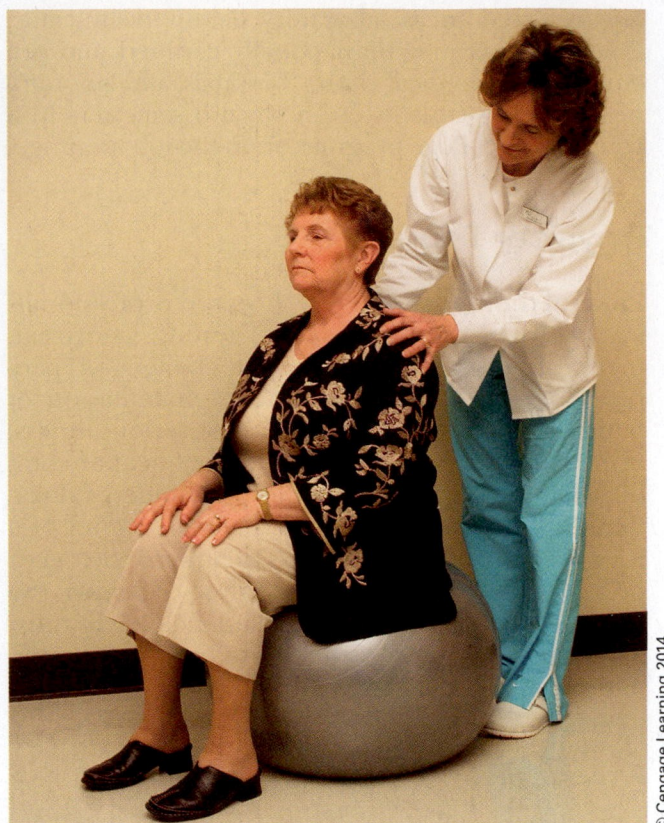

© Cengage Learning 2014

Figure 2-4 Physical therapist working with a patient requiring physical rehabilitation.

Licensed Practical Nurse. A licensed practical nurse (LPN) is a professional trained in basic nursing techniques and direct patient care. LPNs practice under the direct supervision of an RN or provider and are employed in similar settings to RNs. Training includes completion of a state-approved program in practical nursing and successful completion of a national licensure examination.

Nurse Practitioner. Sometimes referred to as an Advanced Registered Nurse Practitioner (ARNP), a nurse practitioner (NP) is an RN who, by advanced education (usually a master's degree) and clinical experience in a branch of nursing, has acquired expert knowledge in a specific medical specialty. Nurse practitioners are employed by providers in private practice or in clinics and sometimes practice independently, especially in rural areas. They are expected to increase in numbers as the number of primary care providers decreases over the next decade. ARNPs may or may not be licensed to prescribe medications.

Physician Assistant

Physician assistants (PAs) receive formal education and training to provide diagnostic, therapeutic, and preventive health care services delegated by and under the supervision of providers and surgeons. PAs take medical histories, examine and treat patients, order and interpret laboratory tests and X-rays, and make diagnoses. They also treat minor injuries by suturing, splinting, and casting. PAs write progress notes, instruct and counsel patients, and order tests and therapy. In 48 states, the District of Columbia, and Guam, PAs may prescribe some medications. They can supervise technicians and medical assistants. PAs may be primary care providers in areas where the supervising physician is not present all the time but is always available for conferring as necessary and required by law.

Most PA programs are two years in length with the added requirement of at least two years of college and some health care experience. For licensure, all states require PAs to complete an accredited, formal education program and to pass the Physician Assistant National Certifying Examination administered by the National Commission on Certification of Physician Assistants (NCCPA). The examination is available only to graduates of an accredited PA education program. Upon successful completion of the examination, the credential "Physician Assistant–Certified" can be used.

THE VALUE OF THE MEDICAL ASSISTANT TO THE HEALTH CARE TEAM

With their broad range of competencies in both administrative and clinical areas, medical assistants are the most valued ambulatory health care team member. Medical assistants are the great communicators, serving as liaison between provider and hospital staff and between provider and any number of allied and other health professionals. Because they often are the first providers to see or speak with patients, they undertake responsibility for directing, informing, and guiding patient care while establishing a professional and caring tone for the entire health care team. The value of a competent, professional, compassionate medical assistant is immeasurable in today's fast-paced and challenging health care environment.

CASE STUDY 2-1

Refer to the scenario at the beginning of the chapter.

CASE STUDY REVIEW

1. Where will you research additional information on being a physical therapy assistant?

2. Compare the working hours, rate of pay, contact with patients, required schooling, and job availability to those of the medical assistant.

3. If other health professions discussed in the chapter are of special interest to you, answer the same questions. This review helps to clarify the position of the medical assistant for you.

CASE STUDY 2-2

You are the medical assistant for a family-practice provider, Dr. Bill Claredon, who is close to retirement. He is much adored by all his patients, but he thinks alternative medicine is outright quackery. Marjorie Johns, a patient with debilitating back pain, tells you she is seeing an acupuncturist and is taking less and less of her prescribed medications. You quietly mention this to Dr. Claredon before he enters the examination room to see Marjorie. He glares at you with disgust at the information and is quite agitated when he enters the examination room.

CASE STUDY REVIEW

1. Describe the discussion that you think will occur between Dr. Claredon and Marjorie.

2. If Marjorie is unhappy when she is ready to leave the facility, what can you do or say to help her?

3. What can you do to help Dr. Claredon?

SUMMARY

The health care environment is a dynamic service that changes rapidly in response to new technology and societal needs. In an effort to provide quality care to the most individuals at a reasonable cost, some form of managed care likely will dominate the health care industry for years to come. A strong health care team is critical in the health care setting, as primary care providers, specialists of all disciplines, alternative care practitioners, and allied and other health professionals collaborate on the best way to provide integrative medicine and quality patient care. In almost any health care environment, but especially the ambulatory care setting, the medical assistant is a vital link in the team and is responsible for a range of responsibilities, both clinical and administrative.

STUDY FOR SUCCESS

To reinforce your knowledge and skills of information presented in this chapter:

- Review the *Key Terms*
- Role-play with other students to apply attributes of professionalism pertinent to this chapter.
- Consider the *Case Studies* and discuss your conclusions
- Answer the questions in the *Certification Review*
- Apply your knowledge by completing the *Activities* in the *Study Guide* and the *Games and Quizzes* in the StudyWARE **StudyWARE** software on the *Premium Website*
- Practice your problem-solving skills with the *Critical Thinking Challenge 3.0* on the *Premium Website*

Additional resources for this chapter include:

- Module 1 of the *Medical Assisting Learning Lab*
- *CourseMate for Delmar's Comprehensive Medical Assisting*
- *WebTutor for Delmar's Comprehensive Medical Assisting*

CERTIFICATION REVIEW

1. Medical assistants are mostly employed in:
   a. hospitals
   b. nursing facilities
   c. ambulatory care settings
   d. insurance companies
2. A health maintenance organization is one kind of:
   a. managed care operation
   b. individual practice
   c. sole proprietorship
   d. hospital
3. With its emphasis on controlling costs, managed care is likely to affect:
   a. only hospitals
   b. all health care settings
   c. only providers in private practice
   d. only patients
4. The health care team:
   a. should exclude the patient as part of the team
   b. is only important in the hospital setting
   c. consists of physicians and nurses
   d. includes physicians, nurses, allied health care professionals, patients, and integrative medicine practitioners
5. Integrative health care approaches are:
   a. increasingly accepted as complementary to traditional health care
   b. always covered by insurance
   c. seldom approved for licensure
   d. not important to understand
6. A medical assistant permitted by law to draw blood for diagnostic laboratory testing performs a procedure similar to those performed by a:
   a. health unit coordinator
   b. health information technician
   c. phlebotomist
   d. respiratory therapist
7. The "boutique" or "concierge" medical practice:
   a. is another form of managed care
   b. allows patients special privileges in their health care
   c. is covered by all major insurance plans
   d. does not require special fees for services
8. Providers just establishing their practice often seek to work with another provider in the same field. When expenses and profits are shared, this form of management is called a/an:
   a. HMO
   b. corporation
   c. sole proprietor
   d. group or partnership
9. Which of the following will the medical assistant *not* do in health care?
   a. code and bill insurance, bookkeeping
   b. diagnose and treat ailments
   c. screen when making appointments
   d. assist provider, perform clinical and laboratory procedures
10. An alternative approach to medicine that treats patients using thin, flexible needles is called:
    a. acupuncture
    b. naturopathy
    c. chiropractic
    d. homeopathy

REFERENCES/BIBLIOGRAPHY

American Board of Medical Specialties & Subspecialties. *Approved ABMS specialty boards & certificate categories.* Retrieved August 3, 2011, from www.abms.org/

Bondurant, S. (2005). Mainstream and alternative medicine: Converging paths require common standards. *Annals of Internal Medicine, 142*(2), 149–150.

Credentialing CAM Providers: Understanding CAM Education, Training, Regulation, and Licensing, NCCAM Publication No. D451. Retrieved June 20, 2010, from http://nccam.nih.gov/health/decisions/credentialing.htm

Eisenberg, D. M., Cohen, M. H., Hrbek, A., Grayzel, J., Van Rompay, M. I., & Cooper, R. A. (2002). Credentialing complementary and alternative medical providers. *Annals of Internal Medicine, 137*(12), 965–973.

Frenkel, M. A., & Borkan, J. M. (2003). An approach for integrating complementary-alternative medicine into primary care. *Family Practice, 20*(3), 324–332.

Health Care Careers Directory, 2009–2010. (2009). Chicago, IL: American Medical Association.

Jorgensen, A. (n.d.) Choosing the right practice for you. Retrieved August 3, 2011, from www.netdoc.com

Tamparo, C. D., & Lewis, M. A. (2011). *Diseases of the human body* (5th ed.). Philadelphia: F. A. Davis Publishers.

CHAPTER 3

History of Medicine

OUTLINE

Cultural Heritage in Medicine

Medical Specialists in History

History of Medical Education

History of Attitudes Toward
  Illness

Historical Medical Treatments
  The Scourge of Epidemics
  Other Threats to Health

Significant Contributions
  to Medicine
    Women in Medicine
Frontiers in Medicine

LEARNING OUTCOMES

1. Define, spell, and pronounce the key terms as presented in the glossary.

2. Evaluate the effects of culture on medicine.

3. Paraphrase the role of religion, magic, and science in medicine's history.

4. Describe how attitudes toward illness are manifested today.

5. List a minimum of three previously used common medical treatments.

6. Critique a minimum of three theories/practices of ancient medicine that are still prevalent today.

7. Name and describe the historical roles of medical specialists.

8. Summarize three major epidemics and their impact on medical care.

9. Analyze the role of women in medicine.

10. Trace the progression of medical education.

11. Name at least five significant contributions to medicine.

12. Describe a minimum of three recent developments in medicine.

13. Analyze the professionalism questions and apply them to this chapter's content.

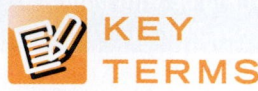

KEY TERMS

allopathic

asepsis

bubonic plague

malaria

moxibustion

pharmacopoeia

pluralistic (pluralism)

septicemia

trephination

typhus (typhoid)

yellow fever

ATTRIBUTES OF PROFESSIONALISM

Communication
- Did you apply active listening skills?
- Does your knowledge allow you to speak easily with all members of the health care team?

Competency
- Did you pay attention to detail?
- Did you ask questions if you were out of your comfort zone or did not have the experience to carry out tasks?
- Were you knowledgeable and accountable?

Initiative
- Did you seek out opportunities to expand your knowledge base?

Integrity
- Did you demonstrate sensitivity to patient's rights?
- Did you protect personal boundaries?
- Did you demonstrate respect for individual diversity?
- Did you demonstrate an appreciation for the patient's attitude toward his or her illness or condition?

SCENARIO

You may recall your mom putting a mentholated salve on your chest when you had a cold. Your cousins had to take a spoonful of cod-liver oil each night before they went to bed. Grandma made chicken soup with homemade noodles when you had the flu. An apple a day, hot or cold steam in a room, and many more traditions are medical practices of years gone by. Many still stand, however, and from them others have developed. Interestingly, medicine has a rich history, and every culture exhibits that history differently. The more you know of and understand that history and its various cultural influences, the more effective and therapeutic your communication will be with patients.

INTRODUCTION

The historical development of medicine has been driven by many and varied events. These include the presence of illness and injury, plagues and widespread epidemics, the dissection first of animals and then of human bodies, the discovery of bacteria, and the experimentation with herbs and potions for medicinal purposes. Medicine as it is known today is the result of multiple revolutions of thought throughout the world. The history of medicine must remind us that more than one discipline and more than one philosophy have contributed to medicine. This is perhaps more true now than ever as our world becomes smaller and our society becomes increasingly pluralistic, ethnically, culturally, and religiously.

CULTURAL HERITAGE IN MEDICINE

Today's health professional will give care to individuals of varied cultures who hold differing philosophical beliefs toward medicine. The informed and caring health professional will recognize that a person's culture and ethnic heritage play an enormous role in any kind of health care. For example, if the patient's culture and history lean toward a more natural, nonmedical form of health care, treating the patient with prescription drugs will necessitate a careful explanation and rationale for the use of medications. Otherwise, the patient may refuse to take all or part of the medications, thus hindering recovery. It would be better to seek a treatment for the patient that embraces both the health care professional's desire to heal and the individual's wish to respect cultural tradition.

In every society, medicine has been an important element for its people. From the earliest time, culture was an important influence on medicine, and modern day medicine is in many ways a reflection of this diverse and rich heritage.

It is certain that religion, magic, and science all played a vital part in the history of medicine. Religion was important because it was perceived that certain gods were to be called on for a cure through ceremonies, prayers, and sacrifices. Magic was practiced because it was such an important part of many societies and was seen as an essential ingredient to chase away evil spirits. The importance of science was demonstrated in the use of plants and minerals for medicinal purposes that are found throughout medicine's history. Unearthed clay tablets reveal hundreds of plants, minerals, and animal substances used for medicinal purposes in ancient Mesopotamia and Babylon. The Chinese pharmacopoeia was rich in the use of herbs.

Skeletal remains of prehistoric cultures show advanced stages of arthritis, a nearly toothless jaw, and only a 20- to 40-year life span for humans. Skull bones reveal round holes referred to as trephination, believed necessary to release the evil spirits thought to be causing a person's illness. Mesopotamian cultures believed that illness was a punishment by the gods for violation of a moral code. Ancient Egyptians believed the body was a system of channels for air, tears, blood, urine, sperm, and feces. All the channels were thought to come together in the rectum and were believed to become easily clogged. Thus, emetics, enemas, and purges of the anus were common treatments. In ancient India, punishment for adultery was cutting off the nose, therefore allowing practitioners many opportunities to practice and refine the art of nose reconstruction or plastic surgery.

The ancient Chinese cultures examined and carefully monitored the pulse in each wrist. It was believed that the pulse had hundreds of characteristics important in medical treatment. There were five methods of treatment to bring a person back to the right track. They were:

1. Cure the spirit.
2. Nourish the body.
3. Give medications.
4. Treat the whole body.
5. Use acupuncture and moxibustion.

Acupuncture is the piercing of the skin by very thin, sterile, flexible needles into any of 365 points along 12 meridians that transverse the body and transmit the active life force called "qi" (pronounced "chee"). Each of these spots is related to a particular organ. **Moxibustion** requires the use of a powdered plant substance that is made into a small mound on the person's skin and then burned, usually raising a blister.

Even today's **allopathic**, or traditional, practitioners would agree that the first four methods of treatment from ancient Chinese culture are excellent guidelines for health care. There also is new awareness that acupuncture has a valid place in allopathic medicine, not only for the control of some types of pain but also for treating some illnesses. A type of moxibustion can be used today with acupuncture treatment. There are many different techniques for moxibustion in which varying substances are used to apply heat to a broad area of the skin. The intense direct heating of points is used to treat some diseases, to relax tense muscles, and to gently relieve aching and mild pain without making skin blisters.

MEDICAL SPECIALISTS IN HISTORY

Medicine's history gives early evidence of many "specialists" in the healing arts. They were known by various names—witch doctors, medicine men and women, shamans or healing priests, and physicians. These healers were more than ancestors of the modern practitioner, however, for they performed many functions that involved the welfare of the entire community or village. By today's standards, they were considered to be equivalent to spiritual advisers, social workers, counselors, and teachers.

These medical specialists were among the world's earliest professionals. They were present at important "rites of passage," such as births and deaths, puberty initiations, and marriages. The role of the healers varied among cultures, but central to all cultures was the belief that the healers had the ability to draw upon some power beyond themselves. Their goal was to help others live and work in harmony with nature and each other.

Evidence also suggests that many ancient healers used a variety of mind-altering drugs. A mythical drug called "soma" is reported in India's religious literature. Primitive tribes of Central, South, and North America used "yage" and "peyote" to induce trance-like experiences. Many ancient healers also practiced certain types of what today might be called yoga and meditation.

These healers were given special status in their culture. Sometimes they were recognized by their dress and the pouch or satchel they carried. They were not expected to work, and their needs were supplied by the members of their tribe. Much later, when medical education was available, a healer was called a "physician" if a university degree was held. Surgeons were part of a lower class because they usually had only apprentice training and included the group of barbering surgeons who used their razors to cut into blood vessels to relieve infection and fever.

Today the more common terms "provider" or "practitioner" are often used because there are so many health professionals who are a part of the patient's health care team providing treatment.

From the earliest times, it appears that some payment was expected for medical services rendered. In many instances, the payment was dependent on the status of the practitioner, as well as the patient. At the same time, some cultures punished a practitioner who was not successful in treatment by forcing that practitioner to treat only those too poor to pay.

HISTORY OF MEDICAL EDUCATION

During the rise of Christianity, emphasis was placed on the soul rather than the body; therefore, early Christian monks held great control over medicine. This is evidenced by St. Benedict of Nursia (480–554), who forbade the study of medicine. The care of the sick was encouraged, but only through prayer and divine intervention. Thus, Christ's healing mission was institutionalized in a fashion that was to control medical care almost completely for the next 500 years, until the seventh century.

At that time the religion of Islam moved to preserve the classical learning that had been achieved in medicine. Not only were practitioners able to return to the same methods as those practiced by earlier Greek and Roman cultures, but also medical study was now encouraged.

Medical education in established universities began in the ninth century. These universities included Salerno in southern Italy, the University of Montpelier in southern France, and the University of Paris. By the time the Renaissance was at its height in the mid-fifteenth century, the practitioner had become licensed, was receiving great status, and was attending the ill in a velvet bonnet and fur-trimmed cloak.

Art and science were more closely related during the Renaissance than at any other period. Michelangelo (1475–1564) spent years on careful human dissection, and this anatomical detail is evident in his paintings in the Sistine Chapel in the Vatican in Rome. Leonardo da Vinci (1452–1519) made anatomical preparations from which he produced drawings representing the skeletal, muscular, nervous, and vascular systems. His accurate sketch of the spinal vertebrae went undiscovered for more than 100 years.

HISTORY OF ATTITUDES TOWARD ILLNESS

Various attitudes prevailed toward the ill person. A sick person might be excused from daily activity but was likely to be shunned if the disease was believed to be a punishment by the gods for mortal sin. This forced isolation may well have been beneficial to the community. In contrast, touching by Jesus was an important component of healing, as was the faith of the individual involved. The New Testament parable of the Good Samaritan helped establish a nexus between the early church and a concern for the sick. It was believed that though the body might be wasted and foul with disease, the purity of the soul guaranteed life everlasting. This was unlike the pagan religions that tended to abandon individuals thought to be ill because they were in disfavor with the gods.

Native Americans had various feelings about illness. The ill were treated with kindness among the Navajo and Cherokee, and some who recovered from serious illness were considered to have extraordinary powers. However, if a tribe was faced with famine, suicide by the aged and infirm was considered the highest form of bravery. The Eskimos put their older adults unprotected onto ice floes. Neither the Romans nor the Greeks treated the hopelessly ill or deformed, and unwanted infants were disposed of quickly or left to die.

 Some of these attitudes are seen even today. The Western medical community and the consumers it serves are heatedly debating the right to choose life or death and the ethics and legality of death with dignity or physician-assisted death, which is acceptable in many other cultures. Even with our vast knowledge of medicine and the disease process, many individuals are still fearful of any illness they do not understand or that they perceive as threatening their health—AIDS is a good example. This fear is often accompanied by public ill treatment of the individuals suffering from certain diseases.

CRITICAL THINKING

What steps are taken today in hospitals and in ambulatory care settings to prevent the spread of harmful bacteria and viruses? Name the antibiotic-resistant bacteria that plague hospitals today. What steps do you personally take?

HISTORICAL MEDICAL TREATMENTS

The writings of ancient Egypt reveal that when a woman suspected she was pregnant, she urinated over a mixture of wheat and barley seeds combined with dates and sand. If any of the grains sprouted, she was surely pregnant. If the wheat grew, she would have a boy. If the barley grew, it would be a girl. Urine is still used in modern tests to determine pregnancy.

During the Ming dynasty (1368–1644), Chinese medicine seemed to reach its peak. This is the time that Li Shih-chen wrote his *Pen ts'ao Kang mu,* "The Great Herbal." This pharmacopoeia summarizes what was known of herbal medicine up to the late-sixteenth century, describing in detail more than 1,800 plants, animal substances, minerals, and metals, together with their medicinal properties and applications.

Early medical treatments were often crude. For a sore throat, a practitioner might mix barley water, vinegar, and mulberry syrup for a gargle. Someone suffering with rheumatism might be given a prescription of chopped mice, lynx claws, and elk hooves. Rhubarb, senna, bitter apple, turpentine, camphor, and mercury were among the practitioners' staples. Some practitioners washed the instruments used in treating the ill; others scoffed at such a practice. **Malaria**, diphtheria, tuberculosis, **typhoid**, and dysentery were commonplace. Leprosy was prevalent, and venereal diseases were rife. Smallpox was frequent in villages; sometimes the sufferer would be placed in a meat pickling vat and fumigated. The death toll from such diseases was particularly high among children. Finally, in the eighteenth century, Edward Jenner made a great contribution to the prevention of disease by discovering a method of vaccination against smallpox.

Medicine progressed rapidly during the nineteenth century. Two important discoveries occurred: anesthesia to alleviate pain during surgery, and the realization that some bacteria cause disease. Once it had been proved that certain bacteria were causes of diseases and were transmissible agents responsible for contagion, greater care was taken to prevent that transmission. **Asepsis** became important to reduce the risk for infection. The Hungarian physician and obstetrician Ignaz Philipp Semmelweis (1818–1865) was able to prove that physicians who came from an autopsy directly to the care of postpartum women, without scrubbing their hands and washing instruments, carried infection with them that often caused puerperal fever (**septicemia** after childbirth) and death to the new mothers.

The names of Louis Pasteur (1822–1895), Joseph Lister (1827–1912), and Robert Koch (1843–1910), are familiar to all bacteriologists. Louis Pasteur has sometimes been referred to as the father of preventive medicine as the result of his work in recognizing the relationship between bacteria and infectious disease (Figure 3-1). Joseph Lister revolutionized surgery because of his belief in Pasteur's theory of using carbolic acid as an antiseptic spray. He insisted that all instruments and physicians' hands be washed with the solution. Robert Koch used the culture-plate method for isolating bacteria and demonstrated how cholera was transmitted by food and water. His discovery changed the way health departments cared for persons with infectious disease.

Fortunately, early in the twentieth century, society was finally liberated from many of the infectious and epidemic diseases that had scourged the human race for millennia. Smallpox vaccinations became common, the causes of **yellow fever**, **typhus**, and **bubonic plague** were determined, and

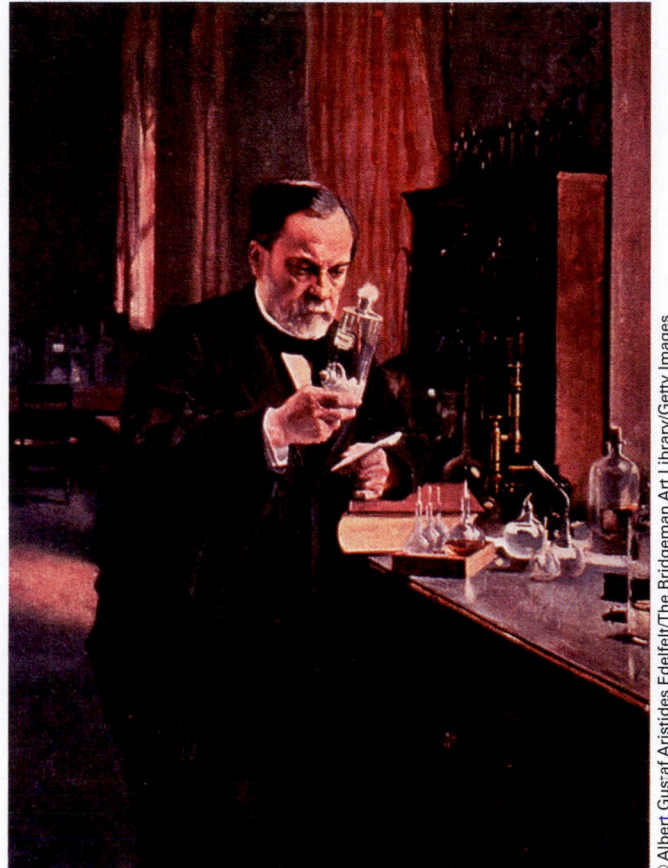

© Albert Gustaf Aristides Edelfelt/The Bridgeman Art Library/Getty Images

Figure 3-1 Louis Pasteur, known for his recognition of the relationship between bacteria and infectious disease.

appropriate measures were taken to eradicate these diseases. Life expectancy increased. Tuberculosis became less frequent. In 1922, Frederick G. Banting and medical student Charles Best were able to isolate and inject insulin into a 14-year-old boy who was dying of diabetes. Two weeks later, the boy was alive and alert. By 1923, insulin was available for general sale in pharmacies throughout the world. Antibiotics were discovered and the Salk and Sabin vaccines were found for poliomyelitis.

The first electrocardiogram machine was invented in 1903. George Papanicolaou discovered cancer cells in 1928, the same year penicillin was discovered by Alexander Fleming. Penicillin, however, required further development, which was accomplished by Howard Florey and Ernst Chain, and was finally brought into production in 1945. C. Walton Lillehei performed the first successful open-heart surgery in 1952. Dr. Christian Barnard performed the first human heart transplant in 1967. Advancing technology enabled medicine to march steadily forward.

The Scourge of Epidemics

There is a saying, "Two steps forward—one step back." At the same time giant strides are made in medicine for one disease, the battle rages for eradication of another. What follows is a discussion of three diseases that have caused much fear in our world, are still a great concern throughout the world, and are still a challenge for medical research.

Paralytic Poliomyelitis. Paralytic poliomyelitis, a virus spread through the fecal-oral route, multiplies in the intestine and invades the nervous system. It is often referred to as infantile paralysis. It mostly affects children under the age of 5 years, and there is no cure.

A 3,000-year-old Egyptian stone carving indicates the presence of the virus in ancient times. There is evidence of polio outbreaks occurring during the summer months in the late 1890s in the United States. During the Great Depression of the 1930s and into the 1950s, infantile paralysis was greatly feared. It struck mostly children, resulted in crippling paralysis within hours, and sometimes caused death. Children were hospitalized and isolated in polio wards. Children were kept from swimming pools and public playgrounds and were reminded not to get too tired or chilled. A practitioner was called if headache, fever, sore throat, stiff neck, or aching muscles occurred.

Those individuals with bulbar polio, a poliomyelitis that affected nerve cells in the medulla oblongata—the lowest portion of the brainstem responsible for regulating heart rate, breathing, and blood pressure—were placed in iron lungs. Iron lungs worked by creating an airtight seal around individuals placed on their backs so that only their heads were visible. A pump alternately raised and lowered the air pressure inside to fill and deflate the lungs, forcing the body to simulate breathing (Figure 3-2). Lying in the iron lung, individuals were fully dependent on their caregivers, relying entirely for their view of the world on a mirror suspended above their face and angled toward the rest of the room.

President Franklin D. Roosevelt, diagnosed with polio in 1921, waged war on the disease. He funded polio research that eventually led to a vaccine. Roosevelt founded the National Foundation for Infantile Paralysis, which later became known as the March of Dimes. Children throughout the United States placed dimes in card folders to take to school to donate to a cure for polio. Dr. Jonas Salk developed the first polio vaccine in 1952, and Dr. Albert Sabin developed an oral polio vaccine in

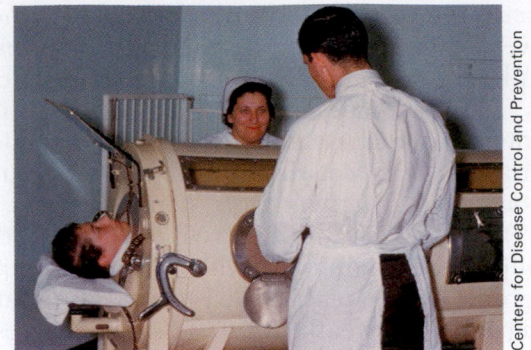

Centers for Disease Control and Prevention

Figure 3-2   A doctor and nurse with a patient in an iron lung during the Rhode Island polio epidemic, 1960.

1961. In 1979 the last case of polio in the United States was reported. Scientists knew that children could have lifelong protection from polio with the polio vaccine given multiple times.

Worldwide, however, polio is still a problem in Asia, Afghanistan, India, Nigeria, and Pakistan. Many agencies, including Rotary International, the World Health Organization (WHO), United Nations International Children's Emergency Fund (UNICEF), and the U.S. Centers for Disease Control and Prevention (CDC), have established programs to vaccinate the world's children. For 20 years, the incidences of polio decreased all around the world. The WHO had hoped to announce as early as 2005 that polio had disappeared from the world. Instead, out of fear and superstition, leaders of a few nations began to counsel against the polio vaccine. Mothers were told the vaccine would make their children infertile and infect them with HIV. Unfortunately, in 2011, there were still 650 cases of polio diagnosed in the world.

Cancer. Cancer was an affliction long before polio was first evidenced. The earliest specimen of cancer was noted in the remains of a skull dated in the Bronze Age (1900–1600 BC). The writings of Hippocrates describe cancers of many body sites. In the nineteenth century, the pathology of cancer was viewed with a microscope, and metastasis was first understood. It was believed that cancer growth was like planting seeds to be carried through the bloodstream into another organ that was hospitable.

Researchers first believed that cancer resulted from excess bile collecting in various body sites. Some believed cancer was the result of fermenting and deteriorating lymph fluid. Today, the inability of the body's immune system to destroy abnormal cell growth, trauma, chronic irritation, and viral and cellular derivations are considered the primary causes of cancer.

Cancerous tumors are often removed through surgery. Radiation and/or chemotherapy may also be used to rid the body of the disease. Today an individual's DNA structure is considered in treatment. Chemotherapy drugs are matched to the specific genetic code of an individual, can be designed to prevent blood vessel growth from surrounding tissue to a solid tumor, or can prevent cancer cells from multiplying and invading other tissues. Recently it was discovered that cancers contain stem cells that produce other cancer cells. Research now turns to identifying markers specific to these stem cells and to creating therapies that can eliminate the reproducing stem cells.

Even with the many years of research and the millions of dollars spent to cure cancer, more than 1.5 million new cancers are diagnosed every year in the United States, and more than half a million people will die of cancer each year, or about 1,500 per day.

HIV Infection/AIDS. In 1981, a rare cancer outbreak known as Kaposi's sarcoma was seen in young gay men in New York and California. In addition, increased cases of a pneumonia called pneumocystitis were reported among the same demographic group. The CDC later coined the term AIDS (acquired immune deficiency syndrome). In 1981, 1,600 cases of AIDS were reported, with close to 700 deaths. As the death rate soared in the next few years, researchers sought the cause of and a cure for the disease. In 1984 the human immunodeficiency virus (HIV) was discovered to be the cause of AIDS.

HIV is a virus that slowly destroys the body's immune system, thus making an individual much more susceptible to infection and other illnesses. There is no cure for AIDS, but with prompt and aggressive treatment, individuals with HIV are living long and productive lives. HIV can be transmitted through bodily fluids during sexual contact; by sharing contaminated needles to inject drugs; by accidental sticks or pokes from HIV-contaminated needles; by transfusion of infected blood products (rare since 1992); and from mother to baby during pregnancy, delivery, and breast-feeding (greatly reduced in the last few years).

Any life-altering, life-threatening disease is a challenge, but HIV infection and AIDS come with awareness that some in society will condemn and shun those infected. Education in the United States has done much to calm the nerves and erase some of the fear that infected individuals face from those who would condemn.

Worldwide HIV/AIDS statistics of 2010 show that since the beginning of the epidemic, nearly 30 million people have died from AIDS-related causes. Statistics for the United States are slow in reporting, but by July 2010 approximately 1 million persons were living with HIV/AIDS, and an estimated 54,000 new diagnoses of HIV infection infections were expected to occur each year. Although HIV infection and AIDS cases show decline in the United States, there are still serious challenges to be met. A large majority of infected persons are unaware they are infected and are passing the virus on to others. Three quarters of new infections in women in the United States are heterosexually transmitted. Cultural differences sometimes create difficulty in preventing the disease if condoms are frowned upon or men have multiple heterosexual partners at the same time they are having sex with other men. Across the world, 2.7 million people were infected with HIV in 2010, causing serious and debilitating physical and mental difficulties, with 1.8 million AIDS-related deaths.

Other Threats to Health

Early in the twenty-first century, we are still quite aware of the limitations of modern medicine. In developing countries torn with war and strife, cholera causes the deaths of thousands simply because there is no proper sanitation. In the microbial world, new drug-resistant strains of malaria, tuberculosis, and other diseases are not responding to known treatments.

Health professionals in hospitals and health care facilities, especially nursing homes and dialysis centers, are very much aware of a new type of bacteria known as health care associated methicillin-resistant *Staphylococcus aureus* (HA-MRSA), which is resistant to many antibiotics. MRSA infection is especially dangerous to individuals with weakened immune systems. It can come from medical facilities or be community based. The latter can be found in athletic locker rooms and in other areas where large numbers of individuals congregate. This form is identified as community associated or CA-MRSA. The use of antibiotics completely changed medicine by providing the ability to cure bacterial-related disease. However, bacteria have now evolved to be resistant to those antibiotics. This is another example of the earlier statement, "Two steps forward—one step back." The challenge of medicine is as strong today as it was 100 years ago.

SIGNIFICANT CONTRIBUTIONS TO MEDICINE

Hippocrates (ca. 460–ca. 377 BC) is the physician most frequently recalled from ancient Greek culture. It is not known why his name surfaces above all other Greek physicians, for some were surely just as prominent. His writings, however, have contributed much to today's medical culture. Hippocrates is remembered by many for his well-known Hippocratic Oath, which established guidelines for a physician's practice of medicine (Figure 3-3). Although few physicians swear to this oath today when they embark on their medical careers, it is still recognized for its validity and wisdom. There are various translations of the Hippocratic Oath, but all communicate the same fundamental message.

It would be impossible to identify all the other individuals who made significant contributions to medicine in this text. However, Table 3-1 lists several notable individuals in the history of medicine. Note that only a few entries are made in the most recent years—not because there are no major medical discoveries occurring, but rather because so many are occurring that they cannot all be listed.

Women in Medicine

Whereas women were accepted as healers in primitive societies, later cultures reduced their status to that of being allowed to care only for women and to assist in childbirth. In any culture that granted women only secondary status, women were also considered unqualified to become physicians. In Chinese culture, the first reference to a female physician mentioned by name is in documents from the Han dynasty (206 BC–AD 220). In Muslim society, the reluctance of Arabic physicians to violate social taboo and touch the genitals of female strangers further encouraged relegating the practice of obstetrics and gynecology to midwives.

Women were not accepted as medical physicians in Western culture until the nineteenth and twentieth centuries. Italy granted women the status earlier than other cultures. In the United States, the first female physician was Elizabeth Blackwell, who was awarded her degree in 1849. Although she was snubbed by the public, she soon earned the respect of her colleagues. When she refused to be absent from class when the male reproductive system was discussed, her fellow male students supported her actions.

In 1860 there were only 200 female practitioners in the United States. In 2012, 31% of U.S. providers were women, and there were ten female deans in U.S. medical schools. Women received 48% of the medical degrees awarded in 2010. Today women are represented in all areas of medicine; however, the majority work in internal medicine, family practice, pediatrics, obstetrics/gynecology, psychiatry, and anesthesiology.

FRONTIERS IN MEDICINE

There has been phenomenal growth in medicine in the past two decades. Only a few advances are mentioned here. Much better imaging that leads

---

THE OATH OF HIPPOCRATES

I swear by Apollo Physician and Aesculapius and Hygeia and Panacea and all the gods and goddesses, making them my witnesses, that I will fulfill according to my ability and judgment this oath and this covenant:

To hold him who has taught me this art as equal to my parents and to live my life in partnership with him, and if he is in need of money to give him a share of mine, and to regard his offspring as equal to my brothers in male lineage and to teach them this art—if they desire to learn it—without fee and covenant; to give a share of precepts and oral instruction and all the other learning to my sons and to the sons of him who has instructed me and to pupils who have signed the covenant and have taken an oath according to the medical law, but to no one else.

I will apply dietetic measures for the benefit of the sick according to my ability and judgment; I will keep them from harm and injustice.

I will neither give a deadly drug to anybody if asked for it nor will I make a suggestion to this effect. Similarly, I will not give to a woman an abortive remedy. In purity and holiness I will guard my life and my art.

I will not use the knife, not even on sufferers from stone, but will withdraw in favor of such men as are engaged in this work.

Whatever houses I may visit, I will come for the benefit of the sick, remaining free of all intentional injustice, of all mischief, and in particular of sexual relations with both female and male persons, be they free or slaves.

© Cengage Learning 2014

Figure 3-3 The Hippocratic Oath.

Table 3-1 Important Persons and Events in the History of Medicine

Moses (1205 BC)	Advocate of health rules in Hebrew religion
1000 BC	Beginnings of ancient Chinese medicine
Hippocrates (460–377 BC)	Greek physician; "father of medicine"
Chang Chung-ching (168–196)	Chinese physician; called the Hippocrates of China
1368–1644	Chinese medicine reaches its peak
Andreas Vesalius (1514–1564)	Brussels physician; wrote first anatomical studies
Anton van Leeuwenhoek (1632–1723)	Dutch lens grinder; discovered lens magnification
John Hunter (1728–1793)	Founder of scientific surgery
Edward Jenner (1749–1823)	Developed smallpox vaccine
Rene Laennec (1781–1826)	Invented the stethoscope
Samuel Hahnemann (1755–1843)	German physician; established homeopathy
Ignaz Semmelweis (1818–1865)	Introduced hand washing to prevent childbed fever
W. T. G. Morton (1819–1868)	U.S. physician; introduced ether as anesthetic
Louis Pasteur (1822–1895)	"Father of bacteriology"
Florence Nightingale (1820–1910)	Founder of modern nursing
Elizabeth Blackwell (1821–1910)	First female physician in the United States
Clara Barton (1821–1912)	Started the American Red Cross in 1881
Joseph Lister (1827–1912)	Laid the groundwork on asepsis
Andrew Taylor (1828–1917)	Established the first school of osteopathy in 1892
Daniel David Palmer (1845–1913)	Founded chiropractic profession in Iowa in 1895
Elizabeth G. Anderson (1836–1917)	First female physician in Great Britain
Frederick G. Banting (1891–1941)	Isolated and injected insulin for diabetes treatment in 1922
1903	First electrocardiogram machine invented
Robert Koch (1843–1910)	Bacteriologist; developed culture-plate method
Wilhelm Roentgen (1845–1923)	Discovered X-rays (roentgenograms)
George Papanicolaou (1883–1962)	Discovered cancer cells in 1928
Sir Alexander Fleming (1881–1955)	Discovered penicillin in 1928
Albert Schatz (1920–2005)	Discovered streptomycin in 1943; cure for tuberculosis
1945	Penicillin brought into production

continues

Table 3-1   Important Persons and Events in the History of Medicine (*Continued*)

Paul Zoll (1911–1999)	Created the first heart pacemaker in 1952
C. Walton Lillehei (1918–1999)	Performed first successful open-heart surgery in 1952
John Gibbon (1903–1973)	First heart–lung machine used for surgery (1953)
Joseph Murray (1919–)	Performed first person-to-person kidney transplant in 1954
Christian Barnard (1922–2001)	Performed first human heart transplant in 1967
Ian Wilmut (1944–)	Cloned a Finn Dorset sheep called Dolly in 1996
1953	Three-dimensional structure of DNA discovered First human heart–lung bypass machine used on human
1950–1960	Vaccines against polio, measles, and rubella developed
1978	First baby born from in vitro fertilization
1982	Hepatitis B vaccine available
1990–2000	Human genome map created by team of scientists
1991	Women's Health Initiative begins 15-year research on cardiovascular disease, cancer, and osteoporosis
1995	Varicella (chickenpox) and hepatitis A vaccines available
2005	Combination vaccine for measles-mumps-rubella and varicella (MMRV) available
2006	Vaccine for adult shingles approved
2007	Diabetics using stem-cell therapy stop taking insulin Minimally invasive procedures performed • Surgeons at University of California/San Diego Medical Center remove diseased gallbladder through vagina • Surgeons at University of Texas Southwestern Medical Center remove diseased kidney through belly button
2009	H1N1 influenza pandemic thwarted
2010	A new pattern of resistance emerges among gram-negative bacteria that threatens to make common infections untreatable; the most resistant genes are NDM-1 and KPC.
2011	Once again, pertussis (whooping cough) becomes an epidemic in some states
2012	Obesity among youth poses threat of type 2 diabetes

© Cengage Learning 2014

to much better diagnoses is now available. Where exploratory surgery might have been performed in the past to determine a diagnosis, today noninvasive ultrasounds, CT scans, and MRIs assist in diagnosis. A 64-slice cardiac CT scan developed in 2004 can capture images of a human heart in just five heartbeats. In a technique known as volume computed tomography (VCT), the VCT system can perform a whole-body trauma scan in less than 10 seconds. People who have worn glasses or contact lenses for many years are turning to laser eye surgery and implantable lenses.

Surgeons have performed the first successful human larynx transplant. Consider the implications of the AIDS saliva test that creates a needle-free way to test for HIV. Needleless injections are now possible. There is a flu prevention inhaler and an osteoporosis pill.

Since 2000 there has been successful use of adult stem cells in the treatment of some diseases. Adult bone marrow stem cells are able to produce multiple tissues, and adult stem cells from various organs of the body have shown amazing abilities to develop into healthy tissue. Adult stem cells can be stimulated to form insulin-secreting pancreatic cells, to repair eye retinal damage, and to stimulate growth in children with bone disease. There is the possibility that adult stem cells will also be able to treat Parkinson's disease and other degenerative neural disorders. In the meantime, the political debate continues over the use of human embryonic stem cells.

A smooth plastic capsule with a tiny camera at each end, known as the PillCam ESO, is able to take as many as 2,600 pictures of the esophagus in less than 20 minutes. This marvel makes it easier to diagnose diseases of the esophagus without sedating a patient as is normally done in traditional endoscopy. Scientists are developing spider silk for extraordinarily fine sutures to be used in nerves and eyes. The combination of the all-encompassing broadband technology and new cellular infrastructure makes it easier for health professionals to stay in touch with patients. Medical Bluetooth (see Chapter 11) makes an easy path for connection of medical devices. For example, remote heart-care diagnostics can be transmitted from a cell phone to providers who can determine if a patient needs to travel to the clinic for further care. Computer chips are being used to create bionic eyes for patients with advanced retinal degeneration, with implanted image sensors taking over the functions of damaged retinal cells.

A new artificial cornea developed by scientists in Sweden, Canada, and California could save the sight of millions of people worldwide. The new cornea, made from artificial collagen, is transplanted into the eye and encourages damaged cells to regenerate and colonize new tissue.

Experimentation with aromatherapy indicates that some aromas actually improve brain function. Research has shown that individuals suffering from dementia often respond favorably to the odor of freshly roasted coffee and bread baking. Inhaling the scents of green apple, banana, and peppermint stimulates positive feelings. It is thought that with aromatherapy we will soon accelerate learning and speed up rehabilitation for people who have had a stroke.

The *British Journal of Psychiatry* recently reported that music therapy can be of value in individuals with schizophrenic illnesses. There also is evidence that music therapy can help to:

- Relieve treatment-related distress in individuals with cancer
- Calm individuals undergoing cardiac catheterization procedures
- Provide pain relief
- Decrease apathy in people with dementia

The American Music Therapy Association notes that extensive use of specifically chosen music during massage, acupuncture, yoga, and t'ai chi ch'uan enhances each type of practice. Some surgeons report better concentration and more relaxed patients when certain music is played during surgery.

Who can possibly predict what the future will bring in medicine?

CASE STUDY 3-1

Refer to the scenario at the beginning of the chapter and recall two or three medical treatments or practices used in your family and culture.

CASE STUDY REVIEW

1. Were these medical treatments helpful? If so, how?
2. Is any part of these treatments still used today? If so, describe.
3. Discuss this case study with a friend or classmate.

CASE STUDY 3-2

You are a male practitioner on call in your hospital's emergency department when a woman, 5 months pregnant, is brought in. She is hemorrhaging. Her husband shuns you and requests a female practitioner. You quickly realize this couple is Muslim. Role-play a solution to this scenario with a classmate.

CASE STUDY REVIEW

1. How can you solve the dilemma?
2. Consider the possibility that your only female practitioner is out of the country on vacation.

CASE STUDY 3-3

Your employer, Dr. Anne Shea, an internist in Southern California, is considering renting office space to an acupuncturist and a naturopath because many of her patients often seek treatment from both. Dr. Shea believes her practice can be integrated, therefore allowing patients one-stop treatment for their illnesses. As the CMA (AAMA) and clinic manager, you are asked to participate in a meeting of all three practitioners to discuss guidelines for the clinic.

CASE STUDY REVIEW

1. What questions will you ask the group?
2. What will be necessary to get the word out to patients?

SUMMARY

Medicine's history leaves us with a rich heritage and a sound basis for the future of health care. Medical history continues to be in the making today. For example, research in gene manipulation has the potential benefit of being able to reverse the progression of many debilitating diseases. One day we will look on the medical discoveries of this decade and be impressed by how much further medicine has advanced.

STUDY FOR SUCCESS

To reinforce your knowledge and skills of information presented in this chapter:

- Review the *Key Terms*
- Role-play with other students to apply attributes of professionalism pertinent to this chapter.
- Consider the *Case Studies* and discuss your conclusions
- Answer the questions in the *Certification Review*
- Apply your knowledge by completing the *Activities* in the *Study Guide* and the *Games and Quizzes* in the StudyWARE **StudyWARE** software on the *Premium Website*
- Practice your problem-solving skills with the *Critical Thinking Challenge 3.0* on the *Premium Website*

Additional resources for this chapter include:

- *CourseMate for Delmar's Comprehensive Medical Assisting*
- *WebTutor for Delmar's Comprehensive Medical Assisting*

CERTIFICATION REVIEW

1. A pharmacopoeia is:
   a. a book describing drugs and their preparation
   b. an ancient religious rite used in medicine
   c. a source of magic
   d. used only by twentieth-century physicians
2. At one time, women were typically allowed to use their health care skills to:
   a. cure everyone in society
   b. care only for women and to assist in childbirth
   c. become physicians
   d. care only for older adults
3. An accurate sketch of the spinal vertebrae was created during the Renaissance by:
   a. Leonardo da Vinci
   b. Michelangelo
   c. early Christian monks
   d. Louis Pasteur
4. Hippocrates is a Greek physician often called:
   a. the founder of scientific surgery
   b. the inventor of the smallpox vaccine
   c. the father of medicine
   d. the father of preventive medicine
5. The first woman physician in the United States was:
   a. Florence Nightingale
   b. Clara Barton
   c. Elizabeth Anderson
   d. Elizabeth Blackwell
6. The physician who introduced hand washing to prevent childbed fever was:
   a. Joseph Lister
   b. John Hunter
   c. Ignaz Semmelweis
   d. Edward Jenner
7. Medicine was greatly influenced by:
   a. Greek and Chinese physicians
   b. Culture and science
   c. Religion and magic
   d. b and c
8. Paralytic poliomyelitis
   a. was first evidenced during the summer of 1890
   b. is cured by childhood vaccinations
   c. caused great fear in the U.S. during the 1970s
   d. has been eradicated from the world
9. Cancer
   a. metastasis was first understood in the nineteenth century
   b. is only treated with chemotherapy
   c. deaths will total 1.5 million per year
   d. is the result of an inherited tendency
10. HIV/AIDS:
    a. was first known in the Bronze Age
    b. is decreasing in the U.S. but rages on in other parts of the world
    c. only infects gay men
    d. is caused by a bacterium transmitted through bodily fluids

REFERENCES/BIBLIOGRAPHY

American Cancer Society. (2011). *Surveillance research.* Retrieved August 9, 2011, from http://www.cancer.org/Research/index

American Medical Association. (2010). *Women in medicine.* Retrieved August 1, 2011, from http://www.ama-assn.org/go/wpc

Centers for Disease Control and Prevention (CDC). Ten Great Public Health Achievements–Worldwide, 2001–2010. *MMWR Weekly 60*(19), 587. Retrieved August 8, 2011 from www.cdc.gov/mmwr/preview/mmwrhtml/mm6019a5.htm

Lewis, M. A., Tamparo, C. D. & Tatro, B. (2012). *Medical law, ethics, and bioethics for health professions* (7th ed.). Philadelphia: F. A. Davis.

Lyons, A. S., & Petrucelli II, J. R. (1978). *Medicine: An illustrated history.* New York: Harry N. Abrams.

Mayo Clinic. (2010, May 29). *MRSA Infection.* Retrieved August 3, 2011, at http://www.mayoclinic.com/health/mrsa/DS00735/

Polio Global Eradication Imitative. (2012, May 2). *Polio This Week.* Retrieved May 6, 2012, from http://www.polioeradication.org/Dataandmonitoring/Poliothisweek.aspx

Until There's a Cure. (2009). *Learn the Facts.* Retrieved October 15, 2012, from https://until.org/learn-the-facts/

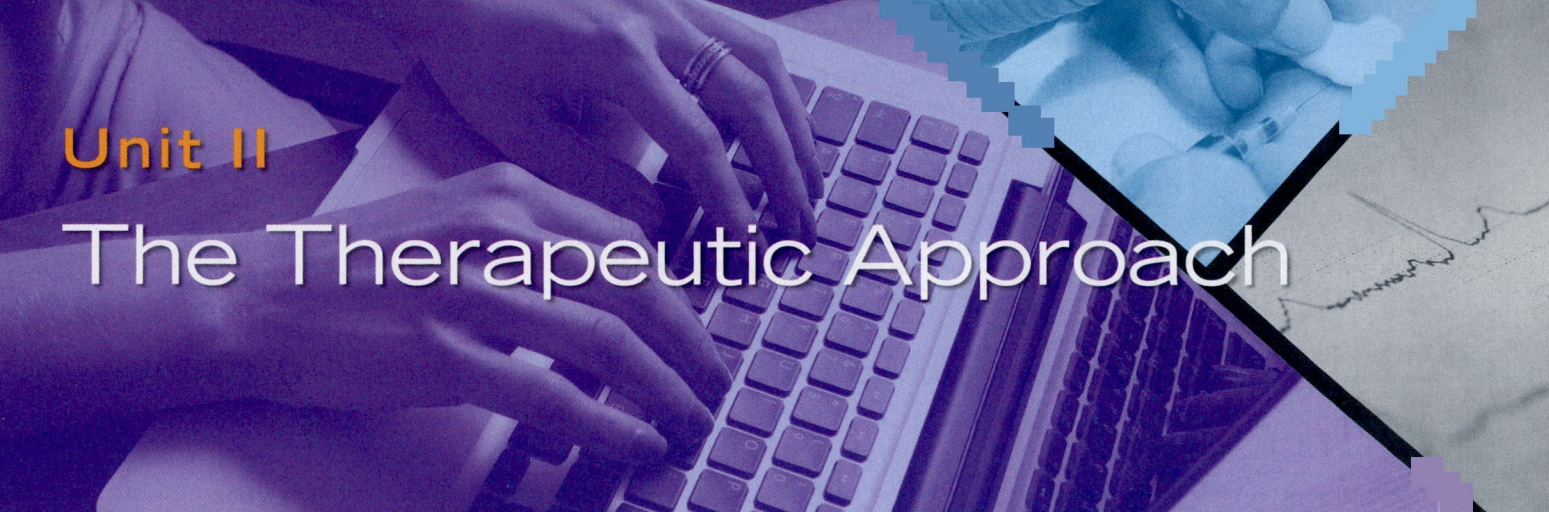

Unit II
The Therapeutic Approach

CHAPTER 4
Coping Skills for the Medical Assistant 56

CHAPTER 5
Therapeutic Communication Skills 68

CHAPTER 6
The Therapeutic Approach to the Patient
with a Life-Threatening Illness 92

Coping Skills for the Medical Assistant

OUTLINE

What Is Stress?
The Body's Response to Stress

Factors Causing Stress
Stress in the Work
Environment

Effect of Prolonged
Stress—Burnout
Persons Most Vulnerable to
Burnout

General Stress Management
Techniques

Goal Setting as a Stress Reliever

LEARNING OUTCOMES

1. Define, spell, and pronounce the key terms as presented in the glossary.
2. Analyze the difference between stress and stressors.
3. Describe the three categories of stressors.
4. Discuss Hans Selye's General Adaptation Syndrome (GAS) theory.
5. Differentiate between short-duration and long-duration stress.
6. Describe the body's response to stress as reflected by the sympathetic and parasympathetic nervous systems.
7. Analyze stress in the work environment and discuss ways to eliminate or cope with it.
8. Model ways a positive attitude may reduce the level and duration of stress.
9. Discuss physical illnesses and psychological symptoms of stress on the body.
10. Describe characteristics of prolonged stress.
11. Describe the four stages of burnout.
12. Identify persons most vulnerable to burnout.
13. Discuss general stress management techniques and identify three that you will implement into your lifestyle.
14. Differentiate between long-range and short-range goals.
15. Analyze the professionalism questions and apply them to this chapter's content.

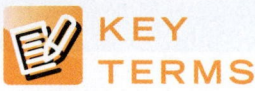

KEY TERMS

burnout
goal
inner-directed people
long-range goals
outer-directed people
parasympathetic
  nervous system
self-actualization
short-range goals
stress
stressors
sympathetic
  nervous system

ATTRIBUTES OF PROFESSIONALISM

Communication
- Did you provide appropriate responses/feedback?
- Did you display appropriate body language?

Presentation
- Did you display a calm, professional, and caring manner?

Competency
- Did you display sound judgment?
- Did you remain calm in a crisis?
- Do you recognize the effect of stress on all persons involved in emergency situations?

Initiative
- Did you show initiative?
- Were you flexible and dependable?
- Were you respectful of others?
- Did you assist coworkers when appropriate?

Integrity
- Did you work within your scope of practice?
- Did you maintain your moral and ethical standards?

SCENARIO

At the clinic of providers Lewis and King, there are four full-time medical assistants who collaborate to make the clinic run smoothly, both administratively and clinically. One day a month, though, clinic manager Marilyn Johnson, CMA (AAMA), is out of town, leaving Ellen Armstrong, CMA (AAMA), the administrative medical assistant, in charge of a busy reception area and an ever-ringing telephone.

On these days, Ellen is particularly careful to organize her work so that things run as they should. Although Ellen cannot anticipate every emergency, she does try to influence the situation rather than let events control her.

INTRODUCTION

Even in the most well-managed ambulatory care setting, medical assistants and other health providers are likely to feel the effects of stress from time to time. They may be overworked on certain days, they may face difficult patient situations, and they may find that the administrative and paperwork load is getting ahead of them.

This chapter helps today's busy, multifaceted medical assistant pinpoint the symptoms of stress and provides ideas for coping with stress as it occurs. The better equipped the medical assistant is to confront and solve the sources of stress, the less likely stressors will become so overwhelming as to lead to burnout on the job. Goal setting, recognizing one's limitations and potentials, setting priorities, and keeping a balanced perspective can work together to reduce stress and enable the medical assistant to take pleasure in working with patients and colleagues.

WHAT IS STRESS?

The body's response to mental and physical change is termed **stress**. Walter Cannon, a neurologist, is credited with first determining that both emotional and physical events act as stressors and that the body reacts in a similar way to either type of event. What constitutes stress is highly individual and depends to a great extent on personality type. Events that may be stressful to one person may be enjoyable to another. A delayed airplane flight may be very stressful to a person who worries about making another connection or missing a meeting. Another person will simply look for an alternative flight or notify the people that he or she was to meet and then take the time to enjoy a good book, experiencing little or no mental or physical change. Stress is neither good nor bad. The key is to learn how to manage stress so that it works for you rather than against you.

Adaptive behavior patterns we assume in response to real physical threats or emotional effects result in either eustress (positive feelings) or distress (negative feelings). Moving to a new city or receiving a promotion usually are perceived as positive events, whereas going through a divorce or losing a job are, conversely, perceived as negative events; however, each of these events can result in inducing stress in the body. These events are called **stressors**. Stressors can be divided into three categories:

1. *Frustrations.* Circumstances that prevent us from doing what we want to do
2. *Conflicts.* Incompatibility between two important things or objectives equally important to us
3. *Pressure.* Demands of schedule, workload, or expectations placed on us by ourselves or others

Complete the "How Stressed Are You????" exercise in Chapter 4 of the Study Guide to help assess your current stress level.

According to Hans Selye, who first conceived the theory of nonspecific reaction as stress, which is the body's response to any demand or stressor, the body does not differentiate between positively and negatively induced stress. It is only the level of the stress and its duration that affect the body. Short-duration stress, sometimes called *acute stress*, can be beneficial. Short-duration stress adds anticipation and a feeling of "being alive." For example, when we experience a roller coaster ride or bungee jump off a cliff, we experience acute stress. The short-lived adrenaline rush brings the world into sharper focus and enhances our lives. It helps us focus on details, achieve difficult goals, and perform at our best.

When we have a last-minute rush in the clinic or are hurrying to get an assignment finished for school, we are experiencing short-duration stress. Short-duration stress is experienced when the telephone rings, the examination rooms are full, and the provider is called to the hospital on an emergency. Immediately, the body's stress mode is activated and adrenaline is produced, enabling you to make quick judgments and decisions, to be organized and efficient, and to accomplish tasks within minimal time limits.

Longer-duration stress is sometimes called *episodic* or *chronic stress*. Examples of episodic stress include taking on too many projects or needlessly worrying. Chronic stress is the result of events over which we have little control, such as long-term unemployment, dysfunctional relationships, or chronic illness. Longer duration stress, normally associated with negative events, can be harmful to the body, resulting in illnesses such as headaches, insomnia, allergies, cancer, acute indigestion, stomach ulcers, hypertension, blood clots, stroke, and immune system disorders. Psychologically, the body also is influenced by long-duration stress. Onsets of depression and anxiety, as well as eating problems resulting in weight loss or gain, are associated with the body's psychological response to stress. Anorexia and bulimia are common eating disorders attributed to long-duration stressful events. Long-duration stress can also affect our ability to think clearly, and objectivity may be impaired. Physical symptoms of these emotional effects include cigarette smoking, obesity, and lack of interest in or excessive sexual activity.

The Body's Response to Stress

The body's response to stress goes back to early human development. That response was designed to help humans survive whatever they were experiencing that caused a fearful response. The **sympathetic nervous system** prepared the body for "fight or flight" to allow humans the best chance of survival. The brain inhibits short-term memory, promotes long-term memory, and releases hormones such as adrenaline into the bloodstream. The respiration rate becomes more rapid, blood flow increases, red and white blood cells are released by the spleen, and the immune system is altered to allow immune-boosting antibodies to be sent to the body. Blood vessels in the skin contract to minimize blood loss from wounds, blood vessels in the muscles dilate to increase circulation, and

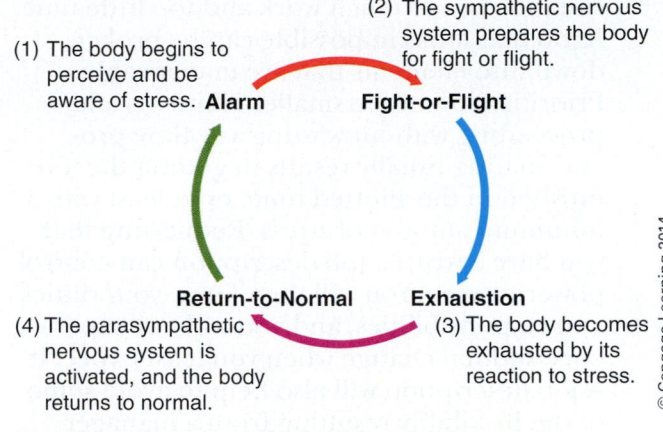

Figure 4-1 Hans Selye's General Adaptation Syndrome (GAS) theory proposes that four stages are involved in adapting to stress.

fluids are diverted from nonessential locations; the metabolism rate is diminished to permit all available energy to be focused on the event that triggered the fight-or-flight response.

All of these caveman responses to stress are with us today. The symptoms of headache, stomachache, diarrhea, cold clammy hands, heart palpitations, indigestion, and short-term memory loss that we experience are the result of our body's reaction to stressors that has been developed over millennia. Short term, these responses are not harmful, and the body's **parasympathetic nervous system** returns the body to normal after the stressor has been removed. Long term, these responses are harmful to the body. See Figure 4-1 for an illustration of the adaptive stages related to stress.

FACTORS CAUSING STRESS

Stress cannot be prevented; in fact, life would be dull without short-duration stress. Anticipating the birth of a child, planning an upcoming wedding, or graduating from school are all stressful changes, albeit pleasant ones, that make life interesting. Long-duration stressful situations are not desirable, but the situations leading to them can be managed if we understand the causes. Some causes of stress are:

- *Overwhelming situations.* Inability to control expectations, workload, and duties; feelings of frustration; and panic because of schedules can all result in feelings of powerlessness and not knowing where to start. Planning and prioritization can help to prevent panic and reduce stress when faced with the inevitable situation of too much work and too little time. A job that looks impossible can be broken down into elements that are manageable. Prioritization of the smaller elements and proceeding without wasting any time procrastinating usually results in getting the job finished in the allotted time, or at least with a minimum amount of stress. Requesting that you have a written job description can control powerlessness. You will then know your duties and responsibilities, and you will not experience sudden change when you least expect it. A job description will also help to avoid some of the instability resulting from a manager who is too sanguine or manages from one crisis to another. If you know what your job entails, you can anticipate the events and take action to prevent a crisis.

- *Round peg in square hole.* Not being emotionally suited or qualified for the position you hold. The only solution for this situation is changing jobs or obtaining training to become qualified for the requirements of the present job. A medical assistant can find himself or herself in emotional stress if the provider asks them to do tasks that they are not allowed to perform under the scope of their education and training. An example of this could be a medical assistant working for a provider who does outpatient surgery and expects the medical assistant to suture the incision after he or she has completed the major part of the procedure.

- *Traumatic events on the job.* Not being emotionally prepared for trauma involved in the job. Not every medical assistant would experience this type of situation, requiring a change in emotional sensitivity. A medical assistant finding himself or herself in this position could be proactive and seek a move from the clinical to administrative duties or take steps to obtain another position having fewer traumatic events.

Stress in the Work Environment

Stress in the work environment may come from many different conditions, some of which you may control by making a few accommodations to resolve the stress. Conditions that cannot be changed may need to be accepted as a part of the job. Examples of work environment conditions that may cause stress include the following, but are not limited to these mentioned.

 Physical Environment. Physical conditions such as noise, lighting, or some other types of stressors are frequently within the control of the worker. Earplugs could be used to combat annoying noise, additional lighting could be added or light shields could be used as suits the situation, and dressing in layers to accommodate temperature changes could mitigate the "too cold" stressor. The main point is not to sit back and become upset about situations over which you have some control. Take proactive steps to alleviate the stress-causing condition.

 Management Style. Your manager's management style may cause uproar or instability in work demands. Talking to the manager might affect the situation, but it is highly unlikely. Obtaining a detailed job description; being able to say "no"; and utilizing goal-setting techniques, as discussed later in this chapter, are the best ways to reduce stress from this cause.

 Difficult Coworkers. Difficult people are all around us; in fact, you may be one to someone else. Maintaining a good interpersonal relationship with fellow employees is important to achieving a satisfying work experience and has a remarkable effect in reducing the problem of difficult people. Before a strong interpersonal relationship is established with others, a positive self-attitude is needed. The choices we make affect our positive attitude. Making positive decisions will affect the work environment, and hence the level and duration of stress experienced. Following are some choices we all make in our lives:

- To be respectful of others
- To be a diligent worker
- To be willing to learn
- To be honest
- To be willing to assume responsibility for one's actions
- To express appropriate humor
- To have an attitude of humility
- To be goal directed
- To understand Maslow's hierarchy of needs (see Chapter 5 for information related to Maslow's hierarchy of needs)

If you do all these things and still have difficult people in your work environment, develop a plan and take steps to have the least contact possible with that person. Taking proactive steps will in itself reduce stress.

Failure to Meet Needs. Certain job conditions do not permit achievement of Maslow's needs. Failure to meet our needs results in frustration, lack of job satisfaction, and ultimately burnout. Failure to meet needs can result from low salary, little opportunity for career growth, and discrimination in opportunities available and perceived distribution of assignments.

Job Instability. Job instability is an example of a stressor capable of causing worry. Worry is excessive concern about situations over which we have no direct control. Ensuring job stability is not directly within the medical assistant's control, but the medical assistant can be proactive in developing an employment plan and working toward its implementation. Taking these proactive steps to alleviate a potentially difficult situation over which you have no direct control will reduce worry and stress.

Technological Changes. Change, even good change, can cause stress. Implementation of a total practice management system (see Chapter 11) into a medical facility is an excellent example of an event that will result in stress for almost all employees; they are divorcing themselves from the familiar and being asked to embrace the unknown. The resulting level and duration of stress would be dependent on the comfort level of each individual with computer technology. For some older employees it may create stress until they retire. The best way to avoid stress from technological change is to remain current with the tools of your profession through continued education programs.

Organization Size. Working in a large organization may lead to less understanding of the total job picture by the worker, resulting in less predictability and less control of the job to which the employee is assigned. This frequently results in feeling overwhelmed and frustrated. As the formalization and centralization of an organization increase, the stress experienced by an employee also increases. Downward delegation by management is the best approach to minimizing this problem.

Overspecialization. This problem results in the employee never seeing the overall picture and receiving little or no satisfaction from his or her work.

EFFECT OF PROLONGED STRESS—BURNOUT

Long-duration stress, normally associated with negative events, can be harmful to the body and, if the situation persists, results in **burnout**. Burnout is a psychological term for the experience of long-term emotional exhaustion and diminished interest that affects job performance, health-related outcomes, and mental health problems. Burnout has four stages:

- *Honeymoon.* Love your job and have unrealistic expectations placed on you either by your manager or by yourself if you are a perfectionist; take work home and look for all the work you can get; cannot say "no" to accepting additional work.

- *Reality.* Begin to have doubts you can meet expectations; feel frustrated with your progress and work harder to meet expectations; begin to feel pulled in many directions; may not have a role model to follow and guidelines may not be established or defined.

- *Dissatisfaction.* Loss of enthusiasm; try to escape frustrations by binges of one sort or another: drinking, partying, shopping, or excessive eating or sex; fatigue and exhaustion develop.

- *Sad state.* Depression, work seems pointless, lethargic with little energy, consider quitting, and look on yourself as a failure; represents full-blown burnout.

All of these stages are part of the process leading to burnout. The honeymoon stage might seem desirable, and it is pleasant; however, the seeds of the illness are present in the unrealistic expectations and the workaholic attitude of the employee. Unless these causes are eliminated, the progression to full burnout is ensured.

Burnout results in physical illnesses such as headaches, insomnia, allergies, cancer, acute indigestion, stomach ulcers, hypertension, blood clots, stroke, and immune system disorders. Psychologically, the body also is influenced by long-duration stress. Onsets of depression and anxiety, as well as eating problems resulting in weight loss or gain, are associated with the body's psychological response to stress. Anorexia and bulimia are common eating disorders attributed to long-duration stressful events. Long-duration stress can also affect our ability to think clearly, and objectivity may be impaired. Animal studies strongly suggest that maternal stress can also affect a fetus in later life. Physical symptoms of these emotional effects include alcohol abuse, drug abuse, cigarette smoking, obesity, depression, and lack of interest in or excessive sexual activity. A person in danger of burnout may also experience loss of energy and make poor exercise and nutritional choices, leading to a further cycle of medical problems and a more serious burnout condition.

Persons Most Vulnerable to Burnout

People with inadequate social support networks who are poorly nourished, sleep deprived, or physically ill have a reduced capacity to handle the pressures and stressors of everyday life and are at greater risk of burnout. Some stressors are particularly associated with certain age groups or life stages. Persons facing life transitions such as children, adolescents, working parents, and seniors are vulnerable simply because of the increased stress associated with these transitional changes.

Personality type can have a role in susceptibility to burnout. When individuals with a high need to achieve do not reach their goals, they are apt to feel angry and frustrated and become negative toward their job. Failing to recognize these signs as symptoms of burnout, they may throw themselves even more fully into work-related goals. Unless there is some type of revitalization outside of the workplace, burnout occurs. Perfectionists try to do everything equally well without setting priorities; thus fatigue and exhaustion associated with burnout begin to set in after time.

GENERAL STRESS MANAGEMENT TECHNIQUES

  If you recognize that you are stressed, or in one of the stages of burnout, you have reached a turning point. It is imperative that you make some changes in your relationship with your job. The following changes are appropriate and helpful in stress management or once you have entered the burnout stage:

- Make a concerted effort to say "No" when asked to assume additional work. Job scope creep is a leading factor in burnout.

- If you have more work than you can realistically accomplish, either prioritize it with the approval of your superior or delegate it within the limits of your authority.

- Change your work-related environment by creating variations. Modify your work routine slightly, rearrange your workstation to make it more personal, or change the computer desktop picture or screensaver to something you find pleasant that generates positive emotions.

- Evaluate the negative feelings you have regarding your job and attempt to replace them with more positive thoughts (i.e., instead of thinking the glass is half empty, think of the glass as half full).

- Try to look on work as a "fun" experience and an adventure.

- Establish some long- and short-term realistic goals and write them down along with a plan to make them happen.

- Develop strong social support networks by promoting friendships with coworkers; with family; or in outside religious, fraternal, or professional organizations. Occasionally going to lunch together with coworkers to laugh a little will promote a strong office support network and may help with that difficult person in your office life. Social networking using Facebook®, Twitter®, or other online sites can be a stress-reducing tool as long as you remember that all that is put online may be published to the whole world, including current and future employers and coworkers. Do not be insulting and do not burn bridges to future employment or associations. Venting frustrations will reduce stress just as removing the valve from a pressure cooker will reduce pressure, but never vent in any recorded media. Remember that audio and video recorders are on most smartphones, and you do not want to be the next star attraction on YouTube®.

- Embark on a program of relaxation and meditation to reduce stress. Relaxation reduces muscle tension resulting from stress and can be achieved in a few minutes. Meditation requires about 20 minutes each day. Meditation affects body processes such as heart rate, blood pressure, metabolic rate, and brain activity and helps to obtain a feeling of "well-being."

- Start an exercise regime. The stress response prepares us to fight or to flee; our bodies are primed for action. Exercise on a regular basis helps to reduce the production of stress hormones and associated neurochemicals. Studies have found that exercise is a potent antidepressant, anxiolytic (i.e., combats anxiety), and sleeping aid for many people. Punching a bag, pumping iron, or abusing the treadmill is a safe way to vent, and it does not broadcast your feelings to the whole world.

Internal factors that influence your ability to handle stress include your nutritional status, overall health and fitness levels, and emotional well-being. The amount of sleep and rest you get can determine your body's ability to respond to, and deal with, external stress-inducing factors.

CRITICAL THINKING

Self-Evaluation

- List several situations in your life that are stressful. Select the one that is most stressful.
- List as many things as possible about the situation that make it stressful to you.
- How would you change each of the things you have listed to make them less stressful?
- List the things you "could do" to effect the changes you listed.
- Rank the items in your "could do" list in terms of achievability.
- Select one or two of the items that are achievable and discuss them with a classmate. Now attempt to put them into practice for a week. Report back to your classmate on how effective these items were in reducing stress in your life.

GOAL SETTING AS A STRESS RELIEVER

 Do you direct your life, or do you allow others to influence and make decisions for you? **Outer-directed people** let events, other people, or environmental factors dictate their behavior. By contrast, **inner-directed people** decide for themselves what they want to do with their lives. Laurence Peter, author of *The Peter Principle*, states, "If you don't know where you are going, you will end up somewhere else" (Wilkes & Crosswait, 1995).

Studies prove that goal-oriented employees are more effective and assertive than are colleagues with no goals or future objectives. Recognizing the value of goal planning, many employers arrange planning sessions or seminars to encourage goal setting as a practical application for coping with stress and burnout and to develop career objectives. If your employer does not offer these outlets, seek your own seminars for goal setting. Such an activity not only "centers" you in your current employment, but also helps you clearly picture your future plans and hopes.

What is a **goal**? According to *Merriam-Webster's Collegiate Dictionary*, a goal is "the result or achievement toward which effort is directed." To reach a desired goal, a person must implement planning supported by a sincere desire to work hard. Skill in goal setting allows the medical assistant to clarify what must be accomplished and to develop a strategic plan to successfully achieve that goal.

A goal must be specific, challenging, realistic, attainable, and measurable. Specific goals are focused and have precise boundaries. A goal that is challenging creates enthusiasm and interest in achievement. Realistic goals are practical or beneficial both for the present and for future **self-actualization**. An attainable goal refers to the fact that the goal is possible to fulfill. Measurable goals achieve some form of progress or success. By reflecting on the process, one is encouraged to establish additional goals.

Long-range goals are achievements that may take three to five years to accomplish. Long-range goals give direction and definition to our lives and serve to keep us "on track," so to speak. Much discipline, perseverance, determination, and hard work will be expended in accomplishing long-range goals. Some adjustment and readjustment to your goals may be necessary, however. The rewards of goal achievement include satisfaction, pride, a sense of accomplishment, and a job well done.

Short-range goals take apart long-range goals and reassemble the required activities into smaller, more manageable time segments. The time segments may be daily, weekly, monthly, quarterly, or yearly periods.

As a graduate and new employee, one of your long-range goals might be to become the clinic manager in the ambulatory care setting in which you are currently employed. You may wish to attain this goal within the next three to five years; by breaking it into three longer range goals and a series of short-range goals, you will be able to measure progress and feel a sense of accomplishment. Examples of long- and short-range goals might include:

Long-range goal 1:
- To become proficient in all clinical skills during the first year of employment.

Short-range goals necessary to achieve this:
- Practice accuracy and proficiency when performing tasks and skills.
- Practice efficiency by planning ahead for the equipment and supplies needed for each task performed.
- Evaluate your progress on a regular basis, and identify areas that need improvement.

Long-range goal 2:
- To add administrative tasks and skills to your routine during the second year of employment.

Short-range goals necessary to achieve this:
- Practice accuracy and proficiency when performing all administrative tasks and skills.
- Practice efficiency by planning ahead for the equipment and supplies needed for each task performed.
- Evaluate your progress on a regular basis, and identify areas that need improvement.

Long-range goal 3:
- To begin to focus on clinic management during the third year of employment.

Short-range goals necessary to achieve this:
- Develop a procedure manual for all clinical and administrative tasks and skills.
- Enroll in clinic management classes.
- Focus on team-building skills.

By the fourth year, you will be ready to move into the clinic manager position.

Long- and short-range goals work together to help make changes in our lives. Goals keep life interesting and give us something for which to strive. We can all reach goals successfully with some planning, hard work, discipline, and dedication.

CASE STUDY 4-1

Refer to the scenario at the beginning of the chapter.

CASE STUDY REVIEW

1. What work can Ellen Armstrong, CMA (AAMA), organize the night before the clinic manager is out of town, leaving Ellen in charge of the reception area and the ever-ringing telephone the next day?

2. How might Ellen relieve stress as the hectic day progresses?

CASE STUDY 4-2

Ellen Armstrong, CMA (AAMA), has been employed for five years as an administrative medical assistant with providers Lewis and King. Ellen is a perfectionist and has pushed herself to achieve many of her short- and long-term goals. The clinic staff has become aware that Ellen does not have a sense of humor lately. She seems frustrated and irritable, and she is becoming critical of herself and others. Ellen has felt physically and emotionally exhausted, yet she continues to focus on her high standard of job performance; however, work is becoming a chore. At the end of the day, if everything has not been completed to her satisfaction, she feels like a failure.

CASE STUDY REVIEW

1. Do you feel Ellen is stressed or experiencing burnout? On what do you base your conclusions?

2. What might Ellen do to differentiate these two conditions?

3. What changes might Ellen implement to resolve this problem?

SUMMARY

Stress is very much a part of the medical profession. Each individual working in a medical career experiences consecutive days of demanding, emotionally and physically draining interactions with patients and staff members. This highly technical and ever-changing career requires its professionals to maintain a high level of skill and training and to be familiar with the newest technology.

Goal setting is one approach to reducing stress and burnout and promoting a sense of pride in the workplace, self-actualization, and possible employment promotion. Both long-range and short-range goal planning work together to help make changes in our lives.

STUDY FOR SUCCESS

To reinforce your knowledge and skills of information presented in this chapter:

- Review the *Key Terms*
- Role-play with other students to apply attributes of professionalism pertinent to this chapter.
- Consider the *Case Studies* and discuss your conclusions
- Answer the questions in the *Certification Review*
- Apply your knowledge by completing the *Activities* in the *Study Guide* and the *Games and Quizzes* in the StudyWARE (StudyWARE) software on the *Premium Website*
- Practice your problem-solving skills with the *Critical Thinking Challenge 3.0* on the *Premium Website*

Additional resources for this chapter include:

- *CourseMate for Delmar's Comprehensive Medical Assisting*
- *WebTutor for Delmar's Comprehensive Medical Assisting*

CERTIFICATION REVIEW

1. Which answer is *not* true about stress?
   a. It does not occur suddenly.
   b. It has physical and emotional effects on the body.
   c. It may be positive or negative in its effects on the body.
   d. It is the body's response to change.

2. Hans Selye's General Adaptation Syndrome theory proposes that adaptation to stress occurs in how many stages?
   a. 2 stages
   b. 3 stages
   c. 4 stages
   d. 5 stages

3. Which is *not* a stage in the General Adaptation Syndrome?
   a. Fight-or-flight
   b. Exhaustion
   c. Burnout
   d. Alarm

4. The four stages of prolonged stress–burnout are:
   a. honeymoon, reality, dissatisfaction, sad state
   b. honeymoon, frustrations, conflicts, pressures
   c. honeymoon, reality, conflicts, pressures
   d. honeymoon, dissatisfactions, frustrations, pressures

5. Signs and symptoms of burnout include all of the following *except:*
   a. emotional and physical exhaustion
   b. hair-trigger display of emotion
   c. feelings of accomplishment and pride in work
   d. irritability and impatience

6. Long-range goals are easy to achieve if:
   a. they are not too challenging
   b. they are divided into a series of short-range goals
   c. they don't involve too much hard work
   d. you never change or adjust them

7. The GAS theory proposes which order for its stages:
   a. fight-or-flight, alarm, exhaustion, return-to-normal
   b. exhaustion, alarm, fight-or-flight, return-to-normal
   c. exhaustion, fight-or-flight, alarm, return-to-normal
   d. alarm, fight-or-flight, exhaustion, return-to-normal

8. Stressors can be divided into which three categories:
   a. frustrations, conflicts, pressure
   b. pressure, anxiety, depression
   c. conflicts, resolution, burnout
   d. frustrations, conflicts, burnout

9. Which of the following is *not* true of the sympathetic nervous system:
   a. Returns the body to normal after the stressor has been removed
   b. Prepares the body for fight-or-flight
   c. Allows humans the best chance of survival
   d. Releases hormones into the bloodstream

10. Signs and symptoms of burnout may include all of the following *except*:
   a. anger
   b. frustration
   c. negativity
   d. experience self-actualization

REFERENCES/BIBLIOGRAPHY

Geil, T. M., Phd. *How Stressed Are You????* PowerPoint Presentation. Retrieved from www.edu/vpsa/nakama/documents/toi_Geil_TalkNakamaWeb.PDF

Keir, L., Wise, B. A., Krebs, C., & Kelly-Arnex, C. (2008). *Medical assisting: Administrative and clinical competencies* (6th ed.). Clifton Park, NY: Delmar Cengage Learning.

Merriam-Webster's collegiate dictionary (11th ed.). (1998). Springfield, MA: Merriam-Webster.

Milliken, M. E., & Honeycutt, A. (2004). *Understanding human behavior: A guide for health care providers.* Clifton Park, NY: Delmar Cengage Learning.

Stoppler, M. C., MD. *Stress.* Retrieved May 13, 2011, from www.medicinenet.com/stress/article.htm

Tamparo, C. D., & Lindh, W. Q. (2008). *Therapeutic communications for health care.* Clifton Park, NY: Delmar Cengage Learning.

Tetrick, L. E., (1998) Organizational Structure. In J. M. Stellman (Ed.), *Encyclopedia of Occupational Health & Safety* (4th Ed., Vol. I, P. 1990). Geneva: International Labour Office.

Understanding Stress. Retrieved May 13, 2011, from www.helpguide.org/mental/stress.htm

What you need to know about stress management. (2004). Retrieved February 27, 2008, from stress.about.com

Wilkes, M., & Crosswait, C. B. (1995). *Professional development: The dynamics of success.* San Diego: Harcourt Brace Jovanovich.

OUTLINE

Importance of Communication

The Communication Cycle
  The Sender
  The Message
  The Receiver
  Feedback
  Listening Skills

Types of Communication
  Verbal Communication
  Nonverbal Communication
  Congruency in Communication

Factors Affecting Therapeutic Communication
  Age Barriers

Economic Barriers

Education and Life Experience Barriers

Bias and Prejudice Barriers

Verbal Roadblocks to Therapeutic Communication

Defense Mechanisms as Barriers

Barriers Caused by Cultural and Religious Diversity

Human Needs as Barriers to Therapeutic Communication

Maslow's Hierarchy of Needs

Patients with Special Needs

Environmental Factors

Time Factors

Establishing Multicultural Communication
  Cultural Brokering

Therapeutic Communication in Action
  Interview Techniques
  Point of Care Techniques

Community Resources

LEARNING OUTCOMES

1. Define, spell, and pronounce the key terms as presented in the glossary.

2. Identify the importance of communication.

3. List and define the four basic elements of the communication cycle.

4. Identify the four modes or channels of communication most pertinent in our everyday exchange.

5. Model the importance of active listening in therapeutic communication.

6. Recognize differences between the terms *verbal* and *nonverbal communication*.

7. Analyze the five Cs of communication and describe their effectiveness in the communication cycle.

8. Demonstrate the following body language or nonverbal communication behaviors: facial expressions, personal space, position, posture, gestures/mannerisms, and touch.

9. Identify and explain congruency in communication.

10. Differentiate between low-context and high-context communication styles.

11. Discuss Table 5-3 and generalizations of cultural/religious effects on health care.

12. Discuss the use of Maslow's hierarchy of needs in therapeutic communication.

13. Demonstrate respect for individual diversity, incorporating awareness of one's own biases in areas including gender, race, religion, age, and economic status.

14. Recall at least three steps to building trust with culturally diverse patients.

15. Discuss cultural brokering and its use in medical facilities.

16. Recognize eight significant roadblocks or barriers to therapeutic communication.

17. Discuss common defense mechanisms.

18. Compare/contrast closed questions, open-ended questions, and indirect statements.

19. Differentiate between adaptive and nonadaptive coping mechanisms.

20. Analyze the professionalism questions and apply them to this chapter's content.

KEY TERMS

active listening
bias
body language
closed questions
clustering
compensation
congruency
cultural brokering
culture
decode
defense mechanism
denial
displacement
encoding
hierarchy of needs
high-context
    communication
indirect statements
interview techniques
kinesics
low-context
    communication
masking
open-ended questions
prejudice
projection
rationalization
regression
repression
roadblocks
sublimation
therapeutic
    communication
time focus
undoing

ATTRIBUTES OF PROFESSIONALISM

Communication

- Did you listen to and acknowledge the patient?
- Did you provide appropriate responses/feedback?
- Did you display appropriate body language?
- Did you respond honestly and diplomatically to the patient's concerns?
- Did you demonstrate empathy in communicating with patients, family, and staff?
- Did you apply active listening skills?
- Did you maintain eye contact with the patient during communication?
- Did you refrain from sharing your personal experiences?

Presentation

- Were you dressed and groomed appropriately?
- Did you do something to bond with the patient?
- Did your actions attend to both the psychological and the physiological aspects of the patient's illness or condition?
- Did you attend to any special needs of the patient? Did you first ask if assistance was needed, rather than taking charge?
- Were you courteous, patient, and respectful to the patient?
- Did you display a positive attitude?
- Did you display a calm, professional, and caring manner?

Competency

- Did you pay attention to detail?
- Did you display sound judgment?
- Were you knowledgeable and accountable?
- Did you apply critical thinking skills in performing patient assessment and care?

Initiative

- Were you flexible and dependable?
- Did you direct the patient to other resources when necessary or helpful, with the approval of the provider?
- Did you assist coworkers when appropriate?

Integrity

- Did you work within your scope of practice?
- Did you demonstrate sensitivity to patients' rights?
- Did you protect personal boundaries?
- Did you demonstrate respect for individual diversity?
- Did you demonstrate an appreciation for the patient's attitude toward the illness or condition?
- Did you protect and maintain confidentiality?

SCENARIO

In the two-provider clinic of Drs. Lewis and King, four medical assistants constantly interact with patients, allaying their concerns, scheduling their appointments, instructing them on medications, and helping them understand their insurance coverage. On any given day, clinic manager Marilyn Johnson, CMA (AAMA), is greeting patients warmly as they arrive for their appointments. Some patients, such as Anna and Joseph Ortiz, are new to the practice. Marilyn's warm manner puts them at ease. Other patients, such as Martin Gordon, who has prostate cancer, may be depressed and anxious. Marilyn tries to create an environment where they feel free to share their concerns and anxieties.

Marilyn demonstrates therapeutic communication by acknowledging each patient as they arrive for appointments and puts them at ease by providing instructions. Medical assistants who project a warm and courteous presence while maintaining composure, even during difficult situations, and who ask the right questions in a nonthreatening manner will achieve therapeutic communication.

INTRODUCTION

Of all the tasks and skills required of the medical assistant in the ambulatory care setting, none is quite so important as communication. Communication is the foundation for every action taken by health care professionals in the care of their patients. Because medical assistants are often the liaison between patient and provider, it is critical to be aware of all the complexities of the communication process.

Every day, Marilyn, Ellen, and the two clinical medical assistants at the clinics of Drs. Lewis and King face many communication challenges. This chapter describes effective communication principles, applies those principles to face-to-face communication, and describes the basic roadblocks to communication. The key word to all communication in the medical setting is therapeutic. In all conversations with patients, the more therapeutic the conversation, the more satisfied the patient will be with the care provided.

IMPORTANCE OF COMMUNICATION

Therapeutic communication differs from normal communication in that it introduces an element of empathy into what can be a traumatic experience for the patient. It imparts a feeling of comfort in the face of even the most horrific news about the patient's prognosis. The patient is made to feel validated and respected. Therapeutic communication uses specific and well–defined professional skills.

Therapeutic communication in the health care setting is the foundation of all patient care and is of the utmost importance. Communication must be in nontechnical language the patient can understand, delivered with feeling for the patient's emotional situation and state of mind, and yet it still must be technically accurate. The medical staff must be alert to the patient's state of stress and whether defense mechanisms have taken over to the extent that the patient has "tuned out" and is no longer communicating with the staff.

Patients seeking an ambulatory care service look for medical professionals with technical skills and a clinical staff capable of communicating with them. Questions frequently asked by individuals seeking a new provider and clinic include: "Will the doctor talk with me so that I understand?" "Will the doctor listen to what I have to say?" and "Can I talk to the doctor honestly and openly?" The answer to all of these questions needs to be "yes." This chapter discusses these issues and presents specific techniques for therapeutic communication.

THE COMMUNICATION CYCLE

All communication, whether social or therapeutic, involves two or more individuals participating in an exchange of information. The communication cycle involves sending and receiving messages even when not consciously aware of them.

Four basic elements are included in the communication cycle. They are (1) the sender, (2) the message and a channel or mode of communication, (3) the receiver, and (4) feedback (Figure 5-1).

The Sender

The sender begins the communication cycle by **encoding** or creating the message to be sent. This is an important step, and much care should be taken in formulating the message. Before creating the message, the sender must observe the receiver to determine the complexity of the words to be used within the message, the receiver's ability to interpret the message, and the best channel by which to send the message.

The Message

The message is the content being communicated. The message must be understood clearly by the receiver. Various levels of complexity in communication are used depending on the ability of the receiver to recognize and understand the words contained within the message. Children do not have the vocabulary base or the cognitive skills to communicate and understand at the same level as adults. The health of the receiver also must be considered. A patient who is experiencing stress or is in pain may find it difficult to concentrate on the message. If the patient is of a different nationality or culture from the sender, verbal communication may require special skill. When visual or hearing acuity is impaired, another challenge must be surmounted.

The four modes of communication, also called channels of communication, most pertinent in our everyday exchange are (1) speaking, (2) listening, (3) gestures or body language, and (4) writing. These modes or channels are affected by our physical and mental development, our culture, our education and life experiences, our impressions from models and mentors, and in general by how we feel and accept ourselves as individuals. Each mode or channel of communication has its appropriateness and must be considered when formulating the message.

The Receiver

The receiver is the recipient of the sender's message. The receiver must **decode**, or interpret, the meaning of the message. The primary sensory skill used in verbal communication is listening. It is hard work to concentrate and listen. When decoding the message, the receiver must be aware that not only the spoken word but the tone and pitch of the voice and the speed at which the words are spoken carry meaning and must be evaluated.

Feedback

Feedback takes place after the receiver has decoded the message sent by the sender. Feedback

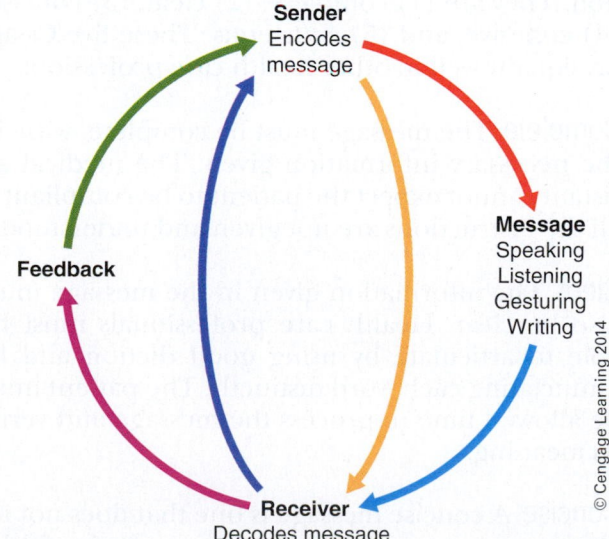

Figure 5-1 The communication cycle and channels of communication.

is the receiver's way of ensuring that the message that is understood is the same as the message that was sent. Feedback also provides an opportunity for the receiver to clarify any misunderstanding regarding the original message and to ask for additional information.

Listening Skills

A vital part of feedback in the communication cycle is listening. A good listener is alert to all aspects of the communication cycle—the verbal and nonverbal message, as well as verification of the message through appropriate feedback.

Active listening is one method used in therapeutic communication. In this technique, the received message is sent back to the sender, worded a little differently, for verification from the sender.

Sender: "How can I possibly pay this fee when I have no insurance?"

Receiver: "You're worried about paying your bill?"

The preceding example illustrates how the receiver is able to validate the sender's concerns at the same time the message is checked for accuracy. The door is then left open for a therapeutic response, such as:

Sender: "Our bookkeeper will be glad to work out a payment plan with you that will fit your resources."

Active listening involves listening with a "third ear," that is, being aware of what the patient is *not* saying or picking up on hints to the real message by observing body language. The health care professional should have three listening goals:

- To improve listening skills sufficiently so that patients are heard accurately
- To listen either for what is *not* being said or for information transmitted only by hints
- To determine how accurately the message has been received

So many health professionals try to "fix" everything with a recommendation, a prescription, even advice. Sometimes, none of those things is necessary. The patient simply needs someone to listen, to acknowledge the difficulty, and to remember that the patient is not helpless in finding a solution to the problem.

Skill in communication takes years of practice and frequent review. It will never become perfect; we can only hope that we will become better at it with each passing day. Communication is and always will be the basis for any therapeutic relationship (Tamparo & Lindh, 2008).

TYPES OF COMMUNICATION

We communicate by what we say, and also by our tone of voice, body movements, and facial expressions. The following paragraphs present the aspects of verbal and nonverbal communication. The importance of maintaining consistency between verbal and nonverbal messages also is stressed.

Verbal Communication

Verbal communication takes place when the message is spoken. However, one must keep in mind that unless the words have meaning, and unless the sender and the receiver apply the same meaning to the spoken words, verbal communication may be misunderstood. If, for example, you overhear a conversation in a language foreign to you, you are indeed a witness to verbal communication, but you may not understand the message. To have any meaning, the spoken word must be understood by all parties of the communication (Tamparo & Lindh, 2008).

The Five Cs of Communication. The book *Legal Nurse Consulting Principles and Practice*, edited by Patricia W. Iyer, identifies the five Cs of communication. They are (1) complete, (2) clear, (3) concise, (4) cohesive, and (5) courteous. These five Cs apply equally well in other health care professions.

Complete. The message must be complete, with all the necessary information given. The medical assistant cannot expect the patient to be compliant if all the instructions are not given and understood.

Clear. The information given in the message must also be clear. Health care professionals must be able to articulate by using good diction and by enunciating each word distinctly. The patient must be allowed time to process the message and verify its meaning.

Concise. A concise message is one that does not include any unnecessary information. It should be brief and to the point (Figure 5-2). Patients must not be overloaded with technical terms that may

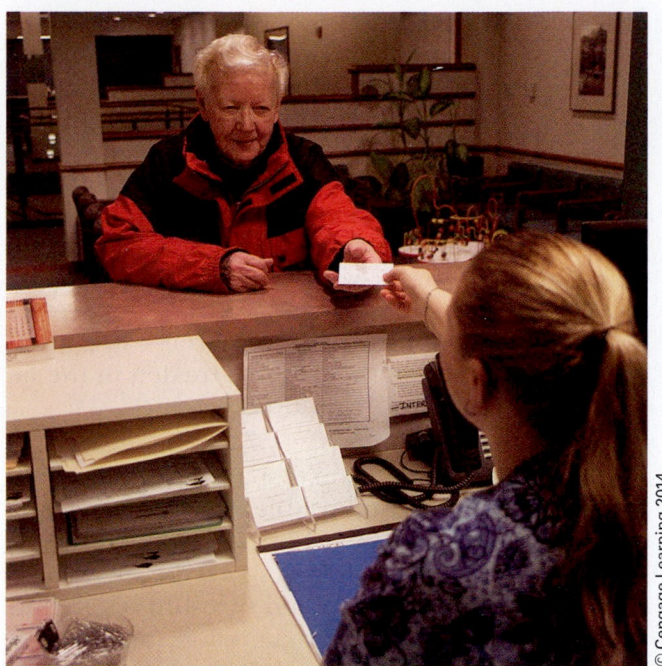

Figure 5-2   To say to the patient after greeting her by name, "I've completed an appointment card to remind you of your next appointment, Tuesday at 2:00 PM" is an example of a concise message that is brief and to the point.

not be understood or that tend to distract them by diverting their attention away from the balance of the message.

Cohesive. A cohesive message is organized and logical in its progression. The cohesive message does not ramble and does not jump from one subject to another. The patient should be able to follow the message easily. The medical assistant should always allow time to summarize detailed messages and use responding skills to verify that the patient fully understands the message.

When communicating within the health professions, keep in mind the following:

1. Good communication skills are necessary in establishing rapport with patients.

2. Patients feel respected and validated when called by their full name, such as Mary O'Keefe or Mrs. O'Keefe.

3. Patients should be encouraged to verbalize their feelings and concerns.

4. Patients should be given technical information in a manner that they can understand.

5. Patients should be allowed to suggest and discuss any personal applications to their health care.

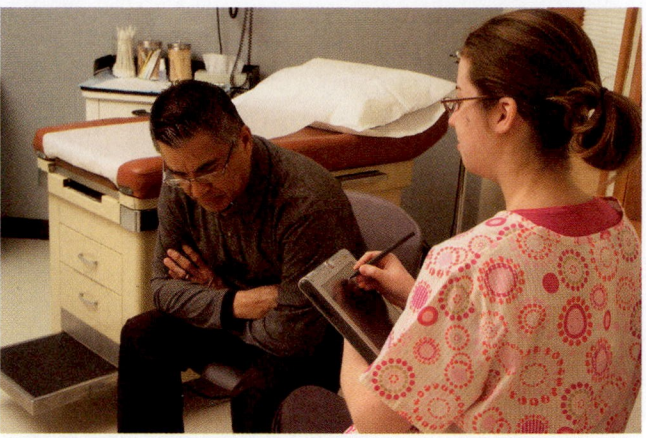

Figure 5-3   Body language can communicate more than spoken words.

Courteous. Courtesy is important in all aspects of communication. It only takes a moment to acknowledge a patient with a smile or by name. Knocking on the examination room door before entering validates the patient's right to privacy and builds self-esteem.

Remember to be courteous to colleagues in the clinic. Good working relationships and professionalism are always enhanced by simple courtesy.

Nonverbal Communication

Verbal communication alone is not always adequate in conveying the message being sent. In most instances, more than one mode or channel of communication is used. Nonverbal communication, often referred to as **body language**, includes the unconscious body movements, gestures, and facial expressions that accompany speech. The study of body language is known as **kinesics** (Figure 5-3).

Nonverbal communication is the language we learn first. It is learned seemingly automatically when infants learn to return a smile or respond to touches on the cheek. Much of our body language is a learned behavior and is greatly influenced by the primary caregivers and the culture in which we are raised.

Feelings and emotions are communicated most often through nonverbal means. The body expresses its true repressed feelings using body language. Most of the negative messages we communicate are also expressed nonverbally and usually are unintentional. Experts tell us that 70% of communication is nonverbal. The tone of voice communicates 23% of the message—only 7% of

PATIENT EDUCATION

Sensitive medical assistants will encourage patients to verbalize their concerns. The ability to ask questions in a nonprobing way and to elicit patient responses is an important function in any ambulatory care setting, because it is critical to know a patient's history, current medications, and other relevant data.

the message is actually communicated by the spoken word.

Facial Expression.

Facial expression is considered one of the most important and observed nonverbal communicators. Each facet or aspect of the anatomy of the face sends a nonverbal message.

Often expressions of joy and happiness or sorrow and grief are reflected through the eyes. The anatomy of the eyes does not change, but the movements of the structures surrounding the eyes enhance or magnify the message being communicated.

Children are told it is not polite to stare at people. It is acceptable to stare at animals in the zoo or art objects in the museum, but not at humans. Staring is dehumanizing and is often interpreted as an invasion of privacy.

The medical assistant must learn not to stare when patients present with ailments that make them "look" different. Patients such as these are individuals who have needs, who perhaps feel pain and discomfort, and who have decreased self-esteem and value. These feelings will only be amplified if the medical assistant and other health professionals are unable to "see" them as humans. A lack of eye contact may also be viewed as avoidance or disinterest in being involved.

The movements of the eyebrow indicate many nonverbal cues as well. Surprise, puzzlement, worry, amusement, and questioning are often nonverbal messages reflected by the position of the eyebrow. Wrinkling of the forehead sends similar messages.

 Cultural influences affect customs and different forms of facial expressions. It is important to remember that there are many cross-cultural similarities in body language, but there are also many differences. Various cultures denote different meanings to various gestures. If your patient is from another culture, never assume that gestures used hold the same meaning for the patient as they do for you. For example, some cultures believe that prolonged eye contact is rude and an invasion of privacy, whereas others consider it a sign of intimacy. Some people stare at the floor when concentrating or thinking through a process. Other cultures avoid eye contact to display modesty, whereas others feel eye contact expresses hostility or aggression. It is important to understand the cultures of the patients treated in the facility in which you are employed.

Personal Space.

Personal space is the distance at which we feel comfortable with others while communicating. In the classroom, for example, students claim their personal space the first day of class. The area is well defined by using books and papers, or by placing the arm, hand, or chair on boundary lines. When another invades the personal space, a shift in body position or the use of eye contact sends the message, "This is my area." Individuals may feel threatened when others invade their personal space without permission. Some examples of comfortable personal space for U.S. culture are as follows:

- Intimate: touching to 1½ feet
- Personal: 1½ to 4 feet
- Social: 4 to 12 feet (most often observed)
- Public: 12 to 15 feet

As with facial expressions, personal space is handled differently by various cultures. For example, there is no word for privacy in the Japanese language. Population numbers require crowding together publicly, as well as privately. Public crowding is often viewed as a sign of warmth and pleasant intimacy in Japan. In the private home, several generations may live together; however, each considers this space to be his own and resents intrusion into it.

Arabs like to touch their companions, to feel and to smell them. To deny a friend your breath is to be ashamed. When two Arabs talk to each other, they look each other in the eyes with great intensity. U.S. businessmen often end a business arrangement with a handshake; however, American Indians may view a handshake as an act of aggression or an offensive behavior. Each culture has its own distinct nonverbal communication cues.

The medical assistant may perform many invasive tasks during the course of a clinic visit. Examples include taking vital signs or giving injections, both of which require touching the patient. It is beneficial to explain procedures that invade another's space before beginning the procedure so that it will not be perceived as threatening. This helps to empower the patient by involving the patient in the decision–making process and builds a sense of trust in the medical assistant.

Posture. Like personal space, posture is important to health care professionals. Posture relates to the position of the body or parts of the body. It is the manner in which we carry ourselves, or pose in situations. We tend to tighten up in threatening or unknown situations and to relax in nonthreatening environments. Those who study kinesics believe that a posture involves at least half the body, and that the position can last for nearly five minutes.

When the patient is seated with the arms and legs crossed, the message of closure or being opinionated may be relayed. In contrast, sitting in a chair relaxed with the hands clasped behind the head indicates an attitude of being open to suggestions. Slumped shoulders may signal depression, discouragement, or, in some cases, even pain.

Position. Position, the physical stance of two individuals while communicating, and, is a key factor to consider while communicating with the patient. Most provider-patient relationships use the face-to-face communication arrangement. When speaking with a patient, the provider or medical assistant will want to maintain a close but comfortable position, enabling observation of all cues being sent, both verbal and nonverbal (Figure 5-4).

Standing over a patient can convey a message of superiority, and too much distance between the two parties may be interpreted as avoidance or exclusivity. Generally, leaning toward the patient expresses warmth, caring, interest, acceptance, and trust. Moving away from the patient may be interpreted as dislike, disinterest, boredom, indifference, suspicion, or impatience.

Whenever possible, it is best to have a chair in the examination room and to have the patient seated comfortably in the chair to begin the communication cycle. The medical assistant or provider can sit on a stool that can be moved easily toward the patient. This arrangement aids the patient in feeling valued, listened to, and cared for as a fellow human being.

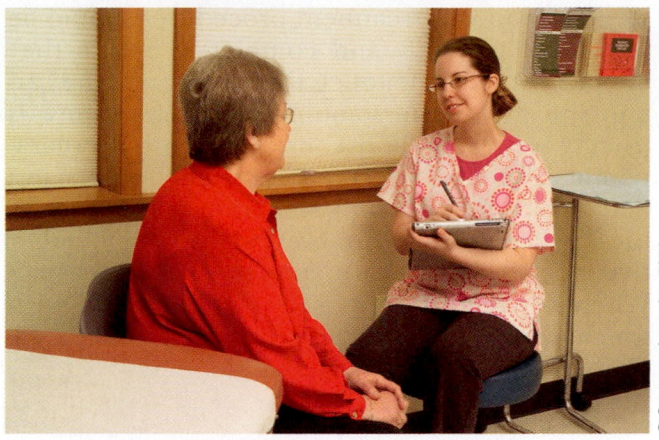

Figure 5-4   Positive posture and position encourage therapeutic communication.

Gestures and Mannerisms. Most of us use gestures and mannerisms when we "talk" with our hands. This form of body language may be useful in enhancing the spoken word by emphasizing ideas, thus creating and holding the attention of others. Some common gestures and their possible meanings are as follows:

Finger-tapping	Impatience, nervousness
Shrugged shoulders	Indifference, discouragement
Rubbing the nose	Puzzlement
Whitened knuckles and clenched fists	Anger
Fidgeting	Nervousness

Touch. Touch is a powerful tool that communicates what cannot be expressed in words. Its appropriateness in the patient–health professional relationship has well–defined boundaries and requires the use of good judgment on the part of the professional. Infants who are not touched, cuddled, and loved do not grow and develop as do those who receive these reassuring gestures. Touch is personal and is linked closely to personal space. Understanding touch as it relates to various cultures must be considered. For example, Vietnamese, Cambodian, Hmong, and Thai families traditionally consider the head to be the site of the soul. During conversation and patient assessment, avoid touching the patient's head unless it is necessary for the examination. Southeast Asian patients may fear bodily intrusion; therefore, physical examination and treatment procedures should be explained carefully and completely before they are performed. The touch that communicates caring, sincerity, understanding, and reassurance is usually welcomed and considered to be a therapeutic response. Most patients will understand and accept the touching behavior as it relates to the medical setting; however, we must remember that not all patients are comfortable with touch. Whenever the patient is not comfortable with touch, ask permission and create as safe and reassuring an environment as possible.

Congruency in Communication

Using some keys to successful communication promotes effective communication. There must be **congruency** between the verbal and nonverbal communication. Shaking your head NO while saying YES verbally sends a mixed message. In most cases, the nonverbal messages will be accepted as the intended message.

It is also important to remember that most nonverbal messages are sent in groups of various forms of body language. The grouping of nonverbal messages into statements or conclusions is known as **clustering**. **Masking** involves an attempt to conceal or repress the true feeling or message. The perceptive professional will be aware of all these messages.

Perception as it relates to communication is the conscious awareness of one's own feelings and the feelings of others. To be most useful and therapeutic as health professionals, we must first explore our own feelings and appreciate and accept ourselves.

Learning to use perception involves the ability to sense another's attitudes, moods, and feelings. It takes practice and experience to develop and use this skill effectively. Being attentive to other professionals and observing their use of perception will yield insight into its usefulness and provide an example to emulate. A word of caution—the use of perception may easily be misinterpreted, especially when going with your feeling or assessment of what is happening regarding the patient. Always follow perceived assessments with verbal validation before assuming your perception of the circumstance is correct.

Nonverbal communication is easily misinterpreted. Careful observation for congruency between verbal and nonverbal communication, and clustering nonverbal cues being sent into non-verbal statements will strengthen your ability to interpret the message accurately.

FACTORS AFFECTING THERAPEUTIC COMMUNICATION

Anything that interferes with the patient's ability to focus has a negative impact on therapeutic communication. The following paragraphs discuss significant barriers. The medical assistant must recognize that until these barriers are dealt with or minimized, therapeutic communication will be significantly affected.

Age Barriers

Professional medical assistants must understand human growth and development and be able to adapt their communications appropriately to any age group. Many scientists and researchers have studied human growth and development and have proposed guidelines for communication with patients during each stage. Erik Erikson (1902–1994) taught that each stage or phase is part of a continuum throughout the life cycle. Table 5-1 lists Erikson's stages of human growth and development and identifies communication problems and suggested actions to be taken during each stage.

Economic Barriers

The influence of economics may reveal a discomfort if the clinic staff and patients have a different perception about how billing is managed and when and how payment is expected. A discussion of billing and payment procedures at the first clinic visit or before a major procedure will be beneficial to all concerned parties.

Education and Life Experience Barriers

Educational and life experiences will, in part, determine how patients react to their care. Patients with family members being treated for a chronic illness will have more knowledge and understanding of that illness in their own lives. Individuals who have already suffered a great deal of loss and

Table 5-1 Stages of Human Growth and Development

Age Group	Communication Problem	Action Taken
Infant 0–1 years Trust versus Mistrust	Total dependence on others for life support	• Respond to social smiles • Provide warm, friendly atmosphere • Consider safety issues • Wear colorful uniform
Toddler 2–3 years Initiative versus Guilt	Limited vocabulary, fear of encounter with medical staff, separation anxiety if separated from caregiver	• Use child's own vocabulary and rephrase • Encourage and praise • Use simple commands • Allow child some control by permitting ambulating • Establish consistent clinic visit routine • Display a cordial relationship with parent to promote trust by child
Preschooler 3–6 years Initiative versus Guilt	Unable to comprehend abstract ideas, cannot tolerate direct eye contact, creative imagination, short attention span, seeks control	• All of the above as appropriate • Physical contact at child's eye level if possible • Role play therapy (give pretend injection to stuffed toy) • Allow control by permitting child to make as many choices as possible (Would you like to be measured to see how tall you are or weighed first?)
School Age 6–11 years Industry versus Inferiority	Developing ability to comprehend, taking some ownership of health care, concern for privacy	• Include child in explanation of treatment and protocols using child's vocabulary • Encourage and praise • Make health care a teaching opportunity • Respect privacy of child
Adolescent 12–18 years Identity versus Role Confusion	Increased comprehension, capable of abstract thought, may be fiercely independent, may use colloquial language, sexually maturing, concerned about confidentiality	• Actively listen, using patient's own language idioms as much as possible • Use abstract thought, but be alert to lack of understanding • Reassure that confidentiality will be protected, but state limits • Recognize peer pressure • Be aware of body image impacts
Early Adulthood 19–40 years Intimacy versus Isolation	Greater comprehension and abstract thought capability, usually more in touch with reality than adolescents	• All of the items listed for adolescent • Provide health care options • Describe benefits and expectations of good health care
Middle Adulthood 40–65 years Generativity versus Stagnation	Established socioeconomically, thinks of charities, concerns for succeeding generation	• Listen • Validate • Provide health care choices when appropriate
Late Adulthood 65 to death Integrity versus Despair	Anxious and stressed, hearing or vision impaired, slow to respond to inquiries, prone to omitting facts, overemphasis on somatic concerns, fear or embarrassed by loss of physical control, fear of being alone at death	• Be in proximity to patient and gently touch as appropriate • Speak slowly and clearly • Pace the encounter to match patient's tolerance • Be gentle and truthful

CRITICAL THINKING

Define in your own words the terms *bias* and *prejudice*. Now identify one bias and one prejudice that you have. How will these impact your ability to respond therapeutically in the medical setting? What steps can you take to become more accepting of the uniqueness of others, thereby improving therapeutic communication?

grief in their lives may handle the information of a life-threatening illness more calmly than someone who has experienced little grief.

Bias and Prejudice Barriers

Personal preferences, biases, and prejudices will enter into many provider-patient relationships. Such biases affect the types of communication possible. When individuals are not aware of their biases or prejudices, hostile attitudes may prevail.

For therapeutic communication to take place, biases must be examined, a person's comfort level with each bias determined, and measures taken to ensure that a hostile attitude is not present. **Bias** is defined as a slant toward a particular belief. **Prejudice** is defined as an opinion or judgment that is formed before all the facts are known; prejudice is a preconceived and unfavorable concept of some other person or group. Common biases and prejudices in today's society include:

1. A preference for Western-style medicine
2. Choosing providers according to gender
3. Prejudice related to a person's sexual preference
4. Discrimination based on race or religion
5. Hostile attitudes toward people with different value systems than one's own
6. A belief that people who cannot afford health care should receive less care than someone who can pay for full services

 Medical assistants must recognize such biases and prejudices so that their own culture with its biases does not prevent them from responding therapeutically in communications with patients. Such recognition requires being aware of the differences among human beings and willingly accepting the uniqueness of each person.

Verbal Roadblocks to Therapeutic Communication

Being sensitive to patients' unique personalities and needs will enable the health care professional to avoid **roadblocks** to communication (Table 5-2).

It must be the concern of each health care professional to facilitate communication by encouraging and enabling patients to express themselves honestly without fear. Roadblocks close communication and prevent quality care of the total person.

Well–intentioned attempts to make the patient feel more comfortable can sometimes have negative effects on therapeutic communication. The following are some examples:

- Attempting to dispel the patient's anxiety by implying that there is not sufficient reason for it to exist is to completely devalue the patient's own feelings. Developing a sincere interpersonal relationship more readily helps the patient. The health care professional should remain neutral in regard to the patient's condition. He or she should remain empathetic, but nonjudgmental.

- Rejection of the patient's ideas or comments causes therapeutic interaction to cease and thwarts the patient's expression.

- Indicating accord with the patient by using statements such as "That's right" or "I agree" can result in the health care professional speaking for the patient and can sometimes unintentionally put the health care professional's conclusions in the patient's mind.

Defense Mechanisms as Barriers

Therapeutic communication becomes difficult if a patient is in a highly emotional state. A patient who is frightened, ashamed, guilty, or threatened often will resort to defense mechanisms as a means of avoiding injury to the ego. We all use defense mechanisms to some limited extent, but they become harmful when they result in a breakdown in therapeutic communication. Failure by the patient to face problems often results in inability to provide satisfactory treatment on the part of the medical practitioner. Recognizing common defense mechanisms enables the medical staff to minimize

Table 5-2   Roadblocks to Communication

Roadblock	Example
Reassuring clichés	"Don't worry about not having a job, Mr. McKay; you'll find another one really soon."
Moralizing/lecturing	"If you were smart, Mrs. Johnson, you'd lose fifty pounds and you wouldn't have such a problem with your diabetes and hypertension."
Requiring explanations	"Why would you not want to have chemotherapy, Mr. Gordon? Seeing your wife die of cancer should surely make you want to seek treatment."
Ridiculing/shaming	"Ha, ha, Mr. Gordon! It's not *prostrate*—it's prostate cancer."
Defending/contradicting	"Mr. Marshal, I assure you the physician is *very busy*. He will not see you until he has finished with his other patients."
Shifting subjects	"Yes, Mrs. Jover, your work is very interesting, but I must ask you to sign this permission form to test for HIV."
Criticizing	"Mrs. O'Keefe, why in the world would you stay with an abusive husband?"
Threatening	"There is no way you will get rid of this cough if you do not stop smoking, Mr. Fowler."

© Cengage Learning 2014

the triggering event and to communicate more effectively.

Defense mechanisms are defined as behavior that is used to protect the ego from guilt, anxiety, or loss of esteem. Use of defense mechanisms is most often subconscious to the person using them. It is the body's way of seeking relief from uncomfortable or painful reality. A mentally healthy person uses defense mechanisms to put a problem on hold until sufficient time has passed to permit him or her to address it without unacceptable emotional pain. Excessive use of defense mechanisms or failure to address a problem even after sufficient time has elapsed may be a sign of mental health issues.

Defense mechanisms are usually readily apparent to the disaffected observer; however, they are difficult to analyze without knowledge of the motive behind the behavior. The following paragraphs describe some commonly observed defense mechanisms.

Regression is an attempt to withdraw from an unpleasant circumstance by retreating to an earlier, more secure stage of life. It is usually used when the person feels powerless to affect the events causing the pain; it can be thought of as a desperation move. A toddler's regression to bedwetting or soiling himself or herself shortly after a new baby arrives in the family is an example of this defense mechanism. Use of a security blanket by an adult or child when faced with something that disrupts his or her life is another example.

Denial is refusal to accept painful information that is readily apparent to others. This defense mechanism commonly is encountered in the case of a person being diagnosed with a disease such as cancer or experiencing the death of a close family member or associate. Denial has a devastating effect on communication. The person will not hear what you say, but will quite frequently acknowledge what you are saying. Careful attention to what the person is saying will reveal that he or she does not accept his or her situation and is not mentally conscious that it is happening. Denial is often the first stage of an emotional response after a traumatic event. The next stage is anger toward the event, the medical staff, God, or others. The stage after anger is frequently depression. A mentally healthy person eventually reaches the final stage of acceptance.

Repression is similar to denial, but it is a totally subconscious reaction. In the case of repression, the person seems to experience temporary amnesia. It is the mind's way of defending itself from mental trauma by forgetting or wiping things out of the conscious memory. A child subconsciously forgetting to tell parents that he or she got into trouble at school is an example. The fear associated with the event becomes overwhelming, causing the mind to forget. Repression should not be confused with outright lying. In severe cases, repression can be related to mental illness.

Projection is attributing unacceptable desires, impulses, and thoughts falsely to others to avoid acknowledging they are actually the person's own experiences. It is a means of defending against feelings or urges the person does not want to admit they are experiencing. A mother who abuses her child might accuse the medical assistant of being rough with the child while performing patient assessment to conceal her feelings of wanting to throttle the child. Projection is an indication of mental illness.

Sublimation is the channeling of a socially unacceptable behavior into a socially acceptable behavior. An overly aggressive person directed to play football to relieve aggression is an example. Constructive behavior is substituted for destructive behavior.

Displacement is the subconscious transfer of unacceptable emotions, thoughts, or feelings from one's self to a more acceptable external substitute. A patient who is angry with the provider for some reason slams the door as he or she leaves the clinic.

Compensation is a conscious or subconscious overemphasizing of a characteristic to offset a real or imagined deficiency. This defense mechanism involves substituting strength for a weakness and may be viewed as healthy. An example is the young boy whose physical stature keeps him from being a football star, so he compensates by achieving an academic award.

Rationalization is the mind's way of making unacceptable behavior or events acceptable by devising a rational reason. The purpose of rationalization is to avoid embarrassment or guilt or to avoid obeying a directive. The rational reason is usually a stretch of the truth and can be quite apparent to disinterested individuals. An example is the patient who tells the provider that he or she did not take his or her blood pressure medication because he or she did not have enough time before leaving for work. The medication easily could have been taken at home or at work. Most people rationalize things to some extent, but excessive rationalization may be construed as unhealthy.

Undoing is acting in ways designed to make amends or to cancel out inappropriate behavior. Showering the abused person with gifts to compensate for unacceptable actions that took place in the past is an example.

Barriers Caused by Cultural and Religious Diversity

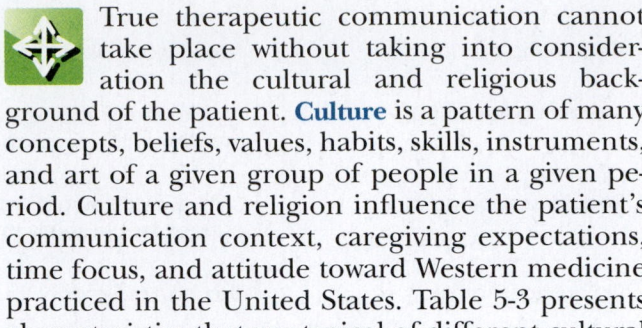 True therapeutic communication cannot take place without taking into consideration the cultural and religious background of the patient. **Culture** is a pattern of many concepts, beliefs, values, habits, skills, instruments, and art of a given group of people in a given period. Culture and religion influence the patient's communication context, caregiving expectations, time focus, and attitude toward Western medicine practiced in the United States. Table 5-3 presents characteristics that are typical of different cultural and religious groups.

Communication Context.
Communication context can be one of two styles: low-context or high-context. **Low-context communication** uses few environmental idioms to convey an idea. It relies on explicit and highly detailed language. **High-context communication** relies on body language, reference to environmental objects, and culturally relevant phraseology to communicate an idea. Neither communication style is superior to the other. It is important, however, that both the speaker and the listener be cognizant of the style being used in the conversation. In the medical clinic, the medical assistant should be aware of communication content and attempt to utilize the style used by the patient to the extent that it is practical.

Persons having different communication styles can easily develop an incorrect impression of the other person. Low–context communication is direct and in-your-face, whereas high-context communication is indirect and seems to take forever to reach a conclusion. The high-context speaker is often thought of as mentally slow or uneducated, and the low-context speaker is thought of as being rude or arrogant. Conclusions based on communication style usually are preconceived misconceptions and should be considered at all times when health care professionals are working with patients.

Caregiving Expectations.
Caregiving expectations refer to the arrangements for taking responsibility for medical requirements. Most persons from the Western culture are individualistic and take personal responsibility for their medical care. However, many other cultures and religions do not share this philosophy. This can result in problems related to privacy requirements and patient compliance.

Table 5-3   Generalization of Cultural/Religious Effects on Health Care

Culture or Religion	Medical Care Background	Caregiving Structure	Communication Traits	Time Focus*
Caucasian, Western Culture	**Western medicine,** rely on prescription medications, practice preventive medicine, may rely on holistic medicine or folk medicine in some rural areas.	**Individual,** immediate family, close friends.	**Low context,** direct, eye contact expected, not adverse to therapeutic touching, may challenge medical opinions, basic English, speaks loudly.	**Future**
African American, Western Culture	**Western medicine,** rely on prescription medications, practice preventive medicine, may rely on holistic medicine or folk medicine in some rural areas.	**Extended family,** relatives, close friends, neighbors, church family.	**Low context,** direct, eye contact expected, not adverse to therapeutic touching, may challenge medical opinions and can distrust medical personnel, basic English sometimes mixed with street language (Ebonics).	**Present/ Future**
Black, African, or Caribbean Culture	**Mixture** of Western and holistic medicine combined with spiritualism.	**Extended family,** relatives, close friends, neighbors, church family, tribal affiliation.	**Low context,** eye contact expected, highly emotional, basic English strongly mixed with local dialect.	**Present**
Asian Culture Asian, Indian, Chinese, Filipino, Japanese, Korean, Thai, Laotian, Vietnamese	**Mixture** of Western and holistic medicine combined with Confucian principals, i.e., mind control of the body and maintaining a balance between natural forces and energy in the body, eating foods designated as having hot and cold properties to cure illness is common, mental illness is considered shameful and is denied.	**Immediate family,** opinions of family and particularly elders are important.	**High context,** indirect, avoid eye contact, show little emotion, avoid therapeutic touching, youth speak basic English, elders may speak little English, may agree with what is said even when they do not understand in order to avoid conflict or to avoid losing face, speak softly.	**Present/ Past**
Native American, South Sea Island Cultures	**Mixture** of Western and folk medicine combined with importance of a balance between the forces of nature.	**Extended family,** relatives, close friends, neighbors, tribal affiliation.	**High context,** avoid eye contact, speak softly and slowly, basic English mixed with tribal dialects.	**Present**
Hispanic and Latino Cultures	**Mixture** of Western and folk medicine combined with a strong belief in intervention by God, eating foods designated as having hot and cold properties to cure illness is common.	**Extended family,** relatives, church family, collective community.	**High context,** be respectful and make direct eye contact, speak softly, some basic English, most speak Spanish.	**Present/ Past**
Judaism	**Western medicine,** religion does not allow eating pork and requires kosher food.	Culturally dependent.	Culturally dependent.	**Future/ Present**
Hinduism/ Buddhism	**Western medicine,** religions do not allow eating meat, modest regarding their body.	Culturally dependent.	Culturally dependent.	**Future/ Present**

(continues)

Table 5-3 Generalization of Cultural/Religious Effects on Health Care (*Continued*)

Culture or Religion	Medical Care Background	Caregiving Structure	Communication Traits	Time Focus*
Islam	**Mixture** of Western and folk medicine combined with a strong belief in intervention by Allah, match gender of caregiver and patient, women may not be permitted to be examined by male medical professional, mental illness denied, do not ingest alcohol, believe complete rest is proper for all illnesses, do not eat pork.	**Immediate family,** opinions of family and particularly male head of household are important.	**High context,** touching between men and women is prohibited for strict believers, do not discuss sexual dysfunction, females do not make direct eye contact, will not discuss many taboo subjects (mental illness, birth defects, contraception, hospice), those from Middle East speak loudly to indicate the importance of what they are saying.	**Future/ Present**

© Cengage Learning 2014

*The bold term represents the predominant focus.

Time Focus. The cultural background as well as the socioeconomic environment of the patient have considerable impact on time focus. **Time focus** relates to whether the patient's attitude toward life is future, present, or past. Time focus is culture and religion related and is not necessarily related to current circumstances.

Future time focus is found in persons whose physical needs have been met and who can sacrifice immediate gratification to achieve perceived greater future returns. Future-oriented persons are time conscious and plan out their daily lives in considerable detail. Persons from affluent Western cultures usually are future oriented.

Present time focus is found in persons who are less assured of being able to meet their physical needs. It is difficult to plan for the future when basic items in the hierarchy of needs have not been met. Punctuality usually is not important to present-focus persons.

Past time focus is associated with persons from cultures having long-standing traditions. Tradition becomes the central focus of their life.

Human Needs as Barriers to Therapeutic Communication

Human needs, such as those discussed in Maslow's hierarchy of needs, are barriers to effective therapeutic communication if they are not met. A patient who does not know where he or she will find food or shelter or who feels rejected and unloved will frequently make these needs first and of primary concern in their mind. It is nearly impossible to focus on communication regarding other concerns until these basic needs have been met. This section discusses human needs and how they can be satisfied by the medical assistant or by referrals provided by health care professionals.

Maslow's Hierarchy of Needs

Abraham Maslow is considered the founder of humanistic psychology and is most well known for his **hierarchy of needs** (Figure 5-5). *Webster's Dictionary* defines hierarchy as "a group of persons or things arranged in order of rank, grade, class, etc." According to Maslow's theory, human needs could be grouped into five levels. He also theorized that each level of need must be satisfied before one could move on to the next level.

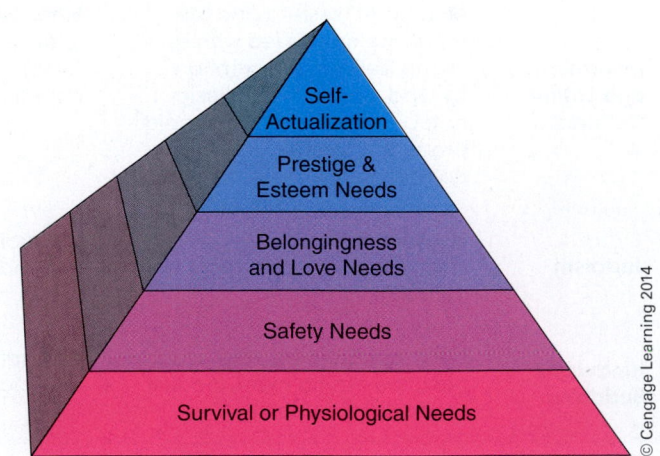

Self-Actualization

Prestige & Esteem Needs

Belongingness and Love Needs

Safety Needs

Survival or Physiological Needs

© Cengage Learning 2014

Figure 5-5 Maslow's hierarchy of needs (Adaptation based on Maslow's Hierarchy of Needs).

CRITICAL THINKING

An established patient arrives 20 minutes early for his appointment. He is in obvious pain and discomfort and tells the administrative medical assistant, "I can't sleep, I can't eat, and I can't go to work today." Which of Maslow's stages most accurately describes this patient? What actions should the medical assistant take to assist this patient?

The needs in the first level include physiologic or survival needs. These needs include food, water, and air to breathe—homeostasis for the body. The second level includes needs of safety and security, that is, the need for security, stability, and protection. Everyone has the desire to be free from fear and anxiety. Safety needs also include the need for structure, law and order, and limits.

The third level involves belonging and love needs. This level of need involves both giving and receiving affection. Additional words that express our connectedness are roots, origins, peers, friends, family, neighborhood, territory, clan, class, and gang. We have a basic animal tendency to herd, flock, join, and belong.

The fourth level, prestige and esteem needs, comes from a basic need for a stable, healthy self-respect for ourselves and others. There is the desire for achievement, strength, and confidence. Also, there is the need for recognition, prestige, reputation, status, and even fame. Satisfaction of these needs leads to feelings of self-confidence and worth. The final level is self-actualization. In this stage, we are at our peak, doing what truly fits us. It is an achievement of potential.

Individuals may move back and forth from one need to another depending on circumstances.

Understanding this hierarchy helps to assess a patient's needs. If the most basic of needs are not met, it is highly unlikely that a patient can be successful with any treatment protocol. Keeping this hierarchy in mind will help to facilitate therapeutic communication.

Patients with Special Needs

Language can be a barrier to communication and can be especially detrimental in the case of therapeutic communication. Using medical terms without defining them as well as using medical jargon or slang can close the door to meaningful communication with the patient. In the case of an English-as-a-second-language patient, the services of an interpreter may be required. The health care provider should be careful to enunciate clearly and speak slowly. A normal conversational tone should be used because speaking loudly serves only to upset the patient and create more stress.

Patients who are audio challenged pose a serious challenge to effective therapeutic communications. In the case of patients who are deaf, the Americans with Disabilities Act requires that appropriate auxiliary aids, including sign language interpreters, be provided in the medical clinic. Some examples of auxiliary aids include note takers, computer-assisted real time transcription services, written materials, and a variety of assistive-listening devices. Therapeutic accommodations for patients with hearing disabilities may also include a quiet environment during the interview process and appropriate lighting to allow for lip-reading. The medical professional should also speak slowly while facing the patient, taking care not to shield his or her mouth.

Patients who are visually challenged may be able to understand the spoken language; however, their vocabulary may be limited because of their disability. Utilize large-print materials and assure adequate lighting in all patient areas. Always speak in a normal voice to the patient as you enter the examination room or before you touch them. Extra caution must be exercised to ensure that patients who are visually impaired understand the message you are attempting to transmit.

Problems with mental cognition will be a deterrent to communication. Dementia or other types of mental impairment, or even a serious illness, may make communication difficult if not impossible. Communication should be with the patient's legal guardian or caregiver. Even so, every attempt should be made to have the patient involved in the conversation so they are not frustrated and feeling powerless and overwhelmed by the situation.

Environmental Factors

Environmental factors such as noise or any visual commotion that causes a distraction for either the patient or the health care professional will be an extreme barrier to communication of any type. Your conversation with the patient should be stopped until you can either move to a more suitable environment or the distraction has stopped. Physical barriers such as a computer screen or a desk between the patient and health care professional should be avoided. The medical professional should attempt to take a position close to the patient and at eye level, taking care not to invade their personal space. Always be vigilant to ensure there are no privacy issues.

Time Factors

Therapeutic communication requires time. Rushing a conversation with a patient and expecting effective conveyance of a message is unrealistic. The patient will listen but not retain your message if he/she perceives a rush situation. The emotional state of the health care professional will be conveyed by body language in such circumstances.

ESTABLISHING MULTICULTURAL COMMUNICATION

 Multicultural communication is the ability to communicate effectively with individuals of other cultures while recognizing one's own personal cultural biases and prejudices and putting them aside.

Approximately one third of the population of the United States comes from a culture other than mainstream American (i.e., Caucasian, English-speaking, Judeo-Christian). Figure 5-6 illustrates the percentage of various cultures living in the United States.

Medical professionals working within a specific cultural community should seek further information relating to that particular culture. In many instances, health care professionals can develop rapport with their ethnically diverse patients by simply demonstrating an interest in their culture and background.

Before multicultural or any therapeutic communication can begin, the patient must first be willing to discuss his or her health care issues, listen to the professional's questions, and give honest answers to those questions. The patient must trust the professional. Several steps to building trust include:

- *Risk/trust.* It is essential for the helping professional to build an atmosphere of trust, making it easier for the patient to risk expressing feelings and attitudes about the problem. Trust has to be earned. Remember to promise no more than you can deliver, be honest, and carefully and thoroughly explain procedures and policies. Answer all questions truthfully and honestly.

- *Empathy.* Empathy is the ability to accept another's private world as if it were your own. Empathy communicates identification with and understanding of another's situation. It states, "I'm available to walk this road with you."

- *Respect.* Respect values another person and considers him or her as a special individual. It is important to respect the patient's personal space, to provide privacy, and to use his or her full name and title when appropriate.

- *Genuineness.* This means being real and honest with others. The health care professional must be able to communicate honestly with others, while being careful not to blame or condemn.

- *Active listening.* Active listening involves verbal and nonverbal clues that send the message you are completely involved in the communication. Sit facing the patient with no barriers, such as a desk, between you. Lean toward the patient slightly to convey genuine concern and interest. Establish and maintain appropriate eye contact to elicit interest and concern. Maintain an open, relaxed posture to establish a nonthreatening environment for the patient. Listen carefully to the words the patient uses to describe problems, and use those terms rather than medical terminology when discussing symptoms.

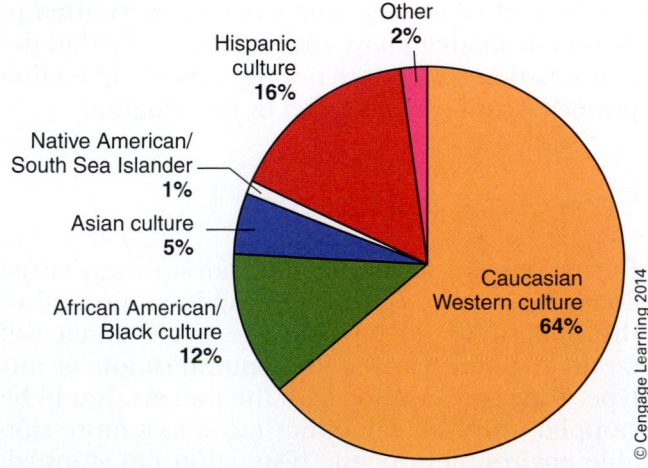

Figure 5-6 United States demographic make-up (2010 Census).

Other 2%

Hispanic culture 16%

Native American/ South Sea Islander 1%

Asian culture 5%

African American/ Black culture 12%

Caucasian Western culture 64%

© Cengage Learning 2014

Cultural Brokering

 Cultural brokering is "the act of bridging, linking, or mediating between groups or persons through the process of reducing conflict or producing change" (National Center for Cultural Competence, Georgetown University Center for Child and Human Development, Georgetown University Medical Center, 2004). A cultural broker serves as a go-between, or one who advocates on behalf of another individual or group within the health care community. The 2010 Census indicates the projected demographic trends in the United States are more complex than ever measured previously. The belief systems related to health, healing, and wellness are diverse, with many cultural variations in the perception of illness and disease and their causes. Cultural brokers respect the values of diverse cultures and health care systems and are knowledgeable of both. They are able to overcome any existing language barriers, so that everyone understands each other clearly. The goal of cultural brokering is to increase the capacity of health care and mental health programs to design, implement, and evaluate culturally and linguistically competent service delivery systems. Cultural and linguistic competence have been determined to be fundamental in the goal of eliminating racial and ethnic disparities in health care.

Cultural brokers may assume the role of medical interpreter. An interpreter is one who takes the spoken message in one language and converts it to another language. Interpreters do not provide word-to-word equivalence, but rather focus on the accurate expression of equivalent meaning. They serve as communicators and liaisons between the patient and the provider in health care facilities. If an interpreter is necessary, it is important to remember to speak directly to the patient, not the interpreter. If English is the second language or a heavy accent is involved, speaking clearly and slowly can greatly enhance communication.

In some cases, a family member may serve as the interpreter. This may not be the best solution because the family member may not understand the medical terminology. It would also be difficult for a family member to be the one to share a life-threatening diagnosis or a poor prognosis report.

THERAPEUTIC COMMUNICATION IN ACTION

The following section identifies the proper communication techniques medical assistants should use as part of the most important communication function they perform: patient interview techniques.

Interview Techniques

 All health professionals must be adept at **interview techniques**—knowing how to encourage the best communication between themselves and the patient. It is important to remember that an unequal relationship exists between the health professional and the patient. The health professional, whether it be the provider or the medical assistant, is in the power position and has a great deal of control over the patient. Therefore, it is important to equalize the relationship as much as possible. That is the reason why some professionals use the term *client* rather than *patient*.

Early in the interview, the patient must feel comfortable enough to risk being honest with the health professional. The health professional must build an atmosphere of trust by showing concern for the patient. A gentle touch and a warm, caring facial expression may be all that is necessary. Always be honest and genuine in your responses to patients. Be sympathetic and empathic and create an environment that is free of hypocrisy.

When the medical assistant is interviewing the patient for the presenting problem or chief complaint, it is important to listen with a "third" ear. Listen to what the patient is not saying but is apt to exhibit through nonverbal communication.

You might choose to share your observation of the nonverbal message with the patient, thus encouraging the patient to verbalize more freely. When feelings are shared, validate and acknowledge those feelings through such statements as "I understand your distress." You can verify the communication by reflecting or paraphrasing what the patient has said.

You will be asking **closed questions** during the interview. Closed questions can be answered with a simple yes or no.

"Are you still taking your medication?"

"Are you in pain now?"

You will also use **open-ended questions** with the patient. These questions encourage therapeutic communication because the patient is required to verbalize more information.

"What kind of help will you have at home during your recovery?"

"How are you coming along on this diet?"

Indirect statements will also prove helpful in facilitating therapeutic communication. An indirect statement will elicit a response from a patient without the patient feeling questioned.

"Tell me what you've been doing since you retired."

"I'd like to know more about your exercise program."

Additional helpful approaches to establishing therapeutic communication include:

- *Silence.* Utilizing the absence of verbal communication gives the patient time to put their feelings and thoughts into words, regain composure, and continue talking. Silence reduces the pace of the encounter and gives the patient time to feel like a human and not an inanimate object. A positive and accepting silence can be a valuable therapeutic tool, particularly for a shy and quiet patient; it shows that he or she has worth and is respected by another person. The medical assistant needs to be alert to what they are communicating by their body language. Even a momentary loss of interest can be interpreted by the patient as indifference. In long periods of silence, the medical assistant must not become bored or allow their attention to wander from the patient. The medical assistant should give a broad opening such as "Where would you like to begin" and avoid small talk. Let the use of silence encourage patients to express themselves.

- *Feedback.* Nodding "Yes," saying "I understand" if you do, or just "uh hmm" are forms of feedback. Not only are words important, but also are our nonverbal cues that communicate feedback such as facial expression, tone and inflection of voice, and posture. Offer general leads and give encouragement to the patient to continue by using statements such as "Go on," "And then?" or "Tell me about it." Acknowledge the patient's right to his or her opinion, to make decisions, and to think for himself or herself. Seeking to make clear that which is not meaningful or that which is vague provides useful feedback. Attempt to verbalize what the patient has hinted at or suggested. Search for mutual understanding and for accord in the meaning of words.

- *Giving recognition.* Give recognition and acknowledge their presence through greeting the patient by name. When the patient makes an effort or accomplishes something, the medical assistant should acknowledge it and give encouragement.

- *Offering comfort.* Help the patient to be comfortable during the medical encounter by showing empathy with the patient's situation. Introduce yourself and explain what is about to happen or to be done to the patient. Make available the facts the patient needs to feel at ease and to make the encounter less stressful.

Refer to Chapter 23 for additional information related to patient interviewing.

Point of Care Techniques

Point of care refers to the location in which the patient and provider or patient and clinic personnel physically interact. This interaction may take place at the reception desk, in the laboratory, or in the examination room. The goal of therapeutic communication at the point of care is varied. It may be to determine the reason for the visit, collect a blood specimen, or explain a course of treatment to the patient. The principal barrier to communication at the point of care is emotional tension, that is, the patient is upset. The patient may be upset due to fear of the illness or diagnosis, pain, or anger as part of the loss of quality of life resulting from the illness. Other barriers to communication less frequently encountered are language, speech or hearing impairment, and were discussed in other sections of this chapter.

If the patient is delivered unpleasant information skillfully, he or she can take in and process the material rather than reject it. Words and statements that promote anxiety or anger should be avoided. Examples are complex medical terminology that the patient may not understand or judgmental statements about lifestyle. Both can instill fear and anger in a patient. Every effort should be made to clarify the information being communicated to the patient. Patients should be encouraged to restate the information in their own words. Under no circumstance should the patient be given false reassurance. This can result in a lack of trust if the patient perceives that he or she is being deceived. The medical assistant should be alert to notice emotional reactions by the patient and be prepared to take appropriate corrective action.

Avoid familiar phrasings and mannerisms—for example, the type we use when unsure of what to say in an uncomfortable situation, such as saying "perhaps," rather than the more usual "maybe," or nervously clearing our throats. All of these are signs of self-protection on the part of the speaker, which

PATIENT EDUCATION

Education of a patient or caregiver should consist of the following fundamentals regardless of the subject:

- Do not attempt to educate the patient while he or she is emotionally upset or distressed. Under these conditions the individual will not be communicative; that is, they are listening but not hearing what is said to them. Make every effort to calm the patient. If necessary, reschedule another time for the educational session.

- Use multiple methods, such as visual, verbal, and action, to convey the

message. This approach ensures that your communication style will be versatile and meet the needs of the patient. Convey information in a clear, concise manner using context that is relevant to the patient.

- Limit the amount of material covered. If necessary, schedule additional sessions so that the patient is not overwhelmed.

- Communicate in simple words, avoiding medical terminology that may not be understood by the patient.

---

the patient may notice. Good communication skills and forethought make such self-protective mechanisms less necessary.

COMMUNITY RESOURCES

 There may be circumstances in which a patient will need a referral to a community resource. These resources range from the more simple acts, such as arranging with Meals on Wheels to deliver a hot meal daily, to making complex arrangements for skilled nursing facilities or hospice care. The medical assistant will need to know the patient's name, address, and telephone number, as well as the particular

resource needed, the diagnosis, and the reason for the service.

It is helpful to have a list of community resources readily available. Using the Internet and telephone directory, compile a list of local community resources. Include the name of the agency, address, phone number, contact person, and instructions for submitting a referral for each agency listed. Contact each agency and request an informational brochure and referral application with instructions. The list may be computerized, or hardcopy information may be filed in a notebook. The information should be put into categories for ease in locating it quickly. See Procedure 5-1 for steps in developing a Community Resources Manual.

PROCEDURE 5-1

Identifying Community Resources

PURPOSE:
To have a list of community resources readily available for referral to patients.

EQUIPMENT/SUPPLIES:
Computer and printer
Following is a list of information sources to consider when beginning to put together a Community Resources Manual:

- Local Public Health Department
- Internet

- Community service numbers in the local telephone directory
- State/federal agencies
- Visiting nurses
- Counselor/social workers at local hospitals
- Nursing home associations
- Local charities

continues

Procedure 5-1 (continued)

PROCEDURE STEPS:

1. With your provider, determine the types of community resources your patients may need. RATIONALE: In order to save time and space, only information on resources useful to your specific clinic clientele should be maintained.

2. Create a listing of each resource including the full name, address, telephone number, and services offered by each agency.

3. *Show initiative* by contacting each agency on the list and requesting the name of a contact person, referral instructions, and a brochure describing the facility.

4. *Pay attention to detail*. Compile the information from steps 2 and 3 to create a Community Resources Manual. RATIONALE: The information may be stored on the computer database or printed and placed in a notebook. Information is readily available when needed.

DOCUMENTATION:

The Community Resources Manual information should be updated on a regular basis. New resources should be added, as they become available. A footnote at the bottom of each page indicating the date each resource was added or updated is very useful.

CASE STUDY 5-1

Refer to the scenario at the beginning of the chapter and respond to the following.

It is a typically active day at the clinics of Drs. Lewis and King. Despite the three emergencies in the early afternoon and the full schedule of patients, everything is running smoothly with Dr. Lewis, and the entire staff is responding quickly but thoroughly to patient concerns.

At 4:00 PM another emergency patient arrives; at the same time, Jim Marshal, an architect in a downtown firm, comes in early for a routine appointment and demands to be seen immediately. Jim, a regular patient, has a history of being difficult and impatient; being a bit arrogant, he tends to put his needs first. However, Dr. Lewis is occupied with another patient. It is critical to treat the patient with the emergency as soon as possible, and Jim is half an hour early.

Joe Guerrero, CMA (AAMA), the clinic's administrative and clinical medical assistant, calmly asks Mr. Marshal to please wait until his scheduled appointment time. When he threatens to leave, Joe explains to Mr. Marshal that there are two patients ahead of him, but that the provider will see him at his scheduled appointment time.

CASE STUDY REVIEW

1. What communication roadblocks did medical assistant Joe Guerrero avoid in reacting to Jim Marshal's demands to see the provider?

2. With another student, role-play the scenario, with one student taking the role of patient and one student the role of the medical assistant. Identify roadblocks to communication imposed by the patient. How is the medical assistant using the five Cs of communication to deal with the situation?

3. Do you think the medical assistant reacted appropriately? What else could he have done? What should he *not* do in this situation?

CASE STUDY 5-2

You have learned in this chapter that communication has not been successful until the cycle is complete. Consider the following scenario.

An 82-year-old woman with moderate dementia and a hearing impairment is brought to the surgeon's clinic for a follow-up appointment after hip replacement surgery. The woman's daughter accompanies her. The goal of the appointment is to make certain the hip is healing nicely and to discuss precautions before the patient returns to her assisted-living apartment. Almost immediately, the conversation is directed toward the daughter because it is so much easier to explain to her what should be done.

CASE STUDY REVIEW

1. What might the staff do to help the patient understand the following?
   - Use the walker consistently.

- Shoes must be leather, tennis-shoe type, or uniform style; consider Velcro closure as opposed to laces that have to be tied.
- Do not wear pantyhose.
- You will not be able to walk your dog on a leash.

2. Should the patient be left out of the conversation? Should the daughter be included?

3. In cases such as these, is something other than verbal communication indicated?

SUMMARY

Throughout this text you are reminded of the importance of effective communication techniques. Good communication takes practice. Use the techniques identified in this chapter with your family and with your peers. Watch for roadblocks, be aware of defense mechanisms, and remember the five Cs of communication.

STUDY FOR SUCCESS

To reinforce your knowledge and skills of information presented in this chapter:

- Review the *Key Terms*
- Role-play with other students to apply attributes of professionalism pertinent to this chapter.
- Consider the *Case Studies* and discuss your conclusions
- Answer the questions in the *Certification Review*
- Apply your knowledge by completing the *Activities* in the *Study Guide* and the *Games* and *Quizzes* in the StudyWARE **StudyWARE** software on the *Premium Website*
- Perform the Procedure using the Competency Assessment Checklist in the *Competency Manual*
- Practice your problem-solving skills with the *Critical Thinking Challenge 3.0* on the *Premium Website*

Additional Resources for this chapter include:

- Module 5 of the *Medical Assisting Learning Lab*
- *CourseMate for Delmar's Comprehensive Medical Assisting*
- *WebTutor for Delmar's Comprehensive Medical Assisting*

CERTIFICATION REVIEW

1. Factors affecting therapeutic communication include which of the following?
   a. Age
   b. Education and experience barriers
   c. Bias and prejudice barriers
   d. All of the above

2. In the cycle of communication, encoding means:
   a. deciphering a message
   b. creating the message to be sent
   c. sending the message
   d. receiving the message

3. Body language:
   a. is used to express feelings and emotions
   b. is not as important as verbal communication
   c. only makes up 7% of the message
   d. is only used in Eastern cultures

4. A comfortable social space is defined as:
   a. touching to 1½ feet
   b. 1½ feet to 4 feet
   c. 12 to 15 feet
   d. 4 to 12 feet

5. A reassuring cliché is:
   a. a way of calming down a patient
   b. a means of rationalizing a decision
   c. a roadblock to communication
   d. always useful in daily communications

6. Redirecting a socially unacceptable impulse into one that is socially acceptable is an example of which of these defense mechanisms?
   a. Sublimation
   b. Rationalization
   c. Projection
   d. Displacement

7. When using an open-ended question with a patient, we expect:
   a. a yes or no answer
   b. him or her to tell us the truth
   c. a response that permits the patient to elaborate
   d. only the right answers

8. High-context communication relies on all of the following *except*:
   a. body language
   b. reference to environmental objects
   c. explicit and highly detailed language
   d. culturally relevant phraseology

9. Which statement is *true* of kinesics?
   a. The study of body language
   b. The study of personal space
   c. The study of touch
   d. The study of congruency

10. Which statement is the definition of defense mechanisms?
   a. Refusal to accept painful information that is readily available to others
   b. The conscious or subconscious overemphasis of a characteristic to offset a real or imagined deficiency
   c. Behavior used to protect the ego from guilt, anxiety, or loss of esteem
   d. The mind's way of making unacceptable behavior or events acceptable by devising a rational reason

11. Auxiliary aids for patients with audio challenges include all of the following *except*:
   a. sign language interpreters
   b. written materials
   c. large print materials
   d. note takers

12. Indirect statements:
   a. statements that elicit a response without asking a direct question
   b. form of an open-ended question
   c. elicit simple yes/no-type questions
   d. are not considered therapeutic

REFERENCES/BIBLIOGRAPHY

Blair, G. M. (January 23, 2000). *Conversation as communication.* Retrieved June 2, 2010, from http://www.ee.ed.ac.uk/~gerard/Management/art7.html

Iyer, P. W. (Ed.) (2002). *Legal nurse consulting principles and practice.* (2nd ed.) Boca Raton, FL: CRC Press.

Luckmann, J. (2000). *Transcultural communication in health care.* Clifton Park, NY: Delmar Cengage Learning.

National Center for Cultural Competence, Georgetown University Center for Child and Human Development, Georgetown University Medical Center. (Spring/Summer 2004). *Bridging the cultural divide in health care settings: The essential role of cultural broker programs.* Washington, DC: Author.

Taber's cyclopedic medical dictionary. (21st ed.). (2009). Philadelphia: F. A. Davis.

Tamparo, C. D., & Lindh, W. Q. (2008). *Therapeutic communications for health care.* Albany, NY: Delmar Cengage Learning.

http://facstaff.gpc.edu/~dhuntley/Fundamental%20 Conceots%20of%20Nsg%201921/TC%20handout.htm accessed June 2, 2010.

http://www.broksidepress.org/Products/Nursing_Fundamentals_1/lesson_1_Section_2.htm accessed June 2, 2010.

CHAPTER 6

The Therapeutic Approach to the Patient with a Life-Threatening Illness

OUTLINE

Life-Threatening Illness

   Cultural Perspective on Life-Threatening Illness

Choices in Life-Threatening Illness

The Range of Psychological Suffering

The Therapeutic Response to the Patient with HIV/AIDS

The Therapeutic Response to the Patient with Cancer

The Therapeutic Response to the Patient with End-Stage Renal Disease

The Stages of Grief

   Denial

   Anger

   Bargaining

Depression

Acceptance

The Challenge for the Medical Assistant

LEARNING OUTCOMES

1. Define, spell, and pronounce the key terms as presented in the glossary.
2. Recognize possible patient perspectives when facing a life-threatening illness.
3. Define "life-threatening" illness.
4. Critique the cultural manifestations of life-threatening illness.
5. Identify the strongest cultural influence in the life of a patient.
6. List at least four choices to be made when facing a life-threatening illness.
7. Analyze the different forms of living wills and health care directives.
8. Explain how a durable power of attorney for health care is used.

9. Discuss the range of psychological suffering that accompanies life-threatening illnesses.
10. Summarize additional concerns/fears when the life-threatening illness is AIDS, cancer, or end-stage renal disease.
11. Explain the five stages of grief and the meaning of the acronym TEAR.
12. Recall a number of challenges faced by the medical assistant when caring for people with life-threatening illnesses.
13. Analyze the professionalism questions and apply them to this chapter's content.

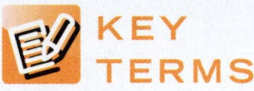

KEY TERMS

durable power
   of attorney for
   health care

health care directive

palliative

psychomotor
   retardation

ATTRIBUTES OF PROFESSIONALISM

Communication

- Did you listen to and acknowledge the patient?
- Did you speak at the patient's level of understanding?
- Did you demonstrate empathy in communication with patients, family, and staff?
- Did you include the patient's support system as indicated?

Presentation

- Did your actions attend to both the psychological and the physiological aspects of the patient's illness or condition?
- Did you attend to any special needs of the patient?
- Were you courteous, patient, and respectful of the patient?
- Did you display a calm, professional, and caring attitude?

Competency

- Were your respectful of others?

Integrity

- Did you demonstrate sensitivity to patient's rights?
- Did you demonstrate respect for individual diversity?
- Did you demonstrate an appreciation for the patient's attitude toward the illness or condition?

SCENARIO

You have seen the medical reports and agonize with your employer who must tell long-time patient Suzanne Markis when she comes in today that she has inoperable pancreatic cancer. When she arrives, you treat her as you normally would, making certain she suspects nothing from you. When she emerges from the provider's room, you make certain to meet her, take her arm, and ask if you can call someone for her. You do not present her with a bill or make another appointment at this time. You recognize that anything you say probably will not be remembered, so you focus entirely on this patient and her immediate needs. In a day or two, as instructed by your employer, you will telephone to make an appointment for Suzanne and anyone she might want present at her next visit with the provider so any questions can be answered.

INTRODUCTION

Everything you learned in Chapter 5 regarding therapeutic communication is heightened and considered more difficult when the patient has a life-threatening illness. If you were told today that your life would probably be shortened because of a serious illness, your perspective would most likely change. What was important yesterday may mean little or nothing now. Something that meant nothing to you yesterday suddenly takes on great importance to you now. It is essential for the medical assistant to remember this difference in perspective and remember what is likely to be important to patients with a life-threatening illness.

It also must be remembered that no two individuals respond to a life-threatening illness in the same way. Some respond with denial and act as if the information had never been shared with them. Others alter their lives radically and drastically change their priorities. Still others quietly continue their lives, changing little outwardly, but recognizing that their choices may now be limited (Figure 6-1).

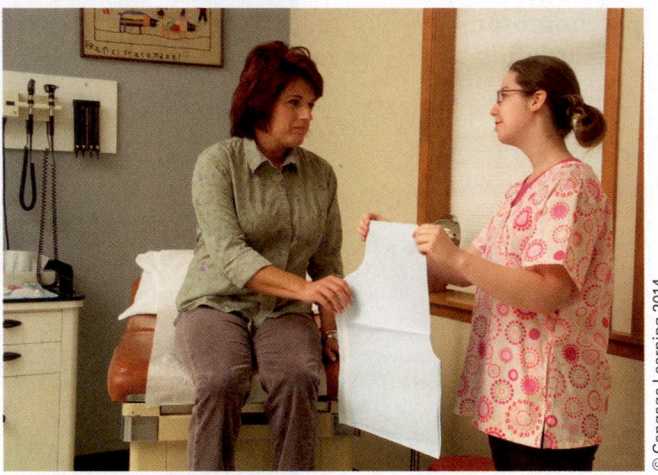

Figure 6-1 Establishing a caring and trusting relationship can help the patient come to terms with a life-threatening illness.

LIFE-THREATENING ILLNESS

A life-threatening illness is not easily defined. Some use the word *terminal*; others refuse to use that word because they believe it removes any hope from the situation. Still others believe even the term *life-threatening* is too hopeless and prefer to use the terms *life-limiting* or *life-altering*. Also, what one individual considers life-threatening may not be the same for another. For our purposes, life-threatening is used to imply a life that in all probability will be shortened because of a serious or debilitating illness or disease. It may be defined as death that is imminent; it may be defined in terms of a serious illness that a person will battle for many years but one that will ultimately shorten his or her life.

Cultural Perspective on Life-Threatening Illness

 Strong cultural manifestations will be seen during the treatment of a life-threatening illness and in anyone facing death. Culture is defined as how we live our lives, how we think, how we speak, and how we behave. Cultures can be accepting, denying, or even defying of death. Death can be considered either as the end of existence or as a transition to another state of being or consciousness. Death can be considered as profane or sacred. In some cultures, a life-threatening illness may be viewed or referred to as a "slow-motion" death because of degenerative diseases that often exhaust the resources and emotions of patients and their families.

SPOTLIGHT ON CERTIFICATION

RMA Content Outline
- Patient relations
- Interpersonal skills
- Develop, assemble, and maintain patient resource materials

CMA (AAMA) Content Outline
- Basic principles (psychology)
- Hereditary, cultural, and environmental influence on behavior
- Communication
- Patient instruction
- Professional communication and behavior
- Medicolegal guidelines and requirements
- Legislation

CMAS Content Outline
- Professionalism
- Patient information and community resources

Some cultures prefer that the life-threatening illness not be shared with the patient in the beginning, but with the family who helps to prepare the patient for the inevitable. A few cultures generally do not seek care for an illness until it is quite advanced; this practice can make pain management and treatment more difficult or impossible in some cases. Some cultures surround the person who is ill with great attention, never leaving the person alone. Other cultures view the illness as something that must be removed from the body, perhaps even believing that the individual has been given this illness because of some past sin or transgression.

Pain is viewed in the same manner. Some cultures believe it is to be endured quietly without complaint; others believe there is to be no pain, and family members will go to great lengths to have health care providers relieve the pain. When questioning a patient about the pain level, it must be within a cultural perspective. For example, cultures with an Asian influence are more likely to describe pain in general terms related to the imbalance of the body rather than in terms such as "piercing, intermittent, or throbbing" or "on a scale from 1 to 10."

The strongest influence in managing any life-threatening illness in the life of the patient is *not* the health care team; it is the family and those closest to the patient. Therefore, great care must be taken to determine and understand the patient's cultural perspective as much as possible, and the patient must be given great respect. Often, the cultural influence may contradict the standard of care preferred by the health care provider. It is better to understand the culture and work within that parameter than to deny it and continually work against the patient's belief system and the influence of family.

CHOICES IN LIFE-THREATENING ILLNESS

Many choices are available to a patient with a life-threatening illness, but there are also many decisions to be made. The urgency of the decisions will depend, in part, on possible life expectancy. Sometimes these decisions may seem contrary to recommended medical intervention.

Patients have the right to choose or to refuse treatment in most cases. Some rush into a treatment protocol only to discover later that their choices have brought them pain, disability, and expense far beyond what originally was assumed. Although it is the health care professional's goal to heal, if healing is not likely or possible, patients ought not to be "urged" into treatment protocols that are likely to be contrary to their personal wishes for the sake of treatment only.

 In fact, there are a number of choices those facing a life-threatening illness might make:

1. **Palliative** care that focuses on quality of life while relieving symptoms of pain and suffering is often requested alongside disease-focused treatment.

2. As stated earlier, patients may choose to forgo any treatment, including medications, transfusions, artificial hydration and feeding, respirators, surgery, chemotherapy, radiation, and dialysis.

3. There is a growing group of individuals who choose not to eat or drink anything by consciously refusing all food and fluids for a more natural death. This choice is referred to as VSED (voluntarily stop eating and drinking) in medical circles.

4. Total sedation may be sought and is used when dying patients experience unbearable suffering and their bodies do not respond to other

treatments. The medication causes unconsciousness and eventually death.

5. In a few states there is the option to seek aid in dying, usually through self-administration of medication prescribed by a personal physician.

Although health care professionals are generally less comfortable with any of these choices and death than they are with saving life, there are some issues appropriate to discuss with patients especially when facing life-threatening illness. Those issues include the following:

1. *Alternative methods of treatment should be discussed, as well as the outcome if no treatment is sought.* At some point, many patients will want to know *all* the treatment protocols that are feasible. This is a logical time to discuss any alternative or integrative medicine therapies that have shown success. Explanations should be made in language that the patient can understand. Illustrations and diagrams can be beneficial. Referrals might be made to integrative medicine practitioners, and patients are to be encouraged to discuss any chosen alternative therapies with their primary care provider. Sometimes treatment alternatives the patient may consider are not within the realm of recognized medical acceptability, but it is better to have that discussion than to ignore the possibility. Patients may also ask what happens if no treatment is chosen. This question can be difficult for health care providers who are anxious to provide some form of treatment for patients, but patients may have a number of reasons not to seek treatment. Remember the earlier statement indicating that family members and friends bring more influence to bear than does the health care professional.

2. *Discussion of pain management and treatment is essential.* The major fears patients have in facing life-threatening illness are pain, loss of self-image, and loss of independence. A frank discussion of pain control and how that can be accomplished can alleviate a fair amount of concern. Loss of self-image is devastating to many. To experience serious gain or loss of weight, loss of mobility, and the inability to perform daily tasks is seen by some as a fate worse than death. Providers will want to be ready to discuss loss of independence related to any life-threatening illness or to make a referral to someone who can be helpful. Patients

have concerns such as wanting to know how long before the disease takes its toll, how long can they drive, what kind of care or assistance will be necessary, whether they can remain in their own home, and how long before they must have someone make decisions for them.

3. *A durable power of attorney for health care or health care proxy allows an individual to make decisions related to health care when the patient is no longer able to do so.* In the best of circumstances, this document will carry out the decisions the patient has already made in some form of a **health care directive** regarding terminal conditions and whether to prolong life. Advances in medicine allow patients' lives to be sustained even when they are unlikely to recover from a persistent and vegetative state. The health care directive and the durable power of attorney for health care allow patients to make decisions before becoming incapacitated on whether life-prolonging medical or surgical procedures are to be continued, withheld, or withdrawn, as well as if or when artificial feeding and fluids are to be used or withheld. These documents can help providers and patients talk about dying and open the door to a positive, caring approach to death. The health care directive and the durable power of attorney for health care documents are legal in all 50 states. Although states may vary somewhat in the wording of these documents, they provide the same overall benefit to patients (see Chapter 7 for more information.) The federal government passed the Patient Self-Determination Act in 1990, which gives all patients receiving care in institutions receiving payments from Medicare and Medicaid written information about their right to accept or refuse medical or surgical treatment. The act also requires that patients be given information about their options to create living wills and to appoint someone to act on their behalf in making health care decisions (durable power of attorney for health care). Any documents of this nature that the patient has should be copied in the medical chart that goes with the patient when admitted to the hospital. At any time the patient makes a change in such a document, the old document is to be replaced with the new one.

4. *Finances are to be considered.* If there is insurance, what will be covered? Who makes the decisions in a managed care environment? What family resources can or will be used?

Finances are no one's favorite subject, especially for providers. However, such a discussion is important. Often, patients fear not being able to meet their financial obligations and leaving large debts to surviving family members almost as much as the life-threatening illness itself. As a medical assistant, you can help patients understand the parameters of their health insurance and any restrictions there might be on particular illnesses or treatments. Can medical insurance be canceled if the patient's employer pays a portion of the health insurance and the patient is no longer able to work? If there is a life insurance policy, help patients determine if any portion of the policy can be used for end-of-life expenses. Any services you can provide to the patient or family members in relieving the financial stress can bring great relief to everyone involved.

5. *Emotional needs of the patient and family members are important.* Emotional support is vital when dealing with a life-threatening illness. Health care professionals will want to determine the source of that support for the patient. Should a support system be suggested for the patient and family members? For some patients and families, an individual giving spiritual guidance is seen as a member of the family and as a member of the health care team. For others, no spiritual influence is recognized or sought.

It is not the responsibility of the health care professionals treating the individual with life-threatening illness to provide all these services, but a health care professional who raises these issues for patients and families to deal with is more closely in tune with a patient's power in the illness.

Life-threatening illnesses are *family* illnesses. There are primary (the person suffering from the illness) and secondary (family and friends) patients. Stress on a spouse or partner is enormous as they think about taking over the other person's role and as they try to deal with their own feelings. Patients and their families and friends often feel angry. The situation is especially tragic if it might have been avoided (for example, a long-time smoker dying of lung cancer). There needs to be time to grieve. Depression is common among patients with life-threatening illness and warning signs should be reported to the provider. Remember that how patients live their last days are just as important as the numbers on the laboratory reports.

THE RANGE OF PSYCHOLOGICAL SUFFERING

The range of suffering associated with a life-threatening illness is extensive. Patients feel extreme distress. Anxiety and depression are common. At the time of diagnosis, patients' responses may include denial, numbness, and an inability to face the facts. Sadness, hopelessness, helplessness, and withdrawal often are exhibited.

The range of psychological suffering often leads to physical symptoms, such as tension, tachycardia, agitation, insomnia, anorexia, and panic attacks. The provider may be so intent on treating the physical ramifications of the illness that the psychological suffering is mostly ignored.

Relationships of individuals with a life-threatening illness often change. Close friends may feel uncomfortable with someone who is dying. Some fear touching or caressing the dying patient and become aloof and distant. However, new friendships can often be made if patients meet others with the same or similar life-threatening issues and help maintain each other's self-esteem. Relationships are important because they provide support and encouragement beyond any other source. Patients experience a loss of self-esteem when they are ill, are in pain, and have a body that is failing them. When self-image is lost, patients feel useless, see themselves as burdens, and have difficulty accepting help from anyone. The psychological effect of this "loss of self" can even hasten death.

It is often helpful to encourage patients to set goals for themselves. These can be small goals such as walking around the block, eating all their dinner, or connecting with a friend. The goals may also be much larger, such as staying alive until a son graduates from college, or putting all financial matters in order for surviving family members. Personal goals give the patient something other than the illness to plan for and work toward.

Carefully listening to patients and seeking clues for what *may not* be said is essential for the medical assistant and support staff caring for patients. Putting yourself in their shoes and asking what would be helpful is often beneficial. Be ready with a list of community resources that may benefit patients at this time.

It is not the intention of this chapter to specifically identify the many life-threatening illnesses and their particular needs. However, three life-threatening illnesses are identified in the following sections along with some specific information (see Chapter 3 for additional information on AIDS and cancer).

THE THERAPEUTIC RESPONSE TO THE PATIENT WITH HIV/AIDS

Patients testing positive for human immunodeficiency virus (HIV) and those with acquired immune deficiency syndrome (AIDS) feel great stress from the infection, the disease, and the fear of other life-threatening illnesses. Some persons with HIV infection may have only a short time before the onset of AIDS; others may have a much longer period. AIDS is a disease that can have many periods of fairly good health and many periods of serious near-death illnesses. Recent developments in the treatment of HIV infection and AIDS help patients to live longer, but their lives are greatly compromised because of their suppressed immune system.

In some cases, guilt develops about past behavior and lifestyles or the possibility of having transmitted the disease to others. Individuals with HIV infection may feel added strain if this is the first knowledge their families have of any high-risk behaviors they have that are associated with the transmission of the disease. When the disease is contracted by individuals who feel they are protected or safe from the disease, anger is paramount. HIV affects mostly individuals who are relatively young. Thus, they are not as likely to have substantial financial resources or permanent housing. Treating HIV is expensive, and many patients have little or no insurance coverage.

Patients with HIV may experience central nervous system involvement. Forgetfulness and poor concentration may be followed by **psychomotor retardation**, or the slowing of physical and mental responses, decreased alertness, apathy, withdrawal, and diminished interest in work. Some patients later experience confusion and progressive impairment of intellectual function or dementia. When HIV-infected patients contract other opportunistic diseases, those symptoms are experienced as well.

THE THERAPEUTIC RESPONSE TO THE PATIENT WITH CANCER

The first reaction patients with cancer usually have is the fear of loss of life. Patients think, "Cancer equals death. Am I going to die?" After that, issues

Complex criteria determine whether a patient's illness is identified as AIDS rather than HIV infection. Some providers prefer not to use the term *AIDS*; rather, they discuss the illness as early or later stage HIV infection. Many providers in the United States and around the world use the term *AIDS* when patients' CD4 counts (healthy T4 lymphocytes) decline to less than 200. (The average healthy individual will have CD4 lymphocyte counts of 800–1,500.) Many developing countries in the world, however, are unable to measure the CD4 counts. AIDS is then diagnosed by the symptoms and any immunodeficient illnesses the patients have. Using only a CD4 count for diagnosis can be quite discouraging for patients who monitor those counts quite closely. Also, a patient's CD4 count can decrease dramatically into the "AIDS zone" one time, and then increase in sufficient numbers to move the patient back into HIV infection another time. Other criteria that may identify an illness as AIDS are a particular type of opportunistic infection or tumor, an AIDS-related brain or lung illness, and severe body wasting. Allied health professionals will need to take the lead from their employers.

begin to differ for each person. A few may choose no treatment and allow life to take its course. Most, however, will wonder about what treatment to choose, how to make that choice, and how effective it will be. Many patients are empowered by taking a major role in the decision making related to their cancer. Research can be helpful in studying the many options that may be available in treatment. The facts are that many patients diagnosed with cancer will die, whereas others diagnosed will live many years after diagnosis and treatment.

The three most likely treatments of cancer are surgery, radiation, and chemotherapy. Often, treatment is a combination of the three. Patients can experience serious side effects from both radiation and chemotherapy. Alternative practitioners have shown that meditation or acupuncture can help relieve the side effects for some patients. Loss of hair, nausea, vomiting, and pain are quite disconcerting to patients trying to cope. The American Cancer Society (http://www.cancer.org) has a number of resources for patients.

CRITICAL THINKING

Many individuals in the end stages of both AIDS and cancer have lost their image of themselves. Their bodies have been diminished; they may have lost a great deal of weight from the disease or gained much weight from the medications taken. They may have no hair. They may have lost their ability to speak or to control bodily functions. What can you do or say to help them feel like a human being?

CRITICAL THINKING

Discuss with a friend what cultural influences might affect each of you if you were facing a life-threatening illness. What choices would each of you make?

The most common signs and symptoms of advanced cancer are weakness, loss of appetite and weight, pain, nausea, constipation, sleepiness or confusion, and shortness of breath. Make certain your patients understand your provider's willingness to relieve and treat these symptoms. Even when there is "nothing more to do" related to the cancer, there is still "much to do" to maintain comfort and to give patients the chance to do the things that are meaningful to them and their families.

THE THERAPEUTIC RESPONSE TO THE PATIENT WITH END-STAGE RENAL DISEASE

Loss of kidney (renal) function leads to a serious illness known as end-stage renal disease (ESRD). When the kidneys fail completely, patients cannot live for long unless they receive dialysis or a kidney transplant. A successful kidney transplant relieves the person of kidney failure. However, there are not enough transplants for every person who needs one, and not all transplants are appropriate or successful. Dialysis is the process of artificially replacing the main functions of the kidneys— filtering blood to remove wastes. Choosing dialysis as a treatment plan can sustain life for years and is covered by Medicare, but it does have complications that burden patients and their caregivers.

Depending on age, a patient's general health, and other circumstances, some patients will opt not to have dialysis and to let death come from kidney failure. The by-products of the body's chemistry accumulate in renal failure and cause an array of symptoms. Mild confusion and disorientation are common. Upsetting hallucinations or agitation can occur. Certain minerals concentrated in the blood can cause muscle twitching, tremors, and shakes.

Some patients experience mild or severe itching. Appetite decreases early, and breathing can be rapid and shallow. Many patients with kidney failure pass little or no urine. Fluid overload results in edema, or swelling of the body, particularly of the legs and abdomen. Patients with some urine output may live for months even after stopping dialysis. People with no urine output are likely to die within a week or two. Patients will lose energy and become sleepy and lethargic. Typically, patients slip into a deeper sleep and gradually lose consciousness. Kidney failure has a reputation for being a gentle death.

THE STAGES OF GRIEF

There are a number of different philosophies on grief and the stages patients are apt to experience when they know their lives are about to end, but none is so widely known as that of Dr. Elisabeth Kübler-Ross, who was one of the first to conduct research and determine possible stages of grief. Those stages are discussed in the following sections.

Denial

This is the stage where patients cannot believe that this is happening. They are likely to experience shock and dismay. If the grief is for the loss of a loved one, it is difficult for them to believe that the loved one is dead. If the grief is for themselves and some incident in their lives, they have a hard time accepting the reality of the loss. Words such as "I can't believe it is true" and "There must be some mistake" are common.

It is difficult to help someone in denial. You may be able to reaffirm the reality of the circumstances, but there is little you can do to move someone from the stage of denial.

Anger

Patients express anger, sometimes openly and assertively. Other times, the anger is turned inward and is difficult to accurately express. Patients ask the question "Why?" and often need explanations of what is occurring. Anger is often expressed to others who have no idea what is happening in patients' lives.

When possible, this type of anger should be realized for what it is and never taken personally. Patients are angry at the event, not at you. Patients can be helped to express the anger in a realistic and nonhurtful manner.

Bargaining

In this stage, patients bargain with God or a higher being and even their providers and express their desire to make a certain milestone in their lives. "If you can just get me through this current crisis so I can make it to my 40th wedding anniversary, I can accept what is happening." Goals can be very helpful to patients, and they can be encouraged to continue to set realistic goals during their grieving.

Depression

Patients who reach this stage are sad and sometimes quiet and withdrawn. There is a feeling that they have given up. They often prefer not to be around anyone. The depression can be and often is treated so that patients' grief is eased somewhat. This is true especially when patients remain in this stage for a very long time.

Acceptance

This is the time that patients accept the loss. If it is death that is being faced, they often feel they are ready. Everything is in place, and peace has been made with the prognosis. If a loss is being suffered, it is the time when patients begin to move on and make other plans for their lives and their future.

Dr. Kübler-Ross reminds health care professionals that while not all patients go through all five stages, some patients go through all five stages over and over again, each time with a little less stress. Others get stuck in one stage, usually denial. Grief and dying are very personal. No two patients will follow the same pattern. Family members also suffer grief and are often in different stages; therefore, it is often difficult for them to communicate and help each other. Remember that grief work is exhausting. So much energy is spent in the grief process that it is often difficult to carry on

day-to-day tasks. Any help that can be made available is appreciated.

The acronym "TEAR" is fairly popular and is often used to describe the grieving process. It has similarities to the five stages of grief:

T: To accept the reality of the loss

E: Experience the pain of the loss

A: Adjust to what was lost

R: Reinvest in a new reality

Although the five stages of grief and the TEAR stages discussed in this chapter are directed toward patients with life-threatening illnesses, remember that the family members and loved ones of patients also will experience grief. Both of these principles can be applied to any kind of serious loss that occurs in one's life—loss of a job, divorce, disaster, war, famine, loss of a limb or important body function, Alzheimer's disease, loss of a friend, or even the death of a beloved pet. The stages of grief and the acronym TEAR can apply just as easily to these situations.

Dr. Kübler-Ross, in her final days before her own death in 2004, reminded her co-author to "Listen to the dying. They will tell you everything you need to know about when they are dying. And it is easy to miss."

THE CHALLENGE FOR THE MEDICAL ASSISTANT

 As a medical assistant, you face the challenge of caring for people with a life-threatening illness; you can comfort those who face great suffering and death. You will become a source of information for patients and their support members. Be sensitive and respectful toward individuals who may be shunned by society. Examine your own beliefs, lifestyle, and biases so that you can be comfortable treating all patients, no matter what the illness is or how it was contracted.

As well as assisting your employer in providing the best possible medical care, you may be required to provide many nonmedical forms of assistance for patients suffering from a life-threatening illness. You may need to make referrals to community-based agencies or service groups. Health departments, social workers, trained hospice volunteers, and AIDS and cancer volunteers may also be helpful to you, your patients, and their families.

The best therapeutic response to the patient with a life-threatening illness will build on the person's own culture and coping abilities, capitalize on strengths, maintain hope, and show continued human care and concern. Patients may want up-to-date information on their disease, its causes, modes of transmission, treatments available, and sources of care and social support. Be prepared to recommend support systems where patients can discuss their feelings and express their concerns. Treat patients with concern and compassion and assure them everything will be done to provide continuity of care and relief from distress. Patients also may be encouraged to call on a spiritual advisor.

CASE STUDY 6-1

Refer to the scenario at the beginning of the chapter. As you prepare for the second visit of Suzanne Markis, you make a mental note of what kind of information you will have available.

CASE STUDY REVIEW

1. What paperwork might be necessary?
2. What questions might you have for Suzanne?
3. What might family members who may accompany Suzanne want to know?
4. As the medical assistant, how does your role differ from that of your employer?

CASE STUDY 6-2

The extended family of Wong Lee is concerned about his illness and his care. Chronic obstructive pulmonary disease (COPD) has ravaged his body. He is on oxygen all the time now. He wants to remain at home to die; his family wants that, too. The family has been with him and has been involved in his care plan all along. However, you are uncertain of how much information to give to members of his extended family when they call.

CASE STUDY REVIEW

1. Are the questions that the extended family members raise intended to harm or help Mr. Lee?
2. Is there a durable power of attorney for health care in place?
3. Which, if any, of the family's desires are related to the culture?
4. What can you and your employer suggest to be of help to everyone involved?

CASE STUDY 6-3

Jeff and Amy live in rural Tennessee. They are expecting their first baby and are excited beyond belief because they had so much trouble getting pregnant. You are the medical assistant for their family practice provider. Test results from their recent ultrasound have been returned to your clinic, and the news is not good. There appears to be some difficulty and one or more apparent birth defects in the developing fetus. You and your employer discuss possible resources.

CASE STUDY REVIEW

1. As the medical assistant, what is your first responsibility to these expectant parents?
2. Where might you look for possible resources?
3. Identify three to five possible resources.
4. If referral to a specialist is to be made, what role might you play in that referral?

SUMMARY

Medical assistants will want to remember that when caring for patients with a life-threatening illness, having even the slightest fear of death can undermine the ability to respond professionally, with empathy and support. If you feel yourself losing the ability to be helpful, it is time to briefly step aside. This does not mean withdrawal from your position or refusal to care for your patients. It means that you do whatever is necessary so that your perspective is not lost. It may mean taking a day off from work to "fill up your psyche" and to give yourself a rest. If the ambulatory care setting has an abundance of patients with life-threatening illnesses, it may require that you spend some time in a support group of your own so that you are better able to cope. Never be afraid to feel sad or weep with your patients. It is better to sense their pain and, at times, feel the pain with them, than it is to be so clinically objective that you miss their true needs.

STUDY FOR SUCCESS

To reinforce your knowledge and skills of information presented in this chapter:

- Review the *Key Terms*
- Role-play with other students to apply attributes of professionalism pertinent to this chapter.
- Consider the *Case Studies* and discuss your conclusions
- Answer the questions in the *Certification Review*
- Apply your knowledge by completing the *Activities* in the *Study Guide* and the *Games and Quizzes* in the StudyWARE StudyWARE software on the *Premium Website*
- Practice your problem-solving skills with the *Critical Thinking Challenge 3.0* on the *Premium Website*

Additional resources for this chapter include:

- *CourseMate for Delmar's Comprehensive Medical Assisting*
- *WebTutor for Delmar's Comprehensive Medical Assisting*

CERTIFICATION REVIEW

1. When a practice treats patients with HIV/AIDS, cancer, or ESRD, it is important for medical assistants to:
   a. warn other patients about the dangers of transmission
   b. segregate these patient reception areas from other patient areas
   c. be supportive and free of prejudice
   d. deny any information to patients regarding the seriousness of the illness

2. The Patient Self-Determination Act:
   a. allows a patient to have a choice of providers
   b. ensures a patient's right to accept or refuse treatment
   c. gives patients the right to formulate advance directives
   d. all of the above
   e. only b and c

3. The strongest influence on a patient with a life-threatening illness is:
   a. the provider
   b. the hospital
   c. the family
   d. the patient

4. Life-threatening illness may be defined as:
   a. a life shortened because of serious illness or disease
   b. death that is imminent
   c. serious illness to battle for many years but may shorten life
   d. all of the above

5. Culture may be defined in part as:
   a. how we choose a friend
   b. how we think and live our lives
   c. how we select a medication
   d. all of the above

6. Therapeutic communication with a patient with a life-threatening illness:
   a. is no different than communicating with any patient
   b. is heightened and considered more difficult
   c. is left to nonmedical support staff
   d. comes naturally and requires no special skill

7. Cultural influence may in part determine:
   a. when/how to involve family members
   b. whether spiritual support is sought
   c. how the illness and its pain are managed
   d. all of the above

8. Durable power of attorney for health care:
   a. enables someone other than the patient to make only health care decisions
   b. enables someone other than the patient to make any decisions for the patient
   c. makes certain that patients' financial responsibilities are met
   d. makes certain an attorney's wishes are followed

9. The confusion, disorientation, and mental deficiency sometimes seen in patients with life-threatening illness:
   a. may make communication difficult or impossible
   b. is a good reason for a durable power of attorney for health care
   c. is made easier if patients expressed earlier their desires in a health care directive
   d. all of the above

10. Effective pain management may depend on:
    a. patient's medical insurance
    b. family wishes and patient's needs
    c. professional nursing criteria
    d. all of the above

REFERENCES/BIBLIOGRAPHY

Compassion & Choices. (2011). How to die in Oregon and across America. Denver, CO.

Kübler-Ross, E., & Kessler, D. (2005). *On grief and grieving.* New York: Scribner.

Lewis, M., Tamparo, C., & Tatro, B. (2012). *Medical law, ethics, and bioethics for the health professions.* Philadelphia: F. A. Davis.

Purnell, L., & Paulanka, B. (2008). *Transcultural health care: A culturally competent approach.* Philadelphia: F. A. Davis.

Tamparo, C., & Lindh, W. (2007). *Therapeutic communications for health care.* Clifton Park, NY: Delmar Cengage Learning.

UNIT III
Responsible Medical Practice

CHAPTER 7
Legal Considerations..106

CHAPTER 8
Ethical Considerations..136

CHAPTER 9
Emergency Procedures and First Aid 156

Legal Considerations

OUTLINE

Sources of Law
  Statutory Law
  Common Law
  Criminal Law
  Civil Law
Administrative Law
  Title VII of the Civil Rights Act
  Equal Pay Act of 1963
  Federal Age Discrimination Act
  Americans with Disabilities Act
  Family and Medical Leave Act
  Health Insurance Portability and Accountability Act
  Occupational Safety and Health Act
  Controlled Substances Act

Uniform Anatomical Gift Act
Regulation Z of the Consumer Protection Act
Medical Practice Acts
Contract Law
  Termination of Contracts
Tort Law
  Standard of Care and Scope of Practice
  Classification of Torts
  Common Torts
Informed Consent
  Implied Consent
  Consent and Legal Incompetence
Risk Management
  Professional Liability Coverage

Civil Litigation Process
  Subpoenas
  Discovery
  Pretrial Conference
  Trial
Statute of Limitations
Public Duties
  Reportable Diseases/Injuries
  Abuse
  Good Samaritan Laws
Advance Directives
  Living Wills/Advance Directives
  Durable Power of Attorney for Health Care
  Patient Self-Determination Act

LEARNING OUTCOMES

1. Define, spell, and pronounce the key terms as presented in the glossary.
2. List and briefly describe the five sources of law.
3. Differentiate between civil and criminal law.
4. Summarize key points of Title VII of the Civil Rights Act.
5. Recall at least seven of the nine administrative law acts important to the medical profession.
6. Outline the implications of HIPAA for the medical assistant.
7. Paraphrase administering, prescribing, and dispensing of controlled substances.
8. Describe the measures to take for disposal of controlled substances.
9. Discuss licensure renewal and revocation for physicians.
10. Outline the differences between expressed and implied contracts.
11. Devise a plan for the three main reasons for a provider/patient contract to be terminated.
12. Follow established policies when initiating or terminating medical treatment.
13. Classify and give examples of torts.
14. Compare/contrast intentional and negligent tort.
15. List and characterize the 4Ds of negligence.
16. Distinguish provider and medical assistant roles in terms of standard of care.
17. Delineate what constitutes battery in the ambulatory care setting.
18. Summarize the two forms of defamation of character and how they might occur.

Continues on page 108

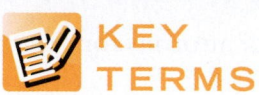

KEY TERMS

administer
administrative law
agent
alternative dispute
   resolution (ADR)
arbitration
civil law
common law
constitutional law
contract law
criminal law
defendant
deposition
discovery
dispense
durable power
   of attorney
   for health care
emancipated minor
expert witness
expressed contract
felony
Health Insurance
   Portability and
   Accountability
   Act (HIPAA)
implied consent
implied contract
incompetence
informed consent
interrogatory
intimate partner
   violence (IPV)
libel
litigation
malfeasance
malpractice
mature minor
mediation
medically indigent

minor
misdemeanor
misfeasance
negligence
noncompliant
nonfeasance

Patient Self-
   Determination
   Act (PSDA)
plaintiff
precedents
prescribe

risk management
slander
statutory law
subpoena
tort
tort law

ATTRIBUTES OF PROFESSIONALISM

Communication
- Did you listen to and acknowledge the patient?
- Did you speak at the patient's level of understanding?
- Did you demonstrate empathy in communicating with patients, family, and staff?
- Did you include the patient's support system as indicated?

Presentation
- Did you do something to bond with the patient?
- Did you attend to any special needs of the patient?
- Were you courteous, patient, and respectful to the patient?
- Did you display a positive attitude?

Competency
- Did you pay attention to detail?
- Did you display sound judgment?
- Did you recognize the importance of local, state, and federal legislation and regulations in the practice setting?
- Did you apply appropriate risk management principles?

Initiative
- Did you show initiative?
- Were you flexible and dependable?
- Were you respectful of others?

Integrity
- Did you work within the scope of your practice?
- Did you demonstrate sensitivity to patient's rights?
- Did you protect personal boundaries?
- Did you demonstrate respect for individual diversity?
- Did you protect and maintain confidentiality?

LEARNING OUTCOMES *(continued)*

19. Recall how medical assistants can help to maintain a patient's privacy.
20. Discuss informed consent and its importance.
21. Classify the types of minors.
22. Evaluate at least 10 practices to help in risk management.
23. Outline the necessary steps in civil litigation and how a medical assistant might be involved.
24. Discuss how and when subpoenas are used.
25. Recall the special considerations for patients related to issues of confidentiality, the statute of limitations, and public duties.

26. Describe procedures to follow in reporting abuse.
27. Discuss Good Samaritan laws.
28. Critique the various forms of advance directives.
29. Recall maintenance of advance directives in the ambulatory care setting.
30. Discuss the durable power of attorney for health care.
31. Analyze the professionalism questions and apply them to this chapter's content.

SCENARIO

Gwen, the office manager in Dr. Gold's clinic, is reviewing legal concerns in a staff meeting. Even though each employee is well aware of privacy, confidentiality, and the many ways their actions are legally binding, Gwen has noticed occasional carelessness creeping into their busy activities. Gwen has heard voices of staff from the hallway discussing confidential matters, has noticed an occasional patient medical history in public view, and wants to review HIPAA compliance.

INTRODUCTION

The law as it relates to health care has grown increasingly complex in the last decade. The agendas of federal and state governments include an investigation of quality health care, a desire to control health care costs (while hoping to ensure equitable access to health care), and an interest in protecting the patient. The Patient Protection and Affordable Care Act of 2010 further added to this complexity. Today's medical assistant must have knowledge of federal, state, and local laws related to health care. A full discussion of health law requires several volumes; therefore, the aim of this chapter is awareness of the law and its implications and establishment of sound practices and procedures to both safeguard patient rights and protect the health care professional.

SOURCES OF LAW

 Law is a binding custom or ruling for conduct that is enforceable by an agency assigned that authority. Laws come from state statutes, common law, both civil and criminal laws, administrative law agencies, and contract and tort law. The highest authority in the United States is the U.S. Constitution. Adopted in 1787, this document provides the framework for the U.S. government. The Constitution includes 27 amendments, 10 of which are known as the Bill of Rights. This authority is sometimes referred to as **constitutional law**. The U.S. Constitution calls for three branches of the federal government:

- *Executive branch.* The president and vice president (elected by U.S. citizens), cabinet officers, and various other departments of the federal government.
- *Legislative branch.* Members of the U.S. Senate and the House of Representatives (elected by U.S. citizens) and the staffs of individual legislators and legislative committees.
- *Judicial branch.* The courts, including the U.S. Supreme Court, courts of appeals for the nine judicial regions, and district courts.

Laws enacted at the federal level are often referred to as acts, laws, or by a specific title. An example is Title XIX of Public Law, the Social Security Act, established in 1967 to provide health care for the **medically indigent**. This program is known as Medicaid. Federal Law is the supreme law of the land.

Statutory Law

The body of laws made by states is known as **statutory law**. Constitutions in the 50 states identify the rights and responsibilities of their citizens and identify how their state is organized. States have a governor as the head and state legislatures (both elected by the state's citizens), as well as their own court systems with a number of levels. All powers that are not conferred specifically on the federal government are retained by the state, yet states vary widely in their interpretation of that power. State law cannot override the power of any laws defined in the U.S. Constitution or its amendments,

although states often attempt to do so. State statutes commonly include practice acts for doctors and nurses. Some identify licensure or certification requirements for medical assistants, also. These practice acts broadly define the scope of practice for the profession as well as licensure and/or certification requirements.

Common Law

Common law is not so easily defined but is essential to understanding law in the United States. Common law was developed by judges in England and France over many centuries and was brought to the United States with the early settlers. Common law is often called judge-made law. The law consists of rulings made by judges who base their decisions on a combination of a number of factors: (1) individual decisions of a court, (2) interpretation of the U.S. Constitution or a particular state constitution, and (3) statutory law. These decisions become known as **precedents** and often lay down the foundation for subsequent legal rulings.

Criminal Law

Criminal law addresses wrongs committed against the welfare and safety of society as a whole. Criminal law affects relationships between individuals and between individuals and the government. Another term that might be used to describe a criminal act is **malfeasance**. Malfeasance is conduct that is illegal or contrary to an official's obligation. Criminal offenses generally are classified into the basic categories of a **felony** or a **misdemeanor** that are specifically defined in statutes.

Felonies are more serious crimes and include murder, larceny or thefts of large amounts of money, assault, and rape. Punishment for a felony is more serious than for a misdemeanor. A convicted felon cannot vote, hold public office, or own any weapons. Felonies often are divided into groups such as first degree (most serious), second degree, and third degree. Sentences are generally for longer than one year and are served in a penitentiary. Misdemeanors are considered lesser offenses and vary from state to state. Punishment may include probation or a time of service to the community, a fine, or a jail sentence in a city or county facility. Misdemeanors also can be divided into groups or classifications, such as A, B, or C class misdemeanors, denoting the seriousness of the crime (Class A is the most serious).

For a person to be found guilty of a crime, a judge or jury must prove the evidence against the individual "beyond a reasonable doubt." In a criminal case, charges are brought against an individual by the state with the intent of preventing any further harm to society. For example, a physician practicing medicine without a proper license may be subject to criminal action by the courts for endangering a patient's life.

Civil Law

Civil law affects relationships between individuals, corporations, government bodies, and other organizations. Terms that may be used in civil law are **misfeasance**, referring to a lawful act that is improperly or unlawfully executed, and **nonfeasance**, referring to the failure to perform an act, official duty, or legal requirement. The punishment for a civil wrong is usually monetary in nature. When a charge is brought against a **defendant** in a civil case, the goal is to reimburse the **plaintiff** or the person bringing charges with a monetary amount for suffering, pain, and any loss of wages. Another goal might be to make certain the defendant is prevented from engaging in similar behavior again. In civil law, cases need to show that a "preponderance of the evidence" is more than likely true against the defendant. The most common forms of civil law that directly affect the medical profession are **administrative law**, **contract law**, and **tort law**.

ADMINISTRATIVE LAW

Administrative law establishes agencies that are given power to specialize and enact regulations that have the force of law. The Internal Revenue Service is an example of an administrative agency that enacts tax laws and regulations. Health care professionals are bound by federal administrative law through the Medicare and Medicaid program rules administered by the Social Security Administration.

There are a number of other regulations in administrative law governing health professionals and their employees. It is important that medical assistants be informed of legislation and any federal or state regulations that are critical to patients and the medical profession. Identified here with a brief description are a number of administrative acts, some of which also are referred to in other chapters in this textbook.

Title VII of the Civil Rights Act

Title VII of the Civil Rights Act of 1964 protects employees from discrimination. The Act states that an employer with 15 or more employees must not discriminate in matters of employment related to age, sex, race, creed, marital status, national origin, color, or disabilities. (Some states are more restrictive in their law and identify employers with eight or more employees.) The Equal Employment Opportunity Commission (EEOC) enforces Title VII and provides oversight of equal employment regulation and policies.

Although some health care settings have fewer than 15 or even 8 employees, it is best to follow state and federal guidelines on all matters of employment.

Currently, 21 states have laws banning employment discrimination because of sexual orientation. Those states are California, Colorado, Connecticut, Delaware, Hawaii, Illinois, Iowa, Maine, Maryland, Massachusetts, Minnesota, Nevada, New Hampshire, New Jersey, New Mexico, New York, Oregon, Rhode Island, Vermont, Washington, and Wisconsin. The District of Columbia passed similar legislation.

Harassment. Included in Title VII is an employee's protection from sexual harassment and a hostile work environment.

Harassment occurs when sexual favors are implied or requested by a supervisor in return for job advancement or special treatment on the job. Another form of harassment and a more common problem that may exist in the workplace is referred to as a "hostile work environment." A hostile work environment exists when pervasive or severe sexual comments, jokes, or inappropriate touching create a workplace so negative that it interferes with an employee's work performance.

A written policy on sexual harassment detailing inappropriate behavior and stating specific steps to be taken to correct an inappropriate situation should be established. The policy will include (1) a statement that harassment is not tolerated, (2) a statement that an employee who feels harassed needs to bring the matter to the immediate attention of a person designated in the policy, (3) a statement about the confidentiality of any incidents and specific disciplinary action against the harasser, and (4) the procedure to follow when harassment occurs.

It is illegal for a supervisor or employer to ignore an employee's complaint. An employer or supervisor who does not take corrective action is liable. The EEOC guidelines make the employer strictly liable for the acts of supervisory employees, as well as for some acts of harassment by coworkers and clients (see Chapter 46).

Equal Pay Act of 1963

Ambulatory health care clinics may not have as much of an issue with this act as some other places of employment, but it is important to note. The Equal Pay Act (EPA) of 1963 protects men and women in the same place of business who perform substantially the same work with substantially equal skill, effort, and responsibility from sex-based wage discrimination. In other words, the starting salary for two medical assistants of the opposite sex is to be the same when they are performing essentially the same job with equal skill and experience under similar working conditions.

Federal Age Discrimination Act

The Federal Age Discrimination in Employment Act of 1967 protects certain individuals 40 years and older from discrimination based on their age in matters of employment, promotion, discharge, compensation, or privileges of employment. This act has become increasingly important as individuals are working longer and seeking employment in their later years. Age restriction may *only* be applied when required by law. For instance, servers of alcohol must be 21 years of age. Valid reasons to decline applicants for employment include (1) health issues that may interfere with the safe and efficient performance of the job, (2) unavailability for the work schedule of the particular job, (3) insufficient training or experience to perform the duties of the particular job, and (4) someone else is better qualified.

Americans with Disabilities Act

The Americans with Disabilities Act (ADA) of 1990 prohibits discrimination preventing individuals who have physical or mental disabilities from accessing public services and accommodations, employment, and telecommunications. A disability implies that a physical or mental impairment substantially limits one or more of an individual's major life activities. ADA is identified in five titles. Title I, enforced by the EEOC, prohibits discrimination in employment (see Chapter 46 for further details). Essentially, Title I requires a potential employer to identify and

prove that certain disabilities cannot be accommodated in performing the job requirements. Employers only have to provide reasonable accommodations rather than anything an employee demands or something that is extraordinarily expensive. Individuals who formerly abused drugs and alcohol and those who are undergoing rehabilitation also are covered by the ADA and cannot be denied employment because of their history of substance abuse.

Titles II, III, and IV mandate disabled individuals' access to public services, public accommodations, and telecommunications. ADA protects persons with HIV infection or AIDS, making certain they cannot be refused treatment by health care professionals because of their health status. Generally speaking, health care professionals with HIV infection or AIDS cannot be kept from providing treatment either, unless that treatment could be found to be a significant risk to others. Title V covers a number of miscellaneous issues such as exclusions from the definition of "disability," retaliation, insurance, and other issues. Again, the ADA applies to businesses with at least 15 employees, but some states have more stringent laws.

Family and Medical Leave Act

The Family and Medical Leave Act (FMLA) of 1993 is important for large ambulatory care centers and hospitals. FMLA requires all public employers and any private employer of 50 or more employees to provide up to 12 weeks of job-protected, unpaid leave each year for the following reasons: (1) birth and care of the employee's child, or placement for adoption or foster care of a child; (2) care of an immediate family member who has a serious health condition; and (3) care of the employee's own serious health issue. Employees must have been employed for at least 12 months and have worked at least 1,250 hours in the 12 months preceding the beginning of the FMLA leave.

CRITICAL THINKING

Using the Internet, determine if or when a medical clinic might be required to follow the federal guidelines of the Family and Medical Leave Act (FMLA). Identify reasons to follow the FMLA guidelines even if not required by federal law.

Health Insurance Portability and Accountability Act

HIPAA The **Health Insurance Portability and Accountability Act (HIPAA)** of 1996 required the Department of Health and Human Services to adopt national standards for electronic health care transactions. The law also required the adoption of privacy and security standards to protect an individual's identifiable health information. This mandate required greater protection of a patient's protected health information (PHI). The privacy of telephone conversations, all verbal exchanges, and all written data regarding a patient must be assured. The goal of HIPAA was also to assist in making health insurance more affordable and accessible to individuals by protecting health insurance coverage for workers and their families when they change or lose their jobs.

HIPAA law is identified in seven titles. They are summarized briefly as follows:

I. Health Insurance Access, Portability, and Renewal: Increases the portability of health insurance, allows continuance and transfer of insurance even with preexisting conditions, and prohibits discrimination based on health status.

II. Preventing Health Care Fraud and Abuse: Establishes a fraud and abuse system and spells out penalty if either event is documented; improves the Medicare program through establishing standards; establishes standards for electronic transmission of health information.

III. Tax-Related Provisions: Promotes the use of medical savings accounts (MSAs) used for medical expenses only. Deposits are tax-deductible for self-employed individuals who are able to draw on the accounts for medical expenses.

IV. Group Health Plan Requirements: Identifies how group health care plans must provide for portability, access, and transferability of health insurance for its members.

V. Revenue Offsets: Details how HIPAA changed the Internal Revenue Code to generate more revenue for HIPAA expenses.

VI. General Provisions: Explains how coordination with Medicare-type plans must be carried out to prevent duplication of coverage.

VII. Assuring Portability: Ensures employee coverage from one plan to another; written specifically for health insurance plans to ensure portability of coverage.

As of April 21, 2006, all covered health care entities were required to be in compliance of HIPAA's privacy regulations. These regulations originally caused concern among providers. However, once the electronic codes and transactions for electronic filing of health insurance claims were identified and put in place, the required security and privacy of all patient information was not so complex.

Government and industry are allocating billions of dollars into electronic medical records software and the transfer of the paper medical record to the digitized format. (See IV above.) Federal stimulus money was approved in 2009 to help underwrite the cost to clinics or hospitals that serve Medicare and Medicaid patients when their electronic medical records software meets the required standards for sharing information between proprietary networks. Strings attached to the funding are designed to create a wider access to medical records. The goal is to make a patient's chronic health care issues, acute incidents, family history, and prescriptions only a click away for providers giving treatment.

Occupational Safety and Health Act

The Occupational Safety and Health (OSH) Act of 1967 is a division of the U.S. Department of Labor. Its mission is to ensure that a workplace is safe and has a healthy environment. Penalties assessed by OSHA can be quite high for repeated and willful violations. (OSH Act refers to the actual law, while OSHA refers to the administration or group of individuals who oversee and govern the law.) Among these guidelines are those that make certain all employees know what chemicals they are handling, know how to reduce any health risks from hazardous chemicals that are labeled 1 to 4 for severity, and have Material Safety Data Sheets (MSDSs) listing every ingredient in the product. Other sections of this law protecting medical assistants and patients are detailed in additional chapters. They include the Clinical Lab Improvement Amendments of 1988 (CLIA) (see Chapter 38), the Bloodborne Pathogens Standard of July 1992 (see Chapter 22), and the Needlestick Prevention Amendment of 2001 (see Chapter 22).

Controlled Substances Act

The Controlled Substances Act of 1970 became effective in 1971. The act is administered by the Drug Enforcement Administration (DEA) under

CRITICAL THINKING

Identify the types of providers or medical specialties most likely to administer and dispense as well as prescribe controlled substances.

CRITICAL THINKING

Research the DEA website to determine the steps required to dispose of contaminated or outdated Schedule II drugs.

the auspices of the U.S. Department of Justice. The Controlled Substances Act lists controlled drugs in five schedules (I, II, III, IV, and V) according to their potential for abuse and dependence, with Schedule I having the greatest abuse potential and no accepted medical use in the United States. This act and the U.S. Code of Federal Regulations regulate individuals who **administer**, **prescribe**, or **dispense** any drug listed in the five schedules. Any individual who administers, prescribes, or dispenses any controlled substance must be registered with the DEA. The DEA supplies a form for registration and mandates that renewal occurs every 3 years.

A provider who only prescribes Schedule II, III, IV, and V controlled substances in the lawful course of professional practice is not required to keep separate records of those transactions. The majority of all providers fall within this category. Providers who regularly administer controlled substances in Schedules II, III, IV, and V or who dispense controlled substances are required to keep specific records of each transaction.

For those providers who dispense or administer controlled substances, an inventory must be taken every 2 years of all stocks of any controlled substances on hand. The inventory must include (1) a list of the name, address, and DEA registration number of the provider; (2) the date and time of the inventory; and (3) the signatures of the individuals taking the inventory. This inventory must be kept at the location identified on the registration certificate for at least 2 years. All Schedule II drug records must be maintained separate from all other controlled substance records. These records must be made available for inspection and copying by duly authorized officials of the DEA. Some states are even more restrictive than the federal requirements.

Any necessary disposal of controlled substances, usually occurring when they become outdated or when a medical practice is closed, requires specific action. The provider's DEA number and registration certificate should be returned to the DEA. Specific guidelines for destruction

of the controlled substances will need to be obtained from the nearest divisional office for the DEA. Using the Internet, search using the words "Controlled Substances Act of 1970" for a listing of sites providing more information. You will find a listing of drugs in each of the five schedules that changes from time to time as new drugs come on the market and are classified. (See Chapter 35 for additional details.)

Uniform Anatomical Gift Act

The Uniform Anatomical Gift Act of 1968 allows persons 18 years and older and of sound mind to make a gift of all or any part of their body (1) to any hospital, surgeon, or physician; (2) to any accredited medical or dental school, college, or university; (3) to any organ bank or storage facility; and (4) to any specified individual for education, research, advancement of medical/dental science, therapy, or transplantation. The gift may be noted in a will or by signing, in the presence of two witnesses, a donor's card. Some states allow these statements on the driver's license. There is no cost to donors or their families for gifts of all or part of the body, and there is a great need for organ donors in this country.

Regulation Z of the Consumer Protection Act

Regulation Z of the Consumer Protection Act of 1967, referred to as the Truth in Lending Act, requires that an agreement by providers and their patients for payment of medical bills in more than four installments must be in writing and must provide information on any finance charge (see Chapter 20). This act is enforced by the Federal Trade Commission. These guidelines are often seen in fee-for-service plans in prearrangements for surgery or prenatal care and delivery, because patients may not be able to pay the entire fee in one payment.

Medical Practice Acts

Each state has medical practice acts that regulate the practice of medicine with the intent of protecting its citizens from harm. These statutes govern licensure, standards of care, professional liability and negligence, confidentiality, and torts. Table 7-1 summarizes licensure, renewal, and revocation rules for medical doctors. Medical assistants sometimes are asked to maintain their employer's records of continuing education for license renewal and to process the renewal at the proper time. In some states, the renewal may be done online if the license is active and in good standing.

States also may regulate personnel who are employed in the ambulatory care setting. Generally, medical assistants perform their duties and responsibilities under the direct supervision of the physician or doctor, and therefore are governed by medical practice acts or the state board of medical examiners. Medical assistants employed and supervised by independent nurse practitioners are governed by the nurse practice acts and the state board of nursing. Other health professionals, such as chiropractors and naturopaths, may have separate practice acts as well. Medical assistants employed by these practitioners will need to be knowledgeable of those laws. Some states require that medical assistants be licensed or certified to perform any invasive procedures. Other states require additional education and training in radiology for the medical assistant to be able to take

Table 7-1   Licensure, Renewal, and Revocation for Medical Doctors

Licensure	Renewal	Revocation
Completion of medical education	Payment of a fee	Conviction of a crime
Completion of internship	Documentation of continuing medical education (CME)	Unprofessional conduct
Passing the U.S. Medical Licensing Examination (USMLE)	CMEs might include appropriate medical reading, teaching health professionals, and attending conferences and workshops	Personal or professional incapacity

© Cengage Learning 2014.

radiographs. Furthermore, there are still a few states so strict in their regulations that medical assistants mostly perform clerical functions and noninvasive clinical duties.

  Certainly, medical assistants desiring to use their skills must be aware of state regulations and always perform only within the scope of those regulations as well as their education and professional preparation. Medical assistants will want to be as diligent as any other health professional about maintaining their certification, registration, and licensure and should monitor any legislation that pertains to licensure or certification.

CONTRACT LAW

The contractual nature of the provider-patient relationship necessitates a discussion of contracts, which are an important part of any medical practice. A contract is a binding agreement between two or more persons. A provider has a legal obligation, or duty, to care for a patient under the principles of contract law. The agreement must be between competent persons to do or not to do something lawful in exchange for a payment.

A contract exists when the patient arrives for treatment and the provider accepts the patient by providing treatment. An example of a valid contract occurs when a patient calls the office or clinic to make an appointment for an annual physical examination. Assuming both provider and patient are competent, and that the provider performs the lawful act of the physical examination and the patient pays a fee, all aspects of the contract exist.

There are two types of contracts: expressed and implied. An **expressed contract** can be written or verbal and specifically describes what each party in the contract will do. A written contract requires that all necessary aspects of the agreement be in writing. Examples of a written contract in the medical environment include a third party's agreement to pay a patient's bill, or the contract between a patient and the provider indicating a bill can be paid in four or more installments. An **implied contract** is indicated by actions, even silence, rather than by words. The majority of provider-patient contracts are implied contracts. It is not required that the contract be written to be enforceable as long as all points of the contract exist. An implied contract can exist either by the circumstances of the situation or by the law. When a patient reports a sore throat and the provider takes a swab for a throat culture to diagnose and treat the ailment, an implied contract exists by the circumstances. An implied contract by law exists when a patient goes into anaphylactic shock and the provider administers epinephrine to counteract shock symptoms. The law says that the provider did what the patient would have requested had there been an expressed contract.

For a contract to be valid and binding, the parties who enter into it must be competent; therefore, the mentally incompetent, the legally insane, individuals under heavy drug or alcohol influences, infants, and some minors cannot enter into a binding contract.

Medical assistants are considered **agents** of the employers they serve, and as such must be cautious that their actions and words may become a binding contract for their employers. For example, to say that the provider can cure the patient may cause serious legal problems when, in fact, a cure may not be possible.

Termination of Contracts

A broken contract or breach of contract occurs when one of the parties does not meet contractual obligations. A provider is legally bound to treat a patient until:

- The patient discharges the provider
- The provider formally withdraws from patient care
- The patient no longer needs treatment and is formally discharged by the provider

Patient Discharges Provider.
When the patient discharges the provider, a letter should be sent to the patient to confirm and document the termination of the contract. The notice is sent by certified mail with return receipt requested. Keep a copy of the letter in the patient's record (Figure 7-1).

Provider Formally Withdraws from the Case.
To avoid any charges of abandonment, the provider should formally withdraw from the case when, for example, the patient becomes **noncompliant** or the provider feels the patient can no longer be served. Again, notice should be sent to the patient by certified mail with return receipt requested, and a copy of the notice should be filed in the patient's record (Figure 7-2 and Figure 7-3).

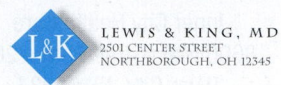

LEWIS & KING, MD
2501 CENTER STREET
NORTHBOROUGH, OH 12345

January 6, 20XX

CERTIFIED MAIL

Jim Marshal
76 Georgia Avenue
Millerton, TX 43912

Dear Mr. Marshal:

This will confirm our telephone conversation today in which you discharged me as your attending physician in your present illness. In my opinion your condition requires continued medical supervision by a physician. If you have not already done so, I suggest that you employ another physician without delay.

You may be assured that after receiving a written request from you, I will furnish the physician of your choice with information regarding the diagnosis and treatment which you have received from me.

Very truly yours,

Winston Lewis

Winston Lewis, MD
WL:ea

© Cengage Learning 2014

Figure 7-1 Letter confirming a physician's discharge by the patient.

The Patient No Longer Needs Treatment.
Unless a formal discharge or withdrawal has occurred, a provider is obligated to care for a patient until the patient's condition no longer requires treatment.

TORT LAW

A **tort** is a wrongful act, other than a breach of contract, resulting in injury to one person by another.

Standard of Care and Scope of Practice

To better understand torts, we must consider the standard of care and the four Ds of negligence. All health care providers have the responsibility and duty to perform within their scope of training and to always do what any reasonable and prudent health care professional in the same specialty or general field of practice

Inner City Health Care
8600 Main Street, Suite 200
River City, NY 01234

May 9, 20XX

CERTIFIED MAIL

Lenny Taylor
260 Second Street
River City, NY 01234

Dear Mr. Taylor:

You will recall that we discussed our professional relationship in my office on May 6, 20XX.

Your son, George Taylor, and Bruce Goldman, my medical assistant, were also present. As you know, the primary difficulty has been your failure to cooperate with the medical plan for your care.

While it is unfortunate that our relationship has reached this stage, I will no longer be able to serve as your physician. I will be available to you on an emergency basis only until June 10, 20XX. Meanwhile, you should immediately call or write the Medical Society, 123 Omega Drive, Carlton, MI 11666, Tel. 123-456-7899 and obtain a list of providers. Any delay could jeopardize your health, so please act quickly.

Your physical (and/or mental) problems include hypertensive heart disease, decreased kidney function, and arteriosclerosis. You could have additional medical problems that may also require professional care. Once you have found a new provider have him or her call my office. I will be happy to discuss your case with the provider assuming your care and will transfer a written summary of your case upon the receipt of a written request from you to do so.

Thank you for your anticipated cooperation and courtesy.

Very truly yours,

James Lewis

James Lewis, MD
JL:kr

© Cengage Learning 2014

Figure 7-2   Letter reiterating "for the record" the osteopath's decision to withdraw from the case discussed during a previous meeting with patient.

Inner City Health Care
8600 Main Street, Suite 200
River City, NY 01234

December 5, 20XX

CERTIFIED MAIL

Rhoda Au
41 Academy Road
River City, NY 01234

Dear Ms. Au:

I find it necessary to inform you that I am withdrawing further professional medical service to you because of your persistent refusal to follow my medical advice and treatment.

Because your condition requires medical attention, I suggest that you place yourself under the care of another provider without delay. If you so desire, I shall be available to attend you for a reasonable time after you have received this letter, but in no event later than January 7, 20XX. This should give you sufficient time to select someone from the many competent practitioners in this area.

You may be assured that, upon receiving your written request, I will make available to the provider of your choice your case history and information regarding the diagnosis and treatment that you have received from me.

Very truly yours,

Mark King

Mark King, MD
MK:kr

© Cengage Learning 2014

Figure 7-3   Letter notifying patient of provider's withdrawal from the case.

would exercise in similar circumstances. Negligence occurs when someone experiences injury because of another's failure to live up to a required duty of care. This is a primary cause of malpractice suits. **Malpractice** is professional negligence or the failure of a medical professional to perform the duty required of the position, causing injury to another.

Four Ds of Negligence. The four elements of negligence, sometimes called the "4 Ds," are:

1. *Duty.* Duty of care
2. *Derelict.* Breach of the duty of care
3. *Direct cause.* A legally recognizable injury occurs as a result of the breach of duty of care
4. *Damage.* Wrongful activity must have caused the injury or harm that occurred

would do. That is what is expected of every provider when a contact is made by a patient. Failure to do what any reasonable and prudent health care professional would do in the same set of circumstances can be seen as a breach of the standard of care.

Negligence is defined as the failure to exercise the standard of care that a reasonable person

If an individual has knowledge, skill, or intelligence superior to that of a layperson, that individual's conduct must be consistent with that status. For instance, medical assistants are held to a high standard of care by virtue of their skills, knowledge, and intelligence. As professionals, medical assistants are required to have a standard minimum level of special knowledge and ability. This is what is known as "duty of care."

The Medical Assistant's Role in Negligence.

Medical assistants must be certain to recall the 4 Ds of Negligence and the standard of care required of their profession at all times. The first rule is to remember to *always* practice within the scope of one's instruction and education. The second rule is to remember that each state is likely different in what is included in the medical assistants' scope of practice. Understanding and performing within that scope of practice is essential.

Medical assistants may commit a tort that can result in **litigation**. When it can be proven that the injury resulted from the medical assistant (or other health care professional) not meeting the standard of care governing their respective professions, then litigation is a possibility. If, however, the medical assistant (or other health care professional) commits a wrongful act but the patient experiences no injury or harm, then no tort exists. For example, if the medical assistant changes a wound dressing, breaks sterile technique, and the patient suffers a severely infected wound, the medical assistant has committed a tort and can be held liable to any legal action taken. In contrast, if the medical assistant changes a wound dressing, breaks sterile technique, and the patient's wound does not become infected, no harm has occurred, and a tort does not exist. If a medical assistant fails to report to the provider an abnormal result on a blood test that prevents the provider from making an early diagnosis of a disease, the assistant's omission of an act has caused a breach in the standard of care.

CRITICAL THINKING

Identify the scope of practice for a medical assistant in your state and explain how this affects the practice in the ambulatory care setting.

Classification of Torts

There are two major classifications of torts: *intentional* and *negligent*. Intentional torts are deliberate acts of violation of another's rights. Negligent torts are not deliberate and are the result of omission and commission of an act. Malpractice is the unintentional tort of professional negligence; that is, a professional either failed to act in a reasonable and prudent manner and caused harm to the patient, or did what a reasonable and prudent person would not have done that caused harm to a patient.

There are two Latin terms that can be used to describe aspects of negligence. These are known as doctrines. *Res ipsa loquitur,* or "the thing speaks for itself," is the term used in cases that involve situations such as a nick made in the bladder when the surgeon is performing a hysterectomy. The negligence is obvious. The other doctrine, *respondeat superior*, or "let the master answer," expresses that providers are responsible for their employees' actions. If a medical assistant violates the standard of care, therein lies the basis for a suit of medical malpractice. For example, the medical assistant used the incorrect solution to clean the patient's wound and the patient sustained injuries to the wound. The provider-employer can be sued under the doctrine of *respondeat superior* because the provider-employer is responsible for the acts of employees committed in the scope of their employment. The medical assistant also can be sued because individuals are responsible for their own actions.

Common Torts

Some common areas of negligence may result in torts when adherence to the standard of care has not been fulfilled. Specific examples of common torts that can occur in the office or clinic are *battery, defamation of character,* and *invasion of privacy.*

Battery.

The basis of the tort of battery is unprivileged touching of one person by another. A patient must consent to being touched. When a procedure is to be performed on a patient, the patient must give consent in full knowledge of all the facts. It does not matter whether the procedure that constitutes the battery improves the patient's health. Patients have the right to withdraw consent at any time.

One example of battery is when a medical assistant insists on giving the patient an injection that was ordered for the patient even though the patient refuses the injection. Another example can be seen when a surgeon performs additional surgery beyond the original procedure (the surgeon performed a hysterectomy, for which consent was given, but is liable for battery for removing a suspicious looking abdominal nevus from the patient's abdomen without consent). It does not matter that the surgeon does not charge for the additional procedure. It also does not matter if the patient would have given consent if asked in advance.

Defamation of Character. The tort of defamation of character consists of injury to another person's reputation, name, or character through spoken or written words for which damages can be recovered. Two kinds of defamation are **libel** and **slander**. Libel is false and malicious writing about another, such as in published materials, pictures, and media. An example can be seen when the medical assistant writes in the patient's record, "Mr. O'Keefe's wife and her negative attitude appear to be the cause of his ulcer." A copy of Mr. O'Keefe's records were later sent to a new provider, who reviewed the record and read the remarks quoted by the medical assistant.

Slander is false and malicious spoken words. Slander can be seen in the following comment directed by a patient to the provider, "Dr. Woo is incompetent. He should have his license revoked." The statement is overheard by the clinic administrative medical assistant and other patients waiting in the reception area.

For a tort of defamation of character (either libel or slander) to exist, a third party must see or hear the words and understand their meaning.

Invasion of Privacy. Invasion of privacy is another kind of tort. It includes unauthorized publicity of patient information, medical records being released without the patient's knowledge and permission, and patients receiving unwanted publicity and exposure to public view. For example, if a minor unmarried girl has been examined for possible pregnancy, and the medical assistant telephones the girl's home and inadvertently gives the laboratory results to someone other than the patient, her privacy has been invaded. A second situation exists when persons other than those providing care and performing examinations and procedures (essential or nonessential personnel) are allowed to be present without the patient's consent. Yet another example of the patient's right to privacy being violated is when the patient is asked to walk from the examination room across the hall to a treatment room while wearing only a patient gown in full view of other patients and personnel.

 Medical assistants and other health care professionals should:

- Close a door, pull a curtain, or provide a screen when looking at, handling, or examining the patient
- Expose only body parts necessary for treatment (drape the patient, exposing only the part that is being treated)
- Discuss the patient with no one except those individuals involved in the patient's care, and then discuss only those aspects of care that relate to the needs of the patient

It is not an invasion of privacy to disclose information required by a court order, subpoena, or by statute to protect the public health and welfare, as in the reporting of violent crime.

INFORMED CONSENT

Documentation of **informed consent** becomes an important part of the patient care process. Every patient has a right to know and understand any procedure to be performed. The patient is to be told in language easily understood:

- The nature of any procedure and how it is to be performed
- Any possible risks involved, as well as expected outcomes of the procedure
- Any other methods of treatment and the risks they involve
- Risks if no treatment is given

It is the responsibility of the health care provider to make certain the patient understands. If an interpreter is necessary, the provider must procure one.

Often, consent forms will be signed if there is to be a surgical or invasive procedure performed (Figure 7-4). The medical assistant may be asked to witness the patient's signature and may be expected to follow through on any of the provider's instructions or explanations, but is not expected to explain the procedure to the patient. The signed consent form is kept with the medical record, and a copy also is given to the patient.

Increasingly, providers who perform invasive procedures on a regular basis (i.e., surgeons, dermatologists, etc.) use video to further explain the procedure(s) to be performed. Some formal consent forms ask patients to explain in their own

CONSENT TO
OPERATION, ADMINISTRATION OF ANESTHETICS AND
RENDERING OF OTHER MEDICAL SERVICES

1. I hereby authorize and direct Dr. _____, my physician, and

    whomever he/she designates as his/her assistants (associates and/or resident physicians), to perform upon

    (state name of patient or myself) _____

    The following procedures: _____

    _____

    _____

    If any unforeseen condition arises in the course of this operation for the physician's judgment to perform procedures in addition to or different from those now contemplated, I further request and authorize him/her to do whatever he/she deems advisable and necessary in these circumstances. Such additional services may include, but are not limited to, the administration and maintenance of anesthesia and the performance of services involving pathology and radiology.

2. The following information has been explained to me to the degree that I wish to have it discussed:
    *   The nature and character of the proposed treatment or procedure;
    *   The anticipated results;
    *   Possible recognized alternative methods of treatment, including non-treatment;
    *   Recognized serious possible risks, complications, and anticipated benefits involved in proposed and alternative treatments, including non-treatment.

    My questions have been answered to my satisfaction. I acknowledge that no guarantee, warrantee, or assurance has been made as to the results or cure that may be obtained.

3. Federal Regulations (21 CFR Part 821) require manufacturers to track certain medical devices, and assist the U.S. Food and Drug Administration (FDA) with notification to individuals in the event that a certain medical device presents serious health risks. I authorize and agree to the release of my contact information to the manufacturer: _____ for this tracking purpose only. I understand that the manufacturer may notify me, if necessary, of important safety information about my medical device, and may release my information to the FDA if ordered to do so. I understand that this consent is valid for the life of the medical device.

    Any sections below that do not apply to the proposed treatment may be crossed out. The patient must initial any section crossed out.

4. I consent to the administration of blood and blood products if deemed medically necessary. I understand that all blood and blood products involve the risk of allergic reaction, fever, hives, and in rare circumstances infectious diseases such as hepatitis and HIV/AIDS. I understand that precautions are taken by the blood bank in screening donors and in matching blood for transfusion to minimize those risks.

5. I hereby consent to the disposal or use for research purposes any tissues, parts, or products of conception, which may be removed.

6. I authorize and agree to the presence of observers during my surgical procedure. These observers may include persons other than the medical staff that are considered appropriate by my health care provider during my care and treatment. The purpose of these individuals observing would be for instruction and medical study.

I certify that I have read this form and understand its contents.

PATIENT NAME & ID #	
	_____
	Signature of Patient or Legally Responsible Party
	_____
	Relationship to patient, if not signed by patient
	_____
	Signature of Witness
	_____
	Printed Name of Witness
	Date _____ Time _____ a.m. / p.m.

MRD: HOSP1
DISTRIBUTION: 1-**WHITE** – CHART   2-**CANARY** – PATIENT COPY

© Cengage Learning 2014

Figure 7-4   Model formal consent for treatment form.

words the procedure to be performed. The explanation given serves as a measure of the patient's understanding of the process.

Implied Consent

Two circumstances related to consent are worth mentioning at this point. **Implied consent** occurs when there is a life-threatening emergency, or when the patient is unconscious or unable to respond. The provider, by law, is allowed to give treatment within his or her scope of practice without a signed consent. Implied consent also occurs in more subtle ways. For example, the patient who rolls up a shirtsleeve for the medical assistant to take a blood pressure reading is implying consent to the procedure by the action taken.

Consent and Legal Incompetence

Consent for treatment is not valid if the patient is legally incompetent to give consent. Legal **incompetence** means that a patient is found by a court to be insane, inadequate, or to not be an adult. In such instances, consent must be obtained from a parent, a legal guardian, or the court on behalf of the patient. Consent for treatment can be given only by the natural parent or legal guardian as determined by the court for a **minor** child. A minor is a person who has not reached the age of majority (18–21 years old), depending on the laws of each state. Generally, a minor is considered unable to give effective consent for medical treatment; therefore, without proper consent from parents or guardians, medical professionals can be held liable for battery if medical treatment is given. Exceptions to this rule are in cases of emergency and for mature and emancipated minors. **Emancipated minors** are minors younger than 18 years who are free of parental care and are financially responsible, married, become parents, or join the armed forces. **Mature minors** are persons, usually younger than 18 years, who are able to understand and appreciate the nature and consequences of treatment despite their young age. Nearly every state allows minors to give consent for treatment for pregnancy, drug or alcohol addiction, and sexually transmitted disease. Some states have passed legislation that name minors as statutory adults at 14 years old for the purpose of receiving medical care. In these states, minors may consent and be protected by confidentiality and privacy even though their parents or legal guardians may still be financially responsible for their medical bills.

Questions related to the ability of minors and emancipated minors to give consent often must be determined on a case-by-case basis because state statutes vary. Placing a telephone call to the state attorney general's office can help clarify issues, questions, and concerns that involve consent and treatment of minors.

RISK MANAGEMENT

Practicing good **risk management** makes the medical assistant and the provider-employer less vulnerable to litigation.

Following are some ways to avoid incidents that may lead to litigation:

- Perform only within the scope of your training and education.
- Comply with all state and federal regulations and statutes.
- Keep the clinic safe and equipment in readiness.
- Never leave a patient unattended; if you must leave, pass the responsibility for the patient's care on to another individual.
- Keep all patient information confidential.
- Follow all policies and procedures established for the clinic.
- Document fully only facts; formally document withdrawing from a case and discharging patients.
- Log telephone calls and return calls to patients within a reasonable time frame.
- Follow up on missed or canceled appointments.
- Never guarantee a cure or diagnosis, and never advise treatment without a provider's order.
- Secure informed consent as necessary.
- Do not criticize other practitioners.
- Explain any appointment delays.
- Be particularly watchful with patients who have special needs, such as the elderly, pediatric patients, and those with physical and emotional disabilities.
- Report any error that may have occurred to your employer.

CRITICAL THINKING

Identify the suggestions in the previous risk management list that are most likely not performed if the staff in the ambulatory care setting find themselves overworked, overwhelmed, and behind. What might be done to prevent carelessness brought on by such circumstances?

Professional Liability Coverage

Providers commonly carry professional liability insurance coverage in order to cover the costs of any litigation that may occur. In today's health care climate, there is a great deal of discussion regarding the cost of such insurance and the dollar amounts of awards being made to plaintiffs. While not recommended, some providers are doing without professional liability coverage and notifying their patients of such action. Others have chosen to limit their practice to procedures that are not high risk. For instance, a family practice provider may choose not to deliver babies because of the high cost of professional liability coverage for deliveries.

Health care employees need their own professional liability coverage. While litigation activities may seek out the "highest-paid" individual to sue, employees can be and are sued quite regularly. Medical assistants can purchase professional liability coverage from the American Association of Medical Assistants (AAMA). Such insurance is designed to help protect personal assets from being taken in order to cover any judgment awarded the plaintiff.

CIVIL LITIGATION PROCESS

Despite all the best efforts of health care professionals and their employees, litigation can occur. Litigation is the process of taking a lawsuit or a criminal case through the courts. It is helpful to understand the steps taken for civil litigation to occur. The greatest amount of any litigation seen in the ambulatory care setting occurs when relationships between individuals break down for one reason or another. When this happens, the party, or plaintiff, bringing the action, usually a patient, seeks an attorney who agrees to bring the complaint to the courts. The provider, or defendant, is summoned to court.

This summons or subpoena notifies the provider of the plaintiff's suit and allows the defendant to file an answer with the court.

Subpoenas

The **subpoena** is an order from the court naming the specific date, time, and reason to appear. A portion of a medical record or the entire medical record may be subpoenaed, the health care provider may be subpoenaed to testify in court, or both the medical record and the provider may be subpoenaed (*subpoena duces tecum*). The staff in the ambulatory care setting usually will have ample time to make certain the record is current and complete before its inclusion in court. Out of courtesy, a provider will notify patients whose records have been subpoenaed. If, for any reason, the patient does not want the record released, the provider must call for legal advice on how to respond to the subpoena.

Certain records, because of their sensitive nature, may require more than a subpoena to be released. These include records related to sexually transmitted diseases, including AIDS and HIV testing; mental health records; substance abuse records; and sexual assault records. For the courts to have access to these records, a *court order* is required in many states.

HIPAA law requires clinics to identify in written policies and procedures what information they will release regarding patients. Before patient information is released, the following must be identified: (1) the purpose or need for the information, (2) the nature or extent of the information to be released, (3) the date of the authorization, and (4) the signature(s) of the person(s) authorized to give consent. Release only what the subpoena or court order specifically requests rather than releasing the entire medical record. Many practitioners keep a patient's consent information in a specific section of the medical record for quick referral and to demonstrate HIPAA compliance.

The care taken with subpoenas and court orders for certain information is to ensure patients of confidentiality. The information in the medical record, including the information a patient shared with the provider and medical assistant, is private.

No patient information can be given to another person or entity (provider, patient's attorney, insurance carrier, or federal or state agency) without the expressed written consent of the patient. Care must be exercised at all times to ensure that the patient's right to confidentiality is not breached. For example, information given to unauthorized personnel associated with the provider's or clinic's practice in regard to the patient's condition, or financial status regarding payment of bills, violates the patient's right to confidentiality. Likewise, when discussing issues over the telephone that can be overheard by others, such as the patient's account being turned over to a collection agency, the patient's right to confidentiality has been violated.

Certain disclosures of information about a patient's conditions and suspected illnesses are required by law. Legally required disclosures are necessary when the public needs to know certain information for its safety and welfare. The disclosures supersede the patient's right to privacy and confidentiality (see the Reportable Diseases/Injuries discussion in the Public Duties section).

Discovery

In the litigation process, the period of **discovery** follows the subpoenas. This is the time in which both parties are allowed access to all the information and evidence related to the case. Rules of discovery vary from state to state but may include the following:

1. An **interrogatory** is a written set of questions that can come from either the plaintiff or the defendant that must be answered, under oath, and within a specific time period.
2. A **deposition** is oral testimony taken with a court reporter present in a location agreed on by both parties. Both attorneys are usually present when depositions are taken.

Medical assistants may be asked to respond to an interrogatory or may be deposed by the plaintiff's attorney. The defendant's attorney will provide specific instructions in both situations. Because both are done under oath, honesty is an absolute. The medical assistant may be asked to refer to certain documents, recall specific information, or identify documentation in a medical record.

Expert Witnesses. Providers and members of their staff may be called to testify in court to the standard of care. In such a case, they are usually considered **expert witnesses**. An expert witness is one who has enough knowledge and experience in a field to be able to testify to what is the reasonable and expected standard of care. Expert witnesses are expected to tell what they know to be

fact and are best counseled to use lay terms rather than complicated medical language. The goal is for jurors and judges to understand the nature of any medical information shared. Visual aids, charts, and computer simulations often are used to illustrate or clarify testimony given by expert witnesses.

Pretrial Conference

A pretrial conference is generally held close to the trial date to decide if there is just cause for the suit, to make certain that both parties are ready, and to determine if there might be an out-of-court settlement. If a trial seems imminent, **alternative dispute resolution (ADR)** may be suggested. ADR saves money, time, and adverse publicity that can come from a trial.

Mediation allows a neutral facilitator to help the two parties settle their differences and come to an acceptable solution. If no settlement is reached, the case can still look to the court for satisfaction. **Arbitration** allows the neutral party to settle the dispute. This arbitration can be binding or nonbinding. In binding arbitration, both parties agree at the outset to accept the neutral party's decision as final. In nonbinding arbitration, the case can look to the court for settlement.

Trial

A trial can be held before a judge or before a judge and a jury. When the trial begins, opening statements outlining the details of the case are made by both sides. The plaintiff's attorney calls witnesses to produce evidence first. This is known as direct examination. In cross examination, the defendant's attorney questions the witness. When the plaintiff's case is finished, the defendant presents the case in the same manner. When all the information has been presented, the case is turned over for judgment.

If the plaintiff's case is successful, the judge or jury may award a specific amount of money or damages. The judge will instruct a jury regarding the kinds of damages that can be considered in that state. A number of states have placed limits on monetary awards in malpractice cases making it impossible to go above the maximum award allowed even when juries determine that the monetary award should be higher than allowed by the state. If the defendant's case is successful, the case is dismissed. After a court decision, the party that

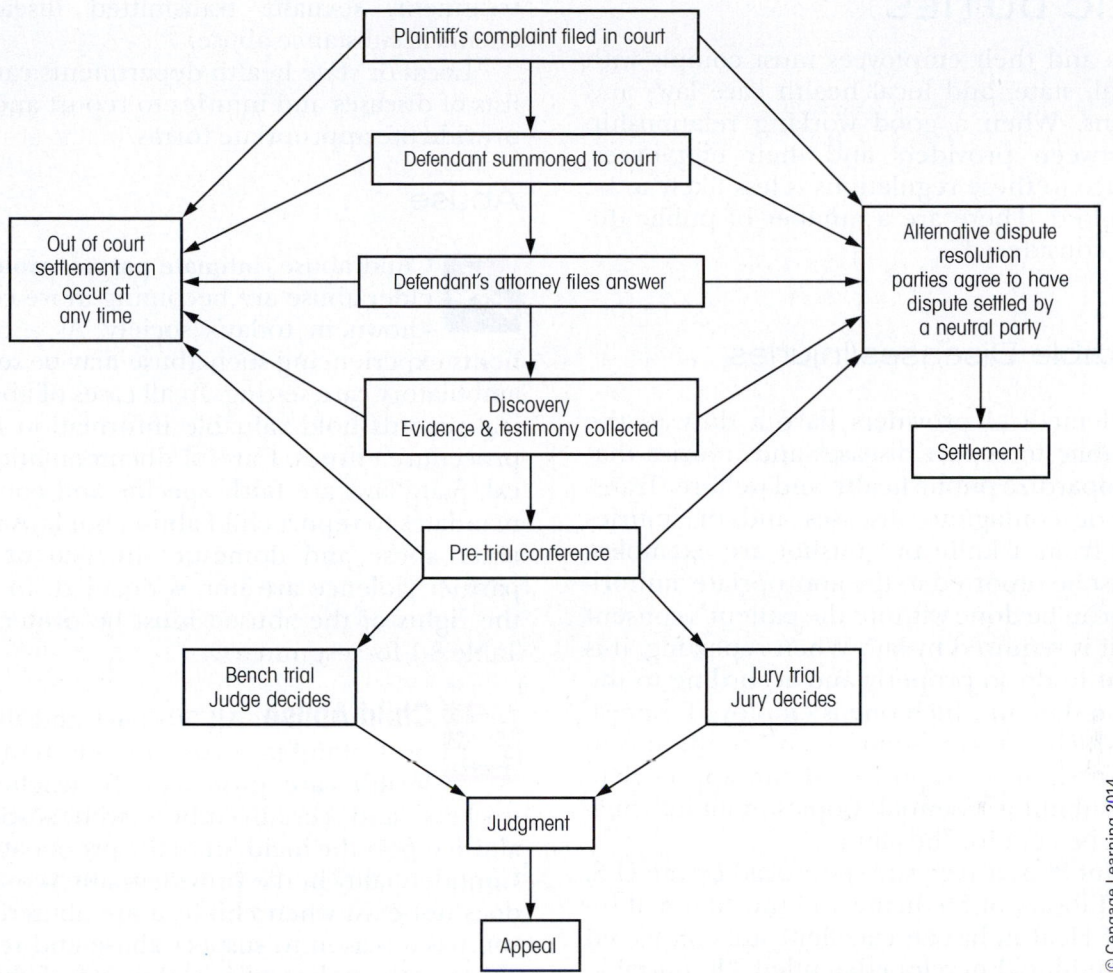

Figure 7-5 Civil litigation process.

© Cengage Learning 2014

has lost the case can begin an appeal process. The appeal requests an opinion from higher courts that review cases usually on the basis of a faulty legal process or action.

Figure 7-5 outlines the civil case process.

STATUTE OF LIMITATIONS

No discussion of negligence, malpractice, or medical records is complete without a brief statement regarding the statute of limitations that will, in part, determine timelines for any litigation and how long medical records are kept. Statutes of limitations most commonly begin at the time a negligent act was committed, when the act was discovered, or when the care of the patient and the provider-patient relationship ended. Therefore, generally all records should be retained until after the statute has run out, usually 3 to 6 years. It is easy to understand why many providers choose to keep their records indefinitely, a plan made much easier with electronic files.

State and federal statutes set maximum time periods during which certain actions can be brought or rights enforced; there is a time limit for individuals to initiate legal action. The statute of limitations varies from one jurisdiction to another, and a lawsuit may not be brought after the statute of limitations has run. For example, in the Commonwealth of Massachusetts, the statute of limitations for an act of medical malpractice committed on an adult is 3 years. If harm to a patient resulted from a medical assistant administering the wrong dose of medication to a patient in Massachusetts, a lawsuit must be brought within 3 years from the time the medication error was made, with the 3 years commencing at the time the negligent act was committed.

PUBLIC DUTIES

Providers and their employees must comply with all federal, state, and local health care laws and regulations. When a good working relationship exists between providers and their employees, compliance to these regulations is less likely to be compromised. There are a number of public duties to be considered.

Reportable Diseases/Injuries

All medical providers have a duty to the public to report diseases and injuries that jeopardize public health and welfare. Transmittable or contagious diseases and/or injuries resulting from a knife or gunshot are examples; these must be reported to the appropriate authorities. This can be done without the patient's consent because it is required by law. When reporting, it is important to do so properly and according to the laws of the state in which one is employed. Knowledge of which illnesses, injuries, and conditions to report, to whom to report, and the appropriate forms to submit is essential. Copies of all information must be kept for the clinic.

MedlinePlus, a Web site sponsored by the U.S. National Library of Medicine and the National Institutes of Health, has an excellent site connected to the Medline Encyclopedia titled "Reportable Diseases" that identifies guidelines for reportable diseases. Local, state, and national agencies such as the Centers for Disease Control and Prevention (CDC) require such diseases to be reported when diagnosed by providers or laboratories. States may vary in the diseases that require reporting, but their lists are likely to include the list of "Nationally Notifiable Infectious Diseases" listed on the CDC's Web site (http://www.cdc.gov). Some diseases require written reports. Others require reporting electronically or by telephone; they include rubeola (measles) and pertussis (whooping cough). Still others ask only for the number of cases to be reported. Such reporting is beneficial to society and all health care managers in tracking and preventing illness. The list changes as new diseases occur and are diagnosed.

Other generally required facts to report include births; deaths; childhood immunizations; rape; and abuse toward a child, elder, or intimate partner.

Some states have laws specific to the release of information relative to mental or psychological treatment, HIV testing, AIDS diagnosis and treatment, sexually transmitted diseases, and chemical substance abuse.

Local or state health departments can provide lists of diseases and injuries to report and will also provide the appropriate forms.

Abuse

Child abuse, **intimate partner violence**, and elder abuse are becoming more commonly known in today's society. As a result, patients experiencing such abuse may be seen in the ambulatory care setting. In all cases of abuse, medical records hold valuable information if a court procedure ensues. Careful documentation is critical. State laws are fairly specific and consistent in mandates to report child abuse, but laws related to elder abuse and domestic violence or intimate partner violence are not as detailed. In any case, the rights of the abused must be protected. (See Table 8-1 for a summary.)

Child Abuse. All 50 states and the District of Columbia mandate, or require, that health care professionals, teachers, social workers, and certain others who suspect child abuse report the incident to the proper authorities. Confidentiality in the provider-patient relationship does not exist when children are abused. If a person has a reason to suspect abuse and reports the abuse to the police and, in the case of child abuse, to the child protective agency, this individual is protected against liability as a result of making the report. Failure to report could result in criminal or civil penalties. Usually, the child protective unit of the state department of social services is called to investigate suspected cases of child abuse. Some injuries that are commonly seen in child abuse are bruises, welts, burns, fractures, and head injuries. Evidence of neglect, intimidation, or sexual abuse also may be seen.

If a suspicion of abuse exists, the provider should:

- Treat the child's injuries
- Send the child to the hospital for further treatment when necessary
- Inform parents of the diagnosis and that it will be reported to the police and social services agency
- Notify the child protective agency (keep phone number posted)
- Document all information
- Provide court testimony if requested

Elder Abuse. Elder abuse may consist of neglect, physical abuse, punishment, physical restraint, or abandonment. Examples are seen when elders are overmedicated or undermedicated, physically restrained, intimidated by shouting or profanity, sexually abused, neglected or abandoned, or in any other way have their rights and dignity violated. The person reporting the abuse is generally a health care professional who observes or suspects the abuse, and the reporting agency is most likely one of a social service or welfare nature. The majority of states have laws protecting vulnerable adults and the elderly from abuse.

Intimate Partner Violence (IPV). The term "domestic violence" has been changed to be more encompassing of an escalating problem. "Intimate partner violence (IPV)" is now used and refers to violence or abuse between a spouse or former spouse; boyfriend, girlfriend, or former boyfriend/girlfriend; and same-sex or heterosexual intimate partner or former same-sex or heterosexual intimate partner. The abuse may include physical or sexual violence, threats of the same, and psychological or emotional violence. Physical violence is a criminal act, and failure to report it is considered a misdemeanor in some states. Victims of IPV should be treated as soon as possible after the assault so that evidence can be preserved for legal purposes. Some forms of IPV are considered acceptable behavior in many cultures, even in the United States. Some cultures believe the woman is chattel, or property, of her spouse; that she has no rights or authority; and that she must submit to her husband's, brother's, or father's demands.

An individual who manages to come to the ambulatory care setting with signs of IPV is courageous and probably is extremely frightened as well, because reporting the violence may increase the risk for continued violence and even death in some instances.

Make certain that community resources are readily available for survivors of IPV, even if they choose to stay in the abusive situation. In many cases, the abused patient's options are so few that leaving is more frightening than staying in the abusive relationship. Do not pass judgment on these survivors; they desperately need understanding and compassion.

Your understanding and compassion are perhaps the only door through which they might feel comfortable enough to leave the abusive relationship.

Good Samaritan Laws

 All 50 states have laws regarding the rendering of first aid by health care professionals at the scene of an accident or sudden injury. Good Samaritan laws, although not always clearly written, encourage health care professionals to provide medical care within the scope of their training without fear of being sued for negligence. In an emergency situation, medical assistants cannot be held liable should an injury result from some form of first aid rendered or from first aid they omitted to render as long as they acted in a reasonable way within the scope of their knowledge. Medical assistants and other health care professionals with skills in cardiopulmonary resuscitation (CPR) who are present when CPR is needed must perform the procedure on the victim or otherwise could be declared negligent. Emergencies that arise in the ambulatory care setting generally are not covered by Good Samaritan laws.

ADVANCE DIRECTIVES

Medical assistants in the ambulatory care setting will be asked to attach advance directives or living wills to patients' medical records (Figure 7-6). These directives are legal documents in which patients indicate their wishes in the case of a life-threatening illness or serious injury.

Health care providers in many states and cities have adopted the Physician Orders for Life-Sustaining Treatment (POLST) (Figure 7-7) form. This form is to be completed by a health care provider based on the patient's preferences regarding the type of life-sustaining treatment wanted and medical indications. POLST is most often brightly colored (neon pink or green). To be valid, the form must be signed by the proper authority. Some states may use another name than POLST, but the intent is quite similar. POLST is appropriate for seriously ill individuals with life-threatening or terminal illnesses. Some providers believe that even with an advance directive in place, it is advisable to complete a POLST form. This form goes with the patient when he or she is moved between care settings. For those in the home, it is recommended that the form be posted on the refrigerator where emergency responders can locate it easily. As of 2011, 33 states had endorsed or are developing POLST documents (http://www.POLST.org). Such documents should always accompany the patients to the hospital for any treatment or care. They may be updated from time to time, and patients can ask to rescind such a document at any

HEALTH CARE DIRECTIVE

Directive made this _____ day of _____ , _____ .
(Year)

I, _____ being of sound mind, willfully, and voluntarily make known my desire that my dying shall not be artificially prolonged under the circumstances set forth below, and do hereby declare that:

(A) If at any time I should have an incurable and irreversible condition certified to be a terminal condition by my attending physician, and where the application of life-sustaining treatment would serve only to artificially prolong the process of my dying, I direct that such treatment be withheld or withdrawn, and that I be permitted to die naturally. I understand "terminal condition" means an incurable and irreversible condition caused by injury, disease or illness that would, within reasonable medical judgment, cause death within a reasonable period of time in accordance with accepted medical standards.

(B) If I should be in an irreversible coma or persistent vegetative state, or other permanent unconscious condition as certified by two physicians, and from which those physicians believe that I have no reasonable probability of recovery, I direct that life-sustaining treatment be withheld or withdrawn.

(C) If I am diagnosed to be in a terminal or permanent unconscious condition, [*Choose one*]

I want _____ do not want _____

artificially administered nutrition and hydration to be withdrawn or withheld the same as other forms of life-sustaining treatment. I understand artificially administered nutrition and hydration is a form of life-sustaining treatment in certain circumstances. I request all health care providers who care for me to honor this directive.

(D) In the absence of my ability to give directions regarding the use of such life-sustaining procedures, it is my intention that this directive shall be honored by my family, physicians and other health care providers as the final expression of my fundamental right to refuse medical or surgical treatment, and also honored by any person appointed to make these decisions for me, whether by durable power of attorney or otherwise. I accept the consequences of such refusal.

(E) If I have been diagnosed as pregnant and that diagnosis is known to my physician, this directive shall have no force or effect during the course of my pregnancy.

(F) I understand the full import of this directive and I am emotionally and mentally competent to make this directive. I also understand that I may amend or revoke this directive at any time.

(G) I make the following additional directions regarding my care:

_____

_____

_____

_____

Signed: _____

The declarer has been personally known to me and I believe him or her to be of sound mind. In addition, I am not the attending physician, an employee of the attending physician or health care facility in which the declarer is a patient, or any person who has a claim against any portion of the estate of the declarer upon the declarer's decease at the time of the execution of the directive.

Witness: _____

Witness: _____

Figure 7-6 Sample health care directive.

HIPAA PERMITS DISCLOSURE OF POLST TO OTHER HEALTH CARE PROVIDERS AS NECESSARY

Physician Orders for Life-Sustaining Treatment

Last Name - First Name - Middle Initial

Date of Birth _____ _____ _____   Last 4 #SSN _____ _____ _____   Gender   M   F

FIRST follow these orders, **THEN** contact physician, nurse practitioner or PA-C. The POLST is a set of medical orders intended to guide emergency medical treatment for persons with advanced life limiting illness based on their current medical condition and goals. Any section not completed implies full treatment for that section. Everyone shall be treated with dignity and respect.

Medical Conditions/Patient Goals:

Agency Info/Sticker

A
Check One

CARDIOPULMONARY RESUSCITATION (CPR): Person has no pulse and is not breathing.

☐ CPR/Attempt Resuscitation   ☐ DNAR/Do Not Attempt Resuscitation (Allow Natural Death)

Choosing DNAR will include appropriate comfort measures and may still include the range of treatments below. When not in cardiopulmonary arrest, go to part B.

B
Check One

MEDICAL INTERVENTIONS: Person has pulse and/or is breathing.

☐ **COMFORT MEASURES ONLY** Use medication by any route, positioning, wound care and other measures to relieve pain and suffering. Use oxygen, oral suction and manual treatment of airway obstruction as needed for comfort.   **Patient prefers no hospital transfer:** *EMS contact medical control to determine if transport indicated to provide adequate comfort.*

☐ **LIMITED ADDITIONAL INTERVENTIONS** Includes care described above. Use medical treatment, IV fluids and cardiac monitor as indicated. Do not use intubation or mechanical ventilation. May use less invasive airway support (e.g. CPAP, BiPAP).   **Transfer** *to hospital if indicated. Avoid intensive care if possible.*

☐ **FULL TREATMENT** Includes care described above. Use intubation, advanced airway interventions, mechanical ventilation, and cardioversion as indicated.   **Transfer** *to hospital if indicated. Includes intensive care.*

Additional Orders: (e.g. dialysis, etc.) _____

C
SIGNATURES: The signatures below verify that these orders are consistent with the patient's medical condition, known preferences and best known information. If signed by a surrogate, the patient must be decisionally incapacitated and the person signing is the legal surrogate.

Discussed with:
☐ Patient   ☐ Parent of Minor
☐ Legal Guardian   ☐ Health Care Agent (DPOAHC)
☐ Spouse/Other:

PRINT — Physician/ARNP/PA-C Name | Phone Number

✗ Physician/ARNP/PA-C Signature *(mandatory)* | Date

PRINT — Patient or Legal Surrogate Name | Phone Number

✗ Patient or Legal Surrogate Signature *(mandatory)* | Date

Person has: ☐ Health Care Directive (living will)   ☐ Living Will Registry   **Encourage all advance care planning documents to accompany POLST**
☐ Durable Power of Attorney for Health Care

SEND ORIGINAL FORM WITH PERSON WHENEVER TRANSFERRED OR DISCHARGED

Revised 2/2011   Photocopies and FAXes of signed POLST forms are legal and valid. May make copies for records

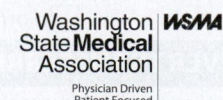
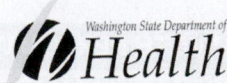

Washington State Medical Association | WSMA
Physician Driven Patient Focused

Washington State Department of Health

Figure 7-7   Physician Orders for Life-Sustaining Treatment (POLST) form. (*continues*)

HIPAA PERMITS DISCLOSURE OF POLST TO OTHER HEALTH CARE PROVIDERS AS NECESSARY

Other Contact Information (Optional)

Name of Guardian, Surrogate or other Contact Person	Relationship	Phone Number	
Name of Health Care Professional Preparing Form	Preparer Title	Phone Number	Date Prepared

D ADDITIONAL PATIENT PREFERENCES (OPTIONAL)

ANTIBIOTICS:

☐ No antibiotics. Use other measures to relieve symptoms.   ☐ Use antibiotics if life can be prolonged.

☐ Determine use or limitation of antibiotics when infection occurs, with comfort as goal.

MEDICALLY ASSISTED NUTRITION:
<u>Always offer food and liquids by mouth if feasible.</u>

☐ Trial period of medically assisted nutrition by tube.
(Goal: _____)

☐ No medically assisted nutrition by tube.   ☐ Long-term medically assisted nutrition by tube.

ADDITIONAL ORDERS: (e.g. dialysis, blood products, etc. Attach additional orders if necessary.)

✗ Physician/ARNP/PA-C Signature	Date

DIRECTIONS FOR HEALTH CARE PROFESSIONALS

Completing POLST

- Must be completed by health care professional.
- Should reflect person's current preferences and medical indications. Encourage completion of an advance directive.
- POLST must be signed by a physician/ARNP/PA-C to be valid. Verbal orders are acceptable with follow-up signature by physician/ARNP/PA-C in accordance with facility/community policy.

Using POLST

Any incomplete section of POLST implies full treatment for that section.

This POLST is effective across all settings including hospitals until replaced by new physicians's orders.

The health care professional should inquire about other advance directives. In the event of a conflict, the most recently completed form takes precedence.

SECTION A:
- No defibrillator should be used on a person who has chosen "Do Not Attempt Resuscitation."

SECTION B:
- When comfort cannot be achieved in the current setting, the person, including someone with "Comfort Measures Only," should be transferred to a setting able to provide comfort (e.g., treatment of a hip fracture).
- An IV medication to enhance comfort may be appropriate for a person who has chosen "Comfort Measures Only."
- Treatment of dehydration is a measure which may prolong life. A person who desires IV fluids should indicate "Limited Additional Interventions" or "Full Treatment."

SECTION D:
- Oral fluids and nutrition must always be offered if medically feasible.

Reviewing POLST

This POLST should be reviewed periodically whenever:

(1) The person is transferred from one care setting or care level to another, or

(2) There is a substantial change in the person's health status, or

(3) The person's treatment preferences change.

A person with capacity or the surrogate of a person without capacity, can void the form and request alternative treatment.

To void this form, draw line through "Physician Orders" and write "VOID" in large letters. Any changes require a new POLST.

Review of this POLST Form

Review Date	Reviewer	Location of Review	Review Outcome
			☐ No Change ☐ Form Voided ☐ New form completed
			☐ No Change ☐ Form Voided ☐ New form completed

SEND ORIGINAL FORM WITH PERSON WHENEVER TRANSFERRED OR DISCHARGED

Photocopies and FAXes of signed POLST forms are legal and valid. May make copies for records

Figure 7-7 (*continued*)

PATIENT EDUCATION

 Because of the increased awareness of confidentiality as a result of HIPAA, medical assistants can be helpful by suggesting that any family member(s) who might be involved and need to know about the patient's care be indicated in the patient's medical record with a signed release from the patient. There have been examples recently of adult children of elder adults who were either not informed when their ailing parent was taken to emergency services in another state or were unable to get any information about their parent from a hospital or provider even though a durable power of attorney for health care was in place. If that directive does not go with the patient, no information can be given. For that reason, it is suggested that patients may want to keep a wallet card containing a notice of the advance directive, any appointed agent named, and any family member(s) who is allowed information.

time. Medical assistants must remember that these documents reflect the choices of their patients and are to be respected as such.

Living Wills/Advance Directives

Patients who desire to make known in advance their choices related to health care, especially when death is near, are likely to have living wills, advance directives, a health care proxy, or a POLST order. The title of such a document is largely determined by the state in which the document is made. These documents are necessary because advances in medicine allow medical professionals to sustain life even if the individual will not recover from a persistent vegetative state. Persons who prefer not to remain in that state can use the living will or advance directive to make decisions about life support and to direct others to implement their wishes in that regard. Such a document allows individuals to indicate to family and health care professionals whether life-prolonging medical or surgical procedures are to be continued, withheld, or withdrawn, and whether artificial feeding and fluids are to be used or withheld. The document allows individuals to make this decision before incapacitation.

To be valid, the proper and particular form, different in each state, must be used, and it must be lawfully executed. States vary in the number of witnesses required and whether a notary public is required for those signatures. The form goes into effect when provided to a patient's health care provider *and* when the patient is no longer capable of making health care decisions. Examples of incapacity include permanent unconsciousness, life-threatening illness in the latter stages, and inability to communicate. The U.S. Legal Forms Web site (http://USlegalforms.com) has samples of living wills for all 50 states and the District of Columbia under the heading "Living Will." A sample from each state is available without a fee.

Durable Power of Attorney for Health Care

Another document seen in the ambulatory care setting is the **durable power of attorney for health care** or designation of health care surrogate (Figure 7-8) or health care proxy. This document allows a patient to name another person as the official spokesperson for that patient should he or she be unable to make health care decisions. A basic durable power of attorney document allows another person to manage finances and personal matters; however, it takes a durable power of attorney for health care for that person to make medical decisions.

Every state has a slightly different version of their living will, advance directive, durable power of attorney for health care, or POLST. Most forms and specific information can be found on the Internet by keying in a particular state and the title of the document wanted. Also, the Web site for Compassion and Choices (http://www.compassionandchoices.org), located in Portland, Oregon, is quite helpful.

Patient Self-Determination Act

In 1991, the federal government passed the **Patient Self-Determination Act (PSDA)**, which applies to all health care institutions receiving payments from Medicare and Medicaid. PSDA requires that all adults receiving health care from these institutions

DURABLE POWER OF ATTORNEY FOR HEALTH CARE

Notice to Person Executing This Document

This is an important legal document. Before executing this document you should know these facts:

- This document gives the person you designate as your Health Care Agent the power to make MOST <u>health</u> care decisions for you if you lose the capability to make informed health care decisions for yourself. This power is effective only when you lose the capacity to make informed health care decisions for yourself. As long as you have the capacity to make informed health care decisions for yourself, you retain the right to make all medical and other health care decisions.

- You may include specific limitations in this document on the authority of the Health Care Agent to make health care decisions for you.

- Subject to any specific limitations you include in this document, if you do lose the capacity to make an informed decision on a health care matter, the Health Care Agent *GENERALLY* will be authorized by this document to make health care decisions for you to the same extent as you could make those decisions yourself, if you had the capacity to do so. The authority of the Health Care Agent to make health care decisions for you *GENERALLY* will include the authority to give informed consent, to refuse to give informed consent, or to withdraw informed consent to any care, treatment, service, or procedure to maintain, diagnose, or treat a physical or mental condition. You can limit that right in this document if you choose.

- A Health Care Agent can only act under state law. "Mercy killing" is not allowed under Washington state law. A Health Care Agent will **NEVER** be allowed to authorize "mercy killing," euthanasia or any procedure which would actually speed up the natural process of dying.

- When exercising his or her authority to make health care decisions for you when deciding on your behalf, the Health Care Agent will have to act consistent with your wishes, or if they are unknown, in your best interest. You may make your wishes known to the Health Care Agent by including them in this document or by making them known in another manner.

- When acting under this document the Health Care Agent *GENERALLY* will have the same rights that you have to receive information about proposed health care, to review health care records, and to consent to the disclosure of health care records.

1. Creation of Durable Power of Attorney for Health Care

I intend to create a power of attorney (Health Care Agent) by appointing the person or persons designated herein to make health care decisions for me to the same extent that I could make such decisions for myself if I was capable of doing so, as recognized by RCW 11.94.010. This designation becomes effective when I cannot make health care decisions for myself as determined by my attending physician or designee, such as if I am unconscious, or if I am otherwise temporarily or permanently incapable of making health care decisions. The Health Care Agent's power shall cease if and when I regain my capacity to make health care decisions.

2. Designation of Health Care Agent and Alternate Agents

If my attending physician or his or her designee determines that I am not capable of giving informed consent to health care, I _____, designate and appoint:

Name_____   Address _____

City _____ State _____ Zip _____ Phone _____

as my attorney-in-fact (Health Care Agent) by granting him or her the Durable Power of Attorney for Health Care recognized in RCW 11.94.010 and authorize her or him to consult with my physicians about the possibility of my regaining the capacity to make treatment decisions and to accept, plan, stop, and refuse treatment on my behalf with the treating physicians and health personnel.

In the event that _____ is unable or unwilling to serve, I grant these powers to

Name_____   Address _____

City _____ State _____ Zip _____ Phone _____

In the event that both _____ and _____

are unable or unwilling to serve, I grant these powers to

Name_____   Address _____

City _____ State _____ Zip _____ Phone _____

Figure 7-8 Durable power of attorney for health care.

Your name (print)_____

3. General Statement of Authority Granted.

My Health Care Agent is specifically authorized to give informed consent for health care treatment when I am not capable of doing so. This includes but is not limited to consent to initiate, continue, discontinue, or forgo medical care and treatment including artificially supplied nutrition and hydration, following and interpreting my instructions for the provision, withholding, or withdrawing of life-sustaining treatment, which are contained in any Health Care Directive or other form of "living will" I may have executed or elsewhere, and to receive and consent to the release of medical information. When the Health Care Agent does not have any stated desires or instructions from me to follow, he or she shall act in my best interest in making health care decisions.

The above authorization to make health care decisions does not include the following absent a court order:

(1)   Therapy or other procedure given for the purpose of inducing convulsion;

(2)   Surgery solely for the purpose of psychosurgery;

(3)   Commitment to or placement in a treatment facility for the mentally ill, except pursuant to the provisions of Chapter 71.05 RCW;

(4)   Sterilization.

I hereby revoke any prior grants of durable power of attorney for health care.

4. Special Provisions

_____

_____

_____

_____

_____

DATED this _____ day of _____ , _____ .

(Year)

GRANTOR _____

STATE OF WASHINGTON   )

)ss.

(COUNTY OF _____)

I certify that I know or have satisfactory evidence that the GRANTOR, _____

signed this instrument and acknowledged it to be his or her free and voluntary act for the uses and purposes mentioned in the instrument.

DATED this _____ day of _____ , _____ .

(Year)

_____

NOTARY PUBLIC in and for the State of Washington,

residing at _____

My commission expires _____

Figure 7-8   (*continued*)

be given the opportunity to provide information about their wishes in an advance directive.

Copies of advance directives are to be given to patients' providers so the documents can be transferred to a hospital or nursing facility as necessary. Any named agent should have a copy, and family members also may have a copy.

CASE STUDY 7-1

Refer to the scenario at the beginning of the chapter. You realize that any breach of confidentiality is a serious matter, whether intentional or accidental.

CASE STUDY REVIEW

1. What corrective measures can you suggest to decrease voices heard in the hallway or from examination rooms?

2. How can private patient information be kept out of public view?

3. What HIPAA regulations apply here?

CASE STUDY 7-2

Three weeks ago, Dr. King treated a new patient, Boris Bolski, for lower back pain, which the patient believed was the result of consistent heavy lifting at his job. Medical assistant Joe Guerrero, CMA (AAMA) assisted Dr. King during the examination. Today, both Joe and Dr. King were served with subpoenas by Mr. Bolski's attorney. Mr. Bolski is alleging that unsafe conditions at his workplace caused severe strain on his back, and he is suing his employer for damages. Dr. King and Joe Guerrero were called as expert witnesses to a civil hearing; Joe, especially, is a bit nervous about this, because he has never been on the witness stand in court and is not sure what is expected of him.

CASE STUDY REVIEW

1. How will Mr. Bolski's medical record help Joe answer questions at the hearing?

2. What information should Joe gather so that he is prepared to testify?

3. As an expert witness, what might Joe be expected to communicate to the judge in this case?

CASE STUDY 7-3

Wanda Hanson, RMA (AMT), is working on a part-time basis in Hudson, Florida, as an administrative medical assistant on the phone desk in the Emergency Department at Hudson Community Hospital when a frantic long-distance call is received. The caller is Larry Nelson from Cheyenne, Wyoming. He received a call from the nursing home where his 95-year-old mother is living informing him that she was taken by ambulance to your hospital. Larry wants to know if Muriel Nelson has arrived and what her condition is. Wanda is aware of a patient's right to privacy, confidentiality, and the new HIPAA regulations. Wanda observed Mrs. Nelson arrive at the emergency department quite incoherent and confused.

CASE STUDY REVIEW

1. What can Wanda tell Mr. Nelson, especially after noting that no records were with the elderly Mrs. Nelson when she arrived at the hospital?

2. What information would Wanda need from Mr. Nelson before complying with his request?

3. How can Wanda put Mr. Nelson at ease? What can Wanda do to help?

SUMMARY

Changing societal values have contributed to an increase of lawsuits in medical practice. Patients are more aware than ever of their rights, especially those of confidentiality and the right to privacy, consent, and records ownership. They are likely to seek redress when they perceive their rights have been violated.

A healthy relationship between all providers and patients and between medical assistants and patients, as well as respect for the patient's rights, reduces the likelihood of any lawsuit.

Additional knowledge of the laws that regulate medical and business practices in your state is necessary to be in compliance. Sources of information regarding state and federal laws can be obtained from the state medical society, the provider's liability insurance company, the state medical assistant society, the state attorney general's office, the Internet, or the public library.

STUDY FOR SUCCESS

To reinforce your knowledge and skills of information presented in this chapter:

- Review the *Key Terms*
- Role-play with other students to apply attributes of professionalism pertinent to this chapter.
- Consider the *Case Studies* and discuss your conclusions
- Answer the questions in the *Certification Review*
- Apply your knowledge by completing the *Activities* in the *Study Guide* and the *Games and Quizzes* in the StudyWARE StudyWARE software on the *Premium Website*
- Practice your problem-solving skills with the *Critical Thinking Challenge 3.0* on the *Premium Website*

Additional resources for this chapter include:

- Module 3 of the *Medical Assisting Learning Lab*
- *CourseMate for Delmar's Comprehensive Medical Assisting*
- *WebTutor for Delmar's Comprehensive Medical Assisting*

CERTIFICATION REVIEW

1. The type of contract that most often exists between provider and patient is:
   a. expressed
   b. implied
   c. privileged
   d. civil

2. The administrative law act that prohibits discrimination, has five sections, and is enforced by the EEOC is called the:
   a. Controlled Substances Act
   b. Federal Age Discrimination Act
   c. Americans with Disabilities Act
   d. Health Insurance Portability and Accountability Act

3. Slander is defamation through:
   a. spoken statements that damage an individual's reputation
   b. written statements that damage a person's reputation
   c. written falsehoods about an individual
   d. all of the above

4. Occasionally, a provider will be sued for the negligence of an employee, even though the provider is not guilty of any negligent act. This is done on the basis of the doctrine of:
   a. *res ipsa loquitur* c. proximate cause
   b. *respondeat superior* d. contract law

5. The standard of care expected of a provider is held by the courts to mean:
   a. on a par with all other providers engaged in the same medical specialty anywhere
   b. reasonable, attentive, diligent care comparable with other providers of the same specialty or general field of practice
   c. the best possible under the circumstances
   d. the same as the national norm
6. Advance directives:
   a. allow patients to direct how their billing is to be handled
   b. are designed to encourage providers to render first aid in an emergency
   c. indicate a patient's wishes in life-threatening circumstances
   d. are not considered legal documents
7. A subpoena:
   a. is a court order requesting data, an appearance in court, or both
   b. is sufficient to enforce a release of any type of medical record or information
   c. may be ignored without consequences
   d. allows the person being served to select a specific date or time to appear

8. The 4 Ds of negligence are:
   a. duty, danger, damage, and disaster
   b. derelict, direct cause, damage, and danger
   c. danger, direct cause, damage, disaster
   d. duty, derelict, direct cause, damage
9. Emancipated minors:
   a. are considered adults and can consent to treatment
   b. live on their own and are self-supporting
   c. may be married or serve in the military
   d. all of the above
   e. only b and c
10. Torts:
    a. include battery, defamation of character, invasion of privacy
    b. are always intentional in nature
    c. do not require that harm has occurred
    d. do not include malpractice

REFERENCES/BIBLIOGRAPHY

Compassion & Choices. Washington durable power of attorney for health care. Retrieved April 4, 2011, from http://compassionindying.org

U.S. Equal Employment Opportunity Commission (n.d.). Federal laws prohibiting job discrimination questions and answers. Retrieved March 14, 2011, from http://www.eeoc.gov/facts/qanda.html

Anderson, H. (2011, February 23). HIPAA Privacy Fine: $4.3 Million: Clinics failed to provide patients with records access. Retrieved March 14, 2011, from http://www.govinfosecurity.com

Lewis, M. A., Tamparo, C. D., & Tatro, B. (2012). *Medical law, ethics, and bioethics for health professions* (7th ed.). Philadelphia: F. A. Davis.

Washington State Medical Association (WSMA). (2007). Durable power of attorney for health care, health care directive, and POLST. Retrieved April 4, 2011, from http://www.wsma.org

CHAPTER 8

Ethical Considerations

OUTLINE

Ethics
  Principle-Centered
  Leadership
  Five Ps of Ethical Power
  Ethics Check Questions
Keys to the AAMA Code of
Ethics
Ethical Guidelines for Health
Care Providers
  Advertising
  Confidentiality
  HIPAA
  Medical Records

Professional Fees and
  Charges
Professional Rights and
  Responsibilities
Disaster Response and
  Emergency Preparedness
Treatment for a Culturally
  Diverse Clientele
Care of the Poor
Abuse
Bioethics
  Allocation of Scarce Medical
  Resources

Health Care: A Right or a
  Privilege?
HIV and AIDS
Reproductive Issues
Abortion and Fetal Tissue
  Research
Genetic Engineering/
  Manipulation
Dying and Death
Hospice

LEARNING OUTCOMES

1. Define, spell, and pronounce the key terms as presented in the glossary.

2. Summarize reasons for Codes of Ethics.

3. Paraphrase the eight characteristics of principle-centered leadership.

4. Describe the five Ps of ethical power.

5. Implement the ethics check questions.

6. Relate the five principles of the AAMA code to patient care in the ambulatory care setting.

7. Discuss the role of ethical codes in ambulatory care.

8. Critique the ethical guidelines for health care providers, giving at least four examples.

9. Summarize professional rights and responsibilities for health care personnel.

10. Categorize the different types of abuse for those individuals at risk.

11. Restate the dilemmas encountered by the following bioethical issues: (a) allocation of scarce medical resources; (b) health care as a right or a privilege; (c) HIV and AIDS; (d) reproductive issues; (e) assisted reproduction; (f) abortion and fetal tissue research; (g) genetic engineering/manipulation; (h) dying and death.

12. Analyze the professionalism questions and apply them to this chapter's content.

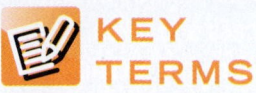

KEY TERMS

bioethics

cryopreservation

ethics

female genital
   mutilation

genetic engineering

in vitro fertilization
   (IVF)

intimate partner
   violence (IPV)

macroallocation

microallocation

surrogate

tubal ligation

vasectomy

ATTRIBUTES OF PROFESSIONALISM

Communication
- Did you listen to and acknowledge the patient?
- Did you speak at the patient's level of understanding?
- Did you display appropriate body language?

Presentation
- Were you dressed and groomed appropriately?
- Did you do something to bond with the patient?
- Did you attend to any special needs of the patient?
- Were you courteous, patient, and respectful to the patient?
- Did you display a positive attitude?

Competency
- Did you pay attention to detail?
- Did you display sound judgment?
- Did you remain calm in a crisis?

Initiative
- Did you show initiative?
- Were you flexible and dependable?
- Were you respectful of others?

Integrity
- Did you work within the scope of your practice?
- Did you demonstrate sensitivity to patient's rights?
- Did you protect personal boundaries?
- Did you demonstrate respect for individual diversity?
- Did you maintain your moral and ethical standards?

SCENARIO

Harley Navarro is a new medical assistant in a busy internist's clinic. He finished school a few months ago and is awaiting the date to take his exam to become a certified medical assistant. He is nervous and scared. All the other medical assistants are female and have many years of experience. Harley wants so much to be accepted and recognized for his skills. Today, however, he twice had a rough time taking a blood pressure reading. In fact, the provider was ready for one of Harley's patients before he was finished with the reading, and the provider stepped in to take the reading. Harley was embarrassed. His current patient is obese. His first attempt at getting a blood pressure reading failed. He gets a larger cuff for his second reading. His patient complains, however, that her arm is hurting about halfway through the reading. Harley hurries the process and takes a guess at the diastolic pressure figure, but he knows it is close.

INTRODUCTION

It is impossible in today's world to function as a medical assistant without an awareness of the impact of ethics and bioethics on health care. Just as an understanding of the law and complying to the law are vital for the medical assistant, it is equally important to understand ethics and bioethics.

From Chapter 7, you have come to realize that there are many circumstances and situations that occur in health care that are guided and directed by state and federal laws. You, personally, are expected to be above reproach in all your actions in this regard. You must also work with your employer and other members of the health care team to ensure that each member of the staff functions within the law—protecting both patients and providers.

Ethics plays a huge role in such an endeavor. To function ethically demands that you never function outside the law. Ethics, however, demands something more—ethics calls for honesty, trustworthiness, integrity, confidentiality, and fairness. To function ethically, you must know yourself well and understand weaknesses and any vulnerability that might prevent you from acting ethically.

The scenario described earlier is just one situation in which medical assistants may need to reflect on their actions and be sure that they are acting ethically and within the range of their skills. Medical assistants also need to recognize the warning signs that they, or some other staff member, may be about to breach a code of ethics. Often, this kind of breach occurs when one has, or seeks to have, too much power; when one attempts to take on too much authority; or when one has too little knowledge and experience and is afraid to ask for help. When a breach seems about to occur, the individuals involved should be encouraged to step back and review their actions and the likely consequences of those actions.

ETHICS

Traditionally, **ethics** is defined in terms of what is considered right or wrong. Sometimes ethics is referred to as "morals." However, morals refer to personal choices of conduct, whereas ethics is more of a philosophy related to making judgments about right and wrong. Professional organizations often identify their ethics in codes, which provide a set of principles and guidelines.

The American Medical Association (AMA) has established such a code of ethics called the Principles of Medical Ethics. This code can be reviewed by accessing the AMA website (http://www.ama-assn.org). Also published every 2 years by the AMA is The Code of Medical Ethics Current Opinions with Annotations; this document provides up-to-date information on a number of ethical dilemmas. A number of other professional medical organizations have well-established ethical codes also. They include such professions as osteopaths, chiropractors, nurses, professional coders, and emergency medical technicians.

The American Association of Medical Assistants (AAMA) has a code of ethics and a creed shown in Figure 8-1. In addition, the AAMA Mission Statement, AAMA Medical Assistant Code of Ethics, and AAMA Medical Assistant Creed appear on the AAMA website (http://www.aama-ntl.org). Clicking on "About AAMA" will detail these statements for you.

SPOTLIGHT ON CERTIFICATION

RMA Content Outline
- Principles of medical ethics
- Ethical conduct

CMA (AAMA) Content Outline
- Displaying professional attitude
- Performing within ethical boundaries
- Maintaining confidentiality
- Complying with legislation
- Working as a team member to achieve goals

CMAS Content Outline
- Legal and ethical considerations
- Professionalism
- Confidentiality

The Hospital Patient Bill of Rights presented by the American Hospital Association (AHA) has long been a standard of many hospitals and can be viewed at http://www.patienttalk.info/AHA-Patient_Bill_of_Rights. Similar statements have been adapted to the ambulatory health care setting as well. See Figure 8-2 for a generic sample.

These codes give additional guidance for making ethical decisions, taking ethical action, and further identifying patient rights.

There are more than 50 different codes of ethics for professional organizations, and most are related to medicine and are designed to offer guidance and direction to health care professionals.

Seven ethical codes that pertain to the entire world are pertinent for review. They include such famous codes as the Declaration of Geneva, Declaration of Helsinki, and the International Code of Medical Ethics. A listing of these codes is found by searching the Internet for "world medical ethics codes." Another fascinating website identifies the characteristics of Traditional Chinese Medical Ethics when you use the Internet to search for "Chinese Medical Ethics." Chinese medical ethics emphasizes self-cultivation and personal ethics of practitioners rather than a strict organizational code of ethics.

Codes of ethics bring standards of moral and ethical behavior together in one place. They assist organizations and individuals in putting words to their expected behaviors and actions. There is a benefit to such codes when they become reminders to everyone regarding appropriate conduct. Codes also can have a limiting effect, however. For instance, if an organization does not have a code of ethics, that organization is not necessarily viewed as unethical. Further, having a code of ethics does not necessarily create an ethical organization, especially if the code is mostly ignored.

 Medical assistants and medical professionals are asked to balance personal and professional areas of their lives in the middle

---

AAMA CODE OF ETHICS

The Code of Ethics of AAMA shall set forth principles of ethical and moral conduct as they relate to the medical profession and the particular practice of medical assisting.

Members of AAMA dedicated to the conscientious pursuit of their profession, and thus desiring to merit the high regard of the entire medical profession and the respect of the general public which they serve, do pledge themselves to strive always to:

A. render service with full respect for the dignity of humanity;
B. respect confidential information obtained through employment unless legally authorized or required by responsible performance of duty to divulge such information;
C. uphold the honor and high principles of the profession and accept its disciplines;
D. seek to continually improve the knowledge and skills of medical assistants for the benefit of patients and professional colleagues;
E. participate in additional service activities aimed toward improving the health and well-being of the community.

(A)

CREED

I believe in the principles and purposes of the Profession of Medical Assisting.
I endeavor to be more effective.
I aspire to render greater service.
I protect the confidence entrusted to me.
I am dedicated to the care and well-being of all people.
I am loyal to my employer.
I am true to the ethics of my profession.
I am strengthened by compassion, courage, and faith.

(B)

Figure 8-1 (A) American Association of Medical Assistants (AAMA) Code of Ethics. (B) AAMA Creed.

*PATIENT BILL OF RIGHTS FOR AMBULATORY CARE

As a patient, you have the right to:

Be treated with courtesy and respect, with appreciation of your dignity and without discrimination at all times.

Participate in your healthcare by receiving a prompt and reasonable response to questions and requests, receiving information concerning diagnosis, course of treatment, alternatives, risks, and prognosis.

Access your medical record and receive a copy upon request. Seek a second opinion and to know who is providing your medical services.

Confidentiality at all times and your privacy protected.

An estimate of charges for medical care.

A reasonably clear and understandable itemized bill and to have the charges explained.

Refuse any treatment.

Have your advance directive on file.

Be informed of any medical treatment for purposes of experimental research and to give consent or refuse to participate.

*Compilation of several clinics across the United States; prepared by Carol D. Tamparo. CMA (AAMA), Ph.D.

© Cengage Learning 2014

Figure 8-2   Patient Bill of Rights for Ambulatory Care.

of constant pressure and crises. At the same time, the quality of one's personal life is going to be shown in the quality of their service to others in their professional life. To be effective in the medical profession, individuals need to demonstrate maturity in both personal and professional selves to create the utmost of ethical conduct and professionalism.

Principle-Centered Leadership

  Stephen R. Covey, author of *The 7 Habits of Highly Effective People* and *Principle-Centered Leadership*, has identified eight characteristics of principle-centered leaders. Leaders who know themselves and understand their principles more easily abide by a code of ethics. Consider the following questions adapted from Covey's book as guides to how you might perform ethically in a medical setting:

- *Are you continually learning?* Do you seek training, take classes, listen to others, and learn from your peers? Are you curious? Do you realize that developing new knowledge and skills is a lifelong endeavor?

- *Are you service-oriented?* Do you see your life as a mission rather than a career? Are you generally a nurturing individual who seeks service in the medical field? Can you see yourself working alongside a coworker and pulling together with that person toward a goal? Can you put yourself in the place of others?

- *Do you radiate positive energy?* Are you cheerful, pleasant, optimistic, and positive? Is your spirit hopeful? If it is, you carry a positive energy field that allows you to neutralize or sidestep a negative energy source. Do you see yourself as a peacemaker or one who can create harmony to undo negative energy?

- *Do you believe in other people?* Can you keep from labeling, stereotyping, or prejudging other people? Can you believe in the unseen potential of others? Can you keep from overreacting to negative behaviors and criticism? Can you put aside any grudges?

The final characteristics of principle-centered leaders identified in Covey's book are more personal. They can help you understand yourself and how you might make ethical decisions in the medical field:

- *Do you lead a balanced life?* Do you keep up with current affairs and events? Do you know what is happening in the medical field and how that affects you? Do you have at least one confidant with whom you can be transparent? Are you physically active within your limits of age and health? Do you enjoy yourself? Do you have a good sense of humor? Are you open to communication?

- *Do you see life as an adventure?* Are you able to rediscover persons each time you meet them? Are you interested in others? Do you listen well? Are you flexible and unflappable? Does your security come from within rather than from without?

- *Are you synergistic?* Synergy is what happens when the whole of something is greater than the sum of its parts. Do you know your weaknesses? Can you complement your weaknesses with the strengths of others on the team? Can you work hard to improve most situations?

Are you trusting? Can you separate the person from the problem?

- *Do you exercise for self-renewal?* In this element, Mr. Covey identifies four dimensions of the human personality that need exercise: physical, mental, emotional, and spiritual dimensions. How do you keep your body in shape? How do you keep your mind alert? Do patience, unconditional love, and accepting responsibility for your own actions keep you emotionally healthy? Do you have a way to meditate, pray, or "draw away" for a period to "fill up your spirit"?

These questions and your responses to them can give you insight into your ability to function ethically and to be successful in the world of medicine.

Covey has a later book entitled *The 8th Habit: From Effectiveness to Greatness* that discusses how individuals can be more excited about their lives and their work when they reach beyond effectiveness toward fulfillment, contribution, and greatness. Individuals who feel fulfilled and excited about their work are more apt to perform ethically than those who do not.

Five Ps of Ethical Power

Another approach to how you might act in an ethical manner comes from Kenneth Blanchard and Norman Vincent Peale, who wrote a simple but powerful little book called *The Power of Ethical Management*. In it they discuss the "Five Ps of Ethical Power." The five Ps are as follows:

1. *Purpose.* Understand your objective or your purpose. Your purpose may change from time to time, but it is something that requires you to behave in a way that makes you feel good about yourself.
2. *Pride.* Have pride in what you do. Feel good about yourself and your accomplishments. Nurture your self-esteem while remaining humble. Be proud to be a medical assistant.
3. *Patience.* It takes time to create an atmosphere in which your objective can be obtained. Strive to believe that no matter what happens, everything is going to work out. Expect results from yourself and your work, but refrain from demanding it "now."
4. *Persistence.* To act in an ethical manner means to strive to act in that manner all the time, not

CRITICAL THINKING

With a peer, identify one or more examples in your life when you truly did not give up on attaining your goals. Describe what you learned from that experience. How might "never giving up" help in your pursuit of a career?

just when you want to or it seems easy to do. Winston Churchill said, "Never, never, never, never give up!" That is what persistence is. If you make a mistake, admit it, correct it, learn from the mistake, and move on, but never give up. An individual who is truly aware of his or her personal ethical power is able to admit an error, does not compromise any procedure or any technique, and does not ever put the patient at risk, even if it means facing reprimand from a supervisor.

5. *Perspective.* Keep your life and your purpose in perspective. Find time each day to maintain balance in your life (perhaps looking again at the eight questions for principle-centered individuals). Plan some quiet time, some fun time, but certainly some reflective time. The constant pressure and the crises will become overwhelming without keeping perspective.

Ethics Check Questions

Finally, when there is uncertainty about a dilemma or there is little or no experience to draw from, those striving to act in an ethical manner can perform a simple test each time there is a question about ethics. This, too, comes from Blanchard and Peale. The questions to ask are:

1. *Is it legal?* Is it against the law or any company policy?
2. *Is it balanced?* Is this the best possible approach for all concerned? Does it promote a win–win situation?
3. *How will it make me feel about myself?* Will I feel good if my decision is published in a newspaper? Will my family and coworkers be proud of my decision?

These questions provide a simple yet profound guide that is easy to recall and to apply to almost any situation. They are used throughout the business world by managers and employees seeking to work and practice legally and ethically.

Ethics are not easy. Performing ethically is hard work. Being ethical means determining who you are and how you will act. Laws are more clearly defined than ethics, but acting in an unethical manner can cause as much pain and difficulty as can acting illegally. The ideas of Covey, Blanchard, and Peale give guidance, thoughts to ponder, and perhaps goals to reach. Keep them in mind both as you review the next section and as you enter into your career as a medical assistant.

KEYS TO THE AAMA CODE OF ETHICS

 Medical assistants might consider the more salient points in the AAMA Code of Ethics (refer to Figure 8-1) and ask themselves the following questions:

A. *Render service with full respect for the dignity of humanity.*

- Will I respect every patient even if I do not approve of his or her morals or choices in health care?

- Will I honor each patient's request for information and explain unfamiliar procedures?

- Will I give my full attention to acknowledging the needs of every patient?

- Will I be able to accept the indigent, the physically and mentally challenged, the infirm, the physically disfigured, and the persons I simply do not like as equal and valid human beings with an equal right to service?

B. *Respect confidential information obtained through employment unless legally authorized or required by responsible performance of duty to divulge such information.*

- Will I refrain from needless comments to a colleague regarding a patient's problem?

- Will I refrain from discussing my day's encounters with patients with my family and friends?

- Will I always protect patients' medical information and records and everything included from unnecessary observation?

- Will I keep patients' names and the circumstances that bring them to my place of employment confidential?

C. *Uphold the honor and high principles of the profession and accept its disciplines.*

- Am I proud to serve as a medical assistant?

- Will I always perform within the scope of my profession, never exceeding the responsibility entrusted to me?

- Will I encourage others to enter the profession and always speak honorably of medical assistants?

D. *Seek to continually improve the knowledge and skills of medical assistants for the benefit of patients and professional colleagues.*

- Will I be willing to learn new skills, to update my skills, and seek improved methods for assisting the provider in the care of patients?

- Will I keep my credentials current and valid?

- Can I remember that I am a member of a group of broad-based health care professionals, and that my goal is to complement rather than to compete with that team?

E. *Participate in additional service activities aimed toward improving the health and well-being of the community.*

- Will I be able to serve in the community where I reside and work to further quality health care?

- Will I promote preventive medicine?

- Will I practice good health care management for myself and be a model for others to follow?

No matter how prepared, experienced, or principled one is in a chosen profession, there will still be times of great stress and wonder about decisions made.

ETHICAL GUIDELINES FOR HEALTH CARE PROVIDERS

As stated earlier, it is fairly common for each professional group of medical practitioners to have its own code of ethics. The AMA's Code of Medical Ethics and the "Current Opinions with Annotations of the Council on Ethical and Judicial Affairs" has been a leader in this field, but by no means is it the only code. The American Osteopathic Association has a Code of Ethics with 19 different sections. The American Chiropractic Association's Code of Ethics is identified in six sections. Other practitioners may consider their mission and policies to be their code of ethics. Some have no specific written code of ethics but rather call on their practitioners to refer to their culture as one based on ethics, mutual respect, and moral evaluation when ethical decisions are made. There are many similarities in these statements on ethics that are important for patients and medical employees. A few prominent statements are provided here.

Advertising

Health care providers and professional people traditionally have not advertised; however, it is not illegal or unethical to do so if claims made are truthful and not misleading. Advertisements may include credentials of providers and a description of the practice, kinds of services rendered, and how fees are determined. Managed care agencies may advertise their services and the names of participating providers.

Confidentiality

Providers must not reveal confidential information about patients without their consent unless the providers are otherwise required to do so by law. Confidentiality must be protected so that patients will feel comfortable and safe in revealing information about themselves that may be important to their health care. The following list contains examples of the kinds of reports that allow or require health professionals to report a confidence:

- A patient threatens another person and there is reason to believe that the threat may be carried out.
- Certain injuries and illnesses *must* be reported. These include injuries such as knife and gunshot wounds, wounds that may be from suspected child abuse, communicable diseases, and sexually transmitted diseases.
- Information that may have been subpoenaed for testimony in a court of law.

When in doubt, it is always recommended that a provider have the patient's permission to reveal any confidential information.

HIPAA

 Extra caution must be taken to protect the confidentiality of any patient's data that are kept on a computer database. As few people as possible should have access to the computer data, and only authorized individuals should be permitted to add or alter data. Adequate security precautions must be used to protect information stored on a computer. HIPAA has specific guidelines for computer privacy (see Chapters 11 and 14).

Medical Records

Medical records and the information in them are the property of the provider and the patient. No information should be revealed without the patient's consent unless required by law. The record is confidential. Providers should not refuse to provide a copy of the record to another provider treating the patient so long as proper authorization has been received from the patient. Also, providers should supply a copy of the record or summary of its contents if a patient requests it. A record cannot be withheld because of an unpaid bill.

On a provider's retirement or death, or when a practice is sold, patients should be notified and given ample time to have their records transferred to another provider of their choice.

Professional Fees and Charges

Illegal or excessive fees should not be charged. Fees should be based on those customary to the locale and should reflect the difficulty of services and the quality of performance rendered. Fee splitting (a provider splits the fee with another provider for services rendered with or without the patient's knowledge) in any form is unethical. Providers may charge for missed appointments (if patients have first been notified of the practice) and may charge for multiple or complex insurance forms. Providers and their employees must be diligent to ensure that only the services actually rendered are charged or indicated on the insurance claim. Only what is documented in the patient's chart is to be billed.

Increasingly, a number of providers refuse any insurance payments and operate strictly on a cash-only basis. There are others who charge a yearly fee to care for a family, providing all services necessary at that flat fee. Providers, upset by the rules and regulations of insurance, find this method of payment creates a simpler form of medical practice. Providers and patients alike will be discussing the ethics of such a move for some time. Although providers may choose whom they wish to serve, the cash-only basis is difficult for low-income families and the poor, thereby creating an ethical dilemma.

Professional Rights and Responsibilities

As stated earlier, providers may choose whom to serve, but they may not refuse a patient on the basis of race, color, religion, national origin, or any other illegal discrimination. It is unethical for providers to deny treatment to HIV-infected individuals on that basis alone if they are qualified to treat the patient's condition. Once a provider takes a case, the patient cannot be neglected or refused treatment unless official notice is given from the provider to withdraw from the case.

Patients have the right to know their diagnoses and the nature and purpose of their treatment and to have enough information to be able to make an informed choice about their treatment protocol. Providers should inform families of a patient's death and not delegate that responsibility to others.

Providers are expected to expose incompetent, corrupt, dishonest, and unethical conduct by other providers to the disciplinary board. It is unethical for any provider to treat patients while under the influence of alcohol, controlled substances, or any other chemical that impairs the provider's ability.

Providers who know they are HIV positive must refrain from any activity that would risk the transmission of the virus to others.

Any activity that might be regarded as a "conflict of interest" (for example, a provider holding stock in a pharmaceutical company and prescribing medications only from that company) is to be avoided. Financial interests are not to influence providers in prescribing medications, devices, or appliances.

Disaster Response and Emergency Preparedness

Medical professionals are essential at the time of any disaster, such as epidemics, floods, fires, weather-related disasters, and terrorist attacks. Care for the sick and injured is of primary concern when disaster strikes. Providers are encouraged to give their medical expertise not only to prepare for any type of disaster but to provide assistance when one occurs. Providers should consider seeking training in emergency preparedness and disaster response and lend their knowledge where it is most beneficial and effective in making certain that medical care is available during such events (see Chapter 10).

Treatment for a Culturally Diverse Clientele

 All providers are reminded to strive to provide the same quality of care to all their patients regardless of race or ethnicity. Providers must remember to eliminate biased behavior toward any group of patients deemed different from themselves. All patients have the right to participatory decision making with their providers based on mutual trust and understanding. Communication factors are to be considered and interpreters provided as necessary so that patients understand the medical information as well as any communication exchanged.

Diversity is to be encouraged in the medical profession and considered when hiring assistants. Ethnically diverse neighborhoods and clientele deserve an ethnically diverse group of medical professionals for their care. If it is not possible to employ an ethnically diverse group of medical professionals, then medical professionals who are keenly aware of and knowledgeable of the ethic group served is of primary importance.

Care of the Poor

From the earliest history of medical treatment, care for the poor has been a concern and a goal for medical practitioners. Today that obligation is still mentioned in most ethical codes and discussions. All medical providers have a responsibility to ensure that the needs of the poor in their communities are met. Caring for the poor should be a regular part of every provider's practice and can be accomplished in a number of ways. Providers can be encouraged to take a certain number of patients on a reduced-cost basis or provide free services. Providers can volunteer their time and efforts to treat patients in reduced-cost, freestanding clinics that treat the poor or provide services to those in homeless shelters for battered and abused individuals. Providers can volunteer their time to lobbying and being advocates for those without medical coverage.

Abuse

Abuse usually is described as neglect, physical injury, emotional/psychological/mental injury, or sexual abuse. In child abuse, there also may be molestation, sexual exploitation, and incest. Elder abuse can come in the form of any other abuse, but financial abuse is included. Stalking and rape are also considered to be forms of abuse.

All 50 states have legislation defining child abuse and mandate who is responsible for reporting such abuse. The majority of states have enacted legislation regarding the abuse of elder adults 60 years of age or older. Intimate partner (or domestic) violence is a criminal offense in some states, but whether a state requires that **intimate partner violence (IPV)** be reported depends in part upon whether a weapon is used.

Stalking is the repeated act of spying upon, following, or making contact with an individual or appearing at an individual's residence or place of employment after being asked not to. It is a crime in some states. *Rape,* also a crime of violence, is forced sexual intercourse or penetration of a body orifice with the penis or some other object. Gang rape involves several individuals. Rape is a reportable criminal act.

Medical assistants must know if their state specifically names them as a reporter for abuse. A discussion should be held with medical providers and employers regarding who, when, and how the abuse will be reported and documented. It is unethical for a medical assistant to fail to report abuse simply because an employer prefers "not to get too involved." For a clearer understanding of some of the factors that constitute abuse, review Table 8-1.

It is the responsibility of medical professionals and their employees to report all cases of suspected child abuse, to protect and care for the abused, and to treat the abuser (if known) as a victim also. This is not an easy task. Abuse is not easy to witness. Although there are

Table 8-1   Descriptions of Abuse

Type of Abuse	Child Abuse	Elder Abuse	Intimate Partner Violence
Neglect	Failure to provide basic food, shelter, care; endangering health of child	Lack of attention that causes harm; withholding basic needs; abandonment; lack of help with hygiene or bathing	Not treating a partner with respect; not recognizing the human worth of an individual
Physical abuse	Causing burns, unusual or severe bruising, lacerations, fractures, injury to internal organs; usually obvious	Assault, beating, whipping, hitting, punching, pushing, pinching, force-feeding, shaking, rough handling during caregiving, causing bodily harm or severe mental stress	Intent to harm; hitting, pushing, grabbing, biting, punching, slapping, restraining, burning; use of a weapon or one's own strength to harm
Emotional/psychological abuse	Causing harm to child's emotional and intellectual growth; not always obvious	Actions that dehumanize; social isolation, name calling, humiliating, insulting; threats to punish; yelling, screaming	Humiliating; controlling; isolating partner from friends/family; denying personal support and encouragement
Sexual abuse	Using a child to engage in any sexual activity; abuse not always obvious	Sexual contact without permission; fondling, touching, kissing, rape, coerced nudity; spying while in bathroom	Sexual contact without permission; abusive sexual contact; sex with one who is unable to say "no"
Sexual exploitation	Pornography, prostitution; use of child's image in media; incest or sexual activity between family members	Showing an elderly person pornographic material; forcing the person to watch sex acts; forcing the elder to undress in presence of others	Forcing a partner to engage in sexual acts with others against that partner's will.
Financial abuse	Refusal to provide the basics of adequate health care or clothing	Exploitation of an elder's resources; forging signature on documents; withholding or cashing funds received	Withholding funds or basic resources; monitoring to the penny funds spent for groceries or expenses of daily living

specific laws regarding suspected child abuse, and in most states medical assistants are mandated to report abuse, the laws are vague or nonexistent for older adults or in cases of IPV. However, whatever form the abuse takes, it is best to treat all forms of abuse in the same manner by providing a safe environment for those abused and seeking treatment for the abused and the abuser.

BIOETHICS

Bioethics brings the entire focus of ethics into the field of health care and into those ethical issues dealing with life. Never before in the history of medical care has bioethics been such a topic of concern. In the past, most bioethical decisions were made by physicians and esteemed members of the medical or legal profession. However, advancing technology giving patients and consumers numerous choices regarding their health care leads everyone to take a more active role in bioethics.

Medical assistants will encounter ethical and bioethical issues across a total lifespan. In Figure 8-3, a few issues are identified for contemplation and discussion. Issues of bioethics common to every medical clinic are the allocation of scarce medical resources; is health care a right or privilege; reproductive issues such as contraception, assisted reproduction, abortion and fetal tissue research; genetic engineering or manipulation; and the many choices surrounding life, dying, and death.

Guidelines for bioethical issues are even harder to define than are guidelines for ethics, because each of the bioethical issues calls for decisions that directly affect a person's life. In some instances, the bioethical issue requires a choice about who lives and requires a definition of the quality of life. Such dilemmas are difficult, if not impossible, to approach from a neutral point of view even though medical professionals should strive not to impose their own moral values on patients or coworkers.

Allocation of Scarce Medical Resources

The issue faced daily by health care workers is the allocation of scarce medical resources or rationing of health care. Even with the government's attempts at health care reform, medical resources are not available to everyone. When the administrative medical assistant determines who receives the only available appointment in a day, when patients are turned away because they have no insurance or financial resources to pay for services, when Medicare and Medicaid patients are denied services because of low return from state and federal insurance programs, medical resources are being rationed and denied.

The Centers for Disease Control and Prevention (CDC) reported that 59 million people were without health insurance coverage in 2011. Although the Health Care Reform Act of 2010 has brought some reform and an end to some issues of rationing, the issue is still a serious one. These reforms have helped more children get health coverage, ended lifetime and most annual limits on care, allows young adults under 26 to stay on their parent's health insurance, and gives some patients access to a number of recommended preventive services such as vaccinations, influenza and pneumonia shots, and blood pressure and diabetes screenings without co-payment or deductible costs. Other reforms are in process. A yearly timeline can be viewed at http://www.healthcare.gov/law/provisions/preventive/index.html to help you determine those most pertinent to the ambulatory care setting.

Hispanic and non-Hispanic black children are still more likely to have no health care than are non-Hispanic white children. Of note, the average waiting time by new patients for a medical appointment is between 14 and 17 days. The elderly, many of whom have both Medicare and supplemental health insurance, have difficulty finding providers who take new Medicare patients. This dilemma can be particularly problematic when the elderly move from their homes and communities to be closer to their children.

Weightier decisions might include who gets the surgery, a kidney transplant, or the bone marrow transplant. These allocations and rationing decisions are being made and will continue to require dedication on the part of the health care team. Rationing of health care will continue to be an issue as politicians, health care providers, and consumers struggle to achieve a balance between providing access to care while still curtailing costs.

Decisions made by Congress, health systems agencies, and insurance companies are termed **macroallocation** of scarce medical resources. Decisions made individually by providers and members of the health care team at the local level are termed **microallocation** of scarce resources. No matter what the level, medical assistants will be involved.

ETHICAL ISSUES FOR CONTEMPLATION AND DISCUSSION

Infants

- Imperiled newborns (those who are seriously disabled, deformed, often premature with low birth weight) have a greater chance for survival with today's medical technology. However, this ability places parents and health care professionals in an uncomfortable position to determine when the costs of expensive intervention outweigh the benefits. Often medical insurance does not cover these costs.
- Vulnerability of infants can lead to negligence, rejection, and even abuse. Parents are vulnerable, too, because of their inability to cope with the entire family's needs. How can families be helped in these challenging situations?

Children

- Children who are not well fed, housed, educated, and clothed exhibit great needs for preventive, curative, and rehabilitative health care. They likely do not have medical coverage, do not see a health care provider regularly, and make more trips to the hospital emergency room than other children.
- Increasing numbers of children are not receiving proper inoculations to protect them from communicable diseases.
- Obesity in children is a serious health issue. Evidence of eating disorders is seen at an earlier age. Many children receive one or two free or low-cost meals at school, share very few meals with their family members, and eat at fast-food restaurants. Sweets are often used as reward or to express love. Even while a move is being made toward healthier choices at the national level, how are children educated to make better choices?
- ADHD and eating disorders often require comprehensive mental health evaluation which is not available to children or inadequately covered by insurance.
- An increasing number of children live within very dysfunctional families where one or more parent is absent, is a substance abuser, has mental health issues, or has very little time to spend with their children. Many children have multiple parents or caregivers. Many spend large portions of the day in a daycare environment. Child abuse is a concern. Children must be protected, but they can be caught in a web of social services so overloaded and understaffed that only the most severe concerns receive attention. How do health professionals protect these children?
- Increased allergies and asthma are seen in young children and often carry into adulthood. Children rarely have control over their environment, often the cause of allergy and asthma.

Adolescents

- The adolescent's growing autonomy, need for independence, changing values, and desire for peer acceptance often lead to the decision to become sexually active, use birth control, or experiment with drugs and alcohol.
- Mental health issues and ADHD often interfere with the adolescent's normal social development, yet adequate mental health assessment and treatment is difficult to find. Eating disorders may be serious issues, especially for teenage girls. Conversely, problems with obesity continue.
- Adolescents as young as 14 to 18 years of age may seek treatment for substance abuse, birth control, even abortion without parental consent. Does this violate parents' right to medical information regarding their children? Should the adolescent, often fearful of parental reaction, have a right to treatment? Who pays?

Adults

- A large number of men and women find that both must be employed in order to provide a home for their families. How is it possible to balance full-time employment, full-time parenting, full-time housekeeping, and full-time partnering, and still take care of oneself?
- Many low-income women lack sufficient access to prenatal care, even though it is a cost-saving medical measure that is critical to the health of both mother and infant.
- Adequate and quality health care is a problem. Some adults have no health care coverage; others are part of managed care programs that keep changing as employers seek lower health insurance premiums. Many adults lack an ongoing provider–patient relationship.
- War, terrorist attacks, and an overburdened military place families in very stressful circumstances. Many who serve in the military are returning with horrendous lifelong and debilitating injuries. Lives are forever changed. How do they cope?
- Even with an advance directive or living will, a dying patient's wishes may not be followed. Technological advances in medicine have created situations where patients may not be able to exercise their wishes.

Senior Adults

- Elderly patients have the right to maintain dignity and privacy, but their dependency on others may deprive them of these basic rights.
- Many senior adults are finding that very few providers accept new Medicare patients. The problem is even more severe when senior adults must rely upon Medicaid for their medical care because of the few number of providers who accept Medicaid.
- Even with health care reform, some elderly patients must choose between food on their tables or prescribed medications they cannot afford.
- Dementia is a common problem that is physically and financially exhausting and heartbreaking to the caregiver who usually is a spouse, partner, or adult child. How do individuals cope in the "sandwich" arrangement of caring for themselves, their children, and elderly parents, some who may have dementia? What happens when there are insufficient funds for assisted living or long-term care?

Figure 8-3 Ethical issues across the life span.

© Cengage Learning 2014. Compiled by Carol D. Tamparo, CMA (AAMA), PhD, and Marilyn Pooler, RN, MEd.

Health Care: A Right or a Privilege?

Very close to the issue of allocation of scarce medical resources is the question whether basic health care is a right or a privilege. There are many countries within the world where health care is a privilege provided only to a few either because of the availability of health care or because of one's financial resources. However, even within the United States, where the best of health care is available, there are health care professionals whose personal ideologies often discriminate and deny basic health care.

For example, consider the following circumstances. How would you choose?

- *For the available kidney.* A young mother of two or a 45-year-old gentleman (a recovering addict) with numerous body piercings?
- *For the next available pediatric appointment.* A 16-year-old who needs an athletic physical or a troubled and combative 13-year-old whose only insurance is Medicaid?
- *For artificial insemination.* The single woman desiring a child of her own or the couple who have been trying to get pregnant for 3 years?
- *Referral to a mental health specialist.* A prominent businessman suffering from depression with symptoms of bipolar disorder or a welfare mom struggling with addiction?

It is often difficult to remain neutral and wait for decisions until all the facts are known. One area of discrimination surrounds the health care issue of AIDS and HIV.

HIV and AIDS

The general public's fear and wariness of AIDS (acquired immunodeficiency syndrome) continues to cause some serious bioethical issues. Patients who suspect they have HIV (human immunodeficiency virus) or AIDS should be tested for the virus. In fact, the CDC recommends that voluntary screening for HIV/AIDS become a routine part of medical care for all patients ages 13 to 64 years. Confidentiality must be safely guarded, however, because individuals with HIV/AIDS have been denied medical insurance, faced loss of employment and housing, and even suffered the loss of family members and friends. It is unethical to deny treatment to individuals because they test positive for HIV.

Although individuals with HIV/AIDS are to be protected, so must the public. Therefore, if providers suspect that an HIV-seropositive patient is infecting an unsuspecting individual, every attempt should be made to protect the individual at risk. Health professionals will first encourage the infected person to cease any activity that endangers that person. If the patient refuses to notify the person at risk, authorities can be contacted. Many states and cities have Partner Notification Programs that will anonymously notify any person at risk, keeping the source confidential. The program informs them that it has been brought to their attention that they are a "person at risk" and provides them with free testing. In some instances, the provider can notify any person at risk.

Reproductive Issues

Reproductive bioethical issues generally affect women more than men. A few are identified here. Most medical assistants will be faced with these issues at some time in their career, even if they are not employed in specialty clinics.

Female Genital Mutilation. The World Health Organization (WHO) reports that there are over 170,000 young girls and women in the United States who have been subjected to **female genital mutilation** (FGM). FGM includes partial or complete removal of the clitoris (female circumcision), partial or total removal of the labia minora or labia majora, infibulation (narrowing the vaginal opening by creating a covering seal), and the pricking, piercing, or cauterizing of genitals. These procedures are performed, in part, to enhance a man's sexual pleasure, but destroy a woman's capacity for sexual pleasure and can cause serious infections. The practice can also cause recurring urinary tract infections, difficulties with menstruation, and pregnancy complications. FGM is illegal in this country, but can be seen in immigrants from countries such as some African, Asian, and Middle Eastern nations where it is regularly practiced.

Contraception. Birth control of any kind, other than *fertility awareness methods (FAM)* that require abstinence from sexual intercourse during ovulation, is still a taboo in some cultures and religions and becomes a bioethical dilemma. Many are opposed to any contraception that destroys a fertilized egg. Therefore, a thorough understanding of how a particular contraception works is essential for some patients.

The controversy gained attention when the RU-486 or mifepristone hormone drug became available for use in the United States in the last decade. RU-486, often referred to as the abortion pill, ends an early pregnancy. In general, it can be used up to 63 days—9 weeks—after the first day of a woman's last period.

Contraception continues to be an issue addressed more by women than their male partners. To date, there is no reliable birth control method for men other than a condom.

Sterilization. When permanent contraception is sought, sterilization has become the choice. It is not only used by those who simply wish to prevent pregnancy, but it may be practiced by those who prefer not to pass on a genetic anomaly. A **tubal ligation** for women and a **vasectomy** for men are considered permanent, even though there have been reversals. Some religious groups oppose permanent sterilization.

Assisted Reproduction. Assistance with reproduction is very common today. Artificial insemination, in vitro fertilization, and surrogacy are most commonly practiced.

For many individuals, *artificial insemination* is the only means by which they are able to conceive a child. Providers are called on to perform artificial insemination for couples and for women who want a child. If artificial insemination is performed, it is recommended that the signed consent of each party involved be obtained. It is also recommended that providers practicing artificial insemination by donor have several donors available for semen collection and that meticulous screening be performed before the insemination.

In vitro fertilization (IVF) is a process that has been shown to be very successful in the past decade. In IVF, the ovum is fertilized in a culture dish, allowed to grow, and then implanted into the uterus. This procedure can be used for women with blocked fallopian tubes or oviducts. Ethically, this procedure faces little controversy when a husband's sperm is used to fertilize his wife's ovum, which is then implanted into her uterus. Other procedures raise ethical concerns for some and are not addressed in law.

A woman can have a donor's egg fertilized by her husband's sperm for implantation. A woman can receive donor embryos (embryo adoption) from successfully completed IVF from two unrelated individuals. Couples who have successfully had a baby through IVF are sometimes willing to donate their additional embryos. A woman can carry an embryo created from a donor egg and donor sperm that will have no genetic relationship to her.

It is possible to screen for genetic flaws among embryos created by IVF; however, the latest medical research indicates that such analysis sometimes causes abnormalities.

Surrogacy is another method of assisted reproduction. Men have been used as **surrogates**, or substitutes, for decades with the practice of artificial insemination. Society seems to have a more difficult time accepting surrogate mothers who are artificially inseminated by a donor and carry the fetus to term for another parent. Men sometimes seek surrogates who are able to provide them a child who represents half their genetic makeup. Women may choose a surrogate if they are unable to carry a pregnancy to term for medical or personal reasons. How should the rights of each individual in the arrangement and exchange be protected? For many of these issues, there is little protection or guidance under the law; therefore, health professionals are often required to make decisions on the basis of their personal belief systems.

Ethical questions are sometimes raised regarding assisted reproduction. Should artificial insemination and in vitro fertilization be performed for individuals who do not fit the "traditional" family model? Who will be a fit mother or father for this infant? Some religious faiths consider artificial insemination by donor to be the same as adultery. Who or what agency carefully protects the selection and screening process of donors and surrogates? How are donors selected? Is there a responsibility to make certain that individuals with the same father through artificial insemination by donor do not marry? Some fertility specialists recommend that a donor be chosen from a city far from where the potential mother lives and that formal adoption occur immediately when the infant is born. Some oppose in vitro fertilization because fertilized ova are destroyed if found to be genetically inappropriate. Others have great difficulty when embryos that are not implanted are often frozen for later use, but sometimes are abandoned and eventually destroyed.

Most assisted reproduction techniques were viewed as experimental and quite controversial just 25 years ago. Today, however, the procedures are widely practiced and available. Assisted reproduction is very costly and can create legal tangles for all involved if careful steps are not taken.

Abortion and Fetal Tissue Research

The issues associated with abortion and fetal tissue research will be with us for quite some time. Although the law as set forth in *Roe v. Wade* is specific on abortion guidelines, there is a continual challenge in the courts of its validity. A number of states continue to press for more restrictions regarding whether and how abortions might be performed in the second and third trimesters of pregnancy, and challenge the U.S. Supreme Court's decision in *Roe v. Wade*. However, the current law stipulates that a woman has a right to an abortion in the first trimester without interference from regulations in any state.

Medical professionals must decide whether to perform abortions within these legal parameters and under what circumstances. Providers cannot be forced to perform abortions, nor can any employee be forced to participate or assist in an abortion. Employees not wishing to participate in abortions are advised to seek employment where they are not performed.

The volatility of the issue is so strong that terrorism on some abortion clinics and their providers has made it difficult for a person wanting an abortion to receive one. Terrorism of any sort is illegal, but providers who perform abortions have been murdered, one even in a church during worship. Such terrorism points to the very passionate debate that is unlikely ever to find a common ground of agreement.

Many unanswered ethical questions related to abortion make the decision difficult for health care professionals. Should abortion be considered a form of birth control? If not, should birth control and abortion be readily available to all who seek it, regardless of age? Should insurance pay for birth control? Is it ethical to deny an abortion to a woman on welfare but provide one to a woman who has money for the procedure or whose insurance pays? Some question if *any* abortion should be legal. And, of course, the major unanswered question that must be considered by every individual is: When does life begin—at conception, when the brain begins to function, quickening, or at birth?

The abortion issue raises the bioethical issue of fetal tissue research and transplantation. As early as the 1950s, fetal tissue research led to the development of polio and rubella vaccines. Today, fetal cells hold promise for medical research into a variety of diseases and medical conditions, including Alzheimer's disease, Huntington's disease, spinal cord injury, diabetes, and multiple sclerosis. Some research indicates that fetal retinal transplants may be a successful treatment of macular degeneration, which is the leading cause of age-related blindness in the United States. This issue is political as well as bioethical, and it changes with each major political shift in the government. About half

CRITICAL THINKING

When fertilization occurs outside the womb, additional embryos are stored and saved for future use. How long should they be stored? To whom do they belong? What happens if no one wants those embryos later? Should they be destroyed, given to some other hopeful parent, or used for genetic research?

of the states have laws regulating fetal research. Some ban research using aborted fetuses. Federal law prohibits the sale of fetal tissue and requires all federally funded fetal tissue research projects to comply with state and local laws. Fetal tissue research is not to be used to encourage women to have abortions; rather, the tissue would be available only after a decision had already been made regarding abortion.

While the debate related to the use of fetal tissues for research marches on, the door has opened for research using umbilical cord blood. The use of cord blood has met with little controversy. In 2005, President George W. Bush signed into legislation a federal program to collect and store cord blood and to expand the current bone marrow registry program to include cord blood. Stem cells in cord blood have shown to be beneficial. For example, they can help restore red blood cells in people with sickle cell anemia. When a small group of children newly diagnosed with type 1 diabetes were transfused with their own stored cord blood, they showed reduced severity of the disease.

Medical assistants who work in fertility clinics must at all times respect the choices made by individuals seeking artificial insemination, IVF, or surrogacy. These procedures are truly private and very personal. Anyone who feels uncomfortable with such procedures is likely to be happier finding employment elsewhere.

Genetic Engineering/Manipulation

So much is possible today in the area of **genetic engineering** and new discoveries increasingly are being made. This biotechnology can be used in the diagnosis of disease, in the production of medicines, for forensic documentation (DNA used in solving crimes), and for research. Some reasons for continuing study in this area include determining if anything can be done to prevent or cure some 4,000 recognized genetic disorders and major diseases that have large genetic components. Few individuals would not like to see a cure for certain illnesses, but there is a fear among many that genetic engineering may lead to choices that should not be made. Deciding what should be done when the unborn is determined to have a severe birth defect, manipulating genes to a more perfect offspring, and discarding defective embryos are just a few of those concerns.

If and when countries move past the dilemma related to the use of embryonic stem cells, a number of significant medical advances might be made. Researchers may be able to create custom-made organs to replace those that are defective or diseased. Although it might be a wonderful thing to create a new pancreas or a semisynthetic liver to replace an organ that is no longer performing its necessary function, the greater fear of some individuals is that of cloning. Scientists already have cloned mice, sheep, rabbits, goats, pigs, and a dog. Where does cloning stop? Will human beings be cloned if science advances further into research with stem cells? Some countries with a different political arena than the one found in the United States are moving into this area. It is interesting to note, however, that in August 2005 the General Assembly of the United Nations voted to prohibit all forms of human cloning.

Dying and Death

The goal for all health professionals is to preserve and enhance life, thus making death an event contrary to the goals of health care. Yet, death cannot be avoided. How death is faced has both legal and ethical dimensions. Legally, individuals can make choices about their death and are often encouraged to do so by health care and legal professionals. When those wishes are indicated in documents such as advance directives and when health professionals disagree or refuse to honor those wishes, a legal problem arises.

The legal aspect was made famous by the cases of Karen Ann Quinlan and Theresa (Terri) Schiavo. Both were young women, without any advance health care directives, whose deaths were caught in battles between family members, the medical staff, and the courts. Quinlan lived for 11 years in a vegetative state after much duress with health professionals and hospital staff who believed she should be kept on a respirator. The family members of Schiavo were in legal battles for 15 years before permission was received to remove her feeding tube; she died 14 days later. When there is conflict among family and those caring for someone near death, even a well-written and executed advance directive can be faced with challenges. Then a legal dilemma becomes an ethical dilemma as well.

Patients continue to make decisions expressing their choices in death. Oregon was the first state to pass legislation allowing physicians to assist patients in death. The Oregon law was voted upon and passed on two separate occasions and was challenged by the U.S. Attorney General before the U.S. Supreme Court determined that the law could stand. Washington state voters approved similar legislation November 2008. Montana was recently added to the list, but Massacuhusetts failed to pass a similar measure in November, 2012. Several other states are struggling with issues to allow those who are dying a death with dignity. Many find comfort in the law that allows them the right to choose the time and place for their own death; however, the number of individuals who choose physician-assisted death still is small. Some make the choice, receive the medications from their physician, and then do not use the medication. Others receive the medication, find much relief in their choice, and do take the medication. Still others believe that any intervention that hastens death is criminal.

The law is changing rapidly as additional states wrestle with the concept of assisted death. For the latest up-to-date information, refer to your state's legislation.

Choices available to patients who are dying create the question, What is "quality of life"? Although the answer to that question is different for everyone, it is a question often in conflict with today's medical technology that can, in many instances, keep a patient alive much longer than the patient might prefer. The benefits of advanced technology will continue to be weighed against what many consider the right to die with dignity and a minimum of medical intervention.

Hospice

Hospice is the term used to describe either a place of residence for those who are dying or an organization whose medical professionals and volunteers are in attendance of someone whose death is imminent. The main objective of hospice is to make patients comfortable and as free from pain as possible and to allow them dignity in their deaths.

Cardiopulmonary resuscitation (CPR), intravenous therapy, and feeding tubes are discouraged. Death is treated as a natural end-of-life experience. Death is neither hastened nor prevented.

Hospice volunteers and their counselors indicate that although most patients will choose hospice, some family members may not be as comfortable in that choice. Family members may not be ready to let go of a loved one; also, they may be uncomfortable if the hospice service is in the home rather than the hospital or a hospice facility. The latter is related to how comfortable family members are in observing or being a part of the death process. The expense of hospice is often covered by medical insurance and is less expensive than inpatient hospital care.

Medical assistants may be involved with the hospice protocol when patients of their employers are referred to and become a client of the hospice.

CASE STUDY 8-1

Refer to the scenario at the beginning of the chapter.

Harley Navarro, the new medical assistant, is especially hesitant to ask for assistance or admit that he is having a problem. Twice today he was unable to get a good blood pressure reading on patients. One patient was very obese, and the other kept trying to carry on a conversation with him.

CASE STUDY REVIEW

1. If Harley's behavior does no harm to the patient, has he acted unethically? Illegally?

2. What might the office manager do if she senses Harley's lack of certainty?

3. Discuss the role of female and male medical assistants working together and how they might complement each other.

CASE STUDY 8-2

Liz Corbin is a medical assistant in the fertility clinic of a large metropolitan medical clinic and hospital. Liz really likes her job and is delighted when parenthood is made possible for many of those seeking the clinic's advanced technology. The clinic also stores and maintains the unused frozen embryos that result from artificial insemination. She is a little alarmed when her provider–employer informs her that four of the embryos are to be destroyed. Her employer has been unable to contact the owners (now parents of more than one child from artificial insemination) for directions, and space for storage is limited. Liz is instructed to destroy the embryos.

CASE STUDY REVIEW

1. Liz is rather hesitant to comply with her employer's orders, so she does a little research. She discovers that most fertility clinics ask couples using **cryopreservation** to decide early in the process how to handle their excess embryos. The choices are to (1) discard the embryos, (2) donate anonymously to other infertile couples, and (3) donate to scientific research. What might Liz do to influence the clinic's policy?

2. Can anything be done to ensure that couples do not abandon their embryos?

3. If embryos are given to other infertile couples, how is a decision made on who should have them?

SUMMARY

As medical technology continues to advance, a greater need for ethical guidelines is necessary. Providers and health care professionals at all levels must stay abreast of the issues and carefully consider all aspects before making any decision.

Medical assistants must, however, keep the following legal and ethical guidelines in mind: (1) always practice within the law; (2) preserve the patient's confidentiality; (3) maintain meticulous records; (4) obtain informed, written consent; (5) do not judge patients whose belief system differs from yours.

STUDY FOR SUCCESS

To reinforce your knowledge and skills of information presented in this chapter:

- Review the *Key Terms*
- Role-play with other students to apply attributes of professionalism pertinent to this chapter.
- Consider the *Case Studies* and discuss your conclusions
- Answer the questions in the *Certification Review*
- Apply your knowledge by completing the *Activities* in the *Study Guide* and the *Games and Quizzes* in the StudyWARE **StudyWARE** software on the *Premium Website*
- Practice your problem-solving skills with the *Critical Thinking Challenge 3.0* on the *Premium Website*

Additional resources for this chapter include:

- Module 3 of the *Medical Assisting Learning Lab*
- *CourseMate for Delmar's Comprehensive Medical Assisting*
- *WebTutor for Delmar's Comprehensive Medical Assisting*

CERTIFICATION REVIEW

1. Typically, ethics has been defined in terms of:
   a. what is right and wrong
   b. whether an action is legal
   c. the expedient thing to do
   d. professionalism in the workplace

2. Bioethics has to do with:
   a. biological reproduction
   b. the act of artificial insemination
   c. genetic engineering
   d. ethical issues that deal with life and health care

3. The AAMA Code of Ethics:
   a. is concerned with principles of ethical and moral conduct
   b. defines the duties the medical assistant can perform
   c. is intended for physicians only
   d. applies only to patient rights

4. When providers or medical assistants suspect child abuse, they should:
   a. give the parent a warning
   b. report it to the proper authorities
   c. not impose their values on the parents
   d. give the child some hints on how to protect against abuse

5. When a patient has HIV:
   a. it is ethical for the provider not to provide treatment
   b. it is unethical for the provider not to provide treatment
   c. other patients should be warned of the possibility of infection
   d. all friends and family members of the patient should be notified

6. Macroallocation of scarce medical resources implies that:
   a. the local health care team makes the decisions
   b. Congress, health systems agencies, and insurance companies make the decisions
   c. medical assistants will not be involved
   d. patients will get the benefit of the best medical care

7. The eight characteristics of principle-centered leaders originates from the following author:
   a. James R. Jones
   b. Stephen R. Covey
   c. Francis H. Ambrose
   d. Jason N. Diamond

8. The five Ps of ethical power are:
   a. personality, performance, purpose, pride, patience
   b. purpose, patience, perfection, personality, procrastination
   c. patience, purpose, pride, persistence, perspective
   d. purpose, pride, patience, perfection, perspective
9. Which of the following is true?
   a. A provider can choose whom to serve.
   b. A provider may charge for completing multiple and complex insurance claims.
   c. Providers and their employees cannot be forced to perform abortions.
   d. All of the above
   e. Only b and c above

10. You are most likely to make ethical decisions correctly when:
    a. you have a clear picture of the situation
    b. you leave emotion out of the decision as much as possible
    c. you understand your weaknesses and vulnerabilities
    d. honesty and integrity are hallmarks of your entire life
    e. all of the above

REFERENCES/BIBLIOGRAPHY

American Medical Association. (2010–2011). Code of medical ethics. *Current opinions of the council on ethical and judicial affairs, 2010.* Chicago: American Medical Association.

Blanchard, K., & Peale, N. V. (1988). *The power of ethical management.* New York: William Morrow and Company, Inc.

Covey, S. R. (1991). *Principle-centered leadership.* New York: Simon & Schuster.

Lewis, M. A., Tamparo, C. D., & Tatro, B. M. (2012). *Medical law, ethics, and bioethics for health professions* (7th ed.). Philadelphia: F. A. Davis.

OUTLINE

Recognizing an Emergency
- Responding to an Emergency
- Primary Survey
- Using the 911 or Emergency Medical Services System
- Good Samaritan Laws
- Blood, Body Fluids, and Disease Transmission

Preparing for an Emergency
- The Medical Crash Tray or Cart

Common Emergencies
- Shock
- Wounds
- Burns
- Musculoskeletal Injuries
- Heat- and Cold-Related Illnesses
- Poisoning
- Sudden Illness

- Cerebral Vascular Accident
- Heart Attack

Breathing Emergencies and Cardiac Arrest
- Rescue Breathing
- Cardiopulmonary Resuscitation

Safety and Emergency Practices

LEARNING OUTCOMES

1. Define, spell, and pronounce the key terms as presented in the glossary.
2. Learn to recognize, prepare for, and respond to emergencies in the ambulatory care setting.
3. Describe basic principles of first aid and demonstrate first aid procedures.
4. Understand the legal and ethical considerations of providing emergency care.
5. Demonstrate appropriate interventions to prevent disease transmission considerations in emergency situations.
6. Perform the primary assessment in emergency situations.
7. Identify and care for different types of wounds.
8. Understand the basics of bandage application.
9. Discriminate among first-, second-, and third-degree burns.
10. Assess injuries to muscles, bones, and joints.
11. Describe heat- and cold-related illnesses.
12. Describe how poisons may enter the body.
13. List the symptoms of a poisonous snake bite.
14. Recall six types of shock.
15. Define a cerebral vascular accident.
16. Describe the signs and symptoms of a heart attack.
17. Discuss potential role(s) of the medical assistant in emergency preparedness.
18. Analyze the professionalism questions and apply them to this chapter's content.

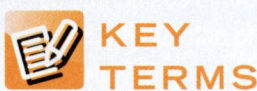

KEY TERMS

abrasions

anaphylactic

automated external
    defibrillator (AED)

avulsion

bandage

cardiogenic

cardiopulmonary
    resuscitation (CPR)

cardioversion

cauterized

constriction band

crash tray or cart

crepitation

dislocation

dressing

emergency medical
    services (EMS)

explicit

first aid

fracture

hypothermia

hypovolemic

implicit

lackluster

myocardial
    infarction (MI)

neurogenic

normal saline

occlusion

rescue breathing

risk management

septic

shock

splint

sprain

Standard Precautions

strain

syncope

triage

universal emergency
    medical identification
    symbol

vasovagal syncope

wound

ATTRIBUTES OF PROFESSIONALISM

Communication
- Did you demonstrate empathy in communicating with patients, family, and staff?

Presentation
- Did you display a calm, professional, and caring manner?

Competency
- Did you display sound judgment?
- Did you remain calm in a crisis?
- Were you knowledgeable and accountable?
- Did you apply critical thinking skills in performing patient assessment and care?
- Did you recognize the importance of local, state, and federal legislation and regulations in the practice setting?
- Did you recognize the effect of stress on all persons involved in emergency situations?
- Did you demonstrate self-awareness in responding to emergency situations?

Initiative
- Did you seek out opportunities to expand your knowledge base?
- Did you direct the patient to other resources when necessary or helpful, with the approval of the provider?

Integrity
- Did you work within your scope of practice?
- Did you demonstrate sensitivity to patient's rights?
- Did you protect and maintain confidentiality?

SCENARIO

It has been a busy day at Tri-City Clinic. The final patient is being seen. Just as Phyllis Cosper, RMA, is closing the door to the lobby, Mr. Keston Edwards enters holding his chest. He states, "Your clinic is closer than the hospital and I needed to see someone. My chest is hurting and I can't catch my breath."

Ms. Cosper knows that Mr. Edwards is exhibiting signs of a heart attack. She immediately notifies the provider and instructs the front desk person to call 911. Ms. Cosper escorts Mr. Edwards to a treatment room, has him lie down, and immediately takes his vital signs. As Ms. Cosper is certified in CPR and first aid, she begins to take the appropriate steps to make sure that the patient is safe and cared for prior to the arrival of EMS. Mr. Edwards is given a full-strength aspirin to chew and oxygen is applied. Mr. Edwards is calm and his chest pain is easing just as the EMS team arrives. It is essential to activate the EMS system as soon as possible when an emergency presents itself in a nonacute care setting. Care is then relinquished to the EMS personnel to provide further intervention.

INTRODUCTION

Although the ambulatory care setting is primarily designed to see patients under nonemergency conditions, occasionally the provider will need to administer emergency care, and the medical assistant will be called on to assist the provider in this care. For the medical assistant who may need to screen or assess the patient's condition, the first and most critical step in responding to an emergency is developing the skill to recognize when emergency measures should be taken.

 Whereas some emergencies can be treated in the clinic, others cannot, and the medical assistant must know when to call for outside help. If the emergency occurs in the ambulatory care setting, the provider usually administers immediate care. It is possible, however, that the medical assistant may be the first emergency caregiver should the provider be out of the clinic. The medical assistant also may be called on to provide care in an emergency outside the clinic environment.

This chapter acquaints the medical assistant with types of emergency situations that may occur either inside or outside the clinic. However, this chapter is merely an introduction to emergency topics and does not substitute for first aid and cardiopulmonary resuscitation (CPR) instruction taught through the American Red Cross, the American Heart Association, the American Safety and Health Institute, or the National Safety Council. Medical assistants in CAAHEP- and ABHES-accredited programs must be certified to a provider-level in CPR and must be taught by instructors who are certified to teach CPR. These hands-on classes are vital teaching tools, and all medical assistants should take them on a regular basis to continually update their skills.

RECOGNIZING AN EMERGENCY

An emergency is considered any instance in which an individual becomes suddenly ill and requires immediate attention. Most emergencies develop quickly and usually without warning. They can occur unexpectedly at any time to anyone. Some may be gradual, as seen with dehydration or slow blood loss, and become an emergency over time. As you mature in your career, you will begin to develop the ability to make quick determinations about the conditions of people around you. Your experiences in medicine will allow you to assess emergency situations simply by using your senses. By using your sense of sight, you will note an abnormal coloring of the skin, an expression of pain or discomfort, or evidence of bleeding or bruising. Your sense of smell will help detect a wound that has become infected or identify the fruity breath that occurs when a patient's blood sugar is very high. Your sense of touch helps to assess a patient's pulse or the temperature of his skin. Your sense of hearing will recognize a wheeze or cough indicting respiratory distress. It is also essential to be acutely sensitive to any unusual behaviors such as screaming, crying, moaning, or staring blankly off in space.

In the ambulatory care setting, medical assistants may encounter a range of emergency situations requiring first aid techniques. **First aid** is designed to render immediate and temporary emergency care to persons injured or otherwise

SPOTLIGHT ON CERTIFICATION

RMA Content Outline

- Anatomy and physiology
- Medical terminology
- Medical law and ethics
- Patient education
- Asepsis
- Vital signs and mensurations
- First aid and emergency response

CMA (AAMA) Content Outline

- Medical terminology
- Anatomy and physiology
- Medicolegal guidelines and requirements
- Principles of infection control
- Patient preparation and assisting the physician
- Emergencies

CMAS Content Outline

- Medical terminology
- Anatomy and physiology
- Legal and ethical considerations
- Vital signs and mensurations
- Medical office or clinic emergencies
- Safety

disabled before the arrival of a health care practitioner or transport to a hospital or other health care agency.

Emergency situations can be minor or severe and can include:

- Choking and breathing crises
- Chest pain
- Bleeding
- Shock
- Stroke
- Poisoning
- Burns
- Wounds
- Sudden illnesses such as fainting/falling
- Illnesses related to heat and cold
- Fractures

 Some of these situations will be life threatening; all will require immediate care. In either case, it is critical to remain calm, to follow the emergency policies and procedures established by the ambulatory care setting, and to be well versed in first aid and be certified in CPR. The patient should not be further endangered.

Responding to an Emergency

Once it has been determined that an emergency exists, it is essential to act quickly. Before making any decisions about how to proceed, it is necessary to assess the nature of the situation. Does it include respiratory or circulatory failure, severe bleeding, burns, poisoning, or severe allergic reaction?

Sometimes, it is possible that more than one type of care must be administered. As a medical assistant approaches any situation, it is imperative to begin with assessment of the ABCs: Airway, Breathing, and Circulation. Based on this information, the next step is to screen the situation so that treatment can be prioritized. When an individual experiences more than one illness or injury, care must be given according to the severity of the situation. When two or more patients present with emergencies simultaneously, screening helps determine which patient is treated first. This process is known as **triage**. Table 9-1 lists the common ordering of screening situations.

To identify the nature of the emergency and respond effectively, it is critical that the patient be assessed. If the patient is conscious, ask for personal identification and identification of next of kin. Try to obtain information about symptoms being experienced to identify the problem. Always check for a **universal emergency medical identification symbol** (Figure 9-1) and accompanying identification card, which will describe any serious or life-threatening health problems that the patient has. Quickly observe the patient's general appearance, including skin color and size and dilation of pupils. Check pulse and blood pressure.

Patient confidentiality must be maintained during an emergency situation, as at any other time. Sometimes, when a situation is urgent and the patient is having trouble breathing, is bleeding heavily, is having a severe allergic reaction or any other kind of emergency, in your eagerness to assist the patient, your voice when speaking to other health care providers might be overheard by other patients. Be certain other patients cannot hear any conversations. Privacy must be maintained

Table 9-1   Examples of Emergency Categories

First Priority	Next Priority	Least Priority
Burns on face	Second-degree burns not on the neck and face	Fractures (simple)
Airway and breathing problems	Major or multiple fractures	Minor injuries
Cardiac arrest	Back injuries	Sprains, strains
Severe bleeding that is uncontrolled	Severe eye injuries	Simple lacerations
Head injuries	Syncope	Dehydration without change in vital signs
Poisoning	Seizure	
Anaphylactic shock	Lacerations involving multiple tissue layers	
Stroke	Hyper/hypoglycemia	
Open chest or abdominal wounds		

© Cengage Learning 2014

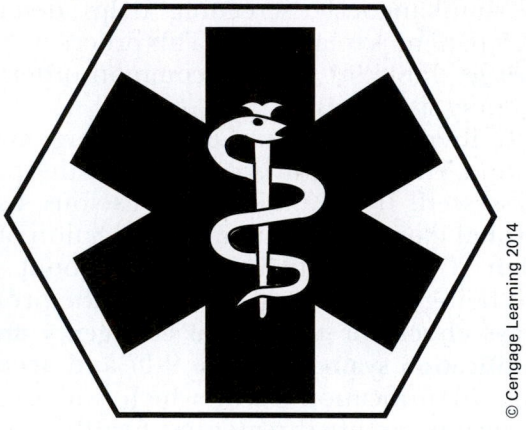

© Cengage Learning 2014

Figure 9-1   The universal emergency medical identification symbol.

when faxing information to the emergency department. Also, be cautious in keeping the patient's anonymity protected.

Primary Survey

A method for assessing life-threatening injuries is known as the primary survey. This is a critical assessment of the ABCDEs, which are listed here:

- Airway
- Breathing
- Circulation
- Disability
- Expose and evaluate

To assess whether the unresponsive patient is breathing and to determine if there is an open airway, place your face close to the patient's face and look, listen, and feel. Observe the patient's chest and notice whether the chest rises and falls with breathing. Listen for air entering and leaving the nose and mouth and feel for moving air.

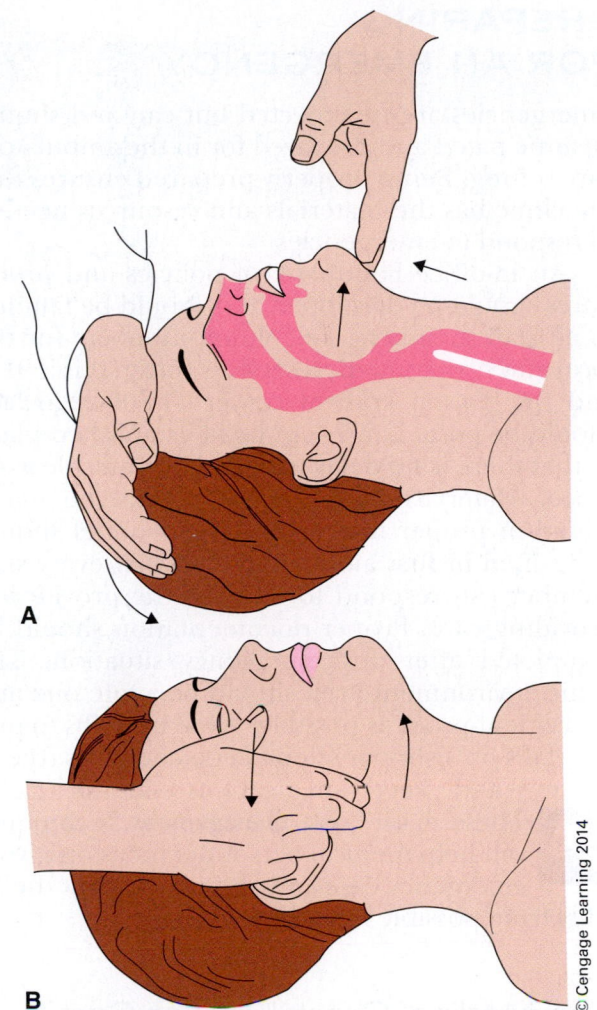

Figure 9-2   If the individual is not breathing, first open the airway (A) by tilting the head and lifting the chin, for victim without head or neck trauma, or (B) by the jaw-thrust maneuver, for victim with cervical spine injury. This involves placing both thumbs on the patient's cheekbones and placing the index and middle fingers on both sides of the lower jaw.

If the individual is not breathing, first open the airway either by tilting the head and lifting the chin (Figure 9-2A) or by the jaw-thrust maneuver, which involves placing both thumbs on the patient's cheekbones and placing the index and middle fingers on both sides of the lower jaw (see Figure 9-2B). **CAUTION:** Do not attempt to tilt the head and lift the chin when the patient has a head, neck, or spinal cord injury.

If the patient still does not breathe after the airway has been opened, rescue breathing must be performed.

To assess circulation, check for the presence of a pulse at the carotid artery on the side of the neck below the ear. If no pulse is present, the patient may be in cardiac arrest and must be given CPR. A trained provider of CPR should initiate compressions if no pulse is detected. A medical assistant should maintain current cardiopulmonary resuscitation certification for management of emergency situations. Use of an **automated external defibrillator (AED)** may be necessary (see Chapter 37).

Using the 911 or Emergency Medical Services System

The **emergency medical services (EMS)** system is a local network of police, fire, and medical personnel who are trained to respond to emergency situations. Other community experts and volunteers also act as resources in an EMS system. In many communities, the network is activated by calling 911. Even when preliminary emergency care is provided by the ambulatory care provider, the patient may still need to be transported to a hospital for follow-up care. It is also possible that the provider may not be equipped to deliver the type of emergency care required, in which case, one person should call for EMS help while another stays with the patient until help arrives. Never leave a seriously ill or unconscious patient unattended.

While waiting for EMS to arrive, continuously check the patient for the following signs: (1) degree of responsiveness, (2) airway/breathing ability, (3) heartbeat (rate and rhythm), (4) bleeding, and (5) signs of shock. Monitor vital signs. Keep patient warm and lying down. If there are no head injuries, the legs can be elevated on pillows.

Good Samaritan Laws

When delivering or assisting in delivering emergency care, the medical assistant may be concerned about professional liability. Most states have enacted Good Samaritan laws, which provide some degree of protection to the health care professional who offers first aid.

Most Good Samaritan laws provide some legal protection to those who provide emergency care to ill or injured persons on a voluntary basis. However, when medical assistants or any other individuals give care during an emergency, they must act as reasonable and prudent individuals and provide care only within the

© Cengage Learning 2014

scope of their abilities. Remember that a primary principle of first aid is to prevent further injury.

Although Good Samaritan laws give some measure of protection against being sued for giving emergency aid, they generally protect *off-duty* health care professionals. Also, conditions of the law vary from state to state. As part of establishing emergency care guidelines, every ambulatory care setting should understand the **explicit** and **implicit** intent of the Good Samaritan law in its state (see Chapter 7 for more information on legal guidelines).

Blood, Body Fluids, and Disease Transmission

When providing any care, including emergency care, medical assistants should always protect themselves and the patient from infectious disease transmission. Serious infectious diseases, such as hepatitis B (HBV), hepatitis C (HCV), and human immunodeficiency virus (HIV) infection, can be transmitted through blood and body fluids (see Chapter 22 for more detailed information).

By establishing and following strict guidelines, the risk for contracting or transmitting an infectious disease while providing emergency care is greatly reduced.

- Always wash hands thoroughly before (if possible) and after every procedure or use hand sanitizer.
- Use protective clothing and other protective equipment (gloves, gown, mask, goggles) during the procedure.
- Avoid contact with blood and body fluids, if possible.
- Do not touch nose, mouth, or eyes with gloved hands.
- Carefully handle and safely dispose of soiled gloves and other objects.

Refer to Chapter 22 for more information on standard precautions. **Standard Precautions** were issued by the Centers for Disease Control and Prevention (CDC) in 1996 and combine many of the basic principles of universal precautions with techniques known as body substance isolation. These augmented 1996 guidelines represent the standard in infection control and are intended to protect both patients and health care professionals.

PREPARING FOR AN EMERGENCY

Emergencies are unexpected but can and should be anticipated and prepared for in the ambulatory care setting. Being properly prepared ensures that the clinic has the materials and resources needed to respond to emergencies.

An in-office handbook of policies and procedures should be developed and should be familiar to all staff members. Telephone numbers for the local emergency medical services (often this is 911) and the poison control center (1-800-222-1222) should be posted and kept in an established place so that there is no delay in calling for outside assistance. Materials and supplies should be maintained in proper inventory. All personnel should be trained in first aid and CPR so that every staff member can respond to or assist the provider in providing care. Proper documentation should be completed after any emergency situation. The clinic environment itself should be a safe one and as accident-proof as possible. Wipe up spills to prevent falls on a slippery floor, keep corridors free of clutter, and keep medications out of sight. These basic **risk management** techniques will help medical personnel focus on giving emergency care and also will protect the facility from possible litigation.

The Medical Crash Tray or Cart

Every health care facility should have a **crash tray or cart**, with a carefully controlled inventory of supplies and equipment (Figure 9-3). The provider should determine the contents of this tray or cart. These first aid supplies should be kept in an accessible place, and the inventory should be routinely monitored to ensure that all supplies are replaced. All medications should be up to date and have not reached their expiration dates.

A smaller practice may require only a portable tray for emergency and first aid supplies. Larger urgent care centers may respond more frequently and to more complex emergencies and thus may need a cart that can hold a larger inventory and variety of supplies. Whether a tray or cart is used, supplies should be customized to the facility and the type of emergencies frequently encountered. Remember that only providers can order medications or treatment.

It is the role of the professional medical assistant to maintain the stock of this cart or tray. There should be a daily check of supplies to determine

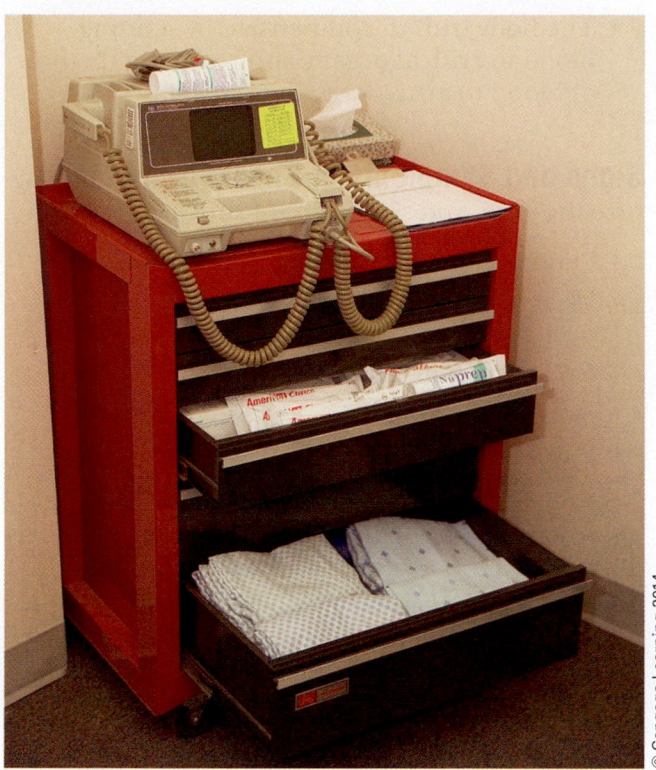

Figure 9-3 Medical crash cart with defibrillator.

© Cengage Learning 2014

their security, expiration dates, and functionality of equipment.

Following is a brief list of some common supplies found on most trays and carts (see Chapter 35 for more information on supplies and medications).

General supplies:
- Adhesive and hypoallergenic tape
- Alcohol wipes
- Bandage scissors
- Bandage material
- Blood pressure cuffs (standard, pediatric, large)
- **Constriction band**
- Defibrillator/AED
- Dressing material
- Flashlight
- Gauze rolls
- Gloves
- Hot/cold packs
- Intravenous (IV) catheters in various sizes
- IV start pack

- IV tubing
- Needles and syringes for injection
- Glucose tabs or gel
- Penlight (with extra batteries)
- Personal protective equipment
- Stethoscope
- Syringes in 1-mL, 3-mL, and 20-mL sizes

Emergency Medications	Uses
Activated charcoal	Poisonings
Aspirin 325 mg	Fever, heart attack
Atropine	Slow heartbeat
Benadryl	IV for treatment of anaphylactic shock
$D_{50}W$	IV solution of dextrose in water (50%) for hypoglycemia
Dextrose	Insulin reaction
Diazepam*	Antianxiety
Diphenhydramine	Antihistamine
Dopamine	Increases blood pressure
Epinephrine	Constricts blood vessels, increases blood pressure
Glucagon	Insulin reaction
Insulin	Hyperglycemia
Lidocaine	IV for cardiac arrhythmia
Narcan	Reversal of narcotic overdose
Nitroglycerin tablets, patches	Chest pain from angina pectoris
Normal saline	IV access and delivery method for emergency drugs
Pepcid 20 mg vial	Treatment of anaphylactic shock
Phenobarbital*	Sedative
SoluMedrol	IV for treatment of anaphylactic shock
Verapamil	Hypertension, angina pectoris, irregular heartbeat, tachycardia
Xylocaine, Marcaine	Local anesthetics

*Controlled substance—must be kept in locked cabinet.

Respiratory supplies:
- Airways of all sizes for nasal and oral use
- McGill forceps
- Ambu bag in infant, pediatric, and adult sizes
- Bulb syringe for suction
- Laryngoscope blades in various shapes and sizes
- Laryngoscope handles with batteries
- Nasal cannulas in infant, pediatric, and adult sizes
- 100% nonrebreather masks in infant, pediatric, and adult sizes
- Oxygen tank with Christmas tree adapter

This list represents many of the supplies to be found on a well-stocked crash cart or tray. 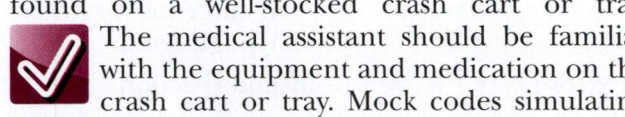 The medical assistant should be familiar with the equipment and medication on the crash cart or tray. Mock codes simulating various emergency situations are helpful for preparing staff members for actual emergencies.

COMMON EMERGENCIES

Included in this discussion of common emergencies are shock, wounds, burns, musculoskeletal injuries, heat- and cold-related illnesses, poisoning, snake bite, sudden illness, cerebral vascular accident, and heart attack.

Shock

When a severe injury or illness occurs, shock is likely to develop. **Shock** is a condition in which the circulatory system is not providing enough blood to all parts of the body, causing the body's organs to fail to function properly.

Shock is always life threatening, and EMS should be activated. The body's attempt to compensate for a massive injury or illness, especially those involving the heart and lungs and severe bleeding, often lead to other problems. During shock, several things occur.

- The heart becomes unable to pump blood properly.
- Consequently, the body's cells, tissues, and organs do not get enough oxygen, which is carried by the blood.

- The body tries to compensate by sending blood to critical organs and reducing the flow of blood to arms, legs, and skin.

Signs and Symptoms of Shock. Learn to recognize the signs and symptoms of shock.

- Patient may be restless or feel irritable.
- Weakness, dizziness, thirst, or nausea may occur.
- Breathing may be shallow and rapid.
- Skin is cool, clammy, and pale.
- Pulse is weak and rapid.
- Blood pressure is low.
- Area around the lips, eyes, and fingernails may turn cyanotic (blue) from lack of oxygen.
- The patient may be confused or become suddenly unconscious, or both.
- Dilated pupils and **lackluster** eyes are obvious.

Types of Shock. Shock can be defined by categories or by the underlying cause. There are several categories of shock. Cardiogenic shock is due to decreased ability of the heart to function as a pump. Another category of shock caused by decreased venous return is hypovolemic shock. High cardiac output hypotension shock is caused by underlying factors such as sepsis. Other types of shock are anaphylactic, neurogenic, traumatic, and compression of the heart. Table 9-2 describes common types of shock seen in an ambulatory care setting.

Treatment for Shock. A person suffering from shock needs immediate medical attention. The focus for intervention in all types of shock is to treat the underlying causative factors. Call for outside emergency help first, then care for the patient until help arrives. **CAUTION:** Shock is progressive, and if not treated immediately, most types can be life threatening. Once shock reaches a certain point, it is irreversible.

To care for a patient in shock (regardless of the type), follow these procedures:

- Activate EMS.
- Lay the patient down. This minimizes pain and decreases stress on the body.
- Loosen the patient's clothing.
- Check for an open airway.
- Check breathing.
- Control any external bleeding.

Table 9-2 Common Types of Shock with Descriptions

Type of Shock	Description
Cardiogenic	The cardiac muscle is unable to contract and adequately provide blood to the body. This can be caused by myocardial infarction, coronary artery disease, arrhythmias, or valve disease.
Hypovolemic	The body has lost blood or fluid volume to such an extent that there is not enough circulating volume to fill the ventricles. The heart attempts to compensate by increasing the heart rate.
Neurogenic	Injury or trauma to the nervous system causes the loss of tone in the vessels, resulting in massive dilation of arterioles and venules. This results in a dramatic drop in blood pressure. This type of shock can be caused by brain or spinal cord injuries, general or spinal anesthesia, or pain and anxiety.
Anaphylactic	In this severe allergic reaction to substances such as drugs, blood products, contrast medium, insect or animal venom, or food products, chemicals are released that cause veins and arteries to vasodilate and decrease the amount of blood returning to the heart. Capillaries dilate and allow proteins and fluids to escape into the soft tissues, causing edema.
Septic	When overwhelming infection occurs in critically ill patients chemicals are released into the blood stream that cause vasodilatation and other organic products that are harmful to the organs and tissues. The vasodilation and decreased ability of the cells and tissues to utilize oxygen form the basis for this type of shock
Respiratory	Trauma to the respiratory tract (trachea, lungs) causes a reduction of oxygen and carbon dioxide exchange. Body cells cannot receive enough oxygen.

© Cengage Learning 2014

- Help the patient maintain normal body temperature. A blanket over and under the patient can help avoid chilling. Do not overheat.
- Reassure the patient.

- Elevate the patient's legs about 12 inches, unless you suspect head injury, spinal injuries, or broken bones involving the hips or legs.
- Do not give the patient anything to eat or drink.
- Ascertain that outside help has been called and stay with the patient until help arrives.
- Monitor vital signs.

Wounds

Typically, **wounds** are classified as open or closed. In the closed wound, there is no break in the skin; a bruise, contusion, and hematoma are common closed wounds. An open wound represents a break in the skin and can be classified as an abrasion, avulsion, incision, laceration, or puncture wound.

Closed Wounds. Most closed wounds do not present an emergency situation. If there is pain and swelling, the application of a cold compress can be effective. Protect the patient's skin by placing a cloth beneath the source of cold; apply the compress for 20 minutes, then remove for 20 minutes; continue for 24 hours. Then apply heat 20 minutes on and 20 minutes off for the next 24 hours. A common procedure for treating closed wounds is to RICE or MICE it. It is generally thought that RICE is the preferred treatment for the first 24–48 hours. Once the signs of inflammation are gone, MICE is the more appropriate treatment.

Rice	*Mice*
• *Rest*	• *Motion* or *Movement*
• *Ice*	• *Ice*
• *Compression*	• *Compression*
• *Elevation*	• *Elevation*

Recently, some providers, especially those who treat sports injuries, advocate motion or movement as a means of treating a closed wound injury. They also advise ice, compression (elastic bandage), and elevation (MICE). Check for provider preference.

Some closed wounds, such as hematomas, can be dangerous and may be associated with internal bleeding. If the patient is in severe pain and was subject to an injury caused by high impact, call for help and keep the patient comfortable until the help arrives. Watch for symptoms of shock and monitor vital signs.

Open Wounds. Open wounds can be minor tears in the skin or more serious skin breaks, but all open wounds represent an opportunity for microorganisms to gain entry to the body and cause an infection. Some major open wounds may involve heavy bleeding, which will need to be controlled, probably by suturing. A tetanus injection is indicated for an open wound if the patient has not had a booster in the last 7 to 10 years (see Chapter 22 for immunization information).

 Common types of open wounds are described as follows:

1. *Abrasions* are a superficial scraping of the epidermis. Because nerve endings are involved, they can be painful. However, they are not usually serious, unless they cover a large area of the body. Administer first aid by cleaning the area carefully with soap and water, apply an antiseptic ointment if prescribed by a provider, and cover with a dressing.

2. In an *avulsion*, the skin is torn off and bleeding is profuse. Avulsion wounds often occur at exposed parts: fingers, toes, ear. First, control bleeding (see Procedure 9-1). Then clean the wound. If there is a skin flap, reposition it. Apply a dressing, then bandage as necessary. Note that pieces of the body may be torn away. If possible, save the body part, keep moist, and transport with the patient.

3. *Incisions* are wounds caused by a sharp object, such as a knife or piece of glass. Incisions may need sutures. The wound must be cleaned with soap and water and a dressing applied.

4. *Lacerations* tear the body tissue and can be difficult to clean; therefore, care must be taken to avoid infection. If there is not severe bleeding, which in itself is a cleansing mechanism, these wounds may need to be soaked in antiseptic soap and water to remove debris. If there is severe bleeding, it must be controlled immediately (see Procedure 9-1). Lacerations with severe bleeding need suturing.

5. *Punctures* pierce and penetrate the skin and may be deep wounds while appearing insignificant. Usually, external bleeding is minimal, but the patient should be assessed for internal bleeding. Because a puncture wound is deep, the risk for infection is great and the patient should be advised to watch for signals of infection, such as pain, swelling, redness, throbbing, and warmth.

Use of Tourniquets in Emergency Care. In the past, tourniquets were regularly used in the field to control hemorrhaging from an extremity when all other attempts to control bleeding were unsuccessful. However, because tourniquet application was meant to completely stop blood flow, many times the complete lack of blood flow resulted in tissue death of the extremity. Often, the affected extremity needed to be amputated.

To remedy the situation, a "constriction band" was substituted for the tourniquet and is now widely used. The constriction band is made of a material similar to that used in the tourniquet. When the band is applied to an extremity to control bleeding, it is applied tightly enough to stem the rapid loss of blood but loosely enough to allow a small amount of blood to continue to flow. A pulse should be felt distally to the constriction band. The use of the constriction band applied in this manner allows a blood supply to the remainder of the extremity, unlike the tourniquet, which cuts off all blood flow. Chapter 31 provides information on wounds and minor surgery.

If the bleeding is controlled, direct pressure is still the best method to handle blood loss.

Dressings and Bandages. After the provider has treated an open wound, it is critical to dress and bandage it properly to curtail infection. Covering of the wound is accomplished by a series of **dressings** and **bandages**.

Typically, dressings are sterile gauze pads placed directly on the wound; they often have nonstick, sterile surfaces, but they are absorbent and will soak up blood and protect the wound from microorganisms. They are often made of a gauze-type material.

Bandages, which are nonsterile, are placed over the dressing. They hold the dressing in place and are made to conform to the area to be covered. Sometimes, as in a Band-Aid, the dressing and bandage are combined. Bandage materials are selected based on the location and type of wound to be covered. Kling is a type of flexible gauze that stretches and clings as it is applied. Roller bandages (sometimes called by their brand name, Ace Bandages), such as those made of elastic, can be placed over a dressing and used to help control bleeding or swelling. Recently, there has been a rise in the utilization of self-adherent elasticized wrap known as Coban.

Bandages and their applications can take many shapes and forms, depending on the type of injury and the injury site. In all cases, a bandage must be secure, but not constricting. Avoid too tight or too loose a wrap.

- Spiral bandages are useful for injuries to the arms or legs (Figure 9-4).
- A figure-eight bandage holds the dressing in place on a wound on the hand or wrist, knee, or ankle (Figure 9-5).
- Fingers, toes, arms, and legs can also be bandaged using a tubular gauze bandage (Figure 9-6, Figure 9-7, and Figure 9-8). Using

a cylindrical applicator, a quantity of gauze is stretched over the wound site.

- Commercial arm slings are used to support injured or fractured arms (Figure 9-9). To apply, support the injured arm above and below the injury site while applying the sling.

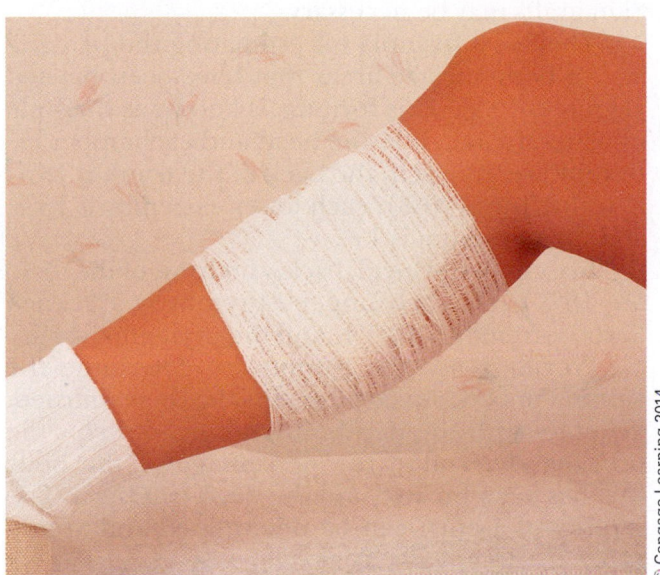

Figure 9-4   The spiral bandage is an option for arm and leg injuries.

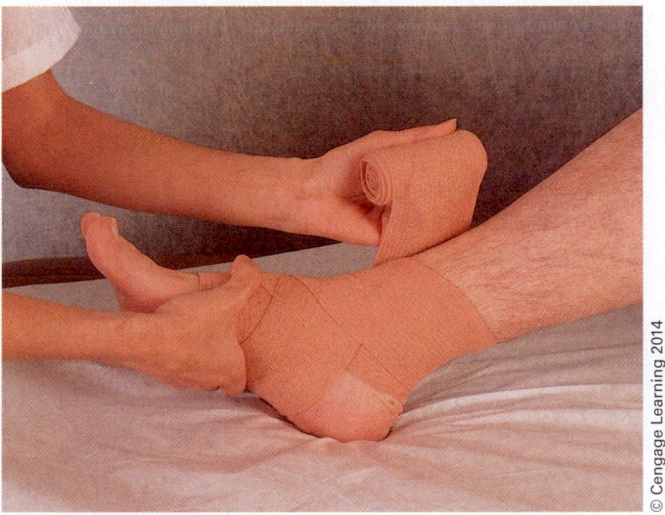

Figure 9-5   An elastic figure-eight bandage holds dressings in place or can be used for immobilization, as with an ankle sprain.

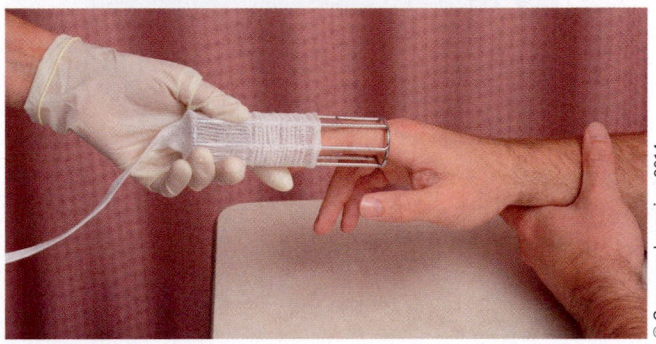

Figure 9-6   The cylindrical applicator is placed over the finger.

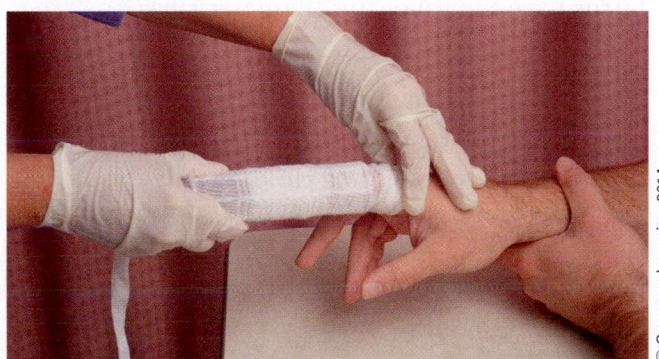

Figure 9-7   Gauze is stretched over the finger.

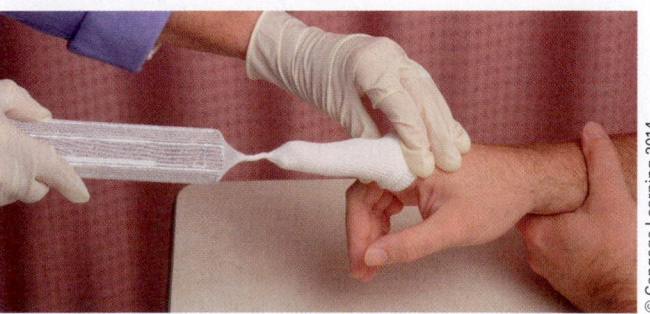

Figure 9-8   Applicator is pulled off, leaving the bandage.

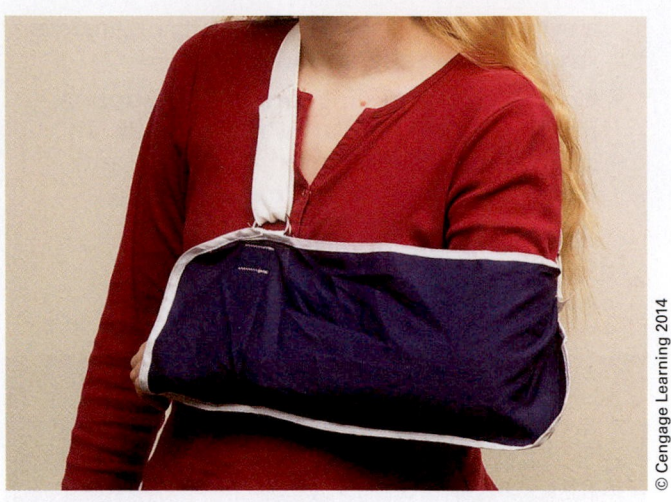

© Cengage Learning 2014

Figure 9-9 A commercial sling is used to support injured or fractured arms.

Burns

Most burns are caused by heat, chemicals, explosions, and electricity. Critical burns can be life threatening and require immediate medical care. According to the American Red Cross, critical burns have the following characteristics:

- Involve breathing difficulty
- Cover more than one body part
- Involve the head, neck, hands, feet, or genitals
- Involve any burns to a child or older adult (other than minor burns)

To distinguish critical from minor burns, it is important to understand the classifications of burns and what they mean.

First-, Second-, and Third-Degree Burns.
First-degree burns are superficial burns that involve only the top layer of skin. The skin appears red, feels dry, is warm to the touch, may be swollen, and is painful. First-degree burns usually heal in a week or so with no permanent scarring. Treatment consists of cleansing the area and protecting it from further damage. First-degree burns are considered minor unless they cover a large area of key body parts such as the face, hands, feet, groin, or buttocks. They may require emergency care if the area is large enough.

In a second-degree burn, the first layer of skin has been burned through and the tissues underneath are involved. The skin is red and blisters are present. Because of the involvement of nerves in the dermal layer, this type of burn is very painful. The healing process is slower, usually a month, and some scarring may occur. Second-degree burns affect the top layers of the skin and are very painful.

Third-degree burns are the most serious, affecting or destroying all layers of tissue. It is not unusual for fat, muscles, bones, and nerves to be involved. These burns can look charred or brown. There may be great pain or, if nerve endings are destroyed, the burn may be painless. Victims of third-degree burns must receive immediate medical attention both for the burn and for shock. Of serious concern with a third-degree burn is the likelihood of infection and the amount of fluid loss. Scarring can result in loss of body function. Skin grafts may be necessary.

There is a formula for estimating the percentage of body surface areas that have been burned (Figure 9-10A). This formula is known as the Rule of Nines. In an adult, the head and each upper extremity are 9% each, the back of the trunk is 18%, as is the front (18%), each lower extremity is 18%, and the perineum is 1%.

In a child, the head, back, and front of the torso are 18% each, each upper extremity is 9%, each lower extremity is 13.5%, and the perineum is 1%.

Providers use the formula to determine the amount of body surface area that has been burned. Together with the depth of the burn, it helps the provider determine the percentage of the body that has been burned and the degree of burn. The severity of a burn can be determined and appropriate treatment given.

Figure 9-10B shows the relative penetration level of each degree of burn into the skin and underlying structures.

General Guidelines for Caring for Burns.
Treatment for burns depends on the type of agent causing the burn. General treatment strategies for any degree of burn include the following:

- Cool the burn with large amounts of cool normal saline, or water if saline is unavailable.
- Cover the burn with a sterile dressing if one is available and burn is minor. Otherwise, cover the burn with a sheet or other smooth-textured cloth for a burn over a large area of the body.
- Be sure the patient is protected from being either chilled or overheated.

However, it is important to refrain from the following:

- Do not apply ice or ice water to a burn.
- Do not touch a burn, except with a sterile dressing.

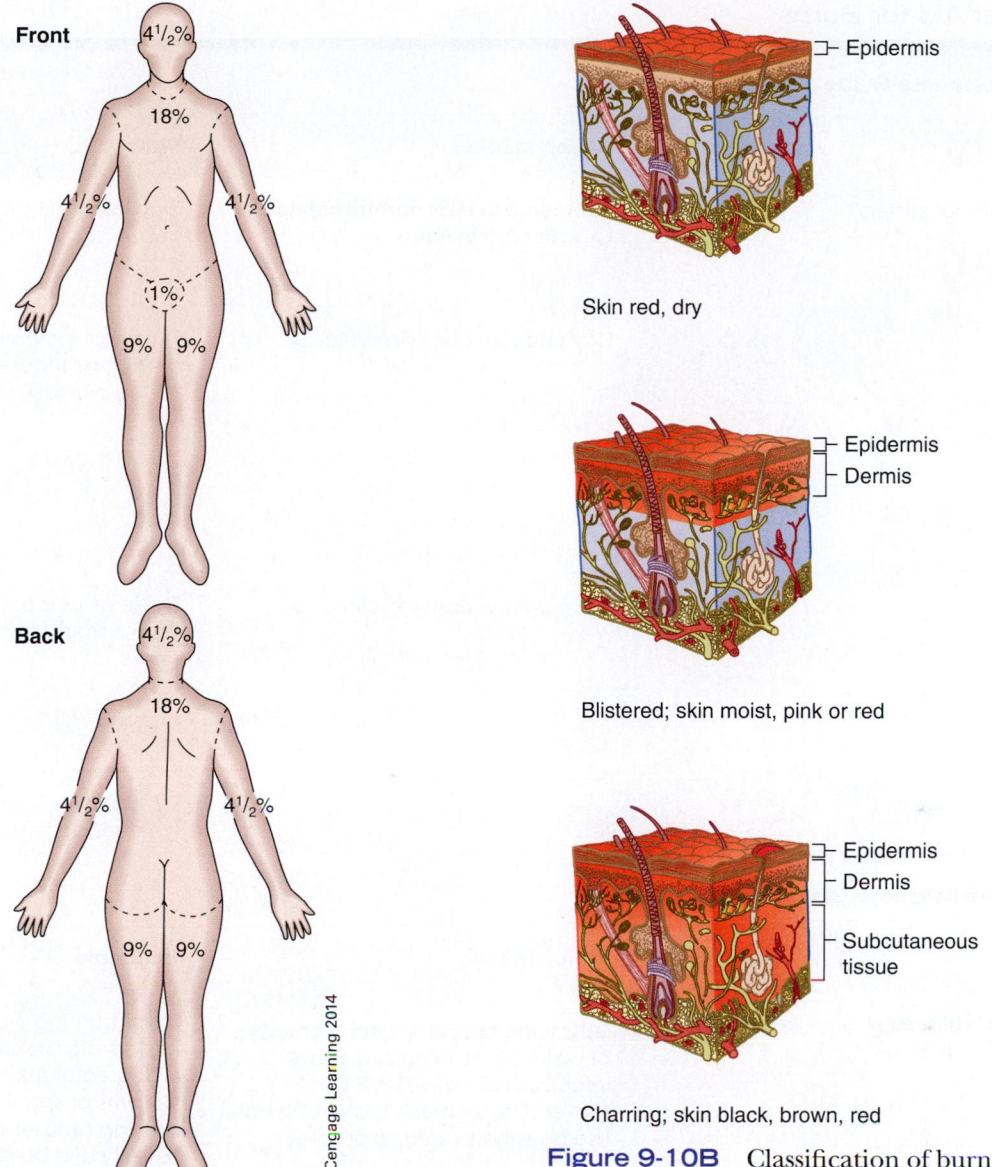

Front

4½%

18%

4½%   4½%

1%

9%   9%

Back

4½%

18%

4½%   4½%

9%   9%

© Cengage Learning 2014

Epidermis

Skin red, dry

First-degree, superficial

Epidermis
Dermis

Blistered; skin moist, pink or red

Second-degree, partial thickness

Epidermis
Dermis
Subcutaneous tissue

Charring; skin black, brown, red

Third-degree, full thickness

© Cengage Learning 2014

Figure 9-10B Classification of burn injuries.

Figure 9-10A Diagram for use in calculating the extent of burns or other injuries in an adult.

- Do not clean a severe burn, break blisters, or use any kind of ointment.
- Do not remove pieces of clothing that may be sticking to the burn.

First Aid for Burns. First aid for burns is outlined in Table 9-3.

Types of Burns. Most burns are caused by heat; however, burns can also be caused by chemicals, electricity, and solar radiation.

Chemical Burns. Chemical burns can occur in the workplace or even in the home with "ordinary"

household chemicals. To stop the burning process, you must remove the chemical from the skin. Have someone call EMS while you flush the skin or eyes with cool water. Remove any clothing contaminated by the chemicals unless they adhere to the skin. If clothing clings to the skin, it can be cut with scissors. Do not attempt to pull clothing away from a burned area.

Electrical Burns. Electrical burns can be caused by power lines, lightning, or faulty electrical equipment in the home or workplace. *It is important to remember never to go near a patient injured by electricity until you are sure the power has been shut off, because you could be injured.* If there is a downed line, call the power company and EMS.

Table 9-3   First Aid for Burns

First-Degree Burn Response Guide

Questions	Responses	Action to Take	Rationale
Is skin reddened without blisters? NO ⬇	YES ⇨	Submerge in cool **normal saline** or ⇨ water 2–5 minutes.	Stops burning process.
Does area involve: • hands? • feet? • genitals? • face? NO ⬇	YES ⇨	Have patient come to clinic. ⇨	These are potential danger areas and require evaluation by the provider.
Is patient: • elderly? • very young? NO ⬇	YES ⇨	Have patient come to clinic. ⇨	These groups are susceptible to burn complications.
Consult provider.			Provider has final decision whether patient is seen.

Second-Degree Burn Response Guide

Questions	Responses	Action to Take	Rationale
Is skin reddened with blisters or splitting of the skin? NO ⬇	YES ⇨	Submerge in cool normal saline ⇨ or water 10–15 minutes if skin is intact. Use compresses if skin is broken. Do not break blisters. Do not use anesthetic creams or sprays.	Stops burning process. If blisters are broken, the area is at greater risk for infection. Creams or spray may slow healing process and increase severity of a burn.
Does area involve: • hands? • feet? • genitals? • face? NO ⬇	YES ⇨	Have patient come to clinic or go ⇨ to the emergency department.	These are potentially dangerous areas and require medical attention.
Is the area involved larger than a child's hand? NO ⬇	YES ⇨	Have patient come to clinic or go ⇨ to the emergency department.	Burns of this size are susceptible to complications.
Is patient experiencing trouble breathing? NO ⬇	YES ⇨	Patient should go to emergency ⇨ department.	There may be swelling of the airways because of heat and noxious fumes.

Table 9-3 First Aid for Burns (*Continued*)

Second-Degree Burn Response Guide

Questions	Responses	Action to Take	Rationale
Consult provider.			Provider has final decision whether patient is seen.

Third-Degree Burn Response Guide

Questions	Responses	Action to Take	Rationale
Does skin appear gray, black, or charred? Can muscle, fat, or bone be seen in wound? NO ⇩	YES ⇨	Tell patient or family to call EMS ⇨ immediately. Do not apply cold; do not remove burned clothing from burn area.	Life-threatening emergency that requires prompt attention.
Is patient experiencing: • pallor • loss of consciousness? • shivering? NO ⇩	YES ⇨	Patient in shock: ⇨ Tell family to call EMS and to: • maintain airway • maintain body temperature • elevate feet if appropriate • monitor breathing Patient may need oxygen and intravenous fluids while waiting for EMS to arrive.	Need to control shock caused by fluid loss.
Consult provider.			Provider has final decision whether patient is seen.

© Cengage Learning 2014

A victim of an electricity burn may be suffering from two burns: one where the power entered the body, and one where it exited. Often, the burns themselves may be minor. Of more serious consequence are the possibilities of shock, breathing difficulties, and other injuries. CPR often is needed in this situation.

Solar Radiation. Most "sunburns," although not advisable or good for the skin, represent minor burns. If the patient has a severe burn, however, he or she should see a provider who will cover the burn area to reduce chance of infection and protect the patient against chill.

Musculoskeletal Injuries

Most injuries to muscles, bones, and joints are not life threatening, but they are painful and, if not

PATIENT EDUCATION

Some burns can be prevented. Advise patients who insist on sunbathing to protect themselves against harmful rays by using a sunscreen with 15 SPF or higher and avoiding the sun between 10 AM and 2 PM.

properly treated, can be disabling. Some injuries, such as those to the spinal cord, can be quite serious and can result in paralysis. These injuries are not typically seen in the ambulatory care setting.

Types of Injuries. A **sprain** is an injury to a joint, often an ankle, knee, or wrist, that involves a tearing of the ligaments. Some sprains are minor and

PATIENT EDUCATION

Advise patients not to run should their clothing catch on fire. They should fall to the ground or wrap themselves in a blanket or rug and roll on the ground to extinguish the flames. This method is known as STOP, DROP, and ROLL.

heal quickly; others are more severe, include swelling, and may not heal properly if the patient continues to put stress on the sprained joint. Signs of a sprain are rapid swelling, discoloration at the site, and limited function. Many times it is difficult to determine whether the patient has sustained a sprain or a fracture because the degree of pain may not be a true indicator of the patient's injury. As with most closed wounds, treating the injury with the RICE or MICE method is beneficial and determined by the provider's choice.

A strain results from the overuse or stretching of a muscle, tendons, or group of muscles, as with improper lifting or moving heavy objects. Applications of ice and heat (as described earlier in "Closed Wounds"), as well as rest, are indicated for treatment of strains. Surgery is not usually required for sprains and strains. Significant injuries (large tears) may need surgery. Slings, crutches, and removable splints help protect the injury from further damage and limit movement until a more specific diagnosis can be made.

Dislocations are painful and involve the separation of a bone from its normal position. These injuries usually result from the kind of wrenching motion that might occur during a fall, automobile accident, or sports injury. Dislocations must be treated urgently and require x-ray studies of the affected joint, and potentially magnetic resonance imaging (MRI) for imaging and relocation by a trained provider.

Fractures involve a break in a bone and can be caused by a fall, a blow, bone disease, or sports activities. There are several types of fractures, but all are classified as either open or closed fractures. An open fracture involves an open wound and is characterized by a protruding bone. In a closed fracture, the skin is not broken. Signs and symptoms that occur with a fracture may include swelling, discoloration, pain, deformity, and immobility of the body part. It is not unusual for patients to tell you

that they heard the bone break or that they sensed a grating feeling. Crepitation is the term that describes the grating sensation experienced or heard when bone fragments rub together. Fractures are further defined as follows:

- *Incomplete or greenstick.* Fracture in which the bone has cracked, but the break is not all the way through; frequently seen in children
- *Simple.* Complete bone break in which there is no involvement with the skin surface
- *Compound.* Fracture in which the bone protrudes though the skin surface, creating the possibility of infection
- *Impacted.* Fracture in which the broken ends are jammed into each other
- *Comminuted.* More than one fracture line and several bone fragments are present
- *Spiral.* Fracture that occurs with a severe twisting action, causing the break to wind around the bone
- *Depressed.* Fracture that occurs with severe head injuries in which a broken piece of skull is driven inward
- *Colles'.* Fracture often caused by falling on an outstretched hand; involves the distal end of the radius and results in displacement, causing a bulge at the wrist

These fractures represent major types of fractures. Figure 9-11 shows examples of these fractures.

Assessing Injuries to Muscles, Bones, and Joints.
Sometimes it is difficult to determine the extent of an injury, especially in closed fractures. There are some assessment techniques to call on, however, to gauge the seriousness of an injury.

- Note the extent of bruising and swelling.
- Pain is a signal of injury.
- There may be noticeable deformity to the bone or joint.
- Use of the injured area is limited.
- Talk to the patient: What was the cause of the injury? What was the sound or sensation at the time of injury?

Caring for Muscle, Bone, and Joint Injuries.
Most injuries to muscles, bones, and joints are treated in a similar way; some require motion, but most require rest, elevation of the injured part, immobilization, and the application of ice to the injury.

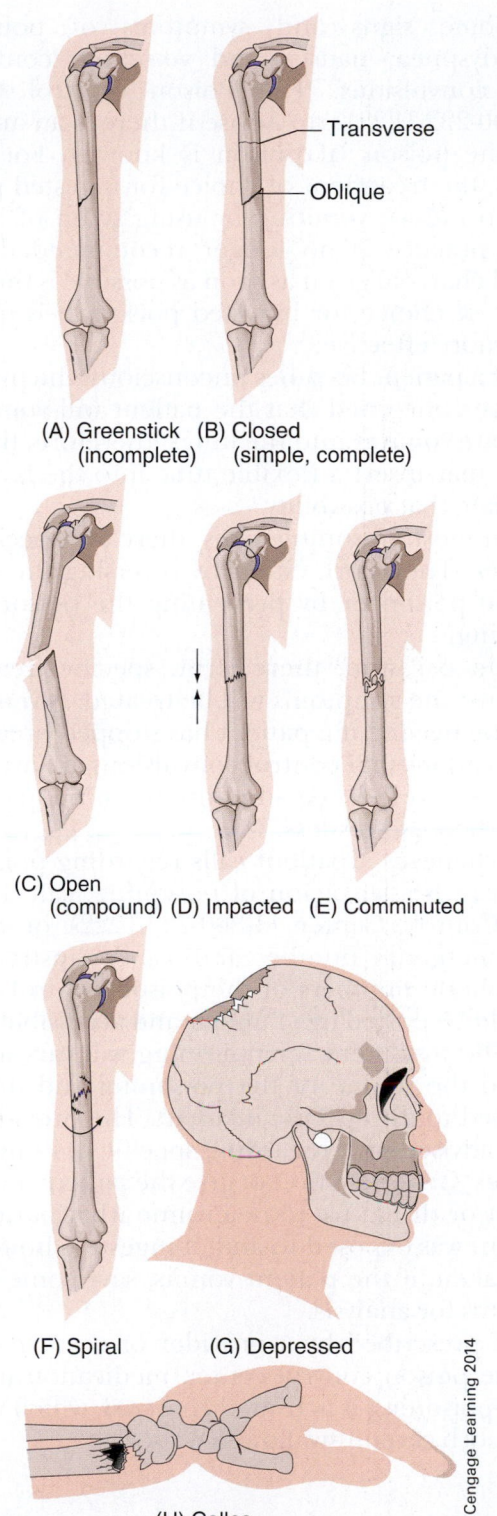

(A) Greenstick (incomplete)   (B) Closed (simple, complete)

Transverse
Oblique

(C) Open (compound)   (D) Impacted   (E) Comminuted

(F) Spiral   (G) Depressed

(H) Colles

© Cengage Learning 2014

Figure 9-11   Types of fractures.

After calling EMS (always check for life-threatening symptoms, such as breathing difficulties; bleeding; or head, neck, or back injuries), it is important to immobilize the injured area if the patient must be moved. EMS personnel use a variety of **splints** to immobilize bones and joints. Some fractures must be treated in the hospital. Compound fractures and fractures with nerve or blood vessel involvement are some examples. Most often, a fracture can be treated with outpatient care. A splint and a cast may be applied to prevent movement and to hold the fracture steady. Procedure 9-2 gives instructions for splinting an arm in the ambulatory care setting.

Heat- and Cold-Related Illnesses

The condition of patients who have been subject to extreme heat and cold can deteriorate rapidly, and either a heat- or cold-related illness can result in death. Individuals especially vulnerable to extreme exposures include the very young and very old, individuals who must work outdoors, and people who suffer from poor circulation.

Heat-Related Illnesses. Illnesses related to heat, in increasing degree of severity, include heat cramps, heat exhaustion, and heat stroke. Heat cramps, the least serious, involve cramping in the legs and abdomen caused by excessive body exposure or exercise in hot weather. Heat cramps should be considered a signal to stop, slow down, rest in a cool place, and drink plenty of water. Salt tablets should not be taken. The individual should lightly stretch the muscles. Heat cramps can progress to heat exhaustion or heat stroke, both of which are more serious conditions.

Heat exhaustion, often experienced by people who work or exercise in extreme heat, is a more serious reaction and is signaled by exhaustion, cold and clammy skin, profuse sweating, headache, and general weakness. The individual should come out of the heat immediately; apply cool, wet towels; and slowly drink cool water. The provider will advise the patient not to resume activity in the heat.

Heat stroke is the least common but the most dangerous of heat-related illnesses and requires immediate medical attention. Heat stroke is characterized by red, dry, hot skin; an abnormal, weak pulse; and breathing that is shallow and fast. In heat stroke, the body systems are extremely taxed. EMS should be alerted; until they arrive, stay with the patient, watch for breathing problems, and attempt to reduce body temperature by applying cool, wet towels or sheets.

Cold-Related Illnesses. Exposure to extreme cold for prolonged periods can lead to frostbite or hypothermia.

Frostbite, which typically affects the extremities such as fingers, toes, ears, and nose, involves the freezing of exposed body parts. Symptoms include skin that becomes off-color, is cold, or takes on a waxy appearance. Severity can range from the superficial (frostnip) to more penetrating stages, which may require amputation.

Individuals with frostbite need immediate medical attention. To care for frostbitten extremities, warm the area of injury by wrapping clothing or blankets around the affected body part. Be careful in handling the frozen part. It is best to have the patient transported as soon as possible to emergency care. This type of facility is better able to properly rewarm the frozen part, preventing further tissue damage.

Hypothermia is a serious condition in which the body temperature decreases to a perilously low level. It can result in death if the individual does not receive care and if the progression of hypothermia is not reversed. Hypothermia occurs when a person falls through the ice or is exposed to cold temperatures, for example, after getting lost in the woods while hiking. Symptoms include shivering, cold skin, and confusion.

After checking for breathing problems and alerting EMS, care for the patient. Make the individual comfortable, provide a source of warmth, such as a blanket, and *gradually* warm the body. If clothing is wet or cold, remove it and put on dry clothing. In extreme cases, it may be necessary to provide rescue breathing.

Poisoning

Poisons can enter the body in four ways:

- *Ingestion.* Ingested poisons enter the body by swallowing. Swallowed poisons may include medications, plant material, household chemicals, contaminated foods, and drugs.

- *Inhalation.* Poisons are inhaled into the body in poorly ventilated areas where cleaning fluids, paints and chemical cleaners, or carbon monoxide may be present.

- *Absorption.* Poisons absorbed through the skin include plant materials such as poison oak or ivy, lawn care products such as chemical pesticides, and other chemical powders or liquids.

- *Injection.* Drug abuse is the most common cause of injected poisons. The stingers of insects inject poisons into the body and can be extremely dangerous and can lead to anaphylactic shock in allergic individuals.

Some signs and symptoms of poisoning are dyspnea, nausea and vomiting, confusion, and convulsions. The Poison Control Center (1-800-222-1222) can advise if there is an antidote for the poison (if poison is known). For many years, the treatment of choice for ingested poison was to induce vomiting by using syrup of ipecac. This practice is no longer recommended. Activated charcoal given as soon as possible is the treatment of choice for ingested poison. It is quicker and more effective.

If a patient becomes unconscious, the provider will be concerned that the patient will vomit and aspirate vomitus into the lungs; therefore, the provider may insert a flexible tube into the larynx to alleviate that possibility.

In most poisoning cases, there are specific antidotes. They work either by reversing the effects of the poison or by preventing the poison from working.

On occasion, there is no specific treatment and just the symptoms will be treated. A ventilator may be needed if a patient has stopped breathing. Medications that control convulsions are available, and sedatives can be administered if the patient is disturbed and restless.

Whenever a patient calls regarding poisoning or there is a suspicion of poisoning, call the Poison Control Center (1-800-222-1222) or the local emergency number and ask for instructions. Telephone numbers of the poison control center should be posted in a familiar and accessible place.

The treatment for poisoning will vary according to the source of the poisoning and must be tailored to the specific incident. The provider will have advised staff regarding specific poisoning antidotes. Generally, do not give the patient anything to eat or drink; try to determine what poison the patient was exposed to and, if ingested, how much was taken; if the patient vomits, save some of the vomitus for analysis.

If prescribed by a provider or recommended by the poison control center, medication used to treat poisoning is activated charcoal, which is used to absorb certain swallowed poisons.

CRITICAL THINKING

Your practice has just received Poison Help Stickers to distribute to the parents of pediatric patients. Create an educational flyer regarding poison prevention.

Insect Stings. The medical assistant in the ambulatory care setting is likely to receive calls every summer from patients who have been stung by insects, typically yellow jackets, hornets, honeybees, or wasps. In the nonallergic patient, the sting is likely to result in localized swelling, tenderness, and slight redness. The provider will recommend that these localized symptoms be managed with a topical cream and oral antihistamines. Swelling can be significant and cause for serious concern if the sting occurred in a vulnerable area of the body such as the mouth or tongue. Swelling in these locations can be frightening and dangerous because it can impair breathing. An antihistamine, administered as soon as possible after the sting, may help to curtail symptoms somewhat. Treatment of insect stings in nonallergic individuals consists of removing the stinger by scraping it off with the edge of something rigid such as a credit card or a fingernail. Tweezers can cause more venom to be dispersed into the patient's body tissues, so this method should not be used. Wash the area with soap and water, apply a cold pack to the site, and watch for a possible severe reaction.

The individual who experiences an allergic reaction or hypersensitivity to a sting needs to be seen immediately, because in severe cases a sting may induce an anaphylactic reaction that can lead to death. If allergic, individuals who have been stung are likely to experience symptoms within a half hour of the incident. Symptoms are generalized throughout the body and may include hives, itching, and lightheadedness and may progress to difficulty breathing, faintness, and eventual loss of consciousness.

For individuals with known allergic reactions, the provider will prescribe epinephrine, which patients should carry with them and self-inject should they not be able to get immediate emergency care. EpiPen is an auto-injector device that delivers epinephrine. The patient should then seek immediate emergency treatment. For individuals who present at the ambulatory care setting with an apparent allergic reaction to a sting, the provider will prescribe epinephrine, an antihistamine, and corticosteroids if necessary. Attempt to allay patient apprehension and monitor vital signs while waiting for EMS personnel to arrive.

Sudden Illness

Sudden illness is, by definition, an unexpected occurrence. Although the cause of the illness may be unexplainable, it is important to respond sensibly and responsibly within the parameters of knowledge and resources.

Sudden illnesses include, but are not limited to, fainting, seizures, diabetic reaction, and hemorrhage.

Fainting. Also known as **syncope**, fainting involves a loss of consciousness, caused by an insufficient supply of blood to the brain. Loss of consciousness may simply be the result of a fainting episode, or it may indicate a more serious medical problem such as diabetic coma or shock. A fall during a fainting incident may result in bodily harm.

If a patient in the office or clinic "feels faint," indicated by lightheadedness, weakness, nausea, or unsteadiness, have the individual lie down or sit down with head level with the knees. This may prevent a fainting episode.

PATIENT EDUCATION

Snake Bite

Most snakes are not poisonous, and snakes usually will not strike unless provoked. Some poisonous snakes are rattlesnake, copper snake, cottonmouth water moccasin, and coral snake. Individuals who live in snake-inhabited areas, campers, hikers, and other outdoor lovers need to be mindful and cautious when outdoors. To avoid a possible snake bite, wear thick high boots, stay on the hiking path, do not reach down to pick up something from the ground unless you have a clear view around the area, and be careful on rocks (snakes like to live in or around piles of rocks).

Common signs and symptoms of a snake bite are rapid pulse, nausea and vomiting, severe pain, swelling, blood and fang marks at wound site, convulsions, thirst, and diaphoresis.

Emergency treatment consists of the following:

- Call for emergency help immediately
- Wash wound with soap and water if possible
- Immobilize body part and keep below heart level if possible
- Apply a constriction band 4 inches above site
- Cover wound with clean cool cloth
- Monitor vital signs

The most common type of fainting episodes occur when the blood pressure drops quickly in response to a highly charged emotional or stressful situation. The name for this common fainting spell is **vasovagal syncope**. The individual's skin feels sweaty and clammy, and lightheadedness is common.

If a patient faints, gradually lower the patient to a flat surface, loosen any tight clothing, check breathing and for any life-threatening emergencies, and apply cool compresses to the forehead. Elevate the legs if there is no back or head injury. If vomiting occurs, place the patient on his or her side. Although fainting is typically not serious in itself, 911 or EMS may need to be called because the problem may be indicative of a more complex medical condition.

Seizures.

Seizures or convulsions occur when normal brain functioning is disrupted, which can occur for a variety of reasons including fever, disease such as diabetes, infections, or injury to the brain. Epilepsy is a common cause of convulsions. Involuntary spasms or contractions of muscles characterize seizures.

To the onlooker, seizures look frightening and painful, which may lead inexperienced individuals to try to stop the seizure when they see it occurring in another person. A patient experiencing a seizure should never be restrained; simply care for the victim with compassion and medical understanding. The goal is to protect the patient from self-injury during the episode. Do not force anything between the patient's clenched teeth—an individual experiencing seizures cannot "swallow" the tongue.

Most patients recover from a seizure in a few minutes. During the seizure, protect the patient from injury, cushion the patient's head, clear the area of any objects that might cause injury, and roll the patient to the side if any fluid is in the mouth. After the seizure subsides, calm and comfort the patient.

If a patient is known to regularly have seizures and the patient's seizure subsides in a matter of minutes, EMS personnel usually do not need to be summoned. Repeated seizures during the same time frame, however, dictate a call to emergency services, as does any seizure if the patient is diabetic, pregnant, or injured, or does not regain consciousness after the incident.

Diabetes.

Diabetes is defined by the American Diabetes Society as the "inability of the body to properly convert sugar from food into energy."

Under normal functioning, the body produces a hormone called insulin, which transports sugars into body cells. In some cases, the body does not produce insulin at all or does not produce enough; this results in diabetes.

Diabetes occurs in two major types:

- Type 1, or insulin-dependent diabetes
- Type 2, or non-insulin-dependent diabetes, which usually occurs in adults; in type 2, the body produces insulin in insufficient quantities

Complications from diabetes, which you may encounter in a medical office or clinic setting, include diabetic coma (acidosis) and insulin shock or reaction. The provider will prescribe either insulin or glucose before the patient is transported to the hospital. Both are serious emergencies that require immediate EMS assistance. Table 9-4 lists common causes and symptoms of diabetic coma or insulin shock (see Chapter 36 for calculation of medication dosage and medication administration).

Hemorrhage. The different sources of bleeding determine the seriousness of hemorrhage, or bleeding.

External Bleeding. External bleeding includes capillary, venous, and arterial bleeding. Capillary bleeding, often from cuts and scratches, usually clots without first aid measures. Bleeding from a vein, which is characterized by dark red blood that flows steadily, needs to be controlled quickly (see Procedure 9-1) to prevent excessive blood loss. Bleeding from an artery produces bright red blood that spurts from the wound; this is the most serious type of bleeding and occurs when an artery is punctured or severed. Like venous bleeding, arterial bleeding requires immediate emergency care because serious loss of blood and profound irreversible shock can happen quickly.

Epistaxis, or nosebleed, may be the result of breathing dry air for a long period; can result from injury or blowing the nose too hard; may be caused by high altitudes; may be caused by hypertension (high blood pressure); or may result from overuse of medications such as aspirin and anticoagulants. The mucous membranes of the nose are vascular and contain many small vessels very close to the surface of the tissues. These vessels are easily damaged.

To control nosebleeds, seat the patient, elevate the patient's head, and pinch the nostrils for at least 10 minutes. Assist the patient to sit with head tilted forward so blood running down the back of the throat will not be swallowed or aspirated. Bleeding should be controlled within 20 minutes. If bleeding cannot be controlled, the provider may request that you activate EMS. The patient's nostril may need to be cauterized or a gauze packing inserted (see Chapter 30). Bleeding associated with a head injury or trauma must be treated in an emergency setting in order to rule out serious underlying causes.

Table 9-4   Causes and Symptoms of Diabetic Coma and Insulin Shock

Diabetic Coma or Acidosis		Insulin Shock or Reaction	
Causes	Too little insulin, ingesting large amounts of carbohydrates, infections, fever, emotional stress	**Causes**	Too much insulin or oral hypoglycemic drug, ingesting too few carbohydrates, an unusual amount of exercise
Symptoms	• Skin: Dry and flushed • Behavior: Drowsy • Mouth: Dry • Thirst: Intense • Hunger: Absent • Vomiting: Common • Respiration: Exaggerated, air hungry • Breath: Fruity odor of acetone • Pulse: Weak and rapid • Vision: Dim • Blood glucose greater than 200 mg/100 mL	**Symptoms**	• Skin: Moist and pale • Behavior: Often excited • Mouth: Drooling • Thirst: Absent • Hunger: Present • Vomiting: Usually absent • Respiration: Normal or shallow • Breath: Usually normal • Pulse: Full and pounding (gives patient feeling of heart pounding) • Vision: Diplopia (double) • Low blood glucose level (40–70 mg/100 mL or less)
First aid	Keep patient warm Obtain medical help immediately	**First aid**	If patient is conscious, give sugar or any food containing sugar (fruit juice, candy, crackers) Obtain medical help immediately

© Cengage Learning 2014

Internal Bleeding. Internal bleeding may be minor or serious, depending on the cause of the injury. A contusion, or bruise, will result in minor internal bleeding. A sharp blow may induce severe internal bleeding.

Because there is no visible blood flow, it is important to recognize other indications of internal bleeding. Signs and symptoms are similar to those of shock and include a rapid and weak pulse, low blood pressure, shallow breathing, cold and clammy skin, dilated pupils, dizziness, faintness, thirst, restlessness, and a feeling of anxiety. There may be pain, tenderness, or swelling at the injury site. The abdomen may be boardlike (stiff and hard to the touch).

If internal bleeding is suspected, ask another staff member to call EMS; until they arrive, stay with the patient and take measures to prevent shock. Monitor vital signs.

Cerebral Vascular Accident

The common term for a cerebral vascular accident (CVA) is stroke. A stroke is the result of a ruptured blood vessel in the brain, or it can be caused by **occlusion** of a blood vessel by a clot. Both of these situations can result in the brain being deprived of oxygen, causing brain cells to die. Symptoms of a stroke include numbness in the face, arm, and leg on one side of the body; loss of vision; severe headache, mental confusion; slurred speech; nausea; vomiting; and difficulty in breathing and swallowing. Paralysis may be present. If a patient is suspected of having a stroke, call EMS, loosen tight clothing, lie the patient down, and keep him or her comfortable. Position the patient's head to facilitate the flow of secretion from the mouth to avoid choking and maintain an open airway. Do not give anything by mouth and monitor vital signs. Immediate emergency care is critical for all individuals experiencing strokes. If the stroke is caused by a clot that blocks blood flow, drugs may be able to protect the individual from permanent injury. Rapid transport to the hospital is important for treatment to be instituted as soon as possible. Treatment with the clot-dissolving drug must be given within 3 hours after onset of symptoms for it to be effective.

Heart Attack

Heart attack, also known as **myocardial infarction (MI)**, is usually caused by blockage of one or more of the coronary arteries. Symptoms include tightness of the chest, pain radiating down one or both arms, or pain radiating into the left shoulder and jaw. Other signs include rapid and weak pulse, excessive perspiration, agitation, nausea, and cold and clammy skin. Heart attack symptoms in a woman may or may not be similar to those experienced by a man. Women may have symptoms such as abdominal discomfort, burning sensation in the chest, discomfort or pain in the lower chest or back, unexplained sudden fatigue, sweating, and breathlessness.

If you suspect the patient is experiencing a heart attack, contact EMS immediately, loosen tight clothing, and keep the patient comfortable. Prepare to give oxygen and other medications such as aspirin, as directed by the provider. Monitor vital signs. If the patient experiences an episode of cardiac fibrillation, **cardioversion** or defibrillation may be necessary with an automatic external defibrillator. Prepare to begin CPR if necessary.

BREATHING EMERGENCIES AND CARDIAC ARREST

Breathing or respiratory emergencies occur for a variety of reasons, including choking, shock, allergies, and other illnesses or injuries such as drowning and electrical shock. When an individual stops breathing, artificial or rescue breathing must be given quickly, for without a constant supply of oxygen, brain damage or death will occur.

When the breathing problem is accompanied by cardiac arrest, the rescue breathing must be accompanied by chest compressions. This procedure is known as **cardiopulmonary resuscitation (CPR)**. Cardiac emergencies may occur in the medical clinic because of the large number of patients who have heart disease.

In order to graduate from a CAAHEP-accredited program, medical assistants must attain provider-level CPR certification and take first aid training courses. Frequent refresher courses and recertification in CPR are necessary.

PATIENT EDUCATION

Lay Person CPR

- The person does not need to be certified.
- Chest compressions alone are sufficient.
- Patients more likely to survive without brain damage with only chest compressions.
- Use 30 compressions per minute to keep blood moving to brain and heart.
- Drowning victims and smoke inhalation victims are the exception. Both need rescue breathing and CPR.

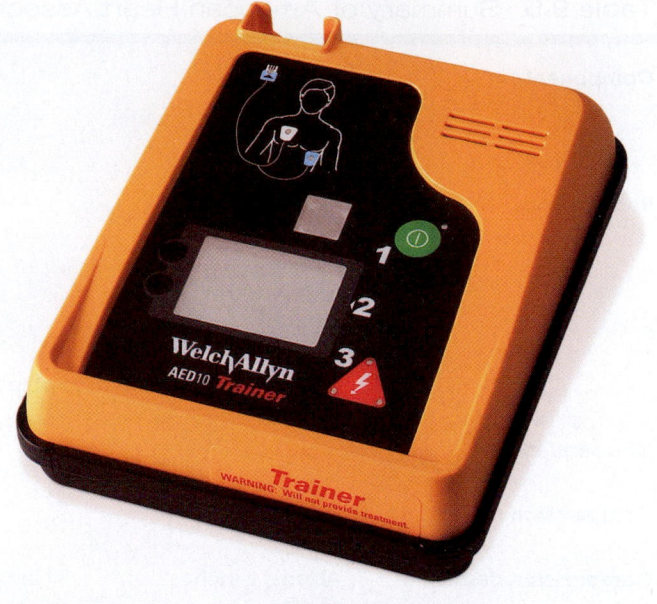

Figure 9-12   Automated external defibrillator.

Rescue Breathing

Individuals in respiratory arrest require immediate emergency care. **Rescue breathing**, previously called mouth-to-mouth resuscitation, provides oxygen to the patient until emergency personnel arrive.

When performing rescue breathing procedures in the ambulatory care setting, it is recommended that resuscitation mouthpieces be used and that direct mouth-to-mouth (i.e., with no personal protective equipment) resuscitation never be used.

Cardiopulmonary Resuscitation

The combination of rescue breathing and chest compressions is known as CPR. Alone, CPR cannot save an individual from cardiac arrest—it represents preliminary care until advanced medical help is available to the heart attack victim.

In 2010, the American Heart Association (AHA) updated their emergency care guidelines for CPR and Emergency Cardiovascular Care (ECC) (http://www.americanheart.org/cpr.html). The new guidelines recommend immediately beginning chest compression rather than opening the airway and beginning ventilations. There is a change in the A-B-C methodology to C-A-B. The emphasis has been placed on high-quality CPR (with chest compressions of adequate rate and depth, allowing complete chest recoil after each compression, minimizing interruptions in the compressions, and avoiding excessive ventilation).

Studies have found that if bystanders act quickly and begin CPR, many more victims could be saved. It was determined that CPR plus a shock with an AED (Figure 9-12) is the most effective immediate treatment for cardiac arrest. The AHA says that early recognition of the emergency, calling EMS, and performing immediate CPR can double or triple a victim's chances of surviving. Furthermore, the AHA says that CPR plus defibrillation (AED) that is started within 3 to 5 minutes of collapse can boost survival significantly. Lay rescuer AEDs are available in airports, sports facilities, airplanes, casinos, and many other locations. The AED is becoming more readily available, is easy to use, and is very accurate. The 2010 Guidelines suggest that an AED be utilized immediately for a witnessed arrest.

The 2010 Guidelines have changed the number of compressions per minute to *at least* 100 from *approximately* 100. The depth of compressions recommended has changed to *at least* 2 inches from 1.5–2 inches. The look, listen, and feel method has been replaced by a new suggested method to assess breathing while checking for responsiveness. Again, the updated AHA guidelines stress that compressions should begin immediately, prior to initiating rescue breathing. Table 9-5 summarizes the AHA 2010 Guidelines for CPR and defibrillation.

Refinements have also been made to recommendations for immediate recognition and activation of the emergency response system once the health care provider identifies the adult victim who is unresponsive as having no breathing or no

Table 9-5 Summary of American Heart Association 2010 CPR Guidelines

Component	Recommendations		
	Adults	**Children**	**Infants**
Recognition	Unresponsive (for all ages)		
	No breathing or no normal breathing (i.e., only gasping)	No breathing or only gasping	
	No pulse palpated within 10 seconds for all ages (HCP only)		
CPR sequence	C – A – B		
Compression rate	At least 100/min		
Compression depth	At least 2 inches (5 cm)	At least ⅓ AP diameter About 2 inches (5 cm)	At least ⅓ AP diameter About 1½ inches (4 cm)
Chest wall recoil	Allow complete recoil between compressions		
	HCPs rotate compressors every 2 minutes		
Compression interruptions	Minimize interruptions in chest compressions Attempt to limit interruptions to < 10 seconds		
Airway	Head tilt-chin lift (HCP suspected trauma: jaw thrust)		
Compression-to-ventilation ratio (until advanced airway is placed)	30:2 1 or 2 rescuers	30:2 Single rescuer 15:2 2 HCP rescuers	
Ventilations: when rescuer untrained and not proficient	Compressions only		
Ventilations with advanced airway (HCP)	1 breath every 6–8 seconds (8–10 breaths/min) Asynchronous with chest compressions About 1 second per breath Visible chest rise		
Defibrillation	Attach and use AED as soon as available. Minimize interruptions in chest compressions before and after shock; resume CPR beginning with compressions immediately after each shock.		

Abbreviations: AED, automated external defibrillator; AP, anterior-posterior; CPR, cardiopulmonary resuscitation; HCP, health care provider.
*Excluding the newly born, in whom the cause of an arrest is nearly always asphyxia.

© Cengage Learning 2014

normal breathing (i.e., only gasping). Once no normal breathing has been identified, the provider then activates the EMS and retrieves the AED (or sends someone to do so). The health care provider should not spend more than 10 seconds checking for a pulse, and if a pulse is not definitively felt within 10 seconds, the provider should begin CPR and use the AED when available.

More information is available from the following sources:

- American Heart Association (http://www.americanheart.org)
- American Red Cross (http://www.redcross.org)
- National Safety Council (http://www.nsc.org)
- National Institutes of Health (http://www.health.nih.gov)

SAFETY AND EMERGENCY PRACTICES

The Commission on Accreditation of Allied Health Programs (CAAHEP) believes allied health students should understand how to respond in an emergency situation, as health care professionals and citizens. Medical assistant programs accredited by CAAHEP have within their Standards and Guidelines a new section requirement for safety and emergency practices. Provider-level CPR and basic first aid are part of these requirements for graduation.

The Accrediting Bureau of Health Education Schools (ABHES) also has a requirement in its competencies under the heading of Medical Office Clinical Procedures.

Health professionals recognize an obligation to use their skills and knowledge in a disaster environment.

There are many kinds of mass disasters, natural and manmade. Some examples are floods, hurricanes, tornadoes, tsunamis, and earthquakes. Others are explosions, structural collapses (I-35W bridge collapse in Minneapolis in 2007), transportation accidents, and war or terrorism (see Chapter 22).

What would a large-scale disaster be like and how could we respond? Disaster threatens public health and safety; disrupts services (gas, water, electricity, transportation); destroys roads, bridges, homes, and other buildings; and makes food and water unsafe or impossible to obtain. Law enforcement, fire departments, hospitals, and military all could be affected. There is a need for collaboration between disaster experts and health professionals to plan for emergencies.

What can medical assistants do to help? How could you use your skills without technology (unavailable due to the disaster)? Some examples are assisting your neighbors at local shelters, using your first aid and CPR skills, helping out at a clinic, giving injections for mass immunizations, supporting overwhelmed providers, working with the American Red Cross, giving emotional support, and filling in at a hospital.

In addition to mass disasters, medical assistants should be prepared to respond to emergency situations in the medical clinic or a home environment. Circumstances in which a patient goes into shock, or an elderly family member has a fall, or the medical clinic needs to be evacuated for a fire are examples of these emergency situations.

Medical assisting curriculum may include related courses to be certain that medical assisting graduates are prepared to help during an emergency situation.

In 2002, President Bush asked for teams of volunteers of medical and health professionals to contribute their skills during times of need in their communities. The Medical Reserve Corps (MRC) was established (http://www.medicalreservecorps.gov), and the teams of volunteers within the MRC work with Health and Human Services of the U.S. government and the American Red Cross. The MRC is community based. Its goal is to organize and use volunteers who want to donate their time and expertise to respond to emergencies and to promote healthy living throughout the year. The MRC supplements existing emergency and public health resources. Volunteers include providers, nurses, respiratory care therapists, massage therapists, pharmacists, dentists, and a wide array of allied health professionals such as medical assistants.

The MRC volunteer units are assigned to specific areas. They work with and support the county and state public health departments. The main office is in the Surgeon General's office in Washington, DC.

PROCEDURE 9-1
Control of Bleeding

STANDARD PRECAUTIONS:

PURPOSE:
To control bleeding from an open wound

EQUIPMENT/SUPPLIES:
Sterile dressings
Sterile gloves
Mask and eye protection
Gown
Biohazard waste container

PROCEDURE STEPS:

1. Wash hands.

2. *Paying attention to detail,* assemble equipment and supplies.

3. Apply eye and mask protection and gown if splashing is likely to occur.

4. Put on gloves.

5. Apply dressing and press firmly (Figure 9-13A).

6. If bleeding continues, elevate arm above heart level (Figure 9-13B). RATIONALE: Raising the arm above the heart level will slow the flow of blood because it is flowing against gravity.

7. *Display sound judgment.* If bleeding continues, press adjacent artery against bone (Figure 9-13C). Notify the provider if bleeding cannot be controlled. *Remain calm in a crisis.* RATIONALE: Pressing the adjacent artery against a bone provides solid pressure to help control bleeding.

8. Apply pressure bandage over the dressing.

9. Dispose of waste in biohazard container.

10. Remove gloves and dispose in biohazard container.

11. Wash hands.

12. Document procedure in patient's chart or electronic medical record.

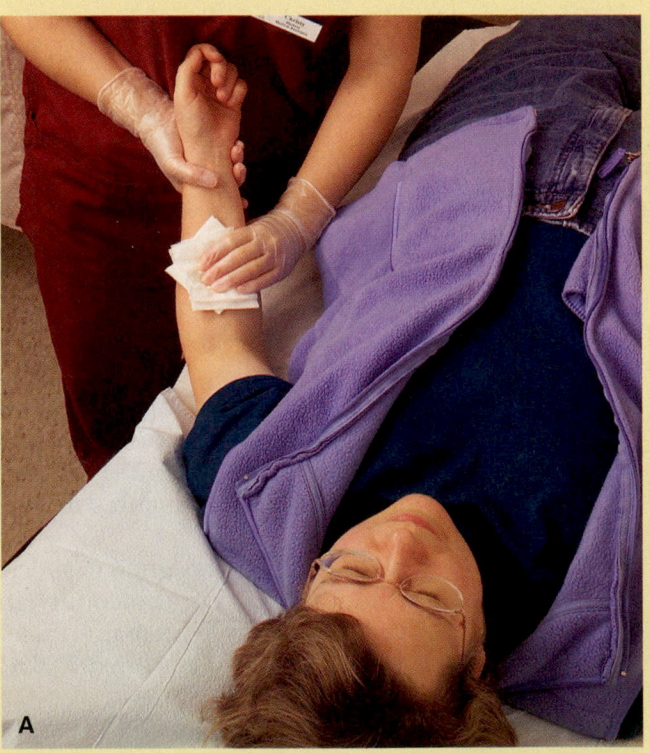
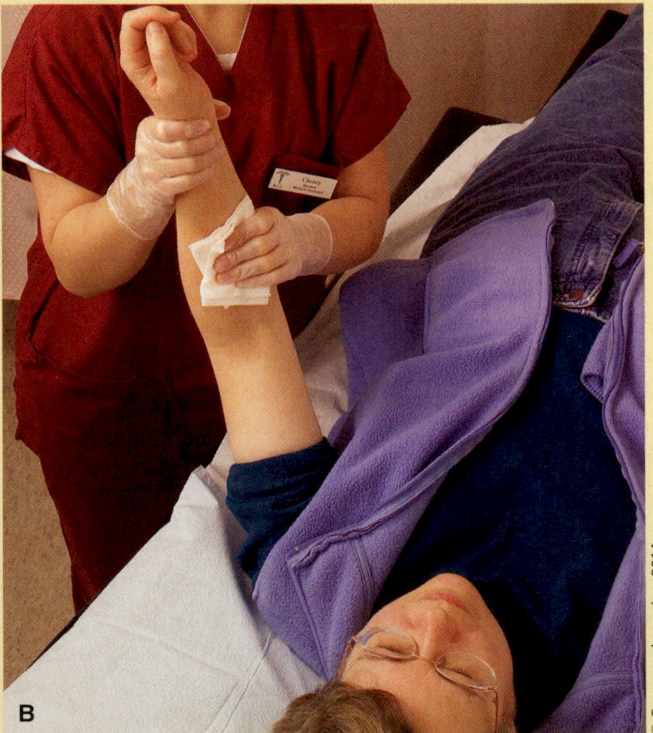

© Cengage Learning 2014

Figure 9-13   (A) Apply dressing and press firmly. (B) Elevate arm above heart level.

Procedure 9-1 (continued)

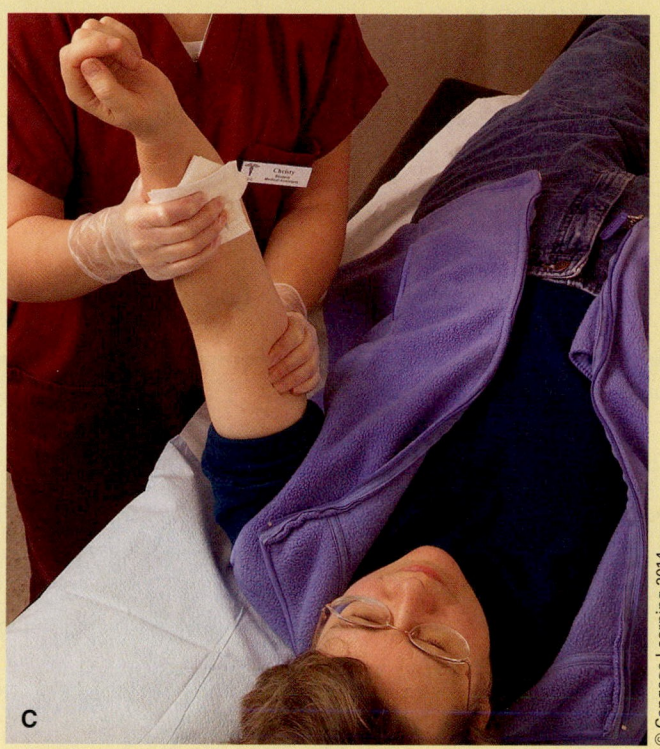

Figure 9-13 (continued) (C) Press artery against bone.

Caution: If wound is large and bleeding is not controlled, the patient may go into hemorrhagic shock. Be prepared to call EMS immediately.

DOCUMENTATION:

4/4/20XX—10:00 AM   Patient sustained small (1 cm) laceration on inside left forearm. Bleeding moderately. Pressure dressing applied to wound, left arm elevated above heart level. Bleeding continued. Pressure applied to brachial artery. Pressure bandage applied over dry sterile dressing. Bleeding seems to have subsided. BP 118/74, P 92. Seen by Dr. King. P. Cosper, RMA (AMT)

PROCEDURE 9-2

Applying an Arm Splint

STANDARD PRECAUTIONS:

PURPOSE:

To immobilize the area above and below the injured part of the arm in order to reduce pain, immobilize, and prevent further injury.

EQUIPMENT/SUPPLIES:

Thin piece of rigid board; cardboard can be used if necessary
Gauze roller bandage

PROCEDURE STEPS:

1. Wash hands.

2. *Introduce yourself and identify patient.* Place the padded splint under the injured area.

3. *While displaying a calm and professional manner,* hold the splint in place with gauze roller bandage. Pad gaps between arm and board (wrist) with gauze pads or other soft material. RATIONALE: More comfortable for patient.

4. After splinting, check circulation (note color and temperature of skin, note color of nails, check pulse) to ascertain that the splint is not too tightly applied. RATIONALE: Checks for impaired circulation.

continues

Procedure 9-2 (continued)

5. Apply a sling to keep the arm elevated, which increases comfort and reduces swelling.

6. Wash hands.

7. ***Accurately and concisely update the provider on the patient's care.*** Document the procedure in patient's chart or electronic medical record.

DOCUMENTATION:

4/4/20XX—2:00 PM   Splint applied to right arm above and below injured area. Sling applied for comfort. Nail beds pink, hand warm, radial pulse easily palpated. Seen by Dr. Woo. J. Guerro, CMA (AAMA)————————————

CASE STUDY 9-1

Refer to the scenario at the beginning of the chapter.

CASE STUDY REVIEW

1. Why is it essential to activate EMS even though Mr. Edwards is being seen in an ambulatory care setting?

2. What would be the next steps after assessing the patient if the chest pain continued and the patient lost consciousness prior to the arrival of EMS?

3. Phyllis Cosper, RMA, is screening patients the morning Mr. Edwards enters the clinic with a complaint of chest pain. What questions should she ask Mr. Edwards?

4. Because Mr. Edwards is obviously having a cardiac event, what are the first measures to be taken?

CASE STUDY 9-2

Annette Samuels, a regular patient at Inner City Health Care, is walking her dog one morning, stops to rest on a grassy knoll, and notices a wasp on her arm. She brushes it away, unthinking, and then realizes it has stung her. She receives two more stings and suddenly notices she is at a nest site. Annette is now a half-hour walk from home but is not really concerned because she has never had an allergic reaction to a wasp sting. However, a few minutes into her walk, her palms become itchy, her ears start to burn, and she feels lightheaded. She is not having difficulty breathing. She is determined to get home and she does, at which point she notices she is covered with hives. She calls Inner City Health Care to ask: Should she come in?

CASE STUDY REVIEW

1. Linda Ludemann, CMA (AAMA) is screening calls the morning that Annette is stung. What questions should she ask Annette?

2. Because Annette obviously is having a hypersensitive or an allergic reaction, she is advised to seek emergency care immediately. What first-aid measures might be taken?

3. To prevent reactions to stings in the future, what patient teaching might be appropriate for Ms. Samuels?

CASE STUDY 9-3

Bryan Mountjoy is a 32-year-old patient of Dr. Osborne. He has been working in the yard throughout the day even though the temperature was over 100°F. Being so focused on the job at hand, Mr. Mountjoy has not taken in enough fluids over the course of the day. He calls out to his wife that he is feeling faint. She finds him with reddened, dry, hot skin; shallow, fast breathing; and a weak pulse. Ms. Mountjoy calls the clinic seeking medical advice.

CASE STUDY REVIEW

1. What immediate questions should you ask Mr. Mountjoy?

2. What would you advise Mr. Mountjoy to do in order to receive the most appropriate level of care?

SUMMARY

Although many of the emergencies covered in this chapter may never be seen by the medical assistant in the ambulatory care setting, it is nonetheless important to develop a broad base of information about the various types of potential emergency situations. This knowledge gives the medical assistant the confidence and the preparation to manage the emergencies that do occur with speed, accuracy, and understanding until outside emergency help arrives. Staff will need to assess their response to emergencies on a continual basis. Was protocol followed? Were there difficulties in the delivery of care? Were staff and equipment prepared and ready to deal with these potentially life-threatening situations?

Staff meetings should be held to discuss these and other questions that may have arisen and to allow staff the opportunity to talk about any fears or concerns they might have. It must be stressed that this chapter is at best an introduction to the topic of emergency procedures and first aid; it is essential that medical assistants in all ambulatory care settings, whether large or small, enroll in an American Red Cross, American Heart Association, American Safety and Health Institute, or National Heart Association first aid and CPR program, attain provider-level CPR certification, and take refresher courses to update skills.

STUDY FOR SUCCESS

To reinforce your knowledge and skills of information presented in this chapter:

- Review the *Key Terms*
- Role-play with other students to apply attributes of professionalism pertinent to this chapter.
- Consider the *Case Studies* and discuss your conclusions
- Answer the questions in the *Certification Review*
- Apply your knowledge by completing the *Activities* in the *Study Guide* and the Games and Quizzes in the StudyWARE **StudyWARE** software on the Premium Website
- Perform the *Procedures* using the *Competency Assessment Checklists* in the Competency Manual
- Practice your problem-solving skills with the *Critical Thinking Challenge 3.0* on the *Premium Website*

Additional resources for this chapter include:

- Modules 11 and 26 of the *Medical Assisting Learning Lab*
- *CourseMate for Delmar's Comprehensive Medical Assisting*
- *WebTutor for Delmar's Comprehensive Medical Assisting*

CERTIFICATION REVIEW

1. Good Samaritan laws:
   a. are designed to protect the public
   b. protect non-health care professionals
   c. require that all individuals providing assistance act within the scope of their knowledge and training
   d. protect health care professionals on the job

2. Which of the following defines an avulsion?
   a. The skin is torn off and bleeding is profuse.
   b. There is superficial scraping of the dermis.
   c. It is an injury that results from a sharp object.
   d. It is a tear of the body tissue.

3. First-degree burns:
   a. are the most serious and penetrate all layers of skin
   b. affect only the top layer of skin
   c. often leave scar tissue
   d. usually take more than a month to heal
4. According to current AHA CPR guidelines, what is the order of steps for cardiopulmonary resuscitation?
   a. Airway, breathing, compressions
   b. Breathing, compressions, airway
   c. Compressions, airway, breathing
   d. None of the above
5. A fracture in which the bone protrudes through the skin is called:
   a. greenstick fracture
   b. compound fracture
   c. depressed fracture
   d. comminuted fracture
6. To control a nosebleed, it is important to:
   a. have the patient lie down
   b. tilt the patient's head back
   c. tilt the patient's head forward
   d. call 911 immediately

7. Another name for a heart attack is:
   a. cerebral vascular accident
   b. cardiac arrest
   c. angina pectoris
   d. myocardial infarction
8. The depth of compressions for adults is:
   a. 0.5 to 1 inch
   b. 1 to 1.5 inches
   c. 1.5 to 2 inches
   d. 2 to 2.5 inches
9. Exposure to extreme cold for prolonged periods can cause which of the following:
   a. hypothermia
   b. hyperthermia
   c. frostbite
   d. both a and c
10. Septic shock is the result of:
    a. a severe allergic reaction
    b. overwhelming infection
    c. trauma to the respiratory system
    d. extreme loss of blood

REFERENCES/BIBLIOGRAPHY

American Heart Association. (2005). Adult basic life support. *Circulation, 112*, IV19–IV34.

American National Red Cross. (2001). *Staywell.* St. Louis, MO: Mosby-Year Book.

American Red Cross. (2005). *CPR and emergency cardiac care: New CPR guidelines for professionals and non-professionals.* Retrieved September 19, 2007, from http://www.redcross.org/cpr.html

Consumer Reports on Health. (2008). *Consumer Unions, 20,* 7, 3.

Medical Reserve Corps. (2008). *Emergency medical care.* Retrieved September 17, 2007, from http://www.medicalreservecorps.gov

National Institutes of Health. (2008). *New CPR guidelines.* Retrieved September 17, 2007, from http://www.health.nih.gov

Taber's cyclopedic medical dictionary (21st ed.). (2003). Philadelphia: F. A. Davis.

http://www.heart.org/HEARTORG/CPRAndECC/HealthcareTraining/AdvancedCardiovascularLifeSupportACLS/Advanced-Cardiovascular-Life-Support-ACLS_UCM_001280_SubHomePage.jsp

http://www.nlm.nih.gov/medlineplus/ency/article/003133.htm

http://www.heart.org/idc/groups/heart-public/@wcm/@ecc/documents/downloadable/ucm_317350.pdf. Accessed April 4, 2012.

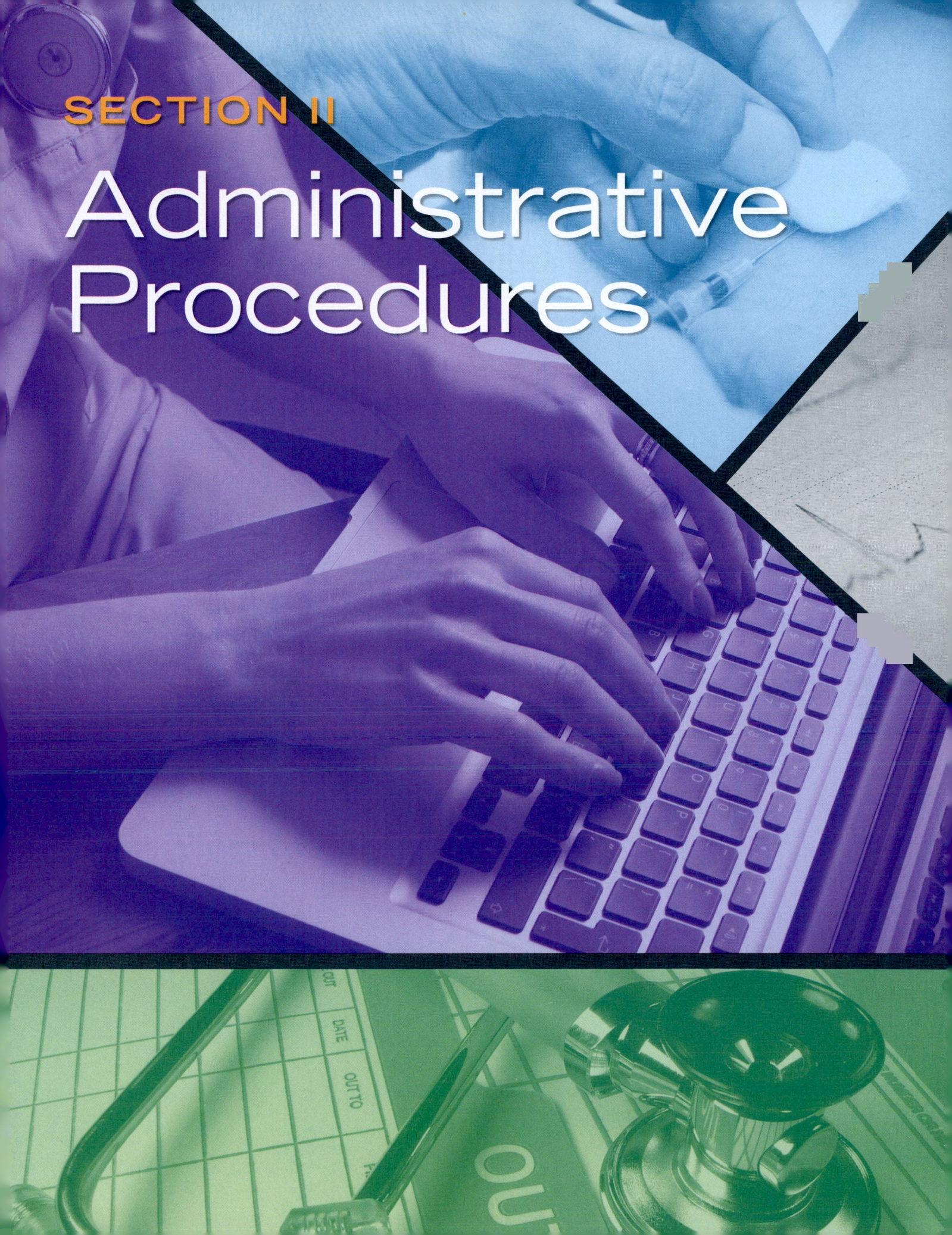

SECTION II
Administrative
Procedures

UNIT IV

Integrated Administrative Procedures

CHAPTER 10
Creating the Facility Environment 187

CHAPTER 11
Computers in the Ambulatory Care Setting 210

CHAPTER 12
Telecommunications 238

CHAPTER 13
Patient Scheduling 270

CHAPTER 14
Medical Records Management 294

CHAPTER 15
Written Communications 324

CHAPTER 16
Medical Documents 352

Creating the Facility Environment

OUTLINE

Creating a Welcoming
  Environment
The Reception Area
  The Receptionist
  Cultural Considerations
  When Children Are
    Patients
  Education in the
    Reception Area
Clinic Design and Environment
  Ventilation and Infection
    Control

Lighting
Nature, Music, Water,
  and Color
Noise Reduction
Legal Compliance in the
  Facility
  HIPAA
  Americans with Disabilities Act
Safety
  Creating a Safe Environment
  Evacuation Procedures

Fire Safety
Response to Natural Disaster
  or Emergency
The Medical Assistant's
  Response to Disaster
  Preparedness
Opening the Facility
Closing the Facility
The Future Environment
  for Ambulatory Care

LEARNING OUTCOMES

1. Define, spell, and pronounce the key terms as presented in the glossary.
2. Illustrate a comfortable, welcoming, and pleasing reception area.
3. Demonstrate important personality characteristics the receptionist should possess.
4. Determine cultural aspects to consider in the reception area.
5. Discuss the needs of children in the reception area.
6. Identify how the reception area can be used for educational purposes.
7. Explain the benefits of lighting, music, color, nature, and water in a facility.
8. Interpret the role of HIPAA in patient privacy and the facility environment.
9. Determine the number of patients a reception area should accommodate.

10. Recall essential elements of the Americans with Disabilities Act.
11. Evaluate the facility for safety and emergency preparedness.
12. Develop a personal and patient safety plan.
13. Explain the components for an evacuation plan of a provider's clinic.
14. Demonstrate proper use of a fire extinguisher.
15. Review steps to take in case of a natural disaster.
16. Outline the role of the medical assistant in emergency preparedness.
17. List at least three tasks to perform on opening and closing the facility.
18. Outline future characteristics of the ambulatory health care environment.
19. Analyze the professionalism questions and apply them to this chapter's content.

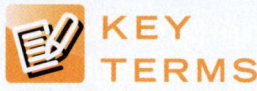

KEY TERMS

LASIK

cataract

ATTRIBUTES OF PROFESSIONALISM

Communication

- Did you introduce yourself?
- Did you listen to and acknowledge the patient?
- Did you allay patients' fears and help them feel safe and comfortable?

Presentation

- Did you attend to any special needs of the patient?
- Did you assist the patient if help was needed?
- Were you courteous to the patient?
- Did you display a positive attitude?
- Did you display a calm, professional, and caring manner?

Competency

- Did you pay attention to detail?
- Did you display sound judgment?
- Did you remain calm in a crisis?
- Were you knowledgeable and accountable?
- Did you ask questions if you were out of your comfort zone or did not have the experience to carry out the task?
- Did you apply appropriate risk management principles?
- Did you demonstrate self-awareness in responding to emergency situations?
- Did you take necessary safety precautions?

Initiative

- Were you proactive?
- Did you develop a strategic plan to achieve your goals?
- Were you respectful of others?

Integrity

- Did you work within your scope of practice?
- Did you demonstrate sensitivity to patients' rights?
- Did you demonstrate respect for individual diversity?
- Did you protect and maintain confidentiality?

SCENARIO

The design of any ambulatory setting often evolves as the needs of the clinic and patients change. In the clinic of Drs. Lewis and King, a two-provider family practice, the environment has always been warm and welcoming, which is particularly important because the providers see many children. However, the clinic was initially designed in the early 1980s, before the Americans with Disabilities Act (ADA) was passed by the U.S. Congress.

Once this act was passed in 1990, the office manager, Marilyn Johnson, CMA (AAMA), was aware of the need to comply with its mandates. In addition, Drs. Lewis and King wanted to make all their patients, including those with disabilities, as comfortable as possible. Working with a local architect, changes were incorporated into the practice's existing space: a ramp was added outside, doorways were widened to provide wheelchair access, and new Braille signage was installed outside for the visually impaired patients. Although the changes were not without expense, the staff of Drs. Lewis and King willingly complied with the ADA not only because it is law, but because it gave better access to more patients.

More recently, while making certain the clinic protocol was in compliance with the Health Insurance Portability and Accountability Act of 1996 (HIPAA), the clinic staff took another look at the facility to ensure it was favorable in light of protecting patient confidentiality. They discovered that the reception area was seriously lacking in providing privacy and confidentiality for patient information and the entire clinic needed serious updating in many other aspects.

INTRODUCTION

The environment of the medical facility contributes almost as much to a patient's well-being as does the medical attention given by providers and their medical assistants. The physical environment can foster a feeling that embraces and welcomes patients or, conversely, can cause them to feel alienated and intimidated. Numerous recent studies reveal that the physical environment of a clinic is linked to the comfort of both patient and staff. In fact, such "evidence-based design" can lead to reduced noise, improved lighting, better ventilation, and ergonomic designs with supportive work spaces and improved layout in medical clinics. These design changes make clinics safer, promote healing, produce fewer errors on the part of staff, and reduce the pain and discomfort of patients.

Dental providers have set a trend in the field of health care design. Dentists recognize that few individuals enjoy visiting a dentist and know that their patients expect to feel discomfort, pain, and extended-length procedures that are stressful. Dentists also realize that about one-fourth of the country's population refuses to see a dentist for any reason because of fear of pain and discomfort. In order to lessen patients' anxiety and to encourage patients to return on a regular basis for dental care, many dentists turned to "spa-like" dental environments.

In this environment, patients can recline in heated chairs, are given blankets for their legs, can listen to soothing music, or may be given video headsets to watch their favorite television programs. Dental assistants may even dip a patient's hands into paraffin and then tuck them into silk mitts to soften the hands while dental work is being done. Other dentists offer foot, hand, or shoulder massages. Patients may choose to undergo Botox procedures, receive facials, or have unwanted facial hair removed. Brief massages and paraffin hand treatments usually are free; other, more complicated procedures are provided for a fee, sometimes in a separate area of the dental clinic. The idea behind the entire "spa-like" environment is to make patients feel comfortable with their dental procedures and want to return.

Does this sound like the future of medical clinic design? Probably not, but careful observation and comparison will reveal an increasing number of medical clinics seeking to attract patients not only with high-quality medical care but also with attention to detail that provides comfort and a more "resort-like" atmosphere. Medical providers understand that their best advertisement is a good word from patients who have had positive experiences of their encounters for medical care. Perhaps the "spa-like" environment might be more welcomed when a patient is not feeling well, suffers from a chronic illness, or is facing a life-threatening disease.

Interior designers and experts who specialize in medical space planning are advising all individuals involved in designing clinics, medical offices, and hospitals that patient comfort must be considered as important as the facility's functional utility and ease of maintenance.

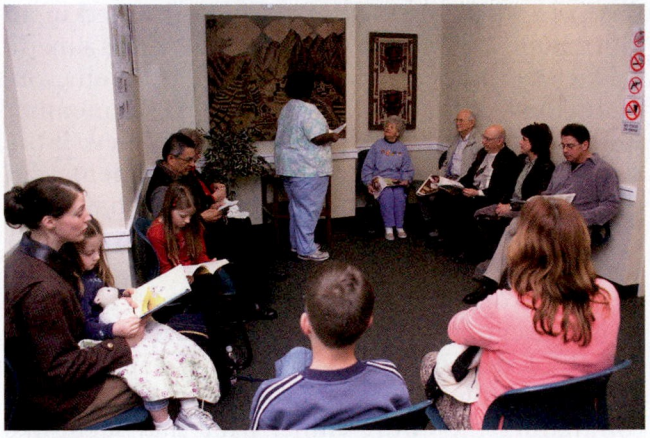

© Cengage Learning 2014

Figure 10-1 A busy reception area can still be pleasant and offer comfortable seating.

CREATING A WELCOMING ENVIRONMENT

The creation of a health care facility involves many variables. Some are tangible elements, such as lighting, color choice, and furniture arrangement. Others are intangible and are expressed in an administrative medical assistant's greeting and attitude toward patients. Important components of patient satisfaction are a warm and caring staff, comfortable surroundings, and the ability of patients and visitors to find their way around the medical clinic without getting lost. Convenience of access and privacy are essential. The ADA (see Chapter 7) also must be taken into account when creating any medical clinic environment by making provisions to accommodate patients who are physically challenged. HIPAA regulations (see Chapter 7) identify how a patient's privacy and confidentiality are to be protected and may also dictate medical clinic space planning. Finally, an environment that demonstrates attention to safety, the prevention of hazards, and effective response to emergency situations further enhances patient and even employee satisfaction. Together, all these elements help make an ambulatory setting the kind of environment where patients will feel comfortable and secure.

THE RECEPTION AREA

A reception area is just that—a place of reception. It should never be thought of as "the waiting room." This is the area first viewed by the patient and this is the first opportunity to make the patient feel welcome, secure, and comfortable. First impressions are lasting. Adequate and comfortable seating, consideration for patients of all ages, proper lighting and ventilation, the use of color, noise reduction, and the influence of nature are all aspects to consider in creating the clinic environment (Figure 10-1).

Space planners who specialize in medical clinics and hospitals and who have spent many hours analyzing patient flow indicate that the reception area should accommodate at least 1 hour's patients per provider plus a friend or relative who may accompany each patient. Another quick rule of thumb to use is 2.5 seats in the reception area for each examination room. Clinics where providers see patients without advance appointments will, of course, need a larger reception area.

Depending on the clientele of the ambulatory care setting, consider the following items to help ease patients' time in any area where waiting is essential (i.e., pending laboratory results, etc.) and to help take their minds off current medical problems: a table and chairs with a "puzzle in progress," Internet access for busy employees, an electronic Sudoku board, or a juice bar. Although these items are not appropriate in every setting, they certainly can be in some (refer to Case Study 10–2).

It is helpful if there is a place for patients to hang heavy coats or wet umbrellas. Accessories and artwork can easily add a special touch to a facility. Nature pictures elicit a more favorable response from patients than abstract art. Although fresh flowers might be a nice touch, they harbor microorganisms, and some patients are allergic to them. There is the tendency to use living plants in the medical facility, but some silk plants and flowers also may be appropriate.

Even when the office or clinic is housed in an older building not originally constructed as a medical facility, much can be done to create an environment that enhances patient comfort. Remember to see things from the patient's point of view. If the facility is a maze of corridors where patients can easily get turned around, make certain that directions are clear and that proper signage is easily understood.

It is worth the investment to have a professional designer specializing in medical space planning look through the facility to make suggestions regarding color, artwork, and the general environment of the entire clinic. What may seem like an unnecessary expense to the clinic operation can result in greater satisfaction on the part of all patients.

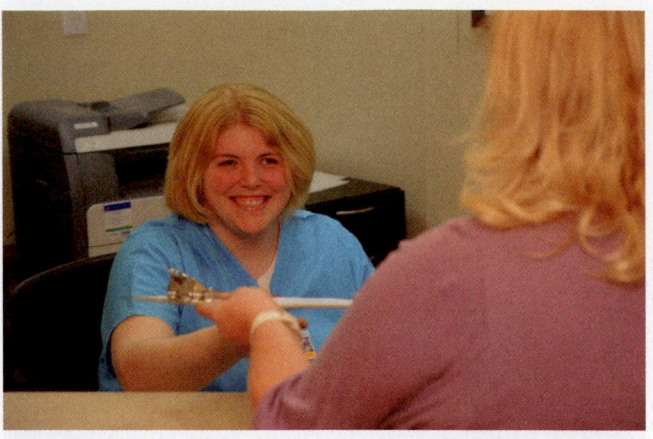

Figure 10-2   A friendly, warm greeting from the medical assistant is reassuring to arriving patients.

The Receptionist

  A receptionist who has a smile and a greeting for every patient, offers assistance, and carefully explains any waiting that might be necessary helps to create that "reception" environment. No matter how "rushed" the reception area may seem with patient activity and ringing telephones, the calm and reassuring attention of the receptionist helps set the stage for satisfied patients (Figure 10-2).

The receptionist must always keep a positive "We can help you" attitude, have a smile for each patient, and exude a genuine "We care about you" personality. This individual—who often has other duties as well—must be able to perform telephone prioritization, retrieve records, greet patients, present a bill, make appointments, and log data into the computer, all the while remembering that the patient's comfort is of primary concern. All medical personnel, but especially the receptionist, must genuinely like people and not react when patients are grumpy, irritable, or depressed and worried about an illness. The employee in the reception area of the clinic is the person who sets the social climate for the interchange between the patient and the provider and the rest of the staff.

Patients who are very ill, injured, or upset should not have to wait in the reception area, but should be shown to an examination room away from other patients. The receptionist may also have to monitor children who may be intent on disrupting patients. This is especially necessary if the parent seems unconcerned about keeping youngsters under control.

Receptionists also are expected to maintain the tidiness of the reception area. Magazines can be straightened, litter picked up, and surface counters attended to. Counters, table surfaces, and toys in medical clinics are among those most infested with microbes; therefore, they should be sanitized daily, or sometimes twice a day, especially when patients may have contagious diseases. Receptionists may be asked to place paper face masks in the reception area and instruct patients when they make their appointments to pick up a paper mask on arrival at the front door if they are experiencing a respiratory illness.

If there are unexpected delays in the provider's schedule, hopefully never more than 20 minutes, receptionists will notify patients of the delay tactfully and graciously and offer them the alternative of making other arrangements. The patient's time is as valuable as the provider's.

CRITICAL THINKING

Discuss the difference between the idea of a "waiting" area and a "reception" area. Which term is used more frequently by patients? Explain your response.

CRITICAL THINKING

With a fellow student, role-play a situation in which a frustrated and angry patient must be calmed by the receptionist. Assume the patient is angry because of a long wait in the reception area.

Cultural Considerations

In consideration of cultural differences, there are some points to recall. Some people do not like to be touched by strangers. Middle Eastern and Latin cultures, by contrast, encourage closeness and touching, and individuals from these cultures may cluster themselves close together in the reception area. Cultural differences also will have an impact on the amount of space necessary for the reception area. Some ethnic populations are likely to bring several relatives with them to an appointment. This is especially common if the patient needs emotional support or a language interpreter.

Many do not like to face other patients in the reception area and prefer anonymity. No one likes to be in close proximity to a stranger who appears to be contagious. Most are more comfortable in close quarters primarily with individuals of the same gender. While some patients are bothered by children, others find them to be a pleasant distraction. Adequate and comfortable seating affords patients their own space and respects these cultural preferences.

When Children Are Patients

If the clinic treats children as patients or if children are apt to accompany adult patients, a children's area is especially helpful and appreciated. A special table and chairs for children, interactive toys (with emphasis on the interactive), and perhaps even a small television placed in a children's corner can be provided. This area needs to be away from doors that swing or hazards on which children might be injured. A children's area should always be in sight of the administrative medical assistant or receptionist who may be charged with keeping order, especially if a parent must be seen unaccompanied by children in an examination room.

A pediatric facility that treats only children and youth might consider a particular theme for its design. Figure 10-3 shows a pediatric clinic with a Hawaiian village theme. Ocean murals and the aquarium are enhanced by the grass hut and palm trees design. There is much in the environment to keep children interested and enthused about their visit to the provider.

Education in the Reception Area

Many providers place educational materials for patients in the reception area. For example, new parents always appreciate pamphlets related to raising children. If the provider is an ophthalmologist, information on **LASIK** or **cataract** surgeries are likely seen in the reception area. It is also

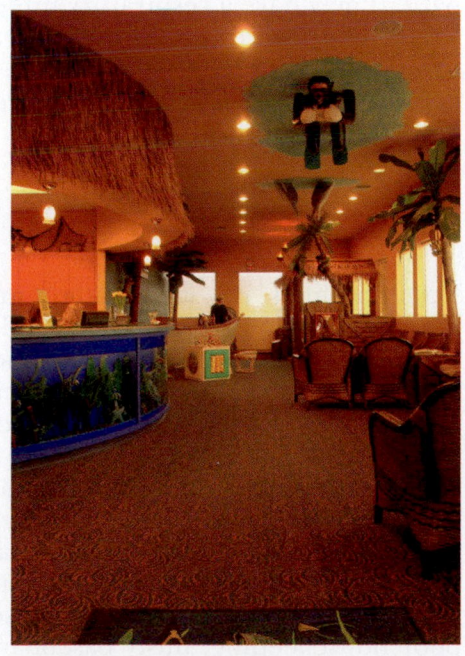
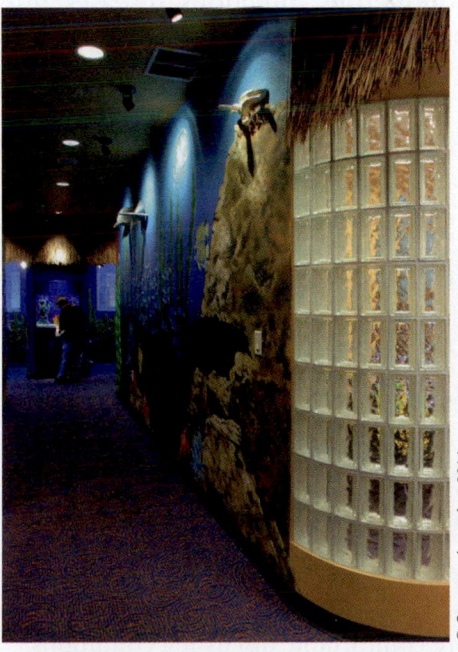

© Cengage Learning 2014

Figure 10-3   A pediatric medical clinic with a Hawaiian village theme provides ample distraction for children, yet is functional and efficient.

appropriate to have available in the reception area a patient information brochure that describes the services of the clinic, the function of medical staff members, measures to take in case of an emergency, and other issues that patients may need to consider (see Chapter 45 for more information on developing brochures for patient use). In some cases, the educational material may be presented in media form on a television screen.

CLINIC DESIGN AND ENVIRONMENT

Clinic environments, by their own definition, are places where persons who are ill gather for support, diagnosis, treatment, and healing. There are a few very important factors that can make the environment more conducive to patient comfort. Some rooms in the facility, by their very nature, may cause patients to feel anxious. Consider, for example, the patient on an examination table who only has on a cloth or paper gown, interacting with the provider who is fully clothed, wearing a white lab coat, and comfortably seated at a counter desk. The patient is at a disadvantage and may feel vulnerable in discussion and negotiation, contrary to the goal in medical care to empower the patient with as much control as possible (Figure 10-4).

Ventilation and Infection Control

The risk of contracting infectious diseases due to airborne and surface contamination is high in

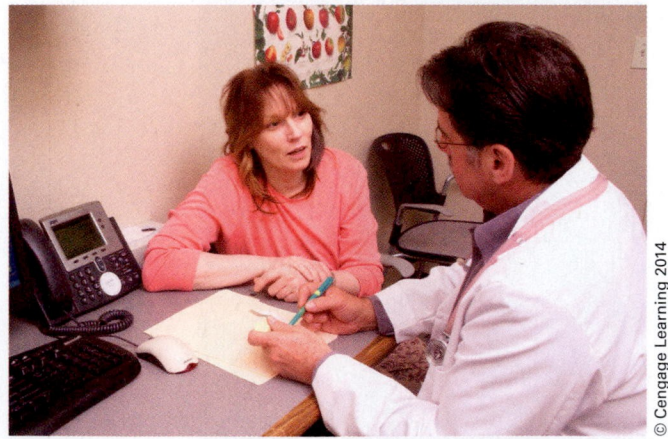

Figure 10-4 Patients should be afforded as much dignity and empowerment as possible. Many patients feel more comfortable discussing conditions, procedures, or treatments in the provider's office rather than in the examination room.

© Cengage Learning 2014

any medical facility; therefore, proper ventilation and effective infection control measures are essential. Many patients will find offensive the common odors that can be present in a medical facility, even when the odors are from necessary antiseptics. Proper ventilation can alleviate this issue. Although ventilation systems are often overlooked in medical clinics, appropriate air filters (usually HEPA), airflow direction, and air pressure are critical elements in reducing airborne infection and are to be considered in the heating and air conditioning design of the facility.

Diligent surface cleaning and the use of alcohol-based hand-rub dispensers that are easily accessible will encourage recommended hand washing and reduce contact contamination. All areas of a clinic are susceptible to contamination and diligence is necessary to curb transmission. As noted earlier, the reception area is one of the most contaminated areas of the clinic—countertops where patients likely check in, computer keyboards, telephone ear pieces, common pens used for writing—all are examples where microorganisms often grow and multiply. Statistics show that the easier the access to the hand-rub dispensers and sinks for hand cleansing, the more likely they are to be used. For example, after the Veterans Affairs Medical Center in Washington D.C. introduced these dispensers, there was a 21 percent drop in antibiotic-resistant staph infections. Many clinics also provide face masks with their use recommended when a patient may have a respiratory infection.

Such measures described here are important in any clinic but absolutely essential when a majority of the provider's clientele have a depressed immune system.

Lighting

Many facilities pay close attention to lighting, use very few fluorescent lights, and allow natural light to penetrate the rooms as much as possible. The use of natural light and images of nature or nature itself in the form of a garden, plants, etc. has shown to be very beneficial to both patients and staff. Sunlight is known to boost serotonin, which helps to lessen pain and depression. The goal is to provide as much peace and relaxation as possible to reduce stress and promote healing. A poorly illuminated room also may suggest poor housekeeping, dusty baseboards, soiled carpets, or faded draperies. Lighting can be soft and inviting while providing proper illumination. Note that fluorescent lighting is not used in the spaces shown in Figure 10-5 and Figure 10-6. Ceiling can lights and lamps provide ample light for both the reception area and many of the work areas. Superior lighting in areas of any close examination, medication preparations, minor surgery, etc. helps to reduce the chance of errors.

Nature, Music, Water, and Color

Some clinics are designed with floor-to-ceiling windows throughout the clinic, especially in the reception area, that overlook a garden of plants, trees, and flowers as well as a waterfall or pool that attracts birds. A professionally maintained built-in aquarium can help to set a calming tone for clinic clientele. Other medical facilities are experimenting with the addition of music in their facilities. There is proof that certain melodious tunes and water sounds such as a babbling brook enhance healing. The use of these sounds reduces the time-space experience of waiting and masks the noise of electronic medical technology and even voices that might otherwise be overheard. As well as reducing stress and anxiety and refreshing the minds of patients, visitors, and caregivers, such an environment emphasizes the facility's focus on compassion and caring. Figure 10-7 shows water cascading quietly down a wall.

Color can do much to establish a comfortable environment. Greens and blues are good in areas that require quiet and extended concentration. Cool colors cause individuals to underestimate time and make heavier items seem lighter, objects smaller, and rooms larger. Warm colors with high illumination cause increased alertness and an outward orientation. The elderly adult may

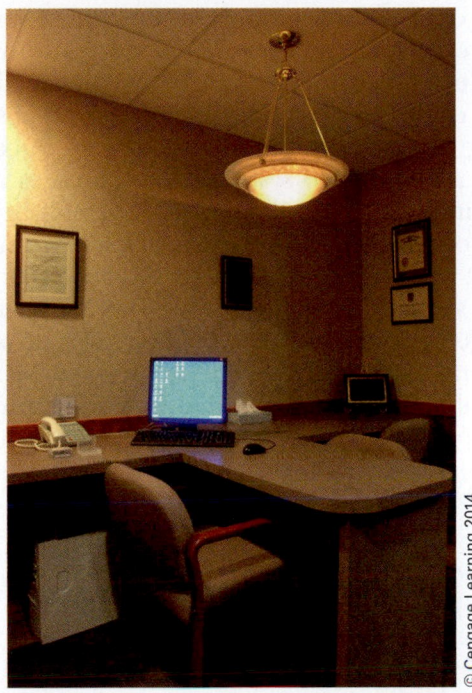

Figure 10-6   Small conference area adjacent to the receptionist area where issues such as insurance coverage, financial arrangements, and surgical plans can be discussed.

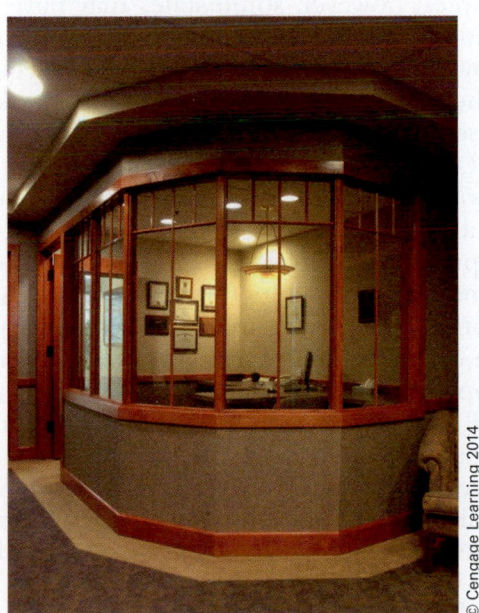

Figure 10-5   Receptionist work space, with favorable lighting, that provides privacy from conversations while offering a view of the entire reception area.

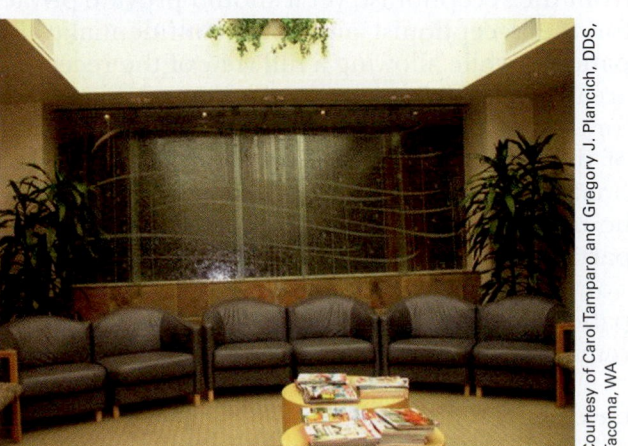

Figure 10-7   Reception area with cascading waterfall on the wall behind chairs. The environment is peaceful and calming.

have difficulty distinguishing pastels because of failing eyesight. Strongly contrasting patterns and extremely bright colors can be overwhelming and even intimidating or threatening to elder adults. Design specialists can assist in color choices that are appropriate in medical facilities.

Noise Reduction

Research has shown that patients and their families are more comfortable in surroundings that provide a quiet withdrawal from the hectic pace of the outside world. The use of sound–absorbing ceiling tiles and surfaces will help reduce clinic noise. A telephone system that produces a pleasing chime is preferred to the traditional shrill ring. Staff voices that are muted and pleasant are preferred; loud laughter and teasing are to be kept to the staff room and out of the hearing range of patients. Also appreciated are appropriate and current magazines and plants or pictures of nature. The fabric and texture of draperies, upholstery, and carpet should be pleasing, comfortable, and easy to maintain as well as assist in noise reduction.

LEGAL COMPLIANCE IN THE FACILITY

HIPAA

It is necessary to ensure HIPAA compliance for protecting patient information and privacy. With this in mind, HIPAA mandates certain building features. A reception window or desk should not make the patient feel closed off from the receptionist, yet it should provide privacy for the receptionist and total confidentiality for patients, while allowing a full view of the reception area. Figure 10-5 shows an efficient working space for the receptionist while still allowing visualization of the entire reception area. Figure 10-6 shows a small conference area in the same space that can be used when issues of privacy with a patient are particularly important. This space allows for discussion about insurance coverage, billing solutions, or patient education; voices cannot be heard in the remainder of the reception area.

To ensure HIPAA compliance, some clinics have the receptionist greet patients on their arrival and then direct them to a more private area where they are checked in, their insurance or payment plan is verified, and follow-up appointments are made. The telephones are located in this more private area so conversations with callers cannot be overheard in the reception area.

In the examination room, privacy is especially important to patients. Remember that privacy implies that the patient's conversation cannot be overheard in any other part of the facility. Studies have shown that when patients fear their voices can be overheard by others nearby, they will not respond to questioning as honestly as they would if their privacy is assured. In the examination room, provide space for patients to hang their clothes and undergarments out of view. Always ask if a patient needs help in disrobing, and always knock before entering a room. A mirror is especially helpful for dressing after the examination.

Americans with Disabilities Act

Accessibility, or making facilities and equipment available to all users, is a major consideration when creating the health care environment. The Americans with Disabilities Act (ADA) was passed by the U.S. Congress in 1990. The purpose of this act is to provide a clear and comprehensive national mandate to end discrimination against individuals with disabilities and to bring them into the economic and social mainstream of life. In addition to accessibility regulations identified in Titles II, III, and IV, this act also provides employment protection for persons with disabilities (Title I). ADA applies to businesses with 15 or more employees; however, some states may have stricter legislation applying to businesses of only 8 or more employees. Even before ADA became legislation, most health care facilities attempted to make their premises barrier free and accessible to patients with special needs. Although many ambulatory care settings will have less than 8–15 employees, accessibility for all patients in all settings is important.

A professional designer not only can make suggestions regarding color, artwork, and the general environment of the clinic, but also can provide advice on how the facility can be made accessible to people who are physically challenged. For example, all doors and hallways must accommodate a wheelchair. Likewise, a bathroom must accommodate individuals with special needs. Signage in Braille assists patients with visual disabilities (Figure 10-8). Elevators must be provided if the facility is on more than one level.

At least one accessible entrance must comply with ADA. It should be protected from the weather by a canopy or overhanging roof. Such entrances are to incorporate an accessible passenger loading

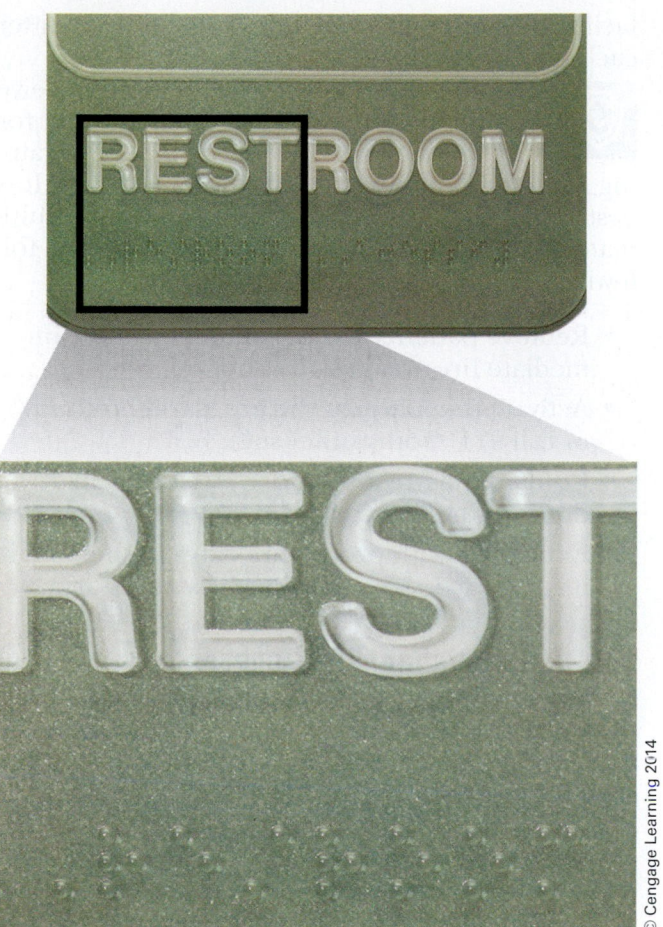

Figure 10-08   A Braille plate allows a blind patient to identify where the bathroom is located.

zone. Ten percent of the total number of parking spaces at outpatient facilities must be accessible. (Visit the ADA Web site at http://www.ada.gov for more information.) Be mindful of patients whose impairments are not obvious—for example, individuals with impaired hearing or vision and individuals whose disability (temporary or permanent) may prevent them from doing certain physical activities.

SAFETY

Safety will always be paramount in any medical environment. Responsibility for a patient's safety begins the instant a patient enters the facility. Every staff member must be alert to any safety issue and be ready to offer assistance to patients at any time. Hazards are to be reported to a supervisor or provider in order to prevent or correct the hazard. On a regular basis, a safety inspection should be made of all areas of the facility. It is often best if one person is in charge of the inspection; some large clinics will have a designated

safety officer. Even the smallest of clinics can maintain a checklist of safety features to be inspected on a regular basis. There are safety references throughout this text identified by the safety icon.

Creating a Safe Environment

Strict adherence to building ADA compliance identified earlier will greatly enhance a safe environment. Keep in mind that all areas must accommodate a wheelchair and provide for persons with special needs. Large multiclinic facilities often have attendants greet patients who arrive and need wheelchair assistance from their car to inside the facility. Other facilities provide parking attendants so that patients are not dropped off and left unattended while a family member parks the car.

In the facility itself, exit signs must be clearly indicated and easily seen. All restrooms should have safety bars and a pull cord that calls for special assistance when needed. The surface of all floors should be nonslippery, and all spills should be promptly cleaned and dried. A multiple-floor facility will need procedures for moving patients from one area to another or to the lower levels when elevators cannot be used. A regular inspection will look for any frayed or loose wires on equipment and uneven surfaces on floors or carpets so that immediate correction can be made.

Evacuation Procedures

Carefully identified procedures for evacuation are essential. Fire; hazardous chemical spills; power outages; earthquake; and threats of tornado, hurricane, or flood—all are examples that might necessitate evacuation of patients and all personnel. Large multiclinic facilities will have a written protocol and individuals assigned to particular areas to assist and manage in any evacuation. Smaller clinics will rely more heavily on providers and every employee for assistance. When the threat of any disaster is known, it is best to close the clinic facility for the period of the threat. Calls can be made to cancel appointments, and patients already in the facility may be directed to return home or to a designated public space prior to the event. When there is no advance warning, as in the case of earthquake or fire, clearly identified evacuation procedures are necessary.

Any necessary evacuation must include a check of every examination room, restroom, and procedure area. A wayfinding system should include

© Cengage Learning 2014

easy-to-understand signs and numbers with clear directions to the exits. Special consideration is given to patients who need assistance or are in wheelchairs. Employees have the responsibility to assist patients and not leave the facility themselves until patients are safe. Any procedures that are underway, even minor surgery, must be stopped as soon as possible to facilitate the evacuation. It is important to turn off any oxygen or compressed gas systems. Never use elevators in a multistory building evacuation; always use the stairs. Close the door when an area is vacated.

Emergency Codes. There are some common emergency codes that can be helpful to understand. They are used primarily in hospitals and large ambulatory medical centers, but are applicable to any medical facility. A few are identified as follows:

- *Code Red.* Fire emergency: Protect patients and staff from fire; it may be necessary to leave the facility.
- *Code Blue.* Adult medical emergency: Specialized personnel respond with necessary equipment.
- *Code Pink.* Infant/child abduction: Protect children and infants; block entrance and exit; notify authorities.
- *Code Gray.* Combative individual/assault: Respond to area; protect patients; notify authorities if necessary.
- *Code Green.* Bomb threat: Notify authorities of suspicious package; evacuate the building if advised.
- *Code Yellow.* Hazardous material spill: Identify unsafe exposure; safely evacuate area and protect others from exposure.
- *Code White.* Evacuation necessary: Move everyone out of the facility as quickly as possible.

Fire Safety

When there is a fire, evacuation must be considered unless the fire is quickly contained without threat to others. All employees must know where fire alarms are located and how they are activated; this is also true of fire extinguishers. Fire hazard has been decreased a great deal in medical facilities through the ban of smoking and smoking materials. Cracked or split electrical cords or plugs should be replaced, and electrical outlets should never be overloaded. If laundry is done within the

facility, emptying the lint filter on the dryer after each use is a must.

 Periodically, all personnel should receive training on the use of a fire extinguisher for a small fire (see Procedure 10-2) and training for a planned evacuation when necessary. It is best remembered that fire prevention is the ultimate goal. However, if there is a fire, take the following emergency actions (**RACE**):

- **Remove** patients and personnel from the immediate fire area if safe to do so.
- Activate the **Alarm** at the fire alarm box and/or call 911. Notify other staff.
- **Contain** the fire and smoke by closing all doors to the fire area.
- **Extinguish** with proper fire extinguisher *only* if it is safe to do so, or **Evacuate** as necessary.

Fire Extinguisher Safety. Remember that all fire extinguishers should be checked periodically, usually monthly, to make certain pressure is at the appropriate level according to the manufacturer's suggestions. An extinguisher should be readily visible and not blocked by any furniture or doors. Make certain hoses and nozzles are free of insects or debris. The outside of the extinguisher should be clean and free of any oil or grease as well as any dents or signs of damage. Dry chemical extinguishers may need to be shaken monthly to prevent the powder from settling or packing. Pressure test the extinguisher periodically to ensure the cylinder is safe to use. Replace an extinguisher immediately after use. Local fire department personnel also check extinguishers and will do so in their regular facility inspections.

Response to Natural Disaster or Emergency

 Disaster can strike quickly and without warning causing evacuation of a home or any building. It can also confine you to a building or home. Knowing what to do and being prepared is the best protection and is your responsibility (see Procedure 10-1). A very valuable resource can be found at http://www.ready.gov/are-you-ready-guide. Prepared by the federal government, this website will direct you to a number of publications following the theme "Are you Ready" that are free to download. The following hazards are covered: floods, tornadoes, hurricanes, thunderstorms, and lightning; winter storms and

USE OF A FIRE EXTINGUISHER

1. **Call for help before extinguishing a fire.** A fire can quickly spread to dangerous levels. The typical extinguisher should never be used on anything but small contained fires that have just started. Remember that all fires produce smoke and carbon monoxide. Some fires also produce toxic gases that often form from burning nylon in carpeting, foam padding, etc. and can be fatal.

2. **Are you strong enough to extinguish a fire?** Some personnel will find any commercial extinguisher too heavy to handle or have difficulty exerting enough pressure to operate it.

3. **Check for a clear exit for escape prior to using the extinguisher.** If the exit is at all threatened, leave immediately.

4. **Know which type of fire extinguisher to use.** The most common classes of extinguishers are often characterized by the class of fire—A, B, or C—or the extinguisher type—APW, Carbon Dioxide, or Dry Chemical.

   - **APW.** APW (air-pressured water) extinguisher has silver casing; suitable for Class A fires of cloth, wood, or paper. Weighs about 25 lbs. and is 2 ft. tall.

   - **Carbon dioxide.** CO_2 extinguisher is filled with pressurized nonflammable CO_2 gas. Has red casing and a horn or spout; suitable for flammable liquid (Class B) and electrical fires (Class C). Should not be used on Class A fires. Weight and size vary.

   - **Dry chemical.** Mainly filled with monoammonium phosphate powder, pressurized by nitrogen. Also known as a DC fire extinguisher; used either for Class B and C fires or for Class A, B, and C fires, and will be labeled as such. Has red casing and can weigh between 5 and 20 lbs. The dry chemical fire extinguisher appropriate for Class A, B, and C fires is the most likely choice for the ambulatory care facility.

5. **Ready the extinguisher.**
   - Break the seal and pull the safety pin or metal ring from the handle.
   - Squeeze the lever to discharge the fire extinguishing agent.
   - Aim for the base of the fire and sweep back and forth.

6. **Remember: P.A.S.S to help you use the extinguisher properly: Pull, Aim, Squeeze, Sweep.**

Refer to OSHA's website on evacuation plans and procedures; see "Extinguisher Basics" at http://www.osha.gov/SLTC/etools/evacuation/portable_about.html#Types for pictures, diagrams, and more detail.

---

extreme cold; extreme heat; earthquakes, volcanoes, landslides, and debris flows (mudslides); tsunamis; fires and wildfires; hazardous materials incidents and household chemical emergencies; nuclear power plant and terrorism (including explosion, biological, chemical, and nuclear and radiological hazards). While it is not the purpose of this chapter to detail responses to each of these disasters, there are some simple guidelines to keep in mind.

Every emergency plan will include information on what to do if there is no access to food, water, or electricity for some time. Most of these plans suggest creating kits to last, if necessary, for as long as two weeks but certainly never less than for 3 days. Kits can be assembled in storage bins or some other sturdy container, but should be readily accessible and regularly updated. Go to http://emergency.cdc.gov/preparedness/kit/disasters/ or http://www.redcross.org for a detailed list of supplies. Kits should be available for use at home, in a vehicle, and at a place of work.

In a disaster emergency it is important to pick two places for family members to meet, perhaps right outside the home or at a particular spot in the neighborhood. Decide how you will communicate with and reach others, especially family members you might be separated from during a disaster. Ask an out-of-town relative or friend to be your "family contact." It is often easier to make a long distance call than a local call. Know the location of your nearest shelter should you be required to evacuate. Make emergency phone numbers readily available

CRITICAL THINKING

Visit the websites indicated in this section to identify what you need to establish a disaster plan. What will you need to purchase for your supply kit for your home or car? What will be readily available to you or easy to supply? Identify special supplies you may want for any additional needs such as medications, pets, etc. Estimate the cost of any purchases as well as any other action to be taken in a safety plan.

to everyone. Teach everyone how to turn off the water, gas, and electricity. Keep necessary tools near gas and water shut-off valves. These safety tips are applicable to your workplace, too.

Sadly, the majority of households or places of employment do not have disaster kits. Mostly this is because it takes a serious warning of a disaster or the experience of a disaster before individuals make the effort to prepare.

The Medical Assistant's Response to Disaster Preparedness

Because medical assistants are individuals with both administrative and clinical education, experience, and training and are able to perform emergency first aid and CPR, they can be very valuable to a community in a time of need. Individuals who respond to emergencies must not only have the skills necessary to attend to those in need, they must also be able to curb the stress they are likely to feel in order to function in a calm, yet "take control" manner. Anyone who responds in an emergency also is to be reminded of the "fallout" or "letdown" that follows a period of severe stress and/or intense care management. That is the time to have some rest to allow the body to function in a less stressful mode.

OPENING THE FACILITY

When the facility is opened in the morning, everything should be in readiness. The receptionist or administrative medical assistant, who arrives at least 20 minutes before the first patient, will make a visual check of each room to be certain it is prepared and ready for the day.

Rooms should be of a comfortable temperature, well organized, pleasantly illuminated, and spotless. The clinical medical assistant will check all necessary supplies and equipment for readiness. At all times, patient comfort and safety should be paramount.

A schedule of the day's activities is printed for all personnel in the facility. It includes patients to be seen by the providers, meetings to be held that day, and any other information important in keeping the day's schedule running smoothly. As cancellations, no shows, or added appointments are made, they can be added to the schedule. This schedule can be posted in a place where staff can view it quickly, but it should never be visible to any patient. Patient charts for the day should be retrieved if not done so the prior evening. Facilities whose records are all electronic will sometimes print the latest laboratory results and information from the most recent visit to the facility for the provider to refer to when seeing the patient. The patient's information, whether paper or electronic, should be checked to make certain all information is up-to-date and accurate. The administrative medical assistant will check the answering service or machine for any telephone messages and follow up as necessary.

An effective way to check a room's readiness is to imagine yourself in the room as a patient. Ask yourself how you feel about being there, what mood the surroundings create for you, and whether you would feel welcome and comfortable as a patient.

CLOSING THE FACILITY

At the close of the day, each room should be checked to make certain all equipment is shut down and doors and windows are secured. Be sure that all materials of a sensitive nature are under lock and key. The preferred method of record storage is a lateral file cabinet with doors that can be closed and locked to ensure patient confidentiality. Any drugs identified in the Controlled Substances Act list of narcotics and non-narcotics must be in a locked and secure cabinet and should also be checked when leaving the clinic. Petty cash kept on the premises must be locked in a safe container. It is best to put each room and area in readiness for the next day. The day's receipts, plus a bank deposit slip, should be taken to the bank to be deposited or locked in a safe for a later deposit.

Local law enforcement officers can advise you on appropriate indoor and outdoor lighting, as well as any other security measures to make both during and after business hours.

Always contact the answering service to notify them that the clinic is closed and where and how the medical staff can be reached in an emergency.

THE FUTURE ENVIRONMENT FOR AMBULATORY CARE

One prediction seems certain for the future of the ambulatory care facilities environment: The number of patients 85 years or older—who are most likely to require medical care for multiple chronic conditions—will greatly increase in the next few years. It is predicted that by 2020, almost 40% of a provider's time will be spent treating members of the population who are aging. The federal government struggles with Medicare's reimbursement policies, which do not adequately cover most costs incurred by providers to care for the elderly population. Ambulatory care centers will continue to struggle to provide facilities and services with environments conducive to the needs of this population.

The number of primary care providers willing to take new patients 65 years and older must increase. Patients will need to access their provider via convenient public transportation, take care of as many of their needs as possible in 1 day, and have prescriptions filled before returning home. The elderly population will need to navigate a wheelchair easily down corridors, into examination rooms, and into laboratories for assessment. Providers can be expected to spend additional time with elderly adults who will ask many questions and will be quite knowledgeable of their medical needs.

Members of the elderly adult's family will have an increasing presence in the care of their parents. Providers will want to give patients the opportunity for family members of their choosing to have access to their health information. HIPAA requires providers to have patients sign a release so that their family members can be kept informed. Providers can expect family members of patients to want the very best for their loved ones, both medically and environmentally.

Discussions with elderly adults regarding their health care experiences reveal that their greatest frustration comes from the lack of clarity of instructions given by *all* health professionals ranging from the administrative medical assistant to the primary provider. The

most successful approaches to solving this dilemma include:

1. Providing clear and concise written instructions whenever possible in easy-to-read print.
2. Creating an environment where ease of movement from one department to another is not confusing.
3. Making certain all patients fully understand their prescription instructions, directions, and orders for additional tests.
4. Identifying for patients under what circumstances to report back to their primary provider for follow-up.

The goal of a medical facility and its staff should be not only to welcome and receive patients with a "we care for you" attitude, but also to have patients leave the facility and staff with a sense of satisfaction for the care received. As higher efficiency is demanded of providers and their staff members in order to reduce medical costs, thoughtful and attentive personalized care must not be forsaken.

The American Medical Association (AMA) predicts that within 5 years, about 50% of providers will treat patients through online methods (see Chapter 12). Electronic mail (email) communication between patients and providers is now commonplace in many areas; however, patients are asked to give written permission for the transmission of information via email because privacy cannot always be guaranteed.

At the same time, medical providers work diligently to decrease the number of medical errors made, and advancing technology creates new patterns of health care. Also, patients are becoming astute consumers. These new consumers are better educated; they seek value and are comparison shoppers. They know that managed care has its limitations, and that providers can be wrong. These patients believe they know their own bodies better than anyone, and that quality of life is important. They know, too, that cost containment and the complexities of the health care system leave them vulnerable to medical difficulties if they do not take responsibility for themselves and their medical care.

Today's patients are exposed to numerous Internet sites and magazine articles that provide medical information to them 24 hours a day, 7 days a week. These patients arrive at their appointments with the ability to discuss potential diagnoses and treatment plans. Hopefully, the health care team welcomes this new partnership, even if health care professionals have to assist patients in weeding out some of the invalid medical information available.

PROCEDURE 10-1

Develop a Personal and/or Employee Safety Plan in Case of a Disaster

PURPOSE:

To develop a plan of action in case of a disaster that promotes personal safety and can also be applied to both employees and patients in ambulatory care.

EQUIPMENT/SUPPLIES:

Computer
Clear plastic protector envelope for plan

PROCEDURE STEPS:

1. *Be proactive* by reviewing state and local recommendations for emergency preparedness. *Pay attention to detail*. RATIONALE: Some areas of the country are prone to particular natural disasters such as floods, tornados, or hurricanes. Your plan should be pertinent to your geographical area.

2. *Show initiative* by gathering family members or other employees together to discuss a disaster plan. RATIONALE: When those close to you are involved in the process, they are more likely to participate in the activity and understand the importance of the actions to be taken.

3. List supplies necessary for your supply kit. Be certain to include any special needs required in your supplies. Allow each person 1 personal item for the kit. Plan your needs for a minimum of 48 hours. RATIONALE: A detailed list of the supply kit items reminds you of what you will need to purchase, when items will expire or lose their usefulness, and what one item is most important to each individual.

4. Plan for evacuation. Where are the exits? Identify the safest route for exit. List the steps to take prior to evacuation. RATIONALE: Planning ahead makes it easier to function in the time of great stress. Who will be responsible for picking up the supply kit? A first aid kit? Who will turn off electricity, gas, water?

5. Determine a communication or contact plan to follow should you be separated from others during the disaster. Where will you meet? Name a "neutral" person or friend in another location who can be a telephone contact. RATIONALE: Following any disaster, the first concern is always for the well-being of your loved ones and those closest to you. Knowing how to reach one another will reduce this stress.

6. Schedule updates to the personal safety plan at least every quarter, *developing strategic plans to achieve your goals*. RATIONALE: This time frame allows for changes that may be necessary in the supply kit, reinforcing the safety protocol you have devised, and the ability to make any other changes necessary.

7. Make certain everyone has a copy of the plan. Post a copy of your plan in a prominent place where it is noticed regularly. RATIONALE: Unless everyone has a copy of the plan and it is posted where everyone is continually reminded, the plan loses its effectiveness.

PROCEDURE 10-2

Demonstrate Proper Use of a Fire Extinguisher

PURPOSE:

To demonstrate the ability to operate a fire extinguisher or help another person operate the extinguisher and to describe the precise steps to take to prevent errors and delay in operation.

EQUIPMENT/SUPPLIES:

Fire extinguisher

PROCEDURE STEPS:

1. Determine the type of fire extinguisher(s) on the premises. RATIONALE: The type of extinguisher will determine the kind of fires it may be able to control.

2. Examine the cylinder and carefully read any instructions supplied from the manufacturer, *paying attention to detail*. RATIONALE: This gives a brief review of how to operate the equipment and tell you what kind of fires to use it on.

Procedure 10-2 (continued)

3. Determine if you are able to handle the weight of the extinguisher, *asking for assistance if you are unable to carry out the task*. RATIONALE: This will tell you if you can move forward or will have to ask another to manage the extinguisher.

4. If a fire is present, *be proactive* by calling 911 before you discharge the extinguisher. RATIONALE: You cannot tell how quickly a fire may be out of your control.

5. Check your nearest exit. If it is blocked, *display sound judgment* by evacuating without discharging the extinguisher. RATIONALE: Trying to fight a fire that threatens a safe exit is dangerous and can cost a life.

6. Break the seal and turn and pull the safety pin from the handle. RATIONALE: This step is necessary before you are able use the extinguisher as it unlocks the mechanism.

7. Aim the nozzle or hose at the base of the fire and squeeze the lever to discharge the extinguishing agent. RATIONALE: The base of the fire is its source and it is vital to stop the fire at the source.

8. Standing several feel back from the fire, sweep side to side to put out the flames. RATIONALE: A side to side motion helps to put out the fire.

9. If the fire does not respond after you have used up the fire extinguisher, *remain calm* and remove yourself to safety immediately. RATIONALE: Do not take a chance in being caught in a fire; allow the professionals to put the fire out.

10. If the area fills with smoke, *remain calm* and leave immediately. RATIONALE: Smoke can be more deadly that the fire and is often very toxic.

11. Replace the depleted fire extinguisher immediately. Never leave an empty extinguisher where someone might believe it is ready for use. RATIONALE: A fire extinguisher that is fully operational and ready for use is the only kind to have in any facility.

CASE STUDY 10-1

Refer to the scenario at the beginning of the chapter.

CASE STUDY REVIEW

1. What is your first reaction to the environment in the medical facility described? Justify your response.

2. List as many solutions as you can to address the lack of privacy and confidentiality in the reception area. Begin with simple solutions and then move to the more complex ideas that surface in your planning.

3. How do you think patients will be affected by each of your solutions?

4. What other improvements might be considered in the updating of the clinic?

CASE STUDY 10-2

The eighth-floor orthopedic surgery department in a large metropolitan clinic has an interesting approach to patient dynamics. Providers and their assistants see patients for diagnosis and preparation for surgery. Patients likely are seen in this department three to five times before and after their procedures. The staff involves their patients to relieve any anxiety they might have.

Addison Burton approaches the reception desk; he is immediately greeted and asked to wait a moment until the administrative medical assistant clears a previous patient. There is a huge box filled with slightly used tennis shoes that patients and staff are collecting for needy children and the homeless. Addison remembers he has a couple of pairs at home he could bring. After checking in, he is directed to a counter where coffee, tea, and water are available, as well as the daily newspapers. Addison can take a seat in a chair, on a couch at a window

that allows him to put his feet and legs up, or at a table with chairs. The window seat gives a view of the city and a terrace garden four floors below. At the table there is an unusual puzzle being put together, and Addison takes a seat there. He is able to put four to five puzzle pieces together before being called for his appointment.

CASE STUDY REVIEW

1. When Jorja Anderson, CMA (AAMA), calls Mr. Burton to the examination room, what might the conversation be? Would this conversation help to dispel anxiety?

2. When the surgeon sees Mr. Burton for his hip problem, everyone has a good laugh—on the bottom of Addison's shoe is a puzzle piece. What kind of mood has been established for this visit?

CASE STUDY 10-3

Even though she appears collected on the outside, Abigail Johnson, who is about 75 years old, is quite nervous about having her annual physical. Clinical medical assistant Audrey Jones senses her patient's underlying tension and wants to do what she can to help Abigail relax. She knows that this patient has hypertension, suffers from occasional dizziness, and says she feels guilty about going off the diet that was designed to help manage both her high blood pressure and her diabetes. At this moment, Audrey is helping Abigail get ready to see Dr. King, her provider. She does not want to intrude on her patient's privacy but does want her to relax a bit.

CASE STUDY REVIEW

1. What are some of the actions Audrey can take to ensure her patient's privacy?

2. In what ways can the physical environment itself become a calming influence for Abigail?

3. How will Audrey's sympathetic attitude affect her patient?

SUMMARY

Keep in mind that the environment in which patient care is given must promote health rather than aggravate illness and feed anxiety. Evidence-based design will help create environments that provide effective, safe, and caring-centered facilities. The environment must be clean, fresh, cheerful, safe, and nonthreatening, with contemporary furnishings, appropriate colors, proper lighting, and soothing textures.

Even if patients are not consciously aware of the message they are getting from the clinic design and environment, they are subconsciously receiving it. The clinic environment reveals things that might subconsciously undermine a patient's confidence in the provider and the health care team.

Safety preparedness may not be obvious to patients, but its importance cannot be minimized. Every space in the facility with its appointed purpose must be designed and maintained to protect patient and employee safety, and every employee must be safety conscious every moment of the day.

STUDY FOR SUCCESS

To reinforce your knowledge and skills of information presented in this chapter:

- Review the *Key Terms*
- Role-play with other students to apply attributes of professionalism pertinent to this chapter.
- Consider the *Case Studies* and discuss your conclusions
- Answer the questions in the *Certification Review*
- Apply your knowledge by completing the *Activities* in the *Study Guide* and the *Games and Quizzes* in the StudyWARE **StudyWARE** software on the *Premium Website*
- Perform the *Procedures* using the *Competency Assessment Checklists* in the *Competency Manual*
- Practice your problem-solving skills with the *Critical Thinking Challenge 3.0* on the *Premium Website*

Additional resources for this chapter include:

- Modules 11 and 12 of the *Medical Assisting Learning Lab*
- *CourseMate for Delmar's Comprehensive Medical Assisting*
- *WebTutor for Delmar's Comprehensive Medical Assisting*

CERTIFICATION REVIEW

1. Which of the following is appropriate for the reception area of an ambulatory care setting?
   a. heavily scented flowers
   b. medical journals with graphic colored pictures
   c. dim lighting
   d. live or silk plants
2. One of the goals in treating patients is:
   a. to give them as much control as possible
   b. to treat them as quickly as possible
   c. to disregard their desire for privacy
   d. to be sure they arrive on time for their appointment
3. One design element to avoid in a medical clinic is:
   a. a mirror for dressing
   b. the colors green and blue
   c. extremely bright, contrasting patterns
   d. accessories and artwork
4. The ADA is mostly concerned with:
   a. segregating individuals according to type of disability
   b. providing access and opportunity for individuals with physical challenges
   c. only the work environment
   d. getting economic benefits for people with physical challenges

5. In any medical facility, the receptionist's KEY responsibility is to:
   a. not keep the provider waiting
   b. make sure all plants are watered
   c. greet patients in a friendly, warm manner
   d. be efficient, even if it means ignoring patient requests
6. Making a visual check of each examination room is a function of:
   a. weekly housekeeping
   b. opening the clinic
   c. closing the clinic
   d. b and c
7. Space planners recommend the following for the reception area:
   a. three to four seats for each examination room
   b. seats to accommodate 1.5 hours of patients
   c. 2.5 seats for each examination room
   d. not bringing family members to appointments
8. ADA requires that _____ of the total number of parking spaces in outpatient facilities be reserved for individuals with disabilities.
   a. 5%
   b. 10%
   c. 12%
   d. 7%

9. The medical environment will be challenged in the future by:
   a. increasing numbers of pediatric patients
   b. increasing numbers of elderly patients
   c. decreasing numbers of hospital patients
   d. decreasing government compliance

10. Safety in a medical facility may include:
    a. working fire extinguishers
    b. an evacuation plan
    c. an emergency supply kit
    d. all the above

REFERENCES/BIBLIOGRAPHY

Azoulay, R. (2009). *Music, the breath and health: Advances in integrative music therapy.* (1st ed.). New York: Satchnote Press.

Cama, R. (2009). *Evidence-based healthcare design* (1st ed.). New York: John Wiley & Sons.

Centers for Disease Control and Prevention. (n.d.). Emergency Preparedness and Response. Retrieved May 17, 2012, from http://emergency.cdc.gov/preparedness/kit/disasters/

Center for Universal Design and The North Carolina Office on Disability and Health (n.d.). Removing barriers to health care: A guide for health professionals. Retrieved August 17, 2011, from http://www.fpg.unc.edu/~NCODH/RBar/

Glaser, G. (2007, June 3). Zenlike comfort in the dentist's chair. *The Sunday Oregonian,* D1, D3.

Palmer, L. D. (2005). The soundtrack of healing. *Spirituality & Health,* March/April 2005, 42–47.

U.S. Department of Labor, Occupational Safety and Health Administration. (n.d.). Evacuation Plans and Procedures. Retrieved May 21, 2012, from http://www.osha.gov/SLTC/etools/evacuation/evac.html

Ulrich, R., & Zimring, C. (2004). *The role of the physical environment in the hospital of the 21st century: A once-in-a-lifetime opportunity.* (Report to the Center for Health Design for the Designing the 21st Century Hospital Project.) Concord, CA: The Center for Health Design.

CHAPTER 11

Computers in the Ambulatory Care Setting

OUTLINE

The Computer System
  Basic System
  Types of Computer Systems
Components of a Computer System
  Hardware
  Software
  Documentation
  Hardware and Software Compatibility
  Computer Networks
  Systems Security
Cloud Computing

Computer Maintenance by Clinic Personnel
Use of Computers in the Medical Clinic
  General Office Procedures
  Electronic Health Records
  Clinical and Laboratory Applications
  Portable Computers in the Medical Office
Design Considerations for a Computerized Medical Clinic
  Software Selection

Hardware Selection
Scheduling the Changeover
Ergonomics
  Eyestrain
  Cumulative Trauma Disorder
  Posture
Patient Confidentiality in the Computerized Medical Clinic
HIPAA Standards for Safeguarding Protected Health Information (PHI)
Professionalism in the Computerized Medical Clinic

LEARNING OUTCOMES

1. Define, spell, and pronounce the key terms as presented in the glossary.
2. Describe the four fundamental elements of a computer system.
3. Identify the four main types of computers.
4. List four input devices and describe the function of each.
5. List three examples of data output devices.
6. Explain how storage devices might be used in ambulatory care settings.
7. Discuss the use of a flash drive and a tape drive and describe how each might be used in ambulatory care settings.
8. Explain the difference between system and application software.
9. Discuss the importance of computer system documentation and how it is upgraded.
10. Describe networking of computers and its purpose.
11. Differentiate the various network and connectivity technologies.
12. Understand the principles and techniques of promoting network and computer security.
13. Discuss design considerations when computerizing a medical clinic.
14. Discuss applications of electronic technology in effective communication.
15. Discuss principles of using electronic medical records (EMR).
16. Discuss the importance of routine maintenance of clinic equipment.
17. Explain why ergonomics is important and recall at least five guidelines for setting up a computer workstation.
18. Discuss patient confidentiality and guidelines for maintaining confidentiality while keeping in mind HIPAA requirements.
19. Analyze the professionalism questions and apply them to this chapter's content.

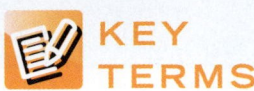

KEY TERMS

application software

apps

back up

central processing unit (CPU)

cloud computing

defragmentation

electronic health record (EHR)

electronic medical record (EMR)

ergonomics

Ethernet

firewall

flash drive

hardware hard drive

input device

Internet

license

man-in-the-middle attack

memory

network interface

networking

operating system (OS)

output device

patch

phishing

random access memory (RAM)

server

Service Sockets Layer (SSL)

smartphones

software

surge protection

system software

total practice management system (TPMS)

Universal Serial Bus (USB) port

WiFi connection

WiMAX

ATTRIBUTES OF PROFESSIONALISM

Competency

- Did you pay attention to detail?
- Did you ask questions if you were out of your comfort zone or did not have the experience to carry out tasks?
- Did you display sound judgment?
- Were you knowledgeable and accountable?
- Did you recognize the importance of local, state, and federal legislation and regulations in the practice setting?
- Did you practice risk management principles?
- Did you follow necessary safety precautions?

Initiative

- Did you develop a strategic plan to achieve your goals? Was your plan realistic?
- Did you seek out opportunities to expand your knowledge base?
- Did you implement time management principles to maintain effective office function?
- Did you assist coworkers when appropriate?

Integrity

- Did you work within your scope of practice?
- Did you acknowledge the scope of practice of other health care professionals?
- Did you demonstrate sensitivity to patients' rights?
- Did you protect personal boundaries?
- Did you protect and maintain confidentiality?
- Did you immediately report any error you had made?
- Did you report situations that were harmful or illegal?
- Did you maintain your moral and ethical standards?
- Did you do "the right thing" even when no one was observing?

SCENARIO

Inner City Health Care, an urgent care center in a large urban area, recently made the transition from a manual to a computerized system. It was a long over-due change, and it required a great deal of fact-finding and research before office manager Walter Seals could convince the center's providers to purchase a network of computers for the five-provider center.

Once he persuaded his employers of the computers' potential value to the center, Walter, an administrative medical assistant, proceeded carefully to research, purchase, and install the new computer system.

INTRODUCTION

Computers have revolutionized our lives. You can order groceries, books, airline reservations, and theater tickets; make motel and car rental arrangements; register for college classes; and possibly find a romantic partner, all using the computer and what is called cyberspace. The medical clinic, hospitals, and even surgical procedures are increasingly dependent on the use of computers.

Computers are no longer a luxury in the ambulatory care setting; they are an essential and sometimes mandatory part of doing business (e.g., filing Medicare statements for service). Today, the medical assistant must be computer literate, able to quickly learn how to use new programs, and knowledgeable of computer procedures that guard against loss or compromise of confidential medical records.

THE COMPUTER SYSTEM

Basic System

All computer systems are composed of four fundamental elements (Figure 11-1):

1. *Input devices* that generate digital data used by the **central processing unit (CPU)** for processing
2. *CPU* that manipulates the data from the **input device** (i.e., addition, subtraction, multiplication, and division)
3. *Software* that instructs the CPU what operations to perform on the data from the input device and send the results to an **output device**
4. *Output devices* that display or store the results from the CPU

The details of each of these fundamental elements are highly technical and involve support systems such as power supplies, time-keeping devices, and **firewalls**, among others. The medical

assistant will, under most circumstances, not need to develop his or her knowledge beyond understanding how to operate the elements, connect them together, ensure they are compatible with other elements in a system, and perform simple maintenance.

Types of Computer Systems

Although the medical assistant will be primarily using a microcomputer system, commonly called a personal computer (PC), it is helpful to understand some of the characteristics of the four major types of computer systems.

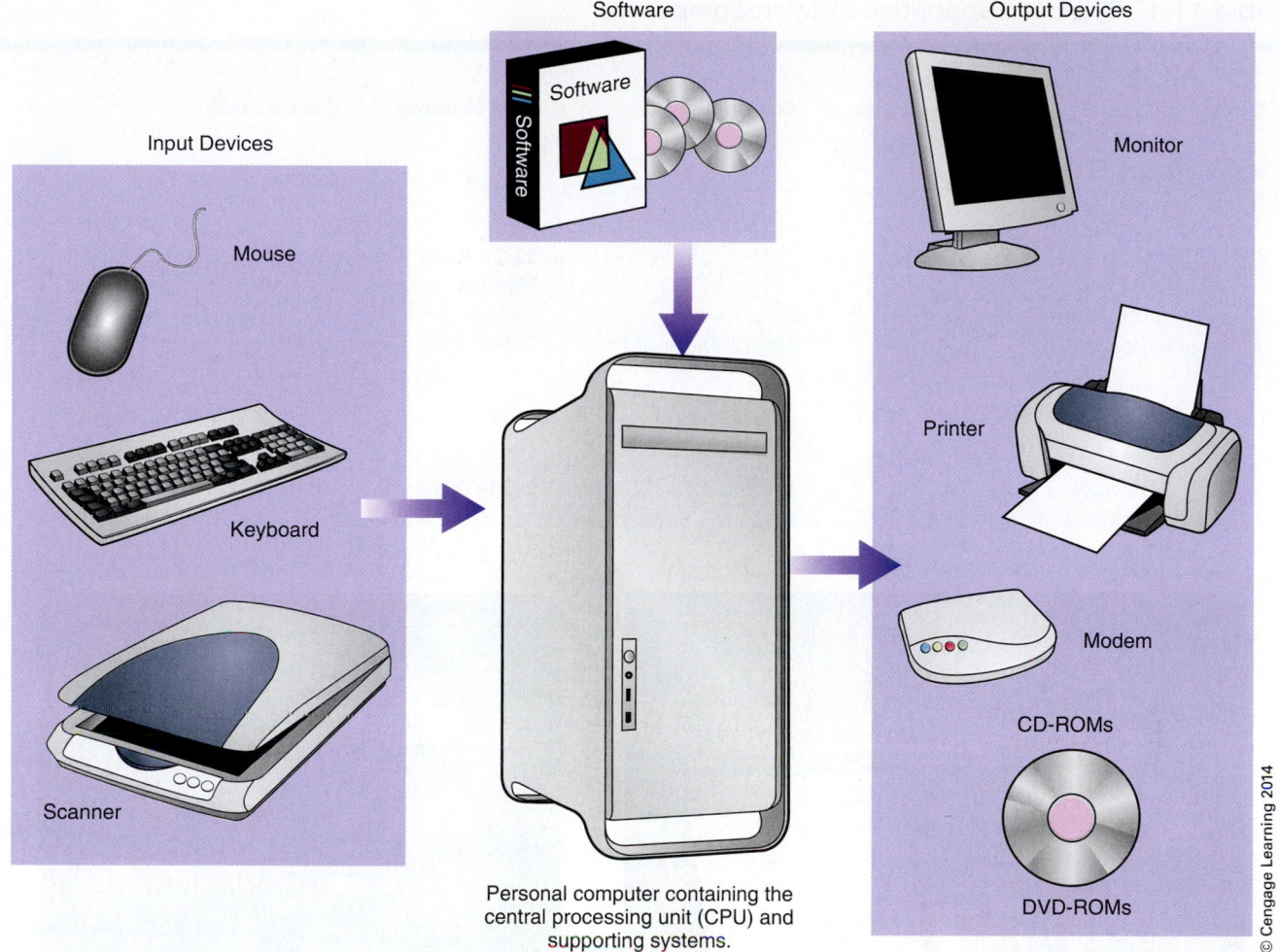

Input Devices

Mouse

Keyboard

Scanner

Software

Software

Output Devices

Monitor

Printer

Modem

CD-ROMs

DVD-ROMs

Personal computer containing the
central processing unit (CPU) and
supporting systems.

© Cengage Learning 2014

Figure 11-1   Components of a computer system.

Supercomputers, the fastest and the most powerful computers, are used in medical research. They are the most expensive and complex of computers, consisting of single computers having multiple processors or multiple computers clustered together. Supercomputer technology is still evolving but holds great promise for the advancement of sophisticated medical interventions.

Mainframe computers, the next largest in size and processing ability, are used for large volumes of repetitive calculations. With their high processing speeds, mainframes are invaluable for large governmental provider service programs such as Medicaid and Medicare.

Minicomputers, grouped between mainframes and microcomputers in terms of size, speed, and capacity, process data in health care facilities in a variety of ways, including patient account processing, insurance claim processing, and statistical analysis of research data. Minicomputers handle large amounts of processing and

challenge the capabilities of older mainframe systems.

Microcomputers are the most widely used type of computer in today's health care facility. The smallest of the four types of computers, they range in size from **smartphones**, which are basically next generation PDAs, to desktop computers often referred to as a personal computer or PC. Smartphones have wireless phone capabilities and are frequently equipped with a camera. In addition to variations in size, microcomputers vary in computing capability, memory storage, and means of communicating with other computers. Table 11-1 lists several types of microcomputers and gives some of their capabilities. Figure 11-2 illustrates variations in computer size. The medical assistant will work with computers on a daily basis performing many clerical and clinical functions. Scheduling appointments and maintaining patient financial records are examples of some of these functions. Today, with the use of an app, it is also possible to receive

Table 11-1 Typical Capabilities of Microcomputers

Computer Type	Processor Speed, GHz	Screen Size	RAM Memory	Connectivity
Personal Data Assistant (PDA)	0.3	2.0″ × 3.0″	100 MB	WiFi, Bluetooth®
Smartphone	1+	2.4″ × 4.0″	32 GB Flash Memory	WiMAX, WiFi, Bluetooth®
Tablet or Netbook	1.2–1.8	10″–12″ Diagonal	256–512 MB	WiMAX, Bluetooth®
Laptop Computer	2.1	14″–17″ Diagonal	4 GB	Ethernet, WiFi, WiMAX, Bluetooth®
Desktop Computer	3.4	Unlimited	6 GB	Ethernet, WiFi, WiMAX, Bluetooth®

© Cengage Learning 2014

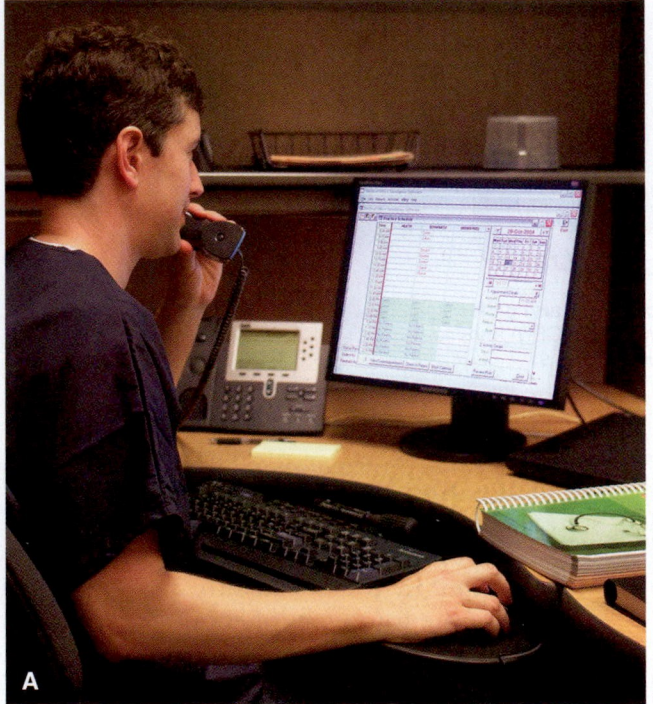
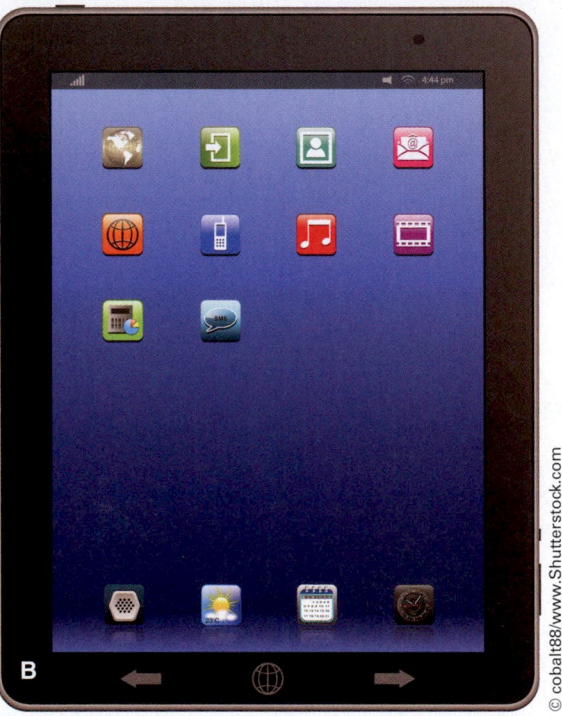

© Cengage Learning 2014

© cobalt88/www.Shutterstock.com

Figure 11-2 Microcomputers come in a variety of sizes and types. (A) Desktop personal computer. (B) Typical pad computer.

EKG and blood pressure data from a patient's smartphone to remotely monitor a patient's condition in real-time for the provider.

The medical assistant will work with the computer on a daily basis in many different ways. Microcomputers may be used in a medical practice to schedule appointments, maintain patient accounts, and process insurance claims. Hand-held micros may be used to input patient information during examination, with data downloaded to a minicomputer, server, or mainframe when it is convenient.

COMPONENTS OF A COMPUTER SYSTEM

A system is an assembly of parts that function together to perform a particular task. A computer system consists of hardware, software, and documentation of the installation.

Hardware

The components of a computer system that you can see, touch, or hear are referred to as **hardware**. Hardware consists of input devices, output devices, and the CPU, as well as some firewalls and modems.

Data Input Devices. A data input device converts analog data such as keyboard keystrokes, motion, temperature, and mouse position into a digital format understandable by the CPU, allowing it to manipulate the data in accordance with the software program. The most common examples of input devices are the keyboard and mouse. In addition to these common examples, touch screens, electronic tablets, scanners, pens, digital cameras, and many electronic clinical laboratory instruments are input devices encountered in medical settings. Input devices usually have their own software called a driver, which must be installed on the computer or provided by the **operating system (OS)** before they will function properly. Data storage devices frequently function as data input devices when raw data, which have been manipulated using the computer, are further processed using a different software program.

Central Processing Unit. The central processing unit (CPU) of a computer is the brain of the system. It carries out instructions defined by the program software on the data input and sends the result to the selected output device. The actual heart of the CPU is a silicon microchip approximately 1.5 inches square with sometimes hundreds of connections to other electronic components. The circuitry printed on the microchip contains logic algorithms for performing functions such as addition, subtraction, and multiplication.

Data Output Devices. The most common data output device is the monitor. The monitor, which looks like a television screen, allows the operator to see the output of the computer and make real-time corrections to the input. The best example of this is in word processing of documents. Printers and fax machines are other examples of output devices used to produce hard-copy output. When hard copy is not required, digital data storage devices are used. As was the case with data input devices, data output devices require a driver, either loaded when the device is installed or provided by the OS.

A modem is a form of an input/output device that alters the digital data from the computer in a manner that allows it to be transmitted over telephone lines or cable installations. A modem is required for dial-up Internet service and some cable services. Computer fax machines also require the use of a modem.

Data Storage Devices. Data storage devices are devices capable of permanently or temporarily storing digital data. Data storage device capacity is often referred to as **memory**. Together with computer speed, this area of the computer has seen the greatest improvement, with capability doubling every few years or less. Computers used by most of us today have no functional limitation for memory, with portable memory cartridges providing unlimited memory expansion. Data storage devices consist of read-only memory (ROM), **random access memory (RAM)**, and data storage memory.

ROM and RAM Memory. The computer manufacturer permanently writes data or instructions into the memory on ROM chips, which are installed directly onto the motherboard. They contain instructions for operations such as booting the computer when the power is turned on. RAM memory is also in the form of chips and is part of the motherboard. It provides the computer with registers in which to store in-process data. RAM memory is erased or "lost" when the computer is turned off or experiences a power failure. RAM memory is important to the user, in that a RAM capacity that is too small will cause the computer to run slow and sometimes will not run some software programs.

Data Storage Memory. Data storage memory is permanent and is not erased when the computer is turned off. It can be either read-only or read-write. Read-only data storage memory is used to store application programs for loading onto the computer. CDs and DVDs are commonly used for this purpose, and Internet servers are increasingly used to store downloadable application programs. The following paragraphs describe several devices for providing data storage.

Magnetic Disk Drives. Magnetic disk drives can be internal or external to the computer unit and are either permanently installed or portable and transportable.

Hard drives are storage devices that are usually installed directly into the computer cabinet that contains the CPU. A hard drive is a read-write device, and the memory is permanent unless the device experiences mechanical failure. Because of failure potential of these devices, it is considered good practice to **back up** frequently the stored data by making a copy of files on a portable data storage device. The frequency of data backup is dependent on the rate at which data are entered into the system. Original records should never be destroyed until the stored data are backed up.

Optical Drives. Two types of optical drives are used in computers: compact disks (CDs) and digital video/versatile disks (DVDs), which are sometimes referred to as digital versatile disks. Currently, Internet storage and advances in flash technology are replacing optical drives.

Compact Disk. Computer data CDs are nearly identical to music CDs commonly used in home and automobile CD players. Whereas music CDs are read-only disks, those used in most computers today have the capability for the computer not only to read a disk (CD-ROM), but to write on them (CD-R) and even erase data and rewrite new data (CD-RW). CD-ROMs are primarily used as data input devices, usually for loading digital code for computer software programs.

Digital Video/Versatile Disk. DVDs are identical to the DVDs used to view home movies. They are similar to CDs, except that the format for writing the data to DVDs is different, permitting storage of up to 26 times more data. Several formats for writing data are used at this time. It is important that the storage media, the disk, and the drive are of the same format for the system to function.

Flash Drive. **Flash drives** are solid-state memory devices with no moving parts. It is usually connected to computers using a **Universal Serial Bus (USB) port** or high-performance serial bus (IEEE 1394). The device is small and can be carried on a key chain. It may be used as a readily transportable data storage device when it is desirable to move data between computers that are not connected on a network. Some flash memory devices have sufficient capacity to replace magnetic hard drives. They are also used for system backup.

Tape Drives. Tape drives are data storage devices capable of storing large amounts of data on replaceable reels of magnetic tape, much like a tape recorder but on a larger scale. Because they are much slower than many other storage devices, they are used when time is not usually too significant, such as in backing up a computer system. The storage media cost is significantly less with this type of storage device.

Servers. **Servers** are not true data storage devices. They usually contain or are connected to massive hard drives, but in many networked systems they become the storage devices for the user workstations. Servers may be located remote from workstations or even on the Internet. When servers are used, special protocols must be used to protect confidentiality of records, which are discussed in "Patient Confidentiality in the Computerized Medical Clinic."

RAID Storage. Redundant array of independent disks (RAID) storage is not a type of storage media like optical or flash. It is a storage system that can use any of the storage media described previously. The storage devices are coupled into a redundant system to minimize loss of data should an equipment malfunction occur.

Software

Software, frequently referred to as a computer program, can be thought of as a set of instructions that a computer follows to control computer hardware and to process data. System software and application software are both required by a computer to accomplish its tasks.

System Software. System software, frequently just called the operating system, tells the computer hardware what to do and when to do it. Most modern systems operate with a graphic interface that uses graphic symbols for input to the system and is much more user friendly than systems requiring alphanumeric inputs. Microsoft Windows® and Macintosh® systems are probably the best known of the graphic interface operating systems.

Application Software. Application software performs a specific data-processing function. Word

CRITICAL THINKING

Your clinic has received legal notification requiring a list of all the software used in the practice and to show proof that all necessary licenses are current. You are successful in showing compliance, but the clinic procedures were disrupted for days in meeting this court mandate. Prepare an clinic protocol designed to ensure that all software is legal and that unauthorized persons have not installed illegal software on any clinic computers.

processing, accounting, scheduling, and insurance coding are examples of application software functions.

Drivers. Drivers are computer programs that are designed to convert data output from one device into a format compatible with another device. They are required for most input and output devices and either are supplied with the device, must be downloaded from the **Internet**, or are contained in the OS software.

Documentation

Computer system documentation consists of the manuals and documents that define how programs operate. Documentation explains how to execute specific functions and gives the specifications for specific hardware, such as the frequency of the internal clock, RAM, and hard drive available memory. Although documentation is more likely provided on an optical disk that contains the specific program, it may also be in printed format or online.

Updates to program documentation are increasingly made available on the Web site of the company providing the program, together with **patches** for glitches discovered in the basic program. The system should always be backed up prior to installing updates and patches in case they cause problems. It is recommended that this work be done when supplier technical support is available. Third-party documents defining how to use application software are becoming increasingly popular and are frequently more user-friendly than documentation from the software supplier. All documentation, including **licenses**, recovery software, and program disks that come with the computer system; add-on hardware; and software, should be maintained in a safe location for the life of the equipment and software, and then disposed of when the system or software is phased out of use.

Hardware and Software Compatibility

The hardware drivers and software of a computer system must be compatible. Many applications programs share files with the OS, and if there is a conflict with files having the same name, either the OS will not allow the applications program to load or it will not function properly. The documentation for most applications programs defines the versions of the operating system for which compatibility has been established and should always be checked before purchase of either a new applications program or a new version of the OS. Hardware driver requirements should also be checked for compatibility with the OS. The amount of RAM memory, CPU clock speed, and available drive storage space can affect whether a program will run satisfactorily.

Computer Networks

Networking is the electronic or optical connection of computers and peripheral equipment for the purpose of sharing information and resources.

Types of Networks. The most common networks encountered in the medical office are:

- Local area network (LAN)
- Wide area network (WAN)
- Internet

Both LAN and WAN are dedicated networks limited to connected computers operated by a single company, clinic, or hospital. They differ principally by the size of the geographic area covered. The LAN usually is limited to a single office or building, whereas the WAN covers a wider geographic area and may be linked by leased telephone lines, fiberoptic cables, microwave links, or even radio. Each computer in the LAN or WAN usually has its own computing power, but it can also access other devices on the network subject to the permissions it has been allowed.

The Internet is a worldwide publicly accessible network of networks and computers. It differs from a LAN or WAN not only in sheer size but also in the manner of data transmission, called *protocols*. Data transmitted on the Internet are broken into packets, which are routed over different networks to the final destination where they are reassembled for use by the client computer. If one network is inoperative the system chooses another. Data that are in transit are almost impossible to intercept, making them immune from most unauthorized users.

Connecting Networks. Connection to a network can be through either a hard-wired system or a wireless system. Hard-wired connections include standard telephone modem (dial-up), digital subscriber phone line (DSL), local area network, or through a modem using either copper wire or fiber-optic cable. Wireless connections include WiFi, Bluetooth®, satellite systems, and cellular technology.

Hard-Wired Connection. Hard-wired connections are often referred to as **Ethernet** connections. Connections can be made using a telephone line–type cable called a *crossover cable* between computers having an installed network interface controller. Most new computers have this feature. Hard-wired systems are capable of higher data transmission rates than wireless systems, but with advanced technology WiFi systems, the difference is not noticeable unless very large files are being transmitted.

WiFi Connection. **WiFi** can be used to connect computers directly or to connect a computer to the Internet. WiFi is a brand originally licensed by the Wi-Fi Alliance to describe the underlying technology of wireless local area networks (WLANs). It was developed to be used for mobile computing devices, such as laptops, but is increasingly used for more services, including Internet, voice over Internet protocol (VoIP) phone access, gaming, PDAs, and basic connectivity of consumer electronics. It has a range of about 300 feet.

Because WiFi uses radio transmission, it is vulnerable to unauthorized users eavesdropping on the transmission. Measures to deter unauthorized users include:

- Suppressing the access point's (AP's) Service Set IDentifier (SSID), which is used by the AP to tell the world that it is online
- Allowing only computers with authorized media access control (MAC) addresses to join the network
- Using various encryption standards (WAP2, WAP, WEP)

WAP2 has the most sophisticated encryption and is almost totally secure. WAP encryption is the next best alternative, and WEP is better than nothing. If the eavesdropper has the ability to change his MAC address he can potentially join the network by forging his MAC to an authorized address that he determines by listening to network activity using a scanning device.

Bluetooth® Connection. A technology called Bluetooth can be used to connect computers to a LAN. Bluetooth is the name given to a radio technology capable of transmitting signals over short distances (30-foot range). This means of connecting networks is primarily used to connect smartphones and PDAs to each other and to a host computer. Because Bluetooth is a radio technology, it is vulnerable to eavesdropping, but because of the short range it is less vulnerable than WiFi. Most systems

that are designed to hold personal data have built-in security in the form of a four or more digit alphanumeric personal identification number (PIN), much like the one used for an ATM at the local bank. Product owners should share PIN numbers only with trusted associates to ensure maintaining security.

WiMAX Connection. **WiMAX** is sometimes referred to as "Wi-Fi on steroids" and can be used for broadband connections requiring connectivity over distances of several miles. Both 3G (third generation) and 4G (fourth generation) networks are in use. 3G networks were designed primarily for voice communications rather than data, and 4G networks were designed especially for data transmission. Typically 4G networks stream data four times faster than 3G networks. Data transmission speeds are in the range of 6 to 40 Mbit/second and are better for streaming video and other data-intensive uses.

While WiMAX networks are much more secure than WiFi networks, they are susceptible to **man-in-the-middle attacks**, exposing subscribers to confidentiality concerns from sophisticated hackers. An amendment added to the WiMAX specification providing for the addition of Extensible Authentication Protocol (EAP) to WiMAX networks resolves much of this problem. Application of EAP protocols is, however, currently optional for service providers. The amendment also makes available the Advanced Encryption Standard (AES) cipher, providing strong support for confidentiality of data traffic when used.

Systems Security

All systems connected to the Internet or to computers that are connected to the Internet are vulnerable to attack by hackers and require strong security measures. Hackers used to limit their activities to gaining notoriety, but that is no longer the case. Their motives have changed; they are now in it for the money. The nuisance-type of attack on a computer system will always be a concern, and the theft of electronic records from a medical practice can be a virtual gold mine to a criminal hacker. Electronic theft of social security records of staff and patients can lead to identity theft. Theft of bank account and credit card information can result in untold consumer fraud, and compromised medical records may lead to blackmail of patients made vulnerable by release of such information.

Protection of sensitive data is a legal responsibility for any business that has such data in its computer system. The Federal Trade Commission takes enforcement actions against corporations or businesses that fail to provide adequate data security. Protection of a computer system from unauthorized access requires defense in depth. Protection can be broken into the following defenses:

- *Operating system:* Select an operating system with as few flaws as possible. The Microsoft Windows 7 operating system is designed with this in mind, but it is not perfect.

- *Firewall:* Protect the network with a firewall, which limits access to the system from outside.

- *Antivirus software:* Have an active, updated virus protection system.

- *Password:* Require passwords to gain access to sensitive medical and financial data.

- *Training:* Train personnel not to open email from unknown sources and not to go to Web sites received in an unsolicited fashion to avoid **phishing**. Phishing is a practice where the recipient of email is directed to go to a Web site to provide information to his bank, the IRS, or other official organization. The Web site is, in fact, a fake, made to resemble the real thing. When information is given, it goes to the consumer-fraud criminal. If you feel you must take action, contact the organization on the phone to verify that the Web site is authentic before releasing sensitive information.

- *Inventory control:* Maintain strict inventory control of laptops, PDAs, memory cards, and other portable devices that contain data. The best network security system in the world can be breached if a laptop is taken home and either is stolen or is used with unprotected Internet access. Unknown to the user, the laptop can have programs downloaded that reveal passwords or provide a free ride into the secure system of the clinic network.

- *Data management:* Purge the system of inactive files containing sensitive data; archive or destroy them as necessary.

- *Data backup:* Back up all clinic systems on a regular basis to permit restoration of the system in case of a catastrophic event.

- *Manual selection of WiFi access points:* Do not let the computer automatically search for and connect to the access point with the strongest signal. Hackers operate access points designed to gain access to your computer. If in doubt, check the address of the access point to be sure it represents a legitimate source or connect only to officially known access points.

- *Personal access points:* The personal access point, which is part of your network system, should be given a unique name that does not reflect the business name or the name of personnel. It should be security protected as previously described.

- *Deactivate file sharing by your computer:* Allowing files to be shared may be convenient for coworkers, but it leaves a wide open door for hackers.

- *Enable email encryption:* Enable the **Service Sockets Layer (SSL)** option for transmission of email by your email service provider.

Virus Protection Programs. Protection from viruses, worms, and malicious software (malware) is extremely important to prevent damage to files; unauthorized access to the files; and slowing, damage, or shutdown of the system. Viruses find their way onto a system principally through downloading materials and programs from the Internet, opening attachments from email files containing a virus, and unauthorized software. Antivirus software is one of the main defenses against computer viruses.

Antivirus software is a computer program that can be used to scan files to identify and eliminate computer viruses and malware. Antivirus software typically uses two different techniques to accomplish this:

- Examining files to look for known viruses by means of a virus dictionary

- Identifying suspicious behavior from any computer program that might indicate infection

Most commercial antivirus software uses both of these approaches.

In the virus dictionary approach, when the antivirus software examines a file, it refers to a dictionary of known viruses that have been identified by the author of the antivirus software. If part of the file matches a virus identified in the dictionary, the software will either delete the file or quarantine it, making it unable to spread. The program may also attempt to repair the file. The virus dictionary approach requires periodic online downloads to update the virus dictionary. The dictionary approach to detecting viruses is often insufficient due to the continual creation of new viruses.

Dictionary-based antivirus software typically examines files when the computer's operating system creates, opens, and closes them and when the files are sent or received as email. A known virus can be detected immediately upon receipt. The software can also typically be scheduled to examine all files on the user's hard disk on a regular basis.

The suspicious behavior approach attempts to monitor the behavior of all programs. If a program tries to write data to an executable program, this action is flagged as suspicious behavior, and the user is alerted and asked how to proceed.

Recognizing Secured Sites. Secure Internet sites are easily discernible by either a small padlock in the Web browser window, not the Web site window itself, or by the site address (Figure 11-3). Secure sites have an address beginning with https://. Sites that are not secure have an address beginning with http://, without the "s."

Secure wireless sites can be identified by the same padlock next to the network name shown when your wireless device searches for a signal. When a padlock is shown, you will have to configure your device to connect to the hotspot. This is usually in the form of a password or passphrase.

Firewalls. Firewalls come in two varieties: hardware and software. Both types function in a similar fashion; namely, they establish a list of acceptable sites based on a profile the device develops on the users of the system. It will then allow these sites access to your computer. All other sites are blocked. Some firewalls limit the type of files that can be transmitted. Other firewalls cloak specific network channels, making them invisible to hackers trying to gain access to your computer. Still others monitor the content of incoming packets of data.

System Backup. Viruses, equipment failure or damage, and hacker attacks make system backup mandatory. System backup devices are basically data storage devices that store the entire content of the nonportable computer memory so it can be recovered if a catastrophic system loss should occur. All clinic systems should use backup on a regularly scheduled basis. The frequency of the backup should be dependent on how much data the user can afford to lose. Magnetic tapes, optical drives, and flash drives are frequently used for this purpose. The backup is frequently done during hours when the system is not being used. Some system backup devices are automatic, requiring only that the tape or disk from the disk drive be changed in the morning and placed in safe storage. Current backup media should be stored in a secure off-site location. A backup system should be tested to ensure it is capable of restoring the computer to the initial state.

Power Outage, Electrical Surge, and Static Discharge Protection Devices. Protection devices must be an integral part of a medical clinic computer system. Computer systems should have an uninterruptible power supply, or battery backup, to prevent power outages from shutting down the system or destroying data. The power supply should also have a **surge protection** capability to prevent voltage surges on the utility line from damaging computer components. Static electricity can also be highly damaging to computers by transferring thousands of volts of electrical charge to components that are damaged by only a few hundred volts. This is the type of charge we all experience during dry weather when we get a shock from touching a grounded object and draw a spark. Nylon stockings, synthetic clothing, and walking on a synthetic fiber carpet all create static charges. To prevent damage from static discharges, grounding mats are required at all workstations.

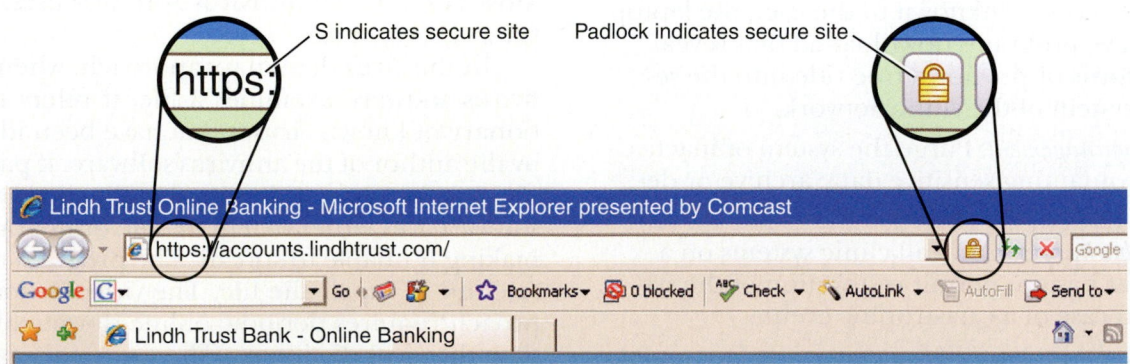

Figure 11-3 Indications of a secure site shown on Web browser.
Source: Used with permission of Microsoft.

CLOUD COMPUTING

Just when you thought you had learned the basics of what is needed for an a clinic computing system, we're going to show the future of computing in the medical clinic. A future where there is no need for concern with CPUs, RAM capacity, data storage devices, and especially software. Everything will come from the **cloud computing**.

The cloud is like a computer rental agency where an order is placed for the applications or **apps** to be performed, such as keying-in a document, or preparing graphics for an a clinic bulletin board, scheduling appointments, coding procedures and billing insurance for services, etc. The computing requirement is sent to the cloud and the app appears on the clinic monitor screen. Hardware and software updates, loading programs, or having to call the Information Technology (IT) person will be a thing of the past. It is done in the cloud. The term "cloud" comes from the vision of cyberspace, where the Internet is represented by a cloud. In cloud computing, the cloud will provide all computing needs for a fixed service price on a pay-for-use-basis. It will securely store data in a manner that all authorized persons in the clinic can access, and provide it as requested. This is not magic of course; behind the service are computer resources and a management system, but the only user concerns will be availability on demand and reliability of the service. Cloud computing is made possible by the commoditization of apps, just like rental cars, airline flights, or utilities. Payment is required for only those services used. The main advantages of cloud computing are:

- Reduced cost resulting from reduction in IT personnel, hardware, software, and service hours
- Improvement in resource availability time, more secure data backup, and better disaster recovery

Some computing equipment will still be required in the medical clinic. A very basic computer and input devices capable of connecting to the Internet, as well as having a graphics capability to produce an image on the monitor, will still be necessary. A printer will still be required. Both the printer and the monitor will have to be selected to meet the requirements of the practice, just as is the case with current computing systems.

Data confidentiality will continue to be a concern to the medical community. Cloud computing services will not be without potential threats to data security, but by using encryption, VLANs, and firewalls, the threats can be minimized. Multiplicity of geographical data storage can reduce the problem of data loss.

Cloud computing will be the development that makes electronic health records a reality. Electronic medical records that are accessible through a single facility or clinic using its servers are not global. Until those records are global, where anyone with authorization, regardless of their geographic location, can obtain access, electronic health records will not be a reality.

COMPUTER MAINTENANCE BY CLINIC PERSONNEL

Maintenance of computer systems is generally limited to cleaning the monitor screens, replacing printer ink or toner cartridges, and refilling paper trays. Procedure 11-1 provides instructions for performing routine maintenance of clinic computers and ancillary equipment with documentation. Other maintenance tasks that are within the capability of a computer-literate member of the health care team are file removal, disk **defragmentation**, and installation of security patches recommended by the supplier of the computer software.

The hard drive of a computer accumulates a host of old files ranging from old emails to obsolete programs and data files. If not removed, they use hard drive storage space and ultimately can slow the speed at which the computer stores and retrieves data. Simply right-clicking on the file with the mouse and then selecting Delete from the menu can remove these old files. After removing files, you should also empty the recycle bin. Be careful with this step, however, because once the recycle bin has been emptied, the files can no longer be recovered without extraordinary means.

When files are deleted from the hard drive, blank spaces are left on the disk. For the computer to save new files it must sort through these blank spaces. The defragmentation process removes the blank spaces similar to the way you move all the books on a shelf to one side so new books can be added to the empty side. Defragmentation is easily done using a disk defragmenter that is included with the OS. Defragmentation takes a significant amount of time and should be performed when the clinic is closed.

The medical assistant may have as one of his or her responsibilities establishing a service agreement for maintenance of computers on a periodic basis as well as any emergency repairs resulting from a major system failure. These agreements may also include personnel training and general technical support services. The medical assistant responsible for this contract should make certain that the vendor has signed the contracts required by the confidentiality protocols established by the medical clinic and that all removable data storage media have been removed and secured before hardware is taken to the service company's facility.

USE OF COMPUTERS IN THE MEDICAL CLINIC

Computers are increasingly used in the medical clinic for:

- Routine clinic tasks
- Maintaining **electronic medical records (EMR)** and **electronic health records (EHR)** and managing the clinic or practice
- Clinical laboratory applications

Specialized software that ties together management of the entire practice is expensive, sometimes costing several hundred thousand dollars per application. Increased revenue resulting from improved productivity and reduction in the amount of undercoding or overcoding during the billing process have been found to more than justify the expenditure.

General Clinic Procedures

General purpose applications include word processing, spreadsheets, graphics, databases, online communication programs, and stand-alone accounting programs. These programs replace the typewriter, adding machine, drafting table, pegboard system, and mechanical file sorting systems. They have resulted in productivity increases, but they still require skilled operators with specialized training and are being displaced by electronic practice management systems. General purpose programs will continue to be used for writing letters, preparing journal articles, compiling unique reports, preparing drawings, and preparing digital photographs and scans for inclusion in manual reports.

Electronic Health Records

 Electronic medical records are rapidly replacing paper charts in the medical clinic. At the present time approximately 30% of medical clinic in the United States have converted to EMRs. Other countries, such as Great Britain and Canada, are already at 88% EMR utilization. Electronic patient records from a single medical practice, hospital, or pharmacy are known as electronic medical records (EMRs). An EMR is created for each individual patient and replaces the paper medical chart. When EMRs from multiple sources are combined into one master database for a patient, the electronic record is known as the patient's electronic health record (EHR). EHRs transcend any one medical provider and in theory encompass the patient's medical universe. The data generated for an EMR are compiled using **total practice management system (TPMS)** software.

TPMS software is a category of software that deals with the day-to-day operations of a medical practice. Practice management systems currently and in the near future will perform all or part of the following functions:

- Enter demographic data, track patient forms and authorizations, schedule and track patient appointments, and schedule appointments or referrals
- Provide medical records and laboratory test results to the provider, document procedures performed and diagnoses and treatment plan selected, and write and forward prescriptions to the patient's pharmacy
- Send insurance claims and patient statements as part of the collection process; process insurance, patient, and third-party payments; and generate reports for the administrative and clinical staff of the practice

Figure 11-4 illustrates an insurance screen from Medical Office Simulation Software (MOSS).

Figure 11-5 generalizes all of the functions of a TPMS. The records stored by a computer include patient records, personnel records, appointment scheduling, financial records, and billing status information for each of the practice functions illustrated. TPMS is gaining increasing use in all practices by decreasing the labor involved in maintaining medical records and minimizing medical liability risks.

 In order to satisfy legal requirements, TPMS must demonstrate their complete functionality by ensuring that the record is complete, accurate, secure, and compatible with all systems from which information about the patient is obtained. The system must meet the preliminary American Recovery and Reinvestment Act of 2009 (ARRA) certification requirements of the

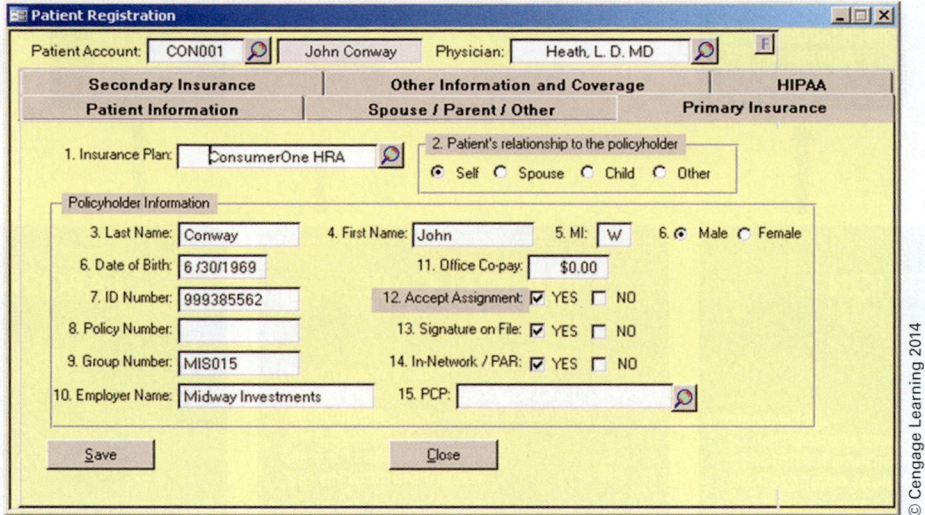

Figure 11-4 An insurance screen from Medical Office Simulation Software (MOSS).

Clinical and Laboratory Applications

Computer usage in the clinical and laboratory setting is well ahead of its use in the area of practice management. It has been used for years to automate medical tests, and many scanning tests would not even be possible without the computer. Probably the greatest impact of computer use in the laboratory environment has been the replacement of film as the recording media for X-ray images and other scanning tests. This application has made possible the electronic transfer of records between facilities on a real-time basis and made laboratory medical records readily available to the provider at the point of care.

Portable Computers in the Medical Clinic

The provider and back-office staff rely heavily on computer monitors in the examination room. Small hand-held personal digital assistants (PDAs) however, are taking the place of the monitor due to their extreme mobility. A PDA is a highly compact computer, the latest version of which is more commonly known as a "smartphone" because it provides easy-to-operate functionality for mobile communications and computing in one small package.

A smartphone accesses small computer programs, called apps, that are designed to meet a multitude of computing functions. The main attribute of a smartphone is its capacity to be a multipurpose device that can multitask. The user can easily move from application to application, take phone calls, take pictures, and email or synchronize data for later use, and then simply return to an earlier app in progress. Smartphones allow medical personnel to carry a data link and mobile communication wherever they go. A photo of a typical smartphone is shown in Figure 11-6.

A larger alternative to a PDA or smartphone is the tablet PC, which provides greater screen size. These devices are gaining in popularity for reviewing laboratory data requiring greater graphic resolution.

With a PDA or tablet PC having the necessary apps installed, medical personnel can access schedules, review patient records, compile notes of the encounter, remotely monitor a patient's EKG and blood pressure in "real time," check drug dosages and interactions, and write prescriptions that are then electronically forwarded. Other apps allow document preparation, downloading email, and searching the Internet. They provide ready access to a personal calendar, phone numbers, and a host of other features.

DESIGN CONSIDERATIONS FOR A COMPUTERIZED MEDICAL CLINIC

Computerization of a medical clinic requires careful consideration of the computer system, software, and the physical layout of the facility. If the change to a computerized system is

Certification Commission for Health Information Technology (CCHIT) (http://www.cchit.org).

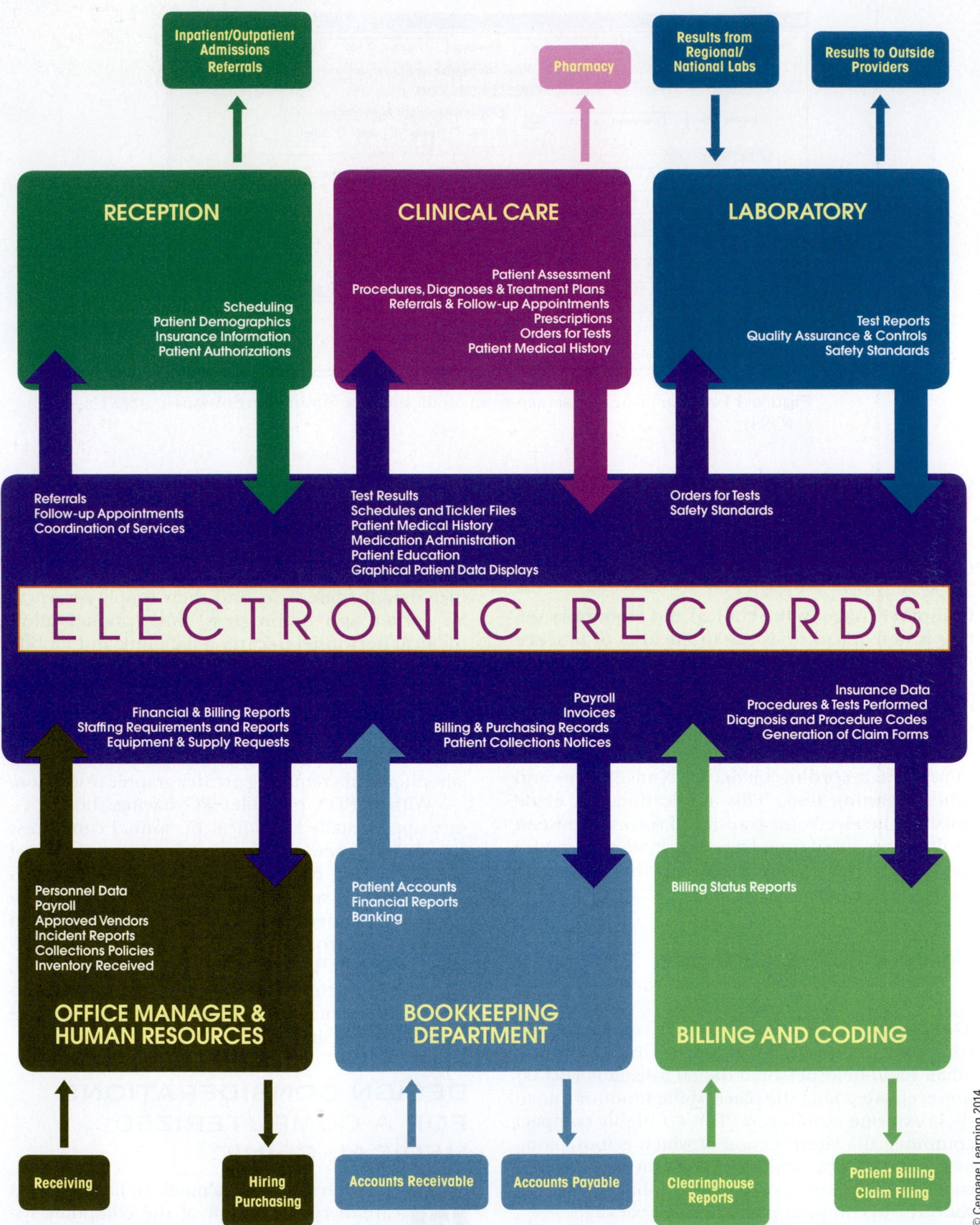

Figure 11-5 Total practice management system (TPMS) data flow.

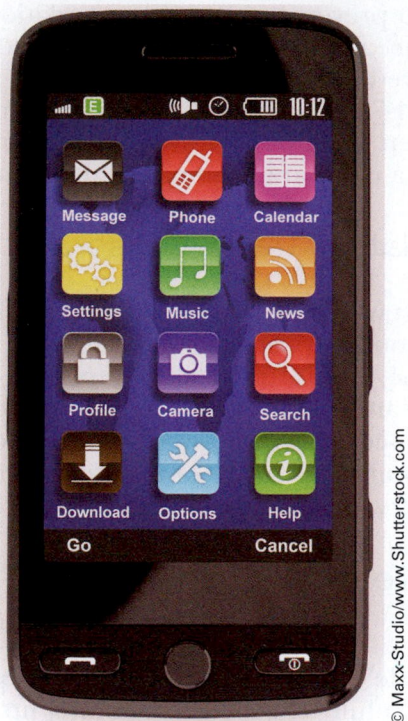

© Maxx-Studio/www.Shutterstock.com

Figure 11-6 Example of a smartphone.

well planned, with input sought from all affected personnel and with time allotted for training, the experience will be less stressful for all concerned. Involvement of all clinic personnel in the design of the system is extremely important because it creates a feeling of ownership and garners more willing support during the disruptive changeover period.

Software Selection

The first step in selection of software is to choose a knowledgeable and trustworthy vendor. The vendor should not only understand computers and software but also the needs of the medical clinic. A reliable vendor should be able to assist in anticipating and allowing for future needs (at least 2 years' future needs) as the medical practice grows and new diagnostic tools are introduced.

The next and most important step in developing a plan for computerization of a medical clinic is to determine what tasks will be computerized and preparing specifications that will become part of the contract with the vendor. This is done in conjunction with the vendor, by seeking input from staff, and by talking with other people in medical clinics similar to your facility. Software available for each of the tasks should be identified and evaluated, preferably by actually using the programs on a trial basis. The best program for each task should be identified, and the hardware requirements for each program should be defined. Keep in mind that the program should be selected with operational commonality with all of the other software taken into consideration. Programs with similar menus and appearance on the monitor screen make training personnel much easier. Packaged programs that perform multiple tasks are commonly available. Microsoft® Office Suite is an example of a packaged program that includes word processing, spreadsheet, scheduling, email, and database programs with commonality in menus and procedures. Similar programs tailored to the medical clinic are available. Procedure 11-2 provides software installation steps.

Hardware Selection

Once the memory capacity (RAM, hard drive data storage capacity), CPU speed, and input and output device requirements have been identified for the software, the next step is to determine whether you are going to network. The type of network selected will be based on data transmission speed requirements and facilities considerations for running cables and the distance between computers and output devices. The hardware you select should meet or exceed the identified minimum requirements and be name brand equipment to ensure future availability of replacement parts. If possible, get a computer system with substantially more memory than required by the software, because inadequate memory or CPU speed may restrict the ability to use future software updates or improved programs. The CPU speed should be as fast as the technology permits at the time you make your purchase. The computer should also have one or more USB 3.0 ports to allow faster connection speeds. The trend is toward using more memory and requiring greater CPU speed, especially if graphic programs will be used in your system. The more memory and CPU speed you can purchase, the longer your system will be viable without replacement of hardware. The size of monitor and screen display resolution limit should be selected to be compatible with the type of work the computer is used to perform. These requirements are necessary to achieve image sharpness and avoid eyestrain of personnel. The computer control panel display settings should also be set to match the monitor display resolution limit. Resolution is usually expressed as pixels in the horizontal and vertical dimensions of the screen. Many inexpensive computer monitors have a resolution of 1280 ×1024 and this is adequate for most clinic work. Persons doing graphic design frequently use a monitor with a resolution of 1600 ×1200, and a resolution of 3280 × 2048 is used in medical diagnostic work. For reference purposes, the most common widescreen HD television has a resolution of 1920 × 1080. Procedure 11-3 provides hardware installation steps.

Scheduling the Changeover

The installation of a computer system is disruptive to the clinic routine. Not only does it take time to install the hardware and load software, but it takes time to transfer files and data. Personnel may be intimidated by the computer and must be well trained to avoid being overly threatened. The installation of hardware should be scheduled during a down period such as a long holiday or vacation period. It is best to introduce the new system while continuing to use the old system. Start by transferring files and data, then when the staff is comfortable with the system and their computer skills, make the changeover. If your staff does not accept ownership for the system and is not trained and comfortable with it, disaster is almost guaranteed. The process cannot be rushed, and the short-term inefficiency must be accepted as a trade-off for the efficiency that will result from a computerized medical clinic.

ERGONOMICS

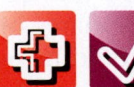 Although **ergonomics** in the medical office is an important consideration even without computerization, specific problems must be addressed when changing over to a computerized office environment. Safety issues and concerns specific to the computer, if addressed, can be minimized or avoided.

Eyestrain

Eyestrain can be a problem associated with the use of computers. The computer monitor should be positioned to prevent excessive glare entering from windows or reflecting from interior lighting. Attachment of an antiglare screen to the monitor further reduces eyestrain by reducing remaining residual glare. Computer operators should take a five-minute break each hour and focus on a distant object to prevent ocular accommodation and the headache and blurred vision associated with it. Using eye drops can minimize dry and itchy eyes. Figure 11-7 illustrates the proper positioning of the flat screen monitor to prevent glare from artificial lights in a room and incoming light from windows.

Cumulative Trauma Disorder

The most widely known injury associated with individuals routinely using a computer is carpal tunnel syndrome. It is attributed to repetitive wrist motion. It can be prevented or the onset delayed by using a special keyboard that conforms to the natural position of the hands or by using a conventional keyboard with wrist support, as show in Figure 11-8.

Posture

Reports of back pain resulting from poor posture while using the computer are quite common. Carefully choosing and setting up computer equipment can minimize this type of injury. Computer operators should use a comfortable chair with lumbar support adjustment. A special chair with ergonomic features should be considered for individuals whose primary duty is keyboarding. Figure 11-9 shows the recommended computer operator position for proper posture to prevent back strain while operating a computer. The desktop

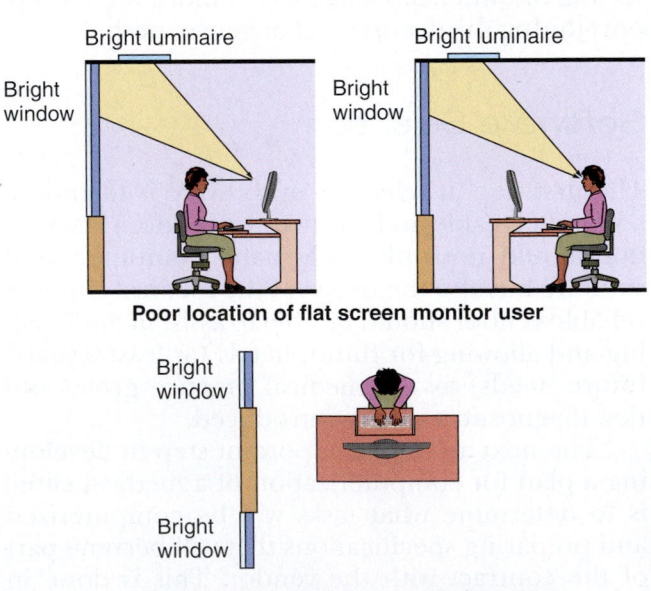

Poor location of flat screen monitor user

Good location of flat screen monitor user (sight line parallel to window)

© Cengage Learning 2014

Figure 11-7 Proper positioning of the flat screen monitor will prevent glare from incoming light from windows and artificial lights in the room.

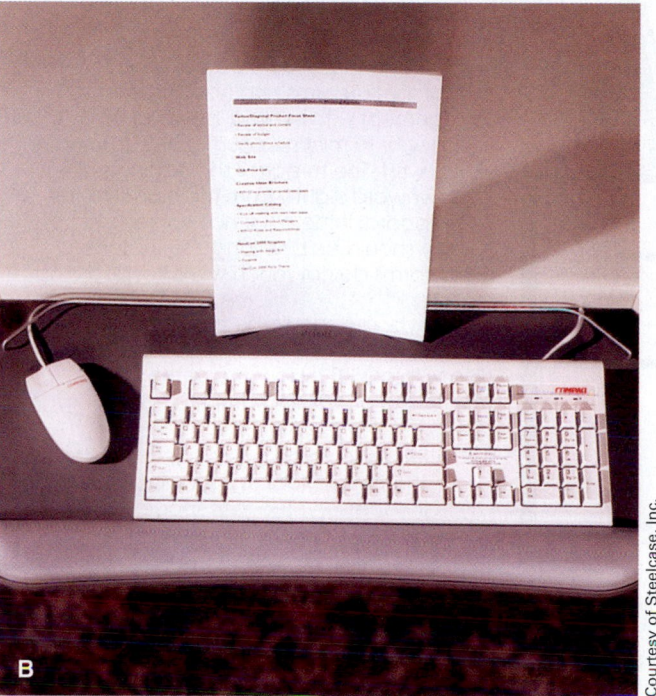

Figure 11-8A Ergonomic keyboard.

Figure 11-8B Keyboard with built-in wrist support.

should be 28 to 30 inches above the floor with an adjustable keyboard holder allowing adjustment for individual operator body size. A footrest may be helpful in further minimizing posture problems (Figure 11-10). A document holder should be used to avoid excessive turning of the neck and looking downward (Figure 11-11). Operators who talk on the telephone while keyboarding or inputting data should use a headset telephone.

CRITICAL THINKING

Your clinic has obtained new medical management software. List as many options you can think of for training clinic personnel to use the management software effectively. Identify the pros and cons for each option.

PATIENT CONFIDENTIALITY IN THE COMPUTERIZED MEDICAL CLINIC

The computer and other electronic transmission media are powerful tools, but they are equally powerful in their potential to jeopardize patient confidentiality.

The starting point for a meaningful information security system is a comprehensive security policy that adheres to HIPAA policies and procedures and that is understood and supported by staff and employees. All staff, employees, and vendors having access to the computer system should be educated on the security policy and asked to sign a contract affirming that they will adhere to the policy before they are given access to confidential data. The signed contract affirms that they have received training and have been instructed in proper procedures to protect medical records. The signed contracts together with the protocols become a part of the facility's documentation showing compliance with HIPAA regulations.

The next essential step is to ensure that computer-literate personnel are employed to set up the system. Protocols should be established defining who can access and modify data, providing identification, dating, and authenticating mechanisms for those changes and additions. Procedures should be in place to ensure that people other than the intended recipient cannot accidentally read misdirected files, and that firewalls are in place or precautions are taken to prevent people from hacking into the system through Internet or **network interfaces**. Antivirus programs should be part of the system to prevent loss of the data or the unintentional dissemination of files.

Passwords incorporating employee personal identification numbers (PINs) or passwords that are specific to individual employees are essential in controlling access to files and providing an authentication mechanism that identifies personnel making changes to files.

Output devices, such as printers and fax machines, should be located where unauthorized personnel cannot view them. Unauthorized persons should not be allowed to wander around the facility unescorted. Data storage media should be secured, and accountability records of persons accessing the media should be maintained.

The American Medical Association (AMA) supports the adoption of standards to protect individual confidential information. Figure 11-12 summarizes AMA Policy E5-07,

This diagram shows the recommended sitting posture for computer operators. The recommendation is based on establishing a posture that is comfortable while minimizing the risk of cumulative trauma injuries. Correct posture also minimizes operator fatigue and increases productivity.

- Distance to the screen should be adjusted so that the chin does not jut forward when the trunk is against the chair back.

- Top of the screen should be slightly below eye level. It should be squarely in front of the body to prevent twisting the body or the neck.

- The chair seat should not be so deep that the front edge is against the calve of the operator's leg, preventing the operator from supporting the back against the chair while in an erect position.

- The keyboard should be adjusted so that the forearms and hands are in alignment with minimal bending of the wrist to minimize cumulative trauma to the wrist. The forearms should angle downward slightly from the elbow to the keyboard. If the chair has armrests, they should be positioned so that the forearms do not touch while keyboarding.

- The chair adjustment should place the thighs level with or slightly above the knees to allow upper body weight to pass directly from the spine into the chair.

- The keyboard should be placed in front of the operator so that the elbows are in line with or slightly forward of the centerline of the body trunk.

- Feet should be in firm contact with the floor. A foot rest should be used if necessary. The foot space should be free from obstructions.

- High seat back with lumbar support is recommended to relive spinal stress. Adjust the back to match the lumbar curve of the spine so that the chair supports some of the body weight. The spine should be as erect as possible to let it support a maximum amount of body weight to reduce fatigue.

© Cengage Learning 2014

Figure 11-9 Recommended computer operator position with ergonomic considerations.

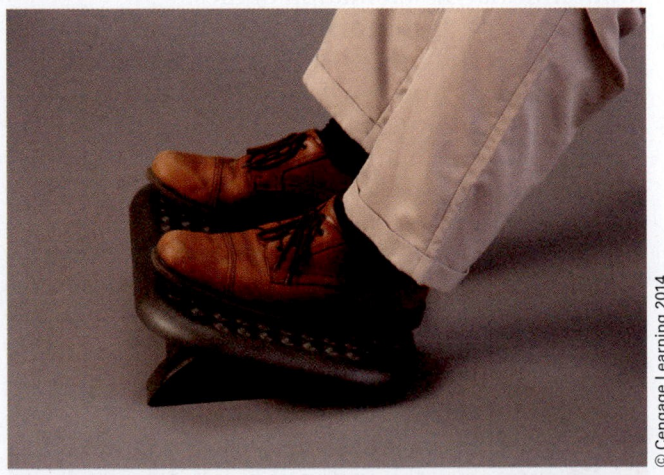

© Cengage Learning 2014

Figure 11-10 Using a footrest may help to prevent posture problems.

"Confidentiality—Computers," issued before April 1977 and updated in 1994, 1998, 2002, and on August 26, 2005.

HIPAA STANDARDS FOR SAFEGUARDING PROTECTED HEALTH INFORMATION (PHI)

HIPAA standards for safeguarding PHI include:

- Preparation and implementation of written confidentiality protocols and procedures regarding PHI
- Staff training in implementation of all protocols

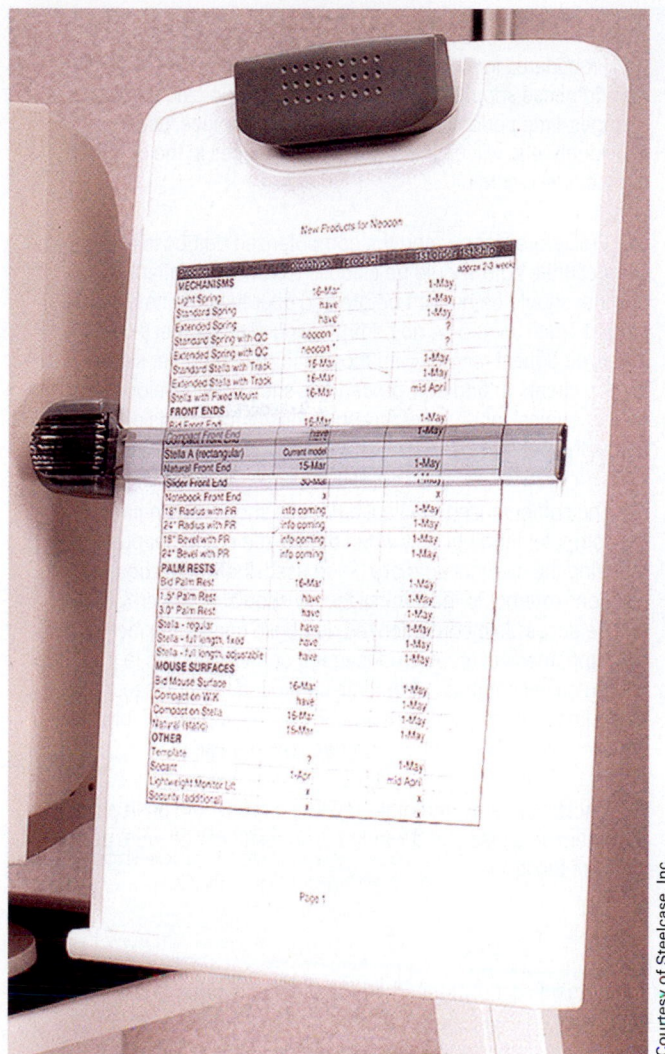

Courtesy of Steelcase, Inc.

FIGURE 11-11 Vertical document holder.

- Identification of authentication protocols for all personnel
- Access control of computer output, modification, or destruction of files
- Security of transmitted data
- Control of discarded records, storage media, and computer hardware

PROFESSIONALISM IN THE COMPUTERIZED MEDICAL CLINIC

Areas of professionalism directly related to the computerized medical clinic may include:

- *Working as a member of the health care team.* The medical assistant should become actively involved in the process of upgrading medical software and implementing policies and procedures related to computerization and should follow all protocols adopted by the employer.
- *Adapt to change.* The medical assistant must adapt to change. Computerization in the medical clinic will stretch the comfort limits facility all personnel. New procedures will result in office inefficiency until everyone is familiar with the new system and it becomes second nature in its use. Always be dependable and follow through with any assigned tasks. Be flexible and consider the schedule of coworkers. Tasks sequence require being performed in a different order than you prefer in order to accommodate others' needs.
- *Work ethic.* The medical assistant should refrain from using the clinic computer for personal use. This includes sending and receiving personal email and searching the Internet. Passwords should never be shared, and unauthorized software should not be loaded onto the clinic computer. Protocols should be carefully followed in transmission of patient confidential information.
- *Enhance skills through continuing education.* Introduction of a computer system and periodic updates to program revisions will require continued education and training on the part of the medical assistant. A professional will approach these minor disruptions with a positive attitude.

EHR The impact of EHRs affects the entire clinic staff as well as patients. Consider customer service at the point of care. When medical assistants are working at a computer, often they are not focused entirely on what the patient is telling them. They are busy keying in information and checking which fields need to be completed or searching for additional screens on which to add information. This situation may occur when the patient enters the clinic and is asked questions to aid in the completion or verification of patient registration information. The computer may be encountered in the examination room when the medical assistant or provider discusses the patient's reason for the visit or reviews the chart. During visits to the lab, again computers come into play.

It is important to the remember the techniques discussed in Chapter 5. Eye contact and personalization are important techniques used during

E-5.07 Confidentiality: Computers. The utmost effort and care must be taken to protect the confidentiality of all medical records, including computerized medical records.

The guidelines below are offered to assist providers and computer service organizations in maintaining the confidentiality of information in medical records when that information is stored in computerized databases:

(1) Confidential medical information should be entered into the computer-based patient record only by authorized personnel. Additions to the record should be time and date stamped, and the person making the additions should be identified in the record.

(2) The patient and provider should be advised about the existence of computerized databases in which medical information concerning the patient is stored. Such information should be communicated to the provider and patient prior to the provider's release of the medical information to the entity or entities maintaining the computer databases. All individuals and organizations with some form of access to the computerized databases, and the level of access permitted, should be specifically identified in advance. Full disclosure of this information to the patient is necessary in obtaining informed consent to treatment. Patient data should be assigned a security level appropriate for the data's degree of sensitivity, which should be used to control who has access to the information.

(3) The provider and patient should be notified of the distribution of all reports reflecting identifiable patient data prior to distribution of the reports by the computer facility. There should be approval by the patient and notification of the provider prior to the release of patient-identifiable clinical and administrative data to individuals or organizations external to the medical care environment. Such information should not be released without the express permission of the patient.

(4) The dissemination of confidential medical data should be limited to only those individuals or agencies with a bona fide use for the data. Only the data necessary for the bona fide use should be released. Patient identifiers should be omitted when appropriate. Release of confidential medical information from the database should be confined to the specific purpose for which the information is requested and limited to the specific time frame requested. All such organizations or individuals should be advised that authorized release of data to them does not authorize their further release of the data to additional individuals or organizations, or subsequent use of the data for other purposes.

(5) Procedures for adding to or changing data on the computerized database should indicate individuals authorized to make changes, time periods in which changes take place, and those individuals who will be informed about changes in the data from the medical records.

(6) Procedures for purging the computerized database of archaic or inaccurate data should be established and the patient and provider should be notified before and after the data has been purged. There should be no commingling of a provider's computerized patient records with those of other computer service bureau clients. In addition, procedures should be developed to protect against inadvertent mixing of individual reports or segments thereof.

(7) The computerized medical database should be on-line to the computer terminal only when authorized computer programs requiring the medical data are being used. Individuals and organizations external to the clinical facility should not be provided on-line access to a computerized database containing identifiable data from medical records concerning patients. Access to the computerized database should be controlled through security measures such as passwords, encryption (encoding) of information, and scannable badges or other user identification.

(8) Backup systems and other mechanisms should be in place to prevent data loss and downtime as a result of hardware or software failure.

(9) Security:

A. Stringent security procedures should be in place to prevent unauthorized access to computer-based patient records. Personnel audit procedures should be developed to establish a record in the event of unauthorized disclosure of medical data. Terminated or former employees in the data processing environment should have no access to data from the medical records concerning patients.

B. Upon termination of computer services for a provider, those computer files maintained for the provider should be physically turned over to the provider. They may be destroyed (erased) only if it is established that the provider has another copy (in some form). In the event of file erasure, the computer service bureau should verify in writing to the provider that the erasure has taken place. Issued prior to April 1977; Updated June 1994, June 1998, and August 26, 2005.

Figure 11-12   Computer confidentiality guidelines. (Source: *Code of Medical Ethics Current Opinions with Annotations,* 1994 Edition, American Medical Association, Copyright 1995–2005.)

therapeutic communication. If possible, have the patient sit next to the medical assistant so that he or she can also view the monitor while providing information. Questions should be directed to the patient, not to the computer monitor. When the task is complete, the medical assistant should look at the patient, thank the patient for his or her help, and provide any additional instructions.

CRITICAL THINKING

The provider–employer has informed the clinic manager that he or she has observed employees visiting Web sites not connected with clinic requirements and is concerned about the practice becoming widespread. You have been asked to prepare a draft guideline for a policy on business and personal Internet use on clinic equipment during business hours. You have been further told that the policy should not be totally prohibitive, but it does need to address performing personal tasks during business hours and exercising propriety in the sites visited.

Prepare a draft policy proposal for computer use, and obtain written comments from several students regarding the policy guidelines. Prepare a final draft incorporating changes made to obtain consensus by the persons making comments and submit the original draft, the comments, and final draft to the instructor, together with your observations on the difficulty in achieving consensus on the policy.

PROCEDURE 11-1

Instructions for Performing Routine Maintenance of Clinic Computers and Ancillary Equipment with Documentation

PURPOSE:
To ensure that all computers in the clinic are serviced according to manufacturer suggestions and that documentation is logged appropriately.

EQUIPMENT/SUPPLIES:
Maintenance log form with location of each computer and its ancillary pieces (modems, printers)
Database identifying all copyright software, product IDs, computer IDs on which software is installed, and renewal dates for all copyright software
Service calendar log form
Clipboard with maintenance log and service calendar log forms attached, pen with black ink, and access to all computers
Disk defragmenter included with the OS

PROCEDURE STEPS:

1. Locate the number assigned by the clinic manager to identify the computer being serviced, verify serial number, manufacturer/maker, technical support phone number, warranty information, and last date of service. RATIONALE: Provides medical assistant with all information needed for maintenance and servicing of equipment.

2. *Paying attention to detail,* visually inspect each piece of equipment associated with the computer setup.

   - *Practice risk management principles.* Check for any frayed electrical cords, loose connections, or safety issues such as tripping hazards associated with electrical cords.

   - Clean monitor screens, replace printer ink or toner cartridges, and refill paper trays. RATIONALE: To ensure proper working order and reduce risk management issues.

3. Remove any unnecessary data files and empty the recycle bin. Next, complete the defragmentation process.

4. Install security patches provided by the provider of the computer software. RATIONALE: To save hard drive storage space, increase the processing speed of the computer, and protect the security of the system. *Using sound judgment and paying attention to detail* are critical factors to consider.

5. Record updated information on the maintenance log and service calendar forms and date and initial. Report to appropriate personnel any personal copyright software that is not on the database list. Verify that the licenses are in the documentation file and properly cover the

continues

Procedure 11-1 (continued)

number of computers on which software is installed. RATIONALE: To ensure accurate maintenance documentation is on file regarding each computer and associated ancillary pieces in the medical office. *Working within the scope of practice* and within the law is critical. *Protect and maintain confidentiality* at all times.

6. Schedule equipment servicing during the current month with an appropriate vendor and let coworkers know that equipment servicing has been scheduled. RATIONALE: Set a specific time with the vendor and the medical office to ensure equipment is available for servicing. Working efficiently and using your time appropriately are important, as are being flexible and dependable. Demonstrate respect for others and assist coworkers when appropriate.

DOCUMENTATION EXAMPLE:

Maintenance Log Form

Name of Equipment	Serial Number	Mfg/ Maker	Technical Support Phone Number	Purchase Date	Service Plan	Last Serviced	Completed By
Computer #6	79031	HP	xxx-xxx-xxxx	1/20xx	On file	6/12/20xx	bql
Printer #10	80462	HP	xxx-xxx-xxxx	7/20xx	On file	6/12/20xx	bql

Service Calendar Log Form

January	February	March	April	May	June
July	August	September	October	November	December

PROCEDURE 11-2
Software Installation

PURPOSE:
To add software programs to the computer system for later call-up and use. RATIONALE: To provide the computer with the necessary software codes to perform the application.

EQUIPMENT/SUPPLIES:
Computer system
Software CD
Software documentation

PROCEDURE STEPS:
Software can be installed on Microsoft Windows® using an automatic "Installation Wizard" or by manual means.

Automatic Installation
- Close all open programs.
- Insert the CD supplied with the program into your CD drive. Shortly after the light on the drive shows activity, the Installation Wizard screen will

Procedure 11-2 (continued)

appear. If more than one disk is supplied (many programs have multiple disks because of the size of the program and files that must be stored to use the program), start with disk number 1 or the one marked "program." Usually, other disks will be marked disk 2, disk 3, or "data."

- Follow the instructions given by your software documentation and the Installation Wizard screens that will appear. The wizard will usually ask for the following:

  1. The product registration number or serial number.

  2. Where you want the files to be stored on your hard drive. (A default address is usually given and should be used unless your organization has a policy of storing programs in a specific drive or server. If that is the case, you probably have a system administrator for your computers and you should not be doing the installation.)

  3. Whether you want the program icon on your desktop to aid in quickly starting the program. (You should say YES to this question unless your desktop is quite cluttered. If you say NO, you will have to use the START button, then select PROGRAMS from the menu that appears, and then find the SOFTWARE NAME and click on it to start the program. If the program is frequently used, this becomes a nuisance.)

- At the completion of the installation, you may be asked to register the program if you are on-line, and then asked to restart your computer before the program will be operational. Just follow the instructions given by the wizard. It is a good idea to register the program so that you receive updates and announcements. If you are not on-line, you can register using ground mail.

Manual Installation

Sometimes the Installation Wizard will not recognize the program or the settings are not such that it will be automatic. In this case, you will need to perform the following steps:

- Close all programs.
- Place CD in desired drive.
- Click START.
- Select My Computer.
- Double click on drive containing CD.
- Follow prompts from Installation Wizzard screens that appear.
- Use suggested defaults.
- Click FINISH and launch the program.

DOCUMENTATION:

All computer documentation including licenses, recovery software, and program disks should be stored in a designated safe place for the life of the equipment and software. A current list of all documentation should be maintained for easy access.

DOCUMENTATION EXAMPLE:

- Software Installation
- (create a table with these 3 headings)
- Software Date Installed Date Uninstalled
- Windows Office June, 20xx

PROCEDURE 11-3
Hardware Installation

PURPOSE:
To add hardware programs to the computer system for later call-up and use. RATIONALE: To provide the computer with the necessary information to install the hardware.

EQUIPMENT/SUPPLIES:
Computer system
Driver for the equipment (on CD or download from the Internet site of manufacturer)

PROCEDURE STEPS:
Microsoft Windows® 7 normally identifies new hardware and asks you if you want to install it, or it simply starts Installation Wizard. In some instances, the wizard will not recognize the new hardware, necessitating manual initiation of the wizard.

The wizard will request all or some of the following information:

- Close all open programs
- Manufacturer and model number of the hardware
- How it is connected to the computer (USB, parallel, or IEEE 1394 cable)

- The driver supplied with the hardware or already registered with Microsoft (if not part of your operating system, you will need to install a CD into the drive for the computer to load into memory)

Follow the directions given by the wiard. If the wizard does not appear, you will need to manually initiate the wizard to install the hardware. In this case, do the following:

- Close all open programs.
- Go to START, CONTROL PANEL, and double-click ADD HARDWARE. The Add Hardware Wizard screen will start. Follow the instructions given on the screen. You may be asked to insert the CD with the driver supplied by the manufacturer.

DOCUMENTATION
The Documentation Log should be updated each time a new piece of technology is added to the practice. The name of the equipment, serial number, mfg/maker, technical support phone number, purchase date, and if there is a service plan should all be included in the log.

CASE STUDY 11-1

Refer to the scenario at the beginning of the chapter.

CASE STUDY REVIEW

1. How will Walter establish benchmarks or comparisons for computer needs?

2. List important considerations when selecting a computer vendor.

3. What steps might Walter implement to ensure a smooth transition from a manual to a computerized system?

CASE STUDY 11-2

Walter Seals, CMA (AAMA), who is employed by Inner City Health Care, has been given approval to computerize the office. Walter is also concerned about confidentiality issues involved with a computerized medical clinic.

CASE STUDY REVIEW

1. Identify the areas where confidentiality is most likely to be jeopardized.

2. Suggest possible solutions to protect confidentiality in each of these areas. Write a one-page summary and submit it to your instructor.

SUMMARY

As the capabilities for networking and communications between computer systems continue to develop, the potential for increasingly sophisticated uses of computer systems is becoming a reality. We have entered the age of global computing, where information is available almost as quickly as it is requested. As these changes occur, the role of the medical assistant will reflect the growing reliance of the medical practice on the capabilities of computers.

It will become the responsibility of all medical assistants to be information managers, taking advantage of the wealth of resources available by computers that can enhance patient care.

Providers will require assistance in retrieving information from medical databases that support diagnosis; clinic staff may need assistance in locating, accessing, and working with applications software.

The medical assistant's professional responsibilities will become even more challenging as computers become indispensible to the ambulatory care setting.

STUDY FOR SUCCESS

To reinforce your knowledge and skills of information presented in this chapter:

- Review the *Key Terms*
- Role-play with other students ways to apply attributes of professionalism pertinent to this chapter
- Consider the *Case Studies* and discuss your conclusions
- Answer the questions in the *Certification Review*
- Apply your knowledge by completing the Activities in the *Study Guide* and the Games and Quizzes in the StudyWARE software on the *Premium Website*
- Perform the Procedures using the Competency Assessment Checklists in the *Competency Manual*
- Practice your problem-solving skills with the Critical Thinking Challenge 3.0 on the *Premium Website*

Additional resources for this chapter include:

- Module 6 of the *Medical Assisting Learning Lab*
- *CourseMate for Delmar's Comprehensive Medical Assisting*
- *WebTutor for Delmar's Comprehensive Medical Assisting*

CERTIFICATION REVIEW

1. Microcomputers:
   a. are the fastest and most powerful computers
   b. handle large amounts of processing and challenge the capabilities of old mainframe systems
   c. are widely used in today's health care facility
   d. are expensive and complex
2. The CPU:
   a. consists of electronic tablets with pointers, scanners, and touch screens
   b. is the brain of the computer system
   c. is often referred to as memory
   d. frequently is referred to as a computer program
3. Data output devices include all of the following except:
   a. the monitor
   b. printers
   c. keystrokes, motion, and temperature
   d. fax machines
4. Data storage devices include:
   a. keystrokes, motion, temperature, and the mouse
   b. ROM, RAM, hard drives, and flash drives
   c. hard copy, ROM, the mouse, and OS
   d. data input devices, hard copy, and OS

5. Documentation:
   a. performs a specific data processing function
   b. is a set of instructions that a computer follows to control computer hardware and to process data
   c. frequently is called the operating system (OS)
   d. consists of the manuals and documents that define how programs or hardware operate

6. Types of networks include:
   a. optical drives, compact disks, and digital video disks
   b. flash drives, tape drives, optical drives, and digital video disks
   c. LANs, WANs, and Internet
   d. CDs, DVDs, and LANs

7. Connection to a network through a hard-wired system includes all of the following *except:*
   a. WiMAX
   b. standard telephone modem (dial-up)
   c. digital subscriber phone line (DSL)
   d. modem using either copper wire or fiber-optic cable

8. Security features of a computer system must protect against two threats:
   a. viruses and worms
   b. selection of an OS with as few security flaws as possible
   c. unauthorized access to the computer
   d. a and c only

9. Computer maintenance by clinic personnel includes:
   a. cleaning monitor screens
   b. replacing printer ink or toner cartridges
   c. refilling paper trays
   d. all of the above

10. Practice management software is capable of performing all of the following functions *except*:
    a. recording results of laboratory tests
    b. tracking patient forms and authorizations
    c. scheduling and tracking patient appointments and referrals
    d. none of the above

11. PDAs provide ready access to perform all of the following functions *except:*
    a. complete all insurance forms
    b. access schedules
    c. connect to the Internet
    d. review patient records

12. When going from a manual to a computerized medical clinic, it is important to do all of the following *except:*
    a. know what the clinic needs in a computer system
    b. install the operation during a down period
    c. work with a trusted, knowledgeable vendor
    d. expect the computer system to be 100% operational immediately

13. The beginning point for a meaningful information security system is a comprehensive security policy that:
    a. involves the use of LANs
    b. adheres to HIPAA policies and procedures
    c. follows office policies and procedures
    d. involves the use of WANs

14. Which is *not* true of smartphones:
    a. Smallest type of microcomputer
    b. Have wireless phone capabilities
    c. Used mainly by governmental provider services
    d. Are basically next generation PDAs

15. Advantages of cloud computing include all of the following *except:*
    a. cloud computing is made possible by WiMAX connections
    b. reduced costs in IT personnel
    c. reduced hardware and software costs
    d. important in secure data backup

REFERENCES/BIBLIOGRAPHY

American Medical Association. (2005). *E-5.07 confidentiality: Computers.* Retrieved March 20, 2011, from http://www.ama-assn.org

Correa, C. (2011). *Getting started in the computerized medical office: Fundamentals and practice* (2nd ed.). Clifton Park, NY: Delmar Cengage Learning.

ingenix. (2003). *HIPAA tool kit.* Salt Lake City, UT: St. Anthony Publishing/Medicode.

Karp, G. (1996). *Preventing computer injury.* Adapted from paper presented at the Association of American Medical Transcriptionists, Baltimore, MD.

Keir, L., Wise, B. A., & Krebs, C. (2008). *Medical administrative and clinical competencies* (6th ed.). Clifton Park, NY: Delmar Cengage Learning.

Krager, D., & Krager, C. (2005). *HIPAA for medical office personnel.* Clifton Park, NY: Delmar Cengage Learning.

Security Standards, Department of Health and Human Services. (2003). *Final rule health insurance reform.* Federal Register/vol 68, No. 34, pp. 8334–8381. Retrieved September 28, 2012, from http://www.himss.org/content/files/CPRIToolkit/version6/v6%20pdf/D15_HIPAA_Final_Standard_for_Data_Security_in_Plain_English.pdf

CHAPTER 12

Telecommunications

OUTLINE

Telecommunications in the Electronic Health Record Environment

Basic Telephone Techniques
- Telephone Personality
- Professional Telephone Etiquette
- Answering Incoming Calls

Routing Calls in the Medical Clinic
- Types of Calls the Medical Assistant Can Take
- Types of Calls Referred to the Provider
- Special Consideration Calls

Telephone Documentation

Using Telephone Directories

Placing Outgoing Calls

Placing Long-Distance Calls

Legal and Ethical Considerations

HIPAA Guidelines for Telephone Communications

Americans with Disabilities Act (ADA)

Telephone Technology
- Automated Routing Units
- Answering Services and Machines

Voice over Internet Protocol (VoIP) Telecommunications

Facsimile (Fax) Machines

Electronic Mail (Email)

Clinical Email

Interactive Videoconferencing

Cellular Service

Professionalism in Telecommunications

LEARNING OUTCOMES

1. Define, spell, and pronounce the key terms as presented in the glossary.
2. Name at least three calls the medical assistant can take, and state the reasons why. Name three calls the medical assistant should refer to the provider, and state the reasons why.
3. Recall six questions that should be asked during telephone screening.
4. Discuss how calls from angry individuals should be handled in a professional manner, and demonstrate steps to follow when this type of call is received.
5. Analyze rules for using proper telephone technique.
6. State at least five common telephone courtesies.
7. Discuss proper screening techniques.
8. Model the proper procedure for answering incoming calls and transferring calls.
9. Describe the information every message should contain.
10. Model the proper procedure for placing outgoing calls.
11. Discuss telephone documentation.
12. Identify ways to ensure patient confidentiality when using the telephone.
13. Discuss the impacts of HIPAA regulations on telecommunications.
14. Identify several security measures to consider before sending a fax containing confidential information.
15. Differentiate between email and clinical email.
16. Recall several risk management considerations to address before implementing clinical email.
17. Discuss VoIP telecommunications.
18. Describe email encryption and its importance.
19. Analyze the professionalism questions and apply them to this chapter's content.

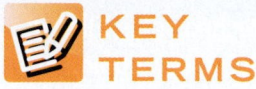

KEY TERMS

answering services

articulating

automated routing
   unit (ARU)

buffer words

cellular phones

clinical email

electronic mail (email)

encryption

enunciation

fax (facsimile)

Good Samaritan laws

jargon

modulated

screening

smartphone

Uniform Resource
   Locator (URL)

Voice over Internet
   Protocol (VoIP)

ATTRIBUTES OF PROFESSIONALISM

Communication

- Did you introduce yourself? Did you identify the patient through name and birth date or other identifying feature?
- Did you listen to and acknowledge the patient?
- Did you speak at the patient's level of understanding?
- Did you provide appropriate responses/feedback?
- Did you respond honestly and diplomatically to the patient's concerns?
- Did you demonstrate empathy in communicating with patients, family, and staff?
- Did you apply active listening skills?

Presentation

- Were you courteous, patient, and respectful to the patient?
- Did you display a positive attitude?
- Did you display a calm, professional, and caring manner?

Competency

- Did you pay attention to detail?
- Did you display sound judgment?
- Did you remain calm in a crisis?
- Did you recognize the importance of local, state, and federal legislation and regulations in the practice setting?

Initiative

- Did you assist coworkers when appropriate?

Integrity

- Did you work within your scope of practice?
- Did you demonstrate sensitivity to patients' rights?
- Did you protect and maintain confidentiality?
- Did you immediately report any error you had made?
- Did you maintain your moral and ethical standards?

SCENARIO

At a busy two-provider family physician's clinic, the telephone lines are rarely quiet. Yet administrative medical assistant Ellen Armstrong has learned to maintain her composure when she is responsible for managing incoming calls. Ellen has in her favor a naturally warm telephone manner, but she has had to cultivate other traits so that she can represent the practice in a professional manner, help patients and other callers feel at ease, and efficiently screen or refer calls as necessary.

Ellen has researched the three different types of Voice over Internet Protocol (VoIP) services and understands the security issues related to this type of service. Other telecommunication technologies new to Ellen include HIPAA requirements associated with facsimile (fax) machines and the use of encryption for electronic mail used in the clinic. Ellen feels organized and prepared to implement her newly acquired skills in telecommunications. To stay abreast of new telecommunication technologies, Ellen attends conferences and seminars to learn how emerging technology can be used effectively in the medical clinic.

INTRODUCTION

As in many clinic settings, the telephone is the lifeline of the ambulatory care setting. By means of telecommunication, which can also include fax, wireless technology, and email transmissions, patient appointments are scheduled, referrals made, critical information related, and the practice personality conveyed.

Medical assistants, more multiskilled than ever, have a wealth of knowledge to bring to telecommunications. Over the telephone, they welcome new patients, reassure current patients, collaborate with other organizations on patient care, and calmly and efficiently deal with emergencies. They will need to draw on their resource of administrative and clinical knowledge; they will also need to cultivate a telephone personality that is warm and accessible while also being efficient and organized.

In this chapter, medical assistants will come to understand the principles basic to successful telecommunications, whether initiating or answering calls; will learn the extent and limits of their authority as medical assistants; will discover how to prepare themselves for making or receiving calls; and will be introduced to telephone systems and new technologies.

TELECOMMUNICATIONS IN THE ELECTRONIC HEALTH RECORD ENVIRONMENT

EHR Electronic health records (EHR) are the wave of the future. A total practice management system (TPMS) permits patients to schedule and manage their appointments, send secure messages to their care team, view lab results, request medication refills, and view a summary of

SPOTLIGHT ON CERTIFICATION

RMA Content Outline

- Human relations
- Patient education
- Medical secretarial–administrative medical assistant
- Oral and written communications
- Use of email applications

CMA (AAMA) Content Outline

- Professionalism
- Adapting communication according to an individual's needs
- Professional communication and behavior
- Receiving, organizing, prioritizing, and transmitting information
- Telephone techniques
- Legislation
- Equipment operation
- Releasing medical information

CMAS Content Outline

- Legal and ethical considerations
- Clinic communications
- Professionalism
- Medical clinic clinical assisting
- Medical records management
- Medical clinic information processing

their medical information. Many medical clinics are still using the telecommunications skills applicable to the paper environment or are implementing computerized approaches one area at a time.

BASIC TELEPHONE TECHNIQUES

Telephone answering techniques are rapidly changing in all clinics, even the smaller single-provider practices. The medical assistant responsible for answering the telephones previously was the first contact most people had with the practice, but today the first contact is usually with an automated phone system. Just as with a human answering the phone, first impressions are lasting. The program setup in the automatic phone system should be user friendly. It is not uncommon for a person unfamiliar with a menu-driven telephone system to be unable to find the menu that applies, and it is extremely frustrating if the person cannot find a way to connect with a human operator. An option to speak with an administrative medical assistant should always be offered. An automatic answering system should begin with a message instructing the caller what to do if the call is an emergency. In most locations, the caller is instructed to hang up and dial 911. After this should be a list of menus for such items as prescription refill, billing, scheduling an appointment, and so forth. If at all possible, the menu system should only be one level deep; for example, the billing selection should not lead to another menu for Medicare, HMO, or other finance categories.

Regardless of whether the automated system or a medical assistant makes first contact with the caller, at some point the medical assistant will speak with the caller. The impression the patient forms of the practice will depend on your telephone personality and how you answer incoming calls. To create a positive impression, answer the telephone by the end of the first ring and certainly within three rings. If your station has more than one incoming line, it may be necessary to interrupt a conversation to answer another call. Some guidelines to follow in this instance include:

- Excuse yourself to the first caller by saying, "Excuse me, another line is ringing. May I put you on hold for a moment?" This may be done only once, not repeatedly during the conversation.
- When, and not before, the first caller has given permission to be put on hold, answer the second call. Determine who is calling and the nature of the call. If it is not an emergency and permission is given, place the caller on hold. Never try to quickly resolve the second call before returning to the first call.
- Return to the first caller and thank the person for holding.
- Explore the possibility of an automated message after three rings to put the calls into a waiting queue with a message that you are on another line and will answer the next call momentarily.

Telephone Personality

First impressions are usually conveyed through verbal and nonverbal communication (see Chapter 5 for a review of these communication modes.) In telephone communications, however, personality and attitudes are conveyed only through the tone in which words are spoken and the words themselves. Remember, callers are not an interruption of your work but the reason for your job. Even in a large practice, it is rare that someone just answers the telephone and has no other duties. No matter what other duties are pressing, the primary responsibility of every employee in a medical clinic is patient care; everything else is secondary. Whoever answers incoming calls should be prepared to give the caller their complete attention.

Use a voice that is pleasant and well **modulated** (i.e., one that varies in pitch and intensity) and conveys interest in the caller's needs. Hold the handpiece correctly, about 1 to 2 inches away from the mouth, and project your voice *at* the mouthpiece, not *over* it. The use of headsets permits the mouthpiece to be positioned appropriately and frees the hands to locate and record information easily.

Volume, enunciation, pronunciation, and speed all have a profound effect on how you sound to the person on the other end of the line.

- Volume should be the same as when speaking conversationally.
- **Enunciation** implies speaking your words clearly and **articulating** carefully.
- Pronunciation involves saying the words correctly.
- Speed should be at a normal rate, neither too fast nor too slow. Err on the side of speaking more slowly.

Posture, the way the body is carried, also affects the voice. If slumped in a chair, the diaphragm (the muscle separating the abdominal and thoracic cavities) is compressed and breathing may be restricted. Using the headset speaker with the phone promotes good ergonomic position because it decreases neck and shoulder stress by allowing you to sit up straight (Figure 12-1). If you are less tired and tense, you can focus more easily on professional alertness, which comes across to the caller in the sound of your voice.

Being organized and prepared in advance for each telephone call enables the medical assistant to respond to each caller as if there is nothing else to do. A pleasant vocal impression can be delivered by taking a deep breath and putting on a smile before answering the call.

Medical assistants who enjoy their work and want to be of assistance to patients communicate enthusiasm. Enthusiasm conveys interest in the caller and projects a sincere, caring attitude that can be "heard" over the telephone (Figure 12-2).

 Though some callers will be upset, frightened, or even angry, the medical assistant must always be patient and in control. Some calls may be life-threatening emergencies; medical assistants need to remain calm to be of help to the caller, remembering their professional role as health care providers.

Professional Telephone Etiquette

 Telephone etiquette, as with all good manners, simply involves treating others with consideration. Medical assistants have chosen a profession in which care and concern for others are paramount, so it is especially important to keep the patient's feelings in the forefront at all times. Basic telephone courtesies should be kept in mind when answering any professional call.

Answering Incoming Calls

Most calls received in an ambulatory care setting are from patients or prospective patients, but some are from other providers or medical facilities. The remaining incoming calls are from family members, salespeople, and miscellaneous others. Personal calls should not be permitted in the medical clinic because the busy lines are intended for business. Occasional personal emergency calls are appropriate.

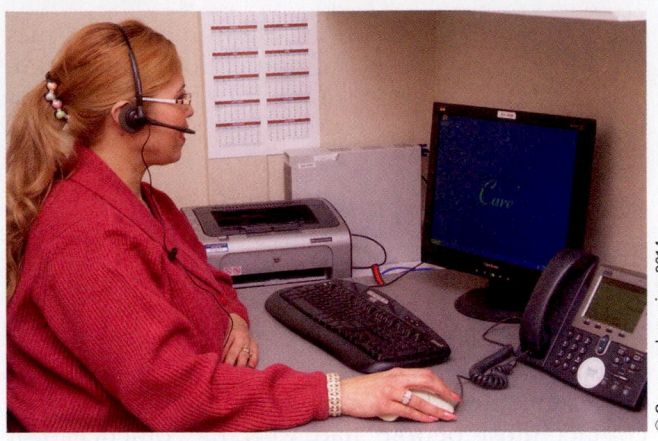

© Cengage Learning 2014

Figure 12-1 The headset-type telephone frees the medical assistant's hands to document and record while maintaining an ergonomic position.

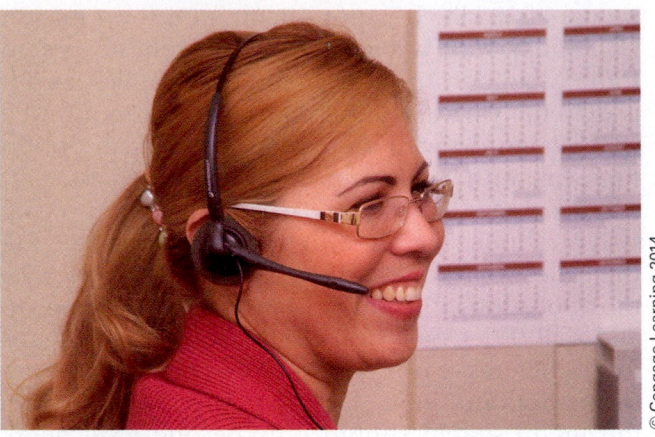

© Cengage Learning 2014

Figure 12-2 Tone of voice can put callers at ease during a telephone conversation.

Preparing to Take Calls. Before answering incoming calls or making outgoing calls, medical assistants should devise a simple system to keep organized throughout the hectic day of telephone communications. If the reception desk is computerized, the first step is to boot up the computer and prepare ready access to the scheduling, patient demographics, and note screens. Figure 12-3 illustrates a scheduling screen from the Medical Clinic Simulation Software (MOSS). If the reception desk is not computerized, collect materials such as message pads, the master schedule book, and prescription refill request forms. Regardless of whether the reception desk is computerized, a list of frequently used telephone numbers and clinic extensions and a supply of sharpened pencils and working pens are needed. A handy reference to

TELEPHONE COURTESIES

- Always use callers' names and titles (e.g., Mrs. O'Keefe or Dr. King) during the course of a conversation when confidentiality is assured; this shows interest in them as individuals.

- Do not use technical terms if simpler ones will convey the information adequately. Using professional jargon, or terminology, is an easy trap to fall into because this terminology is used daily with coworkers. Jargon only confuses people outside the profession; the goal in communication is mutual understanding.

- Do not use slang or nonstandard terms in a business setting. Slang terms may have entirely different meanings to individuals from another generation or cultural background. However, patients may use slang in their communications. It is important not to be offended by slang terms; also, be certain that patients who use slang understand any common medical terminology you may use.

- The "hold" button on the telephone is probably the most misused piece of equipment in the practice; always use it sparingly. Never put a caller on hold until you know who is calling and why. Never place an urgent or emergency call on hold. Never put a caller on hold without asking for and receiving permission to do so. No call should be left unattended for more than 20 to 30 seconds. If it is necessary to keep callers waiting longer, go back to the caller and give the option of continuing to hold or receiving a call back in a few minutes.

- When it is necessary to get additional information and call back later, let the person know when to expect the call. If for some reason the information is not available when the time for the call back arrives, call anyway to let the person know when to expect another call.

- When taking a message for someone in the clinic, give the caller an idea of when to expect a return call. If the person will be out of the clinic for an extended period, see if someone else can help or if the caller would rather wait to hear from that specific individual. Never promise to have someone call back when you cannot control if or when this will happen.

- Pay attention to what the person is saying and how they sound. Do not interrupt or finish sentences for slow talkers. The caller may have difficulty putting some things into words, but give the person a chance to explain the problem or question. Listen with empathy for the caller. Also listen to what the tone of voice expresses.

- Never talk to someone in the clinic while on an open line. This is confusing to the caller, and confidential information could be inadvertently overheard.

- Do not attempt to work on other things while talking on the telephone.

- Never eat or chew gum when talking on the telephone. This impedes enunciation and is distracting to the caller.

- Say "good-bye" when closing the call, and allow the caller to hang up first.

practice protocols would be helpful, as would a supply of new patient registration forms, release of information, and confidentiality information forms required by HIPAA.

Answering Calls. When answering incoming calls, the name of the facility should be clearly identified, as well as the name of the person with whom the caller is speaking. The name of the clinic is important because the caller wants to know the correct number has been reached. To avoid clipping off the clinic name, practice using **buffer words**. Buffer words are expendable words and may consist of introductory words, phrases, or statements such as "Good morning." They allow a caller to realize they have reached the desired number and to collect his or her thoughts.

Obtain the caller's full name and correct spelling, and ask if this is an emergency call. Ask for the caller's telephone number, street address, and date of birth (DOB). This information is necessary for retrieval of the caller's correct medical chart. Determine how you can be of assistance, and

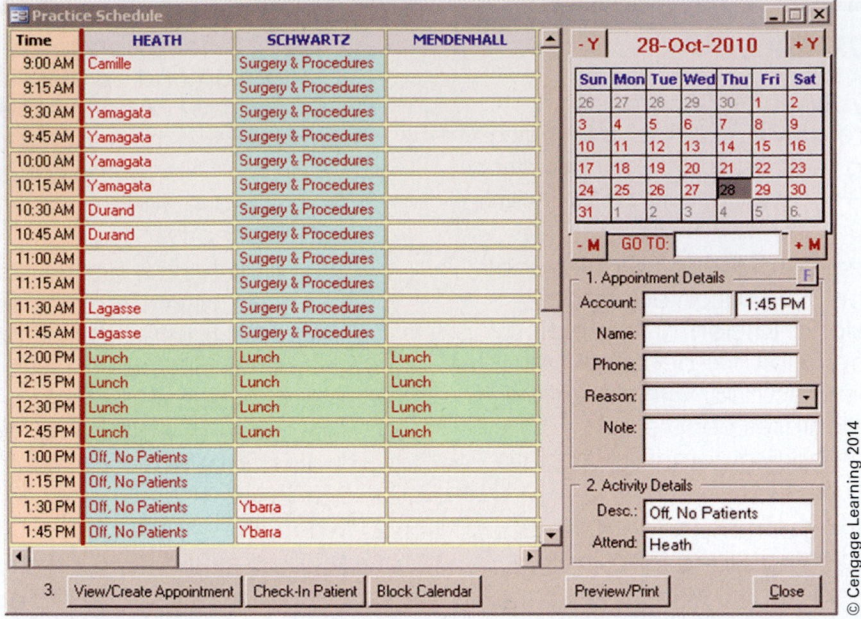

Figure 12-3   Scheduling screen from MOSS.

complete the call efficiently by following all established clinic protocols.

Screening Calls.
One of the medical assistant's responsibilities is to screen incoming calls. The purpose of screening is twofold: (1) to be sure the caller talks to the person who will be most helpful (this is not necessarily the person asked for); and (2) to ensure the provider's time with calls is efficiently managed.

Many people who call an ambulatory care setting will ask to speak to the provider. Patients calling for appointments or with billing problems or insurance questions will sometimes ask to speak to their provider, assuming he or she is the person in charge, and therefore should answer any question or solve any problem. In most practices, this is not the case. Medical assistants and other administrative employees are equipped to deal with administrative functions; usually, providers are not involved in these procedures and sometimes may not be aware of administrative routines.

Screening Techniques. Screening is usually a simple process of asking the caller's name and the reason for the call. There are situations, however, that will require tactful persistence to get the information needed to properly direct the caller. Sometimes callers hesitate to give information because the questions are of a confidential and possibly even embarrassing nature.

Occasionally, a caller flatly refuses to give any information or will just say, "I'm a friend." If it is a patient who refuses to give information after gentle prodding, respect the patient's privacy and take a message. If you do not know who the caller is and you are unable to get any information, take the message and give it to the provider. If the provider does not know the person, he or she can decide whether to return the call. In any event, do not argue with the caller. Be polite and professional at all times. Procedure 12-1 provides steps for answering and screening calls.

Transferring a Call.
During the screening process, calls may mistakenly be directed to someone who is unable to assist the caller adequately. This call will need to be transferred to someone with more expertise in a particular area. Guidelines that ensure successful transfer of calls include:

- Get the caller's full name, telephone number, and any other situation-associated information before attempting to transfer the call.

- Determine who would be the best person to assist with this situation.

- Ask if you may place the caller on hold while you collect any pertinent data and make a call to confirm that the person best suited to assist is available.

- Return to the caller, thank him or her for holding, and give the name and extension of the person to whom you will be transferring the call.
- Follow your telephone system's procedure for transferring the call.
- Follow up to be sure the call transferred correctly.

Taking a Message. When taking messages, it is advisable to use a standard telephone message pad with a carbonless copy that allows the clinic to maintain a record of all incoming calls or the appropriate TPMS screen (Figure 12-4). The information that should be recorded for *every* message includes:

1. Date and time call is received
2. Who the call is for
3. Caller's name, telephone number, and DOB
4. When the caller can be reached
5. Nature and urgency of the call
6. Action to be taken (e.g., will call back, returned your call, please call back)
7. Message, if any
8. Your name or initials (in case there are questions)

Be sure to repeat the information back to the caller to verify that you have heard and copied it correctly. When taking a message, give callers an approximate time when they might expect to receive a call back if there is an established policy and all staff understand and follow that policy. ("Dr. King will be returning calls between 4:30 and 5:00." "Ellen is out of the clinic today, but I'll ask her to call you before 10 AM tomorrow.")

 Always attach a message from a patient to the patient's chart before placing the message on the provider's desk. The provider

cannot discuss the patient's condition or answer questions without this information. Clinics using TPMS can send and receive messages via the computer and can have immediate access to the EMR. Procedure 12-2 identifies the steps and rationales in taking a telephone message.

Ending the Call. Ending the telephone call is as important as answering the call promptly. Bring the conversation to a courteous close and repeat any pertinent information back to the caller. ("Your appointment is scheduled for Friday, January 12, at 9 AM with Doctor King.") Pause just a moment to see if the caller has any additional questions. If not, say "Good-bye." Never use slang terms such as *bye-bye, see you later,* or *so long.* These terms do not reflect a positive professional image. You should always stay on the line until the caller hangs up. The caller might think of something else he or she wanted to ask or verify, and staying on the line gives the caller the opportunity to verbalize a thought rather than having to call back.

ROUTING CALLS IN THE MEDICAL CLINIC

The administrative medical assistant staffing the reception desk is responsible for greeting each patient, whether in person or via telephone, with a warm, friendly response. Incoming calls in the

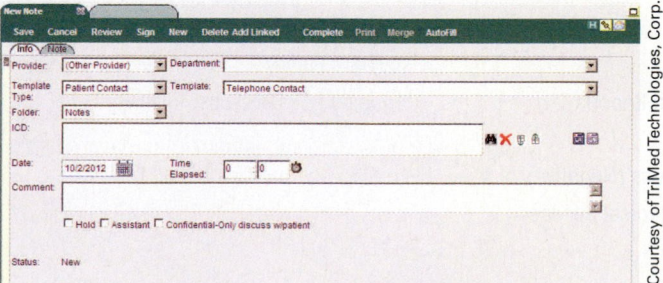

Figure 12-4A   An electronic message template.

Courtesy of TriMed Technologies, Corp.

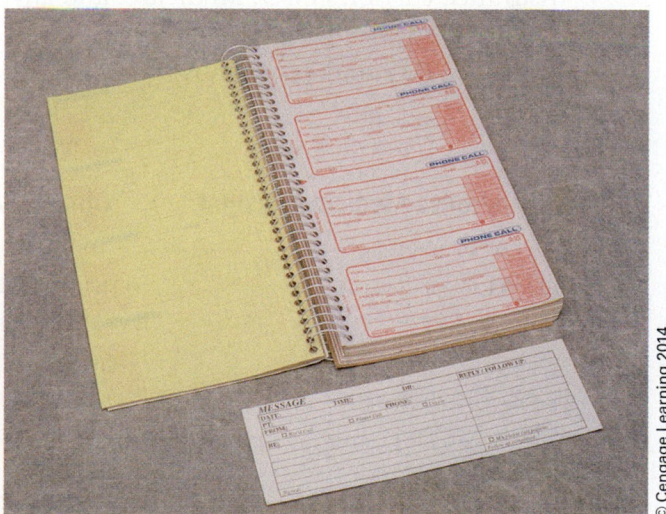

© Cengage Learning 2014

Figure 12-4B   Message pads with a carbonless copy allow the clinic to maintain a written record of all incoming calls.

medical clinic typically are routed by the administrative medical assistant according to subject and who can best respond. The administrative medical assistant, as well as clinical medical assistants, must always follow the provider-approved protocols when screening and responding to telephone calls. Figure 12-5 illustrates examples of routing calls in the medical clinic.

Types of Calls the Medical Assistant Can Take

Keep in mind that, no matter how experienced, the medical assistant has definite limitations of authority and knowledge. Most calls can be handled by the knowledgeable medical assistant, but there are situations that only the provider should manage simply because the provider ultimately is responsible for what happens in the practice. Examples of calls the administrative or clinical medical assistant can take are as follows:

1. *Established patients.* When an established patient calls to set up an appointment, record the patient's name, daytime telephone number, and the reason for the appointment.

2. *New patients.* Require the same information as the established patient plus some additional information, including:
   - Address
   - Age/DOB
   - Employer
   - Insurance carrier, HMO, Medicare, and any secondary insurance
   - Insurance ID numbers of subscriber

- Name of insured (self, spouse, or parent)
- Name of referral source

This information serves as a source for the establishment of the chart and may lead to a discussion regarding payment of fees. Information for both new and established patients should be entered into the TPMS or appointment book if not a computerized clinic.

3. *Scheduling appointments.* A major portion of telephone communications is spent scheduling patient appointments. (See Chapter 13 for detailed information on patient scheduling and rescheduling).

4. *Scheduling patient tests.* Scheduling tests for patients can involve a great deal of coordination. Often appointment times need to be arranged among providers, the patient, and the facility where a test may be conducted.

5. *Billing questions.* Billing questions can be involved and complex, and medical assistants should be prepared to answer questions by retrieving information on the patient's insurance and billing status.

6. *Insurance information.* Calls will come from patients about insurance, as well as from insurance carriers and HMOs with questions about patients or their treatment. Prior to responding to insurance carrier requests for patient records, authenticate that the call is from the carrier using established clinic protocols and ensure that a signed release of information form is on file.

7. *Requests for prescription refills.* If a patient or family member is requesting that a prescription be refilled, medical assistants may take the call.

Administrative Medical Assistant	Clinical Medical Assistant	Provider
Scheduling Appointments	Scheduling Tests and Procedures	Other Providers
Changing Appointments	Prescription Refills	STAT Reports
Cancelling Appointments	Progress Reports	Provider's Family
Fees and Billing Questions	Radiological and Lab Reports	Request for Test Results (Positive)
Insurance Questions	Patient Referrals	
Information Requests	Request for Test Results (Negative)	
General Questions about Practice	Complaints about Medical Service	
Salespeople	Salespeople	

Figure 12-5 Routing calls in the medical clinic.

However, they may not authorize a refill or tell the patient that a prescription will be refilled without the provider's approval. Most clinics ask that the patient call their refill requests directly into the pharmacy; the pharmacy then calls or faxes the provider's clinic for approval. Messages taken on these calls should be attached to the patient's chart or entered into the TPMS and given to the provider for review and for permission to refill. When the provider approves the refill, the pharmacy may be called with an approval. Some practice protocols give authority to the CMA and RMA to refill standard medications with appropriate guidelines, for example, oral contraceptives and blood pressure medications, among others.

 Procedure 12-3 identifies the steps for calling a pharmacy to refill an authorized prescription.

8. *Receiving routine progress reports.* Frequently, providers will ask patients to report on their progress. *If the patient is doing well,* it is acceptable for the medical assistant to take that information on a message form or enter the message into the patient's EMR.

9. *General information about the practice.* People may call requesting information about hours, location, financial protocols, or areas of practice.

10. *Salespeople.* The medical clinic should have policies regarding the scheduling of pharmaceutical and medical supply representatives.

EHR Today, many medical clinics take advantage of options offered through their computerized TPMS when responding to telephone calls. The medical assistant will screen calls and forward messages to other personnel as "tasks." These tasks or messages can go back and forth between administrative and clinical medical assistants as necessary, or they may include the provider if his or her professional judgment is required to handle the call. An example of this screening procedure is as follows: (1) The administrative medical assistant answers a call from a patient wishing to have a prescription refilled. (2) The administrative medical assistant collects all of the pertinent information and sends a message to the clinical medical assistant. (3) When checking the patient's chart, the clinical medical assistant sees there are no additional refills authorized by the provider.

(4) The clinical medical assistant forwards the pertinent information to the provider. (5) The provider, having complete access to the EMR of the patient, authorizes the refill, documents the order, and sends the notice to the clinical medical assistant. (6) The clinical medical assistant calls or sends a fax to the pharmacy to authorize the prescription refill.

Types of Calls Referred to the Provider

Providers have many demands on their time: surgeries, hospital rounds, patient appointments, documentation, and consultations with other providers, to name a few. Therefore, their time is extremely valuable, and misuse of time impacts the clinic in many ways. It is important to carefully screen calls going to providers to ensure that they receive only the calls that are necessary.

Examples of calls that should be referred to the provider include the following:

1. *Other providers.* When other providers call, always ask if they need to speak to the provider immediately or if they would like a call back. Be sure to ask if the call is regarding a specific patient; if so, attach a message to the chart.

2. *STAT reports.* In most cases the provider will only initiate STAT reports when the results are needed immediately.

3. *Provider's family.* Most providers will have an established protocol related to calls from family members. Family members generally do not call unless it is necessary, so in most cases their calls are put through directly.

EHR Many other calls coming into the clinic may require the provider's professional judgment. Generally the majority of these calls can be handled with the TPMS task/message feature. When the provider has a minute between patients, he or she can respond or provide specific instructions.

CRITICAL THINKING

Discuss other appropriate ways to handle the Example: Calls to Other Facilities.

EXAMPLE: CALLS TO OTHER FACILITIES

Herb Fowler needs to have a glucose tolerance test done at the laboratory next door and needs to make an appointment in your clinic for one week after the test is done.

Poor Technique

Medical Assistant: Mr. Fowler, you need to call Johnston Labs to arrange for those tests. We'll see you after the tests are done.

Correct Technique

Medical Assistant: Mr. Fowler, Dr. King has ordered a glucose tolerance test for you with Johnston Laboratory in Suite 516 of this building. Since you are working, we felt it would be better to have you call them yourself to make the appointment. If you have a paper and pencil, I'll give you the information you need.

The lab is open from 6:30 AM to 7 PM Monday through Friday. The phone number is (800) 555-1234 and you should ask for Susan at Extension 23; she makes the appointments. She will need your name, address, phone number, age, Social Security number, the name and address of your insurance company, and your insurance ID and Plan numbers.

After you make your appointment with Susan, please call me back so we can make an appointment for you here for one week later. Dr. King will have your test results by then and will want to go over them with you at that time.

Do you have any questions or do you need any of the information repeated? Fine, I'll speak to you after you talk to Susan and we'll set up your appointment with Dr. King.

Special Consideration Calls

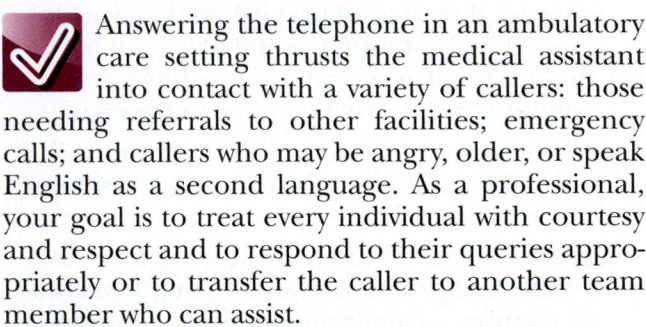 Answering the telephone in an ambulatory care setting thrusts the medical assistant into contact with a variety of callers: those needing referrals to other facilities; emergency calls; and callers who may be angry, older, or speak English as a second language. As a professional, your goal is to treat every individual with courtesy and respect and to respond to their queries appropriately or to transfer the caller to another team member who can assist.

Referral Calls to Other Facilities. If it is necessary to refer the caller to someone outside the clinic, such as to a laboratory or another provider, be sure to tell the caller:

- Why he or she should speak to someone else
- The telephone number to call (be sure to include the area code and extension)
- Who, specifically, to speak with at that number
- What information to have ready when he or she makes the call
- When to call
- If you would like a call back after the other contact is made

Review the example of calls to other facilities.

 Emergency/Urgent Calls. The medical assistant must be careful when handling emergency or urgent calls to ensure that he or she works within the scope of his or her education and training. Donald A. Balassa, JD, MBS, Executive Director and Legal Counsel for the AAMA, states: "Procedures which constitute the practice of medicine, or which state law specifically delegates to licensed professionals to perform, may not be delegated to unlicensed professionals such as medical assistants." Therefore, prior to screening calls the medical assistant should always direct the caller to call 911 if the caller believes they may be experiencing a life-threatening emergency. Every attempt should be made to obtain the caller's name and telephone number before assisting with making the 911 call if it appears the person is confused or unable to dial for himself or herself.

Screening is the act of evaluating the urgency of a medical situation and prioritizing the call. Telephone screening is one of the most important functions for the person answering the telephone. Telephone screening requires skill and experience. An urgent condition is one that requires medical intervention that can be handled in a timely manner at an ambulatory care center.

To determine if a call is truly a medical emergency, keep a list of provider-approved questions near the telephone to assist in evaluating the situation. Standard screening questions can determine the nature of an emergency. Not all questions are appropriate to every call; suitable questions depend on the nature of the situation. Screening questions to ask may include:

- What happened?
- Who is the patient? (Ask name and age.)
- Is the patient breathing?
- Is there bleeding? How much? From where?
- Is the patient conscious?
- What is the patient's temperature?
- If the patient ingested something:
  - What did the patient take?
  - How much?
  - Are there poison or overdose instructions on the bottle?

Screening does not only pertain to emergency calls. Screening techniques can also help determine when a patient with symptoms should be seen by asking the caller questions such as:

- How long have you had the symptoms?
- Is there any fever?
- Are you taking any medications?

This information helps determine whether an appointment should be scheduled immediately or if it can wait a few days.

 The practice should periodically review procedures for handling emergency/urgent calls. If an clinic situation involves a great deal of telephone screening, the staff should enroll in an advanced first-aid course. This will enable all participants to more accurately give instructions or to handle these calls if there is no provider in the clinic at that moment. In-service training provided by the providers is a great tool to make telephone screening run smoothly. Remember, you should only render aid *within the areas of your training and expertise*. **Good Samaritan laws** do not cover paid employees, only uncompensated situations. All ambulatory settings should also post a list of numbers to be used in case of emergencies, such as the poison control telephone number (see Chapter 9 for more information on screening).

Angry Callers.
Medical assistants will probably have occasion to speak with callers who are upset or angry. Although these calls eventually may need to be referred to the clinic manager or the provider, medical assistants need techniques for managing problem calls.

 The first priority is to defuse the situation. This cannot be accomplished if you become upset or angry. As a professional, it is important to remain calm and in control at all times.

Like most skills, defusing a difficult situation becomes easier with practice (see Procedure 12-4).

Older Adult Callers.
Several issues may arise when dealing with older adult patients, such as impaired hearing, confusion, and an inability to understand procedures or technical information.

Do not assume that all older adults are senile or hard of hearing. This is a dangerous pitfall into which many people stumble.

If the individual has a hearing impairment, speak more slowly, more clearly, and a little louder than normal. Do not shout. If uncertain that the person has heard everything, ask if there are any questions, or ask the person to repeat information back to you.

If the person has difficulty understanding you, simplify the information, ask frequently if there are any questions, and try to explain in simple, concrete terms. At times, if it is difficult to communicate with an older adult patient, someone from the patient's family should be given certain information. Discuss this option with the clinic manager or provider first, and be sure signed documentation is on file.

English as a Second Language Callers.
 In any ambulatory care setting, it is possible to have contact with many patients whose primary language is not English.

It is extremely helpful to have at least one person in the clinic who is bilingual. For the nonbilingual medical assistant, certain techniques may help when communicating with all but totally non-English speaking patients.

- A patient who does not *speak* fluent English may still *understand* as well as anyone. Do not assume that individuals with strong accents cannot understand you.
- Speak at a normal volume; raising the voice does not increase the other person's ability to comprehend.
- If the other person has difficulty understanding, speak more slowly. Avoid complicated words when simple ones will express the meaning just as well.

- Ask the person if clarification is needed. Be willing to review the information again.
- Be patient.

If these techniques are not successful, it is the responsibility of your provider–employer to supply an interpreter.

TELEPHONE DOCUMENTATION

Requests for medical information over the telephone should be discouraged. A provider or facility that needs the information to treat the patient usually places an emergency request. A call-back verification procedure should be implemented for this type of request. Request the caller's name and telephone number, and state that you will call back with the necessary information. Then call back to verify the identity of the caller and provide or fax the information. It is important to follow this procedure during routine telephone interchanges that take place between facilities/provider clinics and laboratories seeking test results or consult findings.

All telephone requests for medical information should be documented either in a log reserved for that purpose or in the patient's medical record. This information is important to protect yourself and the medical practice in case of litigation. Documentation includes the following:

- Date of the request
- Name of the requestor
- The information requested
- Patient's name (and patient number)
- Name of the treating provider
- The information released
- To whom the call was referred (if applicable)

When a patient telephones the clinic to request prescription refills, is displeased with medical treatment, or expresses some form of a complaint, documentation of the call should always be recorded in the medical chart. Follow established clinic protocols when handling each and every telephone call. Document every call you have with a patient including all pertinent information.

USING TELEPHONE DIRECTORIES

The medical assistant should have on hand in the clinic a variety of print and online telephone directories and be skilled in their use. The telephone directory contains an organized, accurate, and complete listing of the name, address, zip code, and area code with telephone number for most individuals with telephone service. Often, the pages within the directory are color-coded; residences are listed on white pages, business numbers on blue pages, and advertisements on yellow pages. The front pages of many directories contain other useful information such as:

- Information that provides emergency and nonemergency numbers.
- The Internet guide makes it easy to get online.
- Information guide and consumer tips provide a variety of free facts and answers about the things you want to buy and the services you need.
- Community pages provide attractions, events, and the general-interest information unique to a particular area. Often, maps are provided on these pages.
- Phone service pages answer questions you may have regarding your phone service.
- Government pages contain information about county, state, tribal, and federal government clinics, as well as information regarding public schools and voter registration information.
- An index makes finding what you need easy.

Many metropolitan medical centers and hospitals produce another type of directory. These directories list important telephone numbers specific to that facility. Examples of information available within these directories include:

- Provider referral information
- Community education services
- Nurse counseling service/nurse line
- Main hospital/facility telephone number

- Automated operator
- TTY line for the hearing impaired
- Medical center departments
- Medical staff including department and photo of providers and their names with credentials

Some of these publications list providers no longer maintaining their active/associate privileges at the facility. Often, a map of the facility is included within the front or back pages. The large facilities also may produce supplements to maintain current information.

Many online telephone directory services are also helpful resources. Examples of these include but are not limited to the following:

http://www.yellowpages.com
http://www.dexonline.com
http://www.switchboard.com
http://www.whitepages.com
http://www.anywho.com

PLACING OUTGOING CALLS

When making calls for the medical clinic, whether to patients, health care facilities, or other providers, know what information is needed and have it at hand before making the calls. For example:

- If arranging for a patient to receive care at another facility, have the patient's health record and insurance information available. Determine provider instructions as to the diagnosis and type of care (specific tests, radiographs, and so on) that need to be ordered.
- If calling insurance companies for claim follow-up, gather copies of all claim forms in question so you can answer specific questions regarding each claim.
- If scheduling meetings or outside appointments for clinic providers, have their schedules in front of you.

Arrange to make outgoing calls from a telephone in a location that is free of distractions. If the calls concern patients (whether bills, insurance, or care), it is mandatory that the calls be made from a telephone where you cannot be overheard by other patients or people in the reception area.

Always choose a time when calls can be made without interruption. Do not make outgoing calls while covering incoming call responsibilities.

It is best to establish a routine for making various types of outgoing calls. Most clinics call the next day's patients to confirm appointments near the end of each day. Collection and insurance calls, as well as pharmacy callbacks, are usually done either before the clinic is open for patients in the morning, during the period from noon to 2 PM when the clinic is closed for lunch, or after the last patient has been seen.

PLACING LONG-DISTANCE CALLS

Most long-distance calls medical assistants make are likely to be direct dialing calls, that is, calls placed without the help of an operator. Operator-assisted calls are more costly and should be handled through other alternatives if possible. Examples of operator-assisted calls include the following:

- Person-to-person calls
- Conference calls
- International calls
- Collect calls

Conference calls may be local or long distance and are convenient for communicating or discussing information with several individuals at the same time. Each person involved in the conference call must be notified about specifics regarding the date, time, and any special instructions related to the call. Many clinics have conference call capabilities on their telephone or computer systems.

International direct distance dialing (IDDD) is available in many parts of the Unites States. Additional numbers or codes may preface the international access, country, and city codes when using IDDD. Station-to-station calls may be dialed following this sequence:

- Dial the international code 011
- Dial the country code
- Dial the city code
- Dial the local telephone number
- Press the pound sign (#) button if the telephone is touchtone

It may take up to 45 seconds after dialing any international code for the ringing to begin. The Internet posts frequent updates on international call procedures and country and city codes.

When making a long-distance call out of the area code, it is possible that a time zone change

CRITICAL THINKING

Your clinic is located in Seattle, WA, and you are calling Charleston, NC. What are some important considerations before placing the call?

may occur (Figure 12-6). When scheduling the day's calls, it is important to keep in mind the location of the call and plan accordingly. Time zones include Pacific, Mountain, Central, and Eastern times and usually span a three-hour difference. If it is noon in New York, it is 11 AM in Illinois, 10 AM in Arizona, and 9 AM in Washington state.

Many conventional telephone companies, wireless services, and Internet providers are competing for long-distance business. Judging the offers and services of long-distance companies can be a complex task, but a wise choice can save an ambulatory care setting hundreds of dollars a year or more in telephone charges. It is important to analyze the medical clinic long-distance requirements and then make comparisons among several long-distance companies. Company representatives usually are more than willing to discuss their services in light of specific needs to help you comparison shop. The decision of which service to use will usually be made by the providers and the clinic manager with feedback from all employees.

LEGAL AND ETHICAL CONSIDERATIONS

 Two of the most important issues in the medical setting are patient confidentiality and the right to privacy. Respecting the confidentiality of all patient information is a legal and ethical obligation. No information about patients is to be discussed outside the clinic, with family or friends, or with other patients. All notes that may be jotted down on paper during telephone calls must be disposed of following clinic protocols. In most cases, this means shredding the notes. Violations of confidentiality leave you and your provider open to lawsuits. More importantly, they are violations of patient trust.

When calling patients, whether to discuss treatment or finances, do so with respect for the patient's privacy at all times. The front desk is certainly not the place to make collection calls when other patients are in the reception room. Either make calls from another location or choose a time when other patients cannot overhear you. Always

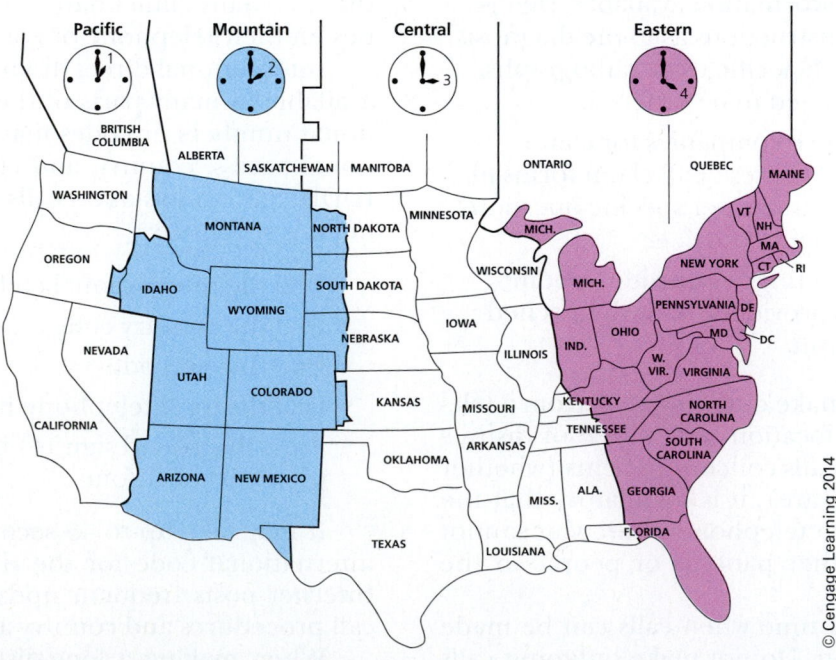

Figure 12-6 Time zone map of the United States.

© Cengage Learning 2014

be aware of the surroundings and who may be able to overhear conversations.

There are many situations when individuals will call the clinic to discuss a patient. Parents, spouses, grandparents, other relatives, significant others, employers, and friends often will have questions about a patient's condition or finances. Usually these people are asking questions out of genuine concern and a desire to help. The information they request may seem harmless, but discussing anything about a patient can turn into an ethical and legal issue (see the "Examples: Legal and Ethical Consequences of Protocol Errors" box).

To ensure patient confidentiality and practice sensible risk management, never discuss a patient with:

- The patient's spouse or family, without specific permission and a signed release

- The patient's employer
- Insurance carriers, HMOs, or attorneys without a signed release
- Credit bureau/collection agencies (reporting a patient to a credit bureau or collection agency is a violation of confidentiality)
- Other patients
- People outside the clinic (friends, family, acquaintances)

When necessary for medical or administrative reasons, you can discuss a patient with:

- Members of the clinic staff as necessary to the patient's care
- The patient's insurance carrier or HMO, if you have a signed release
- The patient's attorney (usually in accident or Workers' Compensation cases), if you have a signed release
- The patient's parent or legal guardian, except concerning issues of birth control, abortion, HIV, or sexually transmitted disease (check the laws in each state regarding minors' right to privacy)
- Another health care provider (provider, laboratory, or hospital) that is providing care to the patient under orders from the patient's provider
- Referring provider's clinic

HIPAA GUIDELINES FOR TELEPHONE COMMUNICATIONS

 The following guidelines should be followed when communicating information to patients by telephone:

- Determine whether the patient has requested confidential communications. Specific instructions should be provided to staff members on how to determine whether the patient has requested and been granted special conditions for keeping communications with the medical practice confidential.
- If the patient has not requested confidential communication, the patient should simply be called at the standard phone number contained in his or her records. If the patient has requested confidential communications and has provided an alternative telephone

EXAMPLES: LEGAL AND ETHICAL CONSEQUENCES OF PROTOCOL ERRORS

Situation 1

A medical assistant called the home of a patient inquiring about the delinquent status of his account. The patient was not home, but his wife answered the phone. The medical assistant discussed the situation with the patient's wife, who wanted to know what the charges were for. On checking the file, it was discovered the patient had been tested for a sexually transmitted disease.

Situation 2

A patient's employer calls to find out "how Boris is doing and when he can come back to work. We really miss that guy!" The medical assistant, who just saw Boris in the reception area yesterday, responds without thinking, "Oh, he seems to be doing great, I'll bet you'll have him back in a few days." If he or she had checked the patient chart, he or she might have seen that Boris was filing a disability claim, as well as a negligence suit against the employer for unsafe working conditions. The medical assistant might also have seen that Boris is still in physical therapy and on pain medication, or that he may have permanent problems as a result of the accident.

number, care should be taken to ensure that only the alternative number is called.

- The caller should identify himself or herself by name and say that he or she is an employee of the medical practice (use the complete official name of the practice).

- If the patient is not available, it is acceptable to leave a live or recorded message asking the patient to return the call. Leave the telephone number, and if the medical practice is returning a call made by the patient, it is acceptable to state this in the message that is left for the patient. However, it is important that the message does not contain any medical information or mention the purpose of the call. Never leave a message containing test results.

- When the patient is contacted, it is acceptable to discuss his or her medical information over the telephone. It is critical, however, that test results and other protected health information (PHI) *not* be given to anyone other than the patient or a person designated as the patient's representative.

AMERICANS WITH DISABILITIES ACT (ADA)

The ADA requires that communication procedures are available for persons with disabilities. Combined with HIPAA requirements, this presents a challenging situation in dealing with patients who are deaf or hearing impaired. The act requires that health care providers give effective communication alternatives using auxiliary aids and services that ensure that communication to people with hearing loss is equal to others without this disability. This includes patients as well as caregivers of patients, guardians, or spouses.

Alternative devices or services include interpreters for individuals with a language problem, assistive hearing devices, note takers for individuals who have difficulty writing, written materials, and so forth. The health care provider can choose the device as long as the result is effective communication. The patient who is deaf or hard of hearing should be consulted on which device he or she finds to be most effective. The cost of alternative devices or services cannot be billed to the patient. The expense must be charged against the overhead of the clinic or practice.

Telephone service for patients who are hearing impaired is required by the ADA. Many individuals who are hearing impaired, deaf, or speech impaired may use a teletype (TTY) or telecommunication device for the deaf (TDD). These devices transmit a keyed-in message via the telephone network just as a voice message would be sent if spoken. The recipient of the message reads the keyed-in message on the TTY's text display. A TTY or TDD device is required at both ends of the conversation in order to communicate. In addition, Internet chat capability that can replace TTY or TDD devices is readily available online.

TELEPHONE TECHNOLOGY

Though much of this chapter has been dedicated to the interpersonal nature of telephone communications, astute medical assistants will also investigate and become knowledgeable about the technology of telecommunications.

Ongoing advances in telecommunications have had a tremendous impact on how the staff of a medical clinic communicates both within the clinic and with patients, hospitals, and others outside the clinic. These advances include telephone systems with automated routing units; Voice over Internet Protocol (VoIP); electronic transmissions (fax and email); and cellular phones.

Automated Routing Units

Many hospitals and larger ambulatory care settings have **automated routing unit (ARU)** telephone systems to manage heavy telephone traffic. The system answers the call, and a recorded voice identifies departments or services the caller can access by pressing a specified number on the touch-tone telephone. If callers indicate they are having a medical emergency, the system can be programmed to immediately route calls to the medical assistant. This saves patients with immediate medical problems from waiting during busy telephone times.

Most automated telephone systems have electronic mailboxes so the caller can leave a message if the person they are calling is unavailable. In many ARU systems, selecting any of the numbered choices often gives the caller a second, third, or fourth menu of choices. If the caller does not select an option, the ARU will usually switch the call automatically to a live operator.

A disadvantage with ARU systems is that the recorded voice may be difficult to hear, especially for older adult or hearing-impaired patients. Many patients may not understand the recorded options. Clinics with an ARU system should provide to all patients an information sheet explaining their options when calling the clinic and how to get through to the clinic quickly in an emergency.

Answering Services and Machines

One responsibility of the clinic manager/medical assistant is to ensure that patient calls are answered after clinic hours, both on evenings and weekends. Although in smaller ambulatory care settings it may not be possible to have staff on telephone duty 24 hours a day, nonetheless calls must be answered and messages taken. **Answering services**—typically staffed by a live operator—and answering machines are two methods of taking calls after hours.

Many ambulatory care centers favor answering services because a live operator is reassuring to patients and other callers. These services also can provide flexibility in routing calls and locating the provider for emergencies. Typically, fees for answering services are by the month or by the number of calls.

Answering machines are convenient but perhaps less reassuring for the caller. The machine must be checked frequently for messages should an emergency occur. Sometimes, the message may leave a telephone number where the provider can be reached, but this system is likely to be cumbersome, because too many nonemergency calls may be directed to the provider. If an answering machine is used, the message often contains a number, other than the provider's, that callers can use for emergencies. That call is answered by a live operator who then screens and refers the call appropriately.

Voice over Internet Protocol (VoIP) Telecommunications

Voice over Internet Protocol (VoIP) is a rapidly growing form of telecommunication. The biggest advantages to VoIP are price and flexibility. On the surface, a VoIP phone appears to be a common telephone, but VoIP services convert a voice into a digital signal that travels over the Internet or a virtual private network. When calling a regular telephone number, the signal is converted to a regular phone signal before it reaches the destination. VoIP calls can be made directly from a computer, a special VoIP phone, or a traditional telephone connected to a special adapter any place having broadband connectivity.

Three different types of VoIP services are in common use:

- *Analog Telephone Adapter (ATA).* The ATA allows connection through a standard telephone using a computer or network connection. The ATA is an analog-to-digital converter. It takes the analog signal from a traditional phone and converts it into digital data for transmission over the network. VoIP providers usually bundle the ATAs free with their service.

- *IP Phone.* These specialized phones look just like normal telephones. They have an RJ-45 Ethernet connector in place of the standard RJ-11 telephone connectors. IP phones connect directly to the cable router with all the hardware and software included. Special WiFi phones allow making VoIP calls from any WiFi hotspot. These devices have all of the security problems associated with WiFi (see Chapter 11).

- *Computer/Computer.* This was the original VoIP form of telecommunication. Several companies offer free or very-low-cost software that can be used for this type of VoIP service. Aside from an Internet-connected computer with audio card, microphone, and speakers, nothing else is required. Except for a normal monthly ISP fee, there usually is no charge for computer/computer calls regardless of distance. This type of VoIP can be vulnerable to security problems depending on the security of the URL employed.

Most VoIP providers bundle call waiting, caller ID, three-way calling, repeat dial, return call, and call transfer with the service plan.

Some of the disadvantages of VoIP telecommunications are as follows:

- Most VoIP services do not work during power outages.
- Emergency services through 911 may not be available.
- Directory assistance/white page listings may not be available.

CRITICAL THINKING

Your clinic has just installed an automated telephone answering system. What steps might you take to aid your patients in understanding and using the system properly?

VoIP Security. Small and medium-sized organizations are increasingly adopting VoIP technology. It is predicted that most will choose to implement it over the next five years. With the increased popularity of this technology, the likelihood of attacks by cyber criminals increases. Cyber criminal attack on a VoIP service could mean the criminal eavesdrops on conversations; interferes with audio streams; or disconnects, reroutes, or even answers other people's phone calls.

VoIP is part of the Internet and is susceptible to disruption of service and SPAM just as are other Internet services. A potentially more serious security problem with VoIP, however, is eavesdropping on sensitive conversations. Hackers can eavesdrop on unprotected media streams and intercept VoIP packets to obtain sensitive information by reassembling the packets into speech. One way for hackers to do this is through a man-in-the-middle attack, where a third party spoofs the unique hardware address (MAC address) of the two speaking parties, forcing the IP packets to flow through the hackers' system. Although eavesdropping is not just a risk for VoIP telecommunications, the nature of IP networks makes access to the phone conversations much easier. Eavesdroppers no longer need to physically put a tap into a phone line; they can simply gain access from a laptop connected to the network. A hacker breaking into a VoIP data stream has access to more calls than he would with a traditional telephone wiretap. As a result, the hacker has a much greater likelihood of getting useful information by tapping a VoIP data stream than from monitoring a traditional phone system. Another security compromise possible with VoIP is the interception of a genuine call to a bank and rerouting it to a bogus bank teller.

The following are a few of the safeguards that can be used to provide in-depth protection to a VoIP system:

- Use dedicated VoIP phone instruments (having a digital certificate), not a *softphone*. A softphone uses software for making telephone calls over the Internet on a general purpose computer.
- Use a stateful packet inspection (SPI) firewall. A firewall technology ensures that all inbound packets are the result of an outbound request.
- Ensure that VoIP service providers have security in place for their internal systems.

- Update security patches for computer operating systems and VoIP software.
- Encrypt voice traffic.
- Use a virtual private network (VPN) to separate the data stream from the public Internet over which it travels. This is accomplished by connecting to a server that is set up to communicate with your device using an encrypted data flow. Any data that may be intercepted by a nearby hacker is rendered totally useless unless the encryption code is known. Most corporations use VPNs they operate, and VPN-for-hire firms are available to provide servers to small organizations and individuals. In the case of VPN-for-hire servers, the connection between your device and the Internet is secure; however, the connection between the server and your traffic's destination is not.

Facsimile (Fax) Machines

Fax machines are common in the ambulatory care settings as they are used to send reports, referrals, insurance approvals, and informal correspondence. A **fax** is a **facsimile** transmission sent over telephone lines from one fax machine to another or from a modem to a fax machine. A fax can be sent as easily as putting the document in the machine, similar to the way a document is put in a copy machine, and dialing the receiving telephone number (see Procedure 12-5). There are several advantages to using the fax machine compared with traditional postal or carrier services. These advantages are listed in Table 12-1.

There are other issues involved in using the fax, especially when sending patient information. Figure 12-7 provides insight on several legal and confidentiality issues that should be considered before sending any communications via the fax.

HIPAA requires all medical practices to implement technical measures to protect against unauthorized access to protected health information (PHI) when it is transmitted over electronic telecommunications networks. Two security measures must be addressed: the integrity of the information transmitted, and the vulnerability of the information to unauthorized use or disclosure.

When information is transmitted over public networks, static and other less benign problems can introduce errors into the information. The security rule requires the implementation

Table 12-1   Advantages of the Fax

Speed	The document is transmitted immediately or within minutes of sending.
Cost	Cost of a fax is the approximate cost of the telephone call. For long-distance faxes, this can be many times less than the cost of an overnight service.
Patient care	Patient care could be enhanced, especially in emergency situations where the receiver may need to make decisions based on information in the document.
Legality	The receiver has the "hard copy" document versus relying on verbal information if the information is needed immediately.

© Cengage Learning 2014

FAX (FACSIMILE) CONSIDERATIONS

- Before releasing medical records to other medical personnel, a signed form authorizing the release must be obtained from the patient or legal guardian.
- If it is not of utmost urgency to transmit data immediately, it should be sent by a more secure means such as carrier or mail.
- Faxed messages should be used only when the telecopiers are located in a secure area, e.g., provider offices or nursing stations rather than mail rooms or open areas, unless they are secured with passwords.
- Always use a cover sheet containing the warning: "The following material is strictly confidential; all persons are advised that they may be prosecuted under federal and state law for sharing this information with unauthorized individuals."
- Always recheck before sending the fax that the fax is being sent to the correct telephone number and that the number was entered correctly.
- After faxing, call the person who is receiving the fax and confirm that it was received.

© Cengage Learning 2014

Figure 12-7   Fax (facsimile) considerations.

of security measures to verify the integrity of the information that is transmitted.

Information transmitted over public networks may be intercepted and used by unauthorized users. In some cases, the interception can be deliberate to access sensitive information. In other instances, the interception may be the result of error by the person making the transmission. For example, a person sending a fax dials the wrong number and sends information to an unintended recipient.

The security rule requires implementation of a mechanism to encrypt PHI when appropriate. Encryption requires the cooperation of both parties to the transaction, and the encryption methods are specified in any agreement between the parties.

Electronic Mail (Email)

Electronic mail (email) is the process of sending, receiving, storing, and forwarding messages in digital form over computer networks. Email is a non–real-time method of communication—it permits us to leave a message at our convenience and allows the other person to read and respond at their convenience. Emails can be sent to multiple people at the same time, something a traditional telephone call does not allow. Keep in mind, however, that there is a professional email etiquette that must be adhered to. It is not acceptable to

forward email messages without the permission of the original author, and caution must be taken to avoid sending information that is not appropriate in a professional setting.

Composing email is similar to composing any written communication. Just as a letter or memo has a particular format, the email transmission should also follow a format style. The subject line should be brief and clearly identify the content of the email body.

If your message is in response to another piece of email, your email software probably will preface the subject line with *Re:* (for "regarding"). If your email software does not do this, it would be polite to key in "RE:". If your message is time critical, starting with "URGENT" is appropriate. If you are referring to a previous email, you should explicitly quote that document to provide context.

If a message is to be sent to several parties, individual email messages may be sent to each, thereby protecting their privacy. In many instances, however, it is useful for parties involved in a group "conversation" to be aware of who the other participants are. In this case, all of the addresses may be included on the same email message. Sending a "bcc," or blind copy, also protects the privacy of your email because it does not show to whom else the message was sent.

The body of the message should contain short and clear sentences. In trying to be brief and to the point, however, it is important to not leave out important facts or information. Remember also that some email software only understands plain text. Italics, bold, and color changes should be used sparingly. Some software recognizes **URLs (Uniform Resource Locators)** or Web site addresses in the text and make them "live." Because different software recognizes different parts of the address, if you include a URL in your email message, it is much safer to use the entire address, including the initial http://. See Figure 12-8 for additional email etiquette.

The advantages of using email as a means of communication include:

- Asynchronous communication—both parties need not be available at the same time for communication to take place
- Providers and patients can prepare, leave, read, and respond to messages at times that are convenient
- Can be used to automate certain tasks such as sending out appointment reminders or normal reports of laboratory results
- Creates a documentation trail of interactions between provider and patient
- Some patients may be more forthcoming using email than in face-to-face discussion
- Reimbursement for time spent receiving and responding to clinical email may be billed under the Online Medical Evaluation section of the Current Procedural Terminology reference (see Chapter 18). CPT code 99444 for online services provided by a physician, and code 98969 for online services by a qualified nonpnysician health care professional should be used. Phone consultations may also be billed using CPT code 98966.

The disadvantages of email communications include:

- Lack of real-time interaction and feedback
- Lack of body language or vocal inflection, which may lead to misunderstanding
- May not be suitable for time-sensitive material because determination of when the message will be delivered or read cannot be assessed

Encryption of Email. To prevent possible compromise of medical data when using email, **encryption** renders the transmission essentially secure. Encryption of email can be accomplished in several ways: The email service provider can employ TLS (transport layer security) protocol or its predecessor SSL (as defined in Chapter 11). The email will automatically be encrypted for transmission. The URL address will

EMAIL ETIQUETTE

Most organizations implement etiquette rules for the following reasons:

- Professionalism: Using correct grammar, spelling, and language conveys a professional image.
- Efficiency: Email is a more effective means of communication.
- Protection from liability: Appropriate, business-like language in all email communications limits liability risks.

Remember that an email message is not delivered with body language. A great deal of human communication comes from nonverbal signals such as facial expressions and tone of voice. These cues help make the message clearer. The following etiquette rules promote professionalism, efficiency, and protection from liability:

- Use proper structure and layout. Use short paragraphs and blank lines between each paragraph. When making points, number or bullet each point. Keep it brief, but give pertinent details.
- Do not attach unnecessary files.
- When sending attachments is necessary, tell the recipient the format of the attachment. If a large attachment must be sent, call the recipient first to be sure his or her Internet service will accept it.
- Do not overuse the high priority option.
- Do not overuse Reply to All. Use this feature only when your message needs to be received by everyone. Do not copy a message or attachment without permission. You could be infringing on copyright laws.
- Use a meaningful subject. This helps the recipient focus immediately.
- As a courtesy to your recipient, include your name at the bottom of the message. The recipient may not know that the return address belongs to you.
- Do not write anything you would not say in public.
- Do not write in CAPITALS. If you write in capitals, it seems as if you are shouting.
- Do not send Flame Emails; that is, insulting messages designed to cause pain, as when someone "gets burned."

When confidential or privileged material is sent via email, it should include a disclaimer stating that any review, retransmission, dissemination, or other use of the material is prohibited. It should also state that if the message is received in error, the recipient should contact the sender and delete the material from the computer.

© Cengage Learning 2014.

Figure 12-8   Email etiquette.

display the HTTPS prefix and a padlock icon when the email provider uses this protocol. If the provider does not use this protocol, the sender can initiate encryption by obtaining and using a digital ID. A digital ID is composed of (1) a public key, (2) a private key, and (3) a digital signature. There are different classes of digital IDs, each certifying to a different level of trustworthiness. When an encoded message is sent, the recipient's public key is used to encode the message, and the recipient uses his private key to decode the message so that it can be read. When a message is digitally signed, the digital signature and public key of the sender are added to the message. The recipient can use the sender's digital signature to verify the sender's identity, and he or she can use the sender's public key to send an encrypted email reply that only the sender can read by using his or her private key.

A digital ID can be obtained by downloading it from a certification authority's Web site (see the Microsoft Internet Explorer Digital ID site for links to certification authorities). Independent certification authorities issue digital IDs. When applying for a digital ID, the requestor's identity is verified before it is issued.

With revocation checking, the validity of a digitally signed message can be verified. When making such a check, Outlook Express requests information on the digital ID from the appropriate certification authority. The certification authority sends back information on the status of the digital ID, including whether the ID has been revoked.

To send encrypted email, the sender must have the recipient's digital ID in the sender's address book under the recipient's name. Outlook Express can automatically add digital IDs into the address book when digitally signed mail is received.

Outlook Express can be configured to automatically add a contact's digital ID to the address book by the following procedure:

1. On the *Tools* menu, click *Options*.
2. Click on the *Security* tab.
3. Click *Advanced*, and select *Add senders' certificates to my address book*.

A digital ID can be manually added to an address book by following the procedure:

1. On the *File* menu, click *Properties*.
2. Open the digitally signed message.
3. Click the *Security* tab, and then click *Add digital ID to the address book*.

When a contact has a digital ID, a red ribbon is added to their card in your address book. To add a digital ID to the address book from another source:

1. In the address book, create a new entry for the contact, or double-click an existing one in the address book list.

2. On the *Digital IDs* tab, click *Import*.
3. Find the digital ID file, and then click *Open*.

The following procedure is used to prepare, sign, and encrypt an email message:

1. Compose a message.
2. To digitally sign the message, on the *Tools* menu, click *Digitally Sign*.
3. To encrypt the message, on the *Tools* menu, click *Encrypt*.

Similar procedures are available for other email systems.

Clinical Email

Clinical email is becoming increasingly common as a means of communication between patients and their primary care provider. It is typically used for communication that is not considered urgent. Scheduling appointments, sending reminder appointment notices, providing follow-up instructions, explaining general medical information, answering questions regarding billing procedures, and refilling prescriptions are procedures handled by clinical email.

It is important to include email in your clinic's confidentiality policy. Confidentiality issues must be considered if the ambulatory care clinic sends or receives clinical email messages on a computer that can be used by more than one person. Many clinics use a privacy disclaimer to establish boundaries and ground rules for clinical email messages. The following is an example of such a disclaimer:

> This message is a privileged and confidential clinical communication intended solely for the person to whom it is addressed. If you are not the intended recipient, please be advised that any disseminating, copying, or distributing of this message is strictly prohibited. If you received this message in error, please forward it back to the sender.

CRITICAL THINKING

What legal and ethical issues should be considered when using clinical email? How might the medical facility protect its employees and the patient with regard to clinical email use?

Clinical email to or from patients should be treated the same as telephone messages or letters. That means they should be printed out and filed in the chart. It is important to remember to file both the initial message and any reply.

Before your clinic begins to use clinical email, a written agreement of understanding should be designed for signature by the patients. In addition to obtaining the patient's permission for you to use clinical email, key elements to incorporate in such an agreement may include:

- Email will be exchanged with established patients only.
- Email communication should be limited to patients within the state in which the provider is licensed to practice.
- Email from the patient will include the patient's full name and number.
- The provider is not responsible for email that is not received or responded to in a timely manner.
- Email may not be private and confidential.
- Email may be read by others, intercepted, or misaddressed.
- Email will be filed in the medical record.
- Email will not be permanently stored on the computer system.
- Urgent issues need to be handled by telephone or in person.

Legal and Ethical Issues. When using clinical email, it is important for the provider to remember that the same ethical responsibilities to patients must be adhered to as for other types of encounters. The same standard of professionalism must also be satisfied. Together with the convenience offered through email communications come some risks. Fortunately, following specific guidelines for use of clinical email can minimize risks to a level considered acceptable by many practices.

Patients who meet criteria for email correspondence established by the practice should be identified, and an informed consent form should be signed by each patient desiring this mode of communication. The form may be part of the form used for handling release of PHI. The form should provide instructions to the patient in the secure use of email, the security risks involved, practice email communication policy, the fee charged for email correspondence if any,

DOCUMENTATION

From: Elizabeth J. Parker
Sent: Tuesday, July 20, 20XX 8:55 am
To: Dr. King [King@doctor.com]
Subject: Prescription refill

Please call in a prescription refill for my thyroid medication. The pharmacy is Inner City Pharmacy and the phone number is 890-271-2600. The prescription number is RX6437350 and I have enough pills for three days_____

and a disclaimer absolving the practice in the event of patient noncompliance or technical failure in the system. The original signed form should be filed in the patient chart and a copy given to the patient for his or her records.

A procedure should be established to automatically respond to patients' email messages informing them they have been received. Patients should also be requested to respond to your messages acknowledging their receipt. An automatic receipt option is available under the tools menu of most email software.

Interactive Videoconferencing

Interactive videoconferencing consultation permits providers at remote locations to practice telemedicine and avail themselves of the services of a specialist at a large medical center, university, or teaching hospital. Using the Internet, computer, and real-time transmission of patient observations, the specialist can examine the patient as if he or she were present in the specialist's examination room. Special stethoscopes, digitized radiographs and electrocardiograms, and digital videos are examples of equipment used to provide the specialist all the information required to make a diagnosis. A technician or a physician assistant is present with the patient and performs the tests and transmits observations to be viewed by the specialist in real time. The conference is frequently recorded for future review by either the specialist or local provider.

HIPAA Care must be exercised when implementing interactive videoconferencing to ensure HIPAA compliance. The procedures outlined in Chapter 11 should be followed;

in addition, the record of the conference must be protected and erased after reports have been written. The patient must give written consent before interactive videoconferencing begins.

Cellular Service

Cellular phones, frequently called smartphones, have become increasingly popular and are now available and used in all populated areas of the country. Cellular communication offers convenient and flexible communication. **Smartphones** are available in many models and sizes and can actually be used as small computers when combined with a keyboard, pointing device, and monitor. Smartphones allow immediate verbal contact with the clinic or hospital staff.

 Cellular signals are not secure, which means that other people may be able to listen to the conversations with certain scanning radios. Therefore, staff and providers should be careful not to use patients' full names or reveal any confidential information over the cellular phone.

PROFESSIONALISM IN TELECOMMUNICATIONS

 Professionalism in telecommunications is crucial in the medical clinic environment. The way in which the telephone is answered conveys either a message of a sincere desire to help or a message of interruption. Callers expect to have the phone answered in a professional manner and their concerns addressed promptly. Forwarding calls to someone else in the clinic who is more specialized in the caller's questions area and following up to see that the situation was resolved is evidence of a responsible attitude and of being a team player. One should always be courteous and diplomatic and work within the scope of one's education, training, ability, and legal boundaries.

Remember that personal telephone calls, other than emergency calls, should be avoided during working hours. When speaking with patients or other health care members, slang terms should not be used. Never eat or chew gum while answering the telephone. When completing a call, say "goodbye" and allow the caller to hang up before you do.

Additional attributes of professionalism include using appropriate guidelines when releasing information. Confidentiality issues must always be followed, with awareness of any ethical or legal responsibilities. Documentation is mandatory for follow-up care and for any legal implications. Continuing education is important to stay on the leading edge of new technologies being implemented in the area of telecommunications.

 PROCEDURE 12-1

Answering and Screening Incoming Calls

PURPOSE:
To answer telephone calls professionally, acquiring all necessary information from the caller, documenting it correctly, and properly acting on it.

EQUIPMENT/SUPPLIES:
Telephone
Computer with message screen
Appointment book
Calendar
Message pad
Pen or pencil
Notepad

PROCEDURE STEPS:
1. Be prepared. Have materials organized and computer with message screen up. *Implement time management principles by* answering the telephone promptly. The phone should not ring more than three times before it is answered. RATIONALE: Being ready for calls conveys professionalism and lets the caller know you are prepared to give them your full attention.

continues

Procedure 12-1 (continued)

2. ***Introduce the clinic and yourself*** by answering the call with the preferred clinic greeting, speaking directly into the mouthpiece. The mouthpiece should be 1 to 2 inches away from the mouth. Sample greeting: "Good morning. Doctors Lewis and King. Ellen speaking. How may I help you?" RATIONALE: Use a pleasant tone of voice to convey a warm greeting. Holding the phone correctly and speaking directly into the mouthpiece aid the caller in hearing your message clearly.

3. Ask the name of the caller as quickly as possible, and ***use sound judgment to*** determine whether this is an emergency call. RATIONALE: Using the caller's name personalizes the call and acknowledges that you heard the name correctly. If this is an emergency call, follow emergency protocols.

4. ***Apply active listening skills.*** You may need additional information to assist or direct the call appropriately. RATIONALE: This gives the caller a sense that you are listening attentively while eliciting additional facts and assures that information will be transmitted correctly.

5. Repeat information back to the caller, ***using appropriate responses/feedback.*** RATIONALE: This technique confirms that facts are complete and accurate. The caller also has an opportunity to hear the message and confirm that it is accurate or add something to modify or clarify the message.

6. Follow established written screening protocols for all telephone calls, ***working within your scope of practice.*** RATIONALE: Assures that you understand your role in the health care practice and that all pertinent information is collected.

7. When using a multiline telephone as shown in Figure 12-9, it is helpful to keep a notepad by the telephone. When you answer the phone and have the caller's name, ***pay attention to detail*** and jot down the caller's name, which line the caller is on, and some quick notes about the content of the call. At the end of your work shift, ***protect and maintain confidentiality*** by shredding all

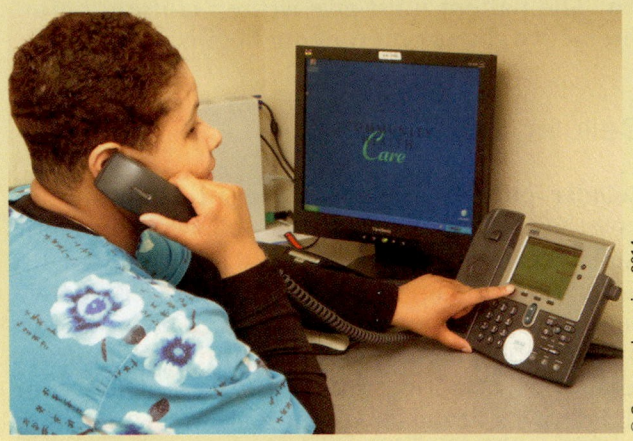

Figure 12-9 An example of a multiline telephone system.

notepapers containing PHI. RATIONALE: Using this simple technique avoids problems if another line rings and you must put the first person on hold. Reviewing your notes allows you to accurately respond to the caller. PHI must be confidential, so disposing of notepapers properly is critical for adherence to HIPAA guidelines.

8. Ask if the caller has any other questions. RATIONALE: This saves you and the caller time. It is frustrating to have to place a second call because you forgot to ask something. It also ties up the telephone lines and is not cost effective.

9. ***End the call courteously.*** Say "thank you" and "good-bye" (not "bye-bye"). Allow the caller to hang up before you disconnect. RATIONALE: Saying good-bye conveys professionalism and leaves the caller with a positive image of the clinic. Often callers think of questions just as they are ready to hang up. It is more time efficient to handle the questions immediately rather than having the caller make another call.

10. Document information and record any necessary actions. RATIONALE: This procedure is necessary for legal reasons. Remember that a deed not documented is a deed not done in a court of law.

© Cengage Learning 2014

PROCEDURE 12-2

Taking a Telephone Message

PURPOSE:
To record an accurate telephone message and follow up as required.

EQUIPMENT/SUPPLIES:
Telephone
Message pad
Black ink pen
Notepad
Medical record if available
Clock or watch

PROCEDURE STEPS:

1. Answer the telephone following the steps outlined in Procedure 12-1. RATIONALE: Being prepared and answering the phone promptly with the preferred clinic greeting prepares the medical assistant mentally to focus on the caller's needs. Using a pleasant tone of voice conveys a warm greeting.

2. Use a message pad, or document directly into the EMR. *Pay attention to detail* when requesting the following information:
   - Date and time call is received
   - Full name and correct spelling of person calling, and daytime and evening telephone numbers, including area code and extension when appropriate

   - Ask for date of birth, clinic number, or social security number to verify correct patient
   - Who the call is for
   - The reason for the call
   - The action to be taken
   - The name or initials of the person taking the call

   RATIONALE: Complete and accurate information is necessary to respond to the caller's requests efficiently.

3. Repeat the above information back to the caller. RATIONALE: To verify that the information was recorded accurately and to allow the caller to acknowledge that the message is correct.

4. If the call is from an established patient or concerns an established patient, pull the medical record/chart and attach the message to it before delivering the message to the intended individual. When using EMR save the message and forward it to the intended recipient. RATIONALE: Information about the patient is available should it be needed, and any required documentation can efficiently be made in the chart.

5. Maintain the old message book with all carbon copies intact. RATIONALE: Documents all telephone calls received by the clinic. This information could be useful in determining the need for additional telephone lines into the clinic.

PROCEDURE 12-3

Calling a Pharmacy to Refill an Authorized Prescription

PURPOSE:
To notify a pharmacy to refill an authorized prescription.

EQUIPMENT/SUPPLIES:
Patient's chart
Provider authorization to refill prescription
Drug name, dosage, and instructions for when and how to take the medication

Pharmacy name and telephone number
Telephone

PROCEDURE STEPS:

1. Receive patient's telephone call asking for a prescription refill. Follow appropriate telephone techniques. RATIONALE: Appropriate

continues

Procedure 12-3 (continued)

telephone techniques demonstrate consistent customer service.

2. *Pay attention to detail.* Obtain the following information from the patient and include it on the message form or EMR message screen:

   - Patient's full name and correct spelling, and patient's DOB

   - Telephone number where the patient can be reached

   - Name of medication and how long patient has been taking it

   - Patient's symptoms and current health condition

   - If patient is a child, ask their weight

   - History of this condition (last clinic visit)

   - Treatments the patient has tried

   - Any known allergies

   - Pharmacy name, telephone number, and address if a chain

RATIONALE: This information is needed by the provider for assessment as to whether a prescription will be refilled, something else prescribed, or if the patient needs to be seen by the provider.

3. Attach the completed message to the patient's chart or EMR and give it to the provider. RATIONALE: The provider may wish to review the patient's history before refilling the prescription.

4. Review comments in the chart by the provider. If the refill is authorized, call the patient's pharmacy with the refill information. Ask the pharmacy to repeat the information back to you. RATIONALE: To verify the pharmacy has recorded the prescription accurately.

5. *Paying attention to detail,* document in the patient's chart the date and time the prescription was called to the pharmacy and the pharmacy address. Verify that the correct drug, dosage, and dosage instructions were provided to the pharmacy. RATIONALE: Provides accurate documentation in the patient's chart.

PROCEDURE 12-4
Handling Problem Calls

PURPOSE:
To handle calls in a positive and professional manner while providing necessary comfort, empathy, and information to the caller to resolve the problem.

EQUIPMENT/SUPPLIES:
Telephone
Message pad
Pen or pencil

PROCEDURE STEPS:

1. Answer the call as outlined in Procedure 12-1.

2. Remain calm and avoid becoming upset with an angry caller. Let the caller say what needs to be said without interruption (unless it is a medical emergency requiring immediate action). RATIONALE: This permits the caller to express

concerns without having to repeat information or possibly forgetting something important.

3. Lower your voice both in pitch and volume. RATIONALE: This technique has a calming effect on an angry caller.

4. *Listen to and acknowledge* what the caller is upset about. Paraphrase information for verification that you have understood the problem. RATIONALE: This technique lets the caller know you are truly listening and have understood the problem.

5. *Be courteous, patient, and respectful.* Use the words "I understand" and show that you are interested in hearing the caller's concerns. RATIONALE: This does not necessarily mean you agree with the caller, but rather that you are willing to empathize and at least accept that, from a particular point of view, there is a reason to be upset.

Procedure 12-4 (continued)

6. Do not take the call personally. RATIONALE: It is the situation that made the caller angry; you have not done so.

7. Offer assistance. RATIONALE: Ask what you can do to help, and then follow through.

8. Document the call accurately and properly. RATIONALE: Complete documentation promotes risk management and prevents lengthy litigation experiences.

9. When dealing with a frightened or hysterical caller, *display a calm, caring, and professional manner* by speaking in a soothing voice; use a slower, lower tone than normal. RATIONALE: This often has a calming effect on the caller.

10. If the call is an emergency, begin screening procedures as needed and *attend to any special needs of the patient.* RATIONALE: Have a list of

screening questions at hand to refer to or instruct the caller to dial 911. Be sure you have the name and telephone number for follow-up.

11. Always have the caller repeat instructions. RATIONALE: People who are upset may not hear or comprehend much of what is said. Your instructions may deal with an emergency situation, thus it is important they are clearly understood.

12. Finalize and follow through on action to be taken, whether it is confirming emergency medical personnel are on the scene or scheduling an emergency appointment. RATIONALE: Ensures quality patient care.

13. Always report problem calls to the provider or clinic manager at once. RATIONALE: This will ensure appropriate action is taken, and it is important for risk management purposes.

PROCEDURE 12-5
Preparing, Sending, and Receiving a Fax

PURPOSE:
To send and receive information quickly and accurately by fax (facsimile).

EQUIPMENT/SUPPLIES:
Fax machine
Telephone

PROCEDURE STEPS:
To send a fax:

1. *Pay attention to detail.* Prepare a cover sheet or use a preprinted cover sheet for the document to be faxed. Include the names of the sender and receiver, the number of pages being sent and whether this includes the cover sheet, and a short message if necessary. RATIONALE: A cover sheet aids in the correct delivery of a fax to the designated person. It also provides a disclaimer should the fax be received in error and what to do if it is misdelivered.

   CAUTION: Fax machines may be located in areas where unauthorized personnel may see

confidential material. Always include a notice of confidentiality on the cover sheet and always ask the receiver for permission to fax a confidential document.

2. Place the document according to machine instructions. RATIONALE: Ensures that content will be read for transmission.

3. Dial the telephone or dedicated fax number of the receiver. If your fax machine has a display showing the number being faxed to, check to be sure the number you dialed is correct. Then press start. RATIONALE: Verify number to be sure fax is being transmitted to correct phone.

4. After the document passes through the fax machine, press the button requesting a receipt. Some fax machines automatically issue a report. RATIONALE: A receipt is your documentation of the date, time, and where the fax was sent.

5. Remove the document from the machine and, when necessary, call the recipient to be sure the fax was received. RATIONALE: Maintains confidentiality and verifies fax was received by intended recipient.

continues

Procedure 12-4 (continued)

To receive a fax:

6. Be sure that the fax machine is turned on and that the telephone line to the machine is not being used. Most clinics have dedicated fax lines. RATIONALE: Enables you to receive a fax.

7. Remove the document from the machine after it is received and immediately deliver it to the addressee. RATIONALE: Maintains confidentiality and enables recipient to take action immediately if necessary.

CASE STUDY 12-1

Refer to the scenario at the beginning of the chapter.

CASE STUDY REVIEW

1. Recall ways to maintain composure when handling and screening incoming telephone calls.

2. Describe the three types of VoIP services and identify safeguards that can be used to provide in-depth protection to a VoIP system.

3. Discuss HIPAA requirements related to fax machine use and PHI.

4. What is encryption, and how is it used with email communication?

CASE STUDY 12-2

Wanda Slawson, a clinical medical assistant at Inner City Health Care, receives a telephone call from Claussen-Mason Laboratories requesting medical information about patient Juanita Hansen. Wanda is told by laboratory personnel that the information is needed to perform the tests scheduled by Dr. King. Wanda is not familiar with this request and asks if she can check the chart and return a call to the laboratory (callback verification procedure).

CASE STUDY REVIEW

1. What information will Wanda need from Claussen-Mason Laboratories?

2. What is the purpose of the callback verification procedure?

3. After the verification has been established, what should Wanda do?

DOCUMENTATION:

In the log reserved for telephone documentation, the following entry could be made based on Case Study 12–2.

07/16/XX   Claussen-Mason Laboratories requested previous laboratory findings from Qwik Lab in Nashville, Tennessee, for Juanita Hansen, patient number 306-30-7840. Juanita is a patient of Dr. King. The information was released to Janet Bailey, employee of Claussen-Mason Laboratories, as directed by Dr. King. W. Slawson, CMA (AAMA)———————————

SUMMARY

Proper telephone techniques require the medical assistant to have excellent communication and listening skills. The ability to convey warmth and reassurance is vital to patient relationships. Efficiency and organization are also key elements in effectively managing the variety of telephone calls answered and placed in the ambulatory care setting. Medical assistants responsible for incoming and outgoing calls need to be able to perform telephone screening, take messages, and refer calls professionally and efficiently.

Medical assistants also need to be aware of telecommunication technology to choose and productively manage the clinic's telecommunication systems. An understanding of technology can result in savings of both time and money for the efficient ambulatory care setting.

STUDY FOR SUCCESS

To reinforce your knowledge and skills of information presented in this chapter:

- Review the *Key Terms*
- Role-play with other students to apply attributes of professionalism pertinent to this chapter.
- Consider the *Case Studies* and discuss your conclusions
- Answer the questions in the *Certification Review*
- Apply your knowledge by completing the *Activities* in the *Study Guide* and the *Games and Quizzes* in the StudyWARE StudyWARE software on the *Premium Website*
- Perform the *Procedures* using the *Competency Assessment Checklists* in the *Competency Manual*
- Practice your problem-solving skills with the *Critical Thinking Challenge 3.0* on the *Premium Website*

Additional resources for this chapter include:

- Module 5 of the *Medical Assisting Learning Lab*
- *CourseMate for Delmar's Comprehensive Medical Assisting*
- *WebTutor for Delmar's Comprehensive Medical Assisting*

CERTIFICATION REVIEW

1. Positive first impressions are conveyed over the telephone by:
   a. using the hold button sparingly
   b. being authoritative with the caller
   c. not permitting the caller too much leeway to speak
   d. working while talking on the telephone
2. Basic telephone techniques involve:
   a. volume, enunciation, pronunciation, and control of speed
   b. being assertive with the caller
   c. not spending too much time talking
   d. referring all calls to the provider
3. Buffer words:
   a. are necessary for clarity
   b. confuse the caller
   c. are used to avoid clipping off the clinic name
   d. are not considered introductory words, phrases, or statements
4. Guidelines that ensure successful transfer of calls include all of the following *except:*
   a. determine who would be the best person to assist
   b. follow your telephone system's procedure for transferring the call
   c. follow up to be sure the call transferred correctly
   d. getting the caller's name and telephone number is not necessary

5. Medical assistants should refer calls to the provider when:
   a. an appointment needs to be scheduled
   b. a patient has a billing question
   c. a salesperson is planning a call
   d. none of the above
6. Screening:
   a. is the act of evaluating the urgency of a medical situation and prioritizing the call
   b. is expressing oneself clearly and distinctly
   c. uses expendable words while answering the telephone
   d. is the ability to be objectively aware of and have insight into others' feelings, emotions, and behaviors
7. In handling a problem call, the medical assistant should:
   a. take it personally
   b. listen calmly to the upset person
   c. become upset to identify with the patient
   d. ask emotionally charged questions to calm down the patient
8. The callback verification procedure:
   a. should never be documented
   b. should always be documented
   c. should sometimes be documented
   d. is not appropriate in the ambulatory clinic setting

9. ARU telephone systems:
   a. transmit over telephone lines via modem
   b. involve transmissions sent from one fax machine to another
   c. use a recorded voice that identifies departments or services the caller can access by pressing a specified number
   d. process messages in digital form through telephone lines

10. Security measures to consider when using a VoIP system include all of the following *except:*
    a. use an SPI firewall
    b. use a softphone
    c. encrypt voice traffic
    d. use a VPN to separate the data stream from the public Internet

11. Security measures to consider when using the fax to send PHI include all of the following *except:*
    a. have a signed form authorizing the release of PHI before releasing the information
    b. faxed messages should only be sent to telecopiers that are located in a secure area
    c. a cover sheet containing warning of confidential information is not necessary when faxing
    d. always recheck before sending the fax that the correct telephone number was selected and entered correctly

12. When using clinical email, all of the following apply *except:*
    a. clinical email to or from patients should be treated differently than telephone messages or letters
    b. print and file the initial message and any reply to clinical email in the patient's chart
    c. have a written agreement of understanding signed by all patients using clinical email
    d. use clinical email protocols in the clinic procedure manual

13. TTY and TDD devices are used by:
    a. individuals with hearing and/or speech impairments
    b. most individuals placing long-distance calls
    c. smartphones
    d. facsimile machines

14. All of the following apply to encryption of email *except*:
    a. may be initiated by obtaining and using a digital ID
    b. renders the email essentially secure
    c. a digital ID may only be added manually to an address book
    d. a digital ID is composed of a public key, a private key, and a digital signature

REFERENCES/BIBLIOGRAPHY

ingenix. (2003). *HIPAA tool kit.* Salt Lake City, UT: St. Anthony's Publishing/Medicode.

Keir, L., Wise, B.A., Krebs, C., & Arney, C. (2008). *Medical assisting: Administrative and clinical competencies* (6th ed.). Clifton Park, NY: Delmar Cengage Learning.

Krager, D., & Krager, C. (2005). *HIPAA for medical clinic personnel.* Clifton Park, NY: Delmar Cengage Learning.

CHAPTER 13

Patient Scheduling

OUTLINE

Tailoring the Scheduling System

Scheduling Styles
  Open Hours
  Double Booking
  Clustering
  Wave Scheduling
  Modified Wave Scheduling
  Stream Scheduling
  Practice-Based Scheduling

Analyzing Patient Flow
  Waiting Time

Legal Issues

Interpersonal Skills

Guidelines for Scheduling Appointments
  Screening Calls
  Referral Appointments
  Recording Information
  Appointment Matrix
  Telephone Appointments
  Patient Check-In
  Patient Cancellation and Appointment Changes

Reminder Systems

Scheduling Pharmaceutical Representatives

Scheduling Software and Materials
  Appointment Schedule
  Computer Scheduling Software

Inpatient and Outpatient Admissions Procedures

LEARNING OUTCOMES

1. Define, spell, and pronounce the key terms as presented in the glossary.
2. Identify pros and cons of six major scheduling systems.
3. Describe the guidelines in scheduling appointments.
4. Explain the importance of screening in scheduling patient appointments.
5. Review proper cancellation procedures and explain the legal necessity of documenting cancellations.
6. List and define three types of reminder systems.
7. Choose an appropriate appointment scheduling tool and describe its advantages.
8. Establish a matrix for a new year and a new practice.
9. Check in patients using a daily appointment sheet.
10. Schedule appointments using a manual system and an electronic system.
11. Schedule outpatient procedures and inpatient admissions.
12. Analyze the professionalism questions and apply them to this chapter's content.

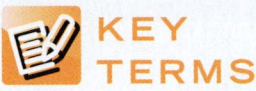

KEY TERMS

encryption technology

matrix

modified wave
  scheduling

screening

stream scheduling

wave scheduling

ATTRIBUTES OF PROFESSIONALISM

Communication

- Did you speak at the patient's level of understanding?
- Did you provide appropriate responses/feedback?
- Did you respond honestly and diplomatically to the patient's concerns?
- Did you apply active listening skills?
- Does your knowledge allow you to speak easily with all members of the health care team?
- Did you demonstrate assertive communication with managed care and/or insurance providers?
- Did you maintain eye contact with the patient during communication?

Presentation

- Did you attend to any special needs of the patient? Did you first ask if assistance was needed, rather than taking charge?
- Were you courteous, patient, and respectful to the patient?
- Did you display a positive attitude?
- Did you display a calm, professional, and caring manner?

Competency

- Did you pay attention to detail?
- Did you display sound judgment?
- Were you knowledgeable and accountable?
- Did you recognize the importance of local, state, and federal legislation and regulations in the practice setting?

Initiative

- Did you show initiative?

Integrity

- Did you immediately report any error you had made?

SCENARIO

At Inner City Health Care, medical assistant Walter Seals, CMA (AAMA), is responsible for efficient patient flow. Because Inner City is an urgent care center, patients are seen as walk-in appointments, on a first-come, first-served basis unless there is an emergency situation. Inner City also operates specialty care clinics, and these clinics require scheduled appointments. Walter has found that the clustering system is most efficient for these specialized care clinics, with certain days dedicated to certain procedures.

Because of the high volume of patients and the need to coordinate multiple provider schedules, Walter's job is not an easy one. However, Inner City is computerized, so paperwork is easy to generate as appointments are made, canceled, or rescheduled. And although Walter manages a smooth patient flow, he makes it a point to remain flexible to accommodate patient needs and keep stress to a minimum.

INTRODUCTION

Patient scheduling has undergone many changes. A medical appointment is most often scheduled over the telephone or in person. Information technology allows appointment scheduling through secure online access using the clinic's Web site. However the appointment is made, the medical staff will need the home telephone number and will want the number of the cellular phone that often accompanies the patient at all times or is used in place of a land-line telephone. In the case of online appointment requests, the patient's email address is necessary. If online appointment scheduling is new to the clinic, the medical assistant may ask if the patient has a computer and is willing to use the computer for online appointment scheduling.

Patient scheduling is an integral part of the daily workload for medical assistants, whether in large family practices, urgent care centers, or sole proprietor clinics. Scheduling becomes more complicated if providers are practicing in more than one location and traveling between them. Scheduling patients can be stressful, especially if the telephone rings constantly and the medical assistant is unable to provide patients a convenient appointment.

Although patient appointment scheduling may seem like a routine function, a smooth patient flow often determines the success of a day in the ambulatory care setting. A variety of administrative skills are used in the performance of this vital function. By effectively scheduling patients to fit a particular practice, it is possible to make profitable use of provider and staff time.

In addition, efficient patient flow pleases the patient. A common patient complaint is the time spent waiting in the reception area or the examination room. Most patients appreciate a clinic that recognizes the value of their time. Accordingly, these patients do not hesitate to advertise their experience (good or bad) to friends and families—a fact of great significance to any medical setting.

In addition to the required administrative skills, medical assistants involved in scheduling patients must put into practice their best interpersonal and communication skills. Scheduling an appointment may be the first contact patients have with the medical facility. They remember and value the treatment they receive from the time of first contact. The personality of the ambulatory care setting is always reflected in the treatment and respect given to patients.

Whether scheduling is done online, through a computerized system, or in the paper appointment book (rare these days), practitioners and their staff must remember the importance of that first impression and make it satisfying for patients.

TAILORING THE SCHEDULING SYSTEM

The patient population of each medical facility will determine the best method for scheduling appointments. A surgeon's clinic will have a much different flow of patients than a pediatrician's clinic. The key is to customize the system to best accommodate the practice. Primary goals in determining this should include:

- A smooth flow of patients with a minimal amount of waiting time
- Flexibility to accommodate acutely ill, STAT (or emergency) appointments, work-ins, cancellations, and no-shows

Medical providers may feel uncomfortable if their days are not busy with patients or they experience idle time. It is also true that patients want access to their medical providers when needed and prefer not to wait several days to be seen. There is no one perfect scheduling style, and some facilities may even be unable to identify their style of scheduling by name. One thing is certain, however; patients, providers, and their staff will know when scheduling is not working successfully.

SCHEDULING STYLES

There are a number of methods for patient scheduling. The best method for a practice is the one that effects good patient flow and proper utilization of staff and physical facilities and meets the needs of the provider(s). Traditionally, all scheduling was done by writing appointments in a book by hand. Increasingly, however, scheduling is done using computer software designed specifically for that purpose or using scheduling programs that are part of total practice management software. Keep in mind that even the most sophisticated computerized system will fail if the scheduling style does not comfortably fit the predetermined and necessary patient flow.

HIPAA Some clinics ask patients to sign in as they arrive. Some legal authorities believe that the only infallible way to prove patients have kept a medical appointment is to have them sign their name upon arrival and give the time.

The Health Insurance Portability and Accountability Act (HIPAA) has ruled that patients can be asked to sign their name upon arrival as long they are not asked to provide any other personal information, such as address, telephone number, Social Security number, or clinic identification number. HIPAA has also ruled that patients cannot be forced to sign if they feel uncomfortable in doing so. A word of caution is important here. The patient's right to privacy ensures that patients do not see confidential information (such as the reason for the visit) of other patients. HIPAA regulations have caused facilities to be more cognizant of patients' rights to privacy and confidentiality.

If the setting and circumstances indicate that a sign-in sheet for patients is the most efficient means of checking in patients, forms can be purchased that meet the privacy and confidentiality expectations of patients.

Figure 13-1 illustrates a carbonized pack with perforations that allows a patient to sign in giving the necessary information. The patient is instructed to remove the top ticket, leaving the information on the bottom form only. The next person to sign in does not see the information of the previous patient. The ticket has a number in the upper right-hand corner that can be used by the medical assistant to call the patient if total confidentiality is preferred. However, many patients believe being called by a number is impersonal and unwelcoming.

Open Hours

In open hours scheduling, patients are seen throughout a particular time frame, for example, 9:00 AM to 11:00 AM or 1:00 PM to 3:00 PM. Patients are seen on a first-come, first-served basis. Many clinics frequently choose this method because they are able, by their nature, to maintain a steady flow of patients. Open hours scheduling is likely a place where a sign-in sheet is helpful, because patients are seen on a first-come, first-served basis. It is important to remember that a sign-in sheet can never replace a warm, welcoming greeting from the administrative medical assistant to set the tone for care given that day.

Double Booking

With the double-booking method, two or more patients are given a particular appointment time. This method is limited to a practice that can

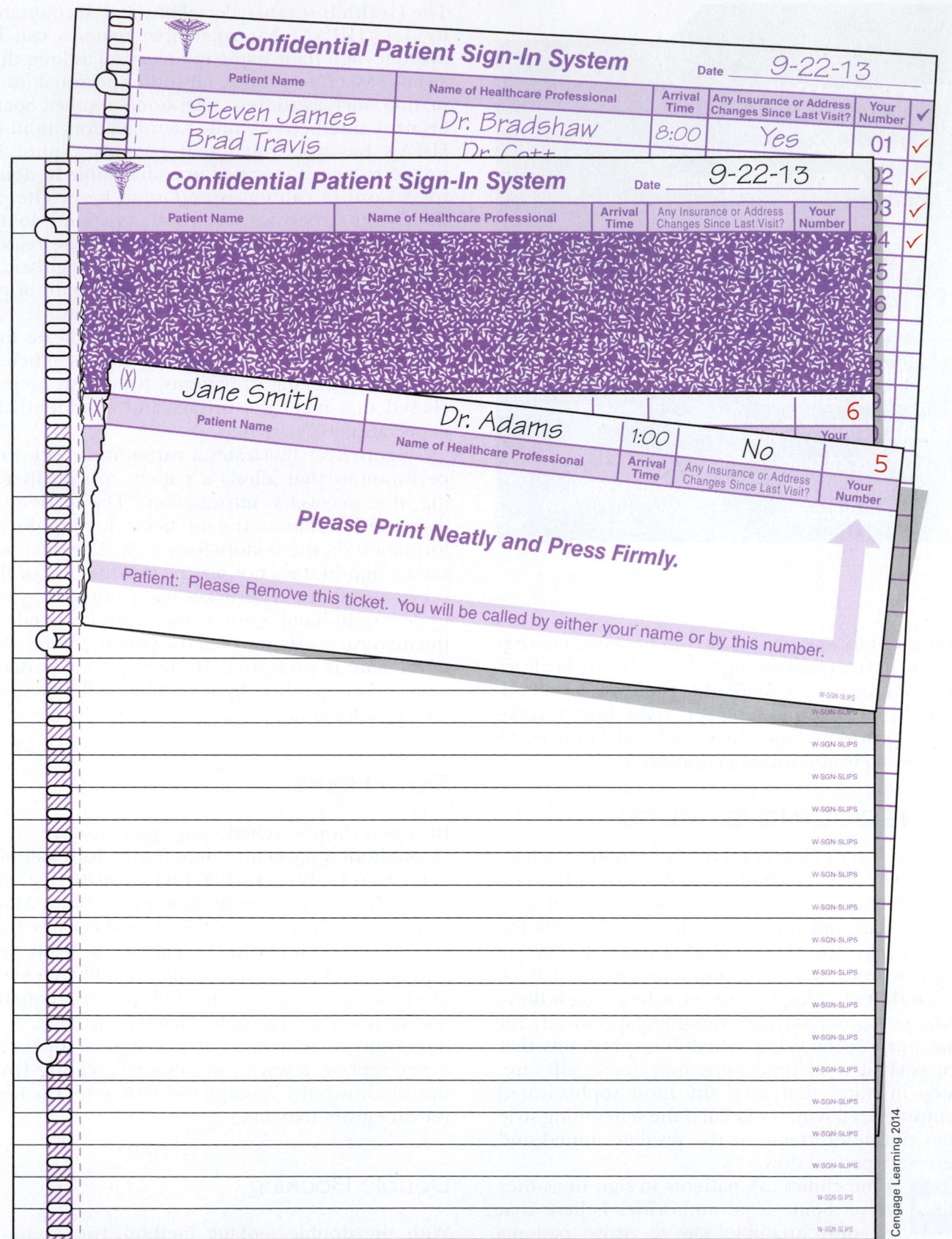

Figure 13-1   Confidential patient sign-in system that offers privacy. Patient can be called by the number of the ticket or by name.

attend to more than one patient at a time. For instance, Maria Jover and Jim Marshal are both given a 9:30 AM appointment. Ms. Jover requires a complete checkup including lab tests, vitals, and provider visit. Mr. Marshal is being seen for suture removal. While the staff conducts the lab tests on Ms. Jover, the primary care provider can see Mr. Marshal. Obviously, this method requires a precise accounting for time, rooms, and adequate staff. A good rule to remember is that if patients consistently have to wait for staff to attend to them, double booking is not a wise choice of scheduling method. Also, patients who do not understand the complex nature of patient scheduling may mistakenly believe that their provider is trying to see two patients at the same time, forcing one of them to wait unnecessarily.

Clustering

The *clustering* method applies the concept used in production line work, namely, that performing only one step or process allows for efficient processing. In the ambulatory care setting, patients with similar problems are booked consecutively. Obstetricians and pediatricians commonly choose this method. A block of time, either hours or days of the week, is set aside for particular types of cases. For instance, an obstetrician might see only patients in their third trimester of pregnancy on Mondays and Fridays and gynecology patients on Tuesdays and Thursdays. A pediatrician's clinic might be organized for immunizations on Tuesday mornings and well-baby checkups on Monday and Friday afternoons.

Wave Scheduling

Wave scheduling is another method that can be used effectively in medical facilities that have several procedure rooms and adequate personnel to staff them. Using the wave scheduling system, patients are scheduled only in the first half hour of each hour. For example, three patients may be given the time of 11 AM. Generally, the first one to arrive is seen first. If they all arrive on time, the one who is most ill is usually seen first, and there will be a waiting time for the other two patients. Depending on the practice, some administrative medical assistants will be instructed to schedule three patients at the top of the hour and another two or three patients at the bottom of the hour (e.g., 11:30 AM). Patients who do not understand this system of scheduling may become irritated if they discover that another patient has the same appointed time with the same provider. This method takes into account that there will be no-shows and late arrivals. It can also accommodate work-in appointments. However, it does require personnel who are able to prioritize patient problems precisely when establishing the appointments.

Modified Wave Scheduling

Modified wave scheduling is a variation of the wave method where patients are scheduled in "waves." In this method, two or three patients are scheduled at the beginning of each hour, followed by single appointments every 10 to 20 minutes the rest of the hour.

A variation of this method assesses major and minor problems. Major time-consuming problems are seen at the beginning of the hour (e.g., new patients). Minor problems are seen from 20 minutes past the hour to half past the hour (e.g., follow-ups, bandage changes, and other minor procedures), and walk-ins (e.g., a child with a 103°F temperature) are accommodated at the end of the hour. Again, good screening will determine the success of this method.

With both the clustering and wave methods, empty or unscheduled periods can be used to catch up on other responsibilities.

Stream Scheduling

Stream scheduling is perhaps the best known and most widely used scheduling system. When this system works as it should, there is a steady stream of patients at set appointment times throughout the workday. There would be, for example, a 30-minute appointment at 9:00 AM; a 15-minute appointment at 9:30 AM; and a 15-minute appointment at 9:45 AM. Each patient is assigned a specific time.

This can best be accomplished by establishing realistic time guidelines for particular types of appointments, such as 45 minutes for consultations, 15 minutes for immunizations, and 30 minutes for hearing tests.

Practice-Based Scheduling

As discussed earlier in this chapter, some ambulatory care settings find it necessary to develop a system unique to their patient load. In these customized systems (practice-based), the practice determines the schedule. An orthopedist might schedule cast removals on Mondays and Fridays using double booking and stream scheduling for new patients, with each patient having a 45-minute appointment. A group of vascular surgeons might use both a double-booking and a modified wave system. They might double book patients for short rechecks and quick procedures but use the modified wave for patients with preoperative and postoperative checks and long specialty procedures.

There are many variations of scheduling styles. An Oregon massage therapist who operates a private practice as a sole proprietor with no staff has found that an online welcome screen and appointment book is the best way for her patients to schedule a massage. Her online system also creates appointment reminder email messages. This massage therapist and her patients are pleased. They believe that the self-service scheduling gives their therapist more time to take care of their needs.

ANALYZING PATIENT FLOW

When reviewing the current scheduling practice, a simple analysis can maximize a clinic's scheduling practices. This entails looking at appointment times, patient arrival times, the actual time a patient is seen, and the time a visit is completed. A simple grid chart can be produced for a given period, for example, 1 to 2 weeks (Figure 13-2). In addition, chart the number of no-shows and cancellations. An electronic scheduling system can automatically provide the detail necessary to analyze the effectiveness of patient scheduling. It has the capability of indicating the scheduled time for specific procedures, for each provider, and for each service given to the patient.

This analysis will provide a clear picture of patient flow and whether personnel are being used efficiently. The data will assist in estimating how

PATIENT FLOW ANALYSIS

February 2, 20XX — Dr. King

Patient Name	Length of Appt.	Appt. Time	Time Seen	Time Out
Martin Gordon	15	10:20	10:22	10:45
Jason Jover	45	11:20	11:20	12:30
Nora Fowler	30	1:00	1:25	1:45
Jim Marshal	15	1:30	1:50	2:10
Herb Fowler	60	2:45	2:15	3:25

© Cengage Learning 2014

Figure 13-2 Patient flow analysis helps a practice determine realistic time frames for appointments.

TYPICAL SCHEDULING TIMES FOR INTERNAL MEDICINE PRACTICE

New patients . . . . 30 minutes

Patients for consultation . . . . 45 minutes

Patients requiring complete physical examinations . . . . 45 minutes

All other patients (minor illnesses, routine checkups, etc.) . . . . 15 minutes

© Cengage Learning 2014

Figure 13-3 Most practices have a list of typical visits with time estimates.

many patients to schedule and realistic time frames for particular problems or procedures. If the staff is scheduling return patients every 15 minutes yet the analysis shows these visits average 24 minutes, then the scheduling method needs adjustment. This may mean either allowing more minutes for follow-up visits or building in slack time when no appointments are made.

Develop a simple list of commonly scheduled visits with time estimates for each. This procedural sheet will be particularly useful when training new employees or when temporary help is used for scheduling (Figure 13-3).

Waiting Time

One of patients' frequently voiced frustrations with medical clinics is excessive waiting time. Obviously, emergencies and other unexpected interruptions cannot be anticipated. However, there are certain measures the medical assistant can take when attempting to keep the schedule on target. If patients are kept waiting, it is a good strategy to explain the reason for the delay and give patients an estimate of how long the delay will be. *Never* ignore the delay hoping patients will not notice; this, in fact, seems to increase perceived waiting time. Find ways to make patients comfortable while they wait; for example, provide an appropriate choice of reading materials (or in the case of children, activities). Refer to Case Study 10-3. If a delay can be anticipated—for example, if the provider is called away for a baby delivery or surgery—attempt to contact patients before they leave home to reschedule the appointments.

If the delay is likely to be a half hour or longer, provide patients with options, for example:

1. Offer patients the opportunity to run an errand, having them return at a specified time.
2. Offer to reschedule appointments for another day, or later that day, or to see another provider in the practice if possible.

In any case, remember that good customer relations dictate your willingness to acknowledge the inconvenience to the patients, and do attempt to provide an acceptable solution. Remember also that some patients simply will not appreciate any efforts to apologize for a delay, in which case you must continue to act professionally toward them.

LEGAL ISSUES

Information provided in any patient scheduling system may be used for legal purposes. A case of malpractice or questions regarding a provider's availability may require a copy of the daily schedule. It might become necessary to identify how many times a particular patient was a no-show or canceled an appointment, never calling to reschedule. The appointment schedule could verify that a patient was seen and treated on a particular day, thus affirming the information in the patient's record. A patient sign-in sheet may serve this purpose, also.

All computerized systems provide a permanent record of patients seen, and any alterations to that schedule are saved on the hard drive or disk and are shown when a printout is produced. If an appointment book is still used, the staff will have to make certain there is a permanent record or daily appointment sheet that indicates cancellations, work-ins, urgent care needs, and no-shows. Any changes to the daily appointment sheet are to be made in pen; therefore, there will be no question regarding accuracy.

Remember that anyone looking into a practice will be looking at the record of documentation. Taking the time to accurately and consistently document all aspects of patient care makes a statement about the providers in the practice and their staff and reflects positively on the presumed quality of patient care.

INTERPERSONAL SKILLS

  Scheduling appointments requires interpersonal skills. Medical assistants convey a great deal to patients through attitude and actions as well as empathy. A hurried or disinterested manner communicates that the patient is not a priority. Because patients are often distraught or anxious when making appointments, it is extremely important to reduce rather than increase anxiety. Also, the medical assistant who schedules appointments may be the first contact a patient has with the clinic; patients do not easily forget rude or insensitive staff. A hurried, disinterested manner toward patients is just as often the basis for legal action as is a negligent act.

If any form of online scheduling is used, be certain that it is user friendly, has a rapid response time of no more than 24 hours, and provides patients an option if the online scheduling proves unsatisfactory for any reason. Make certain that staff are ready for online scheduling and that those responsible for assignments and backups are carefully prepared. It is important that patients not be made to feel inadequate if they choose not to use online scheduling.

The patient should always be made to feel worthy of attention. This validates his or her reason for calling. If you are scheduling a patient in the clinic and the phone rings, answer the call but excuse yourself first. Ask the caller to please hold for a moment. If you are on the telephone scheduling a patient and another patient walks in, acknowledge with a nod or signal that you will be right there—never let the person feel ignored (see Chapter 12). Today, patients have a variety of options for health care and tend to be much more consumer conscious of the treatment they receive.

GUIDELINES FOR SCHEDULING APPOINTMENTS

Whether completed by manual methods or computer technology, the process of scheduling appointments for patients and other visitors to the ambulatory care setting involves a number of variables, including (1) the urgency of the need for an appointment; (2) whether the patient is a referral from another provider; (3) recording methods for new and established patients; (4) implementation of check-in, cancellation, and rescheduling policies; (5) use of reminder systems; and (6) accommodating visits from medical supply and pharmaceutical company representatives.

Providers in some health maintenance organizations who are paid by a salary rather than by patient visit are experimenting with group scheduling. The group visits may be established around patients with specific chronic ailments such as diabetes, hypertension, or geriatric complaints. This is one method to provide patient education, support, and interaction while using time efficiently and keeping costs down. At the same time, patient-provider relationships are maintained in providing health care.

Screening Calls

Urgent calls will need to be **screened** or assessed, before they can be scheduled. In other words, the person making the appointment will need to determine the actual urgency of that call and determine how the patient can best be scheduled. This requires both communication skills and medical knowledge.

Appropriate questions will be asked to determine the actual urgency. Is the patient in immediate need of medical assistance? Is there any bleeding? If so, where? How profuse is the bleeding? Are there chest pains? How intense is the pain? Is the pain localized? How long have the symptoms been present? The medical assistant needs to determine whether this is a life-threatening matter, or whether the problem is urgent in the patient's eyes but not a medical emergency. Precise information will help to determine the critical or noncritical nature of the call.

In screening the patient's urgency of care, be tactful in questioning and avoid making the patient feel that the need is insignificant. If questioning indicates this is a medical emergency, follow the policy for having the patient seen (whether it be an emergency appointment or referral to the emergency department). If referral to the emergency department or a call to 911 is necessary, make the call for the patient, being certain you have the correct address and telephone number available. Such a referral minimizes disruption to patients being seen in the ambulatory care setting. If it is determined that the best method in handling this emergency is to see the patient in the clinic, let scheduled patients know of the emergency and offer them the opportunity of rescheduling or waiting until the emergency has been resolved. A built-in slack time of 30 minutes in the morning and 30 minutes in the afternoon can provide some flexibility in last-minute emergency scheduling. If it is determined that the situation is not an emergency, work the patient into the schedule as the situation warrants and time allows, and make certain the patient is comfortable with the scheduled time. Be sure to leave the patient with the understanding that you have done your best to address the situation. (See Chapters 9 and 12 for more information on screening.)

Referral Appointments

One of the primary sources of patients for any provider is referrals from other providers. This is especially true in a managed care climate, where patients usually must have a referral from their primary care provider and where providers are part of an HMO network. It is important that these appointments be given special consideration and that referred patients are given an appointment as soon as possible.

Adequate information needs to be obtained to determine the urgency of scheduling. If the referring provider or clinic staff calls directly, the situation can be assessed at that time. However, if the referred patient calls, it is best to obtain necessary records and information from the referring provider's clinic to determine the urgency and appropriateness of an appointment. This can be done by obtaining general information from the patient and then scheduling an appointment after the provider's clinic is contacted for complete information regarding the patient's condition. Be polite and assure the patient of an appointment as soon as the referring provider's clinic is contacted.

Recording Information

Patients can be sensitive to the amount of information they are required to provide to make an initial appointment. Keep the information as simple as possible and obtain only essential information. It should be tailored to fit the practice; for example, an obstetrician and a pediatrician will have different questions for the first-time patient.

When patients schedule an appointment online via the clinic's Web site, they are directed to a patient preregistration and health history that can be completed online prior to coming to the facility. The information provided in this format is often more detailed than what is obtained over the telephone. Nevertheless, the following basic items should be obtained from a new patient:

1. The patient's full legal name (with the correct spelling)
2. A daytime telephone number
3. The chief complaint or reason for the visit
4. The referring provider, if relevant

In privacy, repeat this information back to the patient to ensure accuracy.

Clinics with computerized scheduling and billing will require a few additional items, such as:

1. Date of birth
2. Type of insurance
3. Insurance number

The critical determination is whether the information is essential to the first contact or whether it can be obtained at the time of the visit.

An established patient, someone who has already been seen in the clinic, should be required to provide only the following information:

1. Full legal name
2. Chief complaint or reason for the visit
3. A daytime telephone number

When the information is recorded, print legibly and accurately if using a manual system and key in the information if using a computer system. Check for accuracy in either system. Record the appointment as soon as it is made—never rely on memory.

When scheduling an appointment time, ask the patient what day and time is most convenient and then make the appointment for the first available time stated. If possible, provide the patient with a choice of appointment times. Finally, confirm that the patient clearly understands the date and time of the appointment; be sure to repeat the date and time to ensure that both of you have recorded the same information. If the patient is making the appointment in person, provide an appointment reminder.

Scheduling an appointment for the clinic's available times for anyone with an extremely busy schedule can require a great deal of patience. If the patient requests a particular appointment that is not possible, courteously offer an explanation.

Many ambulatory care settings, especially those specializing in family practice and pediatrics, provide alternative hours for scheduling appointments. Having evening appointments at least one day a week or Saturday morning appointments can be helpful for individuals whose work schedule does not permit weekday appointments.

Appointment Matrix

The appointment **matrix** must be established before patients can be scheduled. The matrix provides a current and accurate record of appointment times available for scheduling patient visits. Clinic hours are noted with times blocked when the facility is closed. Provider's schedules, vacations, holidays, hospital rounds, and any responsibilities that make providers unavailable for appointments are recorded. The matrix of the scheduling plan might include slots for patients who need to see only staff members for their appointment; therefore, times when they are unavailable are important to the matrix. Any evening or weekend appointment slots available also are noted (see Procedure 13-1).

Typically, when using an electronic system for scheduling, the program will search through a database of appointments, find an open appointment, and allocate an appointment time according to your instructions. These instructions can include finding an open appointment with a specific time length, on a specific day, or within a specified time frame. Once the appointment time is confirmed with the patient, patient data are keyed in, and the appointment is automatically scheduled (see Procedure 13-2).

Telephone Appointments

More appointments are made by telephone than by any other method. Remember the guidelines for appointment scheduling, appropriate screening of all calls to determine urgency and need, and to follow your provider–employer's instructions regarding patient referrals for appointments. Make certain that you get all the necessary information from the patient when the appointment is made. Procedures 13-3 and 13-4 provide practice for telephone appointments in both a manual system and an electronic system. The professional manner in which telephone appointments are made for patients sets the tone for their satisfaction with the clinic, its providers, and their care.

Patient Check-In

Records of patient appointments serve a legal purpose. Establishing a procedure for checking in appointments simplifies tracking the arrival of patients (see Procedures 13-5 and 13-6). This is particularly true in multiprovider settings where patients are attended by a number of staff before, or instead of, seeing the primary care provider.

As mentioned earlier, more than one method can be used to check in patients. A sign-in sheet might be used, especially in a facility with open hours scheduling. The administrative medical assistant can place a check mark (usually in red) by the patient's name in the appointment book or make an indication electronically (usually an **X**) in scheduling software (Figure 13-4).

The check-in procedure serves the additional purpose of alerting the staff when a patient has arrived and is available to be seen. Communication among the administrative medical assistants and the clinical medical assistants is important for a smooth patient flow and to save time for both patients and providers (Figure 13-5).

Computer scheduling systems include a space to indicate when a patient arrives for an appointment. Some clinics use the printed activity schedule to check when patients arrive. Other clinics rely upon a copy of the day's schedule and the patient's chart indicating a consultation or visit to legally verify the patient's presence in the clinic.

Unfortunately, even the best of electronic systems may fail temporarily. In that case, the manual system is used as a backup. If the day's schedule has already been printed, it can be used to monitor the patient flow and to check in patients. It may also serve as adequate information for any work-in patients to be accommodated that day. However, for appointments to be made in the future, the administrative medical assistant may have to return a call to the patient when the computer is back up and running properly.

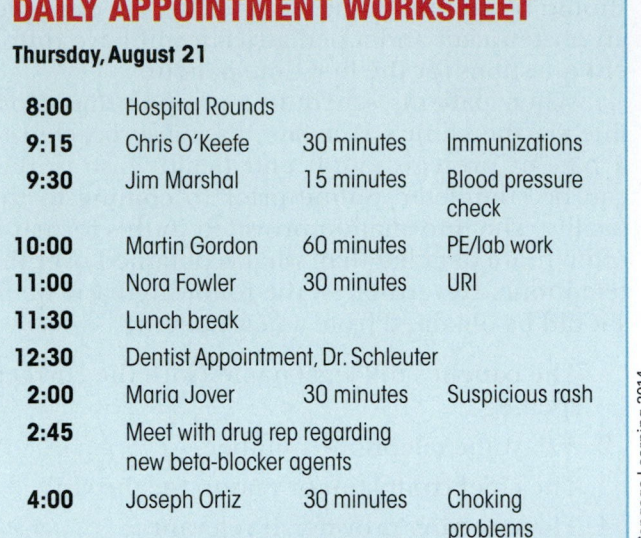

DAILY APPOINTMENT WORKSHEET

Thursday, August 21

8:00	Hospital Rounds		
9:15	Chris O'Keefe	30 minutes	Immunizations
9:30	Jim Marshal	15 minutes	Blood pressure check
10:00	Martin Gordon	60 minutes	PE/lab work
11:00	Nora Fowler	30 minutes	URI
11:30	Lunch break		
12:30	Dentist Appointment, Dr. Schleuter		
2:00	Maria Jover	30 minutes	Suspicious rash
2:45	Meet with drug rep regarding new beta-blocker agents		
4:00	Joseph Ortiz	30 minutes	Choking problems

© Cengage Learning 2014

Figure 13-4 Daily appointment worksheet.

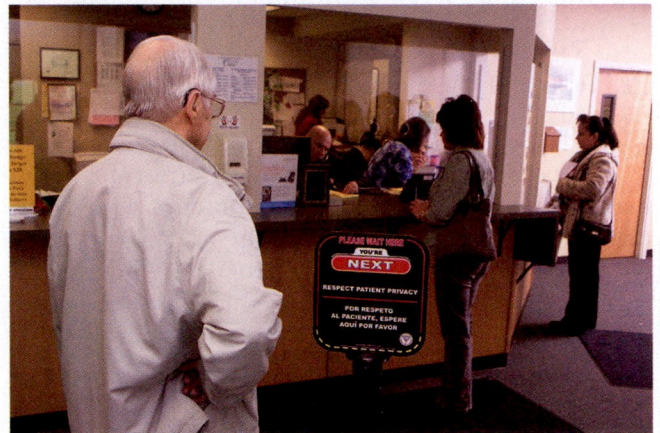

© Cengage Learning 2014

Figure 13-5 The administrative medical assistant checks in a patient and keeps the patient check-in list current.

Patient Cancellation and Appointment Changes

A permanent record of no-shows should be designated on the appointment sheet with a red **X** or some other distinctive mark. Cancellations should be marked through on the appointment sheet with a single red line (Figure 13-6). Some facilities place a notation next to the patient's name. Computer scheduling will also provide an area to indicate no-shows and cancellations. No-shows and cancellations should always be noted in the patient's

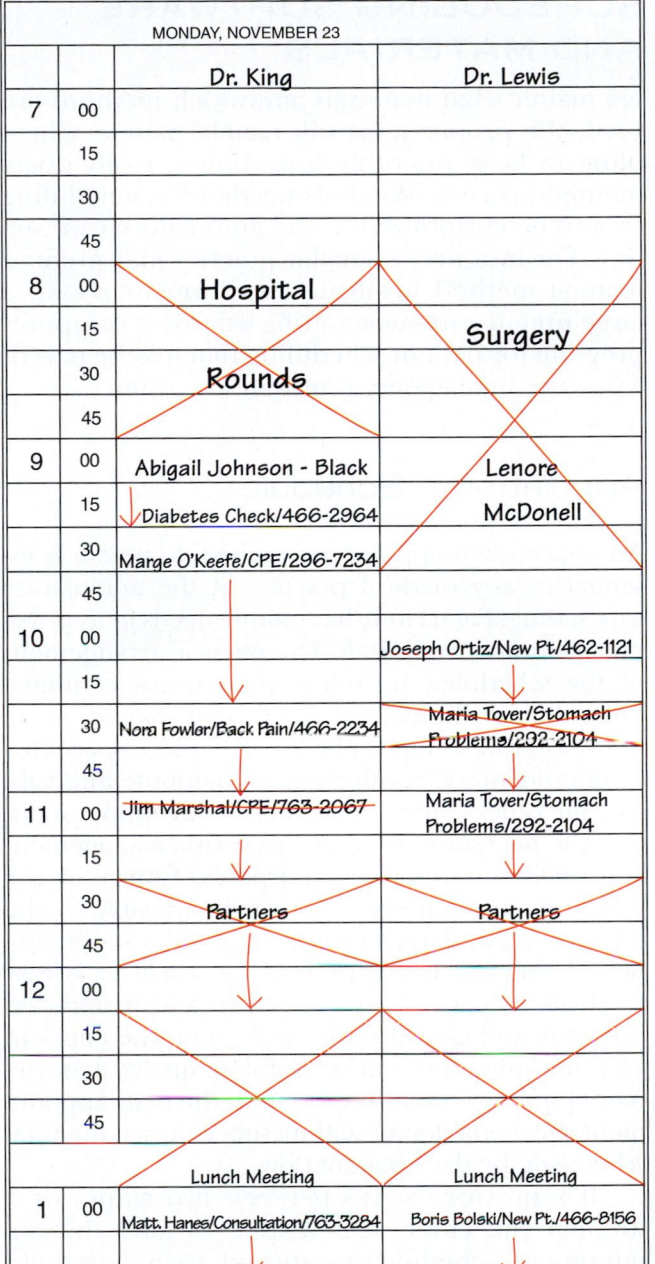

Figure 13-6 Multiprovider clinic where providers' commitments and no-shows are marked with a red X and cancellations are marked with a single red line. Computer systems have slightly different tracking systems, but all no-shows and cancellations also should be marked in the patient's record.

individual chart. Again, it is imperative that the provider's care of the patient be thoroughly documented. Should a patient develop complications and claim a provider was unavailable, the daily appointment sheet and chart would document the patient's failure to show.

Occasionally, patients do not arrive for an appointment because they simply forgot, or sometimes they come on the wrong day or at the wrong time. That can happen simply by human error or miscommunication. However, if one patient begins a pattern of getting the dates and times mixed up or forgets the appointment entirely, the primary care provider should be made aware of the fact. Sometimes, a pattern of missed and mixed-up appointments is a first sign that the patient may be experiencing memory loss and mental confusion.

Many clinics have established firm policies for multiple no-shows and cancellations. The general rule is that after three no-shows or cancellations in a row, the provider will review the records. For the provider to adequately treat a patient, the patient's cooperation is necessary. A no-show pattern may indicate that the patient is not truly committed to assisting in treatment. If a patient routinely cancels or does not show, the provider may write a letter terminating services and explaining why the provider is discontinuing care. This should be sent by certified mail, return receipt requested, to ensure that the patient received the notice (see Chapter 7 for more information on termination of services). Procedure 13-7 outlines the proper cancellation procedures.

Although software programs differ, cancellations are typically performed by deleting the patient's name from the time slot; if the appointment is to be rescheduled, the name is then keyed in to the appropriate time, usually the first time open for other appointments (see Procedure 13-8).

When canceling appointments by computer, be certain that the program maintains a list of canceled appointments including patient name, date, and time. This documentation is necessary for legal purposes. Also, be certain to record canceled appointments in the patients' charts.

Reminder Systems

Studies show that the national average of missed appointments is more than 10%. When patients are reminded of their scheduled appointments, it results in a greater rate of fulfilled appointments. Give patients appointment card reminders when appointments are made at the medical facility. Those cards may easily be tucked in a wallet and forgotten, however. Many clinics notify patients the day before the appointment with a reminder of their choice for the communication—telephone, text message, or email.

 However, keep in mind that the reminder is confidential information and should not be left on a recording device without the patient's express permission to do so. (When initially seeing the patient, obtain a number where a personal message could be left.) Finally, reminders can be mailed. This would be most appropriate for patients who come in on a regular basis (e.g., once every 6 months).

Scheduling Pharmaceutical Representatives

Some medical facilities schedule time with representatives of pharmaceutical and medical supply companies. On the other hand, there are some medical clinics that refuse to see any pharmaceutical representatives. When representatives are seen, however, they can provide a valuable service to providers and staff, and with clear guidelines regarding when and how often representatives can visit, a working partnership can develop. Providers may set aside a specific time during the week to meet with these representatives; generally, a time allotment of 15 to 20 minutes is sufficient for these appointments. Some representatives try to establish a standard appointment once a month. If this is a representative your provider desires to see on a regular basis, that policy can be helpful to both the provider and the representative. However, this practice might not allow adequate time for other representatives; therefore, it is often discouraged.

SCHEDULING SOFTWARE AND MATERIALS

No matter what materials and which methods are used, the proper tools will enable patient scheduling to be a smoothly functioning, easily documented process. Materials needed for scheduling should be customized to the ambulatory care setting. For instance, a smaller practice may prefer a manual method involving appointment books; a large urgent care–type setting will use a computer program for patient scheduling that may be part of a practice management software program.

Appointment Schedule

An appropriate appointment schedule system is essential to any medical practice in the ambulatory care setting. Each clinic has unique needs in its physical facility and for its staff. The physical arrangement of the scheduler, including the various combinations of time allotments, must be determined. Some have major headings for hours with minor spaces for 15-minute intervals, others have 10-minute intervals, and still others only hour intervals. An appointment sheet is necessary for both legal risk management and quality management purposes. Copies of the daily appointment sheet are made available to the doctors, medical assistants, and any other staff members. Using the daily appointment sheet, it is easy to check in patients as they arrive and to indicate no-shows and cancellations. Indicating the check-in and checkout times can be useful for quality management purposes. More importantly, the daily appointment sheet enables all staff members to see the total scheme of the day's patient flow.

If a provider works between two clinics or a hospital and clinic, it is helpful to have this appointment schedule transferred to a handheld computer device for immediate referral. If a handheld computer is not used by the provider, reduce the dimensions of the appointment schedule sheet to pocket-size for the provider's easy access. Generally, if the provider makes hospital visits before coming to the clinic in the morning, this schedule is printed the previous evening before closing.

These daily appointment sheets can also be used to include other provider commitments such as meetings and visits from pharmaceutical representatives. Such a complete record of time ensures that no patient appointments will be booked when, in fact, the provider is not available.

Computer Scheduling Software

Even the smallest of medical facilities today will benefit from the use of information technology. Numerous software programs for the ambulatory care setting require only basic computer hardware that can save time for providers and their staff members. Other programs are more sophisticated and may require on-site technical support.

Some scheduling software programs will schedule resources, equipment, examination rooms, and specialty staff, as well as patients and providers. Some will show copayments due, authorization expiration dates, and insurance expiration dates. They can select the next available appointment, search for appointments by provider, copy and paste appointments, and specify minimum time increments between appointments. The staff can view multiple schedules daily, weekly, monthly, or even yearly. Reminder notes can be created for both providers and patients.

EHR Computerized scheduling systems that are a component of a complete practice management facility, including medical records, are able to indicate no-shows and cancellations in the system and the patient's chart at the same time. Facilities that are partially computerized will still want to indicate patients who do not keep their appointments on the daily worksheet and in the patients' medical records.

Online systems can handle prescription refill requests, patient-provider email messages, and laboratory results. Some will allow patients to update insurance data and complete registration forms. All of the online systems are done within the provider's Web site, which includes security measures and sophisticated **encryption technology**. Therefore, security is less of a concern.

With America's ongoing goal of giving patients increased access to their electronic health record (EHR) and Congress pushing to have prescriptions transferred electronically, electronic scheduling has become the "entry" to the entire field of computerized medical information. Employers in ambulatory care settings who make certain that patients understand computerized scheduling, who have put time and effort into determining the best program for their use, and who have trained their staff well will not be disappointed with the outcome. Whatever system is chosen, keep in mind that the patient's time, the staff's time, and the provider's time are extremely valuable. The goal is to manage that time as efficiently as possible.

INPATIENT AND OUTPATIENT ADMISSIONS PROCEDURES

Often, patients are scheduled for either outpatient or inpatient hospital admissions or for special procedures performed in another facility. These appointments are most likely made while the patient is present in the ambulatory care center and has just been seen by the primary care provider. It will be especially helpful if the patient has an appointment book identifying current responsibilities. Have a calendar handy for visualization of the days discussed.

Outpatient procedures may include endoscopy examinations and specialized radiologic examinations such as mammography, bone scans, and ultrasounds. Computerized tomography (CT) scans and magnetic resonance imaging (MRI) procedures will also require specialized admissions. If a patient prefers to make his or her own arrangements for a procedure, indicate that the following information is necessary:

- Name, address, and telephone number of patient
- Name of provider ordering the procedure
- Name of the procedure and preoperative diagnosis
- Name of patient's insurance, ID number, and Social Security number

 Follow up in a day or two to make certain the required procedure has been scheduled (see Procedure 13-9). In addition, please be certain that the patient has been given and understands any special instructions they must follow prior to the procedure. This includes but is not limited to fasting (no eating or drinking after midnight), withholding the consumption of certain medications (such as anything that can interfere with the anesthesia), having a spouse or loved one available to speak with the provider and staff, or not using lotions, oils, or powders prior to the procedure.

Generally, a real service is done for the patients and staff when the medical assistant schedules the procedure. With the patient present, place a telephone call to the facility where procedures are to be performed. Identify yourself, your provider, and the clinic from which you are calling. Identify any urgency to the request and ask for the next available appointment. As dates and times are discussed, your patient is able to give an immediate response. Consider travel time for your patient and whether there is apt to be any uncomfortable pre-examination procedures that might make travel difficult. Be certain to advise the patient if someone is needed to provide transportation home after the procedure. Often, there is a paperwork follow-up that indicates the nature of the illness and the reason for the specialty examination. Your employer will tell you if a phone response to the examination is required, or if it is acceptable to wait for the written test results.

Once a date has been established, make certain the patient knows the correct date and time, as well as how to get to the place where the examination is to be performed. Inform the patient how and when he or she will receive test results.

Scheduling inpatient admissions to the hospital is similar. However, the provider may want the patient in the hospital as quickly as possible. Call the preferred or designated hospital. Expect to provide pertinent patient and insurance information required by the hospital. Assist the patient in determining whether it is permissible to return home for some personal belongings and to make home arrangements or whether admission is immediate. Some large facilities have a surgery

scheduler to make all these arrangements. In primary care, the medical assistant will do this kind of scheduling.

When a surgery is being scheduled, the medical assistant must sometimes coordinate several entities. Arrangements must be coordinated with an assistant in the surgeon's clinic, with the hospital or outpatient surgery center where the surgery will be performed, and occasionally for scheduling specialty equipment and personnel to be available, as well as with the patient's schedule. If any one of these entities is not available at the time requested, the process needs to begin again and can become quite convoluted. If the scheduling of the surgery is especially complex, the medical assistant should consider obtaining the patient's scheduling preferences and limitations and letting the patient go home to be contacted later when all the parts are in place.

Be sensitive to the patient's needs at this time. Scheduling a specialty examination or a hospital admission is rarely a convenience. More likely it is a great inconvenience to the patient, even when necessary. Anything that makes the scheduling more accommodating or pleasant for the patient will help in creating a beneficial atmosphere for all involved.

PROCEDURE 13-1
Establishing the Appointment Matrix in a Paper System

PURPOSE:
To have a current and accurate record of appointment times available for scheduling patient visits.

EQUIPMENT/SUPPLIES:
Appointment scheduler
Clinic schedule and calendar
Provider and staff schedule

PROCEDURE STEPS:
1. Block off times in the appointment scheduler when patients are not to be scheduled by marking a large *X* through these time slots. This establishes the matrix. Ideally, the whole year can be mapped out to avoid scheduling patients when the provider has other commitments or when the clinic is closed. RATIONALE: Identifies

visually when patients cannot be scheduled for an appointment.

2. Indicate all vacations, holidays, and other clinic closures as soon as they are known. It may be helpful to indicate absences that might affect patient scheduling; for example, the vascular laboratory technician is gone April 20–23, so no Doppler procedures will be scheduled. RATIONALE: Informs all staff members of absences from the facility and indicates when these members are not available to see patients.

3. *Pay attention to detail.* Note all provider meetings, hospital rounds, appointments, conferences, vacations, and other prescheduled provider commitments. If the provider has routine items, such as a Medical Society meeting that is always held on the first Thursday of the month at 7:00 PM or daily hospital rounds at 8:00 AM, write these in. RATIONALE: Informs all staff members of

Procedure 13-1 (continued)

prescheduled commitments when a provider is unavailable to see patients.

4. If the clinic has a scheduling system for certain examinations or procedures (e.g., all cast removals are done in the morning before 10:30 AM), these can be color coded with highlighters. This way it is easily and quickly evident where particular types of appointments are available

to be scheduled. RATIONALE: Allows all staff members to see at a glance where certain examinations or procedures can be scheduled. The color-coded highlighting helps prevent errors in establishing such specific times for certain procedures. *The completed matrix provides proof of the completed task.*

PROCEDURE 13-2
Establishing the Appointment Matrix Using Medical Office Simulation Software (MOSS)

PURPOSE:
To designate and block time for provider commitments outside the clinic on an electronic appointment matrix.

EQUIPMENT/SUPPLIES:
Computer with MOSS installed

PROCEDURE STEPS:
1. Open MOSS and select Appointment Scheduling from the Main Menu.
2. Using the calendar on the top right, select a date. Hint: Use the –M and +M and –Y and +Y to navigate to the correct month and year, and then click on the date.

3. Click on the time slot in the applicable provider column and then click on *Block Calendar*.
4. Click *Yes* to create a new calendar block. In Field 1 of the *Block Calendar* window, enter the name of the time block in the *Description* field. Complete Fields 2–9 with information as applicable to the block.
5. Click on *Save* to post the block to the appointment matrix. A confirmation message will verify the information was posted.
6. Check the appointment matrix to be sure the blocks are in place correctly.
7. Close the Practice Schedule and return to the Main Menu.

PROCEDURE 13-3
Making an Appointment Using Paper Scheduling

PURPOSE:
To schedule an appointment, entering information in the appointment schedule according to clinic policy.

EQUIPMENT/SUPPLIES:
Telephone
Black ink pen
Appointment matrix
Calendar

PROCEDURE STEPS:
1. In a private and quiet location, answer the ringing telephone before the third ring. Identify the facility and yourself. RATIONALE: Assures the patient calling that he or she has the correct number; sets the tone for the conversation. The private location ensures that others will not hear any information said during the telephone call.

continues

Procedure 13-3 (continued)

2. As the patient begins to speak, make notes on your personal log sheet of the patient's name and reason for the call. RATIONALE: Makes certain you are focusing on the call and will not have to ask the patient to repeat something you missed.

3. *Apply active listening skills.* Determine whether the patient is new or established, the provider to be seen, and the reason for the appointment. RATIONALE: Provides necessary information to determine when the patient should be seen and how much time will likely be necessary.

4. *Discuss with the patient any special appointment needs*, and search your appointment schedule (using appointment book or appointment worksheet) for an available time. RATIONALE: Tells the patient that his or her needs and the needs of the clinic are essential to this conversation.

5. Once that patient has agreed to an appropriate time, enter the patient's name in the schedule. Enter last name first, followed by the first name, telephone number (home, work, or cell), and the chief complaint (reason for the visit). Write or print legibly with a black pen in the appointment book or worksheet so that any staff member needing the information will be able to read it. RATIONALE: Provides necessary information for staff to pull a record or to make a chart; chief complaint helps identify the length of time to allot for the appointment. The telephone number provides immediate information without having to pull the chart should there be a need to change the appointment.

6. Repeat the date and time for the appointment, using the patient's name. Provide any necessary instructions about coming to the facility. RATIONALE: Confirms the appointment date and time with the patient and gives information about how to get to the facility.

7. *End the call politely*, perhaps saying, "Thank you for calling. We will see you at 3:45 PM Monday. Good-bye."

8. Make certain you transferred all necessary information from your telephone log to the appropriate appointment schedule. Draw a diagonal line through your notes on the log. This indicates you have completed the task.

PROCEDURE 13-4
Making an Appointment Using Medical Office Simulation Software (MOSS)

PURPOSE:
To schedule clinic visit appointments for new and established patients.

EQUIPMENT/SUPPLIES:
Computer and MOSS

PROCEDURE STEPS:

1. Open MOSS and select Appointment Scheduling from the Main Menu.

2. Using the calendar on the top right, select a date. Hint: Use the −M and +M and −Y and +Y to navigate to the correct month and year, and then click on the date.

3. Click on the time slot in the applicable physician column and then click on *View/Create Appointment*. As an alternate, the time slot may be *double clicked*.

4. Click the patient name to be scheduled, and then click *Add* from the *Appointment Scheduling* window. If a new patient, click on *Add New Patient*, and complete basic registration information and save the record before returning to scheduling.

5. On the *Patient Appointment Form* window, enter data in the fields indicating the physician and duration in minutes and the *Reason* field with the appointment information.

6. In the *Note* field, enter the patient's chief complaint or reason for visiting the provider.

7. When all data is entered, click on *Save Appointment*. Check the Practice Schedule for accuracy when completed.

8. Schedule the next patient, or close the Practice Schedule and return to the Main Menu.

PROCEDURE 13-5
Checking in Patients in a Paper System

PURPOSE:
To ensure the patient is given prompt and proper care; to meet legal safeguards for documentation.

EQUIPMENT/SUPPLIES:
Patient chart
Black ink pen
Required forms
Check-in list or appointment book

PROCEDURE STEPS:

1. The previous evening or before opening the ambulatory care setting, prepare a list of patients to be seen and assemble the charts. RATIONALE: Provides a patient list to use as a guide through the day's schedule; charts are ready before patient arrival. If the task is left to the last minute, it may not get done.

2. Check charts to see that everything is up to date, *paying attention to detail*. RATIONALE: Ensures that providers and staff have all the necessary data before seeing a patient.

3. *When patients arrive, acknowledge their presence.* If you cannot assist them immediately, gesture toward a chair; thank them for waiting as soon as you are available. RATIONALE: Patients feel welcomed, their time is valued, and their presence is noted.

4. Check in the patient and review vital information, such as address, telephone number, insurance, and reason for visit. Be certain to *protect the patient's privacy* by reviewing this information where doing so cannot be overheard by others. RATIONALE: Ensures that you have the latest personal information regarding your patient; provides patients with the privacy and confidentiality to which they are entitled.

5. Use a pen to check off the patient's name from the daily worksheet if one is used for the permanent record. RATIONALE: Ensures that there is a permanent record of the patient's arrival in the facility for an appointment. *Provides documentation for later referral if necessary.*

6. Politely ask the patient to be seated and indicate the appropriate wait time, if any. RATIONALE: Provides direction to the patient and indicates how long a wait might be.

7. Following clinic policy, place the chart where it can be picked up to route the patient to the appropriate location for the visit. RATIONALE: The patient's chart is in readiness when the clinical medical assistant, laboratory personnel, or provider is ready for the patient.

PROCEDURE 13-6
Checking in Patients Using Medical Office Simulation Software (MOSS)

PURPOSE:
To check in patients as they arrive for clinic appointments.

EQUIPMENT/SUPPLIES:
Computer and MOSS

PROCEDURE STEPS:

1. Open MOSS and select Appointment Scheduling from the Main Menu.

2. Using the calendar on the top right, select a date. Hint: Use the −M and +M and −Y and +Y to navigate to the correct month and year, and then click on the date.

3. Click on the time slot for the patient's appointment and click on *View/Create Appointment*. As an alternate, the appointment time slot may be *double clicked*.

4. On the *Patient Appointment Form* window, click in the box in front of *Checked In*. In a clinic environment, after obtaining patient information, signatures, insurance card copies, and/or updating information, the patient file or

continues

Procedure 13-6 (continued)

electronic record is made ready for the clinical staff and provider.

5. Click on the *Close* button to exit the *Patient Appointment Form*.

6. Check in the next patient, or close the Practice Schedule and return to the Main Menu.

PROCEDURE 13-7
Cancelling and Rescheduling Procedures Using Paper Scheduling

PURPOSE:
To protect the provider from legal complications; to free up care time for other patients; and to ensure quality patient care.

EQUIPMENT/SUPPLIES:
Appointment sheet
Red ink pen
Patient chart

PROCEDURE STEPS:
Develop a system so it is evident to staff making appointments that, because of cancellations, time is now open to schedule other appointments.

1. Indicate on the appointment sheet all appointments that were changed, canceled, or no-shows by:

   - *Changes:* Note rescheduling in the appointment sheet margin and directly in the patient's chart; indicate new appointment time. RATIONALE: Notifies all staff of a schedule change; *documents same information in patient's chart.*

   - *Cancellations:* Note on both the appointment sheet and the patient's chart. Draw a single red line through canceled appointments. Date and initial cancellation in the patient chart. RATIONALE: Notifies staff of a schedule change; *documents cancellation in patient's chart, thus identifying a change in the patient's plans.* A cancellation may initiate a follow-up call from a staff member to determine the reason for the cancellation.

   - *No-shows:* Note on both the appointment sheet and the patient's chart. Date and initial notations in the chart. No-shows can be indicated with a red **X** on the appointment sheet. RATIONALE: Notifies the staff of a schedule change; *documents the no-show in the patient's chart.* Provides a reminder to a staff member to follow up on the reason for the no-show.

PROCEDURE 13-8
Cancelling a Patient Appointment Using MOSS

PURPOSE:
To cancel visits already on the practice schedule and provide a reason.

EQUIPMENT/SUPPLIES:
Computer and MOSS

PROCEDURE STEPS:
1. Open MOSS and select Appointment Scheduling from the Main Menu.

2. Using the calendar on the top right, select a date. Hint: Use the –M and +M and –Y and +Y to navigate to the correct month and year, and then click on the date.

3. Click on the time slot for the patient's appointment and click on *View/Create Appointment*. As an alternate, the appointment time slot may be *double clicked.*

Procedure 13-8 (continued)

4. On the *Patient Appointment Form* window, click in the box in front of *Cancelled*.

5. Click the drop down box directly to the right and select the reason code for the patient's cancellation.

6. In the next field to the right, enter the date of cancellation.

7. Click on *Save Appointment*.

8. Click on the *Close* button to exit the *Patient Appointment Form*.

9. Cancel the next patient, or close the Practice Schedule and return to the Main Menu.

PROCEDURE 13-9
Rescheduling a Patient Appointment Using MOSS

PURPOSE:
To reschedule visits already on the practice schedule to another date and time.

EQUIPMENT/SUPPLIES:
Computer and MOSS

PROCEDURE STEPS:

1. Open MOSS and select Appointment Scheduling from the Main Menu.

2. Using the calendar on the top right, select a date. Hint: Use the –M and +M and –Y and +Y to navigate to the correct month and year, and then click on the date.

3. Click on the time slot for the patient's appointment and click on *View/Create Appointment*. As an alternate, the appointment time slot may be *double clicked*.

4. On the *Patient Appointment Form* window, click in the box in front of *Rescheduled*.

5. Click the drop down box directly to the right and select the reason code for the reschedule.

6. In the next field to the right, click on the *View Practice Reschedule* calendar icon. This will open the Practice Calendar.

7. Select the new date, physician column, and time by double clicking in the time slot. Next, click on the *Close* button.

8. On the *Patient Appointment Form*, click on *Save Appointment* to execute the rescheduled appointment.

9. Click *OK* to complete the task.

10. The updated *Patient Appointment Form* will display the rescheduled appointment in Fields 3 and 4. Check appointment for accuracy.

11. Click on the *Close* button to exit the *Patient Appointment Form*.

12. Reschedule the next patient, or close the Practice Schedule and return to the Main Menu.

PROCEDURE 13-10
Scheduling Inpatient and Outpatient Admissions and Procedures

PURPOSE:
To assist patients in scheduling inpatient and outpatient admissions and procedures ordered by the provider.

EQUIPMENT/SUPPLIES:
Calendar
Black ink pen
Telephones
Referral slip
Patient's calendar or schedule (helpful, but not critical)
Provider requests/orders regarding procedures/admissions being scheduled

continues

Procedure 13-10 (continued)

PROCEDURE STEPS:

1. In a private and quiet location, discuss with the patient the inpatient admission or outpatient procedure ordered by the provider. RATIONALE: Helps the patient identify the time necessary for this appointment and the reason for it.

2. If required, seek permission from the patient's insurance company for the procedure or admission. RATIONALE: Clearly identifies for the patient who is responsible for the bill and how it is to be paid.

3. Produce a large, easily read calendar and check to see if the patient has one also. RATIONALE: Visualization of the calendar is easier for determining available time for the appointment. Patient's calendar further identifies available days and times for the appointment(s).

4. Place telephone call to the facility where the appointment is to be scheduled. Identify yourself, your provider, the clinic from where you are calling, and the reason for the call. RATIONALE: Alerts the receiver of the call that a provider's office is calling to schedule an appointment. NOTE: *The more familiar the medical assistant is with the specific procedure to be scheduled or a hospital admission, the easier it is to make certain the patient has all the information necessary. It can be helpful for medical assistants to discuss such arrangements with specialty clinics and hospitals.*

5. ***Display sound judgment*** and identify any urgency. Request the next available appointment for the particular appointment to be scheduled and provide the patient's diagnosis. Identify any time that is not possible for the patient. RATIONALE: Tells the receiver how quickly an appointment is to be made, for what reason, and if any dates or times are not possible.

6. As a time is suggested, confer with the patient for an immediate response.

7. Once the appointment has been scheduled, provide receiver pertinent information related to the patient (e.g., full name, insurance information, Social Security number, telephone number). RATIONALE: Provides essential information to secure the appointment for the proper patient.

8. Request any special instructions or advanced data necessary for the patient. RATIONALE: Helps to ensure that a smooth transition is made from the provider's clinic to the facility where the referral is made and provides the patient with any special instructions.

9. Complete the referral slip for the patient; send or fax a copy to the referral facility. RATIONALE: Ensures that the patient, the referral facility, and the patient's chart have a copy of the reason for the appointment, any specific instructions, and the date and time of the appointment.

10. If an immediate hospital admission is to be made, ***attend to special needs of patient*** by providing him or her time on the telephone to call family members to make arrangements to receive personal items and any other arrangements necessitated by the appointment. RATIONALE: Provides patients a little time to notify a family member and make necessary arrangements.

11. Place a reminder notice to yourself on the calendar or in a tickler file. RATIONALE: To check to make certain the appointment was completed and a report is received from the appointment facility.

12. Document the referral in the patient's chart. A copy of the referral slip and all pertinent data are to be included. Document in the chart when the appointment is completed and a report is received from the referral facility. Date and initial.

DOCUMENTATION:

11/30/20XX—10:45 AM   Referral to Eastside Radiology for breast ultrasound made. A. Rein, RMA (AMT)——————

12/01/20XX—1 PM   Patient given instructions and copy of referral slip. Original referral slip sent to Eastside Radiology. A. Rein, RMA (AMT)——————

CASE STUDY 13-1

Refer to the scenario at the beginning of the chapter. It appears that this clinic has a smooth-flowing scheduling system and that Walter Seals has everything under control.

1. What personal traits might Walter need to possess in order for this scenario to be true?

2. What factors, if any, might make the scheduling at Inner City Health Care work well?

3. If clients are seen on a first-come, first-served basis, how does the clustering system work if patients need to be referred to one of the specialty care clinics?

CASE STUDY 13-2

Rhoda Au has persistently canceled her appointments at Inner City Health Care. Although she always reschedules, she has canceled her last four appointments. Today, she did not call to cancel nor did she arrive for her fifth appointment. Walter Seals, CMA (AAMA), who is responsible for scheduling and patient flow, is concerned that Rhoda is canceling because she is afraid to come in for some reason. Rhoda has been a patient for a few years now, and she was always responsible about keeping her appointments.

CASE STUDY REVIEW

1. From the point of view of the urgent care center, why should Walter be concerned that Rhoda is canceling appointments? What action might be taken?

2. From the patient's point of view, why should Walter be concerned?

3. How should Walter record these cancellations and no-shows?

CASE STUDY 13-3

Audrey Jones, RMA, is a clinical medical assistant in Drs. Lewis and King's clinic. In the past 3 weeks, Audrey has been doing phone screening, primarily because the clinic has been so busy and the providers believe screening calls will help. In fact, Audrey discovered that the administrative medical assistant was screening quite well, but that there does not seem to be sufficient appointment slots to meet the patient demand.

CASE STUDY REVIEW

1. What might be done to determine whether there is a better scheduling style to fit the current demands?

2. What happens when professional staff, providers, and patients view this medical facility as "too busy"?

3. What are some solutions that you can identify?

SUMMARY

Today's ambulatory care setting needs to function efficiently to provide quality care, ensure adequate patient flow, and maintain positive patient relationships. Proper scheduling of patients and other visitors is key to an efficient operation, and the well-organized medical assistant will design a system that meets with both provider and patient satisfaction.

There are at least six common methods of scheduling; ambulatory care settings should use the one that is most appropriate to their patient population, practice areas, and provider preferences. Scheduling methods can and should be customized to the setting, for this usually provides the most adaptable, workable system.

Patient scheduling tools also vary and can be tailored to facility needs. All ambulatory care settings must carefully document appointments, cancellations, and no-shows. The goal is to use scheduling tools wisely and consistently in all scheduling activities while making the patient feel valued.

CERTIFICATION REVIEW

1. Appointment scheduling should always be:
   a. recorded only in pencil
   b. current, accurate, and saved as documentation
   c. left on the front desk for patient viewing
   d. recorded only in red ink

2. Patient screening:
   a. involves taking only emergencies
   b. is assessing the urgency of a call and need for appointment
   c. means sorting appointments by specialized procedure
   d. is only performed by providers

3. Representatives from medical supply and drug companies:
   a. should only be seen as a last resort
   b. should not be scheduled, but seen only if the provider has time
   c. can provide a valuable service and should be scheduled for short visits
   d. have complex information to communicate and need 1-hour appointments

4. The double-booking method:
   a. gives two or more patients the same appointment time
   b. keeps patients waiting unnecessarily
   c. is never the system of choice
   d. is purely for the provider's convenience

5. The stream method:
   a. gives patients appointments as they walk in
   b. schedules appointments at set times throughout the workday
   c. only works in sole-proprietor clinics
   d. refers to streamlining paperwork for each appointment

6. Daily appointment sheets:
   a. indicate when providers and staff take lunch
   b. provide a permanent record for legal risk management and quality management
   c. are available only in computerized scheduling
   d. both a and b

7. Analyzing patient flow:
   a. can maximize a clinic's scheduling practice
   b. often reveals why patient flow is not efficient
   c. may indicate a change in pattern for patient scheduling
   d. all of the above

8. One principle above all else to be observed in scheduling is:
   a. always schedule in ink
   b. schedule for the patient's convenience
   c. be flexible and sensitive
   d. referral patients are first

9. If a patient must wait for an appointment:
   a. it is best to say nothing about the delay
   b. explain the delay and offer options when possible
   c. find ways to make the patient comfortable
   d. both b and c

10. Scheduling outpatient procedures is:
    a. best done by patients who understand their availability
    b. coordinated and completed by the clinic's staff
    c. an important way to enhance patient satisfaction
    d. both b and c

REFERENCE/BIBLIOGRAPHY

Lewis, M. A., & Tamparo, C. D. (2007). *Medical law, ethics, and bioethics for health professions* (6th ed.). Philadelphia: F. A. Davis.

Medical Records Management

OUTLINE

The Purpose of Medical Records

Ownership of Medical Records

Authorization to Release
Information

Manual or Electronic Medical
Records

The Importance of Accurate
Medical Records

   Creating Paper and
   Electronic Charts

   Correcting Medical Records

Types of Medical Records

   Problem-Oriented Medical
   Record

   Source-Oriented Medical
   Record

   Strict Chronological
   Arrangement

Equipment and Supplies

   Vertical Files

   Open-Shelf Lateral Files

Movable File Units

File Folders

Identification Labels

Guides and Positions

Out Guides

Basic Rules for Filing

   Indexing Units

   Filing Patient Charts

   Filing Identical Names

Steps for Filing Medical
Documentation in Patient Files

   Inspect

   Index

   Code

   Sort

   File

Filing Techniques and Common
Filing Systems

   Color Coding

   Alphabetic Filing

Numeric Filing

Subject Filing

Choosing a Filing System

Filing Procedures

   Cross-Referencing

   Tickler Files

   Release Marks

   Checkout System

   Locating Missing Files or Data

   Filing Chart Data

   Retention and Purging

Correspondence

   Filing Procedures for
   Correspondence

Electronic Medical Records

   Archival Storage

   Transfer of Data

   Confidentiality

LEARNING OUTCOMES

1. Define, spell, and pronounce the key terms as presented in the glossary.
2. List the purpose of medical records.
3. Discuss the ownership of medical records.
4. State the reasons for accurately maintaining ambulatory care files.
5. Describe how and when information is released from the medical record.
6. State the pros and cons of the manual medical record and the electronic medical record.
7. Correct a medical record, manually and electronically.
8. Recall eight common supplies used in medical records management.
9. Identify the rules described under Basic Rules for Filing.
10. Describe the five steps commonly used when filing any documentation.
11. Name the two filing systems most often used in the ambulatory care setting.
12. State the purpose of cross-referencing.
13. Recall four common documents kept in the patient's medical record.
14. Discuss storage and purging of medical records.

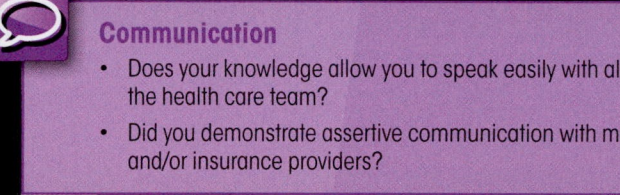

ATTRIBUTES OF PROFESSIONALISM

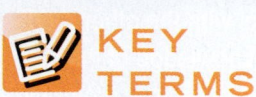
KEY TERMS

accession record

caption

cross-reference

indexing

key unit

out guide

problem-oriented medical record (POMR)

purging

SOAP/SOAPER

source-oriented medical record (SOMR)

tickler file

unit

Communication
- Does your knowledge allow you to speak easily with all members of the health care team?
- Did you demonstrate assertive communication with managed care and/or insurance providers?

Presentation
- Were you courteous, patient, and respectful to the patient?
- Did you display a positive attitude?
- Did you display a calm, professional, and caring manner?

Competency
- Did you display sound judgment?
- Were you knowledgeable and accountable?
- Did you recognize the importance of local, state, and federal legislation and regulations in the practice setting?

Initiative
- Did you show initiative?

LEARNING OUTCOMES (*continued*)

15. Describe electronic medical records and their usefulness to the ambulatory care setting.

16. Discuss confidentiality and privacy as related to medical records.

17. Explain HIPAA security standards for electronic medical records.

18. Analyze the professionalism questions and apply them to this chapter's content.

SCENARIO

Consider a situation that might arise at the multiprovider Inner City Health Care. Patient Juanita Hansen was seen on Tuesday morning by Dr. Whitney for acute stomach pain. She was given a thorough examination and sent for appropriate testing that afternoon. She was then scheduled to return to Inner City on Friday to see Dr. Whitney.

After she was seen Tuesday morning, Juanita received an upper and lower gastrointestinal series; the results were then sent to Dr. Whitney's clinic. However, because Karen Ritter, RMA (AMT), the medical assistant, could not locate Juanita's chart to file the test results, she just set

them aside. Friday arrived and Juanita came back to Inner City for her appointment, anxious to know the results of her tests. Dr. Whitney found Juanita's chart, which was inadvertently left on his stack of dictation, and realized the patient's test results had not been filed.

This left Dr. Whitney with an anxious patient. Karen Ritter is off today, so the provider checks with the other medical assistants on duty. They have no knowledge of the test results. Two acts—not replacing the file, and not promptly filing Juanita's test results—cause undue stress for the provider, medical assistants, and patient.

INTRODUCTION

Every medical facility generates a large amount of information. Business, insurance, personnel, and financial records must be maintained. Supplies and equipment records must be managed. Licensures and certifications must be current. Some records are kept for the life of the practice. The greatest bulk of information, however, comes from patient medical records. A vital function of any medical facility is the maintenance of patient records identifying the care given. Medical assistants, both administrative and clinical, will spend a fair amount of time managing patients' records. Medical records potentially record all medical data about an individual from birth until death.

Even in medical facilities where patient records are managed electronically, there are ample paper records to be stored and retrieved manually. A number of functions essential to proper records management are discussed in this chapter. A clear understanding of the proper methods used to manage the records in a medical facility is an important and necessary skill for medical assistants.

Chapter 11 defined electronic medical records (EMRs) as those coming from a single medical practice, hospital, or pharmacy. When EMRs from multiple sources are combined into one database for a patient, the term electronic health record (EHR) is used (Figure 14-1).

THE PURPOSE OF MEDICAL RECORDS

The primary purposes of medical records in the ambulatory care setting are to:

1. Provide a base for managing patient care
2. Provide interoffice and intraoffice communication as necessary

3. Determine any patterns that surface to signal the provider of patient needs
4. Serve as a basis for legal information necessary to protect providers, staff, and patients
5. Provide clinical data for research

OWNERSHIP OF MEDICAL RECORDS

State statutes have ruled that medical records are the property of those who create them. The information within the medical record, however, belongs to the patient, and that information is always to be protected with the utmost privacy and confidentiality. Patients can be allowed access to their medical records, ask for notes or information to be added to their files, and request that certain information not be included in their files.

Providers who include their patients in their medical record keeping foster trust and respect with their patients. For example, a provider who enters patient data into the electronic patient record while sitting at a computer monitor in the examination room beside the patient has the opportunity to explain that the information is entered now so there is no room for error in reporting or in the provider not accurately recalling the patient information if entered at a later time. A patient who asks a primary care provider to put the pen aside while discussing possible depression symptoms is concerned about privacy, especially if the patient is the pediatrics department manager in the same large metropolitan medical center/hospital as the provider. The provider should realize that a discussion of how to keep this information confidential so that other employees are not aware of the patient's concern is in order.

AUTHORIZATION TO RELEASE INFORMATION

It is recommended that before any information is released from the medical record, the patient be notified and written approval received. Medical facilities will have appropriate forms for such release of information. A sample release of information form is given in Chapter 23. The form should identify the reason for the release of information and what information is specifically requested. Only that information should be released. This does not include the release of information to a patient's chosen insurance carrier. A number of different methods exist to release that information. For some insurance carriers, the release is granted when the patient accepts the insurance coverage. For others, a yearly release form must be signed by the patient.

MANUAL OR ELECTRONIC MEDICAL RECORDS

Today's medical environment has a mixture of manual, or paper, medical records and the electronic form of medical records. The world is changing, however. Some medical providers

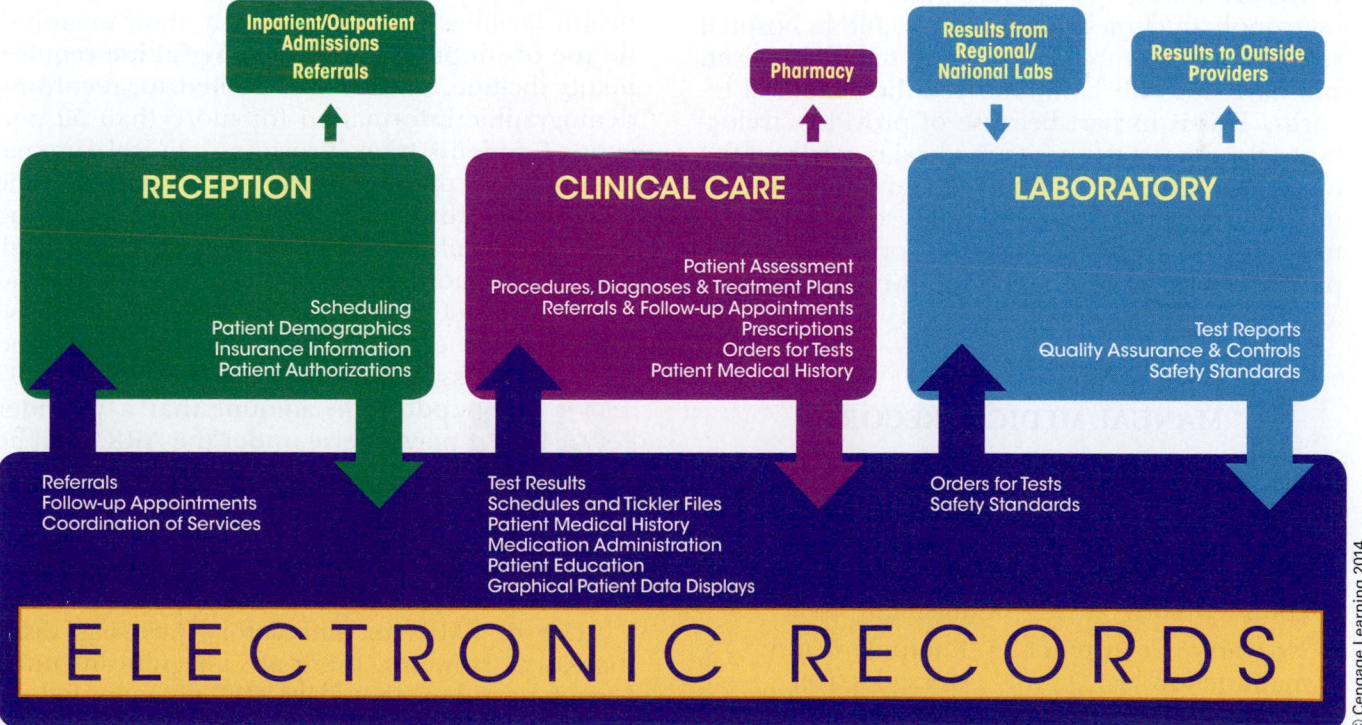

Figure 14-1 Medical records management relates to the laboratory, reception, and clinical care components in a total practice management system.

continue to have difficulty with including the necessary information that is considered vital in documentation for further enhancing the transition to EHR. Key medical data has been either improperly documented or has been omitted from some patients' records, which can create numerous compliance and billing issues when corresponding with insurance companies. By becoming more specific in documentation, providers will ensure that all of a patient's data is included in the electronic record and further enhance the transition to EHR. During his presidency, President George W. Bush announced his Health Information Technology Plan, which included the goal of ensuring that most Americans would have electronic health records by 2014. Planned projects include transmitting X-rays and laboratory results electronically to providers for immediate analysis and standardizing electronic prescriptions, hopefully decreasing errors in patient care. Medical clinics have scrambled to comply. Many have been successful; others have not and were hoping for federal funds to assist in the transition to electronic records. Although the complete transition to electronic health records by 2014 may not occur, it certainly will occur in the next decade.

Frustrated by the slow response of medical providers, lawmakers in the U.S. Senate and the House of Representatives introduced legislation in 2007 to require electronic prescribing (e-prescribing) of medications for Medicare no later than 2011. EMRs are widely seen in large medical clinics, in metropolitan clinics with hospitals, and in hospital settings. Many ambulatory care settings, however, still have not fully computerized their medical records. This is in part because of providers' reluctance to let go of the paper medical record and the incredible expense of switching to computerized medical records. Also, there is the concern of how to transfer the current paper record to the computer record. Consider the following advantages and disadvantages of both records:

MANUAL MEDICAL RECORD

Advantages	Disadvantages
• Currently established and understood	• Can be used by only one person at a time
• Easier to protect confidentiality	• Easily misplaced or misfiled
• No worry of computer malfunction	• Equipment and storage space required
	• More susceptible to error

ELECTRONIC MEDICAL RECORD

Advantages	Disadvantages
• Multiple users are possible	• Needs protection to prevent loss of data
• Not easily misplaced or misfiled	• Expensive to establish and maintain
• Errors less likely	• May require on-site assistance
• Patterns and data more easily accessed	• Can require up to 12 weeks for staff to prove productive after installation
• Quickly available in emergencies	
• Office storage space not required	
• Legible, organized patient documentation	
• Improved medication management	
• Improved quality of care	

In 2009, President Barack Obama signed off on the American Reinvestment and Recovery Act (ARRA). This law provides numerous incentives for providers and hospitals to make the transition to EMR. For example, a specified amount of money has been designated to be disbursed to health facilities that can properly show meaningful use of adopting EMR. Meaningful use requirements include, but are not limited to, recording demographic information for more than 50 percent of patients seen, providing clinical summaries for more than 50 percent of requested clinic visits within three business days, and providing electronic health information within three business days to more than 50 percent of patients who make the request. The final list of meaningful use requirements can be found at http://www.gpo.gov/fdsys/pkg/FR-2010-07-28/pdf/2010-17207 .pdf. The amount that a provider may receive under the ARRA can be as high as $44,000.00. Therefore, it would be highly beneficial for a provider to make this transition—not only for the sake of his or her patients, but for the financial benefits that would be given to the practice.

Use of EMRs in ambulatory care has vastly increased. However, there are a significant number of providers that have still not adopted an EMR system, even though the aforementioned incentives are being provided. Solo practitioners are least likely to use EMRs; EMRs grow at faster

CRITICAL THINKING

Your clinic is planning to implement an electronic medical records system. What steps must you take to ensure the transition goes smoothly? What factors should be considered when selecting an EMR system? How does the implementation of such a system affect overall patient care?

rates in larger, multi-provider clinics. It is interesting to note that most patients believe they have greater access to and more control over their medical records when they are in electronic form, and they believe their primary care providers would be able to give more comprehensive patient care with EMRs. The medical record system must be one that fits the facility and satisfies the needs of the providers. Usually, medical record systems are adapted for a particular facility using certain common components.

Whatever system is used, the management of the medical records must provide easy retrieval of information. All documentation must be complete and correct. Wording must be easily understood and grammatically correct. How corrections are made in the chart, how documents are removed from or added to the chart, and the format of the chart must be predetermined and understood by all users of the information.

THE IMPORTANCE OF ACCURATE MEDICAL RECORDS

Accurate medical records are essential to patient care in any health care setting. One incorrect digit in a patient's Social Security number causes reimbursement problems. An incorrect address or telephone number or a misspelling of a name makes it difficult to contact patients about test results and prescription refills. Medical treatment documentation errors are even more disastrous and can cause serious medical problems for patients. Patient files are critical to the facility's smooth functioning and are important when referring the patient to outside specialists with whom the facility may need to coordinate care. Each treating primary care provider must be aware of tests, procedures, and diagnoses. Maintaining a conscientious record of patient care is also absolutely essential in controlling the costs of medical care.

 Medical records management is also important because of the legal issues that every medical clinic and health care professional must face today. The standard in court is that if there is no record of any piece of information related to a patient and that patient's care and treatment, then it did not happen. The question to ask yourself about any piece of information is: "Does this relate to the patient's care, and should it be in the chart?" To be prepared in the event of medical litigation, you must document all medical treatment. No matter how competently a provider has performed treatment, if a written record cannot prove how and what was done, there is no basis for a defense in a court of law.

Creating Paper and Electronic Charts

The patient's medical chart is prepared on or before the day of the patient's first visit in the medical facility. Paper medical records require the assembly of appropriate file folders, divider pages labeled with identifying tabs, and a number of essential forms to be completed by the patient. Included forms provide demographic information, social and family medical history, previous surgeries, HIPAA guidelines, and release of information details. Often, paper charts include adhesive twin prong fasteners to ensure that sheets of paper are securely held within the chart. Electronic patient medical charts are prepared in much the same manner with the exception being that all information is stored electronically. Patient information that is collected via the paper route will have to be scanned and entered into the record. The EMR will provide an orderly arrangement of patient information according to the particular software design or a predetermined plan selected by the providers and their staff. Procedures 14-1 and 14-2 allow creation of both a paper and an electronic chart.

Correcting Medical Records

The medical record must be readable and accurate; however, errors do occur and may not be discovered immediately. Any corrections necessary to a paper medical record should be corrected using the following method: draw a single line using a red ink pen through the error, make the correction, write "Corr." or "Correction" above the area corrected, and indicate your initials and the current date. The red line through the information indicates the "error" portion of the report. The words "Corr." or "Correction" by the correction indicate the change. The date and initials identify when the correction was made and by whom. Obliterations should never occur. When the medical record becomes the center of attention in malpractice litigation, forensic experts will be able to tell if a record has been tampered with or if information or pages have been added later. When not properly done, altered records become a detriment to any provider's defense in court (see Procedure 14-3).

Errors discovered immediately after the fact in an electronic medical record are corrected differently. Although it could be easy to do so, the error is *not corrected* by simple word processing. In a truly paperless clinic, a notation is entered at the place of the error, a line is drawn through the error (using the tracking device in the word processing software), and the correction is made immediately after the information lined out. "Corr." or "Correction" is indicated and your initials and the date added. The finished product will look similar to a correction in a paper medical chart (see Procedure 14-4). To ensure accuracy and prevent tampering with the information in a patient's record, EMR software locks out any additions to a chart entry after a specific period of time. After the lockout has occurred and a correction is necessary, a new entry is created that identifies the error and the correction to be made. It is dated, signed, and inserted in the document. It will be clear to the reader the error that occurred, the correction made, who made the correction, and when.

If any correction is necessary of any information after either a paper chart or an electronic chart has been sent to another provider or facility, make a copy of the corrected information and send it to the provider or facility as quickly as possible.

TYPES OF MEDICAL RECORDS

Whether patient charts are kept manually or electronically, there are common threads that run throughout medical records. How material is stored within records is important. The choice of method must be in accordance with how the information needs to be accessed and used for each individual clinic. No one method is best. In the examples that follow, arrangement of materials is also discussed.

Problem-Oriented Medical Record

The **problem-oriented medical record (POMR)** places in a prominent location vital identification data, immunizations, allergies, medications, and problems. The problems are identified by a number that corresponds to the charting relevant to that problem number, that is, bronchitis #1, broken wrist #2, and so forth. If the patient returns in 9 months with recurring bronchitis, the same number (#1) is used.

The patient chart is then further built by adding a numbered and titled section for each problem the patient experiences, for example, bronchitis #1, broken wrist #2.

Each problem is then followed with the **SOAP** approach for all progress notes:

S Subjective impressions

O Objective clinical evidence

A Assessment or diagnosis

P Plans for further studies, treatment, or management

Some medical facilities have added two additional letters to the SOAP approach, creating **SOAPER**. This additional charting tool can be especially useful in large teaching hospitals with medical clinics:

E Education for patient

R Response of patient to education and care given

This process makes the chart easier to review and helps in follow-up of all the patient's medical needs. The SOAP/SOAPER approach also allows medical personnel to be aware of the patient's current medications. Starting and resolution dates for each problem also are noted on the tracking page.

Internists, family practitioners, and pediatricians use the POMR system more commonly than do specialists because they see their patients for a variety of problems over a long span of time. It is commonly used in manual medical records as well as EMRs.

A number of medical supply companies produce various formats for POMR manual charts. There are flip-up folder styles and book-style folders made of 125-1b manila or white stock with twin prong fasteners. Divider pages may come with tabs that are preprinted to specific needs or have adhesive labels that can be printed on a printer exactly as you want them. Sometimes, the inside front and back covers are printed with information to be filled in. These areas are often used to provide essential personal information such as name, address, telephone numbers, insurance information, and responsible party. Over a period of time, however, because the information changes, entries on the inside cover are less desirable. A patient demographic form (see Chapter 23) can be attached to the inside cover. It can be updated annually and changed easily. In a prominent place, usually on the inside front cover, is the word "ALLERGIES" in big letters (often preprinted in red). Any allergies that patients have are listed here. Also prominently displayed should be any forms the patient has signed granting release of information, as well as any forms signed to comply with HIPAA regulations.

The problem list may be entered on a divider flap or on specially printed paper. Other dividers may be used for laboratory reports, progress notes, history and physicals, hospital admissions, and medications. Depending on the practice and the wishes of the provider, tab dividers are available for consultations, correspondence, insurance data, hospital notes, pathology reports, and electrocardiogram reports. The problem list is most likely the first divider used, followed by laboratory reports and progress notes, usually in the SOAP/SOAPER format.

SOAP/SOAPER is easily adapted to the EMR. There are a number of methods of indicating SOAP/SOAPER in the EMR. For a brief look at different models, use a computer search engine to key in "SOAP charting in EMRs." You will be able to compare a number of examples.

Source-Oriented Medical Record

The manual **source-oriented medical record (SOMR)** groups information according to its source; for example, from laboratories, examinations, provider notes, consulting providers, and other sources. Facilities use this method because it makes different types of information quickly accessible. A fastener folder is used that contains several partitions with their own fasteners. This allows for a separate section for laboratory reports, pathology, progress notes, physical examinations, and correspondence to be filed chronologically within each section. In the SOMR system, many providers use the SOAP/SOAPER method to record their chart notes.

The organization of the SOMR is quite similar to that of the POMR chart with the one exception that the SOMR does not have the problem list. Also, the SOMR may continually add sheets of identifying information with appropriate sections in the chart rather than transferring any data. Many EMR software packages use either the POMR or the SOMR format and are easily adapted to a particular provider's practice.

Strict Chronological Arrangement

Using strict chronology, data are filed strictly with the most recently charted materials to the top of the folder. For instance, a patient is treated from 2008 to the present. To locate information recorded in 2009, it is necessary to flip through the chart until the material for the year 2009 is located. This method makes it difficult for a provider or medical assistant to quickly assess a patient's clinical picture. This type of arrangement may seem confusing, but it may fit a specialty clinic such as a dietitian, radiologist, or physical therapist where patients are usually seen on a short-term basis.

EQUIPMENT AND SUPPLIES

Three primary types of file cabinets are used in medical clinics where manual files are stored: vertical, lateral, and movable.

Vertical Files

Vertical files are cabinets that have pullout drawers where files are stored (Figure 14-2). Files are retrieved by lifting the appropriate file up and out. These are likely used for business records and document, and should include a locking device.

The best vertical files have a center trough in the bottom of each drawer with a rod running through for holding divider guides. The rod and guides help keep file folders from slipping down underneath other file folders and getting misplaced or lost.

Open-Shelf Lateral Files

Open-shelf lateral file cabinets make quick retrieval of files possible (Figure 14-3). The records are retrieved by pulling them out laterally from the shelf. They are used most often with color-coded filing systems where visual inspection makes it possible to ensure files are kept in the proper order. Open-shelf lateral files are the most popular manual patient record system. It is necessary to be able

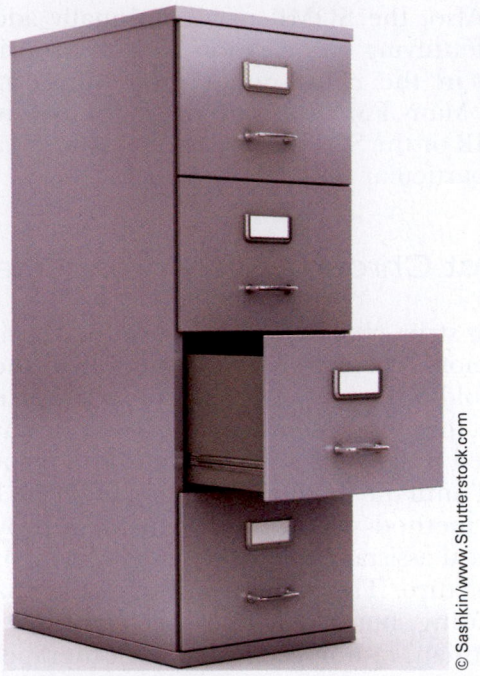

Figure 14-2   Vertical file cabinet.

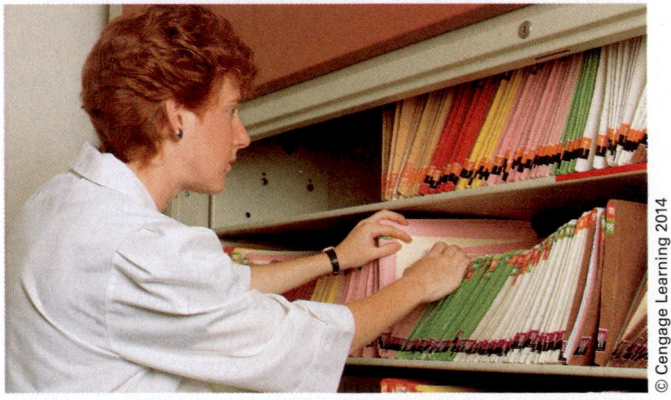

Figure 14-3   Open-shelf lateral file cabinet.

to close and lock the open-shelf lateral files to protect confidentiality.

Movable File Units

Movable file units allow easy access to large record systems and require less space than vertical or lateral files. These units may be electrically powered to move on floor tracks or may be physically moved with an easy-to-turn handle mechanism. The movable shelving unit is electrically powered to open aisles for accessing files or to close aisles when those files do not need to be accessed. There are also movable file storage units that will

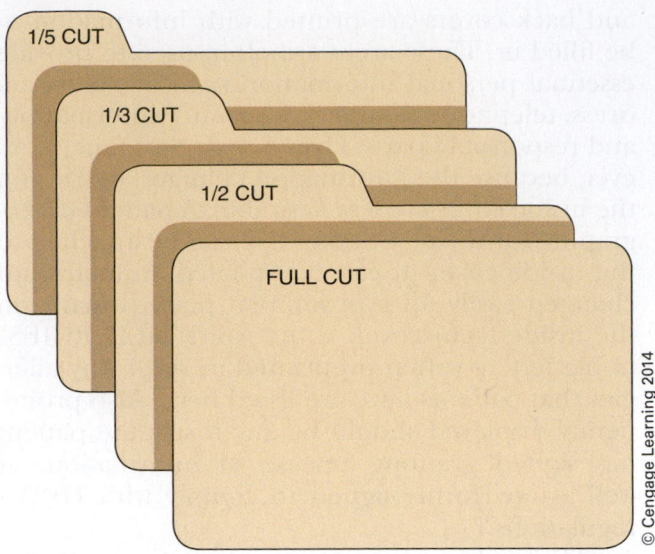

Figure 14-4   Types of cuts, or tabs, on file folders.

automatically travel on a computer-controlled carousel track, moving files around until the required section reaches the operator.

File Folders

File folders are designed for different types of labels. Extending along the top edge (the edge that will be visible when filing) are tabs that are cut in varying sizes and positions to allow for different methods of labeling. Figure 14-4 shows the types of cuts, or tabs, found on file folders. File folders should be constructed of good-quality card stock. If they are too light in weight, they will soon be bent, torn, and battered from use. They need to be sturdy enough for years of use.

Identification Labels

A variety of labels are used to display the information required to select the correct name or number designation for a particular file. The identification label is adhered either along the top of the file folder (top tab) in vertical file cabinets or along the side of the file folder (side tab) in lateral file cabinets.

Guides and Positions

Guides are used to separate file folders. Guides are somewhat larger than file folders and are of heavier stock. Guides are described by the position

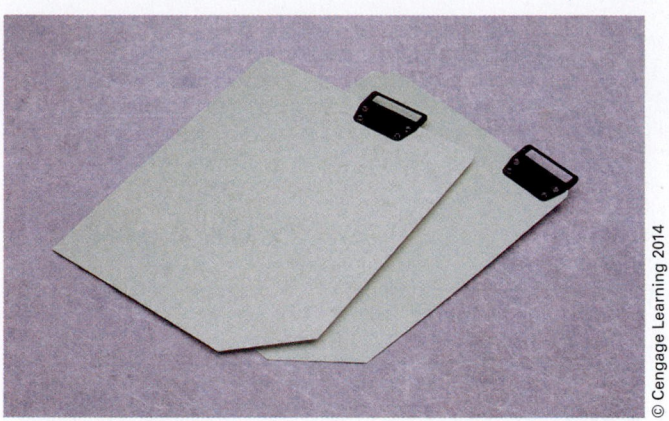

© Cengage Learning 2014

Figure 14-5 Guides separating file folders into subsections. Captions such as A, B, C (single captions) or Ab-Be, Co-Dy (double captions) are placed on the tabs of the guides to identify the sections.

of the tab, designated according to its location. For instance, a tab located at the far left would be in the first position, the next one to the right would be in the second position, and so forth. If using third-cut file folders, there are three positions of guides; if using fifth-cut file folders, there are five positions. Guides are used in vertical and lateral systems.

Captions are used to identify major sections of file folders by more manageable subunits (AA–AC, A, B, Office Supplies). Captions are marked on the tabs of the guides (Figure 14-5). These are denoted as single caption and double caption:

- *Single captions* contain just one letter, number, or unit:
  - A, B, C, D

- *Double captions* contain a double notation to denote a range of files:
  - Ab–Be, Co–Dy, Ho–Le

Out Guides

Out guides or out sheets are devices to help in tracking charts. An out guide is a piece of card stock or a plastic/paper sheet kept in place of the patient chart when the chart is removed from the filing storage (Figure 14-6).

BASIC RULES FOR FILING

Regardless of the type of filing system used, alphabetizing is the key to organizing all files and charts. It is necessary to know more than just the alphabetic order of the letters *A* to *Z*. Thus, certain indexing rules have been developed by the Association of Medical Records Administrators (AMRA) to facilitate the alphabetic process in maintaining files in the medical clinic.

Indexing Units

There must be an organized method of identifying and separating items to be filed into small subunits. This is accomplished with the use of **indexing** units. A unit identifies each part of a name. In this process, each **unit** is identified according to unit 1 (the **key unit**), unit 2, unit 3, and so forth, with each segment of the filing label identified. This

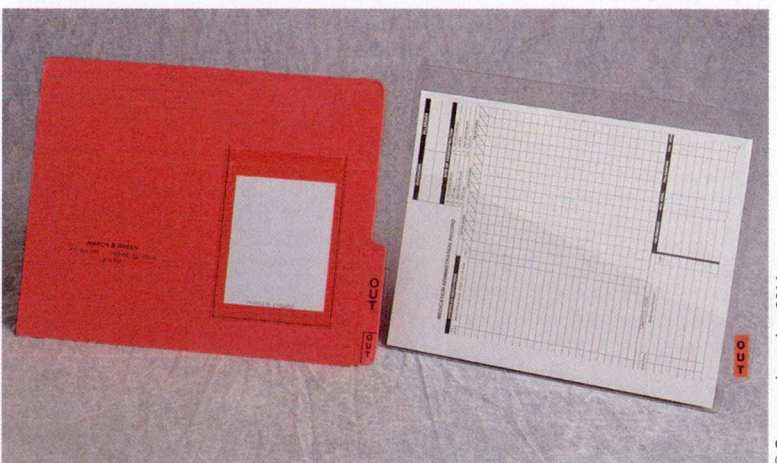

© Cengage Learning 2014

Figure 14-6 An out guide indicating the name of the person who has possession of the file should always be put in place of a patient's record when it is removed from the file.

process can be applied to individual names, organizations, or clinics. Accepted filing rules describe how to assign unit numbers to each element.

Example: Annette Barbara Samuels

Unit 1	Samuels
Unit 2	Annette
Unit 3	Barbara

When working in a medical setting with patient charts, the patient's legal name is always used for the chart rather than a nickname or abbreviation. If the clinic has a practice of calling patients by preferred names, a note of name preferences and nicknames may be noted on the chart. However, the filing label should use the proper name.

Example: The following items to be filed would be assigned units as illustrated:

	Units Assigned		
	1	**2**	**3**
Cole Blanche Little	Little	Cole	Blanche
Wayne Lee Elder	Elder	Wayne	Lee
Kelso Medical Supply	Kelso	Medical	Supply

Filing Patient Charts

Rule 1.   The names of individuals are assigned indexing units, respectively: last name (surname), first name, middle, and succeeding names.

	Units Assigned		
	1	**2**	**3**
Jaime Renae Carrera	Carrera	Jaime	Renae
Lee Allen Au	Au	Lee	Allen
Bill Hugo Schwartz	Schwartz	Bill	Hugo

Rule 2.   Names that include a single letter are indexed as the legal name and are placed before full names beginning with the same letter. "Nothing comes before something."

	Units Assigned		
	1	**2**	**3**
J. Larson	Larson	J	—
James R. Larson	Larson	James	R

Rule 3.   Foreign language prefixes are indexed as one unit with the unit that follows. Spacing, punctuation, and capitalization are ignored. Such prefixes include *d, da, de, de la, del, des, di, du, el, fitz, l, la, las, le, les, lu, m, mac, mc, o, saint, sainte, san, santa, sao, st, te, ten, ter, van, van de, van der,* and *von der* (*st, sainte,* and *saint* are indexed as written).

	Units Assigned		
	1	**2**	**3**
Gerald Steven St. Simon	Stsimon	Gerald	Steven
Carol Louise del Rio	Delrio	Carol	Louise

Rule 4.   When titles are used, they are considered as separate indexing units. If the title appears with first and last names, the title is considered to be the last indexing unit. When dealing with patient charts, the first name always accompanies the title and last name.

	Units Assigned			
	1	**2**	**3**	**4**
Dr. Marlene Elaine Smith	Smith	Marlene	Elaine	Dr
Prof. Marcia Tai Lewis	Lewis	Marcia	Tai	Prof

Rule 5.   Names that are hyphenated are considered as one unit.

	Units Assigned		
	1	**2**	**3**
Adele Marie Johnson-Smith	Johnsonsmith	Adele	Marie
Ray Steven Reynolds-Martin	Reynoldsmartin	Ray	Steven

Rule 6.   When indexing names of married women, the name is indexed by the legal name. Remember that patient charts are legal documents, making this practice necessary (use cross-referencing as necessary).

	Units Assigned			
	1	**2**	**3**	**4**
Amy Sue Sung (Mrs. John)	Sung	Amy	Sue	Mrs John
Tami Jo Strizver (Mrs. Todd)	Strizver	Tami	Jo	Mrs Todd

Rule 7.   Seniority and professional or academic degrees are the last indexing unit and are used only to distinguish identical names.

	Units Assigned			
	1	**2**	**3**	**4**
James Edward Brown, Jr.	Brown	James	Edward	Jr
James Edward Brown, Sr.	Brown	James	Edward	Sr

Rule 8. Mac and Mc are filed in their regular place alphabetically. Some clinics will provide a special guide for both Mac and Mc for ease in filing.

> Mabbott
> MacDonald
> Mazziotti
> McAffe

Rule 9. Numeric units are broken down such that numeric seniority terms are filed before alphabetic terms.

	Edward Lee Kletka, IV
BEFORE	Edward Lee Kletka, Jr.
	George Lee Curtis, II
BEFORE	George Lee Curtis, Sr.

Filing Identical Names

When names are identical, the address may be used to order files. The address is indexed by:

First	City
SECOND	STATE
Third	Street Name
Fourth	**Address #**

Therefore, the following Acme Drug Supply files would be arranged from first to last as follows:

1. Acme Drug Supply, 839 *Kentucky Boulevard*, Crawford, MISSOURI
2. Acme Drug Supply, 683 *Wildflower Avenue*, Fairbanks, ALASKA
3. Acme Drug Supply, 1539 *Wildflower Avenue*, Fairbanks, ALASKA
4. Acme Drug Supply, 742 *Terminal Street West*, Fairbanks, ARIZONA
5. Acme Drug Supply, 731 *Terminal Street East*, New York, NEW YORK

Although this is the official indexing rule, most medical facilities prefer alternative methods for filing identical charts. The primary consideration here is that patient addresses often change frequently. Therefore, preferred methods include date of birth or Social Security number.

STEPS FOR FILING MEDICAL DOCUMENTATION IN PATIENT FILES

Before a discussion of the common filing systems, it is helpful to review procedural steps that accurately and efficiently process data sheets, laboratory requests, dictation, and so forth from the time they are generated to the time the file is returned to the medical records section. Efficiently following these steps will save considerable time in the ambulatory care setting.

Inspect

Carefully inspect the report to identify the patient, subject, or file to whom the information belongs. Remove clips and staples. Make certain the information is complete.

Index

Use the indexing process to determine how the chart would be located, properly identifying indexing units and their order.

Code

Coding in medical records is the process of marking data to indicate how information is to be filed. If using a system other than a strict alphabetic system, determine the proper coding for the chart so it can be retrieved. Otherwise, identify the indexed units by underlining or highlighting. This makes refiling more effective and assures that the item will always be filed in the same place. If a cross-reference is required, identify the cross-reference by double underlining and placing an *X* nearby. This chapter includes detailed information on coding and cross-referencing.

Sort

If there are a number of reports/documents to be filed, sort them into units according to the captions on the charts. This will eliminate wasted time in working back and forth through the alphabet or numbers. Figure 14-7 shows a medical assistant using a desk sorter to put files and reports in alphabetic order.

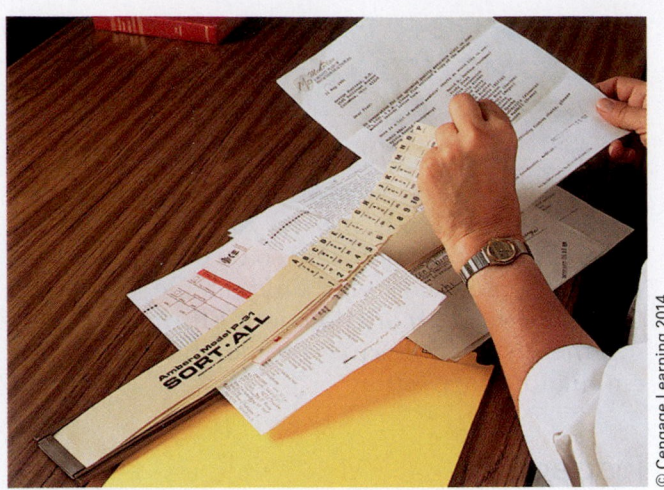

Figure 14-7 Medical assistant using a desk sorter to alphabetize reports to make filing easier.

File

The papers are placed in the proper charts and the charts returned to their proper place in the medical records section. Be alert to the labels and refile any information or charts that have been misfiled.

FILING TECHNIQUES AND COMMON FILING SYSTEMS

Three major filing systems are commonly used in the ambulatory care setting: alphabetic, numeric, and subject. The alphabet is intrinsic to all methods, and the basic rules for filing, covered previously, are used in all systems.

Color coding is used a high percentage of the time in all three systems to minimize filing errors. Another system, geographic, is seldom used in the ambulatory care setting unless there are multiple clinics. Even then, a form of color coding may be used.

Color Coding

Color coding is a technique often used in the three major filing systems. Numerous color-coding systems are available. Patient charts most often use an alphabetic system of color coding, although color coding can be used in numeric filing as well. Smead Manufacturing, Kardex, Bibbero, and American Corporate Services are companies widely known in medical and dental fields for their

color systems and records management systems. Color coding may seem complicated at first, but once medical assistants understand the principles behind it and practice its application a number of times, the task becomes much easier, and there is immediate recognition if a chart is misfiled.

Color coding makes retrieval of files more efficient with the use of visible color differences that facilitate easier maintenance of the files. Color-coding filing systems also use an alphabetic system; after they are coded by color, that designation is used to order the files alphabetically.

Tab-Alpha System. The various forms of the Tab-Alpha system are designed primarily for filing systems in small clinics that use vertical files where all individual charts are clearly visible in one unit.

Each alphabetic letter is assigned a different color. Each folder has a color-coded label. Only full-cut folders are used:

- Colored labels are applied over the edge of the full cut for the first two letters of the key indexing unit (Winston, Paul Lewis: WI).
- A third white label is placed over the tab edge, which contains all of the indexing units (Winston, Paul Lewis).
- In addition, some clinics use a color-coded label to indicate the last year the patient was seen. This makes an efficient method for easily identifying active and inactive files.
- Any additional labels (e.g., allergies, last year seen, or industrial claim) are attached to the chart according to the clinic procedure.

Alpha-Z System. Forms of the Alpha-Z system are designed for use with either open lateral files or vertical drawer files (Figure 14-8A). Alphabetic letters are used as the primary guides. Breakdowns of alphabetic combinations are added as determined by the needs of a particular facility.

A combination of 13 colors is used in the Alpha-Z system with white letters on a solid colored background for the first half of the alphabet and white letters on a colored background with white stripes for the second half of the alphabet (Figure 14-8B).

The 13 colors used are shown in Table 14-1. Folders have three labels:

- The first label contains the typed name, a color block, and the letter of the alphabet for the first letter of the first indexing unit:

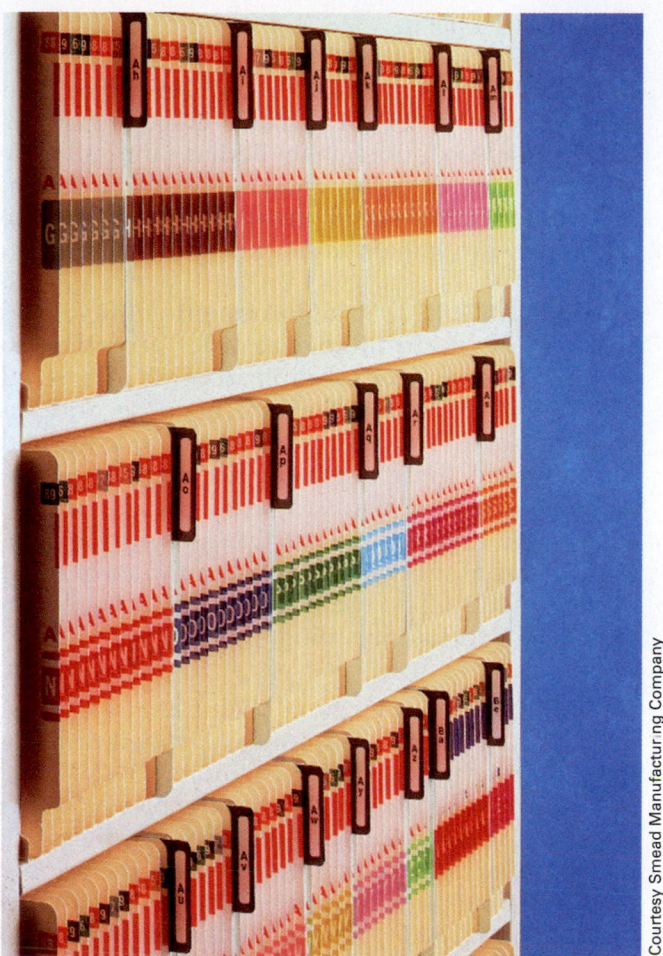

Figure 14-8A Color-coding filing system uses open-lateral shelving unit with color-coded files.

Courtesy Smead Manufacturing Company

Table 14-1 Thirteen Colors Are Used in the Alpha-Z System

White Letter Colored Background	White Letter Striped Colored Background	Color
A	N	Red
B	O	Dark Blue
C	P	Dark Green
D	Q	Light Blue
E	R	Purple
F	S	Orange
G	T	Gray
H	U	Dark Brown
I	V	Pink
J	W	Yellow
K	X	Light Brown
L	Y	Lavender
M	Z	Light Green

© Cengage Learning 2014

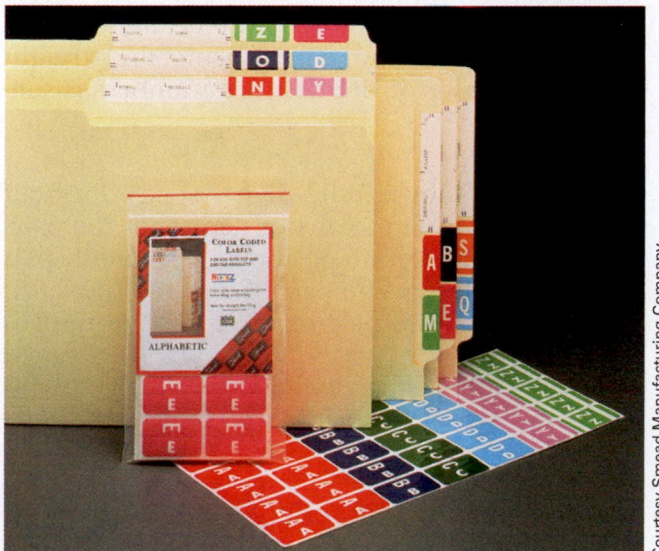

Figure 14-8B Alpha-Z-color-coded labels shown on top- and side-cut files.

Courtesy Smead Manufacturing Company

Winston, Lewis Paul YELLOW "W"

- The second and third labels are color-coded to correspond to the second and third letters of the first unit:

"I" on pink background and "N" on red-striped background

Customized Color-Coding Systems. Many clinics use color systems to meet specific needs.

Colored File Folders by First Name. One method color codes the first letter of the first name. The folders then are filed alphabetically by last name.

Example: A is assigned red folders; M is assigned green folders; S is assigned blue folders

Annette Samuels	Red Folder
Michael Taylor	Green Folder
Susan Boyer	Blue Folder

Many small medical clinics use this system and find it quite effective. In the multiprovider urgent care center, this would be quite time-consuming when locating files for patients of all providers.

Colored File Folders by Last Name. Another method using this system assigns colored folders according to the first letter of the last name. The folders are then filed alphabetically.

Example: *S* is assigned pink folders; *B* is assigned gray folders.

Bill Schwartz	Pink Folder
Corey Boyer	Gray Folder

This system makes it easy to spot folders that have been misfiled under an incorrect first letter, but it does not break it down further for misfiling within the first-letter guides.

Color-Coded Numbers. The color-coded number system is used in a numeric filing system and operates in the same way as alphabetic systems. Numbers from 0 to 9 are color coded. The appropriate colored numbers are then placed on the tabs of the patient's folder.

Alphabetic Filing

Strict alphabetic filing is one of the simplest filing methods, as files are strictly maintained by assigning a label to each file. The first letter of that label (e.g., Jones, Invoices, or Pharmacies) is then used to alphabetize the files from A to Z. When a limited number of files are accessed, this is an acceptable method of maintaining records. Also note that every filing system will utilize the alphabet somewhere. Procedure 14-5 provides steps for manual filing with an alphabetic system.

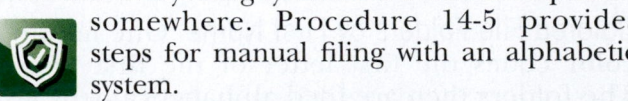

Numeric Filing

Numeric filing is organized by number rather than by letter. A key benefit of numeric filing is that it preserves patient confidentiality because the individual's name is not obviously apparent on the file folder. The numeric filing systems most likely used in medical facilities are straight numeric and terminal digit.

Straight Numeric. Straight numeric filing places charts in exact chronological order according to assigned number. For example, records numbered 45023, 45024, and 45025 will be in consecutive order on a shelf. This is an easy system to learn and use; however, there are some disadvantages. The greater number of digits to recall, the greater the chance for error. Numbers transposition is common. Chart number 45024 can be misfiled as chart number 54024. The use of color with straight numeric can decrease misfiling.

Terminal Digit. In terminal digit filing, a six-digit number is most often used with a hyphen dividing three parts of two digits, for example, 85-32-07 and 86-32-07. Within these numbers, the primary units are the last two numbers; the middle digits are the secondary units; the first two numbers are the third and final units considered. In a terminal digit file, there are 100 primary sections from 00 to 99 to be considered. The medical assistant will consider the primary section first, match the record with the same group to the secondary set of digits next, and then file in numerical order by the third unit.

The advantage to this system is that files and numbers are equally distributed. Only every 100th new medical record will be filed in the same primary section. Filing using the straight numerical order of the first two numbers is simple to learn.

Middle Digit. In middle digit systems, the staff still files according to pairs of digits, but the pairs of digits are in different positions. The middle pair of digits is primary, the pair of digits to the left is secondary, and the pair of digits on the right is third.

The terminal digit and middle digit systems are most likely seen in hospitals and large multiprovider clinics.

Components of Numeric Filing. Four essential components are used with a numeric system, whether it is a manual or computerized system.

Serially Numbered Dividers with Guides. Consecutive numeric guides (5, 10, etc.; 50, 100, etc.) separate the individual file folders into smaller groups of files.

Miscellaneous (General) Numeric File Section. This is reserved for records that have not been assigned numbers. Patients should automatically be assigned a number on the first visit. However, on occasion patients cannot be assigned a number initially. The miscellaneous section is generally in front of all the numeric folders for ease of locating items. Files in the miscellaneous section are filed alphabetically by patient name. This is the best place for the miscellaneous file(s) for two reasons:

1. They do not have to be moved each time a numbered file is added to the back of the order.

2. In a large system of files, retrieval from the front is quick and easy.

Alphabetic Card File. This alphabetic file is necessary as a source to locate numeric files or records. A card contains name, address, and file number (or an *M* if located in the miscellaneous section); any **cross-reference** is here rather than in the numeric files.

The alphabetic card file in a manual system would be equivalent to the computerized record of the patient and whatever number is assigned to him or her in that computer record. If using a computerized system, the program generally will automatically cross-reference the number with the alphabetic list that was generated with the initial entry. If laboratory data on Leo M. McKay come into the clinic, there will need to be a method to know where to locate his chart to file the report, that is, the alphabetic listing.

With a manual system, the alphabetic file is kept in an index card fashion. This file will contain the complete name and address (and any other information denoted by the clinic policy, e.g., insurance and emergency numbers).

Noted with this information there needs to be either an *M* for miscellaneous (for those items not assigned a number) or an assigned number (Figure 14-9A and Figure 14-9B).

If a cross-reference is required, prepare a cross-reference card and include an *X* next to the file number (or *M*) to indicate this is the cross-reference card and not the primary location (Figure 14-9C).

Accession Record. The **accession record** is a journal (or computer listing) where numbers are preassigned. Each new item to be assigned is written on the line next to the number (Figure 14-10). Each new entry for which a chart will be created must be assigned a number. A computerized system would have an accession record in its memory bank. Procedure 14-6 provides numeric filing steps.

Subject Filing

There are many reasons why material would be filed using a system of subjects in a medical clinic.

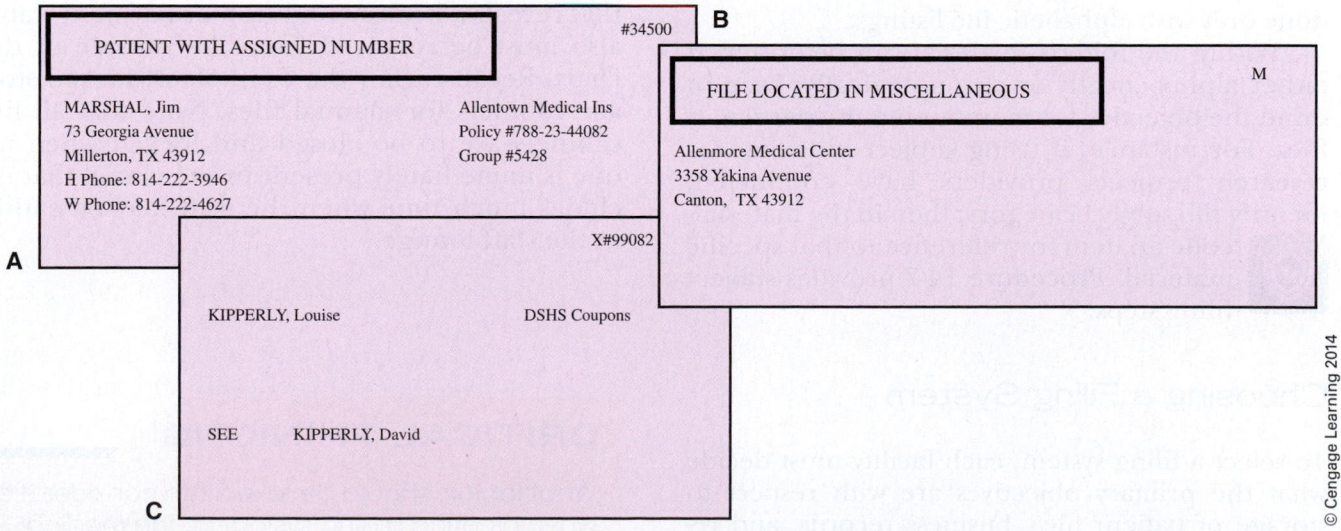

Figure 14-9 Card files used in numeric filing system: (A) Patient with an assigned number. (B) Business record has not had a number assigned and is located in miscellaneous section. (C) Cross-reference card.

© Cengage Learning 2014

ACCESSION LOG BOOK

#	File Name
800	CARRERA, Jaime
801	AU, Rhoda
802	TREMONT Drug Supply
803	
804	
805	
806	
807	

© Cengage Learning 2014

Figure 14-10 Accession record or log sequentially lists predetermined numbers to be used to assign to numeric records. The next number available in this system is 803.

If providers are doing research, they might wish to index research according to diseases. Subject files are convenient for locating frequently used services or for filing reference materials for patient needs. Insurance company information also might be filed by subject.

When using a subject filing system, scan the material to determine the subject or theme. As with color-coding and numeric filing, an alphabetic file is necessary. This can be either a subject list or an index card file listing the subjects. Also, as with numeric filing, all cross-reference cards are done only with alphabetic file listings.

Within the folders, material can be arranged either alphabetically or chronologically; keep in mind the objective for maintaining the particular files. For instance, if using subject indexing for research projects providers have conducted, identify the subject category; then in the material, code an item for reference to that specific material. Procedure 14-7 provides subject filing steps.

Choosing a Filing System

To select a filing system, each facility must decide what the primary objectives are with respect to storage of patient files, business records, and research files. How will the charts be used primarily? Will information need to be tracked by others not familiar with the records? Often more than one filing system will be used, such as alphabetic filing for patient charts, a numeric system for research subjects, and a subject system for miscellaneous correspondence.

The number of documents to be filed is one primary determinant in selecting an alphabetic or numeric system. Alphabetic filing is quite manageable for many clinics. However, when the number of patients is quite large, a numeric system becomes practical because an infinite set of numbers is available. With the numeric system, there is only one of each assigned designation. However, with an alphabetic system, there are a number of common names (e.g., Smith, Jones, Adams, and Johnson) that can have many multiples requiring additional sorting to narrow the search for the correct chart. In addition, with multiple charts of the same last name, the chance for misfiling increases.

Confidentiality is another reason to select a numeric filing system. Confidentiality of charts is maintained more easily with numeric files because no name is visible on the outside of the chart. In addition, numerically referenced records can be used in research activities where random sampling and anonymity are required.

To make the medical facility HIPAA compliant when traditional paper-based or manual charts are used, you need to ensure that no patient-identifiable information is located on the outside of the chart. This includes the patient address or any other information that might be used to determine the identity of the patient, including Social Security number, birth date, or phone number. Any information that reveals a health condition or payment status also must be removed from the outside of the chart. Recall earlier the example of locked storage cabinets for manual files. Note that all file cabinets are to be closed and locked when no one is immediately present in the clinic; that includes lunch time when the staff may be eating in the staff lounge.

CRITICAL THINKING

What factors should be taken into consideration when creating a filing system for the medical practice?

FILING PROCEDURES

By adhering to some common principles in medical records management, any filing system will be more effective and will enable the medical assistant to store, identify, retrieve, and maintain medical records efficiently.

Cross-Referencing

In running an efficient medical facility, files must be stored for quick and accurate retrieval. If there is any doubt as to where a particular file would be located, cross-reference the file. Many clinics fail to take the extra time it requires to do this. However, with the growing number of foreign names, hyphenated names, and stepfamilies, it is well worth the effort. When the clinic receives a letter and a release of information form inquiring about medical facts on Mr. David Kipperly's four stepchildren who were involved in an accident, how will these files be located? If they are cross-referenced under the stepfather's name, this will be a relatively easy procedure. However, if the medical assistant is unfamiliar with the family (as in a larger urgent care center with a large volume of patients), this may become a time-consuming job. Another scenario might involve insurance information on Janet Morgan. A search of the records does not produce a file for any Janet Morgan. The reason for this is that Janet Morgan is married, and her chart has been filed under Janet Hill-Morgan. Time spent cross-referencing contributes to a more efficient method of retrieving information.

A cross-referencing system does not need to be elaborate. It is quite sufficient to use inserts with labels attached that are inserted in the appropriate place in the storage units. For instance, a plain piece of cardstock, rather than a file or chart, could be inserted for "Janet Morgan." This insert would simply have a label directing one to the location of the primary file.

The proper steps for cross-referencing, together with several examples where cross-referencing might be used, are discussed in the next section.

Steps for Cross-Referencing.

1. Identify the primary filing label.
2. Make a proper file to be used as the primary location for all medical records.
3. Identify one (or more) alternatives where one might find the file.
4. For the alternative filings, make a cross-reference sheet, card, or dummy chart that lists the primary reference and refers back to the location of the primary file.

Example: The patient, Jaime Renae Carrera, has made it known to the clinic that most of his information received will refer to the name Renny Carrera, as this is his preference. The SEE reference will identify where the primary file is located.

PRIMARY FILE:	Carrera, Jaime Renae
X-REFERENCE FILE:	Carrera, Renny
	SEE Carrera, Jaime Renae

Rule 1. **Married Individuals.** When taking a spouse's name, the primary file would be the patient's legal name with the cross-reference listed under the spouse's.

PRIMARY FILE:	Au, Rhoda A. (Mrs.)
	Lee Au
X-REFERENCE FILE:	Au, Mrs. Lee
	SEE Au, Rhoda A. (Mrs.)

Rule 2. **Foreign Names.** The primary file would be located under the patient's legal name. It is important, therefore, that you identify the first, middle, and surname (last name) when the patient comes for the first visit. Unless people are familiar with a particular group of names, the first, middle, and surnames are often confused with one another. Again, your experience will teach you which cross-references should be set up.

PRIMARY FILE:	Sing, Yange Teah
X-REFERENCE FILE:	Yange, Sing Teah
	SEE Sing, Yange Teah
X-REFERENCE FILE:	Teah, Yange Sing
	SEE Sing, Yange Teah

Rule 3. **Hyphenated Names.** With the proliferation of hyphenated names, it is common for materials to be listed under different combinations of the hyphenated name. For instance, a married woman may have records under her maiden name, her husband's surname, and her hyphenated name. Therefore, it is necessary to make two cross-references.

PRIMARY FILE:	Krenshaw-Skiple, Rose Marie
X-REFERENCE FILE:	Skiple, Rose Marie
	SEE Krenshaw-Skiple, Rose Marie
X-REFERENCE FILE:	Krenshaw, Rose Marie
	SEE Krenshaw-Skiple, Rose Marie

Rule 4. **Multiple Listings.** A great deal of correspondence is received with multiple listings of names. At times, the medical clinic may receive correspondence from only one of the involved parties. Rather than keep a separate file for each, maintain a primary file as listed on the letter and then cross-reference file(s) for the individual names.

PRIMARY FILE:	Olsen, Piper, and Dillard Associates
X-REFERENCE FILE:	Piper, Richard C., M.D. **SEE** Olsen, Piper, and Dillard Associates
X-REFERENCE FILE:	Olsen, Francis William, M.D. **SEE** Olsen, Piper, and Dillard Associates
X-REFERENCE FILE:	Dillard, Thomas E., M.D. **SEE** Olsen, Piper, and Dillard Associates

Figure 14-11 Tickler files should be reviewed daily or weekly to follow up on activities and actions that must be taken.

Tickler Files

Sticky notes and writing notes on the calendar are popular methods of reminding clinic personnel to follow up with some required action. However, a well-organized, efficient clinic will maintain what is known as a **tickler file**, a method that serves as a reminder that some action needs to be taken at a date in the future.

EHR Some systems have a calendar that pops up to allow reminders to be placed on the calendar. The computer system reminds you of the note when that particular day arrives. Some EMR systems have built-in reminders that automatically give a reminder for such things as annual physical examinations, monthly blood pressure checks, medication checks, and anything else that might be beneficial to both patient and provider. Some systems automatically pick up these reminders from the progress notes that are a part of the electronic medical record.

Most computer systems today have provisions for establishing ticklers on files. However, a standard practice of using index cards for tickler files is easy to maintain (Figure 14-11).

The tickler card should contain the following information:

- Patient name
- Tickler date (when action should be taken)
- Required action (e.g., schedule surgery or mail reminder)

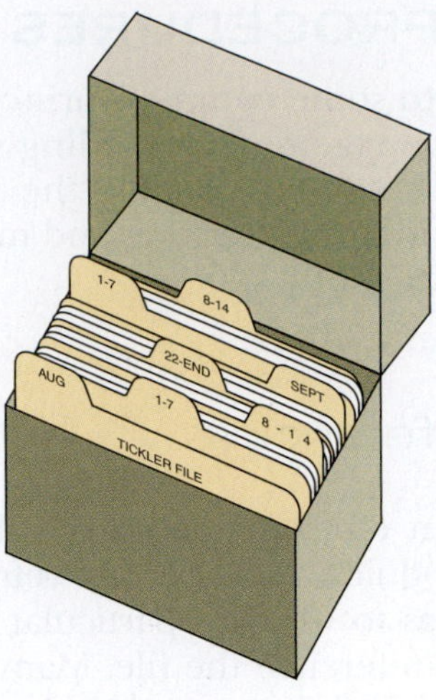

- Additional relevant information (telephone number)

If action is to be taken with a patient or on behalf of the patient (e.g., scheduling a hospital admittance or sending a reminder of a checkup visit), place the information on the tickler card as soon as possible so this task is not forgotten.

When filing records, be sure to look for words such as "on _____ date we will," "pending action," or "follow-up," indicating that some course of action needs to be taken.

It is important to remember that any tickler system, whether manual or computerized, is worthless if the reminder is not adhered to and appropriate action taken.

Release Marks

It is a good practice to use some type of release mark (date stamp, initials, check mark) on every item that is filed. Ideally, the provider should initial the document after it has been read. Then, if action is required by the medical assistant, a release mark is in a consistently identified place on every document. If no action is required after the provider has signed or initialed, place a release mark on the document. A release mark on every piece of information serves as an excellent quality-control measure.

Checkout System

Many clinics have developed dummy charts or files labeled "out sheets" or "out guides" for use when the chart is removed. Most of these guides are identified by an OUT label or metal holder, but they could be assigned a particular color; the key is that they stand out as different from the primary folders (see Figure 14-6).

On the out guide, there should be a minimum of the following information:

- A record of when the chart was removed
- Where the chart can be located

Other information that is useful to note includes:

- Expected date of return
- Actual date the chart was returned
- Signature of the individual checking out the record
- Notation on what section of the chart file was borrowed, such as a laboratory report or specialty examination

Some clinics prefer to have *temporary folders* rather than just an out guide. There are also out guides with pockets to file data in the absence of a chart. This allows for data storage on a temporary basis until the primary file is returned. The data can then be filed permanently when the primary folder is returned. If these folders are of a different color or have a different type of tab/label, they can be spotted easily so the staff can track the temporary files to be sure they do not become permanent folders.

Locating Missing Files or Data

Misfiling can occur for a number of reasons. When this situation occurs, a specific procedure must be established to conduct a search for the missing information. By systematically searching, the missing data usually can be located. This systematic search can be aided by making a mental note of the particular items that commonly are misplaced, such as thin-paper laboratory reports, small laboratory slips, and look-alike names such as "Ward" filed under "Wart" or "Adam" filed under "Adams." Make a note of what was misfiled and where the information was located to more easily locate similar items in the future.

To locate missing pieces of information when the correct file is located but not the particular item within that file:

- Check all of the items within the file.
- Check other files with similar labels.

To locate missing files:

- Check the folders filed before and after the proper location of the misplaced file.
- Look at folders with similar labels.
- Check the provider's desk, the desk tray, and with other clinic personnel.
- If using a color-coding system, look for folders with the same coding as the misplaced file.
- If using a numeric system, look for possible transposition of combinations of numbers.
- Check for transposition of first and last names.
- Check for alternative spellings of names or look-alike names.

Misplaced files can be frustrating and time-consuming to locate. The best strategy is to check files for the proper filing order whenever returning or retrieving a file folder. When removing a file to answer a question, leave the file following it sticking out slightly to make its return easy and correct. Most importantly, when finished with a record, refile it immediately.

Filing Chart Data

Types of Reports. The patient's chart is the key source of information relating to treatment. A number of reports are kept in the chart, all serving to provide a total picture of patient care. Following are the most common documents that are part of the patient's medical record (see Chapter 16 for other documents).

Clinical Notes. Clinical notes include documentation such as the medical history, the physical examination, and the follow-up notes. They track the patient's course of treatment.

Correspondence. Filing of correspondence varies. Some file all types of correspondence together. Others file correspondence about the patient's treatment with the clinical notes.

Laboratory Reports. Included in laboratory reports are X-ray reports, CT scans, ultrasound reports, blood work, urinalysis, EEGs, ECGs, physical therapy–related reports, and pathology reports—information related to clinical data that assess the patient's condition.

Miscellaneous. The miscellaneous category includes insurance-related papers, requests for transfer of medical records, and personal notes from/to patients. In general, miscellaneous encompasses matters not related to direct treatment.

Retention and Purging

As information accumulates, it is necessary to maintain files by the process known as **purging**. Purging can involve several forms of action.

Record Purging. Record purging requires sorting through records and removing those not in active use. Each facility should establish a standard policy for control and processing of records. States have different time requirements for retention of various types of records that will take into account the statute of limitations (see Chapter 7). Table 14-2 lists general guidelines. As a way of controlling risk and practicing responsible risk management, many facilities choose to maintain large numbers of inactive files rather than to destroy any records. Some keep them on computer disks or CDs (discussed later in this chapter). Check with the Medical Practice Act in your state to determine record-keeping requirements.

Active Files. Active files include records that need to be readily accessible for retrieval of information.

Inactive Files. Inactive files consist of records that need to be retained for possible retrieval of information. Files not currently being accessed for information would thus become inactive. Often, the type of practice dictates the relevant time period when files are determined to be inactive (generally 2 to 3 years).

Closed Files. Closed files are those that are no longer required. Again, patient files are

Table 14-2 Records for Retention

Patient Index Files

These include appointment books or daily appointment sheets. They are kept for an indefinite period. They may be required for litigation or research.

Case Histories

The length of storage depends on state requirements and individual practice requirements. Product liability cases have deemed long-term storage of these records necessary (20+ years). The records of minors must be retained at least until the age of majority. The statute of limitations is a deciding factor as well, usually 3 to 6 years.

If records are to be destroyed because of the death of a provider or closure of a practice, the following procedure is required: Each patient should be notified of the circumstances and given the opportunity to have his or her records forwarded to another provider. After notification, the records must be retained for a "reasonable" period (determined by state regulations). A period of 3 to 6 months is generally determined to be a "reasonable" period. The records must be destroyed by burning or shredding to protect confidentiality.

Laboratory and X-ray Data

Originals should be retained permanently with the patient's case history.

Personal/Professional Records

Professional licenses should be stored permanently in a secure location.

Office Equipment Records

These records are generally kept until the warranties and depreciation are no longer valid. They should be kept in an easily accessible location if under maintenance contract.

Insurance Records

Professional liability policies are kept permanently. Other policies are kept in active files while in force.

Financial Records

Bank records are kept in active files for up to 3 years and then placed in inactive storage. Tax records must be retained permanently.

© Cengage Learning 2014

retained for significantly longer periods of time because of litigation and research considerations, usually 3 to 6 years beyond the statute of limitations.

CORRESPONDENCE

Most ambulatory care settings process a considerable amount of correspondence not directly related to patient care. Such items include employment applications, letters from/to pharmaceutical representatives, advertisements for medical supplies, magazine subscription information, and letters to/from other providers on a variety of subjects. This correspondence is processed using alphabetic filing rules. However, an additional step is necessary to determine whether the correspondence is incoming or outgoing. The correspondence must be filed under some aspect that will be distinctly identifiable; that is, what idea, subject, or name would most likely be thought of if someone wanted to retrieve that correspondence or file additional relevant correspondence.

Filing Procedures for Correspondence

Once it is determined whether correspondence is incoming or outgoing, follow the basic rules for filing. In addition:

- Remove paper clips and staple items together.
- Inspect to see if the item is ready to be filed; that is, if any appropriate action has been taken. If not, take care of copies and enclosures, and then place notes in the tickler file for future action before proceeding with the indexing.
- On incoming correspondence, be sure the letterhead is in direct relation to the letter.

Example: A personal letter written by a patient on hotel stationery—index the signature on the letter.

Example: When both the company name and the signature are important, index the company name. A letter from Preston Industries written by the company president—index Preston Industries, not the president's name, which may change.

Example: If there is no letterhead and you have determined the material is not relevant to a patient, index the name on the signature line. A letter received from Carlton Fiske, RPT, advising your clinic of services his firm has to offer your patients—index Fiske.

- On outgoing correspondence, look at the inside address and the reference line.

Example: A letter to the District Court regarding Karen Ritter, an employee who is summoned to jury duty—index Karen Ritter rather than District Court.

Example: If the correspondence is relevant to a patient, index the patient's name. A letter RE: Wayne Elder—index under Elder.

Example: If the correspondence is not relevant to a patient, look to the inside address for the indexing information. A letter inquiring about cost estimates for redecorating the clinic reception room—index the firm in the inside address.

Example: When the inside address is relevant and contains both a company name and a person's name, index the company name. (This avoids the problem of personnel changes.) Cross-referencing would be done under the individual name. A letter to Marvin Fairchild, President of Brandex Pharmaceuticals—index Brandex Pharmaceuticals with a cross-reference for "Morgan Fairchild, President, SEE Brandex Pharmaceuticals."

Example: If the letter is personal, the name of the person to whom the letter is written would be used for indexing purposes. Dr. Whitney writes a letter to Dr. Lewis, one of his colleagues, asking if he plans to attend an upcoming conference—index Dr. Lewis.

- On incoming or outgoing correspondence, code the indexing units of the designated label. If the correspondence is being cross-referenced, be sure to note the cross-referencing unit and place the *X* in a visible place. You may find that the body of the letter contains an important name or subject.

- Create a miscellaneous folder for items that do not have enough in number to warrant an individual folder. Items in the miscellaneous folder are filed alphabetically first, and then identical items are filed with the most recent piece on top. An individual folder is then created when enough pieces accumulate on a particular item.

ELECTRONIC MEDICAL RECORDS

EHR Total electronic automation in any medical facility is a major undertaking. It can be both frightening and exhilarating. Careful study of systems available, impact on providers and staff, time necessary for moving from manual to electronic files, and costs involved are measured against the benefits incurred.

With the government's mandate to have EMRs for most patients and Congress pushing to make all Medicare-covered prescriptions transferred electronically, EMRs are here to stay and one day will replace all paper/manual medical records. Evidence shows that fewer errors are created in EMRs because the "human element" is decreased. If all the data are entered correctly, the computer software "does all the thinking" to find the chart, store information appropriately, create reminder notices, check all medications for any contraindications, and flag any warning to providers, such as high cholesterol or blood pressure readings moving into the "alert" zone. The EMR will keep a record of all patient appointments and any missed appointments as well as any piece of information that might be found in a manual patient record. EMR software creates, stores, edits, and retrieves patient data. It has the added advantage of allowing more than one person to access a chart at the same time.

Electronic automation in the medical facility is discussed in several other chapters (in particular, see Unit 5: Managing Facility Finances). For purposes of this chapter and after reading about the fairly detailed "manual" records management tasks, consider the case for EMRs.

EMR software can be purchased as a single-computer application or as part of a larger "practice management" software package. Often, medical facilities start with one aspect of a practice management software package (usually not EMRs) and

then gradually add the other pieces. EMRs are capable of the following:

- Create and print customized encounter forms and superbills
- View patient records of all provider encounters and laboratory results, transcription notes, radiologic images, and so forth
- Utilize predefined templates to make examination notes, procedures, review of systems, and postoperative checks quicker and more efficient
- Indicate or choose medications (from a predetermined list of those most prescribed), with specific instructions that can be electronically admitted into the chart and to the pharmacy
- Flag any drug interactions, contraindications, or allergies related to the patient
- Give providers pen units or small computers in which to enter data with a simple touch of the pen
- Provide immediate access of the patient record to providers and necessary staff members
- Be easily retrieved and never lost or misplaced
- Eliminate the manual coding and filing of medical charts
- Store medical charts for as long as necessary in a small space on computer disks or CDs
- Reduce the amount of phone tag retrieving necessary information from a paper file
- Create reminders for follow-up as necessary
- Provide a more efficient method of signing charts
- Can be emailed to a referring provider or easily printed, whether part of or the whole chart

EMRs require that providers use computers to open and view charts and write prescriptions. Progress notes can be created using clinical templates and a point-and-click form of entry. Commonly used clinical phrases can be dropped into the progress note with a push of a button. If providers prefer to dictate and have their notes transcribed, that can also be done. The transcribed and entered note will automatically update relevant information such as problem lists, vital signs, laboratory results, and so on. As voice recognition improves, it will become possible for the provider to speak the entries normally keyed into the system (see Chapter 11).

Confidentiality is often mentioned as a concern in EMRs, but with network access limitations, system administrators can identify access and privileges according to the desired policy of the clinic. The EMR is fully recognized as a legal document, is able to track any changes made, and can be presented to a court of law. Because a standard part of any EMR installation is a system backup, you should never be without a medical chart even if the system goes down for a brief period.

Most medical assistants working in facilities that are fully computerized say they hardly remember how they could function any differently. They also report that moving from the manual to the electronic system can be frustrating at times, but it is worth the effort in the long run.

Archival Storage

Most providers preserve patient medical records for at least the life of their practice. This obviously is a space-consuming prospect, particularly in today's large practices. Computers help to solve this dilemma through EMRs. Records are copied onto optical disks or CDs. This method not only eliminates the bulky storage problems encountered with traditional records, but records can be retrieved and viewed almost instantaneously on a computer screen.

One of the advantages of the EMR is the small amount of storage needed for all the patient charts; but remember that computer files, including patient charts, should have a backup system that stores the information in a secure place should there be a computer problem. Some systems provide for automatic backup every 30 minutes or less. Some systems include a second hard drive that stores data as they are being created or as often as determined by facility policy. With an effective and efficient backup system, no one on the clinic staff will ever be without a patient chart when it is needed.

Transfer of Data

EMRs are easily emailed in whole or in part. Computers also streamline transfer of records from one medical facility to another. Faxing is an everyday part of the medical clinic. Gone is the time when it took a provider days to obtain information vital to treating a patient. Within minutes, a patient's entire medical record can be sent electronically from one clinic to another. Scanners (optical character recognition) are devices that allow information to be converted to an image on the computer screen. For instance, a patient's entire medical record can be scanned by the device and then recreated as a computer file exactly as it was in paper form.

Confidentiality

 Maintaining confidentiality is a major issue in using the computer and online devices for storage and transfer of medical information. Not enough emphasis can be placed on the confidentiality issue. Medical assistants employed in a medical facility will hear and see information that is completely private. It is never appropriate to discuss any of that information outside the clinic with any individual unless it is a person who needs that information for medical reasons. It is also unwise to discuss private information within the facility if it is not your concern, and especially if your voice might be overheard by someone waiting in an examination room, a patient using the restroom, or individuals in the reception area. An appropriate situation in which information can be shared is when giving the name, address, and Social Security number or clinic number to the radiology department that will be performing the X-rays ordered by the provider.

 ## PROCEDURE 14-1

Establishing a Paper Medical Chart for a New Patient

PURPOSE:
To demonstrate an understanding of the principles for establishing a paper medical chart.

EQUIPMENT/SUPPLIES:
File folder used in the facility (flip-up or book-style)

Divider pages used in the facility (SOAP/SOAPER laboratory reports, HIPAA information sheets, and so forth)
Adhesive twin prong fasteners for divider pages
Twin hole punch for twin prong fasteners

continues

Procedure 14-1 (continued)

Selected tabs to identify folder and divider pages
Demographic patient information completed before or at the first appointment

PROCEDURE STEPS:

1. Assemble all supplies at a desk or table. RATIONALE: Everything is in one place for efficient use.

2. Punch holes in the manila file folder and any necessary divider pages. RATIONALE: Creates holes for the twin prong fasteners.

3. Affix the adhesive twin prong fasteners. RATIONALE: Places fasteners as appropriate for material to be attached.

4. Assemble the divider pages dictated by the practice and the clinic policy in the proper location of the chart over the twin prong fasteners. RATIONALE: Ensures that items are placed in the same place as in all other charts in the facility.

5. Securely fasten twin prong fasteners over the divider pages. RATIONALE: Ensures that no pages will fall out of the chart.

6. Index and code the patient's name according to the filing system to be used (i.e., alphabetic, numeric, or color). RATIONALE: Determines where the chart will be placed.

7. Affix appropriately labeled tabs to the folder cut. RATIONALE: Prepares the chart for patient information.

8. Transfer demographic data in black ink pen or affix the demographic divider sheet to the inside front cover of the chart. RATIONALE: Identifying patient information is readily available inside the chart cover.

9. Affix HIPAA required information to the chart, after it has been read and signed by the patient, as determined by clinic policy. RATIONALE: Ensures that this task not omitted.

10. Place prepared chart in proper location for pickup by the provider or clinical medical assistant. RATIONALE: Signals to all staff that the chart is ready for the patient's visit.

PROCEDURE 14-2

Registering a New Patient Using Medical Office Simulation Software (MOSS)

PURPOSE:
To register new patients using MOSS by entering information from the Patient Information Form and insurance cards.

EQUIPMENT/SUPPLIES:
Computer and MOSS
Source documents

PROCEDURE STEPS:

1. Open MOSS and select *Patient Registration* from the Main Menu.

2. Select the patient from the *Patient Registration* window.

3. Using the Patient Information Form in Source Document 14_1A_Abbot, enter data for the *Patient Information Tab* from the form. When complete, click *Save*.

4. Click on the *Primary Insurance Tab*. Enter information for the patient's primary insurance. When complete, click *Save*. Enter information about the provider accepting assignment, signature on file, and in-network status. Hint: Refer to the copy of the insurance card for other required information to enter.

5. Click on the *Secondary Insurance Tab*. Enter information for the patient's secondary insurance. Be sure to check the box in Field 11 to bill the secondary after the primary. Enter information about the provider accepting assignment, signature on file, and in-network status. When complete, click *Save*. Hint: Refer to the copy of the insurance card for other required information to enter.

6. Click on the *HIPAA Tab*. Check the box in front of *Yes* indicating that the HIPAA form was given and signed. Enter the date forms were signed. When complete, click *Save*.

7. Click on the *Close* button to exit the *Patient Registration* window.

8. Register the next patient, or close the patient selection window and return to the Main Menu.

PROCEDURE 14-3

Correcting a Paper Medical Record

PURPOSE:
To demonstrate the appropriate method of correcting an error in a paper medical chart.

EQUIPMENT/SUPPLIES:
Document containing error
Document containing correction
Red ink pen

PROCEDURE STEPS:
1. Review information on correcting medical records. RATIONALE: Ensures you know the rules for correcting paper records.

2. Draw a single line through the error using a red ink pen. RATIONALE: Identifies the portion of the record in error.

3. Write in the correction. RATIONALE: Corrects the noted error.

4. Write "Corr." or "Correction" above the corrected information. RATIONALE: Identifies the information as a correction of an error.

5. Initial and date the correction. RATIONALE: Identifies the person who made the correction and the date it was made.

PROCEDURE 14-4

Updating Patient Registration Information Using Medical Office Simulation Software (MOSS)

PURPOSE:
To update patient registration information when changes are required.

EQUIPMENT/SUPPLIES:
Computer and MOSS

PROCEDURE STEPS:
1. Open MOSS and select *Patient Registration* from the Main Menu.

2. Select the patient from the *Patient Registration* window.

3. Select the tab(s) to display the area in which information needs to be updated, deleted, or added. Enter information as applicable.

4. When complete, click *Save*, and then close the *Patient Registration* window.

5. Update the next patient, or close the patient selection window and return to the Main Menu.

PROCEDURE 14-5

Steps for Manual Filing with an Alphabetic System

PURPOSE:
To demonstrate an understanding of the principles of alphabetic filing.

EQUIPMENT/SUPPLIES:
Documents to be filed
Dividers with guides

Miscellaneous number file section
Alphabetic card file and cards
Accession journal, if needed

continues

Procedure 14-5 (continued)

PROCEDURE STEPS:

1. Inspect and index. RATIONALE: Ensures that the chart is ready for filing and determines the order in which the chart will be filed.

2. Sort the charts alphabetically. RATIONALE: Determines the order and placement of the record; allows for a second assessment for placement.

3. Create cross-reference files according to clinic policy.

4. File the charts appropriately.

5. Check the placement with the charts immediately before and after the chart being filed. RATIONALE: Makes certain the chart is filed in the correct location.

PROCEDURE 14-6

Steps for Manual Filing with a Numeric System

PURPOSE:

To demonstrate an understanding of the principles of the numeric filing system.

EQUIPMENT/SUPPLIES:

Documents to be filed
Dividers with guides
Miscellaneous numeric file section
Alphabetic card file and cards
Accession journal, if needed

PROCEDURE STEPS:

1. Inspect and index. RATIONALE: Ensures that the information is ready for filing and determines how the chart will be located.

2. Code for filing units. Check the alphabetic card file for each piece to see if the card has already been prepared. RATIONALE: Determines the number under which the chart will be filed.

3. Write the number in the upper right-hand corner if the piece has been assigned a number. RATIONALE: Tells you the number to be used in filing.

4. If no number is assigned (i.e., it has an *M* for miscellaneous), check the miscellaneous file. If a miscellaneous item is ready to be assigned a number, make a card and note the number in the right-hand corner of the card file, cross out the *M*, and make a chart file. RATIONALE: Tells you if a number should be prepared because of numerous items in the miscellaneous file, or if the piece to be filed should stay in the miscellaneous file.

5. If there is no card, make up an alphabetic card including a complete name and address, and then write either *M* or assign a number. RATIONALE: Ensures that there is always an alphabetic card with necessary demographic information and an assigned number or *M* for each piece of information and chart.

6. Cross-reference if necessary and file the card properly. You are then ready to file the document in the appropriate file folder/chart. RATIONALE: Ensures less likelihood of misfiling if necessary cross-references are prepared.

7. File in ascending order. RATIONALE: Establishes a pattern for filing.

PROCEDURE 14-7

Steps for Manual Filing with a Subject Filing System

PURPOSE:
To demonstrate an understanding of the principles of the subject filing system.

EQUIPMENT/SUPPLIES:
Documents to be filed by subject
Subject index list or index card file listing subjects
Alphabetic card file and cards

PROCEDURE STEPS:

1. Review the item to find the subject. RATIONALE: Checks the item for the main topic of information to determine where piece will be filed.

2. Match the subject of the item with an appropriate category on the subject index list. RATIONALE: Saves you time so that you do not create an unnecessary subject index list.

3. If the item contains information that may pertain to more than one subject, decide on the proper cross-reference. RATIONALE: Ensures that any confusion will be checked with a cross-reference.

4. If the subject title is written on the material, underline it. RATIONALE: Readily identifies the subject used for filing.

5. If the subject title is not written on the item, write it clearly in the upper right-hand corner and underline (_____) it. RATIONALE: Indicates the subject used for filing; consistently places the subject in the expected place.

6. Use a wavy (___) line for cross-referencing and an X as with alphabetic and numeric filing. RATIONALE: Clearly identifies any cross-referencing.

7. Underline the first indexing unit of the coded units. RATIONALE: Ensures the correct order for filing.

CASE STUDY 14-1

Refer to the scenario at the beginning of the chapter.

CASE STUDY REVIEW

1. Juanita Hansen is waiting in the clinic. Dr. Whitney and the staff are scrambling for her medical record. They find the record on the provider's dictation stack, but they cannot find Juanita's test results.

   What can be done now to make certain Juanita has not made the trip unnecessarily?

2. Identify steps to be taken to prevent this situation from happening another time.

CASE STUDY 14-2

Karen Ritter, RMA (AMT), administrative medical assistant at Inner City Health Care, has been chiefly responsible for managing this urgent care center's medical records. However, because Karen is only a part-time employee, the office manager feels she needs to delegate some of the responsibility of maintaining all clinic files to Liz Corbin, CMA (AAMA), a medical assistant who also works part-time. Karen knows the system well and had a hand in designing an effective numeric filing method that both ensures patient confidentiality and satisfies the needs of Inner City and its large volume of patients. Now she is trying to orient Liz, who has little experience with the filing system, to the intricacies of medical records management.

CASE STUDY REVIEW

1. What is a good starting point for Liz Corbin's education in medical records management?

2. What are the basic procedures for filing any piece of documentation that Liz needs to learn?

3. Under the direction of the office manager, Inner City is gradually shifting to a computerized system for all operations. Eventually, patient files will be computerized. What can Karen and Liz do to prepare for this eventuality?

CASE STUDY 14-3

Dr. King is notorious for misplacing files. Often, Dr. King, who does not want to bother busy staff, walks to the lateral file shelves and removes a file or two. Likewise, he may decide to refile a chart that he has had on his desk. He has been known to take charts home when he wants to do some research.

CASE STUDY REVIEW

1. What might the staff do to ensure that Dr. King does not remove charts or refile them without proper use of out guides?

2. Devise a plan to give Dr. King the comfort he desires in the medical clinic where he is a founding partner, yet still protect the patients' charts and ensure the staff knows of the charts' locations.

SUMMARY

Records management plays an ever-increasing role in the ambulatory care setting today. With the need for thorough and proper documentation, a majority of interaction on the patient's behalf is concerned with proper information processing. It is imperative that medical records be managed efficiently, and that the medical assistant possesses the skills required for sorting, filing, retrieving, and maintaining information effectively.

A key aspect of managing patient records is selecting a filing system that achieves the goals of information access and storage. Once an alphabetic, numeric, or subject filing system is chosen, patient charts must be assembled and maintained accurately. As electronic medical records are more widely used, technology and computer applications increasingly play a prominent and varied role in the organization and utilization of charts in the medical facility. The medical assistant who is knowledgeable of procedures/rules related to the management of manual/paper medical records will find the transition to electronic medical records exciting and much easier to organize and control.

STUDY FOR SUCCESS

To reinforce your knowledge and skills of information presented in this chapter:

- Review the *Key Terms*
- Role-play with other students to apply attributes of professionalism pertinent to this chapter.
- Consider the *Case Studies* and discuss your conclusions
- Answer the questions in the *Certification Review*
- Apply your knowledge by completing the *Activities* in the *Study Guide* and the *Games and Quizzes* in the StudyWARE **StudyWARE** insert studyware icon here software on the *Premium Website*
- Perform the *Procedures* using the *Competency Assessment Checklists* in the *Competency Manual*
- Practice your problem-solving skills with the *Critical Thinking Challenge 3.0* on the *Premium Website*

Additional resources for this chapter include:

- Module 7 of the *Medical Assisting Learning Lab*
- *CourseMate for Delmar's Comprehensive Medical Assisting*
- *WebTutor for Delmar's Comprehensive Medical Assisting*

CERTIFICATION REVIEW

1. Maintaining order in files by separating active from inactive files is:
   a. indexing
   b. coding
   c. purging
   d. alphabetizing

2. A system used as a reminder of action to be taken on a certain date is called:
   a. accession log
   b. tickler file or reminder note
   c. release mark
   d. purging system

3. To maintain an accurate filing system, select from the following list the tool used to ensure that records are tracked when borrowed:
   a. release mark
   b. out guide
   c. alphabetic card file
   d. cross-reference file

4. The correct indexing from first to last for assigning units to the name John Porter O'Keefe II would be:
   a. O'Keefe John Porter II
   b. John Porter O'Keefe II
   c. II O'Keefe John Porter
   d. the "II" would be disregarded

5. Of the four systems of filing, the best for every ambulatory care setting is:
   a. the numeric system
   b. the color-coding system
   c. one customized to the needs of the clinic
   d. the alphabetic system

6. Medical records are the property of:
   a. the patients for whom the record is about
   b. insurance carriers who help to pay medical costs
   c. the providers who create the record
   d. a and c

7. Corrections to medical records:
   a. are made by erasing the error and replacing it with the correction
   b. are made by placing a single line through the error and replacing it with the correction
   c. are never made to charts because of the legal nature of the information
   d. are made only by the provider

8. The following statements about EMRs are all true except one:
   a. are initially more expensive than paper medical records
   b. should be available to most Americans by 2014
   c. eliminate coding and filing of medical charts
   d. create reminders for follow-up as necessary

9. When identical names are being indexed, the system for indexing most preferred in a medical clinic is:
   a. the address
   b. the telephone number
   c. the birth date or Social Security number
   d. a preassigned clinic number

10. The preferred order for steps in filing medical documentation is:
    a. code, index, sort, inspect, file
    b. inspect, code, index, sort, file
    c. sort, inspect, index, code, file
    d. inspect, index, code, sort, file

REFERENCES/BIBLIOGRAPHY

Burt, C. W., Hing, E., & Woodwell, D. (2005). *Electronic medical record use by office-based physicians: United States, 2005.* Hyattsville, MD: U.S. Department of Health and Human Services, Centers for Disease Control and Prevention.

Fordney, M. T., French, L., & Follis, J. J. (2004). *Administrative medical assisting* (5th ed.). Clifton Park, NY: Delmar Cengage Learning.

Hansen, D. (2008). *Congress considers mandate for Medicare e-prescribing.* Retrieved February 2008, from http://ww.ama-assn.org/amednews/2008/01/07/gvsb0107.htm

Johnson, J. (1994). *Basic filing procedures for health information management.* Clifton Park, NY: Delmar Cengage Learning.

Lewis, M. A., & Tamparo, C. D. (2007). *Medical law, ethics, & bioethics for health professionals* (6th ed.). Philadelphia: F. A. Davis.

CHAPTER 15

Written Communications

OUTLINE

Composing Correspondence
Writing Tips
Spelling
Proofreading
Proofreading in the Cloud
Components of a Business
Letter
Date Line
Inside Address
Salutation
Subject Line
Body of Letter
Complimentary Closing
Keyed Signature
Reference Initials
Enclosure Notation

Copy Notation
Postscripts
Continuation Page Heading
Letter Styles
Full Block
Modified Block
Simplified
Supplies for Written
Communication
Letterhead
Second Sheets
Printing Multipage Business
Letters
Envelopes
Mail Merge

Other Types of Correspondence
Memoranda
Meeting Agendas
Meeting Minutes
Processing Incoming
and Outgoing Mail
Incoming Mail
and Shipments
Outgoing Mail
and Shipments
Postal Classes
Formats for Efficient
Mail Processing
International Mail
Legal and Ethical Issues

LEARNING OUTCOMES

1. Define, spell, and pronounce the key terms as presented in the glossary.
2. Identify the role of the medical assistant in producing written communications.
3. List the four major letter styles.
4. Compose and key letters using appropriate components of a business letter.
5. Identify various types of form letters that may be written by the medical assistant.
6. Proofread a letter for grammar, spelling, and content.
7. Use proper proofreading marks to correct a document.
8. Describe the various classifications of mail and determine when each class should be used.
9. Address envelopes to satisfy postal regulations.
10. Discuss legal and ethical issues relating to written communications, as well as HIPAA regulations.
11. Analyze the professionalism questions and apply them to this chapter's content.

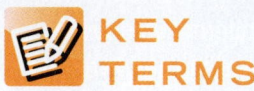

KEY TERMS

agenda

blind copy

bond paper

form letter

full block letter

keyed

memorandum (memo)

minutes

modified block
  letter, indented

modified block
  letter, standard

optical character
  reader (OCR)

portfolio

proofread

simplified letter

watermark

ZIP+4

ATTRIBUTES OF PROFESSIONALISM

Communication

- Did you respond honestly and diplomatically to the patient's concerns?
- Did you accurately and concisely update the provider on any aspect of the patient's care?
- Did you follow up with collateral allied health professionals to optimize the patient's plan of care?
- Did you include the patient's support system as indicated?

Presentation

- Were you courteous, patient, and respectful to the patient?
- Did you display a positive attitude?

Competency

- Did you pay attention to detail?
- Did you ask questions if you were out of your comfort zone or did not have the experience to carry out tasks?
- Did you display sound judgment?
- Were you knowledgeable and accountable?
- Did you recognize the importance of local, state, and federal legislation and regulations in the practice setting?

Initiative

- Did you show initiative?
- Did you direct the patient to other resources when necessary or helpful, with the approval of the provider?
- Did you implement time management principles to maintain effective clinic function?

Integrity

- Did you work within the scope of your practice?
- Did you acknowledge the scope of practice of other health care professionals?
- Did you demonstrate sensitivity to patient's rights?
- Did you demonstrate respect for individual diversity?
- Did you protect and maintain confidentiality?
- Did you immediately report any error you had made?

SCENARIO

When they are produced with care, written communications can be a time-consuming part of the administrative medical assistant's day. This is why Marilyn Johnson, CMA (AAMA), the clinic manager at Drs. Lewis and King's clinic, has compiled a style manual for the two-provider practice. Marilyn is clearly aware that professional appearing and worded letters send a positive message to all recipients. Yet, she wants to make correspondence writing and producing as efficient as possible; her style manual provides an easy-to-use resource for anyone in the clinic responsible for composing or sending written documents.

In her style manual, Marilyn has included examples of the "house" letter format, which is block style; a list of commonly used medical terms for easy spelling reference; answers to common questions staff have in regard to word usage; proofreader's marks; proper addressing procedures for envelopes and packages, depending on whether they are being sent by U.S. mail or by an alternative delivery method; and a quick list of the best ways to send various types of correspondence. Marilyn has also included a list of "Do Nots" to help her staff avoid mistakes in their written communications.

INTRODUCTION

One of the key responsibilities of the administrative medical assistant is written communication. Letters to patients, to referring providers, to other health care organizations, and even interoffice correspondence should be thoughtfully composed, carefully produced according to the style selected by the clinic manager, and mailed and delivered in a way that is both time and cost efficient.

Written correspondence is important in conveying a professional image of the ambulatory care setting and impacts public relations either positively or negatively. It must also be remembered that written documents provide a permanent or legal record in the event of any litigation and thus must be carefully and accurately worded.

In most ambulatory care settings, medical assistants are responsible for creating many forms of written communications. Examples of these forms of communications include:

- *Various types of letters, such as letters to order supplies and equipment, letters replying to various types of inquiries, collection letters, promotional letters*
- *Memoranda and interoffice communications*
- *Referrals, consultation, and surgical report letters*
- *Written instructions for patients*
- *Meeting agendas and minutes*
- *Promotional brochures*
- *Policy and procedure documents*

COMPOSING CORRESPONDENCE

The medical assistant must always remember that the quality of the correspondence reflects the standards of the medical clinic. It is important to also remember that there is a difference between social correspondence and business correspondence. Social correspondence tends to be lengthy and personal in nature, whereas business correspondence should be clear, concise, courteous, and accurate. It is best to keep business letters to one page in length whenever possible.

Writing Tips

Rosemary Fruehling, a writer and lecturer, states, "Business writing is good when it achieves the purpose the author intended." Practice and careful attention to detail are required to write effective business letters. Writing tips for consideration include:

- Follow the style and format determined by your provider–employer. Providers often prefer a professional, formal style of letter composition.
- Think about key points to be addressed in the letter and organize them before beginning composition. The first paragraph should identify what the letter is about and focus the reader's attention.
- Establish a tone of voice. Be personable and cordial in tone while remaining professional.
- Use only language that the reader will understand.
- Most sentences should be short and contain only one idea or thought.

SPOTLIGHT ON CERTIFICATION

RMA Content Outline

- Spelling

CMA (AAMA) Content Outline

- Uses of terminology
- Receiving, organizing, prioritizing, and transmitting information
- Fundamental writing skills
- Equipment operation
- Computer applications
- Screening and processing mail

CMAS Content Outline

- Communications

Table 15-1 Frequently Misspelled Words

abscess	ischium
aneurysm	larynx
arrhythmia	malaise
calcaneus	ophthalmology
cirrhosis	palliative
clavicle	parenteral
curettage	pharynx
hemorrhage	pneumonia
hemorrhoids	psychiatrist
homeostasis	pyrexia
humerus	rheumatic
ileum	roentgenology
ilium	sphygmomanometer
ischemia	staphylococcus

Spelling

It is important that all correspondence contain no misspelled or incorrectly used words. When in doubt, always look the word up in a dictionary (Table 15-1). When checking spelling in a dictionary, develop the habit of reading the definition as well. This will help imprint the correct spelling and meaning of the word.

Be careful about relying on the spell check function of your computer; many medical words are not formatted into the computer. The computer does not recognize if you have used the wrong word, only that the word is spelled incorrectly. For example, the words *to, too,* and *two* may all be spelled correctly but may be misused within the sentence structure.

It may be helpful to develop a list of frequently misused words in an alphabetized notebook, card index, or special file on your computer (Table 15-2). Several computer word processing software packages contain English/medical spell check features. A new word that is not currently identified in the spell check or medical check package may be added to the program.

Proofreading

Before presenting any correspondence to the provider for signature or mailing, the document should be **proofread**. Proofreading is the process of reading the document and checking for accuracy. Accuracy involves checking to be sure that the correct grammar, spelling, punctuation, and capitalization have been used and that the message is clear and concise and presented in a logical organization.

Proofreading marks most commonly used are shown in Figure 15-1. Standard proofreading marks used to indicate corrections hasten the editing process. Some proofreading tips that may be useful include:

- Proofread each document twice, once on the screen checking for obvious errors and then on a hard copy to be sure everything is accurate and makes sense.
- Prepare the document, set it aside, and proofread a third time later. Inaccuracies or errors may "jump" out in a later review.
- Do not proofread when tired.
- If the document is long, proofread in several short intervals.
- Read a long document to another person and have him or her check sentence structure and content accuracy.
- Use a card or ruler as a guide to maintain your place within the document.
- Use a piece of colored clear plastic over the document to rest your eyes. This is especially helpful when proofing a long document.

Proofreading in the Cloud

When several persons are involved in preparing a complex document, proofreading involves one

Table 15-2   *Frequently Misused Words*

advice	advise		hear	here	
affect	effect		hole	whole	
capital	capitol		knew	new	
coarse	course		know	no	
coma	comma		lean	lien	
command	commend		patience	patients	
complement	compliment		personal	personnel	
comprehensible	comprehensive		plain	plane	
council	counsel		precede	proceed	
conscience	conscious		principal	principle	
deposition	disposition		right	write	
device	devise		stationary	stationery	
elicit	illicit		taught	taut	
eligible	illegible		their	there	they are
elude	allude		to	too	two
ensure	insure	assure	vain	vein	
explicit	implicit		weak	week	
farther	further		weather	whether	
heal	heel		you	your	you are

© Cengage Learning 2014

person reviewing and making changes and then sending it to the other author for their concurrence. If changes are made the cycle is repeated. The Cloud (See Chapter 11) has changed the need for the back and forth transferring of a document from one author to another or between the author and an assistant. As of 2012, both Google Apps and Microsoft Office 365 Apps are available on Cloud allowing composition of documents on a server that is available to multiple users having access via a password. The Microsoft Office 365 App allows sharing of documents by several users for modification and review, but not interactively. The Google documents sharing feature allows multiple users to change a document interactively during the same session. This makes the proofreading process much simpler and if combined with a conference call, simplifies obtaining agreement on changes to text. Other Apps can perform some of the same functions and others are on the horizon. The features and capabilities will only improve with time.

COMPONENTS OF A BUSINESS LETTER

 The following sections describe the components of most business letters. Procedure 15-1 provides steps for Preparing and Composing Business Correspondence Using All Components (Computerized Approach). Figure 15-2 graphically illustrates the placement of business letter components, Table 15-3 provides guidelines for preventing errors in letter placement, and Figure 15-3 illustrates how placement can be altered to suit letter size.

Date Line

The date is usually **keyed** on line 15 or two to three lines below the letterhead. In keying, data are input by keystrokes on a computer. The date should be completely written out as January 15, 20XX, rather than 1/15/20XX. (If military style is used, the format would be 01 January 20XX.)

Inside Address

The inside address is keyed flush with the left margin. This address may be two, three, or four lines. Some rural areas only require two lines. If the letter is addressed to a provider, the credentials appear after the name. Do not type Dr. John Jones, M.D. (Both Dr. and M.D. are titles; use one or the other.)

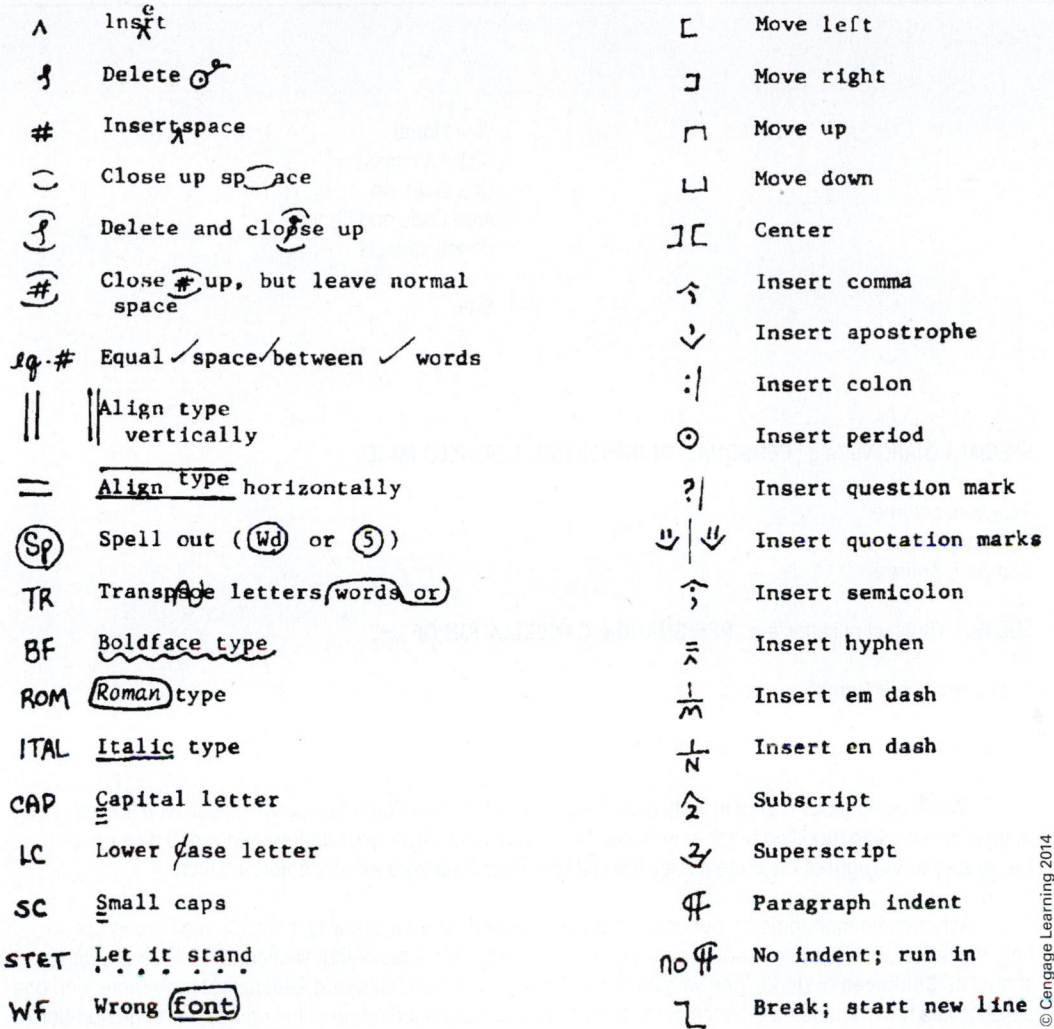

Figure 15-1 Common proofreader's marks.

Salutation

The salutation is keyed flush with the left margin on the second line below the inside address. A colon follows the salutation. The formal salutation should refer to the receiver of the letter using title and last name (e.g., "Dear Mr. Marshal:"). If the receiver and sender know each other well, the receiver's first name may be used (e.g., "Dear Jim:").

Subject Line

If used, the subject line is keyed on the second line below the salutation starting at the left margin.

This may begin flush with the left margin, indented five spaces, or centered. The patient's name or subject (meeting or topic) may be used on the subject line.

Body of Letter

The body of the letter should begin on the second line below the salutation unless a subject line is used that precedes two lines above the body. The body format will depend on the style of letter used. Paragraphs will begin flush with the left margin in full block letter style, or they may be indented five spaces when using the modified block letter style.

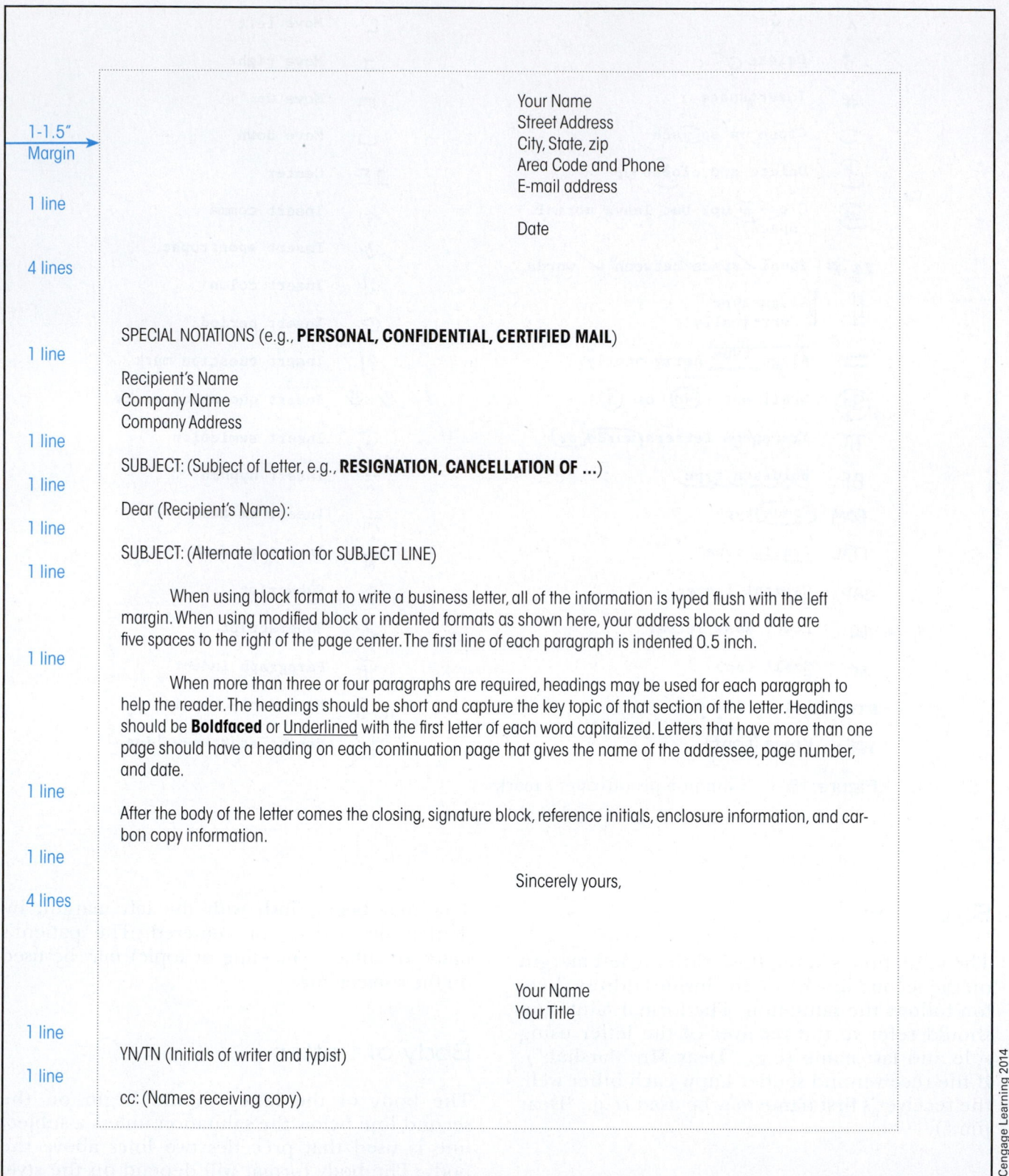

1-1.5"
Margin

1 line

4 lines

1 line

1 line

1 line

1 line

1 line

1 line

1 line

1 line

1 line

4 lines

1 line

1 line

Your Name
Street Address
City, State, zip
Area Code and Phone
E-mail address

Date

SPECIAL NOTATIONS (e.g., **PERSONAL, CONFIDENTIAL, CERTIFIED MAIL**)

Recipient's Name
Company Name
Company Address

SUBJECT: (Subject of Letter, e.g., **RESIGNATION, CANCELLATION OF ...**)

Dear (Recipient's Name):

SUBJECT: (Alternate location for SUBJECT LINE)

When using block format to write a business letter, all of the information is typed flush with the left margin. When using modified block or indented formats as shown here, your address block and date are five spaces to the right of the page center. The first line of each paragraph is indented 0.5 inch.

When more than three or four paragraphs are required, headings may be used for each paragraph to help the reader. The headings should be short and capture the key topic of that section of the letter. Headings should be **Boldfaced** or Underlined with the first letter of each word capitalized. Letters that have more than one page should have a heading on each continuation page that gives the name of the addressee, page number, and date.

After the body of the letter comes the closing, signature block, reference initials, enclosure information, and carbon copy information.

Sincerely yours,

Your Name
Your Title

YN/TN (Initials of writer and typist)

cc: (Names receiving copy)

Figure 15-2   Placement of business letter components.

Table 15-3 Guidelines for Letter Placement

The following guidelines are helpful in preventing errors in placement:

1. An imaginary picture frame should surround the letter. Margins may be 1, 1.5, or 2 inches (see Figure 15-2).
2. The last line of the letter should end no less than 1 inch from the bottom of the page.
3. Do not divide the last word on a page.
4. A minimum of three lines should be keyed on the second page of a letter. When dividing a paragraph at the bottom of a page, keep a minimum of two lines on the bottom of the page and two lines at the top of the next page.
5. If using a computer to prepare letters, it is easy to make adjustments to create a professional letter.
6. Use single space within paragraphs.
7. Use double space between paragraphs.

© Cengage Learning 2014

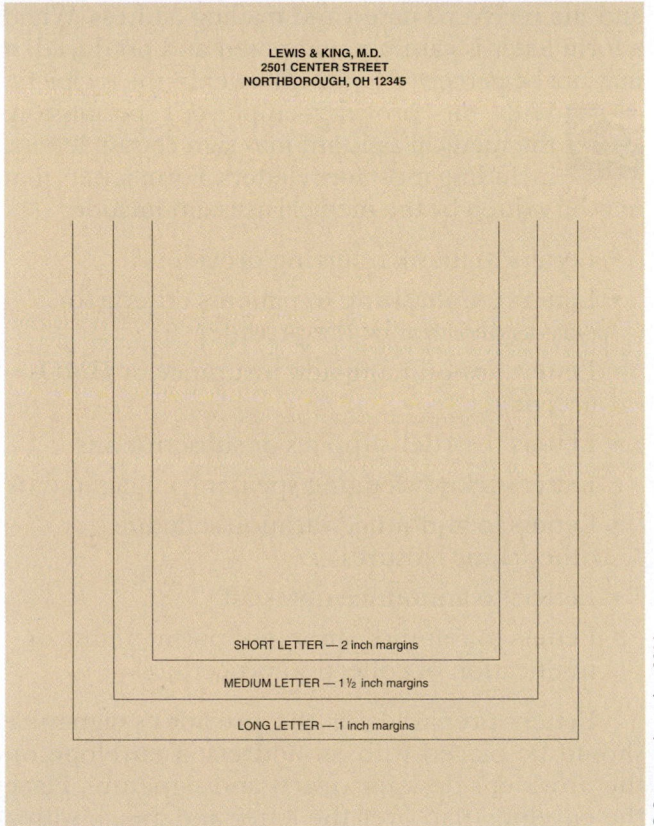

Figure 15-3 Letter length spacing.

Complimentary Closing

The complimentary closure begins on the second line below the body of the letter. The closure depends on the formality of the letter. Only the first letter of the first word of the complimentary closure is uppercase.

The style used in the complimentary closure should correspond with the salutation.

Letter Style	Complimentary Closing
Formal	Respectfully yours or Respectfully
General	Very truly yours or
	Yours truly or
	Sincerely or
	Sincerely yours
Informal (used when reader and writer are on first-name basis)	Regards or Best wishes

Keyed Signature

A keyed signature is a professional courtesy to the reader. Often, a letter is received in which the signature of the sender is not legible. The keyed signature should be at least four lines below the complimentary closing. This space may be lengthened to six lines if you are keying a short letter.

Reference Initials

The keyed signature may be the only initials used if the same person composed and signed the letter. If reference initials are used, the name of the individual composing the letter should be in uppercase letters with the medical assistant's initials keyed in lowercase letters.

Example:

WL:jg or WL/jg

Enclosure Notation

The enclosure indication can be either one or two lines below the keyed reference initials.

The number of enclosures may be indicated using one of several methods:

- Enclosures
- Enc.
- 1 Enc.
- 2 Enclosures
- Enclosures (2)

Some enclosures should be identified specifically, that is, a check for $84. Enclosures also may be sent under separate cover. If this method is used, state that the enclosure is under separate cover. It may be written as Enclosure under separate cover: Sarah Jones's medical record.

Copy Notation

If copies of the letter are to be sent to other parties, the copy notation should be one or two lines below the reference initials. The notation "c" (copy) or "pc" (photocopy) should be followed by the name of the person receiving the copy. When more than one person is to receive a copy of the original letter, key "c:" by the first name. Align the other names under the first person identified alphabetically or by rank.

Example:

c:	Joseph Brown, MD
	John Smith, MD

A **blind copy** notation "bcc:" may be used to send copies of the letter to individuals without the recipient's knowledge. This message is only keyed on the copy of the individual receiving the blind copy. The use of blind copies has decreased and in some practices is no longer used.

Postscripts

Postscripts (abbreviated as P.S.) may be used to:

1. Express an afterthought
2. Identify a thought that has been intentionally deleted from the body of the letter
3. Make a strong significant point

Postscripts are keyed two spaces below reference initials and enclosures.

Continuation Page Heading

There are two methods used to begin the continuation page heading. There should be at least a 1-inch space at the top of each continuing page of the letter. Plain paper matching the color, weight, size, and quality of the letterhead should be used. The following are examples of appropriate continuation page headings.

Example:

(1 inch from top of page)			
Jeremy Brown, MD		-2-	May 4, 20XX
or			
Jeremy Brown, MD			
Page 2			
May 4, 20XX			

LETTER STYLES

The administrative medical assistant may be responsible for creating a variety of letters that support the needs of the ambulatory care facility. Word processing software has business letter and memo templates useful in creating these documents.

One efficient approach to letter composition is to create a **portfolio** or database of frequently used **form letters**. Individualize letters by using the current date and the receiver's name and mailing address. When a form letter is carefully composed and produced, it may not be perceived as a form letter by the recipient. With the provider–employer's permission, the medical assistant may sign certain letters, including most form letters. Form letters that may be written by the medical assistant include:

- Letters to thank referring providers
- Letters emphasizing to patients criteria for care as directed by the provider
- Letters announcing new insurance or HMOs accepted
- Letters to order supplies or subscriptions
- Letters acknowledging speaking engagements
- Letters to announce vacation schedules or other clinic closures
- Letters to announce new staff
- Letters to remind patients of payment due or notification of collection procedures

Letters prepared for the provider's signature should be placed with an addressed envelope on the provider's desk for review and signature. Place the envelope flap over the letter and attach with a paper clip. Also include with the letter any enclosures for the provider's approval.

Four major styles of letters are used by medical and professional clinics:

1. Full block
2. Modified block, standard
3. Modified block, indented
4. Simplified

Full Block

The **full block letter** is the most time efficient for the ambulatory care setting because the medical assistant does not have to use excessive motion to tab indentions or to place address, complimentary close, or keyed signature. When using the full block style, all lines begin flush with the left margin. This style is suggested when desiring a contemporary-looking efficient letter.

Modified Block

In the **standard modified block** style letter, all lines begin at the left margin with the exception of the date line, complimentary closure, and keyed signature, which usually begin at the center position or a few spaces to the right of center. Figure 15-4 illustrates a modified block style letter without indention.

The assistant may choose to use the **indented modified block** style letter. In this format, paragraphs may be indented five spaces. Figure 15-5 illustrates a modified block style letter with indented paragraphs.

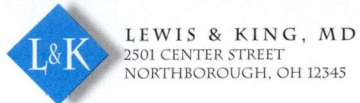

LEWIS & KING, MD
2501 CENTER STREET
NORTHBOROUGH, OH 12345

NORTHBOROUGH
FAMILY MEDICAL GROUP

January 12, 20XX (approximately 15th line)

Jeremy Brown, MD   (approximately 20th line)
111 S Main
Blossom, UT 10283-1120

Dear Dr. Brown:

Blossom Medical Society Meeting

Thank you for inviting me to speak at the Blossom Medical Society Meeting June 15, 20XX. As requested, my topic will describe the use of the MRI in assisting physicians to make a more accurate diagnosis without resorting to invasive procedures. The exact title of my speech will be sent by next Friday.

Please have your clinic manager send information regarding the number of participants expected, time of meeting, location, and any other details that will assist me in preparing my speech.

I will write or call if I have any additional questions.

Yours truly,

Winston Lewis, MD

Winston Lewis, MD

WL:jg

Enclosure: Handout on MRI

© Cengage Learning 2014

Figure 15-4   Sample standard modified block style letter; all elements start at left margin, except date, complimentary closing, and keyed signature.

LEWIS & KING, MD
2501 CENTER STREET
NORTHBOROUGH, OH 12345

NORTHBOROUGH
FAMILY MEDICAL GROUP

January 12, 20XX (approximately 15th line)

Jeremy Brown, MD (approximately 20th line)
111 S Main
Blossom, UT 10283-1120

Dear Dr. Brown:

Blossom Medical Society Meeting

Thank you for inviting me to speak at the Blossom Medical Society Meeting June 15, 20XX. As requested, my topic will describe the use of the MRI in assisting physicians to make a more accurate diagnosis without resorting to invasive procedures. The exact title of my speech will be sent by next Friday.

Please have your office manager send information regarding the number of participants expected, time of meeting, location, and any other details that will assist me in preparing my speech.

I will write or call if I have any additional questions.

Yours truly,

Winston Lewis, MD

Winston Lewis, MD

WL:jg

Enclosure: Handout on MRI

© Cengage Learning 2014

Figure 15-5 Sample modified block style letter with indented paragraphs. This format is the same as the standard modified except that the subject line and paragraphs are also indented.

Simplified

The **simplified letter** style omits the salutation and complimentary closure. All lines are keyed (input by keystroke) flush with the left margin. The subject line is keyed in capital letters three lines below the inside address. The body of the letter begins three lines below the subject line. The signature line is keyed in all capital letters four lines below the body of the letter. The Administrative Management Society recommends this style of letter. However, in medical clinics, this style is most often used when sending a form letter. Figure 15-6 illustrates a simplified style letter.

SUPPLIES FOR WRITTEN COMMUNICATION

Begin written communication at the computer workstation by checking to see that all supplies required to prepare the document are at hand. Check the computer settings and turn the printer on, making sure it is properly loaded with the correct letter stock. The paper should be **bond**, of good quality, and at least 20 to 24 pound stock with a watermark. A **watermark** is legible when paper is held to the light. Choose a shade of white, cream, or gray bond paper.

Although colored paper may be more eye-catching, it does not display a professional image.

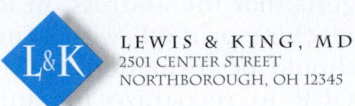

LEWIS & KING, MD
2501 CENTER STREET
NORTHBOROUGH, OH 12345

NORTHBOROUGH
FAMILY MEDICAL GROUP

January 12, 20XX (approximately 15th line)

Jeremy Brown, MD   (approximately 20th line)
111 S Main
Blossom, UT 10283-1120

(triple-space)

Blossom Medical Society Meeting

(triple-space)

Thank you for inviting me to speak at the Blossom Medical Society Meeting June 15, 20XX. As requested, my topic will describe the use of the MRI in assisting physicians to make a more accurate diagnosis without resorting to invasive procedures. The exact title of my speech will be sent by next Friday.

Please have your office manager send information regarding the number of participants expected, time of meeting, location, and any other details that will assist me in preparing my speech.

I will write or call if I have any additional questions.

Winston Lewis, MD   (4 line spaces)

WINSTON LEWIS, MD

WL:jg

Enclosure: Handout on MRI

© Cengage Learning 2014

Figure 15-6   The simplified style letter has no salutation or complimentary closing. The subject line and keyed signature are all upper case.

Also, be sure that the paper stock is compatible with printers used in the ambulatory care center.

Letterhead

The letterhead style and design is usually chosen by the provider(s) and may include a specially designed logo for the practice. The provider/practice name, street address or post office box number, city, state, ZIP code, and telephone number with area code are usually printed on the letterhead. Many clinics also add their fax number and email address. Letterhead information may be placed at either side or in the center of the paper.

Second Sheets

When an order is placed for letterhead, the medical assistant should order additional plain paper of the same stock as the letterhead to be used for second page sheets. The number of sheets will vary from clinic to clinic. If providers normally dictate long letters, this must be taken into consideration when ordering quantities.

Printing Multipage Business Letters

Printing multipage business letters on letterhead stationery requires use of more than one tray in the printer, unless you want to collate the letterhead or hand feed it into the printer. The simplest procedure is to place the letterhead stationery into a tray other than the default tray. Then go to "File," "Page Setup," "Paper Source," and from the menu that appears, specify the tray containing the letterhead stationery. The menu lets you choose the tray for the first page and the tray for the rest of the document. Make sure that the "Apply To" box is set for "Whole Document."

Envelopes

The stock and quality of the envelopes should match the stationery used in the clinic. With the use of **ZIP+4** and City State Files, mail is processed more efficiently and effectively. The address should be standardized so that it contains all delivery address elements. The correct name, city, state, and ZIP+4 codes must be used.

Example:

JEREMY BROWN MD
111 S MAIN
BLOSSOM UT 10283-1120

If Dr. Brown uses a post office box for the delivery of his mail, that address should be used. The postal service delivers to the last line before the city, state, and ZIP code.

Example:

JEREMY BROWN MD
PO BOX 1453
BLOSSOM UT 10283-1120

Place the intended delivery address on the line immediately above the city, state, and ZIP+4 code. The other address may be placed on a separate line above the delivery line.

Example:

JEREMY BROWN MD
111 S MAIN
PO BOX 1453
BLOSSOM UT 10283-1120

This letter would be received at the post office box, not the street address.

General Standards for Addressing Envelopes.
For successful processing by **optical character readers (OCRs)**, the U.S. Postal Service suggests that the address on letter mail needs to be machine-printed, with a uniform left margin. It should be formatted in a manner that allows an OCR to recognize the information and find a match in its address files.

A scanner reads the ZIP code on the bottom line and prints a bar code in the lower right corner of the envelope. Envelopes that are handwritten cannot be read by the OCR. These letters must wait for more costly and slower manual sorting.

To conform to standards, eliminate all punctuation in the envelope address with the exception of a hyphen in the ZIP+4 code. Leave a minimum of one space between the city name and two-character state abbreviations and the ZIP+4 code. The OCR can read a combination of uppercase and lowercase characters in addresses but prefers all uppercase characters (see Procedure 15-2).

Dark ink on a light background using uppercase letters is the suggested method in preparing a keyed address. There should be a uniform left margin on all lines of the address. An imaginary rectangle that extends 5/8 to 2¾ inches from the bottom of the envelope with 1 inch on each side should contain the address. The lower right edge should be kept free of any marks. This area will contain the bar code, whether it is preapplied or printed by an OCR. The bar code area is 5/8 inch from the bottom and 4½ inches from the right side of the envelope.

The U.S. Postal Service publishes several pamphlets and booklets that describe the format to be used when sending any mail. Check with the postal service regarding the latest publications. Service and deliverability will be improved if these standards are used.

Types of Envelopes.
Number 6¾ and number 10 are the envelopes most often used. A window envelope may also be used, especially when mailing statements.

Number	Size
6¾	6½" long × 3" wide
10	9½" long × 4" wide
7	7½" long × 3" wide

The address on the statement need only be keyed once. The entire address is capitalized with no punctuation. Only one space should be used between the state abbreviation and the ZIP code.

you want to insert. You are now ready to print the form letters. Select "Mail Merge-Mail Merge Helper" from the "Tools" menu and select "Printer" from the "Merge To" box. Your printer should show the documents in the queue. Procedure 15-4 gives step-by-step instructions for using mail merge.

CRITICAL THINKING

Using a computer and printer, correctly address a number 10 envelope to a provider following all of the U.S. postal regulations. Print the envelope.

When this statement is folded with the address in view, it may be inserted into a window envelope. Make certain that the entire address is visible through the window.

To prepare envelopes for mailing, lay all envelopes facing upward in a row with the flaps displayed. Moisten all the envelopes with a sponge. With the dominant hand, seal the flap; with the nondominant hand, push the envelope aside while the next flap is closed. Procedure 15-3 illustrates letter folding and placement of envelopes for closure. The use of premoistened or peel-off strips helps speed up the process.

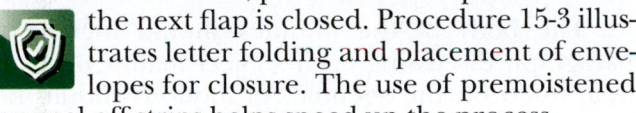

Mail Merge

Mail merge lets you create form letters, envelopes, or mailing labels using data from a data source. You would use this feature to send mailings to your client base or to a list of prospects, among others. Mail merge permits sending a form letter with envelopes to hundreds of recipients in a matter of minutes.

The client names and addresses are first stored in a Mail Merge data source, which can be a table or database such as Microsoft Excel. For Microsoft Word, a Mail Merge data source can be created by selecting "Mail Merge" in the "Tools" menu, selecting "Mail Merge Helper," and following the instructions given in Helper. Almost all word processor programs let you carry out a mail merge with an external database. You will need to consult the program manual for details.

Separate fields are suggested in the database for first name, last name, title, address, city, state, and postal code. To preclude time-consuming changes, three fields should be used for address, to accommodate clients with complex addresses. If a field is not required, leave it blank.

The Mail Merge Helper will give you the choice of editing the main document. Compose the document you want to send, and for each field where you want a new name or address, select "Insert Merge Field," and then select the name of the field

OTHER TYPES OF CORRESPONDENCE

Other specialized types of correspondence the medical assistant may be involved in preparing include memoranda, meeting agendas, and meeting minutes.

Memoranda

A type of interoffice correspondence is the **memorandum**, or **memo** for short. The use of memos permits messages to be sent quickly and without labor-intensive preparation. The memo format may already be preformatted on your computer software. If not, it is easy to design your own memo format.

The side margins should be set for 1 inch. Begin to key the memo heading 2 inches from the top of the page (line 13). The heading includes the words *date, to, from,* and *subject,* which should be boldfaced and capitalized. The words should each be keyed on a separate line with a double space between each line. By setting a tab stop 10 spaces in from the left margin, you will be able to tab to each entry and clear the headings to add the appropriate information. Triple space after the entry for the subject heading.

The body of the memo may begin at the left margin or may be set 10 spaces in so that the text starts directly beneath the typed headings. No salutation is required in a memo. Figure 15-7 provides a sample memo.

Meeting Agendas

Most meetings operate by following *Robert's Rules of Order, Newly Revised* as their parliamentary authority. The outlined order of business is as follows:

- Reading and approval of the minutes
- Reports of officers, boards, and standing committees
- Reports of special committees (ad hoc)
- Special orders

DATE: August 25, 20XX (key heading 2 inches from top
                of page, line 13)
TO: Staff of Doctors Lewis & King (embolden and
                capitalize headings and double space
                between them)
FROM: Walter Seals, Clinic Manager

SUBJECT: Vacation Schedule (triple space after the
                subject)

Doctors Lewis & King will be on vacation January 1–15.
Please do not schedule appointments during that time for
either doctor. Clinic personnel should report to work as usual.
During this two-week period, we will be preparing for the
annual audit.

© Cengage Learning 2014

Figure 15-7   Sample memorandum.

AGENDA
STAFF MEETING
Tuesday, September 1, 20XX
Location–Conference Room

Reading and approval of last months' minutes
Reports
    Risk Management Committee
    Personnel
Unfinished business
    Purchase of new X-ray machine
New business
    Doctors Lewis & King vacation January 1–15
    Annual Audit
Date and time for next meeting
Adjournment

© Cengage Learning 2014

Figure 15-8   Sample meeting agenda.

- Unfinished business and general orders
- New business
- Date and time of next scheduled meeting

The **agenda** lists the specific items that the group plans to discuss at the meeting under each of the above-mentioned divisions. The medical assistant preparing the agenda must determine the topics that are to be discussed. Copies of the agenda should be sent to each group member before the meeting date, and extra copies should be taken to the meeting for those who may have misplaced or forgotten to bring the agenda with them to the meeting. Figure 15-8 provides a sample meeting agenda.

Meeting Minutes

A written record of what transpired during a meeting is called the **minutes**. The minutes should record what business actions were taken during the meeting, who made each motion and what it was, who seconded the motion, any pertinent discussion, and whether the motion was passed.

The first paragraph of the minutes should contain the following information:

- Kind of meeting (regular, special, emergency)
- Name of the group or association
- Date, time, and place of the meeting
- Who officiated at the meeting and names of members present and absent
- Whether the previous meeting minutes were read and approved

The body of the minutes should include a paragraph discussing each subject matter or each item listed on the agenda. All motions should be recorded including the exact wording of the motion, the name of the person making the motion, the person seconding the motion, and whether the motion passed or failed. If the meeting had a guest speaker, the speaker's name and title and the subject of the presentation may be included in the minutes.

The last paragraph should contain the next meeting date, time, and place and the time of adjournment for this meeting. The person recording the minutes should sign them, and a copy of all minutes should be maintained in a notebook designated for that purpose. Corporations are required to have regular meetings with recorded minutes for legal purposes. Figure 15-9 provides a sample of recorded minutes.

PROCESSING INCOMING AND OUTGOING MAIL

The management of written communications also involves developing procedures for sorting, distributing, and otherwise processing incoming mail. It also includes posting and shipping outgoing items by the most cost-and time-effective method.

Incoming Mail and Shipments

All mail should be sorted by type before opening. Incoming mail includes telegrams, faxes, certified or registered letters, personal letters, emails,

---

STAFF MEETING MINUTES

The monthly staff meeting of Doctors Lewis & King was held Tuesday, September 1, 20XX, in the conference room. The meeting was called to order by Walter Seals, Clinic Manager. Those members present included: Dr. Lewis, Dr. King, Marilyn Johnson, Ellen Armstrong, Jane O'Hara, Wanda Slawson, and Bruce Goldman.

The previous meeting's minutes were read and approved as published.

Marilyn Johnson, CMA (AAMA), heading the Risk Management Committee, reported that a thorough walk through of the clinic had taken place to assess for safety issues. It was determined that the pull cords on the blinds could pose a potential hazard to small children. Marilyn made a motion that the blinds be upgraded with new vinyl louvered blinds with the plastic rod-type louver adjuster. Wanda Slawson seconded the motion. After discussion, a unanimous vote was cast to replace the blinds at the earliest time possible.

Walter Seals, Human Resource Manager, announced that he would be posting an opening for a CMA (AAMA) to work in the lab. All staff personnel were asked to share information about this opening with professionals who might be interested in working with Doctors Lewis & King.

Discussion was presented by Doctors Lewis & King regarding the purchase of a new X-ray machine. A committee consisting of Wanda Slawson, Bruce Goldman, and Marilyn Johnson was appointed to investigate the specific needs of the clinic and to locate appropriate vendors. They will present their findings at the next scheduled staff meeting.

New Business items include the fact that Doctors Lewis & King will be on vacation January 1–15, 20XX. We are asked to not schedule appointments during that time.

Walter Seals discussed preparations for the annual audit during the vacation period of Doctors Lewis & King. He will provide a schedule and timeline at the next staff meeting.

The next scheduled meeting will be October 3 at 12:30 PM in the conference room.

The meeting adjourned at 1:45 PM.

Ellen Armstrong

Figure 15-9 Sample meeting minutes.

checks from patients, insurance forms, invoices, medical journals, newspapers, magazines for the reception area, and advertisements regarding equipment and supplies.

Once it is categorized, incoming mail is directed to the appropriate personnel in the clinic. Checks from patients and invoices may be distributed to the bookkeeper, insurance forms to the insurance clerk, medical journals and advertisements can be placed on the provider's desk, and magazines and newspapers can be placed in the reception area.

Personal or confidential letters should not be opened unless the medical assistant has been given this responsibility by the provider or clinic manager.

Use a letter opener to open all mail before taking out the contents and reading the document. After removing the contents:

- Stamp the date it was received in the clinic.

- If the address is not included on the letter, write the address on the letter, as identified on the envelope or on the bank check (if patient is making a payment).

- When a colored reply envelope is sent with the statement to the patient, payments returned in these envelopes can speed up the sorting process.

- Look into the envelope to make certain that all contents have been removed.

- Attach the letter to the envelope with a paper clip, preferably on the left side.

Reply promptly to all requests, answering letters according to date of arrival; emergency situations need to be managed immediately.

Outgoing Mail and Shipments

Before placing postage on outgoing mail, weigh the item to be mailed, using a manual or electronic

CRITICAL THINKING

For the next week, practice sorting and prioritizing your personal incoming mail. If you live with others, ask permission to sort their mail and deliver it to them. Follow procedures outlined in this chapter. Write a paragraph about what you have learned by completing this exercise and how this experience might translate to a medical facility.

scale. A manual scale will read ounces. The assistant will then affix the appropriate postage, either stamps or postal meter. An electronic scale will automatically display the correct postage. If your clinic has a postal meter, this should be used to expedite mail. Metered mail does not have to be canceled or postmarked at the post office.

A postage meter is leased or purchased from a manufacturing company recommended by the postal service. However, the postage meter must be taken to the post office to purchase postage. The meter is locked for the amount of postage

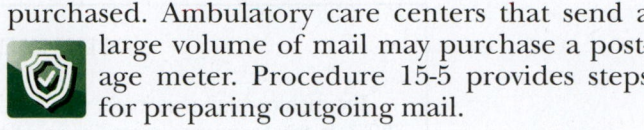 purchased. Ambulatory care centers that send a large volume of mail may purchase a postage meter. Procedure 15-5 provides steps for preparing outgoing mail.

Postal Classes

The Postal Service provides a range of mail classes to accommodate most user needs. Table 15-4 provides information that was in effect as of 2012. Prices reflect continental domestic delivery and are provided for reference only.

Check with the post office to determine costs and anticipated turnaround time to a specific destination.

Formats for Efficient Mail Processing

Certified, registered, and special delivery markings should be placed below the stamp or approximately nine lines from the right top edge of the envelope. "Personal" or "confidential" notation

Table 15-4 Price Comparison for U.S. Postal Rates

Class	Type	Delivery	Weight	Size, Inches	Cost
Express	Cards, letters*	Next day		12½ × 9½	$18.30
Priority	• Envelopes • Small box • Medium box • Medium box • Large box • Large box	2nd or 3rd day	<70 lb	• 12½ × 9½ • 8⅝ × 5⅜ × 1⅝ • 11 × 8½ × 5½ • 13⅝ × 11⅞ × 3⅜ • 12 × 12 × 5½ • 23¹¹⁄₁₆ × 11¾ × 8⅜	• $4.95 • $5.20 • $10.95 • $10.95 • $14.95 • $14.95
First	Cards Letters, envelopes	3 to 7 days	<3.5 oz	>3½ × 5 × .007 thick <6⅛ × 11½ × ¼ thick	• $0.29 • $0.44 1st oz + $0.20/oz over
First	Large envelopes	3 to 7 days	<13 oz	<15 × 12 × 0.75 thick	$0.88 1st oz + $0.20/oz over
First	Package	3 to 7 days	<13 oz	Length + width < 108	$1.71 < 3 oz + $0.17/oz over
Media	Books, manuscripts, video tapes, film, computer disks	3 to 7 days	<70 lb	Length + width < 108	$2.41 1st lb + $0.41/lb over up to 7 lb + $0.39/lb up to 70 lb

*Express mail includes $100 insurance on contents.

Source: http://www.usps.com/tools/calculatepostage/welcome.htm

should be keyed in all caps three lines below the return address. Adherence to other regulations will ensure accurate, timely delivery.

ZIP+4. ZIP+4 consists of the basic five ZIP code digits followed by a hyphen and four additional digits. The use of ZIP+4 will expedite the delivery of mail. If the envelope has been prepared properly to be read through OCR, the digits will be converted to a bar code. This piece of mail then goes to the bar code sorter, which rapidly sorts for the final destination.

Abbreviations. When addressing mail, use the abbreviations for states and U.S. possessions (Figure 15-10) and use official postal service abbreviations for street suffixes, directionals, and locators (Figure 15-11).

International Mail

Classes of international mail include letters and letter packages, postcards and postal cards, aerograms (airmail letters), printed matter, direct sacks of printed matter, matter for the blind, small packets, and parcel post. Special services such as insurance, recorded delivery, registered mail, restricted delivery, return receipt, special delivery, cash on delivery mail, and certified mail are also available. For the most current information on rates and services, inquire at the local postal service.

LEGAL AND ETHICAL ISSUES

Written communication, no matter what form is used, must take into consideration legal and ethical issues. A copy of all written communication should be maintained in the patient medical record or in clinic files should it be needed at a later date.

AL	Alabama	NE	Nebraska
AK	Alaska	NV	Nevada
AS	American Samoa	NH	New Hampshire
AZ	Arizona	NJ	New Jersey
AR	Arkansas	NM	New Mexico
CA	California	NY	New York
CO	Colorado	NC	North Carolina
CT	Connecticut	ND	North Dakota
DE	Delaware	MP	No. Mariana Islands
DC	Dist. of Columbia	OH	Ohio
FL	Florida	OK	Oklahoma
GA	Georgia	OR	Oregon
GU	Guam	PA	Pennsylvania
HI	Hawaii	PR	Puerto Rico
ID	Idaho	RI	Rhode Island
IL	Illinois	SC	South Carolina
IN	Indiana	SD	South Dakota
IA	Iowa	TN	Tennessee
KS	Kansas	TX	Texas
KY	Kentucky	TT	Trust Territory
LA	Louisiana	UT	Utah
ME	Maine	VT	Vermont
MD	Maryland	VI	Virgin Islands, U.S.
MA	Massachusetts	VA	Virginia
MI	Michigan	WA	Washington
MN	Minnesota	WV	West Virginia
MS	Mississippi	WI	Wisconsin
MO	Missouri	WY	Wyoming
MT	Montana		

© Cengage Learning 2014

Figure 15-10 Abbreviations for states, territories, and the District of Columbia.

AVE	Avenue	PL	Place
BLVD	Boulevard	RD	Road
CT	Court	STA	Station
CTR	Center	ST	Street
CIR	Circle	TPKE	Turnpike
DR	Drive	VLY	Valley
EXPY	Expressway		
HTS	Heights	APT	Apartment
HWY	Highway	RM	Room
IS	Island	STE	Suite
JCT	Junction	PLZ	Plaza
LK	Lake		
LN	Lane	N	North
MTN	Mountain	E	East
PKY	Parkway	S	South
		W	West

© Cengage Learning 2014

Figure 15-11 Abbreviations for street suffixes, directionals, and locators.

PROCEDURE 15-1

Preparing and Composing Business Correspondence Using All Components (Computerized Approach)

PURPOSE:
Prepare and compose a rough draft and final-copy letter using appropriate language and letter style to convey a clear and accurate message to the recipient.

EQUIPMENT/SUPPLIES:
Computer or word processor and printer
Printed letterhead and plain second sheet
Dictionary
Thesaurus
Medical dictionary
Style manual

PROCEDURE STEPS:

1. Organize key points to be addressed in a logical sequence. To assist in writing an effective letter.

2. Go to "Page Setup" and set document margins, paper size and source, and the layout. ***Pay attention to detail.*** Set the fonts to be used and paragraph parameters. Name and save the document. RATIONALE: Saves time and loss of formatting.

3. Compose a rough draft of the letter. With time and experience, these outlining steps may be eliminated before drafting the letter. RATIONALE: Business correspondence should be clear, concise, courteous, and accurate. A draft letter aids in checking that the letter is logical and achieves the intended purpose.

4. Use language that is easily understood. State the reason for the letter in the first paragraph and encourage action in the last paragraph. RATIONALE: For communication to take place, both parties must understand the message. The letter must be written so that the recipient understands the language and responds appropriately.

5. Read the draft for obvious errors in grammar, spelling, and punctuation. Use the appropriate reference material (dictionary, style manual, spell check, and so on) to check any inaccuracies. Read again for content. Is the message accurate, logical, and organized appropriately? Save the document again if any changes were made. Lay the letter aside and read it a third time at a

later time. RATIONALE: Reading several times allows you to concentrate on different elements of the letter. Errors may jump out when reading for the third time.

6. Choose the letter format that is customary to the ambulatory care setting. Established templates saved on the computer or provided on computer software are time savers. RATIONALE: The letter style should be efficient to prepare and professional in appearance and content to represent the provider–employer in a professional manner.

7. Key in the date or use the computer's auto date feature on line 15 or two to three lines below the letterhead. RATIONALE: Using the component parts of a business letter ensures that the letter is professional in appearance and represents the provider–employer in a professional manner.

8. Key the recipient's name and address flush with the left margin beginning on line 20. RATIONALE: Using the component parts of a business letter ensures that the letter is professional in appearance and represents the provider–employer in a professional manner.

9. On the second line below the recipient's address, key the salutation flush with the left margin. Follow the salutation with a colon unless you are using open punctuation. RATIONALE: Using the component parts of a business letter ensures that the letter is professional in appearance and represents the provider–employer in a professional manner.

10. Key the subject of the letter on the second line below the salutation flush with the left margin, if the subject line is being used. RATIONALE: Using the component parts of a business letter ensures that the letter is professional in appearance and represents the provider–employer in a professional manner.

11. Begin the body of the letter on the second line below the salutation or subject line. The body format will depend on the style of letter used. For example, if the full block format is used, paragraphs will begin flush with the left margin. Single space within paragraphs; double space between paragraphs. RATIONALE: Using the

Procedure 15-1 (continued)

component parts of a business letter ensures that the letter is professional in appearance and represents the provider–employer in a professional manner.

12. Key the complimentary closure on the second line below the body of the letter. Capitalize only the first letter of the first word of the complimentary closure (e.g., Respectfully yours). RATIONALE: Using the component parts of a business letter ensures that the letter is professional in appearance and represents the provider–employer in a professional manner.

13. Key the signature four to six lines below the complimentary closing. RATIONALE: This ensures that the recipient will be able to determine who sent the letter.

14. If reference initials are used, key the initials two lines below the keyed signature (e.g., WL:jg). RATIONALE: Using the component parts of a business letter ensures that the letter is professional in appearance and represents the provider–employer in a professional manner.

15. Key the enclosure or copy notation one or two lines below the reference initials. RATIONALE: Using the component parts of a business letter ensures that the letter is professional in appearance and represents the provider–employer in a professional manner.

16. ***Pay attention to detail.*** Proofread the document and make corrections as necessary. RATIONALE: All information contained in the letter must be accurate and written in a clear and concise manner with logical organization. The grammar, spelling, punctuation, and capitalization must be correct to ensure a professional appearance and represent the provider–employer in a positive manner.

17. Save the document again and print two copies. RATIONALE: Document is saved on the computer, and a copy for signature and mailing is produced. A hard copy for the file is also established.

18. Prepare the envelope. Place the envelope flap over the letter and attach it with a paper clip. RATIONALE: Prepare the envelope using U.S. postal regulations to ensure delivery in a timely manner. Proofread to be sure the address is accurate to ensure deliverability. By placing the envelope flap over the letter and attaching it with a paper clip, the two will not become separated.

19. Place the letter on the provider's desk for review and signature. RATIONALE: The provider's signature signifies the letter is accurate, sends the intended message, and represents the clinic in a professional manner.

20. File a copy of the letter in an appropriate filing system. RATIONALE: May be needed in the future for reference or as documentation.

PROCEDURE 15-2
Addressing Envelopes According to United States Postal Regulations

PURPOSE:
To address envelopes according to U.S. Postal Service regulations to ensure timely delivery.

EQUIPMENT/SUPPLIES:
Computer or word processor and printer with envelope tray
Envelopes
Address labels
U.S. Postal Service Publication 221, *Addressing for Success*

PROCEDURE STEPS:
1. Insert the envelope in the printer and select the envelope format from the software program. When using a word processor or computer, labels may be used rather than printing directly on the envelope. The label is then adhered to the envelope. Many printers have an envelope

continues

Procedure 15-2 (continued)

tray and software that will transfer the address from the letter to the envelope. This feature is a time saver because you key the address only once. RATIONALE: U.S. postal regulations suggest that the address on letter mail should be machine-printed, with a uniform left margin.

2. Visualize an imaginary rectangle on the envelope. The rectangle extends ⅝ inch to 2¾ inches from the bottom of the envelope, with 1 inch on each side. The address is placed within this rectangle (Figure 15-12). RATIONALE: U.S. postal regulations suggest that the address on letter mail should be machine-printed, with a uniform left margin.

3. Key the address in uppercase letters. Be sure to maintain a uniform left margin on all lines. Eliminate all punctuation in the address except the hyphen in the ZIP+4 code. RATIONALE: Leave a minimum of one space between the city name and the two-character state abbreviation and the ZIP+4 code. A scanner reads the ZIP code on the bottom line and prints a bar code in the lower right corner of the envelope. The OCR prefers all uppercase characters.

4. If you are not using preprinted envelopes, key the return address in uppercase letters in the upper left corner of the envelope. Include the name on the first line; address on the second line; and city, state, and ZIP+4 code on the third line. RATIONALE: The return address should be printed in the upper left corner of the envelope should the letter need to be returned to the sender for any reason.

5. **Pay attention to detail**. Proofread the envelope and make corrections as necessary. RATIONALE: When all information is correct, processing will take place efficiently and correctly.

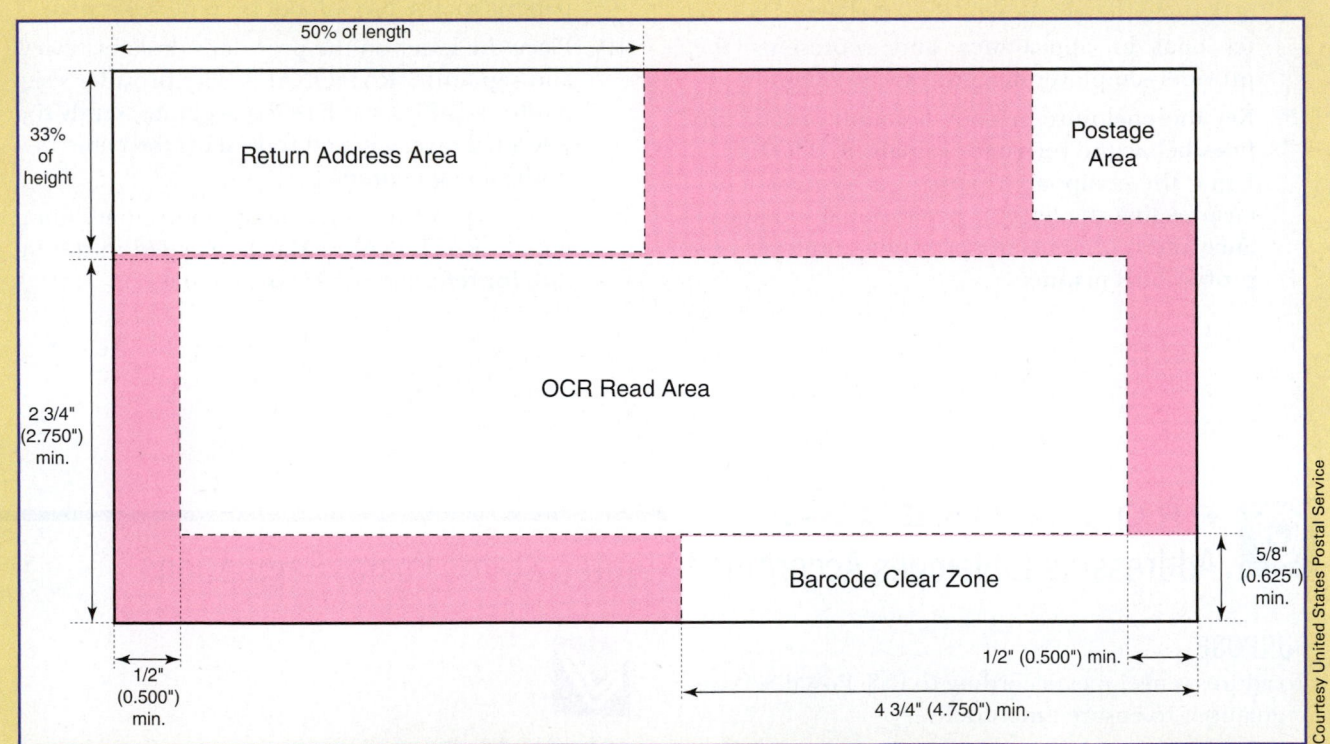

Figure 15-12 Designated zones for accurate reading of envelopes by optical character reader (OCR), the U.S Postal Service's computerized scanner.

PROCEDURE 15-3
Folding Letters for Standard Envelopes

PURPOSE:
To fold and insert letters into envelopes so that the letters fit properly in the envelopes.

EQUIPMENT/SUPPLIES:
Letters to be mailed
Number 6¾ envelope
Number 10 envelope
Window envelope

PROCEDURE STEPS:

1. To fit a standard-size letter into a number 6¾ envelope, fold the letter up from the bottom, leaving ¼ to ½ inch at the top, and crease it. Then fold the letter from the right edge about one third the width of the letter. Fold the left edge over to within ¼ to ½ inch of the right-edge crease. Insert the left creased edge first into the envelope (Figure 15-13A). RATIONALE: Ensures a proper fit of the letter into the envelope with a minimum of folds. The last crease made enters the envelope first. This enables the recipient to begin to read the letter with minimal effort.

2. To fit a standard-size letter into a number 10 envelope, fold the letter up about one third the length of the sheet and crease it. Then fold the top of the letter down to within ¼ to ½ inch of the bottom crease, and crease the top. Insert the top creased edge first into the envelope (Figure 15-13B). RATIONALE: Ensures a proper fit of the letter into the envelope with a minimum of folds. The last crease made enters the envelope first. This enables the recipient to begin to read the letter with minimal effort.

3. To fit a standard-size letter into a window envelope, turn the letter over and fold the top of the letter up about one third the length of the page so that

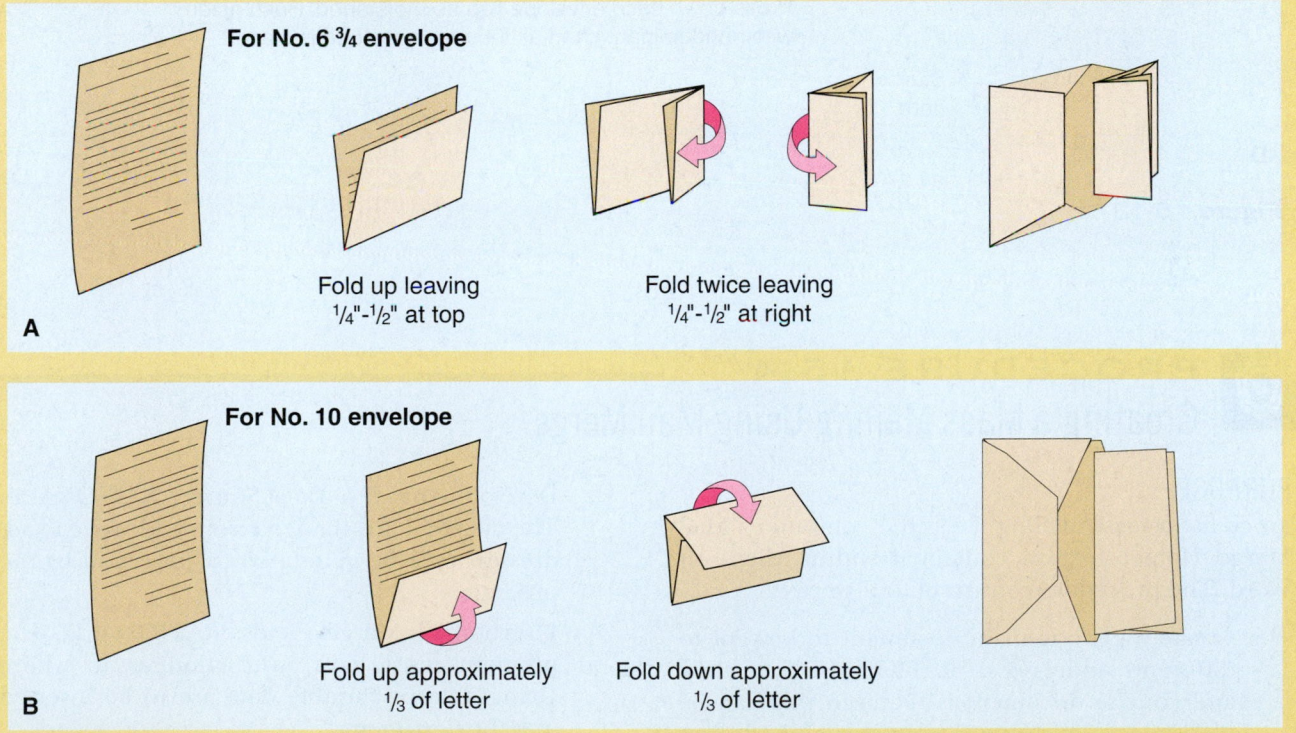

For No. 6 ¾ envelope

Fold up leaving
¼"-½" at top

Fold twice leaving
¼"-½" at right

A

For No. 10 envelope

Fold up approximately
⅓ of letter

Fold down approximately
⅓ of letter

B

Figure 15-13 Proper letter-folding procedures for various envelope type (A–C) and bulk placement of envelopes for moistening before closure (D).

continues

Procedure 15-3 (continued)

the address is facing you. Then fold the bottom of the letter back to the first crease. Insert the letter into the envelope bottom first (Figure 15-13C). ***Pay attention to detail.*** You should be able to read the entire address through the window. RATIONALE: Ensures that the entire address can be read through the window envelope and be delivered correctly.

4. Place envelopes as shown in Figure 15-13D to moisten before sealing. RATIONALE: Efficient method of sealing multiple letters for mailing.

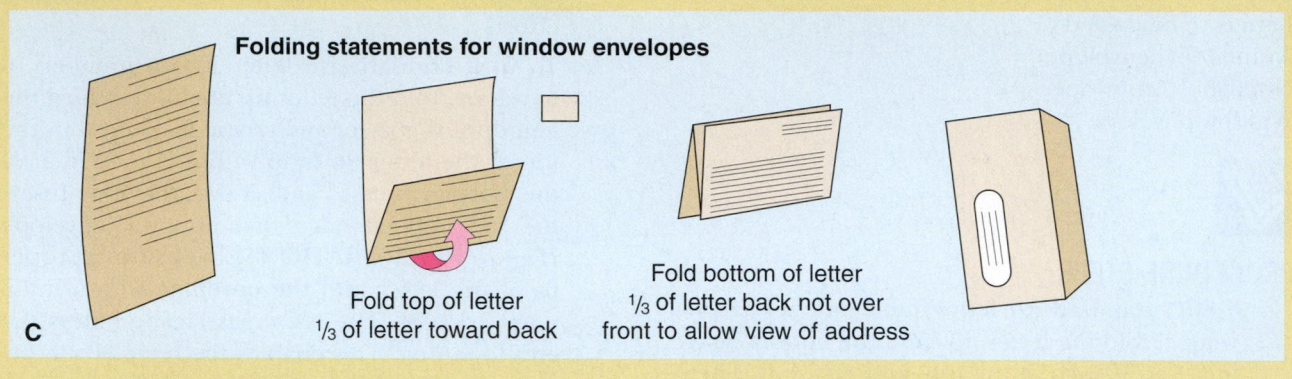

Folding statements for window envelopes

Fold top of letter
⅓ of letter toward back

Fold bottom of letter
⅓ of letter back not over
front to allow view of address

C

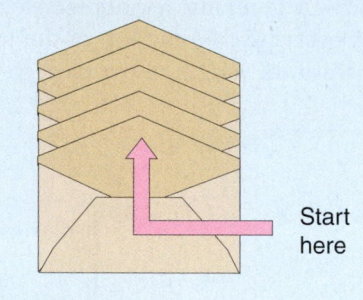

Place envelopes one behind the other. Moisten all flaps. Press down each envelope flap as moistened. Push aside with nondominant hand as the next envelope is closed.

Start here

D

© Cengage Learning 2014

Figure 15-13

PROCEDURE 15-4
Creating a Mass Mailing Using Mail Merge

PURPOSE:

To create a mass mailing using the computer's Mail Merge Helper feature contained within Microsoft Word. The procedure consists of four steps:

1. Create a generic main document to be sent to different addressees. RATIONALE: A clear and concise document is required that can be used to transmit your message for all addresses by changing only the name, address, and title within the document.

2. Development of a Data Source. RATIONALE: The data that are changed from addressee to addressee must be generated for insertion by the program.

3. Insertion of Merge Fields. RATIONALE: The program must have instruction as to where changeable or variable data are to be inserted into the document.

4. Merge the main document and variable data and send it to an output device such as a printer.

Procedure 15-4 (continued)

RATIONALE: The program must be told how to output the final merged document.

EQUIPMENT/SUPPLIES:
Computer and printer
Composed correspondence keyed and saved as a
   Word document
A developed data source

PROCEDURE STEPS:

1. Create main document:
   - The first step in creating a mass mailing is to compose and type the document in Microsoft Word. ***Pay attention to detail.*** At this step, identify each data field (name, address, and so forth) that will be variable to personalize the document for each addressee by inserting a readily identifiable character such as a "?" or "&." For use in Step 2, note the different unique data fields that are required.

2. Develop a data source:
   - Select "Tools" from the menu bar, and then select "Mail Merge" from the drop-down menu that appears.
   - Mail Merge Helper appears, displaying a screen that shows a checklist of actions required by you. You must first identify the type of main document being prepared. Select "Create" from item 1 on the screen and a drop-down menu will appear with several types of documents listed for selection. Select "Form Letter" for this exercise.
   - A new window immediately appears asking where to look for the main document. Because you have already typed the main document in the active window, click on "Active Window." You will notice that the screen displays your choices below the "Create" button.
   - Go to item 2 on the screen and select "Get Data." A drop-down menu immediately appears listing several options. Select "Create Data."
   - A screen appears showing data field titles. It is possible to add additional fields or to eliminate some of the fields in the list. We will want to have three fields for complex addresses, so

type into the upper left block entitled "Field Name" the word "Address3." Immediately, a new button appears below it saying "Add Field Name." Click this button; the name you just typed has been added to the existing list. If it is at the bottom of the list, move it to after "Address2" by first highlighting it and then moving it using the up and down arrows at the right of the screen.
   - All of the field names will not be needed, so delete work phone, home phone, country, and job title. Fields are deleted by first highlighting them, and then clicking the button "Remove Field Names." Check if everything is OK and click "OK."
   - A new screen appears and you are asked where to store your data file. Give it a name "Merge Data" and store it on your "Desktop." You do this by left-clicking with your mouse on the arrow to the right of the "Save In" window. Click the arrow adjacent to select "Desktop." Click the "Save" button from the drop-down menu.
   - A new screen now appears saying that no data are in your file and allowing you to edit your data. Select "Edit Data Source."
   - A data form now appears with the field titles you previously selected and empty boxes are adjacent to each title. Fill in the boxes with the data you have made up for this problem. Any boxes where data do not exist should be left blank. After completing the first record (addressee), click the "Add New" button and a new blank form will appear. Continue until you have added data for at least three records. Click "OK" when finished.

3. Insert merge fields into the main document:
   - You should be back in your main document. You will now insert the field names in the appropriate locations you have marked in the original document with a "?" or "&" character. Insert your cursor and highlight one of the characters. Using your mouse, click on the toolbar entitled "Insert Merge Field." A drop-down menu will appear listing all of the field titles you selected while developing the data source in Step 2. Select the field appropriate to the location of your cursor and left-click. The field name will immediately appear in the

continues

Procedure 15-4 (continued)

main document with double curly brackets ({{ and }}) on either end. Continue until you have replaced all of the characters with field names.

- Check to make sure that the spacing and punctuation are correct. Each field name will be just as if you typed the actual data, with no additional spaces or commas.

4. Sending the merged document to the output device (printer):

- Select "Tools," "Mail Merge," putting you back in Mail Merge Helper. Select "Merge" and a "Merge To" block appears. Select "Printer."

- The printer screen appears. Make sure the printer connected to your computer is

selected, the "Page Range" is set to "All," and the number of copies is set to 1. Click "OK." Three letters should print with the variable data you input to your data file.

- If you have any errors in the data or in spacing, make the necessary changes. To edit your data file, get back to Mail Merge Helper and select "Edit Data Source," followed by clicking the file location suggested by a button that appears below the one you just clicked.

- To move from record to record, use the arrows at the bottom of the screen. When you have finished editing, click "OK" and repeat printing as described earlier in this step.

PROCEDURE 15-5
Preparing Outgoing Mail According to United States Postal Regulations

PURPOSE:
To prepare outgoing mail for expeditious delivery.

EQUIPMENT/SUPPLIES:
Manual or electronic scale
Postage meter or stamps
Envelope or package to be mailed

PROCEDURE STEPS:

1. Sort the mail according to postal class. For example, all single-piece letters that weigh less than 11 ounces are included in first-class mail. Correspondence and statements are sent in this classification. RATIONALE: Sorting by postal class expedites processing at the post office.

2. Using the manual or electronic scale, weigh the item to be mailed. *Pay attention to detail.* If

you are using a manual scale, read the weight in ounces and compute the amount of postage due. If you are using an electronic scale, the correct postage will be displayed on the scale. RATIONALE: Correct postage on each postal item is essential to ensure faster delivery service.

3. Using a postal meter or stamps, affix the appropriate postage to the piece to be mailed. Use of a postal meter expedites delivery of mail because metered mail does not have to be canceled or postmarked at the post office. RATIONALE: Correct postage on each postal item is essential to ensure faster delivery service.

4. Place the prepared mail in the area of the clinic designated for outgoing mail or deliver the mail to the post office according to clinic policy. RATIONALE: Ensures that all mail going out is centrally located and that the postal worker can pick up outgoing mail and deliver incoming mail efficiently.

CASE STUDY 15-1

Refer to the scenario at the beginning of the chapter.

When she was assembling the style manual for all written communications generated by the clinic of Drs. Lewis and King, clinic manager Marilyn Johnson wanted it to be as comprehensive as possible. Therefore, she gathered research over a period of months, noting problems the clinic had experienced in written communications, such as letters going out without the provider's signature. She became familiar with proofreading devices that would ensure letter-perfect correspondence. She also developed source materials on the different classes of mail and the services of the U.S. Postal Service.

CASE STUDY REVIEW

1. Marilyn is ready to outline the manual. Review the chapter information and create an outline indicating major topic headings for the Lewis and King style manual.

2. Because a few of the medical assistants are not comfortable with composing, what writing tips can Marilyn include to make them more confident?

3. Marilyn wants all letters to look alike. What information should she include to educate the manual users about the components of a standard letter?

CASE STUDY 15-2

Drs. Lewis and King are considering adopting the use of clinical email because many of their patients have home computers and use email in their day-to-day communications. Clinic manager Marilyn Johnson is concerned about maintaining patient confidentiality and appropriate use of clinical email. She has decided to develop a written agreement of understanding and plans to ask each patient to sign the agreement before transmission of any clinical email is instituted. Marilyn also believes a privacy disclaimer could be of legal value to the clinic. Review Chapter 12's section regarding clinical email.

CASE STUDY REVIEW

1. Marilyn is developing the agreement of understanding. What are some key elements that should be included in the agreement?

2. Responding to patients using email correspondence is different than social communication. What are some guidelines for email correspondence that will be helpful to remember?

3. List several advantages and disadvantages to using email in the ambulatory health care setting.

SUMMARY

Communication is vital in any ambulatory care setting, and the proper management of written communications ensures both a professional image and an efficient operation. Because of our ability to write letters, send reports, transcribe provider notes, and otherwise communicate with others, the quality of patient care is enhanced, because communication is at the core of much patient treatment.

As well as becoming knowledgeable about the techniques of written communication, it is important for the medical assistant to become comfortable with the act of composition and writing. Proper techniques in letter formatting and proofreading ensure quality control and the maintenance of high administrative standards. Ease in writing and communicating on paper ensures that information is accurate, reliable, and capable of being held up in a court of law if this becomes necessary.

The administrative medical assistant must be skilled in the use of technologies and understand and follow confidentiality and legal policies and procedures.

STUDY FOR SUCCESS

To reinforce your knowledge and skills of information presented in this chapter:

- Review the *Key Terms*
- Role-play with other students to apply attributes of professionalism pertinent to this chapter.
- Consider the *Case Studies* and discuss your conclusions
- Answer the questions in the *Certification* Review
- Apply your knowledge by completing the Activities in the *Study Guide* and the Games and Quizzes in the StudyWARE **StudyWARE** software on the *Premium Website*
- Perform the Procedures using the *Competency Assessment Checklists* in the *Competency Manual*
- Practice your problem-solving skills with the *Critical Thinking Challenge 3.0* on the *Premium Website*

Additional resources for this chapter include:

- Module 6 of the *Medical Assisting Learning Lab*
- *CourseMate for Delmar's Comprehensive Medical Assisting*
- *WebTutor for Delmar's Comprehensive Medical Assisting*

CERTIFICATION REVIEW

1. When proofreading a letter, you should:
   a. never read it against the document
   b. always proof it only on the computer screen
   c. read long documents a section at a time
   d. always finish the job no matter how tired you may be
2. Form letters should be used:
   a. for all patients
   b. for all referring providers
   c. only for pharmaceutical salespeople
   d. with individualized addressing when possible
3. Of the four major letter styles, which is the most contemporary?
   a. Full block
   b. Modified block, standard
   c. Modified block, indented
   d. Simplified
4. Form letters may be written for each of the following *except*:
   a. letters containing laboratory or diagnostic results
   b. letters announcing new insurance or HMOs accepted
   c. letters to announce new staff
   d. letters to order supplies or subscriptions
5. The subject line is keyed:
   a. on line 15 or two to three lines below the letterhead
   b. on the second line below the inside address
   c. four lines below the complimentary closing
   d. on the second line below the salutation
6. Which of the following is a guideline for letter placement?
   a. Use single line space within paragraphs.
   b. When dividing a paragraph at the bottom of a page, keep two lines on the bottom of the page and two lines at the top of the next page.
   c. A minimum of three lines should be keyed on the second page of a letter.
   d. All of the above.
7. After removing the contents from incoming mail, what should you do?
   a. Stamp the date it was received in the clinic.
   b. Look in the envelope to make certain that all contents have been removed.
   c. If the address is not included on the letter, write it on the letter as it appeared on the envelope.
   d. All of the above.

8. Newspapers and periodicals are sent in which postal class?
   a. Express
   b. First class
   c. Bulk rate
   d. Second class
9. First-class mail is divided into which two subclasses:
   a. automation and nonautomation
   b. periodical and standard mail
   c. standard A and standard B
   d. bulk and parcel post mail

10. According to the USPS Domestic Mail Manual, which mail class is the most secure?
    a. Priority mail
    b. Express mail
    c. Standard mail
    d. Registered mail

REFERENCES/BIBLIOGRAPHY

Humphrey, D. D. (2004). *Contemporary medical office procedures* (3rd ed.). Clifton Park, NY: Delmar Cengage Learning.

ingenix. (2003). *HIPAA toolkit*. Salt Lake City, UT: St. Anthony's Publishing/Medicode.

Keir, L., Wise, B. A., Krebs, C., Kelly-Arney, C. (2008). *Medical assisting administrative and clinical competencies* (6th ed.). Clifton Park, NY: Delmar Cengage Learning.

Robert, H. M., III, Evans, W. J., Honemann, D. H., & Balch, T. J. (2000). *Robert's rules of order newly revised* (10th ed.). Cambridge, MA: Perseus Publishing.

Terryberry, K. (2005). *Writing for the Health Profession.* Clifton Park, NY: Delmar Cengage Learning.

Villemarie, D., & Villemarie, L. (2005). *Grammar and writing skills for the health professional.* Clifton Park, NY: Delmar Cengage Learning.

CHAPTER 16

Medical Documents

OUTLINE

The Changing Role of Medical Transcription
- Electronic Medical Records
- Outsourcing
- Voice Recognition Software
- Medical Transcriptionist as Editor
- Authentication

Confidentiality and Legal Issues
- Health Insurance Portability and Accountability Act Regulations
- Protocols

Types of Medical Documents
- Chart Notes and Progress Notes
- History and Physical Examination Reports
- Radiology and Imaging Reports
- Operative Reports
- Pathology Reports
- Consultation

Discharge Summaries
Autopsy Reports
Correspondence

Turnaround Time and Productivity

Medical Transcription as a Career
- Professionalism Related to Medical Transcription

LEARNING OUTCOMES

1. Define, spell, and pronounce the key terms as presented in the glossary.
2. Discuss the changing role of medical transcription.
3. Discuss the impact of electronic health records on medical transcription.
4. List a minimum of three reasons for justifying outsourcing medical transcription.
5. Discuss voice recognition software and its impact upon medical transcription.
6. List responsibilities of the medical transcriptionist serving as editor of medical documents.
7. Review the importance of quality assurance and risk management.
8. Describe the process of flagging and its significance.

9. Discuss what is meant by the term *authentication* and identify three ways it may be done related to medical reports.
10. State what is meant by *privileged* information.
11. Identify four ways the medical transcriptionist can be compliant with the Health Insurance Portability and Accountability Act (HIPAA).
12. Differentiate among chart notes, history and physical examination reports, radiology and imaging reports, operative reports, pathology reports, consultations, discharge summaries, autopsy reports, and correspondence.
13. Discuss turnaround time and its importance to medical records.
14. Analyze the professionalism questions and apply them to this chapter's content.

ATTRIBUTES OF PROFESSIONALISM

KEY TERMS

Association for Healthcare Documentation Integrity (AHDI)

auditor

autopsy report

certified medical transcriptionist (CMT)

chart notes

chief complaint (CC)

confidentiality agreement

consultation report

current reports

discharge summary (DS)

editor

electronic medical record (EMR)

flag

gross examination

Health Insurance Portability and Accountability Act (HIPAA)

history and physical examination (H&P) report

history of the present illness (HPI)

microscopic examination

old report or aged report

operative report (OR)

outsourcing

pathology report

present problem (PP)

privileged

progress notes

quality assurance (QA)

radiology report

registered medical transcriptionist (RMT)

review of systems (ROS)

risk management

stat report

turnaround time (TAT)

voice recognition software (VRS)

Competency

- Did you pay attention to detail?
- Did you ask questions if you were out of your comfort zone or did not have the experience to carry out tasks?
- Did you display sound judgment?
- Were you knowledgeable and accountable?
- Were you respectful of others?
- Did you apply critical thinking skills in performing patient assessment and care?
- Did you recognize the importance of local, state, and federal legislation and regulations in the practice setting?

Initiative

- Did you show initiative?
- Did you develop a strategic plan to achieve your goals? Was your plan realistic?
- Did you seek out opportunities to expand your knowledge base?
- Were you flexible and dependable?
- Did you implement time management principles to maintain effective clinic function?
- Did you assist coworkers when appropriate?
- Did you seek ways to improve the morale of your workplace?

Integrity

- Did you work within your scope of practice?
- Did you acknowledge the scope of practice of other health care professionals?
- Did you demonstrate sensitivity to patient's rights?
- Did you protect personal boundaries?
- Did you demonstrate respect for individual diversity?
- Did you protect and maintain confidentiality?
- Did you immediately report any error you had made?
- Did you report situations that were harmful or illegal?
- Did you maintain your moral and ethical standards?
- Did you do the "right thing" even when no one was observing?

SCENARIO

Inner City Health Care, a multispecialty clinic, employs two full-time medical transcriptionists. Marilyn Johnson, CMA (AAMA), is the clinic manager and has former training and experience as a medical transcriptionist. This experience provides her with the basic understanding necessary to manage the medical transcription and medical records department of the clinic. Marilyn is very cost conscious and is exploring outsourcing all medical transcription.

INTRODUCTION

The development of new technology over the last few years is impacting medical facilities in a variety of ways. Computerized medical facilities have implemented electronic health records (EHR), may use voice recognition software (VRS) and electronic signatures, or may outsource transcription to other areas of the United States or to foreign countries. These changes have a direct impact on the position medical transcriptionists (MTs) once held in the medical environment. Today, the MT may be more involved with quality assurance (QA), risk management, and editing the completed document rather than transcribing written or dictated medical information.

THE CHANGING ROLE OF MEDICAL TRANSCRIPTION

MTs have been responsible for transforming written or dictated medical information into an accurate, permanent document that is legible and uniform in format. The resulting medical record describes the encounter between the patient and health care provider and is extremely important from both a health care and a legal standpoint.

Today's cost-conscious and rapidly changing economy along with new technology has brought about many changes in the profession. The following paragraphs discuss major changes impacting medical transcription today.

Electronic Medical Records

EHR Clinics using **electronic medical records (EMR)** rather than paper-based medical records may delegate much of the MT's responsibility to other medical personnel. For example, the MA may record directly into the EMR the reason for the visit, medications the patient is currently taking, including over-the-counter and herbal products; height and weight; vital signs; and any observations. The provider, using the computer, has access to the entire patient medical record and may call up test results, various images, diagnoses, and treatment plans for verification or comparison. The provider may add to the EMR document by directly keying in chart notes or by dictating to a digital recording system or may use voice recognition software. The provider may complete and transmit prescriptions directly to a pharmacy or forward all or part of the medical record to a referring provider. Refer back to Chapter 11, Figure 11-6 which illustrates the use of electronic health record (EHR) as it relates to EMR.

Each entry into the EMR is automatically date and time stamped, which facilitates documentation and tracking of patient care and outcomes. The EMR provides easy access to quickly locate accurate and readily usable information about the patient at the point of care. EMRs are much more efficient in the clinical decision-making process than the old cumbersome paper-based patient records. EMRs may be sent to all medical personnel involved in the care of a patient in a matter of seconds.

We have covered the process of changeover to a computerized system in the medical clinic in Chapter 11, but we have not covered the process of the physical transition from existing paper medical records to electronic health records. Two issues must be resolved: how much of the paper chart do we convert to a digital format and how do we make the majority of the existing clinical history available to the physician. Several options are available:

- *All patient charts are scanned into the EHR system.* This choice is the most attractive option, but it is also the most costly. Although the basic scanning can be performed by a relatively unskilled worker, a trained medical professional must file the data in the appropriate category of the new medical record so that it can be readily located by the medical provider.

- *Partial scanning of patient charts.* Charts are pulled for existing patients scheduled for the coming week and only the clinically pertinent information from the past three to six visits as identified by the medical provider are scanned and filed in the new system. This process is repeated until partial paper records for all patients are included in the EHR system. This approach requires that paper records be actively retained for a period before they are archived.

- *Do not scan any old information.* Develop an EHR record for all patients from a given date and have the old paper record for existing patients available for the medical provider for as long as the provider feels necessary. At some point the provider will no longer have a need for the paper record and it can be archived.

Some practices receive a lot of calls regarding patient questions or pharmacy requests. The summary page of the paper record can be scanned for all patients to establish an EHR that is useful in fulfilling these types of requests. One of the options for transitioning paper records can then be used to develop a more complete EHR for each patient.

The conversion of paper records to electronic records is most readily accomplished by scanning. It could be done using practice personnel; however, it is more cost effective for an outside firm that will come onsite to do the work. Care must be exercised to follow all HIPAA regulations. A trained medical professional will still be required to ensure that the records are filed appropriately in the EHR system.

The file system used in establishing an EHR system must be carefully thought out to ensure that the medical provider can easily retrieve data. The EHR program being used is a good place to begin in planning the details of the file system while tailoring it to the specific type of medical practice. Documentation of the file system and the conversion procedure is a first step to maintaining consistent nomenclature and data format throughout the conversion.

Outsourcing

Transcription is a task that is presently outsourced by many large clinics and hospitals. **Outsourcing** is the practice of contracting with a service outside the clinic or hospital to a company where the task can be accomplished at a lower cost and with a faster turnaround time. Outsourcing companies usually are located in countries where a source of English-speaking educated labor is present, the pay rate is low, and a stable business climate exists. Currently, outsourcing organizations are located in areas of the United States and Canada as well as offshore at companies primarily located in the United Kingdom, India, and the Philippines.

Today's medical clinics must keep a keen eye on the bottom line—cost. Some advantages given to support outsourcing of medical transcription include the following:

- Outsourcing transcription frees administrative and support personnel to complete tasks that often are delayed because of time crunch factors.

- Outsourcing companies are on the job 24/7 and 365 days of the year, so the medical clinic need not be concerned about vacation periods or sick leave. Someone is always on the job.

- Outsourcing companies focus on transcription without having to answer telephones, schedule appointments, or deal with any number of interruptions encountered in the medical clinic. Therefore, documents are more accurate, standardized, and completed with less turnaround time.

- Outsourcing transcription frees floor space (real estate) previously used to support a line item expense and converts it to a source of revenue.
- Outsourcing saves on costly employee benefits packages.

Digital dictation by the provider can be readily sent to the outsource organization that performs the transcription using the Internet, with the completed document returned in similar fashion. Some important considerations before outsourcing transcription include the following:

- Be sure the medical clinic and the transcription service are using compatible hardware and software.
- Investigate quality assurance, security, HIPAA, and confidentiality measures.
- Be cost conscious. Most transcription fees are calculated by the line, but it may be more cost effective to pay by the minute of recorded dictation time. A digital dictation system allows one to measure to the 10th or 100th of a minute.
- A transcription service that uses a digital dictation system should have a user-friendly method of tracking transcribed documents. The work should be able to be located in less than 3 minutes.
- When using a digital dictation system, a provider's dictation is available to the transcriptionist as soon as the provider hangs up the phone, allowing for no lost time, which equates to cost containment.

Outsourcing is rapidly eliminating the need for the traditional transcriptionist in medical facilities. This practice is in turn being replaced by the use of voice recognition software.

Voice Recognition Software

Voice recognition software (VRS), also known as speech recognition, automatic speech recognition (ASR), or natural language recognition software, converts voice to text using a computer. In essence, the software "translates" the sounds spoken into written words. This type of program has improved greatly in recent years, translating with little error.

Specialized programs are capable of translating highly technical medical terminology.

The latest generation of VRS uses continuous speech technology, which allows the speaker to speak more naturally. All VRS systems require an enrollment process, during which a person sits at the computer and reads sample text out loud to help train the speech recognition software to understand the particular voice pattern. VRS integrates easily with Windows applications, including Microsoft Word, Outlook Express, Internet Explorer, and AOL Instant Messenger. Some VRS products are marketed that work with personal digital assistants (PDAs) and smartphones.

Medical Transcriptionist as Editor

With the use of EHR, outsourcing, or VRS methods of transcription, the MT professional is now serving as the **quality assurance (QA)** manager, responsible for **risk management**, and the **editor** or **auditor** of transcribed documents. A QA manager establishes a process that provides accurate, complete, consistent health care documentation in a timely manner. Figure 16-1 shows data flow for transcribed medical records produced using outsourcing and speech recognition software.

Editing is the process of reviewing the transcribed document for accuracy and clarity. It is important to remember that one must not change the dictator's style or meaning when editing. Common errors are usually in sentence structure, punctuation, and spelling. They are easily changed without altering the dictator's style or meaning. Sound-alike words are another area where errors occur.

The **Association for Healthcare Documentation Integrity (AHDI)** recommends the following principles when reviewing a document:

- Compare the transcribed report against dictation. Do not just read the document.
- Use industry-specific standards for style, punctuation, and grammar (*The Book of Style for Medical Transcription*).
- Consider risk management issues.

CRITICAL THINKING

How will you determine which medication was prescribed for a patient: digitoxin or digoxin?

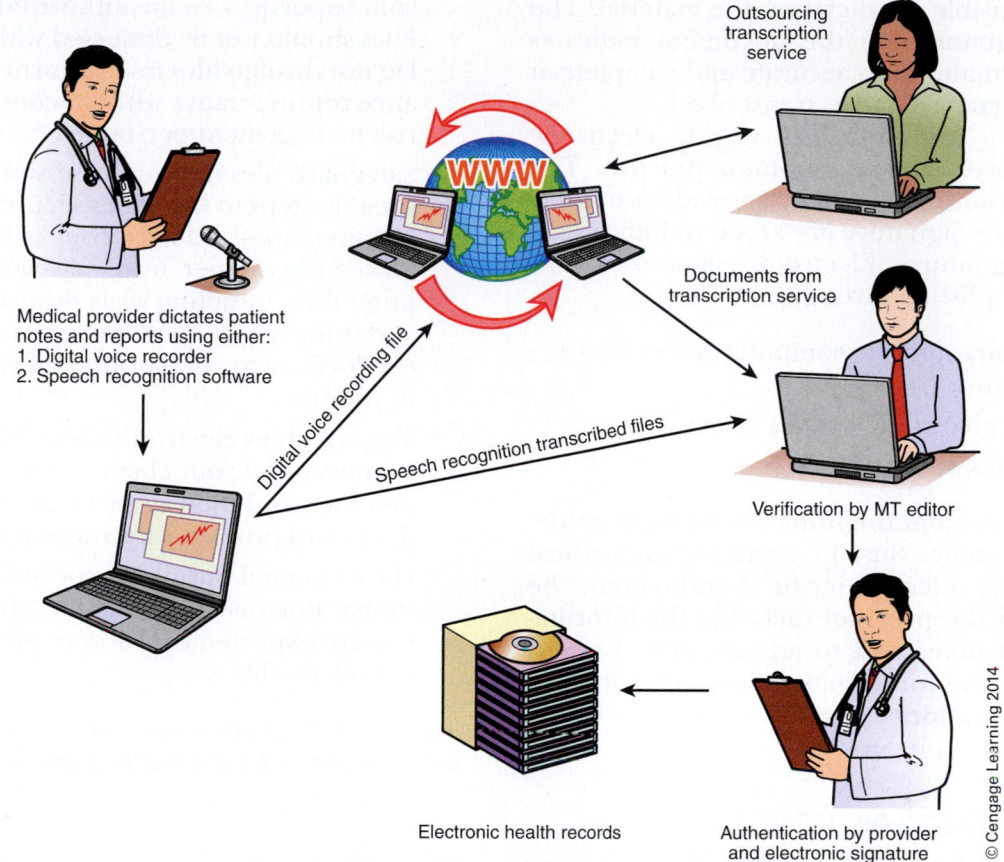

Medical provider dictates patient notes and reports using either:
1. Digital voice recorder
2. Speech recognition software

Outsourcing transcription service

Documents from transcription service

Verification by MT editor

Digital voice recording file

Speech recognition transcribed files

Electronic health records

Authentication by provider and electronic signature

© Cengage Learning 2014

Figure 16-1   Data flow for transcribed medical records produced using outsourcing and speech recognition software.

- Third parties, such as the QA person, proofing a document should provide feedback to the transcriptionist. Although 100% accuracy is desired, accuracy of audited documents should not be less than 98%. Accuracy less than this figure requires corrective action.

If the MT encounters a term that cannot be interpreted or something new that cannot be referenced, the MT should **flag** that section of the document to alert the dictator that something needs to be corrected or resolved. The flagged message may indicate the provider is cut off, what the term sounds like, or the message is incomprehensible. Provide as much information as you can to assist the dictator in recalling the dictated area in question.

Flagging procedures vary from one facility to another and may depend upon the method used to transcribe documents. In large facilities using EHR, VRS, or outsourcing, the flagged documents may be referred directly to QA personnel. The notation may be incorporated into the computerized document using a color-code approach with a flag message. The correct information then can be added to the document and the color coding removed. In-house flagging may simply consist of a sticky note or a preprinted flag attachment.

Authentication

In most cases, the provider dictating the information will sign or authenticate the document. At times an attending provider or physician assistant will be responsible for dictating the material. The provider's signature on the document indicates that the information was accurate and complete at the time of dictation and as transcribed.

In today's technological world, electronic signatures have become common practice. The words "electronically signed by [provider's name]" underneath the signature are keyed to indicate an electronic signature. Electronic signatures may also be accomplished through:

- Use of alphanumeric computer key entries as identification
- Use of an electronic writing device
- Use of a biometric system

Medicare and the Joint Commission guidelines require that the signature on medical reports, electronic or handwritten, be completed by the provider dictating the information and not delegated to anyone else. Federal law, state law, and Joint Commission accreditation standards all address the issue of electronic signatures.

CONFIDENTIALITY AND LEGAL ISSUES

  Confidentiality means treating the patient's medical information as private and not for publication. The patient has a right to privacy; therefore, medical information is **privileged**. Privileged information may only be communicated with the patient's permission or by court order. The MT must learn to follow the motto: *What you see here and what you hear here must stay here when you leave here.*

Health Insurance Portability and Accountability Act Regulations

  Health Insurance Portability and Accountability Act (HIPAA) regulations are government rules and procedures that have resulted from legislation designed to protect the confidentiality of patient information ranging from medical records to personal identification numbers that, if divulged, could result in identity theft.

The MT can meet most HIPAA regulations by adhering to the following simple rules:

- Do not divulge medical records you transcribe to anyone other than the dictator,

your supervisor, or an authorized QA person. Files should not be discussed with the patient. Do not divulge files to an attorney or insurance representative without consulting with risk management personnel.

- Safeguard files in your possession. Take reasonable steps to keep files secure, such as keeping tapes and hard copy of reports in a locked file cabinet, using passwords for computer files, installing virus protection software, and using a firewall if appropriate. Do not carelessly carry files around on your person or in your car.
- Transmit files electronically only with the permission of your client or the dictating provider, and then agree on the proper procedures and protocols for transmission.
- Have a signed business associate agreement or similar document that defines the protocols you are expected to follow to protect patient confidentiality.

These general rules do not constitute legal advice; consult with appropriate legal counsel for specific questions.

Protocols

Protocols are the procedures your clinic has in place to ensure patient confidentiality. You are usually required to sign a **confidentiality agreement** stating that you will comply with the established procedures. Your contracts, together with the protocols, become a part of the institution's documentation demonstrating compliance with HIPAA regulations. The purpose of your signing a contract is to substantiate that you have received training and have been instructed in proper procedures to protect medical records.

From the MT's viewpoint, risk management involves protecting the confidentiality of the medical records and ensuring the accuracy of those records.

MTs are in an excellent position to assist the risk management officer, through their commitment to quality and their awareness of confidentiality procedures and possible medical errors indicated in the dictated data. Should a problem or error be detected that could be a risk management problem, the MT should immediately notify his or her superior, clinic manager, risk management officer, or the employer's or client's legal staff according to clinic policy.

You will recall from Chapter 8 that ethics are not laws but rather standards of conduct. These standards vary from state to state, so you should research your specific state's standards. The AHDI adopted a Code of Ethics (see the AHDI website for the AHDI Code of Ethics available at: http://www.ahdionline.org/MemberCenter/CodeofEthics/tabid/279/Default.aspx) for professional MTs.

Although, in certain cases, the MT can be held financially responsible for errors and omissions, the MT usually is under the jurisdiction of *respondeat superior,* meaning that the provider–director or clinic manager is responsible for the wrongful acts of the MT working under his or her supervision. This is not meant to imply that MTs should not protect themselves by instituting some personal risk management, such as carrying errors and omissions insurance. Insurance should be considered particularly if the MT is operating a home business and contracting transcription work.

Medical records are documents governed by laws and may be subpoenaed for review by various courts. The medical report may play a major role in substantiating injury or malpractice claims.

TYPES OF MEDICAL DOCUMENTS

Medical reports become part of the patient's permanent medical record and are vital to continued patient care. Other providers, attorneys, insurance companies, or the court may review the medical reports in part or in their entirety. Therefore, the medical report must be neat, accurate, and complete. *Neat* refers to a medical report that is legible and assembled to permit easy access to information as needed. *Accurate* means that the dictation has been transcribed as dictated, and *complete* indicates that the document has been dated correctly and signed or initialed by the dictator.

Complete documentation of medical reports is also important for payment or reimbursement of services for which the provider expects to be paid. The billing and diagnosis codes reported on the health insurance claim form must be supported by the documentation contained within the medical report.

A new trend in transcription is the integration of digital images directly into the transcribed record. The response to inputting digital images (photographs, scans, and radiographs) has been positive from both the local health care community and patients themselves. This is attributed to easier understanding of a picture by patients and more precise presentation using both pictures and written text to medical professionals.

The tools required for integrating digital images into word processing programs is already available to most MTs in their current Microsoft Word software packages. They only have to obtain a disk containing digital images from their provider–employer. If the transcribed record is included in the EHR, digital images can be attached, allowing other providers to view, enlarge, and manipulate the images at will.

The transcribed medical report may be formatted in a variety of styles similar to business correspondence. Common transcribed reports include:

1. Chart notes and progress notes
2. History and physical examination reports
3. Radiology reports
4. Operative reports
5. Pathology reports
6. Consultations
7. Discharge summaries
8. Autopsy reports
9. Correspondence

Hospitals and practices may require a specific format for reports different from those described in the following examples. A few helpful formatting rules are:

- Use section headings that clarify the report.
- Do not add sections left out by the dictator.
- Do not include unnecessary confidential information unless specifically instructed to do so.
- Note who dictated the report, if not the attending provider, and provide space for both to sign. The initials of the transcriptionist should be on the signature page.
- Use 1-inch margins all around, unless the document is to be filed in a chart that has a top opening, then use a 1.25-inch margin at the top only. If using sticky paper for chart notes, use 0.5-inch margins.
- Use paragraph format (see the following examples).

```
1/4/20XX                                          HANSEN, HENRY

RV following treatment for fx of the left wrist. The cast was removed
last week. The skin texture and turgor are returning to normal. Range
of motion has increased with physical therapy, and strength is slightly
improved at -4/5. PLAN: Continue whirlpool and ROM exercises. RV 4 weeks.
                                              AE MD/rf CMA(AAMA)
```

© Cengage Learning 2014

Figure 16-2   Sample chart/progress notes.

Chart Notes and Progress Notes

Chart notes, sometimes referred to as **progress notes**, are a concise description of the patient's encounter with the medical clinic. They are chronologically listed and may include in-person visits to the clinic and telephone and electronic mail (email) inquiries. Chart notes should be filed in the chart within 24 hours of the encounter. The present problem, the provider's physical findings, and the treatment plan should be identified within the chart note. Laboratory test results also may be included. The provider or clinic personnel may enter chart note information as informal handwritten notes, or keyed notes affixed to the appropriate space. All notes documented must include the date, time, and signature of the person entering the data along with his or her credential. This information is pertinent for follow-up questions or for litigation purposes. Figure 16-2 shows a sample chart/progress note.

History and Physical Examination Reports

The **history and physical examination (H&P) report** documents information relating to the patient's main reason for treatment. The report is divided into two sections. The first is the history, which includes the **chief complaint (CC)** or **present problem (PP)**, a description of symptoms, problems, or conditions that brought the patient to the clinic; **history of the present illness (HPI)**, a chronological description of the development of the patient's illness; past medical and surgical history; family history; and social history.

The second section is the **review of systems (ROS)** and inquiry about the system directly related to the problems identified in the HPI. The provider determines the extent of the examination performed and documented based on the problems presented. The findings of the actual physical examination make up the documentation for the physical examination section of the report.

The Joint Commission accredits and regulates all policies and procedures of hospitals and provider's clinics owned by hospital organizations. The Joint Commission requires that hospitals provide H&P reports to be filed in patient charts within 24 hours of admission. Occasionally, the patient is seen in the provider's clinic and a decision is made to admit the patient to the hospital. In this case, the examination is performed in the clinic, but the report is dictated to the hospital that transcribes the document and files it within the patient's chart. The H&P format may also be used to document a patient's annual physical examination in the clinic. Figure 16-3 shows a sample H&P Report.

Radiology and Imaging Reports

A **radiology report** is a description of the findings and interpretations of the radiologist who studies the diagnostic procedure. Examples of radiology reports are x-ray studies, computed tomography (CT) scans, magnetic resonance image (MRI) scans, nuclear medicine procedures and fluoroscopic studies. In some cases, a contrast medium is administered either orally or by injection before the procedure is performed. A scan is a procedure that requires the use of radioactive isotopes.

When dictating, the radiologist may switch from present to past tense; that is, the procedure was performed in the past tense, and the findings are given in the present tense.

Stereoscopy and tomography are technologies that view structures within the body in dimensions or layers. Computed tomography uses radiography with computers to visualize a slice of the body part. Sonograms and echograms are another imaging technology that uses high-frequency sound waves to compose a picture of an area of the body. Magnetic resonance imaging produces sectional images of the body without the use of radiology. New technologies create the need for understanding the imaging process and appropriate documentation of patient information.

HISTORY AND PHYSICAL EXAMINATION

PATIENT: Donald Waite
CHART #: 97223

HISTORY: The patient is a 72-year-old male who was admitted because of intermittent, moderately severe chest pain starting from the substernal region radiating to the back and to the left arm and associated with a choking sensation. The pain lasted from minutes to half an hour and was relieved by two nitroglycerin tablets.

This condition has been going on for the last two weeks. The patient has known arteriosclerotic heart disease and since his discharge in July 20XX, has been doing reasonably well on Procardia, nitrates, Persantine, and digoxin.

PAST HISTORY: The patient had a pacemaker implantation for sick sinus syndrome four years ago. He has a history of angina and myocardial infarction. He also has essential hypertension.

His past surgical history includes an appendectomy and bilateral herniorrhaphies. He has no allergies.

The patient still works as a projectionist in a movie house. He does not smoke but drinks occasionally. He denies any history of diabetes, liver, or kidney disease. There is no evidence of claudication. There is dyspnea on exertion and fatigability. GI is negative; GU is negative.

PHYSICAL EXAMINATION: The patient is out of distress right now. He has been given two injections of Demerol. Blood pressure is 120/68, ventricular rate is 72 per minute, and respiratory rate is 60 per minute. Color is good. Skin is warm. Examination of the head shows that right lenticular opacity is greater than the left. Neck veins are flat. There are no bruits. Carotids are brisk, and there is no evidence of thyroid enlargement. The heart is regular with no S3 gallops. There is a systolic ejection murmur at the base III/VI. The lungs are clear. The abdomen showed surgical scars. Extremities have no edema. Pulses are 2+, and there is no calf tenderness.

IMPRESSION: Unstable angina secondary to coronary artery disease with obstructive and mixed pattern spasm on an affixed lesion. Status postpacemaker implantation and degenerative joint disease with cervical degenerative arthritis.

Review of the EKG shows nonspecific ST-T wave changes in II, III, and aVF and in the anterolateral leads. Chest X-ray showed cardiomegaly, and the enzymes are pending.

RECOMMENDATIONS: The patient should be hospitalized in the coronary care unit and monitored. The nifedipine should be increased up to 60 mg—slowly. Continue Persantine. Continue transderm nitro—increase to 10. Monitor the blood level. Consider angiogram when he is stabilized.

Electronically signed by Elizabeth M. King, MD 11/3/20XX   5:37 PM

EMK/urs

d:11/2/XX
t: 11/2/XX

Figure 16-3   Sample history and physical examination report.

When transcribing radiology or imaging reports, the date of service should be used rather than the date of dictation. Other details to be included within the report may include:

- Number and type of views taken
- Any special circumstances that could affect the examination
- Quality of the study (clear or blurry)
- Abnormal findings
- Normal findings
- Radiologist's impression, interpretation, diagnosis, and recommendations
- Signature of the radiologist

The report should be filed in the patient's chart within 4 to 8 hours of the procedure. Sufficient documentation must be in the report for the provider to use if he or she must prove that the study was medically necessary or if justification for reimbursement is required. Figure 16-4 shows an example of a radiology report.

Operative Reports

The **operative report (OR)** chronicles the details of a surgical procedure performed in a hospital, outpatient surgical center, or clinic. The surgeon or assistant dictates the OR immediately after the

MERCY MEDICAL CENTER
300 Main Street
Denver, CO 80201

RADIOLOGY #: 23445

PA & LATERAL CHEST   Date 10/07/XX

The pulmonary vessels are clearly outlined and are not distended. There are not any typical signs of redistribution. A few increased interstitial markings persist, but there are no typical acute Kerley B-lines. There may be a little residual pleural effusion at the costophrenic sinus and posterior gutters. Most of the pulmonary edema and effusion has otherwise cleared. The chest is not hyperexpanded. The thoracic vertebrae show spurring but no compression.

IMPRESSION:
1. No signs of elevated pulmonary venous pressure or frank failure at this time.
2. Residual pleural effusion is seen in the costophrenic sinus and posterior gutters, either residual or recent congestive failure.

BILATERAL MAMMOGRAMS   Date: 10/07/XX

Bilateral xeromammograms were obtained in both the mediolateral and craniocaudal projections. There is no previous exam for comparison. There is slight asymmetry of the ductal tissue in the lower outer quadrant of the right breast. There are no dominant masses, clusters of microcalcifications or pathologic skin changes identified.

IMPRESSION: Normal bilateral mammogram.

Electronically signed by
Renny Genray, MD 10/08/20XX 11:21 AM

JOHN DOE, M.D.   SMITH, HARRIET #123456-7
Dictated by: Renny Genray, M.D.
D&T: 10/07/XX | 10/07/XX | RG/mt

RADIOLOGY REPORT

Figure 16-4 Sample radiology report.

PATIENT: Joseph Oritz

DATE: 6/25/XX

SURGEON: Raja Rao

PREOPERATIVE DIAGNOSIS: Crohn's disease requiring central venous access for hyperalimentation.

POSTOPERATIVE DIAGNOSIS: Crohn's disease requiring central venous access for hyperalimentation.

OPERATION: Insertion of left-sided subclavian double-lumen central venous catheter.

ANESTHESIA: 1% lidocaine.

PROCEDURE: The patient was placed in the supine position with the neck extended to the right side. The left side of the chest was prepared and draped in the usual manner using Betadine solution. The subclavian vein on the left side was percutaneously and easily entered, and the guide wire was advanced into the superior vena cava. The double-lumen central venous catheter with VitaCuff was placed through the guide wire into the superior vena cava. Good blood flow was obtained. The catheter was sutured to the skin using 2-0 silk sutures and connected to IV solution.

A dry sterile dressing was applied.

The patient tolerated the procedure well.

Electronically signed by
Juan Esposito, MD 06/25/20XX
4:15 PM

JE/urs

d: 6/25/XX
t: 6/27/XX

Figure 16-5 Sample operative report.

report should be filed in the chart as soon as possible after surgery so that other staff members caring for the patient will have needed information. Figure 16-5 shows a sample OR.

operation. The OR describes the surgical procedure, preoperative and postoperative diagnoses, and specimens removed. It sometimes includes a sponge count and instrument inventory, an estimate of blood loss, and the condition of the patient on leaving the operating room. The report should also include the name of the primary surgeon and any assistants. The type of anesthesia and name of the anesthesiologist should also be included in the report. Often the report will end with disposition or where the patient was transferred when he or she left the operating room and the condition of the patient at the time of transfer. The authenticated

Pathology Reports

A **pathology report** is generated to describe the **gross** and **microscopic examinations** performed on organs, lesions, tissue samples, or body fluid removed during a surgical procedure. In some cases, the pathologist examines the specimen before the patient is sutured to determine if a more extensive surgical procedure is required (e.g., in the case of malignant tumors).

Pathologists generally dictate the report in the present tense because they interpret the pathologic findings as they view the specimens. The

```
                        PATHOLOGY REPORT
PATHOLOGY NO.:     792 304
DATE:              12/20/XX
CHART NO.:         56 84 20
NAME:              Lee Allen Au          AGE: 15 Female
DEPARTMENT:        Surgery               MD: Dr. Raja Rao

TISSUE:            Appendix

HISTORY:           Right Lower Quadrant Pain

CLINICAL DIAGNOSIS: RLQ Pain

PATHOLOGICAL REPORT: The specimen is labeled appendix and
is received in formalin. The specimen consists of an appendix
that measures 6 × 1 × 0.5 cm in greatest dimension. The
serosa surface has some white fibrinoid material attached
to it and on a cross section. Some purulent fibrinous material
can also be seen. Representative sections are submitted in
1 cassette.

DIAGNOSIS: Acute suppurative appendicitis with periappendi-
citis and mesoappendicitis.


                        Electronically signed by
                        Thomas A. King, MD 12/20/20XX
                        2:22 PM

TAK/rp

d: 12/20/XX
t: 12/20/XX
```

© Cengage Learning 2014

Figure 16-6 Sample pathology report.

report must be completed within 24 hours of receipt with a copy maintained by the laboratory and copies sent to each provider involved in the case. The original is maintained in the patient's chart. Figure 16-6 shows a sample pathology report.

Consultation

When one provider requests the services of another provider in the care and treatment of a patient, a **consultation report** is generated. The information may be disseminated in the form of a report or within the body of a letter. The contents of the consultation report/letter usually contain all of the elements of an H&P with a focused history of the patient's illness and the body system directly related to the consultant's area of specialty. The consultant also includes within the report/letter the findings, supporting laboratory data, diagnosis, and suggested course of treatment. The report/letter usually ends with a comment from the consulting provider thanking the admitting

provider for the referral. It should be filed in the patient's medical record within 24 hours of receipt. Figure 16-7 shows a sample consultation report.

Discharge Summaries

The **discharge summary (DS)** documents the patient's history of hospital admissions. The DS includes the reason for hospital admission, a description of what transpired while the patient was in the hospital, the final diagnosis, follow-up instructions, discharge medications, patient's condition at discharge, and prognosis for recovery. If the patient is transferred to another facility such as a skilled nursing facility, the report is changed from DS to transfer summary. If the patient has expired during the stay, the report is usually called a death summary. The Joint Commission requires that the completed DS be filed in the patient's chart within 48 to 72 hours of discharge from the hospital. Figure 16-8 shows a sample DS.

Autopsy Reports

An **autopsy report** may also be called an autopsy protocol, a necropsy report, or a medical examiner report. Autopsies are performed to determine the cause of death or to ascertain and confirm presence of disease. It is important to understand that state law requires that autopsies be performed in certain situations. For example, an autopsy report is required when someone dies suddenly, when someone dies while unattended, or in the case of suspicion of crime.

When transcribing an autopsy report, more words should be spelled out and abbreviation use kept to a minimum because these records may be entered into a court of law and must be accurate and clearly understood. Many states require that military time be used when documenting the time a body arrives at the coroner's office. Temporary anatomic diagnoses should be placed in the medical report within 72 hours and in the completed report within 60 days. Figure 16-9 shows a sample autopsy report.

Correspondence

It is important for the MT to remember that all forms of medical correspondence also are considered medical documents and must be transcribed with the same care as any other medical

LEWIS & KING, MD
2501 CENTER STREET
NORTHBOROUGH, OH 12345

NORTHBOROUGH
FAMILY MEDICAL GROUP

January 4, 20XX

Margaret Holly, MD
Metroma Medical Center
900 Union Street, Suite 208
Metroma, MI 11666

RE: MARY O'KEEFE

Dear Dr. Holly:

Thank you for referring Mary O'Keefe to our clinic. She presented today stating that she recently relocated to Clinton with her husband and children to be closer to her parents. Mary has been experiencing symptoms suggestive of pregnancy and is here for evaluation. Over the past three weeks, she has noticed increased tenderness of her breasts, fatigue, and a feeling of being bloated. A home pregnancy test was positive.

Her past medical history is positive for the usual childhood diseases and the births of two children, following normal pregnancies. She has a negative past surgical history.

She has no allergies to medications and takes Tylenol for occasional headaches. She is married and has two children, ages 3 years and 12 months. She is employed part-time in an insurance office. She does not smoke or drink.

The family history is noncontributory.

On review of systems, her complaints are limited to those described above. She has had no nausea or vomiting, and no change in bowel habits. She has no dizziness, no fevers, and no urinary symptoms.

Physical examination revealed a 32-year-old white female in no acute distress. HEENT normocephalic, atraumatic. PERRLA, EOMI. The thyroid was not enlarged, and there was no cervical adenopathy. The lungs were clear. The heart had a regular rate and rhythm. The abdomen was soft and nontender. Bowel sounds were normal. The extremities revealed trace ankle edema. The neurological examination was within normal limits. Pelvic examination confirmed a gravid uterus, compatible with a very early pregnancy.

An abdominal ultrasound has been ordered and a beta HCG was drawn.

I believe Mary is pregnant and I will put her on our OB regimen starting with monthly visits. Thank you for your kind referral.

Sincerely,

Elizabeth M. King, MD

EMK/lmb

Figure 16-7 Sample consultation report.

PATIENT: Kelly Cohen
CHART #: 29324

ADMITTED: 9/26/XX
DISCHARGED: 11/19/XX

HISTORY/LAB: This infant was born on 09/26/XX to a 30-year-old, gravida II, para 1 female, with a last menstrual period of 3/22/XX estimated date of confinement 2/29/XX. The mother had been observed regularly during her pregnancy. However, she did develop preterm labor necessitating early hospitalization. At that time, the mother was placed on antibiotics and dexamethasone and delivered at approximately 26 weeks' gestation. At the time of delivery, the membranes ruptured spontaneously and fluid was clear. The infant had an Apgar score of 5 and 8 at 1 and 5 minutes, respectively. The infant required intubation in the delivery room and was then transferred to the NICU. On admission, weight was 1,159 grams, length 38.5 cm, head circumference 25.5 cm, chest circumference 26 cm. Assessment was 26 weeks' gestation.

COURSE/CONDITION ON DISCHARGE/DISPOSITION: At the time of admission the infant had respiratory distress, was intubated, and required Survanta. The infant was placed on IV fluid and antibiotics, and appropriate blood work was done. During the hospitalization, the infant improved with regard to the respiratory distress. However, the infant developed bronchopulmonary dysplasia, hyperbilirubinemia, and apnea of prematurity. The infant was placed on the appropriate medications and improved steadily. Her weight increased gradually. During the hospitalization, the infant was evaluated by Dr. Lally of Ophthalmology who will follow up on an outpatient basis.

The infant was discharged home on 11/20/XX. She had a hearing test, eye examination as stated, and was going to receive home physical therapy three times a week. She was on Fer In Sol drops and was feeding on Neosure and breast milk. The overall prognosis was guarded to good.

FINAL DIAGNOSIS: Preterm, 26-week female infant, appropriate for gestational age, apnea of prematurity, anemia, respiratory distress syndrome, bronchopulmonary dysplasia, hyperbilirubinemia, and presumed sepsis.

Electronically signed by Elizabeth M. King, MD 09/27/20XX   8:15 AM

EMK/vs

d: 11/20/XX
t: 11/20/XX

© Cengage Learning 2014

Figure 16-8   Sample discharge summary report.

report would. Review Chapter 15 for information regarding various styles and formats for business correspondence. Figure 16-10 shows a sample of medical correspondence.

TURNAROUND TIME AND PRODUCTIVITY

Specific time limits are often established for completion of medical reports. **Turnaround time (TAT)** indicates the specific time period in which a document is expected to be completed from the time it is received by the transcriptionist until it is returned to the provider to sign and made a part of the permanent medical record.

Turnaround times for hospital reports fall into three categories:

1. *Stat reports:* Should be completed within 2 to 4 hours.
2. *Current reports:* Should be completed within 24 hours or less.
3. *Old reports or aged reports:* DS reports are an example, except when the patient is being transferred to another facility. Old reports should be completed within 48 to 72 hours or less.
4. *When requesting copies of your medical record* the usual TAT is 7–10 business days.

Different facilities have different requirements; however, the transcriptionist or clinic personnel responsible for medical records should be aware that failure to meet deadlines could result in disciplinary or legal action. The reason for this stringent adherence to turnaround time is that stat and current reports can influence timely treatment of the patient.

Workload, as well as productivity of the transcriptionist, affects turnaround time. When workload is too great to meet turnaround times, the medical records administrator must be notified immediately. Once a job has been accepted, the transcriptionist or transcription service is legally bound to meet the schedule short of a major catastrophe of the type legally considered to be an "act of nature."

AUTOPSY REPORT

Patient Name:	George Matthews
Hospital No.:	11509
Necropsy No.:	98-A-19
Admitting Physician:	Joe Abbott, M.C.
Pathologist:	Loraine Muir, M.D.
Date of Death:	04/05/20XX, 9 PM
Date of Autopsy:	04/06/20XX, 8 AM
Admitting Diagnosis:	Adenocarcinoma, maxilla.
Prosector:	Keith Johnson, P.A.

FINAL ANATOMIC DIAGNOSIS

1. Old fibrotic myocardial infarction of the anterior and septal walls of the left ventricle with anterior ventricular aneurysm, 4.5×3.0 cm.
2. Patchy old fibrotic myocardial infarction of the lateral and posterior septal walls of the left ventricle.
3. Probable recent ischemic changes, especially of the anterior and septal walls of the left ventricle.
4. Severe calcified atherosclerotic coronary vascular disease with up to 95% stenosis of the right coronary artery (RCA), up to 70% stenosis of the left anterior descending (LAD) coronary artery, and greater than 95% stenosis of the left circumflex coronary artery (LCCA).
5. Bilateral arterionephrosclerosis.
6. Atherosclerotic vascular disease, aorta, moderate to severe; circle of Willis, moderate.
7. Old infarct of right inner and inferior occipital lobe; small lacunar infarct, right caudate nucleus.
8. Bilateral pulmonary congestion, moderate.
9. Chronic passive congestion, liver, mild.
10. Simple cysts, right and left kidneys, up to 5.5 cm.
11. Diverticulum, 2.5 cm, duodenum.
12. Diverticulosis, sigmoid colon.
13. Status post partial left maxillectomy for adenocarcinoma, recent.

Electronically signed by Elizabeth M. King, MD 04/26/20XX   6:17 PM

EMK:xx

D:04/26/XX
T:04/26/XX

© Cengage Learning 2014

Figure 16-9 Sample autopsy report.

DOCUMENTATION

8/28/XX   Removed cast from right wrist and instructed patient to make an appointment with PT. Radiology, BQL/ CMA (AAMA) 9/12/XX ——————————

MEDICAL TRANSCRIPTION AS A CAREER

The medical transcription career has changed significantly in the United States. The career continues to evolve with the introduction of new technology and outsourcing. Most health-care providers use either digital or analog dictating equipment to transmit dictation to medical transcriptionists. The Internet has grown to be a popular mode for transmitting documentation and allows for faster turnaround time. Speech recognition technology electronically translates sound into text and creates drafts of reports. The MTs serve as QA managers, to oversee risk management, and to function as editors or auditors of medical documents. Medical transcriptionists are invisible, and yet invaluable, members of the patient care team.

MTs serving as editors enjoy detective work and are curious; if terminology is new to them, they use references to research and learn more. MTs must be self-disciplined, detail oriented, and independent, and usually they are perfectionists. They are dedicated to professional development and enthusiastically committed to learning. MTs possess integrity and understand the importance and legal implications of medical confidentiality.

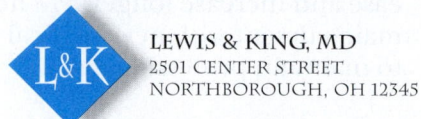

LEWIS & KING, MD
2501 CENTER STREET
NORTHBOROUGH, OH 12345

NORTHBOROUGH
FAMILY MEDICAL GROUP

January 4, 20XX

Susan Smith, Coordinator
Special Project Division
American Drug Company
90058 Northover Road
Welfond, PA 44578

Dear Ms. Smith:

It is my understanding that your department oversees the Aid for
Patients program, which provides Glucogenasin for indigent patients.
I am interested in learning more about this.

I have a 74-year-old female patient who would be greatly helped by this
medication. She suffers with hypertension, adult onset diabetes mellitus,
and moderate angina. Medication compliance has been a problem; however,
we feel that this new drug, with its q.d. dosage, will be easy for her
to deal with.

Any information you could forward would be appreciated.

Yours truly,

Winston Lewis, MD

WL/bk

Figure 16-10   Sample medical correspondence.

Professionalism Related to Medical Transcription

  Professionalism as related to medical transcription has many requirements. Following is advice on how to maintain a professional attitude.

- *Display a professional manner and image.* Working as an MT requires good hygiene practices and dress attire appropriate to the surroundings. The MT should always respect others and use good communication skills.

- *Demonstrate initiative and responsibility.* Demonstrating initiative means being to work early enough to organize and begin the workday at the appointed time. All deadlines must be met or changes approved.

- *Work as a member of the health care team.* The MT is a member of the health care team and as such must sign a business associate agreement and a confidentiality agreement. The MT should report incidents of confidentiality discrepancies and any perceived medical procedural errors to appropriate risk management personnel.

- *Prioritize and perform multiple tasks.* The MT must prioritize the documents to be edited to satisfy turnaround time and maintain productivity standards.

- *Adapt to change.* The MT must be flexible and willing to change. Technological advances require being open to new ways of handling medical documents. The MT's role and job description are changing to meet today's new demands.

- *Enhance skills through continuing education.* New technology, breakthroughs in medicine, and new medications are recognized daily as researchers explore ways in which to treat disease and increase longevity. The MT must remain current with new medical developments to maintain professionalism.

 A qualified MT, described as one with a minimum of 2 years' experience in performing medical transcription in a variety of medical and surgical specialties, may wish to become a **certified medical transcriptionist (CMT)**, through a voluntary examination from the AHDI. Recent graduates, or MTs with less than 2 years' experience, may apply to become **registered medical transcriptionists (RMT)**. For additional information regarding AHDI credentialing, visit AHDI's website at: http://www.ahdionline.org.

According to the Occupational Outlook Handbook, 2010–2011 Edition, medical transcriptionists held about 105,200 jobs in 2008. Of those, 36% worked in hospitals and another 23% worked in clinics of providers. Others worked for business support services; medical and diagnostic laboratories; outpatient care centers; offices of physical, occupational, and speech therapists; and offices of audiologists.

Job opportunities should remain good for those transcriptionists who are certified. Employment opportunities are projected to grow by 11% from 2008 through 2018. Earnings for MTs vary with some paid based on the number of hours they work or the number of lines they transcribe. Employees of transcription services and independent contractors almost always receive production-based pay. In 2008 the salary range for MTs was $10.76 to $21.81 per hour.

PROCEDURE 16-1

Transcribe Medical Referral Letters Using Medical Office Simulation Software (MOSS)

PURPOSE:
To transcribe (type) medical referral letters using MOSS based on physician dictation.

EQUIPMENT/SUPPLIES
Computer and MOSS
Source Documents

PROCEDURE STEPS:
1. After setting up the transcription equipment and inserting the tape, click on the Billing drop down menu option in MOSS (along the top left) and click on Patient Ledger.

Procedure 16-1 (continued)

2. Select the patient from the *Patient Account* list and click on *View*. This will display the patient's ledger.Hint: Click on the magnifying glass icon to drop down the list of patients.

3. At the bottom left of the ledger screen, click on the *Correspondence* button.

4. The *Output To* dialog box will open. Select a location to save your letter and name it as follows: patientlastname_letter_yourlastname. Click *OK* to save the letter.

5. After a short pause, the letterhead for Douglasville Medicine Associates opens. Change the date of the letter to the desired date and put your own last name in the *Student No.* field.

6. Delete the patient's name and address from the inside address area and replace with the name and address of the applicable recipient.

7. If applicable, include a reference line with patient name before the salutation. With the cursor, click at *Type Message Here* and delete that line. Start the body of the letter at that location.

8. Transcribe (type) the physician's dictation as shown on the source document. Be sure to format the letter, use punctuation, and use proper grammar.

9. When complete, save the document by clicking on the *Save* button on the word processor.

10. Print the letter so the physician may sign it and turn in a copy to your instructor. Prepare a mailing envelope(s).

11. Close the word processor and return to the Main Menu in MOSS.

CASE STUDY 16-1

Refer to the scenario at the beginning of the chapter.

CASE STUDY REVIEW

1. List important issues Marilyn will want to consider before outsourcing medical transcription.

2. Using your favorite search engine, research outsourcing as well as VRS options. Write a summary of your findings and state your rationale for supporting either outsourcing, VRS, or keeping the transcription in-house.

CASE STUDY 16-2

At the clinic of Drs. Lewis and King, the MT has just completed the following content in a document: "This patient developed a persistent lesion on the inner aspect of the left upper lip. This lesion was at the junction of the vermilion and mucous membrane. A punch biopsy was obtained of this 1-cm lesion and was read as a probable verrucous squamous cell carcinoma of the lower lip."

CASE STUDY REVIEW

1. What inconsistencies, if any, do you find within this document?

2. What should the MT do to verify inconsistencies and inaccuracies?

3. How should these inconsistencies and inaccuracies be corrected?

SUMMARY

Medical transcription is a vital part of patient health care. Without appropriate medical documentation it is impossible to provide quality health care, to bill insurance carriers properly to ensure providers are reimbursed for services rendered, and to support and protect the provider should records be subpoenaed. The MT must keep all patient information strictly confidential and may be asked to sign a confidentiality agreement. A breach of confidentiality is one of the few areas in which the MT can be held liable.

Professional MTs often become CMTs and recertify every 3 years. A current credential indicates active involvement in continuing education activities that keep the transcriptionist knowledgeable of new technologies, techniques, procedures, and drugs being used. MTs will continue to be medical language specialists. Their role and job description may change, however, with the innovation and use of new technology.

STUDY FOR SUCCESS

To reinforce your knowledge and skills of information presented in this chapter:

- Review the *Key Terms*
- Role-play with other students to apply attributes of professionalism pertinent to this chapter.
- Consider the *Case Studies* and discuss your conclusions
- Answer the questions in the *Certification Review*
- Apply your knowledge by completing the *Activities* in the *Study Guide* and the *Games and Quizzes* in the StudyWARE *StudyWARE* software on the *Premium Website*
- Perform the *Procedures* using the *Competency Assessment Checklists* in the *Competency Manual*
- Practice your problem-solving-skills with the *Critical Thinking Challenge 3.0* on the *Premium Website*

Additional resources for this chapter include:

- *CourseMate for Delmar's Comprehensive Medical Assisting*
- *WebTutor for Delmar's Comprehensive Medical Assisting*

CERTIFICATION REVIEW

1. Three factors influencing the changing role of medical transcription include:
   a. cost
   b. changing economy
   c. new technology
   d. all of the above
2. New technology used in medical transcription include:
   a. EHR   c. VRS
   b. outsourcing   d. all of the above
3. A flag located within a medical document indicates:
   a. the dictator made a mistake
   b. the dictator could not be understood
   c. the transcriptionist made an error
   d. none of the above

4. Authentication means:
   a. use of an electronic signature
   b. the information was accurate and complete at the time of dictation and as transcribed, and has been signed and dated by the dictating provider
   c. use of a biometric system
   d. use of an alphanumeric computer key entry as identification
5. MTs with a question that cannot be resolved should:
   a. guess at what is being dictated
   b. edit the document and exclude what cannot be understood
   c. flag the document
   d. refuse to transcribe documents for that provider

6. QA measures documents for all of the following
   except:
   a. line length of document
   b. accuracy and completeness
   c. consistency in health care documentation
   d. timely preparation

7. Turnaround time for most stat reports should be:
   a. same as aged reports
   b. current
   c. within 2–4 hours
   d. both a and b

8. An H&P report:
   a. is divided into a history section and the ROS
      section
   b. is sometimes referred to as a progress note
   c. describes gross and microscopic examinations
   d. documents the patient's history of hospital
      admission

9. Autopsy reports:
   a. are also called narcolepsy reports
   b. determine cause of death, ascertain and confirm
      presence of disease
   c. should be brief and contain many abbreviations
   d. always are required to use military time

10. Chart notes should be filed within:
    a. 12 hours
    b. 24 hours
    c. 4–8 hours
    d. 48–72 hours

11. When requesting copies of your medical record the
    usual TAT is:
    a. 48–72 hours
    b. 30 days
    c. 7–10 business days
    d. 24 hours

12. The CMT:
    a. is a requirement
    b. is voluntary
    c. requires a minimum of 2 years' experience in a
       variety of specialties
    d. b and c only are correct

REFERENCES/BIBLIOGRAPHY

American Association for Medical Transcription.
(1990). *AAMT model job description: Medical transcriptionist.* Modesto, CA: American Association for
Medical Transcription.

Burns, L., & Maloney, F. (2003). *Medical transcription
and terminology: An integrated approach* (2nd ed.).
Clifton Park, NY: Delmar Cengage Learning.

Conerly-Stewart, D. L., & Lott, W. L. (2004). *Forrest
General Medical Center. Advanced medical transcription
course* (3rd ed.). Clifton Park, NY: Delmar Cengage
Learning.

ingenix. (2003). *HIPAA tool kit.* Salt Lake City, UT:
St. Anthony Publishing/Medicode.

Ireland, P. A., & Novak, M. A. (2005). *Hillcrest medical
center. Beginning medical transcription course* (6th ed.).
Clifton Park, NY: Delmar Cengage Learning.

Tossey, K. L. (1998). The integration of digital photographs into medical transcription. *Journal of the
American Association for Medical Transcription,
17*(6), 19–21.

UNIT V
Managing Facility Finances

CHAPTER 17
Medical Insurance 374

CHAPTER 18
Medical Insurance Coding.. 400

CHAPTER 19
Daily Financial Practices 430

CHAPTER 20
Billing and Collections... 462

CHAPTER 21
Accounting Practices... 484

OUTLINE

Understanding the Role
of Health Insurance

Medical Insurance Terminology

Terminology Specific
to Insurance Policies

Terminology Specific to
Billing Insurance Carriers

Types of Medical Insurance
Coverage

Traditional Insurance

Managed Care Insurance

Medicare

Medicare Supplemental
Insurance

Medicaid Insurance

TRICARE

Civilian Health and Medical
Program of the Veterans
Administration

Workers' Compensation
Insurance

Self-Insurance

Medical Tourism Insurance

Screening for Insurance

Referrals and Authorizations

Determining Fee Schedules

Usual, Customary, and
Reasonable Fees

Resource-Based Relative
Value Scale (RBRVS)

Diagnosis-Related Groups
(DRGs)

Hospital Inpatient
Prospective Payment
System

Hospital Outpatient
Prospective Payment
System

Capitation

Legal and Ethical Issues

Insurance Fraud and Abuse

Professional Careers
in Insurance

LEARNING OUTCOMES

1. Define, spell, and pronounce the key terms as presented in the glossary.
2. Define the terminology necessary to understand and submit medical insurance claims.
3. List at least five examples of medical insurance coverage and discuss their differences.
4. Identify models of managed care.
5. Screen patients for insurance, verifying eligibility for managed care services.
6. Obtain managed care referrals, precertification, and preauthorization, including documentation.
7. Discuss workers' compensation as it applies to patients.
8. Discuss types of provider fee schedules.
9. Define diagnosis-related groups.
10. Discuss legal and ethical issues related to medical insurance and the provider's office.
11. Explore career opportunities in the insurance profession.
12. Describe procedures for implementing managed care and insurance plans.
13. Analyze the professionalism questions and apply them to this chapter's content.

ATTRIBUTES OF PROFESSIONALISM

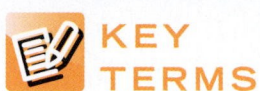

KEY TERMS

abuse

adjustment

assignment of benefits

beneficiary

benefit period

birthday rule

capitation

Centers for Medicare and Medicaid Services (CMS)

coinsurance

coordination of benefits (COB)

co-payment

deductible

Defense Enrollment Eligible Reporting System (DEERS)

diagnosis-related groups (DRGs)

donut hole

exclusion

exclusive provider organization (EPO)

explanation of benefits (EOB)

fiscal intermediary

fraud

health maintenance organization (HMO)

hospital outpatient prospective payment system (OPPS)

integrated delivery system (IDS)

managed care organization (MCO)

Medicare Part A

Communication

- Did you speak at the patient's level of understanding?
- Did you provide appropriate responses/feedback?
- Did you respond honestly and diplomatically to the patient's concern?
- Did you apply active listening skills?
- Does your knowledge allow you to speak easily with all members of the health care team?
- Did you demonstrate assertive communication with managed care and insurance providers?
- Did you maintain eye contact with the patient during communication?

Presentation

- Did you attend to any special needs of the patient? Did you ask first if assistance was needed, rather than taking charge?
- Were you courteous, patient, and respectful to the patient?
- Did you display a positive attitude?
- Did you display a calm, professional, and caring manner?

Competency

- Did you pay attention to detail?
- Did you display sound judgment?
- Were you knowledgeable and accountable?
- Did you recognize the importance of local, state, and federal legislation and regulations in the practice setting?
- Did you demonstrate sensitivity and professionalism in handling accounts receivable activities with patients?

Initiative

- Did you show initiative?
- Did you direct the patient to other resources when necessary or helpful, with the approval of the provider?
- Did you work with the provider to achieve the maximum reimbursement?

Integrity

- Did you demonstrate sensitivity to the patient's rights?
- Did you protect and maintain confidentiality?
- Did you immediately report any error you had made?
- Did you maintain your moral and ethical standards?

KEY TERMS *(continued)*

Medicare Part B

Medicare Part C

Medicare Part D

Medigap policy

point-of-service
 (POS) plan

preauthorization

preferred provider
 organization (PPO)

primary care
 provider (PCP)

referral

remittance advice (remit)

resource-based relative
 value scale (RBRVS)

self-insurance

TRICARE

triple option plan

usual, customary, and
 reasonable (UCR)

workers' compensation
 insurance

SCENARIO

At Inner City Health Care, a multi-provider urgent care center in a large city, medical assistant Jane O'Hara, CMA (AAMA), is responsible for all patient billing procedures. Inner City participates in a number of insurance plans, so Jane must stay abreast of policy changes regarding reimbursement, preauthorizations, and claims filing. She also tries to become acquainted with the conditions of each patient's insurance coverage and helps patients understand their responsibility, if any, for payment. Finally, Jane holds periodic meetings with her assistants to update them; she continually stresses to them the importance of timeliness in filing claims and the need for absolute accuracy in diagnosis and procedure codes, which must always reflect services actually performed.

INTRODUCTION

An understanding of medical insurance and proper coding techniques is absolutely critical to the survival of the ambulatory care setting. In recent years, much has changed in medical insurance coverage: more patients are choosing health maintenance organizations (HMOs) and other managed care options, and even traditional insurance carriers such as Blue Cross and Blue Shield are modifying their insurance plans to include some aspect of managed benefits.

In some ways, managed care coverage has simplified the patient's responsibility for payment, but it is more important than ever for the medical assistant to be accurate, timely, and conscientious in both filing insurance claim forms and understanding—and helping the patient to understand—the conditions of individual insurance policies.

The increasing complexity of health insurance today means that medical assistants must continually update their base of information. This chapter provides the groundwork for understanding the role of insurance, its terminology, and its various forms, and it gives the medical assistant the confidence to take responsibility for claim filing in the ambulatory care setting.

UNDERSTANDING THE ROLE OF HEALTH INSURANCE

Health insurance was designed to help individuals and families compensate for the high costs of medical care. Medical care consists of the diagnosis of diseases/disorders and the care and treatment provided by the health care team of professionals to individuals who are ill or injured. Medical care, which also includes preventive services, is designed to help individuals avoid health or injury problems and is termed *health care.*

Health care insurance is a contract between an individual policyholder and a third-party or government program that reimburses the medical provider or the policyholder for medically necessary treatment or preventive care covered by that specific health care provider.

There is much discussion today about changes in the health care insurance industry. Foremost is the goal that health care insurance should be available to all citizens of the United States. In the past, health insurance was usually tied to the employment package that covers the employee, and possibly the spouse and dependent children. One problem with work-related coverage is that some part-time employees are not eligible for health insurance and thus often go uninsured. Another problem is if an employee takes a position elsewhere, medical benefits may not transfer equally. If a family member is ill with a preexisting condition such as cancer or diabetes mellitus, the new insurance policy may not cover that disease or condition for a fixed time period. This time-dependent limitation of coverage is known as an **exclusion**. If health insurance has previously been in effect for at least 18 months and any lapse in coverage between policies did not exceed 63 days, a preexisting condition cannot be given as a reason for exclusion. Some states have laws limiting the length of an exclusion period; otherwise it is at the discretion of the carrier. An exclusion also may include illnesses or conditions for injury specifically not covered by the policy.

The Patient Protection and Affordable Care Act (PPACA), signed into law by President Barack Obama in 2010, is intended to help resolve many of these concerns. It will require all individuals who do not already have medical insurance coverage through a group plan with their employer or coverage through Medicare or Medicaid to purchase health coverage. There are many parts to the PPACA, which altogether will be making many changes to our health insurance industry over the next 10 years. For example, as of January 2014, insurance companies will no longer be permitted to charge policyholders a higher premium if they have a preexisting condition. It is also stated in the PPACA that by 2018, insurance plans are not to charge a co-payment if the office visit is for preventive medicine, such as well-women and well-child visits.

Another controversial aspect of health insurance is refusal to provide coverage for certain procedures because they have not been sufficiently proved to be effective. Although more insurance companies are beginning to cover procedures such as in vitro fertilization, there remain many other plans that do not agree. Because most insurance carriers will not extend coverage to experimental treatment, family and friends of patients often gather for fund-raising drives to ensure that medical costs would be covered.

Not all insurance carriers cover the same exposures equally, and few carriers pay at the same rate. Similarly, not many carriers charge the same premiums to policyholders. Some insurance companies cover individuals, families, or employee groups through work or through groups such as the American Association of Retired Persons (AARP). Some premiums reflect the insured person's past medical history and the company's exposure in covering the person. Premiums may be less if the insured person selects a higher annual deductible. Other premiums represent the rate that a group is able to obtain based on the group's claim history.

MEDICAL INSURANCE TERMINOLOGY

Before discussing the types of insurance coverage, one must understand the language used by the insurance industry. The terminology is specific in meaning and has been tested in courts of law to further define its meanings.

Terminology Specific to Insurance Policies

A policy is an agreement between an insurance company or government program and the insured, or **beneficiary**, that is, the person covered under the terms of the policy. The insured person may include as beneficiaries a spouse and dependent minor children; others may be included if related by blood and dependent on the insured for more than 50% of their support. The insurance carrier pays a percentage **(coinsurance)** of the cost of the services covered under the policy in exchange for a monthly premium or charge. This premium is paid by the insured or the employer, or it is shared by both.

At the inception or beginning of the policy, the insured is given an identification card, which must be presented before receiving medical treatment. This card contains the insured person's name, identification number, group number, and any co-payment amount or restrictions for treatment.

The back of the insurance card contains an address where claims should be submitted and telephone numbers needed to receive prior authorization for treatment when required.

Deductible.
The language of the policy spells out the terms of the coverage. Usually there is an annual **deductible**, or an amount of money that the insured must incur for medical services before the policy begins to pay. This deductible can range from $100 to $1,000, or an even greater amount, depending on the language of the policy. The deductible must be met each calendar year by medical charges that are incurred after the inception or anniversary date of the policy.

For instance, if Boris Bolski went to the provider on January 22 and incurred $258 in charges but his policy did not go into effect until February 1, none of these charges would apply toward his deductible. If, however, he returned to the doctor on February 3 and incurred another $85 charge, that amount could be applied against his deductible.

Coinsurance.
After application of the deductible to the submitted bills, the insurance policy pays a percentage of the remaining amount. This percentage or coinsurance can vary from 50% to 100% depending on the language in a specific policy. Most traditional plans pay 80%.

Co-payment.
Some insurance policies, especially **health maintenance organizations (HMOs)** and other managed care policies, require the patient to make a payment of a specified amount, for instance, $5 or $10, at the time of treatment. This payment must be collected at the time of the office visit. Some policies have both a **co-payment** and a coinsurance clause. In addition, co-payment amounts may differ between a primary physician and a specialist. For example, the co-payment to the primary physician may be only $20 per office visit. However, when a patient visits a specialist, the co-payment may increase to $35. Co-payments may also be applied in the emergency room (ER) setting. Often, the ER co-payment is waived if the patient is admitted to the hospital. The co-payment may be possibly waived in other situations, such as when a patient is coming in for a follow-up visit after surgery for suture removal.

Preexisting Condition.
The earlier example of Boris Bolski presents another problem. If a person had an illness, disease, or injury before the inception of the insurance, regardless of whether treatment was received, there is a good chance that most insurance policies will not cover any charges related to that specific illness, injury, or disease because it is considered a preexisting condition. Many policies have a specific waiting period before coverage is extended to those preexisting conditions. This waiting period can be a matter of months, years, or the lifetime of the policy. If the person had a previous insurance policy that was not as inclusive as the new policy, often the new policy would still consider this a preexisting condition and will deny payment until the waiting period requirement is met. However, if the new policy has similar benefits and the person had no lapse in coverage, legally, the company must cover those conditions without applying a preexisting condition or waiting period to the policy.

Exclusions.
Exclusions are noncovered services and are an important part of a policy. Some policies exclude elective procedures (procedures that are not medically necessary) such as cosmetic surgery, whereas other policies may allow some elective procedures. Other examples of exclusions or noncovered services might be preexisting conditions, dental services, chiropractic services, or routine eye examinations. Not every policy has the same exclusions.

Coordination of Benefits.
When more than one policy covers an individual, the policy language provides for **coordination of benefits (COB)**. This is determined by the policy language and coordinates payments between the policies so that the final total benefit is not greater than the original charge (does not exceed 100%). Policy language again determines which of the two policies is primary or will pay first.

The employee's policy will pay first for the employee. For instance, if John O'Keefe is covered by an insurance policy where he works and is also covered by his wife's medical coverage, the policy Mr. O'Keefe gets from his employer will pay benefits first for him. The coverage under his spouse's policy will pay second because John is considered a dependent under that policy. Even if the inception date of his wife's policy came first, John's policy will still be the primary insurance plan.

Whichever insurance is primary pays for their covered services up to the maximum allowed under the plan, less the deductible and co-payment. The secondary insurance will coordinate the benefits and pay as appropriate, but the amount is never to exceed the total amount of the services. If the secondary insurance offers a COB, it will only consider the percentage paid as if it were primary; that is, Boris's $258 claim was allowed at 80% by both his primary and his secondary insurances. His primary insurance would pay $206.40, and if his secondary plan offered COB, they would pay 80% as well. Because $206.40 and $206.40 total $412.80, which is more than the total bill of $258, Boris's secondary insurance will pay the balance left by the primary insurance, in this case, $51.60 (which may cover the co-payment, too). If Boris's secondary insurance does not offer COB, it would cover the same 80% the primary covered, and therefore would pay nothing. This is assuming that his deductibles have been satisfied and that Boris has received treatment from a participating provider with his insurance plan.

The issue of which insurance is primary and which is secondary applies when there are dependents covered under two policies. In this case, the **birthday rule** usually applies. When children of married parents are covered under both parents' policies, the birthday rule is used to determine which policy is primary. This rule simply states that the policy of the parent with the birthday falling earlier in the year is primary. Thus, if the father's birthday is October 17 and the mother's birthday

is May 12, the mother's policy is primary. The year of the birth date is not relevant.

If the parents share the same birthday, then the policy with the earlier inception date is primary. If John and Mary both have birthdays on July 12, and the policy for John started August 1, 2004, and the policy for Mary started December 1, 2003, Mary's policy is primary for their dependent children.

For children of divorced parents who are covered under both parents' policies, the policy of the custodial parent usually is primary unless divorce papers stipulate which parent is responsible.

Explanation of Benefits. The insurance carrier generates an **explanation of benefits (EOB)**, which is mailed to each patient. The EOB is a statement summarizing how the insurance carrier determined the reimbursement for services received by the patient. The backside of the EOB addresses questions frequently asked and defines the terms used within the EOB. The EOB is not to be considered a bill; it simply details information as to how the claim was processed by the insurance carrier. Figure 17-1 shows an example of an EOB.

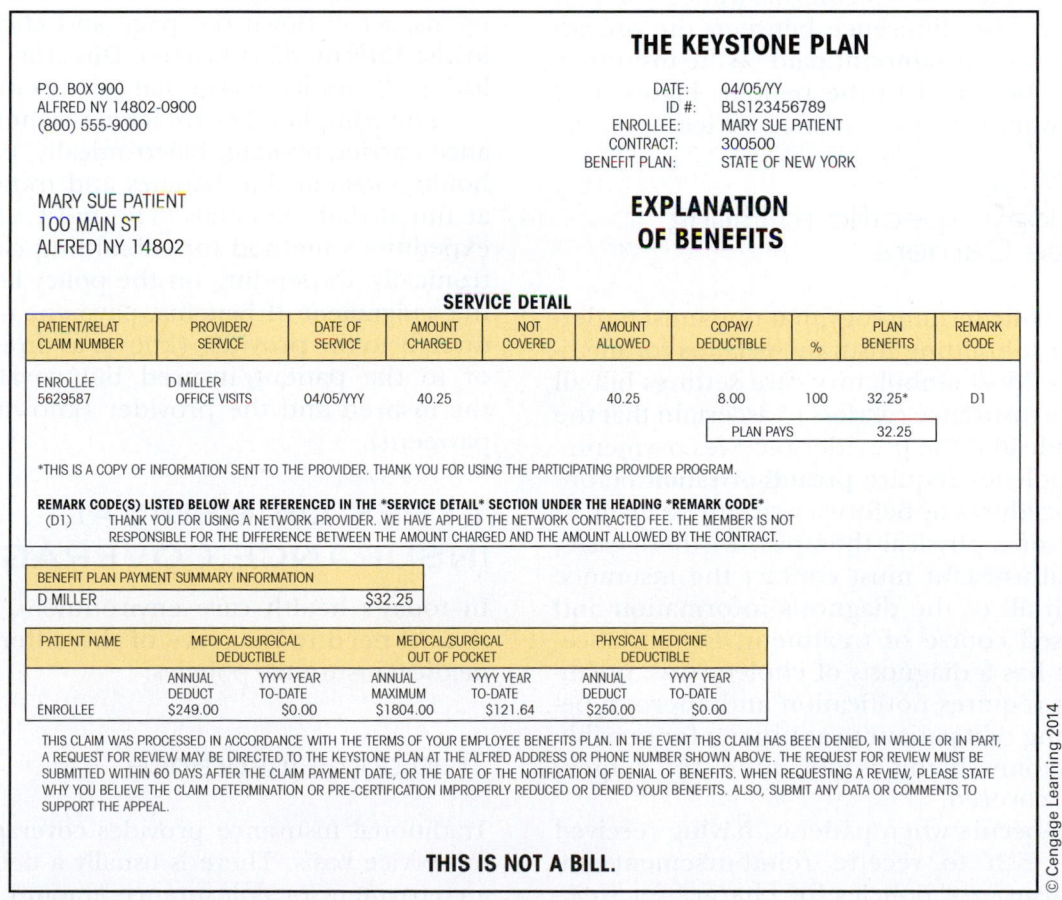

Figure 17-1 Explanation of benefits (EOB) sample.

ABC INSURANCE COMPANY
100 MAIN STREET
ALFRED NY 14802
1-800-555-1234

REMITTANCE ADVICE

DAVID MILLER, M.D.
101 NORTH STREET

ALFRED, NY 14802

PROVIDER #: 123456
PAGE #: 1 OF 1
DATE: 04/05/YY
CHECK/EFT #: 000235698

PERF PROV SERV DATE POS NOS PROC MODS BILLED ALLOWED DEDUCT COINS GRP/RC AMT PROV PD

NAME BAKER, JENNY HIC 235962541 ACNT BAKE1234567-01 ICN 1235626589651 ASG Y MOA MA01
236592ABC 0405 0405YY 11 1 99213 75.00 50.00 0.25 0.00 CO-42 15.00 50.00
PT RESP 10.31 CLAIM TOTALS 75.00 50.00 0.25 0.00 15.00

NET 50.00

TOTALS	# OF CLAIMS	BILLED AMT	ALLOWED AMT	DEDUCT AMT	COINS RC AMT	TOTAL AMT	PROV PD ADJ AMT	PROV AMT	CHECK AMT
	1	75.00	50.00	0.25	15.00	65.25	50.00	0.00	50.00

Figure 17-2 Remittance advice (single claim) sample.

Remittance Advice. The provider's office receives a **remittance advice** (or **remit**) from the insurance carrier. The provider's remit summarizes all of the benefits paid to the provider within a particular period of time. The remit includes all of the patients covered by a specific insurance for that time period. The difference between the provider's charges and the amount paid by the insurance carrier may be billed to the patient. Figure 17-2 shows an example of a remittance advice.

Terminology Specific to Billing Insurance Carriers

There is specific terminology that one must understand when submitting insurance claims for medical benefits. Most ambulatory care settings bill all appropriate insurance carriers to ascertain that the claim is made and the provider receives payment.

Many policies require **preauthorization** before certain procedures or before a visit can be made to a specialist or a physical therapist. In these cases, the medical assistant must contact the insurance carrier with all of the diagnosis information and the proposed course of treatment. For instance, if a patient has a diagnosis of cholecystitis, preauthorization requires notification and approval before referring that patient to a surgeon for possible cholecystectomy. If this is not done, the surgery may not be covered.

A claim occurs when patients, having received treatment, wish to receive reimbursement under their insurance policies for charges for treatment. The patient (or the center's billing office) sends the claim to the insurance carrier for the amount of the treatment. This is done via a claim form, the most common of which is the CMS-1500 (08-05) (Figure 17-3). The Medicare regional carrier can be found at http://www.cms.hhs.gov/contractinggeneralinformation/. When this page opens, scroll down the page and click on Downloads: Intermediary-Carrier Directory. A PDF file listing all Medicare regional carriers will open.

The completed claim form is sent to the insurance carrier by mail, electronically, or through a holding system that batches and transmits claims at timed daily intervals. The most common and expeditious method for submitting claims is electronically. Depending on the policy language and the **assignment of benefits**, payment is sent either directly to the provider (known as direct payment) or to the patient/insured but payable to both the insured and the provider (known as indirect payment).

TYPES OF MEDICAL INSURANCE COVERAGE

In today's health care environment, medical assistants need to be aware of the different types of medical insurance policies.

Traditional Insurance

Traditional insurance provides coverage on a fee-for-service basis. There is usually a deductible and a co-payment or coinsurance amount. The health care provider submits bills to the insurance carrier,

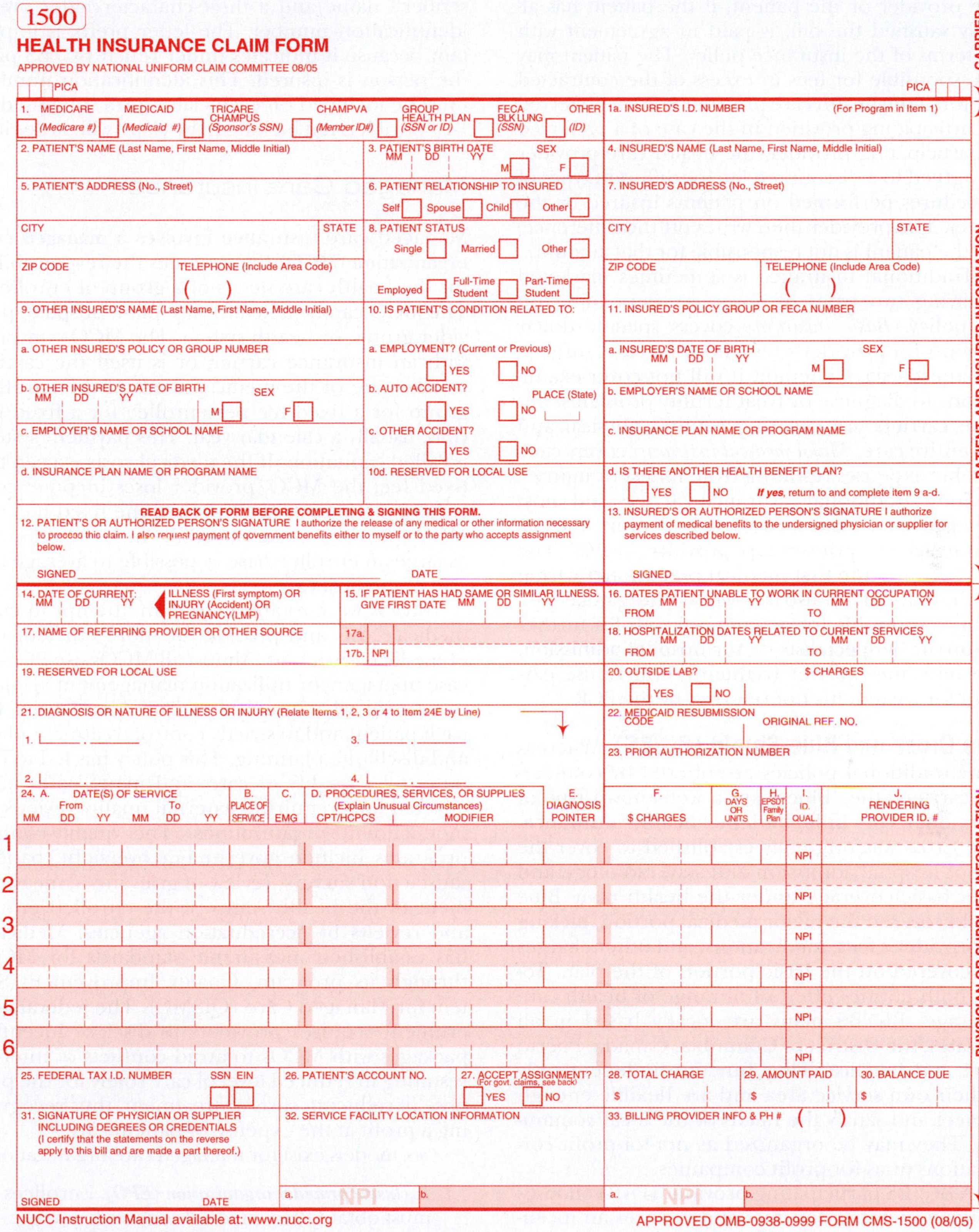

Figure 17-3   CMS-1500 (08/05) claim form.

and after any deductible has been met, the health care provider or the patient, if the patient has already satisfied the bill, is paid in agreement with the terms of the insurance policy. The patient may be responsible for fees in excess of the contracted amount if the health care provider is not a preferred or participating provider. In the case of a preferred or participating provider, the health care provider has agreed to a discounted fee for different types of procedures performed on patients insured by the carrier. The provider then writes off the difference, and the patient is not responsible for that amount.

Traditional insurance is sometimes marketed as having two types of coverage, depending on the policy. *Basic insurance* covers specific dollar amounts for provider's fees, hospital care, surgery, and anesthesia. Generally, it will not cover examinations to diagnose or treat fertility problems, but more carriers are covering routine physical and preventive care. *Major medical insurance* covers catastrophic expenses resulting from illness or injury.

Some traditional insurance carriers and most managed care insurance carriers require the patient to select a **primary care provider**, or **PCP**. The PCP becomes the first medical practitioner caring for the patient, is also known as the gatekeeper, and is responsible for making referrals for further treatment by specialists or for hospital admission. The insurance carrier frequently will refuse payment for treatments not referred by the PCP.

Blue Cross and Blue Shield (BC/BS).
Whereas many traditional policies are offered by commercial carriers, the "Blues" are a well-known type of traditional, or independent, health insurance. Blue Cross was originally established to cover the cost of hospital admission and stay, radiology, and other basic coverage under the health plan. Blue Shield covered the major medical portion, picking up provider's fees, medications, and other charges not covered on the basic portion of the plan. Today, both entities offer a full range of health care coverage. BC/BS plans are locally based in all 50 states, the District of Columbia, Canada, Puerto Rico, and Jamaica. They function independently in their own service area and are flexible enough to meet and satisfy the needs of the local community. They may be organized as not-for-profit corporations or as for-profit companies.

A BC/BS participating provider (PAR) chooses to sign a member contract and receives an incentive. PARs agree to accept the BC/BS reimbursement as payment in full for covered services. BC/BS agrees to reimburse providers directly and in a shorter turnaround time.

Each policyholder is given a card with the subscriber's name and a three-character letter prefix identification number. The letter prefix is important because it indicates under which BC/BS plan the person is insured. This identification number must be included on each claim form submitted to BC/BS; if it is not included, the claim will be denied.

Managed Care Insurance

Managed care insurance involves a **managed care organization (MCO)** that assumes the responsibility for the health care needs of a group of enrollees. The MCO can be a health care plan, hospital, provider group, or health system. The MCO contracts with an insurance carrier, or is itself the carrier, to take care of the medical needs of the enrolled group for a fixed fee per enrollee for a fixed period, usually a calendar year. This payment system is called capitation. If the medical costs exceed the fixed fee, the MCO/provider loses income; conversely, if the costs are less than the fixed fee, the MCO/provider makes a profit. An MCO relies on as large an enrollee base as possible to average the cost of medical care.

MCOs were established in an attempt to curb medical costs and provide for more efficient use of medical resources. Almost all MCOs use PCPs as case managers or utilization management services to control what medical resources are used for each patient and to strictly control treatment plans and discharge planning. This policy has led to disputes over quality of care, and many states have enacted laws requiring external quality reviews by independent organizations. The quality-control programs include government oversight, patient satisfaction surveys, review of grievances, measurement of the health status of the enrolled group, and reviews by accreditation agencies. Medicare has established measurable standards for MCOs through its program, Quality Improvement System for Managed Care (QISMC). The federal government requires providers to disclose incentive packages with MCOs to avoid conflicts of interest resulting in reduced level of care solely for the purpose of reducing costs or treatment, thus recognizing a profit at the expense of patient care.

Six models exist for managed care organizations:

1. *Exclusive provider organization (EPO).* Enrollees must obtain their medical services from a network of providers or health care facilities that are under exclusive contract to the EPO. The state insurance commissioner regulates EPOs.

2. *Integrated delivery system (IDS)*. Enrollees obtain medical services from an affiliated group of service providers. The service providers consist of private practices and hospitals that share practice management and services to reduce overhead. An IDS may also be called one of the following: integrated service network, delivery system, horizontally integrated system, vertically integrated system or plan, health delivery network, and accountable health plan.

3. *Health maintenance organization*. Enrollees obtain medical services from a network of providers who agree to fixed fees for services but are not under exclusive contract to the insurance carrier.

4. *Point-of-service (POS) plan*. The enrollee has the freedom of obtaining medical services from an HMO provider or by self-referral to non-HMO providers. In the case of self-referral, the enrollee will have to pay greater deductibles and coinsurance charges.

5. *Preferred provider organization (PPO)*. Enrollees obtain services from a network of providers and hospitals that have contracted their services at a discounted fee to an insurance company on a nonexclusive basis.

6. *Triple option plan*. Enrollees have the option of traditional, HMO, or PPO health plans.

Table 17-1 lists differences between traditional and managed care policies.

Table 17-1 Differences between Traditional and Managed Care Policies

Traditional	Managed Care
Usually can go outside provider network	Usually must stay inside provider network
Coinsurance	Co-pay each visit
Annual deductible	No annual deductible
Illness or injury only	Preventive treatment, as well as illness and injury
Premium paid monthly to company by employer or subscriber	Premium paid monthly to company by employer or subscriber
Provider paid by fee for service	Provider paid by capitation

© Cengage Learning 2014

Health maintenance organizations, or HMOs, are probably the most familiar managed care organizations. Originally, HMOs were designed to provide a full range of health care services under one roof. More recently, the HMO without walls has become established, which is typically a network of participating providers within a defined geographic area.

Today, as managed care and managed competition sweep the health care industry, other arrangements include the preferred provider organization (PPO), in which providers network to offer discounts to employers and other purchasers of health insurance, and the Independent Physician Association (IPA), of which the members agree to treat patients for an agreed-upon fee.

The Impact of Managed Care. The emergence of managed care in today's society provides new administrative and clinical challenges to members of the health care team as they struggle to provide the best health care while working within limitations often imposed by insurance carriers. Virtually all health care settings, whether they are individual practices or urgent care centers, are experiencing the impact of managed care, where providers network and compete to serve patients better and more cost-efficiently.

Under managed care, critics charge, health care dollars have grown scarce, providers must strive to provide the same quality for reduced reimbursement, preapprovals must be obtained for many services, and some services may be denied because they are not considered cost-effective.

Clinically, managed care may set limits on services or length of services. Second opinions are encouraged and sometimes required. In some systems, the patient selects a primary care provider, who is considered the *gatekeeper* and who must provide a referral for specialist care. Critics of managed care point out that restricting or denying services may lead to an increase in professional liability.

Administratively, paperwork and documentation have become increasingly important to ensure proper reimbursement. Although it is the patient's responsibility to understand the conditions of the insurance policy, these are often difficult to understand or interpret. The medical staff must be fully aware of when a preapproval or treatment plan is required, when a second opinion is necessary for reimbursement, and other clauses and restrictions that affect care and reimbursement for care.

At the same time, although managed care is challenging even the most resilient of providers,

CRITICAL THINKING

Do you agree with the policy that managed care may set limits on services or length of services? Why or why not? Give your rationale.

the very real need to keep costs down has also generated considerable creativity and energy among the health care profession as providers seek to use technology more efficiently; as they collaborate on new, cost-effective delivery methods; and as everyone involved in health care—insurers, providers, and patients—works together to contain costs by emphasizing prevention and lifestyle changes. Procedure 17-1 provides the steps involved in applying managed care policies and procedures.

Medicare

Medicare, established in 1966, is the largest medical insurance program in the United States. Most individuals 65 years and older, individuals with a disability that keeps them from working, and individuals with chronic kidney disease are eligible for Medicare. Medicare coverage consists of Parts A, B, C, and D. Part A is the original Medicare program for hospitalization and requires no monthly premiums. Parts B, C, and D require monthly premiums to be paid by the patient, with the amount depending upon income and specific plans selected. Medicare and Medicaid are administered

by **Centers for Medicare and Medicaid Services (CMS)** which is an agency within the U.S. Department of Health and Human Services.

Medicare Part A. **Medicare Part A** covers hospital admission and stay, home health care, and hospice care. It has a substantial deductible and a limit to the number of hospital days per stay and the total number of hospitalizations per year. Medicare Part A pays only a portion of a patient's hospital expenses, which are calculated on a **benefit period** basis. A benefit period begins with the first day of hospital stay and ends when the patient has been out of the hospital for 60 consecutive days. Many individuals subscribe to supplemental insurance (called Medigap policies) to cover the substantial deductible.

Individuals not yet 65 years old who already receive retirement benefits from Social Security, the Railroad Retirement Board, or disability are automatically enrolled in Part A and Part B. For all other qualified individuals, Medicare becomes effective the month of their 65th birthday. Three months before their 65th birthday, or the 24th month of disability, individuals are sent an initial enrollment package containing information about Medicare and a Medicare card. If both Medicare Parts A and B are desired, they simply sign the Medicare card and keep it in a safe place for use when needed. Figure 17-4 shows a sample Medicare card.

Medicare Part B. **Medicare Part B** covers outpatient expenses that include providers' fees, physical therapy, laboratory tests, radiologic studies, ambulance services, and charges for durable medical equipment. Durable medical equipment (DME) charges are for

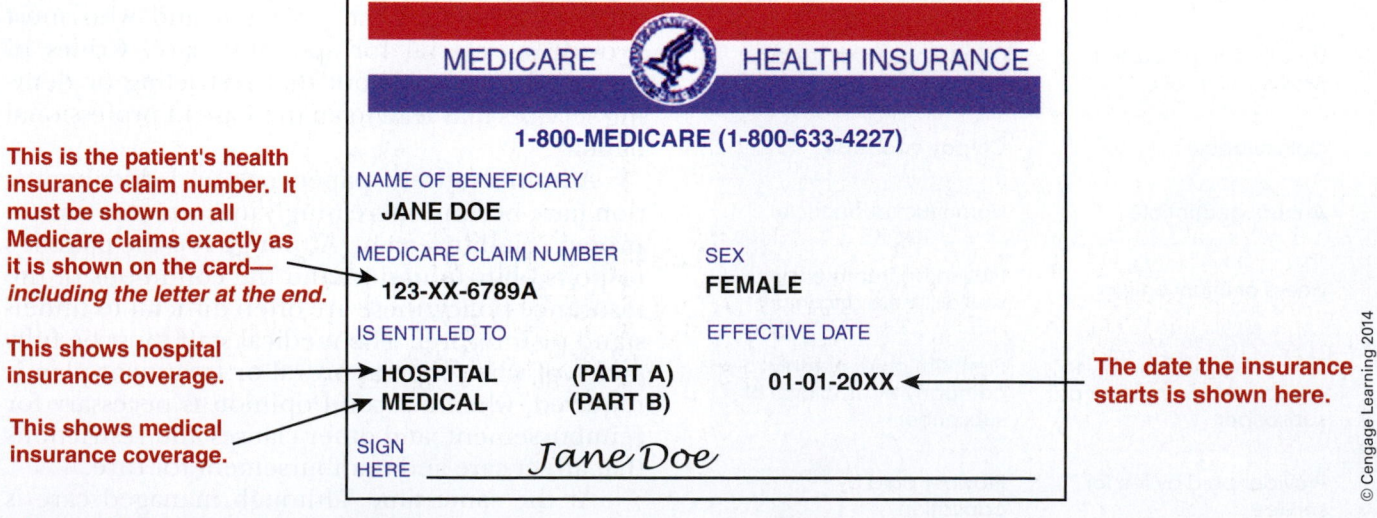

This is the patient's health insurance claim number. It must be shown on all Medicare claims exactly as it is shown on the card—*including the letter at the end.*

This shows hospital insurance coverage.

This shows medical insurance coverage.

The date the insurance starts is shown here.

MEDICARE   HEALTH INSURANCE
1-800-MEDICARE (1-800-633-4227)
NAME OF BENEFICIARY
JANE DOE
MEDICARE CLAIM NUMBER   SEX
123-XX-6789A   FEMALE
IS ENTITLED TO   EFFECTIVE DATE
HOSPITAL   (PART A)   01-01-20XX
MEDICAL   (PART B)
SIGN HERE   Jane Doe

© Cengage Learning 2014

Figure 17-4 Medicare health insurance card.

items that can withstand repeated use, and are meant to serve only a medical purpose (meaning they are not needed in the absence of illness or injury). Such equipment includes such items as canes, crutches, walkers, commode chairs, and blood glucose monitors. Part B does not cover medications *except* certain diabetic testing supplies. Medicare Part B requires a monthly premium, which is adjusted annually and can be dependent on income level.

In 2012, the patient must pay an annual deductible of $131 before Medicare Part B will begin to pay its share of the bills. Medicare then reimburses 80% of the Medicare fee schedule for medical care and 100% for laboratory fees. Medicare's fee schedule was adopted in 1992 and is based on the **resource-based relative value scale (RBRVS)**. The RBRVS was developed using values for each medical and surgical procedure based on work, practice, and malpractice expenses and is factored for regional differences.

Figure 17-5 shows how the Medicare worksheet would look if there were no exclusions or deductions.

Medical service providers can elect to accept Medicare fee schedules and become a PAR, or they may accept assignment on a case-by-case basis as a nonparticipating provider (non-PAR). Billing of Medicare is done through the regional carrier that is selected by a competitive bidding process. Medical providers are required to bill Medicare as a service to the patient. The regional carrier will file claims with supplemental insurers for PARs, but non-PARs must file claims with the supplemental insurer. The patient cannot be billed for the difference between the participating provider's charges and the Medicare allowed fee. Providers can drop out of Medicare and enter into a contract with their Medicare patients that allows them to charge what they wish for services, but they must not bill

Allowed Charges	
Office visit	$105.00
Return visit	+ 50.00
Total Charges	$155.00
Less deductible	-131.00
Subtotal	$ 24.00
Apply 80% coinsurance	x 80%
Insurance Payment	$ 19.20
Patient Owes	$ 4.80*

*In addition to the annual Medicare deductible

© Cengage Learning 2014

Figure 17-5   Sample Medicare worksheet with no exclusions or deductions.

Medicare for any services for the next 2 years, except in cases of emergency or urgent care.

In the example shown in Figure 17-6 the RBRVS allowed charge is applicable to both the participating and nonparticipating provider in computing the benefits Medicare pays to the provider. However, the non-PAR provider is limited to 95% of the RBRVS allowed charge in computing the amount of coinsurance. The difference between the provider charge in the case of non-PAR, and the RBRVS allowed charge in the case of PAR provider, less the coinsurance, is the amount the patient must pay. The PAR provider must write off the difference between what the provider charges for the procedure and the Medicare allowed charge as a courtesy adjustment. In the case of the non-PAR provider, the patient must pay the amount of the courtesy adjustment out of pocket in addition to the amount owed after Medicare has paid its share. This example assumes the yearly Medicare deductible has been met. The yearly deductible is the patient's responsibility to pay out of pocket.

Medicare Part C.   **Medicare Part C** is commonly referred to as Medicare advantage plans. The

CRITICAL THINKING

A Medicare patient has an office visit and is seen by a PAR provider. The allowed charge for the visit is $150. An insurance claim form is submitted to the local Medicare **fiscal intermediary** to apply against the deductible. At the next visit, the allowed charge is $75. This bill also is submitted to Medicare. How much of the bill will insurance pay after the deductible has been subtracted? How much does the patient owe?

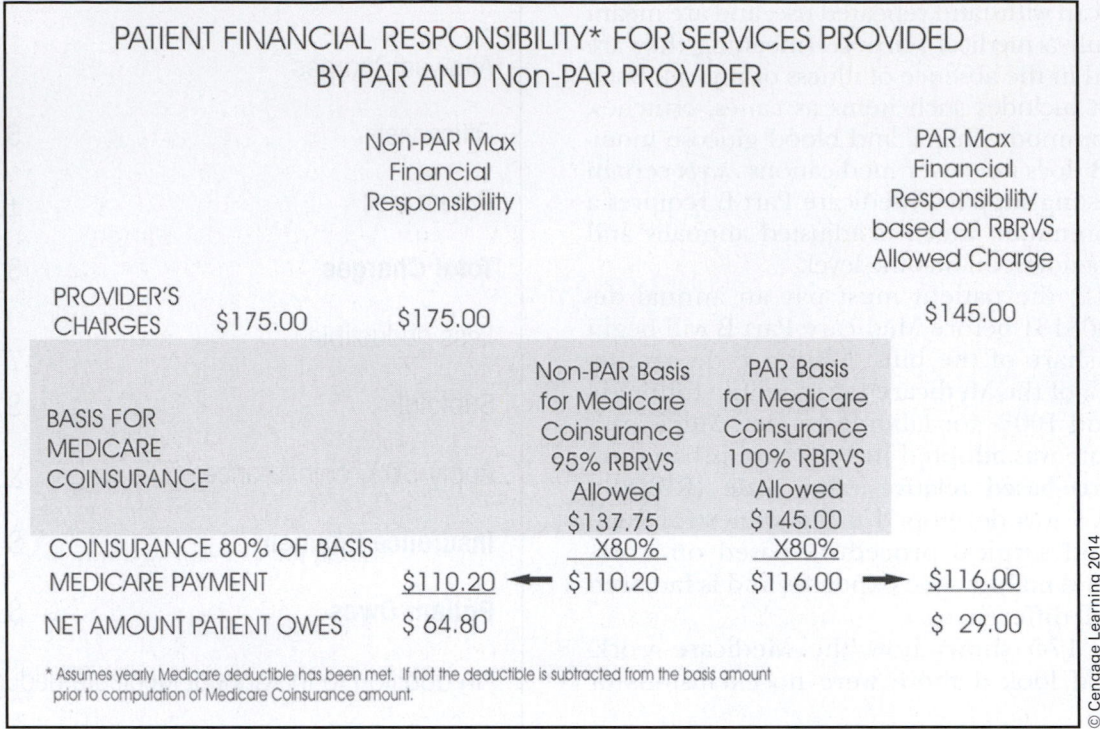

Figure 17-6   RBRVS allowed charge applicable to both the participating and the nonparticipating provider in computing the benefits Medicare pays to the provider.

plans are approved by Medicare and are run by private companies. Advantage plans provide Part A and Part B coverage and may also include Part D coverage. They require a monthly premium and may have restrictions on approved providers and hospital facilities. The medical office should always check the patient's Medicare card to verify the type of plan and effectiveness as this can affect billing procedures.

Medicare Part D. Medicare Part D offers prescription drug coverage for everyone covered by Medicare. Part D requires a monthly premium that varies depending on the plan selected. In the case of advantage plans, the cost of Part D may be administered by private companies.

Part D prescription drug coverage plans have a unique feature called the **donut hole** or coverage gap. All plans provide coverage until the total drug costs reach $2,400, then the patient is totally responsible for the next $3,051.25 of drug costs, after which the patient only pays a small co-payment for each prescription until the end of the calendar year. Drug coverage plans vary greatly. Selection should be based on convenience, cost, and drugs covered by the plan.

Medicare Supplemental Insurance

Medicare supplemental insurance is a secondary insurance that covers Medicare deductibles, coinsurance requirements, and additional procedures not covered by Medicare. It is purchased by the patient through an insurance carrier or is provided as part of an employee retirement package. Supplemental **Medigap policies** are filed with the carrier by the Medicare regional carrier. The regional carrier is not required to file claims for employee retirement plan supplemental packages on behalf of the patient. Supplemental insurance frequently requires the patient to seek treatment with specific providers and hospitals. Different programs have different coverage, which is dependent on the carrier and state requirements and should be determined when scheduling an appointment.

Medicaid Insurance

Medicaid insurance covers medical care for certain qualifying low-income individuals. It is funded by the federal government and is administered

CRITICAL THINKING

A patient has an office visit and is seen by a provider whose office does not accept the Medicare assignment. The charges are $150; however, the Medicare allowable amount is $100. A return office visit is charged at $90, with a Medicare allowable amount of $70. The $131 deductible has not yet been satisfied for the year. How much does the patient owe?

by each state's department of Supplemental Security Income (SSI). Pregnant single women with income below the poverty level; those who cannot work because of emotional, mental, or physical difficulties; and people who are on Aid to Families with Dependent Children qualify for this program. Recipients have an identification card for the program. Not all providers accept Medicaid patients. When referring a patient to a specialist or another provider, it is wise to ascertain whether that provider accepts Medicaid patients. A referral form prepared by the PCP or referring provider usually is required.

Because Medicaid is always secondary to any supplemental insurance, billings to Medicaid are considered only after all other insurance payments have been made. When a person has both Medicare and Medicaid, charges are submitted first to Medicare and last to Medicaid.

Both Medicare and Medicaid are federal programs, and errors in billing could be construed as fraud, for which there are criminal penalties. It is therefore imperative that all billing practices conform to the legal requirements of these programs.

TRICARE

TRICARE, formerly the Civilian Health and Medical Program for Uniformed Services (CHAMPUS), is medical insurance for active duty, activated guard, reserves, and retired members of the military, and their families and survivors. Active duty, guard, and reserve service members are automatically enrolled in TRICARE Prime. Retirees and dependents must enroll in one of the three TRICARE options: Prime, Extra, or Standard (originally CHAMPUS). TRICARE Prime provides treatment mainly through military hospital

facilities. TRICARE Extra provides care primarily through contracted civilian providers called *preferred providers.* TRICARE Standard provides care through traditional fee-for-service providers. Preferred providers receive a fee based on TRICARE Allowable Charges (TAC). Fee-for-service providers can charge up to 15% more than the TAC values, for which the patient is responsible. Primary care managers direct the care of TRICARE Prime and Extra patients, and referrals are required for treatment by a specialist. TRICARE Extra and Standard options usually require a deductible and co-payments. TRICARE patients are issued identification cards providing information on the type of plan in which they are enrolled. Qualifying subscribers must be listed in the Defense Department's **Defense Enrollment Eligible Reporting System (DEERS)**. The TRICARE insurance program is managed by three regional centers in the United States and by a TRICARE overseas center.

Civilian Health and Medical Program of the Veterans Administration

Civilian Health and Medical Program of the Veterans Administration (CHAMPVA) is medical insurance for spouses and unmarried dependent children of a veteran with permanent total disability resulting from a service-related injury and for the surviving spouse and children of a veteran who died of a service-related disability. The patient has an identification card for the program. The program is administered by the Health Administration Center in Denver, Colorado.

Workers' Compensation Insurance

Workers' compensation insurance is medical and paycheck insurance for workers who sustain injuries associated with their employment. In some instances, the insurance covers family members in the case of death of the worker. The employer usually pays the premium to the state or an insurance carrier designated by the state. Some large employers assume the insurance risk and are self-insured. Federal and state laws define minimum standards for workers' compensation programs. Workers' compensation covers 100% of associated medical expenses. Claims are filed with the insurance carrier. Although most workers are insured under state programs, federal programs exist for the following specific groups:

- Office Workers' Compensation Programs (OWCP)
- Energy Workers' Occupational Illness Compensation Program
- Federal Black Lung Program
- Federal Employees' Compensation Act Program (FECA)
- Longshore and Harbor Workers' Compensation Program
- Mine Safety and Health Administration (MSHA)

Self-Insurance

Large companies, nonprofit organizations, and governments frequently use **self-insurance** to reduce costs and gain more control of their finances. Each self-insured plan differs in coverage and claim filing requirements. The plan administrator should be contacted before scheduling a patient appointment.

Medical Tourism Insurance

Medical tourism is an unusual option being added to conventional insurance plans in an effort to control rising health care costs. It consists of health-provider networks paying the insured client to go abroad for treatment at internationally accredited hospitals. This insurance option has several potential disadvantages that may outweigh the reduced costs. Safety of blood supplies for transfusions and tissue for bone grafts are questionable in some countries, long distance travel may be dangerous to some patients, and returning patients may find it difficult to obtain follow-up care due to concerns of providers about exposure to possible malpractice lawsuits. Medical tourism options are quite new to the industry. At this time, whether it will become the new wave in insurance or will disappear from the future of insurance is uncertain.

SCREENING FOR INSURANCE

It is the responsibility of the medical assistant to screen all new patients for their insurance. New patients should be asked to arrive 15 to 20 minutes earlier than their appointment time to complete a patient registration form. The form requests vital information that enables the medical office to contact the patient, process their billing and insurance claims, know who to contact in case of emergency, authorize payment of insurance benefits, and record method of payment. Commercial forms are available for purchase or can be designed by office management personnel for this purpose.

The medical assistant should review each section of the patient registration form to verify that all information is complete and legible. Many offices make a photocopy of the patient's driver's license and attach it to the registration form. This procedure helps in identifying the correct person through photo identification should it be necessary. It is important to verify the spelling of all patient names: first, middle, and last.

Ask the patient to show his or her health insurance card and verify the effective date and pertinent information. All medical offices should make a photocopy of both sides of the card to maintain in the patient's chart, or scan both sides of the card and upload to the patient's electronic medical record. In most cases, the back of the card contains information about any deductible, co-payment, and preapproval requirements, as well as the insurance company's name, address, and telephone number. It also shows any special claim submission instructions.

Each time a patient checks in, the medical assistant should ask questions to verify the following insurance information:

- Request DOB (date of birth) to establish correct patient.
- Confirm the patient's current address.
- Confirm the patient's insurance carrier and plan.
- Ask for the patient's insurance card and verify information and effective dates.
- Determine whether the insurance carrier covers the procedure.
- Determine that the patient's PCP is performing the procedure.
- Confirm whether a referral is required and whether an authorization number or authorization code is required. Confirm evidence of qualifying has been secured.
- Establish proof of eligibility.

When screening patients for insurance, it is important to understand the philosophy of the medical office. Some see patients regardless of ability to pay; responsible medical assistants will investigate all avenues for reimbursement first. Some situations include the patient who is eligible for Medicaid but has not yet applied, or the patient who has applied for Medicaid but has not yet received notification of qualification. Procedure 17-2 provides the steps for screening for insurance.

The medical assistant should investigate and verify that all avenues have been taken to achieve the proof of eligibility that the office needs to receive reimbursement from Medicaid. This may include calling the Medicaid office to verify eligibility or going online and printing a proof of eligibility directly from the Medicaid system. This electronic data exchange system is called an *envoy*. Proof of eligibility cards are distributed to recipients and are in effect for at least 1 year. However, the most common avenue to ensure that services will be reimbursed is not to see any patient who does not have proof of Medicaid coverage. Medicaid sends an eligibility Medical Assistance Identification (MAID) (medical coupons) to the patient the first day of the month. This coupon guarantees the ambulatory care center payment for the services provided. Unless it is an emergency, some offices will not schedule Medicaid patients before the fifth of each month. This allows ample time for the beneficiary to receive the medical coupon. If the patient presents for an appointment without a medical coupon, and proof of eligibility cannot be determined elsewhere, it is common practice to have that patient reschedule the appointment. The exception is an emergency.

Medical assistants with responsibility for billing are vital to the success of a thriving ambulatory care center. Billing the insurance carriers promptly, completing claim forms properly, billing patients as needed, and keeping track of aging accounts will do much to ensure a flow of adequate income. In all insurance matters, be available to patients with questions regarding their insurance or accounts because a friendly attitude helps patients feel positive about the care they receive and establishes a long-term relationship.

REFERRALS AND AUTHORIZATIONS

When a PCP refers a patient to a specialist, the term **referral** is used by managed care facilities. Referrals may be denied because of incomplete information contained on the referral form or because a medical necessity was not established. Referrals are generally categorized as one of three types:

- *Regular.* Usually takes 3 to 10 working days to review procedures and approve
- *Urgent.* Usually takes about 24 hours for approval
- *Stat.* May be approved via telephone after faxing the information to the utilization review department

The most common referral used by managed care plans is the regular referral. The member services department must be contacted to check the status of a referral. It is important to never tell the patient that the referral has been approved until you have obtained a hard copy of the *authorization* (a managed care term for approved referrals). Be sure to review the content of the referral carefully. The typical referral will contain important information regarding its limitations, such as:

- Amount of authorized visits to the provider
- The type of services authorized
- Expiration date (i.e., most will last for only 90 days)

Preauthorizations and *precertifications* are terms used to determine whether a service or procedure is covered and if the insurance plan approves it as medically necessary. Preauthorization is required for some services, hospital admissions, inpatient and outpatient surgeries, and most elective procedures (Procedure 17-4). Once approved, an authorization number will be provided. The patient also receives a letter containing the authorization number and the approved services. The patient must present this letter to the specialist's office on the day the service is provided.

When questions arise regarding preauthorization, precertification, or referral procedures, the medical assistant should call the plan's contact number for specific information. Many offices find it helpful to maintain a reference log regarding these requirements. Information to maintain includes:

- Name of the insurance plan
- Address and telephone number
- Name and telephone number of contact person or the person with whom you spoke
- Co-payment amount and deductible information
- Inpatient and outpatient surgery benefits

- Preauthorization requirements, second-opinion options
- Participating hospitals, radiology service providers, laboratories, and physicians

The authorization number and referral numbers are entered in Box 23 of the CMS-1500 form when billing for services.

DETERMINING FEE SCHEDULES

A provider charges for services using a variety of means for computing a fee schedule. Although all of the fee computation plans vary and give somewhat different results, they all have common elements. Note the following examples:

- *The overhead or practice expenses for the clinic or office.* This category includes rental of the physical building or office space and equipment; utilities; cost of medical supplies inventory; and salaries of nurses, medical assistants, bookkeepers, and other personnel who are paid on a salary or contract basis. It also includes cost of employee benefits such as retirement plans, sick leave, and vacation time.
- *The cost of medical malpractice insurance.* This cost is separated from the charge for general insurance, which is included in the preceding category, because of the significant portion of the fee attributed to this item and because it varies greatly for different types of services. Obstetric/gynecologic procedures are probably the greatest for the entire medical community, including surgical procedures.
- *Hourly rate for the services provided by the provider.* This rate varies depending on the skill and training required for the procedure, the cost of living in the area, and the rate charged by other providers in the area. (The law of supply and demand applies here as in any other economic arena.) Surgeons charge a greater rate than providers in general practice, rates are greater in a metropolitan area than in a rural area, and experience level commands greater rates.

All of these cost elements are derived on an hourly basis. The sum of the above elements combined with the time required is used to arrive at the fee schedule for a procedure or service.

The advent of insurance plans, Medicare, and managed care plans has resulted in specific formulas being developed and accepted by the different plans to establish a fee schedule acceptable to the carrier. Several of the fee schedule systems in common usage are discussed in the following sections. All of them, however, incorporate the preceding three elements (practice expenses, malpractice expenses, and provider's experience).

Usual, Customary, and Reasonable Fees

Usual, customary, and reasonable (UCR) fee schedule is a fee system that defines allowable charges that will be accepted by insurance carriers. The actual rate may vary from one carrier to another, but the process is the same.

- Usual fee is the provider's average fee for a service or procedure. This fee is based on the economic analysis of the practice described earlier in this section.
- Customary fee is the average or range of fees within the geographic area that an insurance carrier will accept. It is frequently tied to a national average for a similar metropolitan or rural setting.
- Reasonable fee is the generally accepted fee for services or procedures that are extraordinarily difficult or complicated and require more time and effort by the provider.

An example of the operation of the UCR system is as follows. An insurance carrier operating on the UCR fee schedule may have determined a customary fee range for a new patient office visit with history taking and physical examination to be $140 to $225 for that region. If the amount billed by the provider were $160, the provider would be reimbursed for the service in full. Had the provider billed $250, the reimbursement would be $225, and the provider would have to write off the $25 nonallowed charge. The amount the provider would have to write off is often referred to as an **adjustment**. Providers who participate in UCR systems cannot bill the patient for the nonallowable charge

Resource-Based Relative Value Scale (RBRVS)

Medicare has used the RBRVS since 1992. Under this system, provider's services are reimbursed based on relative value units (RVUs). Each service, procedure, and medication is assigned a code compiled from the *Current Procedural Terminology*

(CPT) manual issued by the American Medical Association for procedures and the *International Classification of Diseases, 9th Revision, Clinical Modification* (ICD-9-CM) manual for diagnoses issued by the World Health Organization. Medicare then issues three RVUs for each code in the *Medicare Fee Schedule* (MFS) manual issued each year. The RVUs are for provider's work, practice expenses, and malpractice expenses. The practice expense is further differentiated based on location, that is, whether the work was done in a hospital (facility) or in a clinic or office (nonfacility). The nonfacility practice expense further differentiates between whether the nonfacility is transitioned or fully implemented. A geographic practice cost index (GPCI) related to the geographic area where the provider is located is issued for each RVU category. The GPCI is based on ZIP code for the address of the practice or wherever the service is performed. The payment for service is then established from the sum of the geographically adjusted RVUs multiplied by a nationally uniform conversion factor for services. The complex formula calculation is given in Table 17-2. RBRVS units and formula for payment are subject to frequent changes. The prudent medical assistant will verify that this information is current.

Diagnosis-Related Groups

In order to consider a claim for accepted reimbursement, Medicare will carefully examine the **diagnosis-related groups (DRGs)**. These designations are part of a reimbursement strategy that is designed to focus upon the diagnoses of the patient instead of the services rendered. It ensures that all given diagnoses are as specific as possible and also justify the length of a patient's stay in the hospital. This concept also brings together conditions that were known to be related to one another and could prove medical necessity, as well as validate the treatments given.

Hospital Inpatient Prospective Payment System

The IPPS is a reimbursement system for hospitals based on similar diagnostically related groups (DRGs) of inpatients discharged. Rather than the traditional method of payment based on actual costs incurred in providing care, DRGs are based on an average cost for treatment of a patient's condition. The hospital is reimbursed for each discharge according to a predetermined rate for each DRG.

Hospital Outpatient Prospective Payment System

The **hospital outpatient prospective payment system (OPPS)** is a reimbursement system for hospital outpatients, certain Part B services furnished to hospital inpatients who have no Part A coverage, and partial hospitalization services furnished by community mental health centers. All services are classified into groups called Ambulatory Payment Classifications

Table 17-2 Medicare Formula for Payment of Services

Code	Description of Procedure	Factor	Work	Practice Expense (PE)	Malpractice (MP)
38206	Stem cell collection @ transitioned nonfacility	RVU	1.5	0.61	0.07
		GPCI 2007 (King County, Seattle, WA)	1.014	1.109	.755

Budget Neutrality Adjuster (BNA) = 0.8806.
RVU Conversion Factor (CF) for 2008 = $38.0870.
GPCI = geographic practice cost index; MA = Medicare allowable; RVU = relative value unit.
MA = [(RVU$_{work}$ × BNA)* × GPCI$_{work}$ 1 RVU$_{PE}$ × GPCI$_{PE}$ 1 RVU$_{MP}$ × GPCI$_{MP}$] × RVU CF
MA = [(1.5 × 0.8806)* × 1.014 1 0.61 × 1.109 1 0.07 × 0.755] × $38.0870 = $78.76
*Rounded to two decimal places = 1.32.

(APCs). Payments are established for each APC, and the hospital is reimbursed for each patient. Depending on the services provided, hospitals may be paid for more than one APC for an encounter.

Capitation

Capitation is a payment system used primarily by managed care organizations. A fixed dollar amount is reimbursed to the provider for patients enrolled during a specific period. The payment per patient is independent of services or procedures provided to a patient. To be financially responsible, this system requires enrollment of a large number of patients so that a few patients do not unduly skew an average cost. This type of system requires extensive practice of preventive medicine to be cost-effective. Procedure 17-5 provides steps for computing the Medicare allowable fee schedule.

LEGAL AND ETHICAL ISSUES

Most Medicare claims are now required to be submitted electronically, and private payers in growing numbers are also using electronic claims submission. In a computerized system, everything related to billing and reimbursement is computerized and transmitted electronically. If the office is participating in CMS's Electronic Data Interchange (EDI), it will be assigned a unique identifier number that constitutes its legal electronic signature. Be cautious with this electronic signature, because the office is responsible for any and all claims made with it. The Health Insurance Portability and Accountability Act (HIPAA) of 1996 (specifically title II, subtitle F) regulates the security and privacy of transmitted health care information. Review HIPAA's regulations in Chapters 11 and 15.

Many legal and ethical issues related to insurance issues face the medical assistant on a daily basis; therefore, it is important that each patient be treated equally and fairly. As mentioned in Chapter 4, it is critical that patients not be stereotyped, regardless of whether they have multiple insurance plans or are not covered by any insurance plan at all. Every patient must be cared for objectively, with respect, and in a professional manner.

Medical personnel are bound by law to maintain the confidentiality of all medical information and must be able to recognize information that is protected by privacy rules and understand how it is to be handled. Protected

health information (PHI) may be considered "individually identifiable health information." This includes information that describes the health status of an individual, including basic demographics and the use of medical services, as well as information that either identifies or can be used to identify an individual. Medical personnel must remember that informed consent is not consent to use and disclose personal information.

Insurance Fraud and Abuse

Insurance **fraud** and **abuse** may be involved in more than 10% of submitted medical claims according to the Insurance Information Institute. These estimates include both intentional as well as accidental coding and billing irregularities and, if detected and proved, can result in legal action against the practice or clinic and personnel responsible for or having knowledge of the irregularities. Personnel involved in coding and billing should be alert for both accidental and intentional coding and billing irregularities and bring them to the attention of responsible managers. If no corrective action is taken, they are legally responsible to report the irregularities to the insurance carrier. Examples of fraudulent insurance activities include but are not limited to:

- Coding to a higher level of service to increase revenue (upcoding)
- Misrepresenting the diagnosis to justify payment
- Billing for services, equipment, or procedures that were never provided
- Unbundling service procedure codes
- Charging uninsured patients less than insured patients
- Receiving rebates or any type of compensation for referrals (kickbacks)

Insurance abuse involves activities that are inconsistent with accepted business practices. Some examples of abuse include but are not limited to:

- Charging for services that are not medically necessary
- Overcharging for services, equipment, or procedures
- Improper billing practices
- Violating participating provider agreements with insurance companies

Heavy penalties, including a $10,000 fine per claim form plus three times the fraudulent claim amount, may be sanctioned on individuals who knowingly and willfully misrepresent information submitted on insurance claim forms to gain greater payments or benefits.

To protect yourself and the medical practice from committing insurance fraud and abuse, you should begin by identifying risk areas based on errors in the past history of billing and insurance claims processing. Practice internal audits to monitor compliance with written protocols. Participate in seminars and in-service programs to keep current with coding and billing practices. Be sure to use only the current year's coding manuals to ensure accuracy. Code only what is documented in the medical record, and ask for clarification when needed.

An auditor should check claim forms, whether submitted electronically or by hard copy, to see that they are completed correctly. Include all pertinent dates and diagnostic and procedural coding information necessary for insurance payers to generate reimbursement. Auditors look specifically for any indicators of insurance fraud and abuse.

PROFESSIONAL CAREERS IN INSURANCE

 To be successful in the field of health insurance specialists, training and entry-level requirements are essential. An opportunity for employment in these specialties is greater for those with a college degree that includes coursework in medical terminology, anatomy and physiology, pharmacology, insurance and coding procedures, and communication skills.

 Personal attributes that enhance employment possibilities as health insurance specialists include, but are not limited to, the following descriptions: self-motivated, works well independently, detail oriented, a critical thinker, ethical, maintains confidentiality, cooperative, reliable, and adaptable.

The following Internet links will help you explore a variety of health insurance specialist career opportunities.

- American Academy of Professional Coders (AAPC) at http://www.aapc.com
- American Health Information Management Association (AHIMA) at http://www.ahima.org
- American Medical Billing Association (AMBA) at http://www.ambanet.net
- National Association of Claims Assistance Professionals (NACAP) at http://www.medical-codingandbilling.com
- National Electronic Billers Alliance (NEBA) at http://www.nebazone.com/part1.html

 PROCEDURE 17-1

Applying Managed Care Policies and Procedures

PURPOSE:
To apply managed care policies and procedures that the provider or medical facility has partnership agreements with.

EQUIPMENT/SUPPLIES:
Managed care contracts
Managed care policies and procedures manuals
Patient record
Authorized forms from managed care organizations
Clerical supplies

PROCEDURE STEPS:
1. Determine which managed care organization the patient has contracted with. RATIONALE: To ensure that the correct policies and procedures are applied to the correct organization.

2. Contact the insurance carrier(s) via telephone to:
   a. verify the patient has insurance in effect and is eligible for benefits
   b. confirm any exclusions or noncovered services
   c. determine deductibles, co-payments, or any other out-of-pocket expenses that the patient is responsible for paying
   d. ask if preauthorization is required for referrals to specialists or for any procedures and/or services. RATIONALE: Ascertains that insurance is viable and what benefits and patient expenses are established within the contract.

continues

Procedure 17-1 (continued)

3. Record the name, title, and telephone number and extension of the insurance person contacted. RATIONALE: Documents the name of the individual providing the information. If questions arise at a later date, a contact is readily available.

4. Collect any forms necessary to process the patient claims. RATIONALE: Submitting correct forms to managed care organization expedites the process.

5. *Pay attention to detail.* Document the information collected in the patient's medical record and on the Verification of Eligibility and Benefits form. RATIONALE: Provides a record of what has taken place.

6. *Show initiative* by attending seminars and workshops offered by managed care organizations or in-service training sessions. RATIONALE: Promotes obtaining up-to-date information regarding managed care policies and procedures.

PROCEDURE 17-2
Screening for Insurance

PURPOSE:
To verify insurance coverage and obtain vital information required for processing and billing insurance claim forms.

EQUIPMENT/SUPPLIES:
Patient registration forms
Clipboard and black ink pen
Patient's chart

PROCEDURE STEPS:

1. When scheduling the first appointment, ask the patient to bring his or her insurance card and to arrive 15 to 20 minutes before the appointment time to complete the patient registration form. RATIONALE: The insurance card is required to verify effective dates and pertinent information relative to insurance coverage. The registration form also requests vital information necessary for patient care and insurance billing.

2. When the patient turns in the completed registration form, review it immediately, *paying attention to detail,* to be sure that all information has been collected and that it is legible. RATIONALE: It is important that all information has been included on the registration form and that

the medical assistant can read it clearly when processing the insurance claim forms. If information is omitted from the claim form or is incorrect, the insurance carrier may deny the claim.

3. Ask the patient for his or her insurance card. Make a photocopy of both sides of the card to be maintained in the patient's chart, or scan the insurance card and upload to the patient's electronic medical record. RATIONALE: The insurance card provides vital information, including correct spelling of patient's name, insurance plan numbers, effective dates, telephone numbers to call regarding referrals and preauthorizations, and information about any deductible and co-payment.

4. Verify proof of eligibility for Medicaid patients. The patient should have his or her proof of eligibility card with him or her, or you may need to make a telephone call directly to Medicaid or use the online electronic data exchange system to determine proof of eligibility. RATIONALE: This information is required for Medicaid reimbursement.

5. Each time a patient checks in, whether established or new, the following information should be verified:

   • Address. Confirm the patient's current address and telephone number. RATIONALE:

Procedure 17-2 (continued)

Patients may have moved and may not realize they had not reported the new address and telephone number to the office.

- Verify insurance coverage. RATIONALE: This information is required for correct claims processing and billing procedures.

- Ask for the patient's insurance card and verify information and effective dates. Also be sure that a photocopy of the card is maintained in the patient's chart. RATIONALE: This is a means of keeping insurance records current for billing purposes.

- Determine whether the insurance carrier covers the procedure. RATIONALE: If the carrier does not cover the procedure,

reimbursement will need to come from a third party or the patient.

- Determine that the patient's PCP is performing the procedure. RATIONALE: This information is needed for reimbursement purposes.

- Determine whether a referral is required and whether an authorization number or code is needed. RATIONALE: Reimbursement by the carrier cannot take place without the proper documentation and authorization number.

- Confirm that evidence of qualifying has been secured. RATIONALE: Proof of eligibility must be verified for reimbursement from Medicaid.

PROCEDURE 17-3

Verifying Insurance Eligibility Using Medical Office Simulation Software (MOSS)

PURPOSE:
To verify insurance benefits electronically by using the Online Eligibility feature in MOSS.

EQUIPMENT/SUPPLIES:
Computer and MOSS

PROCEDURE STEPS:

1. Open MOSS and select *Online Eligibility* from the Main Menu.

2. Select the patient from the *Online Eligibility* window.

3. Review the patient's data in the *Online Eligibility* window, and then click on the *Send to Payer* button.

4. The *Online Eligibility Status* window will display the progress of electronically verifying the benefits. When complete, click on *View*.

5. Review that data on the *Online Eligibility Report,* and then click on *Print (or Save, as directed by your instructor).*

6. Click on the *Close* button to exit the *Online Eligibility Report* window. Return to the *Main Menu,* and click on Online Eligibility once more.

7. Select the patient from the *Online Eligibility* window.

8. Verify benefits for the secondary insurance. First, click on the record bar at the bottom left to display the secondary insurance plan.

9. Review the patient's data in the *Online Eligibility* window, and then click on the *Send to Payer* button.

10. The *Online Eligibility Status* window will display the progress of electronically verifying the benefits. When complete, click on *View.*

11. Review the data on the *Online Eligibility Report,* and then click on *Print (or Save, as directed by your instructor).*

12. Click on the *Close* button to exit the *Online Eligibility Report* window.

13. Verify eligibility for the next patient, or return to the Main Menu.

PROCEDURE 17-4
Obtaining Referrals and Authorizations

PURPOSE:
To ascertain coverage by the insurance carrier for specific medical services, hospital admissions, inpatient or outpatient surgeries, elective procedures, or when the PCP elects to refer the patient to another provider.

EQUIPMENT/SUPPLIES:
Patient's medical chart and copy of his or her insurance card
Name and telephone number of the contact person for the carrier
Completed referral form
Telephone/fax machine
Pen/pencil

PROCEDURE STEPS:
1. Collect all necessary documents and equipment (patient's chart/record, insurance carrier's information and telephone number). RATIONALE: Allows for efficient use of time in acquiring the referral or authorization.

2. Determine the service or procedure requiring preauthorization. You will also need to know the name and telephone number of the specialist involved and the reason the request is being sought. RATIONALE: This information is required to complete the referral form to obtain authorization from the patient's insurance carrier.

3. Complete the referral form, being sure to include all pertinent information. RATIONALE: The request may be denied if all information has not been included.

4. Proofread the completed form, *paying attention to detail*. RATIONALE: Because of the importance of this step, accuracy is critical.

5. Fax the completed form to the insurance carrier. RATIONALE: It apprises the carrier of the patient's medical condition, requests preauthorization for treatment, requests a verification or authorization number, and confirms the treatment plan.

6. Maintain a completed copy of the referral form in the patient's chart. RATIONALE: The form can be accessed in the future should questions arise.

PROCEDURE 17-5
Computing the Medicare Fee Schedule

PURPOSE:
To compute the Medicare allowable (MA) payment for services.

EQUIPMENT/SUPPLIES:
CPT book
Computer
Calculator

PROCEDURE STEPS:
1. Using the *Current Procedural Terminology* (CPT) book, obtain the CPT code for the exact procedure or service for which a fee schedule is being computed. RATIONALE: Accurate code must be obtained to ensure correct billing.

2. Using the Medicare Fee Schedule, which is issued each year, determine the relative value units for (a) provider's time (work), (b) practice expense (PE), and (c) costs of malpractice insurance (MP) listed for the CPT code in Step 1. These factors represent the relative amount of a fee allocated to each item.

3. Using the Medicare Fee Schedule, determine the geographic practice cost index (GPCI). This factor accounts for different cost of living values for urban versus rural and geographic locations in the United States.

4. Using the Medicare Fee Schedule, determine the Budget Neutrality Adjuster (BNA). This number is a factor that attempts to reduce Medicare fees to match the amount budgeted by Congress.

> **Procedure 17-5 (continued)**
>
> 5. Using the Medicare Fee Schedule, determine the relative value unit (RVU) conversion factor (CF). This factor converts RVU units to dollars based on an average for the entire United States.
>
> 6. Compute the Medicare allowable fee for the procedure or service using the following equation:
>
> $$MA = [(RVU_{work} \times BNA)* \times GPCI_{work} + RVU_{PE} \times GPCI_{PE} + RVU_{MP} \times GPCI_{MP}] \times CF$$
>
> *Round product of numbers to two decimal places.

CASE STUDY 17-1

Refer to the scenario at the beginning of the chapter.

CASE STUDY REVIEW

1. Identify ways that Jane O'Hara, CMA (AAMA), can stay abreast of policy changes regarding reimbursement.

2. List options for Jane to take in order to be up to date with insurance coverage so that she can help patients understand their responsibility, if any, for payment.

3. Recall steps for screening patients for insurance. Why is this so important?

CASE STUDY 17-2

Jane O'Hara, CMA (AAMA), is responsible for all patient insurance billing procedures. Jane has the following information:

	Total Charges	Allowed Charges
Office visit	$100.00	$90.00
Return visit	$70.00	$65.00

Deductible has not been satisfied.

CASE STUDY REVIEW

1. Calculate the patient's correct billing if the provider accepts assignment.
2. Calculate the patient's correct billing if the provider does not accept assignment.

SUMMARY

An understanding of medical insurance terminology and various types of coverage is vital to a thriving ambulatory care setting. The astute medical assistant will perceive the challenges involved in understanding his or her role in the management of medical office insurance. The medical assistant must be able to explain insurance procedures to the patient and know how to make contact with appropriate representatives to determine eligibility and coverage questions.

STUDY FOR SUCCESS

To reinforce your knowledge and skills of information presented in this chapter:

- Review the *Key Terms*
- Role-play with other students to apply attributes of professionalism pertinent to this chapter.
- Consider the *Case Studies* and discuss your conclusions
- Answer the questions in the *Certification Review*
- Apply your knowledge by completing the *Activities* in the *Study Guide* and the *Games and Quizzes* in the StudyWARE StudyWARE software on the *Premium Website*
- Perform the *Procedures* using the *Competency Manual Checklists* in the *Competency Manual*
- Practice your problem-solving skills with the *Critical Thinking Challenge 3.0* on the *Premium Website*

Additional resources for this chapter include:

- Module 8 of the *Medical Assisting Learning Lab*
- *CourseMate for Delmar's Comprehensive Medical Assisting*
- *WebTutor for Delmar's Comprehensive Medical Assisting*

CERTIFICATION REVIEW

1. The most common avenue to ensure that services will be reimbursed is:
   a. not see any patient who does not have proof of Medicaid coverage
   b. complete an envoy
   c. go online and print a proof of eligibility directly from the system
   d. ask patients if they are covered

2. The most common insurance claim form is the:
   a. UB04 form
   b. ICD-9-CM
   c. CMS-1500 (08-05) form
   d. assignment of benefits

3. Medicare:
   a. was created by Title 19 of the Social Security Act
   b. covers most persons age 65 years and older
   c. is designed to cover prescriptions
   d. is handled separately by each state

4. If the RBRVS allowable is $150 and the deductible has not been met, Medicare will pay:
   a. $20
   b. $40
   c. $120
   d. 80% of RBRVS allowable after $131 deductible

5. There are primary _____ MCO models operating across the country.
   a. four
   b. three
   c. six
   d. eight

6. Medicaid insurance:
   a. is funded by the federal government and administered by each state's department of SSI
   b. requires a Medigap policy
   c. consists of Part A, Part B, Part C, and Part D
   d. requires PARs to accept assignment

7. BC/BS:
   a. are locally based in all 50 states in the United States
   b. operate like MCOs
   c. recognize Medicare Part B
   d. are part of CHAMPVA

8. TRICARE:
   a. is part of CHAMPVA
   b. is part of OWCP, MSHA, and FECA programs
   c. is a self-insurance program
   d. was formerly the Civilian Health and Medical Program for Uniformed Services

9. All of the following are examples of insurance fraud EXCEPT for:
   a. charging uninsured patients less than insured patients
   b. charging for services that are not medically necessary
   c. coding to a higher level of service to increase revenue
   d. receiving rebates or any type of compensation for referrals

10. According to the birthday rule, the following is TRUE:
    a. The father's insurance policy will always be the primary insurance plan.
    b. The policy with the later effective date will be the primary plan.
    c. The mother's policy will always be the primary insurance plan.
    d. The parent with the earlier DOB will carry the primary plan.

REFERENCES/BIBLIOGRAPHY

Green, M. A. (2012). *3-2-1 Code It!* (3rd ed.) Clifton Park, NY: Delmar Cengage Learning.

Green, M. A., & Rowell, J. C. (2006). *Understanding health insurance: A guide to billing and reimbursement* (8th ed.). Clifton Park, NY: Delmar Cengage Learning.

ingenix. (2003). *HIPAA tool kit.* Salt Lake City, UT: St. Anthony Publishing/Medicode.

Moisio, M. A. (2011). *A guide to health insurance billing* (3rd ed.). Clifton Park, NY: Delmar Cengage Learning.

CHAPTER 18
Medical Insurance Coding

OUTLINE

Insurance Coding Systems
  Overview
    ICD-10-CM and ICD-10-PCS
Coding of Medical Procedures
    CPT Manual Organization
    and Use
    Modifiers
Healthcare Common Procedure
  Coding System (HCPCS)
Coding of Medical Diagnoses
    ICD-9-CM Manual
    Organization and Use
    External Cause Codes
    (E Codes)

Supplementary Health Factor
  Codes (V Codes)
  Morphology Codes
  (M Codes)
  Code References
Coding Accuracy
Coding the Claim Form
Third-Party Guidelines
Completing the CMS-1500
  (08-05)
    Uniform Bill 04 Form
    Using the Computer
    to Complete Forms

Common Errors in
  Completing Claim Forms
Benefits of Submitting Claims
  Electronically
Managing the Claims Process
    Documentation of Referrals
    Point-of-Service Device
    Maintaining a Claims Registry
    Following Up on Claims
The Insurance Carrier's Role
    Explanation of Benefits
Legal and Ethical Issues
    Compliance Programs

LEARNING OUTCOMES

1. Define, spell, and pronounce the key terms as presented in the glossary.

2. Define terminology necessary to understand and code medical insurance claim forms.

3. Describe how to use the most current procedural and diagnostic coding systems.

4. Code a sample claim form.

5. Apply third-party guidelines.

6. Recognize common errors in completing insurance claim forms.

7. Explain the difference between the CMS-1500 (08-05) and the UB-04 forms.

8. Compare processes for filing insurance claims both manually and electronically.

9. Discuss why claims follow-up is important to the ambulatory care setting.

10. Discuss legal and ethical issues related to coding and insurance claims processing.

11. Analyze the professionalism questions and apply them to this chapter's content.

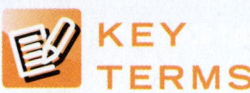

KEY TERMS

bundled codes

claim register

CMS-1500 (08-05)

Current Procedural
Terminology (CPT)

down-coding

E codes

encounter form

explanation of
benefits (EOB)

Healthcare Common
Procedure Coding
System (HCPCS)

International
Classification of
Diseases, 9th Revision,
Clinical Modification
(ICD-9-CM)

M codes

modifier

point-of-service
(POS) device

unbundling

Uniform Bill 04 (UB-04)

up-coding

V codes

ATTRIBUTES OF PROFESSIONALISM

Communication
- Did you apply active listening skills?
- Does your knowledge allow you to speak easily with all members of the health care team?
- Did you demonstrate assertive communication with managed care and insurance providers?

Competency
- Did you pay attention to detail?
- Did you display sound judgment?
- Were you knowledgeable and accountable?
- Did you recognize the importance of local, state, and federal legislation and regulations in the practice setting?

Initiative
- Did you show initiative?
- Did you seek opportunities to expand your knowledge base?
- Did you work with the provider to achieve the maximum reimbursement?

Integrity
- Did you protect and maintain confidentiality?
- Did you immediately report any error you had made?
- Did you maintain your moral and ethical standards?

SCENARIO

At Inner City Health Care, a multiprovider urgent care center in a large city, medical assistant Jane O'Hara, CMA (AAMA), is responsible for all patient billing procedures, including insurance claim forms. Jane stresses with her assistants the fact that coding is the basis for information exchanged between the health care providers and various agencies that compile health care statistics as well as third-party payers for health care services rendered to patients. Understanding medical terminology, anatomy, physiology, and how to code medical procedures and diagnoses accurately is a must. Using the computer to complete insurance forms, while considering common errors that may lead to denial of a claim, and transmitting the claims electronically are reviewed during in-service meetings. Jane emphasizes that accurate coding must always reflect services actually performed and documented within the patient's chart.

INTRODUCTION

Coding is the basis for the information on the claim form. Medical coding is mandatory for the accurate transmission of procedures and diagnosis information between health care providers and various agencies that compile health care statistics and the insurance companies that act as third-party payers for health care services rendered to patients. To code accurately, the medical assistant must have a good understanding of medical terminology, especially of those medical specialties found in the ambulatory care setting.

The use of computers to generate the insurance claim form and to transmit the form to the third-party payer is commonplace today. Computers are able to compute and compare numbers only. Letters that are in a sequence, such as the alphabet, are able to be compared as to their relativity to each other. For instance, A comes before B in the alphabet, and thus, a computer can compare those two values. For that reason, all charges, patient accounts, insurances, diagnoses and procedures, and even various categories are assigned letters or numbers (alphanumeric). The letters/numbers assigned to diagnoses and procedures (services) are called insurance codes. People whose jobs are to check accuracy of insurance codes and assign billing parameters (such as code modifiers) are called medical coders. (See Professional Careers in Insurance section at the end of Chapter 17 for more information.)

INSURANCE CODING SYSTEMS OVERVIEW

The process of translating written or spoken description of diseases, injuries, medical procedures, services, and supplies into numeric or alphanumeric format is called *coding*. The following coding systems are used within the United States:

- **Current Procedural Terminology (CPT)** system was developed by the American Medical Association (AMA) to convert commonly accepted descriptions of medical procedures into a five-digit numeric code with two-digit numeric **modifiers** when required. This system is used to code medical procedures such as clinic visits, x-rays, laboratory tests, and professional fees for providers after having performed surgery.

- **Healthcare Common Procedure Coding System (HCPCS)** was developed by Medicare as a supplement to the CPT system for procedures not defined with sufficient specificity. This system uses a five-digit alphanumeric code (one letter followed by four numbers) with an additional two-digit alphanumeric modifier if required.

- **International Classification of Diseases, 9th Revision, Clinical Modification (ICD-9-CM)** system was developed by the World Health Organization (WHO) to classify all known diseases and disorders to assist in maintaining statistical records of morbidity (sickness) and mortality (death). This system is used for both diagnostic coding (for all health care settings) and procedure coding (for inpatient services only). The current ICD-9-CM code consists of a three-digit code (called a *category*) with one or two numeric digits following a decimal point. The ICD-9-CM coding manual is revised periodically and is updated yearly. The book is in its ninth revision.

ICD-10-CM and ICD-10-PCS

The *International Classification of Diseases, 10th Revision, Clinical Modification* (ICD-10-CM) is in the process of being finalized. Implementation will be based on the process for adoption of standards under the Health Insurance Portability and Accountability Act (HIPAA). The mandatory implementation date for all health care facilities to convert to ICD-10-CM is set for October 1, 2014, and it will replace the ICD-9-CM code set that has been in use since 1979. The ICD-10-CM will use alphanumeric codes consisting of up to seven characters. This format results in a much more detailed description of medical conditions and increases the number of codes from approximately 14,000 to 69,000. The descriptions of the codes will be a lot more specific than many of the currently used code descriptions. Many of the ICD-10-CM codes will be in a combination format, which will decrease the need to use multiple codes on a claim. In addition, some of the codes will specify laterality (right versus left) within their descriptions. The amount of chapters included in the Tabular List will increase from 17 to 21. Some of the names of the current chapters in ICD-9-CM will change in the ICD-10-CM, and a few others are being added. Many of the coding rules and conventions will remain the same, whereas others are being added in order to successfully navigate through the ICD-10-CM manual. Many credentialing organizations, such as AHIMA and the AAPC, have already been providing training and resources to their members so they are prepared by the time the transition to ICD-10-CM takes place.

ICD-10-PCS, the inpatient hospital procedural coding system, is connected to the implementation of ICD-10-CM. The amount of available codes is going to dramatically increase from over 3,000 to over 80,000. There will be a unique code available for almost every procedure performed (instead of having to use the same code to represent several procedures). Individual characters within the code will help to identify important aspects of the procedure itself, and will be a lot more specific to the procedure that was performed. Organizations such as the NCHS (National Center for Health Statistics) will have tools available that will assist medical professionals with being able to convert an ICD-9 code into an ICD-10-PCS code until they become more familiar with the new system.

As previously mentioned, the United States has continued to use ICD-9-CM codes for some time, even though other countries have already made the conversion to ICD-10-CM/PCS. There are continuing concerns among the health care professionals of today, who are wondering what type of impact this conversion will have on their facility. Although this may seem like an uphill battle to many individuals, the implementation of ICD-10-CM/PCS will provide many benefits. The new system will help to ensure that all patients will receive the best possible quality of care. It will help to expedite the processing of insurance claims and will eventually lead to more accurate reimbursement. Because both diagnosis and procedure codes will be so much more specific, ICD-10-CM/PCS will help to better identify those cases that turn out to be fraudulent.

The most important thing that medical providers must realize is that they should not procrastinate in preparing for the numerous changes on the way. All encounter forms will have to completely be reprinted, and providers will also have to make sure that their medical software has the capabilities to support all of the extra codes and code characters needed.

CODING OF MEDICAL PROCEDURES

When performing billing procedures, medical assistants are expected to adhere to ethical standards and legal practices. All diagnostic and procedural codes reported must be supported by documentation in the patient's chart. Understanding medical terminology, anatomy, physiology, and procedures is critical to coding accuracy.

It is also important to maintain coding skills by attending continuing education activities that discuss changes in codes and present guidelines and regulation requirements necessary for accurate coding. Networking with other medical coders is another valuable method of staying current with what is happening in this profession.

CPT Manual Organization and Use

The CPT manual, published every November and released the following January, is used to code medical procedures and services of all kinds—clinic, hospital, nursing facility, and home services. The current volume, which is the fourth edition, is divided into six main sections and an index, which are discussed in the following paragraphs.

To determine the CPT code, turn to the Category I section of the CPT codebook and select one of the sections that constitutes the general classification of the procedure being coded (e.g., Surgery, Radiology). Then select the name of the procedure or service that accurately identifies what you are looking for. Do not select a CPT code that only approximately defines the service performed. If you cannot find a name that exactly defines the service provided, report the service using the appropriate unlisted code. Unlisted codes are found at the end of each subsection in the CPT codebook, and are also listed within the guidelines that precede each of the main sections. Most unlisted CPT codes end in 99. When using an unlisted code, a special report must be submitted with an insurance claim form to avoid denial or rejection. A special report will contain the nature, extent, and need of the procedure performed. An example of a special report would be the provider's operative note. Unlisted codes should not be used if a Category III code is available. This section is found in the back of the codebook and gives temporary codes for emerging technologies, services, and procedures.

Evaluation and Management. The Evaluation and Management section takes every possible combination of visits into consideration and assigns each its own number. For instance, Mary O'Keefe, a new patient, is seen for a period of 45 minutes during which the provider takes a detailed history, examines the patient, and makes a medical decision of moderate complexity. The CPT code for this visit (99204) is found by looking under "Office and Other Outpatient Services, New Patient." In another instance, Abigail Johnson, an established patient, is seen in the hospital for several days. These visits (99231, 99232, or 99233) would be found under "Hospital Services, Subsequent

Hospital Care." Codes for any type of evaluation and management are found in this section. In many clinics, the provider determines the level or charge for visits; however, the medical assistant must be familiar with all of the codes to make certain that billings are correct and that codes match the provider's documentation.

Anesthesia. The Anesthesia section includes all codes for anesthesia required for any procedure (with the exception of local anesthesia). The codes listed begin with the head and continue down the body to the legs and feet, concluding with anesthesia for radiologic procedures. If you want to find the correct code for anesthesia during a total hip replacement (arthroplasty), you will find "Anesthesia" in the index, look for the subterm "hip," and refer to the range of codes listed: 01200–01215. When you refer back to the Anesthesia section, you find:

01200 Anesthesia for all closed procedures involving hip joint

01202 Anesthesia for arthroscopic procedures of hip joint

01210 Anesthesia for open procedures involving hip joint; not otherwise specified

01212 hip disarticulation

01214 total hip arthroplasty

01215 revision of total hip arthroplasty

As you read through the codes, you see that the correct code is 01214. Please note that this CPT code represents only the services provided by the anesthesiologist, not the surgical procedure itself.

Surgery. The section on Surgery divides the codes according to body system. It begins with the Integumentary system, and continues through subsequent systems ending with the Ocular and Auditory systems. The codes are very specific in this section, and care must be taken at all times to ensure the selection of the correct code. For example, a simple laceration repair of the neck is found as:

12001 Simple repair of superficial wounds of scalp, neck, axillae, external genitalia, trunk and/or extremities (including hands and feet): 2.5 cm or less

12002 2.6 cm to 7.5 cm

12004 7.6 cm to 12.5 cm

12005 12.6 cm to 20.0 cm

12006 20.1 cm to 30.0 cm

12007 over 30.0 cm

Thus, the exact length of the laceration and complexity of the repair can be found and coded correctly on the claim form. However, the aforementioned code description illustrates three important points. First, the code selected must represent the site of the laceration. Second, the code must represent the correct level of complexity for the repair. Third, the code must specify the correct length of the repair. If the medical assistant selects a code that is off by even just one digit, there would be a delay in reimbursement. The insurance claim would have to be corrected and resubmitted to the insurance company.

Radiology.
Coding in the Radiology section covers each procedure done and each specific alteration to the procedure. For instance,

75889 Hepatic venography, wedged or free, *with* hemodynamic evaluation, radiological supervision, and interpretation

75891 Hepatic venography, wedged or free, *without* hemodynamic evaluation, radiological supervision, and interpretation

Radiologic procedures are not often done in the provider's clinic, although they may be in larger urgent care centers. Occasionally, chest x-rays are done or, in an orthopedic specialty, many skeletal x-rays may be done. More often, though, radiologic studies are ordered by the provider through a local facility that bills the insurance company directly, using the diagnosis the provider has provided.

Pathology and Laboratory.
The Pathology and Laboratory section includes every test and combination of laboratory tests that can be ordered, as well as a section on surgical pathologic evaluation. This latter section includes specimens sent for examination, such as Pap smears, analysis of biopsy tissue from surgical sites, and tissue typing. Following is an example of a laboratory procedure code for hepatitis B that illustrates the complete selection of tests that may be ordered:

87340 Hepatitis B surface antigen (HBsAg)

86704 Hepatitis B core antibody (HBcAb); total

86705 IgM antibody

86706 Hepatitis B surface antibody (HBsAb)

87350 Hepatitis Be antigen (HBeAg)

86707 Hepatitis Be antibody (HBeAb)

Once again, it is very important that the code for the exact service be selected. The medical assistant should be aware of laboratory codes because when a laboratory test is ordered, the laboratory may call to clarify the order. If the coding is correct, the laboratory should have no questions.

For surgical pathologic evaluation, the codes are different. The level of examination (gross and microscopic) for the item determines the code. The provider usually determines these levels or the charge for these services based on the type of tissue obtained, and the reason for the service.

Medicine.
The section of the CPT entitled Medicine includes codes for immunizations, injections, dialysis, allergen immunotherapy, and chemotherapy, as well as ophthalmologic, cardiovascular, pulmonary, and neurologic procedures, to name a few. Some of the procedures are considered invasive, although others are not. As in the earlier sections, there is a comprehensive breakdown of each procedure. For example:

Cardiography

93000 Electrocardiogram, routine ECG with at least 12 leads; with interpretation and report

93005 tracing only, without interpretation and report

93010 interpretation and report only

Chemotherapy Administration

96409 Chemotherapy administration, intravenous, push technique

96413 infusion technique, up to one hour

+96415 infusion technique, one to eight hours, each additional hour

96416 infusion technique, initiation of prolonged infusion (more than eight hours), requiring the use of a portable or implantable pump

The plus symbol before the CPT code indicates that the procedure is an add-on to a previously described procedure. For example, 96413 would be used to describe the service and the time administered up to 1 hour. Anything longer than 1 hour would be listed as +96415 for each additional 1 hour of administration that took place.

Index.
The final portion of the CPT codebook is a comprehensive index listing every procedure alphabetically. The proper use of the CPT codebook involves looking for the procedure in the index by its main term and then checking the number given to determine the precise code.

Category I codes found in the CPT have five numeric digits. This is the level of codes that are used the most to describe procedures and other professional services. Category II and Category III codes are made of four numeric digits and are followed by an alpha character. These codes would be used when no specific Category I code is available. Note that there are no decimal points in any of the codes. Each five-digit code stands for a specific procedure not duplicated elsewhere.

Modifiers

Occasionally, a service or procedure needs to be modified or altered in a certain way. In that case, there are two-digit numeric modifiers that can be applied to the five-digit CPT code. These modifiers can indicate unusual procedural services (–22), bilateral procedures (–50), multiple procedures (–51), two surgeons (–62), surgical team (–66), or repeat procedure by same provider (–76). The modifiers are listed in the inside front cover of each of the CPT code books as well as Appendix A of the book to alert the coder to modifiers available for that section. In addition, there are other modifiers of an alpha or alphanumeric nature that are also listed in the front of the CPT codebook. These modifiers come from the HCPCS codebook, and are commonly used with CPT codes. Review the following examples that illustrate the use of modifiers:

Surgical arthroscopy of the right shoulder with rotator cuff repair: 29827-RT

Bilateral otoplasty of protruding ears with size reduction: 69300-50

Blepharoplasty of the lower right eyelid; extensive herniated fat pad: 15821-E4

 See Procedure 18-1 for instructions on CPT coding.

CRITICAL THINKING

In which code book would you look to find the code for upper gastrointestinal endoscopy, simple primary examination (e.g., with small-diameter flexible endoscope) (separate procedure)? Which code did you select?

HEALTHCARE COMMON PROCEDURE CODING SYSTEM (HCPCS)

In 1983, Medicare created HCPCS (pronounced "hick picks"), the Healthcare Common Procedure Coding System. These codes are used as supplements to the basic CPT system and are required when reporting services and procedures provided to Medicare and Medicaid beneficiaries (patients). HCPCS uses the basic system (Level I) with two additional levels (II and III) as required. Level II provides codes to enable the provider to report nonprovider services such as durable medical equipment, supplies and medications (particularly injectable drugs), and ambulance services. Two-digit alphanumeric or alpha modifiers are used in Level II codes to provide greater detail on procedures and medical supplies. (*NOTE:* The use of CPT code 99070 defining supplies and materials provided by the provider over and above those normally included in the clinic visit should be avoided, and Level II codes, which are more detailed, should be used.) Level III codes are defined by the Medicare regional Part B carriers. Local codes are five-digit alphanumeric codes and use letters *S* and *W* through *Z*.

CODING OF MEDICAL DIAGNOSES

The ICD-9-CM is published annually, available October 1, by the National Center for Health Statistics (NCHS) and Centers for Medicare and Medicaid (CMS).

ICD-9-CM Manual Organization and Use

The ICD-9-CM was created by the WHO to provide a diagnostic coding system for the compilation and reporting of morbidity and mortality statistics for ICD-9-CM reimbursement purposes in the United States. A quarterly publication, *Coding Clinic for ICD-9-CM*, is available as the official guideline for ICD-9-CM. A similar publication will become available when ICD-10 is officially implemented. The *Official ICD-9-CM Guidelines for Coding and Reporting* are provided in the front of every ICD-9-CM codebook and are applicable to all settings; provider's clinic and hospital inpatient, outpatient, and clinical settings.

ICD-9-CM is broken into three volumes:

- *Volume I*, also known as the Tabular List, lists all diagnostic codes in numeric order. This area of the codebook is used to confirm codes prior to official code assignment.

- *Volume II* is an alphabetic index of all known diagnoses (Index to Diseases). It includes symptoms, accidents and their causes, and concurrent diagnosis. Volume II also contains a table of drugs and chemicals, a neoplasm table, and a list of external causes for injuries. Volume II is the recommended starting point to identify diagnostic codes; each code must be confirmed within Volume I after using this index.

- *Volume III* lists inpatient procedures in tabular form. It is never used in the outpatient setting, where the procedure codes of the CPT are used. Information in Volume III can, however, be helpful in identifying a procedure in the CPT.

The first step in coding a diagnosis is to enter Volume II using the main reason or condition (main term) that brought the patient into the medical facility. This could be a "soreness in the throat" or a "broken leg," among other symptoms. The lookup entry (main term) in Volume II would never include the anatomic term of "throat" or "leg," but would list "sore" or "fracture." The main term is shown in boldface type in the upper left of the page in the margin. Information in parentheses following the main term is called a nonessential modifier. The presence or absence of nonessential modifiers does not affect the code assignment.

Step 2 is to identify subterms that further identify the condition. Subterms are indented two spaces from the main term identified in step 1. Sometimes there is too much information to fit on the subterm line and it will be included on a carryover line that is indented two spaces from the subterm line.

Step 3 consists of selecting the main term or subterm that matches the diagnosis and obtaining the code. The code is then verified within the tabular list of Volume I (Classification of Diseases and Injuries) to reveal that it identifies the proper diagnosis. The tabular listing is broken into 17 chapters that are grouped according to cause or body system. Sometimes more specific identification is provided in the tabular list in the form of fourth or fifth digits. The more digits an ICD-9-CM code contains, the more specific the code turns out to be. When a more specific code is found, it must be used. Consider the following example:

Category 250: Diabetes mellitus

Subcategory 250.4: Diabetes with renal manifestations

Subclassification 250.42: Uncontrolled Type I diabetes with renal manifestations

The information given in the tabular list about a particular code takes precedence over the information given in the Volume II index. All ICD-9-CM codes must be confirmed in the tabular list before being assigned to a claim.

External Cause Codes (E Codes)

When the cause of a patient's visit is not due to a disease but rather to an injury or poisoning, an additional code is required to identify the reason for the visit or the cause of the injury. These codes are called **E codes**. The E codes have their own area within the Volume II index as well as their own area within the tabular list of Volume I. The most important thing to remember about E codes is that they are never listed before the actual diagnosis; E codes only serve as supplemental information for a claim.

In the case of the broken leg, listed earlier, if the patient had fallen from a ladder, the code would be E881.0; if the patient had fallen from a scaffold, the code would be E881.1. Like diagnosis codes, E codes must be as specific as possible.

Supplementary Health Factor Codes (V Codes)

When the patient comes to the medical facility for a reason other than sickness or injury, a supplementary health factor code is used. These are called **V codes**. Had the patient simply come in for a test, such as a tuberculin skin test, a supplementary health factor code would be required. In this case, the V code from ICD-9-CM would be V74.1, Screening for Pulmonary Tuberculosis. In addition, V codes can provide information about a patient's medical history, such as family history of breast cancer (V16.3), or long-term (current) use of insulin (V58.67).

CRITICAL THINKING

In which code book would you look to determine the code for hypoparathyroidism that is induced surgically? Which code did you select?

Morphology Codes (M Codes)

M codes (morphology codes) are used primarily with cancer registries. They are used to further identify the behavior and the cell type of a neoplasm. This code is used in conjunction with neoplasm codes for the main classification.

Code References

Sometimes a diagnostic code has the notation NEC or NOS attached to it. NEC means "not elsewhere classified" and is used if there is not enough information to find a more specific code. NOS means "not otherwise specified." An ICD-9-CM code with this notation is used when there is absolutely no other code available to fully describe the patient's diagnosis.

 See Procedure 18-2 for instructions on ICD-9-CM coding.

CODING ACCURACY

Accuracy in coding is vitally important. Imprecise coding can affect how quickly the provider is reimbursed and also the amount of the reimbursement. Codes must be appropriate to the documentation. Insurance carriers always **down-code** if documentation or codes are ambiguous and reimburse the provider for the lowest possible fee. Following are the three primary reasons why down-coding happens:

- The coding system used on the claim form does not match the coding system used by the insurance carrier. The carrier's computer will convert the submitted claim code to the closest recognized code. In most cases, the reimbursement amount will be less.

- If a worker's compensation claims examiner has to convert a CPT code to a relative value scale (RVS) code, the examiner will select the lowest-paying code. When billing worker's compensation, always use the RVS system used by that carrier and match the code to the best description of the CPT code.

- When attached documentation does not match the written description of the procedure, the reimbursement will always be the lowest paying code that fits the written description.

    Up-coding, also known as *code creep, overcoding,* or *overbilling,* occurs when the insurance carrier is

deliberately billed a higher rate service than what was performed to obtain greater reimbursements. Computer software programs have been developed to detect this practice easily. Often, complete audits are performed to assess the extent of upcoding practices. Sanctions and penalties are imposed on offenders.

The Medicare program, in particular, uses CPT codes, which are **bundled codes**. A bundled code is a grouping of several services that are directly related to a specific procedure and are paid as one. For example, surgical dressings and reading test results may be bundled into evaluation and management codes. **Unbundling** refers to separating the components of a procedure and reporting them as billable codes with charges to increase reimbursement rates. This procedure may also be termed *fragmentation, exploding,* or *à la carte medicine.* This practice is considered fraud and may lead to audit, sanctions, and penalties.

The more accurate the coding on the claim form, the less chance there is for error, the more

CRITICAL THINKING

The provider operates as part of a clinic in an integrated medical facility with radiology, laboratory, and surgical facilities in the same building. The clinic is located in Philadelphia, Pennsylvania, with the provider operating as a participating provider in the Medicare system.

A healthy, 65-year-old man presents at the clinic with a chief complaint of a badly bruised left hand and an apparent dislocation of the metacarpophalangeal joint. He had been putting up Christmas lights at his home using a 20-foot aluminum ladder. The ladder had fallen, striking his left thumb as he tried to catch the ladder. He is an established patient.

The provider orders anteroposterior, lateral, and oblique radiographs of the hand to rule out fractures. The radiographs show no evidence of fractures. The diagnosis is dislocation of the metacarpophalangeal joint. The joint is bruised and extremely painful. The procedure performed is a closed treatment of the metacarpophalangeal dislocation with manipulation and requires anesthesia.

Determine the diagnostic and procedures codes. Should you consider E codes? Why or why not? Determine the provider's fee to be billed to Medicare.

quickly the provider is reimbursed, and the better the chance that the provider's reimbursement will reflect the actual charge. Many insurance carriers keep a fee profile of each provider's charges. This profile reflects the amount of each charge for each service and can affect the provider's reimbursement for those services.

Do not guess when coding. The coding that is used becomes a permanent part of the patient's medical record with the insurance carrier. If an incorrect code is used, that coded diagnosis will stay with that patient. This can be a difficult problem for insured persons if they change insurance carriers or if other health problems occur.

Consider a patient with hip pain. She has a history of ovarian cancer for which she has had radiology treatments. The hip pain is thought to be possible metastases from the original cancer site. When ruling out this possibility, the provider indicates the following code for the claim form:

198.89 Secondary malignant neoplasm of other specified sites: hip.

When the pain is finally discovered to be arthritis and it is determined that the patient needs a hip replacement, the insurance carrier denies coverage for this operation for the following reason: The patient's condition is terminal, and the company does not want her to spend her last months having surgery and recovering from surgery when she is already in poor health. And, of course, there is the cost factor to consider in the eyes of the insurance carrier.

Incorrect coding can be a problem with ruling out a diagnosis. For instance, a patient presents many symptoms of peptic ulcer disease. Do not immediately code that patient as having that disease until the diagnosis is confirmed. Instead, code the symptoms. When the tests come back and a specific diagnosis of peptic ulcer can be made, then code the disease as:

533.70 chronic without mention of hemorrhage or perforation without mention of obstruction.

When coding:

- Be as precise as possible.
- Do not guess.
- Do not code what is not there.

CODING THE CLAIM FORM

For the insurance company to understand what is being billed, the claim form is completed by the medical assistant or billing clerk in the ambulatory care setting. The provider completes an **encounter form** at the time of the visit. This encounter form (Figure 18-1) includes the date of service, the visit or consultation code, diagnoses for this visit, procedures done and laboratory tests ordered, and if necessary, the date the patient is to return. This information is then translated onto the claim form.

The **CMS-1500 (08-05)** is the claim form accepted by all insurance carriers (Figure 18-2). This form is prepared using words and CPT codes for procedures performed and ICD-9-CM codes for diagnoses. Keep in mind that the codes must correlate; for instance, if a person had an ICD-9-CM diagnosis code of earache, otitis media, or 382.9, and the CPT procedure code indicated was 69090, ear piercing, the insurance company would question the claim and reject it for payment. The person completing the claim form must be *as precise as possible*. If the coding is wrong, the claim will be denied and the provider will not receive payment. Coding must correlate with the provider's note in the chart; otherwise, fraud is committed.

Coding the claim form is a precise way to communicate with the insurance carrier. Coding indicates the complexity of the visit, the diagnosis for the visit, and the specific procedures performed during the visit. This results in little confusion, and a minimum of communication is needed between the carrier and the provider's clinic because all information is contained in the codes.

For instance, Leo McKay, an established patient, is seen for an extended visit to determine the cause of his abdominal pain. Symptoms include diarrhea, fever, nausea, and anorexia. An abdominal ultrasound is ordered, as well as laboratory tests, and the results are unknown at the time of the insurance billing. The visit lasts 30 minutes and includes a full physical examination and a history of the present illness.

The CPT procedure coding for this visit is 99214, which reflects the examination and time spent with the patient, the history taken of this illness, and a medical decision of moderate complexity.

The ICD-9-CM diagnosis coding for abdominal pain is 789.00, for diarrhea 787.91, for nausea 787.02, and for anorexia 783.0. The claim form is submitted to the insurance carrier with these codes, and even though they are all symptoms, the claim will be paid because the visit and the tests ordered interrelate.

When the test results are known, they show a positive diagnosis of *Giardia lamblia*. The diagnosis

PLEASE RETURN THIS FORM TO RECEPTIONIST

NAME _____

Receipt No: _____

PLACE OF SERVICE:
( ) OFFICE
( ) NEW YORK COUNTY HOSPITAL
( ) COMMUNITY GENERAL HOSPITAL
( ) RETIREMENT INN NURSING HOME
( ) _____

DATE OF SERVICE _____

A. OFFICE VISITS - New Patient

Code	History	Exam	Dec.	Time
___ 99201	Prob. Foc.	Prob. Foc.	Straight	10 min. ____
___ 99202	Ex. Prob. Foc.	Ex. Prob. Foc.	Straight	20 min. ____
___ 99203	Detail	Detail	Low	30 min. ____
___ 99204	Comp.	Comp.	Mod.	45 min. ____
___ 99205	Comp.	Comp.	High	60 min. ____

B. OFFICE VISIT - Established Patient

Code	History	Exam	Dec.	Time
___ 99211	Minimal	Minimal	Minimal	5 min. ____
___ 99212	Prob. Foc.	Prob. Foc.	Straight	10min. ____
___ 99213	Ex. Prob. Foc.	Ex. Prob. Foc.	Low	15 min. ____
___ 99214	Detail	Detail	Mod.	25 min. ____
___ 99215	Comp.	Comp.	High	40 min. ____

C. HOSPITAL CARE   Dx Units

1. Initial Hospital Care (30 min) ____ ____ 99221
2. Subsequent Care ____ ____ 99231
3. Critical Care (30-74 min) ____ ____ 99291
4. each additional 30 min. ____ ____ 99292
5. Discharge Services ____ ____ 99238
6. Emergency Room ____ ____ 99282

D. NURSING HOME CARE   Dx Units

Initial Care - New Pt.
1. Expanded ____ ____ 99322
2. Detailed ____ ____ 99323

Subsequent Care - Estab. Pt.
3. Problem Focused ____ ____ 99307
4. Expanded ____ ____ 99308
5. Detailed ____ ____ 99309
5. Comprehensive ____ ____ 99310

E. PROCEDURES

1. Arthrocentesis, Small Jt. ____ 20600
2. Colonoscopy ____ 45378
3. EKG w/interpretation ____ 93000
4. X-Ray Chest, PA/LAT ____ 71020

F. LAB

1. Blood Sugar ____ 82947 ____
2. CBC w/differential ____ 85031 ____
3. Cholesterol ____ 82465 ____
4. Comprehensive Metabolic Panel ____ 80053 ____
5. ESR ____ 85651 ____
6. Hematocrit ____ 85014 ____
7. Mono Screen ____ 86308 ____
8. Pap Smear ____ 88150 ____
9. Potassium ____ 84132 ____
10. Preg. Test, Quantitative ____ 84702 ____
11. Routine Venipuncture ____ 36415 ____

F. Cont'd   Dx Units

12. Strep Screen ____ 87081
13. UA, Routine w/Micro ____ 81000
14. UA, Routine w/o Micro ____ 81002
15. Uric Acid ____ 84550
16. VDRL ____ 86592
17. Wet Prep ____ 82710
18. _____ ____ ____

G. INJECTIONS

1. Influenza Virus Vaccine ____ 90658 ____
2. Pneumoccocal Vaccine ____ 90772 ____
3. Tetanus Toxoids ____ 90703 ____
4. Therapeutic Subcut/IM ____ 90732 ____
5. Vaccine Administration ____ 90471 ____
6. Vaccine - each additional ____ 90472 ____

H. MISCELLANEOUS

1. _____ ____ ____
2. _____ ____ ____

AMOUNT PAID $ _____

Mark diagnosis with (1=Primary, 2=Secondary, 3=Tertiary)	DIAGNOSIS NOT LISTED BELOW _____

DIAGNOSIS	ICD-9-CM 1, 2, 3	DIAGNOSIS	ICD-9-CM 1, 2, 3	DIAGNOSIS	ICD-9-CM 1, 2, 3
Abdominal Pain	789.0_	Dehydration	276.51	Otitis Media, Acute NOS	382.9
Allergic Rhinitis, Unspec.	477.9	Depression, NOS	311	Peptic Ulcer Disease	536.9
Angina Pectoris, Unspec.	413.9	Diabetes Mellitus, Type II Controlled	250.00	Peripheral Vascular Disease NOS	443.9
Anemia, Iron Deficiency, Unspec.	280.9	Diabetes Mellitus, Type II Controlled	250.02	Pharyngitis, Acute	462
Anemia, NOS	285.9	Drug Reaction, NOS	995.29	Pneumonia, Organism Unspec.	486
Anemia, Pernicious	281.0	Dysuria	788.1	Prostatitis, NOS	601.9
Asthma w/ Exacerbation	493.92	Eczema, NOS	692.2	PVC	427.69
Asthmatic Bronchitis, Unspec.	493.90	Edema	782.3	Rash, Non Specific	782.1
Atrial Fibrillation	427.31	Fever, Unknown Origin	780.6	Seizure Disorder NOS	780.39
Atypical Chest Pain, Unspec.	786.59	Gastritis, Acute w/o Hemorrhage	535.00	Serous Otitis Media, Chronic, Unspec.	381.10
Bronchiolitis, due to RSV	466.11	Gastroenteritis, NOS	558.9	Sinusitis, Acute NOS	461.9
Bronchitis, Acute	466.0	Gastroesophageal Reflux	530.81	Tonsillitis, Acute	463.
Bronchitis, NOS	490	Hepatitis A, Infectious	070.1	Upper Respiratory Infection, Acute NOS	465.9
Cardiac Arrest	427.5	Hypercholesterolemia, Pure	272.0	Urinary Tract Infection, Unspec.	599.0
Cardiopulmonary Disease, Chronic, Unspec.	416.9	Hypertension, Unspec.	401.9	Urticaria, Unspec.	708.9
Cellulitis, NOS	682.9	Hypoglycemia NOS	251.2	Vertigo, NOS	780.4
Congestive Heart Failure, Unspec.	428.0	Hypokalemia	276.8	Viral Infection NOS	079.99
Contact Dermatitis NOS	692.9	Impetigo	684	Weakness, Generalized	780.79
COPD NOS	496	Lymphadenitis, Unspec.	289.3	Weight Loss, Abnormal	783.21
CVA, Acute, NOS	434.91	Mononucleosis	075		
CVA, Old or Healed	438.9	Myocardial Infarction, Acute, NOS	410.9		
Degenerative Arthritis		Organic Brain Syndrome	310.9		
(Specify Site)	715.9	Otitis Externa, Acute NOS	380.10		

ABN: I UNDERSTAND THAT MEDICARE PROBABLY WILL NOT COVER THE SERVICES LISTED BELOW

A. _____ B. _____ C. _____

Patient

Date _____ Signature _____

Doctor's Signature _____

RETURN: _____ Days _____ Weeks _____ Months

INNER CITY HEALTH CARE
8600 MAIN STREET, SUITE 201
RIVER CITY, NY 01234
PHONE No. (123) 555-0326
EIN# 00-1234560

❑ S.RICE, M.D.
NPI# 9995010111

❑ J.S. LEWIS, M.D.
NPI# 9995020212

❑ M.M KING, M.D.
NPI #9995030313

Figure 18-1 Encounter form.

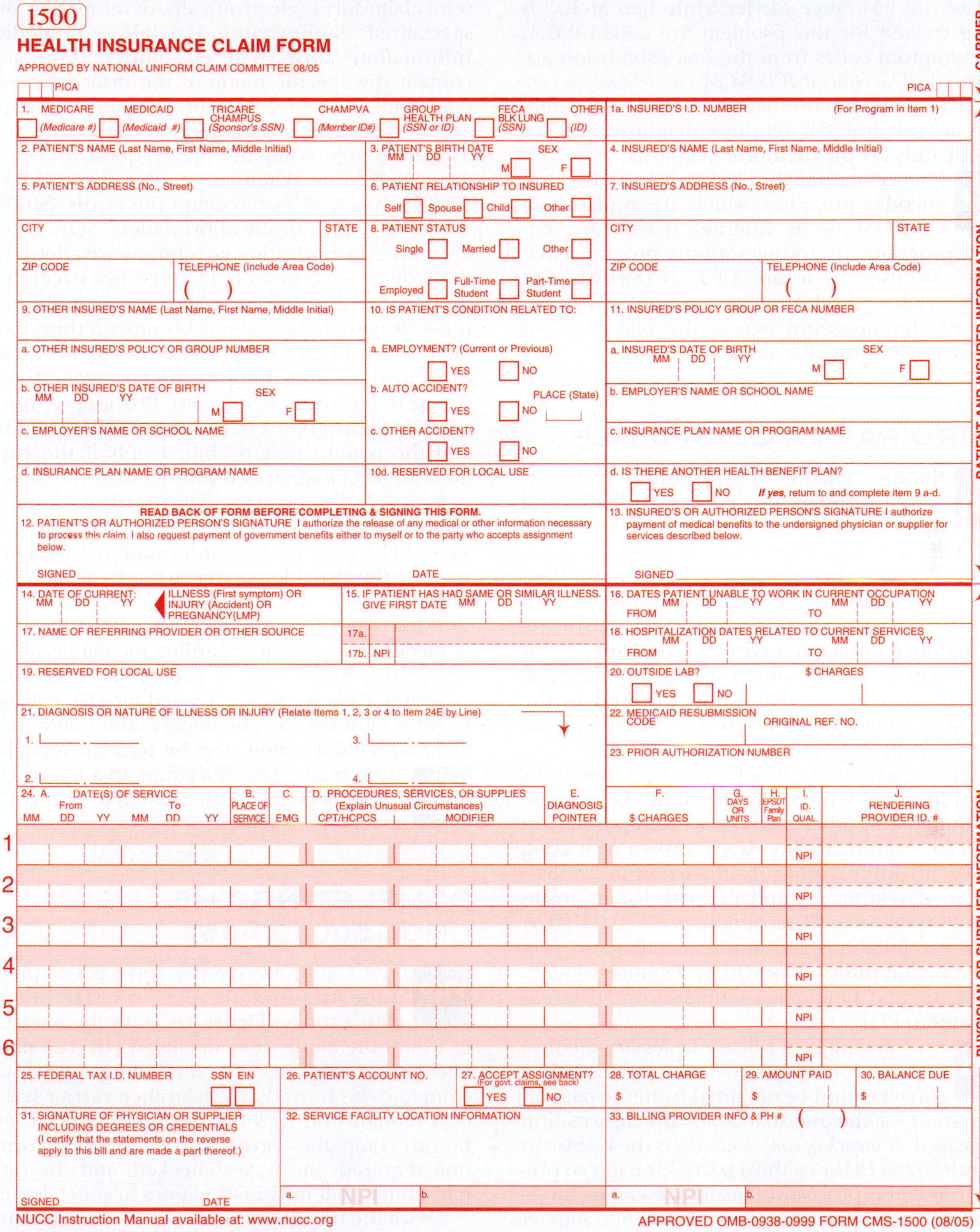

1500

HEALTH INSURANCE CLAIM FORM

APPROVED BY NATIONAL UNIFORM CLAIM COMMITTEE 08/05

Courtesy of the Centers for Medicare and Medicaid Services. Reprinted according to www.cms.gov website content reuse policy.

Figure 18-2   CMS-1500 health insurance claim form.

code is changed to 007.1. Any further charges sent to the insurance carrier while Leo McKay is being treated for this problem are coded 007.1. The symptom codes from the first submission are dropped. *The Official ICD-9-CM Guidelines for Coding and Reporting* state that when signs and symptoms are integral to a definitive diagnosis, you are to code only for the definitive diagnosis.

EHR Many electronic health records (EHRs) use encoder programs, which are available on CD-ROM or as Internet downloads. Encoder programs are coding software programs that allow the user to locate CPT, ICD-9-CM, and HCPCS codes quickly using the computer. Many of the encoder programs permit the placement of bookmarks or notes for quick reference.

THIRD-PARTY GUIDELINES

Because patient information is easily accessed through medical charts, EHRs, and the human factor, security and confidentiality measures must be in place in medical clinics. When patients schedule an appointment and are seen by the provider, they enter into a contract for specific services. The first party is the person receiving the contracted service. The second party is the person or organization providing the service. A third party is one that is not involved in the patient–provider relationship but rather with reimbursement procedures.

HIPAA The patient has a right to expect that his or her health information will not be disseminated to others without written permission to do so. Confidentiality issues involve restricting the health information to only those individuals who need to know. Compliance with Health Insurance Portability and Accountability Act (HIPAA) of 1996 regulations is one way to safeguard protected health information (PHI). Chapters 11, 12, 13, 14, 15, and 17 all place emphasis on HIPAA as it relates to PHI.

Authorization to release necessary medical information to payers, such as insurance carriers, must be obtained from the patient, the parent, or the guardian *before* any information is released. A *breach of confidentiality* is the release of unauthorized PHI to a third party. One way to prevent this when processing insurance claims forms is to ask the patient, parent, or guardian to sign an "Authorization to Release Medical Information" statement *before* the claim form is completed. The CMS-1500 (08-05) form provides space for this signature in Block 12.

Some medical clinics, especially those that send claim forms electronically, develop their own specialized "Authorization for Release of Medical Information" form. The customized form must contain the specific name of the insurance company and must be signed by the patient, parent, or guardian. This form is generally valid for 1 year. The insurance company may request a copy of the signed form. When completing the CMS-1500 (08-05), Block 12 may contain the words "SIGNATURE ON FILE" or the abbreviation "SOF."

Three authorization exceptions are allowed by the federal government. The first two exceptions apply to Medicaid and worker's compensation. In these instances, the patient becomes a third-party beneficiary in the contract between the health care provider and the government agency sponsoring the insurance program. Providers agree to accept the program's payment as payment in full, and the patient may be billed only if the payer does not cover services rendered or if the patient is ineligible for benefits. The third exception is related to hospital admission. The patient must sign a release of medical information *before* being seen by the provider or receiving treatment in a hospital.

Most states have specific laws related to release of medical information regarding mental health services and federally assisted alcohol and drug abuse programs. Patients being screened for HIV infection or AIDS must sign an additional authorization statement *before* information may be released regarding their status. See Procedure 18-3 for specific steps involved in authorization to release PHI to third-party payers.

COMPLETING THE CMS-1500 (08-05)

EHR The CMS-1500 (08-05) form is completed using data from the patient's EHR in most clinics today (Figure 18-3). In the few cases in which the clinic does not use EHR, the paper encounter form is used by the billing specialist to complete the form. Each insurance carrier has its own thoughts on how the form is completed and no two companies agree entirely on the information required, the boxes checked, and the rationale about what information goes in which boxes.

With the transition to an increase in electronic claims submission and the HIPAA regulations, the National Uniform Claim Committee (NUCC) established a standardized dataset for use in an electronic environment as well as with paper claim

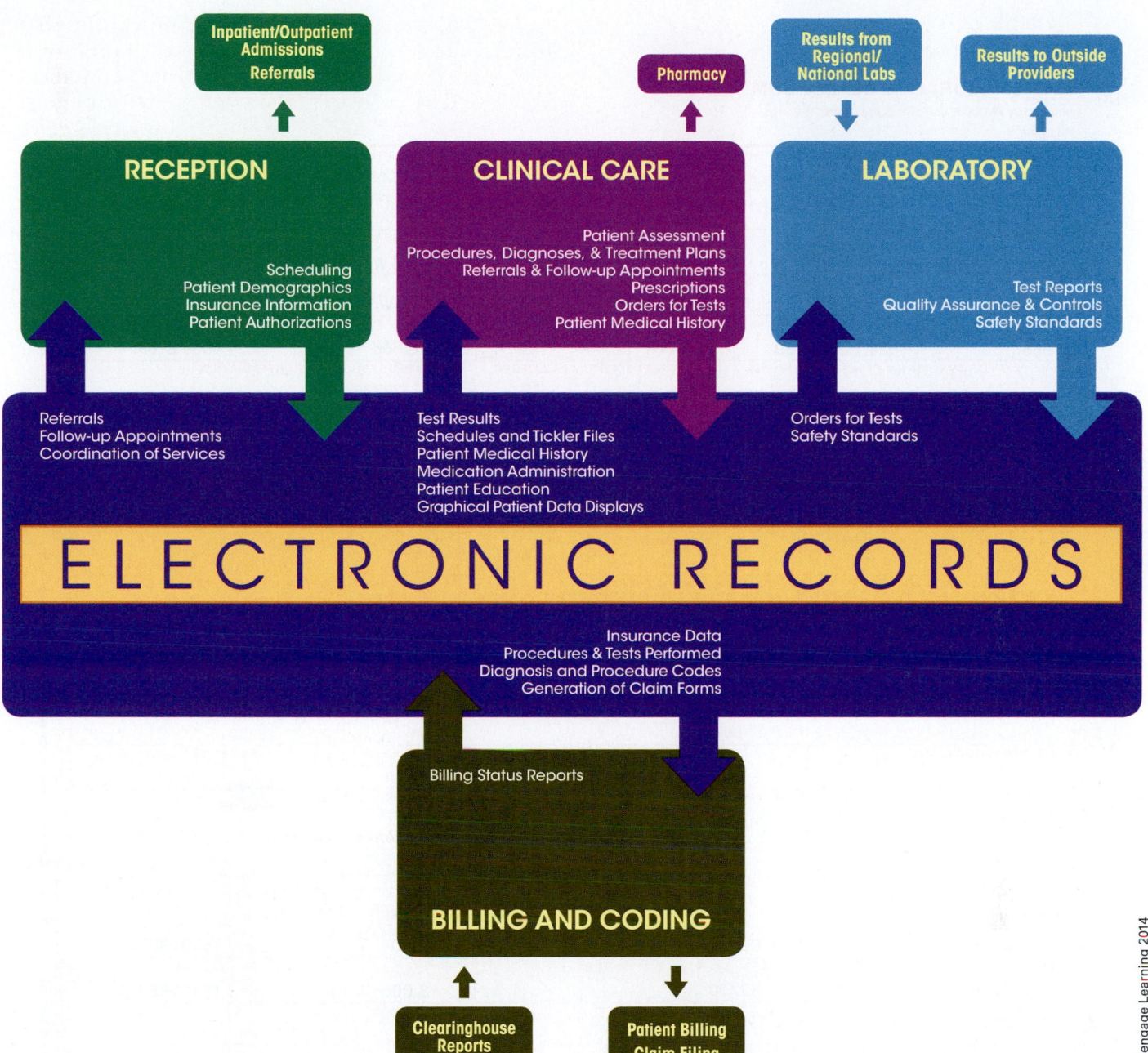

Figure 18-3   How the EHR can be used in processing insurance procedures.

form standards. The NUCC continues to monitor how insurance carriers use the various claim form fields. Additional changes to the CMS-1500 (08-05) form may be required in the future as the NUCC works to create standardized national instructions for completing the form.

To illustrate the completion of a claim form, a fictitious insurance carrier will be used. Insurance carriers often change their rules and regulations for submitting claims constantly. To avoid

out-of-date material, we sent this claim for payment to How Much Insurance Company. Using the example given of Leo McKay in the coding section, the CMS-1500 (08-05) in Figure 18-4 shows the properly completed claim form.

Remember, many insurance carriers require some of the boxes to be filled in and others left blank. The billing person for the medical clinic needs to comply with the current requirements of the insurance carrier that is being billed. There is

1500

HEALTH INSURANCE CLAIM FORM

APPROVED BY NATIONAL UNIFORM CLAIM COMMITTEE 08/05

PICA | PICA

CARRIER

1. MEDICARE (Medicare #) | MEDICAID (Medicaid #) | TRICARE CHAMPUS (Sponsor's SSN) | CHAMPVA (Member ID#) | GROUP HEALTH PLAN (SSN or ID) | FECA BLK LUNG (SSN) | OTHER (ID) [X]

1a. INSURED'S I.D. NUMBER (For Program in Item 1): 555-55-555

2. PATIENT'S NAME (Last Name, First Name, Middle Initial): MCKAY LEO M

3. PATIENT'S BIRTH DATE MM DD YY: 04 01 1963 — SEX: M [X] F [ ]

4. INSURED'S NAME (Last Name, First Name, Middle Initial): MCKAY, LEO M.

5. PATIENT'S ADDRESS (No., Street): 123 W FIRST STREET

CITY: ANYWHERE — STATE: PA

ZIP CODE: 11666 — TELEPHONE (Include Area Code): (824) 556-6189

6. PATIENT RELATIONSHIP TO INSURED: Self [X] Spouse [ ] Child [ ] Other [ ]

7. INSURED'S ADDRESS (No., Street): 123 W FIRST STREET

CITY: ANYWHERE — STATE: PA

ZIP CODE: 11666 — TELEPHONE (Include Area Code): (824) 556-6789

8. PATIENT STATUS: Single [X] Married [ ] Other [ ]; Employed [ ] Full-Time Student [ ] Part-Time Student [ ]

9. OTHER INSURED'S NAME (Last Name, First Name, Middle Initial):

a. OTHER INSURED'S POLICY OR GROUP NUMBER

b. OTHER INSURED'S DATE OF BIRTH MM DD YY — SEX M [ ] F [ ]

c. EMPLOYER'S NAME OR SCHOOL NAME

d. INSURANCE PLAN NAME OR PROGRAM NAME

10. IS PATIENT'S CONDITION RELATED TO:

a. EMPLOYMENT? (Current or Previous) YES [ ] NO [X]

b. AUTO ACCIDENT? YES [ ] NO [X] PLACE (State)

c. OTHER ACCIDENT? YES [ ] NO [X]

10d. RESERVED FOR LOCAL USE

11. INSURED'S POLICY GROUP OR FECA NUMBER: 1122334

a. INSURED'S DATE OF BIRTH MM DD YY: 04 01 1963 — SEX: M [X] F [ ]

b. EMPLOYER'S NAME OR SCHOOL NAME: ABC MANUFACTURING COMPANY

c. INSURANCE PLAN NAME OR PROGRAM NAME: HOW MUCH INSURANCE COMPANY

d. IS THERE ANOTHER HEALTH BENEFIT PLAN? YES [ ] NO [X] *If yes*, return to and complete item 9 a-d.

READ BACK OF FORM BEFORE COMPLETING & SIGNING THIS FORM.

12. PATIENT'S OR AUTHORIZED PERSON'S SIGNATURE I authorize the release of any medical or other information necessary to process this claim. I also request payment of government benefits either to myself or to the party who accepts assignment below.

SIGNED: SIGNATURE ON FILE — DATE: 01 14 XXXX

13. INSURED'S OR AUTHORIZED PERSON'S SIGNATURE I authorize payment of medical benefits to the undersigned physician or supplier for services described below.

SIGNED: SIGNATURE ON FILE

PATIENT AND INSURED INFORMATION

14. DATE OF CURRENT: ILLNESS (First symptom) OR INJURY (Accident) OR PREGNANCY(LMP) MM DD YY: 01 10 XXXX

15. IF PATIENT HAS HAD SAME OR SIMILAR ILLNESS. GIVE FIRST DATE MM DD YY

16. DATES PATIENT UNABLE TO WORK IN CURRENT OCCUPATION FROM MM DD YY TO MM DD YY

17. NAME OF REFERRING PROVIDER OR OTHER SOURCE — 17a. — 17b. NPI

18. HOSPITALIZATION DATES RELATED TO CURRENT SERVICES FROM MM DD YY TO MM DD YY

19. RESERVED FOR LOCAL USE

20. OUTSIDE LAB? YES [ ] NO [ ] — $ CHARGES

21. DIAGNOSIS OR NATURE OF ILLNESS OR INJURY (Relate Items 1, 2, 3 or 4 to Item 24E by Line)

1. 789 . 0 — 3. 783 . 0

2. 558 . 9 — 4.

22. MEDICAID RESUBMISSION CODE — ORIGINAL REF. NO.

23. PRIOR AUTHORIZATION NUMBER

	24. A. DATE(S) OF SERVICE From MM DD YY	To MM DD YY	B. PLACE OF SERVICE	C. EMG	D. PROCEDURES, SERVICES, OR SUPPLIES (Explain Unusual Circumstances) CPT/HCPCS	MODIFIER	E. DIAGNOSIS POINTER	F. $ CHARGES	G. DAYS OR UNITS	H. EPSDT Family Plan	I. ID. QUAL.	J. RENDERING PROVIDER ID. #
1	01 10 XXXX		3		99214		1 2 3	85 00	1		NPI	1543298760
2	01 10 XXXX		3		82270		1 2	13 00	1		NPI	1543298760
3											NPI	
4											NPI	
5											NPI	
6											NPI	

25. FEDERAL TAX I.D. NUMBER: 91-1234432 — SSN [ ] EIN [X]

26. PATIENT'S ACCOUNT NO.: MCK111

27. ACCEPT ASSIGNMENT? (For govt. claims, see back) YES [ ] NO [X]

28. TOTAL CHARGE: $ 98 00

29. AMOUNT PAID: $

30. BALANCE DUE: $ 98 00

31. SIGNATURE OF PHYSICIAN OR SUPPLIER INCLUDING DEGREES OR CREDENTIALS (I certify that the statements on the reverse apply to this bill and are made a part thereof.)

SIGNED: MARK WOS MD — DATE: 01 14 XXX

32. SERVICE FACILITY LOCATION INFORMATION — a. NPI b.

33. BILLING PROVIDER INFO & PH #: (814) 555-1155

INNER CITY HEALTH CARE
222 S FIRST AVE
CANTON PA 11666

a. R09876543 b.

PHYSICIAN OR SUPPLIER INFORMATION

NUCC Instruction Manual available at: www.nucc.org — APPROVED OMB-0938-0999 FORM CMS-1500 (08/05)

Figure 18-4 Completed CMS-1500 claim form.

no right or wrong answer for every insurance carrier. If there is a question about billing, check with that carrier about its requirements. There are certain formatting guidelines when completing the claim form that will remain consistent, no matter which insurance company you are dealing with:

- The form must ALWAYS be completed in black ink.
- The form must ALWAYS be completed using all capital letters.
- The form must NEVER contain any punctuation or symbols of any kind; only letters and numbers may be used.
- Any date entered on the form (DOS, DOB, etc.), must be in eight-digit format. For example, the DOB for our previously mentioned patient, Leo McKay, is April 1, 1963. Therefore, his DOB on the form should appear as 04011963. (Notice there are no hyphens or slashes.)

The CMS-1500 (08-05) claim form contains all of the identification information that the carrier needs to process or analyze the claim for payment. The new form is distinguishable from the old form in that the 1500 symbol and the date approved by the NUCC appear in the top left margin. When completing the PATIENT AND INSURED INFORMATION section, do not use commas to separate the last name, first name, and middle initial. Do not use periods within the name. Do not use commas, periods, or other punctuation in the address. When entering the nine-digit ZIP code, you may include the hyphen. This is the only exception to the punctuation rule. Do not use a hyphen or space as a separator within the telephone number. The top right-hand space, identified as CARRIER, provides space for the carrier's name and address 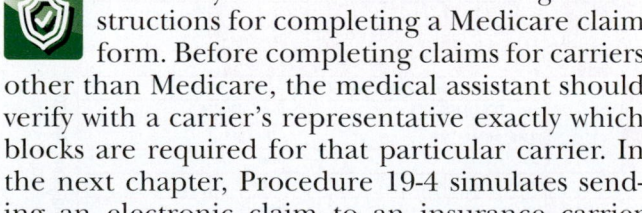 to be keyed in. Procedure 18-4 gives instructions for completing a Medicare claim form. Before completing claims for carriers other than Medicare, the medical assistant should verify with a carrier's representative exactly which blocks are required for that particular carrier. In the next chapter, Procedure 19-4 simulates sending an electronic claim to an insurance carrier after procedure and diagnostic codes have been posted to a patient's account.

Uniform Bill 04 Form

The NUCC has also updated the CMS-1450 claim form, also known as **Uniform Bill 04 (UB-04)**, to accommodate reporting the National Provider Identifier (NPI) number. The NPI, a requirement of HIPAA legislation, must be used by all HIPAA-covered entities. Figure 18-5 shows a sample of the UB-04 form.

The UB-04 form is the standard form used for inpatient admissions, outpatient and emergency department services and procedures, psychiatric facilities, drug and alcohol facilities, clinical and laboratory services, walk-in centers, nursing facilities, home health care agencies, hospice centers, and long-term care benefits under a health plan.

Using the Computer to Complete Forms

The CMS-1500 (08-05) claim form is designed to accommodate optical scanning of paper claims. A scanner is used to convert printed characters into text that can be viewed by the optical character reader (OCR). This technology greatly increases claims processing productivity, with some claims being paid within 7 to 10 days.

Practice management software may require data to be entered using uppercase and lowercase letters and other data be entered without regard to OCR guidelines. The computer program converts the data to the OCR format when the claim is printed or electronically transmitted to the carrier. Always use the software program's test pattern program to verify alignment of forms. Be sure the Xs are completely within the designated boxes. You may need to check this alignment each time a new batch of claims is inserted into the printer.

While completing the claim form on the computer, remember not to interchange a zero (0) with the alpha character (o). A substitute space should be used in place of the following keystrokes:

- Dollar sign or decimal in all charges or totals
- Decimal point in a diagnosis code number
- Dash in front of a procedure code modifier
- Parentheses surrounding the area code in a telephone number
- Hyphens in Social Security numbers

When a fee is expressed in whole dollars, always enter two zeros in the cent column. Birth dates should be entered using eight digits (MMDDYYYY). Two-digit code numbers are used for months (January 01, February 02, and so on). If the day of the month number is less than 10, add a zero before the day (i.e., 03 for the third day of the month).

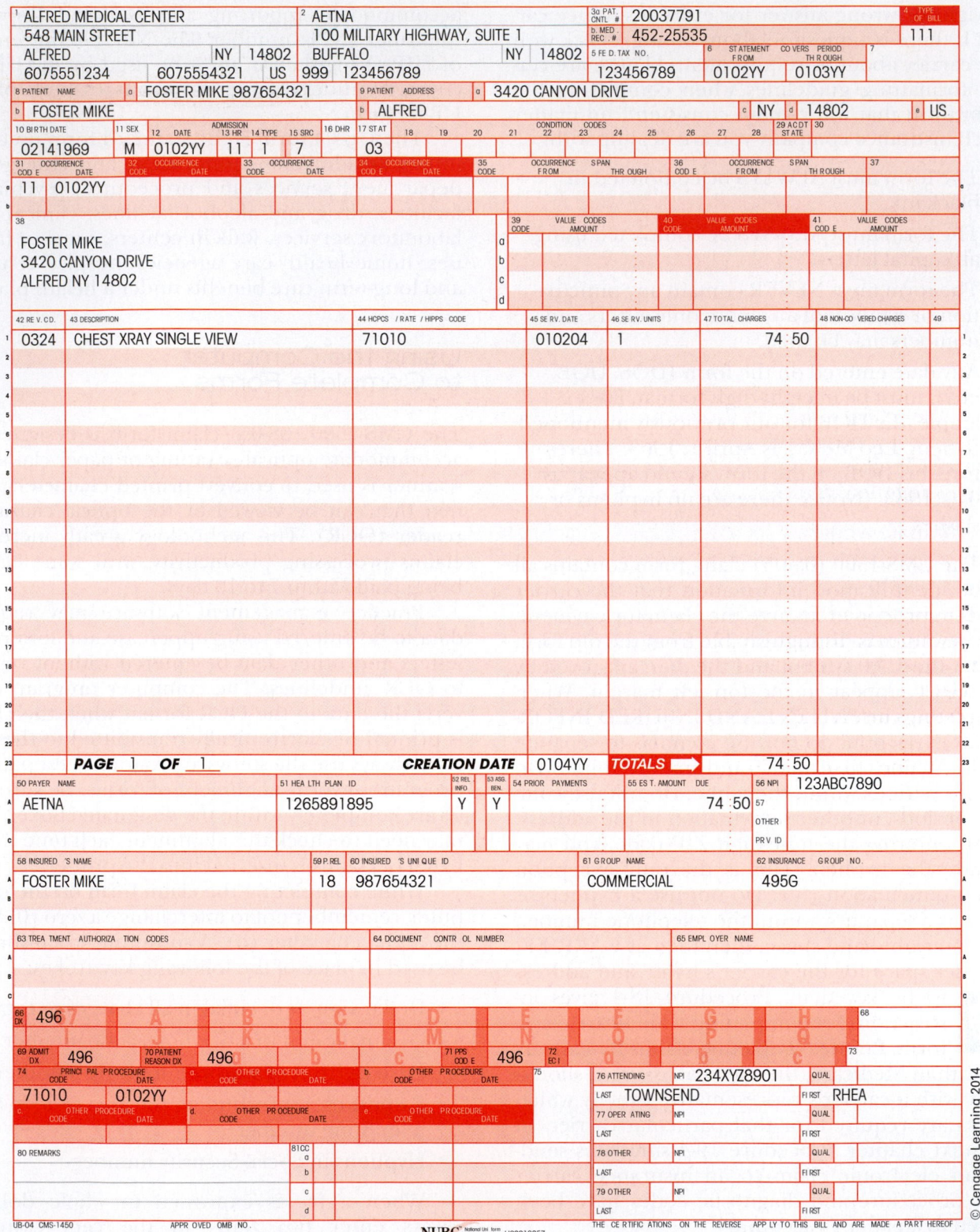

Figure 18-5   UB-04 claim containing sample patient data (with highlighted form locators that contain ICD-9-CM and CPT codes).

EHR The Administrative Simplification Compliance Act (ASCA), which went into effect July 5, 2005, specifies that no payment may be made under Part A or Part B of the Medicare program for any expenses incurred for items or services for which a claim is submitted in a nonelectronic form. Simply stated, paper claims submitted to Medicare will not be paid. Some exceptions to this rule can be found in the *Medlearn Matters* article MM3440 available at the CMS website (http://cms.hhs.gov/medlearn/matters).

Common Errors in Completing Claim Forms

Once the claim form has been completed, it should be proofread for accuracy and to make certain that all information has been filled in correctly. The following list provides common errors:

- Eliminate typographic errors. Check all numbers carefully to be sure they have not been transposed or entered incorrectly.
- Eliminate incorrect information. The name of the patient and the name of the policyholder must be the same (unless a wife is covered under a husband's insurance, a child under a parent's insurance, etc.).
- Verify that all blanks have been completed accurately. Specifically check that units of service are entered, hospital admission and discharge dates are included, and procedure service date is provided.
- Verify that each procedure links correctly with the correct diagnosis (Block 24E).
- Verify that the procedure was medically necessary.
- Include the patient's name and policy identification information on each page of all attachments.
- Do not use staples when submitting paper claims because the form cannot feed through the OCR if it is defaced or creased.
- Verify that the printer alignment was properly set and that all claim information is contained within its proper field.
- Be sure the claim form is signed appropriately.

BENEFITS OF SUBMITTING CLAIMS ELECTRONICALLY

Submitting claims electronically has many benefits, which may include, but are not limited to, the following:

- Standardized electronic claim format ensures consistency, reducing errors.
- Submitters can exchange electronic data with multiple payers using the same data format.
- Supplies required (e.g., paper, postage) and administrative costs are reduced.
- Cash flow can be significantly improved because Medicare pays 14 days after receipt of electronically submitted claims (paper claims may take a minimum of 29 days to process).

MANAGING THE CLAIMS PROCESS

Once the claim form has been coded, a series of events take place. The medical assistant, who may have used a referral number generated by a point-of-service device, enters the claim into the office register of submitted claims; the insurance carrier processes the claim; an explanation of benefits is sent to the insured person and the medical provider; and, if necessary, follow-up procedures are instituted if payment is not received from the carrier within a specified time period. Each of these events is discussed in detail in the following sections.

Documentation of Referrals

Many insurance plans require that a referral be preapproved by the plan before scheduling an appointment with someone other than the primary care provider. This is particularly true for managed care plans, especially HMOs. The medical assistant working in both the primary care facility and specialist facility must make sure that when an approval is required, the necessary authorization has been obtained and the referral number is recorded in the patient's file. The referral number must be submitted as part of the claim submitted to the carrier by the specialist. This piece of information would be entered in Block 23 of the CMS-1500 (08-05).

Point-of-Service Device

An electronic device available to some health care providers is a **point-of-service (POS) device**. This device provides immediate and direct access to patient eligibility information and managed care functions through an electronic network connecting the medical clinic and the health plan's computer.

The POS device is a small card-swipe box similar in design and function to a credit card terminal (Figure 18-6). It allows medical clinic personnel to:

- Record a patient visit
- Check eligibility for patients in the health plan
- Enter referrals for patients in managed care plans
- Verify referral information
- Check authorization status
- Enter inpatient authorization requests
- Enter outpatient authorization requests

After the necessary information is entered by the medical assistant, the POS device communicates with the health plan's computer system. The computer then returns an acknowledgment to the medical clinic confirming the transaction or giving an error message code. For example, when visits are recorded accurately, a reference number is generated that is used as the medical clinic's confirmation that the transaction is complete. On successful entry of a referral, a referral number is generated. Specialists may use this number on claims they submit for services they render under the referral.

Maintaining a Claims Registry

When claim forms are sent to the appropriate insurance carrier, it is wise and necessary for the medical clinic personnel to keep a diary or register of submitted claims (Figure 18-7). This **claim register** should include the patient's name, the insured's name if it is different from the patient's name, the dates of service for which the claim is being made, the amount of the claim, and the date the claim is submitted. When payment is received, the date of payment should be entered. When aging and reconciling accounts, the bookkeeper then can check the diary to note where the claim is in the process.

Following Up on Claims

Occasionally, claims are denied because the claim form was not properly coded. However, if there is no payment from the carrier and no other notification after a period of 4 to 6 weeks, it is necessary to follow up on the claim. The claim register will enable the clinic to keep track of the progress of claims (Figure 18-7).

To follow up, a toll-free number is provided by most carriers. The necessary information to have on hand before making the call includes a copy of the claim form and the patient's name

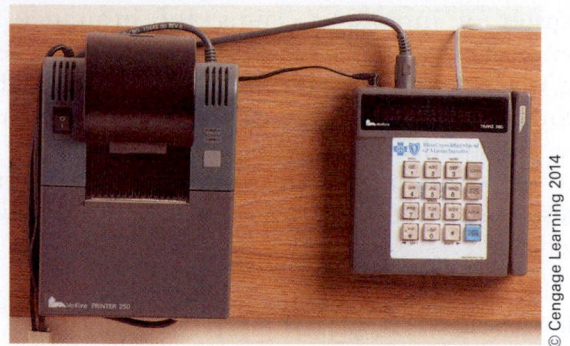

Figure 18-6 Point-of-service device. (Right) To enter information, the patient's insurance card is swiped through the machine, or the patient's identification number is entered on the keypad together with specific transaction code numbers. (Left) Responses from the plan's computer are printed directly in the medical office.

© Cengage Learning 2014

INSURANCE CLAIMS STATUS

ACTION DATE	LAST NAME	FIRST NAME	INSURANCE COMPANY	ORIGINAL BILLING DATE	TOTAL CHARGES $	AMOUNT RECEIVED	STATUS / ACTION TAKEN
1/30/2008	McKay	Leo	Nationwide	1/30/2008	$ 88.00	$ -	Submitted
2/14/2008	Lovelace	Terry	World Health	9/24/2007	$ 128.00	$ -	Add'l data submitted
4/15/2008	Taxman	William	US Health	12/15/2007	$ 640.00	$ 640.00	Paid in full
5/1/2008	Fooler	April	Surprise Health	4/1/2007	$ 375.98	$ -	Collection
5/16/2008	Zonker	James	Gotcha Covered	4/3/2008	$ 236.00	$ 136.00	Patient billed $100.00
7/5/2008	Stripes	Stanley	Bangor Insurance				

© Cengage Learning 2014

Figure 18-7 Sample claim register.

and insurance identification number. The carrier should be able to give the status of the claim. If payment is delayed, the carrier should be able to give the date when it can be expected. It is possible that payment was sent to the insured person, in which case a statement should be sent to the patient. If there is a problem with the claim, the medical assistant may need to investigate the cause of the error and submit a revised claim.

See Chapter 20 for information on billing and collection procedures.

THE INSURANCE CARRIER'S ROLE

On receipt of the claim form, the claims processor at the insurance carrier checks the codes to confirm that the procedures and accompanying diagnoses link properly with one another. The processor then analyzes the information to confirm that:

1. The coverage was in force at the time of treatment.
2. The provider has contracted with the insurance carrier.
3. There are no exclusions or restrictions on the policy for payment of that diagnosis.
4. There are no preexisting condition restrictions.
5. The diagnosis and procedures done are medically necessary and reasonable.

The processor also checks to make sure that the billed amount falls within the usual, customary, and reasonable fee that the insurance carrier has developed for that specific procedure.

Explanation of Benefits

On completion of the processing of the claim, the insurance company sends an **explanation of benefits (EOB)** to the insured person. Figure 17-1 shows a sample EOB. This form includes the dates; charges; amounts applied toward the deductible; amounts not covered either because of an exclusion or excess over the usual, customary, and reasonable charge; and the amount the company is paying for this claim. Some EOB forms even serve as a "bill" or "notice" in that they indicate the amount the insured must forward to the provider for payment of the account in full.

LEGAL AND ETHICAL ISSUES

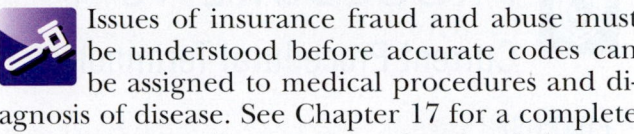

Issues of insurance fraud and abuse must be understood before accurate codes can be assigned to medical procedures and diagnosis of disease. See Chapter 17 for a complete discussion regarding insurance fraud and abuse.

Coding errors pose another type of legal and ethical issue. The Omnibus Budget Reconciliation Acts of 1986 and 1987 state that providers can be assessed civil penalties if they "know of or should know that claims filed with Medicare or Medicaid on their behalf are not true and accurate representations of the items or services actually provided." This means that providers can be held responsible not only for negligent mistakes they make but also for mistakes made on their behalf by their medical assistants who complete insurance claim forms. The penalties assessed are usually in the form of a monetary fine and may also involve exclusion from Medicare and Medicaid programs for a specified period of time.

Compliance Programs

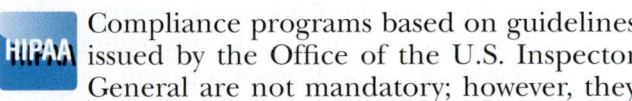

Compliance programs based on guidelines issued by the Office of the U.S. Inspector General are not mandatory; however, they help prevent violations that can be financially costly and that may carry criminal penalties for the provider and clinic personnel. Participation in a compliance program demonstrates that the practice is making a good-faith effort to submit claims appropriately and is considered equivalent to practicing preventative medicine. The following are basic elements of a compliance program:

1. Have a designated compliance officer.
2. Develop and use written standards and procedures for coding.
3. Develop a plan for communicating coding standards and procedures.
4. Train personnel in standards and procedures.
5. Conduct periodic audits.
6. Respond to detected violations and notify appropriate government agencies.
7. Make personnel aware that they have an ethical duty to report suspected or observed fraudulent or erroneous coding practices so that they can be corrected. Publicize and enforce disciplinary standards on coding violations.

PROCEDURE 18-1

Current Procedural Terminology Coding

PURPOSE:

To convert commonly accepted descriptions of medical procedures (services) and visits of all types—clinic, hospital, nursing facility, home services—into a five-digit numeric code with two-digit numeric modifiers when required.

EQUIPMENT/SUPPLIES:

CPT code book for the current year
Copy of the encounter form and access to the patient's chart
Pencil and paper

CASE SCENARIO:

Mary O'Keefe, a new patient, is seen for 10 minutes, during which the provider takes a focused history and completes a problem-focused examination. A routine urinalysis, nonautomated and without microscopy, is performed and a straightforward medical decision is made. Mary's preliminary diagnosis is painful urination. The urinalysis confirms a urinary tract infection. The provider writes her a prescription for an antibiotic and asks her to make an appointment in 10 days for another urinalysis to confirm the infection has cleared.

PROCEDURE STEPS:

1. Using the CPT code book, look in the Evaluation and Management section, Office or Other Outpatient Services, New Patient. Carefully read through the options until the code matching the described scenario has been found. RATIONALE: This section of the CPT code book provides codes used to report evaluation and management services provided in the provider's clinic or in an outpatient or other ambulatory care facility. You should have selected 99201.

2. Continue with the CPT code book, turn to the Index again, and look up Urinalysis, Routine. The code given is 81002. RATIONALE: This provides you with a code to investigate and determine its appropriateness.

3. Continue in the CPT code book and turn to the Pathology and Laboratory section. Follow the codes until you locate code 81002. Be sure the description provided there matches what the provider has documented in the patient's chart. RATIONALE: To verify that the code is correct and matches documentation.

PROCEDURE 18-2

International Classification of Diseases, 9th Revision, Clinical Modification Coding

PURPOSE:

The ICD-9-CM code books provide a diagnostic coding system for the compilation and reporting of morbidity and mortality statistics for reimbursement purposes.

EQUIPMENT/SUPPLIES:

Volumes 1 and 2 of the ICD-9-CM code books for the current year
Copy of the encounter form and access to the patient's chart
Pencil and paper

CASE SCENARIO:

Mary O'Keefe, a new patient, presents at the clinic today reporting painful, frequent urination. She is seen for 10 minutes, during which time the provider takes a focused history and completes a problem-focused examination. A routine urinalysis, nonautomated and without microscopy, is performed and a straightforward medical decision is made. Mary's preliminary diagnosis is painful urination. The urinalysis confirms a urinary tract infection. The provider writes her a prescription for an antibiotic and asks her to make an appointment in 10 days for another urinalysis to confirm the infection has cleared.

PROCEDURE STEPS:

1. Using Volume II of the ICD-9-CM code book, the alphanumeric Index to Diseases, look up

Procedure 18-2 (continued)

the main symptom or condition that brought the patient to the facility or the specific diagnosis confirmed by test results. In this case, the laboratory results confirmed a urinary tract infection. Code 599.0. RATIONALE: Use alphanumeric Volume II first to close in on the section of Volume I for specificity. *NOTE:* Enter the Tabular List, Volume I, with the first three digits of the code determined (599).

2. Using Volume I, look up code 599. Read through all of the 599 listings to determine the appropriate code having the highest level of specificity. RATIONALE: To establish the most accurate code: urinary tract infection, site not specified. 599.0.

PROCEDURE 18–3

Applying Third-Party Guidelines

PURPOSE:
To obtain written authorization to release necessary medical information to third-party payers.

EQUIPMENT/SUPPLIES:
Patient chart
CMS-1500 (08-05) claim form

PROCEDURE STEPS:
1. When the patient signs in at the reception desk, check his or her chart to ascertain whether an "Authorization to Release Medical Information" form has been signed and is currently valid. RATIONALE: PHI cannot be released without written authorization from the patient.

2. If there is no record of SIGNATURE ON FILE, have the patient sign Block 12 of the CMS-1500 (08-05) claim form or the offices' customized "AUTHORIZATION TO RELEASE MEDICAL INFORMATION" form. RATIONALE: PHI cannot be released without written authorization from the patient.

Courtesy of the Centers for Medicare and Medicaid Services. Reprinted according to www.cms.gov website content reuse policy.

PROCEDURE 18-4

Completing a Medicare CMS-1500 (08-05) Claim Form

PURPOSE:
To complete the CMS-1500 (08-05) insurance claim form for Medicare for reimbursement.

EQUIPMENT/SUPPLIES:
Patient information
Patient account or ledger card
Copy of patient's insurance card
Insurance claim form
Computer and printer

PROCEDURE STEPS:
1. The CARRIER section of the CMS-1500 (08-05) is in the upper portion of the form. The bar code that contained the carrier's name and address has been eliminated. Use the blank space at the top right of the section marked CARRIER to enter the name and address of the payer to whom this claim is being sent. The payer is the carrier, health plan, third-party administrator, or other payer who will handle the claim. The format for this information should be as follows:

   Key on line 4: first line — Name

   Key on line 5: second line — First line of address

   Key on line 6: third line — Second line of address

   Key on line 7: fourth line — City, state (2 letters) and zip code

   Do not use commas, periods, or other punctuation in the address. When entering a nine-digit ZIP code, do not include the hyphen. When printing page numbers on multiple-page claims (generally done by clearinghouses when converting the electronic claim form to the CMS 1500 claim form), print the page numbers in the Carrier Block on Line 8 beginning at column 32. Page numbers are to be printed as Page XX of YY. RATIONALE: The claims processor must know who the claim is from.

2. The PATIENT AND INSURED INFORMATION section asks for specific information related to the patient and his or her health insurance plan. The following information is required for this section. Complete each block as directed. RATIONALE: These blocks must be accurately completed or the claim may be denied.

   Block 1   Indicate the type of health insurance coverage applicable to this claim by placing an X in the Medicare box. Only one box can be marked.

   Block 1a   Enter insured's ID number as shown on insured's ID card for the payer to whom the claim is being submitted. RATIONALE: The insured's ID number is the identification number of the person who holds the policy. This information identifies the patient to the payer. (For Medicare beneficiaries, this appears as a nine-digit number followed by a letter.)

   Block 2   Enter the patient's full last name, first name, and middle initial in this block.

   Block 3   Enter the patient's eight-digit birth date (MMDDYYYY). Enter an X in the correct box to indicate sex of the patient. Only one box can be marked. If gender is unknown, leave blank.

   Block 4   Enter the insured's full last name, first name, and middle initial.

   Block 5   Enter the patient's mailing address and telephone number.

   Block 6   Enter an X in the correct box to indicate the patient's relationship to insured when Block 4 has been completed. Only one box can be marked.

1500

HEALTH INSURANCE CLAIM FORM
APPROVED BY NATIONAL UNIFORM CLAIM COMMITTEE 08/05
PICA   PICA

CARRIER

Courtesy of the Centers for Medicare and Medicaid Services. Reprinted according to www.cms.gov website content reuse policy.

Procedure 18-4 (continued)

CMS-1500 health insurance claim form — Patient and Insured Information section, including blocks 1–13. Courtesy of the Centers for Medicare and Medicaid Services. Reprinted according to www.cms.gov website content reuse policy.

Block 7	Enter the insured's address and telephone number. If Block 4 has been completed, then this field should also be completed.
Block 8	Enter an X in the box for the patient's marital status and in the box for the patient's employment or student status. Only one box on each line can be marked.
Block 9	If Block 11d is marked yes (to indicate that the patient carries a secondary insurance plan), complete fields 9 and 9a–d with the patient's secondary insurance information, otherwise leave blank. When additional group health coverage exists, enter other insured's full last name, first name, and middle initial of the enrollee in another health plan if it is different from that shown in Block 2.
Block 9a	Enter the policy or group number of the other insured. Do not use a hyphen or space as a separator within the policy or group number.
Block 9b	Enter the eight-digit date of birth (MMDDYYYY) of the other insured and an X to indicate the sex of the other insured. Only one box can be marked. If gender is unknown, leave blank.
Block 9c	Enter the name of the other insured's employer or school.
Block 9d	Enter the other insured's insurance plan or program name.
Blocks 10a–10c	When appropriate, enter an X in the correct box to indicate whether one or more of the services described in Block 24 are for a condition or injury that occurred on the job or as a result of an automobile or other accident. Only one box on each line can be marked. The two-letter state abbreviation must be shown if YES is marked in 10b. RATIONALE: Any item marked YES indicates there may be other applicable insurance coverage that would be primary.
Block 10d	Refer to the most current instructions from the applicable public or private payer regarding the use of this field.
Block 11	Enter the insured's policy or group number as it appears on the insured's health care ID card. If Block 4 has been completed, then this field should also be completed.

continues

Procedure 18-4 (continued)

Block 11a   Enter the eight-digit date of birth (MMDDYYYY) of the insured and an X to indicate the sex of the insured. Only one box can be marked. If gender is unknown, leave blank.

Block 11b   Enter the name of the insured's employer or school.

Block 11c   Enter the insurance plan or program name of the insured. (Some payers require an ID number of the primary insurer rather than the name in this field.)

Block 11d   When appropriate, enter an X in the correct box. If marked YES, complete Blocks 9 and 9a–d. Only one box can be marked.

Block 12   Enter "Signature on File," "SOF," or legal signature. When legal signature, enter date signed in the proper eight-digit format. If there is no signature on file, leave blank or enter "No Signature on File."

RATIONALE: The patient's or authorized person's signature indicates there is an authorization on file for the release of any medical or other information necessary to process or adjudicate the claim.

Block 13   Enter "Signature on File," "SOF," or legal signature. If there is no signature on file, leave blank or enter "No Signature on File." RATIONALE: The insured's or authorized person's signature indicates that there is a signature on file authorizing payment of medical benefits.

3. The PHYSICIAN OR SUPPLIER INFORMATION section must be accurately completed or the claim may be denied.

Block 14   Enter the eight-digit date of the first date of the present illness, injury, or pregnancy. For pregnancy, use the date of the last menstrual period (LMP) as the first date. Leave blank if unknown.

Courtesy of the Centers for Medicare and Medicaid Services. Reprinted according to www.cms.gov website content reuse policy.

Procedure 18-4 (continued)

Block 15	Enter the first date the patient had the same or a similar illness. Enter the date in the eight-digit format. Previous pregnancies are not a similar illness. Leave blank if unknown.
Block 16	If the patient is employed and is unable to work in current occupation, an eight-digit date must be shown for the "from–to" dates that the patient is unable to work. RATIONALE: An entry in this field may indicate employment-related insurance coverage.
Block 17	Enter the name (first name, middle initial, last name) and credentials of the professional who referred, ordered, or supervised the service(s) or supply(ies) on the claim. Do not use periods or commas within the name. A hyphen can be used for hyphenated names.
Block 17a	The two-digit qualifier code is entered in the small box. Qualifiers are as follows:

0B State License Number

1B Blue Shield Provider Number

1C Medicare Provider Number

1D Medicaid Provider Number

1G Provider UPIN Number

1H CHAMPUS Identification Number

E1 Employer's Identification Number

G2 Provider Commercial Number

LU Location Number

N5 Provider Plan Network Identification Number

SY Social Security Number (the Social Security number may not be used for Medicare)

X5 State Industrial Accident Provider Number

ZZ Provider Taxonomy

The other ID number of the referring, ordering, or supervising provider is reported in the larger space.

Block 17b	Enter the NPI number of the referring, ordering, or supervising provider. RATIONALE: The NPI number refers to the HIPAA National Provider Identifier number.
Block 18	Enter the inpatient eight-digit hospital admission date followed by the discharge date (if discharge has occurred). If not discharged, leave discharge date blank.
Block 19	Refer to the most current instruction from the applicable public or private payer regarding the use of this field.
Block 20	Complete this field when billing for purchased services. Enter an X in "YES" if the reported service(s) was performed by an entity other than the billing provider. If "YES," enter the purchased price under charges. RATIONALE: A "YES" indicates that an entity other than the entity billing for the service performed the purchased services. A "NO" indicates that no purchased services are included on the claim. Only one box can be marked.
Block 21	Enter the patient's diagnosis/condition. You may list up to four ICD-9-CM diagnosis codes. Relate lines 1, 2, 3, and 4 to the lines of service in Block 24E by line number. Use the highest level of specificity. Do not provide a narrative description in this field. When entering the number, include a space between the two sets of numbers.
Block 22	Enter the original reference number for resubmitted claims. Refer to the most current instruction from the applicable public or private payer regarding the use of this field. If it is not a resubmitted claim, leave this block blank.
Block 23	Enter any of the following: prior authorization number, referral number, mammography precertification number, or CLIA number, as assigned by the payer for the current service. Do not enter hyphens or spaces within the number.

continues

Procedure 18-4 (continued)

Block 24A Enter date(s) of service, from and to. If there is one date of service only (such as a clinic visit), enter that date within the "From" blank as well as the "To" blank. Both the "From" and "To" areas must be completed in order to comply with proper completion rules.

Block 24B Enter the appropriate two-digit code from the Place of Service Code list for each item used or service performed. Place of Service Codes are available at www.cms.hhs.gov/PlaceofService Codes/Downloads/POSDataBase .pdf.

Block 24C This block was originally titled "Type of Service" and is no longer used. Check with trading partner to determine if emergency indicator is necessary. If required, enter Y for "YES" or leave blank if "NO." RATIONALE: The definition of emergency would be defined by either federal or state regulations or programs or payer contracts, or as defined in the electronic 837 Professional 4010A1 implementation guide.

Block 24D Enter the CPT or HCPCS code(s) and modifier(s), if applicable, from the appropriate code set in effect on the date of service.

Block 24E Enter the diagnosis code reference number as shown in Block 21 to relate the date of service and the procedures performed to the primary diagnosis. When multiple services are performed, the primary reference number for each service should be listed first; other applicable services should follow. Enter the numbers left justified in the field. Do not use commas between the numbers.

Block 24F Enter number right justified in the dollar area of the field. Do not use commas when reporting dollar amounts. Negative dollar amounts are not allowed. Dollar signs should not be entered. Enter 00 in the cents area if the amount is a whole number.

Block 24G Enter the number of days or units. This field is most commonly used for multiple visits, units of supplies, anesthesia units or minutes, or oxygen volume. If only one service is performed, the numeral 1 must be entered. Enter numbers right justified in the field.

Block 24H For Early and Periodic Screening, Diagnosis and Treatment-related services, enter the response as follows: If there is no requirement to report a reason code for EPDST, enter Y for "YES" if the service applies to EPDST. If "NO," leave blank.

Block 24I Enter the qualifier identifying if the number is a non-NPI. The Other ID# of the rendering provider is reported in Block 24J. The NUCC defines the same qualifiers as listed for Block 17a.

Block 24J Enter the non-NPI ID number in the top portion of the field if applicable. Enter the NPI number of the service provider in the lower area of the field.

Block 25 Enter the provider of service or supplier federal tax ID or Social Security number. Enter an X in the appropriate box to indicate which number is being reported. Only one box can be marked. Do not enter hyphens with numbers. Enter numbers left justified in the field.

Block 26 Enter the patient's account number assigned by the provider of service's or supplier's accounting system. Do not enter hyphens with numbers. Enter numbers left justified in the field.

Block 27 Enter an X in the correct box. Only one box can be marked.

Procedure 18-4 (continued)

Block 28 Enter total charges for the services (total of all charges in Block 24F). Enter number right justified in the dollar area of the field. Do not use commas when reporting dollar amounts. Negative dollar amounts are not allowed. Dollar signs should not be entered. Enter 00 in the cents area if the amount is a whole number.

Block 29 Enter the total amount the patient or other payers paid on the covered services only (such as a co-payment given on the date of service). Enter number right justified in the dollar area of the field. Do not use commas when reporting dollar amounts. Negative dollar amounts are not allowed. Dollar signs should not be entered. Enter 00 in the cents area if the amount is a whole number.

Block 30 Enter the total amount due. Enter number right justified in the dollar area of the field. Do not use commas when reporting dollar amounts. Negative dollar amounts are not allowed. Dollar signs should not be entered. Enter 00 in the cents area if the amount is a whole number.

Block 31 Enter the legal signature of the practitioner or supplier, signature of the practitioner or supplier representative, "Signature on File," or "SOF."

Enter either the eight-digit date the form was signed. RATIONALE: The signature refers to the authorized or accountable person and the degree, credentials, or title.

Block 32 Enter the name, address, city, state, and ZIP code of the location where the services were rendered. Providers of service must identify the supplier's name, address, ZIP code, and NPI number when billing for purchased diagnostic tests. When more than one supplier is used, a separate claim form should be used to bill for each supplier. Follow previously outlined format for entering address information.

Block 32a Enter the NPI number of the service facility location.

Block 32b Enter the two-digit qualifier identifying the non-NPI number followed by the ID number. Use the same qualifiers as listed in Block 17a.

Block 33 Enter the provider's or supplier's billing name, address, ZIP code, and phone number. The phone number is to be entered in the area to the right of the field title. Follow previously outlined format for entering address information.

Block 33a Enter the NPI number of the billing provider.

Block 33b Enter the two-digit qualifier identifying the non-NPI number followed by the ID number as listed in Block 17a.

CASE STUDY 18-1

Refer to the scenario at the beginning of the chapter.

CASE STUDY REVIEW

1. Explain why coding accurately is important to health care providers and insurance companies that act as third-party payers for health care services rendered to patients.

2. List ways to ensure accurate coding.

3. Recall common errors in completing insurance claim forms.

CASE STUDY 18-2

Leo McKay, an established patient at Inner City Health Care, schedules a visit, reporting nausea and severe abdominal pain. Dr. Mark Woo spends 30 minutes taking a history and doing an examination. He suspects an ulcer and orders laboratory tests (complete blood count [CBC], guaiac, lipid panel, and urinalysis [UA]) to be done in the clinic and sends Mr. McKay for an upper GI series. Mr. McKay returns in 10 days to learn that the test results show a duodenal ulcer.

CASE STUDY REVIEW

1. What are the proper diagnosis codes for Mr. McKay?
2. What are the proper procedure codes for Mr. McKay?
3. In coding the claim form for Mr. McKay's visit, what ethical principle and legal principle should guide the medical assistant?

SUMMARY

Much material has been covered in this chapter. Remember, you can be the person to make a difference in insurance billing. By checking and double-checking your work, you make certain that the provider's time is being billed at the appropriate rate, that all procedures are billed with the proper diagnoses and CPT codes, and that the billing is sent to the correct insurance carrier. It takes much less time to double-check this work and have it correct *before* it is sent out than to send it out with errors that cause difficulty in the future.

An understanding of medical insurance coverages and coding procedures is vital to a thriving ambulatory care setting. The astute medical assistant will perceive the challenges involved in proper coding techniques and will understand his or her role in the management of the provider's clinic.

STUDY FOR SUCCESS

To reinforce your knowledge and skills of information presented in this chapter:

- Review the *Key Terms*
- Role-play with other students to apply attributes of professionalism pertinent to this chapter.
- Consider the *Case Studies* and discuss your conclusions
- Answer the questions in the *Certification Review*
- Apply your knowledge by completing the *Activities* in the *Study Guide* and the *Games and Quizzes* in the StudyWARE StudyWARE software on the *Premium Website*
- Perform the *Procedures* using the *Competency Manual Checklists* in the *Competency Manual*
- Practice your problem-solving skills with the *Critical Thinking Challenge 3.0* on the *Premium Website*

Additional resources for this chapter include:

- Module 8 of the *Medical Assisting Learning Lab*
- *CourseMate for Delmar's Comprehensive Medical Assisting*
- *WebTutor for Delmar's Comprehensive Medical Assisting*

CERTIFICATION REVIEW

1. CPT codes:
   a. are for diagnosis coding
   b. have five digits and may have two-digit modifiers
   c. have three-digit codes with a decimal point and one to two additional digits
   d. are updated semiannually

2. When coding a diagnosis, go first to:
   a. CPT
   b. Volume I of ICD-9-CM
   c. Volume II of ICD-9-CM
   d. E codes in ICD-9-CM

3. Level II of HCPCS:
   a. provides codes to enable the provider to report nonprovider services
   b. is the same as the regular CPT system
   c. is assigned by the fiscal intermediary
   d. uses the letter codes W, X, Y, and Z

4. The ICD-9-CM codes:
   a. were developed by the AMA as uniform descriptions of medical, surgical, and diagnostic services
   b. are divided into seven sections
   c. use modifiers
   d. code every disease, illness, condition, injury, and cause of injury known

5. Most insurance carriers accept which claim form?
   a. UB-04
   b. CMS-1500 (08-05)
   c. CPT
   d. HCFA-1450

6. Claim registers are used to:
   a. anticipate claims to be sent to insurance companies for processing
   b. check how many claims are sent to Medicare
   c. monitor claims that have been sent to insurance companies for processing
   d. help in aging accounts

7. Information to be included in the CARRIER section of the CMS-1500 (08-05) insurance claim form includes all of the following *except:*
   a. the payer's name
   b. the patient's name
   c. the payer's address
   d. the payer's city, state, and ZIP code

8. Information to be included in the PATIENT AND INSURED section of the CMS-1500 (08-05) insurance claim form includes all of the following *except*:
   a. health insurance plan
   b. patient's name and address
   c. insured's name and address
   d. NPI number of the billing provider

9. Differentiate the following as either CPT or ICD-9-CM codes and list the code you assign to each:
   a. irregular menstrual cycle
   b. biopsy, soft tissue of neck
   c. dissection of the renal artery
   d. adenitis, lymph gland, except mesenteric
   e. thyroid hormone (T_3 or T_4) uptake
   f. hearing aid examination and selection; monaural

REFERENCES/BIBLIOGRAPHY

American Medical Association. (2011). *Current procedural terminology.* Chicago: American Medical Association.

American Medical Association. (2011). *International classification of diseases, clinical modifications* (ICD-9) (2nd ed., 9th rev.). Chicago: American Medical Association.

Bowie, M. J., & Schaffer, R. (2011). *Understanding ICD-10-CM and ICD-10-PCS: a worktext.* Clifton Park, NY: Delmar Cengage Learning.

Greene, M. A. (2012). *3–2–1 Code it!* (3rd ed.). Clifton Park, NY: Delmar Cengage Learning.

ingenix. (2003). *HIPAA tool kit.* Salt Lake City: St. Anthony Publishing/Medicode.

ingenix. (2011). *HCPCS level II.* Salt Lake City: St. Anthony Publishing/Medicode.

Moisio, M. A. (2011). *A guide to health insurance billing* (3rd ed.). Clifton Park, NY: Delmar Cengage Learning.

Office of Inspector General, U.S. Department of Health and Human Services. (2000). *Compliance program guide for individual and small group physician practices.* Retrieved March 1, 2003, from http://oig.hhs.gov/authorities/docs/physcian.pdf

CHAPTER 19
Daily Financial Practices

OUTLINE

Patient Fees
Helping Patients Who
  Cannot Pay
Determining Patient Fees
Discussion of Fees
Adjustment of Fees
Credit Arrangements
Payment Planning
The Bookkeeping Function
Managing Patient Accounts
Recording Patient Transactions
Encounter Form
Patient Account or Ledger

Day Sheet
Receipts
Month-End Activities
Computerized Patient
  Accounts
Banking Procedures
Online Banking
Types of Accounts
Types of Checks
Depositing Checks
Cash on Hand
Accepting Checks
Lost or Stolen Checks

Writing and Recording
  Checks
Reconciling a Bank Statement
**Purchasing Supplies and
Equipment**
Preparing a Purchase Order
Verifying Goods Received
Petty Cash
Establishing a Petty Cash
  Fund
Tracking, Balancing, and
  Replenishing Petty Cash

LEARNING OUTCOMES

1. Define, spell, and pronounce the key terms as presented in the glossary.
2. Practice the importance of effective communication in regard to establishing patient fees.
3. Identify circumstances that require adjustment of fees and post accordingly.
4. Develop knowledge of various credit arrangements for patient fees.
5. Differentiate between bookkeeping and accounting.
6. Compare manual and computerized bookkeeping systems in ambulatory healthcare.
7. Describe the pegboard system.
8. State the advantages of computerized systems for financial practices.
9. List six good working habits for financial records.

10. Describe the encounter form.
11. Identify the parts of the patient account or ledger.
12. Discuss preparation of patient receipts.
13. Describe month-end activities.
14. Describe banking procedures, including types of accounts and services.
15. Show proficiency in preparing deposits and checks and reconciling accounts.
16. Explain the process of purchasing equipment and supplies for the ambulatory care setting.
17. Demonstrate proficiency in establishing and maintaining a petty cash system.
18. Analyze the professionalism questions and apply them to this chapter's content.

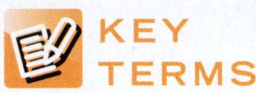

KEY TERMS

accounts payable

accounts receivable

adjustments

balance

cashier's check

certified check

credit

day sheet

debit

electronic check

encounter form

guarantor

ledger

money market account

notary

payee

pegboard system

petty cash

posting

traveler's check

voucher check

ATTRIBUTES OF PROFESSIONALISM

Communication
- Did you speak at the patient's level of understanding?
- Did you provide appropriate responses/feedback?
- Did you respond honestly and diplomatically to the patient's concerns?
- Did you apply active listening skills?
- Does your knowledge allow you to speak easily with all members of the health care team?
- Did you demonstrate assertive communication with managed care and/or insurance providers?

Presentation
- Did you attend to any special needs of the patient? Did you first ask if assistance was needed, rather than taking charge?
- Were you courteous, patient, and respectful to the patient?
- Did you display a positive attitude?
- Did you display a calm, professional, and caring manner?

Competency
- Did you pay attention to detail?
- Did you display sound judgment?
- Were you knowledgeable and accountable?
- Did you recognize the importance of local, state, and federal legislation and regulations in the practice setting?
- Did you demonstrate sensitivity and professionalism in handling accounts receivable with patients?

Initiative
- Did you show initiative?
- Did you direct the patient to other resources when necessary or helpful, with the approval of the provider?
- Did you work with the provider to achieve maximum reimbursement?

Integrity
- Did you protect and maintain confidentiality?
- Did you immediately report any error you had made?
- Did you maintain your moral and ethical standards?

SCENARIO

At the clinic of Drs. Lewis and King, many different types of patients are seen. Most have some kind of insurance, either a traditional plan or an HMO plan; some are on Medicare; a few are on Medicaid; and occasionally a patient does not have any insurance or any financial resources to pay for treatment. Whoever schedules the first patient appointment also opens a courteous discussion with the patient about provider fees and the patient's anticipated method of payment. Initiating this discussion of fees at the beginning of the provider–patient relationship keeps patients informed of their responsibility for payment and helps the medical assistants at Drs. Lewis and King's practice make any necessary credit arrangements with the patient before treatment begins.

INTRODUCTION

Ambulatory care settings are primarily designed to serve the patient. However, without sound financial practices, patient care will suffer and the practice will not thrive and grow. The health care industry is complex and complicated. The impact of managed care and the many detailed insurance plans affect not only the way patients receive treatment, but the manner in which the ambulatory care center is administered from a financial point of view.

The discussion of fees is only a small part of the ambulatory care setting's daily financial practices. Selecting an appropriate system for tracking patient accounts, overseeing banking procedures, managing the purchase of supplies, controlling patient accounts, and establishing a petty cash system all are important to the smooth functioning of today's ambulatory care setting.

PATIENT FEES

All providers receive education, training, and experience in diagnosing and treating the concerns of their patients. That is their major concern; therefore, the management of the business details usually becomes the responsibility of the medical assisting staff. This includes but is not limited to: informing the patients about charges, collecting payments, making credit arrangements if necessary, and making certain that patients and their providers receive the full benefit of medical insurance. An attitude that anticipates that the majority of patients pay their medical bills in a timely and responsible manner is helpful in completing these tasks.

Helping Patients Who Cannot Pay

   There are times when patients may have difficulty paying their bills. The economy is constantly changing, and with its fluctuations, individuals lose their jobs and often their medical insurance. The majority of today's employment force does not recall a time without medical insurance when patients expected to pay the total fee for medical services. These same patients may not fully comprehend what medical services cost. They likely do not understand the explanation of benefits (EOB) from their insurance reports. There is also a growing number of "working poor" in society, who may work two or more part-time jobs but never qualify for company insurance benefits and struggle daily to pay necessary bills. Some patients must decide whether to put food on the table or pay the provider. Emergencies can deplete an individual's financial resources as well. These are the times when the administrative medical assistant might make financial arrangements with patients allowing full payment for the services provided. Patients will appreciate the assistance, and the administrative medical assistant can expect the patient to abide by the agreed plan. Such an agreement fosters a climate where patients are less likely to withdraw from any necessary medical treatment when their finances are low.

Determining Patient Fees

Providers place a value on their services. In today's managed care environment, ambulatory care settings have many different arrangements with patients, insurance carriers, and health maintenance organization (HMO) insurance contracts. Managed care contracts pay predetermined fees for specific procedures and services. Providers who practice in a concierge-type medical group collect an additional fee. This usually is a flat fee at the beginning of each year for the specialized service; many do not accept the insurance carrier's required co-payment. Patients who choose concierge medical services are willing to pay the additional fee and generally have the resources to do so. Provider fees for procedures, however, are billed and reimbursed according to standard insurance guidelines. Chapter 17 provides further details on fees.

Discussion of Fees

The manner in which billing is done and fees are established varies depending on the type of medical facility, the needs of the practice, and the professional services rendered. Today, the fee for the visit is simply stated, and if a person does not have cash or a check, the option of credit or debit card payment is often provided. If a patient is a member of an HMO, the patient is expected to pay any established co-payment amount at the time of service.

Inherent to the total billing process is the necessity of informing patients of charges and exactly what portion of the bill they are expected to pay. Ideally, the patient should be told the approximate cost of the procedures at the start of treatment. For Medicare and Medicaid patients, a form officially known by Medicare as an Advanced Beneficiary Notification (ABN) or by Medicaid as a waiver is the only legal means a clinic has to collect payment on charges not allowed by Medicare or Medicaid. These forms are to be in writing, should indicate the type of procedure(s), the total responsibility of the patient, and the reason why this payment is the patient's responsibility.

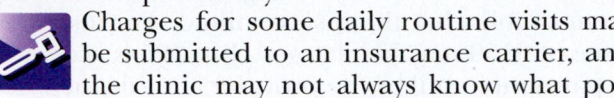 Charges for some daily routine visits may be submitted to an insurance carrier, and the clinic may not always know what portions are covered until information is received from the carrier. The facility may contract with numerous insurance plans, including private carriers, and participation in these plans determines the amount the patient owes. Many misunderstandings can be prevented and subsequent collection of delinquent accounts expedited when the clinic staff is well informed about insurance reimbursement and carefully explains fees to the patients.

Adjustment of Fees

Providers who accept assignment with Medicare and Medicaid are mandated to charge every patient the same amount for similar services rendered. If a professional courtesy is extended, then it is considered insurance fraud, because the clinic would be billing insurance an increased rate over what others are charged. Deductibles are to be collected from patients as part of their premium expectation. Unless you follow government guidelines for establishing when patients are financially unable to pay their portion of the bill, you cannot give discounts to patients for cash payments.

Adjustments may be made for patients with limited income. For example, for patients who recently lost a job or ran into unfortunate financial circumstances, the provider may write off a portion of the bill. This sum will be written off against the provider's income, and the patients do not pay that portion.

Adjustments also may occur with Medicare, Medicaid, Blue Cross/Blue Shield, and private

PATIENT EDUCATION

One way to easily provide information to patients regarding fees is to include in the clinic brochure policies regarding fees, insurance, co-payments, and how third-party payments are handled. If credit and debit cards are allowed, include that information as well.

health insurance patients. Providers who accept assignment in these programs agree to accept as payment in full what the insurer allows. For instance, a fee of $150 may be charged, but $95 is accepted as payment in full by the provider after deductibles and co-payments are satisfied. The remainder of the bill, $55, is written off so that the patient is not responsible for the nonallowed amount.

Medical assistants must be aware, however, of the pitfalls of adjusting or reducing fees. It is difficult to accept all hardship cases and still remain a viable practice. It is always a helpful resource to patients who cannot pay to be given the names and telephone numbers of local health care clinics that may be able to accept them as patients on a sliding scale or no-fee basis.

Refunds. On rare occasion, a refund will be necessary. It usually occurs when the insurance carrier pays more than anticipated. Notably, there are a few members of the older adult population who may still be a little uncomfortable with Medicare and are accustomed to paying for all their medical expenses out of pocket; therefore, they will pay their entire bill when the statement is received. When Medicare payments arrive, an overpayment is created. The financial transaction required is to prepare a check for the amount due to the patient and enter the transaction on the **day sheet** and patient account or ledger.

CREDIT ARRANGEMENTS

 If the patient will need to pay a substantial out-of-pocket amount, it is beneficial to make the patient aware of this and discuss different credit arrangements that can be made. Many ambulatory care settings will accept prearranged installment payments, usually without finance charges, to spread the cost of services over a pre-agreed period. This eases the financial burden on the patient and also makes it more likely that the balance due will be collected.

Payment Planning

Medical assistants can help patients plan for anticipated medical expenses (having a baby, surgery, extensive therapy). When patient and provider know in advance that there will be costly medical expenses, the medical assistant should review the patient's insurance coverage. It is helpful to prepare an estimate sheet, which will give the patient an idea of the cost of the medical services for the planned treatment. The estimate may also include the anticipated cost of anesthetist, consultants, and hospital charges.

Many ambulatory care settings accept credit and debit cards as a means of payment. Remember, this service is strictly for the convenience of the patient, and providers cannot increase their charges for patients who wish to use these cards even though the provider is charged a fee for this service. Credit and debit cards are convenient and ensure payment; therefore, the practice may wish to encourage their use.

The one advantage to the ambulatory care setting that accepts credit/debit cards is that monies for fees charged usually are available within 24 hours. Also, the provider is relieved of the responsibility of collection. However, credit card companies do assess a fee for every charge made, which the ambulatory care center must pay.

 When a patient decides to use a credit or debit card, it is extremely important that confidentiality be maintained to the fullest extent possible. When writing a description of the services on the credit card receipt, the medical assistant should be as vague as possible to preserve patient confidentiality. For example, "medical services" is often used.

THE BOOKKEEPING FUNCTION

Daily financial management in the ambulatory care setting is important to the functioning of the clinic, because it directly affects overall accounting and bookkeeping procedures. *Accounting* generates financial information for the ambulatory care setting and is defined as a system of monitoring the financial status of a facility and the specific results of its activities. Accounting provides financial information for decision making (see Chapter 21). *Bookkeeping*, the actual daily recording of the accounts or transactions of the business, is a major part of this accounting process. This chapter deals with daily bookkeeping (or recording) functions necessary to manage the income and expenses of an ambulatory care setting.

Managing Patient Accounts

All businesses must keep careful records of income and expenses for tax and legal purposes. One aspect of this recordkeeping in a medical practice is maintaining patient accounts. Because few patients are able to pay in full each time they are seen by the provider, it is necessary to maintain account records for each individual or family as opposed to simply keeping a record of cash received, as is done in many other types of business. The total amount of money owed to the medical facility by patients is known as **accounts receivable**; this must be carefully monitored to ensure that the provider is paid for services provided in a timely manner and that patients are properly credited for payments made.

There are various ways to track patients' balances. This chapter discusses the two most common methods:

- Computerized financial systems
- The **pegboard system** (also known as the write-it-once method)

Although the financial records of most practices are fully automated, many practices probably started with some sort of manual system (generally pegboard). Converting from manual to computerized recordkeeping seems cumbersome at the beginning, but it offers great versatility and reduces the need to record and re-record entries. A knowledgeable medical assistant will understand both the manual and computerized systems.

The Importance of Good Working Habits in Financial Transactions.

In managing the day-to-day finances of the ambulatory care setting, always observe the following guidelines:

1. Always work with care and accuracy; it is extremely easy to transpose numbers (e.g., entering 23 instead of 32) or make other posting errors. A moment of carelessness can result in hours spent trying to find the mistake.
2. The work must be kept current or it may become an overwhelming chore.
3. Double-check all entries made for accuracy.

In a manual bookkeeping system, follow these additional rules:

- Use a consistent ink color; black or blue is preferred.
- Form your numbers and letters carefully, using neat and clear writing.
- Align your columns carefully, preferably using paper with grid lines.

- Write small enough to stay within the columns.
- Be careful when placing or carrying decimal points.
- Double-check all math.
- If a mistake is found, draw one line through the error and write "Corr." or "Correction" above it. Red ink may be used in correcting errors on a paper copy.

Pegboard System. A complete pegboard or write-it-once system consists of day sheets, ledger cards, **encounter forms** or charge slips, and receipt forms. The forms are designed to work together to simplify the task and to avoid mistakes in patient accounts. All forms have matching columns that align and are held in place on the pegboard when the system is in use (Figure 19-1). The forms are on NCR (no carbon required) paper, which permits entering of charges, credits, or adjustments, called **posting**, onto the day sheet, encounter form, or receipt and the patient's ledger simultaneously. The day sheet provides complete and up-to-date information about accounts receivable status at a glance. Also, a pegboard system is relatively inexpensive.

Computerized Financial Systems. The majority of medical facilities use computers for bookkeeping. A number of medical practice software packages are available on the market. These ready-made systems are available for both single or multiple-provider partnerships and large group practices. Occasionally, a consultant is hired to design a customized program, although this can be more expensive than purchasing mass-produced software. When selecting and using any computer system:

- Be sure the system will meet current needs, and will grow with the practice.
- Consider adopting a system that allows the practice to start with one component, such as scheduling, and to add another component, such as bookkeeping and medical records, at a later date until the entire practice is fully automated (Figure 19-2).

CRITICAL THINKING

Discuss with another student the advantages and disadvantages of adopting a computer system that allows the practice to start with one component and add more components at a later time.

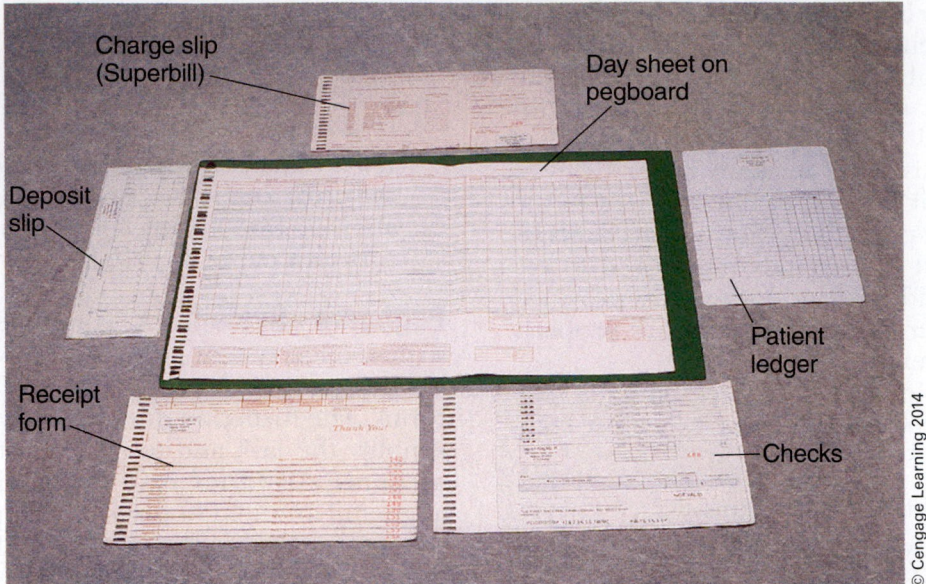

Charge slip
(Superbill)

Day sheet on
pegboard

Deposit
slip

Patient
ledger

Receipt
form

Checks

© Cengage Learning 2014

Figure 19-1 An example of a pegboard system and possible overlays.

RECORDING PATIENT TRANSACTIONS

The administrative medical assistant is largely responsible for recording patient transactions for the practice. Bookkeeping activities must be exact. Either they are right or they are wrong, and in any form of business, they have to be right to be correct and to be "in balance." In the pegboard or manual system, if an error is made during entry, it will carry through to all the other documents, thus compounding the error. In a computerized system, there is the old but true statement, "garbage in, garbage out." All entries must be correct; there is no room for just a "slight" mistake.

In one way or another, the forms and procedures discussed in the following sections are common elements to any system of bookkeeping for a medical practice.

Encounter Form

The encounter form, also known as the charge slip, superbill, or multipurpose billing form, is used in both manual and computerized bookkeeping systems. It often is a three-part form that has the following functions:

1. Provides patients one copy with a record of account activity for the day (usually a pink form)
2. Provides a second copy of account activity for possible insurance submission (usually a yellow form)

3. Provides a third copy that serves as the clinic's permanent copy of account activity (usually a white form)

The encounter forms can be custom designed to fit the particular practice, computer system, or pegboard. Information on the form includes the patient's name, address, account number, and necessary insurance information, as well as any previous balance. Often, the encounter form is attached to the patient's chart so that the provider is able to indicate the day's activities and charges; the provider can also use this form to indicate a requested return visit. The encounter form will typically include procedure and diagnosis codes. The most applicable procedure codes can be preselected and printed on the encounter form to fit the practice, with blank lines added for infrequently used procedures. Often, providers use the form to check the appropriate procedures and diagnoses while they are still with the patient in the examination room. The encounter form also will carry the name, address, and telephone number of the practice and the attending provider's 10-digit National Provider Identifier (NPI).

Encounter forms are designed to fit over the pegs of a pegboard system when a manual system is used. In a computerized system, an encounter form carrying the same information is prepared for the patient, printed, and attached to the patient chart. Some computer systems automatically match the correct charge to the procedure code identified. When a facility is totally automated (including medical records), the provider identifies

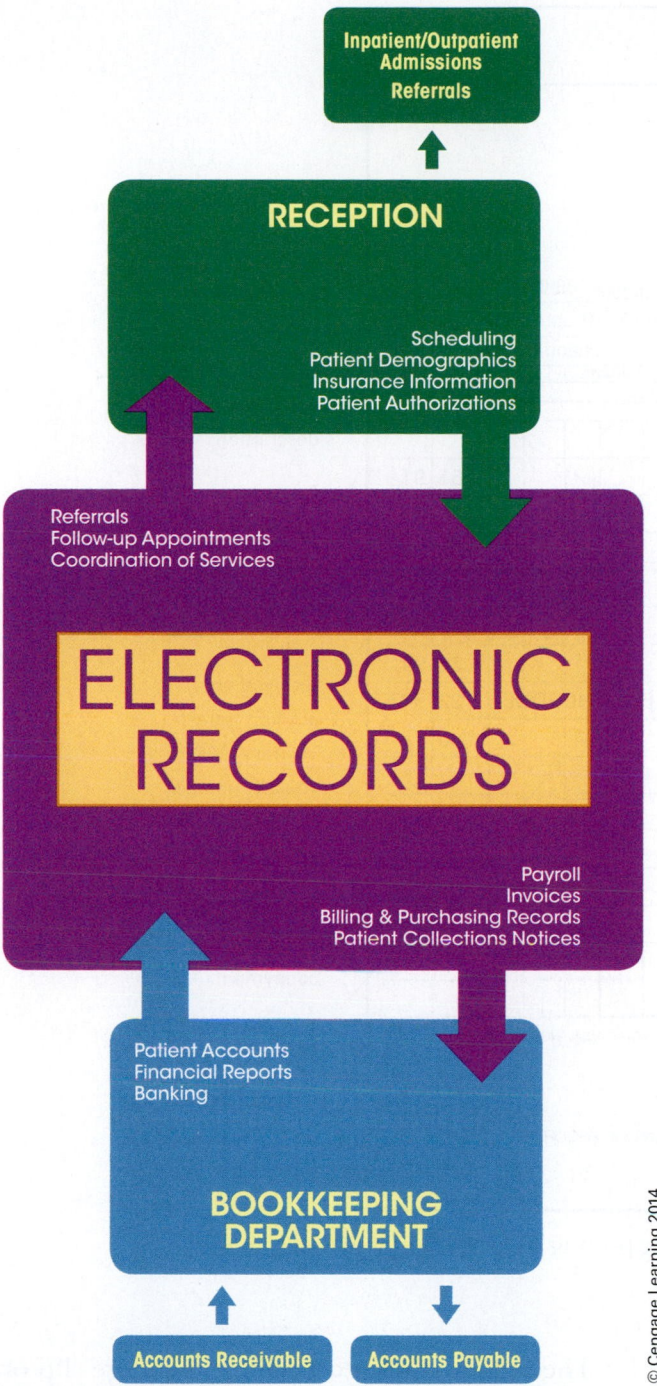

Figure 19-2   Total practice management system diagram illustrating the connection between daily financial practices, patients' electronic medical records, and reception/scheduling activities.

patient procedures in the medical record on the computer. The computer software assigns appropriate codes and charges to create the encounter form, which can be printed for the patient at the completion of the service.

Patient Account or Ledger

The financial record of the patient is known as that patient's account. All the patient accounts with outstanding balances make up the accounts receivable. Patient accounts are recorded in an accounts receivable **ledger**. (Figure 19-3 illustrates a typewritten ledger.) The ledger, or record of services, lists payments and balances due. In family practice, each adult has his or her own ledger or account that carries insurance information, name of subscriber, and patient's relationship to the subscriber. A responsible party is identified for each minor or patient who does not have insurance, and that name also appears on the ledger. Charges for any members of the family seen in the clinic are entered on their own ledger. It is important that charges and credits be applied to the correct family member for insurance purposes and accurate bookkeeping practices.

In cases of divorced parents and blended families, the parent with physical custody of the child is considered to be the **guarantor** and the one responsible for payment if the child is not insured with a contracted insurance carrier or if there is any amount leftover once the insurance has paid. This prevents the staff from having to interpret divorce decrees and parenting plan documents. This information should be clearly identified and discussed with the parent when appointments are made.

In the manual system of bookkeeping, ledger cards are used. They have a minimum of three columns for entering figures:

1. **Debit** column is on the left and is used for entering charges and a brief description of services, including a procedure code.
2. **Credit** column is to the right of the debit column and is used for entering payments.
3. **Balance** column is at the far right and is used to record the difference between the debit and credit columns and shows any amount due.

Most ledger cards have space for another column called **adjustments**, which are used to indicate any insurance payments, personal discounts or write-offs, or any other subtractions for the account that need to be recorded.

The adjustment column is a credit column; therefore, entries here normally reduce the balance due. When making an adjustment intended to increase the balance, a negative entry (in parentheses) is made to show that you reverse the function when you balance. (Add instead of subtract

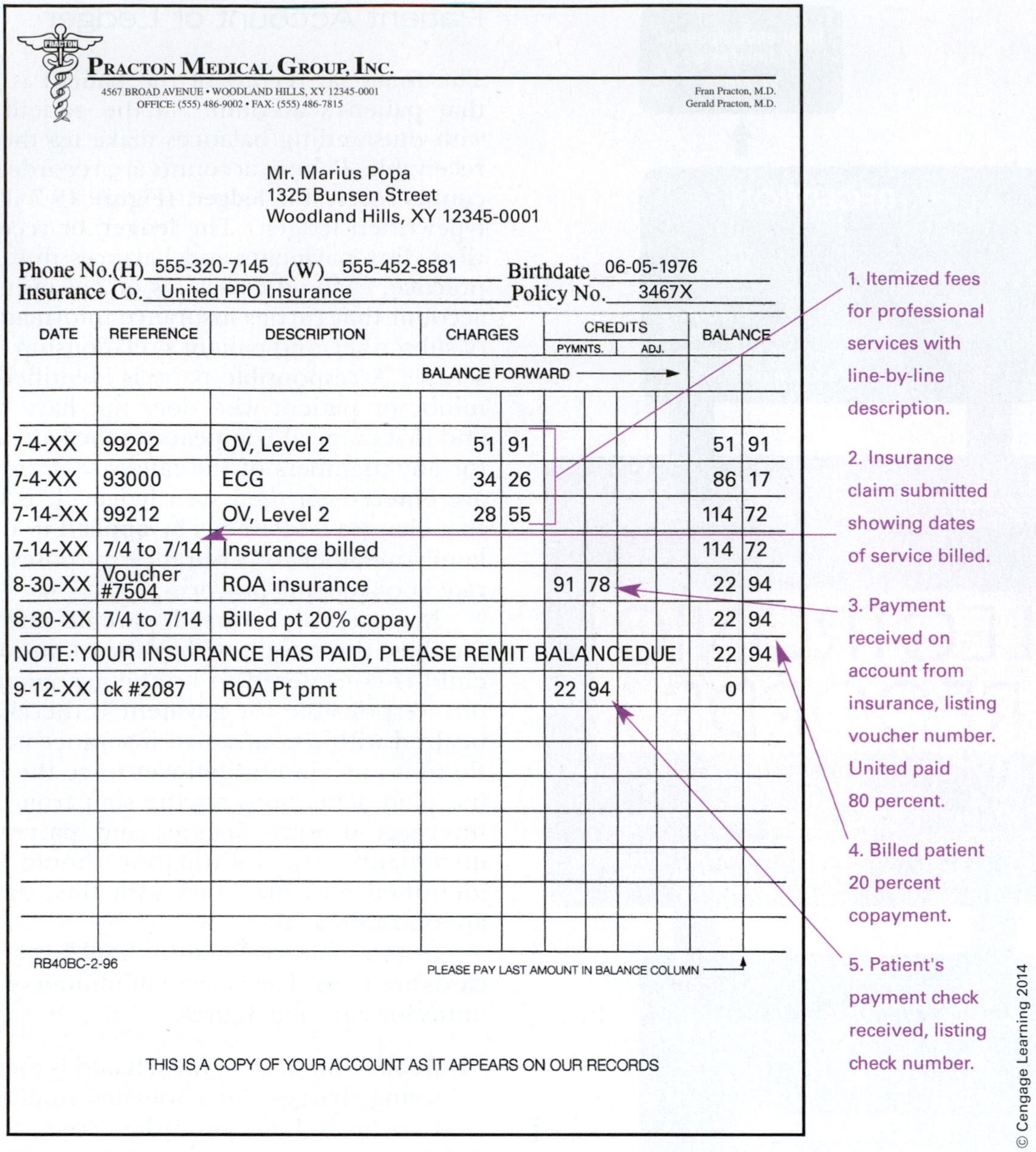

PRACTON MEDICAL GROUP, INC.

4567 BROAD AVENUE • WOODLAND HILLS, XY 12345-0001
OFFICE: (555) 486-9002 • FAX: (555) 486-7815

Fran Practon, M.D.
Gerald Practon, M.D.

Mr. Marius Popa
1325 Bunsen Street
Woodland Hills, XY 12345-0001

Phone No.(H) 555-320-7145 (W) 555-452-8581   Birthdate 06-05-1976
Insurance Co. United PPO Insurance   Policy No.   3467X

DATE	REFERENCE	DESCRIPTION	CHARGES	CREDITS PYMNTS.	CREDITS ADJ.	BALANCE
		BALANCE FORWARD ⟶				
7-4-XX	99202	OV, Level 2	51 91			51 91
7-4-XX	93000	ECG	34 26			86 17
7-14-XX	99212	OV, Level 2	28 55			114 72
7-14-XX	7/4 to 7/14	Insurance billed				114 72
8-30-XX	Voucher #7504	ROA insurance		91 78		22 94
8-30-XX	7/4 to 7/14	Billed pt 20% copay				22 94
NOTE: YOUR INSURANCE HAS PAID, PLEASE REMIT BALANCE DUE						22 94
9-12-XX	ck #2087	ROA Pt pmt		22 94		0

RB40BC-2-96

PLEASE PAY LAST AMOUNT IN BALANCE COLUMN ⟶

THIS IS A COPY OF YOUR ACCOUNT AS IT APPEARS ON OUR RECORDS

1. Itemized fees for professional services with line-by-line description.

2. Insurance claim submitted showing dates of service billed.

3. Payment received on account from insurance, listing voucher number. United paid 80 percent.

4. Billed patient 20 percent copayment.

5. Patient's payment check received, listing check number.

© Cengage Learning 2014

Figure 19-3   Typewritten ledger card illustrating posting of professional services, fees, payments, and balance due.

the amount.) For example, Edith Leonard had surgery, and because of a hardship, the provider agreed to reduce the fee by half of the balance remaining after insurance has paid. At the time of surgery, a charge of $2,500 is entered on her ledger and the day sheet. Today, payment is received from her insurance company in the amount of $2,000, which would normally leave a balance of $500. However, because the provider agreed to write off half of that amount ($250), you enter $250 in the adjustment column when posting the insurance payment. That amount is subtracted from the previous balance to get the new total of $250.

The ledger is placed under the charge slip or encounter form in a pegboard system and aligned before posting. Never post any patient entry in this manual system without the patient's ledger in place. This prevents recording information on the day sheet while inadvertently omitting it from the patient's ledger. Procedure 19-1 identifies steps in recording/posting patient charges and adjustments in a manual system.

In the computerized system, a patient's account or ledger can be printed with the same information by just entering the patient's name and usually an identification number. The computerized patient account ledger provides more room for helpful detail and is much faster to create than the manual paper ledger.

Day Sheet

All financial transactions for professional services are posted daily on a day sheet or daily ledger. This is an important part of the overall bookkeeping process, so absolute accuracy is critical. At the close of each business day, the day sheet is balanced to provide a complete picture of all patient financial activity for that day. Those balances carry over from day to day to provide the accumulated data needed for month-end closing. If more than one day sheet is required to record all the transactions in the pegboard system, pages are numbered and the information is carried forward just as if it were a new day.

There are a number of different styles for the day sheet; some provide a deposit portion to use as a deposit slip and a section used for business analysis. For example, if the provider wants to know the amount of income generated from laboratory services performed in the clinic, the totals can be obtained from the day sheet columns where only laboratory charges were posted. Over time, the laboratory income totals can be compared with the cost for running the laboratory.

The pegboard write-it-once section is where individual transactions are posted, using the ledger card and encounter form on top of the day sheet. The information in this section includes the date, patient name, description of transaction or service, charges, credits, and previous and current balances. At the bottom of the day sheet, transactions are totaled and balanced at the end of the day. This total section includes space to bring forward the previous page balance for a month-to-date total. These totals allow the provider and office manager to monitor totals that assist in predicting the financial status for the practice. The total accounts receivable figure shows how much is owed to the provider by all patients to date, allowing management to see the total outstanding balance at a glance. A major disadvantage to this system, as mentioned earlier, is that an error made in one place is going to carry through to all the other forms. When balancing this financial information, always use a calculator's print function to create a tape of the calculations. These tapes are an invaluable time saver if the initial balance is incorrect and you need to search for mistakes. Procedure 19-2 describes the process for balancing a day sheet in a manual system.

Daily sheets or ledgers in a computerized system require the same data. The patient's name, date, diagnosis, and services provided are posted. The computer system or database matches the correct charge and posts it to the patient account and the accounts receivable ledger. Any error made is quickly changed and corrected throughout. Totals are automatically created for the day-end total, month-end total, and cumulative total from the beginning of the year.

Receipts

Unlike encounter forms, receipt forms used for payments on accounts usually are not customized with other than the name, address, and telephone number of the practice preprinted. The receipt form is used only when someone makes a payment on an account on a day when no services were rendered. In the pegboard system, this transaction is entered on the day sheet and the ledger card at the same time the receipt is filled out. When payments are received by mail, the same system is followed; however, there is no need to create a receipt.

In a computerized system, the receipt is easily printed for the patient as soon as the information has been entered and the patient account updated. If the patient needs a receipt and the payment is not posted right away, a handwritten receipt is acceptable.

The provider may have charges created from emergency department visits, patient hospital visits, surgeries, visits in a convalescent nursing facility, or other out-of-clinic services. These charges are to be entered on the day sheet and the ledger or patient's account. Some providers produce information manually in a pocket-size notebook, in a calendar, or on a personal handheld computer and give it to the medical assistant on their return to the clinic. The medical assistant then enters the data into the daily sheet and the patient's account. If the provider uses the handheld computer for tracking and recording of clinic charges, the medical assistant can electronically download the billing information.

Month-End Activities

In the pegboard system, when the last day sheet for the month has been balanced, it is then necessary to verify that the month-end figures on the day sheet agree with patient accounts. Although this may be a time-consuming process in the manual system, it will find mistakes before they grow into major accounting or collection problems.

Reconciling the month-end sheet to the patient ledgers is accomplished by adding all the open balances on the ledgers and verifying that the total agrees with the end-of-month accounts receivable balance on the last day sheet of the month. When these figures agree, the accounts receivable balance is correct.

By following these procedures of "checks and balances," it is likely that all payments have been properly credited to patient accounts and deposited, and that all charges shown as outstanding on the day sheet agree with the outstanding balances of the individual patient accounts. If a payment is somehow misplaced, the deposits will not agree with the credits or with the patient ledgers, and an error will be revealed immediately. Not only does this catch errors, it also eliminates the possibility of loss of a check or undetected theft of funds, because when a mistake is caught immediately, the payer can stop payment on the missing check or credit or debit card slip and a new payment can be made.

Computerized Patient Accounts

A total practice management system offers many advantages in managing patient accounts. The program automatically creates an encounter form the day before the patient is seen or when the administrative medical assistant prints out the schedule. After the patient's examination, the program calculates the charges for the monthly billing statement (Figure 19-4). The management program also creates and updates the patient account, adds new names to the list of patients and to the daily log, and transfers data to produce insurance forms, statements, a list of checks received each day, and deposit slips. In addition, the program automatically ages accounts at each billing cycle and creates billing statements (Figure 19-5). As a result, when patient accounts are computerized, practice collections usually increase.

The computerized patient account contains personal information about each patient, including name, address, and telephone number; email address; the person responsible for payment; and all insurance carriers. The account also lists all previous clinic visits and the procedures, procedure codes, charges, payments, and adjustments for each visit. Most account management software can be customized to meet the special needs of the individual ambulatory care setting.

As billing information is entered from the encounter forms, the computer automatically updates the account by adding a description of each procedure and procedure code and each diagnosis and diagnosis code. The computer software automatically posts the charges and calculates the balance after credits and adjustments are entered.

Once charges and payments have been entered and the day has been closed, they are not easily removed or changed. This is an important software design because it ensures that monies are not removed from receivables credited to a previous month. This procedure would cause the practice year-end balance to be unresolved. Procedures 19-3, 19-4, 19-5, and 19-6 describe the electronic process for recording patient charges, billing insurance, posting payments and adjustments, credit balances, and refunds.

As useful and efficient as a computerized bookkeeping system can be, it is important to recognize that an inadequate manual system will not get better once computerized. Also, it takes time to move to a computerized system, train personnel, and enter existing patient data. Manual and computer systems may need to run concurrently for a month or two.

BANKING PROCEDURES

Understanding bank accounts and services, making deposits, preparing checks, and reconciling accounts are all a part of daily financial practices. Although many banking services are similar from one bank to another, it is a good idea for the medical assistant in charge of maintaining daily accounts to investigate the banking resources of the local community. In an effort to secure new business, many banks compete for customers by offering special services that can be of use to the ambulatory care setting.

Online Banking

Use of the Internet has changed banking and the services it provides. Online banking allows individuals to check account balances, transfer funds between accounts, pay bills electronically, check credit card balances, view images of checks and deposits, and download account information 24 hours a day, 7 days a week. Considerable time and expense can be saved with online banking, but remember that any online banking should be completed only through the use of secure and unique passwords granted to only those individuals deemed necessary.

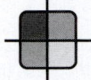

Douglasville Medicine Associates
5076 Brand Blvd., Suite 401
Douglasville, NY 01234
Ph: (123) 456-7890
Fax: (123) 456-7891
E-mail: admin@dfma.com
Web site: www.dfma.com

STATEMENT OF ACCOUNT

MANUEL RAMIREZ
1211 Gravel Way
Douglasville, NY 01234

Date: 1/3/20XX
Account No: RAM001

Date	Patient	Description of Service	Total Charges	Patient Payment	Insurance Payment	Adjust-ments	Deduct-ible	Current Balance
18-Oct-XX	Manuel Ramirez	Established Patient - Level 3 99213	$78.00	$0.00	$47.20	$19.00	$0	$11.80
29-Oct-XX	Manuel Ramirez	Colonoscopy 44389	$750.00	$0.00	$0.00	$0.00	$0	$750.00
29-Oct-XX	Manuel Ramirez	Established Patient - Level 5 99215	$176.00	$0.00	$0.00	$0.00	$0	$176.00
		Totals:	$569.00	$0.00	$47.20	$19.00	$0	$937.80

0 to 30 Days Current	31 to 60 Days Past Due	61 to 90 Days Past Due	91+ Days Past Due	BALANCE DUE	$937.80
$0.00	$0.00	$937.80	$0.00		

Important Note:

Figure 19-4 Computerized patient statement.

Types of Accounts

Checking and savings accounts are the two primary types of accounts used in the medical practice.

Checking Accounts. The checking account is the primary account type the medical assistant will use in the ambulatory care setting. Today, there are many variations on checking accounts. In the event that the medical assistant is responsible for establishing a new account, it is worthwhile to investigate features of different checking accounts both within the same bank and at competing banks.

Some features that may differ include:

- Interest paid
- Monthly fees
- Check charges

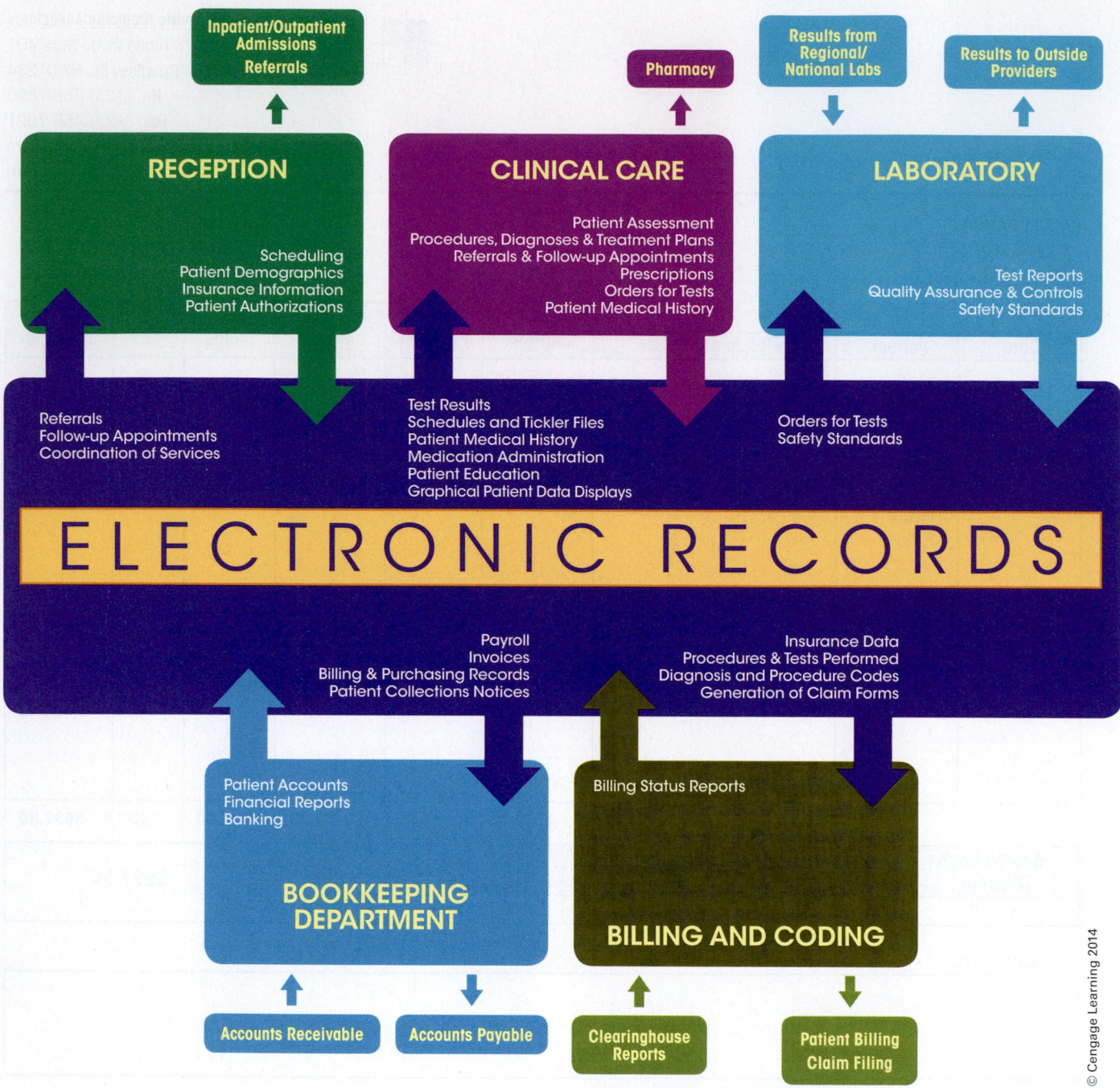

Figure 19-5   Diagram of total practice management system indicating the connection of daily financial practices to insurance billing, clinical care of the patient, reception activities, and laboratory testing.

- Automated teller machine (ATM) access and fees
- After-hours deposit capabilities
- Initial deposit and balance requirements
- Overdraft protection
- Fees for checks

- Special services extended free of charge such as **notary**, cashier's checks, traveler's checks, and online banking

When selecting an account, rather than choosing the account with the lowest fees, consider convenience, the relationship possible with a given bank, bank hours, number of bank locations, and other factors.

Savings Accounts. Savings accounts initially were distinguished from checking accounts because they paid interest on the money deposited. However, many checking accounts now pay interest as well. In either case, the interest is minimal on accounts that give immediate access to the deposit. **Money market accounts** often pay a higher rate of interest, although they may require a higher initial deposit and maintenance of a higher balance. Access to the account may require 24-hour turnaround time. Such accounts are useful when access to money is not needed frequently or when accumulating an amount necessary to invest for long-term goals.

Types of Checks

For the most part, the ambulatory care setting uses a standard business check. However, for special purposes, it is useful to understand the other check types available:

- A **cashier's check** is occasionally used when a check must be guaranteed for the amount in which it is written. Because a cashier's check is the bank's own check drawn against the bank's accounts, the recipient has the assurance that the check will clear. Cashier's checks are obtained at the bank by paying the bank representative cash or sometimes a personal check for the amount of the cashier's check. It is important to understand, however, that not all facilities will accept a cashier's check. Be sure to check with the office manager about accepted policy.

- A **certified check** is the depositor's own check that the bank has "certified" with a date and signature to indicate that the check is good for the amount in which it is written.

- Money orders are available from a number of places, even online. The U.S. Postal Service and Western Union are common sites for the purchase of money orders. They are purchased with cash and are similar to cashier's checks. A few patients may use money orders to pay their bill.

- A **voucher check** is a type of check with a stub attached that can be used to indicate invoice dates, services provided, and so on. Some payroll checks are written on voucher checks.

- **Traveler's checks** are available in most banks and are convenient and safer to use than cash when traveling. They are written in specific denominations ($20, $50, $100) and require a signature when purchased and when used. However, many banks today advise customers to use ATM machines for necessary cash if traveling to areas where ATM machines are readily available.

- **Electronic checks** have become widely used in ambulatory care settings. Although performing the same purpose as a paper check, electronic checks give the added convenience of faster processing, security, and guaranteed value.

Depositing Checks

Deposits are usually made daily because they serve as another proof of posting and because leaving large sums of money in the facility overnight is unwise. A rubber endorsement stamp from the bank should be used to immediately imprint the back of all checks received directly from patients and in the mail. Be sure all checks are stamped before depositing them. Scanning or photocopying all checks before deposit is one way to ensure accuracy.

Because the endorsement transfers rights to whoever holds the check, it is important to take certain precautions. A blank endorsement consists of a signature only (whether in pen or with a stamp) and presents a danger in that, if the check is lost or stolen, someone else could endorse the check below the signature and cash it. A restrictive endorsement should be used on all checks received in the ambulatory care setting. Restrictive endorsements include the signature and the words "for deposit only" or "pay to the order of…" (include the name of bank and account number; in addition, all possible payees' names should be listed under the company name, with the clinic address). This restricts the use of the check should it be lost or stolen.

Cash on Hand

Most medical practices need to have cash available on a daily basis. If it is the practice to collect co-payments and any coinsurance at the time of

CRITICAL THINKING

What factors make money market funds a good investment during one period, but provide little return for the investment at another time?

service, some patients will pay in cash and need change. Cash usually is kept in a locked change drawer that contains up to $200 in small bills at the beginning of each day. Any time a patient pays cash for the service, a receipt is prepared. Receipts are prenumbered, thus monitoring loss or theft. Cash amounts paid by patients must also be noted in their account or ledger. The term *received on account (ROA) cash* is usually indicated in the description column. If payment is made by check, follow the same procedure except the word *check* is used instead of *cash*.

At the end of each day, the cash drawer is balanced. The amount of cash received will be noted on the deposit slip as "currency." The remaining amount in the cash drawer will be the same as the beginning amount. Also, the day's cash received must match the cash control on the daily sheet. It is a good idea for only one person to handle the cash in the cash drawer; thus, it is not necessary for more than one person to balance the cash drawer at the end of the day. The cash drawer is not to be confused with petty cash, which is discussed later in this chapter. Petty cash is used to purchase small items such as postage, clinic refreshments, and so on. Checks are always written for major purchases, with the cash drawer used only to accommodate patient needs when payment is made in cash.

Most business accounts use deposit slips similar to the one shown in Figure 19-6. They are always completed in duplicate or a copy is made—one copy to accompany the deposit and one to be retained for clinic records. As shown, these deposit slips are longer than those generally used for personal accounts and have room for more entries and more information. If your manual day sheet has a built-in duplicate deposit slip, it will have been completed during posting.

A computerized system of financial records can provide deposit slips that may be used. The same procedure is followed as previously discussed. Procedure 19-7 outlines the steps in preparing a deposit.

Accepting Checks

When accepting checks from patients and other individuals, take time to inspect the check. This may eliminate checks returned from the bank for various reasons:

- Inspect the check for correct date, amount, and signature.
- Do not accept a third-party check (a check written to the patient from another person or company) unless it is from the insurance carrier.
- If a deposited check is returned marked "non-sufficient funds" (NSF), call the bank that

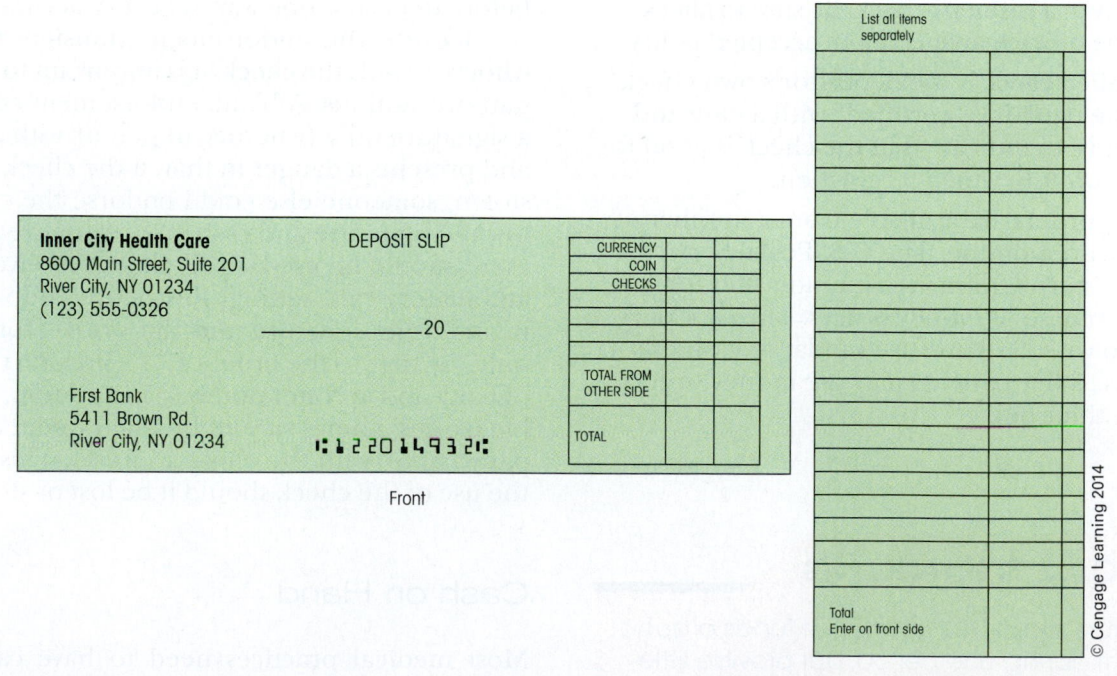

Figure 19-6 Sample deposit slip.

returned it and verify availability of funds. If funds are available, immediately redeposit the check for processing. If the check is returned a second time marked NSF, it is necessary to perform two bookkeeping functions. First, deduct the amount from the checking account balance of the practice. Second, add the amount back into the amount due by the patient in his or her account balance by entering the amount in the paid column in parentheses and increase the balance by the same amount. Place a brief explanation in the description column. Follow the clinic procedure for notifying the patient that the check was returned. See Procedure 19-8.

Lost or Stolen Checks

In the event that a check is missing and is thought to be lost or stolen, report this to your bank immediately. In some cases, you may be advised to stop payment to prevent unauthorized cashing of the check. In other situations, the bank may place a warning on the account, advising bank representatives to be especially careful about checking signatures to detect any attempt at a forged signature.

Writing and Recording Checks

Part of daily financial practices includes writing checks to pay bills (**accounts payable**), refunds of overpayment, and replenishment of petty cash. Writing the checks and paying the bills is usually done systematically. Chapter 21 discusses accounts payable and disbursement records in greater

detail. It is important that checks be prepared either electronically or written legibly to avoid bank errors. Checks should be dated and must include the name of the **payee** and the amount of payment entered both in figures and in words. It is also advisable that the "memo" line indicates what the check is for and includes any account or invoice number for reference. Figure 19-7 shows a sample of a properly completed check.

 Rules for Preparing Checks. Follow these rules to ensure that checks are properly prepared and recorded (see Procedure 19-9).

- Confirm that the numeric and written amounts agree.
- Confirm that everything is spelled correctly.
- Follow clinic procedure for having the provider or office manager approve all expenditures and sign all outgoing checks.
- Determine that the check has been signed by an individual with signature privileges.
- Confirm that the check is payable to the correct payee and that the current date is used.

Chapter 21 provides information on electronic check writing.

Reconciling a Bank Statement

Each month the bank will send a statement for the checking account (Figure 19-8). With online banking, a bank statement can be accessed electronically at any time. It also can be printed and used similar to a standard printed bank statement. The statement will show the account balance according

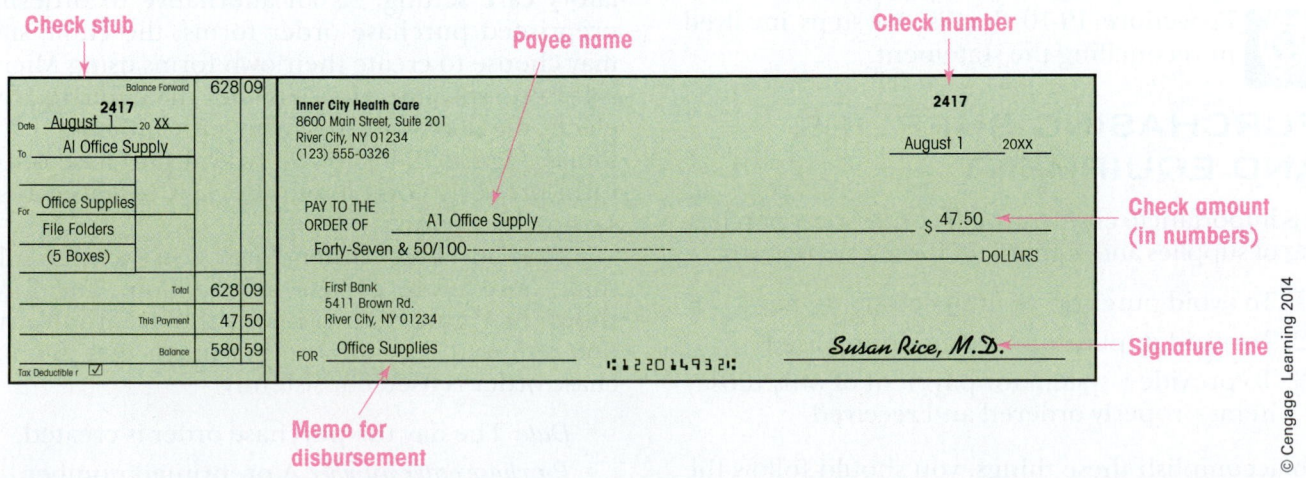

Figure 19-7 Sample of properly completed check and check stub.

Summary of Account Balance			Closing Date 1/15/XX		
Account # 1257-164013			Ending Balance $8,347.62		
Beginning Balance	$7,152.18				
Total Deposits and Additions	$8,643.86				
Total Withdrawals	$7,433.21				
Service Charge	$ 15.24				
Number	Date	Amount	Number	Date	Amount
201	12/18/XX	173.82	234	1/4/XX	96.31
223*	12/18/XX	44.12	235	1/4/XX	73.48
224	12/20/XX	586.00	236	1/6/XX	325.40
225	12/21/XX	24.15	237	1/7/XX	40.00
226	12/22/XX	33.90	238	1/8/XX	66.77
228*	12/23/XX	1250.00	241*	1/9/XX	15.55
229	12/24/XX	11.75	242	1/10/XX	12.45
230	12/24/XX	19.02	243	1/10/XX	4441.25
231	1/2/XX	43.80	244	1/10/XX	64.55
232	1/3/XX	39.00			
233	1/4/XX	71.50			

*Denotes gap in check sequence

Date	Deposit Amount	Date	Deposit Amount
18-Dec	361.75	4-Jan	825.00
19-Dec	586.00	5-Jan	1286.71
20-Dec	918.21	7-Jan	608.00
21-Dec	201.00	8-Jan	811.15
2-Jan	475.00	9-Jan	1092.68
3-Jan	1478.36		

Front

1. Enter Ending Balance from the front of this statement
$ 8,347.62

2. Enter deposits not shown on this statement
$ 3,162.50

3. Subtotal (add 1 & 2)
$ 11,510.12

4. List outstanding checks or other withdrawals here

Check #	Amount
222	37.89
227	161.15
239	11.50
240	92.12
245	835.17
246	21.75
247	586.00

5. Total outstanding checks
$ 1,745.58

Balance (subtract #5 from #3)
$ 9,764.54
This should equal your checkbook balance

Back

© Cengage Learning 2014

Figure 19-8   Sample bank statement with check reconciliation.

to the bank's records, a listing of all checks that have cleared the bank, deposits received by the bank, and any service charges deducted from the account. It is necessary to reconcile the entries in the checkbook against this statement to be sure there are no errors either in the checkbook or in the bank's records. Your bank statement is another means of ensuring that the accounts receivable is accurate for the previous month. If you use an accounting software package, this will also have a computerized option for reconciling.

Procedure 19-10 details the steps involved in reconciling the statement.

PURCHASING SUPPLIES AND EQUIPMENT

It is important to ensure proper control over purchasing of supplies and equipment for several reasons:

1. To avoid purchase of unnecessary items
2. To avoid duplication of items purchased
3. To provide a system for payment of only those items properly ordered and received

To accomplish these things, you should follow the first rule of purchasing: nothing is ordered or paid for without a purchase order or purchase order number. A copy of the purchase order is sent to the supplier and a copy is retained by the clinic for verification of shipment and payment of invoice.

Preparing a Purchase Order

Purchase order forms are available from office supply companies or can be ordered from a printer and customized to the needs of the ambulatory care setting. As an alternative to ordering preprinted purchase order forms, the clinic staff may choose to create their own forms using Microsoft Excel software. This enables the clinic to have electronic access to the form with imbedded formulas. Figure 19-9 shows a typical purchase order form properly completed, which is reviewed here section by section.

The purchase order form can vary greatly; some have more or less information. The form shown in Figure 19-9 contains the usual information required. The important thing is that the purchase order is used consistently.

- *Date.* The day the purchase order is created.
- *Purchase order number.* A preprinted number that is used on invoices and statements from

PURCHASE ORDER

NO. 1742

Date:

Bill To:	Ship To:	Vendor:
Inner City Health Care 8600 Main Street, Suite 201 River City, NY 01234 (123) 555-0326	**Inner City Health Care** 8600 Main Street, Suite 201 River City, NY 01234 (123) 555-0326	**AZ Medical Supply** 4721 E. Camelback Rd. Phoenix, AZ 85252 (602) 555-3246

REQ BY	BUYER	TERMS
Karen Ritter	Walter Seals	Net 30

QTY	ITEM	UNITS	DESCRIPTION	UNIT PR	TOTAL
10	427A	Box	Surgical Gloves - Sz 7	9.20	92.00
1	327DC	Case	2" gauze pads	60.30	60.30
5	1943C	Box	Tongue Depressors	5.80	29.00
15	7433	Ea	Examination Table paper (roll)	10.50	159.50

SUBTOTAL	338.80
TAX	28.80
FREIGHT	Prepaid
BAL DUE	376.60

Figure 19-9   Purchase order form.

the supplier and on the check used to pay the invoice. It is also important for tracking the status of the order. In smaller practices, the purchase order number may simply be the name of the person ordering with the date the order was placed immediately following.

- *Bill to address*. This is generally used when items are to be shipped to an address different from the address where the supplier will send the bill for goods or services.
- *Ship to address*. When items are to be sent by supplier, this must always be completed.
- *Vendor information*. The name and address of supplier where purchase order is to be sent.
- *Req. by* ("Requested by"). States which individual or department has requested the item(s).
- *Buyer*. States the individual in the clinic who is authorized to issue a purchase order.
- *Terms*. Agreement between buyer and seller as to when payment is due.

- *Qty*. Quantity of item being ordered (number of units).
- *Item*. Vendor's catalogue part or item number.
- *Units*. How the item is sold—individually (ea.), by the box, case, or dozen. Many suppliers will not split units (i.e., will not sell less than a full case).
- *Description*. Brief description of item (helps as a cross-check for vendor in the event that an item number is entered incorrectly).
- *Unit price*. How much *one* unit (ea., box, case, dozen) costs.
- *Total*. Cost of one unit multiplied by the number of units being ordered.
- *Discount*. If any discount is allowed for quick and early payment, it is noted here. For instance, there might be a 10% discount for paying within 10 days. The discount amount is entered before the Total column is summed.
- *Subtotal*. Sum of the Total column.

- *Tax.* Sales tax required by the state.
- *Freight.* How much the customer must pay to have the order delivered (not always applicable).
- *Bal. Due.* The sum of the subtotal, tax, and freight charges; this is how much the clinic will be billed.

Verifying Goods Received

Proper purchasing procedure does not stop with the completion and mailing of the purchase order. When goods are received, it is necessary to verify that the correct items and quantities were shipped by the vendor. Chapter 21 discusses accounts payable.

PETTY CASH

Petty cash is money kept in the clinic for minor, routine, or unexpected expenses such as postage-due mail or coffee supplies. Keep petty cash totally separate from the cash drawer that is used to make change for patients paying their co-payment. Keeping this cash on hand eliminates the necessity of the provider or office manager having to sign checks for such items. Petty cash is not used to pay bills or make large routine purchases.

The amount of cash on hand for this purpose is small, usually $75 to $100, and is usually kept in small denominations. However, records must be as carefully maintained as for any other financial transactions and balanced each day before closing.

Establishing a Petty Cash Fund

If your clinic does not already have a petty cash fund or if you are in a new practice that has not yet established a fund, determine how much the fund should be and write a check to "Cash" for that amount. The amount should be enough to cover several days of incidental expenses.

Tracking, Balancing, and Replenishing Petty Cash

Tracking. Keep a supply of petty cash vouchers on hand to track how petty cash is used. When money is taken from petty cash, a voucher must always be completed and the receipt from the purchase attached. Vouchers and receipts are kept in the petty cash box with the money until the fund is replenished.

Balancing and Replenishing. When the fund gets low, write another check to "Cash" to bring it back up to the original amount. To determine the amount of the check, it is necessary to first balance the account. After the account is balanced, list how funds were spent in such a way that the bookkeeper can disburse the check properly.

 Procedure 19-11 outlines the steps involved in establishing and maintaining a petty cash account.

DOCUMENTATION

Financial records of patients are to be kept separate from the patients' medical charts. Except for the attachment of the encounter form or superbill at the time of the visit, they rarely are seen together. Often, only the patient's medical record is necessary for documentation; other times, only the financial information is necessary. This policy also serves as a reminder that the care given to patients has nothing to do with their ability to pay.

 PROCEDURE 19-1

Recording/Posting Patient Charges, Payments, and Adjustments in a Manual System

PURPOSE:
To record information including services rendered, fees charged, any adjustments made, and balances pertaining to a patient's visit to the provider and patient's account.

EQUIPMENT/SUPPLIES:
Calculator
Patient's account or ledger

Procedure 19-1 (continued)

PROCEDURE STEPS:

1. Check the patient's account before the patient's appointment to make certain it is current. The account will indicate any recent insurance payments, any amount received on the account, and any balance due. RATIONALE: Allows the medical assistant to focus entirely on the patient at arrival time and gives a current picture of the patient's account.

2. When the patient arrives, check for name, address, telephone numbers, and any changes regarding medical insurance. Make any changes in the account or on the ledger. RATIONALE: Ensures that information is current and up to date.

3. On the encounter form or superbill, complete any necessary items such as the date of service and the responsible party's name. Then attach it to the patient's medical chart that is now ready for the clinical medical assistant to take with the patient to the examination room. RATIONALE: The encounter form allows the provider to indicate appropriate procedure and diagnosis codes.

4. When the provider completes the treatment or examination, he or she will check the procedures and diagnosis on the encounter form. RATIONALE: Provider marks the appropriate codes and signs the encounter form, indicating it is correct. The provider or licensed caregiver is the only one authorized to select the appropriate procedure codes.

5. When the patient returns to the front desk, refer to the provider's fee schedule, enter the charge next to each procedure, and calculate the total. If the procedure description is not indicated, one is to be provided. A description is necessary for each service. Check to see if the codes match the services provided. If they do not match, refer it back to the provider or licensed caregiver for correction. RATIONALE: Medical clinic staff and the patient can identify the charge to the particular service given and know that the coding and charges will match.

6. In the *manual pegboard system,* post each service or procedure as a charge or debit. Post any payments received today in the payment column as a credit. RATIONALE: Clearly indicates charges made and payments received, creating an updated account.

7. If any adjustment applies to the account, enter the amount in the adjustment column. If there is no adjustment column and the adjustment will *reduce* the bill, enter the amount in the payment column enclosed by parentheses. If the adjustment will *increase* the bill, place the amount in the charge column (no parentheses) with an explanation in the description column. In the *manual system,* the adjustment amount will be either added to or subtracted from the totaled figures. RATIONALE: Adjustment is shown as separate from basic charge so that the provider's fee profile is unaffected.

8. Determine current balance by adding credits and subtracting debits to the running balance and determine the amount in the current balance. Always use a calculator (one with a tape is recommended) to calculate and verify your mathematics. RATIONALE: Completes the recording of patient charges, payments, and adjustments.

9. If the recording is a payment from the patient, place a restrictive endorsement on the check. RATIONALE: Ensures that the check can only be cashed by the authorized party.

10. Enter the amount in the payment column. In the description column, identify as cash, check, or insurance payment. If payment is a check, enter the number of the check. RATIONALE: This information is necessary in making the bank deposit slip.

11. Place the cash or processed check in the appointed secure place awaiting deposit. RATIONALE: Keeps receivables together and ready for deposit.

PROCEDURE 19–2

Balancing Day Sheets in a Manual System

PURPOSE:
To verify that all entries to the day sheet are correct and that the totals balance.

EQUIPMENT/SUPPLIES:
Day sheet
Calculator

PROCEDURE STEPS:

1. *Column totals.* The first step in balancing a day sheet is to total columns A, B_1, B_2, C, and D, and enter the total for each column in the boxes marked "Totals This Page." The column totals are then added to the figures entered in the "Previous Page" column boxes to arrive at the "Month to Date" totals, which provide the total charges, credits, and so forth entered from the first working day of the month to the present. RATIONALE: Establishes column totals.

2. *Proof of posting.* This box is used to verify that entries have been made correctly and that the column totals are accurate. *All figures entered here are taken from the "Totals This Page" column boxes.*

   a. Enter today's column D total, which shows the sum of all the previous balances entered when the transactions were posted.

   b. Added to this is the column A total of all charges for that day, to arrive at a subtotal. Enter the amount where indicated in the box.

   c. Because columns B_1 and B_2 are both credit columns that reduce balances, they are added together and entered in the box labeled "Less Cols B_1 and B_2"; the total of credits is subtracted from the subtotal. If all entries and addition are correct in the posting area, the result should equal the amount in column C and the transactions for that day are balanced. RATIONALE: Verifies entries have been made correctly and that the totals are accurate.

   Overview: When an individual transaction is entered, the patient's previous balance (D) is added to the charges for the day (A). If there are any payments or adjustments made at that time, they are entered in the B columns and subtracted from the A + D amount to achieve

the new balance (C). Because each transaction is actually D + A − B = C, the column totals of D + A − B will always equal the C total.

D		A		B		C
10	+	5	−	2	=	13
2	+	7	−	1	=	8
Column Totals 12	+	12	−	3	=	21

3. *Accounts Receivable (A/R) Control.* This box simply adds the previous day's A/R balance to the current day's totals to include the current day's business and arrive at the new A/R total.

   a. The column A and column B totals are carried straight across from the Proof of Posting box to the corresponding blanks in the A/R Control box.

   b. Add the amount already entered in the Previous Day's Total space to the Column A amount to arrive at a subtotal.

   c. Subtract the amount carried over from the "Less Columns B_1 and B_2" box to find the new A/R amount. RATIONALE: Determines new accounts receivable balance.

4. *A/R Proof* verifies, or proves, the A/R balance in the A/R Control box. *The figure entered on the first line of this box will not change during a calendar month because it shows how much the A/R balance was on the first working day of the month. All other figures entered will be taken from the "Month-To-Date" column boxes.*

   a. Enter the amount from column A (month-to-date) where shown.

   b. Add the column A amount to the "A/R 1st of Month" figure and enter the sum in the subtotal space.

   c. Enter the B_1 and B_2 month-to-date amounts and subtract from the subtotal. This amount goes in the Total A/R space.

   If all posting and addition are correct, the Total A/R amounts in the A/R Control and A/R Proof boxes will match and the day is balanced. RATIONALE: Verifies the accounts receivable balance in the accounts receivable control box.

Procedure 19-2 (continued)

5. *Deposit verification* involves totaling the columns in Section 2 and entering the sum of the columns in the space marked "Total Deposit." *NOTE:* The Total Deposit and the Total of Payments Received in column B_1 should match. RATIONALE: Verifies deposit total.

6. *Business Analysis Summary.* If this section is used, total each column in the summary section. *NOTE:* If the Business Analysis Summary is used to break out charges by type or by provider, the sum of the columns should equal today's column A total. If it is used to credit payments to different providers, the sum of the columns will equal today's payment column. RATIONALE: The total deposit and the total of payments received in column B_1 should match to prove totals.

7. *After the day sheet is balanced,* there is one step remaining: the transfer of balances.

   a. Take out a new day sheet for the next day.

   b. Transfer the "Month-To-Date" column totals to the "Previous Page" columns boxes on the new sheet.

   c. Enter the Total A/R amount from the last day sheet in the "Previous Day's Total" space of the A/R Control box on the new day sheet.

   d. Enter the A/R 1st of Month Amount in the A/R Proof box on the new sheet. RATIONALE: Transfers balances to prepare a new day sheet for the next day's activities.

The new day sheet is now ready for posting.

PROCEDURE 19-3

Posting Procedure Charges and Payments Using Medical Office Simulation Software (MOSS)

PURPOSE:
To post service charges to a patient account and apply a payment during the check out.

EQUIPMENT/SUPPLIES:
Computer and MOSS
Source documents

PROCEDURE STEPS:

1. Open MOSS and select *Procedure Posting* from the Main Menu.

2. Select the patient from the *Procedure Posting* patient list, and then click *Add.*

3. Enter the Encounter Form Reference Number in Field 1. *Hint:* See Encounter Form.

4. Enter the Date of Service in Field 5. *Hint:* See Encounter Form.

5. Enter the first CPT service code in Field 8. *Hint:* See Encounter Form.

6. Enter the ICD (diagnostic codes) in Field 12, using up to four codes as applicable.

7. Click *Post* to apply the charges to the patient account.

8. Enter additional services in the same manner until all service charges have been posted.

9. Click the *Post Payment* button to apply a payment during the time of procedure posting.

10. Click on the line item for the required procedure, and then click on the *Select/Edit* button.

11. Enter the date of posting in Field 3 and the payment information in Fields 4 through 12 as applicable to the payment.

12. Click on *Post* to apply the payment.

13. Click on the *View Ledger* button.

14. Review all postings on the patient's ledger.

15. Click *Close* to close all open windows and return to the *Procedure Posting* patient selection window.

16. Post charges for the next patient, or close the Posting Procedures patient selection window and return to the Main Menu.

PROCEDURE 19-4

Insurance Billing Using Medical Office Simulation Software (MOSS)

PURPOSE:
To submit claims electronically to insurance carriers using MOSS.

EQUIPMENT/SUPPLIES:
Computer and MOSS

PROCEDURE STEPS:

1. Open MOSS and select *Insurance Billing* from the Main Menu.

2. In the *Claim Preparation* window, drop down the list for Field 1 and select *Patient Name*.

3. In Field 2, *Settings*, select the specific provider name or *ALL*, enter the *From/Through* Service dates, and select an individual patient or *ALL* for *Patient Name* and *Patient Account*.

4. In Field 3, *Transmit Type*, click in front of the box for the type of claim to be submitted, *Electronic* or *Paper (1500)*.

5. In Field 4, *Billing Options*, select whether claim is primary insurance, secondary, or other.

6. In Field 5, click on the insurance carrier to be billed, or *ALL*.

7. Click on the *Prebilling Worksheet* button.

8. Review claims to be billed on the *Prebilling Worksheet* report.

9. Print the *Prebilling Worksheet* report.

10. Close the *Prebilling Worksheet* report and return to the *Claims Preparation* window. *Hint:* Be careful not to close the entire MOSS software program.

11. Click on the *Generate Claims* button.

12. Before sending the claims electronically or printing paper claims, preview the CMS 1500 claims forms for each patient. *Hint:* Use the record bar at the bottom left to see each patient's claim.

13. Click on *Transmit EMC* (or *Print Forms* for paper claims) to execute the claims submissions.

14. After the electronic transmission is completed, click on *View* to review the *Transmission Report*, or collect printed claim forms from printer, as applicable.

15. Print the *Claims Submission Report*, or prepare mailing envelopes for the paper claims, as applicable.

16. Close the *Claims Submission Report* and click *Close* to exit the *Transmission* window, or return to the *Main Menu* if paper claims were printer by closing all windows. *Hint:* Be careful not to close the entire MOSS software program.

PROCEDURE 19-5

Posting Insurance Payments and Adjustments Using Medical Office Simulation Software (MOSS)

PURPOSE:
To post insurance payments and adjustments to patient accounts using MOSS.

EQUIPMENT/SUPPLIES:
Computer and MOSS
Source documents

PROCEDURE STEPS:

1. Read the EOB/RA from the insurance carrier and prepare information before applying a payment to the patient's account. Use the guidelines below to read the EOB/RA:

   How much did the insurance allow?

   How much was disallowed?

   How much did the insurance pay?

2. Click on the *Posting Payments* button on the *Main Menu*. Select the patient and then click *Apply Payment*.

Procedure 19-5 (continued)

3. Click on the line item for the date and procedure for which a payment shall be posted in the *Procedure Charge History* area (Field 1), and then click on the *Select/Edit* button. Make certain Field 13 shows the correct *Balance Due.*

4. Input the date of posting and the following insurance payment information as follows:

   Payment by Insurance, Field 4 (Click the drop down box)

   Reference #, Field 5 (Enter claim number, check number, or other reference number)

   Amount of payment, Field 6

   Press *Enter* when finished to update the *Balance Due* in Field 13.

5. Input the disallowed amount as an insurance adjustment as follows: Select *Adjustment Insurance* from the drop down box, Field 10, and then enter the Adjustment Amount in Field 11. Press *Enter* when finished to update the Balance Due in Field 13.

6. Click *Post* when payment is ready to be posted to the account.

7. If there is more than one service on the EOB/RA, prepare the information for the next service before applying a payment to the patient's account. Use the guidelines below:

   How much did the insurance allow?

   How much was disallowed?

   How much did the insurance pay?

8. Enter the payment information as before for the next service. *Hint:* Click on the line item for the applicable date and procedure.

9. Click *Post* when payment is ready to be posted to the account.

10. Click *View Ledger* to review payment posting.

11. When complete, either *View* and print a report, or click on *Close* and return to the patient selection window.

12. Post payment for the next patient, or return to the *Main Menu.*

PROCEDURE 19-6

Processing Credit Balances and Refunds Using Medical Office Simulation Software (MOSS)

PURPOSE:
To post overpayment refunds to patient accounts with a credit balance.

EQUIPMENT/SUPPLIES:
Computer and MOSS

PROCEDURE STEPS:
To post overpayment refunds to patient accounts with a credit balance.

1. Click on the *Posting Payments* button on the *Main Menu.* Select the patient and then click *Apply Payment.*

2. Select the patient and then click *Apply Payment.*

3. Click on the line item for the date and procedure for which a refund shall be posted in the *Procedure Charge History* area (Field 1), and then click on the *Select/Edit* button. Make certain Field 13 shows the correct *Balance Due. Hint:* If more than one service needs to be refunded, apply it to each separately.

4. In Field 10, drop down the list of adjustment types and select *Refund Overpayment.*

5. In Field 11, enter the amount to be refunded. Press *Enter* to apply the refund to the balance. Make certain Field 13 shows the correct *Balance Due $0.00* (or balance if only a portion was refunded).

6. Click *Post* to enter the refund to the account.

7. If applicable, apply a refund to the next service. Click on the line item for the procedure (Field 1), and then click on the *Select/Edit* button. Make certain Field 13 shows the correct *Balance Due.*

continues

Procedure 19-6 (continued)

8. In Field 10, drop down the list of adjustment types and select *Refund Overpayment*.

9. In Field 11, enter the amount to be refunded. Press enter to apply the refund to the balance. Make certain Field 13 shows the correct *Balance*

Due $0.00 (or balance if only a portion was refunded).

10. Click *Post* to enter the refund to the account.

11. When complete, click *Close* and select the next patient, or return to the *Main Menu*.

PROCEDURE 19–7

Preparing a Deposit

PURPOSE:
To create a deposit slip for the day's receipts.

EQUIPMENT/SUPPLIES:
New deposit slip
Check endorsement stamp
Calculator
Cash and checks received for the day

PROCEDURE STEPS:
1. Separate all checks from currency (paper money). RATIONALE: Each must be entered as a separate total.

2. Count all currency to be deposited and enter the amount in the space provided. Gather bills facing the same direction in order (i.e., 50s, 20s, 10s, and so on). RATIONALE: Follows bank procedure.

3. Count all coins to be deposited and enter the amount in the space provided. Coins may need to be wrapped. RATIONALE: Follows bank procedure.

4. On the back of the deposit slip list each check separately. Include the patient name in the left-hand column and enter the amount of the check in the right-hand column. RATIONALE: Follows bank procedure.

5. Total the checks listed and copy the total on the front where it is indicated to place the total from the other side. RATIONALE: Follows bank procedure.

6. The sum of currency, coins, and checks should always equal the total in the Payments column on that day's day sheet. RATIONALE: Proof of accuracy.

7. Attach the top copy of the deposit slip to the deposit, leaving the carbon on the pad. RATIONALE: Provides the clinic and bank with record of deposit.

8. Enter the date and amount of the deposit in the space provided on the checkbook stubs. RATIONALE: Keeps checkbook register current with money in account.

9. Add the amount of the deposit to the checkbook balance. RATIONALE: Keeps checkbook register current with money in account.

10. Deposit at the bank, either in person or at the night deposit. In either case, be sure a record of deposit is received (it will be mailed if the night deposit is used). It is not recommended that deposits be made through ATMs; currency should never be deposited in an ATM. RATIONALE: Proof bank processed the deposit as indicated.

PROCEDURE 19–8

Recording a Nonsufficient Funds Check in a Manual System

PURPOSE:
To perform bookkeeping functions that keep account in proper balance.

EQUIPMENT/SUPPLIES:
The practice's account balance
Manual day sheet

Procedure 19-8 (continued)

Manual ledger

Nonsufficient funds (NSF) check

PROCEDURE STEPS:

1. Follow the clinic policy for notifying the patient of the returned check. RATIONALE: Policy may vary from clinic to clinic.

2. When the NSF check has been returned the second time, deduct the check amount from the account balance of the practice. RATIONALE: The funds can no longer be counted as earnings received.

3. Add the amount of the NSF check back into the patient's ledger. Place the amount in parentheses in the paid column and increase the total by the same amount. In a manual system, the entry and math are performed by the medical assistant. RATIONALE: The amount is still owed by the patient, is not considered paid, and must be reflected in the amount due.

4. Place a brief explanation in the description of the column such as "NSF 12/09/2012."

PROCEDURE 19-9

Writing a Check

PURPOSE:

To write a check to pay for expenses incurred and provide proof of payment. (Never written a check before? Go to http://www.thebeehive.org for practice.)

EQUIPMENT/SUPPLIES:

Checkbook and check register with balance of
    $7,298.35

Pen with black ink

Calculator

CHECKING WRITING EXERCISES:

Write checks for the following invoices using the current date:

1. $54.99 for case of printer paper to Landau Products

2. $450.00 for last month's janitorial services to MJB Services

3. $1,335.38 for clinical supplies to Redding Medical Supply House

4. $687.19 to Atlantic Electric for last month's heat and electricity

5. $350 to American Association of Medical Assistants for AAMA membership for the four medical assistants in the clinic

PROCEDURE STEPS:

1. Gather all invoices to be paid.

2. For the check register, use black ink:

   a. Enter check number 101 in the register if not preprinted.

   b. Enter the current date and year (usually in numbers, i.e., 02/14/2012).

   c. Enter the individual or company the check is to be paid to: Landau Products.

   d. Enter the amount to be paid on the check: $54.99.

   e. Subtract check amount from the present balance. Total $7,243.36 appears as the available balance. RATIONALE: These steps ensure that the check register is not overlooked when writing a check and establishes a well-recognized routine.

3. To write the check, use black ink:

   a. Enter check number 101 if not preprinted.

   b. Enter the current date and year (usually written out, i.e., February 14, 2012).

   c. Enter the individual or company the check is to be paid to: Landau Products.

   d. Enter the amount to be paid on the check: $54.99. Do not leave spaces between numbers or between the dollar sign and the first number. RATIONALE: This helps to prevent any tampering of the check by adding numbers.

continues

Procedure 19-9 (continued)

e. Write out the amount to be paid by check (Fifty-four dollars and 99/100). Fill in any space left between the last number or word and draw a wiggly line over to the amount entered in numbers. RATIONALE: When the written amount and the number amount match, errors are prevented. The wiggly line makes it more difficult for anyone to tamper with the check.

f. Describe what the check is written for in the bottom left corner (Printer paper, case). RATIONALE: Explains the purpose of the check.

g. If you have check-writing authority in the clinic, sign the check with your name the same as indicated on the bank's records. If you do not have check-writing authority, hold this check and the others to give to the individual with that authority. RATIONALE: The person responsible can review the checks with the invoices to verify valid expenses.

4. Continue writing checks for items 2 through 5 in the Check Writing Exercises, being certain to number checks consecutively and to subtract each check. Submit checks and check register with final balance to your instructor for evaluation.

PROCEDURE 19-10
Reconciling a Bank Statement

PURPOSE:
To verify that the balance listed in the checkbook agrees with the balance shown by the bank.

EQUIPMENT/SUPPLIES:
Checkbook
Bank statement
Calculator

PROCEDURE STEPS:
1. Make sure the balance in the checkbook is current (all deposits and checks entered have been added or subtracted). RATIONALE: Ensures totals are accurate.

2. If a service charge is listed on the statement, subtract that amount from the last balance listed in the checkbook. RATIONALE: Reconciles current balance.

3. In the checkbook, check off each check listed on the statement and verify the amount against the check stub. RATIONALE: Verifies accuracy.

4. In the checkbook, check off each deposit listed on the statement. RATIONALE: Verifies accuracy.

5. The back of the statement contains a worksheet to be used for balancing.

6. Copy the ending balance from the front of the statement to the area indicated on the back.

7. Go through the check stubs and list on the back of the statement in the area provided any checks that have not cleared and any deposits that were not shown as received on the statement.

8. Total the checks not cleared on the statement worksheet.

9. Total the deposits not credited on the worksheet.

10. Add together the statement balance and the total of deposits not credited.

11. Subtract the total of checks not cleared. This amount should agree with the balance in the checkbook. If so, the checkbook is balanced and the statement should be filed in the appropriate place. RATIONALE: Following procedure steps 5 through 11 completes verification of accuracy.

PROCEDURE 19-11

Establishing and Maintaining a Petty Cash Fund

PURPOSE:

To establish and maintain a petty cash fund for incidental expenses, making certain that receipts match the difference between the beginning and ending balance of the fund.

EQUIPMENT/SUPPLIES:

Petty cash box with cash balance
Vouchers
Calculator

Petty Cash Exercises:

1. Write a check for $100 cash at the bank.

2. Vouchers are made for the following incidentals:

    a. $20 to staff employee to purchase coffee supplies. Actual amount for supplies is $13.87; employee returns $6.13 cash

    b. $2.24 for postage due to postal employee

    c. $3.18 to postal employee for guaranteed forwarding address

    d. $35.00 to Shannon's Pizza delivery for staff meeting lunch

PROCEDURE STEPS:

Establish the Fund:

1. Write a check at the bank to "Cash" for $100 (or other predetermined amount). Receive the cash in denominations of 1s, 5s, 10s, and 20s. Place the cash in the cash box. RATIONALE: The amount establishes petty cash and provides bills for the incidental purchases.

2. When cash is needed for an incidental expense, such as postage due, prepare a voucher for the amount needed. No cash is taken from the fund without a voucher. RATIONALE: The written voucher indicates what the money is used for.

3. After the purchase, attach the receipt for the purchase to the voucher. RATIONALE: This step provides proof of the purchase.

Balance Petty Cash Fund:

1. After the activity identified in the Petty Cash Exercises, count the money remaining in the box. RATIONALE: Verifies the amount of cash remaining in petty cash.

2. Total the amounts of all vouchers in the petty cash box. RATIONALE: Determines amount of expenditures.

3. Subtract the amount of receipts from the original amount in petty cash. This should equal the amount of cash remaining in the box. RATIONALE: Proves that the amount of expenditures deducted from the beginning amount equals the amount left in the box.

4. When the cash has been balanced against the receipts, write a check *only for the amount that was used*. RATIONALE: Brings dollar amount back to original petty cash amount.

Petty Cash Check Disbursement:

1. Sort all vouchers by account.

2. On a sheet of paper list the accounts involved.

3. Total vouchers for each account and record individual totals on the list.

4. Copy this list with its totals on the memo portion of the stub for the check written to replenish petty cash.

5. File the list with the vouchers and receipts attached, after noting the check number on the list.

CASE STUDY 19-1

Refer to the scenario at the beginning of the chapter. As you consider the discussion of patient fees, determine what steps to take in the following situations.

CASE STUDY REVIEW

1. The clinic's patient has been diagnosed with non-Hodgkin's lymphoma (diffuse large B-cell lymphoma) in stage 3. Surgery and aggressive chemotherapy are in process. The patient has Medicare and a small Medigap policy. You know there are expenses coming soon that neither insurance will cover. What can you suggest?

2. This patient has been with the clinic for 11 years and was covered most of the time by excellent private insurance. The circumstances have changed, however. Today the patient works part time, has only Medicaid insurance, and has very few private funds. The provider's diagnosis is severe depression, and the provider instructs the patient to make two appointments weekly until the medication prescribed begins to make a significant difference in this patient's life. You know there are severe limitations to reimbursement from the state regarding this diagnosis. What steps will you take?

CASE STUDY 19-2

Joann Crier has completed her 3-month probation period with Drs. Lewis and King. She is doing quite well and has demonstrated skill in accurate financial documentation. She has been asked to take over reconciling the monthly bank statements and managing all the accounts payable, including getting the checks ready for the provider's signature. She has difficulty, however, completing these tasks until after hours when the clinic is closed and quiet. Marilyn Johnson has told her that it must be done within normal working hours unless special permission is granted.

CASE STUDY REVIEW

1. What suggestions can you make to Joann to allow her to complete these tasks during normal working hours?

2. What impact does the time of day, day(s) of the month, or place where the tasks are completed have on your suggestions?

3. Are there any circumstances you can identify when overtime might be warranted to allow Joann to complete the tasks after hours?

SUMMARY

In this chapter, we discussed the daily financial duties in an ambulatory care setting: patient bookkeeping, working with the checkbook, purchasing supplies and equipment, and petty cash. By becoming proficient in these functions, you will be prepared to handle the day-to-day financial aspects of any ambulatory care setting.

Patient bookkeeping involves not only a responsibility to your employer (you are keeping track of income) but also to the patient, to be certain that charges for services rendered are correct and that payments are properly credited. The pegboard system is a comprehensive manual system for posting and tracking these data. Computerized bookkeeping offers many advantages of speed, high accuracy, and elimination of some routine tasks while providing the same important financial data.

It is important to maintain a scrupulous accounts payable system to ensure that bills are paid on time and that payments are properly documented for tax purposes. To accomplish this, checks are prepared properly, prepared on time, and recorded to effectively track expenditures.

Accuracy is important at all times. To ensure maximum accuracy in all bookkeeping functions, observe a few rules: record all charges and receipts immediately; make deposits of checks and currency the same day they are received; always verify and recheck totals of all deposits and expenditures; stay current with all checking account duties such as account reconciliation; and be prompt with all accounts payable.

STUDY FOR SUCCESS

To reinforce your knowledge and skills of information presented in this chapter:

- Review the *Key Terms*
- Role-play with other students to apply attributes of professionalism pertinent to this chapter.
- Consider the *Case Studies* and discuss your conclusions
- Answer the questions in the *Certification Review*
- Apply your knowledge by completing the *Activities* in the *Study Guide* and the *Games and Quizzes* in the StudyWARE (StudyWARE) software on the *Premium Website*
- Perform the *Procedures* using the *Competency Assessment Checklists* in the *Competency Manual*
- Practice your problem-solving skills with the *Critical Thinking Challenge 3.0* on the *Premium Website*

Additional resources for this chapter include:

- Module 10 of the *Medical Assisting Learning Lab*
- *CourseMate for Delmar's Comprehensive Medical Assisting*
- *WebTutor for Delmar's Comprehensive Medical Assisting*

CERTIFICATION REVIEW

1. The debit column of a ledger is:
   a. the column to the right of the balance column
   b. the column on the left; used to enter charges, procedure codes, and description of services
   c. the column at the far right that records the difference between the debit and credit columns
   d. the column that indicates the patient's debt to the practice

2. The use of debit/credit cards by patients to pay for services in ambulatory care settings is:
   a. never done
   b. unethical
   c. sure to compromise the integrity of the clinic
   d. a financial arrangement increasingly being used

3. The first section of the manual day sheet is used:
   a. to record deposits
   b. for business analysis
   c. to post individual transactions
   d. to total transactions

4. Good working habits for bookkeeping functions include:
   a. double-checking all entries for accuracy
   b. keeping the bookkeeping tasks current and up to date
   c. allowing the computer to create all the entries
   d. a and b

5. Petty cash:
   a. is necessary to give patients change when they pay in cash.
   b. is used by the provider when taking a colleague to lunch
   c. pays for routine and unexpected minor expenses of the clinic
   d. comes from the provider's personal account

6. Encounter forms:
   a. can be ordered to fit the practice
   b. provide a separate ledger for each patient household
   c. list common services provided, procedural code, and diagnosis code
   d. a and c

7. Receipts:
   a. are used for payments on accounts
   b. are not given unless services are rendered the same day
   c. are mailed to patients when payment is made by mail
   d. are unnecessary, especially in the computerized system

8. When accepting checks from patients:
   a. inspect for correct date, amount, and signature
   b. immediately stamp with a restrictive endorsement
   c. third-party checks are acceptable
   d. a and b
9. A check with an attached stub for recording information is called a:
   a. certified check
   b. cashier's check
   c. voucher check
   d. money order

10. It is important to ensure proper control over purchasing of supplies and equipment for the following reasons:
    a. to avoid purchase of unnecessary items
    b. to avoid duplication of items purchased
    c. to provide a system for payment of only those items properly ordered and received
    d. all of the above

REFERENCES/BIBLIOGRAPHY

Centers for Medicare and Medicaid Services. (2007). *CMS clarifies guidelines for national provider identifier (NPI) deadline implementation.* Retrieved April 12, 2007, from http://www.cms.hhs.gov

Electronic prescriptions. Retrieved February 2008, from http://www.medisoft.com

Fordney, M. T., French, L., & Follis, J. (2008). *Administrative medical assisting* (6th ed.). Clifton Park, NY: Delmar Cengage Learning.

How to write a personal check. Retrieved February 2008, from http://www.thebeehive.org

CHAPTER 20

Billing and Collections

OUTLINE

Billing Procedures

Credit and Collection Policies

Payment at Time of Service

Truth-in-Lending Act

Components of a Complete Statement
  Computerized Statements

Monthly and Cycle Billing
  Monthly Billing
  Cycle Billing

Past-Due Accounts

Collection Process
  Collection Ratio
  Accounts Receivable Ratio

Aging Accounts
  Computerized Aging

Collection Techniques
  Billing Insurance Carriers
  Telephone Collections
  Collection Letters

Use of an Outside Collection Agency

Use of Small Claims Court

Special Collection Situations
  Bankruptcy
  Estates
  Tracing "Skips"

Statute of Limitations

Maintain a Professional Attitude

LEARNING OUTCOMES

1. Define, spell, and pronounce the key terms as presented in the glossary.

2. Analyze the importance of billing and collections to the ambulatory care setting.

3. Describe the advantages of billing at least the co-payment and coinsurance at time of service.

4. Describe the impact of the Truth-In-Lending Act as it applies to collections.

5. Compare computerized billing and manual billing.

6. Recall the components of a complete statement.

7. Differentiate between monthly and cycle billing.

8. Explain the process of aging accounts.

9. Describe the importance of a courteous manner in telephone collections.

10. State legal and ethical guidelines for telephone collections.

11. Describe the impact of the Fair Debt Collection Practice Act as it applies to collections.

12. Describe the process of sending a series of collection letters.

13. List points to consider when using a collection agency.

14. Recall three special collections problems encountered in the ambulatory care setting.

15. Explain how the statute of limitations impacts the medical assistant's practice.

16. Discuss the merits of a professional attitude in collections.

17. Analyze the professionalism questions and apply them to this chapter's content.

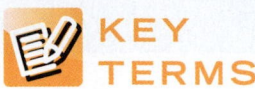

KEY TERMS

accounts receivable ratio

collection ratio

Fair Debt Collection Practice Act (FDCPA)

probate court

statute of limitations

Truth-in-Lending Act

ATTRIBUTES OF PROFESSIONALISM

Communication

- Did you listen to and acknowledge the patient?
- Did you speak at the patient's level of understanding?
- Did you provide appropriate responses/feedback?
- Did you respond honestly and diplomatically to the patient's concerns?
- Did you apply active listening skills?
- Does your knowledge allow you to speak easily with all members of the health care team?
- Did you demonstrate assertive communication with managed care and/or insurance providers?
- Did you maintain eye contact with the patient during communication?

Presentation

- Did you attend to any special needs of the patient? Did you first ask if assistance was needed, rather than taking charge?
- Were you courteous, patient, and respectful to the patient?
- Did you display a positive attitude?
- Did you display a calm, professional, and caring manner?

Competency

- Did you pay attention to detail?
- Did you display sound judgment?
- Were you knowledgeable and accountable?
- Did you recognize the importance of local, state, and federal legislation and regulations in the practice setting?
- Did you demonstrate sensitivity and professionalism in handling accounts receivable with patients?

Initiative

- Did you show initiative?
- Did you direct the patient to other resources when necessary or helpful, with the approval of the provider?
- Did you work with the provider to achieve maximum reimbursement?

Integrity

- Did you demonstrate sensitivity to patient's rights?
- Did you protect and maintain confidentiality?
- Did you immediately report any error you had made?
- Did you maintain your moral and ethical standards?

SCENARIO

At Drs. Lewis and King, patient billing is typically done at time of service, and a charge slip noting date, description of charges, and fees is given to the patient on leaving the clinic. Clinic policy states that, if possible, patients should pay their part of the fee, or their co-pay, at time of service. Marilyn Johnson, the office manager, has found that this is the most efficient way to ensure timely payment and eliminates the need to mail a separate statement. However, the clinic is flexible, and if the patient cannot pay all or part of the charge at the visit, Marilyn works out a payment schedule that is acceptable to both the clinic and the patient.

INTRODUCTION

In the ambulatory care setting, patient billing is a critical administrative function that helps to maintain a healthy, viable practice. Timeliness is essential in billing, because the ambulatory care setting depends on its accounts receivable to pay its bills in a responsible manner. Billing need not be a complex activity, but it must be completely accurate. In the few clinics still using pegboard accounting, billing and collection procedures are done manually, often using the patient's ledger as the basis for the statement. When the facility is computerized, patient bills and collection notices are computer generated.

The best method of patient billing and collections is a method that is customized to the practice and that regards the patient as a consumer who should be respected. Patients appreciate knowing in advance what charges and fees to expect. Many facilities include these in their informational brochures or post them in a prominent place on the premises.

SPOTLIGHT ON CERTIFICATION

RMA Content Outline
- Financial and bookkeeping

CMA (AAMA) Content Outline
- Professional communication and behavior
- Legislation
- Bookkeeping systems
- Computer applications

CMAS Content Outline
- Fundamental financial management
- Patient accounts

BILLING PROCEDURES

The ambulatory care setting's cash flow and collection process are dependent on up-to-date and accurate billing techniques. The financial status of the practice is reflected in monthly statements indicating unpaid patient balances, which, if they persist, are reviewed for appropriate action, including possible referral to a collection agency. Copies of all billing forms will be retained in the patient account record.

Timeliness and accuracy have a significant influence on prompt payment and how soon collection of the patient account will be finalized. In other words, billing performance can be measured by the time it takes to generate and submit a complete statement, that is, a statement with full documentation. If a facility is experiencing problems generating patient bills, a billing timeliness analysis worksheet can be constructed to identify internal delays that affect how quickly an account is billed, and thus paid. By focusing on inefficiencies in the revenue cycle, processes may be identified that need to be streamlined. For example, the date of service and insurance verification, the date the bill was generated, and the date the bill was submitted to the patient or third party can determine the efficiency of the billing process.

A billing efficiency report is another instrument that may be used to monitor the efficiency of the billing process. This report lists the previous month's billing backlog, which is added to the number of new accounts. The number of processed accounts is then subtracted. The weekly number of accounts that were rebilled also is noted, and the amount of time billing personnel spent on billing accounts is recorded. Production efficiency is calculated from these data. Inherent to this system is the careful monitoring of follow-up bills, including whether they were paid, whether the insurance paid, and an assessment of the patient's responsibility for payment.

CREDIT AND COLLECTION POLICIES

It is important that patients understand the billing policy and are educated about their accounts, how they are paid, and what their responsibility is toward payment. This is most easily accomplished in a patient-information brochure (see Chapter 45) identifying all aspects of the medical practice, including how bills are paid. The clinic staff also must have a well-defined policy related to patient billing and collecting.

Even uncomplicated patient billing should be done according to credit and collection policies established by the provider–employers of the ambulatory care setting. Having a formalized policy makes decision making easier and gives the medical assistant or office manager responsible for billing and collections authority to act. For example, some questions the providers and office manager may want to address include:

- When will payment be due from the patient?
- What kind of payment arrangements can be made if the patient does not pay at time of service?
- At what point should a patient be reminded of an overdue bill?
- How is the reminder initially managed: by telephone, a note on the statement, or a letter?
- At what point will a patient bill be considered delinquent?
- Will a collection agency be used? Who decides?
- If exceptions to the policy are to be made, who makes these exceptions and what steps are taken?

By answering these and other questions, a straightforward credit and collection policy can be devised that is a guide to both patients and the medical assistant in charge of billing.

PAYMENT AT TIME OF SERVICE

The best opportunity for collection is at the time of service. This process begins with the medical assistant who schedules appointments. Make certain all patients have the information they need. After determining the urgency and reason for the appointment, collecting in-formation regarding a chief complaint, and assigning a time for the appointment, it is

appropriate to discuss the financial concerns of patients (Procedure 20-1). Patients may be shy in asking certain questions, but they have questions about most of the following issues:

- Whether the providers contract with their insurance carrier
- How payment is made if insurance does not cover certain procedures
- Whether they can be billed for co-payments and coinsurance
- How payment is made for services if they have no insurance
- An approximate cost of a particular service

Do not tell a patient, "We do not take your insurance." It is much better to make a statement such as, "Our providers do not contract with that insurance. However, we can work with you on a fee-for-service basis and help make finances workable for you." The atmosphere has now been created to ensure prompt collection and increased cash flow for the practice. To accommodate patients, clinics now increasingly accept debit and credit card payments. Remember, also, that if your facility does use a sign-in method as patients arrive, then the all-important personal contact may be missed. With that missed opportunity also goes the opportunity to discuss finances.

Most insurance contracts require the provider to bill the insurance company *before* billing the patient, except for the co-payment. It is critical to abide by each contract to protect the provider. If the patient is a member of a health maintenance organization (HMO) and the ambulatory care center is a participating provider, it is bound to the terms of that agreement. If not restricted by the insurance contract, be certain to explain to the patient at the time of service that any payment owed will be adjusted according to the patient's insurance and the terms of that policy. Also remember that all patients must be treated the same and charged the same for services.

With the knowledge of what portion of the fee can be collected at the time of service, the medical assistant says to the patient prior to leaving the facility, "The fee for your services today is $85. Will you be paying by cash, check, or credit/debit card?" When the policy for collecting fees is shared when the appointment is made, patients are not surprised by this approach. Allow the patient to be the next person to speak in response to the question asked. If for some reason a fee cannot be immediately paid, the patient will respond by asking what kind of arrangements might be made. Even if financial arrangements are necessary, the discussion of the day's fee for the service is in process.

TRUTH-IN-LENDING ACT

In those situations where a payment schedule is arranged, clinic policy will dictate if any interest is charged. Although it is not illegal to charge interest on patient accounts, many providers still prefer not to assign any interest on installment payments or past-due accounts.

For installment payments (such as prenatal care or surgery), medical assistants need to be aware of the conditions of the **Truth-in-Lending Act**, Regulation Z of the Consumer Protection Act of 1967 (see Chapter 7). If there is bilateral agreement between providers and their patients for payment of medical services in more than four installments, that agreement must be in writing and must provide information on any finance charge. The information must be in writing even if there are no finance charges made (Figure 20-1). The patient is given the original copy of the disclosure statement; a second copy is kept in the clinic.

COMPONENTS OF A COMPLETE STATEMENT

Once a patient has been accepted for treatment, it is important to maintain accurate and timely records of his or her account and payment history. That information is just as vital to the healthy management of the practice as the patient's medical record. Invoice patient services promptly according to the clinic policy, send statements regularly, and make certain they are complete and accurate. Statements to patients must be professional looking, neat, inclusive of all services and charges, and

CAPITAL AREA HEALTH CARE
839 Sycamore Park
Boise, ID 83725
(208) 863-4210

FEDERAL TRUTH-IN-LENDING STATEMENT
For Professional Services

Patient _____Cari R. Jacobson_____

Address _____913 Swanson Street_____

_____Boise, ID 61820_____

Parent _____

1. Cost of services rendered	$1,500.00
2. Down Payment	225.00
3. Unpaid Balance	1,275.00
4. Amount Financed	1,275.00
5. Finance Charge	-0-
6. Annual Percentage Rate of Finance Charge	-0-
7. Total of Payments (4 + 5 above)	1,275.00
8. Total Amount After Payments	1,500.00

Total payment due is payable to _Dr. Leslie Swaggert_ at above address in _5_ monthly installments of $ _255_ .The first installment is payable on _August 1, 20XX_ , and each subsequent payment is due on the same day of each consecutive month until paid in full.

____07-24-XX____   _____
Date of Agreement   Signature of Patient;
                          Parent if Patient is Minor

© Cengage Learning 2014

Figure 20-1 Truth-in-Lending Act document showing installment and interest agreement.

easily understood. Procedure and diagnosis codes are necessary for insurance and reimbursement, but they usually mean nothing to patients. Make certain patients can understand the terminology used to explain the procedures they received.

Billing occurs in a number of different ways, with the computer-generated statement the most widely used. As mentioned in Chapter 19, an encounter form may be used as the statement, especially if payment is made at the time of the service (Figure 20-2). Typewritten statements will likely use the continuous-form billing statement that is printed on a roll with perforated edges for separation. Photocopied statements are often used with a pegboard system. The ledger cards are coordinated with the same-size copy paper. These

DATE	PATIENT	SERVICE CODE	FEES CHARGED	PAID		ADJ.	BALANCE DUE		PREVIOUS BALANCE	NAME	RECEIPT NO.
				CREDITS							

THIS IS YOUR RECEIPT AND/OR A STATEMENT OF YOUR ACCOUNT TO DATE

PATIENTS NAME ☐ M ☐ F

ADDRESS

CITY   STATE   ZIP

RELATIONSHIP   BIRTHDATE

SUBSCRIBER OR POLICY HOLDER

☐ MEDICARE ☐ MEDICAID ☐ BLUE SHIELD ☐ 65-SP.

INSURANCE CARRIER

AGREEMENT #

GROUP #

OFFICE VISITS AND PROCEDURES

99211	EST PT - MINIMAL OV	1			HOSPITAL VISIT	14	
99212	EST PT - BRIEF OV	2			EMERGENCY	15	
99213	EST PT - INTERMEDIATE OV	3			CONSULTATION	16	
99214	EST PT - EXTENDED OV	4		93000	EKG	17	
99215	EST PT - COMPREHENSIVE OV	5		93224	ELECTROCARDIOGRAPHIC MONITORING	18	
99201	NEW PT - BRIEF OV	6		93307	ECHOCARDIOGRAPHY	19	
99202	NEW PT - INTERMEDIATE OV	7		85025	CBC	20	
99203	NEW PT - EXTENDED OV	8		81000	URINALYSIS WITH MICROSCOPY	21	
99204	NEW PT - COMPLEX OV	9		36415	ROUTINE VENIPUNCTURE	22	
99205	NEW PT - COMPREHENSIVE OV	10		71020	RADIOLOGY EXAM-CHEST-2 VIEWS	23	
99238	HOSPITAL DISCHARGE	11		30300	REMOVE FOR. BODY-INTRANASAL	24	
99025	NEW PT - SURGERY PROC. PRIMARY	12				25	
	NURSING HOME VISIT	13				26	

D - OTHER SERVICES

AUTHORIZATION TO RELEASE INFORMATION: I HEREBY AUTHORIZE THE UNDERSIGNED PHYSICIAN TO RELEASE ANY INFORMATION ACQUIRED IN THE COURSE OF MY EXAMINATION OR TREATMENT.
SIGNED (PATIENT, OR PARENT IF MINOR) _____ DATE _____

NEXT APPOINTMENT _____ AT _____ AM PM
RETURN _____ DAYS _____ WEEKS _____ MONTHS

PLACE OF SERVICE ☐ OFFICE ☐ OTHER _____
DIAGNOSIS OR SYMPTOMS _____

DOCTOR'S SIGNATURE _____

CAPITAL AREA HEALTH CARE
839 SYCAMORE PARK
BOISE, ID 83725
(208) 863-4210

03626

© Cengage Learning 2014

Figure 20-2 The sample encounter form (charge slip) is a multipurpose form used to document information for insurance claims as well as to provide the patient with a receipt and documentation of procedures, diagnoses, and fees. It can be used as the patient's first bill.

photocopied ledgers are placed in a window envelope so that the address on the ledger card shows through the window.

If the statement is to be mailed, an enclosed self-addressed envelope is appreciated by the patient and may result in a faster turnaround of payment. Stamp the words "Address Service Requested" on the envelope just below the return address. When this statement is stamped on the envelope, a valuable tool in collections is available at minimum cost. If the statement cannot be delivered as addressed (the patient has moved or "skipped" and has left no forwarding address), the post office researches this information and returns the envelope to you with a yellow sticker providing the new address and any other updated information. If the patient has ordered that mail be forwarded, the post office will forward the statement to the patient and send the medical facility a form with the new address. There is a fee for this service.

 A well-prepared patient statement should contain not only information for the patient but information needed to process medical insurance claims as well. The following information should be included (see Procedure 20-2):

- Patient's name and address
- Patient's insurance carrier and identification number
- Date and place of service
- Description of service and fee for each service
- Accurate procedure and diagnosis codes for insurance processing (see Chapters 17 and 18)
- Provider's signature and identification code or National Provider Identifier (NPI)
- Clinic name, address, telephone number, fax number, and Web site when applicable

Computerized Statements

By far the most common statements are computer generated. Typically, the medical assistant keys the computer command to search the patient database for outstanding balances and directs the computer to print statements.

Financial management software will age accounts (see Aging Accounts section) and can generate collection letters that have been specifically designed for the practice, allowing the medical assistant to key in the appropriate specific information (Figure 20-3).

All provider orders, prescriptions, recommendations, and a copy of the visit and health summary can be waiting for the patient at the time of checkout, if desired. With a single key entry, an electronic invoice is generated with appropriate diagnostic and procedural codes already applied. If insurance is to be billed, the claim is automatically placed in the insurance queue to be uploaded electronically to third-party payers.

Any payments made can be posted electronically and statements can then be printed for the patient. The collection portion of the financial management software keeps up with the daily billing tasks. Procedures 20-3 and 20-4 identify accounts receivable and prepare itemized patient statements for billing using an electronic system.

MONTHLY AND CYCLE BILLING

The billing schedule is often determined by the size of the medical practice. Monthly billing is a system in which all accounts are billed at the same time each month. In a smaller ambulatory care setting, monthly billing may be the most efficient method. Cycle billing staggers bills during the month and is a flexible system for larger practices.

Monthly Billing

In a monthly billing system, one or two days are devoted to billing and mailing all statements. Typically, statements should leave the clinic no later than the 25th of the month to be received by the first of the month. The major disadvantage of monthly billing is that a medical assistant may neglect other activities during this time-consuming period. To avoid these problems, billing statements may be prepared intermittently

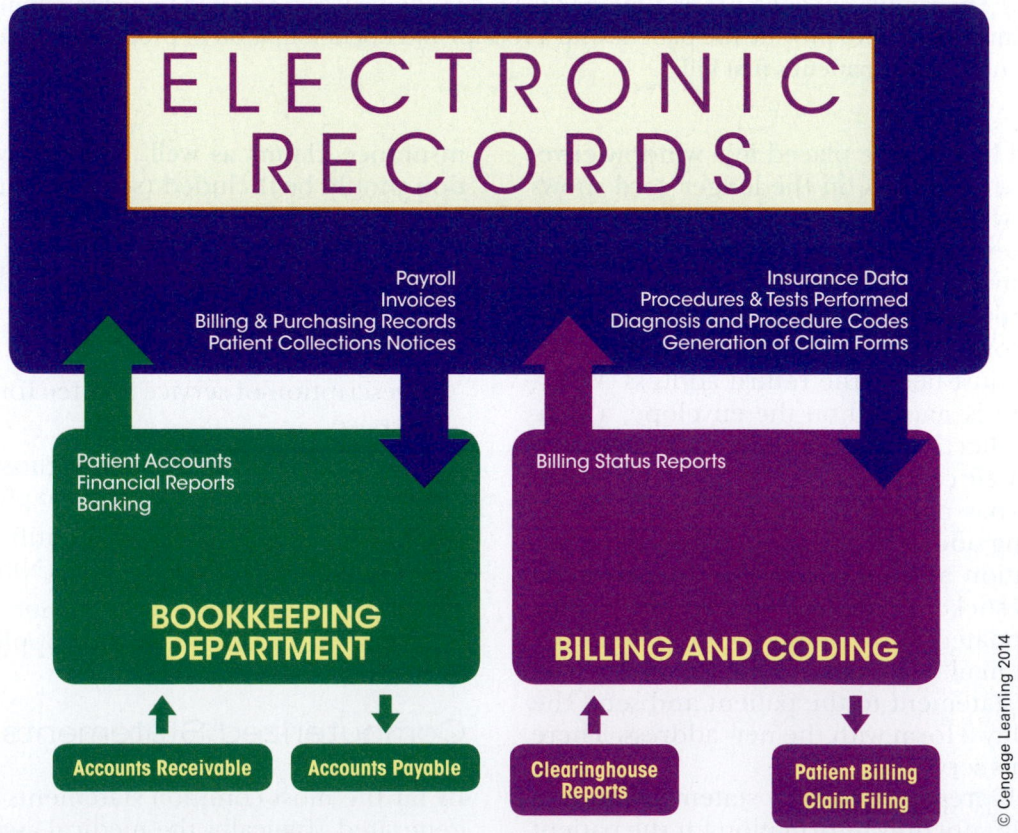

© Cengage Learning 2014

Figure 20-3 Total practice management system diagram illustrating billing and collection activities.

Sample of Cycle Billing

1. Divide the alphabet into four sections: A–F, G–L, M–R, S–Z.
2. Prepare statements for patients whose last names begin with A through F on Wednesday and mail them on Thursday of Week 1.
3. Prepare statements for patients whose last names begin with G through L on Wednesday and mail them on Thursday of Week 2.
4. Prepare statements for patients whose last names begin with M through R on Wednesday and mail them on Thursday of Week 3.
5. Prepare statements for patients whose last names begin with S through Z on Wednesday and mail them on Thursday of Week 4.

© Cengage Learning 2014

Figure 20-4 Typical schedule for cycle billing system.

over a one- or two-week period and stored until the mailing date. To avoid confusion caused by delays in mailing, a message to "Disregard if payment has already been made" should be printed on the form. Patients become annoyed and the practice appears disorganized if a statement arrives several days after payment has been made.

Cycle Billing

In a cycle billing system, all accounts usually are divided alphabetically into groups, with each group billed at a different time. In this way, administrative personnel with numerous bills to process each month will be able to handle them in a more efficient manner. Statements are prepared on the same schedule each month. They can be mailed as they are completed, or held and mailed at one time. A typical cycle billing schedule is shown in Figure 20-4. The system can be varied to suit the needs of the individual practice.

PAST-DUE ACCOUNTS

As efficient and effective as the billing process may be, there will still be collections on some accounts. The most common reasons for past-due accounts include:

- *Inability to pay.* People may have financial hardships from time to time (see Chapter 19).

- *Negligence.* People may forget to make a payment because they have been away or dealing with a family emergency.
- *Unwillingness to pay.* When a patient complains about a charge or refuses to pay, it may have nothing to do with finances. Often, they are dissatisfied with the care or treatment they have received. These patients should be referred to the provider or office manager for immediate attention.
- *Third-party payers.* Past-due accounts may result because of inaccurate or insufficient insurance information. Claims can be rejected because of many varied reasons, and time limits must be observed.
- *Minors.* Minors who are not legally emancipated may seek and receive treatment, but they are not responsible for paying the bill (see Chapter 7). If the medical practice treats minors who are not emancipated, a clinic policy should determine how these minors pay for their services. Emancipated minors are responsible for their bills. Many facilities ask for cash at the time of the service.

COLLECTION PROCESS

The process of collecting delinquent accounts begins with first establishing how much has been owed and for how long.

Ideally, collection of accounts receivable should be prompt and conducted in a timely fashion. Management consultants recommend collecting at least a portion of the fees at the time of service and that a **collection ratio** of 90% or better should be maintained. Another important factor is the **accounts receivable ratio** that measures the speed with which outstanding accounts are paid. The desirable accounts receivable ratio is less than 2 months for collection of accounts receivable.

Collection Ratio

A collection ratio is a method used to gauge the effectiveness of the ambulatory care setting's billing practices. This ratio shows the status of collections and the possible losses in the medical facility. It is a good idea to obtain the ratio monthly, quarterly, and yearly. Typically, the collection ratio is calculated by dividing the total collections by the net charges (gross or total charges minus any adjustments). This yields a percentage that is referred to as the collection ratio. See the following example:

$$\frac{\text{Total Amount Collected this Month}}{\text{Total Monthly Charges Minus Adjustments}} = \text{Monthly Collection Ratio}$$

$$\frac{\$34,650}{\$44,928} = .7712 \text{ or } 77\%$$

In this sample, you can determine that more time and energy needs to be spent in collecting accounts. The practice is losing almost 25% of its income potential. Not only is the income potential being lost but also the ability to invest that income is lost, making the potential loss even greater.

Accounts Receivable Ratio

An accounts receivable ratio indicates how quickly outstanding accounts are paid. It can also be a measure of how effective the collections are. To calculate the accounts receivable ratio, divide the current accounts receivable balance by the average monthly gross charges. This yields the typical turnaround for collecting accounts receivable. See the following example:

$$\frac{\text{Current Accounts Receivable}}{\text{Average Monthly Gross Charges}} = \text{Accounts Receivable Ratio}$$

$$\frac{\$145,048}{\$44,928} = 3.2$$

Because the goal of the accounts receivable ratio is payment in less than 2 months, you can quickly observe that this practice is over 1 month behind in collections. Chapter 21 gives additional information on accounts receivable and collection ratios.

The longer a practice delays attempting to collect delinquent accounts, the less chance there is of receiving payment. Statistics show that the value of the dollar decreases rapidly in the collection process. That is, the more time and energy put into collections, the less value received in return. You may manage to collect the full amount due, but when you consider the time and expense involved, it may not have been worth the effort and expense. Therefore, the value of the debt to be received after successful collection must be considered when determining how aggressive to be in debt collections.

AGING ACCOUNTS

Account aging is a method of identifying how long an account has been overdue. This means that past-due accounts are identified according to the length of time they have been unpaid. When using a peg-board bookkeeping system, color-coded strips are attached to the ledger cards to show the age of an account, or the cards can be stored behind a color-coded divider in a separate file labeled "Unpaid." For example, a red strip might be used for accounts 1 month overdue, a blue strip for accounts 2 months overdue, and other colors for additional months overdue. A written code such as "OD3/2/23" should be written on the ledger card to indicate when the overdue notice was mailed, meaning "Overdue notice No. 3 mailed on February 23."

Depending on the type of patient served, different aging systems are used. In a computerized billing system, the accounts are automatically aged, and the aging schedule or process is shown on the computerized ledger.

Computerized Aging

Aging accounts using a computer software system is simple. Before printing billing statements, the medical assistant keys the appropriate commands to age the accounts. The program can age accounts according to several criteria: for example, by past due balance, zero balance, or credit balance accounts. Accounts can also be aged by government agency category or by insurance carrier. All Medicare or Medicaid accounts might be aged separately from other accounts. Sorting out Medicare and Medicaid accounts may also be done when computing the accounts receivable ratio and the collection ratio.

The computer can also generate and print an accounts receivable report showing each overdue account, the balance overdue, and a breakdown showing how long the account has been overdue. This breakdown is usually divided into accounts 0 to 30 days overdue, 31 to 60 days overdue, 61 to 90 days overdue, and 90 days or more overdue. Additional reports can be generated from the accounts receivable report. For example, the clinic staff may wish to print a report showing accounts that have been delinquent for more than 90 days or accounts that are delinquent by more than a certain dollar amount.

COLLECTION TECHNIQUES

Ambulatory care settings use both telephone and written communications in their collection techniques. Although both have some measure of effectiveness, some practices prefer to call the patient with a past-due account before officially initiating collection proceedings. The patient may have misplaced the statement, forgotten a payment, or been away on an extended vacation; a quick telephone call can often resolve the situation without the time and expense involved in collections. Also, the patient usually appreciates the courtesy and personal approach.

Many patients work part or full time, sometimes making telephone calls difficult to complete. It is often beneficial for providers to ask the office manager or the medical assistant in charge of collections to work 2 or more hours one evening a week for the purpose of making collection telephone calls. Calls are more likely to be answered in the time period from 5 PM to 8 PM than during the middle of the day. Figure 20-5 shows a sample collections policy.

SAMPLE COLLECTION POLICY SCHEDULE

- Encounter form (if used) given to patient at time of visit.
- Itemized statement sent no later than the end of that month.
- Itemized statement with overdue notice no later than the end of the second month.
- Telephone call reminding the patient of the bill. "We've sent two statements and we haven't received payment. Do you need more information from us?" Offer help at this point in establishing a payment schedule, and seek to get a commitment from the patient.
- If a financial schedule is to be established, prepare it and mail to the patient within a day of the phone conversation. Follow up on that commitment within 15 days. The follow-up message may be a thank you for sending the first payment. Carefully monitor payments and their timeliness.
- If no payment schedule is made by the patient, send a letter stating the amount due before the account is past due three months. Discuss with office manager and/or physician regarding the merit of continued collection at this time.
- If collections are to continue, notify the patient one more time of their responsibility and ask for payment.
- If no payment is received, send a letter stating that "Your account has been turned over to a collection agency" if outside collectors are used. Make no more phone calls.*

*Some physicians send a letter of discharge to patients at this time via certified mail. (See Chapter 7.)

© Cengage Learning 2014

Figure 20-5 Sample collection policy.

Billing Insurance Carriers

Many patients have some form of medical insurance (see Chapter 17). Make it a practice to send each computer claim within 2 days or less of the patient account data being entered into the computer. Batches of claims to insurance carriers should be forwarded at the end of each day. In the era of electronic claims processing, much time is saved in not having to prepare hard copies of the forms for mailing. Electronic claims transmission (ECT; also known as electronic medic claims, or EMC, and electronic claims submission, or ECS) dictates that the practice's computer system must be able to communicate with the insurance carrier's computer. This paperless process yields fewer errors than the manual process because ECT software includes some built-in checks to determine any invalid codes, sex or age conflicts, and correct procedure and diagnostic code linkages to the services provided. Sending insurance claims via the paper process will take more time to process, and the turnaround time for payment is also longer. Most claim departments of insurance carriers and government agencies have large numbers of employees with varying levels of experience. Payment can be delayed because of an overburdened claim department, a form that has been lost in transit, a misfiled form, an inexperienced employee, or numerous other reasons.

The medical assistant should maintain an up-to-date claims register or insurance-pending report and take firm control of the practice's collection procedures to ensure that claims are paid promptly.

This claims register or insurance-pending report may be a part of the computerized billing system. If so, the printout will show how much the practice charged insurance carriers and how much was received. This clearly shows which carriers are slower than others and where other problems might arise. For any claim pending more than 45 days, it is a good idea to make a call to the carrier to find out whether the claim has been received, where it is in the process, and whether the clinic staff might have done something to delay the process. Such phone calls can become carefully cultivated personal contacts with insurance representatives to pave the way for cooperation in the future.

In clinics where the medical assistant files claims for patients, a follow-up collection policy is important to maintain strong cash flow. When carriers do not pay in full or question or deny a claim, the medical assistant should determine the nature of the problem and rebill or appeal the decision, whichever action is appropriate.

Telephone Collections

The medical assistant is likely to use the telephone for collection procedures. Telephoning is often an effective measure because a patient may respond to a call more than to a bill received in the mail.

 A successful telephone collection call is enhanced by keeping to the facts and being tactful, pleasant, and diplomatic. When making calls to patients regarding past-due accounts, there are some things to keep in mind to maintain the desired relationship with patients. Always remain courteous and respectful. Do not treat patients with suspicion or threats. Remember, the health profession is dedicated to helping people; avoid antagonizing patients.

Most people do not let their bills become past due on purpose or out of spite. Keep this in mind when making calls. Work with patients to encourage and enable them to pay any fees they owe.

  Certain legal rules and ethical guidelines govern telephone collections:

- When making collection calls, callers must identify themselves and ascertain that they are talking to the person who is responsible for the account.
- A collection call could be embarrassing to the patient; therefore, it should not be made to the patient's place of employment.
- In most states, a debtor may be contacted only between 8 AM and 8 PM.
- Do not make telephone calls at odd hours or make repeated calls to the debtor's friends, employers, or relatives.
- If a contact must be made to the debtor's place of business, do not reveal to any third party the nature of the call. Patients have a right to confidentiality and privacy.
- Do not threaten to turn the person's account over to collection agencies.

When collecting by telephone, it is helpful to keep complete, accurate records of the process indicating who said what and how much was promised as payment. If after 2 weeks nothing has been resolved as a result of the calls, then another course of action may be the solution, especially for large sums of money owed. Collection letters may be necessary.

Fair Debt Collection Practices Act. Violating rules regarding harassment makes the caller vulnerable to charges under the **Fair Debt Collection Practices Act (FDCPA)**. According to the guidelines set by the FDCPA, which is overseen by the Federal Trade Commission (FTC), debt collectors are not allowed to use their positions to collect a debt using any manner of work performance that is found to be abusive, deceptive, or unethical. The collectors must abide by certain guidelines, such as not calling a debtor at work without written consent and keeping calls to debtors between the hours of 8:00 AM and 9:00 PM. Under the FDCPA, debts that are created by medical expenses are a type of debt that can be sent to collection agencies and subsequently collected upon. The collectors are strictly prohibited from using profane language or any language that indicates a threat (such as wage or tax refund garnishment). It is very important that the administrative medical assistant abide by such guidelines as given within the FDCPA.

Collection Letters

Collection letters are sent to encourage patients to pay overdue balances. After two statements are mailed to patients and the charge slip or encounter form has brought no response, the ambulatory care setting begins sending collection letters.

Lack of payment from a patient may not be considered serious until after 60 days. When the patient fails to respond to the encounter form, to the statement, or to a 60-day statement with an "Overdue" remark, a series of collection letters begins. One typical collection letter series is shown in Figure 20-6A through Figure 20-6C. Collection letters and notes are kept separate from a patient's chart.

USE OF AN OUTSIDE COLLECTION AGENCY

Occasionally, the ambulatory care setting turns over highly delinquent accounts to an outside collection agency. Discretion is always advised here, however, because the fees to be collected may not justify the expense of collection. For unpaid accounts with large balances, however, this is often a viable solution.

One service provided by a collection agency is an intercept letter. For a nominal fee, this letter may be sent from the agency as the last resort before the account is turned over to collection. This communication alerts patients to the fact that if a response is not received, their account will go to collection. This often is the only action needed

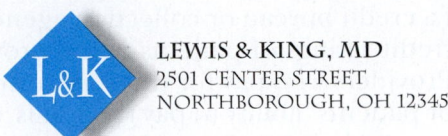

LEWIS & KING, MD
2501 CENTER STREET
NORTHBOROUGH, OH 12345

June 14, 20XX

Mr. John O'Keefe
12 Gravers Lane
Northborough, OH 12345

Dear Mr. O'Keefe:

Your account with our office is three months past due, and you have not responded to our previous requests for payment. Please pay your balance of $852 at this time, or contact us with a plan for payment.

Please call me at 312-824-6925 if you have a question about your account or a plan for payment. Otherwise, we expect your payment immediately.

Sincerely,

Marilyn Johnson
Office Manager

NORTHBOROUGH
FAMILY MEDICAL GROUP

A

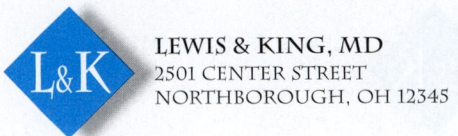

LEWIS & KING, MD
2501 CENTER STREET
NORTHBOROUGH, OH 12345

July 15, 20XX

Mr. John O'Keefe
12 Gravers Lane
Northborough, OH 12345

Dear Mr. O'Keefe:

Your son, Chris, was seriously ill in March when he was seen by Dr. King. Dr. King used her experience and education to treat Chris, believing you would pay your account within a reasonable amount of time.

Four months have passed and you have still not remitted the $852 outstanding balance on your account. We cannot continue to keep your unpaid account on our books. If you are experiencing financial difficulties, please call the office at 312-824-6925 so we can arrange a payment schedule that is agreeable to both of us.

Sincerely,

Marilyn Johnson
Office Manager

NORTHBOROUGH
FAMILY MEDICAL GROUP

B

Figure 20-6   Sample collection letters: (A) First letter. (B) Second letter. *(continues)*

LEWIS & KING, MD
2501 CENTER STREET
NORTHBOROUGH, OH 12345

August 17, 20XX

CERTIFIED MAIL

Mr. John O'Keefe
12 Gravers Lane
Northborough, OH 12345

Dear Mr. O'Keefe:

This is our final attempt to collect your account of $852, which is five months past due. You have not responded to all our previous letters [or letters and phone calls], so we have no alternative but to turn over your account to a collection company.

Your account is being assigned to Ambler Medical Collection Service, which will pursue whatever legal means is necessary to collect this debt. If you contact me at 312-824-6925 within seven days, we can prevent the account from this assignment and resolve the balance.

Sincerely,

Marilyn Johnson
Office Manager

NORTHBOROUGH
FAMILY MEDICAL GROUP

C

© Cengage Learning 2014

Figure 20-6 (continued) (C) Third letter.

for the patient to pay the outstanding bill. Another service of a credit bureau or collection agency is to provide credit ratings of patients at the provider's request. Providers who pay for this service are able to monitor patients' ability to pay their bills, as well as to trace a "skip," someone who leaves with an outstanding bill and no forwarding address.

When selecting a collection agency, be certain to hire one that is compatible with the medical practice's philosophy. Questions that might be asked of potential collection agencies include the following:

- Does the agency handle only medical and dental accounts?
- What methods are used to make collections?
- Is the agency fee a flat charge per account or a percentage of the account recovered?
- How promptly does the agency settle accounts?
- Will the agency supply a list of satisfied customers or references?
- What ability does the medical practice have to end the agency's collection efforts?

Once a collection agency has been selected, carefully follow their instructions about any contact patients make with the medical clinic regarding their account as well as any other guidelines in their contract with the practice. Keep a record of accounts given to the agency, as well as their rate of return. Hopefully, the agency will be able to motivate patients to pay for the health care services they have received while still maintaining the practice's good reputation and increasing your profit margin. Medical collections let your patients know that the practice is serious about collecting past-due accounts.

There is often a question about how payments from collection agencies are posted. This is one purpose of the adjustment column. Place the amount received in the adjustment column because it is a subtraction from the amount due. If there is no adjustment column, put the amount in the charge column and put red parentheses around it or circle in red so the amount is actually subtracted from the balance. The remaining balance after collections are paid is written off (Procedures 20-5 and 20-6).

USE OF SMALL CLAIMS COURT

 In certain circumstances, a clinic's office manager may consider bringing a case to small claims court. Typically, small claims courts handle cases that involve only limited amounts of debt (these vary from state to state), they usually do not permit representation by an attorney, and they are generally efficient and streamlined in their proceedings. Nonetheless, preparing for small claims courts and taking time to appear will require a certain investment of staff. It is important to note that, if the court finds in the clinic's favor, the clinic still must collect the money from the defendant. An account assigned to a collection agency cannot be filed in small claims court.

SPECIAL COLLECTION SITUATIONS

In patient billing and collections, a number of special situations may arise.

Bankruptcy

If a patient has declared bankruptcy, statements may no longer be sent nor may any attempts be made to collect delinquent accounts. A patient declaring bankruptcy usually does so under Chapter 7 or Chapter 13 bankruptcy law. In a Chapter 7 bankruptcy, a patient declares bankruptcy to all debtors and is allowed to clear all debts and start fresh. The medical clinic should file a proof-of-claim form and provide a copy of the patient's outstanding account to the bankruptcy court. In a Chapter 13 bankruptcy, also known as a "wage-earner's bankruptcy," patients (wage-earners) are protected from bill collectors and are allowed to pay their bills over a specified time. The court determines a monthly amount that the debtor can pay, collects that sum, and parcels it out to the creditors over a period as long as five years. The clinic must file a claim as directed by the debtor's attorney to collect any fees outstanding. Because a provider's fee is an unsecured debt, it is one of the last to be paid. Bankruptcy laws are federal and are subject to the Federal Wage Garnishment Law regarding attaching property to satisfy debt.

Estates

Collection of fees when a patient has died must be directed to the executor of the estate or the one responsible for overseeing the estate. Some general guidelines to follow include:

- Show courtesy by not sending a statement in the first week or so after a death.

- Prepare an itemized statement of the deceased patient's account. (In some cases, a special form is required for this.)
- Mail the account information via certified mail with a return receipt requested to the administrator of the estate. The name can be obtained by calling the probate department of the superior court.
- If there is no known or identified administrator, send a copy of the itemized statement to the "Estate of (name of patient)" at the patient's last known address. Often, a family member has assumed the responsibility for paying the patient's account balances.
- If unsure of how to proceed, contact the clinic's attorney or the clerk of the **probate court** for advice.

Tracing "Skips"

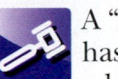 A "skip" is a patient with an unpaid bill who has apparently moved with no forwarding address. If a statement is returned to your clinic marked "no forwarding address," first determine if any internal errors were made in addressing the envelope. If the address is determined to be correct, the medical assistant may try to call the patient at the telephone number on the patient ledger; it is possible that the patient has retained the same number, or there may be a new number given. If the medical assistant is unable to secure a telephone number, the facility needs to decide whether to pursue the unpaid debt. This will depend on clinic policy and the amount that is owed. If it is decided to pursue an unpaid account, it can be turned over to a collection agency. If the medical assistant attempts to trace the skip by calling employers or relatives, it is important not to violate any laws in doing so and to maintain the patient's confidentiality.

STATUTE OF LIMITATIONS

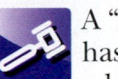 A **statute of limitations** is a statute that defines the period in which legal action may take place. When applying this concept to collections, the time period is usually defined by the class into which the account falls. These include open book accounts, which may have periodic charges against them; written contracts; and single-entry accounts, which have only one charge against them. The time period in which legal action must take place against any of these accounts

varies from state to state. If an unpaid account is more than 3 years old, it is wise to investigate the statute of limitations in your state before spending time and effort in collections. (For state-by-state information on the statute of limitations on debts, see www.creditinfocenter.com, under "Debts.")

MAINTAIN A PROFESSIONAL ATTITUDE

 Collecting past-due accounts is one of the most difficult tasks delegated to medical assistants. Not everyone is able to perform this task. Placing calls can be discouraging, especially if the results seem less than anticipated. Not all accounts can be collected. Identify these accounts early, write them off, and save the medical practice time and money. Keep any bias and your emotions out of the process. Rely only on your information, the aged account, and the realization that the clinic policy is well thought out and provides a win-win solution for both the patient and the provider as much as possible. When dealing with a "true deadbeat" who has no intention of paying the bill, be proud of your provider's attention to that patient's need, but discuss with the provider the possibility of discharging the patient. Staff may need additional training and education from time to time to update skills on patient service and how to maintain goodwill during the collection process.

PROCEDURE 20-1

Explaining Fees in the First Telephone Interview

PURPOSE:
To establish rapport with patients, to discuss providers' fees, and to identify the patient's responsibility before the first visit.

EQUIPMENT/SUPPLIES:
Provider's fee schedule
Appointment schedule
Telephone

PROCEDURE STEPS:

1. Place the providers' fee schedule and the appointment schedule close to the telephone. RATIONALE: The clinic staff that is prepared does not have to search for something vital to the phone conversation.

2. Answer the phone before the third ring. *Identify the name of the clinic and yourself.* RATIONALE: The person calling feels attended to and knows the call has been correctly placed.

3. *Acknowledge the patient* and offer assistance; for example, a comment such as "How can I help you?" RATIONALE: Sets the tone for the patient to continue with the request.

4. After the patient is identified as a new patient and the nature of the visit is determined appropriate, discuss possible dates for the appointment. A statement such as, "Our next available appointment is Thursday at 11:30 AM. Can you make it then?" is a good way to begin.

5. Tell the patient that you will be discussing clinic policies briefly now and will mail the Patient Information Brochure before the appointment. RATIONALE: The patient brochure details some of the information discussed in the telephone conversation and further verifies the clinic's policies.

6. Ask about medical insurance. If the patient is insured, get the identification number, the name of the subscriber, the employer, and a telephone number of the insurance carrier if possible. RATIONALE: This allows you to check for any preauthorization required and for the currency of the plan.

7. Explain that the clinic policy requires any co-payment and coinsurance to be paid at the time of the visit. RATIONALE: Establishes patient's financial responsibility immediately.

8. Check to see if the patient has transportation and knows how to get to the clinic, and provide directions if necessary. RATIONALE: Ensures that there is no confusion about location and accessibility.

9. Request that the patient arrive about 15 minutes before the appointment to complete some forms. RATIONALE: Ensures that the patient has time to complete information and can ask any questions that might occur.

10. After closing the telephone interview, promptly mail the Patient Information Brochure.

PROCEDURE 20-2

Prepare Itemized Patient Accounts for Billing in a Manual System

PURPOSE:
To notify patients of the fees for services rendered and collect on those accounts.

EQUIPMENT/SUPPLIES:
Computer
Calculator
Patient account or ledger cards
Billing statement forms

PROCEDURE STEPS:

1. Gather all accounts and ledgers with outstanding balances. RATIONALE: Everything in one place saves time and energy.

2. Separate any accounts that are labeled as overdue. RATIONALE: Individual decisions on these accounts are necessary before taking action.

3. *Pay attention to detail,* and for each account, perform the following:

   a. Verify the name and address of the patient and the person responsible for payment.

   b. Place current date on the statement.

   c. Scan the account information for any possible errors.

   d. Itemize the procedures in terms patients understand and indicate charges.

   e. Identify and subtract any payments (co-payment, coinsurance, down payment) that have been made.

   f. Use the calculator to verify the unpaid balance that is carried forward and is due.

4. *Discuss with the office manager* any action to be taken on past-due accounts. Follow through with those instructions. RATIONALE: More than one person is involved in the collection process.

5. Place statements in envelopes and mail. RATIONALE: Ensures timely delivery of statements.

PROCEDURE 20-3

Identifying Accounts Receivable Using Medical Office Simulation Software (MOSS)

PURPOSE:
To identify accounts receivable for patient billing or secondary insurance billing.

EQUIPMENT/SUPPLIES:
Computer and MOSS

PROCEDURE STEPS:

1. Click on the *Report Generation* button on the *Main Menu.*

2. Select the *Billing and Payment Report,* option 5.

3. Enter start date of the report needed, then click *OK.*

4. Enter end date of the report needed, then click *OK.*

5. Size the report to a comfortable viewing size.

6. Print the *Billing and Payment Report.*

7. Review the report and identify all patients and the balance due for each.

8. When necessary to view the patient ledger while analyzing the report, click on *Billing* from the drop-down menu along the top left of MOSS, and select *Patient Ledger.*

9. Select the patient name in the ledger to view details of the financial transactions against the *Billing and Payment Report.*

10. Close the report and return to the *Main Menu.* Hint: Be careful to close the report only, and not the entire MOSS software.

PROCEDURE 20-4

Preparing Itemized Patient Statements Using Medical Office Simulation Software (MOSS)

PURPOSE:
To prepare statements for patients with balances due on account.

EQUIPMENT/SUPPLIES:
Computer and MOSS

PROCEDURE STEPS:
1. Click on the *Patient Billing* button on the *Main Menu*.
2. Select the following items on the *Patient Billing* window:

    Field 1: 30-60-90 Standard Statement (or Remainder Statement, as applicable)

    Field 2: Provider: All

    Field 3: Service Dates: Enter from/through dates

    Field 3: Report Date: Date of billing

    Field 3: Patient Name: Select Patient

    Field 3: Account Number: Select Account Number

3. In Field 6, enter the dunning message, if required to explain the balance.
4. In Field 7, select the patient name(s) from the list of accounts that will get the dunning message.
5. Click *Process* to produce the statement(s).
6. Print the statement(s) and prepare mailing envelopes.
7. Close the statement window and return to the *Patient Billing* window. Input data for another statement, or close the window and return to the *Main Menu*.

PROCEDURE 20-5

Preparing Collection Letters Using Medical Office Simulation Software (MOSS)

PURPOSE:
To transcribe (type) medical collection letters using MOSS based on office manager dictation.

EQUIPMENT/SUPPLIES:
Computer and MOSS
Source documents

PROCEDURE STEPS:
1. After setting up the transcription equipment and inserting the tape, click on the *Billing* drop-down menu option in MOSS (along the top left) and click on *Patient Ledger*.
2. Select the patient from the *Patient Account* list and click on *View*. This will display the patient's ledger. Hint: Click on the magnifying glass icon to drop down the list of patients.
3. At the bottom left of the ledger screen, click on the *Correspondence* button.
4. The *Output To* dialog box will open. Select a location to save your letter and name it as follows: patientlastname_collection letter_yourlastname. Click *OK* to save the letter.
5. After a short pause, the letterhead for Douglasville Medicine Associates opens. Change the date of the letter to the desired date and put your own last name in the *Student No.* field.
6. Include a subject line with the date(s) of service and balance due amount before the salutation, as indicated in the dictation. Next, with the cursor, click at *Type Message Here* and delete that line. Start the body of the letter at that location.
7. Transcribe (type) the office manager's dictation as shown on the source document. Be sure to format the letter, use punctuation, and use proper grammar.
8. When complete, save the document by clicking on the *Save* button on the word processor.
9. Print the letter so the office manager may sign it and turn in a copy to your instructor. Prepare a mailing envelope.
10. Close the word processor and return to the Main Menu in MOSS.

PROCEDURE 20-6

Posting Non-Sufficient Fund (NSF) Checks Using Medical Office Simulation Software (MOSS)

PURPOSE:
To post and charge back NSF checks to patient accounts, including bank fees.

EQUIPMENT/SUPPLIES:
Computer and MOSS

PROCEDURE STEPS:

1. Click on the *Posting Payments* button on the *Main Menu.*

2. Select the patient and then click the *Apply Payment* button.

3. Select the line item for service date to be charged back and then click on *Select/Edit.*

4. Change the date to the date of posting and then drop down the box for Field 10, *Adjustments* and select *Adjustment Debit.*

5. In Field 11, enter the amount to be charged back to the account. Include the original amount and add any additional fees, if applicable.

6. Write a note in Field 14 regarding the adjustment so that the reason for the charge back is documented for the line item.

7. Click *Post* to apply the charges.

8. Click *Close* and return to the *Main Menu.*

PROCEDURE 20-7

Post/Record Collection Agency Adjustments in a Manual System

PURPOSE:
To keep track of financial adjustments.

EQUIPMENT/SUPPLIES:
Manual bookkeeping system
Patient's account
Black and red ink pens for use in manual
  bookkeeping system

PROCEDURE STEPS:

1. With the daily schedule of services/charges in front of you (the manual daily sheet), enter amount received from the collection agency on a patient's account and a note such as "Payment from ABC Collection Agency" in the explanation section. RATIONALE: Indicates funds received on a collection contract.

2. Record the amount received and the explanation in the patient's account as well. The amount received is *subtracted* from the account balance. The balance amount of the account is placed in the "adjustment" column. If there is no adjustment column, put the amount in the charge column with parentheses around it or circle the amount in red. These data are copied to the patient's account in the write-it-once system. RATIONALE: Demonstrates the activity and the amount from the collection agency on a patient's account in the patient account documents.

3. Subtract the amount paid by the collection agency from the total charges to create the new balance. RATIONALE: Clearly indicates what portion of the account the patient has paid and the amount that is not collectible.

4. Write off this balance, indicating a zero balance on the patient's account. In the daily sheet, the difference between the amount collected and the amount paid by the collection agency (plus the agency's fee) is entered as a negative adjustment. RATIONALE: At the end of the year, totals can be obtained indicating the amount of uncollected charges for the practice's income tax preparation.

PROCEDURE 20-8

Post/Record Collection Agency Adjustments Using Medical Office Simulation Software (MOSS)

PURPOSE:
To post payments collected by a collection agency to patient accounts and adjust commission fees and uncollectable amounts.

EQUIPMENT/SUPPLIES:
Computer and MOSS
Source documents

PROCEDURE STEPS:

1. Click on *Posting Payments* from the *Main Menu*.

2. Select the patient from the *Posting Payments* patient selection window.

3. Select the line item for the service for which a payment will be posted.

4. Change the date of posting to the date the payment is being applied.

5. In Field 7, drop down the box and select *Other* as the payment option.

6. Input the check number and payment amount in Fields 8 and 9. Hint: See the Monthly Collection Report for the check number.

7. In Field 10, enter the adjustment amount, which includes the agency's commission and, if applicable, remaining balances.

8. In the Note, Field 14, enter the collection agency's business name and the date of the statement.

9. Click on the *Post* button to apply the payment and adjustment.

10. Close the posting window and select another patient, or return to the *Main Menu*.

CASE STUDY 20-1

Refer to the scenario at the beginning of the chapter. For patient accounts more than 60 days overdue, the clinic of Drs. Lewis and King begins a series of collection proceedings to attempt to collect the monies. Initially, they place a telephone call to the patient to determine whether a billing problem might be present that can be clarified over the telephone. If they cannot reach the patient or the patient does not respond to the call, then collections begin. Marilyn has assigned this function of the billing process to Ellen Armstrong, because Ellen has a warm telephone manner and is good with patients.

CASE STUDY REVIEW

1. Why is Ellen's telephone manner important in the collection process?

2. In addition to telephone collections, what patient letters might Ellen send?

3. Ellen has come across an account that is delinquent and discovers that the patient has declared bankruptcy. What can Ellen do now?

CASE STUDY 20-2

Morgan Bryant is the custodial parent and single mother of her 5-year-old son Custer, who has been a patient of the Valley Pediatric Clinic since his birth. Custer's father's insurance covered his medical expenses. During a separation and the resulting divorce, the medical bills continued to go to Custer's father. Morgan comes to the reception desk to discuss the collection letter she received. Her parenting plan requires her former husband to provide medical coverage for their son. However, it appears he canceled his policy coverage on his son 4 months ago and Morgan did not know this until she received the letter. Morgan is in tears.

CASE STUDY REVIEW

1. What is the first step the administrative medical assistant should take?

2. Is there anything the clinic staff might have done differently in collecting this account?

3. What might be done for Morgan now? Are any resources available to Morgan?

SUMMARY

Billing and collection activities in the ambulatory care setting are intricately linked to daily financial practices and claims processing, and the medical assistant responsible for billing should also be well aware of these other functions. Billing need not entail a complex or elaborate system, but whether accomplished by a manual or computer methodology, it needs to be precise, professional, and comprehensive—as all communications with patients should be. If collections become necessary, courteous and straightforward letters and telephone exchanges are the most effective. In the ambulatory care setting, the goal of all billing and collections is to maintain the relationship with the patient, while ensuring good cash flow and payment of accounts receivable.

STUDY FOR SUCCESS

To reinforce your knowledge and skills of information presented in this chapter:

- Review the *Key Terms*
- Role-play with other students to apply attributes of professionalism pertinent to this chapter.
- Consider the *Case Studies* and discuss your conclusions
- Answer the questions in the *Certification Review*
- Apply your knowledge by completing the *Activities* in the *Study Guide* and the *Games and Quizzes* in the StudyWARE **StudyWARE** software on the *Premium Website*
- Perform the *Procedures* using the *Competency Manual Checklists* in the *Competency Manual*
- Practice your problem-solving skills with the *Critical Thinking Challenge 3.0* on the *Premium Website*

Additional resources for this chapter include:

- Module 9 of the *Medical Assisting Learning Lab*
- *CourseMate for Delmar's Comprehensive Medical Assisting*
- *WebTutor for Delmar's Comprehensive Medical Assisting*

CERTIFICATION REVIEW

1. The Truth-In-Lending Act:
   a. is designed to place limits on the amount of debt for which consumers are liable
   b. is also known as the statute of limitations
   c. is also known as Regulation Z
   d. does not apply to medical facilities
2. Cycle billing is a system of billing:
   a. completed every fourth month
   b. done only by computer
   c. completed by the 25th of the month
   d. in which accounts are divided into sections for billing purposes
3. One of the most common reasons patient bills go unpaid is:
   a. inability to pay because of financial hardship
   b. patients consider the cost of medical care too high
   c. patients think their insurance should cover all medical bills
   d. patients think providers make too much money

4. Aging accounts:
   a. is a process of identifying overdue patient accounts
   b. describes patients who have a long-term relationship with the ambulatory care center
   c. describes older adult patients with Medicare
   d. applies to accounts considered inactive
5. If an unpaid account goes to small claims court:
   a. the medical clinic must engage an attorney representative
   b. the medical clinic is still responsible for collecting even if the court finds in its favor
   c. there is no need to show up at court
   d. a large sum of money must be at issue
6. A collection ratio:
   a. shows status of collections and possible losses
   b. divides the current accounts receivable by the average monthly gross charges
   c. should be 90% or better
   d. a and c
7. A claims register:
   a. identifies how many past-due claims have been collected
   b. may also be called the insurance-pending report
   c. is maintained by each insurance carrier for the provider
   d. is a tickler file that maintains all patients' insurance information

8. Telephone collections:
   a. are best made after 8 PM when patients are home
   b. must abide by the Fair Debt Collection Practice Act
   c. are usually successful after numerous calls at the patient's place of employment
   d. will require overtime pay for the medical clinic staff
9. A "skip" is defined as:
   a. the time period when legal action cannot be taken
   b. an estate involved in probate
   c. one who moves without a forwarding address and leaves an unpaid bill
   d. one who has paid a portion of a debt
10. For patient accounts, a collection agency:
   a. is better if it handles only medical and dental accounts
   b. creates a bad feeling between patients and providers
   c. cannot possibly do as good a job as the medical clinic staff
   d. seldom describes its methods for collections

REFERENCES/BIBLIOGRAPHY

Fordney, M. T., French, L. L., & Follis, J. J. (2008). *Administrative medical assisting* (6th ed.). Clifton Park, NY: Cengage Delmar Learning.

Lewis, M. A., & Tamparo, C. D. (2007). *Medical law, ethics, and bioethics for the health professions* (6th ed.). Philadelphia: F. A. Davis Company.

CHAPTER 21
Accounting Practices

OUTLINE

Bookkeeping and Accounting Systems
Single-Entry System
Pegboard System
Double-Entry System
Total Practice Management System
Computer and Billing Service Bureaus
Day-End Summary
Tips for Finding Errors

Accounts Receivable Trial Balance
Accounts Payable
Disbursement Records
The Accounting Function
Cost Analysis
Fixed Costs
Variable Costs
Financial Records
Income Statement
Balance Sheet

Useful Financial Data
Accounts Receivable Ratio
Collection Ratio
Cost Ratio
Legal and Ethical Guidelines
Bonding
Payroll

LEARNING OUTCOMES

1. Define, spell, and pronounce the key terms as presented in the glossary.
2. Explain basic bookkeeping computations.
3. Explain the purpose and range of the accounting function in the ambulatory care setting.
4. Describe the four different types of bookkeeping and accounting systems.
5. Recall the importance of the day-end summary and the accounts receivable trial balance.
6. Compare and contrast financial, managerial, and cost accounting.
7. Explain the use and validity of the income statement and the balance sheet.
8. Recall three useful financial ratios and explain them in detail.
9. Identify the proper steps in accounts payable management.
10. Discuss the impact of utilization review on reimbursement.
11. Discuss legal and ethical guidelines in accounting practices.
12. Analyze the professionalism questions and apply them to this chapter's content.

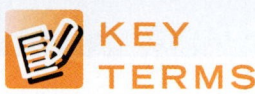

KEY TERMS

accounting

accounts payable

accounts receivable
 (A/R) ratio

accrual basis

assets

balance sheet

cash basis

check register

collection ratio

cost accounting

cost analysis

cost ratio

financial accounting

fixed cost

income statement

liability

managerial accounting

owner's equity

trial balance

utilization review (UR)

variable cost

ATTRIBUTES OF PROFESSIONALISM

Competency
- Did you pay attention to detail?
- Did you display sound judgment?
- Were you knowledgeable and accountable?
- Did you recognize the importance of local, state, and federal legislation and regulations in the practice setting?
- Did you demonstrate sensitivity and professionalism in handling accounts receivable with patients?

Initiative
- Did you show initiative?
- Did you direct the patient to other resources when necessary or helpful, with the approval of the provider?
- Did you work with the provider to achieve maximum reimbursement?

Integrity
- Did you protect and maintain confidentiality?
- Did you immediately report any error you had made?

SCENARIO

When James Whitney, one of the owners at Inner City Health Care, and office manager Jane O'Hara, CMA (AAMA), decided to add a new medical assistant to the staff, they first reviewed the financial records for the previous year. Although the volume of work in the center generated the need for an additional employee, Whitney and O'Hara had to be sure it was financially feasible. In addition to past records, they also had to make some projections for the upcoming year; with certain new managed care fees, they had to be sure that anticipated revenues would be sufficient to sustain the salary of a new employee.

INTRODUCTION

Medical financial management in the ambulatory care setting is vitally important in the daily functioning of the medical clinic business. It directly affects overall bookkeeping and accounting procedures. Accounting generates financial information for the ambulatory care setting and is defined as a system of monitoring the financial status of a facility and the specific results of its activities. It provides financial information for decision making.

Previous chapters have included the topics of proper daily bookkeeping financial practices (see Chapter 19), the accurate coding and the specific processing of insurance forms (see Chapters 17 and 18), and the efficient management of collecting on accounts (see Chapter 20). All of these functions are essential to obtaining maximum reimbursement and creating profitability for the practice.

This chapter ties many of these elements together and creates a total picture of their interdependence. Each element is critical to accurate accounting practices in the ambulatory care setting.

SPOTLIGHT ON CERTIFICATION

RMA Content Outline

- Financial bookkeeping

CMA (AAMA) Content Outline

- Computer applications
- Bookkeeping systems
- Accounting and banking procedures
- Employee payroll

CMAS Content Outline

- Fundamental financial management
- Patient accounts

BOOKKEEPING AND ACCOUNTING SYSTEMS

Medical practices use a variety of methods to monitor their financial accounts and the total financial operations of the business. Although some clinics still use the single-entry bookkeeping and pegboard systems, the majority prefer double-entry or computerized systems, or a combination.

Financial records should provide the following information at all times:

- Amount earned in a given period
- Amount collected in a given period
- Amount owed in a given period
- Where the expenses were incurred in a given period

The financial records can show these data as often as you like, usually on a monthly, quarterly, or yearly basis. Comparisons can be made with similar periods. Analysis of the financial data can help to determine if some services are not profitable, whether the practice is experiencing healthy growth, or why a loss might be realized. The accounts receivable and accounts payable data are vital to this information.

Single-Entry System

The single-entry system has been used in medical practices for many years. This includes a daily journal or log, patients' statements or accounts, ledgers, checks, and disbursement (expenditure) records. Information is first recorded in the journal, which provides a chronological record of financial transactions. Information from the journal is then transferred to the ledger through the process of posting. All amounts entered in the journal must be posted to the accounts kept in the ledger to summarize the results. This system has been used because of its simplicity and inexpensive nature. However, it is difficult to find errors because there are no internal controls, and financial analysis information is inadequate.

Pegboard System

As discussed in Chapter 19, the pegboard, or "write-it-once," system is easier to use than the single-entry system and has greater internal controls. The pegboard system provides control over collections, payments, and charges. It uses No Carbon Required (NCR©) forms that are layered or shingled on pegs on the left of the board so that both income and disbursement entries need to be written only once. Many pegboard plans include a charge slip (or encounter form), which simplifies third-party payment processing for both the medical practice and the patients. The charge slip is used to record the input needed during the patient's visit, while serving as the patient's receipt for services performed and fees charged. An advantage of the pegboard system is its accuracy, because data are entered at the time of service and not recopied, so fewer errors can creep in.

Double-Entry System

The double-entry system is based on the fact that each transaction has two aspects, that is, a dual effect on the accounting elements. This system is based on the accounting principle that assets equal liabilities plus owner's equity.

$$\text{Assets} = \text{Liabilities} + \text{Owner's Equity}$$

Assets are the properties owned by the business (supplies, equipment, accounts receivable, and so on). **Liabilities** include what is owed to creditors. **Owner's equity** is the amount by which the business assets exceed the business liabilities. Net worth, proprietorship, and capital are often used as synonyms for owner's equity.

The double-entry system requires that the two aspects involved in every transaction be recorded on each side of the equation and that the two sides always be in balance. Although this accounting system requires time and skill, it provides a comprehensive financial picture and has built-in accuracy controls. It is orderly, fairly simple, flexible, and accurate, making it impossible for certain

types of errors to remain undetected for long. For example, if one aspect of a transaction is properly recorded but the other aspect is overlooked, the records are out of balance. This occurrence may be easily discovered and subsequently corrected.

Total Practice Management System

EHR The majority of medical practices rely on accounting software packages to prepare financial records, such as ledgers and reports, and to retrieve patient information. An increasing number of practices are using financial management software that is part of a total practice management system (TPMS) (Figure 21-1). TPMS is a system of computerizing the entire facility and likely includes:

- Patient information data and scheduling
- Electronic medical records (EMRs) and electronic health records (EHRs)
- Insurance coding and billing; processing claims electronically
- Management and human resources; payroll, purchases, personnel records
- Bookkeeping and accounting; generation of financial records including business income and expenses

A computerized accounting system is most likely to be based on the principles of either the pegboard (write-it-once) or a double-entry bookkeeping system, or a combination of both.

A computer financial system can be customized to meet the needs of the practice. Most large multispeciality clinics have a computer system designed particularly for their needs. TPMS has the capability of including the most common procedure and diagnostic codes within a database to be recalled when completing insurance claim forms. The software will assist in matching the charges with the appropriate diagnosis codes.

TPMS has the flexibility of assigning codes in other categories to indicate whether a bill has been paid with cash, with a check, or by a third-party payer. Codes may also be assigned to identify the place of service and the professional performing the service. This facilitates the tracking of payments and also allows for the analysis of specific sources that generate income for the practice. Adjustments to reflect discounts or reduced fees may also be entered into the computer. The software is used in the preparation of billing statements, insurance forms, collection letters, and a

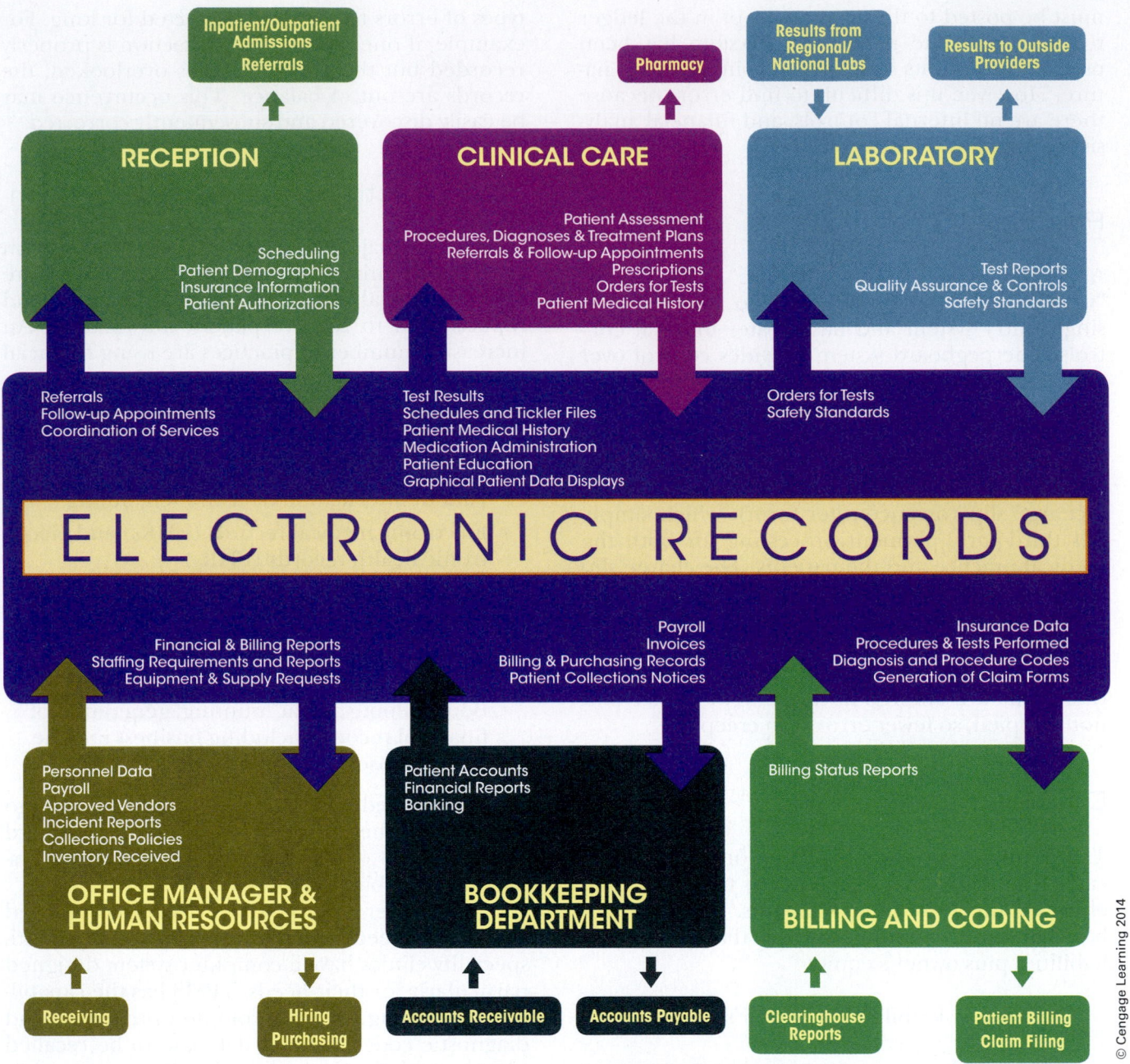

Figure 21-1 Diagram of a total practice management system (TPMS) showing the many aspects of a total electronic medical clinic system.

number of financial ratios and statements to assist in monitoring the practice's financial stability.

Computer and Billing Service Bureaus

An option for ambulatory care settings that choose not to purchase accounting software or a TPMS in their practice is to use a computer service bureau for billing purposes and the creation of many

financial records. In this case, the ambulatory care setting provides the data, and the bureau provides basic billing and accounting services, furnishing financial statements, completed insurance forms, payroll materials, and checks.

Service bureaus handle accounts from the medical facilities in one of three ways:

1. Through the clinic's own computer terminal, online sharing occurs where the clinic is tied directly to the bureau's mainframe computer

2. Through online servicing, by which the clinic has its own terminal that allows direct communication with the service bureau's computer

3. Through off-line batch processing, where the medical assistant or bookkeeper sends daily batches of data to the bureau to process

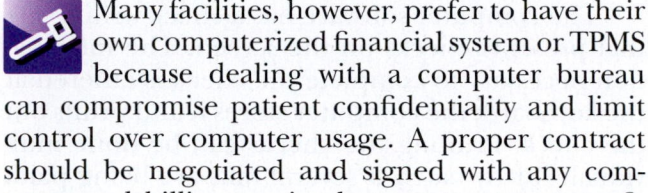 Many facilities, however, prefer to have their own computerized financial system or TPMS because dealing with a computer bureau can compromise patient confidentiality and limit control over computer usage. A proper contract should be negotiated and signed with any computer and billing service bureau to ensure confidentiality, HIPAA compliance, and strict privacy of all patient information.

DAY-END SUMMARY

The financial summary at the end of the day is a helpful tool for a quick financial analysis. Computer accounting systems automatically create the day-end summaries. Pegboard systems require the administrative medical assistant to total the summaries that are shown at the bottom of the day sheet.

The first section of the day sheet identifies all the financial transactions of the day. The second section includes the month-to-date totals. This is where today's totals are added to the month-to-date totals; this must be in perfect balance. The third section identifies the year-to-date accounts, which includes all accounts to obtain the year-to-date total. A deposit slip included with most systems enables the assistant to verify the cash receipts with the checks received. This is helpful in preparing the day's bank deposit.

 When the totals do not balance at the end of the day, the medical assistant must begin the search for errors.

Tips for Finding Errors

Some tips for finding errors are as follows:

- Check the addition of each column, both horizontally and vertically. If a calculator is used, check the tape for entry errors.
- Compute the difference in the totals that are out of balance. Search the day sheet and patient accounts for that exact amount.
- If the amount of the error is divisible by 9, there may be an error in transposition of numbers.

- If the amount of the error is divisible by 2, the amount may have been posted in the wrong column.
- Check your entries when manually carrying forward previous balances. It is quite easy to carry forward an incorrect amount or to place numbers incorrectly. For example, the number $750 might be carried forward as $75.

Anyone who has worked with a manual pegboard system can report horror stories of chasing errors around for several days before finding them. It might be one error in one patient's account that creates the havoc. Also, a search for an error can continue at great length even as the assistant keeps seeing and missing the error. Set the problem aside for a bit, or even a day if you are not pressed with month-end billing deadlines. Have another person check for you. Often that individual sees the error in just a few minutes.

Errors in an electronic financial system can create almost as much havoc but often can be caught earlier. If all data are entered accurately and kept up-to-date, an error that occurs when keying in certain data will create a warning notice that indicates the data are incorrect. Computers do not automatically update all information when fees for services are changed, reimbursement adjustments are changed, salaries are increased, or new data from the laboratory or clinical area are determined. Any time there is a person who is entering data into the system, errors can occur. All medical professionals entering any data into the system must be reminded not to rush through the process and to carefully check for accuracy.

ACCOUNTS RECEIVABLE TRIAL BALANCE

Before preparing monthly statements, a **trial balance** should be done on the accounts receivable in either a pegboard system or a computer system. The trial balance is created by totaling debit balances and credit balances to confirm that total debits equal total credits. The trial balance will indicate any problem between the daily journal and the ledger. Use the following steps to create the trial balance:

1. Pull all patient accounts that have a balance.
2. Total the balance of those accounts.
3. Create an accounts receivable total.
   a. Enter the accounts receivable at the first of the month.

b. Add the total charges for the month and subtotal.

c. Subtract the total payments for the month and subtotal.

d. Subtract the total adjustments for the month.

e. The final total is the accounts receivable at the end of the month.

 This final total, the end of the month accounts receivable, must be the same as the figure received when adding all the patient account balances. If they match, the accounts are then in balance. If they do not balance, the error must be found (see Procedure 21-1).

ACCOUNTS PAYABLE

Accounts payable are an unwritten promise to pay a supplier for property or merchandise purchased on credit or for a service rendered. Accounts payable are the most common liability or financial obligation in a provider's clinic. These include expenses such as medical and office supplies, salaries, equipment, and services. Payments for these expenses are made by check to ensure complete, accurate records of all money received and disbursed.

Supplies and equipment purchased usually come with a packing slip that describes the items purchased and their cost. An invoice may also be enclosed that serves as a bill for the items ordered; however, another invoice is sent to the business later as well. Take time to note on the invoice whether there is a discount for early payment. Some financial managers suggest attaching the invoice and packing slip to the purchase order (see Chapter 19). File in your tickler file or reminder file on the computer so that payment is made in a timely fashion to receive any discount. Some vendors prefer that payment not be made until a statement (or request for payment) is received from them. This is particularly the case if the practice uses that vendor more than once a month. When the statement arrives, check the invoice for accuracy before sending payment. Prepare the check for the accounts payable as appropriate, either monthly or as necessary to receive a discount (see Chapter 19). Write the check number on the invoice, as well as the amount paid, and place in a file for accounts paid according to the practice's filing system.

Disbursement Records

Computerized accounts payable systems track the disbursements and post to appropriate established accounts similar to a manual system. Computer accounts payable systems have a **check register** that records all checks written and categorizes them into separate columns, such as rent, insurance, office supplies, utilities, and so forth. These categories can be designed to be as general or detailed as preferred. The computer system also can create entries for bank deposits and payroll records.

The computer software has a check-writing file that presents checks on the screen. The information necessary to complete the check is entered at the keyboard; the computer stores it and prints out the check. Printing the checks can be done individually or by batch if several bills are being paid. The amount is automatically subtracted from the account's balance. The computer system also can recall data that need to be entered on the checks each time there is a payment. For example, the name of the company where most supplies are purchased can be recalled from the database; thus the assistant does not have to key in that information again. This feature is a particular timesaver when payroll checks are prepared (see Chapter 45).

The manual or pegboard system uses a check register page to record checks written. The check is aligned on the pegboard over the check register before completion. The pegboard checks have an NCR transfer strip that copies the date, the payee, the check number, and the amount to the check register. Pegboard checks can be designed so that the address is entered beneath the payee line and mailed in a window envelope. This check register has a number of columns to categorize expenses. All entries are totaled on the check register when completed, and these totals are carried forward. A balanced check register provides a way to verify the bank statement when it arrives. The check register can also be used for bank deposits and for payroll records.

THE ACCOUNTING FUNCTION

Accounting is a system of monitoring the financial status of a facility and the financial results of its activities. Accounting may be divided into two major categories: financial and managerial. **Financial accounting** provides information primarily for entities external to the organization such as the government. In contrast, **managerial accounting** generates financial information that can enable more efficient internal management. **Cost accounting** helps to determine what it costs the ambulatory care setting to perform particular services and is an integral part of managerial accounting.

A hospital cost report for Medicare is essentially a part of financial accounting because the report is generated for an external user—the Centers for Medicare & Medicaid Services (CMS), which administers the Medicare program. However, it is also a part of cost accounting because a cost report on Medicare will show what it costs to care for patients on Medicare.

COST ANALYSIS

An important aspect of the practice is **cost analysis**. The purpose of the analysis is to determine the costs of each service. There are two factors to consider: fixed costs and variable costs.

Fixed Costs

Fixed costs are costs that do not vary in total as the number of patients vary. For example, the annual depreciation cost of the equipment is fixed because it will remain the same regardless of the number of patients who use it.

Variable Costs

Variable costs are those that vary in direct proportion to patient volume, such as clinical supplies and laboratory procedures. Average costs to treat patients decline because of fixed costs, not variable costs. The greater the volume, the more widely the fixed costs are spread and the less cost any one unit is responsible for.

Patient cost factors include administrative costs, such as the cost of billing and collections, personnel costs for clinic staff providing patient care, equipment costs, and costs for clinical supplies. The provider cost will include costs for interpreting tests, diagnosing illnesses, and maintaining professional liability insurance.

Calculating and reviewing costs provide the ambulatory care setting with data to set fees, market the practice, determine profit, and monitor the practice's performance.

FINANCIAL RECORDS

Indicators of the financial status of the medical facility include financial statements that reflect the daily operations of the business. These records comprise an accounting information system that is maintained for numerous reasons, one of which is to provide source data for use in the preparation of various reports. Two financial statements common to the ambulatory care setting are the income/expense statement and the balance sheet.

Income Statement

Figure 21-2 shows a sample **income statement**, the most commonly generated year-end report. The sample shows the profit and expenses for a given month. The income statement shows the cumulative profit and total expenses by reporting patient income, outside revenue sources, and overhead expenses such as office and medical expenses. Provider's compensation and benefits and employees' compensation, benefits, and withholding taxes can be itemized as well.

Balance Sheet

Sometimes called the statement of financial condition or statement of financial position, the **balance sheet** is an itemized statement of the assets, liabilities, and owner's equity of a medical facility as of a specified date. Its purpose is to provide information regarding the status of these basic accounting elements.

The balance sheet is made possible through the double-entry system of accounting because every transaction is recorded by two sets of entries made in a ledger or journal. Increases in assets are recorded as debits; decreases are recorded as credits. Increases in liabilities and owner's equity are recorded as credits; decreases are recorded as debits.

Debit and credit entries to one or more accounts make up the system. In any recording, the total dollar amount of the debit entries must equal the total dollar amount of the credit entries. Each ledger or journal entry should have the following elements:

1. Date of transaction
2. Journal or ledger account names involved
3. Dollar amount of the charges
4. Brief explanation of the transaction

USEFUL FINANCIAL DATA

A business must determine how and when it will report income earned. There are two systems for doing this. The **accrual basis** reports income at the time charges are generated. This is used mainly in commercial environments. The **cash basis** is most often used in medical practices. In the cash basis, income is recognized when money is collected.

INNER CITY HEALTH CARE
INCOME STATEMENT

	Month of ___, 20XX	Year-to-Date	Budget for Year	Overhead Percentages
A. Revenue:				
1. Office #1	$	$	$	
2. Office #2	$	$	$	
B. Total Revenue:	$	$	$	100%
C. Expenses:				
1. Non–provider (staff) salaries—gross	$	$	$	___%
2. Staff fringes:				
– Payroll taxes	$	$	$	
– Empl. benefits	$	$	$	
– Empl. seminars	$	$	$	
– Uniforms	$	$	$	
– Retirement plan	$	$	$	
	$	$	$	___%
3. Occupancy costs:				
– Rent—Off. #1	$	$	$	
– Rent—Off. #2	$	$	$	
– Property taxes	$	$	$	
– Insurance	$	$	$	
– Utilities	$	$	$	
– Janitor/Grounds	$	$	$	
	$	$	$	___%
4. Medical expenses:				
– Medications	$	$	$	
– Supplies	$	$	$	
– Lab fees	$	$	$	
	$	$	$	___%
5. Office expenses:				
– Office supplies	$	$	$	
– Postage	$	$	$	
– Telephone	$	$	$	
	$	$	$	___%
6. Malpractice ins.	$	$	$	___%
7. Professional expenses:				
– Auto expenses (Providers')	$	$	$	
– Dues/subscriptions	$	$	$	
– Books and videos	$	$	$	
– Dues/memberships	$	$	$	
– Entertainment	$	$	$	
– Professional development	$	$	$	
– Travel	$	$	$	
	$	$	$	___%

Figure 21-2   A sample income statement that can show profit and expenses for 1 month.

A few financial ratios can help evaluate how the practice is doing. Data from the current year and the previous year's financial statements can be converted into ratios to highlight different financial characteristics. However, ratios should always be viewed in relation to the total financial picture.

Ratios are not difficult to calculate, but they can be time consuming when using a manual system. They are quick to create in a computer system

	Month of ___ , 20XX	Year-to-Date	Budget for Year	Overhead Percentages
8. Equipment costs:				
– Depreciation/amortization	$	$	$	
– Rent	$	$	$	
– Service/maintenance	$	$	$	
– Interest (if on equipment purchase loans)	$	$	$	
	$	$	$	%
9. Marketing expenses:				
– Advertising	$	$	$	
– Other fees	$	$	$	
	$	$	$	%
10. Professional expenses:				
– Accounting	$	$	$	
– Legal	$	$	$	
– Consulting	$	$	$	
– Ret. Plan Admin.	$	$	$	
	$	$	$	%
11.				
12.				
13.				
14.				
D. Total Non–Provider Expenses:	$	$	$	%
E. Operating New Income Before Provider's Costs (B minus C)	$	$	$	%
F. Associate Provider's Costs:				
– Salaries—gross:	$	$	$	
– Benefits	$	$	$	
–	$	$	$	
–	$	$	$	
G. Total Non–Owner Provider's Costs	$	$	$	%
H. New Income Available to Owner–Providers (E minus G)	$	$	$	%
I. Owner–Providers' Costs:				
1. Salaries—gross:				
–Dr. A	$	$	$	
–Dr. B	$	$	$	
2. Bonuses—gross:				
–Dr. A	$	$	$	
–Dr. B	$	$	$	
3. Retirement contributions:				
–Dr. A	$	$	$	
–Dr. B	$	$	$	
4. "Semi-personal" expenses:				
–Dr. A	$	$	$	
–Dr. B	$	$	$	
J. Total Owner–Providers' Costs	$	$	$	
K. Net Income (H minus J)	$	$	$	

Figure 21-2   (*continued*)

because all the data are readily available, already totaled, and sometimes created automatically. It is helpful to understand the concept, however, and not rely too heavily on computer-generated reports.

Data that have been entered incorrectly at some point will be reflected in reports generated. The user of accounting software must train his or her mind to think about the sensibility of the report.

CRITICAL THINKING

What are some steps a medical clinic should take to resolve any discrepancies found when calculating ratios?

Although two of these ratios were discussed in Chapter 20, some elaboration is in order in the context of this chapter.

Accounts Receivable Ratio

The **accounts receivable (A/R) ratio** formula measures the speed in which outstanding accounts are paid. The accounts receivable ratio provides a picture of the state of collections and probable losses. The longer an account is past due, the less the likelihood is of successfully making the collection.

$$\frac{\text{Total Accounts Receivable}}{\text{Monthly Receipts}} = \text{Turnaround Time}$$

Example:

$$\frac{\$120,000}{\$60,000} = 2 \text{ Months Turnaround Time for Payment on an Account}$$

The goal of an efficient billing and collecting policy should be a turnaround time of 2 months or less.

Collection Ratio

The **collection ratio** shows the percentage of outstanding debt collected. The goal should be a 90% collection ratio. Total receipts divided by total charges gives the unadjusted collection ratio, but adjustments may include federal and state insurance programs (Medicare and Medicaid, Workers Compensation), managed care adjustments, and any other adjustments as directed by the provider.

Total Receipts	= $40,000
+ Managed Care Adjustments	$3,000
+ Medicare Adjustments	$2,000
TOTAL	$45,000
Total Charges	$52,000

$$\frac{\text{Total Receipts} \; \$45,000}{\text{Total Charges} \; \$52,000} = 86.5\% \text{ Collection Ratio after Adjustments}$$

Cost Ratio

The **cost ratio** formula shows the cost of a procedure or service and can help in determining, for instance, the cost effectiveness of maintaining a laboratory in the ambulatory care setting. The ratio is:

$$\frac{\text{Total Expenses}}{\text{Total Number of Procedures for 1 Month}}$$

$$\frac{\text{Total Laboratory Expenses for September}}{\text{Total Number of Procedures Performed for September}}$$

$$\frac{\$48,000}{240} = \$200 \text{ per Procedure}$$

A conclusion might be reached that the laboratory is too costly because each procedure is not billed at $200.00.

LEGAL AND ETHICAL GUIDELINES

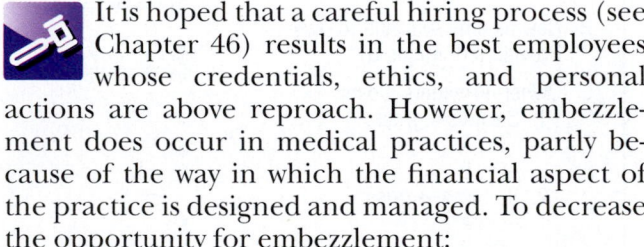 It is hoped that a careful hiring process (see Chapter 46) results in the best employees whose credentials, ethics, and personal actions are above reproach. However, embezzlement does occur in medical practices, partly because of the way in which the financial aspect of the practice is designed and managed. To decrease the opportunity for embezzlement:

- The accountant and the managing provider(s) should conduct regular and irregular audits of the practice accounts. Seek an accountant who is available at any time, not just when it is time to report wages or compute the yearly taxes. The accountant also becomes a valuable asset to the practice in providing essential information to the clinic staff.

- Separate duties among several employees. Consider having one employee open the mail and post checks received. A second employee handles all the cash transactions and prepares the deposit slips. A third employee might order the supplies and prepare all the checks. Many providers choose to sign the checks;

however, this is also a task that can be assigned to the office manager.

- Only one person should use the signature stamp; better yet, consider not using a signature stamp at all.
- The signature card on file at the bank must include the names of each individual authorized to sign the checks.
- Seek employees whose personal honesty sets a good example for everyone.

Providers who demonstrate the same personal honesty and integrity expected of their staff are less likely to be victims of embezzlement.

Bonding

There is another recommended step to take. To protect the practice from embezzlement or other financial loss, providers can purchase fidelity bonds. These bonds reimburse the practice for any monetary loss caused by the practice's employees. There are three types of bonds to consider, and it is reasonable to have more than one type. These bonds include:

1. Position-schedule bonds cover the position rather than a specific individual. For instance, the bookkeeper, office manager, and receptionist might be covered.
2. Blanket-position bonds cover all employees. If the staff members often share duties, cover for one another when there are absences, or work really well together as a team during busy periods, this type of bond might be most beneficial.
3. Personal bonds are designed to cover specific individuals by name and generally require a personal background investigation. This type of bond may give the most assurance.

Bonding not only protects the providers and the practice, but it assures employees that they are covered by a bond should there be a problem with the finances during their shift. Bonding service companies will require implementation of certain procedures and security measures as outlined in their contracts. Costs depend on risk levels, but they are well worth the protection.

Payroll

 The administrative medical assistant is likely to be involved in making certain the W-4 form, the Employee's Withholding

UTILIZATION REVIEW

In the present health care climate, in which there are many managed care plans, more attention has been focused on how the billing and financial management process should proceed. Because of the influence of governmental mandates in the practice of medicine and because of the growth of the **utilization review (UR)** industry, more accurate recordkeeping and documentation in all facets of the ambulatory care setting have become necessary. There are numerous UR firms throughout the country. These companies aggressively sell their services to employers and to insurance carriers. UR is actually a review of the patient service required before the actual service may be performed. If the reviewer determines that the procedure or treatment is not needed, then it will not be approved or covered under the patient's insurance plan. Policies that once permitted medical decisions to be made solely by the provider often are now made by other health professionals who are employed by UR firms. Some clinics may find it beneficial to have one medical assistant whose main responsibility is to present procedures to UR for acceptance or denial. Because of the increasing concern for quality of health care at low cost, more providers also are realizing that they need more documentation of both medical and financial information with more accessible means for retrieval.

Allowance Certificate, is completed by all employees. However, salary calculations, withholding taxes, and Social Security calculations are the responsibility of the office manager. Payroll tasks usually are assigned to the office manager because of the privacy of salary issues, Social Security numbers, and confidentiality of the employees' tax information. Manual systems for managing payroll are available, but the most efficient systems are computerized. The financial management of the payroll responsibilities in the ambulatory care setting is detailed in Chapter 45.

PROCEDURE 21-1

Preparing Accounts Receivable Trial Balance in a Manual System

PURPOSE:
A trial balance will determine if there is any problem between the daily journal and the ledger or patient accounts.

EQUIPMENT/SUPPLIES:
Patient accounts
Calculator

PROCEDURE STEPS:

1. Pull all patient accounts that have a balance due. RATIONALE: Provides only amount due information.

2. Enter the balance of those accounts into the calculator.

3. Add the balances and total. (A calculator with tape can make it quicker to check for errors.) RATIONALE: Gives you the total amount due to date.

4. Create an accounts receivable total:

   a. Enter the accounts receivable total from the first of the month into the calculator.

   b. Add total charges for this month and subtotal.

   c. Total the amount of all payments received this month.

   d. Subtract the total of payments from subtotal of "b" above and subtotal.

   e. Total the amount of the month's adjustments and subtract from the subtotal in "d" above.

   f. This total is the accounts receivable amount. RATIONALE: The end-of-the month accounts receivable total ("f") above must match the total in Step 3. If these totals do not match, an error has been made. If they do match, the trial balance is in order.

PROCEDURE 21-2

Preparing Accounts Receivable Trial Balance Using Medical Office Simulation Software (MOSS)

PURPOSE:
To generate a trial balance using a monthly summary report showing all transactions for a given month.

EQUIPMENT/SUPPLIES:
Computer and MOSS

PROCEDURE STEPS:

1. Click on the *Report Generation* button on the *Main Menu*.

2. Select Option 4, *Monthly Summary*.

3. Enter the *Start Date*.

4. Enter the *End Date*, and then Click *OK*.

5. Print the *Monthly Summary* report.

6. Close the report and *Reports Panel*, and return to the *Main Menu*.

CASE STUDY 21-1

Refer to the scenario at the beginning of the chapter.

CASE STUDY REVIEW

1. Identify the financial records most likely reviewed by James Whitney and Jane O'Hara.

2. What information will be considered when projecting future income?

3. Identify other concerns to consider when hiring an additional medical assistant.

CASE STUDY 21-2

Richard Saxton is a newly licensed acupuncturist who has been in practice for less than a year. He is renting space for his procedures and services with an established doctor of osteopathy. Richard is using a simple pegboard system, makes his own appointments, and collects for most procedures at the time services are rendered unless the patients have medical insurance covering acupuncture. Richard has done fairly well, likes working in the environment the facility offers, and is beginning to show some profit. He would like to purchase a new table, chair, and stool for his acupuncture room.

CASE STUDY REVIEW

1. What facts might Richard want to consider before making the purchases?
2. Consider the variable costs versus the fixed costs of the practice of acupuncture. (You may need to do a little research to determine supplies and other factors.)
3. What information will his pegboard system give him?

SUMMARY

Medical financial management is crucial to the profitability of the ambulatory care setting. It is necessary for each medical facility to decide on which accounting system best serves the individual practice. Careful monitoring of billing procedures and aging accounts, and accurately documenting both the medical and financial record, will help in providing a sound financial analysis and a strong financial foundation for the ambulatory care setting. Just as it is essential that patients receive the best of care and that accuracy be maintained in all patient records, so too must the accuracy of all financial records be maintained in the ambulatory care setting.

STUDY FOR SUCCESS

To reinforce your knowledge and skills of information presented in this chapter:

- Review the *Key Terms*
- Role-play with other students to apply attributes of professionalism pertinent to this chapter.
- Consider the *Case Studies* and discuss your conclusions
- Answer the questions in the *Certification Review*
- Apply your knowledge by completing the *Activities* in the *Study Guide* and the *Games and Quizzes* in the StudyWARE **StudyWARE** software on the *Premium Website*
- Perform the *Procedures* using the *Competency Assessment Checklists* in the *Competency Manual*
- Practice your problem-solving skills with the *Critical Thinking Challenge 3.0* on the *Premium Website*

Additional resources for this chapter include:

- Module 10 of the *Medical Assisting Learning Lab*
- *CourseMate for Delmar's Comprehensive Medical Assisting*
- *WebTutor for Delmar's Comprehensive Medical Assisting*

CERTIFICATION REVIEW

1. If a number has been transposed in financial reports:
   a. the error is divisible by 4
   b. the error is divisible by 2
   c. the error is divisible by 9
   d. none of the above
2. An example of a fixed cost is:
   a. salaries
   b. cost of supplies
   c. depreciation of equipment
   d. cost of treating patients
3. An itemized statement of financial position is the:
   a. income statement
   b. balance sheet
   c. trial balance
   d. collection ratio
4. A check register:
   a. records all checks and categorizes them into separate columns
   b. is used when taking cash from patients
   c. is an accounts receivable record
   d. a and c
5. Utilization review:
   a. looks at the utility of all personnel
   b. examines how useful the ambulatory care center is to patients
   c. is a review of a procedure before it is performed to determine if it is necessary
   d. only affects hospitals

6. Assets include:
   a. equipment and supplies on hand
   b. building or property
   c. accounts receivable
   d. all the above
7. A computer billing and service bureau:
   a. is the service you hire to care for the clinic computer system
   b. may compromise patient confidentiality
   c. can function through linkage of computers, online servicing, or off-line batch processing
   d. b and c
8. In a medical facility where the total receipts including any adjustments are $83,500 and the total charges equal $97,750, the collection ratio:
   a. would be great at 94%
   b. would be quite good at 88%
   c. shows a fair return at 85%
   d. shows a modest return at 75%
9. Money can be saved with accounts payable when:
   a. bills are paid promptly
   b. discounts are realized
   c. supplies are not purchased in bulk
   d. a and b
10. Bonding:
   a. binds providers to the safe caretaking of their patients
   b. protects medical clinic staff and providers if embezzlement occurs
   c. can be purchased in three different types
   d. b and c

REFERENCES/BIBLIOGRAPHY

Droms, W. G. (2003). *Finance and accounting for nonfinancial managers* (2nd ed.). Cambridge, MA: Perseus Publishers.

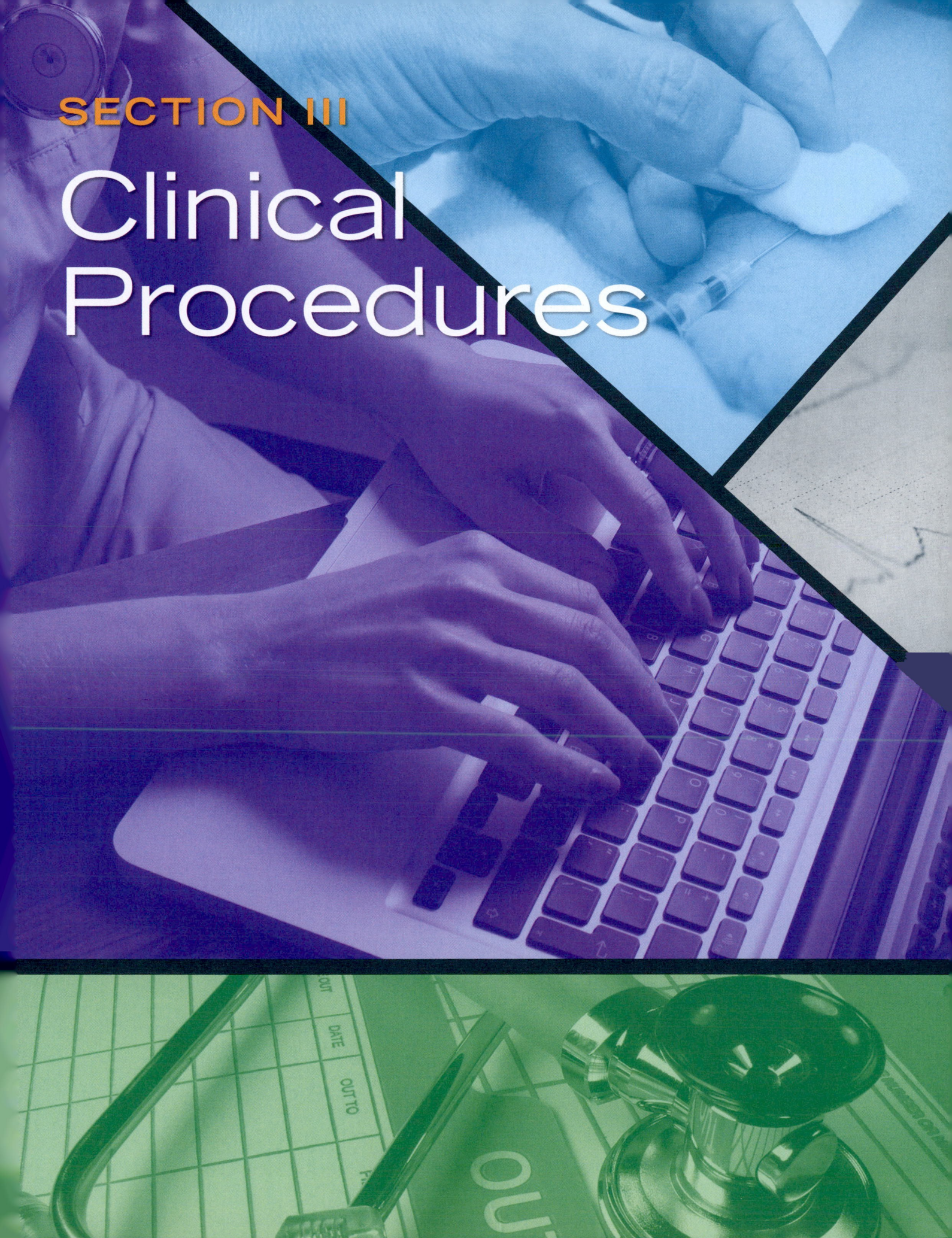

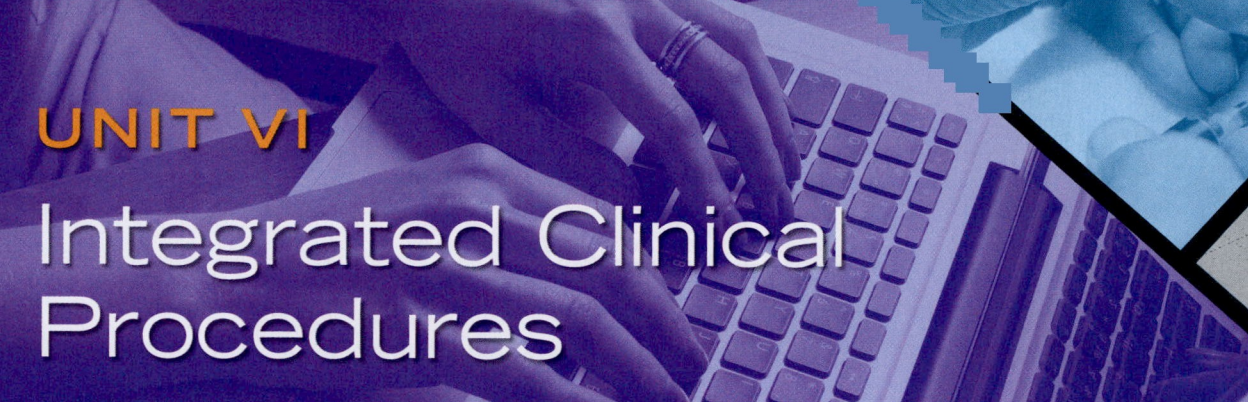

UNIT VI
Integrated Clinical Procedures

CHAPTER 22
Infection Control and Medical Asepsis 502

CHAPTER 23
The Patient History and Documentation........................ 564

CHAPTER 24
Vital Signs and Measurements 592

CHAPTER 25
The Physical Examination... 628

Infection Control and Medical Asepsis

OUTLINE

Impact of Infectious Diseases
The Process of Infection
 Growth Requirements for
  Microorganisms
Infection Cycle
 Infectious Agents
 Reservoir
 Portal of Exit
 Modes of Transmission
 Portal of Entry
 Susceptible Host
The Body's Defense Mechanisms
 for Fighting Infection and
 Disease
 The Body's Natural Barriers
 Inflammatory Response
 The Immune System and
  Immunity
Stages of Infectious Diseases

Incubation Stage
Prodromal Stage
Acute Stage
Acme
Declining Stage
Convalescent Stage
Sequelae
Disease Transmission
Human Immunodeficiency
 Virus and Hepatitis B and C
 HIV and AIDS
 Acute Viral Hepatitis Diseases
Reporting Infectious Disease
Standard Precautions
 Transmission-Based
  Precautions
 Blood and Body Fluids
 Personal Protective
  Equipment

Needlestick
Disposal of Infectious Waste
Federal Organizations and
 Infection Control
OSHA Regulations
 The Bloodborne Pathogen
  Standard
OSHA Regulations and Students
 Avoiding Exposure to
  Bloodborne Pathogens
Principles of Infection Control
Medical Asepsis
 Hand Washing
 Sanitization
 Disinfection
 Sterilization
Bioterrorism

LEARNING OUTCOMES

1. Define, spell, and pronounce the key terms as presented in the glossary.
2. Define and state the critical importance of infection control in the ambulatory care setting.
3. Outline the six stages in the infection cycle.
4. Define the five classifications of infectious microorganisms.
5. Recall and elaborate on the four phases the immune system uses to defend against infectious disease.
6. State the four stages of infectious diseases.
7. Recall at least five infectious diseases, their agents of transmission, and their symptoms.
8. Compare the routes of transmission of AIDS and hepatitis B and C and discuss the risk for infection from needlestick.
9. Describe the purpose of Standard Precautions and give six examples of ways health care providers should practice Standard Precautions.

10. Differentiate among the three types of Transmission-Based Precautions, defining what they are and how they are applied.
11. List eight types of body fluids and give an example of each.
12. Identify appropriate personal protective equipment for potentially infectious situations.
13. Recognize five situations in which exposure to a patient's blood can occur, and discuss why Standard Precautions are important.
14. Describe proper disposal of infectious waste.
15. Identify the role of the Centers for Disease Control regulations in health care settings.
16. List human fluids that may contain HIV, HBV, and HCV.
17. Define medical asepsis.
18. Define bioterrorism and describe five agents that could be used in a bioterrorism attack.
19. Analyze the professionalism questions and apply them to this chapter's content.

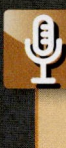
ATTRIBUTES OF PROFESSIONALISM

Presentation
- Did your actions attend to both the psychological and the physiological aspects of the patient's illness or condition?

Competency
- Did you pay attention to detail?
- Were you knowledgeable and accountable?
- Did you apply critical thinking skills in performing patient assessment and care?
- Did you recognize the importance of local, state, and federal legislation and regulations in the practice setting?

Initiative
- Did you seek out opportunities to expand your knowledge base?
- Did you direct the patient to other resources when necessary or helpful, with the approval of the provider?

Integrity
- Did you work within your scope of practice?
- Did you protect and maintain confidentiality?

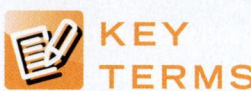
KEY TERMS

acquired immunodeficiency syndrome (AIDS)
airborne transmission
amoebic dysentery
antibodies
aseptic
bacilli
barrier
bloodborne pathogen
carrier
caustic
cell-mediated immunity
cocci
communicable
Contact Precautions
contact transmission
contracting
coryza
debris
declination form
droplet transmission
epidemic
epidemiology
excoriated
excretion
expectorated
fomite
gross contamination
human immunodeficiency virus (HIV)
humoral immunity
immune system
immunoglobulins
immunomodulator
immunosuppressed
infection control
infectious agent

inflammatory response
isolation
isolation categories
jet injection
lymphadenopathy
malaise
malaria
medical asepsis
microorganism
morbidity
mortality
normal flora
nosocomial

opportunistic infections
palliative
parenteral
pathogen
pruritus
regulated waste
resistance
rickettsiae
scabies
scoop technique
secretion
severe acute respiratory syndrome (SARS)

sharps
solvent
spill kit
sputum
Standard Precautions
Transmission-Based Precautions
trichomoniasis
ultrasonic cleaner
Universal Precautions
vaccine
vector
virulence

SCENARIO

Armando Miccoli, RMA, works in a busy internal medicine clinic in a major city in the Southeast. It is flu season again. Dr. Krull sees 25 to 30 patients a day and a large majority of them are complaining of symptoms of the flu. Mr. Miccoli knows that because of the number of patients with influenza seen in the clinic and in order to protect the non-infected patients, it is imperative that he adhere to infection control precautions for all patient-care activities as well as aerosol-generating procedures, such as sputum collection and treatments that deliver medications using a nebulizer. He organizes a staff meeting to make sure that all staff members are aware of their role in preventing the spread of infection in the health care setting. Front desk staff, medical records staff, and business office personnel are all included in this meeting. Mr. Miccoli provides information from the CDC that recommends immunization of the influenza vaccine, implementation of cough etiquette, and management of ill staff members, He spends extra time focusing on the importance of hand washing and the use of hand sanitizer to limit the spread of this virus. He has the approval of the provider to offer masks to persons who are coughing. By implementing these precautions, Mr. Miccoli limits the risk of health care–associated infection.

INTRODUCTION

Infectious diseases have plagued humans since the beginning of time. Recent scientific advances have changed our thoughts and behaviors regarding infectious disease. Advances such as antibiotic therapy and vaccination have significantly reduced risks for mortality from some previously fatal or debilitating infectious diseases. Infectious diseases that once were highly feared because of their likelihood of causing premature death are now preventable or treatable. Removing the deadly impact of many of these common diseases has allowed the public to forget the virulence *and destructive potential of epidemics of infectious disease. The presence of acquired immunodeficiency syndrome (AIDS) as an incurable and fatal infectious disease (although people are living with HIV and AIDS for many years), as well as* severe acute respiratory syndrome (SARS), *West Nile virus, avian flu, hepatitis C virus (HCV), and others, have caused the world to realize the enduring impact of pathogens on the human race.*

Although these medical advances have reduced the incidence of mortality *and* morbidity *from infectious diseases, humans must never underestimate the potential of resurgent infectious diseases. Tuberculosis has been the single leading cause of death in the history of humankind, yet was drastically reduced with the discovery of* antituberculosis drugs. *Today, however, the tuberculosis organism may be found that has adapted to the drugs, thereby becoming resistant to our only line of defense. Medical assistants must pay close attention to the prevention of infectious diseases.*

This chapter addresses the principles of the process of infection and control measures for use in ambulatory care settings. Because medical assistants deal directly with patients and other health care professionals, stringent adherence to the principles can greatly reduce transmission, or spread, of infectious disease. Continuous reliance on infection control measures ensures a clinical environment that is as safe as possible for employees, patients, and families. When infection control principles are not followed, infectious diseases may be transmitted to self, coworkers, or patients. The goals of infection control are to limit the presence of infectious agents, *to create barriers against transmission, and to decrease the risk to others for contracting infectious diseases. These goals can be achieved through medical asepsis and sterilization, by observation of all Standard Precautions and Transmission-Based Precautions set forth by the CDC, and by following the Occupational Safety and Health Administration (OSHA) guidelines.*

IMPACT OF INFECTIOUS DISEASES

Since the discovery of the germ theory by Louis Pasteur and Robert Koch in the nineteenth century, we have seen dramatic changes in global mortality and morbidity statistics from infectious diseases. Many scientists devoted their professional lives to the quest for the prevention and cure of infectious diseases, which were the main cause of death in earlier centuries. In developed countries, deaths from diseases such as tuberculosis, pneumonia, and smallpox have been significantly reduced because of pharmacologic agents such as antibiotics and **vaccines**. Antibiotic agents were widely introduced during World War II, reducing deaths from traumatic wound infections. Edward Jenner is credited with the discovery of the first vaccine to protect against the deadly disease smallpox. Because of the vaccine, smallpox is considered to have been eradicated worldwide.

Epidemiology is the science that studies the history, causes, and patterns of infectious diseases. This field of medicine is credited to a Japanese bacteriologist in the late nineteenth century who recognized the connection between bubonic plague and rat infestation. Recent epidemiological studies have traced infectious diseases such as AIDS from the beginning of the epidemic. The future of studies in infectious diseases will focus on increasing the pharmacologic (drugs) war against infectious diseases.

 Reliance only on treatment of infectious disease does not address the crucial step in halting the spread of infectious diseases, that is, of prevention, or **infection control**. Emerging issues related to infectious diseases involve microorganisms that are resistant to present technology, **bloodborne pathogen** transmission, increased **immunosuppressed** populations, and global access to infection control and treatment. Developed countries become accustomed to anti-infective medications, clean water, and laws that protect the public from infectious agents found in food and other consumables. These safety measures may not be present in other countries where political or economic factors limit access to infection-control measures.

In the future, drug-resistant infectious diseases will place greater emphasis on prevention because there may never be a safe and universally effective drug for all infectious diseases.

 Study of the history of infectious diseases allows us to realize the impact these diseases have on the lifestyles of people in various cultures. Infectious diseases such as AIDS and other sexually transmitted diseases have differing levels of social or cultural impact. Medical assistants should be aware of facts regarding the infectious process of specific diseases to reduce cultural isolation for the patient and to dispel myths regarding infectious diseases (see Chapter 6).

THE PROCESS OF INFECTION

Infectious diseases are caused by pathogenic microorganisms that are capable of causing disease. **Microorganisms** are microscopic living creatures capable of reproduction and transmission in specific circumstances. **Pathogens** are microorganisms that can cause infectious disease. Although all pathogens are capable of causing disease, not all microorganisms cause disease. Many microorganisms are necessary for human, animal, and plant life survival. In the absence of microorganisms, life would not be possible. The term **normal flora** is used to recognize the beneficial role of microorganisms in certain parts of the body, in which microorganisms normally occupy space and use nutrients, thus retarding the potential of pathogenic growth in that specific body area. A fundamental concept in the study of infectious disease is that similar steps or phases occur in all infectious diseases; however, each specific microorganism causes unique characteristics and alterations in the process of infection. Medical assistants must apply the theoretical process of infectious disease growth and transmission to relate to specific pathogens. The goal is to reduce transmission and incidence of infectious diseases in patients, employees, and families.

Growth Requirements for Microorganisms

For microorganisms to survive and thrive, a suitable environment must be available to them. Following is a list of growth requirements for microorganisms:

- *Oxygen.* An aerobic microorganism needs oxygen to live; most pathogenic microorganisms need oxygen to survive: for example, *streptococcus* as in a "strep" throat
- *Lack of or no oxygen.* An anaerobic microorganism needs little or no oxygen to live; two examples are tetanus and gas gangrene
- *Moisture.* Microorganisms grow well in a moist environment; the body provides moisture
- *Nutrition.* The body supplies plenty of nutrients
- *Temperature.* The body's temperature of approximately 98.6°F is an optimum temperature for growth of microorganisms
- *Darkness.* The body's cavities and organs provide darkness
- *Time.* A single cell of bacteria can grow to approximately 150,000 cells within 6 hours
- *Neutral or slightly alkaline pH.* The body's fluids are neutral when in a healthy state

Through the understanding of the optimum growth requirements for microorganisms to grow and multiply, elimination of any or all of the factors helps keep microorganisms from growing and causing infection.

INFECTION CYCLE

For infectious diseases to spread, several necessary steps must occur. These steps, or stages, are known as the "infection cycle." Each stage or step in the infectious process must occur for the spread of infection to take place. Infection control is based on the fact that the transmission of infectious diseases will be prevented when any of the levels in the cycle are broken or interrupted (Figure 22-1). The steps are:

1. Infectious agent
2. Reservoir
3. Portal of exit
4. Means of transmission
5. Portal of entry
6. Susceptible host

Infectious Agents

Infectious agents are microorganisms that can be grouped into five classifications: viruses, bacteria, fungi, parasites, and rickettsia. For an infection to occur, an infectious agent or microorganism must be present. When infectious diseases are identified according to the specific disease-causing microorganism, the disease may be prevented with the use of anti-infective drugs or infection control practices. Each of the five classifications of infectious microorganisms will be explored.

Viruses. Viruses are pathogens that require a living cell for reproduction and activity. These microorganisms are considered intracellular parasites, because they must live inside cells to multiply. They do so by altering particles of genetic material, such as DNA (deoxyribonucleic acid) or RNA (ribonucleic acid). Because viruses live inside cells, they are protected against agents such as chemical disinfectants and antibiotics. To survive, viruses have a notable characteristic of being able to change specific characteristics over time. For instance, viruses can adapt to their environment so they remain resistant to efforts to limit their growth. Viral infections have only a few pharmacologic treatment agents, and usually these agents are **palliative** because they only relieve symptoms of the disease instead of curing the infection. Some viral infections can be prevented by vaccination (Table 22-1). Figure 22-2A and Figure 22-2B show the CDC's recommended adult immunization schedules.

Bacteria. Bacteria are single-celled microorganisms that live in tissues rather than in body cells and are identified by characteristic shapes, or morphology. Bacteria may also be grouped according to ability to accept laboratory staining agents.

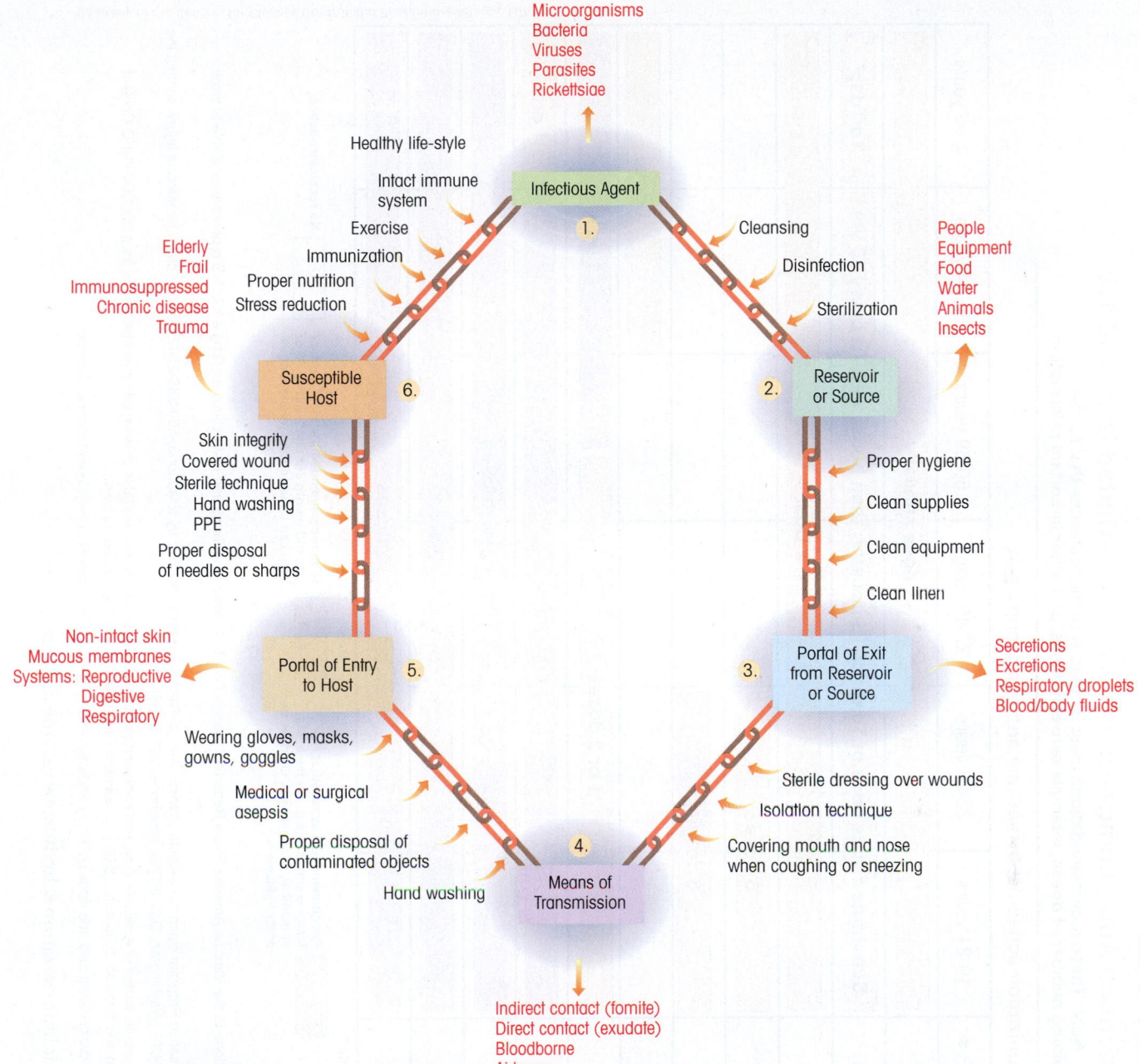

Figure 22-1   Health care worker's interventions used to break the chain of infection transmission.

Gram-negative bacteria stain visibly red under the microscope, whereas gram-positive bacteria stain purple. The bacteria that do not accept stain are considered spores, which are bacteria with a covering that protects them from many chemical disinfectants and higher levels of heat. The three classifications of bacteria are **cocci** (sphere or dot shaped), **bacilli** (rod shaped), and spirilla (spiral shaped). Bacteria are either pathogenic or nonpathogenic. Nonpathogenic bacteria normally reside on the skin of humans and in mucous membrane areas of the body. These are known as *normal flora*. Nonpathogenic bacteria use nutrients and occupy space, competing with the pathogenic bacteria. When nonpathogenic bacteria are reduced, the opportunity exists for pathogenic organisms to take over and cause infectious disease. A common cause of the reduction of nonpathogenic

Recommended Adult Immunization Schedule—United States - 2012

Note: These recommendations must be read with the footnotes that follow containing number of doses, intervals between doses, and other important information.

Figure 1. Recommended adult immunization schedule, by vaccine and age group[1]

VACCINE ▼ AGE GROUP ►	19-21 years	22-26 years	27-49 years	50-59 years	60-64 years	≥ 65 years
Influenza [2]	1 dose annually					
Tetanus, diphtheria, pertussis (Td/Tdap) [3],*	Substitute 1-time dose of Tdap for Td booster; then boost with Td every 10 yrs					Td/Tdap[3]
Varicella [4],*	2 Doses					
Human papillomavirus (HPV) Female [5],*	3 doses					
Human papillomavirus (HPV) Male [5],*	3 doses					
Zoster [6]					1 dose	
Measles, mumps, rubella (MMR) [7],*	1 or 2 doses			1 dose		
Pneumococcal (polysaccharide) [8,9]	1 or 2 doses					1 dose
Meningococcal [10],*	1 or more doses					
Hepatitis A [11],*	2 doses					
Hepatitis B [12],*	3 doses					

*Covered by the Vaccine Injury Compensation Program

For all persons in this category who meet the age requirements and who lack documentation of vaccination or have no evidence of previous infection	**Recommended if some other risk factor is present (e.g., on the basis of medical, occupational, lifestyle, or other indications)**
Tdap recommended for ≥65 if contact with <12 month old child. Either Td or Tdap can be used if no infant contact	**No recommendation**

Report all clinically significant postvaccination reactions to the Vaccine Adverse Event Reporting System (VAERS). Reporting forms and instructions on filing a VAERS report are available at www.vaers.hhs.gov or by telephone, 800-822-7967.

Information on how to file a Vaccine Injury Compensation Program claim is available at www.hrsa.gov/vaccinecompensation or by telephone, 800-338-2382. To file a claim for vaccine injury, contact the U.S. Court of Federal Claims, 717 Madison Place, N.W., Washington, D.C. 20005; telephone, 202-357-6400.

Additional information about the vaccines in this schedule, extent of available data, and contraindications for vaccination is also available at www.cdc.gov/vaccines or from the CDC-INFO Contact Center at 800-CDC-INFO (800-232-4636) in English and Spanish, 8:00 a.m. - 8:00 p.m. Eastern Time, Monday - Friday, excluding holidays.

Use of trade names and commercial sources is for identification only and does not imply endorsement by the U.S. Department of Health and Human Services.

Figure 22-2A   Recommended adult immunization schedule, by vaccine and age group.

Courtesy of the Centers for Disease Control and Prevention, Atlanta, GA

Figure 2. Vaccines that might be indicated for adults based on medical and other indications[1]

VACCINE ▼ INDICATION ▶	Pregnancy	Immunocompromising conditions (excluding human immunodeficiency virus [HIV])[4,6,7,14]	HIV infection[4,7,13,14] CD4+ T lymphocyte count		Men who have sex with men (MSM)	Heart disease, chronic lung disease, chronic alcoholism	Asplenia[13] (including elective splenectomy and persistent complement component deficiencies)	Chronic liver disease	Diabetes, kidney failure, end-stage renal disease, receipt of hemodialysis	Health-care personnel
			< 200 cells/μL	≥ 200 cells/μL						
Influenza [2]	1 dose TIV annually	1 dose TIV annually	1 dose TIV annually		1 dose TIV or LAIV annually	1 dose TIV annually				1 dose TIV or LAIV annually
Tetanus, diphtheria, pertussis (Td/Tdap) [3,*]	Substitute 1-time dose of Tdap for Td booster; then boost with Td every 10 yrs									
Varicella [4,*]	Contraindicated	Contraindicated	Contraindicated		2 doses					
Human papillomavirus (HPV) Female [5,*]	3 doses through age 26 yrs	3 doses through age 26 yrs	3 doses through age 26 yrs		3 doses through age 26 yrs					
Human papillomavirus (HPV) Male [5,*]	3 doses through age 26 yrs	3 doses through age 26 yrs			3 doses through age 21 yrs					
Zoster [6]	Contraindicated	Contraindicated	Contraindicated		1 dose					
Measles, mumps, rubella (MMR) [7,*]	Contraindicated	Contraindicated	Contraindicated		1 or 2 doses					
Pneumococcal (polysaccharide) [8,9]		1 or 2 doses								
Meningococcal [10,*]	1 or more doses									
Hepatitis A [11,*]	2 doses									
Hepatitis B [12,*]	3 doses									

Legend:

Covered | **For all persons in this category who meet the age requirements and who lack documentation of vaccination or have no evidence of previous infection** | **Recommended if some other risk factor is present (e.g., on the basis of medical, occupational, lifestyle, or other indications)** | Contraindicated | No recommendation

*Covered by the Vaccine Injury Compensation Program

The recommendations in this schedule were approved by the Centers for Disease Control and Prevention's (CDC) Advisory Committee on Immunization Practices (ACIP), the American Academy of Family Physicians (AAFP), the American College of Physicians (ACP), American College of Obstetricians and Gynecologists (ACOG) and American College of Nurse-Midwives (ACNM).

These schedules indicate the recommended age groups and medical indications for which administration of currently licensed vaccines is commonly indicated for adults ages 19 years and older, as of January 1, 2012. For all vaccines being recommended on the Adult Immunization Schedule: a vaccine series does not need to be restarted, regardless of the time that has elapsed between doses. Licensed combination vaccines may be used whenever any components of the combination are indicated and when the vaccine's other components are not contraindicated. For detailed recommendations on all vaccines, including those used primarily for travelers or that are issued during the year, consult the manufacturers' package inserts and the complete statements from the Advisory Committee on Immunization Practices (www.cdc.gov/vaccines/pubs/acip-list.htm). Use of trade names and commercial sources is for identification only and does not imply endorsement by the U.S. Department of Health and Human Services.

CDC

U.S. Department of Health and Human Services
Centers for Disease Control and Prevention

Figure 22-2B Recommended adult immunization schedule, by vaccine and medical and other indications.

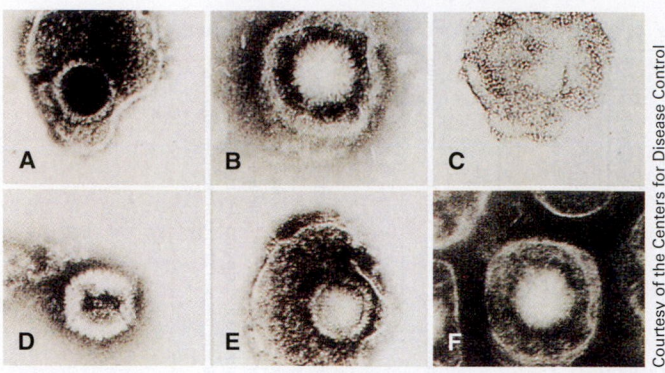

Courtesy of the Centers for Disease Control and Prevention, Atlanta, GA

Figure 22-3   Electron micrographs of various types of herpes simplex virus.

microorganisms is the use of antibiotic drugs. Examples of some bacterial pathogens are listed in Table 22-2 and shown in Figure 22-4.

Fungi. Fungi are microorganisms that may be unicellular (single-cell) or multicellular (many cells). Mushrooms and molds are examples of fungi that are nonpathogenic. Pathogenic fungi cause athlete's foot, ringworm, and candida infections

(Figure 22-5). Other pathogenic fungi include histoplasmosis and toxoplasmosis, which are fungal infections spread through the air from infected fowl and bird waste.

Parasites. Organisms that live in or on another organism are classified as parasites. They may be single-celled or multicelled. Examples include protozoa (single-cell microscopic organisms that cause **malaria**, **amoebic dysentery**, and **trichomoniasis** [Figure 22-6]); metazoa (multicellular organisms that cause pinworms, hookworms, and tapeworms); and ectoparasites (multicellular organisms that live superficially on another host, such as lice and **scabies**).

Rickettsiae. **Rickettsiae** are intracellular parasitic, small nonmotile bacteria. They are larger than viruses and can be seen under conventional microscopes after staining procedures. These microorganisms are susceptible to antibiotic therapy. Examples of rickettsial infections include typhus (transmitted by the body louse); Lyme disease (transmitted by ticks); and Rocky Mountain spotted fever (transmitted by ticks). Characteristic of

Table 22-1   Common Viral Diseases

Disease/Agent	Type of Infection and Site	Vaccine Availability
Herpes groups		
Herpes Simplex Virus 1 (HSV-1) (Figure 22-3)	Cold sores/keratitis	No
Herpes Simplex Virus 2 (HSV-2) (Figure 22-3)	Genital herpes	No
Herpes zoster	Shingles (neurons)	Yes*
Rubeola	Measles	Yes
Rubella	German measles	Yes
Poliovirus	Poliomyelitis	Yes
Influenza (ABC)	Flu, pneumonia	Yes
Human papillomavirus	Genital warts, cervical cancer	Yes
Hepatitis (A, B, C, D, E)	Liver	A, B
Epstein-Barr	Infectious mononucleosis	No
Varicella zoster	Chickenpox (skin)	Yes

*The Advisory Council on Immunization Practice (ACIP) recommended to the CDC that adults over age 60 years receive the Zostavax vaccine. The CDC has given provisional approval.

© Cengage Learning 2014

rickettsia infections is a skin rash caused by the rickettsia invading the small blood vessels. This appears on the skin as a small hemorrhagic rash.

Prions. Prions are abnormal pathogenic agents. Unlike other infectious agents, prions are not living organisms. Prions are transmissible, but unlike bacteria or viruses, prions must be ingested. These agents exist as abnormally folded proteins that are found most abundantly in brain tissue. In humans, they result in diseases of the brain that are degenerative and fatal. Examples of such diseases are bovine spongiform encephalopathy (BSE), or mad cow disease, and Creutzfeldt-Jakob disease (CJD).

Reservoir

The second stage in the infection cycle is the reservoir or location of the infectious agent. The reservoir is the source of a pathogen. Reservoirs are people, equipment, supplies, water, food, and animals or insects (known as vectors). Methods of infection control in the reservoir stage include hand washing, environmental hygiene, disinfection, sterilization, and maintenance of employee health standards, such as annual tuberculosis skin testing and seasonal vaccines.

Portal of Exit

Although the infectious agent is housed or living in the reservoir, it must leave the reservoir in order to infect another person. The portal of exit is the method by which an infectious agent leaves the reservoir. Microorganisms may leave the human body with normally occurring body fluids, such as excretions, secretions, skin cells, respiratory droplets, blood, or any body fluid. The portal of exit

Table 22-2 Examples of Infectious Bacterial Diseases

Disease	Infectious Agent	Mode of Transmission
Anthrax	*Bacillus anthracis*	Inhalation
Chlamydia (sexually transmitted disease)	*Chlamydia trachomatis*	Sexual contact
Clostridial myonecrosis (gas gangrene)	Species of gram-positive clostridia	Wound entry
Escherichia coli	Gram-negative bacilli	Ingestion, wound entry
Gonorrhea (sexually transmitted disease)	*Neisseria gonorrhoeae*	Sexual contact
Legionnaire's disease (pneumonia)	*Legionella pneumophila*	Inhalation
Nosocomial (hospital-acquired) infection	Gram-negative bacteria	Normal flora transmitted during illness/procedures; opportunistic pathogens transmitted during debilitated condition
Pneumococci	*Streptococcus pneumoniae*	Respiratory (inhalation)
Staphylococcal infection (abscesses, food poisoning, urinary tract infections)	*Staphylococci*	Direct contact, ingestion, inhalation, bloodborne, vectors (animals)
Streptococcal infection (strep throat, otitis media, pneumonia)	Hemolytic *streptococci* (usually beta-hemolytic group A)	Inhalation
Syphilis (sexually transmitted disease)	*Treponema pallidum*	Sexual contact
Tetanus (lockjaw)	*Clostridium tetani*	Wound entry
Typhoid fever (enteric fever)	*Salmonella typhi*	Fecal-oral

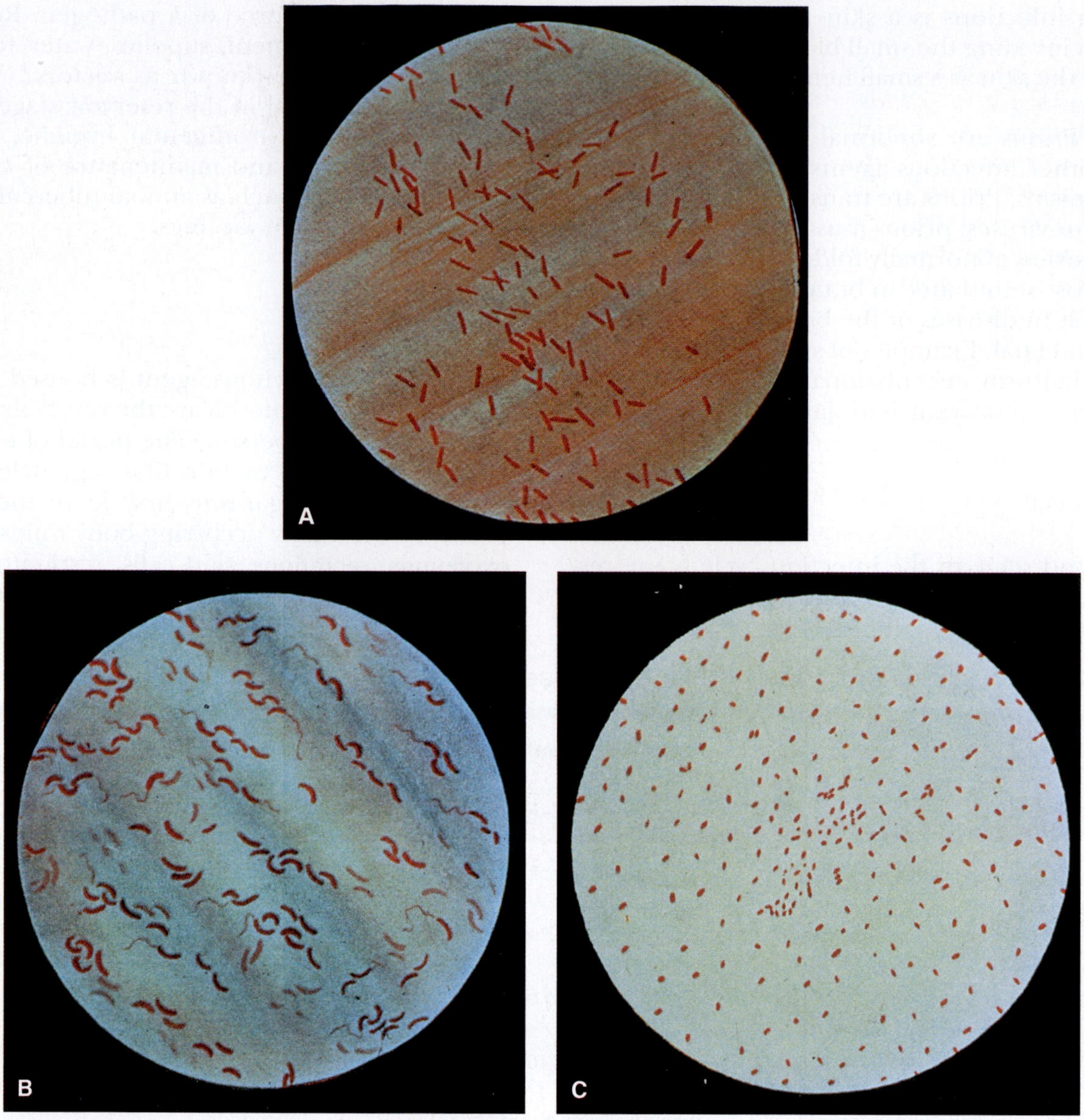

Figure 22-4   Bacterial forms: (A) *Escherichia coli*, (B) *Haemophilus pertussis*, (C) *Vibria cholerae*.

Courtesy of the Centers for Disease Control and Prevention, Atlanta, GA

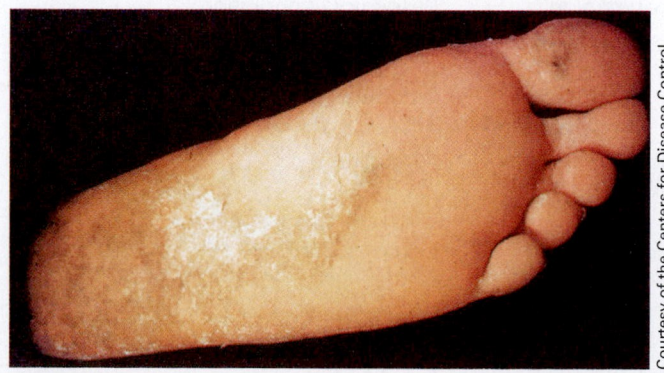

Figure 22-5   Ringworm of the foot (tinea pedis).

Courtesy of the Centers for Disease Control and Prevention, Atlanta, GA

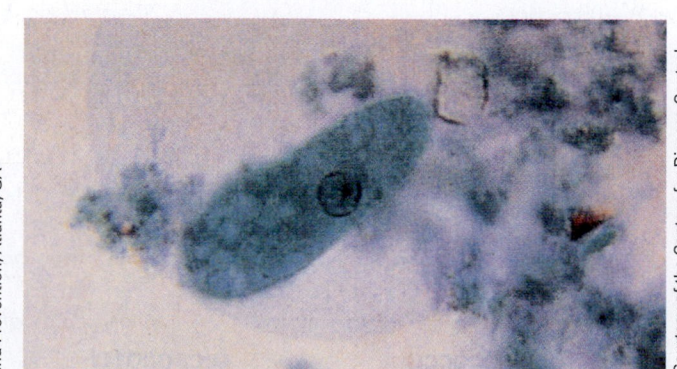

Figure 22-6   Intestinal protozoa, *Entamoeba coli*.

Courtesy of the Centers for Disease Control and Prevention, Atlanta, GA

may be continuous, such as with respiratory droplets, or dependent on the body fluid exiting the body under unusual circumstances, such as when blood leaves the body during a surgical procedure or phlebotomy. The portals of exit in humans are the respiratory, genitourinary, gastrointestinal, integumentary, and transplacental routes.

Standard Precautions and **Contact Precautions** are infection control methods based on the knowledge that infectious diseases exiting the body can be spread to others. These precautions attempt to control the spread of infectious diseases as infectious agents leave or exit the reservoir.

Modes of Transmission

The modes of transmission are specific ways in which microorganisms travel from one place (reservoir) to another (susceptible host). Transmission depends on the characteristics of the microorganisms. There are several modes of transmission.

Direct **contact transmission** occurs when there is physical contact between an infected person, or their body fluids, and a susceptible person that results in a transfer of microorganisms. This mode of transmission usually occurs between members of the same household or among close friends and family, as this type of transmission requires close contact with an infected individual. Examples of direct contact include:

- Touching an infected individual, especially touching body fluids
- Kissing, sexual contact, contact with oral secretions, or contact with body lesions

Indirect contact transmission occurs when there are microorganisms living on a surface that a susceptible person comes into contact with. Some organisms can survive for extended periods of time outside of a host. These are usually found on frequently touched surfaces such as doorknobs, tables, washroom surfaces, medical instruments, computer keyboards, clothing, uniforms, lab coats, and children's toys. These surfaces are referred to as **fomites**.

Droplet transmission delivers organisms via the air. Technically, droplet transmission is a form of contact transmission. Talking, coughing, and sneezing deliver microorganisms that can travel over a short distance. When these droplets come into contact with a susceptible host's eyes, nose, or mouth, the microorganism has found a route of entry. Droplets can also be generated during medical procedures such as nebulizer treatments, oral and endotracheal suctioning, or bronchoscopy.

Airborne transmission occurs when microorganisms are suspended in the air for long periods of time. Only organisms that can survive outside of the host for extended periods and are resistant to drying are a hazard for this mode of transmission. The upper and lower respiratory tracts are the portal of entry for this type of microorganism.

In the fecal-oral mode of transmission, pathogens enter the susceptible host by ingestion of contaminated food or water. These microorganisms multiply rapidly in the digestive tract and are shed in fecal material. To break this infection cycle, there must be adequate sanitation measures in place. An infected person working in the food industry is at risk for contaminating food that they come into contact with if basic sanitation guidelines are not followed stringently. Important measures include:

- Frequent hand washing, especially following washroom use
- Public awareness of the importance of hand washing and proper food handling
- Sanitation practices that include disinfection of frequently touched surfaces
- Following proper food storage techniques
- Cooking food to adequate internal temperatures

Vector transmission involves animals and insects that are capable of transmitting diseases. Well-known vectors include mice, ticks, fleas, rats, and dogs. Vectors allow diseases to be transmitted over a wide area due to the mobility of the animal or insect. The most common vector for disease worldwide is the mosquito. Typically, disease is spread by a bite from the vector; however, feces from the vector can spread certain diseases as well. Vectors can also transmit disease just by contacting food or a susceptible host's skin, as vectors can carry microorganisms on their outer surfaces.

Infection control measures in the ambulatory care area specifically address the transmission stage of the process of infection.

Methods that reduce the transmission of pathogens include adherence to Standard and Contact Precautions, hand washing, sanitization, disinfection, and sterilization. Methods of infection control are used in health care, food handling, water and sewage processing, humanitarian aid work, and child care.

Portal of Entry

Once an organism has found a useful mode of transmission, the next step in the infection cycle is to enter a susceptible host. Common entrance sites to the human body include nonintact skin, mucous membranes, and systems of the body exposed to the external environment, such as the respiratory, gastrointestinal, and reproductive systems. Breathing in airborne microorganisms allows infectious diseases to be spread to the lungs. Eating or drinking contaminated water is a cause of gastrointestinal infectious diseases. Sexually transmitted diseases spread through vaginal, oral, and anal intercourse. Care of patients with infectious diseases includes careful consideration of infection control to limit further spread of the microorganism. Methods such as correct wound care, transmission-based precautions, and **aseptic** technique limit the transmission of infectious microorganisms. The portals of exit and entry need not be the same for infection to be transmitted.

Susceptible Host

The complex relationship between the potential host and the infective agent may or may not result in infection. The person who has come into contact with the microorganism may already have immunity or have the ability to resist colonization. Those without these abilities are considered a susceptible host and can develop a clinical disease. Some can become asymptomatically infected with the microorganism and become a carrier of the disease without ever actually being ill. Resistance to infection relies on several factors such as age, immune integrity, underlying disease, and situations such as surgery when the body's first line of defense is interrupted and the body is bombarded by microorganisms via various pathways of entry. The susceptibility of a person depends on several factors, including:

1. Number and specific type of pathogen
2. Duration of exposure to the pathogen
3. General physical condition
4. Psychological health status
5. Occupation or lifestyle environment
6. Presence of underlying diseases or conditions
7. Youth or advanced age (young and old at greater risk)

 The goal of infection control at this stage in the infection cycle is to identify patients at risk for susceptibility, treat their underlying

PATIENT EDUCATION

Drug-Resistant Bacteria

Antibiotic resistance occurs because bacteria can change their characteristics, thus reducing or eliminating the effectiveness of antibiotics. The resistant microorganisms survive, multiply, and cause a longer illness, necessitating more visits to the provider and more powerful and expensive antibiotics. Death can result from resistant bacteria. The number of antibiotic-resistant bacteria has increased significantly in the past 10 years. For example:

- MRSA (methicillin-resistant *Staphylococcus aureus*)
- Tuberculosis
- VRE (vancomycin-resistant *Enterococcus*)
- PRSP (penicillin-resistant *Streptococcus pneumonia*)
- XDR-TB (extensively drug-resistant TB)

These and other infectious diseases are becoming more resistant to standard antibiotic treatment. Drug options are increasingly limited, are expensive, or simply do not exist. An example of drug-resistant bacteria is the extensively drug-resistant tuberculosis (XDR-TB) bacteria. These bacteria are resistant to almost all antibiotics used to treat TB, including the two best first-line antibiotics, the second-line antibiotics, and at least one of three injectable antibiotics. Because XDR-TB is resistant to several antibiotics, providers are left with much less effective treatment options that frequently have worse treatment outcomes.

In order to prevent the development of other drug resistant pathogens, it is important to educate patients with the following key information:

- Antibiotics should be prescribed by a licensed provider and should be taken only when prescribed to treat a bacterial infection.
- Antibiotics should be taken exactly as directed for the entire course.
- Do not demand antibiotics from your provider. They do not cure a viral infection.

conditions if possible, and isolate them from those reservoirs that could be hazardous to the susceptible person.

Hospitalized patients are at risk for contracting a **nosocomial** infection or healthcare-associated infections (HAI). These infections are caused by a wide variety of organisms. Some of these organisms are common viruses, bacteria, and fungi. Others are more resistant to intervention. In recent years, many strides have been made to limit the risk to those seeking health care. Strict adherence to infection prevention guidelines is the key to limiting patient risk. It is the responsibility of health care providers to maintain surveillance and gather information about HAIs. This data must be reported appropriately to various agencies on the local, state, and federal levels.

In your role as a patient advocate, it is your responsibility to assure that you are aware of infection control practices, use personal protective equipment appropriately, and observe Standard Precautions at all times. Infection prevention is the role of every health care provider. It protects those you care for, your peers, and yourself from exposure to pathogens. Remember that hand washing is the primary tool in prevention of infection!

Key recommendations from the CDC to control the risk of HAIs in the ambulatory care setting include:

- Developing and maintaining infection prevention programs
- Providing sufficient supplies to allow all staff to adhere to Standard Precautions
- Selecting a lead employee to maintain current training in infection prevention and appointing them to lead regular training sessions with other staff
- Assuring that someone with current training is on staff during all clinic hours that include interaction with patients
- Developing a written policy and procedures that address infection control in your particular care setting and adhering to them rigorously

A number of different pathogens are present in the hospital and other health care settings, and as new patients arrive, new pathogens are introduced to the facility. The overuse of antibiotics contributes to microorganisms becoming resistant to them. Some health care staff become carriers of these microorganisms.

In the last decade there has been a continuous rise in antibiotic-resistant bacteria. Since antibiotics were discovered by Alexander Fleming in 1928, antibiotic therapy has saved millions of lives. However, the overuse of antibiotics has led to the severe health care issue of antibiotic-resistant bacteria. Common antibiotic-resistant organisms that are found in the health care setting include methicillin-resistant *Staphylococcus aureus* (MRSA), vancomycin-resistant *enterococcus* (VRE), and extensively drug-resistant tuberculosis (XDR-TB). These organisms have become a major public health problem and research demonstrates that they affect certain populations disproportionately. Those most vulnerable are people receiving health care in an ambulatory or inpatient care setting. It is essential that health care providers do all that is in their power to break the infection cycle to protect those in their care.

CRITICAL THINKING

View Figure 22-1, the diagram of the infection cycle. Which stage most appropriately relates to you as a health care provider?

THE BODY'S DEFENSE MECHANISMS FOR FIGHTING INFECTION AND DISEASE

The Body's Natural Barriers

The body has many natural barriers and defenses in place to help us avoid exposure to pathogens and infection. These barriers can be categorized under physical/mechanical, chemical, and cellular factors.

Physical barriers are the first line of defense. The skin and associated accessories, such as hair and nails, form an anatomical barrier from pathogens. Physical/mechanical factors include eyelashes and eyebrows, cilia (tiny hairs in the respiratory tract), and barriers such as eyelids and intact skin/mucous membranes. Mucous membranes are found in the lining of the mouth, nose, and eyelids, and they function to trap and fight invasion by microorganisms.

Chemical barriers include tears, sweat, mucus, saliva, gastrointestinal secretions, and vaginal secretions. Tears contain active enzymes that attack bacteria. Inhaled pathogens are trapped in the mucus secreted by the respiratory tract. This mucus contains enzymes that serve as antibiotics to protect the body from bacterial infection. Inside the gastrointestinal tract there are various protective devices. The stomach contains strong acid that serves the dual purposes of digesting food and killing pathogens. Bile and pancreatic secretions also have anti-infective properties. The bladder is protected from infection by the mucous membrane lining of the urethra, and the normal acidic environment of the vagina protects from most infections.

Cellular barriers are also called body defenses and consist of white blood cells, which defend against infection in tissues in many ways; the bloodstream; and the lymphatic system. Cellular defenses are explained in more detail in the following two sections.

Inflammatory Response

Inflammation is the body's natural way of responding when invaded by a pathogen or physical trauma. Inflammation is a nonspecific response, meaning that it can occur with any threat to the body, not just in reaction to a particular pathogen. Inflammation can occur regardless of whether it is caused by an agent that is pathogenic, a trauma, a foreign body, or extremes in temperature. If a pathogen is present, the body goes through a distinct process in an attempt to destroy and eliminate the pathogenic microorganisms and their by-products and, if that is not possible, to restrict the amount of damage done.

The cardinal signs of inflammation are redness, heat, swelling, and pain. These symptoms may be slight, almost unnoticed, or quite evident. Remember, inflammation is a natural response and does not necessarily indicate infection. The two should not be confused. Inflammation can occur without infection, but infection does not occur without inflammation.

The steps in the inflammatory process are:

- Blood flow increases to the affected area and the vessels in this area become more permeable, allowing fluid and white blood cells to transfer in and out of the vessel.
- Plasma moves into the tissue causing swelling and pain due to pressure on nerve endings.
- White blood cells move into injured tissue to fight infection, and phagocytes destroy invading pathogens. This occurs within the first several hours after exposure to the pathogen. The bone marrow "turns on" and an increased number of specific white blood cells are released into the blood stream.

After destruction of the pathogen, tissue repair can begin. If the **inflammatory response** is not effective, the specific immune response is necessary.

Indications that an inflammatory process is inadequate are: (1) the accumulation of purulent matter (pus) in the area (due to destroyed pathogens, white blood cells, and body cells); (2) lymph node enlargement (swollen glands); and (3) septicemia, which may result because pathogens have spread to the bloodstream.

Immediate antibiotic therapy is indicated in these circumstances because of the inadequacy of the inflammatory response.

The Immune System and Immunity

To fight infectious diseases, our bodies are equipped with several effective physical and chemical **barriers** such as the skin, mucous membranes, body excretions and secretions, and a complex, highly specific **immune system**. The immune system's purpose is to protect against pathogens and abnormal cell growth. The system is composed of various cells that collectively recognize, subdue, attack, and eliminate pathogens. The human immune system is very complicated and is comprised of numerous pathways that allow the body to defend against attacks.

The two types of immune responses include cell-mediated immunity and humoral immunity; they work interdependently inside the human body to nullify threats from the environment. **Cell-mediated immunity** is usually involved in attacks against viruses, fungi, organ transplants, or cancer cells. The process of cell-mediated immunity begins with the mobilization of various immune cells. Therefore, it is also termed cellular immunity. A group of "attack cells" is produced in the bone marrow and matured in the thymus gland. Known as T cells or T lymphocytes, these cells are members of the white blood cell family. These cells keep the body safe and secure from pathogens and foreign particles. T cells are the core of cell-mediated immunity, but there are innumerable and varied cell types that have specific assignments in the army that defends the body.

Humoral immunity is known as the antibody-mediated system because it deals with immune system structures called antibodies. This type of immunity is a result of the stimulation of B lymphocytes and plasma cells to produce antibodies. Antibodies are proteins that are produced by the immune system when the body detects harmful substances called antigens. Humoral immunity consists of two responses: primary and secondary. During primary immune response, an antigen is encountered by the susceptible host for the very first time. B cells are then activated and multiply. When this first exposure occurs, it may take a prolonged period of time for adequate numbers of cells to be produced. With a secondary exposure, there is already the "pattern" for response and the B cells can be produced much more quickly. Vaccination induces a primary immune response. This allows a more effective secondary response when a body is exposed to a known pathogen. This is known as passive immunity.

Generally, both types of immune responses occur in four phases:

1. *Recognition of the invader.* The immune system is equipped with cells that identify agents, pathogens, and abnormal cell growth as foreign substances. Macrophages and helper T cells recognize foreign invaders, whether they are pathogens, cancer cells, or transplanted tissues.

2. *Growth of defenses, which allows for multiplication of helper T cells and B cells.* After foreign substance recognition, the immune system alerts T and B cells to multiply and move to the site of the foreign substance. In cell-mediated immunity, activation of helper T cells means that the T cells are specifically oriented to a unique antigen, a substance such as bacteria the body recognizes as foreign. Activated T cells divide, forming memory T cells and killer T cells. In humoral immunity, activated B cells are antigen specific and divide into memory B cells and plasma cells.

3. *Attack against the infection.* Cell-mediated immunity uses killer T cells and macrophages to phagocytize, or engulf and destroy the pathogens. Humoral plasma cells have the ability to produce specific **antibodies** that lock on to specific antigens, which prevents the disease-producing characteristics of the pathogen from forming. These antibodies are called **immunoglobulins** and they render the pathogen unable to reproduce or continue growth.

4. *Slowdown of the immune response after death of the infectious agent.* After the death of the foreign substance, the immune response is halted. T and B cells return to normal levels, and in the case of humoral immunity, the presence of antibody production causes the immune system to resist the specific infectious pathogen in future contacts with the pathogen.

Susceptibility to some infectious diseases is closely linked to the person's unique resistance, or immunity. Immunity is the ability of the body to resist specific pathogens and their toxins. **Resistance** occurs after an exposure to a pathogen, which is the antigen–antibody reaction. This natural body defense to fight infectious disease occurs gradually and over time as pathogens and other foreign substances such as antigens enter the human body. When the antigen enters the body, the immune system recognizes the antigen as foreign and attempts to contain and subdue the foreign invader. Specific chemical antibodies to the antigen are produced by B cells, which attempt to prevent the antigen from further growth. After the completion of the stages of that infectious disease, the body retains the ability to produce antibodies in response to that specific microorganism or antigen. Therefore, immunity can last for some length of time, possibly to provide lifetime protection against specific infectious microorganisms. Several forms of immunity can occur in response to specific antigens:

- Naturally acquired active immunity results from contracting an infectious agent and experiencing either an acute or subclinical infectious disease. This immunity is usually permanent.

- Artificially acquired active immunity is achieved after administration of vaccines. This immunity is semi-permanent to permanent.

- Naturally, congenitally acquired passive immunity occurs when antibodies pass to a fetus from the mother providing short-term immunity for the newborn. This immunity is temporary.

- Artificially acquired passive immunity may be achieved through administration of ready-made antibodies, such as gamma globulin, used to treat or prevent infectious diseases. This immunity is temporary.

Our defenses against diseases can be categorized as specific and nonspecific. Specific defenses include those things that protect us against a specific pathogen, whereas nonspecific defenses are not so particular. Some examples of specific defenses are:

- *Vaccines/immunizations.* Designed for specific pathogen

- *Antibodies.* Created against a specific pathogen

- *Tetanus shot.* Protects individuals from tetanus
- *Active immunities.* Created against a specific pathogen
- *Globulin.* Antibodies for exposure to a specific pathogen

Some examples of nonspecific defenses are:

- *Tears.* Contain chemical harmful to a variety of pathogens
- *Skin.* Creates a barrier against many different pathogens
- *Saliva.* Contains chemicals harmful to a variety of pathogens
- *Species resistance.* Being human protects us from many diseases to which other animals are susceptible

Immunization. Immunizing individuals against specific infectious diseases provides immunity with active or passive vaccines. Vaccines have extended the life span of Americans by more than thirty years and reduced the mortality from infectious disease significantly. Globally, vaccination saves two to three million lives per year. A child born in the United States has the opportunity to be immunized against 17 serious diseases and conditions according to the U.S. Department of Health and Human Services (HHS). HHS developed the 2010 National Vaccine Plan to provide guidelines for the U.S. vaccine and immunization schedule for the next ten years.

Several factors influence vaccination compliance rates, such as access to health care, cost of vaccinations, and irregularity or confusion in maintaining young children on the recommended schedule. There are pockets within large cities of significant numbers of underimmunized children. According to the Office of Minority Health, African Americans and Hispanics, across the age continuum, have a lower immunization rate than non-Hispanic whites. An outbreak could cause an **epidemic** of diseases that are preventable with vaccines (see Chapter 27). The Department of Health and Human Services has created a plan to address this issue. It is called the HHS Action Plan to Reduce Racial and Ethnic Health Disparities.

An Anti-Vaccination Movement has influenced compliance with recommended immunization schedules since 1998 when a study linked autism to vaccines, although there has been subsequent research that disputes those findings. Even though all states have immunization requirements for school admission, there is a significant number of parents and caregivers who are resisting the mandated childhood immunizations. These groups want state laws changed and feel that they, as parents and caregivers, should be allowed to decide if they want their children immunized.

Exemptions from mandated immunizations are allowed in all states if there are medical reasons. Some states will exempt children for religious reasons and some on philosophical grounds.

In general, children would more likely suffer greater complications associated with childhood diseases than from the immunizations given to prevent them. Because most of the vaccinations are administered in ambulatory health care settings, medical assistants may have the responsibility to administer, document, and monitor immunizations (see Chapter 27).

There are various classifications of vaccines, depending on the method of immune stimulation:

1. *Live attenuated (changed) pathogens.* These pathogens stimulate the body's own antibody production. However, the patient does not contract the infectious disease (or only a mild or subclinical case) because the pathogen has been altered in some mechanical or chemical means by the manufacturer. Examples of live attenuated pathogens include measles and varicella.

2. *Pathogenic toxins.* Some pathogens produce toxins (poisonous substances) that can stimulate antibody production. Examples of toxin vaccines include tetanus and diphtheria.

3. *Killed pathogens.* Inactivated pathogens stimulate antibody production; however, several vaccines may be required to provide sustained protection. Examples include pertussis, rabies, and poliomyelitis.

STAGES OF INFECTIOUS DISEASES

Depending on the specific pathogen causing an infectious disease, several stages occur from the time of exposure until full recovery and the absence of infection. These stages are often predictable and offer guidelines for patient education and treatment opportunities.

Incubation Stage

The incubation stage is the interval of time between exposure to a pathogenic microorganism and the first appearance of signs and symptoms of the disease. Some infectious diseases have short incubation stages, whereas other infections have lengthy stages, lasting for years. If an exposure to an infectious agent occurs, the patient will manifest (reveal in an obvious way) the disease if the patient's immune system cannot contain the agent. If therapeutic medications are available, it can help to prevent disease progression. Not all infectious agents are treatable or preventable.

Prodromal Stage

The prodromal stage is the initial stage of the disease. There may be signs and symptoms but full-blown illness is not present. It is characterized by common, general complaints of illness, such as **malaise** and fever. It is the interval between the earliest symptoms and the appearance of fever or rash that suggest an impending disease process is occurring.

Acute Stage

This stage is also known as the invasive phase or the period of illness. Disease processes reach their peak during the acute stage. Symptoms are fully developed and can often be differentiated from other specific symptoms. In this stage the host is experiencing full mobilization of their immune system. Treatment modalities are useful to reduce patient discomfort, to reduce possibilities of debilitation and adverse effects, and to promote healing and recovery.

The inflammatory process is the body's natural defensive reaction to the invasion by a foreign substance such as a pathogen, and it is in this acute state that the response is evident.

Acme

This is the peak stage of the disease symptoms. Resolution of the infection depends on the activity of the immune system, intervention by medical science, or the self-limiting aspect of the disease.

Declining Stage

Patient symptoms begin to subside or wane during the declining stage. The infectious disease remains, however, though the patient will demonstrate improving levels of health. It is often during the declining phase of an illness, when patients begin to feel better, that they prematurely discontinue taking the antibiotic that may have been prescribed. This premature discontinuance can result in microorganisms becoming resistant to antibiotics. It is important to educate patients in the proper use of antibiotics.

Convalescent Stage

Recovery and recuperation from the effects of a specific infectious disease are called the convalescent stage. The patient regains strength and stamina. The overall goal of this stage is returning the patient to as close as possible the original state of health.

Sequelae

If the body cannot fully repair the damage from the infectious disease, the pathological conditions that result are referred to as sequelae. Examples of sequelae of untreated strep throat include rheumatic fever, meningitis, and tonsillitis.

DISEASE TRANSMISSION

When providing patients with health care, medical assistants run the risk for **contracting**, or acquiring, an infection from pathogens that are causing patients' illnesses. Such pathogens are viruses, bacteria, fungi, and others that can be found in patients' blood and body fluids. In medical clinics, ambulatory care centers, and hospitals, many ill patients are seen every day. Pathogens can be easily transmitted to another person if care is not taken to prevent such an occurrence.

Consistent use and adherence to infection control measures significantly reduce the risk for disease transmission. The CDC recommends that health care providers consider each patient to be potentially infectious for AIDS, hepatitis B and C, and other bloodborne pathogens and that they routinely and conscientiously apply the techniques of Standard Precautions as a means of infection control.

Infectious diseases are caused by unique infectious agents, are characterized by various symptoms, are transmitted by differing means, and have unique treatments and prognoses. Medical assistants must recognize the unique characteristics of specific infectious diseases to prevent their transmission and help patients suffering from these infections. Table 22-3 classifies several

Table 22-3 Examples of Infectious Diseases

Disease	Agent	Transmission	Symptoms	Diagnosis	Treatment	Comments	Patient Education
Acquired immunodeficiency syndrome (AIDS)	Human immunodeficiency virus (HIV)	• Bloodborne • Sexual contact • Intrauterine • Lactation	Opportunistic infections, lymphadenopathy, fatigue, malaise, fever	CD4 T-cell level less than 200/mm^3, Viral count Chest X-ray CBC	Palliative care and treatment for opportunistic infections, antiviral drugs	World Health Organization global statistics estimate that 37.4 to 40 million adults and children are living with HIV/AIDS (2010)	1. Careful infection control and asepsis to reduce contact with pathogens that cause opportunistic infections. 2. Use of latex condoms in conjunction with effective spermicide. 3. Support groups/education.
Foodborne illnesses	Bacteria or viruses (i.e., staphylococci, clostridium, botulinum, E. coli, shigella)	• Ingestion of contaminated food or water	Nausea, stomach pain, vomiting, bloody diarrhea, dehydration, respiratory failure, death	Culture of feces, vomitus, or suspected food or water	Fluid balance restoration, medications, emergency treatment as required	Report outbreaks to local authorities; especially dangerous in children and older adults; undercooked meat and vegetables and fruits washed in dirty water can carry E. coli.	1. Teach proper food handling. 2. Carefully wash hands before handling all food. 3. Report to provider all signs of dehydration. 4. Gastroenteritis usually communicable via feces for up to 7 weeks after exposure.
Impetigo	Streptococcus	• Direct contact with moist discharges of the lesions	Vesicles become pustular, rupture, and form crusts; pruritus	Culture of discharge	Antibiotics po or IV if severe; local antibiotic ointment	Good hygiene is necessary to help prevent transmission; gloves should be worn when cleaning lesions; expose lesions to air to help dry; can be fatal if not treated properly	1. Good hygiene necessary to help prevent transmission. 2. Can be fatal to newborns if not treated promptly. 3. Wear gloves when touching lesions.
Influenza	Influenza viruses A, B, or C; Haemophilus (bacteria)	• Inhalation • Aerosolized • Mucous droplets	Acute upper/lower respiratory infection, severe cough, fever, malaise, sore throat, coryza	Tissue culture of nasal or pharyngeal secretions	Palliative therapy, active immunization (annual vaccine recommended for persons at risk [older adults, heart patients] for complications from infection)	Report cases to local health authority; may be fatal in older adults and children; may cause meningitis; may easily become epidemic; 80% of elderly who contract the flu die	1. Bed rest for 2–3 days after fever declines. 2. Force fluids. 3. Report signs of secondary infections (pneumonia, otitis media). 4. Vaccine available. 5. Practice cough etiquette.

Disease	Cause	Transmission	Symptoms	Diagnosis	Treatment	Description	Prevention/Notes
Lyme disease	Bacteria (*Borrelia burgdorferi*)	• Transmitted by the bite of infected tick	Rash, flu-like symptoms, headache, fatigue, joint pain	Presence of symptoms; laboratory tests may be inconclusive, taking 6 weeks or more for antibodies to appear in the blood; erythrocyte sedimentation rate; total serum; Ig M level; aspartate aminotransferase level	Antibiotics, po or IV	The tick is so small and bite so mild, patients may not realize they were bitten for a few days to weeks later; bacteria spread to other sites, causing symptoms to heart, joints, and nervous system; arthritis develops and may become chronic	1. Use insect repellant. 2. Remove tick promptly (save for laboratory testing if possible). 3. Wear pants tucked into socks when in wooded areas or where ticks are present. 4. Complete recovery usually occurs if treated with antibiotics. 5. Disease has exacerbations and remissions.
Meningitis	Bacteria*** (more severe; *Neisseria meningitides* is one type) Virus	• Bacterial through exchange of respiratory and throat secretions (coughing, sneezing, shared drinking glasses, bottles, cans, cigarettes)	High fever, severe headache, stiff neck, nausea, rash, vomiting, confusion, sleepiness, seizures	Culture and sensitivity of cerebral spinal fluid	Appropriate antibiotics; vaccine available for the bacteria responsible for 75% of the disease (vaccine lasts 3–5 years)	Rare but potentially fatal disease; there are two forms of meningitis: (1) inflammation of brain and spinal cord, and (2) meningococcemia (infection in the blood). Bacterial meningitis is contagious but not spread by casual contact or by breathing the air where an infected person is present; leading cause of meningitis in older children and young adults; cases have doubled since 1991.	1. Meningitis usually peaks in late winter and early spring and can be mistaken for the flu. 2. High-risk persons are college students living in dorms, immunosuppressed individuals, and persons traveling to areas of world where meningitis is prevalent (these people should get vaccine). 3. The CDC can advise travelers about areas for which they recommend the vaccine be given.

continues

521

Table 22-3 Examples of Infectious Diseases (*Continued*)

Disease	Agent	Transmission	Symptoms	Diagnosis	Treatment	Comments	Patient Education
Methicillin-resistant *Staphylococcus aureus* infections** (MRSA skin infections)	Bacteria (*Staphylococcus aureus*—"Staph") commonly found on skin and in nose of healthy persons	• Direct skin-to-skin contact (e.g., shaking hands, wrestling, other direct skin contact) • Shared towels or shared athletic equipment • Bacteria gain entrance to the body through any break in the skin	Pus-filled boils, pimples, and rashes; same symptoms as other "Staph" infections	Culture and sensitivity of discharge from infected site; blood and other body fluids can be tested by culture and sensitivity	Good wound and skin care; keep area clean and dry; wear gloves and wash hands after caring for site; antibiotics, but MRSA is resistant to many common antibiotics	In the past MRSA was primarily seen in hospitalized patients; now, MRSA is seen in healthy younger people; these infections commonly are not acquired in a hospital but rather in the community; children in day care, athletes, prisoners, IV drug users, men who have sex with men are at higher risk; can cause surgical wound infections, septicemia, pneumonia; use Standard Precautions	1. Regular hand washing helps prevent acquiring and spreading Staph, including MRSA. 2. Keep open sores and breaks in the skin covered until healed. 3. Avoid contact with other person's wounds or dressings. 4. Avoid sharing towels, toothbrushes, washcloths, razors. 5. Keep skin healthy to help avoid Staph on skin surface from causing an infection in nonintact skin and tissues. 6. Take all doses of antibiotic prescribed and do not share them with another person.
Pertussis*	*Bordetella pertussis* (bacteria)	• Direct contact with discharge from respiratory mucous membrane	Primarily seen in the pediatric population; severe coughing, whooping, and vomiting; apnea, pneumonia, seizures	Presence of whooping-type cough; nasal pharyngeal culture PCR (polymer chain reaction) in patient younger than 11 years; serology in patient older than 11 years	DPT vaccine prevents disease; antibiotics may be given for secondary infection of pneumonia	High rate of morbidity and mortality in many countries; incidence in U.S. has increased steadily since the 1980s. In U.S., epidemics occur every 3–5 years; increase seen in adolescents and adults	1. Highly contagious. 2. Adolescents and adults become susceptible when immunity wanes. 3. Practice cough hygiene****.

Disease	Cause	Transmission	Symptoms	Diagnosis	Treatment	Notes	Prevention
Pneumonia	Bacteria**** Viruses***** Fungi Protozoa Rickettsia Aspirations of chemicals and dust	• Cough, sneeze, droplets in air	Cough with sputum, chills, fever, chest pain, dyspnea, fatigue	Chest X-ray, blood culture, sputum culture, CBC	Antibiotics if bacterial; treatment of symptoms if viral; oxygen therapy, bed rest	Elderly, immunosuppressed, and patients with chronic illness are more susceptible; vaccine available; practice cough hygiene	1. Get vaccine. 2. Practice proper respiratory hygiene (cover nose and mouth when coughing or sneezing). 3. Use tissues to contain secretions and expectorations; dispose of used tissues in nearest waste receptacle. 4. If no tissues available, cover nose and mouth with bend of the elbow. 5. Practice proper hand hygiene.
Rubella (German measles)	Virus	• Spread by contact with infected person through coughing and sneezing	Rash, fever for 2–3 days, lymph node enlargement in head and neck	Rubella titer; presence of rubella antibodies in blood	None other than treatment of symptoms; pain and fever medications as needed; treat for shock; practice cough etiquette.	Rubella vaccine can prevent disease; part of the MMR vaccine; birth defects if a pregnant woman acquires rubella (deafness, mental retardation, liver and spleen damage to fetus)	1. The following individuals should get the MMR vaccine: college students or any student beyond high school, people employed in a medical facility, people who travel internationally, people who are a passenger on a cruise ship, females of childbearing age. 2. Vaccine not given during pregnancy.
Toxic shock syndrome (TSS)	Staphylococcus aureus Streptococcus	• Associated with use of tampons and intravaginal contraceptive devices • Can occur post operationally with staphylococcal wound infections	Sudden onset of fever, chills, vomiting, muscle aches, and rash; progresses rapidly to hypotension and multisystem breakdown, shock, and death	Presence of symptoms, vaginal culture, CBC, blood culture	IV fluids and antibiotics; management of respiratory disease, renal impairment, gastrointestinal problems	CDS says TSS could be stopped if use of vaginal tampons ceases; menstruating women, women using barrier contraceptives, and persons with post-operative Staphylococcus infections are at risk.	1. A woman who has had TSS is at risk for recurrence and should not use tampons at all. 2. Women should wash hands carefully before inserting a tampon. 3. Tampon should be changed every 6–8 hours.

continues

Table 22-3 Examples of Infectious Diseases (*Continued*)

Disease	Agent	Transmission	Symptoms	Diagnosis	Treatment	Comments	Patient Education
Tuberculosis (TB)*	*Mycobacterium tuberculosis* bacillus	• Inhalation of contaminated airborne mucous droplets • Possibly ingestion	Productive cough, fatigue, fever, weight loss (behavioral changes, anorexia), night sweats	Sputum culture for *M. tuberculosis*, Mantoux skin test (PPD), chest X-ray, pleural needle biopsy	Antituberculosis agents, airborne transmission-based precautions until drug agents started	Increase in incidence of TB, especially among persons with AIDS and the homeless; may become drug resistant; health care professionals should have annual skin testing; report outbreaks	1. Encourage hand washing, proper sputum tissue disposal. 2. Promote compliance with medications. 3. Encourage close contacts to have skin tests. 4. Encourage a well-balanced diet. 5. Practice cough etiquette.
Vancomycin-resistant *Enterococcus* (VRE)**	Bacteria (enterococci) normally found in intestines and female genital tract	• Direct contact with blood, urine, feces • Indirect contact with contaminated surfaces and from health care worker's hands	VRE can cause infections seen as: septicemia, pelvic, neonatal, and urinary disorders, otitis media	Culture and sensitivity of stool, urine, and/or blood	Antibiotics other than vancomycin	Spread directly by contact with feces, urine, or blood; spread indirectly from hands of health care workers or on contaminated surfaces; Standard Precautions used when caring for patients	1. Wash hands thoroughly after using toilet and before touching food. 2. Wear gloves if handling body fluids containing VRE.

Disease	Causative Agent	Transmission	Signs and Symptoms	Diagnosis	Treatment	Prognosis	Prevention
Varicella (chicken-pox)	Varicella-zoster virus	• Direct and indirect contact with respiratory droplets	Sudden-onset fever, malaise, maculo-papular-vesicular skin rash	Vesicular fluid tissue culture during first 3 days after eruption; serology: increased antibodies 2 weeks after rash; lesion appearance characteristic of varicella	Acyclovir helpful to reduce severity of disease; zoster immunoglobulin (ZIG) for high-risk persons only within 96 hours of exposure; palliative therapy	Vaccine (varicella virus vaccine live) available in United States for children older than 12 months	1. Communicable 1–2 days before rash until lesions crust. 2. Avoid scratching lesions to prevent secondary infection and scarring. 3. Benadryl and calamine lotion can be used for itch. 4. Acetaminophen can be used for fever. 5. Practice cough etiquette.
West Nile virus	Virus	• Infected mosquito	Central nervous system; fever, headache, coma, convulsions, paralysis; 80% of people infected show no signs or symptoms	West Nile virus IgM capture, PRNT (plaque reduction neutralization test)	None—supportive only; if hospitalized IV fluids, ventilator	Potentially serious illness; may have permanent neurologic effects	1. Use insect repellent with DEET. 2. Wear long sleeves and pants when outside, especially at dawn and dusk. 3. Get rid of mosquito breeding sites by emptying standing water in flowerpots, buckets, and barrels. 4. Keep children's pools empty and on their sides when not in use. 5. A small number of cases are spread through blood transfusions, organ transplants, intrauterine, and breast feeding.

* Resurgent Diseases: Case rates of recent years have reversed and are now increasing.

** Emerging Diseases: Have become recognized in recent years.

*** Although meningitis can be bacterial or viral, the information in this table applies to bacterial meningitis because it is the more severe of the two.

**** Bacteria and viruses are the two main causes of pneumonia. Of the two, bacterial is more serious.

common infectious diseases by critical components. When patients have contracted an infectious disease or are exposed to the risk for transmission, patient education plays an important role in infection control. Although a family member may have an infectious disease, proper training and education may protect other family members and close contacts.

Medical assistants are in a unique position to educate patients and the public about disease control. These measures become even more important with the increase in drug-resistant pathogens. All health care professionals must consistently and diligently use every infection control measure available, as well as teach our patients to do the same.

HUMAN IMMUNODEFICIENCY VIRUS AND HEPATITIS B AND C

A great deal of attention has been focused on the **human immunodeficiency virus (HIV)** that causes AIDS, and yet there remains no cure for the disease, although great advances have been made. With the focus on AIDS, other potentially life-threatening and fatal illnesses may seem less dangerous. In reality, hepatitis B and C are examples of other diseases that place health care providers at great risk for serious illness or death. Acute viral hepatitis deserves close attention.

HIV and AIDS

AIDS is caused by the bloodborne virus HIV. The viral infection directly affects the immune response. The HIV is responsible for T-cell destruction; T cells are the white blood cells that provide immunity.

HIV is carried in semen, blood, and other body fluids, and the virus can penetrate mucous membranes. Once HIV is inside the body, the reduced number of helper T cells leaves the patient vulnerable to a wide range of infections and malignancies. The infections that the patient contracts can be devastating. When people are positive for HIV infection, their T-cell counts must be regularly and closely monitored, and they must live their lives with careful consideration toward preventing opportunistic infections. If their T-cell count decreases to less than 200, they are considered to have AIDS. There is no curative treatment of HIV infections, but antiviral drugs such as lamivudine, azidothymidine, zidovudine, stavudine, and others

are used to slow cell processes and weaken cell protein, which is important in the virus's reproduction. Many people are living for many years with HIV and AIDS. Table 22-4 provides information about HIV and AIDS.

Acute Viral Hepatitis Diseases

In any of the acute viral hepatitis diseases, the liver becomes inflamed, and hepatic cells can be destroyed. Healthy persons can regenerate cells, but older adult patients usually cannot. There are several types of viral hepatitis: hepatitis A (HAV), hepatitis B (HBV), hepatitis C (HCV), hepatitis D (HDV), hepatitis E (HEV), and others. HAV, HBV, and HCV are the more common viruses; HDV and HEV are less common (see Table 22-5).

Despite the similarities among HIV, HBV, and HCV, the risk for contracting HBV and HCV is greater than for contracting HIV (Figure 22-7). Statistics provided by the CDC indicate that the risk of contracting HBV from a cut or needlestick exposure ranges from 6%–30%. The risk of contracting HIV from a cut or needlestick exposure is only 0.3%. The Hepatitis B virus can survive outside the body for up to 7 days and still be capable of producing an infection. HIV does not survive outside the body for more than a few hours even in high concentrations.

Medical assistants and all other health care providers must understand the importance of protecting themselves from the viruses that cause AIDS, HBV, HCV, and other pathogenic microorganisms. Through strict adherence to safety precautions and routine infectious disease control measures such as those found in **medical asepsis**, the risk for contracting an infectious disease can be minimized.

There is no vaccine to prevent HCV and no treatment after an exposure to prevent infection. Neither immunoglobulin nor antiviral drugs are recommended. It is a chronic disease, and patients carry the virus for the remainder of their lives. The virus is spread through blood and body fluids, sharing needles, IV drug use, needlesticks or sharps exposure, or from mother to baby during delivery. HCV patients may be at risk for infection with HAV, HBV, and/or HIV. Patients with HCV should be vaccinated for HAV and HBV. Infection control practices (Standard Precautions) are necessary to prevent infection with HCV through blood and body fluids. Patients exposed to HCV should be tested for HCV antibodies and liver enzyme levels

Table 22-4 Facts About HIV and AIDS

Signs and symptoms*	
Early (weeks to months after exposure)	• Flu-like illness • Swollen lymph nodes • Persistent fevers
Late (years after exposure)	• Night sweats • Prolonged diarrhea • Unexplained weight loss • Purple bumps on skin or inside mouth and nose • Chronic fatigue • Swollen lymph nodes • Recurrent respiratory infections
Transmission	
HIV is spread by:	• Vaginal sex • Oral sex • Anal sex • Sharing needles to inject drugs, body piercing or tattooing • Contaminated blood products (rare) • Infected mother to newborn
HIV *cannot* be spread by:	• Shaking hands • A social kiss • Cups • Animals • Hugging • Swimming pools • Toilet seats • Food • Insects • Coughing
Complications/consequences	• Currently no cure available; most people eventually die of the disease (most live about 10 years after infection) • Spread to other sex partners and persons sharing needles
Pregnancy and HIV/AIDS	• HIV can be passed to unborn children from infected mother during pregnancy or childbirth. • Infected mother may infect infant through breast milk (rare).
Prevention	• Always use latex condoms during oral, vaginal, and anal sex. Latex condoms, when used consistently and correctly, are highly effective in preventing the transmission of HIV, the virus that causes AIDS. • Use a latex barrier (dental dam or condom cut in half) on a vagina or anus for oral sex. • Limit or avoid use of drugs and alcohol. • Do not share drug needles, cotton, or cookers. • Do not share needles for tattooing or body piercing. • Limit the number of sex partners.

continues

Table 22-4   Facts About HIV and AIDS (*Continued*)

	• Tests are available to detect antibodies for HIV through providers, STD clinics, and HIV counseling and testing sites. • Notify sex and needle-sharing partners immediately if HIV infected.
Treatment	• No treatment or medication available to cure HIV/AIDS. • Early diagnosis and treatment can prolong life for years. • Medications and treatments available to keep immune system working. • Antiviral drugs slow cell processes and weaken cell protein. • Medications available to treat AIDS-related illnesses. • Medications available for HIV-infected pregnant women to greatly reduce the chance of passing infection to newborn. • Experimental drug trials are testing new medications.

© Cengage Learning 2014

*NOTE: These symptoms are not specific for HIV and may have other causes. Most persons with HIV have no symptoms at all for several years.

Table 22-5   Hepatitis Viruses A to C

	A	B	C
Causative agent	• Hepatitis A virus (HAV) • Fecal-oral; person to person	• Hepatitis B virus (HBV) • Blood; sexual contact; perinatal; breast milk; drug use (sharing needles); tattooing and body piercing	• Hepatitis C virus (HCV) • Blood or body fluids; intravenous drug use; mother to fetus; tattoo and body piercing; needle exchange
Risk groups	• Household/sexual contact with infected persons • International travelers • Men having sex with men • Drug users	• Injection drug users • Household/sexual contact with infected persons • Infants born to infected mothers • Health care workers • Multiple sex partners	• Recipients of blood transfusions or organ transplants before 1992 • People sharing needles • People exposed to blood and blood products • HBV- and HIV-infected persons
Incubation period	• 15–50 days	• 45–160 days	• 14–180 days
Infectious periods	• Usually less than 2 months	• Before symptoms appear; lifetime if carrier	• Before symptoms appear; lifetime if carrier
Diagnostic tests	• IgM anti-HAV	• HBsAg • HBeAg	• Anti-HCV • Serum ALT increased 10× • HCV RNA
Symptoms	• Flu-like • Jaundice • Dark yellow urine • Light-colored stools • Anorexia • Fatigue	• Flu-like • May have jaundice • Dark yellow urine • Light-colored stools • Malaise	• 80% have no symptoms • Flu-like • Jaundice • Anorexia

Prevention	• Hepatitis A vaccine (entire series) • Standard Precautions • Enteric precautions • Good personal hygiene, sanitization • Immunoglobulin (for short term)	• Hepatitis B vaccine (entire series) • Standard Precautions • Reduce risk behaviors • Good personal hygiene, sanitization • Immunoglobulin (for short term)	• Standard Precautions • Reduce risk behaviors • No vaccine
Treatment	• Immunoglobulin within 2 weeks of exposure	• Immunoglobulin (HBIg) • Alpha-interferon • Lamivudine	• Alpha-interferon • Ribavirin (Virazole)
Prognosis	• Rarely fatal • Not a carrier	• No cure • May become a carrier • Liver cancer may develop	• 85% or less have chronic infection • Chronic liver disease or cancer develop in 70%

© Cengage Learning 2014

ALT, alanine aminotransferase; HBeAg, hepatitis Be antigen; HBIg, hepatitis B immunoglobulin; HBsAg, hepatitis B surface antigen.

as soon as possible after exposure and again in 4 to 6 months.

Medication known as **immunomodulators** (i.e., that have the ability to change immune responses) are used to treat some patients who have chronic HCV. Two examples are peginterferon (Pegasys) and ribavirin (Copegus). Patients being treated with these medications must be closely monitored with periodic clinical and laboratory evaluations because the medications cause decreases in leukocyte and platelet counts. There are numerous side effects. The medications are used to prevent progressive liver destruction from the virus.

REPORTING INFECTIOUS DISEASE

Certain infectious diseases must be reported to the state and county health departments. The CDC requires that the information be reported to them. This helps the CDC control the spread of infection. Each state health department has forms for reportable diseases. Each disease has an identification number from the health department, and together with the appropriate form, the information is sent to the state health department and then to the CDC. Table 22-6 lists some of the diseases to be reported to the CDC's Notifiable Disease Surveillance System. Disease reports can be sent via the computer to the appropriate agencies, which will reply with orders for tests and procedures and follow-up orders.

STANDARD PRECAUTIONS

The CDC spent several years researching, improving, and developing recommendations to protect health care providers, patients, and their visitors from infectious diseases. This intensive period of research resulted in Standard Precautions, a set of infection control guidelines that are now used by all health care professionals for all patients. According to the CDC, Standard Precautions are "designed to reduce the risk of transmission of microorganisms from both recognized and unrecognized sources of infection in hospitals." They apply to:

1. Blood
2. All body fluids, secretions, and excretions regardless of whether they contain visible blood
3. Nonintact skin
4. Mucous membranes

To be effective, Standard Precautions must be practiced conscientiously at all times. Although the Standard Precautions include many criteria specific to inpatient settings such as hospitals and skilled nursing facilities, they are absolutely applicable to any medical facility, including ambulatory care settings where medical assistants are more likely to work.

Figure 22-8 provides a comprehensive review of Standard Precautions.

BLOODBORNE FACTS

WHAT IS HBV?

Hepatitis B virus (HBV) is a potentially life-threatening bloodborne pathogen. Centers for Disease Control estimates there are approximately 280,000 HBV infections each year in the United States.

Approximately 8,700 health care workers each year contract hepatitis B, and about 200 will die as a result. In addition, some who contract HBV will become carriers, passing the disease on to others. Carriers also face a significantly higher risk for other liver ailments which can be fatal, including cirrhosis of the liver and primary liver cancer.

HBV infection is transmitted through exposure to blood and other infectious body fluids and tissues. Anyone with occupational exposure to blood is at risk of contracting the infection.

Employers must provide engineering controls; workers must use work practices and protective clothing and equipment to prevent exposure to potentially infectious materials. However, the best defense against hepatitis B is vaccination.

WHO NEEDS VACCINATION?

The new OSHA standard covering bloodborne pathogens requires employers to offer the three-injection vaccination series free to all employees who are exposed to blood or other potentially infectious materials as part of their job duties. This includes health care workers, emergency responders, morticians, first-aid personnel, law enforcement officers, correctional facilities staff, launderers, as well as others.

The vaccination must be offered within 10 days of initial assignment to a job where exposure to blood or other potentially infectious materials can be "reasonably anticipated." The requirements for vaccinations of those already on the job took effect July 6, 1992.

WHAT DOES VACCINATION INVOLVE?

The hepatitis B vaccination is a noninfectious, yeast-based vaccine given in three injections in the arm. It is prepared from recombinant yeast cultures, rather than human blood or plasma. Thus, there is no risk of contamination from other bloodborne pathogens nor is there any chance of developing HBV from the vaccine.

The second injection should be given one month after the first, and the third injection six months after the initial dose. More than 90 percent of those vaccinated will develop immunity to the hepatitis B virus. To ensure immunity, it is important for individuals to receive all three injections. At this point it is unclear how long the immunity lasts, so booster shots may be required at some point in the future.

The vaccine causes no harm to those who are already immune or to those who may be HBV carriers. Although employees may opt to have their blood tested for antibodies to determine need for the vaccine, employers may not make such screening a condition of receiving vaccination nor are employers required to provide prescreening.

Each employee should receive counseling from a health care professional when vaccination is offered. This discussion will help an employee determine whether inoculation is necessary.

WHAT IF I DECLINE VACCINATION?

Workers who decide to decline vaccination must complete a declination form. Employers must keep these forms on file so that they know the vaccination status of everyone who is exposed to blood. At any time after a worker initially declines to receive the vaccine, he or she may opt to take it.

WHAT IF I AM EXPOSED BUT HAVE NOT YET BEEN VACCINATED?

If a worker experiences an exposure incident, such as a needle-stick or a blood splash in the eye, he or she must receive confidential medical evaluation from a licensed health care professional with appropriate follow-up. To the extent possible by law, the employer is to determine the source individual for HBV as well as human immunodeficiency virus (HIV) infectivity. The worker's blood will also be screened if he or she agrees.

The health care professional is to follow the guidelines of the U.S. Public Health Service in providing treatment. This would include hepatitis B vaccination. The health care professional must give a written opinion on whether or not vaccination is recommended and whether the employee received it. Only this information is reported to the employer. Employee medical records must remain confidential. HIV or HBV status must NOT be reported to the employer.

U.S. Department of Labor
Occupational Safety and Health Administration

Single copies of fact sheets are available from OSHA Publications, Room N3101, 200 Constitution Ave. N.W., Washington, D.C. 20210 and from OSHA regional offices.

Courtesy of the U.S. Department of Labor

Figure 22-7 *Bloodborne Facts,* published by the U.S. Department of Labor, Occupational Safety and Health Administration (OSHA). This publication includes facts about hepatitis B virus, declination, and steps to be taken by the employer should exposure to blood, body fluids, or other potentially infectious material occur.

Table 22-6 Partial Listing of Diseases That Must Be Reported to the CDC

AIDS	Poliomyelitis
Anthrax	Rabies (animal and human)
Botulism	Rheumatic Fever
Cholera	Rocky Mountain Spotted Fever
Diphtheria	Rubella
Encephalitis	Salmonella
Giardiasis	Streptococcal toxic-shock syndrome
Gonorrhea	Streptococcus pneumonia
Hepatitis A, B, C	Syphilis
HIV	Tetanus
Legionellosis	Toxic shock syndrome
Lyme disease	Tuberculosis
Malaria	Typhoid Fever
Measles	Varicella
Meningitis	Yellow Fever
Pertussis	

© Cengage Learning 2014

LATEX SENSITIVITY

Health care providers should be aware that some people, including professionals and patients, can be allergic to latex products. Some personal protective equipment (PPE) is made from latex; medical and surgical products also are often made from this product.

The allergic reaction can be a localized one such as dermatitis or a more severe systemic reaction such as anaphylaxis (see Chapter 9), a form of shock marked by vascular collapse, respiratory failure, hypotension, arrhythmia, and laryngeal edema. Vinyl gloves can be worn in place of latex for hypersensitive individuals. Any person with an allergy to latex should wear a bracelet or other form of identification indicating this fact because, in any emergency, medical personnel wear latex gloves (see Chapter 9).

Transmission-Based Precautions

When the CDC was in the process of developing a new guideline for isolation precautions in hospitals, the agency arrived at what it terms two tiers of precautions. The first tier is called the Standard Precautions, discussed earlier, designed for all patients regardless of their diagnosis or presumed infection status. The second tier of precautions is intended for patients diagnosed with or suspected of having specific highly transmissible diseases. These are known as Transmission-Based Precautions.

Transmission-Based Precautions reduce the risk for **airborne**, **droplet**, and contact transmission of pathogens and are always to be used *in addition to* Standard Precautions.

These airborne, contact, and droplet precautions also list specific syndromes that can appear in adult and pediatric patients who are highly suspicious for infection. They identify the appropriate Transmission-Based Precautions to be used until a diagnosis can be made. Figure 22-9, Figure 22-10, and Figure 22-11 provide specific information on these three Transmission-Based Precautions. Remember that these precautions are for specific categories of patients and are to be used in addition to Standard Precautions, which are used for all patients.

Some medical assistants' practicum experiences take place in a hospital setting. For example, the electrocardiography and clinical laboratory departments of the hospital are areas some students rotate through during their practicums. It is important for medical assistants to know and understand how to protect themselves from infectious diseases. Transmission-Based Precautions (isolation) reduce the risk for airborne, droplet, and contact transmission of pathogens. Procedure 22-4 describes the use of barriers (gown, mask, goggles, gloves, and cap) that are used when entering an isolation room to perform an electrocardiogram or phlebotomy on a patient with an infectious disease such as tuberculosis (airborne contact), meningitis (respiratory droplets contact), and wound drainage (direct contact).

STANDARD PRECAUTIONS

Assume that every person is potentially infected or colonized with an organism that could be transmitted in the healthcare setting.

Hand Hygiene

Avoid unnecessary touching of surfaces in close proximity to the patient.

When hands are visibly dirty, contaminated with proteinaceous material, or visibly soiled with blood or body fluids, wash hands with soap and water.

If hands are not visibly soiled, or after removing visible material with soap and water, decontaminate hands with an alcohol-based hand rub. Alternatively, hands may be washed with an antimicrobial soap and water.

Perform hand hygiene:
   Before having direct contact with patients.
   After contact with blood, body fluids or excretions, mucous membranes, nonintact skin, or wound dressings.
   After contact with a patient's intact skin (e.g., when taking a pulse or blood pressure or lifting a patient).
   If hands will be moving from a contaminated-body site to a clean-body site during patient care.
   After contact with inanimate objects (including medical equipment) in the immediate vicinity of the patient.
   After removing gloves.

Personal protective equipment (PPE)

Wear PPE when the nature of the anticipated patient interaction indicates that contact with blood or body fluids may occur.

Before leaving the patient's room or cubicle, remove and discard PPE.

Gloves

Wear gloves when contact with blood or other potentially infectious materials, mucous membranes, nonintact skin, or potentially contaminated intact skin (e.g., of a patient incontinent of stool or urine) could occur.

Remove gloves after contact with a patient and/or the surrounding environment using proper technique to prevent hand contamination. Do not wear the same pair of gloves for the care of more than one patient.

Change gloves during patient care if the hands will move from a contaminated body-site (e.g., perineal area) to a clean body-site (e.g., face).

Gowns

Wear a gown to protect skin and prevent soiling or contamination of clothing during procedures and patient-care activities when contact with blood, body fluids, secretions, or excretions is anticipated.

Wear a gown for direct patient contact if the patient has uncontained secretions or excretions.

Remove gown and perform hand hygiene before leaving the patient's environment.

Mouth, nose, eye protection

Use PPE to protect the mucous membranes of the eyes, nose and mouth during procedures and patient-care activities that are likely to generate splashes or sprays of blood, body fluids, secretions and excretions.

During aerosol-generating procedures wear one of the following: a face shield that fully covers the front and sides of the face, a mask with attached shield, or a mask and goggles.

Respiratory Hygiene/Cough Etiquette

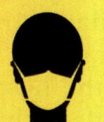

Educate healthcare personnel to contain respiratory secretions to prevent droplet and fomite transmission of respiratory pathogens, especially during seasonal outbreaks of viral respiratory tract infections.

Offer masks to coughing patients and other symptomatic persons (e.g., persons who accompany ill patients) upon entry into the facility.

Patient-care equipment and instruments/devices

Wear PPE (e.g., gloves, gown), according to the level of anticipated contamination, when handling patient-care equipment and instruments/devices that are visibly soiled or may have been in contact with blood or body fluids.

Care of the environment

Include multi-use electronic equipment in policies and procedures for preventing contamination and for cleaning and disinfection, especially those items that are used by patients, those used during delivery of patient care, and mobile devices that are moved in and out of patient rooms frequently (e.g., daily).

Textiles and laundry

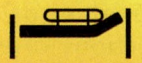

Handle used textiles and fabrics with minimum agitation to avoid contamination of air, surfaces and persons.

SPR

©2007 Brevis Corporation www.brevis.com

Reprinted with permission from Brevis Corporation, www.brevis.com

Figure 22-8   Standard Precautions for Infection Control issued by the Centers for Disease Control and Prevention.

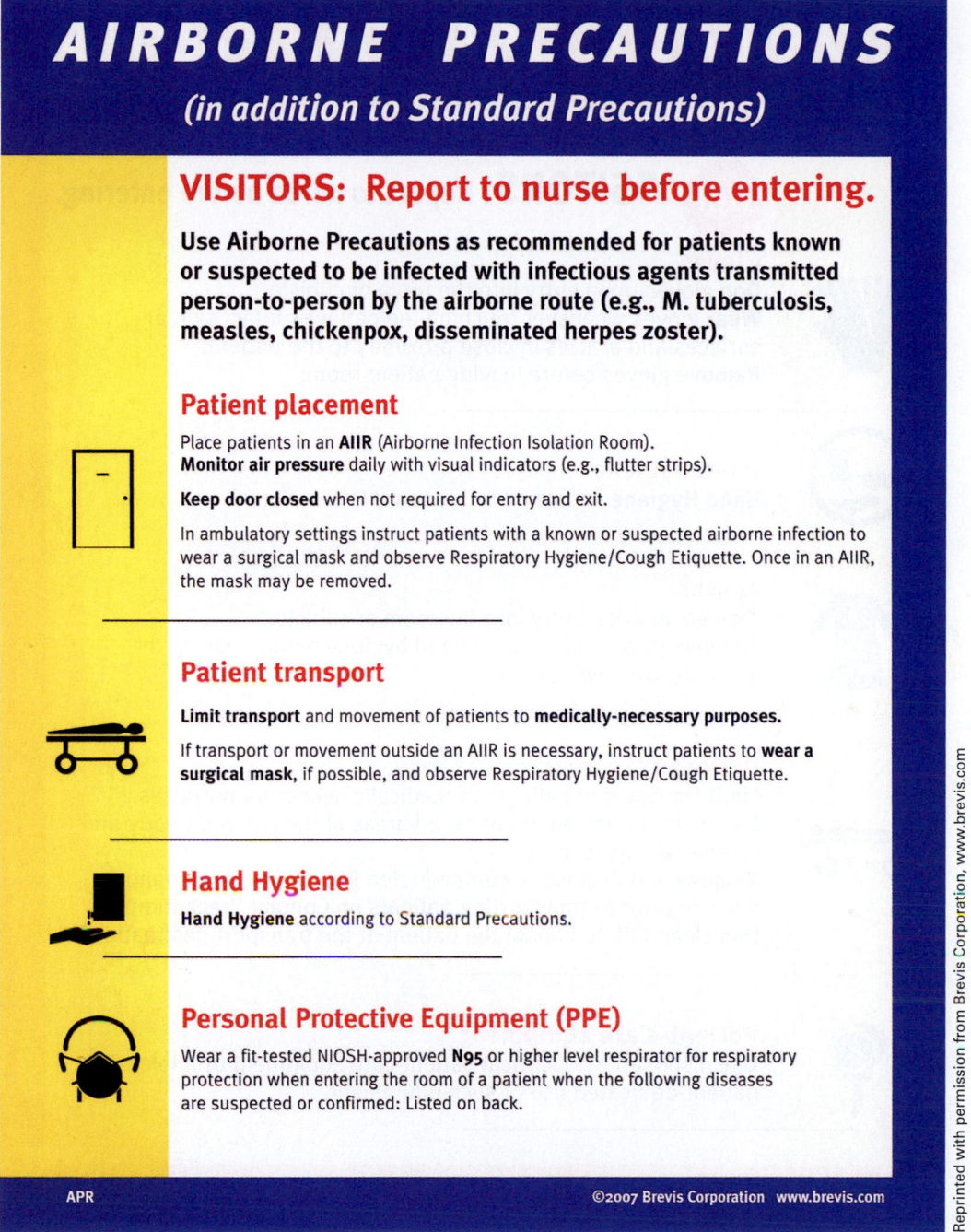

Figure 22-9 Airborne Precautions, one category of Transmission-Based Precautions, for use in hospital settings.

Blood and Body Fluids

In all infection control efforts, it is important to understand what is meant by blood and body fluids. Specifically, they are described as the blood, secretions, and excretions of a patient. Examples of blood and body fluids and some of the areas in which medical assistants may become exposed to them are:

Blood:

• Specimens drawn during venipuncture
• Open wounds or lesions of any kind
• Epistaxes, or nosebleeds
• Vaginal bleeding, including menses (menstruation), lochia (discharge after childbirth), and hemorrhage
• Feces and vomit or other body fluids with or without visible blood

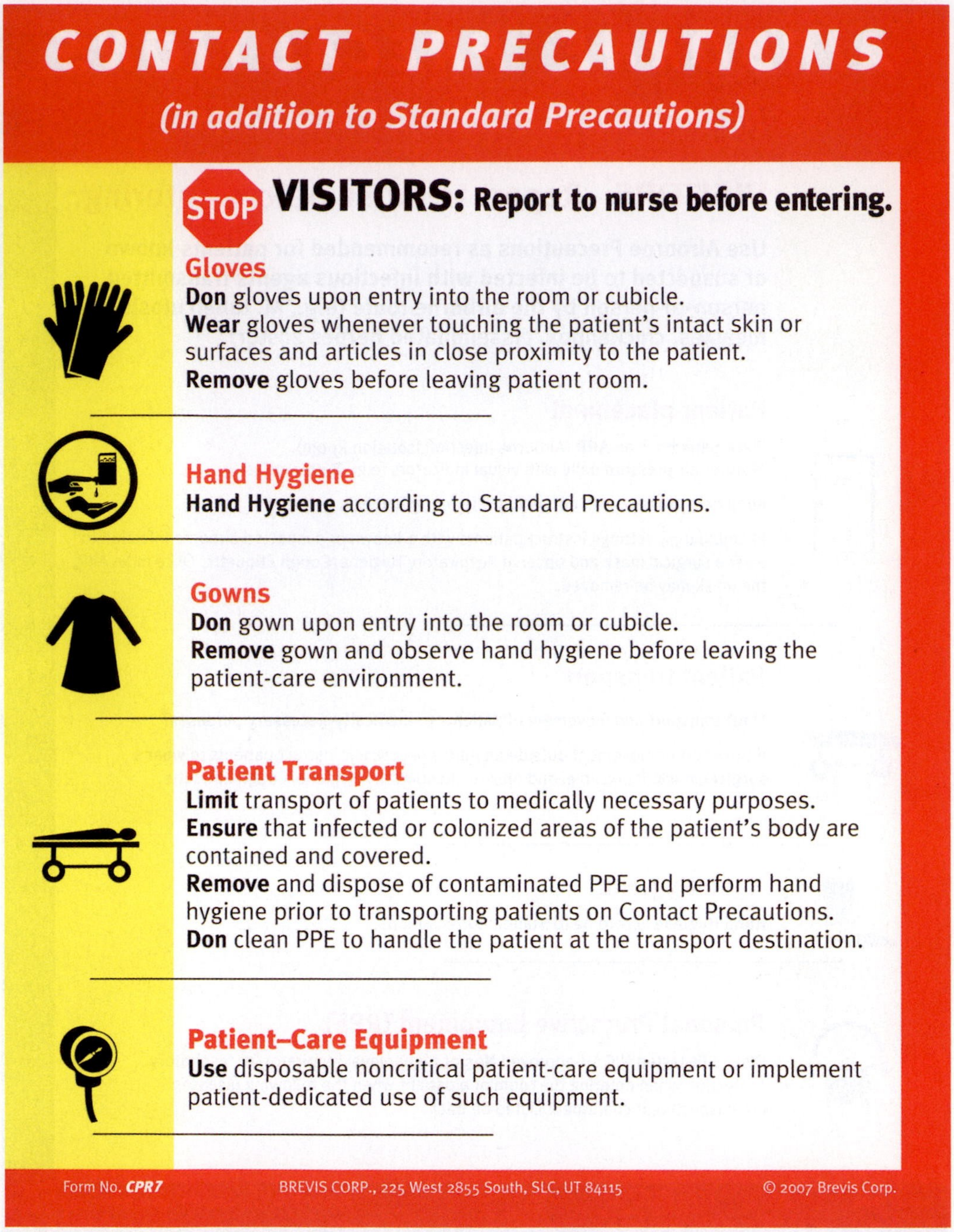

Figure 22-10 Contact Precautions, one category of Transmission-Based Precautions, for use in hospital settings.

Vaginal secretions:

- Physiologic leukorrhea (normal vaginal discharge)
- Vaginitis with discharge

Cerebrospinal fluid:

- Fluid aspirated, or withdrawn, during a lumbar puncture (spinal tap)
- Leakage of fluid due to trauma to the brain or spinal cord (through ear, nose)

Synovial fluid:

- Fluid aspirated during arthroscopic procedures

Pleural fluid:

- Fluid aspirated during thoracentesis, a surgical puncture of the thoracic cavity
- Fluid leakage caused by chest trauma

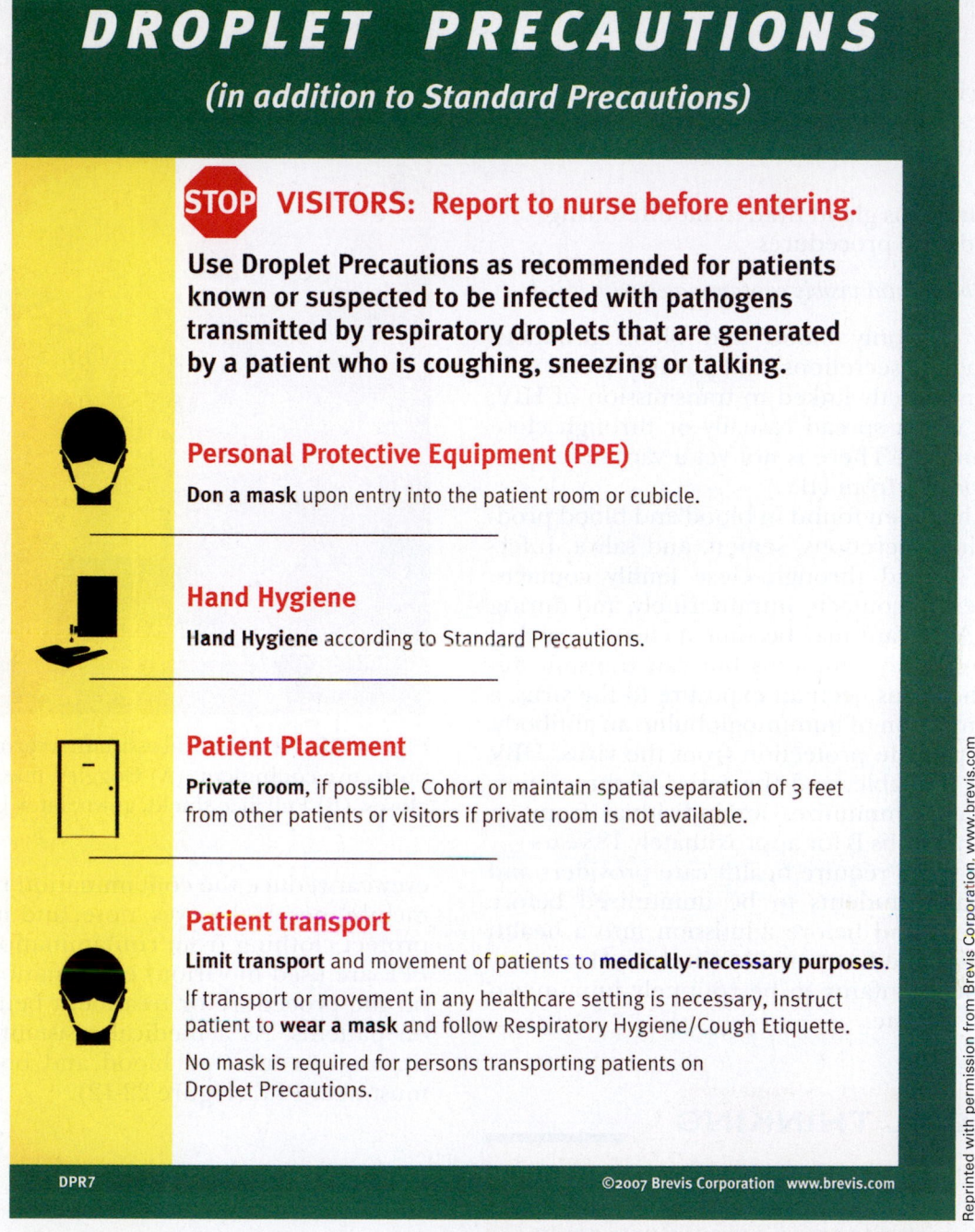

DROPLET PRECAUTIONS
(in addition to Standard Precautions)

STOP VISITORS: Report to nurse before entering.

Use Droplet Precautions as recommended for patients known or suspected to be infected with pathogens transmitted by respiratory droplets that are generated by a patient who is coughing, sneezing or talking.

Personal Protective Equipment (PPE)

Don a mask upon entry into the patient room or cubicle.

Hand Hygiene

Hand Hygiene according to Standard Precautions.

Patient Placement

Private room, if possible. Cohort or maintain spatial separation of 3 feet from other patients or visitors if private room is not available.

Patient transport

Limit transport and movement of patients to **medically-necessary purposes.**

If transport or movement in any healthcare setting is necessary, instruct patient to **wear a mask** and follow Respiratory Hygiene/Cough Etiquette.

No mask is required for persons transporting patients on Droplet Precautions.

DPR7   ©2007 Brevis Corporation www.brevis.com

Reprinted with permission from Brevis Corporation, www.brevis.com

Figure 22-11 Droplet Precautions, one category of Transmission-Based Precautions, for use in hospital settings.

Pericardial fluid:

- Fluid around the heart exposed during cardiac surgery or caused by cardiac trauma

Peritoneal fluid:

- Fluid exposed during abdominal surgery (least likely fluid with which medical assistant will come into contact), but exposure can occur during a paracentesis

Semen:

- Seminal fluid as a laboratory specimen for sperm count in examination for fertility level

Amniotic fluid:

- Fluid aspirated during amniocentesis, a surgical puncture of the amniotic sac
- Vaginal leakage during pregnancy, labor, and delivery

Breast milk (possibility exists)

Sputum:

- Material coughed up and **expectorated** from the respiratory tract

Saliva:

- Oral mucous gland fluid in mouth during oral/dental procedures

Any other body fluid visibly contaminated with blood

Thus far, only blood and blood products, semen, vaginal secretions, and possibly breast milk have been directly linked to transmission of HIV; the virus is not spread casually or through close family contacts. There is not yet a vaccine to protect individuals from HIV.

HBV has been found in blood and blood products, vaginal secretions, semen, and saliva. Infection can spread through close family contacts, kissing, sexual contacts, intrauterinely, and during delivery. An infant may become a chronic **carrier**, one who has no symptoms but can transmit disease. If there has been an exposure to the virus, a prompt injection of immunoglobulin, an antibody, will help provide protection from the virus. HBV vaccine is available, and the series of three injections usually immunizes an individual from an attack of hepatitis B for approximately 18 years.

Some states require health care providers and allied health students to be immunized before employment and before admission into a health program in an educational institution. Also, many states require infants to be routinely immunized with HBV vaccine.

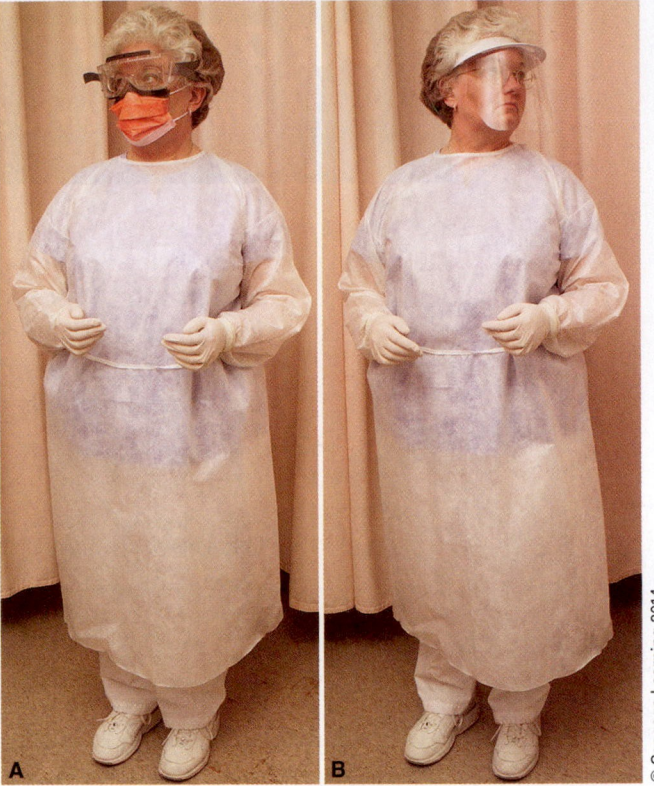

© Cengage Learning 2014

Figure 22-12 Medical assistant wearing personal protective equipment. (A) Goggles, mask, gown, latex gloves. (B) Full-face shield, gown, latex gloves.

CRITICAL THINKING

Give eight examples of body fluids considered to be biohazardous substances. Explain under what circumstances medical assistants could become exposed to blood and body fluids.

Personal Protective Equipment

Standard and **Transmission-Based Precautions** all make use of barriers or personal protective equipment (PPE). The barriers consist of gloves, mask, gown, and goggles/face shield. Gloves reduce the risk for contamination to hands but do not prevent needles or other sharp instruments from penetrating the skin. Masks and protective eyewear reduce the contamination risk to mucous membranes of the eyes, nose, and mouth. Gowns protect clothing from contamination. Barriers or PPE are used in various combinations depending on the procedure or treatment being performed on patients. As a medical assistant, you may be exposed to infected blood and body fluids and must wear PPE (Figure 22-12).

Needlestick

One reason for exposure to blood is caused by accidentally sticking oneself with a dirty (used) needle after performing invasive procedures such as injections, venipuncture, and attempted venipuncture. A needle should be considered contaminated if it has entered the skin of a patient, regardless of the reason. In the past, needlesticks were common because of the practice of needle recapping. Contaminated (used) needles should never be recapped, broken off, removed from syringes, or manipulated by hand in any way. They are disposed of in the approved puncture-proof container designated for **sharps** (Figure 22-13). The disposal

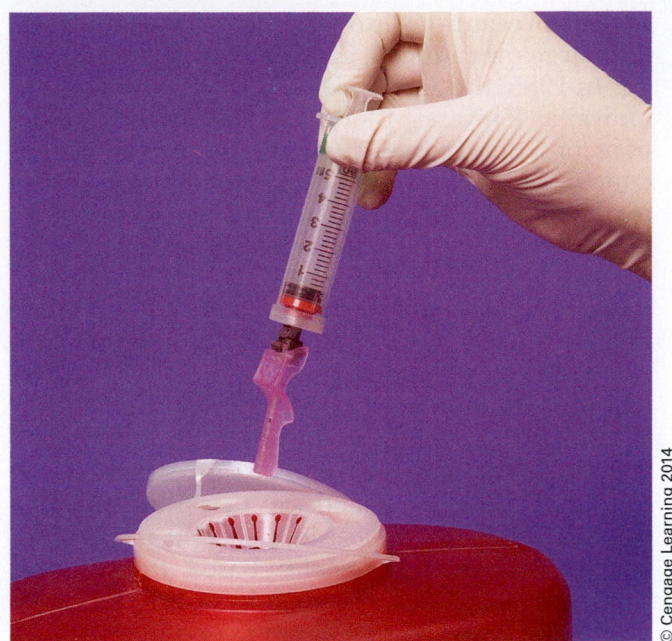

© Cengage Learning 2014

Figure 22-13 Discard the entire disposable safety syringe and needle into the biohazard puncture-proof sharps container.

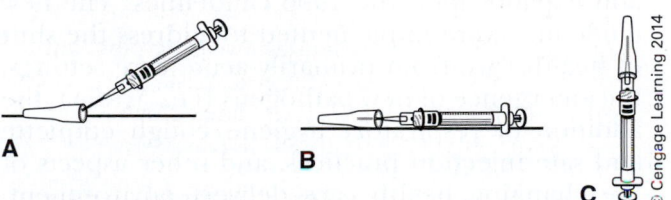

A   **B**   **C**

© Cengage Learning 2014

Figure 22-14 (A) Scoop into cap using one hand. Do not touch the cap with the other hand. (B) Slide needle into cap resting on table. (C) Holding the barrel of the syringe in one hand, carry to the sharps container. **Do not push the cap onto the syringe.**

container for sharps must be in the closest proximity as practical to the area where sharps are used. If a needle is used and an appropriate disposal container is not nearby ("point-of-use disposal"), the **scoop technique** of recapping may be used, but only in this circumstance (i.e., no appropriate container nearby): the cap may be "scooped up" with the needle, using one hand, and then carried to the sharps container. The cap is not, under any circumstances, pushed into place over the needle (Figure 22-14). The risk to a health care provider of HIV infection caused by a needlestick is slight; however, the risk for HBV or HCV infection caused by a needlestick can be significantly greater.

OSHA mandates that (1) employers select the safest needle device available, (2) employers must involve employees in identifying these devices, and

(3) employers maintain a log of injuries caused by contaminated sharps ([66FR5325] OSHA 1910.1030). This is known as the "Needlestick Safety and Prevention Act." The act was added to the original act regarding engineering controls of the OSHA Bloodborne Pathogens Standard.

Desirable characteristics of safety devices include:

- The device is **jet injection**.
- The safety feature is built into the device.
- The device works passively (i.e., requires no activation by the user). If user activation is necessary, the safety feature can be engaged with a single-handed technique, allowing the worker's hands to remain behind the exposed sharp.
- The user can easily tell whether the safety feature has been activated. Some safety features have a sound, such as a click, indicating that the feature is engaged.
- The safety feature cannot be deactivated and remains protective through disposal.
- If the device uses needles, it performs reliably with all needle sizes.
- The device is easy to use and practical.
- The device is safe and effective in patient care.

Additional information regarding specific procedures to follow should an accidental needlestick occur, as well as other safety procedures included in the OSHA and Clinical Laboratory Improvement Amendments or CLIA rules and regulations, will be found later in this chapter and in Chapter 38.

Disposal of Infectious Waste

Infectious waste (contaminated items) is any item that has come in contact with patient blood or body fluids. These items must be handled with gloves and disposed of by placing them in the appropriate biohazard containers that are provided by an agency with which your employer has contracted (Figure 22-15). Infectious waste is either incinerated (burned) or subjected to sterilization by autoclave to render it harmless before it is disposed of in a sanitary landfill. For local rules and regulations of how to dispose of sharps and biohazard/infectious waste, contact your local department of health. Their staff can refer you to companies that specialize in the proper disposal of infectious waste and

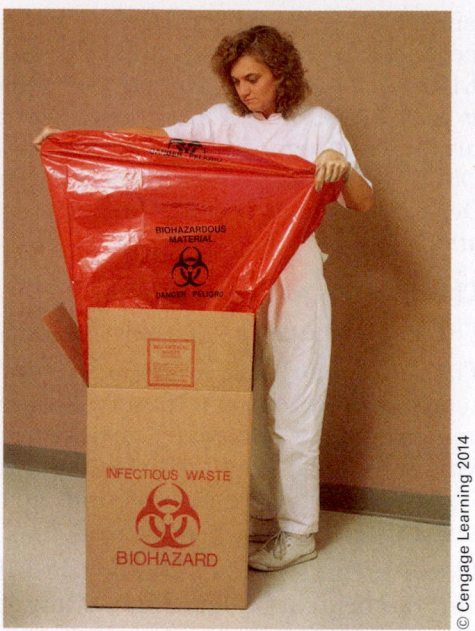

© Cengage Learning 2014

Figure 22-15   The medical assistant is placing a sturdy disposable plastic bag marked with the biohazard waste symbol into a durable cardboard box for collection of infectious waste material. When full, an authorized, licensed waste hauler will dispose of the box (usually by incineration) and provide documentation of its disposal.

sharps. These companies follow strict state and federal regulations and can provide your clinic with containers, labels, and instructions. They will often work out a schedule for pickups, such as daily, weekly, monthly, or "on-call." Charges will usually be based on the amount of infectious waste that requires disposal.

Federal Organizations and Infection Control

The CDC is responsible for studying pathogens and diseases in an effort to prevent their spread. A division of the U.S. Public Health Department, the CDC has issued a number of guidelines over the last 25 years that have enabled health care professionals to practice responsible infection control. As diseases evolve and as new diseases are introduced into our society, the CDC revises and updates existing guidelines or issues new control measures to contain the spread of infection.

In 1970, the CDC developed a system of seven **isolation categories** for patients with known infectious diseases. This category system included strict **isolation**, respiratory isolation, protective isolation,

enteric precautions, wound and skin precautions, discharge precautions, and blood precautions.

In 1985, the agency released a set of guidelines known as Universal Blood and Body Fluid Precautions, or simply **Universal Precautions**. These infection-control practices were written in response to the increase in AIDS and HBV, both bloodborne diseases, and other infectious diseases as well.

Beginning in 1991, the CDC infection control guidelines were reviewed and subsequently revised. In 1996, a new set of guidelines was released. Standard Precautions reflect improved recommendations intended to protect all health care providers, patients, and their visitors from a wide range of **communicable** diseases. At the same time that the CDC issued the new Standard Precautions, they also released a second tier of precautions called Transmission-Based Precautions. These are intended to be used in addition to Standard Precautions when caring for patients with known specific infectious diseases.

In 2007, the CDC published the *Guideline for Isolation Precautions: Preventing Transmission of Infectious Agents in Healthcare Settings* to update and expand upon the 1996 Guidelines. The new guidelines were implemented to address the shift of health care from primarily acute care settings, the emergence of new pathogens (i.e., MRSA), the addition of respiratory hygiene/cough etiquette and safe injection practices, and other aspects of the changing health care delivery environment. This document added a set of prevention measures termed "Protective Environment" that outline methods to prevent HAIs.

The 2007 Guidelines specifically address transmission risks associated with each type of health care setting. There are different needs identified based on the location where care is delivered. Hospitals, intensive care units, burn units, pediatrics, nonacute health care settings, long-term care, ambulatory care, and home care are addressed based on the unique needs of each. A focus is placed on the fundamental elements needed to prevent transmission of infectious agents in each of the above health care settings. Initially, administrative measures are to be enacted to make sure the system of care delivery recognizes the importance of disrupting the infection cycle in order to protect patients. Further guidelines are outlined based on the role of the health care provider.

Hand hygiene is recognized as the single most important practice to reduce the transmission of infectious agents in health care settings. Personal protective equipment (PPE) selection is also addressed item by item.

The 2007 Guidelines also address precautions to prevent transmission of infectious agents. Several additions were made to the recommendations for Standard Precautions. Three areas of practice that were added are: respiratory hygiene/cough etiquette, safe injection practices, and the use of masks for the insertion of catheters or injection of material into spinal or epidural spaces via lumbar puncture procedures.

The most commonly applicable new guideline is Respiratory Hygiene/Cough Etiquette, which includes such elements as:

- Education of health care staff, patients, and visitors
- Posting signs in language(s) appropriate to the population being served
- Covering the mouth and nose with a tissue when coughing and prompt disposal of used tissues, and use of surgical masks by the coughing person
- Practicing proper hand hygiene after contact with respiratory secretions
- Physical separation of at least three feet from persons with respiratory infections for other patients in a waiting room setting

The CDC strives to maintain the health and safety of the community, as well as patients and health care providers. It is their mission to continue educating, researching, and promoting healthy behaviors.

OSHA REGULATIONS

The Occupational Safety and Health Administration (OSHA) has a mission of saving lives, preventing injuries, and protecting the health of America's workers. OSHA establishes guidelines and standards to promote worker safety and health. It is the responsibility of employers to obtain all applicable OSHA standards and fulfill the requirements outlined.

The Bloodborne Pathogen Standard

The OSHA *Bloodborne Pathogen Standard* became effective in March 1992. It came about principally in the hope of reducing occupational-related cases of HIV and HBV infections among health care workers. This standard was updated in 2003.

It covers all employees who can be "reasonably anticipated" to come into contact, as a result of performing their job duties, with blood and other potentially infectious materials. The OSHA *Bloodborne Pathogen Standard* seeks to limit exposure to bloodborne pathogens. An important aspect of this standard is an exposure control plan. This requires employers to identify tasks and procedures where occupational exposure to blood occurs. This plan must be accessible to employees and available to OSHA. Key to this exposure control plan are methods of compliance that mandate the use of universal precautions treating all body fluids/materials as if infectious. The mandate stipulates that employers provide, at no cost to employees, the full component of PPE, and access to facilities for hand hygiene. It also includes the requirement for a written schedule outlining the cleaning, decontamination, and other cleaning for items that routinely come into contact with blood or body fluids. Hepatitis B vaccination is required to be made available to all employees that have occupational exposure to blood within 10 days of hire. There must also be post-exposure evaluation and follow-up for all employees.

OSHA published *Model Plans and Programs for the OSHA Bloodborne Pathogens and Hazard Communications Standards* in 2003, which can be found at http://www.osha.gov/Publications/osha3186.pdf. This publication contains model exposure control plans, model documents, and general guidance for meeting OSHA standards in this important area.

Methods of Compliance to Prevent Exposure. There are several major strategies mandated by OSHA for the prevention of exposure to bloodborne pathogens and other potentially infective material.

1. *Universal precautions.* These are procedures that must be followed by staff when caring for a patient thought to be the host to a pathogenic microorganism. This method extends beyond Standard Precautions and includes the use of PPEs to provide a barrier to prevent the mode of transmission of the pathogen. It includes the selection of appropriate PPEs; appropriate cleaning and disposal of potentially contaminated surgical equipment, needles, and laundry; and the disposal of contaminated waste.

2. *Engineering and work practice controls.* Engineering controls and work practice controls consist of the physical equipment and mechanical devices an employer provides in an attempt to safeguard and minimize employee exposure. A common example of an engineering control

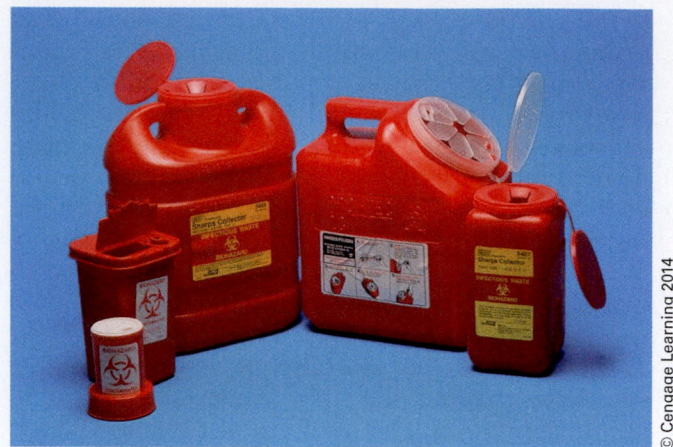

© Cengage Learning 2014

Figure 22-16 Various sizes of puncture-proof sharps containers. These and other biohazard waste containers are autoclaved when full and sent out to a biohazard agency for safe disposal.

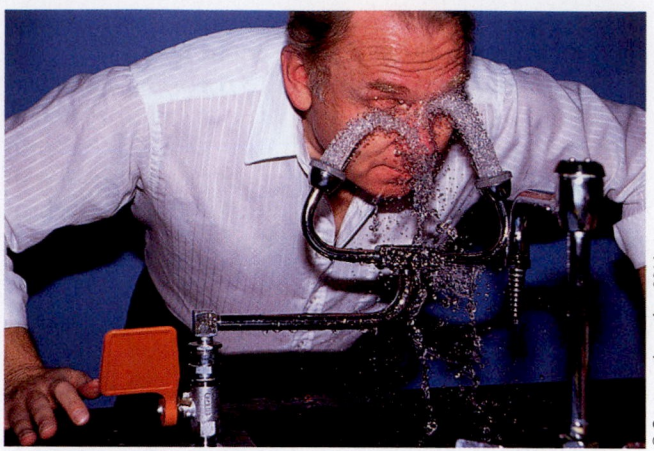

© Cengage Learning 2014

Figure 22-17 Emergency eyewash station: two streams of water or saline wash both eyes simultaneously and continuously.

is a sharps disposal container (Figure 22-16). Others are mechanical pipettes, fume hoods, splash guards, and eyewash stations (Figure 22-17). If and when occupational exposure continues after the engineering controls are in place, PPE must be used. Hand washing facilities or appropriate antiseptic hand cleanser (when hand washing facilities are not accessible) must be readily available.

3. *Personal protective equipment* (*PPE*). The employer must be certain that PPE is available and accessible and must provide an alternative type of glove if an employee is allergic to those originally provided (see "Latex Sensitivity" box earlier in this chapter.) Cleaning and laundering and disposal of PPE are the responsibility of the employer, and the employee does not incur any expense for them.

    All PPE must be removed before the employee leaves the work site and placed in an appropriate container that is supplied by the employer. Figure 22-18 shows PPE.

4. *Cleanliness of work areas.* The employer must maintain a work site that is clean and sanitary and have a written schedule for cleaning and decontaminating the work area after contact with blood and other potentially infectious material. **Spill kits** must be readily accessible (Figure 22-19).

    Broken glass is placed in a sharps container after using cardboard or a dust pan and brush to remove it.

    Laundry that is contaminated is handled with gloves and placed in a labeled container.

If the laundry is damp or wet, gloves and other appropriate PPE must be worn, and the damp or wet laundry must be placed in a plastic bag(s) to prevent blood or other potentially infectious material from leaking through it. PPE cannot be laundered at home. All other Standard Precautions must be adhered to.

5. *Hepatitis B vaccine.* HBV vaccine must be made available free of charge to every employee, full-time, part-time, or temporary, within 10 days of work assignment (Figure 22-20). This refers to employees who have the potential for occupational exposure, and who can "reasonably" be expected to have skin, eye, mucous membrane, or **parenteral** contact with blood or other potentially infectious material. The vaccine is given in three doses over a six-month period and is used to protect the employee from infection with HBV. It is an intramuscular injection with an approximate 96% rate of effectiveness.

    An employee has the right to decline taking the vaccine but must sign a **declination form**. There is the option to reconsider receiving the vaccine at a later time.

6. *Follow-up after exposure.* An accidental exposure is broadly defined as one in which blood, blood-contaminated body fluids, or body fluids or tissues to which Standard Precautions apply are introduced into a mucous surface, into nonintact skin, or into the conjunctiva via a needlestick, skin cut, or direct splash. If an incident exposes an employee to any of these, the employer must make available a confidential medical evaluation in which the following are documented:

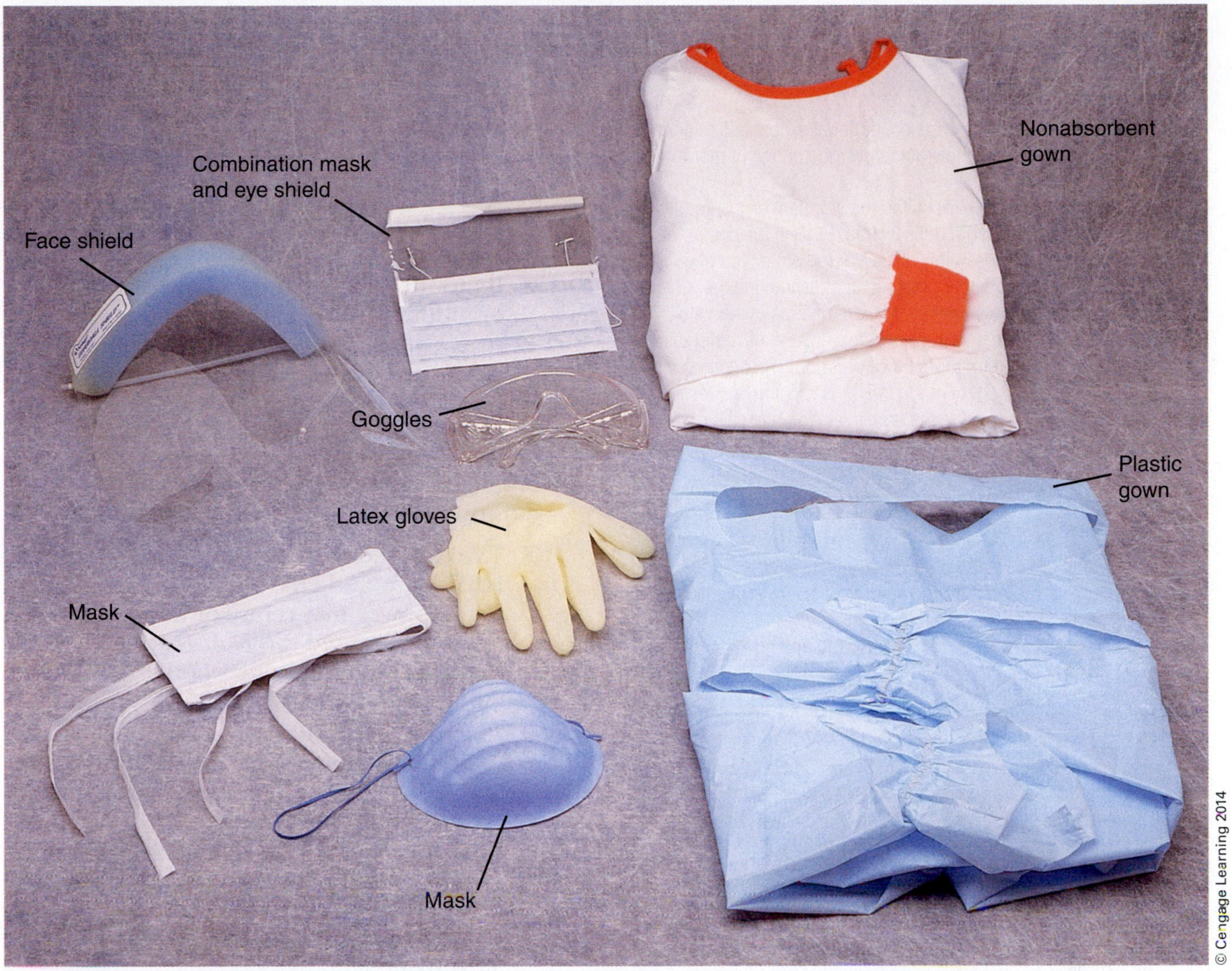

Face shield

Combination mask
and eye shield

Nonabsorbent
gown

Goggles

Plastic
gown

Latex gloves

Mask

Mask

© Cengage Learning 2014

Figure 22-18 Personal protective equipment.

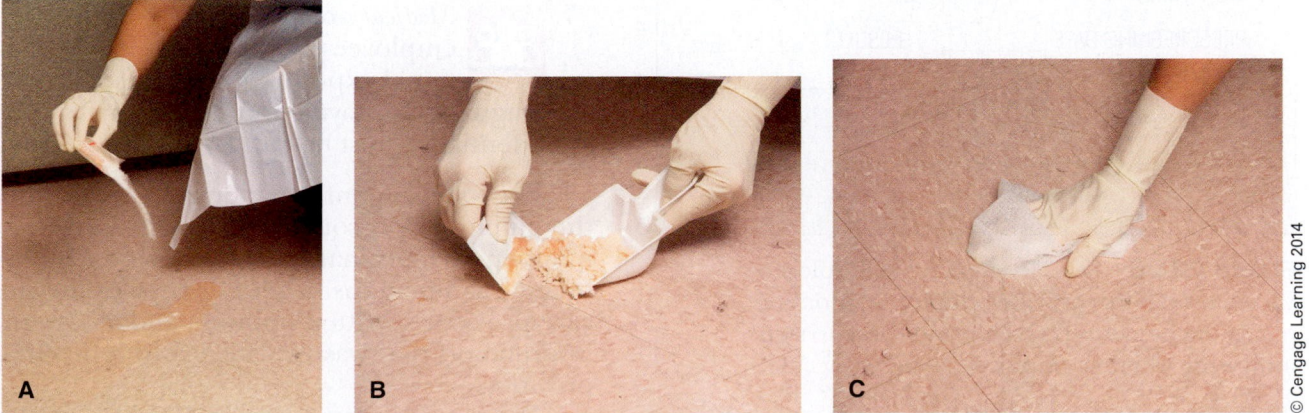

A   B   C

© Cengage Learning 2014

Figure 22-19 (A) Sprinkle coagulating powder over spill wearing protective clothing and gloves. (B) Scoop up spill with scoop from kit. (C) The spill area is then cleaned with a 10 percent bleach solution.

SAMPLE

Hepatitis B Employee Vaccination Form

MEMO: To all employees with occupational exposure to blood or other infectious materials on an average of one or more times per month.

OSHA and the CDC have identified the potential exposure of health care workers to hepatitis B virus (HBV) in the course of performing their duties in this office. For the protection of our employees, we are offering prescreening testing and the HBV vaccination with follow-up evaluation to all employees who are exposed to blood or other potentially infectious materials on an average of one or more times per month. *In accordance with recommended OSHA guidelines, this vaccine and testing will be offered at no cost to the employee.* You have the ability to decide whether or not you want the testing and/or vaccine. At the bottom of this memo, you may indicate your choice. Please return this memo with your signature and date to your immediate supervisor.

[ ]   I want to receive the prescreening (optional)
[ ]   I want to receive the vaccine and follow-up evaluation testing
[ ]   I *do not* want the vaccine and testing and have read the following statement:

I understand that due to my occupational exposure to blood or other potentially infectious materials I may be at risk of acquiring hepatitis B virus (HBV) infection. I have been given the opportunity to be vaccinated with hepatitis B vaccine at no charge to myself. However, I decline hepatitis B vaccination at this time. I understand that by declining this vaccine I continue to be at risk of acquiring hepatitis B, a serious disease. If in the future I continue to have occupational exposure to blood or other potentially infectious materials and I want to be vaccinated with hepatitis B vaccine, I can receive the vaccination series at no charge to me.

_____   _____
NAME   DATE

_____   _____
SIGNATURE   SS#

PRESCREENING DATE _____ RESULTS _____
DATE OF VACCINATIONS _____
DATE OF FOLLOW-UP EVALUATION _____
RESULTS _____
NOTES:

Courtesy of POL Consultants, Inc., 2 Russ Farm Way, Delanco, NJ 08075, 856-824-0800

Figure 22-20   Sample Hepatitis B Employee Vaccination Form provides employee information regarding hepatitis B vaccine and space to sign indicating whether employee declines vaccine.

- The circumstances surrounding the event
- The route or routes of exposure
- The identification of the person who was the source of the exposure

The following procedure describes the steps to take following an exposure incident:

- Immediately wash exposed area with soap and warm water.
- If mouth area is exposed, rinse with water or mouthwash.
- If eyes are exposed, flush with large amounts of warm water.
- Report incident to a supervisor immediately for documentation (Figure 22-21).

In addition, OSHA requires the following information:

- The exposed employee must be tested for HBV, HCV, and HIV only if consent is given. An employee may refuse or may have blood drawn and stored for 90 days at which time the choice can be made whether to have the blood tested.
- The source individual's blood, if permission is granted, is tested for HBV, HCV, and HIV and the employee shall know the results (unless protected by the law).
- The employee is offered prophylaxis, gamma globulin, or HB vaccine after the exposure to HBV or HIV according to the current recommendation of the U.S. Public Health Service.
- The employee is counseled regarding precautions to take to avoid possible transmission and is provided information on potential illnesses for which to be alert.
- An OSHA 301 form must be filed.

7.  *Medical records.* Medical records of an employee who has suffered an occupational exposure must be kept for the length of employment plus 30 years, and confidentiality must be guaranteed.

The following information is to be included in the employee's record: name and Social Security number, HB vaccination status with dates, results of any examinations or tests, a copy of the health care provider's written opinion, and a copy of the information that was provided to the health care provider.

The records must be available to the employee, to OSHA, and anyone with the written consent of the employee, but *not* the employer.

SAMPLE

Post-Exposure Management Record

The following employee was the subject of an infectious exposure incident on (date) _____ and was examined and treated as follows:

Employee Name: _____ SS#_____

Type of Incident (describe) _____

_____

Route of Exposure: _____

Source Patient Information:

_____ Source patient could not be identified.
_____ Source patient was identified but refused to contribute blood.
_____ Source patient was identified and blood was secured from such patient. Results of blood testing of source patient's blood are attached to this form.

Employee hereby grants permission for tests for antibodies of human immunodeficiency virus (HIV-1) and/or hepatitis B virus and acknowledges that the employee has been counseled concerning such tests.

Employee Signature _____ Date _____

The following test(s) were administered under supervision of a qualified provider:

_____ Human Immunodeficiency Virus (HIV-1) Antibodies
_____ Hepatitis B Virus Antibodies

Date(s) of Tests(s): _____ Results of Test(s)—
See attached Provider's or Laboratory statement/report.

Employee hereby acknowledges that the employee was counseled and a written copy(ies) of the results of the above test(s) were furnished to such employee on (date):

_____

Employee Signature _____ Date _____

_____ Additional follow-up was performed as indicated by attached reports.

NOTE: This record should be retained for length of employment PLUS thirty years.

Courtesy of POL Consultants, Inc., 2 Russ Farm Way, Delanco, NJ 08075, 856-824-080C

Figure 22-21   Sample Post-Exposure Management Record can be used to document employee exposure to blood, body fluids, or other potentially infectious material; tests performed on the employee by a qualified provider; and test results.

BIOHAZARD LABELS

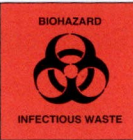

Containers that hold biohazardous materials must be properly labeled. Biohazardous materials include blood and body fluids as well as garments, gloves, masks, needles, gauze, wipes, aprons, and so on that may be contaminated with blood or other potentially contaminated body fluids. Labels shall be used to identify the presence of an actual or potential biological hazard.

CONSIDERATIONS:

- Labels shall be fluorescent orange or orange-red, with lettering or symbols in a contrasting color.
- Labels should be affixed onto or as close as feasible to the container by adhesive, string, wire, or other method.
- Red bags or red containers may be substituted for labels.
- If blood or control serum is stored in a refrigerator, the refrigerator shall be marked with a biohazard label.
- If blood is stored in a refrigerator for transport or same-day shipment, it does not need to be labeled but should be put in containment bags.

© Cengage Learning 2014

Figure 22-22   Biohazard labels alert employees to biohazardous materials, such as blood, body fluids, and other potentially infectious material.

Hazard Communication for Blood.
The employer is required to label containers of **regulated waste**, refrigerators, freezers, and other containers that are used to keep or transport blood or other potentially infectious material with warning labels that are orange or orange-red and have the biohazard symbol affixed to them. The labeling serves to warn employees of the hazard possibility of container contents (Figure 22-22).

Information and Training for Employees.
Employers must ensure and maintaining documentation that employees take part in training sessions during working hours at no cost to employees. The initial session must be provided when occupational exposure may occur and annually thereafter. If employee tasks and job description change, training must take place at that time.

Training components are listed in Figure 22-23. Documentation of training sessions must be available and kept for 3 years.

TRAINING COMPONENTS OF THE BLOODBORNE PATHOGEN STANDARD

Scope and Application

- The Standard applies to all occupational exposure to blood and other potentially infectious materials (OPIM), and includes part-time employees, designated first aiders, and mental health workers as well as exposed medical personnel.
- OPIM includes saliva in dental procedures, cerebrospinal fluid, unfixed tissue, semen, vaginal secretions, and body fluids visibly contaminated with blood.

Methods of Compliance

- General—standard precautions.
- Engineering and work practice controls.
- Personal protective equipment.
- Housekeeping.

Standard Precautions

- *All* human blood and OPIM are considered to be infectious.
- The *same* precautions must be taken with *all* blood and OPIM.

Engineering Controls

- Whenever feasible, engineering controls (devices that isolate or remove health hazards from the workplace) must be the primary method used to control exposure.
- Examples include needleless IVs, self-sheathing needles, sharps disposal containers, covered centrifuge buckets, aerosol-free tubes, and leak-proof containers.
- Engineering controls must be evaluated and documented on a regular basis.

Sharps Containers

- Readily accessible and as close as practical to work area.
- Puncture-resistant.
- Labeled or color-coded.
- Leak-proof.
- Closeable.
- *Routinely replaced* so there is no overflow.

Work Practice Controls

- Hand washing following glove removal.
- No recapping, breaking, or bending of needles.
- No eating, drinking, smoking, and so on in work area.
- No storage of food or drink where blood or OPIM are stored.
- Minimize splashing, splattering of blood, and OPIM.
- No mouth pipetting.
- Specimens must be transported in leak-proof, labeled containers. They must be placed in a secondary container if outside contamination of primary container occurs.
- Equipment must be decontaminated prior to servicing or shipping. Areas that cannot be decontaminated must be labeled.

Personal Protective Equipment (PPE)

- Includes eye protection, gloves, protective clothing, resuscitation equipment.
- Must be readily accessible and employers must require their use.
- Must be stored at work site.

Eye Protection

- Is required whenever there is potential for splashing, spraying, or splattering to the eyes or mucous membranes.
- If necessary, use eye protection in conjunction with a mask or use a chin-length face shield.
- Prescription glasses may be fitted with solid sideshields.
- Decontamination procedures must be developed.

Gloves

- Must be worn whenever hand contact with blood, OPIM, mucous membranes, nonintact skin, contaminated surfaces/items, or when performing vascular access procedures (phlebotomy).
- Type required   —Vinyl or latex for general use.
            —Alternatives must be available if employee has allergic reactions (i.e., powderless).
            —Utility gloves for surface disinfection.
            —Puncture-resistant when handling sharps (i.e., Central Supply).

Protective Clothing

- Must be worn whenever splashing or splattering to skin or clothing may occur.
- Type required depends on exposure. Prevention of contamination of skin and clothes is the key.
- Examples   —Low-level exposure lab coats.
            —Moderate-level exposure fluid-resistant gown.
            —High-level exposure fluid-proof apron, head and foot covering.
- *Note:* If PPE is considered protective clothing, then the *employer must* launder it.

Housekeeping

- There must be a written schedule for cleaning and disinfection.
- Contaminated equipment and surfaces must be cleaned as soon as feasible for obvious contamination or at end of work shift if no contamination has occurred.
- Protective coverings may be used over equipment.

Regulated Waste Containers (non-sharp)

- Closeable.
- Leak-proof.
- Labeled or color-coded.
- Placed in secondary container if outside of container is contaminated.

Figure 22-23   Overview of the *Bloodborne Pathogen Standard.*

TRAINING COMPONENTS OF THE BLOODBORNE PATHOGEN STANDARD

Laundry

- Handled as little as possible.
- Bagged at location of use.
- Labeled or color-coded.
- Transported in bags that prevent soak-through or leakage.

Laundry Facility

- Two options:
  1. Standard precautions for all laundry (alternative color coding allowed if recognized).
  2. Precautions only for contaminated laundry (must be red bags or biohazard labels).
- Laundry personnel must use PPE and have a sharps container accessible.

Hepatitis B Vaccination

- Made available within ten days to all employees with occupational exposure.
- At no cost to employees.
- May be required for student to be admitted to college health program as well as for externship.
- Given in accordance with United States Public Health Service guidelines.
- Employee must first be evaluated by health care professional.
- Health care professional gives a written opinion.
- If the vaccine is refused, the employee signs a declination form.
- Vaccine must be available at a future date if initially refused.

Post-Exposure Follow-Up

- Document exposure incident.
- Identify source individual (if possible).
- Attempt to test source if consent obtained.
- Provide results to exposed employee.

Labels

- Biohazard symbol and word *Biohazard* must be visible.
- Fluorescent orange/orange-red with contrasting letters may also be used.
- Red bags/containers may be substituted for labels.
- Labels required on —Regulated waste.
  —Refrigerators/freezers with blood of OPIM.
  —Transport/storage containers.
  —Contaminated equipment.

Information and Training

- Required for all employees with occupational exposure.
- Training required initially, annually, and if there are new procedures.

- Training material must be appropriate for literacy and education level of employee.
- Training must be interactive and allow for questions and answers.

Training Components

- Explanation of bloodborne standard.
- Epidemiology and symptoms of bloodborne disease.
- Modes of HIV/HBV transmission.
- Explanation of exposure control plan.
- Explanation of engineering, work practice controls.
- How to select the proper PPE.
- How to decontaminate equipment, surfaces, and so on.
- Information about hepatitis B vaccine.
- Post-exposure follow-up procedures.
- Label/color code system.

Medical Records

Records must be kept for each employee with occupational exposure and include:

- A copy of employee's vaccination status and date.
- A copy of post-exposure follow-up evaluation procedures.
- Health care professional's written opinions.
- Confidentiality must be maintained.
- Records must be maintained for thirty years plus the duration of employment.

Training Records

Records are kept for three years from date of training and include:

- Date of training.
- Summary of contents of training program.
- Name and qualifications of trainer.
- Name and job title of all persons attending.

Exposure Control Plan Components

- A written plan for each workplace with occupational exposure.
- Written policies/procedures for complying with the standard.
- A cohesive document or a guiding document referencing existing policies/procedures.

Exposure Control Plan

- A list of job classifications where occupational exposure control occurs (e.g., medical assistant, clinical laboratory scientist, dental hygienist).
- A list of tasks where exposure occurs (e.g., medical assistant who performs venipuncture).
- Methods/policies/procedures for compliance.
- Procedures for sharps disposal.
- Disinfection policies/procedures.

Figure 22-23   (*continues*)

TRAINING COMPONENTS OF THE BLOODBORNE PATHOGEN STANDARD

- Procedures for selection of PPE.
- Regulated waste disposal procedures.
- Laundry procedures.
- Hepatitis B vaccination procedures.
- Post-exposure follow-up procedures.
- Training procedures.
- Plan must be accessible to employees and be updated annually.

Employee Responsibilities

- Go through training and cooperate.
- Obey policies.
- Use universal precaution techniques.
- Use PPE.

- Use safe work practices.
- Use engineering controls.
- Report unsafe work conditions to employer.
- Maintain clean work areas.

Cooperation between employer and employees regarding *The Bloodborne Pathogen Standard* will facilitate understanding of the law, thereby benefiting all persons who are exposed to HIV, HBV, HCV, and OPIM by minimizing the risk of exposure to the pathogens.

Meeting the OSHA standard is not optional and failure to comply can result in a fine that may total $10,000 for each employee.

To obtain copies of *The Bloodborne Pathogen Standard*, contact OSHA at 800-321-6742 or www.osha.gov.

Courtesy of the Occupational Safety and Health Administration, U.S. Department of Labor.

Figure 22-23   (*continued*)

OSHA REGULATIONS AND STUDENTS

✓ With the passage of the OSHA law, all students with potential exposure to chemicals and bloodborne pathogens should follow all safety procedures as outlined by OSHA. Because students are not considered employees of a health care facility and are attending an educational institution, they do not fall under the OSHA guidelines. They should, however, take precautions to avoid contact with potentially infectious materials and toxic chemicals wherever learning is taking place (Figure 22-24).

Avoiding Exposure to Bloodborne Pathogens

Students can come into contact with blood and other potentially infectious material during laboratory practices and practicums. The potential for exposure and contact increases whenever invasive procedures are being performed. Some examples of invasive procedures are:

- Phlebotomy, the process of withdrawing blood
- Administering an injection
- Performing or assisting with medical/surgical procedures such as suturing of wounds or removal of sutures; assisting with certain procedures such as Pap smears, arthroscopies, amniocentesis, thoracentesis, or lumbar puncture; and dressing changes, colposcopies, vaginal

Student Safety Precautions

Gloves must be worn:
- During phlebotomy
- When giving injections
- When performing or assisting with invasive procedures
- When processing blood specimens

Eye protection with side projections must be worn:
- Whenever there is the potential for chemical exposure or the possibility of spray, splash, or splatter from blood or body fluids

Face shields or masks must be worn:
- When there is a chance of spray, splash, or splatter from blood or body fluids

Gowns or **aprons** must be worn:
- Where there exists any potential for exposure to contaminated materials

Lab coats must be worn and buttoned:
- When performing laboratory procedures

Figure 22-24   Student safety precautions.

© Cengage Learning 2014

exams, obstetrical care, vasectomies, biopsies, sigmoidoscopies, and colonoscopies are other examples in which students can contact blood and other potentially infectious material

Students must be aware of and think about the procedures they are involved in and be certain that they use essential safety equipment (PPE) and procedures when necessary. Students should adhere to the same responsibilities that employees do.

PPE should be available in the student laboratory and used as necessary. Standard Precautions must be strictly adhered to.

Students should always be on guard and make safety a priority by taking all precautions to avoid injuries. Some of the precautions are:

- Needles and other sharps (such as microscope slides and coverslips, sharp surgical instruments, and glass containers) should be handled with the same strict guidelines as outlined in the OSHA *Bloodborne Pathogen Standard* and the CDC's Standard Precautions.
- Obey all safety rules and know where the spill kits are located and how to clean up biohazard spills (see Figure 22-19).
- Know where the eyewash stations are and know how to operate them.
- Be familiar with all the information about solutions and chemicals used in the laboratory as outlined in the Material Safety Data Sheet (MSDS) (see Chapter 38).

An exposure to blood or other potentially infectious material experienced by a student must be immediately reported to the instructor if the accident occurs at the college or to the supervisor of the clinical agency and the practicum coordinator if the student is exposed during practicum. OSHA procedures as outlined earlier in this chapter should be followed with the exception of the filing of the OSHA 301 form.

Colleges require students studying the health professions to obtain the hepatitis B vaccine because it is approximately 95% effective against HBV. Because the vaccine is given in three doses over a period of 6 months, students should plan to have the injections in a timely fashion to be prepared for college laboratory courses and the practicum period.

PRINCIPLES OF INFECTION CONTROL

By understanding the dependent nature of the infection cycle, which holds that each step in the process must occur for infectious disease to occur, medical assistants can apply principles of infection control to eliminate or reduce the transmission of infectious microorganisms in the health care setting. Conscious and continual reliance on infection control is a professional standard and protects employees, patients, families, and the public from contracting infectious diseases. There are two general types of infection control: medical asepsis and surgical asepsis. Each is indicated in specific circumstances and each is achieved by the various techniques that are described in this chapter and in Chapter 31.

MEDICAL ASEPSIS

Medical asepsis is the use of practices such as hand washing, general cleaning and disinfecting of contaminated surfaces, and adherence to Standard and Transmission-Based Precautions. These measures are aimed at destroying pathologic organisms. These techniques are used to decrease the risk for transmission to others. Objects should be medically aseptic if they are to be used in procedures that are on the external body or if they will enter a usually contaminated body part, such as the mouth. Many things, such as our hands, cannot be sterilized or even disinfected, but they can be rendered clean of **gross contamination** and most pathogens by simple hand washing. Many items, such as stethoscopes or sphygmomanometers, do not need to be sterile to be used on a variety of patients. These items do not enter into the body or into sterile areas of the body. These items should, however, be either cleaned or disinfected routinely. Sphygmomanometers and stethoscopes are used continuously throughout the day on different patients. Patients with hypertension, postsurgery patients, and patients having physical examinations routinely have blood pressure monitored. Both pieces of equipment contact patients' skin, clothing, or both, making the blood pressure equipment an indirect source of pathogens. Alcohol-based wipes or a simplified method of detergent cleaning should be used regularly to decontaminate blood pressure equipment. Medical asepsis also involves environmental hygiene measures such as equipment cleaning and disinfection procedures. Careful attention to methods of medical asepsis greatly reduces the presence of pathogens that could cause disease in others. Specific procedures to achieve medical asepsis include adherence to Standard and Transmission-Based Precautions. Standard Precautions and Transmission-Based Precautions are considered methods of medical asepsis. These precautions should be followed stringently to provide barriers between potentially infectious blood and body fluids and those people who may come into contact with the fluids. Use of PPE, disinfection, and waste control are crucial steps in practicing these precautions. Hand washing, sanitization, and disinfection of instruments or equipment are also essential.

Some specific examples of appropriate use of medical asepsis include:

- Wash hands before and after handling equipment and supplies, on arrival and before leaving, and before and after working with each patient, even when gloves are worn.

- Handle all specimens as if they were contaminated.

- Use disposable equipment whenever possible and dispose of it properly in a biohazard waste container. All equipment is contaminated after patient use.

- Use PPE as outlined in Standard Precautions and wash hands after removal of any PPE, including gloves.

- Keep contaminated equipment and supplies away from clothing to prevent transmission of pathogens to self and others.

- Place dressing materials, gauze, cotton balls, and any other damp or wet contaminated absorbable material in a waterproof bag before disposal in the biohazard waste container.

- Any break in the medical assistant's skin should be covered with a sterile dressing.

- Items that fall to the floor are contaminated. Either discard or (wash) and then disinfect them before using.

- If uncertain whether equipment or supplies are clean or sterile, consider them contaminated. Clean or sterilize them before use.

Hand Washing

There have been tremendous advances in the last two centuries in the overall hygiene of the human race. This has added to the quality and duration of our lives on earth. General cleanliness has assisted with the eradication of widespread infection outbreaks and epidemics. Hand washing continues to be the most important aspect of all of the infectious control procedures. Proper hand washing removes gross contamination and reduces pathogens that could be transmitted by direct or indirect contact to others. Because hand washing is frequently required, the use of a good lotion is advised to reduce the possibility of skin breaks caused by dryness. Infectious diseases continue to present serious challenges. One of the biggest concerns is the spread of HIV, HBV, and HCV. In May 2007, the WHO issued nine patient safety solution recommendations. The Joint Commission has adopted the nine recommendations. Patient Safety Solutions No. 9 is entitled "Improved Hand Hygiene to Prevent Healthcare Associated Infection (HAI)." It can be applied to this chapter and to others because, according to the WHO, millions of people worldwide are suffering from hospital-acquired infections. "Effective hand hygiene is the primary measure for avoiding this problem," say the WHO and the Joint Commission.

Hand washing is the single, most effective way to lower the incidence of infectious disease transmission.

The CDC recommends that, as part of hand hygiene, when hands are visibly soiled with blood or other body fluids, they should be washed with either a nonantimicrobial soap or an antimicrobial soap and water. Procedure 22-1 describes medical asepsis hand washing. If hands are not visibly soiled, an alcohol-based hand rub or gel can be used routinely for decontaminating hands. These formulations must contain 60%–90% alcohol to be most effective. Early data suggests that the activity of alcohol-based hand sanitizers is less against viral pathogens than against bacterial pathogens. When decontaminating hands with an alcohol-based hand rub, apply to palms of one hand and rub hands together covering all surfaces of hands and fingers, palms, back of hands, fingertips, and between fingers, wrists, and thumbs until hands are dry. The use of alcohol-based hand sanitizers **does not** replace a solid practice of hand washing, using traditional soap and water, by health care providers.

The World Health Organization (WHO) has published the *Hand Hygiene Technical Reference Manual.* This document clearly outlines "My five moments for hand hygiene." These are logical, practical, and useful guidelines for the use of hand hygiene (Table 22-7).

Antimicrobial wipes *cannot* be used as a substitute for an alcohol-based hand rub. Wearing gloves is *not* a substitute for hand decontamination. Artificial fingernails or nail extenders cannot be worn when in direct contact with patients at high risk. Natural nails should be kept less than ¼ inch long.

Sanitization

Sanitization (washing) of instruments and equipment rids them of gross contamination and blood, body fluids, tissue, and other contaminated **debris**. Enzymatic detergent especially designed for medical instruments and a soft scrub brush are used to

Table 22-7   Recommendations for Hand Hygiene*

The 5 Moments	Consensus recommendations
1. Before touching a patient	• Before and after touching the patient
2. Before clean/aseptic procedure	• Before handling an invasive device for patient care, regardless of whether or not gloves are used • If moving from a contaminated body site to another body site during care of the same patient
3. After body-fluid exposure risk	• After contact with body fluids or excretions, mucous membrane, non-intact skin, or wound dressing • If moving from a contaminated body site to another body site during care of the same patient • After removing sterile or nonsterile gloves
4. After touching a patient	• Before and after touching the patient • After removing sterile or nonsterile gloves
5. After touching a patient's surroundings	• After contact with inanimate surfaces and objects (including medical equipment) in the immediate vicinity of the patient • After removing sterile or nonsterile gloves

© Cengage Learning 2014

*Overview of the 2009 *WHO Guidelines on Hand Hygiene in Health Care*

remove all contaminates from surfaces, crevices, hinges, and serrations. Use of enzymatic detergents will help break down the proteins found in body fluids and tissues. Water temperature should be warm but not hot. Heat coagulates protein, making it more difficult to remove. A critical component to promoting effective sanitization is to complete the procedure as soon as possible after contamination so that tissue or body fluids do not have the opportunity to dry on the instruments. Dried debris is more difficult to remove and may require much scrubbing. Instruments may be left to soak in disinfectant solution or water with a **solvent** if sanitization cannot be performed immediately after use (Figure 22-25).

To avoid the risk for punctures or cuts from sharp instruments during sanitization, heavy-duty gloves should be worn. Some facilities use an **ultrasonic cleaner** (Figure 22-26). It uses high-frequency sound waves and agitates the instruments (sanitizes them) before sterilizing them. Goggles are worn to protect eyes from splashing of contaminated debris during the scrubbing procedure. A plastic apron provides protection from splashing of clothing (see Chapter 31). Hot water may be used for rinsing to remove all residue and aid in the drying

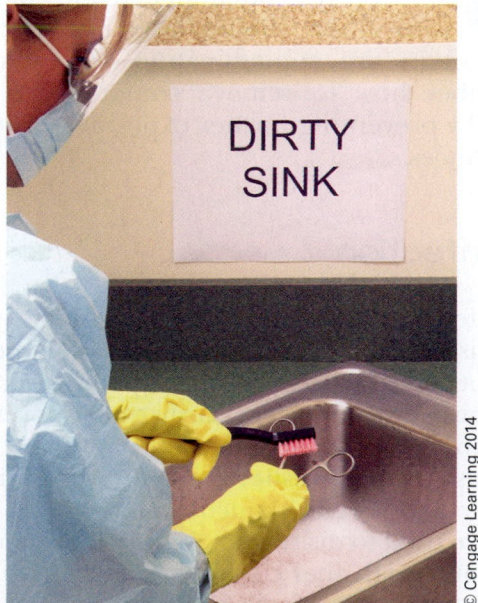

© Cengage Learning 2014

Figure 22-25   Medical assistant sanitizing an instrument.

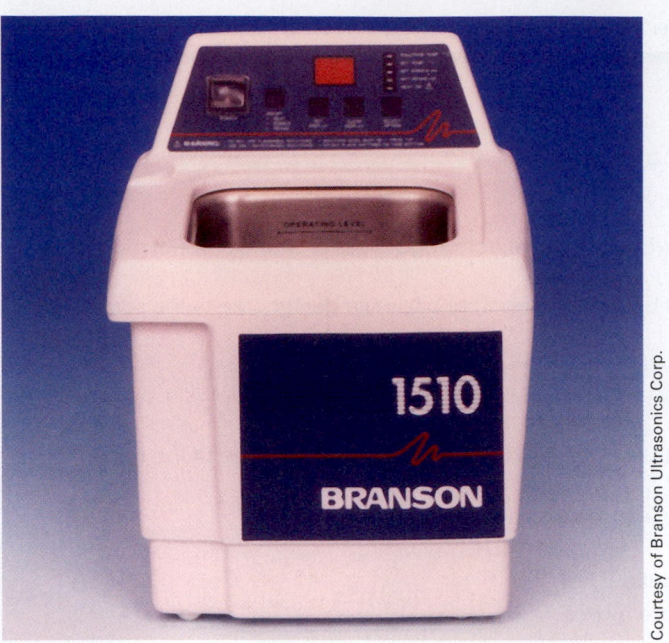

Courtesy of Branson Ultrasonics Corp.

Figure 22-26 The Branson Ultrasonic Cleaner, model 1510.

process. Check instruments for working condition. Drying thoroughly will prevent damage from rust or water spots.

Larger items such as instrument trays or Mayo stands, stools, chairs, examination tables, and lamps should also have a decontaminating sanitization process with thorough washing, rinsing, and drying.

 See Procedure 22-5 for instrument sanitization. Gloves contaminated with blood and body fluids should be removed carefully to contain the contamination. Procedure 22-3 describes how to remove contaminated gloves, thereby preventing further exposure to biohazard substances.

Disinfection

Disinfection, a third procedure used in medical asepsis practices, consists of various chemicals that can be used to destroy many pathogenic microorganisms but not necessarily their spores. Disinfection chemicals are used on inanimate objects. Because of their **caustic** nature, these chemicals can irritate the skin and mucous membranes. Chemicals are used to disinfect items or equipment made from materials that could be damaged by heat or that are too large to fit into an autoclave such as stethoscopes, percussion hammers, examination tables, and Mayo trays and stands. These and other

items that are chemically disinfected are used during *external* physical examination or procedures.

Boiling water (temperature 212°F) is considered a form of disinfection because it will kill some forms of microorganisms. It is important to note that this method *cannot* be considered a sterilization technique because the temperature is not high enough to kill the hepatitis virus, tuberculosis bacteria, or microbial spores. Articles such as nasal and ear specula can be sanitized and disinfected by vigorous boiling for at least 15 minutes, or soaked in a disinfectant according to manufacturer's instructions. The only reasonable use for boiling as a means of disinfection in today's medical setting is for items that:

1. Will *not* be used in invasive procedures
2. Will *not* be inserted into body orifices nor be used in a sterile procedure

Before either chemical disinfection or disinfection by boiling, articles must first be thoroughly sanitized and dried. Of special note are stainless steel gynecologic and proctologic examination instruments. These instruments are not sanitized with other instruments because of the risk for transmission of sexually transmitted diseases (STDs). They are sterilized in the autoclave after sanitization to eliminate transmission of microorganisms.

Chemical disinfectant solutions must be carefully prepared and used according to the manufacturer's instructions to ensure effective disinfectant properties. Medical clinics should use the disinfectant solution that best meets the needs of the ambulatory care setting as to the quantity of instruments to be disinfected, cost, preparation requirements, storage needs, and handling procedures. When choosing a chemical disinfectant solution, pay close attention to the manufacturer's report of the chemical disinfectant properties of the product. Some solutions are effective against a wide spectrum of microorganisms, whereas other solutions may be selective for certain common microorganisms. When chemically disinfecting, items must first be thoroughly sanitized and dried. Any debris or water left on the item being chemically treated will affect the chemical solution, thereby decreasing its effectiveness and compromising the disinfecting process.

For surfaces such as countertops, the least expensive and most readily available chemical is a 1:10 solution of ordinary household bleach (sodium hypochlorite). However, besides the obvious disadvantage of bleaching clothing, bleach is not easily rinsed, and it is only effective if the

Table 22-8   Maximum Process for Infection Control

Maximum Process	Stethoscope	Chair	Ear Speculum	Vaginal Speculum	Fiberoptic Endoscope	Surgical Instrument	Skin
Sanitization	X	X	X	X	X	X	X
Chemical disinfection by wiping	X	X	X				
Chemical disinfection by soaking			X				
Boiling			X				
Sterilization					X	X	

© Cengage Learning 2014

solution is mixed fresh daily. Nevertheless, its effectiveness is so highly respected that many medical laboratories depend almost entirely on bleach to chemically kill pathogens on countertops.

In summary, medical asepsis includes procedures for which all medical assistants must be responsible and qualified to incorporate into daily work practices. The responsibility for maintaining medical asepsis is the combined goal of the clinic staff and providers.

Sterilization

Instrument care includes sterilization. This is the most important part of infection control in any clinic or treatment facility. One of the cardinal rules of infection control is "Do not disinfect when you can sterilize." The process of sterilization kills all microorganisms that are present on the surfaces and the working parts of instruments. Effectiveness of any sterilization process relies on several factors. Conditions must be present to effectively destroy living organisms. The design and operation of the equipment and the combination of temperature and sterilant must be effective to kill pathogens. Any devices or instruments that are to be sterilized must be sanitized first to reduce any biologic material that is present.

The CDC advocates the use of several sterilization methods. Those methods most commonly found in an ambulatory care setting are:

- *Steam.* Autoclaves are a common tool utilized in the ambulatory care setting. These devices utilize steam under pressure to deliver moist heat at a high temperature to kill all microorganisms by coagulating and changing the cellular

proteins. There are strict guidelines that must be followed regarding the wrapping of instruments and the temperature, time, and pressure that are required to assure 100% sterilization.

- *Liquid chemical sterilization.* This method is used to sterilize delicate or heat-sensitive devices that can be immersed. A germicidal solution and complete immersion for a prescribed period of time result in the death of microorganisms. There are a number of liquid chemicals that are commonly used. These include peracetic acid and glutaraldehyde. There is a risk to health care providers who come into contact with these chemicals. Precautions should be taken to limit exposure to these hazardous materials. There are devices that are closed-processing systems that limit exposure to the liquid chemicals.

BIOTERRORISM

Bioterrorism is the use of biologic weapons (pathogenic microorganisms) to create fear in people. A bioterrorism attack is the deliberate release of biologic agents (weapons) such as bacteria, viruses, and toxins to cause death or illness in people, plants, or animals. The agents can spread through the air, food, and water. Terrorists can easily obtain and use biologic agents. The agents can be very difficult to detect and difficult to protect against. They have no odor, are invisible, have no taste, and can be spread quietly. Only small amounts are needed to kill or cause serious illness to hundreds of thousands of people. The agents can be put into food and/or water, absorbed through or injected into the skin, and dispensed as aerosols. Some diseases can be treated with pharmaceutical agents such as antibiotics and antitoxins.

Table 22-9   Example of Six Agents That Could Be Used in a Bioterrorism Attack

Disease	Agent	Transmission	Vaccine Availability	Treatment
Anthrax	Bacterium	Inhalation Not spread person to person	Yes, but not readily available	Antibiotics
Botulism (severe food poisoning)	Toxin	Toxin in food Not spread person to person	Antitoxin (state, local health departments, and CDC have)	Antitoxin should be given as soon as disease is suspected
Plague (2 types: bubonic, pneumonic)	Bacterium found in rodents and their fleas	An infected flea bites someone Materials that are contaminated with bacteria can enter through nonintact skin Bubonic plague does not spread person to person Pneumonic plague occurs when bacteria are inhaled because it spreads through the air and from person to person	None	Antibiotics
Smallpox	Virus	Skin eruptions occur on arms, legs, feet, and face Virus settles in the nose and throat and spreads when infected person coughs, talks, or sneezes Can spread through ventilation systems Contaminated clothes and bedding Highly contagious	After disease was eradicated, supplies of the virus were to be destroyed or locked away in two laboratories, one in the U.S. and the other in Russia Last immunization for smallpox was 1980 Immunity lasts for about 10 years	Symptomatic FDA has approved a new smallpox vaccine that will be used in the event of a bioterrorist attack
Tularemia	Bacterium (infected rabbits and ticks spread bacteria)	Human to human spread uncommon Bacterium can enter nonintact skin, mucous membranes of eyes, respiratory tract, gastrointestinal tract	Yes	Antibiotics

© Cengage Learning 2014

The most dangerous disease threats are anthrax, botulism, pneumonic/bubonic plague, smallpox, and tularemia.

Anthrax, pneumonic/bubonic plague, and tularemia all can be treated with antibiotics. Smallpox is treated by early vaccination (within 4 days). The CDC has the vaccine (Table 22-9).

Education plays a vital role in raising awareness and increasing the knowledge of health care professionals to aid them in being better prepared for threats to the public health. Protection against the agents should be started early. PPE and high-efficiency particulate air (HEPA) filters will filter most biologic agents from the air. Antibiotics given even before the agent is identified helps protect people, as do vaccines.

The Food and Drug Administration (FDA) has approved a new smallpox vaccine. The FDA said it is intended to inoculate people who are at high risk for exposure to smallpox, a highly contagious disease. The FDA said the vaccine could be used to protect people during a bioterrorist attack. There is no FDA-approved treatment for smallpox.

According to the CDC, the threat that biologic agents will be used is more likely now than it has been throughout history. The WHO, the CDC, the Department of Homeland Security, and state and local public health departments are excellent resources for more information about bioterrorism (see Chapter 9).

PROCEDURE 22-1

Medical Asepsis Hand Wash (Hand Hygiene)

STANDARD PRECAUTIONS:

PURPOSE:

To reduce pathogens on the hands and wrists, thereby decreasing direct and indirect transmission of infectious microorganisms. Average duration is 1 minute before beginning to work with patients, 15 seconds (CDC Hand Hygiene recommendation) following each patient contact.

EQUIPMENT/SUPPLIES:

Sink (preferably with foot-operated controls)
Soap (preferably liquid soap in foot-operated container; bar soap discouraged)
Water-based antibacterial lotion
Disposable paper towels
Nail stick or brush

PROCEDURE STEPS:

1. Remove all jewelry (plain wedding band is only acceptable jewelry). Push watch up on arm or remove. RATIONALE: Jewelry harbors microorganisms on the hands.

2. Ensure that nails are clipped short. RATIONALE: Longer nails have been proven to harbor larger colony counts of microorganisms.

3. Roll sleeves to above the elbow. RATIONALE: Clothing harbors microorganisms and can be a vector in the transmission of disease.

4. Prepare disposable paper towel (if using pull-down dispenser, prepare the amount of paper towel necessary for drying hands after wash; if using folded towels, have accessible). RATIONALE: After the hand washing, you may not touch any contaminated surface, such as the handle on a paper-towel dispenser or the water faucets.

5. Never allow your clothing to touch the sink; never touch the inside of the sink with your hands. RATIONALE: The sink is considered contaminated at all times. (*NOTE:* Sinks must be sanitized and disinfected at the end of each day.)

6. Turn on the faucet with a dry paper towel (Figure 22-27A). Discard paper towel after adjusting water temperature to lukewarm. RATIONALE: Lukewarm water is best for hand washing

because excessively hot water may overdry the skin and cause cracking, thereby interrupting the caregiver's first line of defense.

7. Wet hands and apply soap using a circular motion and friction; rub into a lather (Figure 22-27B). RATIONALE: This initial hand wash is to remove visible soil and some microorganisms. Interlace fingers to clean between them (Figure 22-27C).

8. Use an orange stick or brush at the first hand washing of each day (Figure 22-27D and Figure 22-27E). RATIONALE: Nails harbor microorganisms. Even with trimmed nails, this step must be performed on a daily basis.

9. Rinse hands with hands pointed down and lower than elbows (Figure 22-27F). RATIONALE: When hands are held lower than elbows, pathogens and contaminated water run off the hands and not up on the forearms.

10. Repeat soap application and lather; interlace fingers well; wash with vigorous, circular motions all parts of hands including wrists; wash for at least one minute or longer depending on degree of contamination. RATIONALE: Appropriate length of hand washing is required to provide enough friction to remove soil and microorganisms.

11. Rinse well, keeping hands pointed downward. RATIONALE: Rinsing removes microorganisms, contaminated water, and soap from the hands.

12. Repeat hand washing for the first hand washing of the day or if necessary for contaminated or visibly soiled hands. Lather wrists using a circular motion and friction. Rinse arms and hands. RATIONALE: When the hands are excessively contaminated or soiled, two hand washings may be necessary to remove microorganisms from the hands.

13. Dry hands and wrists with disposable paper towel; do not touch towel dispenser after hand washing; blot instead of rubbing with towel; if sink is not foot operated, use a clean disposable towel to turn off water faucet. RATIONALE: Touching the towel dispenser contaminates the hands. Blotting the hands dry reduces drying of the skin. Turning faucet off with paper towel prevents recontamination from dirty faucet.

continues

Procedure 22-1 (continued)

14. Discard paper towel in waste container. Do not leave contaminated towels for repeated use. *NOTE*: Repeat hand washing procedure before and after each patient contact, procedure, or meal. RATIONALE: Hand washing must be performed on a regular and frequent basis to ensure the reduction of microorganisms transmitted by hands.

Water-based antibacterial lotion can be applied to prevent chapped, **excoriated** skin. If skin is excoriated, the medical assistant may not be able to work because of breaks in the skin or may have to wear gloves during any patient contact.

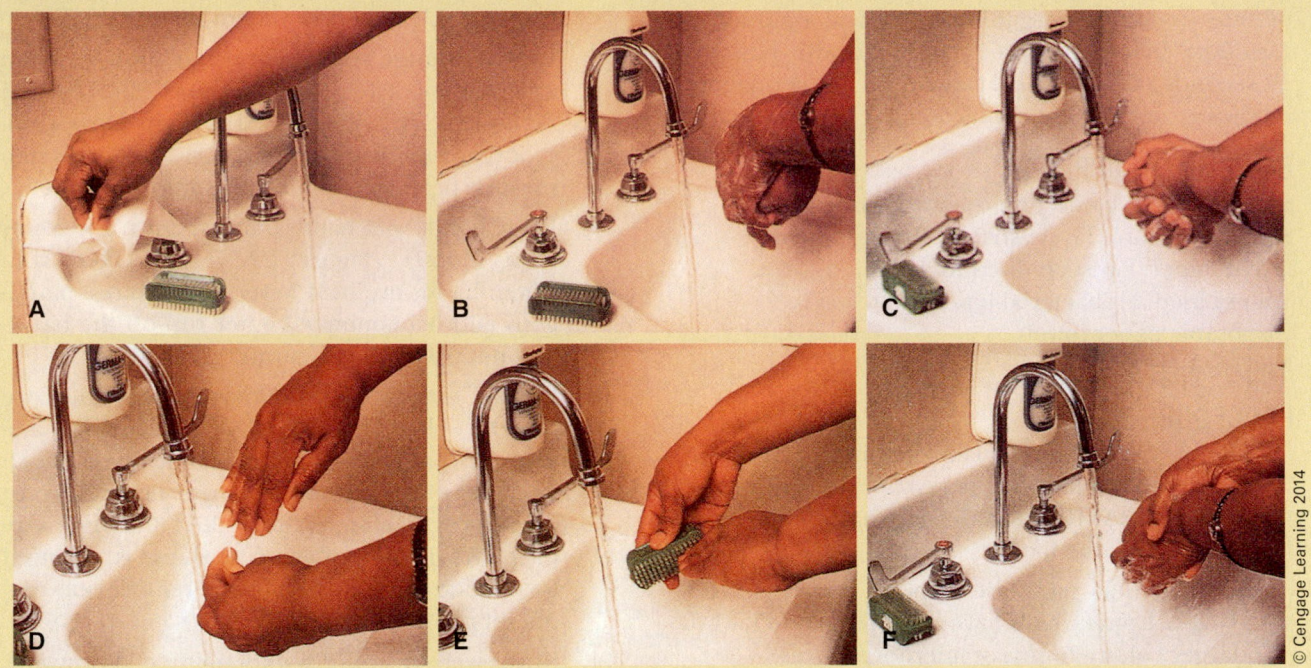

© Cengage Learning 2014

Figure 22-27 (A) Prepare towels for use. Turn on the faucet and adjust water to a lukewarm temperature. (B) Wet hands. Let water flow downward off hands and fingertips. (C) Use a circular motion to create friction and wash the palms and back of hands. Interlace the fingers to clean between them. (D) Use an orange stick to clean under fingernails. (E) A hand brush may also be used to clean under fingernails. (F) Rinse hands thoroughly, letting the water flow downward off your hands and fingertips.

PROCEDURE 22-2

Correct Use of Alcohol-Based Hand Rubs (ABHR)

PURPOSE:
To avoid transmission of pathogens via the hands of health care personnel

EQUIMENT/SUPPLIES:
Alcohol-based hand rub containing 60% to 90% alcohol

PROCEDURE STEPS:
1. Assure there is no gross contamination of hands. RATIONALE: ABHR are ineffective when used in the presence of biologic material that is visible on the hands.

Procedure 22-2 (continued)

2. Dispense 2–3 mL into the palm of your hand. RATIONALE: The health care provider must use enough ABHR to cover all the surfaces of both hands.

3. The ABHR must be applied in the following manner:

   a. Palms rubbed together

   b. Right palm over the dorsal aspect of the left hand and vice versa

   c. Palm to palm with fingers interlaced

   d. Backs of fingers to opposing palms with fingers interlocked

   e. Rotational rubbing of left thumb clasped in right palm and vice versa

   f. Rotational rubbing, backwards and forwards, with clasped fingers of right hand in the left palm and vice versa

   RATIONALE: All surfaces and aspects of the hand must be covered with the ABHR to assure contact with any microorganisms present.

4. Hands should be rubbed together for at least 30 seconds until the hands are dry. RATIONALE: The antimicrobial activity of the ABHR is assured if the application is allowed to dry.

PROCEDURE 22-3
Removing Contaminated Gloves

STANDARD PRECAUTIONS:

PURPOSE:
To carefully remove and dispose of contaminated gloves to contain exposure.

EQUIPMENT/SUPPLIES:
Biohazard waste container

PROCEDURE STEPS:

1. Grasp the palm of the used left glove with the right hand to begin removing the first glove. Notice hands are held away from the body and pointed downward (Figure 22-28A and Figure 22-28B). RATIONALE: Holding the hands away from the body will further prevent exposure to biological contaminants.

2. Turn the used left glove inside out and hold it in the right gloved hand. Be careful not to touch your bare left hand on the contaminated right glove (Figure 22-28C through Figure 22-28E). RATIONALE: Turning the glove inside out helps isolate the biological contaminants.

3. Holding the glove that has been removed with the hand that still has the glove on, insert two fingers of the ungloved hand between your arm and the inside of the dirty glove (Figure 22-28F).

4. Turn the right dirty glove inside out over the other. One glove is inside the other and you can handle the gloves because the dirty, contaminated area is inside the gloves (Figure 22-28G and Figure 22-28H). RATIONALE: Both gloves are inverted with the biological contaminates isolated.

5. Dispose of the inverted gloves into a biological waste receptacle. RATIONALE: All biological waste should be placed into a red biohazard bag.

6. Wash hands thoroughly. RATIONALE: Immediate washing of hands is an additional precaution.

continues

Procedure 22-3 (continued)

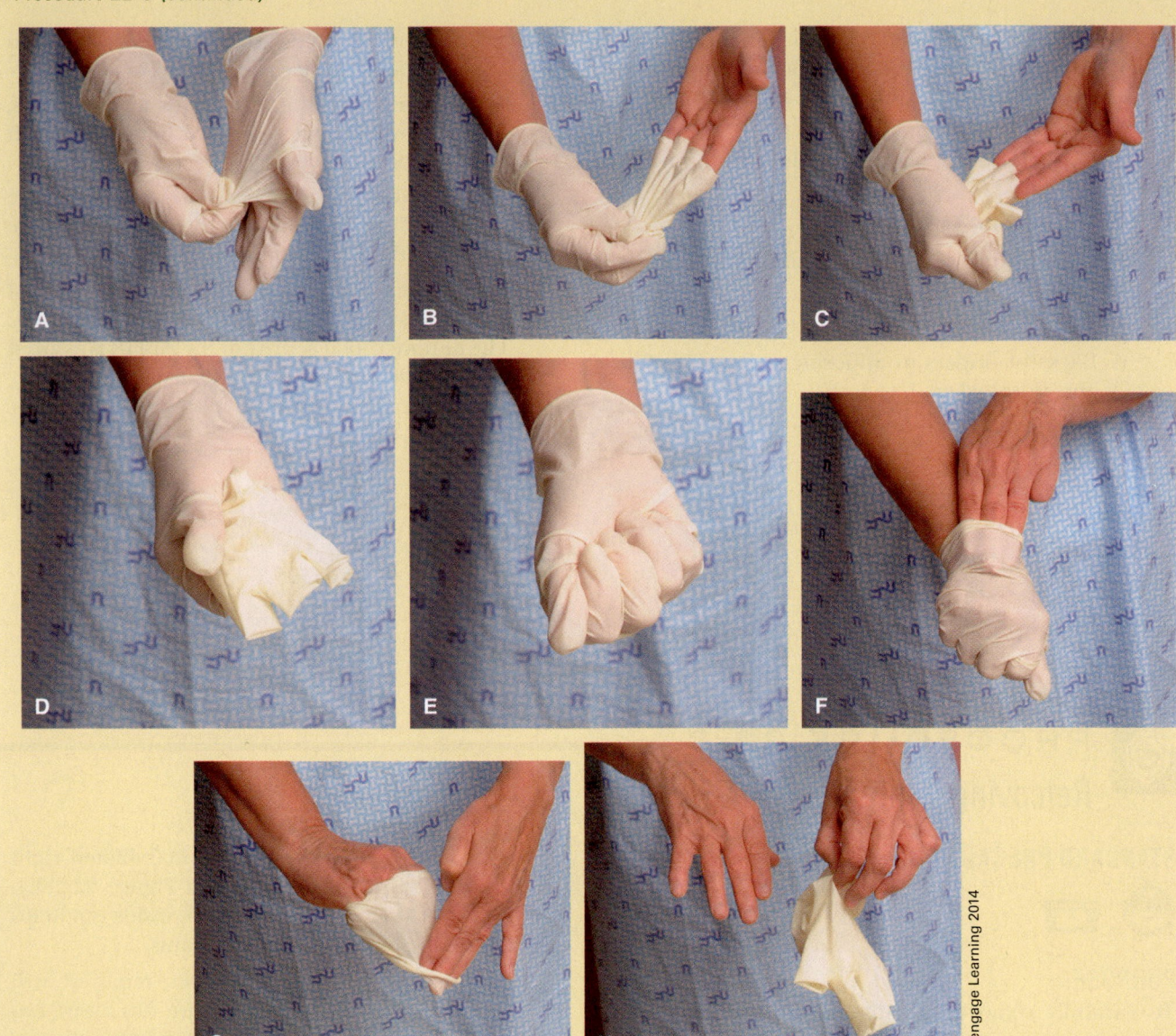

© Cengage Learning 2014

Figure 22-28   (A) Grasp the palm of the used glove with the right hand. (B) Begin removing the first glove. (C) Glove is turned inside out as it is being removed. Take care not to touch bare skin on the contaminated glove. (D) Inverted glove is completely removed into the contaminated glove. (E) Contain the inverted glove completely in the gloved hand. (F) Insert three fingers of the ungloved hand inside the back of the contaminated glove and turn it inside out over the other. (G) Invert the second glove over the first. (H) One glove is now inside the other.

PROCEDURE 22-4

Transmission-Based Precautions: Donning a Gown, Mask, Gloves, and Cap (Isolation Technique)

STANDARD PRECAUTIONS:

PURPOSE:
To provide barriers for medical assistant to be protected from airborne, contact, or droplet infectious diseases.

EQUIPMENT/SUPPLIES:
Disposable gowns
Disposable caps if needed
Disposable masks
Gloves (nonsterile and sterile)
Room with sink and running water
Paper towels
Other supplies relative to patient's condition

PROCEDURE STEPS:

1. Review provider orders and agency protocols relative to the type of isolation precautions. RATIONALE: Provides for patient comfort and decreases the spread of microorganisms. Limits the number of personnel coming into the patient's room and the patient's exposure to microorganisms.

2. Place appropriate isolation supplies outside the patient's room and note type of isolation sign on the door (e.g., airborne, droplet, or contact). RATIONALE: Ensures staff follows isolation protocol and alerts visitors to check with the nurses' station before entering the room.

3. Remove jewelry, laboratory coat, and other items not necessary in providing patient care. RATIONALE: Decreases the spread of microorganisms.

4. Wash hands and don disposable clothing:

   a. Apply cap to cover hair and ears completely.

   b. Apply gown to cover outer garments completely. Hold gown in front of body and place arms through sleeves (Figure 22-29A). Pull sleeves down to wrist. Tie gown securely at neck and waist (Figure 22-29B and Figure 22-29C).

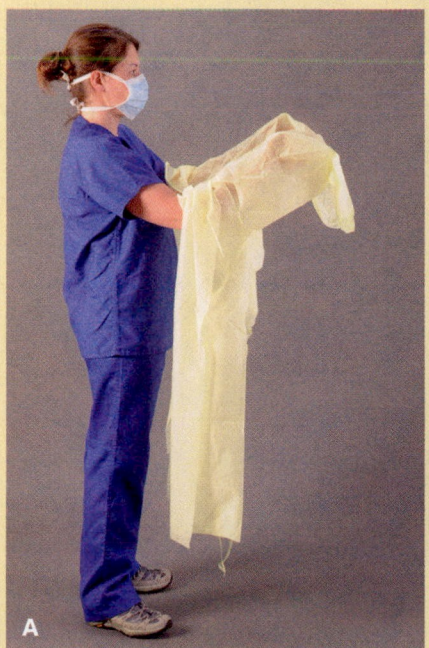 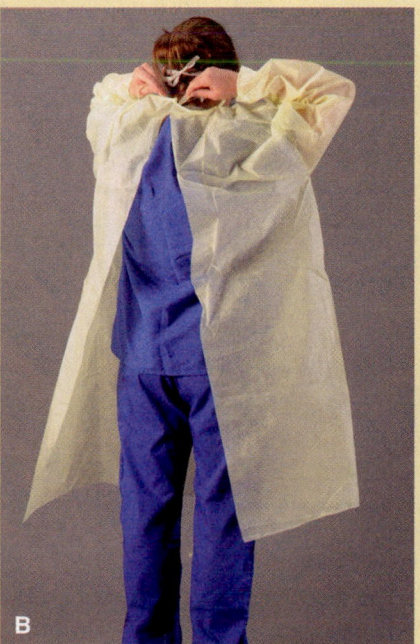 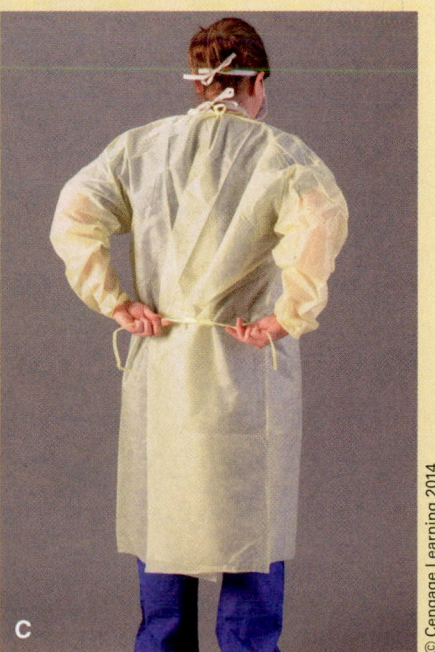

© Cengage Learning 2014

Figure 22-29   (A) Medical assistant has put on a mask and is donning the gown, pulling on the sleeves. (B) The neck of the gown is tied first and (C) the back of the gown, last.

continues

Procedure 22-4 (continued)

c. Don nonsterile gloves and pull gloves over the cuff to cover completely.

d. Apply mask by placing the top of the mask over the bridge of your nose (top part of mask has a metal strip) and pinch the metal strip to fit snugly against the skin of the nose.

RATIONALE: Disposable garments act as a barrier in preventing the transmission of microorganisms from medical assistant to patient and protect the medical assistant from contact with pathogens.

5. Enter patient's room with all gathered supplies. RATIONALE: Prevents trips into and out of the patient's room and keeps supplies clean.

6. Assess vital signs and perform other functions (ECG, phlebotomy) of care to meet the needs of the patient. Record assessment data on a piece of paper, avoiding contact with any articles in the patient room. RATIONALE: Allows for data collection and the performance of patient care.

7. Dispose of soiled articles in the impermeable biohazard bags, which should be labeled correctly according to contents. If soiled, reusable equipment is removed from the room; label bag accordingly. RATIONALE: Impermeable biohazard bags prevent the leakage of contaminated materials, thereby preventing the transmission of infection. Labeling is a warning to other personnel that the contents are infectious.

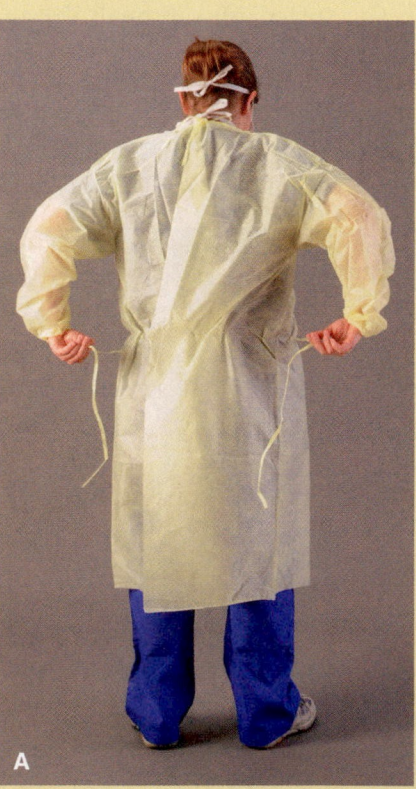

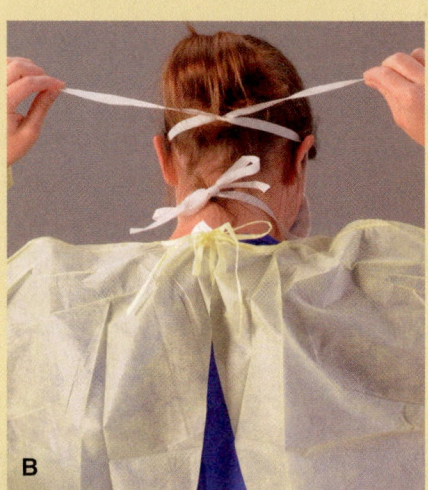

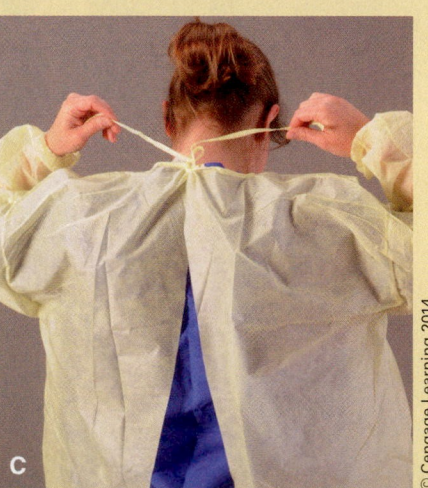

© Cengage Learning 2014

Figure 22-30 (A) When finished in the isolation room, the medical assistant removes the contaminated gloves (see Procedure 22-3), washes hands (see Procedure 22-1), and then unties waist tie of gown. Remove mask by untying bottom ties first, then top ties. (B) Holding mask by ties, place in biohazard container. (C) Untie neck ties of gown. Wash hands.

Exiting the Isolation Room: Removing Gown, Gloves, Mask, and Cap

1. Remove contaminated gloves (see Procedure 22-3). Wash hands and then untie waist tie of gown (Figure 22-30A).

2. Remove mask by untying bottom ties first, then top ties (Figure 22-30B). Holding mask by ties, place in contaminated waste.

3. Untie neckties of gown (Figure 22-30C). Wash hands. RATIONALE: Removes microorganisms from hands before proceeding.

4. Slip fingers of one hand inside cuff (Figure 22-30D) of the other hand. Pull the gown over the hand, being careful not to touch the outside of the gown.

5. Using the hand covered by the gown, pull down the gown over the other hand (Figure 22-30E).

6. Pull gown off your arms. Hold gown away from yourself and roll into a ball with the contaminated side inside (Figure 22-30F). RATIONALE: The gown is removed and folded, touching only the inside of the gown to prevent transmission of microorganisms to yourself.

7. Dispose of gown in biohazard container.

8. Wash hands thoroughly.

9. Document procedures performed on patient (vital signs, EKG, phlebotomy) in patient record or electronic medical record.

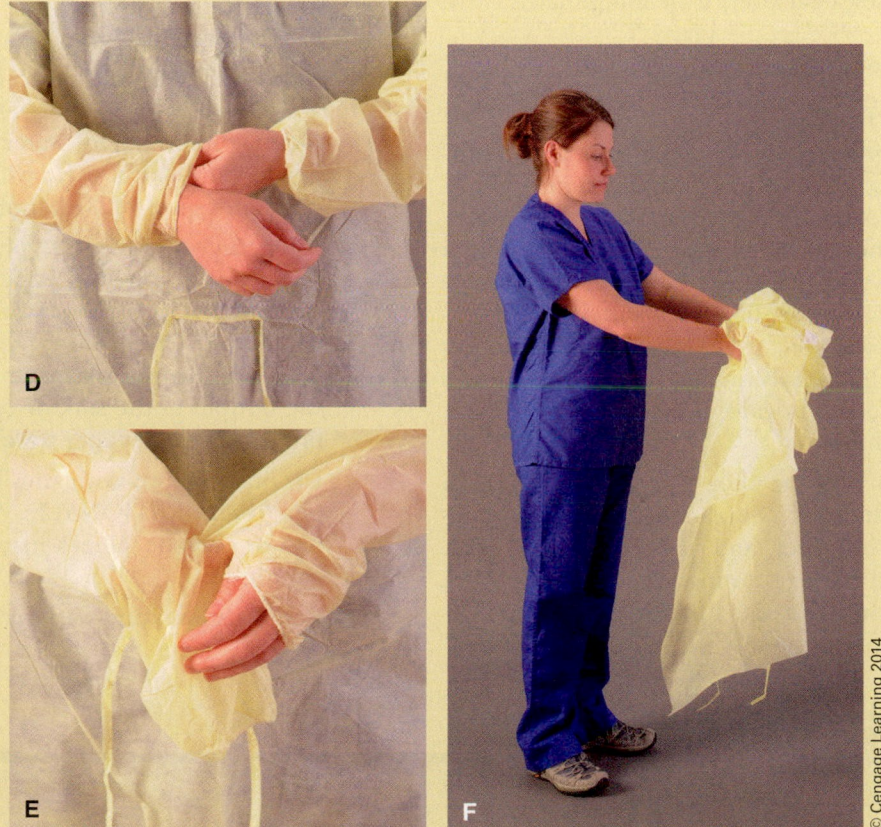

© Cengage Learning 2014

Figure 22-30   *(continued)* (D) Slip fingers of one hand inside cuff of the other hand. Pull gown over the hand, being careful not to touch the outside of the gown. (E) Using the hand covered by the gown, pull down the gown over the other hand. (F) Pull gown off arms and hold away from body and clothing. Roll into a ball with the contaminated side of gown on the inside. Wash hands thoroughly.

PROCEDURE 22-5

Sanitization of Instruments

STANDARD PRECAUTIONS:

PURPOSE:

To properly clean contaminated instruments to remove tissue and debris.

EQUIPMENT/SUPPLIES:

Sink (or ultrasonic cleaner: follow manufacturer's instructions)

Sanitizing agent (low-sudsing detergent, approved chemical disinfectant, or blood solvent)

Brush

Disposable paper towels

Plastic apron

Disposable gloves, heavy-duty if cleaning sharps

Goggles

Biohazard waste container

PROCEDURE STEPS:

1. Wear heavy duty gloves, goggles, and apron. RATIONALE: Contaminated instruments pose a blood and body fluid precaution as indicated by OSHA standards. Disposable gloves must always be worn to sanitize instruments. Wear heavy-duty gloves if cleaning sharp instruments. Goggles are worn to protect eyes from splashing of contaminated debris during scrubbing procedure. A plastic apron provides protection from splashing of clothing.

2. As soon as possible after a procedure in which an instrument is contaminated, rinse the instrument in water and disinfectant solution; rinse again under running water. RATIONALE: Rinsing contaminated instruments as soon as possible after use removes debris and tissue that could quickly dry onto the instrument, making sanitization more difficult.

3. If contaminated instrument must be carried from one place to another for sanitization, place the instrument in a basin labeled "Biohazard." RATIONALE: Do not carry contaminated instruments in your hands. Biohazard basins must be sanitized and disinfected daily according to procedures for Standard Precautions.

4. Scrub each instrument well with detergent and water; scrub under running water, and be sure to scrub inside any edges, serrations, and all surfaces. RATIONALE: Thorough scrubbing removes tissue and debris from all areas of the contaminated instrument. If all tissue is not removed with scrubbing, the instrument may not be sterilized during sterilization procedures.

5. Rinse well with hot water. RATIONALE: Tissue and debris, as well as detergent, must be completely removed. Hot water will help remove all residue and aid in the drying process while rust and water spots will be eliminated.

6. After they are rinsed, place instruments on muslin or disposable paper towel until all instruments have been scrubbed and rinsed. RATIONALE: Often more than one instrument is sanitized; do not place sanitized instrument in the bottom of the sink or on a countertop without a disposable paper towel or muslin towel.

7. Dry instruments with muslin or disposable paper towels. RATIONALE: Wet instruments may rust or corrode. Check instruments for working condition.

8. Remove gloves and wash hands.

CASE STUDY 22-1

Refer to the scenario at the beginning of the chapter.

CASE STUDY REVIEW

1. Explain the importance of including the entire staff at the health care provider's clinic in the educational activity regarding infection control.

2. Make a list of websites that provide important information that is updated regularly on the current "best practices" for Healthcare Associated Infections and infection control.

CASE STUDY 22-2

Your provider has asked you to take the lead in educating the staff on a monthly basis regarding cleaning and proper care of the instruments commonly used in the practice. Identify the appropriate care and methods of preventing the spread of pathogens and prepare one update that is appropriate for a general medicine practice.

CASE STUDY REVIEW

1. How often should this information be updated?

SUMMARY

Effective infection control measures are the first defense against the transmission of infectious diseases in the ambulatory care setting. Reliance on Standard and Transmission-Based Precautions, protective barriers, and basic principles of disinfection promotes professional and responsible clinical care for patients. When the processes of infection control are applied to all clinical procedures, the infection cycle may be broken by many varied means. Remember that an infectious disease will not spread to another person if the cycle is sufficiently broken at any stage.

Infectious diseases spread and accidents occur through lack of education and carelessness. Medical assistants must understand the importance of the regulations and guidelines set forth by the federal government and follow through by helping employers and fellow employees implement them. In doing so, the health and safety of patients and health care workers can be protected; the spread of infectious diseases can be kept under control; and the risk for contracting a serious infectious disease such as HIV, HBV, or HCV will be greatly minimized.

Every medical clinic and ambulatory care setting must, by law, have clearly written and readily available manuals containing information about Standard Precautions and OSHA for the safe handling, storage, and disposal of blood, body fluids, and chemicals.

Through consistent use of Standard Precautions and adherence to OSHA laws, health care providers can acquire the behaviors and techniques needed to safeguard themselves and their patients.

Because of frequent changes in the laws, it is necessary for medical assistants and all other health care providers to keep abreast of the government mandates.

It is essential that all members of the health care team have responsibility to protect their patients and themselves from infectious diseases. This responsibility has many aspects. The medical assistant is an important part of the overall protection picture. As a professional medical assistant, you must stay informed of changes in the practice of infection control. It is also imperative that you conduct yourself with the highest level of integrity in regard to limiting the spread of infection by utilizing all of the skills and interventions that have been reviewed in this chapter. Remember that breaking the infection cycle is everyone's responsibility.

STUDY FOR SUCCESS

To reinforce your knowledge and skills of information presented in this chapter:

- Review the *Key Terms*
- Role-play with other students to apply attributes of professionalism pertinent to this chapter.
- Consider the *Case Studies* and discuss your conclusions
- Answer the questions in the *Certification Review*
- Apply your knowledge by completing the *Activities* in the *Study Guide* and the *Games and Quizzes* in the StudyWARE **StudyWARE** software on the *Premium Website*
- Perform the *Procedures* using the *Competency Assessment Checklists* in the *Competency Manual*

continues

CERTIFICATION REVIEW

1. Standard Precautions are issued by:
   a. Health and Human Services
   b. Centers for Disease Control and Prevention
   c. Food & Drug Administration
   d. Occupational Safety and Health Administration

2. The *Bloodborne Pathogen Standard* is primarily concerned with:
   a. reducing the transmission of HIV, HBV, and HCV infections
   b. protecting the employer from lawsuits
   c. regulating the use of personal protective equipment
   d. taking blood samples from patients

3. In the infection cycle, the location of the infectious agent is known as the:
   a. reservoir
   b. portal of exit
   c. portal of entry
   d. means of transmission

4. The stage in infectious disease in which symptoms are vague and undifferentiated is called the:
   a. incubation stage
   b. prodromal stage
   c. acute stage
   d. onset of disease stage

5. There are several types of infectious organisms. Which of the following are considered pathogens?
   a. Fomite
   b. Virus
   c. Bacteria
   d. b and c

6. Choose the correct order for the stages of infection:
   a. prodromal, incubation, acute, declining, convalescent
   b. incubation, prodromal, acute, declining, convalescent
   c. acute, incubation, prodromal, convalescent, declining
   d. declining, convalescent, acute, prodromal, incubation

7. Sneezing, coughing, and talking can produce which type of disease transmission?
   a. Contact
   b. Airborne
   c. Droplet
   d. Standard

8. Use of handwashing and cleaning and disinfection of contaminated surfaces is known as:
   a. surgical asepsis
   b. medical asepsis
   c. sterilization
   d. all of the above

9. The CDC quotes the risk of infection with HIV from a single needlestick as:
   a. 3%
   b. 30%
   c. 0.3%
   d. 10%

10. A cut on a healthy provider's finger would be considered which of the following stages in the infection cycle?
    a. Susceptible host
    b. Infectious agent
    c. Portal of entry
    d. All of the above

REFERENCES/BIBLIOGRAPHY

Abedon, Stephen T. (2003). Important words and concepts from Chapter 14, Black, 1999. Retrieved May 21, 2012, from http://www.mansfield.ohio-state.edu/~sabedon/black14.htm

Altman, G. B. (2004). *Delmar's fundamentals and advanced nursing skills* (2nd ed.). Clifton Park, NY: Delmar Cengage Learning.

American Academy of Pediatrics. (2009). Prologue. In L. K. Pickering (Ed.), *Red Book: 2009 Report of the Committee on Infectious Diseases*. (28th ed., pp. 1–2). Elk Grove Village, IL: American Academy of Pediatrics.

Arbique, J. (2006). Fingernail length and microbes. *Suite 101*. Retrieved May 15, 2012, from http://judy-arbique.suite101.com/fingernail-length-and-microbes-a9646#ixzz1pVeYmdye

Bloomfield, S. F., et al. (2007). Extensively drug-resistant tuberculosis.

Goldmann, Donald A., MD, et al. (1996). Strategies to prevent and control the emergence and spread of antimicrobial-resistant microorganisms in hospitals: A challenge to hospital leadership. *AMA, 275*(3), 234–240.

Growth requirements for microorganisms. (n.d.). Retrieved May 20, 2012, from http://www.cliffsnotes.com/study_guide/Growth-Requirements-for-Microorganisms.topicArticleId-8524,articleId-8423.html

Infectious Disease Epidemiology, Prevention and Control Division, STD and HIV Section, Minnesota Department of Health. (2007). Hepatitis B and HIV/AIDS. Retrieved June 9, 2007, from http://www.health.state.mn.us

Josephson, D. L. (2004). *Intravenous infusion therapy for nurses: Principles and practices* (2nd ed.). Clifton Park, NY: Delmar Cengage Learning.

Keir, L., Wise, B. A., & Krebs, C. (2008). *Medical assisting: Administrative and clinical competencies* (6th ed.). Clifton Park, NY: Delmar Cengage Learning.

McNeil, S. A., Phelps, A., Barnes, A., & Kauffman, C. A. (2001). The effect of fingernail length on microbial colonization of the hands of health care workers (HCW). *39th Annual Meeting of the Infectious Diseases Society of America (IDSA), 2001.*

Merck. (2009). Host defense mechanisms against infection. In *The Merck Manual for Health Care Professionals.* Retrieved May 21, 2012, from http://www.merckmanuals.com/professional/infectious_diseases/biology_of_infectious_disease/host_defense_mechanisms_against_infection.html

Mount Sinai Hospital, Department of Microbiology. (2007). FAQ: Methods of disease transmission. Retrieved May 18, 2012, from http://microbiology.mtsinai.on.ca/faq/transmission.shtml

Occupational Safety and Health Administration. Bloodborne Pathogens–1910.1030 (Regulations [Standards–29CFR]). Retrieved June 11, 2007, from http://osha.gov

Pommerville, J. C. (2004). *Alcamo's fundamentals of microbiology* (7th ed.). Sudbury, MA: Jones and Bartlett Publishers.

Siegel, J. D., et al., and the Healthcare Infection Control Practices Advisory Committee. (2007). *2007 Guidelines for isolation precautions: preventing transmission of infectious agents in healthcare settings.* Retrieved May 18, 2012, from http://www.cdc.gov/hicpac/pdf/isolation/Isolation2007.pdf

Simmers, L. (2004). *Diversified health occupations* (6th ed.). Clifton Park, NY: Delmar Cengage Learning.

Venes, D., (Ed.). (2002). *Taber's cyclopedic medical dictionary* (21st ed.). Philadelphia: F. A. Davis.

Tamparo, C. D. & Lewis, M. A. (2005). *Diseases of the human body* (4th ed.). Philadelphia: F. A. Davis.

U.S. Department of Health and Human Services, Centers for Disease Control and Prevention. (2001). (Federal Register). Washington, DC: U.S. Government Printing Office. Retrieved June 11, 2007, from U.S. Department of Health and Human Services. (2010). *2010 National vaccine plan: Protecting the nation's health through immunization.* Retrieved May 18, 2012, from http://www.hhs.gov/nvpo/vacc_plan/2010%20Plan/nationalvaccineplan.pdf

U.S. Department of Health and Human Services, Centers for Disease Control and Prevention. (2004). *Facts about pneumonic plague.* Retrieved June 14, 2007, from http://www.emergency.cdc.gov/agent/plague/factsheet.asp

U.S. Department of Health and Human Services, Centers for Disease Control and Prevention. (2002). Guideline for hand hygiene in health-care settings: Recommendations of the Healthcare Infection Control Practices Advisory Committee and the HICPAC/SHEA/APIC/IDSA Hand Hygiene Task Force. *MMWR, 51*(16), 1–44.

U.S. Department of Health and Human Services, Centers for Disease Control and Prevention. (2012). *Healthcare associated infections (HAI).* Retrieved May 18, 2012, from http://www.cdc.gov/hai

U.S. Department of Health and Human Services, Centers for Disease Control and Prevention. (2010). *Precautions to prevent the spread of MRSA in healthcare settings.* Retrieved May 22, 2012, from http://www.cdc.gov/mrsa/prevent/healthcare/precautions.html

U.S. Department of Health and Human Services, Centers for Disease Control and Prevention. (2010). *Prevention strategies for seasonal influenza in healthcare settings.* Retrieved May 21, 2012, from http://www.cdc.gov/flu/professionals/infectioncontrol/healthcaresettings.htm

U.S. Department of Health and Human Services, Centers for Disease Control and Prevention. (n.d.). *Respiratory hygiene/cough etiquette in healthcare settings.* Retrieved May 21, 2012, from http://www.cdc.gov/flu/professionals/infectioncontrol/resphygiene.htm

World Health Organization. (2012). Hepatitis B. Retrieved Jul 22, 2012, from http://www.who.int/mediacentre/factsheets/fs204/en/

Weissman, C., et al. (2002). Transmission of prions. *Proceedings of the National Academy of Sciences, 99*(4), 16378–16383. Retrieved May 22, 2012, from http://www.pnas.org/content/99/suppl.4/16378.full.pdf

CHAPTER 23

The Patient History and Documentation

OUTLINE

The Purpose of the Medical History

Preparing for the Patient

A Cross-Cultural Model

Patient Information Forms

    Demographic Data Form

    Financial Information Form

    Privacy Information Form

    Release of Information Form

    Medical History Form

Computerized Health History

The Patient Intake Interview

    Interacting with the Patient

    Displaying Cultural Awareness

Being Sensitive to Patient Needs

    Approaching Sensitive Topics

Communication across the Life Span

The Medical Health History

    SOAP/SOAPER and CHEDDAR

    Chief Complaint

    History of Present Illness

    Medical History

    Family History

    Social History

    Review of Systems (ROS)

The Patient Record and Its Importance

    HIPAA Compliance

    Contents of Medical Records

    Continuity of Care Record

Methods of Charting/Documentation

    Source-Oriented Medical Records

    Problem-Oriented Medical Records

Electronic Medical Records (EMR)

Rules of Charting

    Abbreviations Used in Charting

    Chart Organization

LEARNING OUTCOMES

1. Define, spell, and pronounce the key terms as presented in the glossary.

2. Explain the purpose of the medical history.

3. Recall three functions to complete prior to a patient's appointment.

4. Compare/contrast the cross-cultural concerns between patients and providers.

5. Describe the four nonmedical information forms to be signed by patients.

6. Discuss the medical assistant's general approach to the patient intake interview.

7. Recall at least four circumstances to address in displaying cultural awareness.

8. Develop a strategy for communicating across the life span with patients.

9. Identify the components of the medical health history and their documentation.

10. Obtain a medical history from a patient.

11. Restate the function and meaning of SOAP/SOAPER and CHEDDAR charting.

12. List the characteristics of the patient's chief complaint and the present illness.

13. Compare/contrast the patient's medical, family, and social histories.

14. Discuss the rationale for including adult immunizations in health histories.

15. Explain how the review of systems is obtained and documented.

16. State five reasons why the medical record is important.

17. Identify three areas of concern regarding HIPAA compliance and the patient's chart.

18. Recall the rules for charting and documenting in the patient's chart.

19. Compare/contrast SOMR and POMR.

20. List the advantages of electronic medical records.

21. Review common charting abbreviations.

22. Describe the organization of a medical record.

23. Analyze the professionalism questions and apply them to this chapter's content.

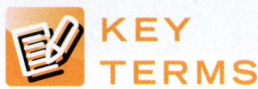

KEY TERMS

allergies

CHEDDAR

chief complaint

clinical diagnosis

objective

problem-oriented medical record (POMR)

SOAP/SOAPER

source-oriented medical record (SOMR)

subjective

ATTRIBUTES OF PROFESSIONALISM

Communication

- Did you introduce yourself? Did you identify the patient through name and birth date or other identifying feature?
- Did you speak at the patient's level of understanding?
- Did you display appropriate body language?
- Did you respond honestly and diplomatically to the patient's concerns?
- Did you apply active listening skills?
- Did you maintain eye contact with the patient during communication?
- Did you refrain from sharing your personal experiences?
- Did you accurately and concisely update the provider on any aspect of the patient's care?

Presentation

- Did you do something to bond with the patient?
- Did your actions attend to both the psychological and the physiologic aspects of the patient's illness or condition?
- Did you attend to any special needs of the patient? Did you first ask if assistance was needed, rather than taking charge?
- Were you courteous, patient, and respectful to the patient?
- Did you display a calm, professional, and caring manner?

Competency

- Did you pay attention to detail?
- Did you apply critical thinking skills in performing patient assessment and care?
- Did you recognize the importance of local, state, and federal legislation and regulations in the practice setting?

Initiative

- Were you flexible and dependable?
- Did you assist coworkers when appropriate?

Integrity

- Did you demonstrate sensitivity to patient's rights?
- Were you respectful of others?
- Did you protect personal boundaries?
- Did you demonstrate respect for individual diversity?
- Did you demonstrate an appreciation for the patient's attitude toward the illness or condition?
- Did you protect and maintain confidentiality?

SCENARIO

When clinical medical assistant Joe Guerrero, CMA (AAMA), of Drs. Lewis and King takes a patient history, he typically uses a form custom designed for the clinic. Joe uses the form as a guideline to be sure he gathers all pertinent information. However, he has learned that he must tailor his questions to the patient and sometimes will rearrange the order of the questions if necessary. Although Joe is adept at gathering specific and necessary patient information, he also is aware of patient concerns and sensitivities and adapts his approach to accomplish the task while making the patient feel at ease.

INTRODUCTION

A patient's medical record and all information in it, including the medical history, are key to competent medical care. Ideally, from the first encounter with the patient to any subsequent visits, all information regarding a patient's medical care is kept in one location—with the primary care provider.

The record created for all new patients will include a number of vital pieces of information. Established patients will have information updated upon each visit. Essential components of a complete medical record include present and past medical history, family and social history, chief complaints or problems, medications, allergies, laboratory results, summaries from other practitioners seen, and a host of other data related to the patient's health. A patient's record will also include demographic data, address, next of kin, and current insurance information.

Often, a family practice or internal medicine clinic will have a broad and rather extensive questionnaire for patients to complete which serves as the basis for the medical history. These questionnaires can be purchased or created on the computer, and they may be unique according to specialty. The questionnaire can be accessed via the clinic website; attached to an email to patients; or mailed to a patient's home address so that questions can be answered in the quiet environment of their homes, where they likely have access to the information requested. When patients are called the day before their appointment, they can be reminded to bring the completed questionnaire with them.

The role of the medical assistant in taking the patient history is to be as thorough as possible and still remain sensitive to the patient. Respect for the patient's privacy is to be balanced with the need for the kind of complete information that results in informed medical treatment and care.

The patient medical record is a collection of confidential patient information. Should a patient's medical record be introduced in court, it becomes a legal record of care given. It is essential that charting in the record be accurate, clear, concise, and complete.

THE PURPOSE OF THE MEDICAL HISTORY

The medical history is the basis for all treatment given by the primary care provider, on-call provider, any other provider, and any specialist consulted to treat the patient. During the history-taking process, information is revealed to help guide treatment for the patient. The medical history makes it easier to recall previous treatment and review notes and laboratory results.

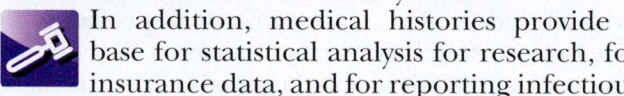 In addition, medical histories provide a base for statistical analysis for research, for insurance data, and for reporting infectious diseases to the health department. The health history and chart notes are a legal record of patient treatment. This is especially important if the patient makes an injury claim against another party or if the patient makes a malpractice claim against the provider. If the records in the chart are precise and correct, the chart becomes a good defense; however, if the charting or documentation is sloppy or incomplete, the entire record may be questioned as insufficient. The best policy is to document everything concerning patient care. See Chapter 14 for information on medical records management.

PREPARING FOR THE PATIENT

Before the patient's visit and obtaining the medical history, perform the following:

1. Make certain the examination room is clean, tidy, and ready for the patient.
2. Check to see that all necessary supplies are available.
3. Review the patient's chart. Note the age, any possible need for assistance, and identified reason for the appointment.

When everything is ready, go to the reception area for the patient. It is preferable to call the patient's full name (John Nichols or Mr. Nichols) unless the patient previously requested the use of the first name or a nickname. Speak clearly and plainly, making certain that your patient will be able to hear. When the patient stands, quickly determine if assistance is necessary. (The physical assessment has begun.) If assistance is warranted, make that offer and accompany the patient to the examination room, remembering later to note in the chart the assistance provided. A friendly greeting is appreciated and helpful; a greeting such as, "How are you today?" may not be appropriate. Patients in the medical clinic generally are not feeling well and take that question seriously. Also, the reception area is not the appropriate place for the patient to begin sharing his or her medical issues. The following comments may be acceptable: "Did you have any trouble finding parking?" or "I really like the colors in the shirt you are wearing. They remind me of summer."

Once in the examination room and the door is closed, seat the patient comfortably and sit face-to-face with the patient to begin the interview. Build rapport with the patient. Use the patient's name often and make certain you pronounce it correctly. Finally, think globally. Ask about factors in the patient's life that might influence health. These topics might be sports, travel, pets, family, and hobbies. Not only does this provide information for the health history, it usually eases and relaxes the patient for the more difficult questions in the interview.

A CROSS-CULTURAL MODEL

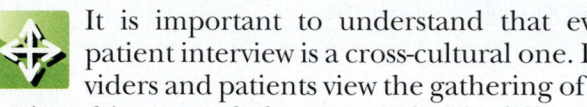 It is important to understand that every patient interview is a cross-cultural one. Providers and patients view the gathering of the patient history and the personal visit differently. Health and illness are inseparable from social and cultural beliefs. Who patients are—their background, their belief system, their family orientation, and their cultural heritage—influences their 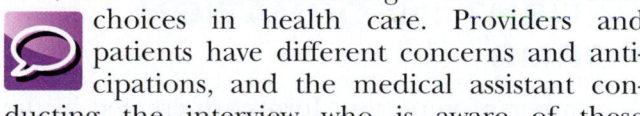 choices in health care. Providers and patients have different concerns and anticipations, and the medical assistant conducting the interview who is aware of these perspectives will keep the following in mind:

- *Patient's chief concern.* The illness. The personal and social significance and the problems created by the illness are important to the patient.
- *Provider's chief concern.* Disease. The provider is concerned with the malfunctioning and maladaptation of biological and psychological processes.
- *Patient's idea of treatment success.* Being able to successfully manage an illness and its problems is often more important to the patient than curing the disease.
- *Provider's idea of treatment success.* Successfully managing treatments, medications, and procedures to control disease problems.

 The medical assistant may find it helpful to ask certain questions of patients to help the medical assistant understand cultural influences for example:

1. What do you think caused your problem?
2. When do you think it started?
3. What effect does it have on you?
4. What are your concerns about this problem?
5. What kind of treatment do you expect?

These questions respect the patient's perceptions while providing helpful information to the provider.

PATIENT INFORMATION FORMS

A number of important forms are created in the medical setting at this time.

Demographic Data Form

The demographic data form (Figure 23-1) registers the patient's full name, address, mailing address if different, home and work telephone numbers, cell phone numbers, date of birth, a portion of the Social Security number, all insurance information, person to be contacted in case of emergency, and a release of information signature.

Financial Information Form

Some facilities include the financial information form (Figure 23-2) to be signed. This form contains information on the financial policy of the practice, including billing, insurance billing, co-payment billing, and any finance charges added to monthly billings.

Privacy Information Form

Since April 2004, the Health Insurance Portability and Accountability Act (HIPAA) privacy rule limited the circumstances in which individuals' protected health information (PHI) could be used or disclosed. It also required medical providers to give notice of their privacy practices to all patients. The notice must describe patients' rights, the facilities' practices related to PHI, and where and how to file a complaint if patients feel their rights have been violated. Health providers must make a good faith effort to obtain written acknowledgment from patients that the privacy notice was received.

HIPAA The privacy notice has a number of components and can be lengthy. Many facilities have printed their notice in a brochure format. Details of the Privacy Rule can be found on the U.S. Department of Health and Human Services Web site (http://www.hhs.gov/ocr/privacy/). Many varieties of privacy notices can be viewed online by searching for "HIPAA privacy notices."

There are civil penalties if a medical facility fails to comply with the Privacy Rule and criminal penalties if a person knowingly obtains or discloses PHI in violation of the HIPAA guidelines.

Release of Information Form

New patients may be asked to complete a Release of Information form (Figure 23-3) that is often created in the clinic. This form is sent to their former providers to obtain past medical records and in some cases can be used to allow sharing of information with family members at the request of the patient.

If the patient has several providers, the examining provider will encourage the patient to choose one person to manage primary medical care so that all medical care and records are concentrated in one location. Under most managed care insurance policies, patients have one primary care provider (women may also have an obstetrician/gynecologist) who coordinates the patient's health care.

Medical History Form

The medical health history form can be as short as one page ($8\frac{1}{2}'' \times 11''$) or as long and detailed as six to eight pages. This form includes information on:

1. Present health history, including why the patient is being seen
2. Health history, both personal and family
3. Social history including marital status, sexual orientation, and occupation

CODE		PATIENT INFORMATION			ACCOUNT

PLEASE PRINT

PATIENT	Mr. Mrs. Miss/Ms. Last	First	MI	HOME PHONE: ( )

Patient's Home Address	Street	City	State	Zip

Patient's Billing Address	Street	City	State	Zip

Social Security #	Date of Birth	Age	Sex	Driver's License #

Patient's Employer	Work Address		Work Phone:

Spouse's Name	Spouse's Employer (Name & Address)	Work Phone:

Emergency Contact:
(Local Relative or Friend) Name   Address   Phone:

REFERRED TO THIS OFFICE BY: _____

WHO IS YOUR PRIMARY PHYSICIAN? _____

INSURANCE	PLEASE LIST ALL HEALTH CARE INSURANCE COMPANIES WHICH COVER THIS PATIENT:

PRIMARY: Name _____ Policy # _____ Subscriber _____

Insurance Address _____

SECONDARY: Name _____ Policy# _____ Subscriber _____

Insurance Address _____

MEDICARE   # _____ (Please Include Letter)

MEDICAID   # _____
(MEDI-CAL)

RESPONSIBLE PARTY	Mr. Mrs. Miss/Ms. Last	First	Middle

Address   Phone:

Occupation   Employers Name & Address   Bus. Phone:

Please remember that insurance is considered a method of reimbursing the patient for fees paid to the doctor and is not a substitute for payment. Some companies pay fixed allowances for certain procedures, and others pay a percentage of the charge. It is your responsibility to pay any deductible amount, co-insurance, or any other balance not paid for by your insurance.

METHOD OF PAYMENT: CASH _____   CHECK _____   CREDIT CARD _____

PLEASE READ & SIGN THE FOLLOWING:
I directly assign all medical / surgical benefits to _____
and understand that I am financially responsible for all charges whether or not paid by insurance. I hereby authorize the doctor to release all information necessary to secure the payment of benefits. I further agree that a photocopy of this agreement shall be as valid as the original.

SIGN HERE _____ DATE: _____

FORM # 58-8421-01 · BIBBERO SYSTEMS, INC. · PETALUMA, CALIFORNIA © 10/85 (REV. 8/93) TO REORDER CALL TOLL FREE: 800-BIBBERO (800 242-2376) OR FAX: (800) 242-9330

Courtesy of Bibbero Systems, Inc., Petaluma, CA, 800-242-2376, www.bibbero.com

Figure 23-1 Sample patient demographic form.

FINANCIAL POLICY

In order to reduce confusion and misunderstanding between our patients and the clinic, we have adopted the following financial policy. If you have any questions about this policy, please discuss them with our Billing Manager. We are dedicated to providing the best possible care and service to you and we regard your complete understanding of your financial responsibilities as an essential element of your care and treatment.

Unless other arrangements have been made in advance by yourself or your health coverage carrier, <u>payment is due at time of service</u>. For your convenience, we accept debit or credit cards or we can arrange a payment schedule.

YOUR INSURANCE:

We accept assignment of benefit from Medicare. We also have direct billing agreements with many insurance companies. We will bill those plans for whom we have an agreement and will only require that you pay the co-payment at the time of service.

If your medical plan determines a service is "not covered," you will be responsible for the entire charge. Payment is due upon receipt of statement from this office.

MINOR PATIENTS:

The adult accompanying the patient and the parent or guardian with custody will be billed for all services rendered to minor patients.

MISSED APPOINTMENTS:

In order to provide the best service and availability to our patients, we ask you to notify us 24 hours in advance if you know that you will be unable to keep the appointment. We reserve the right to charge for missed appointments.

I have read the financial policy and I understand it and agree to be bound by its terms.

_____   Date _____

© Cengage Learning 2014

Figure 23-2   Sample financial information form.

AUTHORIZATION TO RELEASE HEALTH CARE INFORMATION

Patient _____ Date of Birth _____
SSN _____ Previous Name _____
I request and authorize _____ to release the health care information of the patient named above to:
Name _____
Address _____
This request and authorization applies to:
(Please initial the appropriate box)
__ Health care information relating to the following treatment, condition, or dates of treatment:

_____

__ All health care information **EXCLUDING** specific information relating to sexually transmitted diseases (including HIV/AIDS), alcohol or drug use, or visits related to psychiatric disorders or mental health.
__ All health care information **INCLUDING** specific information relating to sexually transmitted diseases (including HIV/AIDS), alcohol or drug use, or visits related to psychiatric disorders or mental health.
__ Other:_____
I understand that my express consent is required to release any health care information relating to testing, diagnosis, and/or treatment of HIV (AIDS virus), sexually transmitted disease, psychiatric disorders/mental health, or drug and/or alcohol use. If I have been tested, diagnosed, or treated for HIV (AIDS virus), sexually transmitted disease, psychiatric disorders/mental health, or drug and/or alcohol use, you are specifically authorized to release all health care information relating to such diagnosis, testing, or treatment.

_____ / _____
Signature of patient or patient's   Relationship
authorized representative   to patient

_____
Date

© Cengage Learning 2014

Figure 23-3   Authorization for release of information.

4. Military service, including dates and assignments (alerts provider to screen for common veteran illnesses and to inquire about Agent Orange exposure)

5. Body systems review/questionnaire

6. Medications currently being taken, including over-the-counter and prescription medications

7. Provider's review of systems (ROS) (completed by the provider)

The best form is neither too long nor too complicated. Patients may feel overwhelmed with a long form and may not finish it, stating they cannot remember all the information. The form that is simple and brief can provide adequate information in many instances. Some patients find a history form intimidating. It is often easier for these patients to talk directly with the medical assistant or the provider about the history, feeling a one-to-one exchange is more personal and private.

Many samples of health history forms can be viewed on the Internet. Facilities often ask patients who regularly use a computer and have Internet access to go online and print their health history form for completion prior to their appointment. Depending on the ambulatory care setting, this form can be tailored to include vaccines and immunizations, usage of recreational drugs, exercise and diet regimens, accident information (especially if patient was hurt on the job), and any other information suited to the provider's specialty. Health history forms can be printed in other languages, such as Spanish.

COMPUTERIZED HEALTH HISTORY

 Health care facilities may use totally computerized health histories. These can be of two types: patient-generated and provider-generated. In patient-generated health histories, the patient responds on the computer to various questions and then reviews information with the medical assistant for completeness. Patients who do not want to use a computer should be given the option of answering the questions face-to-face. When using a provider-generated health history, the medical assistant completes the information on the screen during the patient interview. These programs are user-friendly and save time for both the patient and medical assistant. The medical assistant should remember to interact with the patient by looking up from the computer from time to time during the entry of information. It is easy to forget to look at patients as you ask questions and enter the information. This habit can make the patient feel disconnected to the process.

THE PATIENT INTAKE INTERVIEW

Interacting with the Patient

When the medical assistant takes the medical history, the first responsibility is to put the patient at ease (Table 23-1). A comfort level must be developed as the medical assistant guides the conversation, keeps it on track, and obtains the most information for the provider. Allowing the conversation to wander, talking about other people, or letting the patient tell anecdotes does not help to complete the history. Explaining a term or concept that the patient does not understand is helpful. The medical assistant must remain professional and not be embarrassed or made uncomfortable by the patient's answers regarding illnesses, actions, or personal choices (Figure 23-4).

If the patient is already an established patient but has not seen the provider for several months or longer, update the medical history by asking if any illnesses have occurred in the time elapsed, if any new allergies to any medications or other substances have occurred, and what the reaction was to each. Document the chief complaint for the current visit. The **chief complaint (CC)** is the problem that brings the patient to the provider. Sometimes patients bring several problems to discuss.

Table 23-1 General Approach to the History

1. Ensure an appropriate environment that is clean, well lit, at a comfortable temperature, quiet, private, and free of distractions.

2. Sit facing the patient at eye level; the patient also should be seated. Ensure that the patient is as comfortable as possible, because obtaining the health history can be a lengthy process. Figure 23-4 illustrates an appropriate setting.

3. Treat the patient respectfully, addressing them by their formal name unless requested by the patient to use their first name or a nickname.

4. Avoid the use of medical jargon. Use terms the patient can understand.

5. Reserve asking intimate and personal questions until rapport is established.

6. Remain flexible in obtaining the health history. It does not need to be obtained in the exact order it is presented in this chapter or on the form.

7. Remember that the primary object of obtaining a health history is to listen to and accurately record the patient's statements.

8. Remind the patient that all information will be treated confidentially.

9. Ask the patient if he or she has any questions.

© Cengage Learning 2014

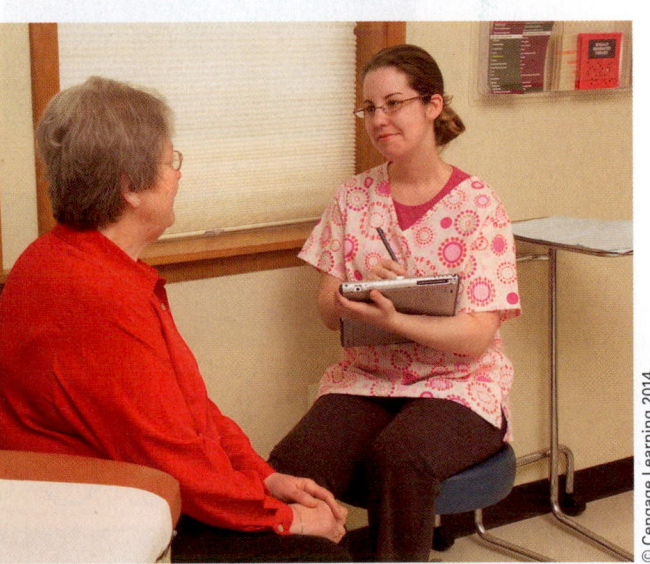

Figure 23-4 The medical assistant reviews the medical history from a computer tablet with a patient while still maintaining eye contact.

Depending on the appointment schedule for the day, this may be difficult to accomplish. If there is time in the schedule, every effort should be made to accommodate patients. However, the medical assistant notes the chief complaint before the provider sees the patient to ensure the main problem is addressed. Use of the electronic medical record (EMR) makes the patient intake process much easier. Little or no handwritten notes are necessary, and the data can be entered during the communication exchange between the medical assistant and the patient. Some settings allow the patient to see the data as they are entered. Figure 23-5 shows the importance of connecting all these data in a Total Practice Management System (TPMS).

Displaying Cultural Awareness

Remembering a cross-cultural model, the medical assistant begins the encounter with the patient aware that cultural differences and other problems may inhibit communication. Any number of situations may arise that the medical assistant must be prepared to address. The medical assistant will overcome major obstacles if it is known in advance the patient does not speak English as a first language or is hearing impaired and requires an interpreter, or that the patient is from a culture in which the female patient does not disrobe for a male provider, or that the patient has a mental disorder that makes communication difficult.

If there is a language difficulty, the medical assistant may be required to arrange for an interpreter. There are language interpreters in most areas; especially in large urban areas, an interpreter might be found for nearly any language. If the patient is receiving medical care through Medicaid, special arrangements can be made for an interpreter through the state agency administering the program. Often the patient will bring a family member to interpret; however, if the matter is personal, the patient may not want to reveal personal matters with the family member present and may prefer an outside, objective interpreter. If the interpreter comes to the clinic as a contractor, a business associate contract should be completed to comply

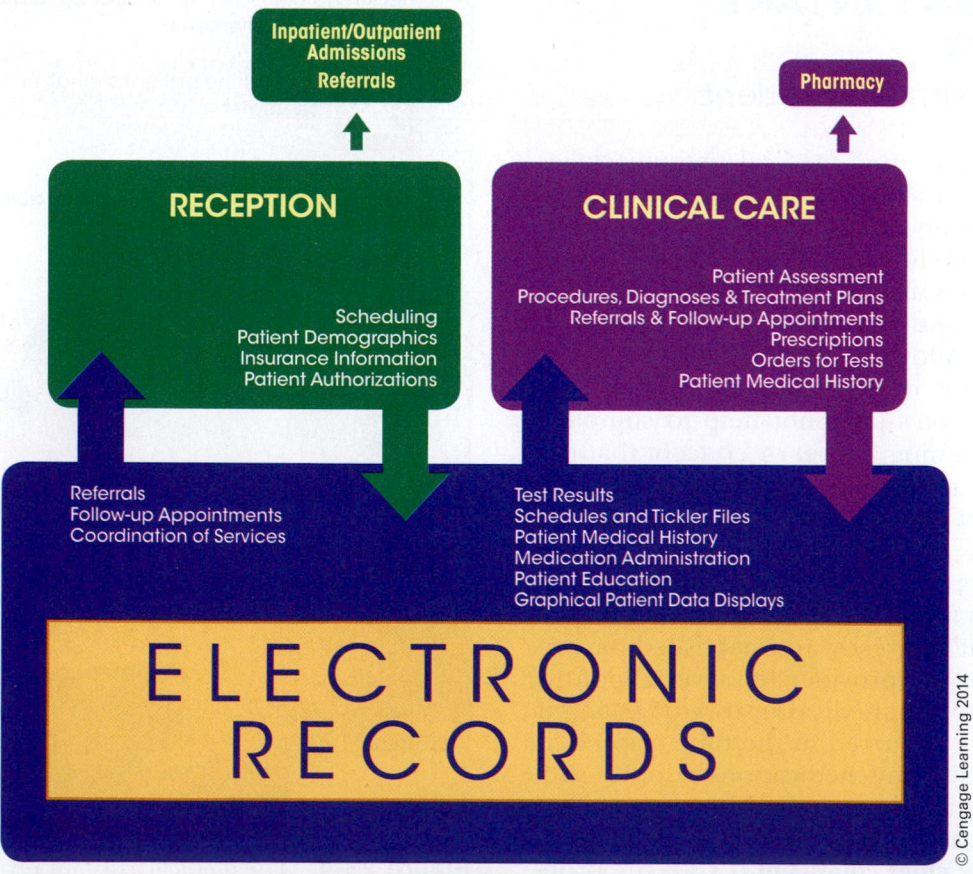

Figure 23-5 TPMS diagram illustrating the relationship between reception and clinical care activities to a patient's medical record.

with HIPAA regulations. The contract is not necessary for a family member, a volunteer, or a clinic employee serving as an interpreter.

The medical assistant will listen attentively to the patient. The patient may be uneasy talking to the provider and may be more comfortable telling the medical assistant about problems. Medical assistants can play an important part in the medical practice by listening and communicating with both the patient and the provider.

Being Sensitive to Patient Needs

Some patients are frightened, hostile, or depressed. It is important to be open to nonverbal and verbal communication in answer to questions. Some patients react positively to a hand placed gently on the forearm; it calms and reassures them. Others have a negative response, pulling away from any such contact. Maintaining a professional boundary with the patient is essential. Boundaries respect the patient's needs for privacy, nurturing, validation, and separation (see Chapter 5 for additional information).

The medical assistant will know when to touch the patient appropriately, always with permission either expressed or implied. If the medical assistant tells the patient a blood pressure reading is next and reaches for the patient's arm and the patient extends an arm, permission to take the reading is implied. If, however, the patient pulls away and states no blood pressure is to be taken, permission is not given, and the reading must not be done at that time. This is charted as "patient refused."

Trying to get information from a reluctant patient can be difficult and requires patience and understanding. If the patient is hesitant to discuss a problem, it is better not to press for information. Pressing for information may make the patient become defensive or angry and can impair communication altogether. Make your provider aware of the patient behaviors that you observe so that he or she may be prepared to interact with the patient.

A patient may come to the clinic upset and crying. This patient must be made to feel more in control, and that no one is going to rush the care being given. Sometimes just taking a few moments to sit with such patients until they feel more settled is enough to calm them and enable the history-taking interview to proceed.

Uncommunicative patients require special questioning techniques. The medical assistant may have to supply a sample of problems to get these patients to acknowledge the health concerns they have. Or they may shrug their shoulders at every question and be unresponsive. Some patients may simply say, "I don't know. I just don't feel well." If a relative has accompanied the patient to the appointment, it may be appropriate initially to have the relative present with the patient. In this way the patient has a familiar face in the unfamiliar, often frightening, clinic. It is always the patient's decision whether anyone else is to be in the room.

Some patients have particular needs that they are willing to express. Meeting these needs is usually a minor matter and makes patients feel more comfortable. For example, "Can you help me undress and get into the gown?"

Approaching Sensitive Topics

Some of the most sensitive topics addressed in the health history include the use of alcohol, recreational drugs or chemicals, smoking, dietary habits, obesity, and sexual practices. An honest reporting on these topics can be important to the patient's well-being and treatment. Consider:

- Assuring the patient that the environment is private and free from distractions.
- Asking these questions in the later stages of the interview after rapport has been established.
- Using casual, direct eye contact without staring; this demonstrates the importance of the topic to the patient and your lack of embarrassment.
- Posing questions in a matter-of-fact tone.
- Adopting a nonjudgmental demeanor.
- Using the communication technique of "normalizing" when appropriate (e.g., "Some high school students drink alcohol/use drugs/engage in sexual relationships on a regular basis. Does this happen at your school? With you?").

If the medical assistant can enhance communication with the patient, communication between the provider and the patient will be more effective.

CRITICAL THINKING

With two others in your class, role-play a scenario where one person is the patient, another is the medical assistant, and the third is an observer. A social history is being taken. As the medical assistant you ask the patient about the use of any recreational drugs or chemicals. The patient responds, "Yes." What additional questions will you ask the patient? What will you include in the medical record?

COMMUNICATION ACROSS THE LIFE SPAN

Keep in mind your patient's age when communicating and seeking information for the medical history. A parent or caregiver often accompanies a child. An infant will want to feel your physical support, your warmth, and a smile. As the child grows, time will be spent communicating with the child as well as the parent. During this time, you may be dealing with two patients, discussing with the parent the problem the child has and assisting the parent in understanding procedures, treatment, and so on. There can come a time, however, when a child may do much better without a parent present. This can be a sensitive issue for parents. Sometimes a couple of simple statements might help; for example, "Dr. Chalmers will want to establish some rapport with your son for a few minutes. Please come with me while I get the literature that she wants you to have. Often these visits can be harder on parents than the children."

Teenagers are old enough to make the decision about being seen alone or with a parent present. Some are comfortable; others are not. Teenagers who have had the same primary care provider since early childhood and have already established a relationship are more likely to feel comfortable without parents. Review a teenager's right to consent in Chapter 7.

Older adults may be accompanied by another adult and may request that the individual be present during the interview. Others may prefer to be alone. Adults who have difficulty hearing, who are memory impaired, who are visually impaired, or whose language may not be understood are likely to be accompanied by another person. Some older adults find it difficult to answer questions in front of their children or even a spouse. Although it is not necessary for relatives, it is a good idea to have a HIPAA waiver signed by the patient, as long as they understand what is being signed. Remember that the intent of HIPAA is *not* to make communication more difficult or cumbersome; it is intended to protect a patient's privacy.

Chapters 27 and 29 have helpful suggestions for communications with children and with older adults.

THE MEDICAL HEALTH HISTORY

The patient's medical health history contains the following components:

- Personal data from the demographic form
- Chief complaint as noted at each visit by the medical assistant
- Present illness
  - Medications
  - Allergies
  - Other providers or alternative therapy practitioners being seen
- Medical history
- Family history
- Social and occupational history
- Review of systems by physician or provider

SOAP/SOAPER and CHEDDAR

The **SOAP/SOAPER** method of charting was introduced in Chapter 14. SOAP charting is very common; SOAPER is increasing in popularity and is often used in clinics attached to teaching and research hospitals (Figure 23-6). **CHEDDAR** is another approach to charting that may be used. These charting methods encourage more comprehensive charting and make evaluating and managing the levels of service easier to document.

SOAP/SOAPER stands for the following:

S Subjective data; patient's complaint in his or her own words

O Objective, observable, measurable findings

A Assessment, probable diagnosis based on subjective and objective factors

P Plan for treatment, medications, instructions, return visit information

E Education for the patient

R Response of patient to education and care given

PATIENT EDUCATION

Some Asian cultures calculate age from conception, not from the actual birth date. For example, a newborn infant is considered to be 1 year old. The medical assistant needs to clarify the chronologic age with the patient or caregiver. This is particularly important for pediatric patients because of the link between age and developmental milestones.

Walter Pethokoukis
Date of Birth: 01/22/1949
Visit Date: 04/04/20XX

S: Patient returns after undergoing upper GI; not in as much discomfort as last visit. States he has been taking clear liquids and soft foods. Says he is hungry.

O: Lab results are back. Chem 7 shows slightly elevated glucose at 133. CBC and UA normal. Upper GI shows two small areas of ulceration.

A: Gastric ulcer.

P: Reduce omeprazole to 10 mg every day. Recheck glucose at return visit in 4 weeks.

E: Patient was advised not to smoke or chew tobacco, limit alcohol intake, and avoid aspirin, ibuprofen, and naproxen. Try acetaminophen instead. No diet restrictions indicated.

R: Patient was relieved; indicates there is no problem following the above plan and recommendation. MM/tim

© Cengage Learning 2014

Figure 23-6 Sample of a SOAP/SOAPER follow-up visit note.

CHEDDAR charting encourages greater detail to SOAP/SOAPER. CHEDDAR stands for the following:

C Chief complaint, presenting problems, subjective information

H History, social and physical, of presenting problem; contributing data

E Examination; body systems reviewed

D Details of problem(s) and complaint(s)

D Drugs and dosages; list of current medications, dosages, frequency

A Assessment; diagnostic evaluation, further testing, medications

R Return visit, if applicable

The medical assistant and the primary care provider in attendance to the patient both contribute to the completeness of the medical history using SOAP/SOAPER and CHEDDAR. A more detailed review of the information in these medical history components follows.

Chief Complaint

The chief complaint (usually abbreviated CC) is the specific reason that brought the patient to see the provider. It should be noted in as few words as possible but be very specific. It can be a direct quote from the patient.

A good example of a chief complaint notation might be: "I've had nausea and vomiting for three days." This is a **subjective** complaint in that it is known by the patient but cannot be seen or measured by the provider. It is specific, however, in relating the patient's condition. Another example is: "I hurt my ankle yesterday when I tripped over a curb." Again this is subjective but specific about cause, time of onset, and complaint. The ankle is visibly swollen and painful to touch. The swelling is an **objective** sign, a manifestation that can be seen, heard, or measured by any observer.

In contrast, a poor example of a chief complaint is "has not been feeling well." This notation tells nothing about what symptoms or problems the patient has been experiencing. It gives no specific clue as to the problem from the patient's perspective. The medical assistant should try to pinpoint a complaint to a body system, to a time frame, and to discomfort in a specific area. The patient usually will respond to questions that offer several options.

Certain characteristics of each chief complaint should be ascertained for a complete history. These characteristics are:

- Location
- Radiation
- Quality
- Severity
- Associated symptoms
- Aggravating factors
- Alleviating factors
- Timing

History of Present Illness

Asking about the history of the present illness is a critical step in allowing the provider to make a diagnosis. The chief complaint is expanded to give more information and detail. Allow the patient to describe the history in their own words.

- *Location* will describe the place where the symptom is located. Ask the patient to be as specific as possible. For instance, "I have pain on the inner thigh of my left leg" is more helpful than "my leg hurts."

- *Radiation* helps describe the symptom more by identifying how large an area the symptom covers. The patient might describe a "tingling sensation all over my left leg," for instance.

- *Quality* addresses the characteristic of the symptom. The description might be "tingling and buzzing," or the pain described as "a dull ache" or "throbbing" or "stabbing."

- *Severity* of symptoms will include such descriptions as "keeps me awake at night," or "causes me to put little or no pressure on the leg." When the symptom is pain, patients may be asked to identify the pain on a scale of 1 to 10, with 10 being the most severe.

- *Associated symptoms* allows the patient to describe what other minor symptoms accompany the chief complaint. "Because I am limping and putting more weight on my right leg, my right hip aches much of the time."

- *Aggravating factors* and *alleviating factors* get at what makes the symptoms worse and what makes the symptoms decrease. "Walking fast or bending forward really hurts. Sitting down with my feet up on a stool makes it all feel better." You will also want to know what the patient has done to treat the problem and if any medications have been taken for the symptoms. The *setting* and *timing* have to do with when the symptoms started and what the patient was doing at symptom onset.

In the preceding example of nausea and vomiting, the patient may indicate inability to eat or take fluids. This would alert the provider to possible dehydration. Often the present illness is based on a prior health problem. For instance, a history of congestive heart failure gives a patient's symptoms of fluid retention, wheezing, and shortness of breath more importance because these are common complications. Without knowledge of the patient's medical history, these symptoms could be confused with bronchitis, asthma, or pneumonia.

Some practitioners will ask the medical assistant to address other topics in the present illness. These questions include the following:

- Are you allergic to anything? Again, the medical chart may note any allergies, but this question alerts the staff to any potential problems and updates the chart. It is a safety measure important to both the patient and provider.

- Are there any other problems you are experiencing at this time? This question allows patients to indicate if there is something other than the chief complaint about which they have concerns.

- What medications are you taking? Even though the patient's chart will indicate some of this information, this is not the case for a new patient. Most patients do not include any over-the-counter medications or alternative therapies they may be using. Some facilities will ask the patients to bring every medication they are currently taking with them to the first visit. Be certain to ask about over-the-counter items such as vitamins, pain medications, herbal remedies, and so on.

Medications and allergies should be reviewed each time the patient is seen in a medical facility. All medications are to be listed. Some patients will benefit from specific questions about over-the-counter medications. If there are no known allergies, it should be noted so the provider knows the topic has been discussed. When there are allergies, they usually are listed on every page of the progress notes or on the summary page in an EMR. Some facilities have begun the practice of printing out the list of all medications and allergies to give to the patient who might want to provide it to any other practitioners.

Medical History

The medical history includes all the patient's health problems, major illnesses, and surgeries. If not included under present illness, all current medications are noted, including dosages and reasons for taking them, as well as all allergies to any medications and the specific allergic reaction to each. These are important to the medical history, because many health problems can overlap and affect the patient in several areas. A patient with a long history of diabetes mellitus may present with an ulcer on his foot. Whereas the same ulcer in an otherwise healthy patient will heal with little intervention, the diabetic patient may require major treatment and attention including debridement (removal of dead or damaged tissue or foreign debris), antibiotics, and close monitoring.

Medications have side effects and contraindications that can affect patients. **Allergies** to medications can be serious and need to be noted in a readily visible part of the chart. A red sticker is often placed in a conspicuous area on the inside cover of the paper chart noting allergies. In a similar fashion, notations will be made in the electronic chart, usually on the summary page, to alert clinic providers and staff members of possible allergies. The information needs to be updated at least annually.

If possible, update immunizations for adults at this time. Childhood immunizations are regularly checked in pediatric examinations. Not all adults recall their records, but some questions can help providers determine if any immunizations are to be given. Refer to Chapter 22 for the immunization schedule for adults.

Family History

The family history can provide clues to the patient's present condition. By asking open-ended questions about medical problems of siblings, parents, and grandparents, the provider is alerted to hereditary and familial diseases and disorders such as coronary artery disease, hypertension, breast cancer, and so forth. Present ages of siblings, parents, and grandparents or causes of their death and age at time of death are noted. For instance,

PATIENT EDUCATION

In some cultures (e.g., Chinese, some Native Americans), it is disrespectful to speak of the dead. Thus, the patient may be reluctant to provide detailed information on the family health history of dead relatives. In these cases, you can ask the patient if there has been any history of specific diseases in the family and not focus on the specific individual if that person is deceased. The patient may be willing to share in which previous generation and on which side of the family the condition existed. If these approaches are unsuccessful, explain to the patient the importance of this information, because it may provide clues to the patient's current health conditions.

a family history of diabetes together with the patient's symptoms of frequent urination and thirst may make a diagnosis of diabetes mellitus a possibility. Be sensitive, however, to cultural variances (see the Patient Education box).

Social History

The social history of patients includes their spouse/partner status; sexual habits; occupation; hobbies; and use of alcohol, tobacco, and recreational drugs or other chemical substances. This part of the history includes those lifestyles and behaviors that may put the patient at greater risk for injury or disease than would normally be found from factors in the family history and medical history.

Patients may not want to answer questions pertaining to sexual history; attempt to return to these questions later. Ask if discussing sexual activity with the provider would make the patient more comfortable.

The adolescent patient may refuse to answer questions of a sexual matter or may provide false answers if the parent or caregiver is present. It may be best to ask the parent or caregiver to leave the room at the completion of the health history so that you can ask the patient if there is anything else to note in the sexual history.

Be alert for cues that demonstrate the patient's desire for knowledge on sexual matters, such as questions or requests for written information. Answer the patient's questions, provide educational materials, and refer the patient to a specialist when indicated.

It may be necessary to inquire about the patient's home environment. Be attentive for clues that signal the necessity of performing an in-depth home environment assessment. Some clues include, but are not limited to, poor hygiene, frequent infections, smoke inhalation, burns, malnutrition, and falls (especially in older adults).

Review of Systems (ROS)

Once the medical history has been taken, it is time to prepare the patient for the examination. Note for the provider any questions for which you were unable to get a complete answer from the patient or any areas where you have concerns. Thank the patient for his or her time and information during the interview. In clear terms and not speaking too rapidly, explain to the patient the need to disrobe, put on a gown, and be seated on the examination table. (Chapter 33 describes how to transfer a patient in a wheelchair to the examination table.) *Always* ask if the patient needs assistance in disrobing. It is also wise to let the patient know that you can return in a few minutes to assist him or her onto the examination table if necessary. This allows you to see that the patient is comfortably settled and to give him or her an estimate of how long it will be before the provider is coming in for the examination.

The ROS is performed during the physical examination. When a patient is seen on a fairly regular basis, only the pertinent body system will be reviewed. In a complete physical examination, an orderly and systematic check of each part of the body is recorded. The provider asks questions concerning each organ and system of the body during the examination of the patient. The ROS, in conjunction with the physical examination, helps elicit information that is essential to the diagnosis of disease. The provider usually begins with an overall assessment and proceeds to check each body system in an organized manner. The order in which this is done may vary by providers, but all will check the cardiovascular, respiratory, gastrointestinal, genitourinary, and neurologic systems, as well as the extremities, the musculoskeletal system, and the skin.

Both positive and pertinent negative findings are documented in the ROS. When a response is positive, the patient is asked to describe it as completely as possible. Table 23-2 lists some symptoms

Table 23-2 Review of Systems

General	Patient's perception of general state of health at the present time; difference from usual state; vitality and energy levels
Neurological	Headache, change in balance, change in coordination, loss of movement, change in sensory perception/feeling in an extremity, change in speech, change in smell, fainting, loss of memory, tremors, involuntary movement, loss of consciousness, seizures, weakness, head injury, disorientation, dizziness
Psychological	Irritability, nervousness, tension, increased stress, difficulty concentrating, mood changes, suicidal thoughts, depression
Skin	Rashes, itching, changes in skin pigmentation, black and blue marks, change in color or size of mole, sores, lumps, change in skin texture, odors, excessive sweating, acne, loss of hair, excessive growth of hair or growth of hair in unusual locations, change in nails, amount of time spent in the sun
Eyes	Blurry vision, visual acuity, glasses, contact lenses, sensitivity to light, excessive tearing, night blindness, double vision, drainage, bloodshot, pain, blind spots, flashing lights, halos around objects, glaucoma, cataracts
Ears	Hearing deficits, hearing aid, pain, discharge, lightheadedness, ringing in the ears, earaches, infection
Nose and Sinuses	Frequent colds, discharge, itching, hay fever, postnasal drip, stuffiness, sinus pain, polyps, obstruction, nosebleed, change in sense of smell
Mouth	Toothache, tooth abscess, dentures, bleeding/swollen gums, difficulty chewing, sore tongue, change in taste, lesions, change in salivation, bad breath
Throat/Neck	Hoarseness, change in voice, frequent sore throats, difficulty swallowing, pain/stiffness, enlarged thyroid
Respiratory	Shortness of breath, shortness of breath on exertion, phlegm, cough, sneezing, wheezing, coughing up blood, frequent upper respiratory tract infections, pneumonia, emphysema, asthma, tuberculosis
Cardiovascular	Shortness of breath that wakes patient up in the night, chest pain, heart murmur, palpitations, fainting, sleep on pillows to breathe better, swelling, cold hands/feet, leg cramps, myocardial infarction, hypertension, valvular disease, pain in calf with walking, varicose veins, inflammation of a vein, blood clot in leg, anemia

Table 23-2   Review of Systems (*Continued*)

Breasts	Pain, tenderness, discharge, lumps, change in size, dimpling
Gastrointestinal	Change in appetite, nausea, vomiting, diarrhea, constipation, usual bowel habits, black and tarry stools, vomiting blood, change in stool color, excessive gas, belching, regurgitation or heartburn, difficulty swallowing, abdominal pain, jaundice, hemorrhoids, hepatitis, peptic ulcers, gallstones
Urinary	Change in urine color, voiding habits, painful urination, hesitancy, urgency, frequency, excessive urination at night, increased urine volume, dribbling, loss in force of stream, bed-wetting, change in urine volume, incontinence, pain in lower abdomen, kidney stones, urinary tract infections
Musculoskeletal	Joint stiffness, muscle pain, back pain, limitation of movement, redness, swelling, weakness, bony deformity, broken bones, dislocations, sprains, gout, arthritis, osteoporosis, herniated disc
Female Reproductive	Vaginal discharge, change in libido, infertility, sterility, pain during intercourse, menses (last menstrual period, age period started, regularity, duration, amount of bleeding, premenstrual symptoms, intermenstrual bleeding, painful periods), menopause (age of onset, duration, symptoms, bleeding), obstetrical (number of pregnancies, number of miscarriages/abortions, number of children, type of delivery, complications), type of birth control, estrogen therapy
Male Reproductive	Change in libido, infertility, sterility, impotence, pain during intercourse, age at onset of puberty, testicular pain, penile discharge, erections, emissions, hernias, enlarged prostate, type of birth control
Nutrition	Present weight, usual weight, food intolerances, food likes, food dislikes, where meals are eaten
Endocrine	Bulging eyes; fatigue; change in size of head, hands, or feet; weight change; heat/cold intolerances; excessive sweating; increased thirst; increased hunger; change in body hair distribution; swelling in the anterior neck; diabetes mellitus
Lymph Nodes	Enlarged, tenderness
Hematological	Easy bruising/bleeding, anemia, sickle cell anemia, blood type

© Cengage Learning 2014

and diseases that can be ascertained during the ROS. Many ambulatory care settings have preprinted ROS sheets. These are convenient, as positive findings can be circled and noted. Negative responses are not circled. In the EMR, the same is available via point and click.

By the completion of this portion of the history, the provider usually has an idea about the patient's condition.

To complete the examination, laboratory tests may be ordered depending on the findings and the probable diagnosis. These results, together with the history, examination, and patient symptoms, help to determine a **clinical diagnosis**.

Each piece of the patient's medical history documents integral parts of the patient's health. If any part is lacking, the current understanding of the patient's health is not complete.

Procedure 23-1 gives the steps for taking a paper medical history. The utilization of an electronic medical record is very similar, with the information recorded digitally.

THE PATIENT RECORD AND ITS IMPORTANCE

The patient's record is a collection of confidential information that concerns the patient, care given to the patient, patient progress, and laboratory and other diagnostic test results that have been completed. This information is secured in a file folder or binder. The EMR is secured in appropriate computer storage, is viewed at the computer screen, and can be printed in part or whole for the provider as necessary. It is used for a variety of purposes, but primarily the record provides a foundation for planning patient care and making decisions about patient care. Other purposes for a medical record include using it as a basis for communication among caregivers, for statistical analysis in research, and for reporting infectious diseases to the health department.

It is also a legal document and belongs to the provider or the agency in which the provider is employed. Chapters 7 and 14 discuss legal guidelines and medical records. Because it is a legal document, the medical record can be used to determine if patient care has been given according to the standards of care that the law recognizes; therefore, it must be complete, concise, accurate, and understandable. Many important items of information must be placed in the patient record and the medical assistant will be one of the professionals making chart entries.

HIPAA Compliance

HIPAA regulations focus on three vulnerable areas with respect to medical records and the patient's chart:

- Paper record storage and computer/server areas
- Fax machines
- Workstations

HIPAA A patient's paper chart must be stored in secure and locked areas. It is important that only those persons with need for access to charts have a key to the storage area. Locks should be changed periodically to ensure security. Sprinkler and fire detection systems should be installed and tested annually to protect paper records. Patients will respect and appreciate all procedures and policies to keep their history and medical records confidential and protected from harm.

EHR Protection of the patient's EMR means that computer workstation terminals should have directional screen filters if they are located in areas where unauthorized individuals may view the screen. Automated screen time-out features should be installed to protect information from passersby. If the clinic connects to the Internet, telecommuters, or hospital networks, a commercial-grade network firewall should be installed, tested, and maintained to ensure security. Antivirus software should be in place and updated regularly. Review Chapters 11, 14, and 15 for additional HIPAA regulations.

Faxing is a growing vulnerability to the threat of unintended disclosure of patient confidential information. Unintentional human, software, and telecommunication carrier code errors contribute to the security problem. Faxes are easily misdirected or intercepted by individuals for whom access was neither intended nor authorized. Only authorized personnel should have access to the fax machine area, and patient information should be faxed only with assurance that the same security is afforded where the fax is being sent.

Contents of Medical Records

Each patient has his or her own medical record. All patients' records hold standard information. In addition to the patient information forms previously mentioned, other important components of the record include:

- Informed consent forms
- Physical examination outcomes
- Laboratory and diagnostic test results
- The provider's diagnosis and plan of treatment
- Surgical reports
- Progress reports
- Follow-up care
- Telephone calls related to care
- Discharge summary
- Other communications (from other providers, laboratories, or agencies)
- Patient records from other providers
- Medication history

Continuity of Care Record

The Continuity of Care Record (CCR) was developed by a number of medical groups including the American Academy of Family Physicians and the American Academy of Pediatrics. This record is a standard for creating electronic records of a patient's health. The CCR makes it easier and more effective to transport patient medical information between providers. The CCR is intended to improve the continuity of patient care, reduce errors, and assure a minimum standard of information that is to be shared with another health care provider. The CCR includes patient and provider information, insurance data, patient's health status, recent care given, recommendations for future care, and the reason for referral or transfer. The patient's health status includes allergies, medications, immunizations, vital signs, pertinent laboratory results and recent procedures, and diagnoses. An expanded CCR likely includes any advanced directives the patient might have. During a time when many referrals take place, especially in managed care, or when patients are transferred from a hospital setting to an assisted living environment where care is likely provided by someone other than the current primary care provider, such a record is most beneficial.

The CCR is likely to be completed by providers, nurses, medical assistants, and ancillary personnel such as social workers and physical therapists, among others. It can include outpatient, community-based, and inpatient services. It should be machine readable, as well as human readable, and can be transferred through a number of electronic formats. At all times, however, the CCR is to be protected and is designed to enhance patient confidentiality.

METHODS OF CHARTING/ DOCUMENTATION

There are two primary ways to maintain chart notes. These methods can be used in both paper and electronic records. They are:

- Source-oriented medical records
- Problem-oriented medical records
  Review Chapter 14 for additional details.

Source-Oriented Medical Records

The traditional or conventional method of charting, the **source-oriented medical record (SOMR)**, consists of a chronologic set of notes for each visit beginning with the patient's first visit (Figure 23-7). This form of charting makes it difficult to follow or track a specific patient problem. The caregiver must search through the record to locate information about a particular patient problem. Source-oriented notes may be typed by the medical transcriptionist from dictation after the provider has seen the patient.

The example of handwritten chart notes (Figure 23-8) shows the complete history taken

Leo McKay
Date of Birth 01/22/1949
Office visit 04/01/20XX

This 57-year-old patient is seen after a several year absence because of abdominal pain which began approximately 2 weeks ago with progressively worsening abdominal pain. He has stopped eating to see if pain would improve, which it did not. Finally yesterday he stopped taking fluids as well. Until this episode, he was drinking several beers daily and smoking approximately 2 ppd.

Weight is 192. BP 152/88 rt. arm sitting P 78 R 18 T 97.6. He is a well-developed, moderately obese male in moderate distress. Abdomen is tense with some guarding at RUQ.

Abdominal pain - pt needs barium swallow, CBC, Chem 7 and UA. To restrict diet to clear liquids until seen in 2 days, omeprazole 20 mg every day.
JW/tlm

© Cengage Learning 2014

Figure 23-7   Sample of dictated and transcribed chart note.

at the time of examination including the present illness (if any), the medical history, allergies, family history, habits (social history), and ROS. The physical examination follows with each area noted. Impressions and changes in medications and plan finish the examination notes.

Problem-Oriented Medical Records

A more efficient way of keeping chart notes is the **problem-oriented medical record (POMR)**. This method is used extensively today, especially by clinics or any medical practice where more than one provider may see the patient (see Chapter 14). This method calls for a list of problems to be made, dated, and assigned numbers. When a patient

Leo McKay 01/22/1949
04/01/XX 3:15 pm abdominal pain × 3 weeks
WT 192   BP 152/88 rt. arm sitting T 97.6   P78   R18
Pt complaining severe abdominal pain for 2 wks getting progressively worse. Describes as burning, pressure.
Past Med. Hist.   chronic Peptic Ulcer Disease
                     quit smoking 3 yr ago – now back to 2 ppd
Allergies–penicillin–hives 1950s
Family Hist   noncontributory
Habits   smokes 2 ppd
              beer–several daily
ROS
HEENT noncontributory–PERRLA OU correct to 20/20
        CR–clear, no rales, ronchi; murmurs
        GI–some guarding. No masses, tenderness lower
        abdomen. No nausea, vomiting, diarrhea
        GU–clear
PE alert; oriented to time & place
      HEENT–pupils   nat teeth
      fundi   thyroid   } ∅
      carotids
      chest–clear
      heart–no murmurs or enlargement
      abdomen–∅ masses
      rectal–soft brown stool in vault
      extremities–neg.
      neuro–reg.
      skin–clear
Impression–Chronic Peptic Ulcer Disease
              Hypertension, mild
Plan–Lab–CBC, Chem 7, UA, barium swallow
Rx–Omeprazole 20 mg every day
Return 3 days
M. Woo, MD 04/01/20XX

© Cengage Learning 2014

Figure 23-8   Sample of handwritten chart note.

Patient: Leo McKay
Date of Birth: 01/22/1949
Visit Date: 04/01/20XX

Chief Complaint: Abdominal pain
History: Has been ill over the last 2 weeks with progressively worsening abdominal pain.
Review of Symptoms: Patient denies the following:
- Chest pain, Chest pressure, Chest heaviness, Circulation problems, Palpitations, Rapid heartbeat, Irregular heartbeat, Ankle swelling
- Cough, Phlegm, Coughing up blood, Shortness of breath, Wheeze, Change in exercise tolerance
- Burning or pain on urination, Difficulty starting or stopping urination, Dribbling after urination, Incontinence of urine, Blood in urine, Cloudiness of urine
- Change in appetite, Unexpected weight loss, Nausea, Vomiting, Difficulty Swallowing, Belly pains, Gas pains, Change in bowel habit: change in frequency, shape, color, consistency, size of stool; Blood, Mucus, or Slime, Rectal pain or discomfort, Hemorrhoids
- Skin rash, New or changing moles, Excess bruising or bleeding
- Mouth sores, Denture problems, Sinus drainage or stuffiness, Facial pain
- Panic attacks, Anxiety, Depression, Sadness, Seizures, Problems with concentration or memory, Disturbance of sleep, Insomnia, Early wakefulness
- Dizziness, Fainting, Lightheadedness on standing, Headaches, Vision problems, Hearing problems, Numbness or tingling in arms or legs, Weakness in arms or legs

Medications, including Herbal, Vitamin, and Mineral Supplements

Drug	Dose	Freq.	Started
none			

Medical Problem List

Problem	When Dx'd	Active?
Peptic Ulcer	1985	no

List of Surgeries

Surgical Procedure	When
none	

Family History: Parents deceased, father died of heart attack, mother of breast cancer.
Social History: Divorced, no children
Habits: Smokes 2 ppd, Several beers daily
Allergies: Penicillin

Physical Examination

GENERAL: Well developed and well nourished gentleman in no distress. No jaundice, cyanosis, clubbing, or edema.
VITALS: Weight = 192, Temp = 97.6, Pulse = 78, R = 18, BP = 152/88
HEENT: Normocephalic and without evidence of trauma, tympanic membranes and external auditory canals are normal. Pharynx and mouth are normal.
NECK: supple, no masses or thyromegaly.
NODES: No cervical nodes palpable. No axillary or inguinal adenopathy.
CARDIOVASCULAR SYSTEM: Heart sounds: no murmurs, rubs or gallops, carotids with good upstrokes, no bruits heard. Peripheral pulses including radials, brachials, and femorals intact. Posterior tibial, and dorsalis pedis pulses intact.
RESPIRATORY SYSTEM: resps 18/min, trachea central, expansion, fremitus, resonance, and breath sounds normal.
ABDOMEN: soft, no masses, organomegaly, or tenderness. No loin or costo-vertebral angle tenderness. Inguinal canals are intact without herniae. Bowel sounds active.
GENITOURINARY: Penis without lesions or discharge, scrotum, testicles, epididymis and cords all normal
RECTAL: no masses, tenderness, or hemorrhoids. Soft brown stool in vault. Prostate normal in size, and shape without nodules or tenderness.
MUSCULOSKELETAL SYSTEM: Joints with full ROM, no joint tenderness or swelling. Muscle bulk symmetric and normal.
SKIN: without masses, skin tags, rash, blisters or ulcerations. Nails are normal without splinter hemorrhages.
NEUROLOGICAL SYSTEM: Alert and oriented to place, person, and time. Communicates with good word recognition and appropriate word usage. Cranial nerves and spinal nerves grossly intact.

Assessment and Plan

Problem	Plan/Status
Abdominal pain	Reports about two weeks of epigastric and retrosternal chest pain radiating up and to the left. Episodes of pain occur usually during the day and last for 3-4 hours. No associated dyspnea, palpitations, sweats, dizziness. No nausea, vomiting or diarrhea. No blood in the stool. To get barium swallow, CBC, Chem 7 and UA. Begin omeprazole 20 every day.

Follow-up appointment: 3 days
Mark Woo MD

© Cengage Learning 2014

Figure 23-9 Sample of electronic medical history and physical examination.

is seen, the problems are identified by number throughout the record. This system makes it easier to follow the patient's progress.

The POMR has four major components:

- *The database.* The patient's medical history, results from laboratory and other diagnostic tests, and results of physical examinations are the core of the record.
- *The problem list.* Each problem is listed individually and assigned a number and dated.
- *The diagnostic and treatment plan.* This component addresses the laboratory and other diagnostic tests completed and the provider's plan for treating the patient.
- *Progress notes.* These notes are entered on every problem initially recorded. Documentation is done chronologically and includes patient's complaints, problems, condition, treatment, and responses to treatment and care given.

The SOAP/SOAPER and CHEDDAR methods of charting can be used in either the source-oriented or the problem-oriented medical record.

Providers may dictate their notes to be typed by a medical transcriptionist and then filed in the chart (see Figure 23-7). These notes may follow the form seen in the handwritten chart note as shown in Figure 23-8.

ELECTRONIC MEDICAL RECORDS (EMR)

The EMR can be viewed as simply a different mode of documenting and saving information related to a patient's care—computer storage versus paper storage. Most practitioners making the transition from paper to electronic records, however, seek a more efficient method for documenting patient care. Because EMRs are the mandate by 2014 paper medical records will be seen increasingly less in the future.

EHR EMRs that are a part of a TPMS can be viewed at a computer terminal by a provider, updated, and saved very quickly. EMRs are available 24 hours per day and can be accessed by the provider from an outside location when necessary. More than one person can view the EMR at the same time. Storage of the EMR is not a serious problem; hundreds of medical records can be stored on one CD or disk. Errors are less likely in EMRs because of the lack of handwritten data. Medication errors are lessened when they are electronically transmitted to the patient's pharmacy, and there is no confusion over the provider's instructions of the

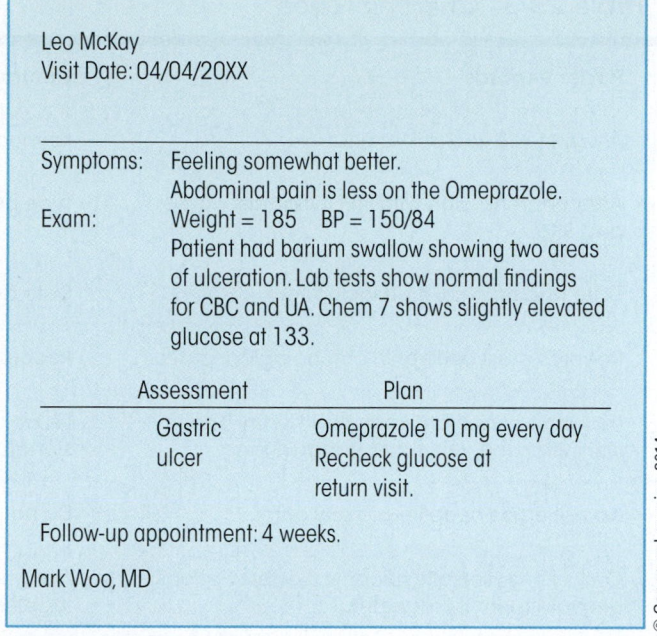

Leo McKay
Visit Date: 04/04/20XX

| Symptoms: | Feeling somewhat better. Abdominal pain is less on the Omeprazole. |
| Exam: | Weight = 185   BP = 150/84 Patient had barium swallow showing two areas of ulceration. Lab tests show normal findings for CBC and UA. Chem 7 shows slightly elevated glucose at 133. |

Assessment	Plan
Gastric ulcer	Omeprazole 10 mg every day Recheck glucose at return visit.

Follow-up appointment: 4 weeks.

Mark Woo, MD

© Cengage Learning 2014

Figure 23-10 Sample of follow-up visit note in EMR.

medication or dosage. EMRs have the capability of "flagging" information or queries to providers to ensure accuracy and completeness.

Figure 23-9 and Figure 23-10 show a sample EMR and follow-up note. The record grows in chronologic order, but problems are noted. Past health problems are shown at the top of each entry, and all current medications are shown on each sheet.

Remember, however, that an improperly implemented EMR is no more effective in supporting quality patient care than is the well-kept paper record. In the EMR, there can be a tendency to rely too much on technology, causing providers to become careless in their entries. There is never room in any medical record system for inattention to detail and accuracy.

Keep in mind the standard accepted rules for charting in both the paper medical record and the EMR. Many of the rules are pertinent to both types of records.

RULES OF CHARTING

Charting is required for each medication, treatment/procedure, or provider and medical assistant action. Accounts of the patient's condition and activities must be charted in a clear and meaningful way. Information charted in the patient's record must be accurate, clear, complete, timely, and entered properly. There is a saying, "If it is not charted, it was not done." Some basic charting rules are given in Table 23-3 and Table 23-4.

Table 23-3 Charting Rules

Paper Records	Electronic Records
Always write in black or blue ink.	Keyboarding must be accurate and appropriate.
After charting, sign with first initial, last name, and title.	Type personal or electronic signature after each chart activity.
Date and time must be included.	Date and time must be included.
Records must be kept in chronological order.	Records must be kept in chronological order.
Leave no space between chart entry and first initial and last name handwritten.	Leave no empty spaces between chart notes and electronic signature.
Do not erase or obliterate any entry.	Do not erase or obliterate any entry.
Only use universally accepted abbreviations or avoid them all together.	Only use universally accepted abbreviations or avoid them all together.
If an error is discovered, draw a single line through the mistake and write the correct information above it.	Errors made at the moment of entry are corrected as usual. Errors discovered later require a new document identifying the error, the correction, the date, and signature of the person making the correction. This document is added to the original document with a note. EMR software programs have variable time lockouts to prevent tampering with the chart.
Never leave a chart unattended in an area that allows those without a need to know access to the contents.	Always close and password protect electronic medical records when they are not in active use.

© Cengage Learning 2014

Table 23-4 Charting Rules That Apply to Both Paper and Electronic Charting

Leave no blank lines in the chart. Enter your data in the next available line.

Ditto marks may not be used.

Use only standard abbreviations that have been determined are not easily misinterpreted. See Abbreviations Common to Medical Charting (Table 23-6).

Avoid medical terminology unless absolutely certain of spelling and definition. Legal authorities advise keeping medical terminology to a minimum. The record must be understandable to the patient and to any authorized user.

Confirm the patient's name is on every page.

Use present tense. Never use future tense, such as "patient to be given a tetanus shot"; instead, wait until the injection is given, then chart the event.

Never chart for another person; chart only what you know, not what someone else has told you.

Describe events and behaviors; do not label them. "Patient was really angry" does not describe the event as well as "Patient yelled and threw the pencil on the counter."

Be as specific as you can. Charting "Patient complained of shoulder pain" is not as clear as "Patient complains of right shoulder pain when reaching overhead."

© Cengage Learning 2014

Abbreviations Used in Charting

Abbreviations are used extensively in charting to document information. Some are used as a shorthand to save time and space, whereas other abbreviations are used to give an exact meaning to a finding. For instance, the abbreviation "N&V" indicates "nausea and vomiting" without having to write out the entire expression. Table 23-5 lists commonly used abbreviations.

Although the use of abbreviations in medical charts is common, remember that there is an increasing expectation that the medical chart should be understandable to any person reading it, especially if it is required in any legal matter. The Joint Commission's *Journal on Quality and Patient Safety*

Table 23-5 Official "Do Not Use" List

Do Not Use	Potential Problem	Use Instead
U, u (unit)	Mistaken for "0" (zero), the number "4" (four) or "cc"	Write "unit"
IU (International Unit)	Mistaken for IV (intravenous) or the number 10 (ten)	Write "International Unit"
Q.D., QD, q.d., qd (daily) Q.O.D., QOD, q.o.d., qod (every other day)	Mistaken for each other Period after the Q mistaken for "I" and the "O" mistaken for "I"	Write "daily" Write "every other day"
Trailing zero (X.0 mg)* Lack of leading zero (.X mg)	Decimal point is missed	Write "X mg" Write "0.X mg"
MS MSO_4 and $MgSO_4$	Can mean morphine sulfate or magnesium sulfate Confused for one another	Write "morphine sulfate" Write "magnesium sulfate"
Additional Abbreviations, Acronyms, and Symbols (For possible future inclusion in the Official "Do Not Use" List)		
Do Not Use	Potential Problem	Use Instead
>(greater than) <(less than)	Misinterpreted as the number "7" (seven) or the letter "L" Confused for one another	Write "greater than" Write "less than"
Abbreviations for drug names	Misinterpreted due to similar abbreviations for multiple drugs	Write drug names in full
Apothecary units	Unfamiliar to many practitioners Confused with metric units	Use metric units
@	Mistaken for the number "2" (two)	Write "at"
cc	Mistaken for U (units) when poorly written	Write "mL" or "milliliters" ("mL" is preferred)
μg	Mistaken for mg (milligrams) resulting in one thousand–fold overdose	Write "mcg" or "micrograms"

Note: Taken from JCAHO "Do Not Use" List.

Source: http://www.jointcommission.org/assets/1/18/Do_Not_Use_List.pdf

Table 23-6 Abbreviations Common to Medical Charting

BP or B/P	blood pressure	NVD	nausea, vomiting, and diarrhea
ac	before meals	OPD	outpatient department
ad lib	at liberty	OR	operating room
b.i.d.	twice a day	P	pulse
c̄	with	PERRLA	pupils equal, round, reactive to light and accommodation
CBC	complete blood count	po	by mouth
CC	chief complaint	prn	as needed
C/O	Complaint of	PT	physical therapy
CPE	complete physical examination	R	respiration
DC or D/C	discontinue or discharge	R/O	rule out
D&C	dilation and curettage	ROM	range of motion
dx	diagnosis	ROS	review of systems
ECG, EKG	electrocardiogram	s̄	without
EEG	electroencephalogram	SOAP	subjective, objective, assessment, plan
ER	emergency room	SOB	short of breath
GI	gastrointestinal	T	temperature
GU	genitourinary	T&A	tonsillectomy and adenoidectomy
GYN	gynecology	t.i.d.	three times a day
HEENT	head, eyes, ears, nose, and throat	UA	urinalysis
H&P	history and physical	UCHD	usual childhood diseases
I&D	incision and drainage	URI	upper respiratory infection
IM	intramuscular	UTI	urinary tract infection
mg	milligram	x̄	without
mL	milliliter	WNL	within normal limits
MI	myocardial infarction	XR	X-ray
npo	nothing by mouth	Δ	change
N&V	nausea and vomiting		

reports that it is best not to use abbreviations when charting medications. As a result, there is an official "do not use" list, as well as a listing of potential abbreviations that are under consideration for exclusion (see Table 23-5). Their findings report that the most common abbreviation resulting in medication error is the use of "qd" rather than "every day or once daily." Their report also noted that medication errors were more likely made during prescribing and were related to improper dose or quantity. Therefore, keep abbreviations to a minimum and use only standard abbreviations. Be prepared to provide any attorney a list of commonly used and accepted abbreviations in your medical practice. The Joint Commission (JCAHO) posts a listing of prohibited abbreviations on their Web site (http://www.jointcommission.org) to further satisfy their goal of patient safety.

Chart Organization

Chart notes in a paper medical record are kept in chronologic order for the primary provider. Laboratory tests results, hospital notes, consultations with other providers, and any correspondence should be kept in an orderly fashion.

The chart order presents current medications followed by laboratory reports and pathology reports, each in chronologic order. In the POMR system, often the list of medical problems is found above the current medications.

The provider's notes are in chronologic order with the most recent first. The radiographs and ECGs follow, including MRIs, mammograms, CT scans, exercise tolerance tests (ETTs), echocardiograms, and other similar tests. Following these are the hospital notes, including the history and physical, hospital consultations, and discharge summary. Consultations by other providers are grouped next, again in chronologic order.

The miscellaneous section may include anything from referrals for insurance companies to orders and updates from nursing homes or home health services. Finally, the correspondence section includes letters, insurance claim forms, and requests for prior medical records.

If a chart is kept in a specific order, information needed is easily gleaned by each member of the clinic staff.

PROCEDURE 23-1

Taking a Medical History for a Paper Medical Record

PURPOSE:
To obtain a medical history from a patient new to the ambulatory care setting.

EQUIPMENT/SUPPLIES:
Patient history forms
Clipboard
Pen

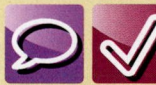

PROCEDURE STEPS:

1. *Introduce yourself to the new patient. Confirm identity of the patient* and escort to the examination room or private area.

2. Make sure the environment is private and there are few distractions.

3. *Make eye contact and use positive body language.* RATIONALE: Puts patient at ease.

4. Explain the purpose and importance of obtaining the patient information, *speaking at the patient's level of understanding.* Ask the questions on the form, trying to get as much information as possible without letting the patient wander from the subject.

5. Ask each question clearly. *Be sure patient understands all questions.* Ask about allergies.

6. Repeat patient answers when needed to confirm. Be specific when documenting answers. Do not just write "yes" for tobacco use. List "2 packs per day." Be specific.

7. Write legibly using dark ink (blue or black).

8. Recheck the medical history form to be sure all parts are complete. *Pay attention to detail.* Note any additional information provided by patient. Make sure numbers, dates, spelling, and other information are accurate and legible. RATIONALE: Ensures that all components of the medical history have been completed.

9. Prepare the patient for the review of systems and physical examination if this is indicated.

10. Document all findings in the patient's chart or EMR. RATIONALE: Identifies person responsible for taking the medical history.

CASE STUDY 23-1

Refer to the scenario at the beginning of the chapter.

Maria Jover, a patient of Dr. Elizabeth King at Drs. Lewis and King, has finally convinced her teenage son to make an appointment for a physical. Adam Jover is 17 years old, outgoing, fun loving, and apparently healthy. But Maria is concerned that he may be engaging in harmful social activities and hopes that by seeing Dr. Winston Lewis, Adam may discover ways to protect himself and his health. Adam agreed to the appointment but is adamant that his mother not accompany him. At the ambulatory care setting, it is decided that Adam might be more forthcoming with a male medical assistant, so Joe Guerrero is scheduled to take Adam's medical history before Dr. Winston does an ROS.

CASE STUDY REVIEW

1. When Joe Guerrero first sits down with Adam to take the history, he notices that Adam is ill at ease and nervous. What can Joe do to reassure Adam that his privacy will be protected?

2. When Joe attempts to take the social history, Adam seems evasive about answering Joe's questions and finally admits that he doesn't want his mother, Maria, to know about his social activities. What is Joe's response?

3. By the end of the interview, it becomes apparent that Adam may be engaging in some behaviors that put him at high risk for contracting the human immunodeficiency virus. How can Joe provide Adam with guidance without alienating him?

CASE STUDY 23-2

Harvey DiAntonio is a 58-year-old patient who lives at 45 W. Smith Avenue, Baltimore, Maryland 21208. His date of birth is July 8, 1954. His phone number is 410-667-1870. He is a Baltimore City fire fighter and has been for 21 years. He has union medical insurance, and Blue Cross/Blue Shield (BC/BS) is his carrier. His number is 211-67-87-56. He also carries major medical and his policy is Diagnostic #4. He has been referred by the fire department practitioner, Dr. Alan Byers. Mr. DiAntonio's complaint is severe "gripping" pain in the anterior mid-chest sometimes radiating to the abdomen, neck, and both arms. Pain seems to occur with strenuous exercise and when walking uphill. Pain usually lasts 20 minutes with each episode. Pain does "ease up" when he ceases activity. Mr. DiAntonio states his episodes have occurred while he was shaving, climbing stairs at work, after a heavy meal, and during sexual intercourse. One episode last week was accompanied with dizziness, nausea, and fatigue. The episodes have been going on now once or twice a month for 5 months. Mr. DiAntonio's history is essentially noncontributory. It is questionable whether this is due to good health or the fact that the patient has not had a physical examination for 8 years. Surgeries include tonsillectomy and adenoidectomy, T&A, 1958, and appendectomy in 1964. Fractured rib, left side, in 1984 due to fire-fighting incident. Usual childhood diseases. Hospitalized for observation, 1962, Sinai Hospital, for an unusually long episode of bronchitis. Social history shows that the patient is a pump operator on the job with much heavy exertion. Smokes 1½ to 2 packs of cigarettes per day and is a moderate drinker. He has a weight problem off and on and tends to eat too much while on duty. Lives in a one-story home. Hobbies include carpentry and music. Some family problems and tension exist as both of his children are in adolescence. Patient describes himself as "fun loving" with a "quick temper" and worries about meeting financial needs of the family. Is in a position to retire from active duty but states he could not tolerate the boredom.

Family history shows both parents deceased—mother of heart attack, age 59, and father of unknown cause at age 49. Has two siblings, one brother with history of hypertension and one sister living and in good health. Has two children both living and well. Family history otherwise negative.

Physical examination revealed a well-nourished, well-developed male in no acute distress at this time. Patient does seem a bit anxious about this examination. T. 98.6 - P. 94 - R. 24 - BP 175/104. Ht. 69", Wt. 198 pounds. HEAD, EYES, EARS, NOSE, THROAT—normal. NECK—supple. Trachea in midline. CHEST—normal in contour. Calcium deposit on left sixth rib probably due to history of fracture. HEART—after careful examination with the patient recumbent and the scope placed lightly on the chest wall near the apex, a left atrial sound was heard (presystolic gallop). ABDOMEN—negative. EXTREMITIES—negative. GENITALIA—negative. SKIN—negative. NEUROLOGIC—negative. Laboratory tests performed show a hemoglobin of 11.0 gms. Awaiting results of serum cholesterol, calcium, phosphorus, and blood urea nitrogen. Chest radiograph essentially negative. EKG report showed atrial sounds occurring presystolically with long P-R intervals. DIAGNOSIS: (1) angina pectoris; (2) anemia; (3) hypertension. TREATMENT: Nitroglycerin tabs, sublingually as needed. To return to clinic in 2 weeks to follow medication effects. In consultation with patient, the patient was advised to control physical activity and quantity of food intake. Avoid extreme cold, 8 hours of sleep/night. Avoid emotional upsets. Attempt four meals/day. Low-fat 1,600-calorie diet. No smoking, moderate alcohol intake.

CASE STUDY 23-2 (CONTINUED)

CASE STUDY REVIEW

1. Identify the following parts of the case study above and extract from the case study the portion that matches the appropriate medical history component.

   - Personal data
   - Chief complaint
   - Present illness
   - Medical history
   - Family history
   - Social history
   - Review of systems

2. Using appropriate terminology and abbreviations, make a charting entry for Mr. DiAntonio by using the SOAPER method of charting.

SUMMARY

The patient's medical history and the information that appears in the medical chart form the base for any and all treatment given to a patient. An efficient and effective medical chart tells the patient's story. It is critical that all information be accurate, documented appropriately, and complete in every way. Taking the medical history, maintaining the patient's chart, and documenting information are major tasks for medical assistants. Increased use of the EMR makes charting easier and quicker for clinic staff personnel and providers. Errors are less likely in the EMR, and information is more readily available when needed. Changing from the paper medical chart to the electronic medical chart is time consuming and often seems overwhelming, but medical personnel using the EMR cannot imagine functioning without them.

STUDY FOR SUCCESS

To reinforce your knowledge and skills of information presented in this chapter:

- Review the *Key Terms*
- Role-play with other students to apply attributes of professionalism pertinent to this chapter.
- Consider the *Case Studies* and discuss your conclusions
- Answer the questions in the *Certification Review*
- Apply your knowledge by completing the *Activities* in the *Study Guide* and the *Games and Quizzes* in the StudyWARE **Study**WARE software on the *Premium Website*
- Perform the *Procedure* using the *Competency Assessment Checklist* in the *Competency Manual*
- Practice your problem-solving skills with the *Critical Thinking Challenge 3.0* on the *Premium Website*

Additional resources for this chapter include:

- Module 20 of the *Medical Assisting Learning Lab*
- *CourseMate for Delmar's Comprehensive Medical Assisting*
- *WebTutor for Delmar's Comprehensive Medical Assisting*

CERTIFICATION REVIEW

1. If the patient has difficulty with English, the medical assistant should:
   a. make the appointment for the patient and obtain the services of an interpreter to be present
   b. set the appointment after contact is made with the interpreter
   c. speak more loudly so the patient will understand
   d. suggest that the patient find a provider who speaks his or her first language

2. A helpful question to ask the returning patient is:
   a. Are you feeling bad today?
   b. Didn't you get better with the treatment prescribed last visit?
   c. Have you noticed any changes in your condition since your last visit?
   d. Do you realize you have gained six pounds since your visit last week?

3. When the patient reports not feeling well, the medical assistant should:
   a. mark the chief complaint as "patient not feeling well"
   b. ask helpful questions to help the patient express specific problems or symptoms
   c. pin down the symptoms by guessing what the problem could be
   d. let the provider work with the patient

4. Source-oriented medical records:
   a. are chronologic notes beginning with the patient's first visit
   b. have four major components
   c. are the best for finding information quickly
   d. are best when many providers see the patient

5. Name, address, telephone numbers, birth date, Social Security number, insurance information, and person to contact in an emergency is information referred to as:
   a. demographic data
   b. CCR of patient information
   c. social history
   d. none of the above

6. The chief complaint:
   a. often is referred to as the CC in the chart
   b. is a statement of objective findings made by the staff
   c. is subjective data as expressed by the patient
   d. a and c

7. Interviewing patients for their medical history requires:
   a. special credentials such as CMA or RMA
   b. cross-cultural interviewing and communication skills
   c. computer skills in medical note taking
   d. a major portion of the receptionist's time and energy

8. The CCR was developed:
   a. by medical groups including the American Academy of Family Physicians and the American Academy of Pediatrics
   b. to reduce errors and ensure certain information is shared among providers
   c. for input from all health care providers, nurses, and medical assistants
   d. all of the above

9. Progress notes include:
   a. medical history and results of laboratory tests
   b. the provider's plan for treating the patient
   c. the CC, problems, conditions, treatment, and responses to care
   d. a and c

10. Subjective, objective, assessment, and plan charting is sometimes referred to as:
    a. SOAP
    b. POMR
    c. SOMR
    d. CCRP

REFERENCES/BIBLIOGRAPHY

California State University–Chico. (n.d.). *JCAHO Do Not Use List.* Retrieved August 8, 2012, from http://www.csuchico.edu

U.S. Department of Health and Human Services, Centers for Disease Control and Prevention.

Recommended adult immunization schedule by age group and medical conditions, United States, 2006–2007. Summary published by the Advisory Committee on Immunization Practices. Retrieved August, 2007, from http://www.cdc.gov

CHAPTER 24

Vital Signs and Measurements

OUTLINE

The Importance of Accuracy

Temperature

    Terms Used to Describe Body
    Temperature

    Phaseout of Mercury
    Thermometers and Other
    Mercury-Containing
    Equipment

    Types of Thermometers

    Measuring Temperature

    Recording Temperature

    Cleaning and Storage of
    Thermometers

Pulse

    Pulse Sites

    Measuring and Evaluating
    a Pulse

    Normal Pulse Rates

    Pulse Abnormalities

    Recording Pulse Rates

Respiration

    Respiration Rate

    Abnormalities

Blood Pressure

    Equipment for Measuring
    Blood Pressure

Measuring Blood Pressure

Recording Blood Pressure
    Measurement

Normal Blood Pressure
    Readings

Blood Pressure Abnormalities

Height and Weight

    Height

    Weight

    Significance of Weight

Measuring Chest Circumference

LEARNING OUTCOMES

1. Define, spell, and pronounce the key terms as presented in the glossary.
2. Discuss normal and abnormal temperatures, including factors affecting temperature.
3. Identify and explain the procedures for using, caring for, and storing the various types of thermometers.
4. Discuss the Environmental Protection Agency's initiative to phase out mercury thermometers and other mercury-containing equipment.
5. Describe the locations and procedure for obtaining pulse rates.
6. Explain the procedure for obtaining respiration rates.
7. Identify and describe normal and abnormal pulse and respiratory rates and the factors affecting each.
8. Describe the appropriate equipment and procedure for obtaining a blood pressure measurement.
9. Identify normal and abnormal blood pressure, including factors affecting blood pressure.
10. Describe the procedures for obtaining height, weight, and chest measurements of adults.
11. Accurately record measurements on the patient's chart or electronic medical record.
12. Explain two reasons why a professional individual shows responsibility by learning about the dangers of mercury.
13. Analyze the professionalism questions and apply them to this chapter's content.

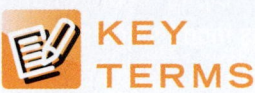

KEY TERMS

afebrile
apical
apnea
arrhythmia
atherosclerosis
baseline
bradycardia
bradypnea
Cheyne–Stokes
diastole
dyspnea
eupnea
febrile
frenulum
hyperpnea
hypertension
hyperventilation
hypotension
hypoventilation
increment
lumen
manometer
meniscus
orthopnea
peripheral
pulse oximeter
pyrexia
rales
stertorous
stridor
systole
tachycardia
tachypnea
wheezes

ATTRIBUTES OF PROFESSIONALISM

Communication
- Did you introduce yourself? Did you identify the patient through name and birth date or other identifying feature?
- Did you listen to and acknowledge the patient?
- Did you speak at the patient's level of understanding?
- Did you provide appropriate responses/feedback?
- Did you allay patients' fears regarding the procedure being performed and help them feel safe and comfortable?
- Did you accurately and concisely update the provider on any aspect of the patient's care?

Presentation
- Did you attend to any special needs of the patient? Did you first ask if assistance was needed, rather than taking charge?
- Were you courteous, patient, and respectful to the patient?
- Did you display a calm, professional, and caring manner?

Competency
- Did you pay attention to detail?
- Did you ask questions if you were out of your comfort zone or did not have the experience to carry out tasks?
- Did you recognize the importance of local, state, and federal legislation and regulations in the practice setting?

Integrity
- Did you protect personal boundaries?
- Did you protect and maintain confidentiality?
- Did you immediately report any error you had made?

SCENARIO

At the medical clinic of Drs. Lewis and King, clinical medical assistant Joe Guerrero, CMA (AAMA), assists both providers in taking patients' vital signs. One of his favorite patients is Abigail Johnson, a friendly woman in her 70s who always has a kind disposition despite her financial and medical difficulties. Abigail is overweight and has hypertension, so her blood pressure is monitored on a regular basis to be certain that it is under control. In reviewing Abigail's chart, Joe notices that her blood pressure has been quite stable for the last few visits. He also checks her weight and notices that Abigail is slowly losing weight. Abigail's chart, with its history of blood pressure and other measurements, informs Joe's perspective and is a helpful record when evaluating the progress Abigail has made since she became a patient 3 years ago.

INTRODUCTION

One of the most important and commonly performed tasks of a medical assistant is obtaining and recording patient vital signs and body measurements. Vital signs, also sometimes referred to as cardinal signs, include temperature, pulse, respiration, and blood pressure, abbreviated TPR B/P. They are indicative of the general health and well-being of a patient and, with regular monitoring, may measure patient response to treatment. Vital signs, in total or in part, are an important component of each patient visit. Height and weight measurements, although not considered vital signs, are often a routine part of a patient visit.

Patients will exhibit vital sign readings that are uniquely their own. As a result, baseline assessments of vital signs are usually obtained during the patient's initial visit. These baseline results are used as a reference point for future readings, differentiating between what is normal and abnormal for the patient.

Two important habits must be developed by the medical assistant before taking a patient's vital signs: aseptic technique in the form of hand washing, and recognition and correction of factors that may influence results of vital signs. Proper hand washing before taking vital signs will assist in preventing cross contamination of patients. Refer to the discussion on Standard Precautions and medical asepsis in Chapter 22. Also, emotional factors of patients must be recognized and addressed. Explaining procedures and allowing the patient the opportunity to relax will ease apprehension that may affect vital sign readings.

THE IMPORTANCE OF ACCURACY

Vital signs may be altered by many factors. Medical assistants must recognize and correct factors that may produce inaccurate results. For example, patients may exhibit anxiety over potential test results or findings of the provider. They may be angry or may have rushed into the clinic. A patient may have had something to eat or drink before the visit or may have had a long wait in the reception area. Patient apprehension and mood must always be considered by the medical assistant, because these factors can affect vital signs. The medical assistant may be required to take vital signs more than once during a clinic visit to ascertain a **baseline** and obtain an impression of overall well-being of the patient. Body measurements such as weight may be influenced by what the patient is wearing; height may be influenced by the patient's shoes and how his or her posture is while being measured.

Accuracy in taking vital signs is necessary because treatment plans are developed according to the measurement of the vital signs. Variations can indicate a new disease process or the patient's response to treatment. They may also indicate the patient's compliance with a treatment plan.

  Although taking vital signs is a task commonly performed by the medical assistant, it is never to be taken casually or lightly, and it should never be rushed or incompletely performed. Concentration and attention to proper procedure will help ensure accurate measurements and quality care of the patient. The following text discusses procedures used to measure the vital signs of children and adults. Procedures used for infant examinations are discussed in Chapter 27.

TEMPERATURE

Body temperature is maintained and regulated by two processes functioning in conjunction with one another: heat production and heat loss.

Body heat is produced by the actions of voluntary and involuntary muscles. As the muscles move, they use energy, which produces heat. Cellular metabolic activities, such as the process of breaking down food sugars into simpler components (catabolism), are another source of heat.

The body loses heat by a combination of five processes:

1. *Convection.* The process by which heat is lost through the skin by being transferred from the skin by air currents flowing across it, such as a fan used on a hot day for cooling purposes.
2. *Conduction.* The transfer of heat from within the body to the surface of the skin and then to surrounding cooler objects touching the skin, such as clothing.
3. *Radiation.* Body heat lost from the surface of the skin to a cooler environment, much like a cool room becoming warm when occupied by many people.
4. *Evaporation.* A heat-loss mechanism that uses heat absorption through vaporization of perspiration.
5. *Elimination.* Heat that is lost through the normal functioning of the intestinal, urinary, and respiratory tracts.

The delicate balance between heat production and heat loss is maintained by the hypothalamus in the brain. The hypothalamus monitors blood temperature and will trigger either the heat loss or heat production mechanism with as little as 0.04°F change in blood temperature.

Body temperature is measured in degrees and is influenced by several factors, including:

- An increase in temperature may result from a bacterial infection, increased physical activity or food intake, exposure to heat, pregnancy, drugs that increase metabolism, stress and severe emotional reactions, and age. Age becomes a factor in that infants have an average body temperature that is one to two degrees higher than adults.
- Decrease in temperature may result from viral infections, decreased muscular activity, fasting, exposure to cold, drugs that decrease metabolic activities, and age. Age in this instance refers to older adults, in that older adults have decreased metabolic activity resulting in a decrease in body temperature.
- Another factor that can increase or decrease body temperature is time of day. During sleep and early morning, the temperature is at its lowest, whereas later in the day, with muscular and metabolic activity, the temperature increases.

Because of the many factors influencing body temperature and the uniqueness of individuals, there is no "normal" temperature. The medical assistant must think of temperatures in terms of the "average," which for an adult is 98.6°F, or 37.0°C.

Terms Used to Describe Body Temperature

The following terms are used to describe body temperature:

- *Afebrile.* absence of fever
- *Febrile.* fever is present
- *Fever.* Body temperature increased beyond normal range; **pyrexia** is another term for fever
- *Onset.* Time when fever begins
- *Lysis.* Body temperature gradually returns to normal after a period of fever
- *Crisis.* Body temperature decreases suddenly to normal levels; the patient may perspire profusely (diaphoresis)
- *Intermittent.* A fluctuating fever that returns to or below baseline, then increases again
- *Remittent.* A fluctuating fever that does not return to the baseline temperature; it fluctuates but remains increased
- *Continuous.* A fever that remains above the baseline; it does not fluctuate but remains fairly constant

Figure 24-1 depicts types of fever.

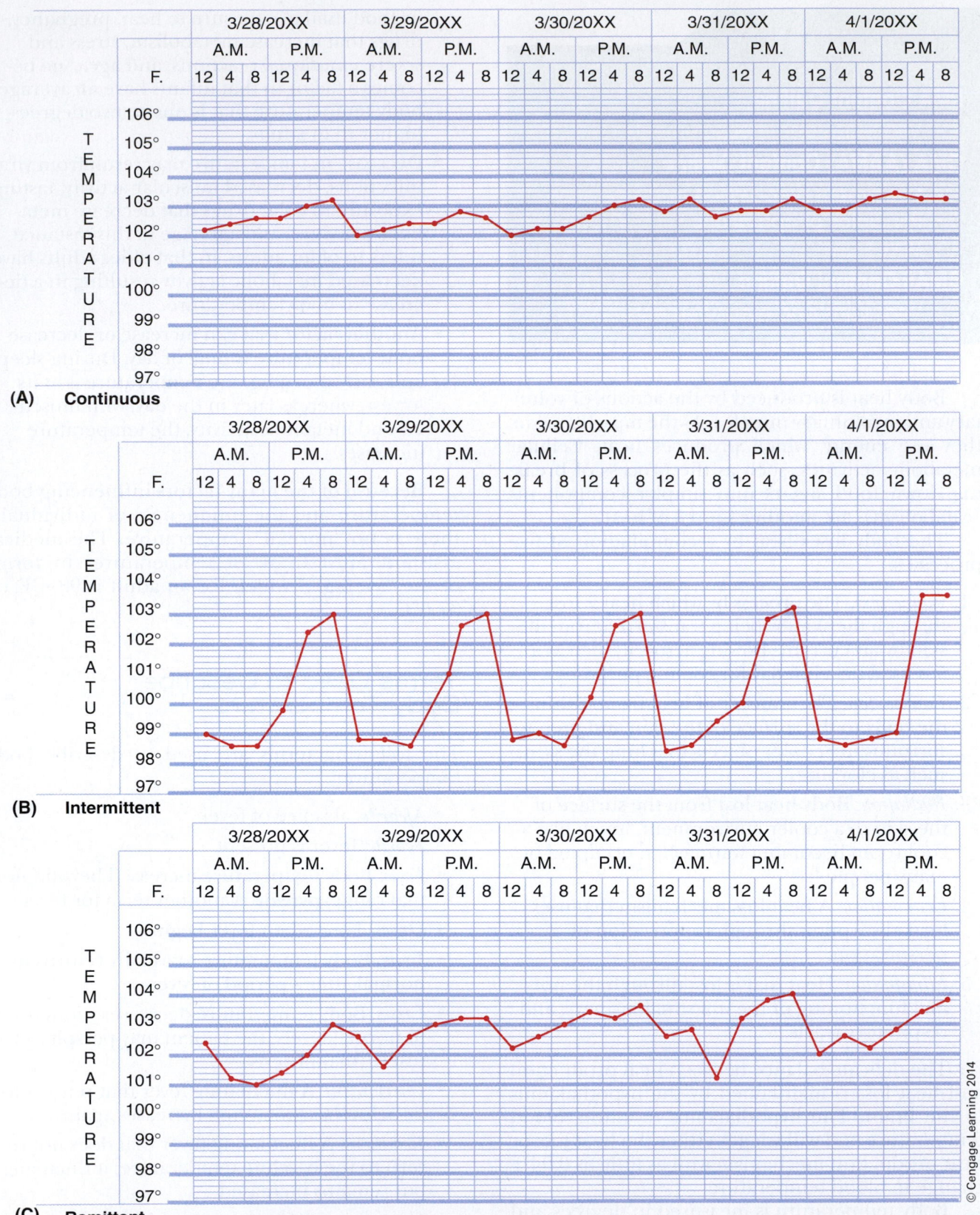

Figure 24-1 Types of fevers. (A) Continuous—remains above baseline. Does not fluctuate. (B) Intermittent—a fluctuating fever. Returns to or below baseline, then rises again. (C) Remittent—a fluctuating fever but does not return to baseline temperature. Remains elevated, but fluctuates.

Phaseout of Mercury Thermometers and Other Mercury-Containing Equipment

Glass mercury thermometers have been used for decades and have been common in health care agencies as well as the home. In recent years, concerns have arisen about mercury toxicity when mercury thermometers or other equipment containing mercury break and spill mercury into the environment.

This can create a mercury vapor in the indoor air, which is a serious problem. The mercury also can cause environmental damage if it enters lakes and rivers where it can contaminate fish, which are part of the food chain. Even small amounts of mercury can do great harm. The fetus is at risk because its developing nervous system is susceptible to mercury toxicity if a pregnant woman eats fish contaminated with mercury. When thermometers break or are disposed of improperly, the mercury can enter the atmosphere, especially if the mercury waste is burned in an incinerator.

If spilled mercury is not cleaned up (perhaps the individual using the thermometer is unaware that it is broken, and the mercury has seeped into a carpet or crevice), the mercury will evaporate and can reach dangerous levels in indoor air. There is medical literature that illustrates some cases of serious illnesses and even death from exposure to mercury from broken thermometers. Most cases involved young children. According to the Environmental Protection Agency (EPA), a 32-month-old child who was exposed to mercury became ill with hypertension, tachycardia, apathy, pulmonary edema, and coma. The mercury from a broken thermometer had not been cleaned up.

Even small mercury spills should be cleaned up as soon as possible. Becton-Dickinson, a thermometer manufacturer, makes the following recommendations for cleaning up a broken thermometer:

- Pick up the mercury with an eyedropper or scoop up the beads of mercury with a piece of heavy paper (cardboard, index card, or playing card).
- Place mercury, the dropper, heavy paper, and any broken glass in a plastic resealable bag. Place this bag into two more resealable bags, zipping each within the other, finishing up with the contents bagged three times. Place this into a wide-mouth, sealable plastic container.

- Call the local health department for the nearest mercury disposal location. If no disposal location is available, dispose of the container according to local and state regulations. The health department can inform you regarding how to obtain the information.
- Leave windows open for about 2 days to ensure complete ventilation.

These recommendations can be applied to mercury spillage caused by other mercury-containing equipment. Do not do the following:

- Do not use household cleaning products. Combinations of some cleansers with mercury can release toxic gases.
- Do not use a broom or brush to clean up mercury; they only spread it around.
- Do not use a vacuum cleaner or shop vacuum. The mercury vapor escapes into the air and increases exposure to individuals in the area.

In 1998, the American Hospital Association signed an agreement with the EPA to eliminate mercury from their hospitals' waste systems. Hospitals and other health care agencies are phasing out the use of mercury thermometers and other medical equipment that contain mercury, such as sphygmomanometers, among others. Many states have recalled mercury thermometers and replaced them with digital ones.

The best alternative is use of nonmercury thermometers, such as digital and electronic. These can be used orally, rectally, or axillary. Also available are tympanic (ear canal); temporal artery; infrared; and flexible, disposable, forehead or oral thermometers (less accurate). There are no known risks with any of the above thermometers.

Types of Thermometers

The following are types of thermometers available for use in the ambulatory care setting:

- Disposable strips
- Electronic/digital
- Tympanic
- Temporal artery

Disposable Thermometers. Disposable thermometers are individually wrapped strips with heat-sensitive dots that change color to indicate temperature. They are used once and then

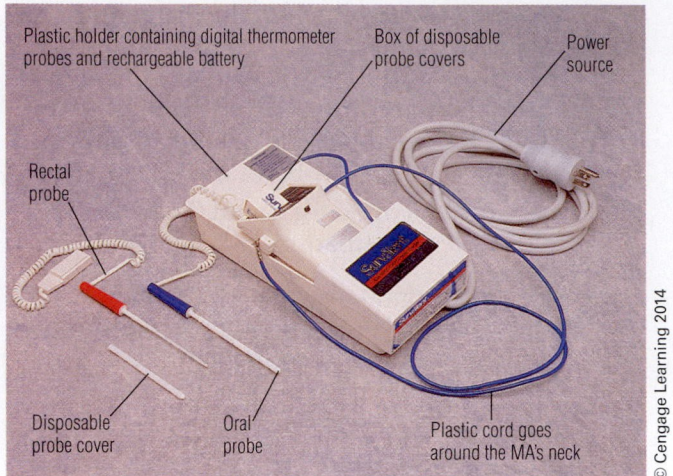

Figure 24-2 Electronic thermometers have interchangeable oral and rectal probes attached to a battery-operated portable unit.

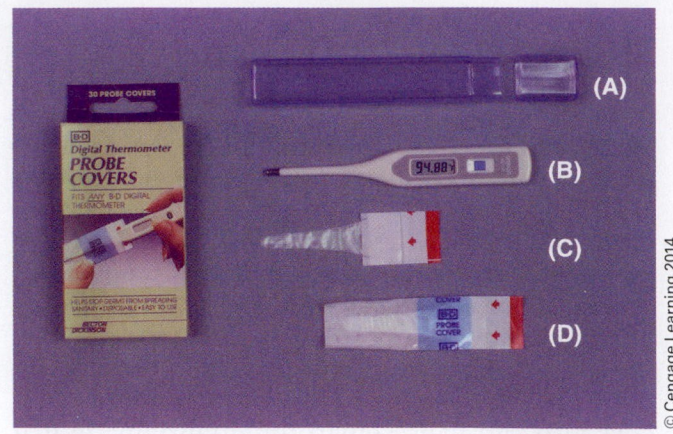

Figure 24-3 Digital thermometer. (A) Carrying case. (B) Digital thermometer. (C) Probe cover without backing. (D) Probe cover with backing.

discarded. There are strips for use on the forehead and others for oral use. Although strips are easy to use and prevent patient cross contamination, accuracy is questionable.

Electronic and Digital Thermometers.
Electronic thermometers are widely used, handheld, battery-operated or plug-in units that have easy-to-read electronic display screens to indicate results (Figure 24-2). Electronic thermometers in Fahrenheit or Celsius scales are available. Probes are attached and are color-coded blue for oral and red for rectal. The probes have disposable plastic covers. The plastic cover acts as a barrier to prevent contamination of the probe and is replaced for each patient to prevent cross contamination. An accurate result can be obtained in approximately 10 seconds.

Inexpensive digital thermometers are widely available for home use (Figure 24-3). They are quick, easy to use, and accurate. Encourage your patients to switch to these from the mercury glass thermometers. These lightweight thermometers do not require recharging; their small imbedded batteries last for years but are not replaceable.

Suggest patients watch for "Turn in Your Mercury Thermometer Days." Some communities, in conjunction with local pharmacies, set aside a day or two each year for residents to take mercury thermometers to their local pharmacy. In exchange for the mercury thermometers, free digital thermometers are given as replacements.

Tympanic Thermometers.
The use of tympanic thermometers is becoming more popular because they are fast, provide no discomfort to the patient, can be used on patients over 2 years of age as well as adults, and usually are accurate. They consist of a handheld unit with a probe tip that is inserted into the ear securely to make a seal. Disposable tips are used to prevent cross contamination. With the tympanic method of measuring body temperature, the procedure is complete in a few seconds. It is comfortable for the patient, nonthreatening to infants and children, and can be used when other methods are inappropriate. It is the thermometer of choice for pediatric patients older than 2 years. However, providers have found that inaccurate readings can result if patients have impacted cerumen in the ear of which they may be unaware. Also, if the patient has otitis media, a middle ear infection, the reading tends to be inaccurate and the procedure is painful.

The most commonly used thermometers are the digital/electronic, tympanic, and temporal artery thermometers.

Temporal Artery Thermometers.
A noninvasive thermometer known as a temporal artery thermometer, or TA thermometer, has been developed and is currently in use. Studies performed at Harvard Medical School and the Hospital for Sick Children found the TA thermometer to be more accurate than the aural (tympanic) and rectal thermometers. It is used on adults and children.

The temporal artery is a major blood vessel in the head. The thermometer measures the temperature of the skin surface over the temporal artery.

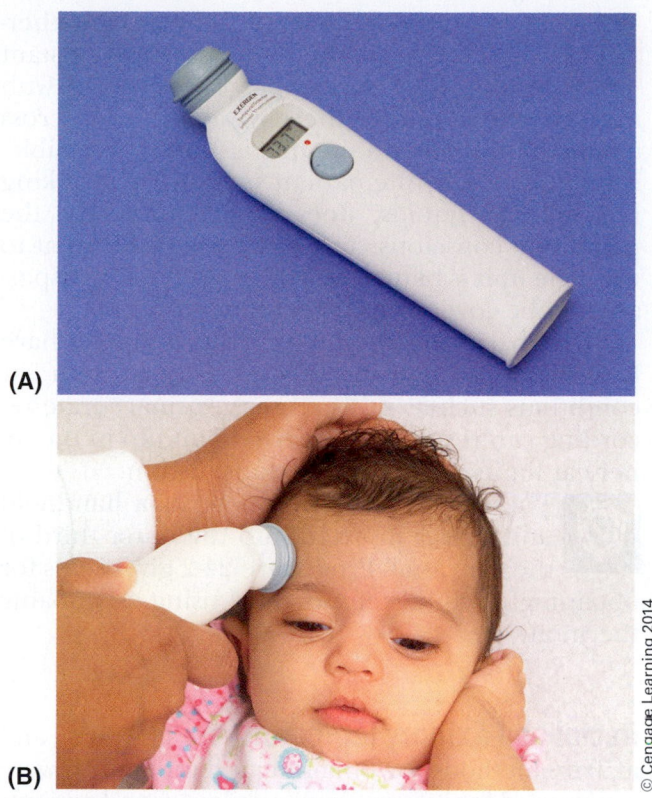

(A)

(B)

© Cengage Learning 2014

Figure 24-4 Using a temporal artery thermometer. (A) Temporal artery thermometer. (B) Slide thermometer across forehead.

The thermometer has a probe that contains a sensor. When the TA thermometer is slid straight across the forehead (midline forehead), the infrared heat from the artery is picked up by the sensor (Figure 24-4). Software accurately determines and displays the temperature. The TA thermometer can also be used behind the ear lobe (if the forehead is wet with perspiration). See Procedure 24-3. There are many advantages to the TA thermometer: It can be used for patients of all ages; it is accurate, painless, fast, convenient, safe, comfortable, and noninvasive; and it can be cleaned with an alcohol wipe between patients.

Some considerations should be kept in mind when using a TA thermometer. If there is perspiration on the forehead, an inaccurate measurement could occur. Other sites that can be used are the femoral, axillary, and behind the ear. Scanning too rapidly can cause a false reading, as can a hat or hair covering the forehead. The TA thermometer must be the same temperature as the room in which it is used. It cannot be stored in the sun or in a room where air-conditioned air has been blowing on the thermometer.

Measuring Temperature

To convert °F to °C:
Subtract 32 from F temperature, then multiply by 5/9.

Example:

$$97°F = 97 - 32 = 65 \qquad 65 \times \frac{5}{9} = 9 \overline{)325.0} = 36.1°C$$

$$\begin{array}{r} 36.1 \\ \hline 9)325.0 \\ 27 \\ \hline 55 \\ 54 \\ \hline 10 \end{array}$$

To convert °C to °F:
Multiply C temperature by 9/5, then add 32.

Example:

$$\frac{36.1°C}{1} \times \frac{9}{5} + 32$$

$$\begin{array}{r} 36.1 \\ \times 9 \\ \hline 324.9 \end{array} \qquad \begin{array}{r} 64.9 \\ 5)324.9 \\ 30 \\ \hline 24 \\ 20 \\ \hline 49 \\ 45 \\ \hline 4 \end{array} \quad or \quad \begin{array}{r} 65 \\ +32 \\ \hline 97°.F \end{array}$$

It is helpful to know and understand the conversion factors from Fahrenheit to Celsius and vice versa. There are numerous websites that explain this calculation such as http://www.wbuf.noaa.gov/tempfc.htm.

Oral Temperatures. To use an oral strip for taking a temperature, make certain that the package is not damaged, then peel it back to reveal the strip. Insert the strip into the patient's mouth. After the appropriate time interval has elapsed, remove the thermometer. The dots that have changed color are read using the scale located on the strip. Although convenient to use, accuracy is not always ensured with the strips, so these strips may not be the best choice for clinical use. Procedure 24-6 gives steps for taking an oral temperature using a disposable oral strip thermometer.

The procedure for obtaining an oral temperature with an electronic thermometer is quick, easy, and accurate (Procedure 24-1). Some electronic thermometers are stored on a recharging base. When removed from the base, they are turned on and ready for use. A disposable cover is placed over the probe, and the probe is placed in the patient's mouth. When temperature measurement is complete, the thermometer beeps and the temperature is displayed on the screen. The probe cover is ejected into a biohazard container without touching the container, and the unit is returned to the base. The temperature is then recorded in the patient's chart. Always read and follow the manufacturer's directions for use and care of a digital unit.

Aural Temperature.

Taking a temperature with a tympanic thermometer is a fast, safe method for obtaining a patient's temperature (Figure 24-5). It is common in ambulatory care settings. Tympanic temperature can be obtained without discomfort for all patients except for children under 2 years of age.

The tympanic thermometer measures the patient's temperature by measuring the infrared waves produced by the tympanic membrane and records the temperature in less than 2 to 3 seconds on a digital screen. The tympanic membrane and the hypothalamus of the brain share the same blood supply, so an accurate measurement of the body temperature can be obtained.

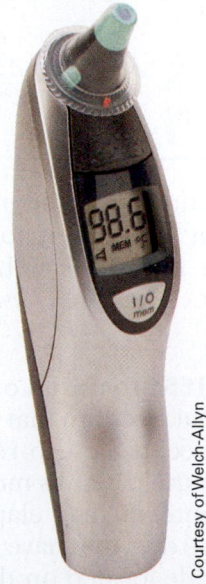

Figure 24-5 Thermo-scan tympanic thermometer.

Courtesy of Welch-Allyn

The greatest benefits of the tympanic thermometer are that it gives nearly instant results; does not come into contact with mucous membranes, thereby minimizing cross contamination; uses a site that is readily accessible; is not affected by the patient smoking or drinking hot or cold liquids; does not require that the patient be conscious; and is an easy instrument to use. The unit is battery operated and uses a disposable probe cover or ear speculum.

Drawbacks to the tympanic thermometer have been demonstrated in pediatric patients with ear conditions such as otitis media. An inaccurate recording can result because fluid buildup in the inner ear limits infrared wave transmission.

The tympanic thermometer is a handheld unit that is inserted into the outer third of the ear canal. Procedure 24-2 gives steps for obtaining an aural temperature using a tympanic thermometer.

Rectal and Axillary Temperatures.

The rectal and axillary methods for obtaining a temperature were widely used for infants, young children, and patients who were unable or uncooperative with oral temperature measurement. The new technologies—tympanic, temporal artery, and electronic and digital thermometers—have simplified temperature measurement. These thermometers are safe, readily accepted by patients, greatly reduce microorganism transmission, are accurate, give a rapid reading, and are widely used in health care settings including ambulatory care. Although the newer eventually will replace the electronic and digital method for measuring temperatures, including the rectal and axillary routes, the steps for obtaining rectal and axillary temperature measurements are included in Procedures 24-4 and 24-5.

Recording Temperature

Temperature may be taken on each visit to the provider's clinic to obtain a baseline for the patient. When recording the temperature in the patient's electronic medical record, the scale used for the results must be designated F for Fahrenheit and C for Celsius. The route used must be labeled as well; methods other than oral must be labeled according to the route used because there is a difference in the measurement. Use R for rectal, A for axillary, Tym for tympanic, and TA for temporal artery.

Temperatures are recorded as shown:

Oral	T 98.6°F
Rectal	T 99.6° (R) F
Axillary	T 97.6° (Ax) F
Tympanic	T 98.6° (Tym) F
Temporal artery	T 99.4° (TA) F

When a facility uses a tympanic thermometer exclusively, the route is known and therefore does not have to be labeled.

 The medical assistant must read all manufacturer's instructions before using any digital, tympanic, or temporal artery thermometer. Each may have a slight difference in operating procedure.

Procedures 24-1 through 24-6 detail steps involved in taking temperature by various routes.

Cleaning and Storage of Thermometers

Oral and rectal thermometers should be separated. Storage depends on the policy of the facility.

Digital, electronic, tympanic, and temporal artery thermometers are cleaned according to the manufacturer's directions. The covers protect the probes from contamination. Each type of thermometer has a storage case or a wall-mounted base made especially for storing the unit. Disinfect these types of thermometers by wiping with a mild disinfectant as instructed by the manufacturer.

PULSE

The pulse rate consists of two phases of the heart action and can be felt when compressing an artery. As the heart contracts, it increases pressure on the arterial walls. The increased pressure passes through the arteries in a wave-like movement resulting in a slight expansion of the arterial wall (contraction). When the heart relaxes, (relaxation) the pressure is decreased in the arteries, resulting in the wall returning to its previous position. One contraction and one relaxation of the heart together is equal to one heart cycle or heartbeat. The pulse and heartbeat rate are usually identical in healthy individuals.

Pulse Sites

The pulse can be felt in areas of the body where an artery is close to the surface and to an underlying

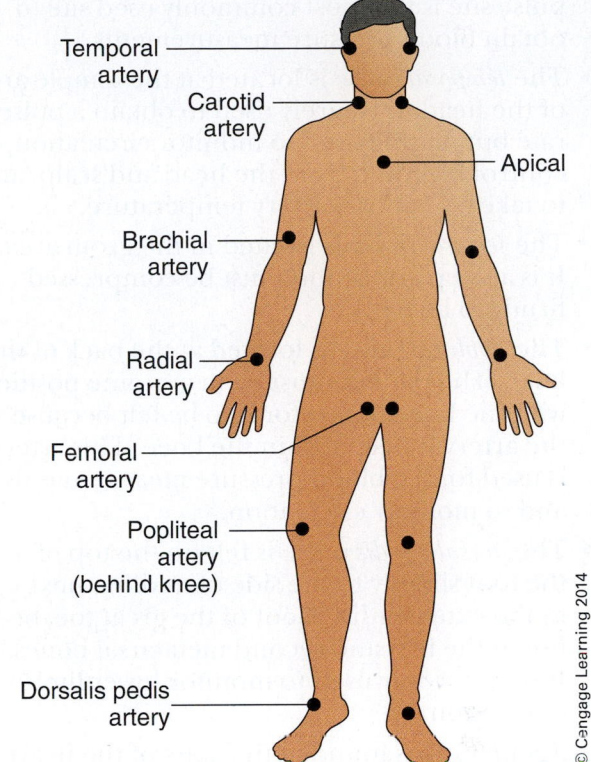

Figure 24-6 Pulse sites in the body.

© Cengage Learning 2014

solid structure such as a bone. Common pulse sites include the radial, carotid, temporal, brachial, femoral, popliteal, and dorsalis pedis arteries (Figure 24-6). An apical pulse, located at the apex of the heart, may also be taken. Although the radial, brachial, and carotid arteries are the most frequently used sites for pulse rates, it is important to recognize pulse beats because circulation may be monitored by palpating the other sites. Pulse sites are also used when necessary as pressure points for controlling severe bleeding.

- The *radial* pulse is located at the thumb side of the wrist approximately 1 inch above the base of the thumb. This is the most commonly used site for obtaining a pulse rate.

- The *carotid* pulse, used during emergency situations and when performing cardiopulmonary resuscitation (CPR), is found between the larynx and sternocleidomastoid muscle in the front side of the neck on either side of the trachea. When measuring the pulse at the carotid site, compress only one side at a time.

- The *brachial* pulse is found in the inner aspect of the elbow called the antecubital space. This pulse site is the most commonly used site to obtain blood pressure measurements.

- The *temporal* pulse is located at the temple area of the head. It is rarely used to obtain a pulse rate but may be used to monitor circulation, control bleeding from the head and scalp, and to take a temporal artery temperature.

- The *femoral* pulse is located in the groin area. It is a deep artery and must be compressed firmly to be felt.

- The *popliteal* pulse is located at the back of the knee. The patient must be in a supine position with the knee flexed for it to be felt because the artery is deep within the knee. This artery is used for leg blood pressure measurements and to monitor circulation.

- The *dorsalis pedis* pulse is felt on the top of the foot slightly to the side of midline next to the extensor ligament of the great toe, between the first and second metatarsal bones. It is commonly used to monitor lower limb circulation.

- *Apical* pulse is found at the apex of the heart, located at the fifth intercostal space left side, midclavicular line, that is, between the fifth and sixth ribs perpendicular to the middle of the clavicle, left of the sternum. A stethoscope is required to obtain an apical pulse. Apical pulse is used for cardiac patients and patients with an arrhythmia, and to obtain infant pulse rates because they are difficult to obtain by the usual methods.

Measuring and Evaluating a Pulse

When measuring a pulse rate, other characteristics besides the rate are noted, such as rhythm, volume of pulse, and condition of the arterial wall.

The rate is the number of pulsations or beats felt in 1 minute. The pulse is counted for 30 seconds, then the number is doubled. Or with practice, the pulse may be counted for 15 seconds and multiplied by four. Pulse rates may vary according to age, activities, general health, sex, emotions, pain, and medications. The rate is lower when sleeping and higher when active or exercising. Rates for infants and children are greater than for adults. Well-conditioned athletes have a lower than average resting rate because their cardiovascular system has been developed to function more efficiently.

Rhythm of the pulse refers to the time between pulsations and regularity of the beat. Normal rhythm occurs when the beats are felt at regular intervals. In abnormal rhythms, **arrhythmias**, the interval between pulsations is altered by either an increased or decreased time span. Arrhythmias must be noted and reported because they may indicate heart disease.

The volume of the pulse refers to the strength of the beat that is felt. The pulsations may feel full, strong, hard, soft, thready, or weak. A pulse may have a regular rate and yet have a variation in intensity or volume. Volume should be noted and reported.

The condition of the arterial wall can be felt as the pulse is taken. The normal artery feels soft and elastic. The abnormal artery may feel hard, knotty, wiry, or a combination of these. These should be noted and reported because they may indicate cardiac disease.

Normal Pulse Rates

Average pulse rates vary from birth to adulthood. At birth, the pulse rate is much higher; as we age, it generally decreases.

NORMAL PULSE RATES

Birth		120–170 beats per minute
Infants		100–150 beats per minute
Children	1 year	120–160 beats per minute
	2 years	80–140 beats per minute
	3 years	70–120 beats per minute
	7–14 years	50–90 beats per minute
Adults		60–100 beats per minute

Pulse Abnormalities

Abnormalities may occur in the rate, rhythm, and feel of the arterial wall. Common pulse rate abnormalities include **bradycardia**, a pulse rate less than 60 beats per minute, and **tachycardia**, a pulse rate greater than 100 beats per minute. Common arrhythmias include a pulsation felt before expected, which is called a premature contraction, and sinus arrhythmia. An occasional premature contraction can occur in response to stress, caffeine, nicotine, alcohol, or lack of sleep. Sinus arrhythmia may occur during respiration and can be found in some children and young adults. The rate increases with inspiration and decreases with expiration. It usually does not require treatment.

 When any pulse rate abnormalities or arrhythmias are felt, take the pulse for 1 full minute, note the frequency of the abnormality, record the abnormality, and alert the provider. The provider may want you to take an apical pulse (see Chapter 37).

Recording Pulse Rates

Pulse rates are normally recorded after the temperature; for example: T 98.6°F P 72 regular. Any unusual findings should be recorded and reported to the provider; for example: P 72 irregular × 2 minutes.

 Procedure 24-7 describes measuring a radial pulse; Procedure 24-8 describes measuring an apical pulse.

RESPIRATION

The function of respiration is the exchange of the gases oxygen and carbon dioxide. External respiration occurs when oxygen is drawn into the lungs when breathing in and carbon dioxide is expelled from the lungs when breathing out. Internal respiration occurs when oxygen is used by the cells for cellular function. Carbon dioxide is a by-product of cellular function and is expelled via exhalation as a waste product. Respiration is an involuntary act controlled by the medulla oblongata of the brain. The medulla oblongata measures blood levels of carbon dioxide and triggers a respiration when the level of carbon dioxide increases. Although it is an involuntary act, respiration may be altered by holding the breath or when hyperventilation occurs. One inspiration (inhalation) drawing in of air and one expiration (exhalation) expelling air together equals one respiration.

Abnormalities in the characteristics of respiration, such as rate, rhythm, and depth, are noted when measuring respiration.

Respiratory rate is the number of respirations per minute. The normal respiratory rate, **eupnea**, varies with age, activities, illness, emotions, and drugs. The average respiration rate to pulse rate is 1:4, one respiration to four pulse beats.

Respiratory rhythm refers to the pattern of breathing. It can vary with age, with adults having a regular pattern, but infants having an irregular pattern. Rhythm may be altered by laughing and sighing.

NORMAL RESPIRATORY RATES

Newborns	30–60 respirations per minute
Infants	24–40 respirations per minute
Children (1–7 years)	22–34 respirations per minute
Adults	14–20 respirations per minute

Depth of respiration is the amount of air that is inspired and expired with each respiration. In the resting state, the amount should be consistent. Depth is noted by watching the degree of rise and fall of the chest wall when measuring respiration rate.

Respiration Rate

Respiratory rate is measured by counting breaths for 30 seconds and doubling the amount. Or with practice, respirations can be counted for 15 seconds and multiplied by four. This will give the number of respirations per minute. It is important that patients not be aware you are measuring their respirations. The best technique requires a good memory. While watching the second hand on your watch, count the pulse rate for 30 seconds. For the next 30 seconds count the respiratory rate. The rate may change if the patient knows they are being counted. Procedure 24-9 gives steps for measuring respiration rate.

Abnormalities

Abnormalities of the respiration rate may be found in the rate, depth, rhythm, and sounds of respiration. Some respiration rate abnormalities include apnea, tachypnea, bradypnea, and Cheyne–Stokes. Sleep apnea and narcolepsy are considered sleep disorders and involve the respiratory system.

Apnea is the complete absence of breathing. It may result from a reduction in stimuli to the respiratory center of the brain. Apnea will occur when the breath is voluntarily held and in Cheyne–Stokes respiration. It can be a serious symptom of other conditions of the cardiovascular and renal systems. It also can result from a head injury such as a concussion.

Tachypnea is a respiratory rate greater than 40 respirations per minute. It may be caused by illness or emotional events or be transient in the newborn. Excessive loss of carbon dioxide may occur if tachypnea is prolonged; there is a potential for this to lead to more serious problems.

Bradypnea is a decrease in the number of respirations to less than 12 breaths per minute and is commonly seen during sleep or because of certain diseases.

Cheyne–Stokes is a breathing pattern that starts with a period of apnea lasting 10 to 60 seconds followed by increasing depth and rate of respiration, which is then followed by a decrease in rate with apnea starting the cycle once again. This cycle may be normal for children but may indicate brain dysfunction in other age groups.

Orthopnea is a respiratory condition of severe **dyspnea** (labored breathing). Breathing is difficult in any position *other* than sitting erect or standing. This condition may be seen in patients with heart failure, angina pectoris, asthma, pulmonary edema, emphysema, pneumonia, and spasmodic coughing. Patients who experience orthopnea must be examined in a sitting position. Other positions will cause discomfort and may not be possible.

Abnormalities in the depth of respiration are divided into shallow abnormalities, such as hypoventilation, and deep abnormalities, such as hyperpnea and hyperventilation.

Hypoventilation occurs when respiration is decreased in rate and shallow in depth. It may result from a depression of nervous stimuli of the respiratory center in the brain.

Hyperpnea is respiration that is increased in both depth and rate. It is commonly seen with activities such as physical exercise. It can also be associated with pain, respiratory diseases, cardiac diseases, hysteria, and use of certain drugs.

Hyperventilation is a type of breathing in which the amount of oxygen drawn in during inspiration is greatly increased, resulting in a decrease in the amount of blood carbon dioxide. Hyperventilation may be associated with asthma, pulmonary embolism or edema, and acute anxiety. The patient can be treated by reducing the amount of oxygen inhaled during an inspiration. The patient may be instructed to hold one nostril closed while breathing or may be instructed to breathe into a paper bag. Either procedure will reduce the amount of inspired oxygen and bring the oxygen and carbon dioxide blood levels back to within normal range.

Sleep Apnea. Airflow during respiration that stops for more than 10 seconds is considered to be sleep apnea. The periods of apnea cause carbon dioxide to accumulate in the blood and oxygen to be depleted. For these reasons, sleep apnea can be dangerous. Oxygen depletion to the brain can cause memory impairment, cognitive changes, and daytime sleepiness. If the condition goes untreated, sleep apnea can result in cardiac arrhythmias, congestive heart failure, cerebral vascular accident (CVA), hypertension, and death.

Sleep apnea is associated with airway obstruction. The soft palate (especially in males who are overweight and who snore) can collapse while the patient is asleep. The result is apnea. The patient usually awakens from sleep enough to resume breathing.

Sleep apnea is diagnosed by sleep laboratory studies when apnea is observed while the patient is sleeping.

Treatment of sleep apnea consists of weight loss and continuous positive airway pressure (CPAP), a device that puts pressure on the airway while the patient sleeps. A mask is placed over the patient's face to keep the airway open. This prevents sleep apnea. A surgical procedure can be performed to remove parts of the soft palate and uvula.

Narcolepsy. Narcolepsy is another type of sleep disorder that causes excessive sleepiness and frequent daytime sleep attacks. The patient can become paralyzed from the sleep, being unable to move, but can still breathe. The cause may be genetic. It is possible that this is an autoimmune disorder. Most commonly, symptoms first appear in 15 to 30 year olds.

The diagnosis is made by ruling out sleep apnea (through sleep studies) and by the history of repeated episodes of daytime sleeping for a few seconds to half an hour. An EEG, EKG, a sleep study, and genetic testing for the narcolepsy gene are all components of testing for narcolepsy. The disorder is not under the patient's control.

Breath Sounds. The presence or absence of breath sounds can be indicative of respiratory problems. Sounds should be listened for and noted when taking the patient's respiratory rate.

Rales (pronounced "rawles") are clicking or rattling sounds heard during inspiration and expiration when the lung passageways contain secretions. The provider uses a stethoscope to auscultate or listen for rales, which are associated with some lung diseases. Rhonchi are sounds similar to snoring, usually produced by a rattle in the throat. These are also heard by auscultation.

Wheezes are high-pitched musical sounds heard on expiration. They can be the result of an obstruction in the bronchi and bronchioles of the lungs. Wheezes are commonly associated with asthma and emphysema, a chronic pulmonary disease characterized by dilated and damaged alveoli.

Stridor is a crowing sound heard on inspiration as a result of an obstruction of the upper airway. It is associated with laryngitis, a foreign body obstruction, and croup in children.

Stertorous respiration is described as a snoring sound with labored breathing. The sound usually is created by partial obstruction of the upper airway.

BLOOD PRESSURE

Blood pressure measures cardiovascular function by measuring the force of blood exerted on **peripheral** arteries during the cardiac cycle or heartbeat. The measurement consists of two components. The first is the force exerted on the arterial walls during cardiac contraction and is called **systole**. The second is the force exerted during cardiac relaxation and is called **diastole**. They represent the highest (systole) and lowest (diastole) amount of pressure exerted during the cardiac cycle. Blood pressure is recorded as a fraction, with the systolic measurement written, followed by a slash, and then the diastolic measurement.

Example:

systole/diastole or 120/80

Blood pressure may be affected by many factors, including blood volume, peripheral resistance, vessel elasticity, condition of the muscle of the heart, genetics, diet and weight, activity, and emotional state.

- Blood volume is the amount of blood within the arteries. Increased volume of blood increases blood pressure, whereas a decrease in blood volume decreases blood pressure, as in the case of a hemorrhage or severe dehydration.

- Peripheral resistance is the resistance to blood flow within the arteries. The resistance is in direct relation to the **lumen** of the arteries. The smaller the lumen, the more pressure needed to push blood through. The reverse is also true: the larger the lumen, the less resistance and less pressure needed to push the blood through. The size of the lumen can become smaller from deposits of fatty cholesterol (plaque), resulting in an increase in blood pressure.

- Vessel elasticity refers to the ability of arteries to expand and contract to provide a steady flow of blood. As a person ages, elasticity of the vessels is reduced. **Atherosclerosis** can cause an increase in arterial wall resistance, resulting in an increase in blood pressure.

- The condition of the heart muscle is extremely important to blood flow and blood pressure. A strong heart muscle provides a forceful pump resulting in efficient blood flow and normal blood pressure. A weak heart muscle results in an inefficient pumping action of the heart leading to a decrease in blood pressure and blood flow (see Chapter 37).

- Uncontrolled hypertension, over time, is responsible for changes in the heart's structure, vessels that supply the heart muscle, and the electrical conduction system of the heart. These changes can lead to life-threatening conditions such as arrhythmias and congestive heart failure.

The viscosity of the blood also is a factor in blood pressure. Viscosity is the property of a fluid that offers resistance to flow. If the blood's viscosity is increased, it acts thicker. Imagine holding a bottle of thin syrup upside down over your pancakes. The thin syrup comes out of the bottle quite readily. Now imagine holding a bottle of thick molasses over the pancakes. Being very viscous, the molasses is thicker and much more difficult to pour. So it is with viscous blood; it is thicker and requires a lot more work for the heart muscle to move it through the vessels, thus increasing the pressure inside the walls of the arteries. In fact, it may be so viscous that it might not be able to reach the tiniest capillaries of the kidney, eyes, and other areas without substantial increase in blood pressure.

Equipment for Measuring Blood Pressure

Blood pressure is measured by the auscultatory method using a sphygmomanometer and a stethoscope (Figure 24-7). Listening carefully is the key to obtaining accurate blood pressure measurement.

Three types of sphygmomanometers are commonly used in the ambulatory care setting: mercury, aneroid, and electronic (digital) manometers (Figure 24-8 through Figure 24-11).

Mercury sphygmomanometers are being phased out with other mercury-containing medical equipment such as mercury thermometers.

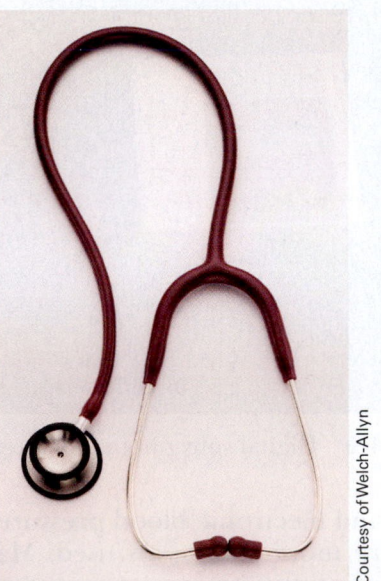

Courtesy of Welch-Allyn

Figure 24-7 Adult stethoscope is used with a sphygmomanometer to measure blood pressure.

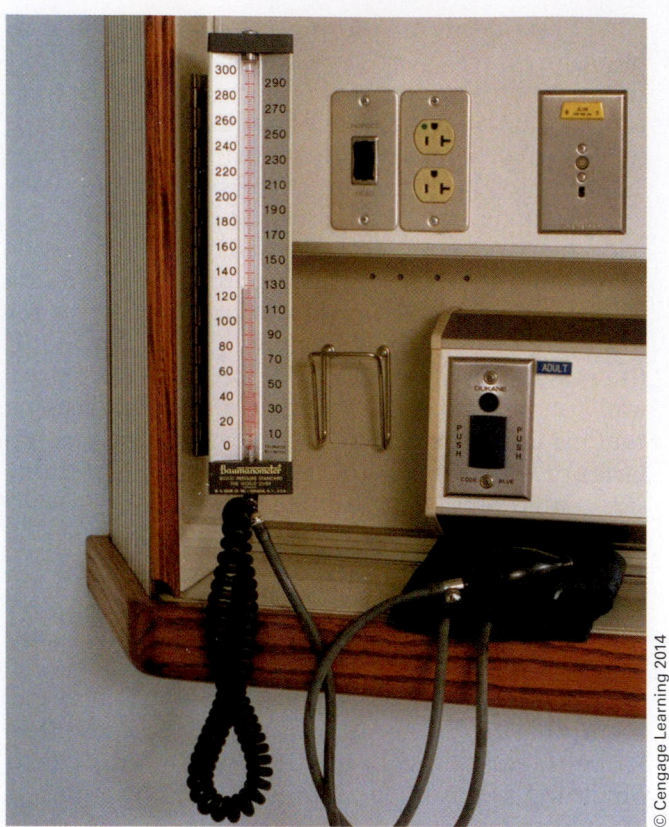

Figure 24-8 A mercury gravity sphygmomanometer.

© Cengage Learning 2014

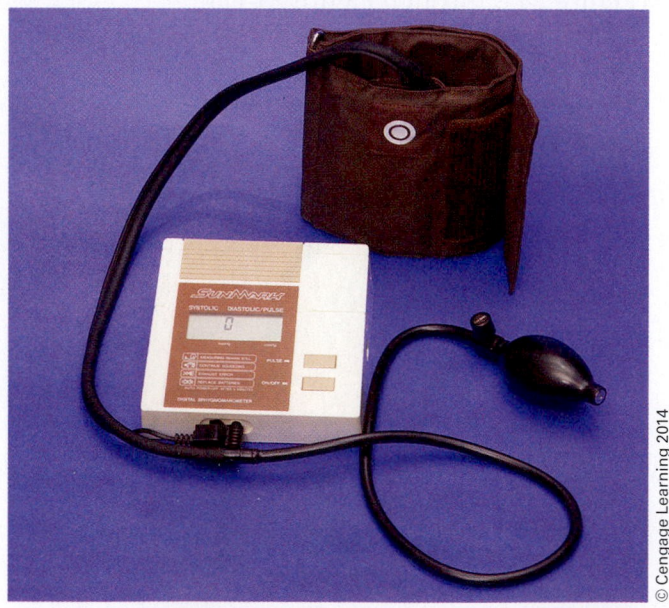

Figure 24-9 Digital sphygmomanometer.

© Cengage Learning 2014

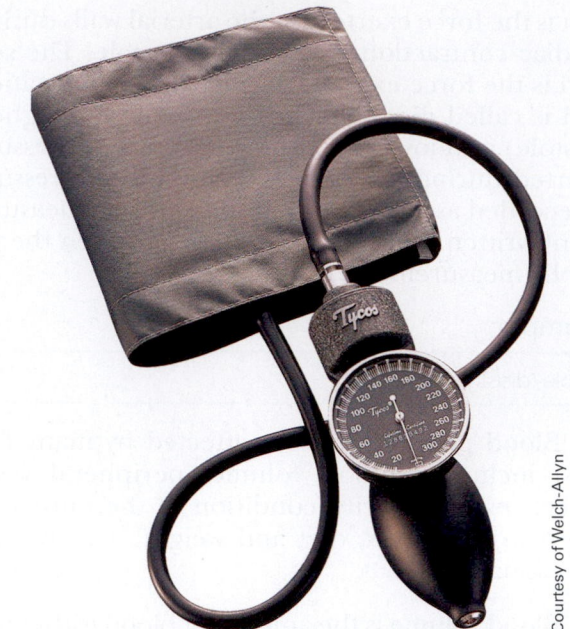

Figure 24-10 Aneroid sphygmomanometer.

Courtesy of Welch-Allyn

Aneroid and electronic blood pressure measuring devices are more commonly used. Many medical facilities continue to use mercury sphygmomanometers while phasing them out in agreement with the EPA, but the process has been slower than the phasing out of mercury thermometers; therefore, information about the mercury sphygmomanometers is provided in this chapter.

The mercury **manometer** consists of a cuff containing a rubber bladder attached by rubber tubing to a glass column of mercury. The blood pressure is read at the **meniscus** of the mercury as it descends the column. The meniscus is the curve seen at the top of a liquid in response to its container. Mercury manometers are the most accurate method of blood pressure measurement and are considered the standard because blood pressure is measured in millimeters of mercury. Although the most accurate, mercury manometers do have disadvantages: they are not as portable as aneroid manometers, and there is always the danger of a mercury spill causing health and environmental problems should the glass column break. Mercury manometers need to be cleaned and checked regularly for accuracy by a professional technician. Care in handling and storage is important to prevent air bubbles and dirt from forming in the column and to prevent breaking the glass containing the mercury.

The aneroid manometer is a cuff containing a rubber bladder attached to a dial. The blood pressure is read at the point of the needle descending the dial. Aneroid manometers need to be calibrated regularly because they do not maintain calibration easily. Care in handling and storage will decrease the loss of calibration. Although not as accurate as a mercury manometer, aneroid

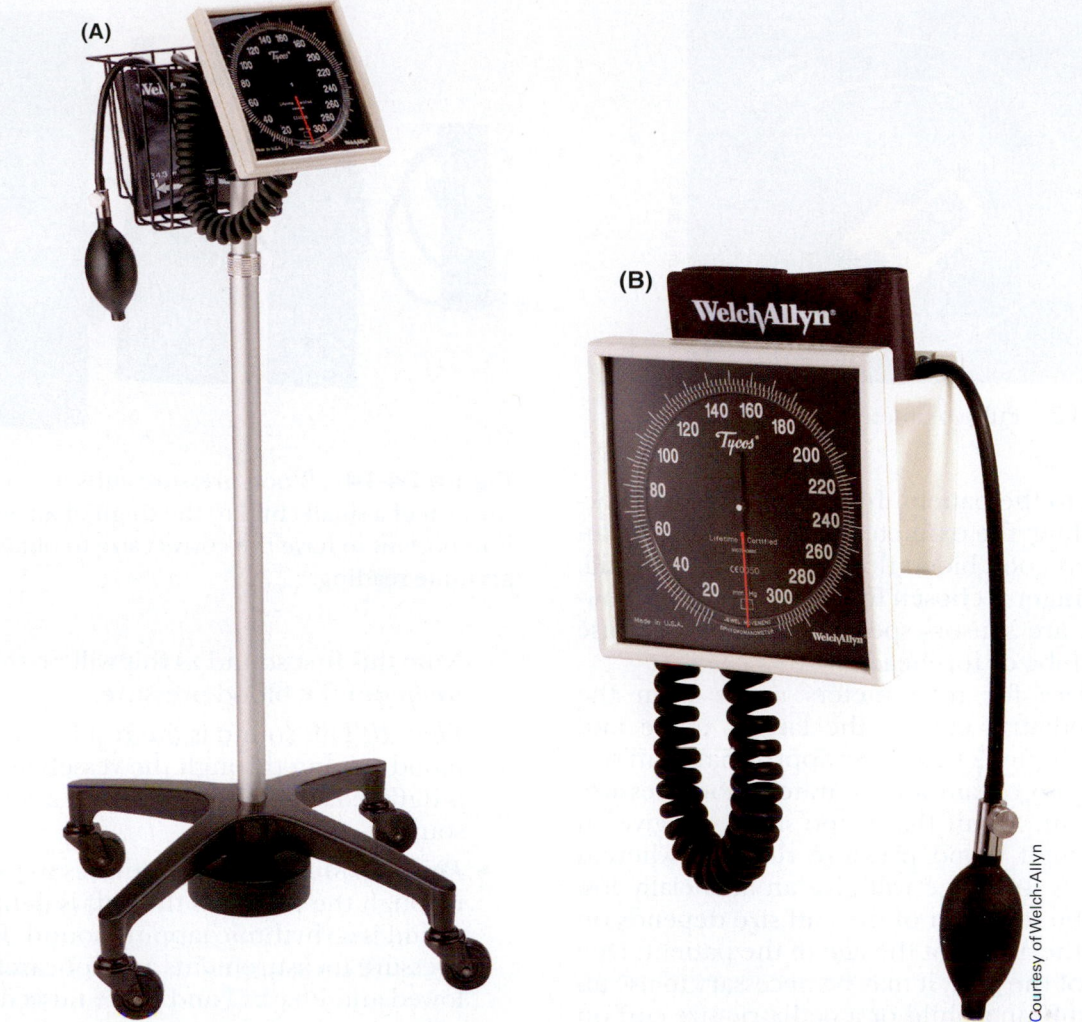

(A)

(B)

Courtesy of Welch-Allyn

Figure 24-11 (A) Mobile aneroid sphygmomanometer. (B) Wall-mounted aneroid sphygmomanometer.

manometers are easily portable and there is no danger of a mercury spill.

An electronic sphygmomanometer is automatic and registers blood pressure in digital form on a screen (Figure 24-12). No stethoscope is needed. Once the cuff is secured on the patient's upper arm, the medical assistant pushes a button and the cuff inflates; the medical assistant then releases the pressure slowly. A readout is visible on the screen (124/75). In addition to blood pressure reading, the unit can automatically measure pulse rate and other vital signs.

A **pulse oximeter** (Figure 24-13) is a noninvasive method for measuring the amount of oxygen that is saturating the hemoglobin molecules contained in a red blood cell. Most pulse oximeters also provide an audible signal for the pulse and display a calculated heart rate. The measurement automatically appears on the screen when the device

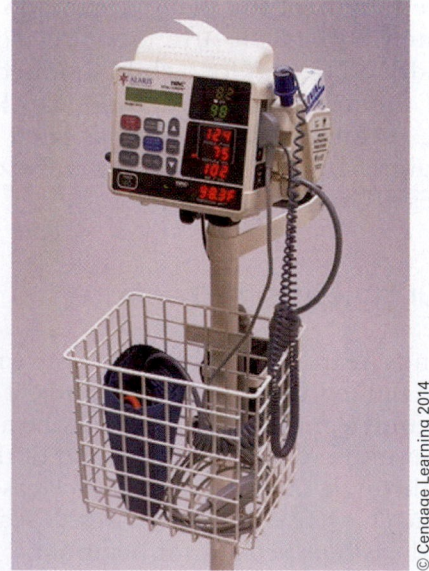

© Cengage Learning 2014

Figure 24-12 An electronic sphygmomanometer can measure pulse and other vital signs simultaneously.

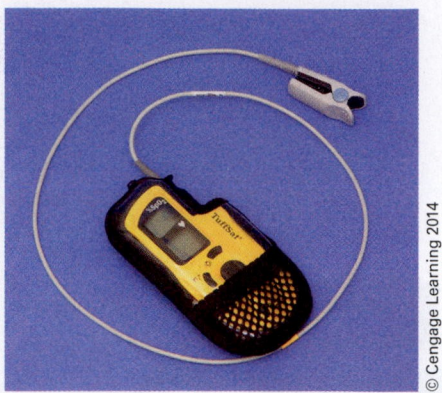

Figure 24-13   Pulse oximeter.

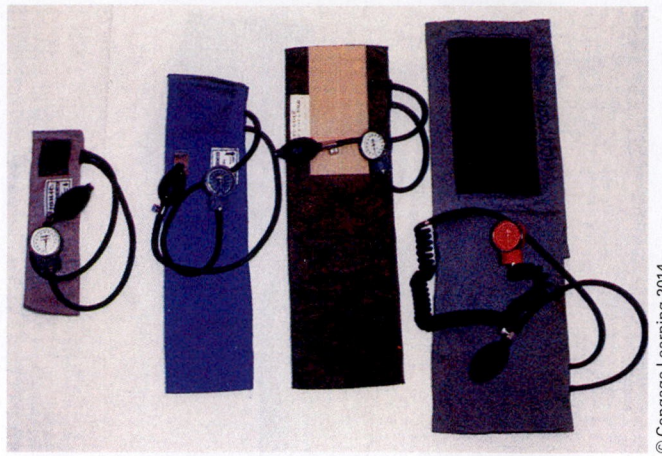

Figure 24-14   Blood pressure cuffs in sizes to fit the arm of a small child to the thigh of an adult. It is important to have the correct size to obtain an accurate reading.

is attached to the patient. In order to obtain an accurate reading, the oximeter must be placed on an area that has good blood flow and can be held still. Usually, a finger is chosen for pulse oximetry. However, there are sensors specially designed for use on the ear lobe or forehead.

Cuff sizes for manometers range from the smallest pediatric cuff to the largest obese and thigh cuff (Figure 24-14). The appropriate cuff size is necessary to obtain an accurate blood pressure measurement. A cuff that is too small will give an artificially high blood pressure reading, whereas a cuff that is too large will give an artificially low reading. The selection of the cuff size depends on the size of the arm, not the age of the patient. Due to the size of the arm, it may be necessary to use an adult-size cuff on a child or a pediatric-size cuff on an adult. Adult cuffs should have a width that covers one third to one half the circumference of the arm. The length of the bladder should cover approximately 80% of the arm (about twice the size of the width). The cuff for a child should cover two thirds of the upper arm. The American Heart Association recommends if there has been a weight loss or gain of 10 pounds, then the cuff size should be reassessed for the appropriate size.

Measuring Blood Pressure

The sounds heard during blood pressure measurement are named the Korotkoff sounds. The cause of the sounds is not known. They may be a result of distention of the vessels or the sound of the blood passing through the vessels. In either case, Korotkoff sounds have five distinct phases. Not all phases are heard easily, especially for beginners.

- *Phase I.* Begins with the first sound heard when deflating the cuff. It is a sharp tapping sound.

Note this first sound as this will be the *systolic reading* of the blood pressure.

- *Phase II.* This sound is the result of more blood passing through the vessels as the cuff is deflated. The sound is that of a soft swishing sound.

- *Phase III.* More blood continues to pass through the vessels as the cuff is deflated. The sound is a rhythmic tapping sound. If blood pressure measurements are not carefully followed and Phases I and II are missed, Phase III may erroneously be reported as the systolic pressure.

- *Phase IV.* Blood is now passing through the vessels fairly easily as the cuff is deflated. The sounds heard will be a muffling and fading of the tapping sounds. This phase may be used to record the diastolic pressure in children and in those patients where a tapping sound is heard throughout the deflation until the mercury reaches zero.

- *Phase V.* Blood is flowing freely at this time; consequently all sounds disappear. The disappearance of sounds is noted and recorded as the *diastolic pressure.*

When measuring blood pressure, keep two things in mind: patient comfort and accuracy.

Auscultatory gap is heard in some patients. It is a time, usually between Phases I and II or III, when all sounds disappear. Within 20 to 30 mm Hg, or 20 to 30 **increments** on the aneroid manometer, the sounds reappear. If the procedures are not followed carefully, the auscultatory gap is easily

Table 24-1   Errors in Blood Pressure Measurement Procedures

Errors in measuring blood pressure must be avoided. Common errors include:

1. Improper cuff size.
2. The arm is not at heart level. Do not hold the arm up or let the patient hold up the arm. Pressure is increased when this is done. It is essential that the arm be at the correct level and supported so that there is minimal muscle tension to obtain a correct reading.
3. Cuff is not completely deflated before use or after palpatory method, resulting in a higher pressure measurement.
4. Deflation of the cuff is faster than 2 to 4 mm Hg per heartbeat or 20–30 increments on the aneroid. Sounds are missed if this happens.
5. Reinflating the cuff during the procedure without allowing the arm to rest for 1 to 2 minutes.
6. Patient is not relaxed and comfortable. An anxious, apprehensive patient will have a reading that is higher than the actual blood pressure.
7. Improper cuff placement. Cuff is too loose, too tight, or not positioned correctly over the brachial artery.
8. Defective equipment in which there are air leaks in the bladder or valve, the mercury column is dirty, or air bubbles are present. Mercury and aneroid sphygmomanometers are not calibrated at zero.
9. Measuring blood pressure with thumb on the head of the stethoscope.

All of these errors are easily corrected by following careful procedure and by having the manometers calibrated and cleaned according to a regular maintenance schedule.

missed, and the blood pressure measurement is incorrect in that systolic and diastolic readings may be in error according to the length of the gap (Table 24-1).

Pulse pressure is the difference between the systolic and diastolic measurements. It is important because it is a better predictor of clinical outcome than either systolic or diastolic pressure alone. An elevated pulse pressure causes more arterial damage and indicates more workload on the left ventricle. The normal range for pulse pressure is 30 to 50 mm Hg. The difference should be no more than one third of the systolic reading. For example, if the blood pressure is 120/80, a normal pulse pressure should be 120 minus 80 or 40. One third of the systolic reading of 120 is 40. Therefore, 40 mm Hg pulse pressure is within the normal range.

Recording Blood Pressure Measurement

The blood pressure is recorded on the patient chart or electronic medical record in a fraction format. The position of the patient (sitting or lying down) may be noted. The arm used is also noted, particularly if the blood pressure was taken in both arms.

Example:

120/80, ® arm, supine or $\frac{120}{80}$ ® arm, supine

For children and those patients whose blood pressure can still be heard to zero, the beginning of Korotkoff Phase IV and zero both are recorded.

Example:

120/70/0 or $\frac{\frac{120}{70}}{0}$

 Procedure 24-10 outlines the procedure for measuring blood pressure.

Normal Blood Pressure Readings

Normal blood pressure is low at birth and gradually increases with age until adulthood, at which point it should remain fairly constant. Blood pressure measurements are taken during yearly physical examinations beginning at age 3.

NORMAL BLOOD PRESSURE READINGS

In a healthy child, blood pressure is taken for the first time during the physical exam when the child is 3 years old. Blood pressure in children varies based on their gender and height percentile.

Child 10 years	100/65
Adolescent 16 years	118/75
Adult	Systolic less than 120
	Diastolic less than 80
Prehypertension	120–139/80–89
High blood pressure	Above 140/90

Blood Pressure Abnormalities

There are only two possible blood pressure abnormalities: hypertension, blood pressure that is consistently above normal, and hypotension, blood pressure that is consistently below normal in which patients are unable to perform their normal activities without dizziness and extreme fatigue. It is

Table 24-2   Blood Pressure Categories

Systolic		Diastolic	American Heart Association B/P Category
Less than 120 mm/Hg	and	Less than 80 mm/Hg	Normal
120 to 139 mm/Hg	or	80–89 mm/Hg	Prehypertension
140 to 159 mm/Hg	or	90–99 mm/Hg	Stage 1 hypertension
160 mm/Hg or higher	or	100 mm/Hg or higher	Stage 2 hypertension
Higher than 180 mm/Hg	or	110 mm/Hg or higher	Hypertensive crisis

Adapted from the American Heart Association 2012 Guidelines. Source: www.heart.org

essential that any blood pressure abnormalities be reported to the provider in a timely manner.

Hypertension. There are five types of **hypertension**: primary or essential, secondary, benign, and malignant.

- The most commonly seen form of hypertension is primary or essential. It is hypertension with no apparent cause or cure but is treatable. Treatment is designed to control hypertension and is a lifelong process. It will not be cured, just controlled. The American Heart Association (AHA) suggests that to diagnose hypertension, the diagnosis is based on the average of three readings at each of three visits to the provider's clinic after the initial baseline screening. According to the AHA, normal blood pressure for adults 18 years and older is less than 120/80, prehypertension is 120–139/80–89, hypertension stage 1 is 140–159/90–99, and hypertension stage 2 is ≥ 160/100 (Table 24-2).

- Secondary hypertension is the result of some underlying problem, such as renal disease, pregnancy, endocrine imbalances, obesity, arteriosclerosis, or atherosclerosis. Once the underlying problem is removed, the blood pressure returns to normal or near normal. Secondary hypertension can be successfully treated.

- Hypertension that has a slow progression but may progress to the same end point as malignant hypertension is referred to as benign hypertension.

- Malignant hypertension (no association with cancer) progresses rapidly with severe damage to the cardiovascular system, possibly to the point of death.

- White coat hypertension is hypertension that can occur in some individuals. It is caused by anxiety or fear when blood pressure measurements are taken by a provider.

PATIENT EDUCATION

Hypertension is at epidemic proportions in the United States, and many patients are not treated because they do not know that they have the problem. It is known as the "silent epidemic" because most people do not experience any symptoms over a span of years. However, untreated or poorly treated hypertension over time can damage the heart, cause myocardial infarction, cause a stroke (cerebrovascular accident), or lead to kidney failure.

There are several nondrug ways to reduce blood pressure, even for people who have inherited hypertensive tendencies. With the provider's advice, there are steps to take that include: eating plenty of produce, grains, and low-fat dairy foods; cutting back on salt; stopping smoking; exercising regularly; maintaining a healthy weight; limiting alcohol intake; and reducing stress. It is easy to see that these recommendations all are lifestyle changes. They can significantly reduce blood pressure if practiced daily. Blood pressure must be monitored regularly by your provider.

Hypotension. Hypotension is blood pressure persistently less than normal, usually less than 90/60, although this may be normal for some healthy adults. Hypotension is defined as a blood pressure so low that the patient is unable to maintain normal function. It is usually a result of various shock-like conditions such as hemorrhage, traumatic or emotional shock, central nervous system disorders, or chronic wasting diseases. With successful treatment of the underlying problems, the blood pressure usually will be in the range of normal readings.

Orthostatic hypotension, sometimes called postural hypotension, occurs when a person rapidly changes position from supine to standing, when standing in one position for too long, or as a side effect of certain medications. In this instance, the blood pressure has momentarily decreased, and the person experiences vertigo (dizziness) and may have blurred vision. These symptoms usually last only a few seconds, just long enough for the blood pressure to return to normal. Care should be taken when helping patients to an upright position from a supine position because orthostatic hypotension can lead to syncope (fainting) and injury from falling.

HEIGHT AND WEIGHT

Although not considered a vital sign, height and weight are routinely measured if warranted by the age and the physical condition of the patient. Many providers prefer that height and weight be measured as part of a yearly physical examination and otherwise may vary the frequency of patient height and weight measurements. Height and weight are normally measured simultaneously.

For children, height and weight are typically measured during each provider visit. The height of adults may be obtained on the initial visit only and weight taken on all visits. An adolescent or young adult may have height measured more frequently to plot body changes. Because older adult patients tend to lose the cushioning between vertebrae through osteoporosis as part of aging, they may need to have their height measured more frequently to check the stage of any degeneration.

Older adult patients require special attention by the medical assistant when measuring height and weight. It is especially important to assist older patients both on and off the scale, because the scale platform is movable, and older patients may lose their balance and fall if unassisted. A stand-alone walker can be placed over the scale platform to aid in stabilizing the patient.

CRITICAL THINKING

Discuss the normal vital signs differences expected between an infant and an adult. Why do they occur?

Height

To measure a patient's height, a scale with a measuring bar is necessary (Figure 24-15A). A paper towel is placed on the scale because the patient's shoes should be removed for accurate measuring. The patient is asked to step on the scale and face away from the measuring bar. Assist the patient onto the scale; the scale platform is movable and the patient could fall.

There are two reasons for having the patient's back to the scale. When the measuring bar is lifted, it could cause face or eye injuries if the patient were facing the bar. Lifting the measuring bar prior to the patient stepping on the scale can also lead to eye and face injuries in that the patient could inadvertently walk into the bar. Another reason to have the patient's back to the scale is if the patient does not look straight ahead, the head is not level, which could result in a less-than-accurate measurement.

After the patient is on the platform, the measuring bar is placed firmly on the patient's head, and the line between where the solid bar and sliding bar meet is read. The bars are measured in quarter inches (Figure 24-15B). Children's heights are recorded in inches, whereas adults are recorded in feet and inches. Conversion from inches to feet is accomplished by taking the number of inches and dividing by 12. Procedure 24-11 gives steps for measuring height.

Weight

Provider preference and patient health dictate the frequency of measuring an adult's weight. Some providers require the patient's weight to be measured on each visit, whereas others do not if there are no health problems that require weight monitoring. Some health conditions that do require weight monitoring include obesity, eating disorders, hormone disorders such as diabetes and thyroid malfunction, hypertension, pregnancy, cancer, and some digestive disorders.

When measuring the weight of a patient, the medical assistant must maintain the patient's privacy. Most people are conscious of their weight and may become embarrassed if the measurement is taken where others may see and

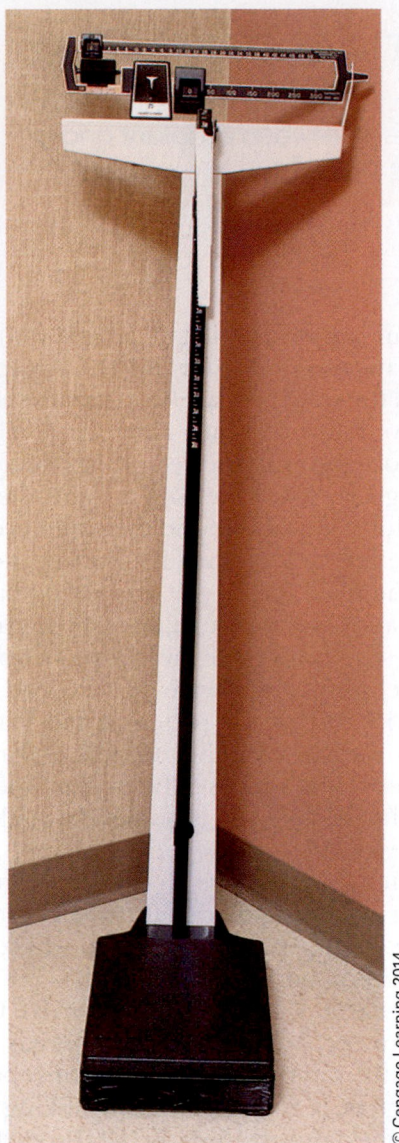

Figure 24-15A   Traditional beam balance scale with measuring bar.

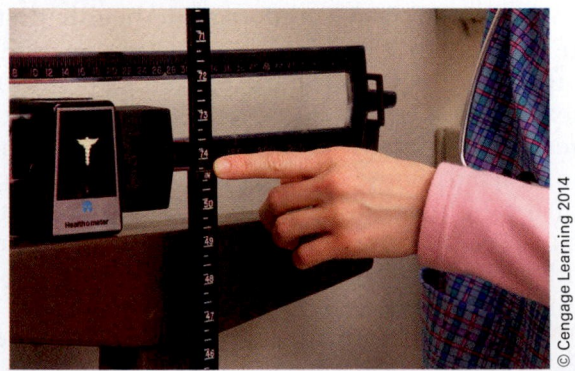

Figure 24-15B   The height is read at the movable point of the ruler. The bars are measured in one-quarter inches. Note the height measurement is 74.25 inches or 6 feet 2¼ inches.

hear. Privacy is important and often overlooked. The medical assistant must also be careful of comments regarding a patient's weight, particularly with the obese patient and with those being treated for eating disorders (see Chapter 34). Encouragement for weight loss for the dieting patient is beneficial but must be done in privacy. Other comments are inappropriate.

Occasionally a patient will be instructed by the provider to monitor weight at home. It is important for the patient to understand the necessity of weighing at the same time each day because weight may vary significantly throughout the day. A normal routine is to measure weight before breakfast.

Before an accurate weight can be obtained, the scale must be calibrated. The point of the balance beam must be floating in the center when no weight is applied to the scale. Some scales are equipped with a screw at the end that can be turned slightly until the beam is in the correct floating position. Once it is centered, it is calibrated and ready for use (Figure 24-16).

An eye-level digital scale with measuring bar measures height in the same way on the measuring bar of the digital scale as it is on the balance beam measuring bar. Weight measurement is quicker, easier, and usually safer taken on the digital scale. The scale platform is stationary, and the patient is assisted as needed onto the scale; the digital reading is ready in a few seconds (Figure 24-17).

The patient can wear normal indoor clothing, rather than disrobing, for weight measurement. Heavy coats or other outerwear should be removed. Heavy objects and purses should not be held during the procedure. A chair or counter should be provided to place these objects on while the procedure is being performed. Shoes should be removed. Procedure 24-12 gives steps for measuring adult weight.

Occasionally, as in the case of medication dosage, the medical assistant is required to convert pound weight into kilogram weight.

1 kilogram = 2.2 pounds
To convert pounds to kilograms:
Take the number of pounds and divide by 2.2

Example:

130 pounds divided by 2.2 = 59.09 kg

To convert from kilograms to pounds:
Take the number of kilograms and multiply by 2.2

Example:

50 kilograms multiplied by 2.2 = 110 lb.

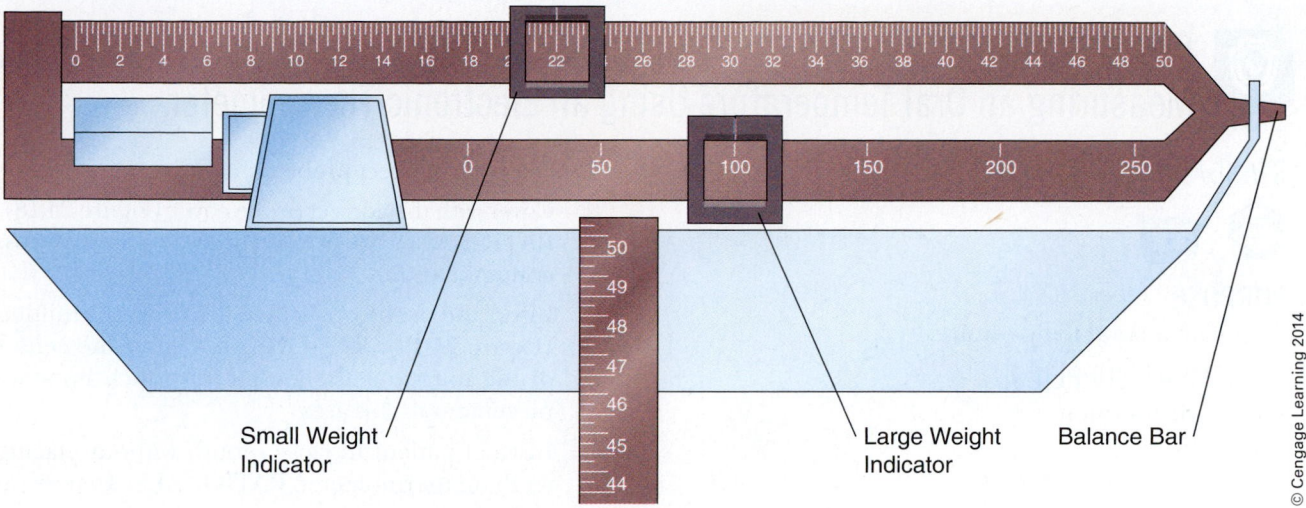

Small Weight Indicator   Large Weight Indicator   Balance Bar

© Cengage Learning 2014

Figure 24-16   The upper bar indicates small pound weights (from 0—50 lb). The weight shown on the lower bar is measured in 50-lb increments. The lower measurement is added to the upper bar amount that is shown. The upper bar shows 22 lb; the lower bar measures 100 lb. Upper bar 22 lb plus lower bar 100 lb equal total weight 122 lb.

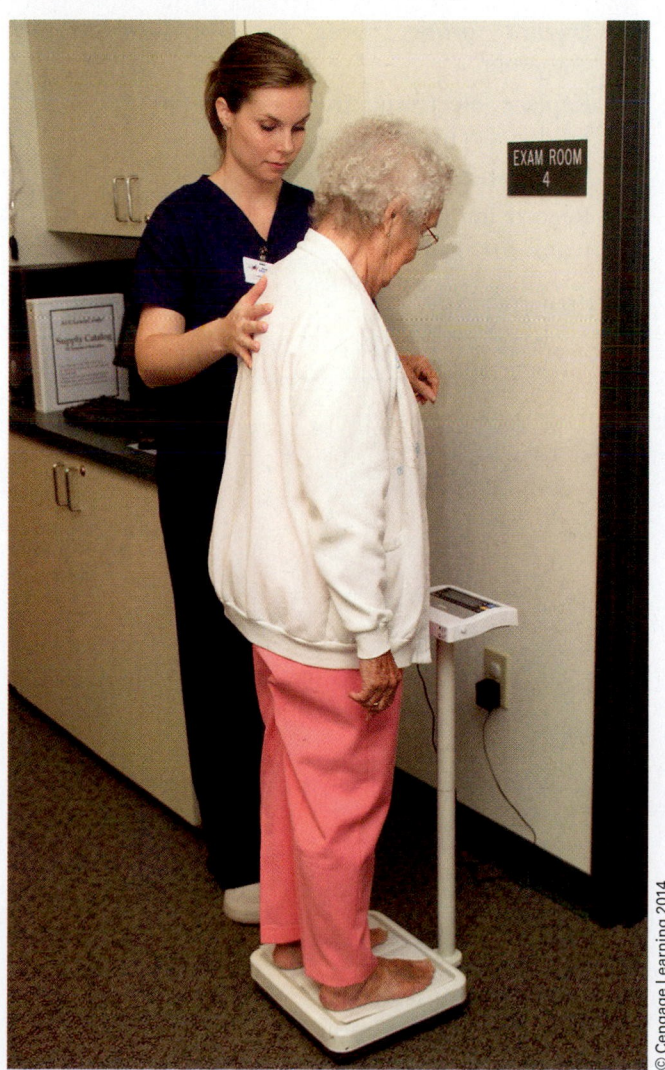

© Cengage Learning 2014

Figure 24-17   An electronic scale.

Significance of Weight

The careful monitoring of a patient's weight may provide an insight into metabolic, nutritional, and emotional problems.

MEASURING CHEST CIRCUMFERENCE

Occasionally, the medical assistant is instructed to measure the chest of an adult. This procedure may be done on patients with emphysema and as a requirement for insurance and truck driver licenses. Two measurements are taken, one on the deepest inspiration and one on the deepest expiration. A comparison is then made to ascertain chest capacity. To perform the procedure, ask the patient to disrobe from the waist up. Place a tape measure around the chest at nipple level. Instruct the patient to inhale deeply while you measure, then ask the patient to exhale completely while you take the second measurement. Record the results as inspiration number and expiration number (see Chapter 30).

CRITICAL THINKING

Discuss the methods the medical assistant may use to obtain patient cooperation when taking vital signs. Describe and demonstrate the appropriate charting procedure for normal vital sign results.

PROCEDURE 24-1

Measuring an Oral Temperature Using an Electronic Thermometer

STANDARD PRECAUTIONS:

PURPOSE:
To obtain an oral temperature.

EQUIPMENT/SUPPLIES:
Electronic thermometer
Probe covers
Biohazard waste container

PROCEDURE STEPS:

1. Wash hands and follow Standard Precautions.
2. *Paying attention to detail,* assemble equipment.
3. *Introduce yourself to the patient. Identify patient.*
4. Position the patient in a comfortable position.
5. Inquire if the patient has ingested hot or cold drinks or food or has been smoking within the previous half hour. RATIONALE: Ingesting hot or cold substances or smoking can result in an arbitrary increase or decrease in temperature results.
6. Being courteous and respectful to the patient, *explain the procedure, speaking at the patient's level of understanding.* RATIONALE: To obtain patient cooperation and consent.
7. Select the correct probe for an oral temperature.
8. Cover with the correct probe cover (Figure 24-18). RATIONALE: To prevent microorganism cross contamination.
9. Insert the probe on either side of the frenulum. (Figure 24-19). RATIONALE: Under the center of the tongue is the **frenulum**, which impedes placement in this area.
10. Instruct patient to close mouth without placing teeth on thermometer. RATIONALE: To prevent air leakage.
11. Leave in place until the beep is heard.
12. Remove the thermometer probe after appropriate time has elapsed.
13. Read the results on the digital display window.
14. Discard probe cover in biohazard waste container.
15. Replace electronic thermometer in the base holder, if required for recharging.
16. Wash hands.
17. Record temperature in patient's chart or electronic medical record.

DOCUMENTATION:
5/26/20XX 11:00 AM   T 99.2°F, P 96, R 14. C. McInnis, RMA (AMT)——————

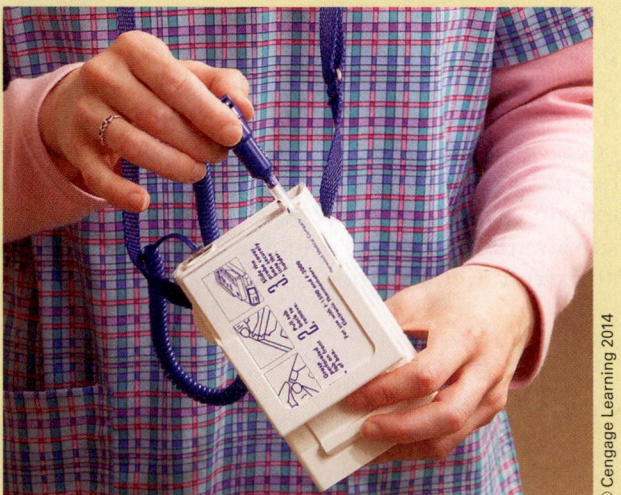

Figure 24-18   Slide the probe into the disposable cover, adjusting if necessary.

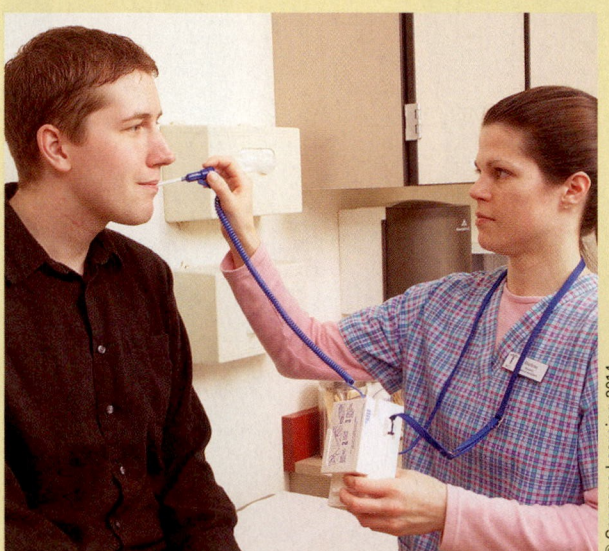

Figure 24-19   Insert the thermometer under tongue to either side of mouth.

© Cengage Learning 2014

PROCEDURE 24-2

Measuring an Aural Temperature Using a Tympanic Thermometer

STANDARD PRECAUTIONS:

PURPOSE:

To obtain an aural temperature using a tympanic thermometer.

EQUIPMENT/SUPPLIES:

Tympanic thermometer (Figure 24-20)
Probe covers or ear speculum
Waste container

PROCEDURE STEPS:

1. Wash hands following Standard Precautions.
2. *Paying attention to detail,* assemble equipment.
3. *Introduce yourself to the patient. Identify the patient.*
4. *Explain procedure, speaking at the patient's level of understanding.* RATIONALE: This will help gain the patient's cooperation and consent.
5. Place cover on thermometer (Figure 24-21).
6. Set thermometer to start.
7. Gently straighten ear canal up and back for adults and place probe into ear canal to seal the area and activate the system (Figure 24-22). RATIONALE: Air leaks will occur if the ear canal is not sealed.
8. Wait until the temperature is displayed on the screen.
9. Remove from the ear.
10. Discard cover into waste container by pressing the release button.
11. Wash hands.
12. Replace thermometer.
13. Record temperature in patient's chart or electronic medical record, indicating tympanic measurement (Tym).

DOCUMENTATION:

*5/26/20XX 4:00 PM   T 99.6° F (Tym), P 100, R 20.
C. McInnis, RMA (AMT)*——————————————

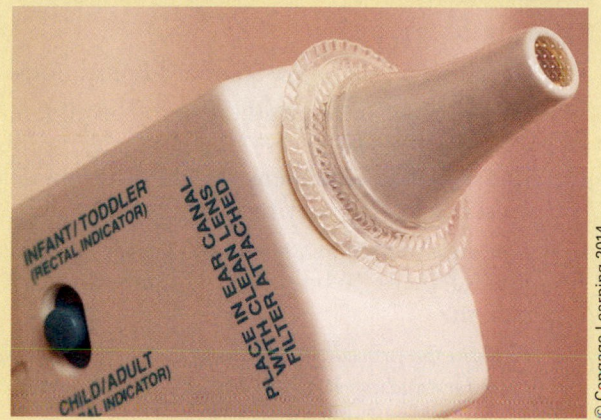

Figure 24-21   Attach the disposable speculum or cover to the tympanic thermometer to prevent spread of microorganisms between patients.

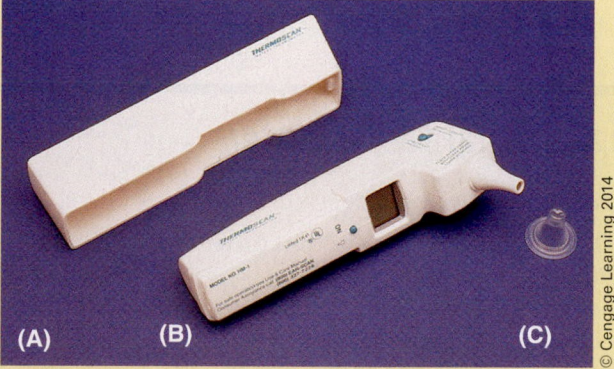

Figure 24-20   Tympanic thermometer: (A) Holder. (B) Tympanic thermometer. (C) Disposable speculum or cover.

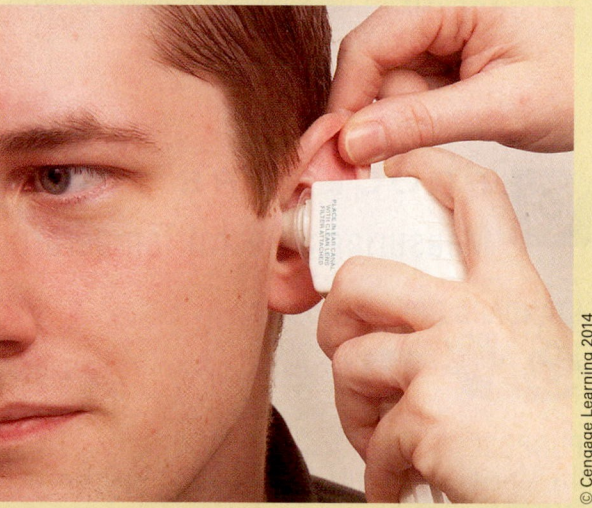

Figure 24-22   Pull up on the ear to straighten the auditory canal for an accurate reading.

PROCEDURE 24-3

Measuring a Temperature Using a Temporal Artery (TA) Thermometer

STANDARD PRECAUTIONS:

PURPOSE:
To obtain a temporal artery temperature using a temporal artery (TA) thermometer.

EQUIPMENT/SUPPLIES:
Temporal artery thermometer
Alcohol wipes, probe cap or cover, or sheath

PROCEDURE STEPS:

1. Wash hands and follow Standard Precautions.
2. *Paying attention to detail,* assemble equipment. Clean probe with alcohol or attach a probe. RATIONALE: The lens of the thermometer must be clean to work properly.
3. *Introduce yourself to the patient. Identify the patient.* RATIONALE: To be certain you have the correct patient.
4. *Explain the procedure, speaking at the patient's level of understanding.* RATIONALE: Gain patient's cooperation and permission.
5. Remove perspiration from forehead, remove hat, push back hair from forehead. RATIONALE: False readings can occur from moisture (perspiration) on forehead cooling the skin or from a hat or hair covering forehead, raising the temperature.
6. Hold the probe in the center of patient's forehead flush against the skin. RATIONALE: Probe must be centered properly for accurate reading over area.
7. Press the scan button and hold while sliding the thermometer slowly across the forehead to the temple area hair line. There will be a tapping or clicking sound that will stop when the temperature has been reached.
8. Release the button and remove the thermometer from the forehead.
9. Read the display for temperature measurement.
10. Turn upside down and wipe probe with alcohol wipe. Let dry. Return to holder. RATIONALE: TA thermometer must be dry to work effectively.
11. Wash hands.
12. Accurately record temperature in patient's chart or electronic medical record, indicating TA temperature.

PRECAUTIONS:
Check the manufacturer's manual. Some models cannot be used when oxygen is being used or when in close proximity to aerosols.

DOCUMENTATION:
8/31/20XX   T. 99.8°F (TA) C. McInnis, RMA (AMT)————

PROCEDURE 24-4

Measuring a Rectal Temperature Using a Digital Thermometer

STANDARD PRECAUTIONS:

PURPOSE:
To obtain a rectal temperature using a digital thermometer.

EQUIPMENT/SUPPLIES:
Digital thermometer with red probe (rectal)
Probe cover
Lubricating jelly on a 4 × 4 gauze or in packet
Gloves
Biohazard waste container

Procedure 24-4 (continued)

PROCEDURE STEPS:

1. Wash hands and don gloves following Standard Precautions.
2. *Paying attention to detail,* assemble equipment.
3. *Introduce yourself to the patient. Identify patient.*
4. *Explain procedure to patient, speaking at the patient's level of understanding.* RATIONALE: Ensures understanding and gains patient cooperation and consent.
5. Remove patient's clothing from the waist down, *protecting patient's personal boundaries;* drape as necessary. RATIONALE: Maintains patient's modesty, privacy, and warmth.
6. Position patient in Sims' position.
7. Place probe cover on red probe (rectal). RATIONALE: To prevent microorganism cross contamination. Red probe indicates rectal thermometer.
8. Lubricate with lubricating jelly. RATIONALE: Easier insertion of thermometer and safety for patient.
9. Spread buttocks and gently insert thermometer into the rectum past the sphincter (1½ inches) for adult.
10. Hold buttocks together while holding the thermometer. Do not let go of thermometer. RATIONALE: Holding buttocks together prevents air leaks and inaccurate recording. Holding onto thermometer ensures patient safety.
11. Hold in place until the beep is heard.
12. Read results on digital display window.
13. Remove from rectum.
14. Discard probe cover into biohazard waste container by pushing the release button.
15. Replace thermometer on holder base.
16. Remove gloves, discard in biohazard waste container, and wash hands.
17. Offer tissue to patient to wipe anus. Assist patient in dressing and position as necessary, *attending to any special needs of the patient.*
18. Accurately record temperature in patient's chart or electronic medical record, indicating a rectal temperature (R).

DOCUMENTATION:

5/28/20XX 8:00 AM   T 99.6° F (R), P 104, R 20. C. McInnis, RMA (AMT)

PROCEDURE 24-5
Measuring an Axillary Temperature

STANDARD PRECAUTIONS:

PURPOSE:
To obtain an axillary temperature using a digital thermometer.

EQUIPMENT/SUPPLIES:
Digital thermometer
Sheath
Towelettes
Paper towels

PROCEDURE STEPS:

1. Wash hands following Standard Precautions.
2. *Paying attention to detail,* assemble equipment; place sheath on thermometer.
3. *Introduce yourself to the patient. Identify patient.*
4. *Explain procedure, speaking at the patient's level of understanding.* RATIONALE: This elicits patient cooperation and consent.
5. Ask patient to remove clothing to provide access to axilla.
6. Cover patient with gown as necessary to maintain patient modesty and warmth.
7. Wipe axillary area with dry towel or towelette to remove moisture. RATIONALE: Moisture in the axilla will cause inaccurate reading.

continues

Procedure 24-5 (continued)

8. Place thermometer in axilla (Figure 24-23).
9. Ask patient to fold arm against chest or abdomen.
10. Hold in place until the beep is heard.
11. Carefully remove from the axillary area.
12. Eject probe cover and appropriately discard.
13. Read temperature in the digital window.
14. Replace thermometer on holder base.
15. Wash hands.
16. Accurately, record temperature in patient's chart or electronic medical record, indicating axillary temperature (A).

DOCUMENTATION:
4/30/20XX 2:00 PM   T97°F (A), P 64, R 12. H. Casey, CMA (AAMA)

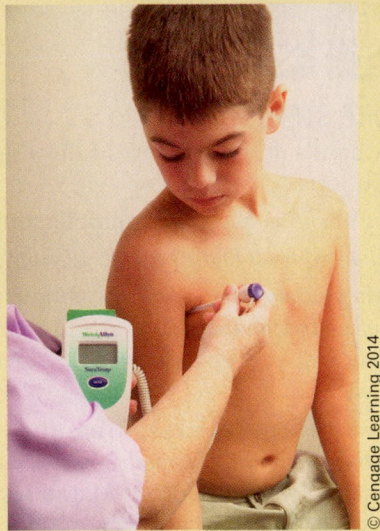

Figure 24-23 After placing thermometer in axilla, ask patient to fold arm against chest or abdomen.

PROCEDURE 24-6
Measuring an Oral Temperature Using a Disposable Oral Strip Thermometer

STANDARD PRECAUTIONS:

PURPOSE:
To obtain an oral temperature.

EQUIPMENT/SUPPLIES:
Oral strip thermometer (Figure 24-24)
Gloves
Biohazard waste container

PROCEDURE STEPS:
1. Wash hands following Standard Precautions.
2. *Paying attention to detail,* assemble equipment.
3. *Introduce yourself to the patient. Identify patient.*
4. Position the patient in a comfortable position.
5. Determine if the patient has ingested hot or cold drinks or food or has smoked within the previous half hour. RATIONALE: Ingesting hot or cold substance or smoking can result in an arbitrary increase or decrease in temperature results.
6. *Explain the procedure, speaking at the patient's level of understanding.* RATIONALE: To obtain patient cooperation and consent.
7. Apply gloves.
8. Insert disposable oral strip thermometer under the tongue to the side of the mouth. RATIONALE: Under the center of the tongue is the frenulum, the fold of mucus membrane that attaches the tongue to the floor of the mouth, which impedes placement in this area.
9. Instruct patient to close mouth tightly. RATIONALE: To prevent air leakage.
10. Leave in place for 60 seconds or according to manufacturer's instructions.
11. Remove thermometer after appropriate time has elapsed.
12. Wait 10 seconds to read the dots.

Procedure 24-6 (continued)

13. Read temperature by locating the last dot that has changed color (Figure 24-25).

14. Discard strip in biohazard waste container.

15. Remove gloves and discard in biohazard waste container.

16. Wash hands.

17. Accurately, record temperature in patient's chart or electronic medical record.

DOCUMENTATION:

4/16/20XX 3:15 PM   T 101°F, P 100, R 22 (disposable oral thermometer reading) H. Casey, CMA (AAMA)————————

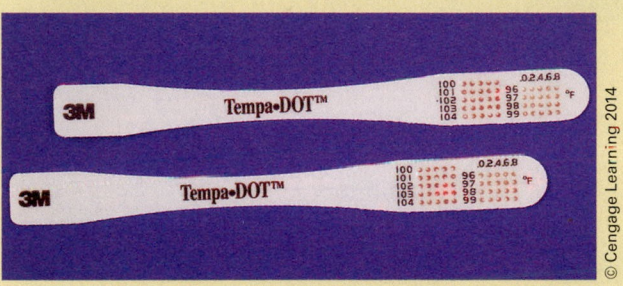

Figure 24-24   Disposable oral strip thermometer.

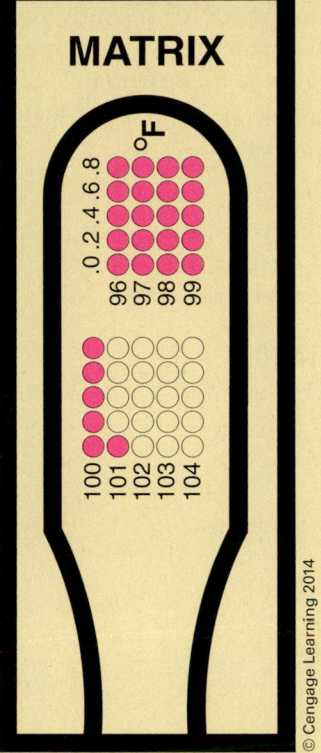

Figure 24-25   The reading on this disposable oral thermometer is 101°F.

PROCEDURE 24-7

Measuring a Radial Pulse

STANDARD PRECAUTIONS:

PURPOSE:
To obtain a radial pulse rate.

EQUIPMENT/SUPPLIES:
Watch with second hand

PROCEDURE STEPS:

1. Wash hands.

2. *Introduce yourself to the patient. Identify patient.*

3. *Explain procedure, speaking at the patient's level of understanding.* RATIONALE: Ensures patient cooperation and consent.

4. Position patient with the wrist resting either on a table or on lap.

5. Locate the radial pulse with the pads of your first three fingers (Figure 24-26). Do not use your thumb; it has its own pulse.

6. Gently compress the radial artery enough to feel the pulse.

7. Count the pulsations for 1 full minute using a watch with a second hand or a digital readout. Counting for a full minute allows for the most accuracy. However, with practice, counting for 30 seconds and multiplying the pulsations by two

continues

Procedure 24-7 (continued)

or counting for 15 seconds and multiplying by four to obtain the beats per minute is allowed as long as the pulse is regular.

8. Note any irregularities in rhythm, volume, and condition of artery.

9. Wash hands.

10. Accurately record pulse in patient chart or electronic medical record after the temperature, noting any irregularities.

DOCUMENTATION:
2/10/20XX 3:00 PM   T98.2°F P80, regular and strong.
D. Kolter, RMA (AMT)——————————————

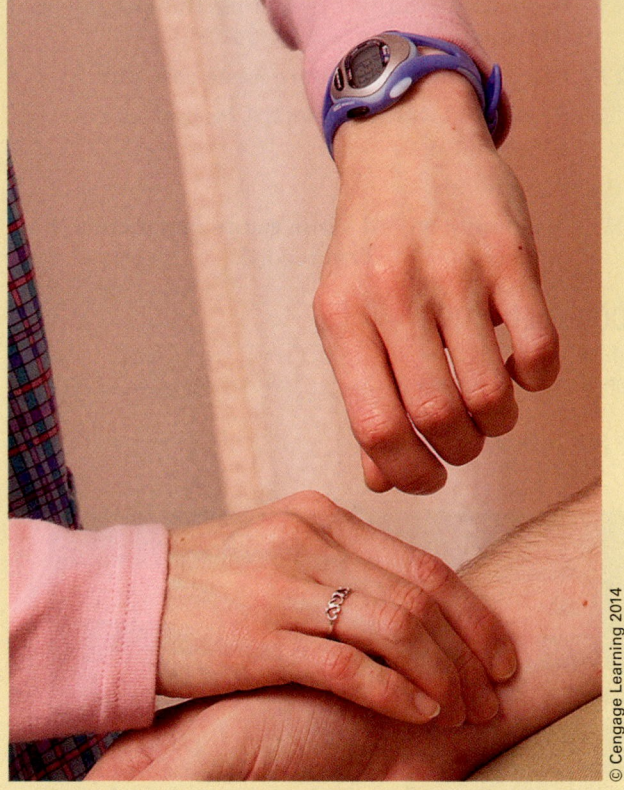

Figure 24-26 Locate the radial pulse with the pads of your first three fingers.

PROCEDURE 24-8
Taking an Apical Pulse

STANDARD PRECAUTIONS:

PURPOSE:
To obtain an apical pulse rate.

EQUIPMENT/SUPPLIES:
Stethoscope
Watch with second hand
Alcohol wipes

PROCEDURE STEPS:
1. Wash hands.

2. *Paying attention to detail,* assemble equipment.

3. Wipe earpiece with alcohol wipes.

4. *Introduce yourself to the patient. Identify patient.*

5. *Explain procedure, speaking at the patient's level of understanding.* RATIONALE: Ensures patient cooperation and consent.

Procedure 24-8 (continued)

6. Assist patient in disrobing, removing clothing from the waist up, *while protecting patient's personal boundaries*.

7. Provide a gown or drape for patient modesty and warmth.

8. Position the patient in a supine position. RATIONALE: Easier access to apex of heart.

9. Locate the fifth intercostal space, midclavicular, left of sternum (Figure 24-27). RATIONALE: Location of apex of heart.

10. Place stethoscope on the site and listen for the lub-dub sound of the heart.

11. Count the pulse for 1 minute; each lub-dub equals one pulse. Note any additional heart sounds or arrhythmias.

12. Assist the patient to sit up and dress, *attending to any special needs of the patient*.

13. Wash hands.

14. Wipe earpieces, diaphragm, and tubing of stethoscope.

15. Accurately, record pulse in patient chart or electronic medical record with the designation of apical pulse (AP) to denote method of obtaining the pulse and note any arrhythmias.

NOTE: Apical pulse and radial pulse are frequently taken simultaneously, with the radial pulse taken by another individual (Figure 24-28). Both pulse rates should be identical. A discrepancy may indicate a cardiac problem.

DOCUMENTATION:

7/8/20XX 12 PM   T 98.6°F, P (AP) 96 reg. (radial)
100 slightly irregular. Dr. King notified. D. Kolter,
RMA (AMT) ─────────────────────

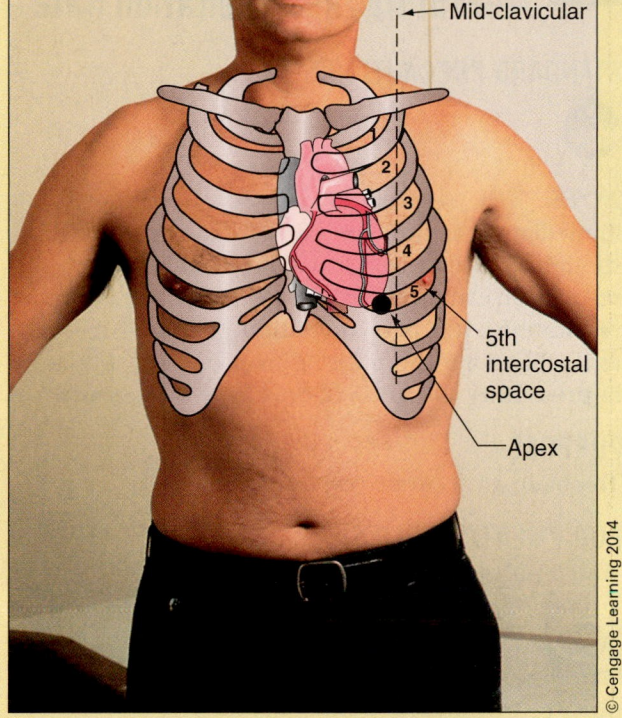

© Cengage Learning 2014

Figure 24-27 Locate the apical pulse by counting intercostal spaces. Locate the fifth intercostal space.

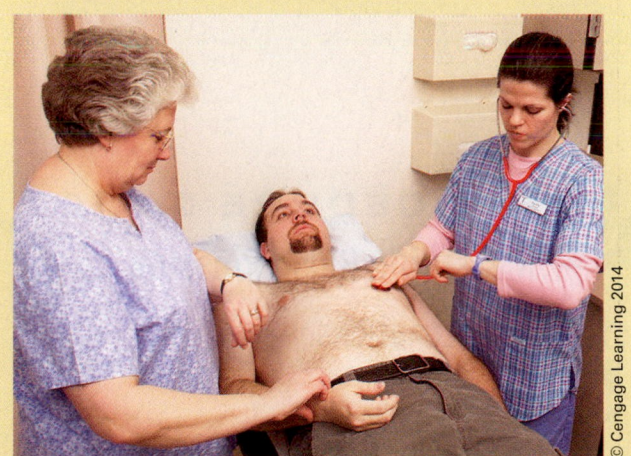

© Cengage Learning 2014

Figure 24-28 Sometimes apical and radial pulses are taken simultaneously.

PROCEDURE 24-9
Measuring the Respiration Rate

STANDARD PRECAUTIONS:

NOTE: The respiration rate is normally taken immediately before or after the pulse rate. It should be taken without patient knowledge because respiration can voluntarily be altered. While counting respirations, it is best to continue grasping the wrist as if still taking the pulse. This procedure will assist in preventing alteration of breathing by the patient.

PURPOSE:
To obtain an accurate respiratory rate.

EQUIPMENT/SUPPLIES:
Watch with second hand

PROCEDURE STEPS:
1. Wash hands.
2. *Introduce yourself to the patient. Identify the patient.*

3. Position patient in a comfortable position.
4. Watch the rise and fall of the chest wall for 1 minute, or while holding the patient's arm, place it across the chest and feel for the rise and fall of chest wall. Alternatively, place a hand on the patient's shoulder and feel and watch for the rise and fall of the chest wall. With practice, counting respirations for 30 seconds and multiplying by 2 or counting for 15 seconds and multiplying by 4 is allowable as long as the respiratory rate is regular.
5. Note depth, rhythm, and breath sounds while counting.
6. Wash hands.
7. Accurately, record respiration rate in patient's chart or electronic medical record, noting any irregularities and sounds.

DOCUMENTATION:
8/7/20XX 2:00 PM   T98.6°F, P 84. Rate and rhythm regular.
H. Casey, CMA (AAMA) —————————————————

PROCEDURE 24-10
Measuring Blood Pressure

STANDARD PRECAUTIONS:

PURPOSE:
To measure blood pressure.

EQUIPMENT/SUPPLIES:
Stethoscope
Sphygmomanometer
Alcohol wipes

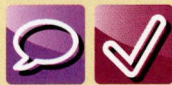

PROCEDURE STEPS:
1. Wash hands.
2. *Paying attention to detail,* assemble equipment, making sure that cuff size is correct. RATIONALE: Inappropriate cuff size will result in inaccurate measurement.
3. Clean earpieces of stethoscope with alcohol wipe.

Procedure 24-10 (continued)

4. *Introduce yourself to the patient. Identify patient.*

5. *Explain procedure, speaking at the patient's level of understanding.* RATIONALE: May be the first instance where blood pressure is measured; to allay anxiety and ensure cooperation and consent.

6. Position patient comfortably; feet flat on the floor, arm resting at heart level on the lap or a table. RATIONALE: Legs crossed may arbitrarily increase blood pressure; arm above heart level may result in inaccurate reading.

7. Bare the right upper arm. If clothing is restricting, have patient remove it. RATIONALE: Tight clothing on the arm can produce inaccurate results. Right arm is used for consistency, but if one arm measures a higher reading, then that arm is used consistently to measure the blood pressure.

8. Position the patient so that the brachial artery is at the level of the heart and the arm is supported so that there is not additional muscular tension.

9. Palpate brachial artery.

10. Securely center the bladder of the cuff over the brachial artery above the bend of the elbow. RATIONALE: Cuff should be high enough so stethoscope does not touch it. Extraneous sounds may be heard. Be certain the gauge is on zero.

11. Locate and palpate the radial pulse and smoothly inflate cuff until the pulse is no longer felt; note the number.

12. Quickly deflate the cuff and allow arm to rest for about one minute. Calculate peak inflation level. RATIONALE: This ensures that an auscultatory gap is not missed.

13. Make sure cuff is completely deflated.

14. Position stethoscope over the brachial artery and hold in position with the fingers only.

15. Inflate cuff smoothly and quickly to the peak inflation level plus 30 mm Hg (Figure 24-29).

16. Deflate the cuff at a rate of 2 to 4 mm Hg per heartbeat. RATIONALE: No matter how experienced you become, accurate blood pressure readings cannot be obtained if the cuff deflation is greater than 2 to 4 mm Hg per heartbeat.

17. Listen for Korotkoff Phase I; note when it appears.

18. Continue deflation, noting the Korotkoff phases.

19. Note when all sounds disappear, Korotkoff Phase V.

20. Continue deflating the cuff at the same rate for at least another 10 mm Hg after sounds have disappeared. RATIONALE: To hear an auscultatory gap should one be present.

21. Deflate the cuff quickly.

22. Remove the cuff.

23. Clean earpieces and diaphragm of stethoscope with alcohol wipes.

24. Wash hands.

25. Accurately, record blood pressure in patient's chart or electronic medical record.

NOTE: On a patient's initial visit and in patients with hypertension, the provider may want the blood pressure taken in both arms. There is normally a slight variation in pressure between the arms. If it is necessary to repeat the procedure, wait approximately 5 minutes before doing so.

DOCUMENTATION:

2/16/20XX 3:00 PM   BP 146/90 in right arm. BP 150/92 in left arm. D. Swingle, CMA (AAMA)————————

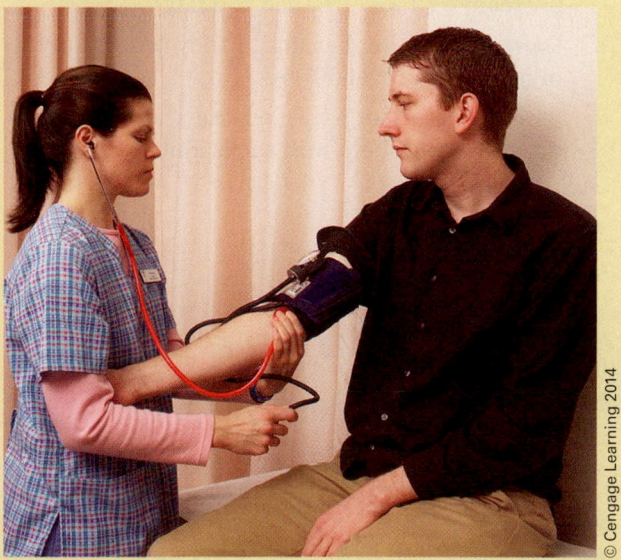

Figure 24-29   Inflate cuff smoothly and quickly.

© Cengage Learning 2014

PROCEDURE 24-11
Measuring Height

STANDARD PRECAUTIONS:

PURPOSE:
To obtain the height of a patient.

EQUIPMENT/SUPPLIES:
Scale with measuring bar
Paper towel

PROCEDURE STEPS:
1. Wash hands.
2. *Introduce yourself to the patient. Identify patient.*
3. *Explain the procedure, speaking at the patient's level of understanding,* to ensure understanding, cooperation, and consent.
4. *Considering any special needs of the patient,* instruct patient to remove shoes and stand on paper towel on scale with back against scale, looking straight ahead. RATIONALE: Back against scale aids patient safety.
5. Assist patient onto scale. RATIONALE: Scale platform is movable, and patient may become unsteady and lose balance and fall.
6. Lower measuring bar until firmly resting on top of head (Figure 24-30).
7. Assist patient's stepping off the scale. Allow patient to sit and help with shoes if necessary.

8. *Paying attention to detail,* read line where measurement falls.
9. Lower measuring bar to its original position.
10. Wash hands.
11. Accurately, record height in patient's chart or electronic medical record.

DOCUMENTATION:
3/4/20XX 2:00 PM   Ht. 59 60. B. Abbott, RMA (AMT)———

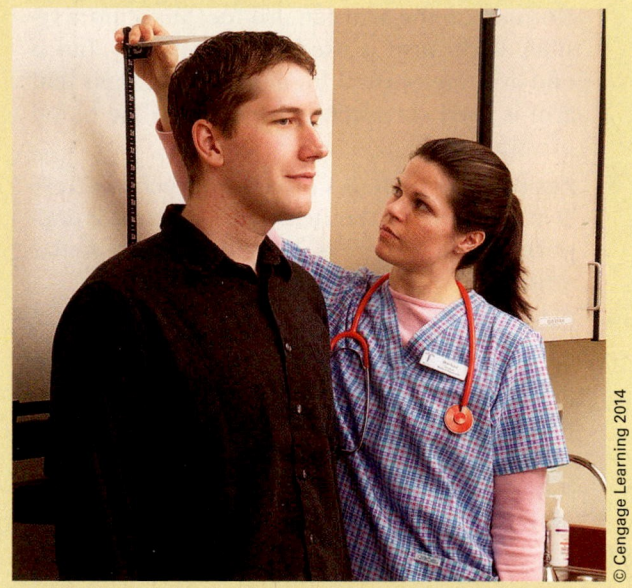

Figure 24-30 To measure height, have the patient stand with back against scale and keep head level.

© Cengage Learning 2014

PROCEDURE 24-12
Measuring Adult Weight

STANDARD PRECAUTIONS:

PURPOSE:
To obtain the weight of the patient.

EQUIPMENT/SUPPLIES:
Balance beam or digital scale
Paper towels

Procedure 24-12 (continued)

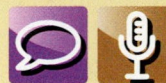

PROCEDURE STEPS:

1. Wash hands.

2. *Introduce yourself. Identify patient.*

3. *Explain the procedure, speaking at the patient's level of understanding,* to ensure understanding and cooperation.

4. Place a paper towel on scale. RATIONALE: Paper towel protects patient's feet from microorganisms.

5. Instruct the patient to place heavy objects on the area provided, including heavy objects that may be in pockets.

6. Zero balance beam or digital scale.

7. *Considering any special needs of the patient,* instruct the patient to remove shoes, jacket, and heavy sweater and step on the scale. Assist patient to the center of the scale. RATIONALE: The scale platform is movable, and the patient may become unsteady, lose balance, and fall. The platform on the digital scale is stationary, but assist the patient onto the scale platform and read the digital reading. If using a balance beam scale, continue with Steps 7 through14.

8. For balance beam scales, move the lower weight bar (measured in 50-pound increments) to the estimated number (the patient may be asked for approximate weight).

9. Slowly slide the upper bar until the balance beam point is centered (Figure 24-31).

10. Read the weight by adding the upper bar measurement to the lower bar measurement (see Figure 24-16). If using a digital scale, simply read and remember the number.

11. *Considering any special needs of the patient,* assist the patient in stepping off the scale.

12. Provide a chair for the patient to sit and put on shoes. Return objects to the patient.

13. If using a balance beam scale, return the weights to zero.

14. Wash hands.

15. Accurately, record weight in patient's chart or electronic medical record.

DOCUMENTATION:

5/2/20XX 3:00 PM   Wt. 142 lbs. B. Abbott, RMA (AMT)——

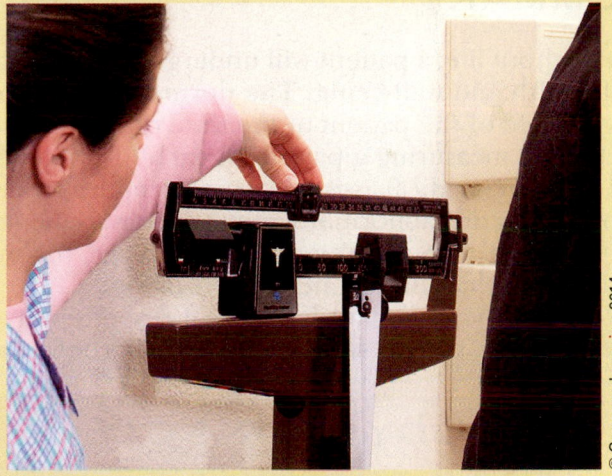

© Cengage Learning 2014

Figure 24–31   When weighing the patient, slide the upper bar until the balance beam point is centered.

CASE STUDY 24-1

Refer to the scenario at the beginning of the chapter.

CASE STUDY REVIEW

1. There are three different kinds of sphygmomanometers. Give advantages and disadvantages of each.

2. When you weigh Mrs. Williams, you notice from her record that she has lost 10 pounds in 6 months. What questions will you ask her about her weight loss?

3. Height and weight measurements are important for many reasons. What do you consider the most important of the many reasons? What do you consider the least important reason? Why?

CASE STUDY 24-2

Herb Fowler, a regular patient of Dr. Lewis at the medical facility of Drs. Lewis and King, is an African American in his 50s. He has smoked for many years and only recently has thought about quitting smoking because of a chronic cough. Herb is significantly overweight but is having a hard time making the decision to give up smoking *and* change his diet. Although his blood pressure has been stable for the last few years, Audrey Jones, CMA (AAMA), is concerned when she takes Herb's vital signs during his most recent checkup. His weight is slightly up, and his blood pressure has jumped from 140/90 to 156/100.

CASE STUDY REVIEW

1. Is a blood pressure reading of 156/100 a cause for concern? Should Audrey take a second reading?

2. In addition to alerting the provider to the change in Mr. Fowler's blood pressure and weight, Audrey feels she may be able to provide advice to the patient (with provider permission). How can Audrey use her communication and medical assisting knowledge to counsel Herb Fowler on lifestyle changes?

3. To follow up, Audrey reviews her knowledge of hypertension and discusses the four types with the provider. What are the four kinds of hypertension and what are their characteristics?

SUMMARY

Throughout life, a patient will undergo various measurements to ascertain growth, development, and general health and well-being. The normal range for each of these measurements will vary according to the stage of life of the patient at the time of examination. The medical assistant must be aware of what to expect when measuring a patient in each life stage. Awareness of normal expectations for each stage of life will help the medical assistant to perform the procedures in a more effective and efficient manner and aid in observing any abnormal signs and measurements.

Together with differences seen with age, the medical assistant will see differences in patients because each patient has unique medical problems.

The medical assistant has a great responsibility when performing patient measurements and must ensure accuracy, patient safety, comfort, and confidentiality while obtaining accurate results.

STUDY FOR SUCCESS

To reinforce your knowledge and skills of information presented in this chapter:

- Review the *Key Terms*
- Role-play with other students to apply attributes of professionalism pertinent to this chapter.
- Consider the *Case Studies* and discuss your conclusions
- Answer the questions in the *Certification Review*
- Apply your knowledge by completing the *Activities* in the *Study Guide* and the *Games and Quizzes* in the StudyWARE **StudyWARE** software on the *Premium Website*
- Perform the *Procedures* using the *Competency Assessment Checklists* in the *Competency Manual*
- Practice your problem-solving skills with the *Critical Thinking Challenge 3.0* on the *Premium Website*

Additional resources for this chapter include:

- Module 20 of the *Medical Assisting Learning Lab*
- *CourseMate for Delmar's Comprehensive Medical Assisting*
- *WebTutor for Delmar's Comprehensive Medical Assisting*

CERTIFICATION REVIEW

1. This type of thermometer measures the temperature of the skin surface over the temporal artery:
   a. aural
   c. tympanic
   b. TA
   d. axillary

2. The artery commonly used for taking a patient's pulse is the:
   a. carotid
   c. radial
   b. brachial
   d. popliteal

3. A blood pressure cuff that is too small for the patient's arm will:
   a. have no effect on the results
   b. give an arbitrarily low result
   c. give an arbitrarily high result
   d. have an effect on certain patients only

4. The term used to indicate a pulse rate significantly above the average is:
   a. bradycardia
   c. arrhythmia
   b. tachycardia
   d. sinus rhythm

5. The absence of respiratory activity is known as:
   a. eupnea
   c. hyperpnea
   b. apnea
   d. dyspnea

6. The medical term for fever is:
   a. pyrexia
   c. afebrile
   b. febrile
   d. both a and b

7. Wheezing can be described as:
   a. a normal breath sound
   b. clicking or rattling sounds heard on inspiration
   c. high-pitched musical sounds heard upon expiration
   d. none of the above

8. Weight is an important measurement to be recorded during a patient assessment. Weight should be recorded in pounds or kilograms. In order to change pounds to kilograms the following is true:
   a. multiply by 2.2
   b. divide by 2.2
   c. use a metric scale and re-weigh the patient
   d. allow the practitioner to calculate the weight in kilograms

9. Which of the following blood pressure results indicates hypertension?
   a. 110/60
   c. 122/86
   b. 148/92
   d. 128/78

10. Things that affect eupnea or normal respiratory rate are:
    a. stress
    b. exertion
    c. disease
    d. all of the above

REFERENCES/BIBLIOGRAPHY

All about heart rate (pulse). (n.d.). American Heart Association. Retrieved April 8, 2012, from http://www.heart.org/HEARTORG/Conditions/More/MyHeartandStrokeNews/All-About-Heart-Rate-Pulse_UCM_438850_Article.jsp

Environmental Protection Agency. (May 18, 2004, Federal Register, page 40517 [40 CFR 273.81(a)]). *Mercury and the environment*. Retrieved from http://www.epa.gov

Michigan State University. *Mercury containment initiative*. Retrieved March 22, 2004, from http://www.aware.msu.edu

Millikan, G. A. (1942). The oximeter: An instrument for measuring continuously oxygen-saturation of arterial blood in man, *Rev. Sci. Instrum, 13*, 434–444.

Narcolepsy: Daytime sleep disorder; cataplexy. (2011). A.D.A.M. Medical Encyclopedia. Retrieved April 8, 2012, from http://www.ncbi.nlm.nih.gov/pubmedhealth/PMH0001805/

National Library of Medicine, National Institutes of Health. *Mercury facts*. Retrieved April 28, 2005, from http://cerhr.niehs.nih.gov/genpub/topics/mercury.html

O' Rourke, M., & Frolich, D. (1999). Pulse Pressure: Is this a clinically useful risk factor? *Hypertension, 34*, 372–374.

Shimbo, D., Muntner, P., Mann, D., Barr, R. G., Tang, W., Post, W., . . . Shea, S. (2011, April 15). Association of left ventricular hypertrophy with incident hypertension: The multi-ethnic study of atherosclerosis. *American Journal of Epidemiology, 173*(8), 898–905.

Taber's cyclopedic medical dictionary (22nd ed.). (2006). Philadelphia: F. A. Davis.

Wilkins, R. L., Dexter J. R., & Smith, J. R. (1984). Survey of adventitious lung sound terminology in case reports. *Chest 85*(4), 523–525. doi:10.1378/chest.85.4.523. PMID 6705583. Retrieved from http://chestjournal.org/cgi/content/abstract/85/4/523

CHAPTER 25

The Physical Examination

OUTLINE

Methods of Examination
  Observation or Inspection
  Palpation
  Percussion
  Auscultation
  Mensuration
  Manipulation
Positioning and Draping
  Examination Positions
Equipment and Supplies for the
  Physical Examination
Basic Components of a Physical
  Examination
  Patient Appearance

Gait
Stature
Posture
Body Movements
Speech
Breath Odors
Weight
Skin and Appendages
The Physical Examination
  Sequence
  Head
  Eyes

Ears
Nose
Mouth and Throat
Neck
Chest
Breast
Abdomen
Genitals
Rectum
Reflexes
After the Examination

LEARNING OUTCOMES

1. Define, spell, and pronounce the key terms as presented in the glossary.
2. Describe the six methods used in physical examinations.
3. Name and describe seven positions used for physical examinations.
4. Discuss the purpose of draping and demonstrate appropriate draping for each position.
5. Identify at least 10 instruments and supplies used for examination of various parts of the body.
6. Identify eight basic components of a physical examination.
7. Describe the sequence followed during a physical examination.
8. Recall method of examination, instrument used, and position for examination of at least eight body parts.
9. Analyze the professionalism questions and apply them to this chapter's content.

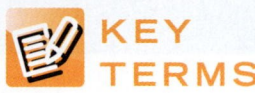

KEY TERMS

ataxia
auscultation
bruits
catheterization
cyanosis
dorsal recumbent
fenestrated drape
Fowler's
jaundice
labyrinthitis
lithotomy
mensuration
pallor
palpation
percussion
proctologic
prone
pyorrhea
scleroderma
Sims'
supine
symmetry
tinnitus
tonometer
Trendelenburg
vertigo
vitiligo

ATTRIBUTES OF PROFESSIONALISM

Communication

- Did you introduce yourself? Did you identify the patient through name and birth date or other identifying feature?
- Did you listen to and acknowledge the patient?
- Did you speak at the patient's level of understanding?
- Did you allay patients' fears regarding the procedure being performed and help them feel safe and comfortable?
- Did you respond honestly and diplomatically to the patient's concerns?
- Did you apply active listening skills?
- Did you accurately and concisely update the provider on any aspect of the patient's care?

Presentation

- Did you do something to bond with the patient?
- Did you attend to any special needs of the patient? Did you first ask if assistance was needed, rather than taking charge?
- Were you courteous, patient, and respectful to the patient?
- Did you display a calm, professional, and caring manner?

Competency

- Did you pay attention to detail?
- Did you ask questions if you were out of your comfort zone or did not have the experience to carry out tasks?
- Were you knowledgeable and accountable?

Initiative

- Were you flexible and dependable?
- Did you assist coworkers when appropriate?

Integrity

- Did you work within your scope of practice?
- Did you demonstrate sensitivity to patient's rights?
- Did you protect personal boundaries?
- Did you demonstrate respect for individual diversity?
- Did you protect and maintain confidentiality?
- Did you do "the right thing" even when no one was observing?

SCENARIO

At the multiprovider Inner City Health Care facility, five providers are employed on a rotating basis, with two or three working at any one time. Clinical medical assistants Wanda Slawson, CMA (AAMA), and Bruce Goldman, CMA (AAMA), have developed a clear understanding of what each provider prefers in both room and patient preparation. Wanda and Bruce also coordinate with each other and with office managers Jane O'Hara and Walter Seals, both CMAs, to ensure patient comfort. Depending on the patient and the type of examination, Wanda will often assist with patient preparation when the patient is female and Walter will assist when the patient is male.

INTRODUCTION

Physical examinations are performed to obtain a picture of the health and well-being of the patient. An initial examination will provide a baseline reference for future examinations. The examination follows a standard routine, usually starting at the head and following through the entire body, including all major organs and body systems. Although the sequence of events for the physical examination is relatively standard, variations occur according to provider preference, type of practice, and patient's chief complaint. Diagnostic procedures such as laboratory tests and X-rays may be ordered or performed in the facility or sent to an outside laboratory. At the conclusion of the physical examination, the provider will have an impression of the patient's general health, a diagnosis if possible, and treatment plans. The provider uses information from three major sources to aid in making a diagnosis: the health history, the physical examination, and laboratory tests and diagnostic procedures.

The role of the medical assistant throughout the physical examination greatly depends on the provider. Some providers delegate many duties to the medical assistant, whereas others require little assistance. Commonly performed clinical medical assisting duties related to physical examinations can be divided into two categories: patient preparation and room preparation. Patient preparation includes patient explanation and preparation, positioning, draping, vital signs, specimen collection such as urine and blood, and electrocardiogram (ECG). Room preparation includes assembling the appropriate instruments and equipment for the provider and ensuring patient privacy and comfort.

When patients arrive for their appointments, the medical assistant will consider confidentiality to be of utmost importance. From the time the patient arrives until the patient leaves, there are multiple occasions to protect patient confidentiality. A patient's medical history, personal finances, and insurance matters must be handled privately, out of the hearing range of others. Pertinent personal information that you may elicit from the patient that will be helpful to the provider during his or her examination also must be kept private. When the patient is undergoing testing such as electrocardiology that requires the patient to undress in preparation for the examination, care must be taken to avoid violating the patient's right to privacy. Respecting the dignity of all patients by protecting their privacy and confidentiality is a sign of a professional who is aware of patient rights.

Additional medical assisting duties include supporting the patient, handing the provider instruments and equipment as required, and taking notes to be entered into the electronic medical record (EMR). Documentation of findings is often a key role for the medical assistant. Throughout and after the examination, the medical assistant adheres to the principles of medical asepsis and Standard Precautions as required by the Occupational Safety and Health Administration (OSHA). The effective *medical assistant establishes an efficient but flexible routine providing for the needs of both the patient and the provider.*

METHODS OF EXAMINATION

There are six methods used by the provider to examine the body. They include observation or inspection, palpation, percussion, auscultation, mensuration, and manipulation. The provider uses all in total or in part, depending on the type of examination being performed.

Observation or Inspection

Observation or inspection is the process of obtaining physical information by observing the patient. Inspection is perhaps the most important tool of examination. Many diagnoses may be made from

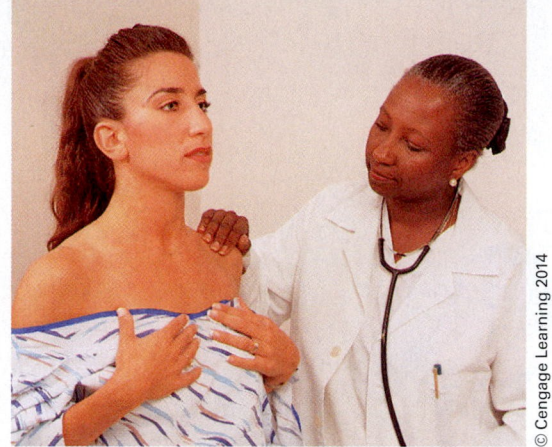

Figure 25-1 The provider uses observation to inspect the body for signs of disease.

the data collected by a skilled practitioner simply using the sense of sight.

General inspection includes taking in the body as a whole. The general health, posture, body movements, skin, mannerisms, and care in grooming are noted. Closer observation focuses on body **symmetry** (correspondence in shape and size of body parts located on opposite sides of the body) and contour. Local inspection is the focus on a specific body area, for example the skin. Deformities and skin rashes are observed. Skin color is noted (Figure 25-1).

Inspection is usually thought of as using the unaided eye. However, there are many instruments that aid in the examination of various body parts. Some examples are the otoscope to examine the ears and the ophthalmoscope for eye exams.

Palpation

Palpation is an examination of the body using touch and may be used to help verify observations. A body part or organ is felt for size and condition. Palpation is especially useful in the examination of the abdomen. Abdominal masses may be felt through the abdominal wall. Skin texture, moisture, and temperature can be felt. The contour of limbs and rigidity and position of bones and joints

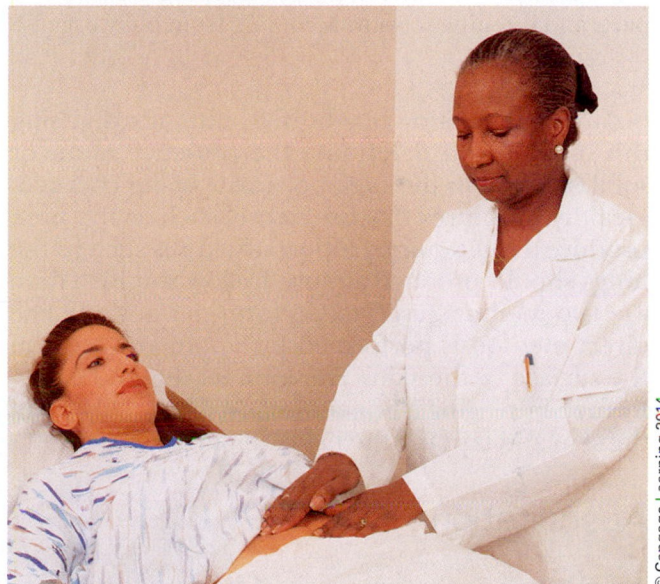

Figure 25-2 For palpation, the provider uses the hands and fingers to feel various body parts.

may be felt. Palpation may be performed with the use of fingertips, one or both hands, or the palm of the hand (Figure 25-2). Palpation is utilized by the professional medical assistant within their scope of practice. Pulse is measured using palpation. The rate, rhythm, and quality of a pulse are all vital components that must be documented in the patient chart.

Percussion

Percussion is the process of eliciting sounds from the body by tapping with either a percussion hammer or fingers. The vibrations and sounds from underlying

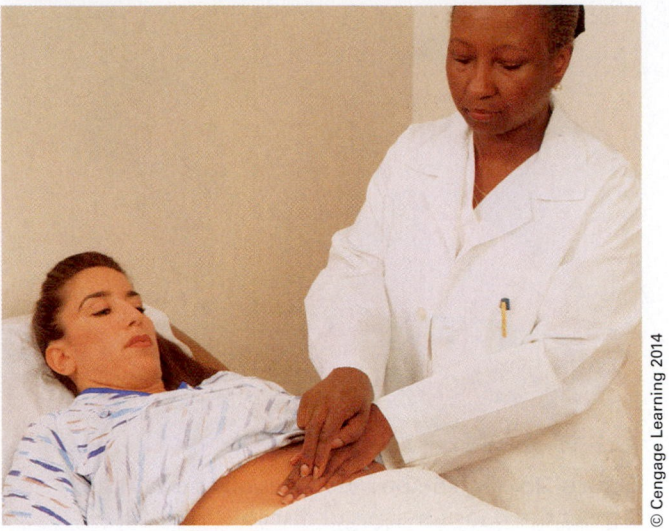

Figure 25-3 Percussion involves tapping on body parts and listening to sounds coming from body organs.

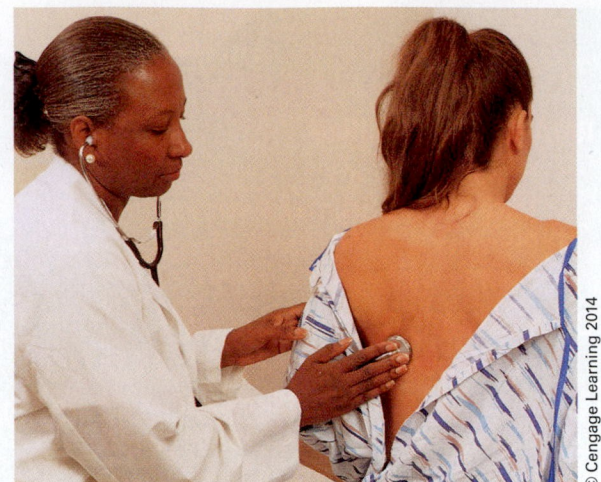

Figure 25-4 The provider is using a stethoscope to listen to heart and lung sounds. This is known as auscultation.

organs and cavities can be felt and heard. Using this method can determine the presence of air or solid material in the organ or cavity being checked. Healthy structures that are dense, such as the liver, produce a dull sound. Hollow structures such as the lungs should produce a more hollow sound. There are two methods used to perform percussion. The direct method is performed by tapping directly on the surface of the skin. The indirect method is performed by placing a finger or hand on the surface of the skin and tapping the hand (Figure 25-3).

Auscultation

Auscultation is the process of listening directly to body sounds, normally with a stethoscope. The provider listens for lung and heart sounds such as murmurs, rales, or **bruits**, which generally are abnormal sounds heard on auscultation of an organ or vessel such as a vein or an artery. The abdomen is examined for bowel sounds that include the clicks and gurgles of normal bowel activity, the sounds that occur with peristalsis (Figure 25-4). Blood pressure is one of the vital signs that are collected by the medical assistant as a part of collecting information. Auscultation using a stethoscope determines the blood pressure reading that is documented in a patient's chart.

Mensuration

The **mensuration** method of examination uses the process of measuring. The measurements of

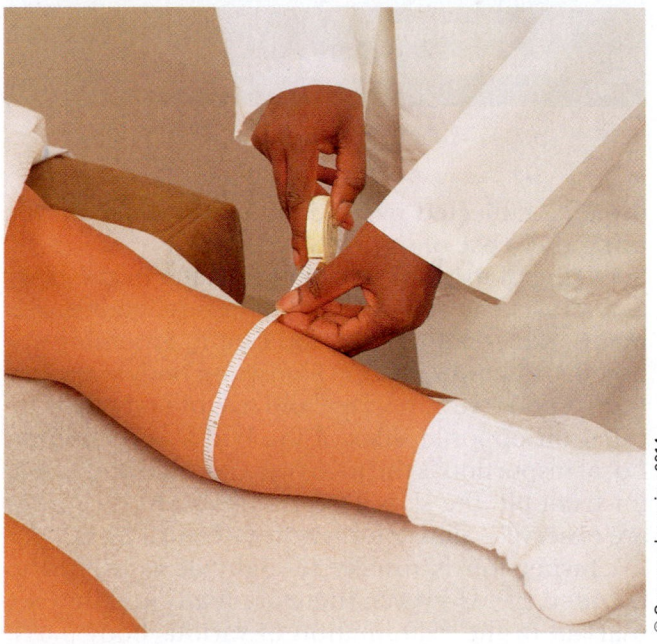

Figure 25-5 A tape measure may be used to measure the circumference of the calf of the patient's leg or other body part. This method of physical examination is known as mensuration.

height and weight, the length of a limb, and the amount of flexion and extension of an extremity are all forms of mensuration (Figure 25-5). Measurements of chest and infant head circumference are also forms of mensuration. In most instances, a tape measure is used to perform mensuration of an infant's head or circumference of a body part.

Manipulation

Manipulation checks the amount of flexion and extension of a joint by applying forceful passive movement on the joint. Range of motion of some joints may be checked using this method.

POSITIONING AND DRAPING

 Physical examinations require patients to be placed in various positions. Each position is designed to make examination of a particular area of the body easier and more efficient. The medical assistant may assist patients in undressing and will provide the appropriate drape and gown. The medical assistant also instructs patients about the appropriate position required for the examination and may assist patients into position by providing support and guidance. Always provide for patient safety.

Proper draping to protect modesty, prevent embarrassment, and provide comfort from chills is essential. If patients are capable of helping themselves, the medical assistant should leave the room while patients undress and put on a gown. If patients are disoriented or extremely ill, the medical assistant must stay in the room; patient privacy can be provided by discreetly removing clothing and covering patients as quickly as possible. When the patient is a child, the medical assistant should note the comfort level of the child while the child undresses. Children develop modesty at an early age and may be embarrassed by sitting on the examination table wearing only underwear. Respect a child's right to privacy by offering a gown or drape. Older adults will need assistance with undressing and draping. Care must be taken to provide as much modesty and privacy as possible as you assist patients of all ages.

Never turn your back on seriously ill or disoriented patients or young children. Ensure patient safety at all times.

Examination Positions

A number of positions may be required of patients during the physical examination. The position used depends on the type of examination. Seven positions can be used:

1. Supine (horizontal recumbent)
2. Dorsal recumbent
3. Lithotomy
4. Fowler's
5. Knee-chest
6. Prone
7. Sims'

Supine (Horizontal Recumbent). The **supine** position is assumed when lying flat facing up (Figure 25-6). It is used for examination of the anterior surface of the body from head to toe. When the provider performs a physical examination on a female patient that includes a breast examination, the patient should be provided with a gown and instructed to wear it with the opening in the front. A drape is then placed over the lap or from the waist own.

Dorsal Recumbent. In the **dorsal recumbent** position, patients lie on their back (dorsal) face up, legs separated, knees flexed with feet flat on the table (Figure 25-7). This is the most comfortable position for patients with back and abdominal problems. Examinations performed in this position include rectal, genital, head, neck, and chest, as well as abdominal palpation. It can also be used for urinary **catheterization**. Preteen and early teen girls requiring a pelvic examination may be placed in this position and will require careful instructions and procedure explanations. The patient is covered with a drape that is diamond shaped. One edge of the diamond can be lifted to examine the genitalia without exposing the rest of the body.

Lithotomy. In order to place a patient in the **lithotomy** position, assist them to lie on their back similar to the dorsal recumbent position except the buttocks should be as close to the bottom edge of the table as possible, and feet are placed in stirrups

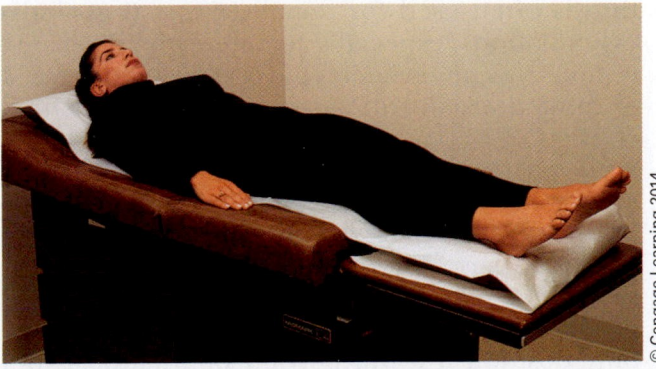

Figure 25-6   Supine or horizontal recumbent position.

© Cengage Learning 2014

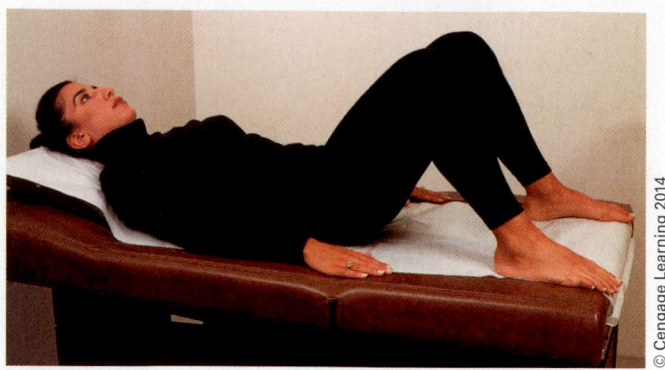

Figure 25-7 Dorsal recumbent position.

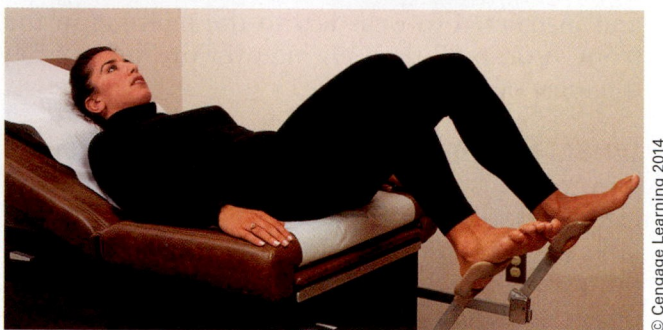

Figure 25-8 Lithotomy position.

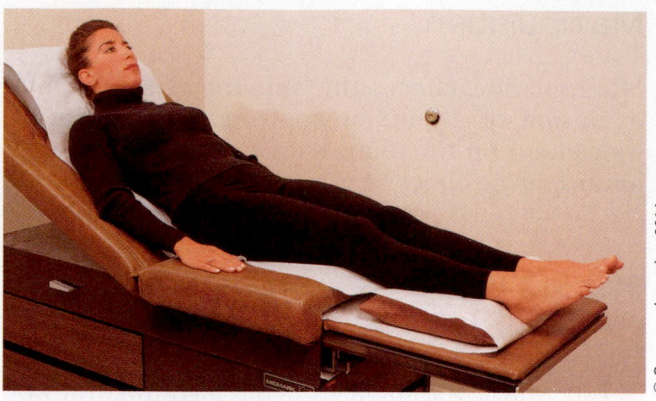

Figure 25-9 Semi-Fowler's position (45-degree angle).

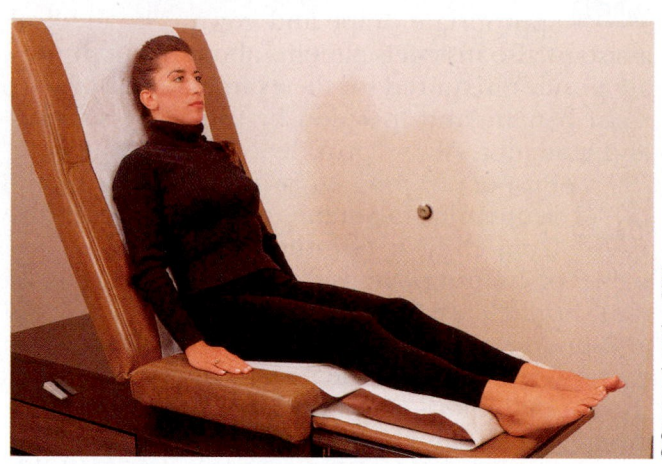

Figure 25-10 High-Fowler's position (90-degree angle).

attached to the foot of the table (Figure 25-8). The lithotomy position is used for genital and pelvic examinations; it can also be used for urinary catheterization. At the conclusion of the examination, the patient should slide toward the head of the table before getting up from this position. Patients with special needs, such as older adults and those physically challenged, as with severe arthritis, may not be able to assume this position. If this is the case, assist patient into the Sims' position or modified dorsal position, and the sigmoidoscopy, proctoscopy, or pelvic exam can be done in this position for these patients.

A modification of the dorsal recumbent position is often used for female external genitalia examinations, especially female urologic examinations, some gynecologic examinations, and examinations during pregnancy. This position consists of the patient lying on the examination table on her back, with her knees bent. The feet are together with the heels pulled up toward the buttocks. During the examination, the knees are relaxed apart. The provider may stand to the side of the patient during the examination. This position has many advantages over the lithotomy position if a full pelvic examination is not required.

Fowler's. There are several **Fowler's** positions. Patients sit in a position with the back of the examination table raised to either 45 degrees (semi-Fowler's, Figure 25-9) or 90 degrees (high-Fowler's, Figure 25-10). Legs rest flat on the table. A pillow may be placed under the knees. This position is used for patients having cardiovascular or respiratory problems to facilitate their breathing, and for examination of the upper body and head.

Knee-Chest. The knee-chest position is rarely used. In this position, patients kneel on the examination table with buttocks elevated, back straight, and chest resting on the table. It is an uncomfortable position to get into, even with assistance, and it is difficult to maintain. Not only is it uncomfortable, but it is embarrassing and risky to place patients in the knee-chest position. The position has been used for proctologic examinations and

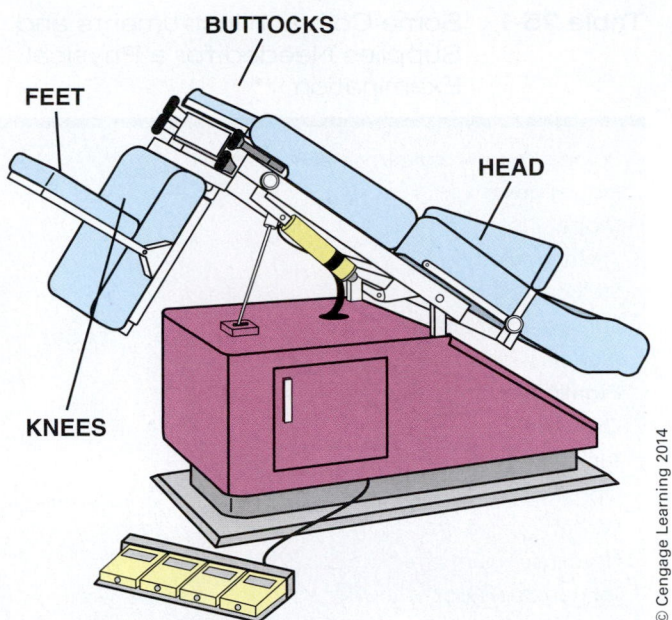

FEET
BUTTOCKS
HEAD
KNEES

Figure 25-11 Proctologic table.

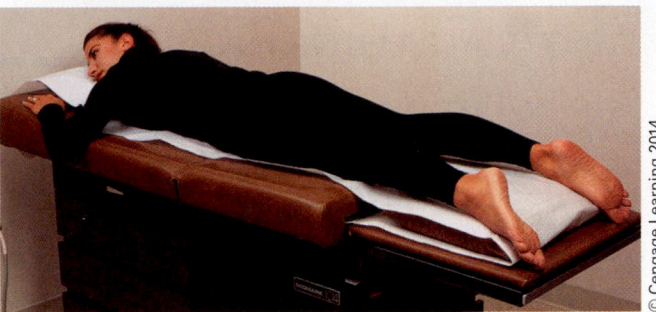

Figure 25-12 Prone position.

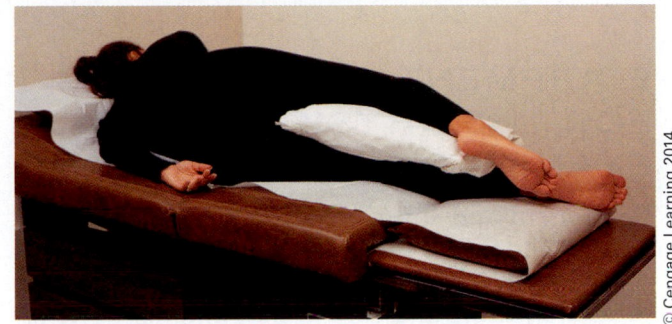

Figure 25-13 Sims' or lateral position.

sigmoidoscopy procedures; however, the procto-logic table (Figure 25-11) has made the position unnecessary. The table is used in specialty clinics, such as gastroenterology and proctology.

Proctologic. This position requires the use of a **proctologic** examination table (Figure 25-11). The patient is instructed to undress from the waist down and to kneel on the knee board of the ta-ble. The patient then bends at the hips and rests the chest on the table. The head is supported by a head board. The table is then turned to elevate the buttocks. A triangular, diamond-shaped, or **fenes-trated drape** covers the patient from the shoulders to the knees. This position is used for proctologic examinations.

Prone. For the **prone** position, the patient is in-structed to lie face down on the table with head turned to side; arms may be placed above the head or along the side of the body (Figure 25-12). The drape must cover from the mid-chest area to the legs. This position may be used for examining the posterior aspect of the body, including the back or spine and legs.

Sims' (Lateral). In the **Sims'** position, the pa-tient is instructed to lie on the left side; the left arm and shoulder may be drawn back behind the body (Figure 25-13). The left knee is slightly flexed to support the body, and the right knee is flexed

sharply. A small pillow is provided for placement under the patient's head. A pillow may also be placed between the patient's legs if it will not inter-fere with the examination being performed. The drape should be large enough to cover the patient from the shoulders to the knees (triangle or dia-mond shape to expose rectum). This position may be used for vaginal or rectal examination, for ob-taining a rectal temperature, for a sigmoidoscopy, or for administering an enema.

Trendelenburg. The **Trendelenburg** position can be used for two reasons. The first is to aid a person who is in shock. By lowering the head and elevat-ing the legs, blood flow from the major vessels in the lower extremities will, by gravity, flow upward toward the brain and major organs. This may help to increase blood pressure enough to sustain the patient until taken to the emergency department (see Chapter 9). The other reason for the Tren-delenburg position is to elevate and incline the legs so that the abdomen and pelvic organs are pushed up toward the chest by gravity, making visibility and maneuverability easier for the pro-vider doing either abdominal or pelvic surgery. In this case, the legs are elevated and inclined (see Chapter 31).

CRITICAL THINKING

Describe a type of examination that may be performed while the patient is placed in each of the following positions: (1) lithotomy, (2) Sims', (3) knee-chest, and (4) supine. Decide in what position you should place a patient and what manner of draping you would use for a Pap smear, examining a patient with shortness of breath, obtaining a rectal temperature, and an examination of the spine.

Table 25-1 Some Common Instruments and Supplies Needed for a Physical Examination

Balance beam, digital, or electronic scale
Patient gown
Drape
Thermometer
Stethoscope
Sphygmomanometer
Alcohol wipes
Examination lights
Otoscope
Tuning fork
Ophthalmoscope
Penlight
Nasal speculum
Tongue depressor
Percussion hammer
Tape measure
Cotton balls
Safety pin
Gloves
Tissues
Lubricant
Emesis basin
Gauze sponges
Specimen bottles/slides—request forms
Biohazard and regular waste containers

EQUIPMENT AND SUPPLIES FOR THE PHYSICAL EXAMINATION

Equipment and supplies used for physical examinations should be properly cleaned and ready for the provider's use (see Chapters 22 and 31 for proper cleaning and care of instruments). The list of instruments and supplies in Table 25-1 includes those that may be used in the physical examination. However, this is a limited list. Actual equipment and supplies needed vary with the provider and with the type of examination. Figure 25-14 shows some common instruments that may be used in the physical examination. (See Chapter 30 for instruments used in specialty examinations.) The medical assistant is responsible for room preparation prior to a physical examination. Equipment must be in working order (bulbs for scopes, good room lighting) and the room properly stocked with gowns, drapes, and other supplies such as gloves, an antibacterial hand washing product, a biohazard container, and any other materials needed to comply with Standard Precautions, such as a sharps container. In addition, the medical assistant is responsible for patient preparation. Urine, blood samples, and an ECG may be performed (if requested by the provider). Vital signs and height and weight will be measured. Signed consent forms, if needed, should be in the patient's record. If the patient needs help undressing and putting on a gown, the medical assistant provides assistance. Patient data can be documented immediately using the computer to electronically record all of the information (vital signs, height and weight, known allergies, any medications the patient is taking) (Figure 25-15). Results of tests and the ECG usually are available within 24 hours and can be accessed in the patient EMR. Ensure patient confidentiality throughout the examination and documentation.

BASIC COMPONENTS OF A PHYSICAL EXAMINATION

The physical examination of the patient begins as soon as the patient enters the clinic. The provider uses information from the health history, physical examination, and laboratory tests to aid in making a diagnosis. Figure 25-16 shows how these components are interrelated in a total practice management system. Although the physical examination is performed by the provider, it is important for the medical assistant to be aware of the various examination components and the significance of each as an indicator of patient well-being.

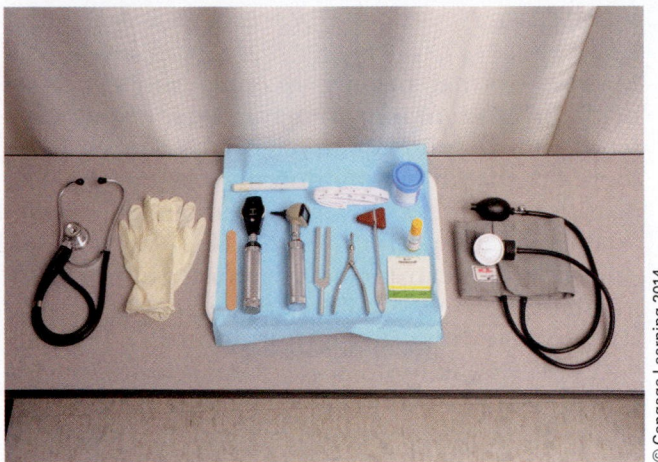

Figure 25-14   Instruments and supplies used in the physical examination: stethoscope and latex gloves; penlight, flexible tape measure, urine specimen container (across top of tray); tongue depressor, ophthalmoscope, otoscope, tuning fork, metal nasal speculum, percussion hammer, guaiac/occult blood slide, guaiac/occult blood slide developer, and sphygmomanometer.

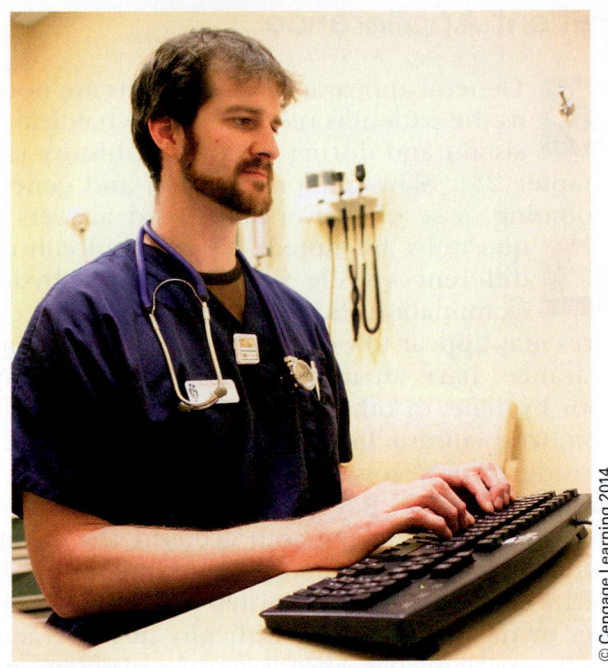

Figure 25-15   The medical assistant is able to document patient data immediately in the exam room computer.

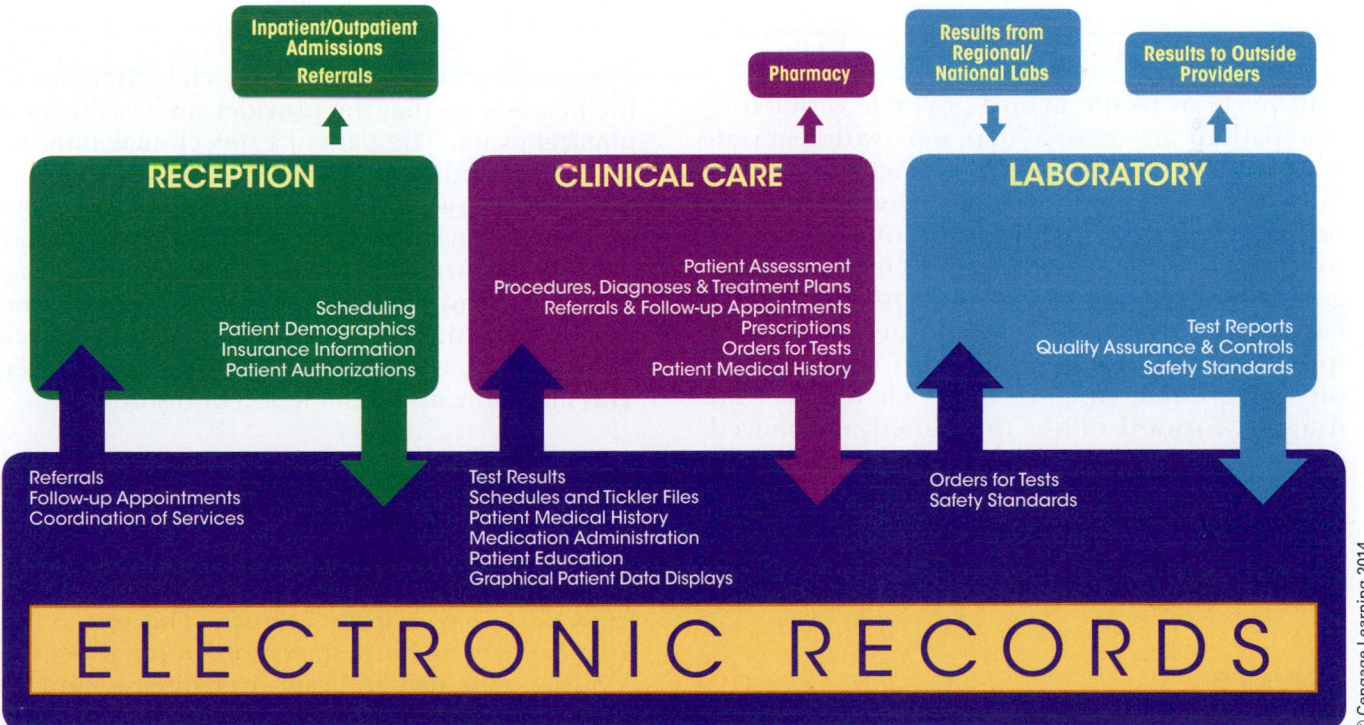

Figure 25-16   The provider uses the health history, physical examination, and lab tests to make a diagnosis. These components are integrated in a total practice management system.

Patient Appearance

 General appearance and actions are noted as the patient is received by the medical assistant and during the patient history (see Chapter 23). Skin color is checked and general grooming, ease of conversation, and answers to questions are noted. Be aware of cultural differences while assisting with a physical examination. Some patients of other cultures may appear to you to be unclean in their appearance, have an unpleasant body order, have poor hygiene, or otherwise appear to be different from your culture. In some cultures, a daily bath is considered unnecessary, and body odor is not considered offensive. Regard your patient in a nonjudgmental way, taking into account the other's cultural beliefs. The medical assistant should be alert to a patient with abnormal skin color, confusion or disorientation, or difficulty in movement. Such a patient may have a serious problem and should be placed in an examination room and the provider contacted immediately.

The following aspects of the patient's health are evaluated by the provider through the method of physical examination known as observation.

Gait

Gait pertains to the manner or style of walking. The patient may have a limp, walk with feet wide apart, appear to be dragging one leg, or have difficulty maintaining balance. The provider observes the patient's gait by instructing the patient to walk on a designated straight line. Abnormal gait can include **ataxia**, an uncoordinated wide-based walk; steppage, in which the leg stepping forward is raised high enough to raise the toes off the ground; drag-to, in which the feet are dragged forward rather than lifted and moved; and spastic, in which the legs are held stiffly together and the feet are slightly dragged forward. Each of these gaits can indicate a disease process or health problem associated with poor neurologic functioning.

Stature

The height of the patient is measured. The provider looks for height, trunk, and limb proportion. Stature is the natural height of a person in an upright position.

Posture

Because normal posture is erect with the head held up, a patient in pain may exhibit postural differences. The spine might be in a fixed position, or there may be limited motion in an extremity. The provider observes spine movement and alignment as the patient performs prescribed movements. Abnormalities can include kyphosis (humpback), which may be seen in older adult patients, particularly women with osteoporosis; lordosis, abnormal curvature of the lumbar area; and scoliosis, curvature of the upper spine.

Body Movements

Body movements may be either voluntary or involuntary. Voluntary body movements describe those movements intended to be made by the patient. Involuntary body movements are movements not controlled by the patient. Tremors are a form of involuntary movement that may be seen in the mouth, fingers, hands, arms, and legs of a patient. Tremors can indicate a neurologic health problem. Involuntary body movements usually are easily observed.

Speech

The quality and regularity of speech is often one of the first aspects that the provider notices during a physical exam. The patient's speech may indicate abnormal conditions. Abnormalities include aphonia, a loss of voice usually because of laryngitis, but which may have other causes; aphasia, the inability to express oneself through speech or writing, which may indicate brain injury or disease; and dysphasia, an inability to use appropriate speech patterns, such as using words in the wrong order. This may indicate a brain lesion or disorder.

Breath Odors

Breath odors may be detected when speaking with the patient or when obtaining vital signs. A sweet fruity odor may indicate acidosis. This may result from diabetes mellitus, starvation, or renal disease. A musty odor may indicate liver disease, and an ammonia odor may indicate uremia.

Poor oral hygiene results in gingivitis (gum disease), caries (cavities), tooth loss, and foul breath odors. Gum disease and caries encourage the growth of microorganisms in the mouth and throat.

Because of the vascularity of the oral cavity, micro-organisms can enter into the circulatory system and travel to the heart, causing endocarditis. Maintaining good oral health is necessary for general health and well-being. Regular dental checkups, cleaning, and daily flossing promote good health.

Weight

Various published charts contain guidelines for normal weight established by height and age. Overweight and underweight are defined as being above or below the published charts. Obesity and underweight are discussed in Chapters 24 and 34. Edema, which is excessive accumulation of fluids in the body tissues, causes weight gain. To test for edema, the provider presses a finger against the skin of the patient in an area over a bony prominence such as the ankle. If edema is present, pitting will be evident when the finger is removed. Fat tissue will not leave an indentation when pressed.

Skin and Appendages

Skin problems include abnormal skin color such as redness, pallor, cyanosis, jaundice, and vitiligo. **Pallor** is defined as lack of color or paleness often seen with anemia; **cyanosis** is a slightly blue or gray discoloration of the skin, often seen in patients with respiratory or cardiac problems; **jaundice** is a yellowing of the skin, often caused by obstructed bile ducts or liver disease; and **vitiligo** is characterized by white patches on the skin, observed against normal pigmentation. Other skin conditions are lesions, ulcers, bruises, and cancer. Skin texture may be smooth, rough, and scaly and have loss of elasticity. These findings may indicate health problems or excessive exposure to the sun. The nails can also indicate some forms of health problems. Infections, either local or systemic, may be observed in nails that are brittle, grooved, or lined. The appearance of the fingertips can be indicators of disorders as seen in clubbing, which may indicate congenital heart disease, and spooning, which may be seen in severe iron-deficiency anemias. Abnormal hair distribution, as in facial hair on a female patient, may indicate hormonal changes.

THE PHYSICAL EXAMINATION SEQUENCE

A sequence is followed for a physical examination, although provider preference and the patient's chief complaint can produce a variation to the sequence.

The physical examination begins with the medical assistant taking and recording the patient's vital signs, height, and weight, and testing visual acuity as well as auditory ability when appropriate. Additional laboratory procedures, such as urinalysis and blood analysis or ECG, may be performed as directed by the provider before the physical examination. Before the examination, the patient is instructed to empty the bladder, saving a urine specimen for analysis. The patient is then told what to expect during the examination. Any questions the patient has should be answered by the medical assistant or referred to the provider. The patient should be instructed about undressing (a private area should be provided for undressing). The medical assistant should be explicit as to what clothing is to be removed and what can be left on. If a complete physical examination is required, all clothing should be removed. A gown and drape are provided for the patient. The medical assistant may leave the room while the patient undresses unless the patient asks for help or is unable to manage alone. It is appropriate to knock before reentering the room.

When the provider is examining a patient, it is customary for the medical assistant to remain in the room for the patient's comfort, to assist the provider, and as a deterrent to potential lawsuits.

The medical assistant places the instruments for the examination on the counter or Mayo stand, according to provider preference, but usually in order of use. When lamps are used for the examination, the medical assistant may turn them on and have them ready for the provider. Make sure that the light is not directed into the patient's eyes. When the patient is comfortably positioned on the examination table, inform the provider that the patient is ready. Normally the physical examination starts at the head and proceeds downward. Table 25-2 gives a detailed review of the components of the physical examination.

Head

The patient is in a sitting position for this examination. The face is checked for puffiness, especially around the eyes. Facial skin is checked for **scleroderma**, a tight and atrophied skin. The older adult patient may have fatty patches that appear raised and yellowish on the eyelids. The face, hair, and

Table 25-2   Components of the Physical Examination

Body Part	Position	Instrument Used	Method of Exam	Provider's Findings	
				Normal	Abnormal
General appearance	Standing	—	Inspection	Patient is cooperative; good hygiene, good skin color, ease of gait	Uncooperative, behavior inappropriate, unkempt appearance
Skin	Supine Prone	Flashlight	Inspection Palpation	Good color, warm to touch; no lesions such as warts, moles, abscesses, rashes	Jaundice, cyanosis, pallor, redness, flakiness of skin, lesions, rashes
Head and neck	Supine or semi-Fowler's or sitting on edge of table	Light source	Inspection Palpation	Symmetry of head; hair not dry or oily and distributed evenly; scalp free of lesions and not dry; no lymph node enlargement	Asymmetry of head; alopecia; dry, flaky scalp; swelling, lumps or pain in head or neck
Eyes	Supine or semi-Fowler's or sitting on edge of table	Ophthalmoscope	Inspection Mensuration	Snellen test shows accurate visual acuity; able to identify color plates; no tearing; equal pupillary reactions to light; retina pink and blood vessels healthy; measurement of intraocular pressure within normal limits; no bulging of eyeballs	Poor visual and color ability; dull-appearing eyes; drainage; unequal pupils; clouded lens; unequal pupillary reaction; intraocular pressure increased; tortuous, unhealthy retinal blood vessels; bulging eyeballs
Ears	Supine or semi-Fowler's or sitting on edge of table	Otoscope Tuning fork Audiometer	Inspection Percussion	Cerumen not impacted on tympanic membrane; tympanic membrane gray and intact; no discharge or pain; able to hear tuning fork or audiometer	Impacted cerumen; red, bulging tympanic membrane; discharge (pus or blood); inability to hear sound from tuning fork; poor auditory ability when checked with audiometer
Nose	Supine or semi-Fowler's or sitting on edge of table	Nasal speculum Flashlight Aromatic substance	Inspection	Mucous membranes moist and pink; able to detect specific odors; septum straight; nostrils equal in size; no abnormal discharge; no lesions	Dry, red, swollen mucous membranes; unable to detect odors; deviated septum; nostrils flaring; discharge, polyps noted
Mouth and throat	Supine or semi-Fowler's or sitting on edge of table	Flashlight Tongue depressors	Inspection	Gag reflex present; mucous membranes moist and pink; teeth intact, pink tongue; tonsils nonswollen, pink	No gag reflex; tongue rough; pallor of mucous membranes; dental caries; swollen tonsils
Arms and hands	Supine or semi-Fowler's or sitting on edge of table	Percussion hammer	Inspection Palpation Percussion	Good muscle tone; normal range of motion; nails pink, smooth; ability to squeeze provider's hands with equal strength; normal reflexes	Poor muscle tone; poor range of motion; nails cyanotic; brittle, ridged nails; abnormal reflexes

Table 25-2   Components of the Physical Examination (*Continued*)

Body Part	Position	Instrument Used	Method of Exam	Provider's Findings	
				Normal	**Abnormal**
Chest and lungs	Supine or semi-Fowler's or sitting on edge of table	Stethoscope Tape measure	Inspection Palpation Auscultation Mensuration Percussion	Axillary lymph nodes not palpable; lungs clear; no cough; ribs nontender; symmetrical chest wall; respirations and heart rate normal; normal chest sounds	Enlarged axillary lymph nodes; asymmetry of chest wall; respiration and heart rate abnormal; abnormal chest sounds
Heart	Supine or semi-Fowler's or sitting on edge of table	Stethoscope Sphygmomanometer Electrocardiogram (ECG)	Auscultation Palpation Mensuration	Normal heart function per ECG; regular rhythm, rate of heart sounds; no murmurs; blood pressure normal range; pulse points good quality	Abnormal heart function per ECG; irregularity of rhythm, rate; murmurs; blood pressure outside normal range; poor pulse quality
Breasts	Supine	—	Inspection Palpation	No lumps, tenderness, swelling, or thickening; no sores or lesions; no bleeding or discharge from nipples; no lymph node swelling in axilla; no dimpling or "orange peel" appearance	Lumps, tenderness, swelling, thickening; sores or lesions; bleeding or discharge from nipple; lymph node enlargement in axilla; "orange peel" appearance to breast tissue; dimpling of skin
Abdomen	Supine	Stethoscope Measuring tape	Inspection Palpation Auscultation Mensuration Percussion	Liver, spleen not palpable; symmetry to abdomen; no abnormal bowel sounds; no abnormal sounds from organs in abdomen; abdomen soft; no abdominal or inguinal hernias	Liver, spleen enlarged; asymmetric abdomen; increased or decreased bowel sounds; unusual sounds elicited from percussion of abdominal organs; abdominal distention; ascites; presence of abdominal, umbilical, or inguinal hernia
Female genitalia and rectum	Lithotomy or dorsal recumbent or Sims'	Vaginal speculum Examination light Slides for occult blood (Hemoccult)	Inspection Palpation	External genitalia without lesions, sores, ulcerations; vaginal mucosa pink and without discharge; nontender ovaries; cervix smooth, noneroded, noninflamed; good muscle tone in perineal floor and rectum; negative stool for occult blood; nonpalpable lymph nodes in groin	Lesions, sores, ulcerations; discharge from vagina, cervix; painful ovaries; cervix ulcerated, inflamed; poor muscle tone in perineal floor and rectum; prolapse of uterus or bladder into vagina; hemorrhoids; positive hemoccult; enlarged inguinal lymph nodes
Male genitalia and rectum	Supine Standing	—	Inspection Palpation	Penis pink, no discharge; no lesions, sores, ulcers; testicles firm, nontender, and movable; rectal musculature intact; nonpalpable prostate; nonpalpable lymph nodes in groin	Discharge from penis; ulcers, sores, other types of lesions; testicles tender, swollen; relaxed anal sphincter; hemorrhoids; positive hemoccult slide; enlarged prostate; enlarged lymph nodes in groin

continues

Table 25-2   Components of the Physical Examination (*Continued*)

Body Part	Position	Instrument Used	Method of Exam	Provider's Findings	
				Normal	**Abnormal**
Legs and feet	Supine Prone	Tape measure	Inspection Mensuration Palpation	Normal muscle tone and range of motion; no edema; pulses normal; no varicosities; toenails smooth; no signs of fungus or other infection; calves equal in size	Muscle weakness; poor range of motion; edema; diminished pulse; varicose veins; toenails ridged, infected; unequal calf measurements
Neuro-logic exami-nation	Supine	Percussion hammer Safety pin Cotton ball	Percussion Inspection	Normal reflexes; oriented to time and place; appropriate responses; normal responses to sensation; alert; steady gait; no vertigo or syncope	All reflexes disoriented; inappropriate responses; dulled response to pain and sensation; lethargic; unsteady gait; poor coordination; vertigo; syncope

© Cengage Learning 2014

scalp are checked for scars, lumps, hair loss, or other lesions. The head and neck are palpated for painful areas, lumps, and swelling.

Eyes

The appearance of the eyes is examined. The pupils of the eyes are checked for light and accommodation. When a penlight or flashlight is placed in front of the pupil, the pupil will constrict. The other pupil should constrict equally. The provider notes whether or not pupils are equal and react to light and accommodation (abbreviated as PERRLA). Pupils that do not constrict and return to normal equally may indicate a problem in the brain. The external eye area is examined for rashes, infection and lesions, and deformity and asymmetry. The sclera and conjunctiva are examined for any abnormalities. Any discolorations, redness, discharge, or lesions are noted. An evaluation of physical fields is a part of the eye exam. A Snellen chart is utilized to assess visual acuity (see Chapter 30).

A **tonometer** may be used to measure the intraocular eye pressure of patients older than 35 years. Normal eye pressure is 13 to 22 mm Hg. An increase above normal will be found in glaucoma. The provider uses an ophthalmoscope to view the blood vessels of the retina. This is done by turning out the lights in the room, allowing the patient's pupils to dilate. The patient is instructed to look straight ahead while the provider looks into the eye. Retinal changes may indicate disease such as hypertension. The sclera are checked for jaundice.

Ears

An otoscope is used by the provider to examine the ears. The external ear is checked for redness in the ear canal and buildup of cerumen. A healthy tympanic membrane has a pearly gray appearance. A red appearance to the tympanic membrane may indicate infection in the middle ear, known as otitis media. **Vertigo** (dizziness) may indicate that the patient has an inner ear infection (**labyrinthitis**). **Tinnitus** (ringing in the ears) may indicate inner ear problems. Other symptoms of ear problems include pain, discharge, and deafness. The tuning fork is used in testing the sensations of hearing, including bone conduction and air conduction.

Nose

The nasal cavity is visualized by the provider with the use of a nasal speculum and flashlight.

Discharge from the nose may indicate a postnasal drip in which the sinuses may be draining into the nose and throat. Other abnormalities may include obstruction because of a deviated septum. Polyps and ulcerations may be found in the nasal cavity. Epistaxis or nosebleed may be seen when the capillaries rupture on the surface of the nasal mucosa.

Mouth and Throat

The provider uses a tongue blade or depressor and a light source. The teeth and gums are checked for dental hygiene conditions such as caries and the gums are checked for signs of **pyorrhea** (discharge of pus from the gums around the teeth). If the tonsils are present, they are checked for signs of infection, such as redness or white pockets of pus. The floor of the mouth is examined both visually and by palpation for indications of swollen glands and ulcerations.

Neck

The provider palpates the neck, looking for swollen lymph nodes. The thyroid gland is palpated anteriorly and posteriorly for size, symmetry, and texture. The patient is asked to swallow several times while the provider feels the thyroid gland. A small glass of water may be given to the patient to aid in swallowing. Range of motion is checked by having the patient turn the head in each direction. Care must be taken with older adult patients. The patient should be instructed to move the head slowly to avoid syncope.

Chest

The symmetry of the chest is observed, both anteriorly and posteriorly. Chest measurement may have been performed before the examination. The chest of a patient with emphysema will appear barrel-like in shape. While the patient is sitting, the provider listens to the lungs with a stethoscope. The patient may be instructed to take several deep breaths during this process. Carefully monitor the patient, particularly the older adult patient, because deep breathing may cause dizziness. The provider is listening for abnormal lung sounds. The provider may examine the lungs by percussion. Heart sounds will be auscultated both anteriorly and posteriorly.

Breast

The patient is placed in a supine position and instructed to place the hand behind the head on the side on which the examination is taking place. The provider examines the breast for masses by using a circular motion, starting at the outer edge of the breast and working toward the center. The nipple is gently squeezed to see if there is any discharge. The patient is then instructed to change arm positions so that the other breast can be examined. With the patient in a sitting position, the provider observes the breasts for symmetry. Female patients should be instructed on the procedure for performing monthly breast self-examination. This may be an embarrassing procedure for the female patient. Maintain as much patient modesty as possible by carefully draping and giving emotional support (see Chapter 26 for more detailed information on breast examination and breast self-examination).

Abdomen

The patient is placed in a dorsal recumbent or supine position with the arms at the sides for examination of the abdomen. The drape is lowered to just above the pubic hair. The female patient wears a gown open in the front that can be pulled to the sides while still covering the breasts. The provider normally stands on the right side of the patient while performing this part of the examination. The abdomen is examined by palpation, percussion, and auscultation. Following the quadrants of the abdomen, the provider gently palpates the organs in each quadrant, working from side to side. The provider feels for organ size and location, as well as the presence of masses; percusses the abdomen listening for sounds from abdominal organs; uses the stethoscope to listen for abdominal sounds; and visually inspects the abdominal area for changes in skin color, scars, or other abnormalities. The contour of the abdomen may be flat or slightly convex. The presence of hernias is checked in both the supine and the standing positions. Patients with abdominal disorders may give a history of dyspepsia, dysphagia or excessive flatulence, nausea, vomiting, bloating, and pain.

Genitals

Refer to Chapters 26 and 28 for more detailed information about genitalia examinations. Care must be taken to protect all patients' modesty and privacy.

Female Genitals. The patient is placed in the lithotomy position. The provider examines both the external genitalia and the reproductive organs. The rectum may be examined and a Hemoccult test done at the conclusion of the pelvic examination. (See Chapters 30 and 44 for information regarding the Hemoccult slide test.) After the examination, the patient is instructed to slide toward the head of the table and may be allowed to sit up slowly. Sitting up quickly may cause orthostatic hypotension and dizziness.

Male Genitals. The provider begins the examination by inspecting and retracting the foreskin of the penis if the patient is uncircumcised. The glans penis is inspected for discharge and redness. The penis and scrotum are palpated for possible tenderness and masses. Because of the seriousness of testicular cancer, the patient will be instructed, usually by the provider, on the procedure for performing monthly testicular examinations (see Chapter 28).

Rectum

The provider may examine the rectum as a part of the male and female genitals examination. The patient may be placed in the Sims' position. The provider performs a manual examination. The prostate gland is examined by digital rectal palpation. The provider inserts the gloved index finger into the rectum and palpates the prostate gland for any masses or swelling (see Chapter 28). A lubricated rectal speculum may then be inserted for visual examination. Because this is uncomfortable for the patient, emotional support is important. The provider can visualize the rectum for bleeding, fissures, polyps, or other lesions.

Reflexes

The patient's reflexes in both the supine and sitting positions are observed by the provider. A percussion hammer is used. While sitting with the arm flexed, the elbow is lightly tapped to elicit movement from the biceps. The patellar or knee-jerk reflex is tested by tapping the area just below the patella at the knee. The Achilles reflex or ankle-jerk is tested by tapping the Achilles tendon. The Babinski reflex is tested on the sole of a relaxed foot (the great toe will flex) with the patient in a supine position. Reflexes determine the integrity of the neurologic system.

 Procedure 25-1 outlines the steps in assisting with the physical examination.

AFTER THE EXAMINATION

  Once the examination has been completed, the patient is instructed to dress. The patient should be given privacy while dressing. Assist the patient as needed. Do not remain in the room to clean it while the patient is dressing. Remain in the room if the patient requires assistance. Further instructions regarding other testing procedures and treatment plans will be given by the provider. Be specific with instructions to patients regarding what they should do after they are completely dressed.

Once the examination is finished and the patient has left the examination room, the equipment and supplies (including the examination table) should be sanitized, disinfected, and sterilized as appropriate.

PATIENT EDUCATION

From the time the patient arrives until the time the patient leaves, including throughout the physical examination, there are many opportunities for patient education. Written instructions should be given when necessary, and provider information should be clarified if needed (Figure 25-17).

Opportunities for teaching the patient how to adopt a healthy lifestyle are abundant. Regular exercise; not smoking; weight control; limiting alcohol consumption; and using stress reduction techniques such as meditation, yoga, massage therapy, and so forth all help to decrease blood pressure and reduce the risk for heart attack, stroke, and other illnesses.

CRITICAL THINKING

At the conclusion of the physical examination, the provider will have an impression of the patient's general health. What specific information can the provider obtain from the examination? From what sources other than the physical examination does the provider gain information to help in making a diagnosis?

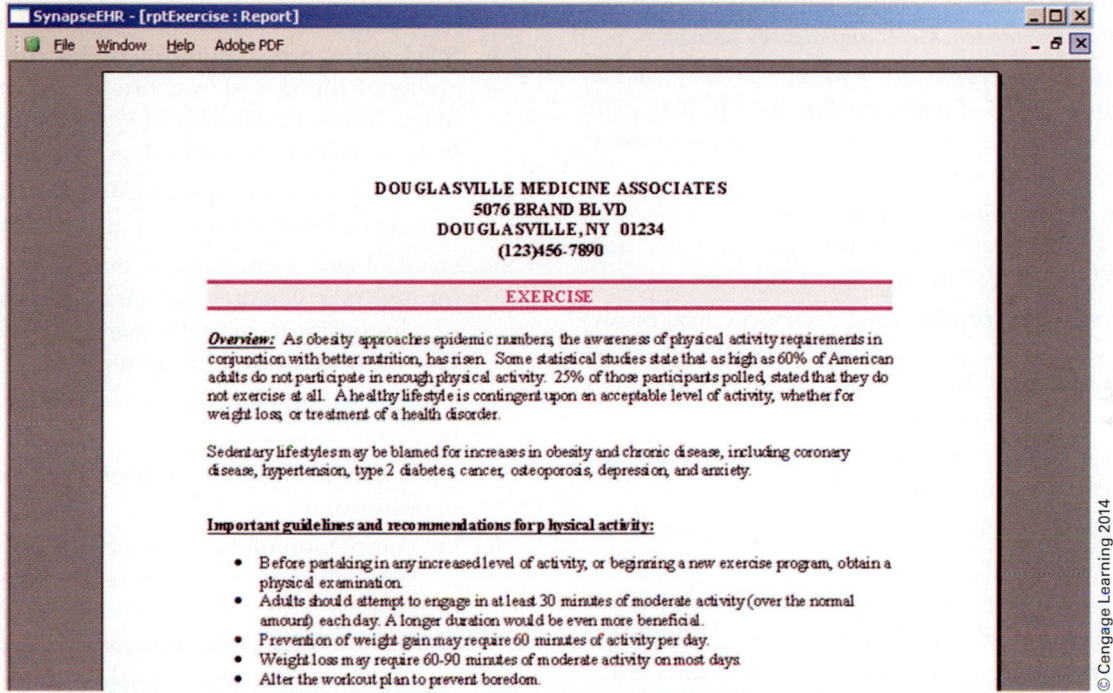

Figure 25-17 Patient education forms can be printed from an electronic medical records software and given to the patient right in the exam room.

PROCEDURE 25-1

Assisting with a Complete Physical Examination

STANDARD PRECAUTIONS:

PURPOSE:

To assist the provider with a complete physical examination.

EQUIPMENT/SUPPLIES:

Balance beam, digital, or electronic scale
Patient gown
Drape
Thermometer
Stethoscope
Sphygmomanometer
Alcohol wipes
Examination lights
Otoscope
Tuning fork
Ophthalmoscope
Penlight
Nasal speculum
Tongue depressor
Percussion hammer
Tape measure
Cotton balls
Safety pin
Gloves
Tissues
Lubricant
Emesis basin
Gauze sponges
Specimen bottles/slides—request forms
Biohazard and regular waste containers

continues

Procedure 25-1 (continued)

PROCEDURE STEPS:
Assisting with a Complete Physical Examination

1. Wash hands. Adhere to Standard Precautions.

2. *Paying attention to detail*, assemble equipment.

3. *Introduce yourself. Greet and identify patient.*

4. *Explain procedure to patient, speaking at the patient's level of understanding.* RATIONALE: To obtain patient cooperation, allay apprehension, and gain consent.

5. *Paying attention to detail*, place instruments in easily accessible sequence for provider use. RATIONALE: Efficient use of time and space.

6. *Using active listening skills*, review medical history with patient (see Chapter 23 for obtaining patient history). RATIONALE: To ensure complete history has been obtained and is current.

7. Take patient vital signs, test visual acuity, and check hearing ability.

8. Obtain a urine specimen (see Chapter 42 for urine collection procedures).

9. Obtain all required blood samples (see Chapters 40 and 41 for blood specimen collection procedures).

10. Perform electrocardiogram (ECG) if directed by provider (see Chapter 37 for ECG procedure).

11. Provide patient with appropriate gown and drape.

12. Assist patient to disrobe completely while *protecting patient's personal boundaries*; explain where the opening for the gown is to be placed. RATIONALE: To assist patient in maintaining modesty, privacy, and warmth.

13. *Attending to any personal needs of the patient*, assist patient in sitting at the end of the table; drape patient across lap and legs. RATIONALE: Always drape patient to maintain modesty.

14. Inform provider when patient is ready.

15. When the provider arrives, *display a calm, professional, and caring manner*, and remain by the patient ready to assist the patient and provider.

16. Position patient in a sitting or supine position for the head, throat, eye, ear, and neck examination.

17. Lights may be turned off to allow pupils to dilate for retinal examination.

18. *Paying attention to detail*, hand the provider instruments as required (some providers do not require the medical assistant to hand the instruments).

19. The sitting position is maintained for auscultation of the chest and heart.

20. Assist the patient into a supine position and drape for examination of the chest. Breast examination is discussed in Chapter 26.

21. Maintain a quiet atmosphere to enhance the ability of the provider in listening to heart and lung sounds. RATIONALE: Quiet is necessary to hear heart and chest sounds accurately.

22. Position patient in supine position and drape for examinations of abdomen and extremities.

23. Gynecologic examination may then be performed (see Chapter 26). Assist female patient into lithotomy position for gynecologic examination. Male genitals are examined.

24. If rectal examination is necessary, assist patient into Sims' position.

25. Place patient in prone position for examination of posterior aspect of body.

26. On completion of the examination, assist patient to sitting position and allow patient to sit at end of table for a few minutes. RATIONALE: Allows patient to recover from potential dizziness.

27. Ensure patient stability (check color of skin, pulse) before allowing patient to stand up. RATIONALE: Prevents the patient from fainting due to orthostatic hypotension.

28. **EHR** Assist patient with dressing; provide privacy.

29. Accurately enter any notes or patient instructions on computer in patient's electronic medical record per provider orders.

30. Escort patient to provider's office for discussion of examination results.

31. Don disposable gloves.

32. Dispose of disposable gown and drape in biohazard waste container if contaminated with blood or body fluids. RATIONALE: Prevents microorganism cross-contamination; gown and drape may have body secretions on them.

33. Dispose of contaminated disposable materials in biohazard waste container. RATIONALE: Prevents microorganism cross-contamination of

Procedure 25-1 (continued)

bloodborne pathogens and other potentially infectious materials (OPIM).

34. Remove table paper and dispose in biohazard waste container. RATIONALE: Prevents microorganism cross-contamination.

35. Disinfect counters and examination table with a solution of 10% bleach. RATIONALE: Prevents microorganism cross-contamination by blood and OPIM.

36. Clean, disinfect, or sterilize reusable instruments as appropriate (see Chapters 22 and 31). RATIONALE: Prevents microorganism cross-contamination.

37. Remove gloves and discard in biohazard waste container. RATIONALE: Prevents microorganism cross-contamination by blood and OPIM.

38. Wash hands.

39. Replace table paper and equipment in preparation for the next patient.

40. **EHR** Document the procedure on computer in patient's electronic medical record.

DOCUMENTATION

11/8/20XX   T 98.2, P 84, R 16 BP 124/76 Complete physical examination performed by Dr. Woo. Urinalysis negative, Hemoccult slide negative. Venipuncture performed and specimens sent to laboratory for complete blood count and electrolytes. Electrocardiogram completed. Patient given written instructions and appointment made for a colonoscopy. Says she understands the preparation for the colonoscopy. W. Slawson, CMA (AAMA)—

CASE STUDY 25-1

Refer to the scenario at the beginning of the chapter.

CASE STUDY REVIEW

1. Why do Wanda and Bruce prepare and assist for physical exams with patients of their own gender?

CASE STUDY 25-2

At Inner City Health Care, clinical medical assistant Wanda Slawson, CMA (AAMA), is helping Liz Corbin, a part-time administrative/clinical medical assistant, to learn to prepare the examination room and patients for the physical examination. In addition to alerting Liz to provider preferences, Wanda wants to be sure that Liz has a solid understanding of the methods of examination, positions and draping, and the components of the physical examination.

CASE STUDY REVIEW

1. In reviewing with Liz the methods of examination used by the providers, what six primary methods would Wanda have Liz describe?
2. What patient positions would Liz need to know?
3. Wanda asks Liz to recall the various examination components and their significance. How should Liz respond?

CASE STUDY 25-3

Mrs. Mason, a 72-year-old somewhat frail woman with arthritis and hypertensive heart disease, has an appointment today for a complete physical examination. It will include a basic physical examination and an examination of the pelvis because she has had bright red vaginal spotting.

CASE STUDY REVIEW

1. Discuss positions and draping for the physical examination, including pelvic examination for this patient.
2. Discuss any special safety needs for Mrs. Mason.
3. What additional supplies and equipment should be available for the provider?

SUMMARY

A complete physical examination will be performed during the patient's initial visit. Findings at this examination, both normal and abnormal, provide a baseline for future examinations.

   The role of the medical assistant throughout the examination is twofold. The assistant assembles the necessary instruments and may hand them to the provider when requested. The medical assistant will also prepare the patient and obtain specimens as required by the examination and provider. Responsibilities to the patient include explanations and careful positioning, protecting modesty by careful draping, and, most important, providing comfort, emotional support, and safety. By performing these duties, the medical assistant can ensure patient compliance and provider efficiency.

STUDY FOR SUCCESS

To reinforce your knowledge and skills of information presented in this chapter:

- Review the *Key Terms*
- Role-play with other students to apply attributes of professionalism pertinent to this chapter.
- Consider the *Case Studies* and discuss your conclusions
- Answer the questions in the *Certification Review*
- Apply your knowledge by completing the *Activities* in the *Study Guide* and the *Games* and *Quizzes* in the StudyWARE StudyWARE software on the *Premium Website*
- Perform the Procedure using the *Competency Assessment* Checklists in the *Competency Manual*
- Practice your problem-solving skills with the *Critical Thinking Challenge 3.0* on the *Premium Website*

Additional resources for this chapter include:

- Module 21 of the *Medical Assisting Learning Lab*
- *CourseMate for Delmar's Comprehensive Medical Assisting*
- *WebTutor for Delmar's Comprehensive Medical Assisting*

CERTIFICATION REVIEW

1. The method of examination that is the process of listening directly to body sounds is called:
   a. percussion
   b. auditory
   c. auscultation
   d. the direct method
2. The supine position is also known as:
   a. horizontal recumbent
   b. dorsal recumbent
   c. knee-chest
   d. Sims'
3. During the physical examination, ataxia might be observed, which relates to:
   a. stature   c. body movement
   b. posture   d. speech

4. When the patient asks a question of the medical assistant, the medical assistant should:
   a. refer all questions to the provider
   b. try to answer all questions, even if uncertain
   c. answer questions to the extent of knowledge; refer others to the provider
   d. ask the patient to please hold all questions until the examination is complete
5. When the abdomen is being examined, the patient is typically in a:
   a. supine position
   b. prone position
   c. Fowler's position
   d. Sims' position

6. A physical exam is usually conducted in which order?
   a. Caudal to cephalad
   b. Cephalad to caudal
   c. Medial to distal
   d. Distal to medial
7. A common supply used during a neurologic exam is:
   a. a cotton ball
   b. a safety pin
   c. a percussion hammer
   d. all of the above
8. An annual GYN exam and PAP smear are conducted in which position?
   a. Dorsal recumbent
   b. Prone
   c. Lithotomy
   d. Fowler's

9. An important method of assessment in which the practitioner observes the patient's appearance, gait, behavior, etc., is which of the following?
   a. Palpation
   b. Percussion
   c. Auscultation
   d. Inspection
10. A common supply used during the examination of the abdomen is:
    a. a drape
    b. a stethoscope
    c. an otoscope
    d. both a and b

REFERENCES/BIBLIOGRAPHY

Hegner, B. R., Acello, B., & Caldwell, E. (2008). *Nursing assistant: A nursing process approach* (10th ed.). Clifton Park, NY: Delmar Cengage Learning.

Keir, L., Wise, B., Krebs, C., & Kelley-Arney, C. (2008). *Medical assisting administration and clinical competencies* (6th ed.). Clifton Park, NY: Delmar Cengage Learning.

Simmers, L. (2004). *Diversified health occupations* (6th ed.). Clifton Park, NY: Delmar Cengage Learning.

Taber's cyclopedic medical dictionary (22nd ed.). (2003). Philadelphia: F. A. Davis.

Tamparo, C., & Lewis, M. (2005). *Diseases of the human body* (4th ed.). Philadelphia: F. A. Davis.

Unit VII

Assisting with Specialty Examinations and Procedures

CHAPTER 26
Obstetrics and Gynecology 652

CHAPTER 27
Pediatrics 706

CHAPTER 28
Male Reproductive System 752

CHAPTER 29
Gerontology 768

CHAPTER 30
Examinations and Procedures of Body Systems 784

CHAPTER 26

Obstetrics and Gynecology

OUTLINE

Obstetrics
   Initial Prenatal Visit
   Subsequent or Return
     Prenatal Visits
   Disorders of Pregnancy
   Parturition
   Postpartum Period

Contraception
Gynecology
   The Gynecologic
     Examination
   Gynecologic Diseases
     and Conditions

Other Diagnostic Tests
   and Treatments for
   Reproductive System
   Diseases
Complementary Therapy in
   Obstetrics and Gynecology

LEARNING OUTCOMES

1. Define, spell, and pronounce the key terms as presented in the glossary.
2. Explain the importance of prenatal care, and discuss what examinations will be performed as part of the initial visit.
3. Explain why the initial prenatal visit is important.
4. List 12 conditions or diseases that can cause a pregnant woman and her fetus to be at greater risk for problems during the pregnancy.
5. List signs and symptoms and their possible corresponding conditions that the provider searches for during the prenatal history and physical examination.
6. Calculate an expected date of confinement (EDC) or expected date of birth (EDB) using Nägele's Rule.
7. Calculate an EDC (EDB) using a gestation wheel.
8. Explain the purpose of ultrasonography and amniocentesis.
9. List and describe six types of abortion.
10. Explain what occurs in each of the three stages of labor.

11. Describe what takes place during the postpartum examination.
12. List and describe the diseases and disorders that can affect the female patient.
13. Describe the laboratory tests and procedures that can help diagnose the diseases and disorders that can affect the female patient.
14. Describe seven sexually transmitted diseases.
15. Explain the medical assistant's responsibilities with a gynecologic examination.
16. Describe breast self-examination and the method of teaching patient breast self-examination.
17. Discuss menopause.
18. Describe the findings and concerns surrounding hormone replacement therapy.
19. Describe several methods of contraception.
20. Explain reasons for impaired fertility.
21. Describe three therapies that assist in reproduction.
22. Analyze the professionalism questions and apply them to this chapter's content.

KEY TERMS

abortion

amniocentesis

amniotomy

bacterial vaginosis

Bartholin gland

bimanual examination

Braxton–Hicks

breast self-exam (BSE)

candidiasis

carcinoma in situ

cervical punch biopsy

Cesarean section

chlamydia

colposcopy

condylomata

congenital anomalies

contraception

coupling agent

cryosurgery

diethylstilbestrol
(DES)

dilation

Down syndrome

dysmenorrhea

dyspareunia

dysplasia

eclampsia

ectopic

effacement

endometriosis

erosion

formalin

fulgurated

genitalia

(continues)

ATTRIBUTES OF PROFESSIONALISM

Communication

- Did you introduce yourself? Did you identify the patient through name and birth date or other identifying feature?
- Did you listen to and acknowledge the patient?
- Did you speak at the patient's level of understanding?
- Did you allay patients' fears regarding the procedure being performed and help them feel safe and comfortable?
- Did you respond honestly and diplomatically to the patient's concerns?
- Did you demonstrate empathy in communicating with patients, family, and staff?
- Does your knowledge allow you to speak easily with all members of the health care team?

Presentation

- Did you attend to any special needs of the patient? Did you ask first if assistance was needed, rather than taking charge?
- Were you courteous, patient, and respectful to the patient?
- Did you display a calm, professional, and caring manner?

Competency

- Did you ask questions if you were out of your comfort zone or did not have the experience to carry out tasks?
- Did you display sound judgment?
- Were you knowledgeable and accountable?
- Did you apply critical thinking skills in performing patient assessment and care?

Initiative

- Did you direct the patient to other resources when necessary or helpful, with the approval of the provider?
- Did you assist coworkers when appropriate?

Integrity

- Did you work within your scope of practice?
- Did you protect personal boundaries?
- Did you demonstrate respect for individual diversity?
- Did you protect and maintain confidentiality?
- Did you immediately report any error you had made?
- Did you maintain your moral and ethical standards?

KEY TERMS   *(continued)*

gestation

gestational diabetes

gravidity

human chorionic
  gonadotropin

hyperemesis gravidarum

hypoxia

hysterosalpingogram

intraepithelium

involute

Lamaze

laparoscopy

lochia

meconium

metrorrhagia

multigravida

Nägele's Rule

neonatal

nullipara

oxytocin

Papanicolaou test (Pap)

parity

parturition

patency

pelvic inflammatory
  disease

placenta abruptio

placenta previa

polycystic

postcoital

preeclampsia

prenatal

primigravida

prostaglandin

puerperium

sickle cell anemia

supine hypotension

Tay–Sachs

thalassemia

titer

trichomoniasis

trimester

ultrasonography

vesicle

viability

wet mount

SCENARIO

Dr. Amy Cox is an OB/GYN in the obstetrics department of Inner City Health Care who has a fully packed schedule today. The morning hours are designated for prenatal visits and the afternoon for in-office GYN procedures.

It is important to understand the kind of prenatal visit that a patient requires. There are varied time requirements based on the patient's progress through her pregnancy. At predetermined gestational stages, there is screening scheduled to detect the risk of birth defects and genetic abnormalities, and to monitor the health of the mother during pregnancy. Other testing, such as ultrasound, monitors the progress of the baby or babies.

First prenatal visits require more of the provider's time than the routine, regularly scheduled visits that occur throughout the pregnancy.

As a professional medical assistant, Ms. Angela Jarreau, RMA (AMT) must be aware of the needs related to each patient visit. She may be required to schedule the visit in an appropriate time slot on Dr. Cox's appointment calendar. She might be assisting Dr. Cox with a screening test or an exam. Ms. Jarreau is the source for all patient teaching materials and handles the scheduling of outside testing for all of Dr. Cox's patients. She is a vital and indispensable part of the health care team.

INTRODUCTION

Obstetrics is the medical specialty in which the provider treats the female patient from the prenatal period through labor, delivery, and during the 6-week postpartum period. Gynecology is the specialty that treats the medical and surgical disorders and diseases of the female reproductive tract. Both specialties are usually combined, and the provider who practices them is known as an obstetrician/ gynecologist, or simply, an OB/GYN provider. Knowledge of the female anatomy, the laboratory tests and procedures for both specialties, the diseases and disorders that affect the female patient during her nonpregnant and pregnant states, and patient education are essential for the medical assistant who will care for these patients. The goal of the

OB/GYN specialty is to promote the health and well-being of the woman and her baby

 HIPAA is important, especially when dealing with the cultural differences in pregnancy. Some cultures demand modesty and protecting their privacy is critical. Infertility is a stigma in some cultures. Maintaining confidentiality is a requirement for all patients.

The patient's partner may be unaware of the patient's obstetrical history such as previous pregnancies, abortions, or sexually transmitted diseases. Confidentiality is of utmost importance, and it is best to be alone with a patient during the collection of this type of medical information.

SPOTLIGHT ON CERTIFICATION

RMA Content Outline

- Anatomy and physiology
- Medical terminology
- Patient relations
- Patient instruction
- Medical asepsis
- Instrument use
- Physical examination
- Laboratory procedures

CMA (AAMA) Content Outline

- Medical terminology
- Anatomy and physiology
- Professional communication and behavior
- Medicolegal guidelines and requirements
- Patient preparation and assisting the physician
- Collecting and processing specimens: diagnostic testing

CMAS Content Outline

- Medical terminology
- Anatomy and physiology
- Examination preparation

OBSTETRICS

Obstetrics is the branch of medicine that provides care to the mother and fetus during pregnancy, labor, delivery, and the postpartum period known as the **puerperium**. Pregnancy is a period of approximately 40 weeks from the day conception takes place (Figure 26-1). The puerperium is the period of 6 weeks after delivery when the mother's body is returning to its prepregnant state. Visits to the provider for prenatal and postnatal care are the initial **prenatal** visit, return visits, and the 6-week postpartum checkup.

Initial Prenatal Visit

The initial prenatal visit is of utmost importance and usually occurs after a woman has missed a second menstrual period or after an at-home pregnancy test result is positive. Some obstetricians recommend prepregnancy or preconception physical examinations. The information gained at this appointment can be used as a baseline on which to compare future tests and procedures. It is a risk assessment of maternal health for identification and prevention of complications. For example, blood pressure measurement performed prepregnancy and not during the first trimester can rule out pregnancy-induced hypertension. The prenatal visit is a time of health promotion for the expectant mother and her baby. It is also the time for diagnosis and treatment of maternal disorders that may have been present before the pregnancy or that may have developed during the course of the pregnancy. Growth and development of the fetus are followed and identification of problems that may impede a normal labor is sought. There is ongoing assessment of the expectant mother and the fetus. Any abnormalities can indicate a problem or complication necessitating further testing and assessment. Early detection and management of conditions such as **gestational diabetes**, urinary tract infections, anemia, and **preeclampsia** can prevent serious complications.

The initial visit requires more time than subsequent visits because a thorough history and physical examination are done, including breast, abdominal, pelvic, and vaginal examinations. Pelvic measurements are taken to help ascertain if the pelvis is adequate for a fetus to be delivered vaginally.

 The initial visit is followed by monthly visits and then, beginning at the 28th week, visits every 2 weeks for weeks 29–36, and visits every week for weeks 37–40. The routine visits consist of checking weight, measuring blood pressure, and testing blood and urine; education about nutrition, activity, and rest; and preparing for childbirth (see Procedure 26-1). Data are entered into the computer each time the patient has an appointment (Figure 26-2). They include findings from the provider's examination, vital signs, weight, blood and urine tests, and patient education for preparing for childbirth. Data are retrievable for comparison purposes and treatment options.

 Many groups of women do not receive prenatal care. Lack of financial resources, insurance, or transportation and poor communication by health care providers are some of the reasons that some women do not participate in prenatal care. Modesty may deter some women from seeking prenatal care. Exposing the body to a man is viewed as a major violation of modesty in some cultures. This is why protecting the privacy of all patients is critical.

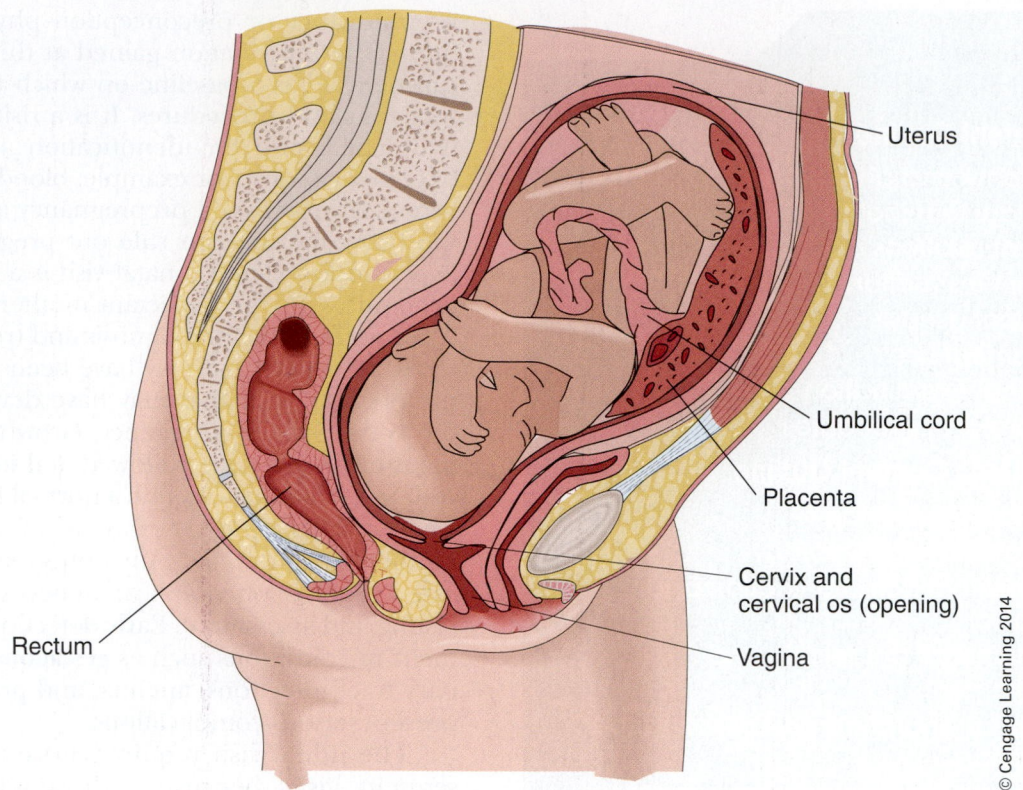

© Cengage Learning 2014

Figure 26-1   Normal uterine pregnancy.

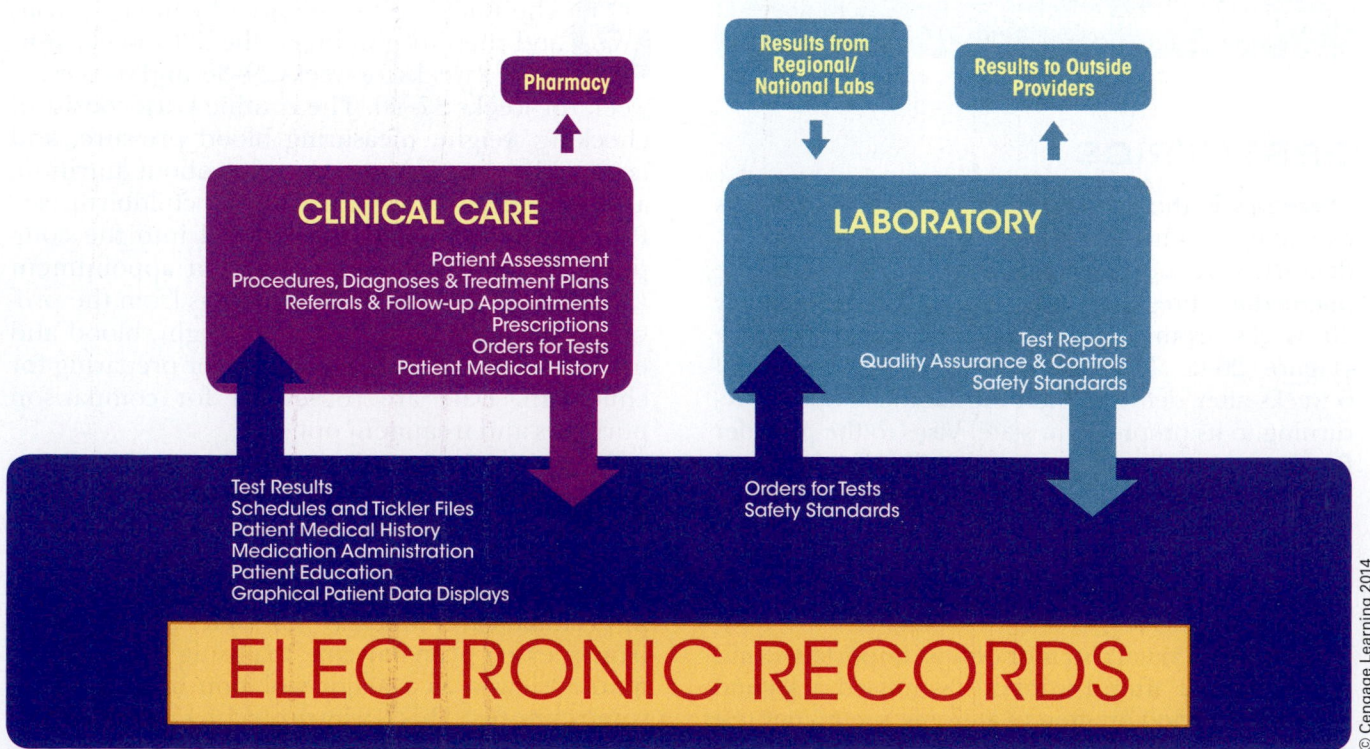

© Cengage Learning 2014

Figure 26-2   Clinical care and laboratory arms of the total practice management system data flow.

Certain cultures expect their women to observe practices believed to ensure a favorable pregnancy. Mexican women are advised not to watch an eclipse of the moon; the belief is that the baby will be born with congenital anomalies. Some Spanish women in the United States wear a braided cord around the midsection to ward off nausea and to ensure safe birth. Medals and beads, often worn by women, are believed to ward off evil spirits. Women of Indian heritage believe that "hot" foods are harmful and "cold" foods are beneficial during pregnancy. Other cultures believe that inactivity during pregnancy will safeguard the mother and baby. There are also many dietary influences within different cultures. (Chapter 34 gives more information on culture, diet, and food choices.) Respect for all cultures is of great importance, and judgments should not be made that some women are ignorant or lazy. Incorporating the patient's customs and beliefs demonstrates that you value cultural diversity and women's self-esteem.

All women should be fully involved in their care. Women with physical or emotional disabilities must have their particular needs addressed. When necessary, make adaptations whenever possible for women who are mentally challenged, blind, deaf, or physically incapacitated.

Laboratory Tests. The laboratory tests and procedures that may be part of the initial prenatal visit are described in Table 26-1.

Patient Education. Patient education includes such topics as nutrition, dental care, rest, and exercise, as well as discussion about over-the-counter (OTC) remedies, prescription medications, and herbal products (Figure 26-3). Alcohol and tobacco and their dangers and potential harm to fetus and mother should also be discussed. Medications, alcohol, cigarettes, and mind-altering substances taken by the mother have harmful effects on the fetus and should not be used.

Before the birth, the expectant couple is encouraged to choose a method of feeding the infant. During the initial prenatal visit, benefits of breast-feeding the newborn are discussed. If the mother is HIV negative, breast-feeding is encouraged because it offers many nutritional, psychological, and immunologic benefits. Because the immune system of newborns is not fully developed, the high level of immunoglobulins in breast milk gives them protection against some pathogenic diseases of the respiratory and gastrointestinal

Table 26-1   Laboratory Tests at the Initial Prenatal Visit

Laboratory Test	Disease or Condition
Complete blood count (CBC), hemoglobin, and hematocrit	To detect anemia or infection
Urinalysis with microscopic examination (pH, specific gravity, color, glucose, albumin, proteins, white and red blood cell counts, casts, acetone, human chorionic gonadotropin [HCG])	To screen for diabetes mellitus, renal disease, infection, hypertensive disease, pregnancy
Blood type, Rh factor	To detect Rh incompatibility
Rubella titer	To determine immunity to rubella
Renal function Alpha-fetoprotein (if initial visit is at 16–18 weeks gestation)	To evaluate renal impairment in women with history of diabetes mellitus, hypertension, or kidney disease
Tuberculin skin test	To screen for tuberculosis
Venereal Disease Research Laboratory (VDRL) and rapid plasma reagin (RPR)	To detect syphilis
Human Immunodeficiency Virus (HIV) with patient permission	To screen for HIV antibodies
Hepatitis B and C virus	To screen for hepatitis B and C viruses
Blood glucose	To screen for gestational diabetes
Cardiac evaluation electrocardiogram (ECG), chest radiograph, or echocardiogram	To evaluate cardiac function in women with history of heart disease or hypertension
Pap smear	To check for cervical dysplasia, herpes simplex virus 2
Vaginal, cervical, or rectal smear or culture for gonorrhea, chlamydia, and *Streptococcus* group B	To check for gonorrhea, chlamydia, human papilloma virus (HPV)

© Cengage Learning 2014

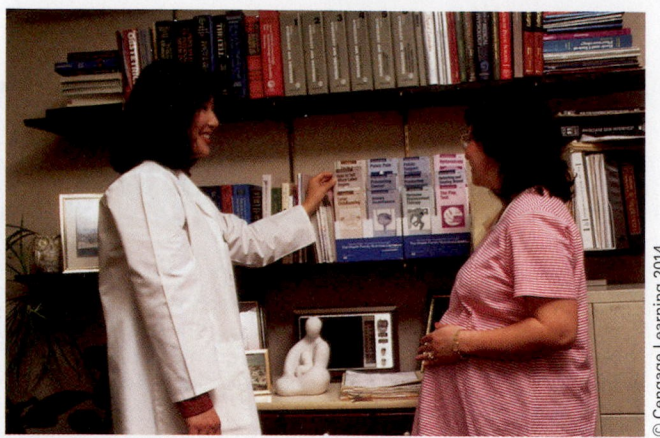

© Cengage Learning 2014

Figure 26-3 Supplying patients with information on a healthy pregnancy and potential risks and danger signs is an important responsibility of the medical assistant.

tracts. Close contact between mother and newborn is certain with breast-feeding, and bonding can readily take place. Breast-fed infants seem to have fewer allergic reactions. For the mother, one benefit of breast-feeding is that the uterus **involutes**, or returns more quickly to the nonpregnant state. Breast-feeding is the optimal way to feed a newborn. The services of a lactation consultant (available in most women's hospitals and some pediatric clinics) can be helpful especially during the initial phase of breast-feeding. The consultant can provide hands-on instructions to the patient to optimize the experience for the mother and baby.

Formal childbirth education classes given in various languages teach the fundamentals of labor, delivery, and newborn care and feeding.

Prenatal History. The prenatal history will be comprehensive and include much of the same information that is obtained during the taking of a regular medical history. However, emphasis will be on identification of the high-risk patient. Particular attention is given to women who have a history of one or more of the following situations or conditions, because they may place a woman and her fetus at greater risk during pregnancy:

- Use of legal drugs (OTC, prescription, tobacco, caffeine, alcohol); illegal drugs (marijuana, cocaine); and herbal products
- Age under 16 years or over 35 years
- Rh-negative blood
- A history of repeated premature labors and deliveries, abortions, or stillbirths

PATIENT EDUCATION

Whatever the pregnant woman ingests or inhales affects the fetus. Smoking during pregnancy poses serious risks to mother and fetus. Low birth weight, placenta abruptio, and deliveries before term are some of the possible effects to the fetus. Lung cancer, emphysema, and cardiovascular disease can affect the mother. Other kinds of substance abuse such as alcohol, cocaine, and other recreational drugs are commonly seen in pregnant women who are abused, such as in a domestic abuse situation; however, women do not have to be in an abusive situation to abuse drugs or alcohol. Ask the patient if she is in immediate danger. If so, a referral can be made to a community resource (e.g., women's shelter, hotline phone number, district attorney's office) or the provider can help devise a safety plan until the community resource steps in to help. (Chapters 7 and 35 provide more information about domestic violence and drug abuse.)

- Genetic diseases in the family
- Previous **Cesarean section**
- Diabetes
- Hypothyroidism or hyperthyroidism
- Sexually transmitted disease
- Hypertension
- Nutritional deficiencies
- Cardiac problems
- Kidney conditions
- Epilepsy
- Headaches

Any of these conditions or diseases can place the woman and fetus at risk for serious complications.

During the initial prenatal visit, an obstetrical history is taken, which includes the **gravidity**, or total number of pregnancies, including the present pregnancy, regardless of duration. The history also includes the **parity**, the number of pregnancies carried to the point of viability regardless of whether the baby was born alive or dead. Multiple births, twins, and triplets count as one pregnancy (gravida) and one delivery (para). For example, a woman pregnant for the first time is referred to as "Gravida 1, Para 0." After this woman delivers, regardless whether the baby is born alive or dead, if it reached the age of **viability**, the history of the woman is "Gravida 1, Para 1." Viability is the ability to grow and develop after birth. The term **multigravida** refers to a woman who has been pregnant more than once. **Nullipara** describes a woman who has not carried a pregnancy to viability.

Para sometimes has four letters that can be used to give more information about past deliveries. It does *not* include the present pregnancy. The four letters are FPAL:

F—number of full-term deliveries (37–40 weeks' gestation)

P—number of preterm or premature deliveries (20–36 weeks' gestation)

A—number of abortions (induced or spontaneous terminations before 20 weeks' gestation)

L—number of living children born to the patient who are still alive at the time of history data collection

For example, a woman has had four term pregnancies, delivered four live infants, but lost a child to leukemia at 7 years of age. This woman is considered to be 4-0-0-3.

The present prenatal history includes information about the present pregnancy. The provider searches for problems indicative of high-risk factors. Identifying high-risk patients helps to limit maternal and newborn deaths and diseases. Some factors that indicate a patient is at high risk are inadequate nutrition; use of drugs such as alcohol, tobacco, or cocaine; existing medical conditions such as high blood pressure or diabetes; sexually transmitted disease; and poverty. The provider watches for signs and symptoms that indicate a potentially serious condition. Examples are listed in Table 26-2.

Subsequent or Return Prenatal Visits

Subsequent visits include weight, blood pressure, urinalysis, complete blood count with hemoglobin and hematocrit, measurement of the height of the uterine fundus (a tape measure is used by placing it on the anterior symphysis pubis and the crest of the uterus) (Figure 26-5), and fetal heart measurements (Figure 26-6). Generally, it is not possible to determine with accuracy the exact date of conception. Many formulas have been used for calculating the EDB (expected date of birth) or EDC

Table 26-2 Signs and Symptoms of Potentially Serious Conditions

Signs and Symptoms	Possible Condition
Rapid weight gain	Preeclampsia
Headaches	Preeclampsia
Hypertension	Preeclampsia
Vision changes	Preeclampsia
Severe nausea and vomiting	Hyperemesis gravidarum/dehydration
Bleeding, discharge, abdominal pain/cramping	Threatened abortion, placenta previa, placenta abruptio, ectopic pregnancy
Edema	Preeclampsia
One-sided pelvic or abdominal pain	Ectopic pregnancy (Figure 26-4)
Chills, fever	Vaginal infection, sexually transmitted disease, other infections

© Cengage Learning 2014

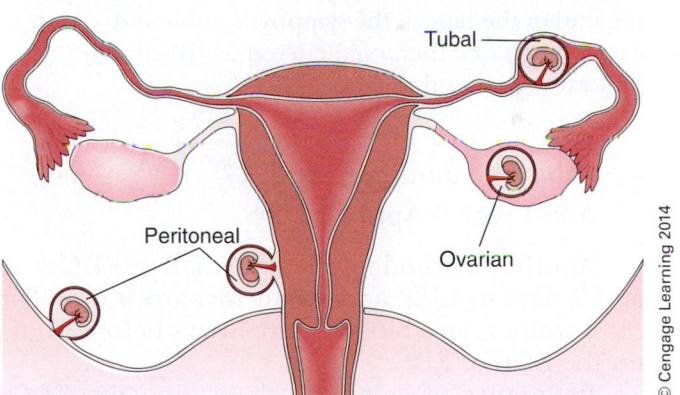

© Cengage Learning 2014

Figure 26-4 Sites of ectopic pregnancy.

(expected date of confinement). Although none is foolproof, **Nägele's Rule** is the usual method used because it is reasonably accurate. Nägele's Rule is to add 7 days to the first day of the last menstrual period (LMP), subtract 3 months, and add 1 year. An example is:

The first day of LMP = July 10, 2007

Add 7 days = July 17

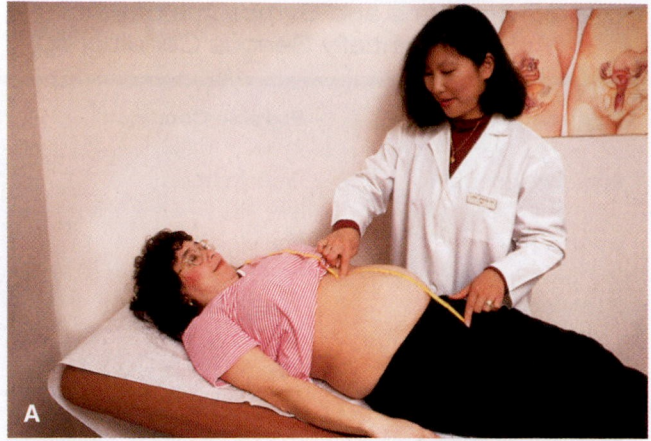

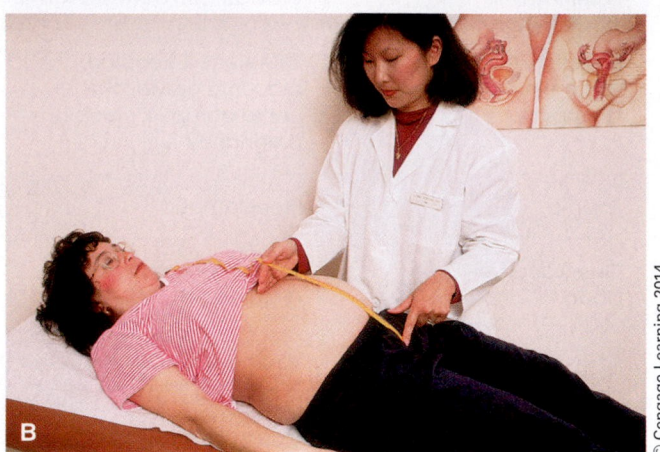

Figure 26-5   Fundal height is measured by placing the end of the tape at the symphysis pubis and extending it in either a (A) curved or (B) straight pattern to the fundus.

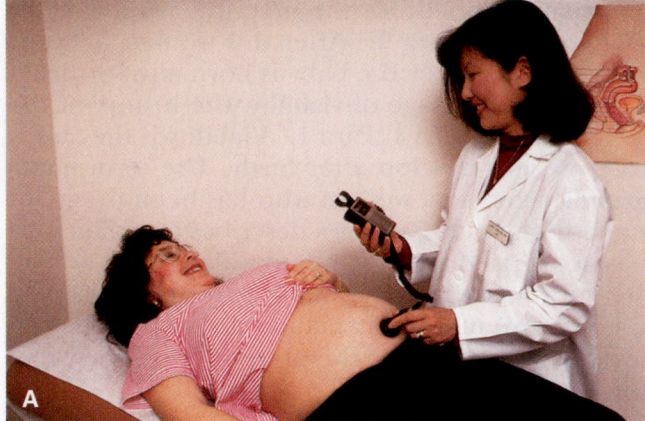

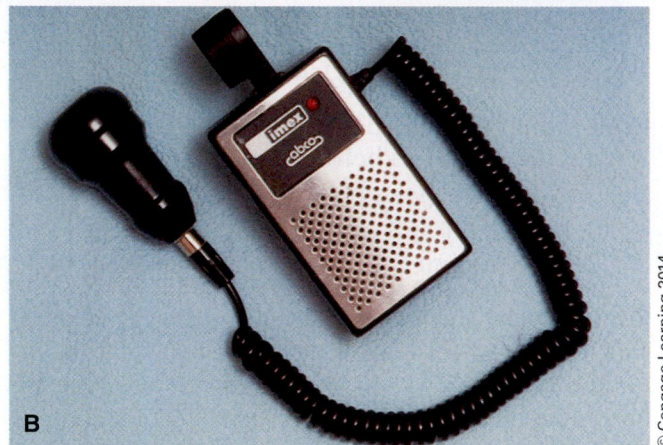

Figure 26-6   (A) Fetal heart tones are measured with a handheld Doppler. (B) Handheld Doppler.

Subtract 3 months = April 17

Add 1 year = April 17, 2008

Another method to calculate EDB or EDC is to add 7 days to LMP and count forward 9 months. Most women give birth within 7 days before or after the EDB or EDC.

Pregnancy wheels help determine the EDC. Line up the arrow of the first day of the LMP, then read off the date that corresponds to the 40-week designation (Figure 26-7).

Vaginal examinations are only done periodically up to 2 to 3 weeks before the EDB or EDC. Patients are encouraged to attend classes in the **Lamaze** method of childbirth, as well as classes in the care of the newborn (Figure 26-8 through Figure 26-10).

Tests and Procedures

Alpha-Fetoprotein. Another test that may be done during a subsequent visit is the mother's serum alpha-fetoprotein (MSAFP) blood test. It is done

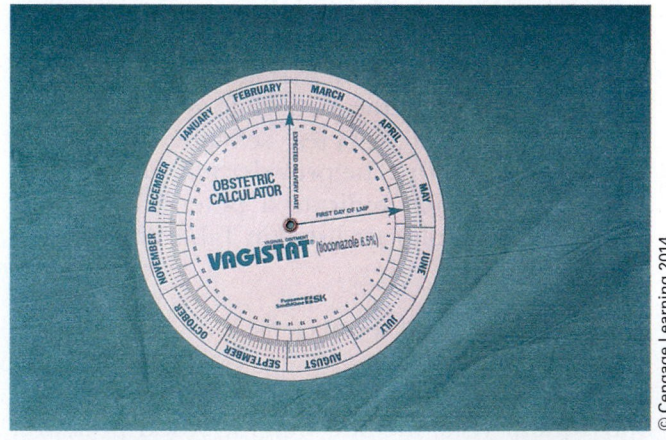

Figure 26-7   Gestation wheel. Place arrow labeled "first day of LMP" on date of last menstrual period (LMP). Read date at arrow labeled "expected delivery date."

about the 16th week of pregnancy. It is a screening test only, done to rule out neural tube defects, abdominal wall defects, and chromosomal problems such as Down syndrome. If the test is positive, additional testing such as an **amniocentesis** or an ultrasound will be used to help make a diagnosis.

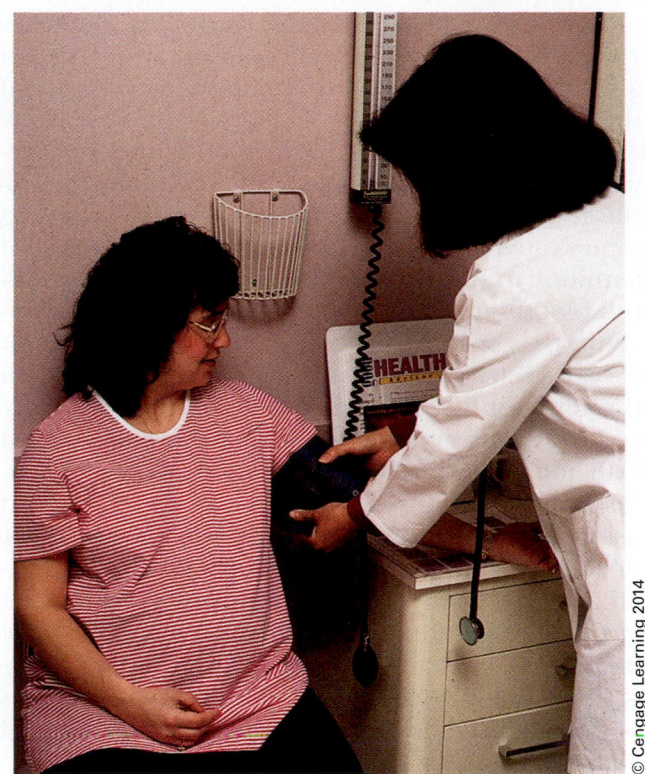

Figure 26-8   Blood pressure is measured at each prenatal visit.

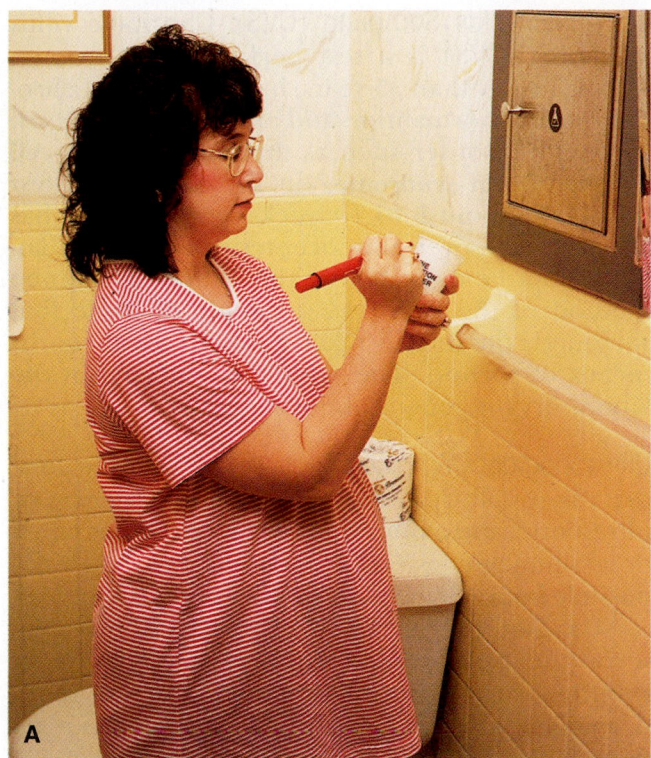

A

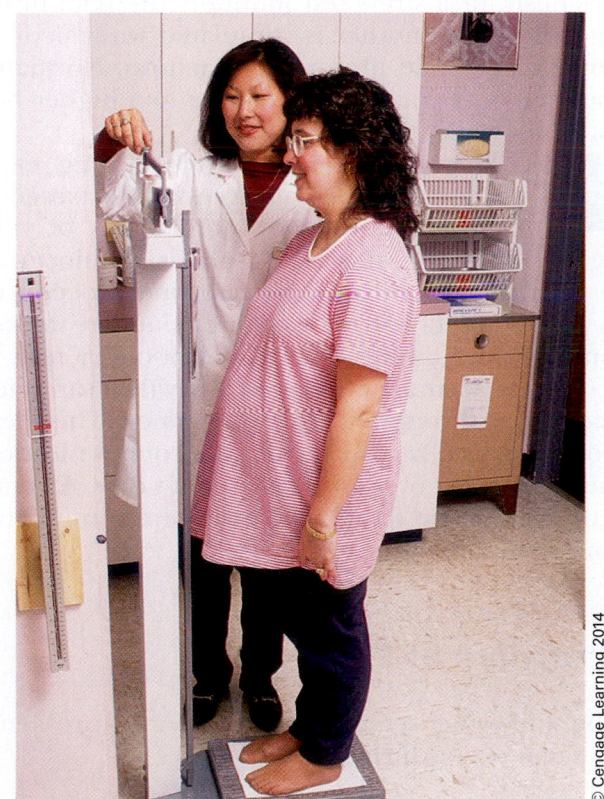

Figure 26-9   Weight gain is tracked throughout the pregnancy.

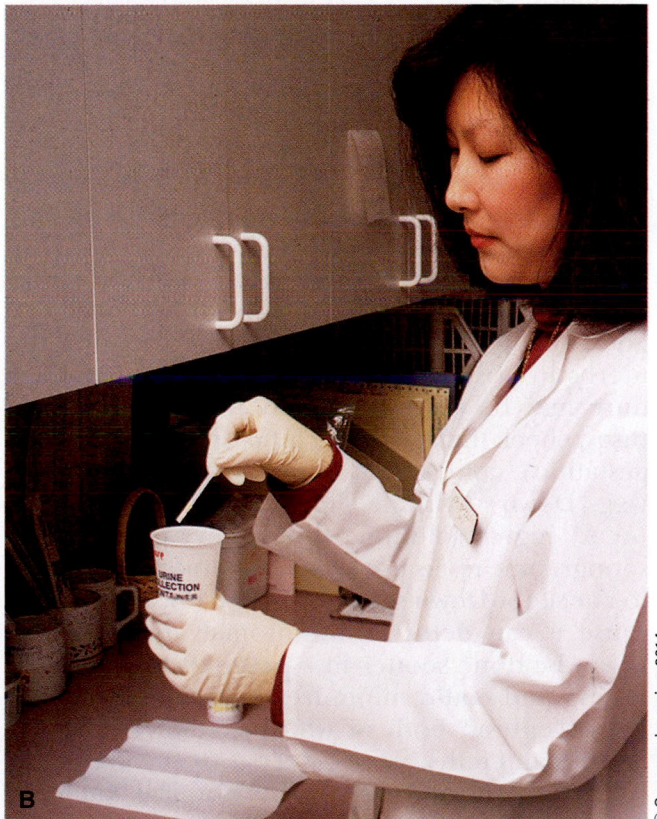

B

Figure 26-10   Urine is tested for glucose and protein at each visit. (A) Client provides a urine sample. (B) Medical assistant uses dipstick to check for glucose and protein.

Chorionic Villus Sampling (CVS). Chorionic villus sampling (CVS) is a test performed on women who are older than 35 years, have a history of chromosomal abnormalities, and are known carriers of a genetic disorder such as **thalassemia**, **sickle cell anemia**, **Down syndrome**, or **Tay–Sachs**. The test is done at about 8 to 10 weeks' **gestation** and has an advantage over amniocentesis because the latter cannot be done before the 14th week. In one method of the CVS test, a sample of tissue that surrounds the fetus is taken through a catheter by means of suction. The sample is analyzed in the laboratory for genetic abnormalities.

Ultrasonography/Amniocentesis. Two tests can be done that can supply vital information: **ultrasonography**, or ultrasound, and amniocentesis. An ultrasonogram is done simultaneously with an amniocentesis to avoid possible injury to the fetus or placenta.

Ultrasound can be performed in the first, second, or third **trimester**. It uses high-frequency sound waves to produce an image of the fetus. A **coupling agent** is spread onto the mother's abdomen to enhance penetration of sound waves through the tissue, and the scanning mechanism is moved over the abdomen. An image of the fetus can be viewed on a screen similar to a television screen. Photos are taken during the examination. The technique usually takes about a half hour. There are no known side effects to the fetus or mother, and ultrasound uses no X-rays. There is no pain involved, but slight discomfort can occur due to a full bladder. (A quart of fluid should be consumed 1 hour before the test and finished within 15 or 20 minutes.) A full bladder is essential to a good-quality ultrasound because it supports the uterus in position for good imaging. This procedure may be used to identify the number of fetuses, check the age of the fetus (number of weeks gestation), and detect some fetal abnormalities (e.g., Down syndrome; Figure 26-11).

A high-resolution three-dimensional ultrasonographic test is used more and more frequently to check for Down syndrome. The test is useful because it can detect chromosomal abnormalities. It can be done sooner in a pregnancy than blood testing and could minimize the need for CVS or amniocentesis, both of which create risks to the mother and fetus.

An amniocentesis is the surgical puncturing, with a long, thin needle, of the amniotic sac through the woman's abdomen. The purpose of this test is to obtain, by aspiration, a sample of amniotic fluid that contains fetal cells. The procedure can be done as early as 14 weeks and helps to diagnose genetic problems, **congenital anomalies** (present at birth), and chromosomal defects. It also can be used to determine the lung capacity of the fetus (Figure 26-12).

Ultrasonography is performed while the provider is doing the amniocentesis to identify the position of the fetus and placenta, thereby avoiding injury to either. There can be bleeding, leaking of amniotic fluid, and infection. Percutaneous umbilical blood sampling (PUBS), also known as cordocentesis, is another procedure that can be done. It accesses fetal circulation by aspirating blood from the fetal umbilical cord vessels. Because the procedure is invasive, it is performed in conjunction with ultrasound. Many blood studies can be performed, and many conditions can be diagnosed using fetal cord blood, such as chromosomal abnormalities, infections within the uterus, and fetal hypoxia. Drug therapy and transfusions can be given through the umbilical vein in the fetal umbilical cord. With either of these procedures, there is a risk of miscarriage. Alerting patients to this potential risk is an important aspect of informed consent.

Fetal heart rate is another test. Monitoring can be done in one of two ways: a nonstress test monitors the fetus's heart rate while it is moving spontaneously, or a stress test monitors the fetal heart rate while the mother is stimulated with medication to have mild uterine contractions. Normally, the fetal heart rate will accelerate to a higher but safe limit while it is being stressed.

EHR Entering data electronically during each visit allows immediate access to the patient's medical record and comparisons of vital signs, laboratory values, ultrasounds, amniocenteses, and all other diagnostic tests and procedures in previous data entries. Baseline values are important, and the timing of certain laboratory tests is crucial for accurate evaluation. Providers can refer back to it throughout the pregnancy. The electronic medical record (EMR) is a communication mechanism for organizing a patient's care. All data entry should be dated and include the time and your signature.

Disorders of Pregnancy

The following sections address some problems that may occur during pregnancy.

Abortion/Interruption of Pregnancy. The interruption of pregnancy before the fetus is viable is

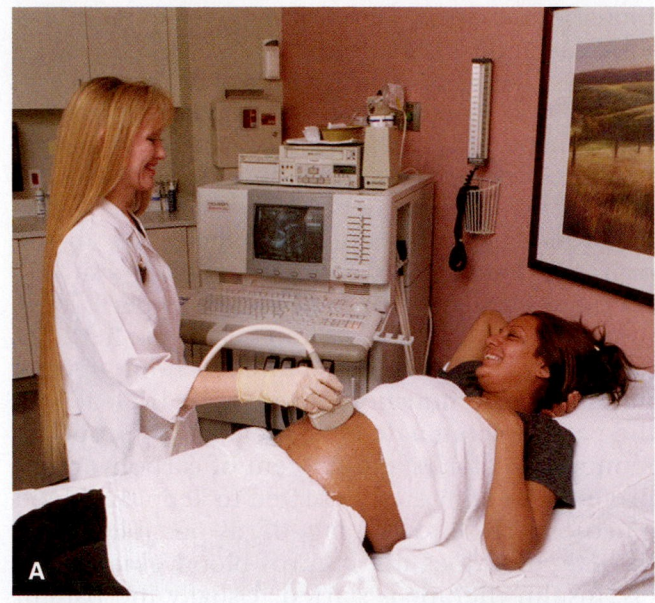

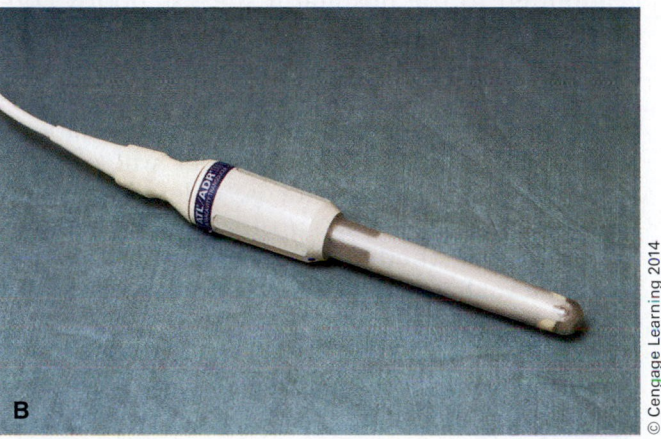

Figure 26-11   (A) Abdominal ultrasound.
(B) Transducer for transvaginal ultrasound.

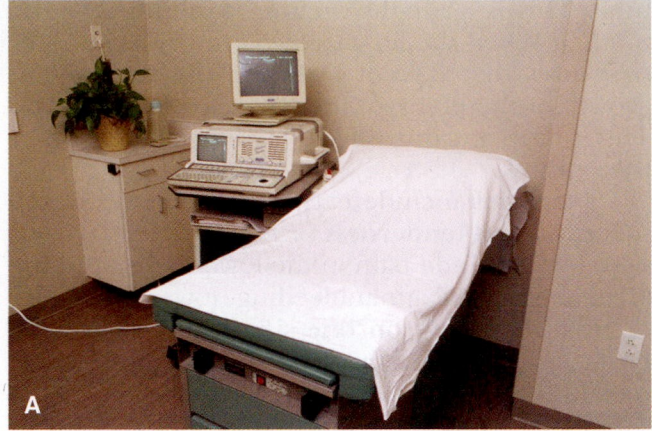

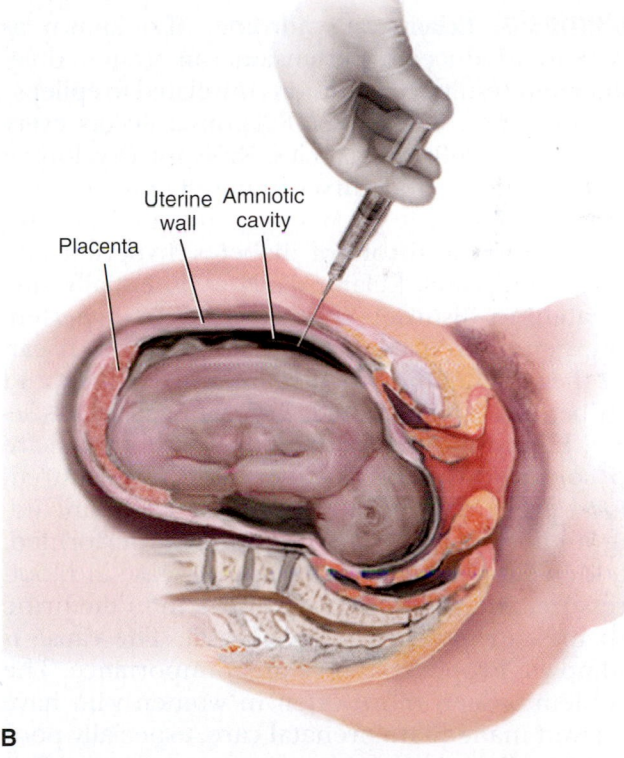

Uterine   Amniotic
wall   cavity

Placenta

B

Figure 26-12   (A) An amniocentesis setup.
(B) During amniocentesis, a sample of amniotic fluid
is aspirated for evaluation. An ultrasonogram is done
simultaneously with an amniocentesis to avoid possible
injury to the fetus or placenta.

known as **abortion**. Six types of abortion are listed
here:

1. *Spontaneous.* Unknown etiology (miscarriage).
2. *Complete.* Expulsion of all products of conception, fetus, and placenta with no surgical
   intervention.
3. *Missed.* Fetus dies in the uterus and must be removed; usually a dilation and curettage (D&C)
   is the surgical procedure performed.
4. *Incomplete.* Only parts of the fetus and placenta
   are expelled. Tissue remains in the uterus and
   a D&C usually must be performed.
5. *Threatened.* Bleeding from the uterus, but
   there are no contractions or dilation of cervix.
   Pregnancy continues.
6. *Induced.* Evacuation of the fetus and placenta
   from the uterus at the mother's request or because mother's health is in jeopardy.

Ectopic Pregnancy. An **ectopic** pregnancy indicates the implantation of an embryo outside of the
uterus. This may occur anywhere in the pelvic region, but occurs most commonly in the fallopian

tube. This is a life-threatening condition for the mother. When the fertilized egg implants in other structures that do not have the capacity for the growth of the embryo, the structure may rupture. This causes uncontrolled bleeding at the site of the rupture.

Symptoms include early pregnancy symptoms such as breast tenderness or nausea. More serious symptoms include pain in the lower belly or pelvic area, abnormal vaginal bleeding, lower back pain, or mild cramping on one side of the abdomen. Post-rupture symptoms include syncope; intense rectal pressure; hypotension; referred pain to the shoulder; and severe, sharp, and sudden pain in the lower abdomen.

Eclampsia. Eclampsia syndrome, also known as pregnancy-induced hypertension, can occur in pregnancy and result in convulsions unrelated to epilepsy or other brain conditions. Eclampsia occurs every 1 in 2,000–3,000 pregnancies. Risks for developing this condition include first or multiple pregnancies; pregnancy after age 35; being of African American heritage; and a history of diabetes, hypertension, or renal disease. Eclampsia is a potentially life-threatening disorder characterized by hypertension, generalized edema, and proteinuria. It can put the woman and her fetus in grave danger and can be fatal if not treated. Preeclampsia is less severe. The symptoms are the same, except there are no convulsions. This is why weight is measured, blood pressure checked, and a urinalysis (including a check for protein) is routinely performed. Sudden significant weight gain, increase in blood pressure, and the presence of protein in the urine can indicate possible preeclampsia. The cause is unknown. Prophylaxis is of great importance. The problem is seen more often in women who have received inadequate prenatal care, especially poor nutrition; in **primigravidas** (pregnant for the first time) younger than 18 years; in women with preexisting cardiovascular and renal conditions; and in women who are diabetic.

Gestational Diabetes. Gestational diabetes first appears during the second or third trimester of the pregnancy and usually disappears after the woman has delivered her baby or when the pregnancy terminates for any other reason. Pregnancy hormones can block the action of insulin resulting in elevated blood glucose. This type of diabetes is usually a milder form of the disease. Prompt detection (through blood and urine glucose testing) and therapy are essential to avoid fetal and **neonatal** (newborn) illness and death. Factors that increase the risk of developing gestational diabetes are a family history of diabetes, pregnancy after age 25, or being overweight before pregnancy.

A blood glucose sample is drawn 1 hour after the patient is given a high-glucose drink. If the test result is elevated, then a 3-hour glucose tolerance test is done. The patient with gestational diabetes requires more frequent prenatal visits to the provider. The fetus is evaluated at each visit. Ultrasound evaluation of fetal growth is performed more often. The patient must control her diet and monitor blood glucose levels at home several times daily. A nutritionist will help by teaching the patient about a diabetic diet. The appropriate number of calories and percent of carbohydrates, proteins, and fats are calculated to keep the blood glucose as close to 100 mg/dL as possible. If the diabetic diet does not control blood glucose levels, insulin therapy is started. Usually the patient is admitted to the hospital if she has poorly controlled diabetes and has the additional factor of hypertension.

Pregnant women with gestational diabetes have a strong possibility of developing diabetes within their lifetime. The provider will order a blood glucose (1-hour glucose tolerance) when the woman is 6 to 8 weeks postpartum. The results will determine whether or not the patient's blood glucose level has dropped to the normal range.

Hyperemesis Gravidarum. Hyperemesis gravidarum, or excessive vomiting during pregnancy, can be harmful and is more than simply morning sickness, which is a common complaint during the first trimester. The cause of the condition is not known, but it is thought to be related to the cells that become the placenta and to the production of pregnancy hormones. The symptoms include uncontrollable nausea and vomiting, inability to eat, and exhaustion from inability to sleep. Severe dehydration can result and starvation may ensue. This complication is usually not fatal, but it is a severe problem that warrants immediate treatment. Treatment includes intravenous fluids to replace those lost through vomiting and mild sedation to aid rest and sleep.

Placenta Previa. Placenta previa occurs when the placenta implants low in the uterus and partially or completely covers the cervical os or opening of the uterus. It is an emergency. The cause is unknown. When labor ensues and the cervix begins to dilate, the placenta is pulled away from the wall of the uterus and causes bleeding. On occasion, the bleeding, which comes on suddenly and is painless, will stop spontaneously. If it continues, significant maternal blood is lost, and the fetus may suffer anoxia and die when the placenta separates from the blood supply (Figure 26-13B).

Ultrasonography can determine where the placenta is attached, at which time the diagnosis can be made and treatment begun. Treatment depends on the gestational age of the fetus and the percent of placenta that covers the cervical os. A Cesarean section may be necessary to remove the placenta, control bleeding, and deliver the fetus safely.

Some of the factors associated with placenta previa are advanced maternal age, maternal smoking, and cocaine use. Maternal exposure to passive smoke and use of tobacco by the mother have been shown to be risky to the fetus, resulting in lower birth weight, premature birth, and infant death.

Placenta Abruptio. **Placenta abruptio** occurs when the placenta prematurely and abruptly separates from the uterine lining (Figure 26-13A). It can result in fetal distress and death and maternal shock and death. It usually occurs late in pregnancy but can occur during labor.

Factors that contribute to this complication are multiple pregnancies, chronic hypertension, trauma to the uterus, and sudden release of amniotic fluid. Delivery as soon as possible either vaginally or by Cesarean section is indicated. The prognosis of the newborn depends on the extent of **hypoxia** suffered during labor and delivery.

The newborn infant should begin to cry and its color turn pink (hands and feet may remain blue for about a week). Abnormalities, if any, are documented. The Apgar score is an indication of the newborn's well-being. Assessments, in numbers from 1 to 10, are made at 1, 5, and 15 minutes. Five aspects of the newborn are evaluated: respiratory ease, heart rate, skin color, reflexes, and muscle tone. Each is assigned a number, which added together determines the newborn's Apgar score. The closer the score is to 10, the closer the newborn is adapting to life outside the uterus. A lower score indicates a problem with the newborn's respirations, heart rate, color, and muscle tone. Oxygen and other measures may be necessary to stabilize a newborn with a low Apgar score (Table 26-3).

Impaired Fertility. The inability to conceive and bear a child after a period of unprotected sex is known as impaired fertility. One reason for this problem is that couples delay pregnancy until later in life when fertility is naturally lower. The increase in the incidence of **pelvic inflammatory disease** (PID), endometriosis, substance abuse, and environmental factors such as pesticides and lead all can contribute to impaired fertility.

Diagnosis and treatment of impaired fertility requires a physical, emotional, and financial investment over a long period. To diagnose impaired fertility in the female patient, a complete history and physical examination are performed. Endocrine system and anatomic and physiologic abnormalities are sought. Laboratory tests on urine and blood are performed. Proof of ovulation can be determined by retrieving an ovum from the uterine tube, performing an endometrial biopsy, assessing mucus characteristics, and taking the basal body temperature. Levels of estrogen, progesterone, follicle-stimulating hormone, and luteinizing hormone are also measured. A **hysterosalpingogram**, a radiograph of the uterus and tubes after the

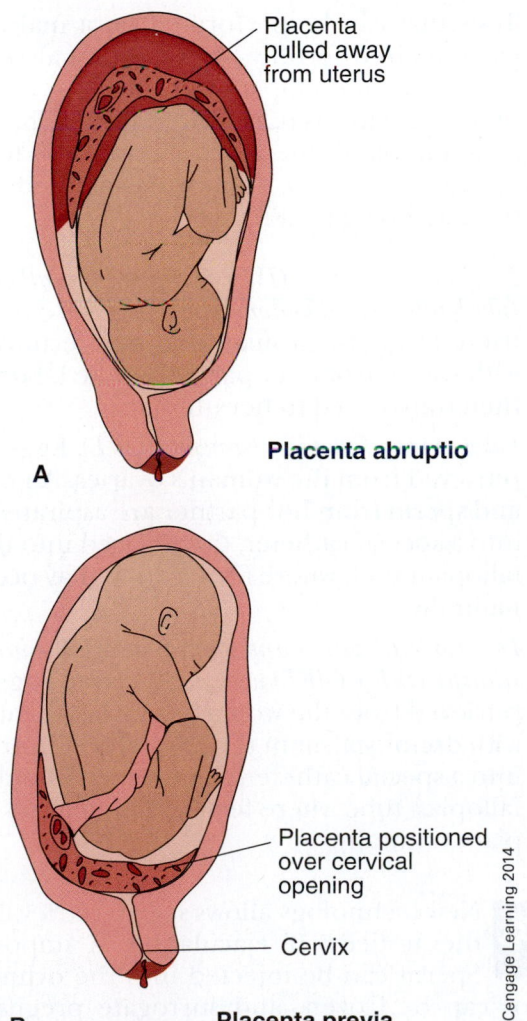

Placenta pulled away from uterus

A

Placenta abruptio

Placenta positioned over cervical opening

Cervix

B

Placenta previa

© Cengage Learning 2014

Figure 26-13   (A) Placenta abruptio. (B) Placenta previa.

Table 26-3 APGAR Score for Assessing Newborns

		APGAR Score		
		0	**1**	**2**
A	Activity	Limp; no movement	Some flexion of arms and legs	Active motion
P	Pulse	No heart rate	Fewer than 100 bpm	At least 100 bpm
G	Grimace	No response to airways being suctioned	Grimace during suctioning	Grimace, pull away, cough, or sneeze during suctioning
A	Appearance	Baby's entire body is bluish-gray or pale	Good body color; bluish hands or feet	Good color on body and extremities
R	Respiration	No respiration	Weak cry, whimpering, slow or irregular breathing	Strong cry and normal respiratory rate

© Cengage Learning 2014

PATIENT EDUCATION

Alcohol Exposure

Alcohol along with tobacco exposure during pregnancy is common. Drinking during pregnancy is the leading cause of childhood mental retardation. Two or more drinks a day while a woman is pregnant increases the risk of the newborn being born with fetal alcohol syndrome (FAS). Birth defects include small brain size; growth retardation; specific facial deformities (e.g., flat middle of the face, wide bridge of the nose, thin upper lip); and heart, kidney, and eye abnormalities. Behavioral problems (e.g., learning and attention difficulties, hyperactivity) occur. No safe amount of alcohol can be consumed during pregnancy, so abstention from all alcohol is necessary.

injection of dye, reveals defects in either the uterus or tubes.

Laparoscopy can be performed to visualize the internal pelvic structures. Tubal patency, **endometriosis**, pelvic adhesions, or **polycystic** ovaries can be seen. Endometrial biopsy is done to examine the tissue and determine whether the endometrium is capable of accepting a fertilized ovum for implantation. Ultrasonography, either abdominal or transvaginal, can assess pelvic organs for abnormalities.

Tests that can be performed on a male to diagnose impaired fertility are semen analysis, hormone analysis, and biopsy of a testicle.

Once a diagnosis of impaired fertility has been made, a number of therapies are available to assist in reproduction. This is known as assisted reproductive technology (ART).

- *In vitro fertilization (IVF), indicated for fallopian tube blockage and endometriosis.* Eggs are retrieved from the woman's ovaries, fertilized with sperm from her partner in the laboratory, then transferred to her uterus.

- *Gamete intrafallopian transfer (GIFT).* Eggs are retrieved from the woman's ovaries. An egg and sperm from her partner are aspirated into a special catheter, then placed into the fallopian tube where fertilization may occur naturally.

- *In vitro fertilization and gamete intrafallopian transfer (IVF + GIFT) with donor sperm.* Eggs are retrieved from the woman's ovaries, fertilized with donor sperm in the laboratory, aspirated into a special catheter, then placed into the fallopian tube where fertilization may take place naturally.

New technology allows sperm retrieval from the testicles if ejaculation is impossible. Sperm can be injected into the ovum, embryos can be frozen, and surrogate pregnancies are possible. With technology come the ethical and legal questions of donor eggs and embryos, pregnancies in older adult women, how to define who the parents are, what to do with frozen embryos after death or divorce, and other issues such as disposal of unused (extra) embryos.

In some cultures, a woman is deemed the responsible party for impaired fertility, and the impairment is thought to be caused by her sins, evil spirits, or her own deficiencies. The virility of a male is questioned unless he is able to manifest his sexual potency by having a child.

Incompatibility. The pregnant woman's blood type and Rh factor are determined at the first prenatal visit. If the woman has Rh-negative blood and the fetus has Rh-positive blood, which will happen if the father of the baby is Rh-positive, problems can occur. When the fetus's blood (red blood cells) leaks into the woman's body during birth, an Rh-negative woman may develop antibodies against the fetus's Rh-positive blood. As it takes time for these antibodies to develop, firstborn infants are not usually affected unless the mother has had previous pregnancies that ended in abortion or miscarriage. The antibodies can pass through the placenta and kill the RBCs in the fetus. The fetus becomes anemic and jaundiced. Death of the fetus is possible if too much fetal blood is destroyed. When an injection of Rh-immune globulin (RhoGAM) is given at around the 28th week of pregnancy and 72 hours postpartum, and after percutaneous umbilical blood sampling (PUBS), CVS, abortion, or amniocentesis, then sensitization is prevented. Rh incompatibility should not occur with any subsequent pregnancy. RhoGAM must be given after every birth, abortion, miscarriage, amniocentesis, CVS, and PUBS to prevent sensitization.

Parturition

Parturition, or labor, is the process during which the uterus, through contractions, expels the fetus and placenta. There are three stages of labor:

- *Stage I—Dilation.* from onset of labor until complete **dilation** (expansion) and **effacement** (thinning and shortening) of cervix

- *Stage II—Expulsion.* from complete dilation and effacement through the birth of fetus (expulsion)

- *Stage III—Placental.* from birth of fetus through expulsion of the placenta

Labor is believed to be triggered by the release of **oxytocin** and **prostaglandins** after the level of other hormones decreases. When the oxytocin is released, it causes the muscles of the uterus to contract. **Braxton–Hicks** contractions, often referred to as false labor, can usually be differentiated from real labor because of their irregularity and tendency to disappear when the woman moves about and changes positions. When the woman is lying in supine position, the heavy, large uterus can press on the inferior vena cava and aorta, reducing blood flow back to the heart. The patient becomes pale, sweaty, and dizzy, and blood pressure drops. The condition is known as **supine hypotension**. When the patient is turned onto her side, the pressure on the vena cava is removed and the hypotension resolves.

If fetal membranes do not spontaneously rupture during labor, an **amniotomy** (artificial rupture of the membranes) can be done. The procedure uses a sterile amniohook, and it may shorten the length of labor (Figure 26-14).

Signs and symptoms to watch for during labor that indicate complications are heavy vaginal bleeding, sudden increase or decrease in blood

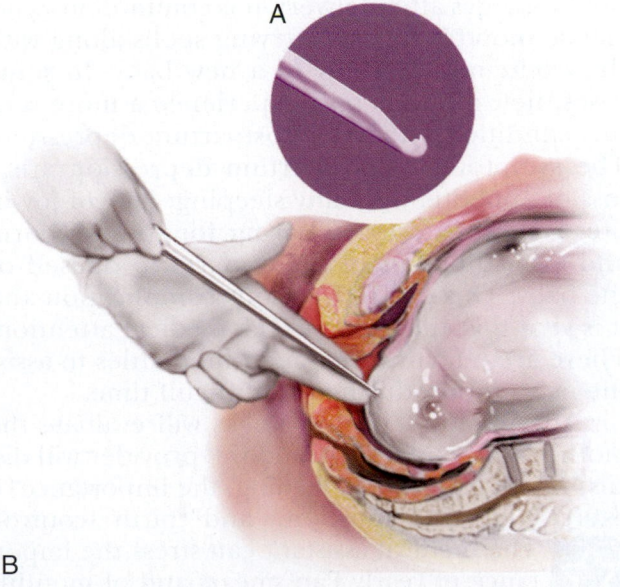

A

B

© Cengage Learning 2014

Figure 26-14 (A) Disposable amniohook used to rupture membranes. (B) Amniotomy technique.

CRITICAL THINKING

A 17-year-old girl has missed her period and has called the clinic describing sharp right quadrant pain. What tests/procedures will help the provider make a diagnosis?

pressure, increased activity by the fetus, headache, extreme restlessness, and visual changes. **Meconium**, the first stool of the newborn, in the vaginal discharge can indicate fetal distress. Care must be taken to assure that the newborn does not aspirate meconium-stained amniotic fluid at birth.

Postpartum Period

The postpartum period is the time known as the puerperium during which the body returns to its nonpregnant state. It is usually 4 to 6 weeks after delivery. The body undergoes changes during this time. The uterus involutes (returns to normal size) and healing of any injuries takes place.

A vaginal discharge, known as **lochia**, appears during the puerperium. It consists of tissue, blood, white blood cells, mucus, and bacteria. It can be described by its appearance. Lochia rubra is bright red and appears the first 3 days after delivery. Lochia serosa is pink or brown and is indicative of less blood. By about 10 days, the flow decreases, becomes whitish-yellow, and is known as lochia alba. Lochia usually disappears by the third week postpartum but may last for up to 6 weeks. Menstruation usually begins in a nursing mother 3 to 6 months after delivery and in nonnursing mothers 2 months after delivery. The mother is told to avoid heavy lifting, not to become fatigued, to eat a well-balanced diet, and to continue to take her prenatal tablets. She is also told to report any feelings of depression as soon as possible. With the rapid shift of hormones and body changes after delivery, it is common to experience mood swings and crying spells along with the excitement and joy of a new baby. In some cases, new mothers may experience a more serious condition known as postpartum depression. The symptoms of postpartum depression are a loss of appetite, difficulty sleeping, lack of joy in life, lack of interest in caring for the newborn, and even thoughts of doing harm to oneself or the baby. This can be a serious complication and it is vital that the mother seek medical attention. There are effective treatment modalities to assist the new mother during this difficult time.

An appointment in 6 weeks will evaluate the mother's general health, and the provider will discuss infant care, breast-feeding, the importance of exercise, good nutrition, and birth control. The medical assistant can stress the importance of yearly Pap smears and of monthly breast self-examinations because these are important aspects of patient education.

Contraception

Voluntary prevention of pregnancy is known as **contraception**. The opportune time to discuss contraception with the mother is soon after delivery and before discharge from the hospital. She should know what method of contraception she and her partner will use before resuming sexual activity. To discuss contraception at the 6-week postpartum checkup can be too late. Sexually transmitted disease (STD) protection should also be reviewed before discharge.

Written instructions about methods of contraception are important and help the patient understand options that are available.

Some nonprescription kinds of contraception are the various barrier methods: condoms, male (latex) and female (nonlatex); contraceptive foam; spermicide (nonoxynol-9) used with a condom to help prevent STDs; vaginal sponges that contain a spermicide; and abstinence.

Many types of prescription contraceptives are available (see Figure 26-15 through Figure 26-19 and Table 26-4). They include hormonal contraception in the form of oral birth control pills; Implanon®, a surgical implant of progestin in the upper arm, which provides up to 3 years of contraception (see Procedure 26-4); a diaphragm used with a spermicide; a cervical cap to fit over the cervix; an intrauterine device (a small device made of copper or progesterone-medicated plastic; see Procedure 26-3); and vaginal rings. The hormonal contraception methods work by changing the complex network of hormonal interactions that allow an ovum to leave the ovary and cause changes in the cervical mucus that allows sperm to enter the cervix. There are also changes that make the lining of the uterus unwelcoming for the implantation.

Sterilization is a surgical procedure that renders the individual infertile. The woman's uterine tubes are **fulgurated** (destroyed by means of an electric current) or bands and clips are placed around the tubes to block them (ligation). Both fulguration and ligation are considered to be permanent methods. Female sterilization can be performed immediately after giving birth or any time afterward during any phase of the menstrual cycle. Laparoscopic surgery is the usual approach. Tubal ligation and oral contraceptives are the top contraceptive choices in the United States (Figure 26-20).

The surgical procedure performed on a male to render him sterile is a vasectomy. It can be performed on an outpatient basis under local anesthesia. Small incisions are made into the scrotum above and to the

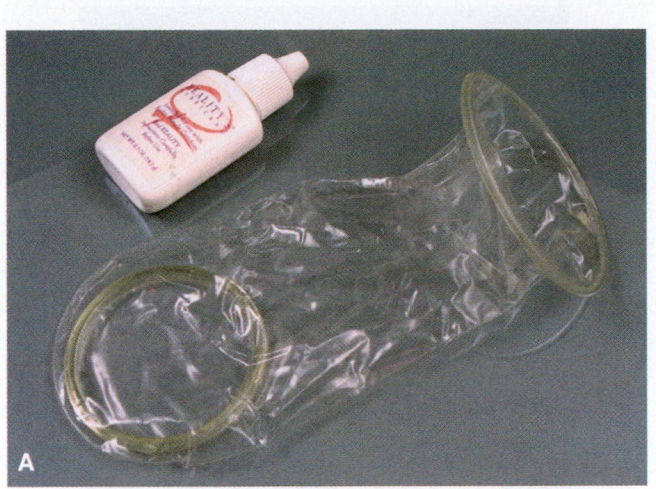

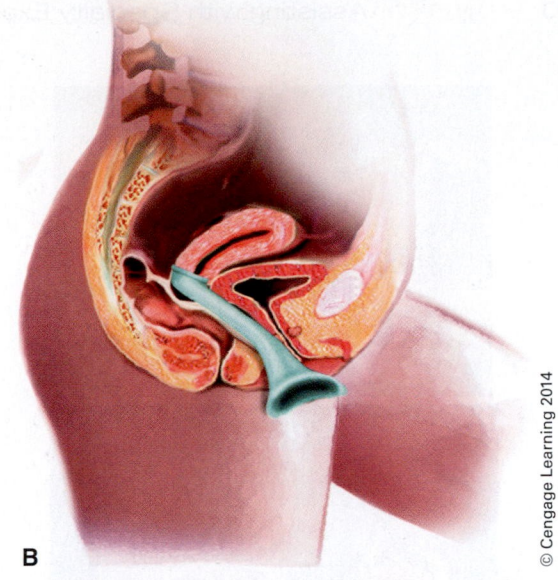

A   **B**   © Cengage Learning 2014

Figure 26-15   (A) Female condom. (B) Proper insertion of female condom.

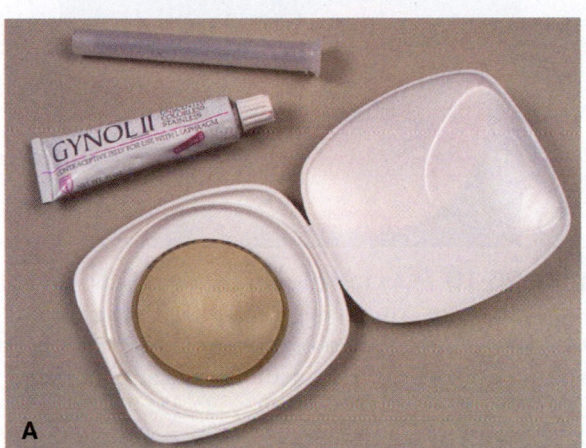

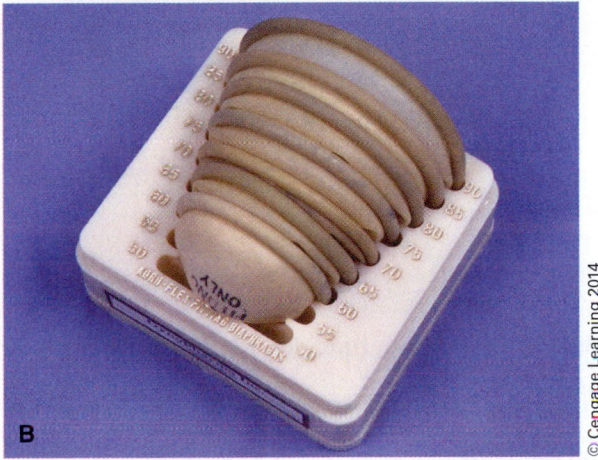

A   **B**   © Cengage Learning 2014

Figure 26-16   (A) Diaphragm with contraceptive jelly. (B) Various sizes of diaphragms. They must be fitted by the provider.

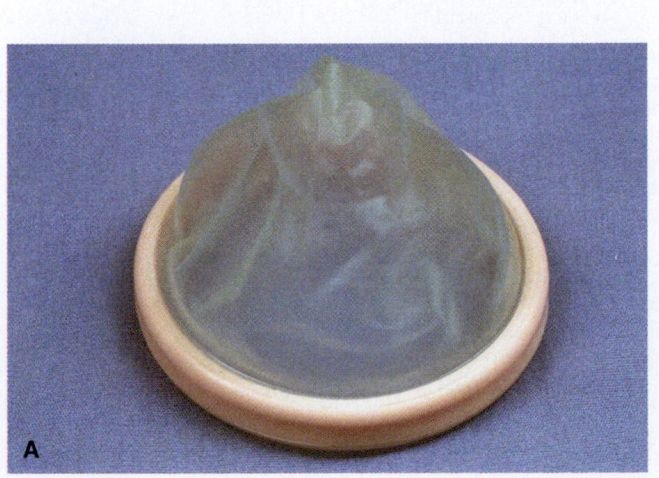

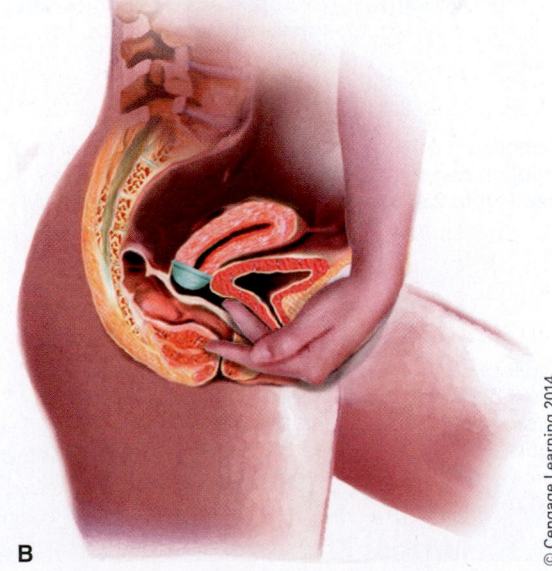

A   **B**   © Cengage Learning 2014

Figure 26-17   (A) Cervical cap. (B) Proper insertion of cervical cap.

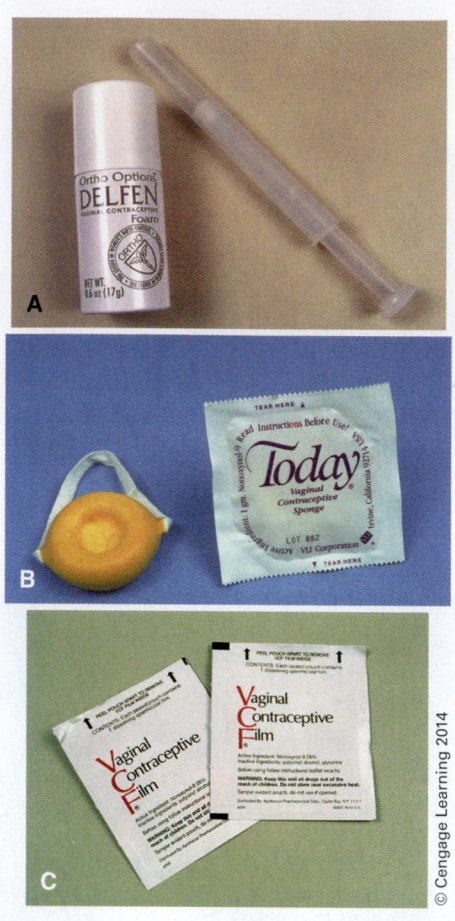

Figure 26-18 Spermicides. (A) Foam. (B) Sponge. (C) Film.

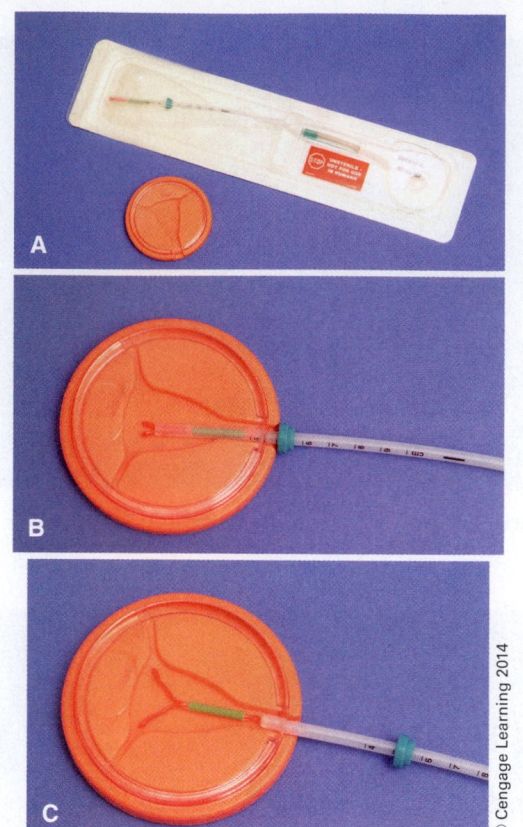

Figure 26-19 (A) Intrauterine device (IUD) and plastic uterus for patient education. (B, C) A plastic uterus can be used to demonstrate proper insertion and placement of IUD during a patient education session.

Table 26-4 Various Contraception (Birth Control) Methods

Method	Description	Effectiveness	Mechanism of Action
Barrier (over-the-counter condom) (see Figure 26-15)	Male and female condoms available. Male condoms are latex; female condoms are nonlatex.	Less effective than hormonal methods or IUD. Use with spermicide. Use to protect from STDs.	Inhibits sperm from entering the vagina. Used only once. To prevent STD and pregnancy, use a condom and another method of contraception.
Diaphragm (prescription needed) (see Figure 26-16)	Use with spermicide. Must be measured and fitted by provider. Fits up against the cervical opening so that cervix is within the cap.	Moderately effective if used correctly. Must fit perfectly. Spermicide is placed inside and around the diaphragm. Must remain in place for 6 hours after intercourse. Will last for years if cared for properly.	Provides barrier between sperm and opening to cervix.
Cervical cap (must be fitted by provider) (see Figure 26-17)	Made of rubber. Fitted to cover the cervix. Folded to insert into the vagina. Must be applied to cervix. Suction keeps the cap in place. Use with spermicide.	Moderately effective if used correctly, similar to diaphragm. Potential for infection because cap can be left in place up to 2 days. Must remain at least 6 hours after intercourse.	Provides rubber barrier between sperm and opening to cervix.

Table 26-4   Various Contraception (Birth Control) Methods (*Continued*)

Method	Description	Effectiveness	Mechanism of Action
Spermicide sponge foam cream/gel (over the counter) (see Figure 26-18)	Chemical known as nonoxynol-9.	When used alone, failure rate is high compared to other methods. Used with condom, diaphragm, or cervical cap, it is more effective. No bathing or douching for 6 hours after intercourse. Must allow 15 minutes before engaging in intercourse. Reapply spermicide with repeated intercourse.	Destroys sperm cells.
Hormonal pills (prescription needed for all hormonal contraceptives)	Various combinations of estrogen and progestin or progestin only.	Highest effectiveness rate when taken correctly. Can help reduce dysmenorrheal and heavy menses.	Prevents ovulation every month.
Injection	Intramuscular injection (Depo-Provera®) every 3 months. Lunelle®, injected once per month.	Highly effective. One of the most effective contraceptives. Best given within first 5 days of menstrual period to be sure patient is not pregnant.	Prevents ovulation for 3 months. Stops ovulation for 1 month.
Patch	Applied to body and contraceptive is absorbed through the skin.	Highly effective. Worn for 1 week and then replaced same day of week for 3 consecutive weeks. Fourth week patch free.	Prevents ovulation for 1 month.
Vaginal ring	Small flexible ring inserted into the vagina. Releases steady flow of hormones. Left in for 3 weeks. Removed for 1 week.	Highly effective.	Prevents ovulation.
Lybrel* Seasonique*	Continuous contraception. No menstrual cycles for indefinite time period. Breakthrough bleeding possible. Continuous contraception for 3 months.	Effective. Highly effective.	Prevents ovulation. Reduces mood swings, migraines, and premenstrual syndrome (PMS). Prevents ovulation for 3 months.
Intrauterine device (IUD) (must be inserted by provider) (see Figure 26-19; Procedure 26-3).	T-shaped device made of copper. Good for 10 years. A second T-shaped device good for 1 year. Mirena® is an IUD that releases hormones. Remains in place for 5 years. To prevent STDs, IUDs should be used in conjunction with a condom.	Both highly effective. One of the most effective contraceptives.	Copper slowly released into uterus and kills sperm. Hormones in Mirena® cause thickening of the mucus in the cervix, so sperm cannot reach the ovum.
Implantable (must be implanted by provider)	Device known as Implanon® is composed of one rod that is implanted. Lasts up to 3 years. Minor surgical procedure is required to implant and remove. Essure® is a spring-like device implanted in fallopian tubes via the cervix.	Highly effective. One of the most effective contraceptives. Becomes more effective as scar tissue grows thicker. Use another form of contraceptive for at least 3 months after implantation.	Inhibits ovulation and changes the cervical and endometrial mucus. Implanted device causes scar tissue to build up within the fallopian tubes, eventually blocking them. When blocked, neither sperm nor ovum can pass through.

continues

Table 26-4   Various Contraception (Birth Control) Methods (*Continued*)

Method	Description	Effectiveness	Mechanism of Action
Tubal ligation or hysterectomy (permanent method) (performed when the woman has a gynecologic problem that requires surgery and she wants permanent sterilization)	Sterilization procedure performed in which the fallopian tubes are tied or bands and/or clips are placed around the tubes to block them (ligation). The tubes can also be burned with electrocautery. Hysterectomy is the surgical removal of the uterus.	Considered permanent, but there is a small failure rate. Permanent sterilization.	Fallopian tubes are severed and/or burned, banded, and/or clipped. Because fallopian tubes now are incapable of transporting either sperm or ovum, fertilization is not possible. Uterus is surgically removed.
Family planning	Ovulation prediction (rhythm method). The woman charts her temperature and her changes in vaginal mucus and abstains from intercourse during the time she is ovulating (as predicted by temperature and mucus changes).	Can be effective if done correctly. However, method must be used consistently and the woman must realize that she may ovulate on a different day each month or at another time.	Prevents conception by avoiding intercourse during the period of ovulation.
Emergency contraception (postcoital contraception) also called Preven® or Plan B (over the counter for age 18 and over, prescription if under 18)	Prevents unintended pregnancy when the woman has had unprotected sexual intercourse. Prevents unwanted pregnancy. Pills (known as "morning after pills") that contain birth control hormones can be taken as soon after unprotected sex as possible and up to 5 days after and still prevent pregnancy. Take a second dose 12 hours after the first dose. Will not interrupt an established pregnancy and will not harm the embryo. No prescription needed.	Very effective.	Not the same as RU-486, an abortion pill. Prevents ovulation or stops fertilization.
IUD made of copper, and the copper helps kill sperm (Mirena® IUD cannot be used as an emergency contraceptive)		Very effective.	Kills sperm or prevents ovum fertilization.

*Newest oral contraceptives called extended hormonal contraceptives

© Cengage Learning 2014

side of each testicle. Each vas deferens is identified, ligated twice, and then severed (Figure 26-21). It is important for the patient to realize that sterility is not immediate because some sperm remain in the sperm ducts after vasectomy. One week to several months may elapse before the ducts are sperm free. Some form of contraception is necessary until two consecutive sperm counts are zero.

Another method of contraception approved by the Food and Drug Administration (FDA) is a medication known as RU-486, which is used to cause or induce an abortion. Its safety has been

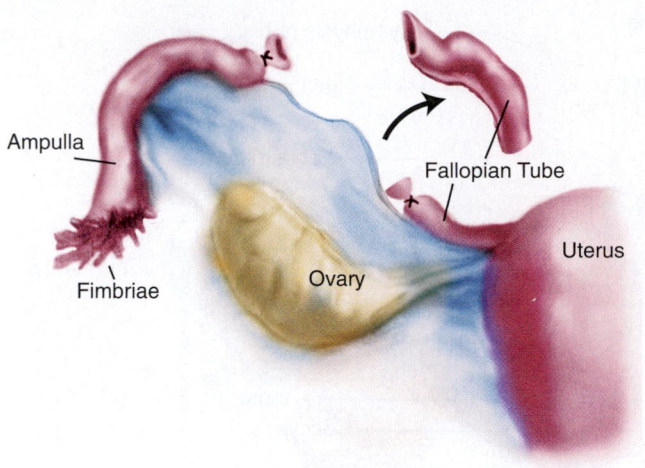

Figure 26-20   Tubal ligation.

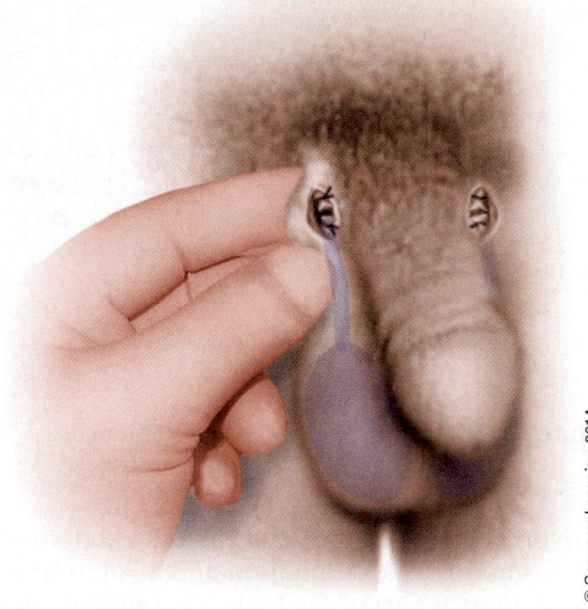

Figure 26-21   Vasectomy.

questioned by experts. Injectable contraceptives are available. Depo-Provera® is given intramuscularly every 3 months. Lunelle® is given intramuscularly monthly. These injectables are best given within the first 5 days of the menstrual cycle to be certain the woman is not pregnant.

The majority of states mandate that health insurance cover the cost of contraception. The Affordable Care Act that was signed into law in March 2010 with the intent of making prevention affordable and accessible for all Americans requires health plans to cover preventative services and eliminate cost sharing. Contraceptive methods and counseling are covered under Health Resources and Services Administration Supported Women's Preventative Services: Required Health Plan Coverage Guidelines. All Food and Drug Administration approved contraceptive methods,

sterilization procedures, and patient education and counseling for all women with reproductive capacity are covered. There is an exception for group health plans sponsored by certain religious employers, and group health coverage in conjunction with such plans are exempt from the requirement to cover contraceptive services.

GYNECOLOGY

Gynecology is the specialty that studies diseases of the female reproductive tract and the breasts. The gynecologic examination is routinely performed

PATIENT EDUCATION

Post IUD Insertion

1. Report any bleeding other than spotting that occurs in the first 2 days.
2. Report fever, vaginal discharge, or pain at once.
3. A small percentage of IUDs are expelled from the uterus into the vagina during the first year. Another contraceptive should be used to prevent pregnancy.
4. There is a risk of perforation of the uterus, but this is most likely to occur during insertion.
5. An IUD does not protect against STDs.

6. Some women experience headaches, breast tenderness, and mood swings. These symptoms usually subside in a few months.
7. It is possible (but rare) to become pregnant with an IUD. It is recommended in this situation that the IUD be removed because it can cause miscarriage or premature birth.
8. The IUD can remain in place for as long as 10 years depending on the type.
9. An IUD must be removed by the provider.
10. An IUD is safe and highly effective.

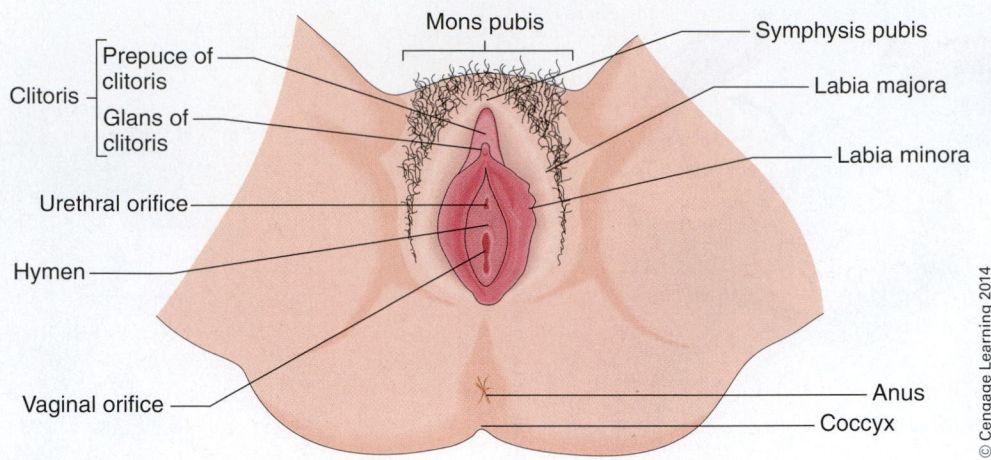

Figure 26-22 External genitalia of the female.

in an office or clinic. It usually includes abdominal, pelvic, and breast examination and a Pap smear. It can be done as part of the female's complete physical examination, or it can be a separate examination performed in the gynecologist's office or gynecology clinic. Early diagnosis and treatment of problems associated with the female reproductive organs help the female to achieve optimum health of these organs and is the goal of the OB/GYN provider (Figure 26-22).

The Gynecologic Examination

It is recommended that a gynecologic examination be done annually on all women beginning when they become sexually active or by age 21 years. It is done to assess the female's health and to screen for cancer of the reproductive organs. It includes a breast examination by the provider and instructions for the patient about how to perform her own **breast self-examination (BSE)**. It also includes a pelvic examination and Pap smear. Pap tests are done to detect cervical cancer. Women should be especially conscientious in scheduling annual Pap tests and mammograms if they have a family history of breast, uterine, ovarian, or cervical cancer. Early detection of cervical and breast cancers and appropriate treatment may cure the disease. Women who have had a hysterectomy because of cancer should continue to be tested for pelvic cancer annually by having a Pap smear. Because the cervix has been removed, the specimen cells are taken from the inner vaginal vault instead. Even after the hysterectomy, the woman still remains at risk for cancer cells to grow within the vagina and she should be encouraged to continue with her

regular pelvic examinations and Pap tests. Others believe that in healthy women a Pap test done every 1 to 3 years is sufficient. The American Cancer Society (ACS) recommends that all women have a **Pap (Papanicolaou) test** about every 3 years, beginning after they become sexually active, or at age 21 years, whichever is sooner; then testing should be done every year with the regular (conventional) Pap test or every 2 years with the newer liquid-based Pap test (e.g., ThinPrep®).

Further, the ACS recommends that at age 30 women who have had three sequential normal Pap tests be tested every 2 to 3 years with either the conventional Pap test or with the liquid-based Pap test and also be tested for human papillomavirus (HPV) DNA.

Women 70 years or older who have had three sequential negative Pap tests in 10 years can stop cervical cancer testing.

Women with a history of cervical cancer, DES exposure before birth, HIV infection, or a weak immune system should continue testing. Risk factors for cervical cancer are first sexual intercourse at an early age, multiple sex partners, sex with partners who have multiple partners, and a history of HPV.

Encourage patients to have regular Pap tests. Women at high risk should have a Pap test and a mammogram according to their provider's recommendations. If the patient is experiencing a vaginal discharge and there is a suspicion of a vaginal infection, smear(s) and cultures of discharge can be done to aid in diagnosis. (Chapter 43 provides more information.)

The American College of Obstetricians and Gynecologists established new guidelines for mammography in July 2011. These guidelines state that women should be offered a screening mammogram annually. Breast magnetic imagining screening is recommended for women at increased risk for breast cancer. This is indicated for women who test positive for the breast cancer type 1 susceptibility protein (*BRCA1*) or breast cancer type 2 susceptibility protein (*BRCA2*) mutations. *BRCA1* and *BRCA2* are human genes that are known as tumor suppressors. When a woman tests positive for this mutation, she is at increased risk for breast and ovarian cancer.

Human Papillomavirus (HPV) and Gardasil®.

There are more than 40 types of HPV that can infect sexually active males and females. Statistics reported by the CDC in march indicates that 50% of sexually active people will contract genital HPV in their lifetime. With these alarming statistics, in June 2006, the FDA approved a vaccine that targets the virus responsible for most cervical cancers and condylomata (genital warts). The vaccine, called Gardasil, protects against four HPVs. According to an article on women's health on Web MD Medical News, two of the four viruses are responsible for 70% of all cervical cancers. The other two viruses are responsible for 90% of condylomata. Gardasil was approved to help prevent vaginal and vulvar cancers, which can be caused by HPV.

HPV is spread through sexual contact. According to the CDC, by age 50 years, at least 80% of women will have had an HPV infection. However, most women with HPV do not get cervical cancer. Gardasil is 100% effective in protecting against two of the HPV strains if the individual has not been exposed to the virus previously. The vaccine will not protect people already exposed to the virus. The vaccine does not contain a live virus. It lasts for at least 5 years. The FDA approved Gardasil for girls and women aged 9 to 26 years. It is on the CDC's recommended vaccine schedule. Screening for cervical cancer (as with the Pap test) still is necessary because Gardasil does not protect against all HPV types. Pap tests also are essential for women who have not been vaccinated or who already are infected with HPV. The vaccine is not recommended during pregnancy.

The Advisory Committee on Immunization Practices (ACIP) recommends that preteen males and females 11 to 12 years of age be immunized with three doses of HPV vaccines, but the series can be started as early as age 9. The second and third doses should be given 2 and 6 months after the first dose. The immunization is most effective if administered prior to any sexual activity, thus the early administration recommendation.

CRITICAL THINKING

A 38-year-old woman has been diagnosed with HPV infection. What patient education materials are appropriate to provide this patient?

HPV vaccines can be administered with other age-appropriate vaccines. Catch-up vaccinations are available for females 13 to 26 years of age who have not been vaccinated previously or who have not completed the full series. The vaccine is licensed only for females 9 to 26 years of age. Each dose is 0.5 mL given intramuscularly.

Scheduling Pap Smear Tests.

Encourage female patients to schedule their Pap smear and annual gynecologic examination on a date that will be easy to remember, such as April Fool's Day, Flag Day, tax day, or the first day of summer. Keep a tickler file to remind patients who "forget." Women may believe that because they have had a hysterectomy, they no longer need their annual examination and Pap smear. Every woman should have an annual (or regular) examination even if the Pap test is not included. A woman who has had a hysterectomy because of cancer should continue to have Pap smears on a regular basis. Many women are not aware of this and need to be educated.

Other gynecologic problems may arise between annual gynecologic examinations and require an appointment. They include symptoms and problems such as severe **dysmenorrhea** (painful menses), lower abdominal pain, **metrorrhagia** (bleeding between menstrual periods), **dyspareunia** (painful intercourse), sexual dysfunction, infertility, discomfort from menstrual symptoms, and infections or the development of STDs. Women experiencing these problems should have a gynecologic examination, and the provider will determine a diagnosis based on the examination, the patient's history, symptoms, signs, and laboratory data. The data from previous appointments are available to the provider via the computer. Comparisons can be made quickly with previous entries, saving time and possibly preventing errors.

It is important to realize that patients' health practices related to culture, values, and belief systems are deeply ingrained and not easily changed. Being aware of some of these practices and beliefs will benefit both you and your patients. You will have a better understanding of their cultural heritage and beliefs that are different from yours, and this will help patients to be more comfortable. At times, it might be necessary to modify care according to the patient's cultural background and practice.

Female Circumcision.
Female circumcision is an ancient cultural custom that has been practiced worldwide for more than 2,000 years. Between 100 and 130 million women in 40 countries have had female circumcisions. Central Africa is one of the main areas where various forms of the procedure are performed. These procedures are performed on females from birth to puberty.

There are four different types of female circumcision: (1) removal of the prepuce of the clitoris; (2) clitoridectomy, removal of prepuce and clitoris; (3) removal of prepuce, clitoris, upper labia minora, and some labia majora; and (4) infibulation, removal of all external genitalia (prepuce, clitoris, labia majora, labia minora). Also known as Female Genital Mutilation (FGM), the World Health Organization defines it as "all procedures that involve partial or total removal of the external female genitalia, or other injury to female genital organs for non-medical reasons." Some reasons given for this practice are that it is a rite of passage, a sign of purity, marriage availability, sexual faithfulness, protection from rape and abortion, and that it is for socialization into the role of a woman. Surgery is usually performed by a lay midwife, and a razor or broken glass is used; infections and hemorrhages are common. If an infibulation is performed, the two sides of the vulva are sewn together. Scar tissue forms over the vagina. A small opening for urination and menstruation is made by inserting a foreign object until the area heals. The most common reason given for this procedure is that it follows customs and tradition. During childbirth, the infibulation is cut to allow for delivery, then resutured after delivery.

 There is opposition to this practice on the basis that it is a human rights violation. However, it is vital that a professional medical assistant always view patients as individuals whose cultural beliefs and practices may differ greatly from your own. Treat them as you would treat all patients, with respect and empathy (see Chapters 27 and 28 for male circumcision).

Breast Examination.
The provider performs a breast examination on the patient as part of a gynecologic examination. As the provider looks for redness, dimpling, and puckering, each breast is palpated and the axillae are felt for lumps or thickening. Part of the medical assistant's responsibility is to teach patients how to perform the breast self-examination (BSE). Figure 26-23 provides illustrations for performing the BSE. The provider may supply several pamphlets and a breast model with lumps and thickening for enhancing patient education and awareness about the importance of the examination (Figure 26-24A and Figure 26-24B).

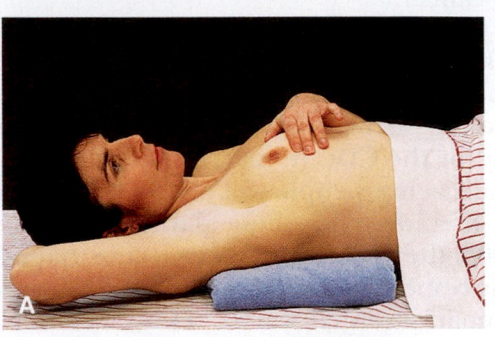

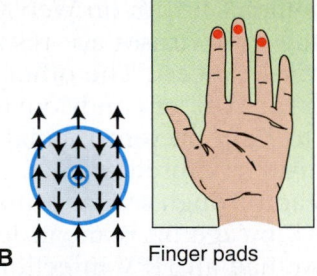

Finger pads

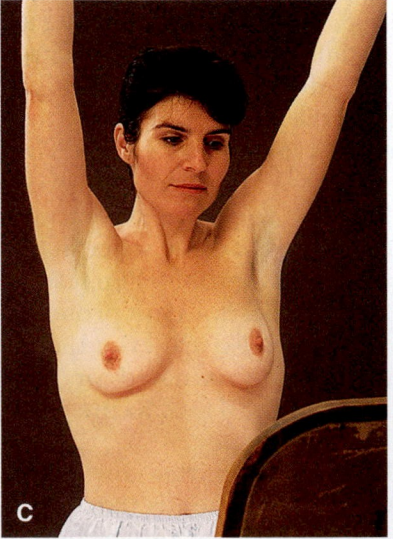

© Cengage Learning 2014

Figure 26-23 Breast self-examination. (A) Lie on your back and put your right arm behind your head. (B) Use the finger pads of your three middle fingers, making up and down pattern to examine the breast. (C) Look in a mirror and observe the breasts for abnormalities.

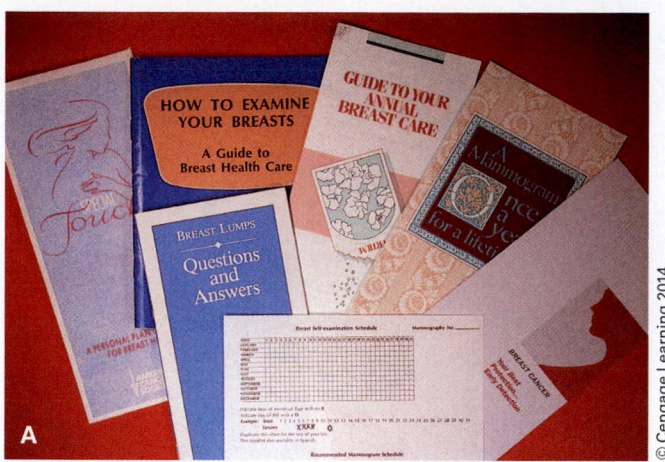

Figure 26-24A Informational pamphlets detailing the breast self-examination and its importance can be helpful to patients.

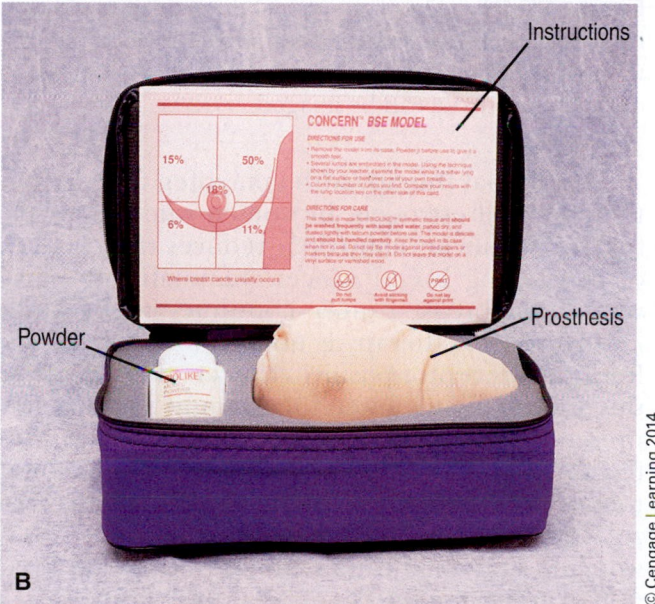

Figure 26-24B Breast self-examination model kit contains instructions for breast self-examination and powder to aid fingers in gliding over the breast prosthesis contains lumps and thickened areas for identification and location.

Breast Self-Examination (BSE). Provide the patient with these steps to follow:

1. Examine your breasts when they are not tender or swollen and at the same time each month, about 1 week after menses.
2. Women who are breast-feeding or pregnant or have breast implants can do a BSE.

3. Ask the medical assistant to review your technique when you have your yearly examination.
4. Lie on your back and put your right arm behind your head. This spreads out the breast tissue, making it easier to feel all of the tissue (Figure 26-23A).
5. Using your left hand and the finger pads of the three middle fingers (Figure 26-23B), feel for lumps or abnormalities in your right breast.
6. Use three degrees of pressure—light, medium, and strong (or firm)—to feel all of the tissue. Light pressure is used for skin and tissue just beneath the surface, and medium pressure is used for tissue in the middle of the breasts, strong pressure is used to feel the tissue closest to the ribs and chest. Use all three degrees of pressure on each spot on your breast before feeling another spot.
7. Use an up-and-down pattern as you move around the breast, starting at your imaginary seam line (straight down from the underarm) and moving up and down to the middle of the chest bone. Be certain you have examined your entire breast, from the collar bone to the ribs.
8. Do the same examination on your left breast, starting with step 4.
9. Looking in a mirror with hands pressing down on your hips, check your breasts for redness; dimpling; and change in shape, size, or contour (Figure 26-23C).
10. Examine each underarm while sitting or standing while your arm is raised slightly so that the area is easily felt.
11. If any of the following are detected, alert your provider immediately:
    - Lump, hard knot, or thickening inside the breast or underarm area
    - Swelling, warmth, redness, or darkening of the breast
    - Change in the size or shape of the breast
    - Dimpling or puckering of the skin
    - Itchy, scaly sore or rash on the nipple
    - Pulling in of your nipple or other parts of the breast
    - Nipple discharge that starts suddenly
    - New pain in one spot that doesn't go away

According to the ACS, breast cancer is the second leading cause of death in women in the United States; the leading cause of death in women is lung cancer.

Diagnosis of breast cancer is made by the provider using some or all of the following diagnostic tools: mammography, tissue biopsy, MRI, ultrasound, and MRI-guided breast biopsies.

The ACS recommends that women without symptoms of breast cancer aged 40 to 49 years have a mammogram every 1 to 2 years, and women aged 50 years and older, once a year (Figure 26-25 and Figure 26-26).

The American College of Obstetricians and Gynecologists (ACOG) endorses the guidelines set forth by the ACS.

Breast cancer risk factors include:

- A family history of breast cancer
- Being female (males can get breast cancer, but there is much less chance)
- A biopsy of a breast lesion that showed atypical hyperplasia
- Early menarche (younger than 12 years)
- Late menopause (after 55 years)
- No children, or first child after 30 years of age
- More than 2 to 5 alcoholic drinks per week
- BRCA1 and BRCA2 gene mutations

The four standard treatment options for patients with breast cancer are surgery, radiation therapy, chemotherapy, and hormone therapy.

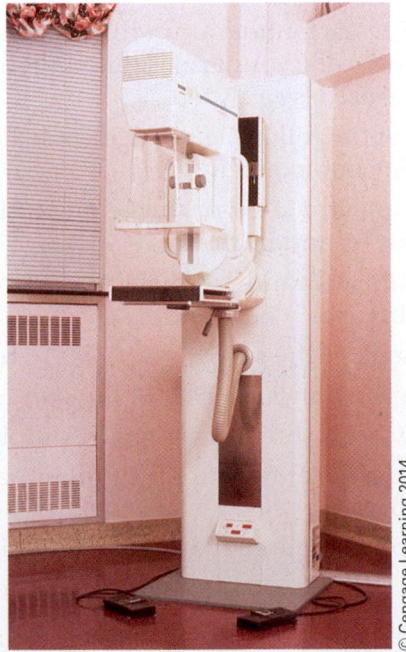

Figure 26-25 Breasts are compressed by the plates of mammographic X-ray unit.

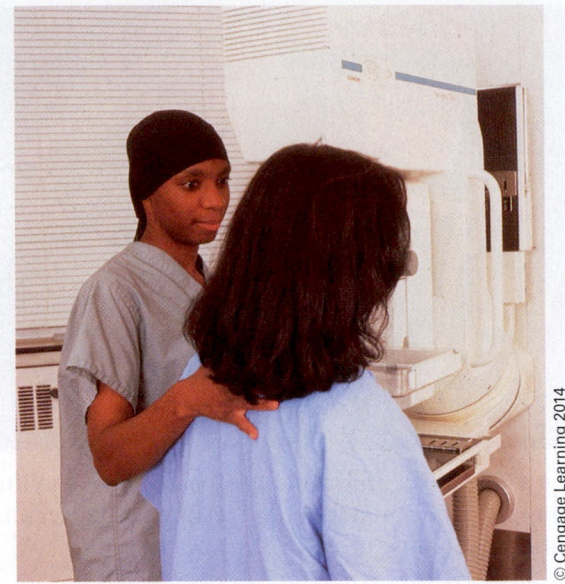

Figure 26-26 The technologist positions the patient for mammography. The procedure requires the patient to move into various positions so that different angles of the breast tissue can be imaged.

Hormonal therapy with tamoxifen acts against the effects of estrogen. In women who are at risk for breast cancer, tamoxifen reduces the chances of developing breast cancer. Tamoxifen for prevention of breast cancer continues to be studied. Hormonal therapy is utilized for people with hormonal-receptor-positive cancer. The goal of this therapy is to lower the amount of estrogen present in the body and to block the estrogen effect on the cancer cells. Another type of hormonal therapy with aromatase inhibitors, such as anastrozole, is particularly beneficial for post-menopausal women. This medication blocks the transformation of androgen into small amounts of estrogen.

Herceptin is a medication (nonhormonal) that can be administered to women with breast cancer if a sample of breast cancer cells shows a particular abnormal protein. Herceptin targets the abnormal protein.

Assisting with a Gynecologic Examination.

The gynecologic examination consists of four parts:

1. Inspection of external **genitalia** (labia minora, labia majora, urinary meatus, clitoris, **Bartholin glands**, and vagina) for swelling, lesions, or ulcerations
2. Pelvic examination of cervix, vagina, uterus, tubes, and ovaries including a **bimanual examination**; may or may not include a Pap test

3. Rectal examination

4. Breast examination

The medical assistant should prepare the patient, equipment, and room before the examination.

Gynecologic Examination with Pap Equipment.

On a Mayo tray near the end of the examination table, place the instruments and supplies the provider needs to perform the gynecologic or pelvic examination with Pap test. Figure 26-27 shows the equipment commonly needed for the examination. To aid in the inspection portion of the examination, you should place a gooseneck lamp at the foot of the table behind the stool on which the provider will sit (see Procedure 26-2).

In preparation for the annual examination, the patient is asked to avoid using tampons, foams, and gels; douching; and sexual intercourse for 2 days before a Pap test. Five days after menses is a good time to have a Pap test. Immediately before a pelvic examination, the patient is encouraged to empty her bladder. The urine may be collected for testing according to the clinic policy or the provider's preference and depending on any urinary tract complaints or symptoms the patient may have. If a Pap test is being performed, take a minute to interview the patient and gather the necessary medical and laboratory information. The data needed include:

- Last normal menstrual period. This question will bring up information about breakthrough bleeding (if patient is taking oral contraceptives), dysmenorrhea, metrorrhagia, postcoital bleeding, perimenopausal irregularities, and other idiosyncrasies of the menstrual patterns.

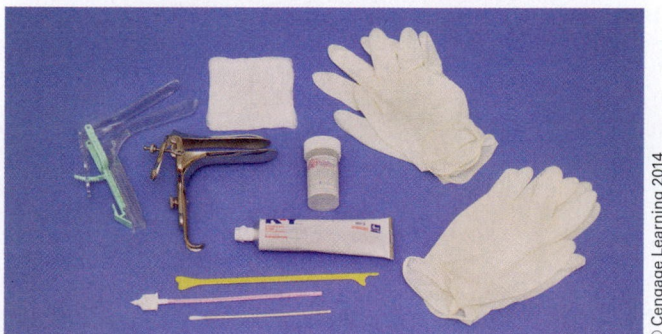

© Cengage Learning 2014

Figure 26-27 Setup for gynecologic examination including equipment for a Thin-Prep© Pap smear: transport medium container spatula, cytology brush and broom, Specula (disposable and reusable), lubricant, gloves, tissues.

- Hormonal therapies, either oral contraceptives or hormone therapy (HT). These are excellent questions for birth control history, successes/failures, and problems/solutions, and menopausal issues, concerns, and problems.

- Surgical history, especially related to the genitourinary tract. These questions will initiate discussions about bladder problems and hysterectomies.

- Sexual history/habits. This will open discussions with the patient about disease prevention, birth control, hormonal problems, and menopausal conditions.

- Symptoms of diseases/disorders, such as pelvic or genital pain or discomfort; vaginal discharge, irritation, or itching; painful intercourse; dysuria; urinary frequency or incontinence; and breast pain or breast conditions/concerns.

EHR All the information gathered during the patient interview can be entered into the patient's medical record on the computer while sitting with the patient. There may be a health form on the computer for the medical assistant to fill out with the patient. The provider then will input the information and any other pertinent data gathered during the examination. The electronic medical record is stored and can be accessed at any time for laboratory and diagnostic tests and procedures, prescriptions, and previous data entry.

In preparation for the examination, have the patient undress and don a patient gown with the opening positioned in the front (for the breast examination) and a drape sheet. The patient is seated on the examination table. Provide the patient with privacy during the undressing. Ensure the patient's comfort by providing her with a blanket if she is cold and have her leave her socks on if her feet are cold.

During the breast and abdominal examinations, the patient is placed into the supine or dorsal recumbent position. Provide a pillow for comfort. For the pelvic examination, the patient is placed into the lithotomy position. Assist the patient into this position, providing leg and back support as needed.

During the pelvic examination and the Pap smear, the medical assistant assists the provider as needed (Figure 26-28). The tray of supplies should be at an appropriate height and position for access by the provider while seated. Ideally, the vaginal speculum (metal or plastic) should be warmed to body temperature. Some examination tables are equipped with warming drawers for storing the specula so that they are warm and ready for use. The medical assistant may set up the pelvic exam/Pap smear supplies on a Mayo tray and position the gooseneck lamp so that the warmth from the light bulb can warm the speculum. The provider may hold the speculum under warm running water just before use. Whichever method is used, the provider will test the speculum to make sure it is not too hot before use. This is often done by touching the speculum on the patient's inner thigh to determine if the temperature is comfortable.

During the examination, the medical assistant will support the patient, hand the provider supplies as needed, and adjust the light source as needed. Cervical cells are obtained when the provider uses a tool called a cytology broom or bush. Once the cells are obtained, the medical assistant will uncap the ThinPrep container, swish the broom or brush vigorously in the ThinPrep solution until all of the specimen has been deposited, dispose of the broom or brush in a biohazard container, reapply the cap, and complete the container label. The label should contain the patient's name, birth date, patient number (if available), and the date and time of collection. If the patient is "status post hysterectomy," the provider will scrape cells (using the spatula) from the inner walls of the vaginal vault rather than from the cervix, which will no longer be present. Those cells are deposited into the ThinPrep solution in the same manner as a cervical specimen.

After the Pap test is performed, the provider will examine the internal organs. This is done using the bimanual (two-handed) examination (Figure 26-29). After applying water-soluble lubricant, two fingers are inserted into the vagina. The other hand is used to press on the outside abdominal wall. Using this method, the shape, consistency, movement, and positioning of the uterus and the ovaries can be felt. If any abnormalities are palpated, further testing may be required. After the bimanual examination, a rectal examination is performed. This examination enables the provider to assess the back side of the uterus, which is not felt during the bimanual examination.

When the pelvic examination is completed, you the medical assistant will help the patient off the table, offer tissue and the sink for her to clean up and wash her hands, and let her know you will be back in a few minutes. When you return, you may take the patient to the provider's office for private discussion. Occasionally, the provider will hold the discussion in the examination room after the patient has dressed.

The ThinPrep container and contents are sent to the cytology laboratory (Figure 26-30).

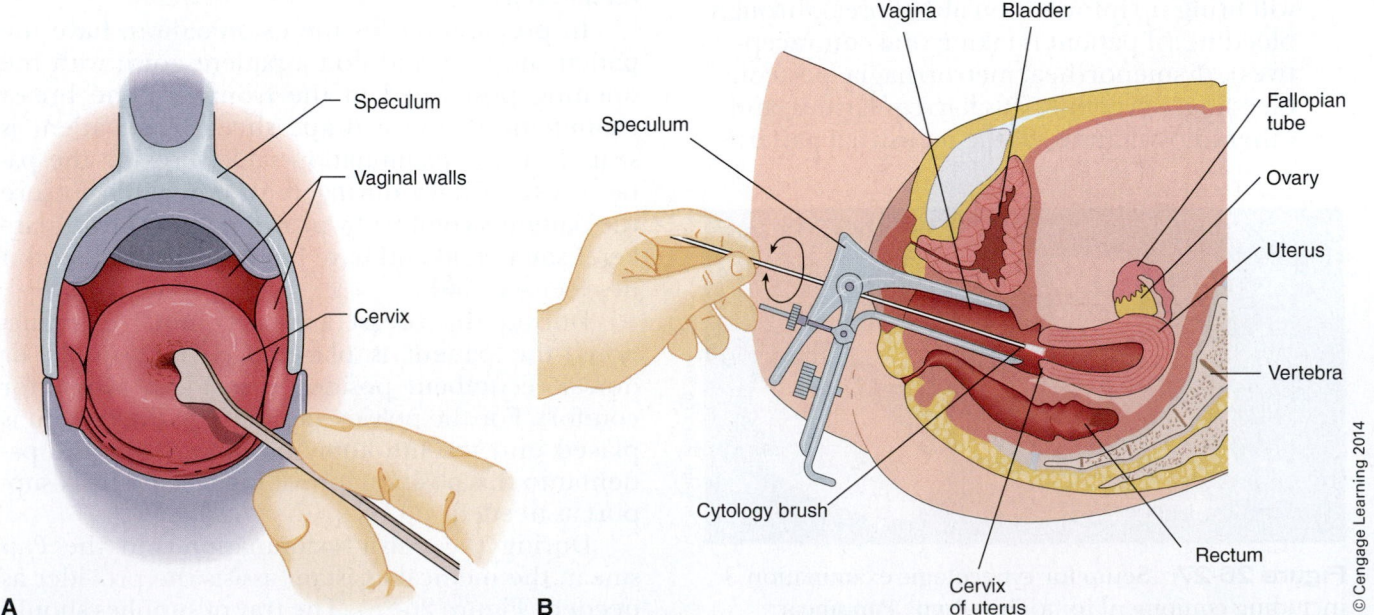

Figure 26-28 Use of speculum, cystology brush, and spatula to obtain material for a Pap smear. (A) The provider uses a spatula to obtain cells from the cervix. (B) The provider uses a cytology brush to obtain cells from the cervix.

© Cengage Learning 2014

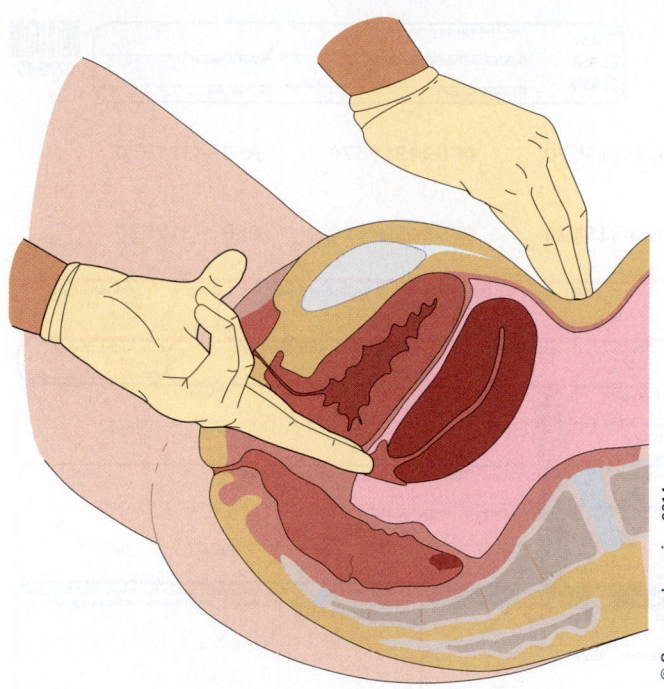

Figure 26-29 Bimanual pelvic examination.

© Cengage Learning 2014

Pap Smear. The conventional Pap smear is performed by scraping the patient's cervix with a spatula and cytology brush and smearing the cells onto a microscopic slide. The slide is then placed into a bottle of Pap fixative or sprayed with Pap fixative and sent to the regional laboratory for viewing. The ThinPrep Pap test differs in that the cells that are obtained on the collecting devices are swished vigorously into a vial of fluid transport medium rather than placed on a slide. The vial is sent to the regional laboratory for processing. Using the conventional method, approximately 80% of the specimen remains on the collecting device, with only about 20% being submitted on the slide. With the ThinPrep Pap test, virtually 100% of the collected cells are rinsed off the collecting device and submitted in the vial. The conventional Pap slide preparation results in an inconsistently distributed specimen containing blood cells, mucus, and other debris that can interfere with the viewing. The ThinPrep Pap test uses a ThinPrep processor to suspend the cervical cells; to eliminate the blood cells, mucus, and other debris; and to distribute a thin and even layer of cells onto a slide for analyzing. The ThinPrep Pap test slide is of better quality, is much clearer and easier to read, and increases accuracy for both the manual assessment and the computerized assessment. It greatly improves detection of precancerous cells.

Although the conventional Pap smear has undoubtedly saved countless lives by detecting cervical cancer, the ThinPrep Pap test is significantly more effective. Another advantage of the ThinPrep Pap test is that the same specimen may be used to determine the presence of HPV or chlamydia/gonorrhea if needed.

The federal government regulates laboratories that perform testing on Pap smears. Requirements are placed on the individuals who study the specimens for malignant cells, and they include specialized training. Limits are placed on the number of slides that can be read in one day. Proficiency testing, mandated by the Clinical Laboratory Improvement Act of 1988 (CLIA '88), ensures accuracy and precision of test results and is a requirement for Pap smear examination (Chapter 38 gives more information about CLIA '88).

A computerized method, known as AutoPap, is used to retest Pap smears that have been analyzed by technologists and found to be normal. The method duplicates the process that the technologists perform. AutoPap can be used for an initial Pap test as long as a technologist examines all abnormal smears.

Another test, known as ViraPap, can be used to screen for HPV in a Pap smear. There is higher incidence of cervical cancer in women who have HPV, and the test can help identify these women. Vaginal cancer can also be detected by a Pap smear. There is an increased risk for both cervical and vaginal cancer in daughters of women who used **diethylstilbestrol (DES)** during pregnancy.

Some advocate "at home" testing. The woman collects her cervical cells by inserting a small plastic applicator into the vagina up the cervix (as far as she can comfortably insert the applicator) and moving it around to collect cells. The applicator is placed in a special container to preserve cells that will be tested by a laboratory. The ACS does not endorse "home" testing. Perhaps in the future "home" testing will become accurate for scientific use and accepted by the medical community.

One system for cytologic reporting of a Pap smear is a descriptive report that tells the provider exactly what cellular changes have taken place. The classification includes the grades of cervical **intraepithelial** neoplasia (CIN).

CIN 1 = mild **dysplasia** (abnormal tissue
   development)

CIN 2 = moderate dysplasia

CIN 3 = severe dysplasia or **carcinoma in situ**

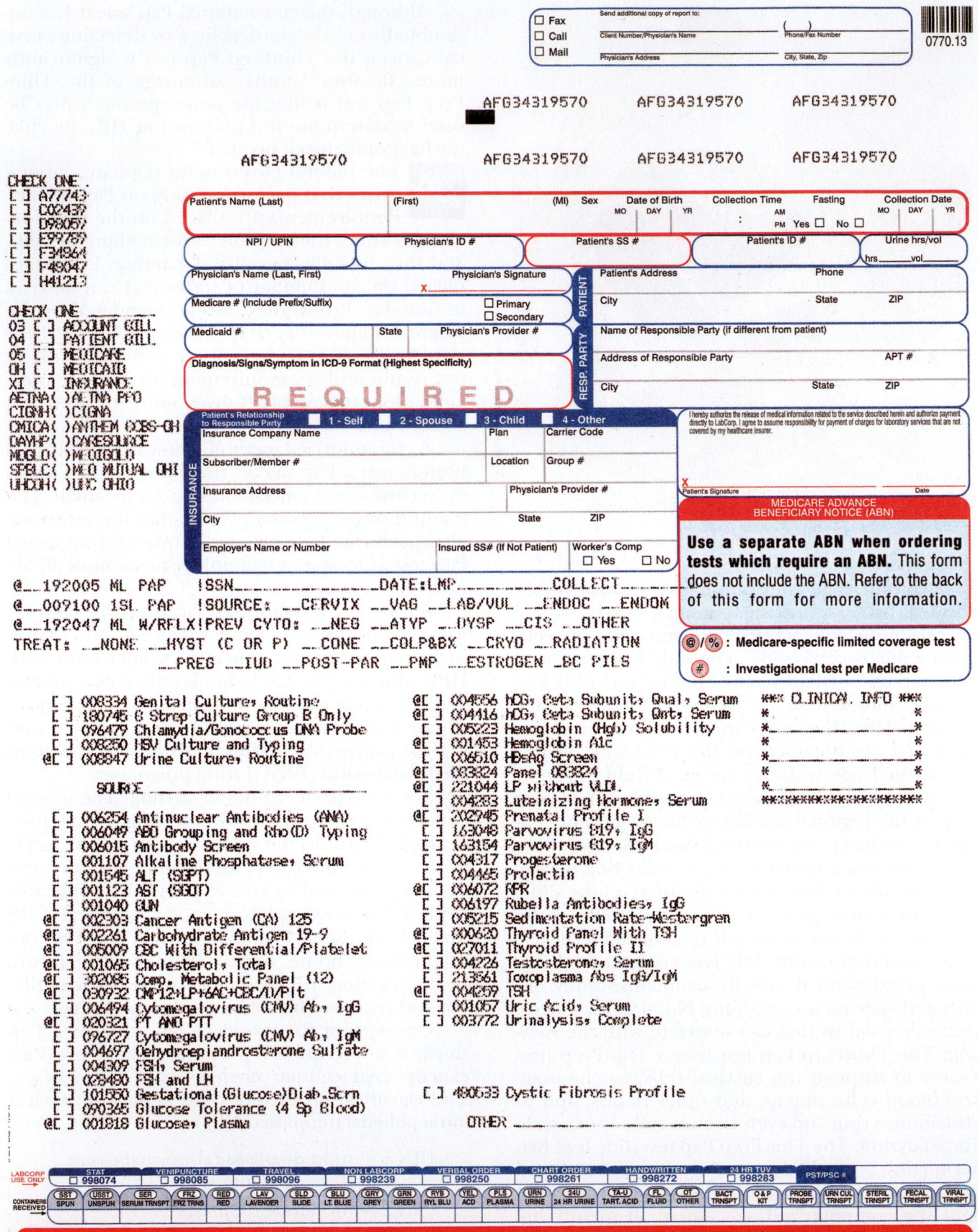

Figure 26-30   Laboratory requisition for OB/GYN practice.

Another system used to report Pap test results is the Bethesda System (TBS). The Bethesda System for reporting results of Pap tests has three main categories, some of which have subcategories:

Category 1 = negative for intraepithelial lesion or malignancy. This indicates that there is no sign of cancer or precancerous cells or other abnormalities found.

Category 2 = epithelial cell abnormalities. The cells of the lining of the cervix show changes that might be cancer or precancerous. There are several subgroups within this group for squamous cells and glandular cells.

1. *Atypical Squamous Cells (ASCs).* The name given to what the cells look like under a microscope. It is difficult to determine whether the abnormal cells are caused by an infection, an irritation, or a precancerous condition. This group is divided again:

   a. *Atypical Squamous Cells of Uncertain Significance (ASC-US)* and *atypical squamous cells where high-grade squamous intraepithelial lesions (SILs) cannot be excluded.* A repeat Pap test is done; biopsy and/or colposcopy and HPV DNA testing may be recommended.

   b. *Squamous Interepithelial Lesions (SILs).* There are low- and high-grade SILs. All patients in this category require a colposcopy. High-grade SILs can develop into cancer if not treated. Treatment can cure both high- and low-grade SILs and prevent cancer from developing. The Pap test does not identify which SIL the patient has; rather, it shows that the results fit into one of the abnormal categories.

   c. *Squamous Cell Carcinoma.* This test result shows that the woman likely has an invasive squamous cell carcinoma. Further testing, colposcopy, and biopsy are needed to be certain of the diagnosis. If the biopsy proves positive, the provider will recommend surgery, radiation, and/or chemotherapy.

   d. *Adenocarcinomas.* These carcinomas are abnormalities of glandular cells. If a clear decision cannot be made by the pathologist as to whether the cells are malignant, the term used is atypical glandular cells (AGS). Further testing is done to decide on a treatment plan.

Category 3 = other malignant neoplasms, including malignant melanoma, carcinoma, and lymphoma. These malignant neoplasms affect the cervix very rarely compared to squamous cell carcinoma and adenocarcinoma.

PATIENT EDUCATION

Many women think that if they have had a hysterectomy because of cancer they no longer need to have Pap smears performed. This is not true, and it is up to health care professionals to educate them. If the hysterectomy was performed because of cancer, the cancer cells can reappear in the vaginal vault after the surgery. During the pelvic examination, because the cervix has been removed, the provider will scrape the inner walls of the vaginal vault for cells to include in the Pap smear.

Pap Smear Results. The Pap smear usually is sent to a reference laboratory where a pathologist examines it and records the results on the cytology report form and in the computer. The form is returned to the provider, and the report can be accessed on the computer. Figure 26-31 lists some of the terms used on the cytology report form.

An abnormal Pap smear result requires intervention by the provider. It is the professional medical assistant's role to assist the provider and the patient in follow up.

atypical—not typical
CIN—cervical intraepithelial neoplasia
CIS—carcinoma in situ
condyloma—a lesion caused by human papillomavirus
dysplasia—precancerous lesion
epithelial—pertaining to epithelium
epithelium—cellular tissue that covers the surface of a body or that lines a body cavity
glandular—the cell making up the epithelium of a body cavity
HPV—human papillomavirus
lesion—a change in the tissue cells or a wound
malignant—a lesion that spreads out of the epithelium into underlying tissues
reactive changes—changes in cells caused by their reaction to infectious agents or a foreign body
reparative changes—changes in cells as they divide rapidly in an attempt to repair damaged tissue
SIL—squamous intraepithelial lesion (that lies within the squamous epithelium)
squamous—a type of cell that makes up the epithelium, the purpose of which is to protect underlying tissues

© Cengage Learning 2014

Figure 26-31 Terms and abbreviations used in cytology Pap test reports.

Gynecologic Diseases and Conditions

The female reproductive system is affected by many diseases and conditions caused by hormonal imbalance, cysts, infection, and tumors. Some of the more common disorders and diseases are covered here.

Infertility. Most women, with unprotected intercourse, will be able to conceive within a year. The inability to conceive can be caused by a problem with either the male or the female individual. Some common causes of infertility in a female patient are:

- Endometriosis
- Certain medications
- Blocked fallopian tubes
- Problems ovulating
- Chronic stress
- Scar tissue from surgery, infection, or ectopic pregnancy
- Tumors

A woman who is having difficulty conceiving and has a history of any of the above will have a physical examination by a provider who specializes in infertility. The specialist will decide what tests and procedures are necessary. Hormone levels may be measured to look for hypothyroidism. Ovarian function can be determined through a surgical procedure, such as laparoscopy. A test for **patency** (openness) of the fallopian tubes can be performed by a hysterosalpingogram, a radiographic procedure done after injection of dye into the vagina, through the cervix, into the uterus, and out the fallopian tubes. The dye will pass through all of these organs if there is no blockage in any of them (see "Impaired Fertility" section earlier in this chapter).

Menopause. The period of time that marks permanent cessation of menstrual activity is known as menopause. It usually occurs between the ages of 35 and 58 years. There may be a gradual decline in monthly menstrual flow, or a woman may suddenly cease to menstruate. Natural menopause occurs when the ovaries produce less and less estrogen. This causes the ovaries to cease ovulation and, therefore, menstruation stops. Surgical menopause is caused by the surgical removal of both ovaries (bilateral oophorectomy). Symptoms occur soon after ovulation ceases with both natural and surgical menopause. Symptoms may last for a few months to several years and include mild to severe symptoms.

Hot flashes, chills, nervousness, fatigue, apathy, mental depression, crying episodes, insomnia, palpitations, and headache are some common symptoms experienced by some women. A long-term effect of lower estrogen levels is osteoporosis. Hormone therapy (HT) was thought to prevent osteoporosis and heart disease. A federally funded HT study, the Women's Health Initiative (WHI), which was slated to run for 15 years, stopped testing in 2002 what had been the most widely prescribed estrogen and progestin combination. Safety concerns brought an early end (5.5 years) to the trial testing the long-term benefits and risks of combined estrogen and progestin therapy (HT). The testing was halted earlier than intended because it was determined that HT, specifically Prempro®, was more harmful than helpful. There were increased risks for breast cancer and cardiovascular incidents; therefore, researchers told the women in the study to stop taking the combination medication. This situation has left many women with few choices for treating menopausal symptoms such as night sweats, hot flashes, dyspareunia, mood swings, fatigue, and osteoporosis. Switching to something else is risky because no other hormones have been as well studied as estrogen and progestin in Prempro®. There are many safe options for prevention and treatment of osteoporosis.

Researchers continued to study the estrogen-only hormone after halting the estrogen–progesterone trial. Because progesterone was initially added to the estrogen to protect women from uterine cancer, the thinking was that healthy postmenopausal women who had a hysterectomy and were given the estrogen-only hormone would not be at risk. However, data showed an increase in stroke in postmenopausal women given estrogen only. As of February 2004, the estrogen-only arm of the WHI study was halted, and the recommendation is for only short-term use of the hormone for women with moderate-to-severe menopausal symptoms. The FDA has urged manufacturers to add warnings to their labels on the estrogen-only hormone about the increased risk for dementia, strokes, abnormal mammograms, and uterine cancer in women who have not had a hysterectomy.

Reanalysis of the data from the WHI found that the risk of heart disease was greatest in women who started HT 10 or more years after menopause began. Women with a history of heart disease or heart attack should not take menopause hormones. Older women also have an increased risk for clot formation around the plaque in their arteries. This plaque can rupture, causing a stroke or heart attack.

The American College of Obstetricians and Gynecologists and the National Institutes of Health recommended that HT is a reasonable choice and likely safe for women to use as short-term treatment of menopausal symptoms. Use of the lowest effective dose for the shortest period of time and yearly reevaluation of women taking HT should be done. However, HT increases the risk of breast cancer in women regardless of when they started HT.

Regardless of whether a woman chooses to use HT (a decision based on discussions with her provider) or decides against HT, the following behaviors are beneficial to all women:

- Do not smoke
- Keep blood pressure within normal limits
- Keep cholesterol level within normal limits
- Exercise regularly
- Maintain a healthy weight
- Get regular mammograms with ultrasound if necessary and Pap tests
- Practice good nutrition (go to the USDA Web site http://www.ChooseMyPlate.gov for information)
- Avoid regular alcohol use

Bioidentical hormone (hormones that are molecularly identical to those naturally occurring in the body) replacement therapy (BHRT) is gaining recognition as an alternative to traditional hormone therapy. While these hormones are derived from plant sources and not synthesized in a laboratory, they still must be synthesized to make them bio-identical. Most of these hormone combinations are specially formulated to the individual's needs. These compounded hormones are not subjected to the same rigid quality control regulations as commercially available prescriptions. Though this therapy is gaining recognition, ACOG's position states that "there is no scientific evidence supporting the safety or efficacy of compounded bioidentical hormones."

Endometriosis. Endometriosis is a painful, common condition characterized by endometrial tissue adhering to tissue and organs outside of the uterus. It is primarily found in the pelvis, adhering to an ovary, fallopian tube, or the pelvic peritoneum. It also can be found outside of the pelvis, even in the abdomen adhering to tissue and organs, such as the bowel. The cause is unknown. The abnormal and engorged endometrial tissue responds to hormonal stimulation (estrogen) and builds up along with the normal endometrium of the menstrual cycle. It sloughs off at time of menstruation and is painful. The blood has no way to leave the body and is discharged into the pelvic or abdominal cavities.

Endometriosis symptoms may respond to contraceptive medication because these pills suppress menstruation and no further treatment may be necessary (Figure 26-32). However, long-term hormonal treatment may help alleviate symptoms. Hysterectomy may be necessary if the woman does not respond to hormonal therapy.

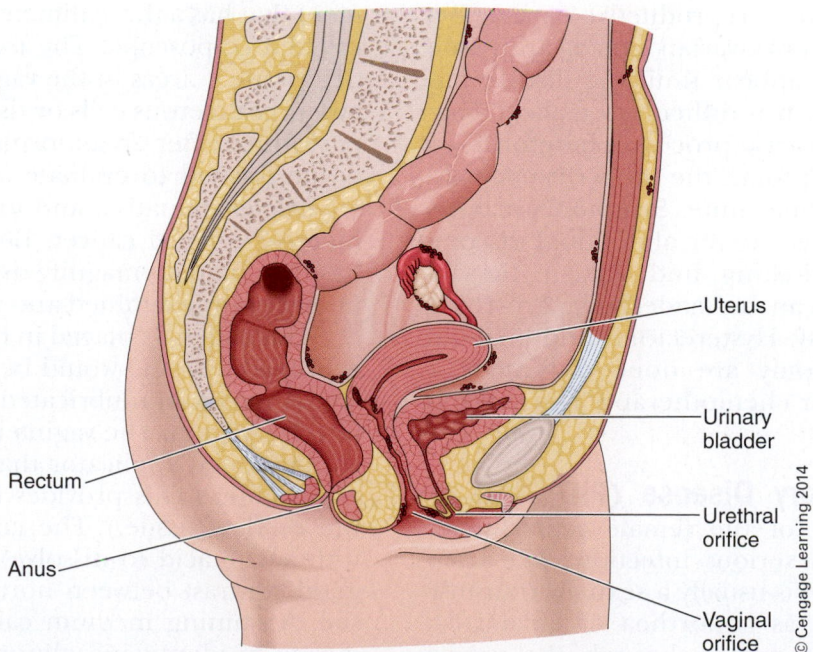

Uterus

Urinary bladder

Urethral orifice

Vaginal orifice

Rectum

Anus

© Cengage Learning 2014

Figure 26-32 Endometriosis–common sites of endometrial implants.

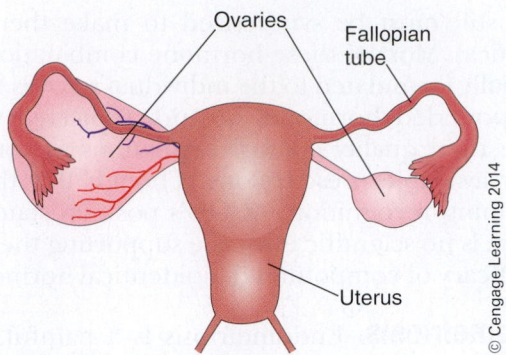

Ovaries

Fallopian tube

Uterus

© Cengage Learning 2014

Figure 26-33 Ovarian cyst.

Ovarian Cysts. Cysts that appear on the ovary are relatively common. As part of the menstrual cycle, the ovarian follicles enlarge and become graafian follicles. Only one graafian follicle ruptures at the time of ovulation. The follicles that do not rupture, but remain, are filled with fluid. They may enlarge and become cysts (Figure 26-33).

Ultrasonography will aid in viewing the ovaries. Most ovarian cysts resolve without treatment. Laparoscopy can be done to either drain or remove the cyst. Contraceptive therapy is often helpful in resolving the cyst without surgery.

Direct viewing of the ovaries and surgery may be necessary because cancer of the ovary must be ruled out.

Ovarian Cancer. Ovarian cancer is the fifth most common cancer in women. It causes more deaths than any other kind of reproductive cancer. Because the symptoms of ovarian cancer are vague and usually do not appear until the disease has become established, it is difficult to make a diagnosis early in the disease process. Therefore, if a woman has any symptoms, the cancer usually has been present for some time. Symptoms may be pressure in the pelvis, lower abdominal discomfort, weight loss, bloating, and fluid in the abdomen. Diagnosis can be made by laparoscopic surgery and a biopsy. Hysterectomy and bilateral salpingo-oophorectomy are done, followed by radiation therapy or chemotherapy. The cause is not known.

Pelvic Inflammatory Disease (PID). PID involves some or all of the female reproductive tract and can be a serious infection. The causative microorganism is usually a sexually transmitted pathogen such as gonorrhea or chlamydia. The microorganism enters through the vagina and ascends through the cervix into the body of the uterus. It can spread out through the fallopian tubes into the pelvic cavity. Culture and sensitivity of the vaginal discharge are performed, and appropriate antibiotics are prescribed. Early treatment helps to lessen damage caused by scar tissue that forms in the pelvis and organs. Delayed treatment can cause septic shock, which can be life-threatening. Infertility and ectopic pregnancy are long-range problems that also can occur (Tables 26-5, 26-6, and 26-7).

Other Diagnostic Tests and Treatments for Reproductive System Diseases

Colposcopy. Colposcopy is examination of the vagina and cervix by means of a lighted instrument that has a three-dimensional magnifying lens called a colposcope. The examination is done to determine if areas in the vagina or the cervix contain precancerous cells or tissue. The procedure is performed after an abnormal Pap test. It can also be performed to evaluate a lesion noted during a pelvic examination and to follow up after treatment of cervical cancer. Because the instrument has the ability to magnify tissue, the cervix can be more readily examined and a biopsy taken.

The patient is placed in lithotomy position and is prepared as she would be for a gynecologic examination. A nonlubricated speculum is inserted into the vagina. The vagina is swabbed with a long cotton-tipped applicator that has been moistened with saline. (This provides better visualization of the cervical tissue.) The cervix is then swabbed with acetic acid to dissolve mucus and provide a good contrast between normal and abnormal tissue. A staining medium can be used as another means of identifying abnormal cells. If the provider finds an area of abnormal tissue, a biopsy can

Table 26-5 Female Reproductive System Laboratory and Diagnostic Tests

Medical Tests or Procedures	Disease/Disorder	Blood	Other	Radiography	Surgery
Pelvic examination	Bartholin gland infection		Exudate culture and sensitivity		Incision and drainage
Monthly breast self-examination	Breast cancer	Breast cancer gene detection BRCA1, BRCA2		Mammography Ultrasonography	Biopsy of breast lesion Lumpectomy
Pelvic examination Colposcopy	Cervical cancer		Pap smear		Cone biopsy Punch biopsy Dilation & curettage (D&C) Cryosurgery LEEP (loop electrosurgical excision procedure) Laser surgery Hysterectomy
Pelvic examination	Endometriosis		Urinalysis	Abdominal ultrasonography Chest radiograph	Laparoscopy Hysterectomy
Monthly breast self-examination	Fibrocystic breasts			Mammography Ultrasonography	Biopsy
Pelvic examination	Pelvic inflammatory disease	Complete blood count and differential (CBC)	Urinalysis Culture and sensitivity of vaginal discharge	Pelvic ultrasonography	Laparoscopy

continues

Table 26-5   Female Reproductive System Laboratory and Diagnostic Tests (*Continued*)

Medical Tests or Procedures	Disease/Disorder	Blood	Other	Radiography	Surgery
Tests for Sexually Transmitted Diseases					
Pelvic examination	Chlamydia	Serology	Urinalysis Direct urethral or cervical smear using monoclonal antibodies ThinPrep Pap Test		
Pelvic examination Pap smear	Condylomata/HPV (genital warts)		ThinPrep Pap Test		Excisional biopsy
Pelvic examination	*Neisseria gonorrhoeae* Hepatitis B and C and HIV	CBC Virology	Urinalysis Direct smear of vaginal discharge, anal canal, and oropharynx Thayer-Martin culture ThinPrep® Pap Test Liver function	Pelvic ultrasonography Abdominal ultrasonography	Liver biopsy
Tests for Vaginitis					
Pelvic examination	Candidiasis	Blood glucose	Urinalysis Wet mount: direct vaginal smear with potassium hydroxide and/or saline (1 drop)		
Pelvic examination	Trichomoniasis		Urinalysis Wet mount: direct vaginal smear with isotonic saline (1 drop) and/or potassium hydroxide (KOH)		
Pelvic examination	Bacterial vaginosis	CBC	Culture and sensitivity of vaginal discharge		

Table 26-6   Female Reproductive System Disorders and Conditions

Bartholin Gland Infection. Infection of the mucous gland(s) that open near the vaginal opening.

Breast Cancer. Most commonly diagnosed cancer in females. A genetic cause has been identified for some breast cancers. Some symptoms are lumps, thickening, swelling, dimpling, pain, and nipple discharge.

Cervical Cancer. A carcinoma of the cervix of the uterus caused by a progressive cervical dysplasia. Most common in women aged 30 to 40 years. A significant risk factor is seen in women who become sexually active early in their lives and who have multiple sex partners. Presence of HPV poses greater risk.

Cystocele. Herniation of the urinary bladder into the vagina. May cause urgency and frequency. Injury to the bladder during delivery of the fetus is one cause.

Endometriosis. Presence of endometrium in sites other than inside the uterus. May be found on the ovaries, fallopian tubes, large bowel, lungs, and pleura. Causes pelvic pain, dysmenorrhea, and infertility.

Endometrial Cancer. A cancer that originates in the endometrial tissue. It is most common in women over the age of 50 and in women who utilize estrogen-only hormone replacement therapy. Obesity and the use of the medication tamoxifen increase the risk.

Fibrocystic Breasts. Benign cysts in breast tissue that increase or decrease in size during menses. Thought to be a normal variation in breast tissue due to monthly hormonal influence.

Pelvic Inflammatory Disease (PID). Pelvic reproductive organs become inflamed and infected by bacteria, viruses, or parasites. An ascending infection can ensue involving the vagina, cervix of uterus, body of uterus, fallopian tubes, and ovaries. Symptoms include vaginal discharge, pain, and fever. May cause infertility. Majority of cases caused by sexually transmitted disease (*Neisseria gonorrhoeae*, chlamydia).

Premenstrual Syndrome (PMS). Cluster of symptoms that occur monthly before the onset of menses thought to be caused by progesterone–estrogen imbalance. Symptoms include fluid retention, weight gain, irritability, and mood swings.

Rectocele. Herniation of the posterial wall of the vagina with the anterior wall of the rectum through the vagina.

Sexually Transmitted Diseases (STDs). Diseases caused by bacteria, viruses, and protozoa that are transmitted through sexual intercourse (vaginal, anal, oral).
  - *Chlamydia.* An invasion by an intracellular parasite causing urethritis, cervicitis, PID, proctitis, infant pneumonia, and conjunctivitis.
  - *Condylomata (HPV).* Genital warts caused by a virus. Grow around the external genitalia, rectum, and cervix. Associated with abnormal Pap smears.
  - *Neisseria gonorrhoeae.* An infection by a bacterium that can involve the cervix, urethra, fallopian tubes and ovaries, rectum, and mouth.

Vaginitis. Inflammation of the vagina that may be caused by bacteria, fungus, protozoa, chemical irritants, irritation from foreign bodies, vitamin deficiency, uncleanliness, and intestinal worms.
  - *Candidiasis.* A yeast (fungal) infection of the vagina caused by prolonged antibiotic therapy, pregnancy, or diabetes, which can change the normal vaginal flora leading to overgrowth of the fungus.
  - *Trichomoniasis.* An infection by a protozoan, most commonly spread through sexual intercourse or may come from fecal contamination of the vagina.

Table 26-7 Common Sexually Transmitted Diseases

Pathology	Symptoms	Test	Treatment
AIDS	Flu-like, lymphadenopathy, infections, malignancies, pneumonia	HIV CBC	Medication: antiretroviral medications such as zidovudine, didanosine, ritonavir
Chlamydia	Usually asymptomatic	Vaginal culture ThinPrep® Pap test Urinalysis	Doxycycline, azithromycin
Condylomata (HPV)	Warts on external and internal genitalia	Visual exam ThinPrep® Pap test HPV	Cryocautery or chemocautery preferred but electrocautery can be used Keratolytic agents such as Podofilox, CO_2 laser
Gonorrhea	Usually asymptomatic; yellowish-green discharge with dysuria in advanced stages	Gram stain or Thayer-Martin culture ThinPrep® Pap test	Ofloxacin, ceftriaxone, cefixine
Herpes simplex I and II	Itching and soreness followed by genital vesicles, which heal in 10 to 14 days	Visual exam Viral isolation by tissue culture	Acyclovir®, Valtrex, Famvir
Syphilis	Stage I: papule develops into ulcer, which develops into chancre on vulva Stage II: fever, general malaise, dermal and mucosal lesions Stage III: degeneration of central nervous system, lesions of internal structures	Venereal Disease Research Laboratory, fluorescent antibody test Dark-field exam Rapid Plasma Reagin (RPR) Culture and sensitivity of spinal fluid	Penicillin
Trichomonas	Milky white, frothy, malodorous discharge with genital burning and itching	Wet mount for microscopic examination	Oral Flagyl®: partner(s) must also be treated

© Cengage Learning 2014

be performed using cervical punch biopsy forceps (Figure 26-34). The specimen is examined by a pathologist to determine whether malignant cells are present.

Endometrial Biopsy/Sampling. An endometrial biopsy/sampling is often performed when patients are experiencing abnormal periods, postmenopausal bleeding, or thickened uterine lining as diagnosed by ultrasound. It is a fairly simple procedure. The sampling device is housed in a long straw-like tube that slides through the cervical os quite easily. Once the end of the tube is inside the uterus, a plunger is pulled back. The action of pulling the plunger suctions a sampling of the endometrial tissue. This is a sterile procedure and

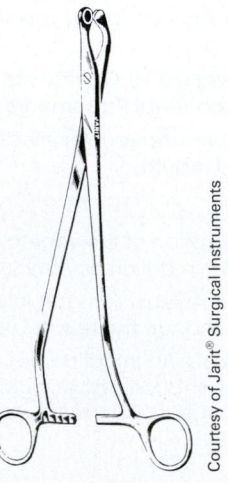

Courtesy of Jarit® Surgical Instruments

Figure 26-34 Toms-Gaylor uterine punch biopsy forceps.

requires an application of a cleansing solution (such as Betadine) to the cervix before performing the biopsy. Endometrial biopsy/sampling is quick and almost painless for the patient. The patient might experience slight cramping.

Cervical Punch Biopsy.

The **cervical punch biopsy** is usually done in conjunction with a colposcopy to obtain a sample of cervical tissue for pathologic examination. The specimen is examined for malignant cells and the biopsy usually follows an abnormal Pap smear report.

The procedure is performed with the patient in lithotomy position and with a vaginal speculum in place. The provider may stain the cervix to aid in identifying abnormal tissue. If the colposcope is being used, it illuminates and magnifies the cervical tissue. The provider takes several tissue samples using the cervical punch biopsy forceps. If bleeding ensues, it can be controlled with a vaginal packing, or the area can be cauterized to stop the bleeding. The specimen is placed in a container with **formalin**, a completed requisition form is attached to the container, and it is sent to the pathology laboratory for examination. The patient may expect a small amount of bleeding and should notify the provider if bleeding ensues that is greater than a menstrual period. A discharge that has a strong, foul odor is to be expected and can last for up to one month after the procedure.

Cervical Cone Biopsy.

Another type of biopsy, known as a cone biopsy, can be performed. An inverted cone of tissue is excised by scalpel or laser under general anesthesia. In this procedure, a larger sample of tissue is excised to rule out invasive cancer and to remove the lesion. It is the most

PATIENT EDUCATION

Post Cervical Biopsy and Cervical Cone Biopsy

1. Rest for 24 hours after the procedure.
2. Do not lift heavy objects for two weeks.
3. Leave packing in place for 24 hours or as directed. Do not insert another tampon unless told to do so by the provider.
4. Report any bleeding greater than a normal menstrual period.

PATIENT EDUCATION

After Cryosurgery of Cervix

1. Expect a clear, watery, heavy discharge for several weeks, eventually tapering off.
2. Use only sanitary pads, not tampons. Change often, cleansing perineal area with each pad change.
3. Report signs of infection: fever, malodorous discharge, pain, nausea, or vomiting.
4. Do not engage in sexual intercourse, douche, or use tampons for 4 weeks (unless instructed otherwise by provider).
5. Expect a somewhat heavier than usual menstrual period the following month.
6. Report excessive bleeding.

comprehensive specimen to diagnose a premalignant or malignant lesion. This is also known as a cold knife biopsy.

Another type of cervical biopsy is the loop electrosurgical excision procedure (LEEP), also called large loop excision of the transformation zone (the border between ectocervix and exocervix). Precancers and cancers commonly develop in this area. Either type of cervical cone biopsy can be used as a treatment to completely remove many precancers and very early cancers.

Cryosurgery.

Cryosurgery is used to treat tissue by freezing temperatures. Chronic cervicitis and cervical **erosion** are two common problems treated in this manner (see Chapter 31 for information about cryosurgery). The freezing temperature causes cells to die; they are then cast off from the cervix and eventually replaced with healthy cells about a month after the procedure.

The procedure is performed with the patient in lithotomy position. The cervix is swabbed to remove mucus. The cryo probe is placed against the affected area of the cervix and the machine is turned on. The liquid nitrogen flows over the area for about 3 minutes and freezes the tissue. The tissue is allowed to thaw, and the treatment is repeated for another 3 minutes. The patient may have some pain similar to dysmenorrhea that may last for about a half hour. There should be no strong, foul odor, but there can be a discharge for up to 1 month. Patients should report any malodorous discharges because this may indicate an infection. Healing usually takes 4 to 6 weeks.

Wet Prep/Wet Mount for Yeast, Bacteria, and Trichomonas.

The wet prep or **wet mount** is a clinic procedure to determine the cause of vaginitis in women and urethritis in men. The provider takes a sample of the discharge on a cotton-tipped applicator. The medical assistant rinses it vigorously in a test tube containing a few drops (about 0.5 mL) of normal saline, pressing the swab against the inside of the test tube to express all the specimen, then places a drop of the solution onto a microscope slide and covers it with a coverslip. The provider then views it microscopically for the following:

- If a yeast infection is present, budding yeast will be seen.

- If a bacterial infection is present, clue cells will be seen. Clue cells are vaginal epithelial cells that appear fuzzy with no clear cell edge. They appear this way because the outside edge is covered with bacteria.

- If trichomonas are present, they appear as motile single-cell protozoa. Movement will be noted. The trichomonas are sometimes identified in a microscopic portion of the urinalysis as well (see Procedure 26-5).

Potassium Hydroxide Prep for Fungus.

After performing the previously mentioned test, a few drops of 10% potassium hydroxide (KOH) may be added to the remaining solution in the test tube and examined microscopically for fungi. The KOH destroys bacteria and vaginal epithelial cells, leaving only the cell walls of the fungus, which makes visualization easier. This slide is prepared in the same way as the wet prep: Place a drop of the solution onto a clean slide; cover with a coverslip. Dispose of all glass slides, coverslips, and test tubes into a sharps container (see Procedure 26-5).

Amplified DNA Probe Test for Chlamydia and Gonorrhea.

The Amplified DNA Probe Test for Chlamydia and Gonorrhea is used as a screening tool for both men and women and on all pregnant women. (See Procedure 26-6.) It is not a culture. Two types of kits are available: the ProbeTec® blue kit for urethral specimens from the male patient (see Chapter 28) and the ProbeTec® pink kit for endocervical specimens from the female

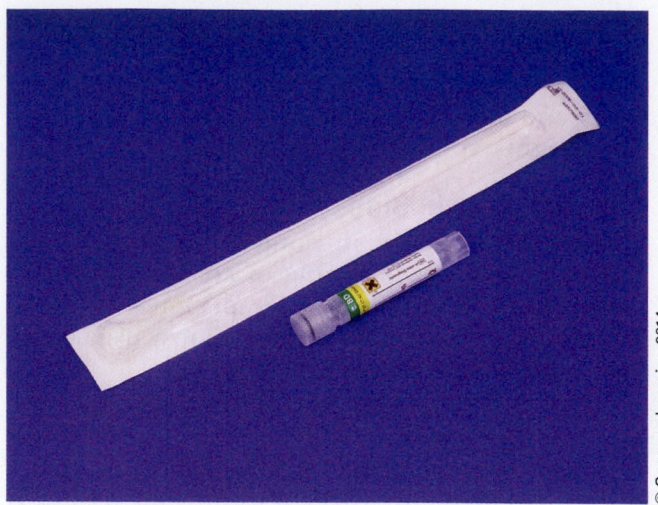

Figure 26-35 BD's ProbeTec Amplified DNA test kit for chlamydia and gonorrhea.

© Cengage Learning 2014

patient. The female kit contains preservative, swabs (one large swab and one small Mini-Tip Culturette Swab), and instructions. This test needs to be performed on the female patient before the digital/bimanual examination so that no lubricating jelly is present. Using the large swab, the provider will clean the cervix of any mucus, blood, and cellular debris and discard the swab. The Mini-Tip Culturette Swab is then inserted into the cervical canal and rotated for 15 to 30 seconds. Immediately, it is placed into the transport tube. If the ProbeTec Wet Transport tube is used (Figure 26-35), the swab is broken off into the liquid before recapping. This test also may be used to test for chlamydia and gonorrhea in a urine specimen, following the manufacturer's instructions for collection and testing (see Procedure 26-5).

Laparoscopy.

Laparoscopy is a procedure in which a lighted instrument is used to view the inside of the pelvic cavity. It can be helpful in diagnosing endometriosis and ovarian cysts or other abnormalities in the pelvic cavity. A tubal ligation, severing of the fallopian tubes, and an oophorectomy can be done laparoscopically. Laparoscopy can be done abdominally or vaginally (Figure 26-36).

Dilation and Curettage.

Dilation and curettage (D&C) is a surgical procedure that involves dilating and scraping the cervix of endometrial tissue. It is commonly performed to remove any remaining tissue after an incomplete abortion or to examine the tissue if the patient has had abnormal uterine bleeding.

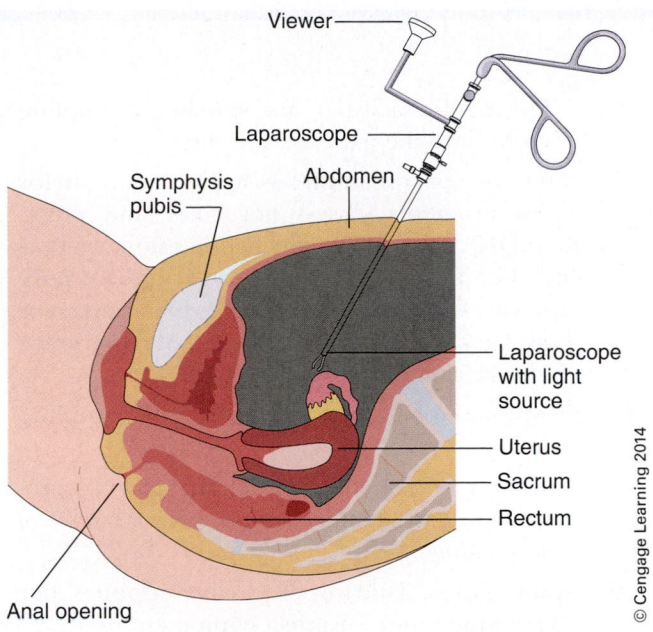

Figure 26-36 Laparoscopy.

Diagnostic ultrasonography is used to help diagnose many gynecologic conditions, such as ovarian masses, fibroids, and endometriosis. The ultrasound can be performed transcervically or transvaginally (see Figure 26-11A and Figure 26-11B).

Complementary Therapy in Obstetrics and Gynecology

Most of the complementary therapy practiced today can be helpful to women in easing the discomforts of pregnancy and labor. In our stress-filled world, emotional calm can be provided through the use of some of these therapies.

Neonatal intensive care unit infants benefit from a calm, warm touch and rocking, hugging, and singing softly.

Information should be obtained from the obstetrics patient at each visit about any form of complementary therapy (stress reduction, imagery, acupuncture, biofeedback, massage therapy, and music therapy, among others). Consultation with the provider concerning their safety during pregnancy is advisable.

Caution is advised when the use of herbal medicine is considered during the pregnancy. Because herbal supplements are available over the counter and little is known about their effects on the fetus, women should be cautioned to avoid using any kind of herbal supplement during their first trimester. Women should ask their provider's advice about the use of the supplements after the first trimester.

PROCEDURE 26-1

Assisting with Routine Prenatal Visits

STANDARD PRECAUTIONS:

PURPOSE:
To monitor the progress of the pregnancy.

EQUIPMENT/SUPPLIES:

Scale	Doppler fetoscope
Disposable gloves	and coupling agent
Patient gown	Urine specimen container
Tape measure	Urinalysis testing supplies
Sphygmomanometer	Biohazard waste container
Stethoscope	

PROCEDURE STEPS:
1. Wash hands and follow Standard Precautions.
2. *Paying attention to detail*, assemble equipment.
3. *Introduce yourself to the patient. Identify patient.*
4. *Explain the procedure, speaking at the patient's level of understanding.*
5. Instruct the patient in the correct method of obtaining a urine specimen. RATIONALE: A urine specimen for analysis is necessary for two reasons: An empty bladder facilitates the examination, and is more comfortable for the patient. The urine sample will be tested.

continues

© Cengage Learning 2014

Procedure 26-1 (continued)

6. ***Considering any special needs of the patient,*** instruct and then assist the patient to remove shoes, jacket or sweater, and step on paper towels on the scale. Assist the patient to the center of the scale. Weigh patient. Accurately record findings. RATIONALE: Assesses gain or loss of weight to help determine fetal development and maternal nutrition.

7. Measure blood pressure and accurately record findings.

8. ***Being courteous and respectful,*** provide patient with gown and drape.

9. ***In a manner that protects the patient's personal boundaries,*** have patient disrobe from waist down and put on a gown, open in the front. RATIONALE: An open gown facilitates access to the abdomen for examination and measurement of the fundal height.

10. Test the urine specimen while waiting for the provider. RATIONALE: Urinalysis is done for detection of glucose and protein, which may indicate disease.

11. ***Attending to any special needs,*** assist patient onto examination table and drape her. RATIONALE: The patient may be off balance and unsteady on her feet because of the enlargement of the abdomen. Provide for her safety.

12. Assist the provider as the examination is performed.
    - Hand the provider the tape measure to measure height of fundus.
    - Hand the provider the Doppler fetal pulse detector for measurement of fetal heart rate.

The medical assistant may spread the coupling agent onto the patient's abdomen.

13. After the examination, assist patient to sit for a few moments. Assess her color and pulse. RATIONALE: Orthostatic hypotension can occur when a patient rises from a recumbent position. Give the patient time for the blood pressure to go back to normal so she will not experience dizziness from decreased blood pressure.

14. Provide towel to patient to wipe off coupling agent.

15. Provide any instructions or clarification of provider's orders, ***speaking at the patient's level of understanding***.

16. Apply gloves. Discard disposable supplies per OSHA guidelines. Disinfect equipment used.

17. Remove gloves.

18. Wash hands.

19. Set up for the next patient.

20. Accurately record all information in patient's chart or electronic medical record.

DOCUMENTATION:

4/14/20XX 2:30 PM   Wt. 148 3/4 lbs., T 98.8°F, P 82, R 16, BP 118/72^L sitting. Urine dipstick negative for glucose and protein. Fundal height at 22 wks. FHR 120. Says she feels well and is sleeping and eating well. C. McInnis, CMA (AAMA)—

PROCEDURE 26-2

Assisting with Pelvic Examination and Pap Test (Conventional and ThinPrep® Methods)

STANDARD PRECAUTIONS:

PURPOSE:

To assist the provider in collecting cervical cells for laboratory analysis for early detection of malignant cells of the cervix and to assess the health of the reproductive organs to detect diseases, leading to early diagnosis and treatment.

EQUIPMENT/SUPPLIES:

Nonsterile gloves (2–3 pair)
Vaginal speculum, disposable or nondisposable
Warm water or warming light
Light source
Drape sheet
Patient gown
Tissues
Vaginal lubricant
Lab requisition (see Figure 26-30)
Urine specimen container

Procedure 26-2 (continued)

Urine testing supplies
Biohazard specimen bag
Biohazard waste container
Adjustable stool for provider

Supplies for the Pap test according to the method used for ThinPrep® Pap:

- Cervical spatula
- Brush and broom
- ThinPrep® container with solution

For conventional Pap test:

- Microscope slides
- Fixative and/or specimen bottle
- Cervical spatula
- Cytology brush

PROCEDURE STEPS:

1. Wash hands and follow Standard Precautions.

2. *Paying attention to detail*, assemble equipment.

3. *Introduce yourself to the patient. Identify patient.*

4. *Explain the procedure, speaking at the patient's level of understanding.*

5. Request that patient empty her bladder. (Instruct patient to save urine specimen and provide specimen container if ordered by provider.) RATIONALE: An empty bladder facilitates examination of the uterus and a urine specimen is frequently used for a urinalysis.

6. *Being courteous and respectful*, provide patient with gown and request her to completely undress, *being sure to protect the patient's personal boundaries*.

7. Instruct patient to sit at end of table when ready for pelvic examination. Drape patient for privacy. If performing conventional Pap test, label the frosted end of the slide with a marking pencil. Include patient's name on slide. Indicate site from where specimen is collected: c = cervix, v = vagina, e = endocervical.

8. Assist patient into lithotomy position. Patient's knees should be relaxed and thighs rotated out as far as comfortable. Drape for privacy and warmth.

9. Encourage patient to breathe slowly and deeply through the mouth during examination. RATIONALE: Allows for relaxation of pelvic muscles and easier insertion of vaginal speculum.

10. Warm vaginal speculum with either warm water or under heat lamp or place on a heating pad. *NOTE:* Do not lubricate speculum. Lubricant obscures exfoliated cervical cells when Pap test is being performed.

11. Hand speculum and spatula, cytology brush, and broom to the provider as needed.

12. Apply gloves.

13. For conventional Pap test, hold slides for provider to apply smear of exfoliated cells, one for vaginal (v), one for cervical (c), and one for endocervical (e), in that order. If spraying Pap fixative, spray it over the slide within 10 seconds at a distance of about 6 inches. Allow to dry for at least 10 minutes. If using Pap fixative in a bottle, place slide directly into bottle. If using ThinPrep®, swish the cytology broom vigorously in the ThinPrep® solution until all of the specimen has been deposited. Dispose of brush into biohazard container. RATIONALE: This maintains cell appearance and avoids contamination of cells. Avoid getting too close to slide with spray because this may destroy or damage cells. Slides must be fixed before they dry to protect the appearance of the cells.

14. For ThinPrep® Pap test, hand the speculum and cytology broom to the provider. Open the ThinPrep® solution container. When the cells have been obtained, take the broom and vigorously swish it into the container of solution until all the cells have been deposited. Replace the cap and label. Dispose of the broom into biohazard waste container. RATIONALE: The ThinPrep® procedure requires that all cells obtained from the cervix be presented in the solution for complete testing.

15. Place lubricant on provider's gloved fingers without touching gloves, for bimanual and rectal examinations. The provider will insert the index and middle fingers into the vagina. The other hand is placed on the lower abdomen. The size, shape, and position of the uterus and ovaries are palpated.

16. The provider will insert one gloved finger into the rectum to check the ovaries and the tone of

continues

Procedure 26-2 (continued)

the rectal and pelvic muscles. Hemorrhoids, rectal fissures, or other lesions may be palpated.

17. Provide the patient tissues to wipe genitalia and rectum.

18. After the examination, assist the patient to a sitting position, allowing her to rest a while. Check her pulse and skin color. RATIONALE: Some patients, especially older adult patients, can experience orthostatic hypotension.

19. Apply disposable gloves. Discard disposable supplies per OSHA guidelines. If stainless steel speculum was used, soak in cool water. Sanitize and sterilize as soon as convenient.

20. Remove gloves and wash hands.

21. Assist patient down and off the table if necessary, *attending to any special needs of the patient.*

22. Assist the patient to dress; provide privacy.

23. Escort the patient to provider's office for discussion of examination results.

24. Prepare laboratory requisition (cytology request) form. Include provider name and address, date, source of specimen, patient's name and address, date of LMP, and hormone therapy, if any. Place slides in slide container or ThinPrep® container into biohazard specimen bag. Place requisition into outer pocket of bag and send to laboratory.

25. Wash hands.

26. Accurately document procedure in patient's chart or electronic medical record.

DOCUMENTATION:

4/14/20XX 11:00 AM   Wt. 138 lbs., T 98°F, P 68, R 20, BP 138/72ᴸ sitting. Urine dipstick negative for protein and glucose. Pap smear performed by Dr. Woo. Slides of vaginal, cervical, endometrial cells sent to lab with requisition. Pelvic and rectal exams performed by Dr. Woo. Patient expressed no complaints of discomfort. BP 142/78 P 80. C. McInnis, RMA (AMT)——————————

PROCEDURE 26-3

Assisting with Insertion of an Intrauterine Device (IUD)

STANDARD PRECAUTIONS:

PURPOSE:

To assist the provider with the insertion of an intrauterine device (see Figure 26-19).

EQUIPMENT/SUPPLIES:

Nonsterile gloves (2–3 pair)
Sterile gloves
Vaginal speculum
Light source and stool for provider
Drape and gown
Tissue
Lubricant
Prepackaged IUD
Biohazard waste container
Local anesthetic
Syringe and needle

Antiseptic such as Betadine® solution or swabs
Emesis basin for used items such as speculum

PROCEDURE STEPS:

1. Wash hands and follow Standard Precautions.

2. *Paying attention to detail*, assemble equipment.

3. *Introduce yourself. Identify the patient.*

4. Draw up local anesthetic into syringe as directed by provider.

5. Request that the patient empty her bladder. Save urine for pregnancy test. RATIONALE: If patient is pregnant, the IUD will not be inserted.

6. *Being courteous and respectful*, ask patient to undress from the waist down and put on a gown, *being sure to protect the patient's personal boundaries.*

Procedure 26-3 (continued)

7. ***Explain procedure to patient, speaking at the patient's level of understanding. Allay the patient's fears regarding the procedure. Help her to feel safe and comfortable.***

8. ***Considering any special needs of the patient,*** assist patient into lithotomy position.

9. Drape for warmth and privacy.

10. Administer medication to patient for pain as prescribed by provider.

11. Hand speculum to provider.

12. Provide nonsterile gloves to the practitioner for the initial pelvic examination.

13. Encourage the patient to breathe slowly and deeply through her mouth during the procedure.

14. The provider does a pelvic examination after donning nonsterile gloves.

15. The provider checks for pelvic infection and position of the uterus. RATIONALE: An IUD cannot be inserted if the woman has a pelvic infection because the procedure can carry microorganisms into the uterus. The position of the uterus is important for the provider to know before insertion.

16. The provider swabs the cervix with an antiseptic and may inject a local anesthetic into the cervix.

17. The provider puts the IUD into the insertion device. The arms of the IUD flatten (the top of the "T").

18. The provider inserts the IUD with the insertion device through the cervix into the uterus.

19. The insertion tube is withdrawn completely.

20. Dispose of insertion device into biohazard waste container or emesis basin. The provider shortens the string on the IUD to 1–2 inches from the cervix and then removes speculum. Dispose of speculum into waste container or emesis basin. RATIONALE: The string is left long enough so the patient can feel for the string through her vagina after every period. The provider will have the patient check the string after the procedure. RATIONALE: Ensures that patient knows how to check for and find the string.

21. Place disposable speculum in biohazard waste container. Place nondisposable speculum into emesis basin.

22. Provide the patient tissues to clean lubricant from exam area.

23. Assist patient to sit for a few moments. Assess her pulse, skin color, and blood pressure if needed. RATIONALE: Some patients can experience orthostatic hypotension and become dizzy if they rise too quickly.

24. Apply nonsterile gloves.

25. Discard disposable supplies according to OSHA guidelines. If stainless steel speculum was used, soak in cool water. Sanitize and sterilize later when convenient.

26. Remove gloves. Dispose in biohazard waster container. Wash hands.

27. ***Considering any special needs of the patient,*** assist patient off table .

28. Assist patient with dressing if needed; provide privacy.

29. Explain to patient that she may experience light cramping and perhaps spotting for 1–2 days.

30. Make an appointment in 4–6 weeks for patient. Inform patient to make a yearly appointment thereafter for a check-up.

31. Accurately document procedure in patient's chart or electronic medical record.

DOCUMENTATION:

8/23/20XX 10:30 AM Pregnancy test negative. 1.0 mL of lidocaine injected into cervix by Dr. King. Pelvic examination done by Dr. King, and a copper IUD was inserted after anesthetic took effect. Small amount (approximately 15 mL) of bright red blood noted after insertion. Patient states she is "having slight cramping." BP 134/88, P 100 immediately after procedure. Patient able to feel string coming out of cervix into vagina. Explained to patient to call the clinic if she cannot feel the string, and that sometimes the string tangles around the cervix and is hard to find. Informed the patient that an ultrasound, if necessary, will show whether the IUD is still in place. Instructed patient to use another form of contraceptive until placement of IUD is confirmed. Blood pressure 10 minutes after procedure 124/82, P 92, color good. Patient left accompanied by her sister. C. McInnis, RMA (AMT)—————————————

PROCEDURE 26-4

Assisting with Insertion of a Hormonal Contraceptive (Implanon®)

STANDARD PRECAUTIONS:

PURPOSE:

To assist the provider with the insertion of an implantable hormonal contraceptive such as Implanon®.

EQUIPMENT/SUPPLIES:

Sterile gloves
Sterile drapes
Skin marker
Drape and gown
Biohazard waste container
Local anesthetic
Syringe and needle
Antiseptic such as Betadine® solution or swabs
Sterile dressing materials

PROCEDURE STEPS:

1. Wash hands and follow Standard Precautions.
2. *Paying attention to detail,* assemble equipment.
3. *Introduce yourself. Identify patient.*
4. Draw up local anesthetic into syringe as directed by provider.
5. *Being courteous and respectful,* provide the patient with a gown and request that the patient to undress from the waist down and put on a gown, *being sure to protect the patient's personal boundaries.*
6. *Explain procedure to patient, speaking at the patient's level of understanding. Allay the patient's fears regarding the procedure. Help her to feel safe and comfortable.*
7. *Considering any special needs of the patient,* assist the patient to recline on the exam table with her non-dominate arm flexed at the elbow and the wrist resting near the ear.

8. Assist the provider with determination and marking the site for subdermal insertion.
9. Assist the provider with cleaning the area with antiseptic and anesthetizing the area.
10. Keep the patient informed during the procedure regarding what is happening and what is expected, *speaking at the patient's level of understanding.*
11. Apply sterile gloves.
12. Place a sterile dressing over the insertion site.
13. Remove gloves. Dispose in biohazard waste container.
14. Wash hands.
15. Apply a pressure dressing to the site. Instruct the patient that it may be removed in 24 hours.
16. *Considering any special needs of the patient,* assist patient off table if she needs help.
17. Assist the patient with dressing; provide privacy.
18. Complete the user ID card and give it to the patient to keep. Apply the Patient Chart Label to the patient's chart.
19. Make an appointment in 4–6 weeks for patient. Inform patient to make a yearly appointment thereafter for a check-up.
20. Accurately document procedure in patient's chart or electronic medical record.

DOCUMENTATION:

8/23/20XX 10:30 AM   Pregnancy test negative. 1.0 mL of lidocaine injected into upper, inner arm by Dr. King. Most appropriate area for insertion determined by Dr. King. Area prepped with Betadine and draped in a sterile fashion. Implanon® inserted following manufacturer's directions. No bleeding or hematoma noted at the site. Sterile dressing applied. BP 134/88, P 100 immediately after procedure. Blood pressure 10 minutes after procedure 124/82, P 92, color good. Patient left accompanied by her husband. Instructed to contact the clinic if there is bleeding, tenderness, or elevated temperature. D. Ragland, RMA (AMT)——————

PROCEDURE 26-5

Wet Prep/Wet Mount and Potassium Hydroxide (KOH) Prep

STANDARD PRECAUTIONS:

PURPOSE:

To test a vaginal specimen to determine the cause of vaginitis. The wet prep/wet mount tests for yeast, bacteria, and trichomonas; the KOH prep tests for yeast.

EQUIPMENT/SUPPLIES:

Cotton-tipped applicator
Small test tube
Normal saline (0.5 mL, or a few drops)
10% potassium hydroxide (KOH; 0.5 mL, or a few drops)
Two microscope slides and coverslips
Microscope
Vaginal speculum
Patient drape
Gloves
Other equipment as necessary for a vaginal examination

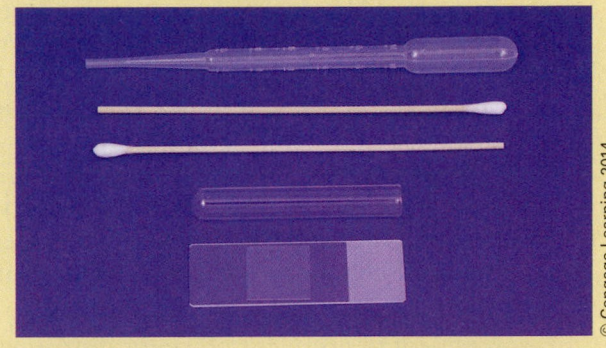

Figure 26-37   Supplies for wet mount and KOH prep: Pipette, cotton-tipped swabs, small test tube, and microscope slide with coverslip (not shown: saline and KOH solution).

PROCEDURE STEPS:

1. Wash hands and follow Standard Precautions.

2. *Paying attention to detail*, assemble equipment for vaginal examination.

3. *Introduce yourself. Identify the patient.*

4. *Being courteous and respectful*, provide patient with a gown and request that the patient undress from the waist down.

5. *Explain the procedure, speaking at the patient's level of understanding. Allay the patient's fears regarding the procedure. Help her to feel safe and comfortable.*

6. *Considering any special needs of the patient*, assist the patient into the lithotomy position.

7. Prepare the patient for a pelvic examination as outlined in Procedure 26-2 (Figure 26-37).

8. Assist the provider with vaginal exam and obtaining the specimen for evaluation.

9. Place several drops of normal saline into a small test tube. RATIONALE: Preparing the test tube for the specimen.

10. Don nonsterile gloves.

11. Using the cotton-tipped applicator, the provider obtains a sampling of discharge from the vagina and hands it to the medical assistant. RATIONALE: The provider will complete the examination of the patient while the medical assistant prepares the sample for viewing.

12. Rinse the swab vigorously in the test tube containing saline, pressing the cotton tip against the inside of the test tube to express all of the specimen. RATIONALE: It is important to get as much of the sample as possible for a more accurate diagnosis.

13. Dispose of the cotton-tipped applicator into a biohazard container. RATIONALE: All body fluid–contaminated supplies should be handled with care and disposed of according to Standard Precautions.

14. Apply a drop on a microscope slide and cover with a coverslip. Hand the slide to the provider

continues

Procedure 26-5 (continued)

for the microscopy examination. RATIONALE: Only a provider may perform the PPMP (Physician Performed Microscopy Procedure) for diagnosis, according to CLIA regulations; *be sure to work within your scope of practice.*

15. *Considering any special needs of the patient,* assist the patient back to a sitting position. Instruct her to dress and offer to assist if needed, *being sure to protect the patient's personal boundaries.* RATIONALE: While the provider is viewing the slide, your responsibility is the safety and comfort of the patient.

16. Escort patient to provider's office for discussion of examination results.

17. In the laboratory, the provider will view the slide for yeast, bacteria, and trichomonas. RATIONALE: The provider will take the slide to the laboratory where the microscope is located.

18. After completion of the wet prep/wet mount, apply a few drops of KOH into the remaining solution in the test tube, place a drop on a fresh slide, and cover with a coverslip. RATIONALE: This is the second part of the microscopy test that can be performed on the vaginal secretion to diagnose the cause of vaginitis.

19. The provider will perform a microscopic examination for yeast. RATIONALE: This is a PPMP.

20. Dispose of all slides and the test tube into a sharps container. RATIONALE: As stated in Standard Precautions, all sharps must be disposed of in a sharps container.

21. Disinfect the laboratory area and equipment. RATIONALE: As stated in Standard Precautions, all biohazard contaminated surfaces must be disinfected after contamination.

22. Return to the patient and assist as needed, *attending to any special needs of the patient.* RATIONALE: The patient may need assistance and direction.

23. Remove gloves and dispose of properly.

24. Wash hands.

25. Accurately document procedure in patient's chart or electronic medical record. Input that a pelvic examination and wet prep were done, and that the provider examined the specimen. The provider will add his or her findings to the patient's electronic medical record. Be sure you sign the entry.

DOCUMENTATION:

6/10/20XX 2:15 PM Wet mount and KOH prep done. Candidiasis identified. Patient given prescription for Gyne-Lotrimin 3 vaginal suppositories (200 mg) at bedtime for three consecutive nights. J. Woo, MD. Patient will call on Monday to tell us how she feels. C. McInnis, RMA (AMT)——————

PROCEDURE 26-6

Amplified DNA ProbeTec Test for Chlamydia and Gonorrhea

STANDARD PRECAUTIONS:

PURPOSE:

To test a vaginal specimen for diagnosis of chlamydia and gonorrhea and as a screening tool for the same for a pregnant woman.

EQUIPMENT/SUPPLIES:

Amplified DNA ProbeTec Kit (pink):

- Transport tube containing preservative

- Swabs (one large and one small Mini-Tip Culturette)

Vaginal speculum
Patient drape
Gloves
Other equipment as necessary for a vaginal examination

PROCEDURE STEPS:

1. Prepare the patient for a pelvic examination as outlined in Procedure 26-2.

2. Don nonsterile gloves.

Procedure 26-6 (continued)

3. Assist the provider with vaginal exam and obtaining the specimen for evaluation.

4. Hand the large swab to the provider, who will use it to clean the cervix. RATIONALE: Mucus or blood on the cervix will interfere with the purity of the specimen.

5. Discard the large swab into the biohazard waste container. RATIONALE: According to Standard Precautions, all biohazard contaminated waste must be handled carefully and disposed of properly.

6. Hand the small Mini-tip Culturette Swab to the provider, who will insert the swab into the cervical os and rotate it for 15 to 20 seconds. RATIONALE: Accurate test results require obtaining adequate endocervical cells and secretions.

7. Immediately place the swab into the transport tube and recap. RATIONALE: The specimen must be placed in the tube with preservative immediately to preserve it.

8. If using the ProbeTec Wet Transport tube, break the tip of the swab off into the liquid before recapping. RATIONALE: The tip of the swab is scored and will snap off easily. This allows the entire specimen to be transported in a small amount of preservative.

9. Remove gloves and dispose of them properly.

10. Wash hands.

11. *Paying attention to detail,* attach requisition to specimen.

12. Attend to your patient, *being sure to address any special needs.*

13. Accurately record all information in patient's chart or electronic medical record. Document pelvic examination and wet prep were preformed and that the provider examined the specimen. The provider will add his or her findings to the patient's electronic medical record. Be sure to sign the entry.

DOCUMENTATION:

6/10/20XX 10:00 AM   DNA ProbeTec test done by Dr. Woo. Entire specimen transported to laboratory.
C. McInnis, RMA (AMT)

CASE STUDY 26-1

Refer to the scenario at the beginning of the chapter.

Mrs. Sanderson has an appointment today in the obstetric clinic at Inner City Health Care. Angela Jarreau, RMA (AMT) is responsible for preparing Mrs. Sanderson for a repeat prenatal visit. Besides getting her patient ready, Angela has other responsibilities to Mrs. Sanderson. Vital signs and certain laboratory tests must be done.

CASE STUDY REVIEW

1. What are some potential problems with Mrs. Sanderson's pregnancy that Angela can discover and relay to Dr. Cox?

CASE STUDY 26-2

Maria Rodriguez has an appointment to see Dr. Cox today. It is her initial prenatal visit. She tells Angela Jarreau, the medical assistant, as she is escorted from the reception area that she has been feeling "pretty good."

CASE STUDY REVIEW

1. List three of the screening exams to be performed during the first prenatal visit.

2. What laboratory and other procedural tests may be performed at the initial visit?

CASE STUDY 26-3

Annette Sanderson has made an appointment with Dr. Cox because she has had symptoms of vaginitis. When she arrives at the clinic, you take her chief complaint and history. She tells you that she has a milky-white, frothy vaginal discharge and that she itches in the genital area.

CASE STUDY REVIEW

1. What tests/procedures will you prepare for Dr. Cox in consideration of Annette's symptoms?
2. What is the most likely causative microorganism for these symptoms?
3. Describe the treatment that Dr. Cox may prescribe.

SUMMARY

Obstetrics and gynecology are two specialties that are usually practiced by the same provider. The OB/GYN provider will care for the health and well-being of the female patient in her pregnant and nonpregnant states.

  Knowledge of the numerous tests and procedures that are performed to diagnose and treat problems in the female patient are essential. Health promotion and patient education are of extreme importance whether the patient is an obstetric patient and scheduled for her initial prenatal visit or a gynecologic patient scheduled for yearly pelvic, Pap, and breast examinations.

STUDY FOR SUCCESS

To reinforce your knowledge and skills of information presented in this chapter:

- Review the *Key Terms*
- Role-play with other students to apply attributes of professionalism pertinent to this chapter.
- Consider the *Case Studies* and discuss your conclusions
- Answer the questions in the *Certification Review*
- Apply your knowledge by completing the *Activities* in the *Study Guide* and the *Games and Quizzes* in the StudyWARE StudyWARE software on the *Premium Website*
- Perform the *Procedures* using the *Competency Assessment Checklists* in the *Competency Manual*
- Practice your problem-solving skills with the *Critical Thinking Challenge 3.0* on the Premium Website

Additional resources for this chapter include:

- Module 21 of the *Medical Assisting Learning Lab*
- *CourseMate for Delmar's Comprehensive Medical Assisting*
- *WebTutor for Delmar's Comprehensive Medical Assisting*

CERTIFICATION REVIEW

1. Which of the following conditions or diseases that an obstetrics patient experiences is considered to place her in the high-risk category?
   a. Urinary tract infection
   b. 19 years of age
   c. Both partners Rh negative
   d. Poor nutritional habits
   e. Poor hygiene

2. Using Nägele's Rule, calculate the expected date of birth of the baby of a patient whose last menstrual period was August 20, 2005.
   a. November 27, 2006
   b. December 13, 2006
   c. May 27, 2006
   d. April 20, 2006

3. The primary test performed at about the 16th week to check the fetus for neural tube defects is known as:
   a. alpha-fetoprotein test
   b. amniocentesis
   c. chorionic villus sampling (CVS)
   d. rubella titer
   e. Rh factor

4. The release of which of the following hormones is thought to cause labor to begin?
   a. Progesterone
   b. Estrogen
   c. Oxytocin
   d. Thyroxine

5. Ultrasonography is done to check for which of the following?
   a. Gestational diabetes
   b. Preeclampsia
   c. Degree of effacement
   d. Number of weeks of gestation

6. After a cervical punch biopsy, it is normal for the patient to experience which of the following?
   a. Bleeding greater than a normal menstrual period
   b. No odor to vaginal discharge
   c. Malodorous vaginal discharge
   d. Severe abdominal cramps

7. To make the diagnosis of trichomoniasis, the medical assistant will need to prepare for which of the following?
   a. Pap smear
   b. Ultrasonography
   c. Wet mount
   d. Culture and sensitivity
   e. Blood glucose

8. To diagnose pelvic inflammatory disease (PID), the provider may order which of the following?
   a. Culture and sensitivity
   b. Pap smear
   c. Urinalysis
   d. Rubella titer
   e. Ultrasonography

9. Which of the following is/are primarily associated with abnormal Pap smears?
   a. Endometriosis
   b. Bartholin cysts
   c. Condylomata
   d. Ovarian cysts
   e. PID

10. The primary purpose of colposcopy is to:
    a. treat advanced cancer of the vagina and cervix
    b. detect dysplastic cells of cervix after an abnormal Pap test
    c. treat PID in the fallopian tube
    d. treat endometriosis of the pelvic cavity

REFERENCES/BIBLIOGRAPHY

American Cancer Society. (2011). Breast cancer: Early detection. Atlanta, GA: American Cancer Society. Retrieved from http://www.cancer.org/cancer/breastcancer/index

American Congress of Obstetricians and Gynecologists. (2009, February). ACOG reiterates stance on so-called "bioidentical" hormones. Retrieved April 14, 2012, from http://www.acog.org/About_ACOG/News_Room/News_Releases/2009/ACOG_Reiterates_Stance_on_So-Called_Bioidentical_Hormones

Centers for Disease Control and Prevention. (n.d.). *Genital HPV infection, CDC fact sheet.* Retrieved August 24, 2008, from http://www.cdc.gov/std/HPV/STDFact-HPV.htm

Centers for Disease Control and Prevention. (n.d.). *Human papillomavirus (HPV).* Accessed April 14, 2012, at http://www.cdc.gov/hpv/vaccine.html

Decision (pp. 165–192). Published by Rodale: Distributed to the trade by Holtzbrinck Publishers, 2007. http://www.who.int/mediacentre/factsheets/fs241/en/

Ghidini, A. (n.d.). Fetal blood sampling: Technique and complications. *UpToDate.* Retrieved April, 13, 2012, from http://www.uptodate.com/home/index.html

Kelly Colihan, reviewed by Louise Change, MD. (2008, August 13). More women ask for birth control. *Web MD, Birth Control Health Center.* Retrieved October 5, 2008, from http://www.webmd.com/sex/birth-control/news/20080813/more-women-ask-for-birth-control

Littleton, L. Y., & Engebretson, J. C. (2002). *Maternal, neonatal, and women's health nursing.* Clifton Park, NY: Delmar Cengage Learning.

Mayo Clinic. (n.d.). Hormone therapy: Is it right for you? Retrieved July 6, 2012, from http://www.mayoclinic.com/health/hormone-therapy/WO00046/

Miranda Hitti, reviewed by Louise Chang, MD. (2008, September 12). Gardasil approved to target more cancers. *Web MD, Medical News Women's Health, Cervical Cancer Vaccine.* Retrieved October 5, 2008.

Morrison, R. W., & Lett, S. M. (2007). *Human papillomavirus (HPV) vaccine for VFC-eligible girls now available (memorandum).* Jamaica Plain, MA: The Commonwealth of Massachusetts, Executive Office of Health and Human Services, Department of Public Health, State Laboratory Institute. Retrieved August 24, 2008, from http://www.cdc.gov/hpv/vaccine.html

National Cancer Institute. (2007). *Tamoxifen: Questions and answers.* Retrieved August 29, 2007, from http://www.cancer.gov/cancertopics/factsheet/therapy/tamoxifen

National Cancer Institute Fact Sheet 4.21. *Human papillomavirus (HPV) vaccines: Questions and answers.* Retrieved October 5, 2008, from www.cancer.gov/cancertopics/factsheet/prevention/HPV-vaccine

Parker-Pope, T. (2007, June 11). The menopause–hormone discussion: How to weigh the risks. *The Wall Street Journal.* Adapted from *The hormone decision.* Published by Rodale: Distributed to the trade by Holtzbrinck Publishers, 2007.

Practice Bulletin. (2011). Breast cancer screening. *Obstetrics and Gynecology, 118,* 372–382.

Roberts, J. M., & Cooper, D. B. (2001). Series, Preeclampsia trio. Pathogenesis and genetics of preeclampsia. *The Lancet 2001, 357,* 53–56.

Rosenberg, M. J., Waugh, M. S., & Long S. (1995). Unintended pregnancies and use, misuse and discontinuation of oral contraceptives. *Journal of Reproductive Medicine, 40,* 355–360.

Spratto, G. R., & Woods, A. L. (2009). *2008/9th edition nurse's drug handbook.* Clifton Park, NY: Delmar Cengage Learning.

Taber's cyclopedic medical dictionary (21st ed.). (2002). Philadelphia: F. A. Davis.

Tamparo, C., & Lewis, M. (2005). *Diseases of the human body* (4th ed.). Philadelphia: F. A. Davis.

Walsh, T., Casadei, S., Coats, K. H., Swisher, E., Stray, S. M., Higgins, J., … King, M-C. (2006). Spectrum of mutations in BRCA1, BRCA2, CHEK2, and TP53 in families at high risk of breast cancer. *Journal of the American Medical Association, 295*(12), 1379–1388.

White, P. (1949). Pregnancy complicating diabetes. *American Journal of Medicine, 7,* 609–616.

CHAPTER 27

Pediatrics

OUTLINE

What Is Pediatrics?
Preparation of Vaccines
for Administration
Recommended Vaccination
Schedule
Considerations for Vaccine
Administration
Giving Injections to Pediatric
Patients
**Theories of Growth
and Development**
Newborns
Infants
Toddlers
Preschoolers
School-Aged Children
Adolescents
Growth Patterns
Length and Weight
Measurements

Infant Holds and Positions
Height and Weight
Measuring Devices
Measuring Head
Circumference
Measuring Chest
Circumference
Infant/Child Failure to
Thrive
Pediatric Vital Signs
Temperature
Pulse
Respirations
Blood Pressure
**Collecting a Urine Specimen
from an Infant**
**Screening Infants for Hearing
Impairment**
**Screening Infant and Child
Visual Acuity**

**Common Disorders
and Diseases**
Otitis Media
The Common Cold
Tonsillitis
Pediculosis
Asthma
Croup
Pertussis (Whooping Cough)
Respiratory Syncytial Virus
Attention Deficit
Hyperactivity Disorder
Child Abuse
Male Circumcision

LEARNING OUTCOMES

1. Define, spell, and pronounce the key terms as presented in the glossary.
2. Describe the various theories of human development.
3. Describe pediatric care including measuring height, weight, head circumference, chest circumference, and vital signs.
4. Maintain growth charts.
5. Explain the process of collecting a urine specimen.
6. Explain the process of screening for hearing and visual impairments.
7. Describe common pediatric diseases and disorders.
8. Explain the importance of immunizations and scheduling of them.
9. Describe infant holds for injections and procedures.
10. Analyze the professionalism questions and apply them to this chapter's content.

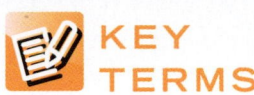

KEY TERMS

aerosolized

circumcision

cochlear implantation

Denver Developmental Screening Test

DTaP (diphtheria, tetanus, pertussis)

exudate

fontanel

hepatitis A vaccine (HAV)

hepatitis B vaccine (HBV)

lyophilized

myringotomy

neonate

organomercurial

phenylketonuria (PKU)

sensorineural

suppurative

tympanostomy

ATTRIBUTES OF PROFESSIONALISM

 Communication

- Did you introduce yourself? Did you identify the patient through name and birth date or other identifying feature?
- Did you speak at the patient's level of understanding?
- Did you provide appropriate responses/feedback?
- Did you allay patients' fears regarding the procedure being performed and help them feel safe and comfortable?
- Did you respond honestly and diplomatically to the patient's concerns?
- Did you demonstrate empathy in communicating with patients, family, and staff?
- Did you accurately and concisely update the provider on any aspect of the patient's care?
- Did you include the patient's support system as indicated?

 Presentation

- Did you do something to bond with the patient?
- Did your actions attend to both the psychological and the physiologic aspects of the patient's illness or condition?
- Did you attend to any special needs of the patient? Did you first ask if assistance was needed, rather than taking charge?
- Did you display a calm, professional, and caring manner?

 Competency

- Did you pay attention to detail?
- Were you knowledgeable and accountable?
- Did you recognize the importance of local, state, and federal legislation and regulations in the practice setting?

 Initiative

- Did you direct the patient to other resources when necessary or helpful, with the approval of the provider?

 Integrity

- Did you demonstrate respect for individual diversity?
- Did you protect and maintain confidentiality?
- Did you immediately report any error you had made?

SCENARIO

At Inner City Health Care, clinical assistant Sarah Thomas, CMA (AAMA), is responsible for encouraging parents to keep track of their children's immunization records. Sarah teaches parents the importance of immunizations for long-term health protection and the importance of following recommended vaccination schedules for maximum benefit.

INTRODUCTION

New techniques and developments occur frequently in medicine, and medical assistants must refine existing skills and learn new ones to be knowledgeable and proficient and to provide the most current, up-to-date quality care to patients. The medical assistant who works in a pediatrician's office or a pediatric ambulatory care setting that treats infants and children will need additional skills when providing pediatric care to patients.

Knowledge of the developmental stages, knowledge of diseases of infants and children, and the ability to gain the child's confidence and trust and the caregivers' cooperation are all skills required to provide for the physiologic, emotional, and psychological needs of the pediatric patient. This chapter covers the specialty examination and the appropriate clinical procedures in pediatrics.

WHAT IS PEDIATRICS?

Pediatrics is the branch of medicine that cares for newborns, infants, children, and adolescents. Pediatricians are providers who diagnose and treat health problems and diseases specific to these age groups. This patient population has special needs, and medical assistants must be knowledgeable about the growth and developmental phases of life and diseases unique to pediatric patients. Children form judgments and have fears about health care providers. They need an atmosphere that is comfortable and one in which their physiologic, emotional, and psychological needs are recognized and addressed.

Medical assistants must gain the confidence and trust of the child and parent(s), allay fear, and help to promote positive relationships between the child and the provider and must themselves develop a positive relationship with the child. Children are likely to be cooperative when being examined or during a procedure if good rapport has been established. It is important to be honest with young patients and approach them at their level of understanding. Allow children to touch and hold a "safe" instrument, such as a stethoscope, and explain its purpose to them.

Doing so can reduce anxiety and fear (Figure 27-1). It is important also for the medical assistant to recognize pediatric patients by their names no matter what their ages.

Taking a history of the child; assessing the child; measuring vital signs, height, weight, vision, and hearing; laboratory work; administration of injections; observing the parent–child interactions; and noting the child's development level are all responsibilities in which a medical assistant takes part.

The first physical examination of a newborn is performed immediately after delivery. The pediatrician assesses the **neonate's** ability to exist outside

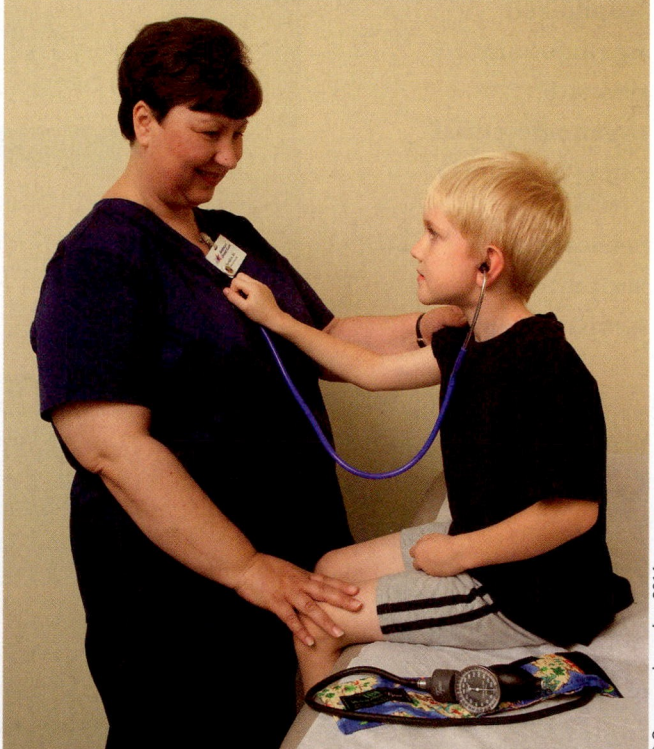

Figure 27-1 The medical assistant allows the child to touch the stethoscope and "listen" to her heartbeat to gain the child's cooperation.

© Cengage Learning 2014

SPOTLIGHT ON CERTIFICATION

RMA Content Outline

- Anatomy and physiology
- Medical terminology
- Patient relations
- Patient education
- Medical asepsis
- Vital signs and mensurations
- Physical examination
- Laboratory procedures

CMA (AAMA) Content Outline

- Medical terminology
- Anatomy and physiology
- Developmental stages of the life cycle
- Adapting communication according to an individual's needs
- Medicolegal guidelines and requirements
- Patient preparation and assisting the provider
- Patient history interview
- Preparing and administering medications

CMAS Content Outline

- Medical terminology
- Anatomy and physiology
- Basic charting
- Examination preparation

considered "well-baby" or "well-child" patients and are having routine checkups. Ill babies or children are often called "sick-child" or "sick-baby" patients. Well-baby appointments are regularly scheduled appointments during which time the provider examines the child and evaluates the growth and development of the child. Most clinics schedule well-baby appointments after birth according to the following time frame: 1, 2, 4, 6, 9, 12, 15, 18, and 24 months, and yearly thereafter.

The goal of well-baby visits or checkups is prevention of health problems and diseases. Typically, immunizations are given during these appointments. The charts shown in Figures 27-2, 27-3, and 27-4 include immunization schedules from the Centers for Disease Control Recommended Immunization Schedule for Persons Aged 0 Through 18 Years. The Advisory Committee on Immunization Practices (ACIP) revises their recommendations every 3 to 5 years. It is the role of this group to help vaccination providers assess risks and benefits of various vaccines. There are 17 vaccine-preventable diseases that occur in infants, children, adolescents, and adults.

Immunizations protect children against hepatitis A and B, poliomyelitis, measles, mumps, rubella, pertussis, diphtheria, tetanus, *Haemophilus influenzae* type b, pneumonia, chickenpox, influenza, rotavirus, meningitis, and human papillomavirus (HPV) (see Chapter 26). Immunizations are given by mouth, injection, and intranasal spray. All of these vaccines need to be given before age 2 years when children are most susceptible to infectious diseases. Vaccines protect children during these periods. HPV is the exception. It is given between ages 13 to 18 with the minimum age 9 years.

Preparation of Vaccines for Administration

Careful attention to both proper storage of vaccines and thorough patient preparation for immunization will promote effective vaccination results. Access to vaccination should be available to all patients, especially to families with young infants and children. Most of the recommended vaccines are administered in the child's first 15 to 18 months of life. Access involves cost of vaccines, appointment requirements, and time required to receive vaccines. Some clinics permit walk-in vaccination administration without cost or with low co-payment fee. Routine well-infant examinations should be

the mother's uterus. A scoring system is used to determine the neonate's physical condition at 1, 5, and 15 minutes after birth. It is known as the APGAR (appearance, pulse, grimace, activity, and respiration) score. Muscle tone, skin color, respiration, heart rate, and response to stimuli are each given a score 0, 1, or 2, the highest total score being 10. Infants with low APGAR scores need immediate attention, such as stimulation, oxygen, medication, and so on. Their condition is monitored closely (see Chapter 26).

Tests are done to detect problems the neonate may have. **Phenylketonuria (PKU)**, iron deficiency anemia, lead poisoning, and hypothyroidism are problems for which neonates are screened shortly after the APGAR scoring is done.

Many patients seen in the pediatric setting are babies or children who are not ill. They are

Recommended immunization schedule for persons aged 0 through 6 years—United States, 2012 (for those who fall behind or start late, see the catch-up schedule

Vaccine ▼ Age ▶	Birth	1 month	2 months	4 months	6 months	9 months	12 months	15 months	18 months	19–23 months	2–3 years	4–6 years	
Hepatitis B[1]	Hep B	HepB			HepB								Range of recommended ages for all children
Rotavirus[2]			RV	RV	RV[2]								
Diphtheria, tetanus, pertussis[3]			DTaP	DTaP	DTaP		see footnote[3]	DTaP				DTaP	
Haemophilus influenzae type b[4]			Hib	Hib	Hib[4]		Hib						Range of recommended ages for certain high-risk groups
Pneumococcal[5]			PCV	PCV	PCV		PCV				PPSV		
Inactivated poliovirus[6]			IPV	IPV	IPV							IPV	
Influenza[7]					Influenza (Yearly)								
Measles, mumps, rubella[8]							MMR		see footnote[8]			MMR	Range of recommended ages for all children and certain high-risk groups
Varicella[9]							Varicella		see footnote[9]			Varicella	
Hepatitis A[10]							Dose 1[10]			HepA Series			
Meningococcal[11]							MCV4 — see footnote[11]						

This schedule includes recommendations in effect as of December 23, 2011. Any dose not administered at the recommended age should be administered at a subsequent visit, when indicated and feasible. The use of a combination vaccine generally is preferred over separate injections of its equivalent component vaccines. Vaccination providers should consult the relevant Advisory Committee on Immunization Practices (ACIP) statement for detailed recommendations, available online at http://www.cdc.gov/vaccines/pubs/acip-list.htm. Clinically significant adverse events that follow vaccination should be reported to the Vaccine Adverse Event Reporting System (VAERS) online (http://www.vaers.hhs.gov) or by telephone (800-822-7967).

1. **Hepatitis B (HepB) vaccine.** (Minimum age: birth)
   At birth:
   • Administer monovalent HepB vaccine to all newborns before hospital discharge.
   • For infants born to hepatitis B surface antigen (HBsAg)–positive mothers, administer HepB vaccine and 0.5 mL of hepatitis B immune globulin (HBIG) within 12 hours of birth. These infants should be tested for HBsAg and antibody to HBsAg (anti-HBs) 1 to 2 months after completion of at least 3 doses of the HepB series, at age 9 through 18 months (generally at the next well-child visit).
   • If mother's HBsAg status is unknown, within 12 hours of birth administer HepB vaccine for infants weighing ≥2,000 grams, and HepB vaccine plus HBIG for infants weighing <2,000 grams. Determine mother's HBsAg status as soon as possible and, if she is HBsAg-positive, administer HBIG for infants weighing ≥2,000 grams (no later than age 1 week).
   Doses after the birth dose:
   • The second dose should be administered at age 1 to 2 months. Monovalent HepB vaccine should be used for doses administered before age 6 weeks.
   • Administration of a total of 4 doses of HepB vaccine is permissible when a combination vaccine containing HepB is administered after the birth dose.
   • Infants who did not receive a birth dose should receive 3 doses of a HepB-containing vaccine starting as soon as feasible (Figure 3).
   • The minimum interval between dose 1 and dose 2 is 4 weeks, and between dose 2 and 3 is 8 weeks. The final (third or fourth) dose in the HepB vaccine series should be administered no earlier than age 24 weeks and at least 16 weeks after the first dose.

2. **Rotavirus (RV) vaccines.** (Minimum age: 6 weeks for both RV-1 [Rotarix] and RV-5 [Rota Teq])
   • The maximum age for the first dose in the series is 14 weeks, 6 days; and 8 months, 0 days for the final dose in the series. Vaccination should not be initiated for infants aged 15 weeks, 0 days or older.
   • If RV-1 (Rotarix) is administered at ages 2 and 4 months, a dose at 6 months is not indicated.

3. **Diphtheria and tetanus toxoids and acellular pertussis (DTaP) vaccine.** (Minimum age: 6 weeks)
   • The fourth dose may be administered as early as age 12 months, provided at least 6 months have elapsed since the third dose.

4. *Haemophilus influenzae* **type b (Hib) conjugate vaccine.** (Minimum age: 6 weeks)
   • If PRP-OMP (PedvaxHIB or Comvax [HepB-Hib]) is administered at ages 2 and 4 months, a dose at age 6 months is not indicated.
   • Hiberix should only be used for the booster (final) dose in children aged 12 months through 4 years.

5. **Pneumococcal vaccines.** (Minimum age: 6 weeks for pneumococcal conjugate vaccine [PCV]; 2 years for pneumococcal polysaccharide vaccine [PPSV])
   • Administer 1 dose of PCV to all healthy children aged 24 through 59 months who are not completely vaccinated for their age.
   • For children who have received an age-appropriate series of 7-valent PCV (PCV7), a single supplemental dose of 13-valent PCV (PCV13) is recommended for:
     — All children aged 14 through 59 months
     — Children aged 60 through 71 months with underlying medical conditions.
   • Administer PPSV at least 8 weeks after last dose of PCV to children aged 2 years or older with certain underlying medical conditions, including a cochlear implant. See *MMWR* 2010:59(No. RR-11), available at http://www.cdc.gov/mmwr/pdf/rr/rr5911.pdf.

6. **Inactivated poliovirus vaccine (IPV).** (Minimum age: 6 weeks)
   • If 4 or more doses are administered before age 4 years, an additional dose should be administered at age 4 through 6 years.
   • The final dose in the series should be administered on or after the fourth birthday and at least 6 months after the previous dose.

7. **Influenza vaccines.** (Minimum age: 6 months for trivalent inactivated influenza vaccine [TIV]; 2 years for live, attenuated influenza vaccine [LAIV])
   • For most healthy children aged 2 years and older, either LAIV or TIV may be used. However, LAIV should not be administered to some children, including 1) children with asthma, 2) children 2 through 4 years who had wheezing in the past 12 months, or 3) children who have any other underlying medical conditions that predispose them to influenza complications. For all other contraindications to use of LAIV, see *MMWR* 2010;59(No. RR-8), available at http://www.cdc.gov/mmwr/pdf/rr/rr5908.pdf.
   • For children aged 6 months through 8 years:
     — For the 2011–12 season, administer 2 doses (separated by at least 4 weeks) to those who did not receive at least 1 dose of the 2010–11 vaccine. Those who received at least 1 dose of the 2010–11 vaccine require 1 dose for the 2011–12 season.
     — For the 2012–13 season, follow dosing guidelines in the 2012 ACIP influenza vaccine recommendations.

8. **Measles, mumps, and rubella (MMR) vaccine.** (Minimum age: 12 months)
   • The second dose may be administered before age 4 years, provided at least 4 weeks have elapsed since the first dose.
   • Administer MMR vaccine to infants aged 6 through 11 months who are traveling internationally. These children should be revaccinated with 2 doses of MMR vaccine, the first at ages 12 through 15 months and at least 4 weeks after the previous dose, and the second at ages 4 through 6 years.

9. **Varicella (VAR) vaccine.** (Minimum age: 12 months)
   • The second dose may be administered before age 4 years, provided at least 3 months have elapsed since the first dose.
   • For children aged 12 months through 12 years, the recommended minimum interval between doses is 3 months. However, if the second dose was administered at least 4 weeks after the first dose, it can be accepted as valid.

10. **Hepatitis A (HepA) vaccine.** (Minimum age: 12 months)
    • Administer the second (final) dose 6 to 18 months after the first.
    • Unvaccinated children 24 months and older at high risk should be vaccinated. See *MMWR* 2006;55(No. RR-7), available at http://www.cdc.gov/mmwr/pdf/rr/rr5507.pdf.
    • A 2-dose HepA vaccine series is recommended for anyone aged 24 months and older, previously unvaccinated, for whom immunity against hepatitis A virus infection is desired.

11. **Meningococcal conjugate vaccines, quadrivalent (MCV4).** (Minimum age: 9 months for Menactra [MCV4-D], 2 years for Menveo [MCV4-CRM])
    • For children aged 9 through 23 months 1) with persistent complement component deficiency; 2) who are residents of or travelers to countries with hyperendemic or epidemic disease; or 3) who are present during outbreaks caused by a vaccine serogroup, administer 2 primary doses of MCV4-D, ideally at ages 9 months and 12 months or at least 8 weeks apart.
    • For children aged 24 months and older with 1) persistent complement component deficiency who have not been previously vaccinated; or 2) anatomic/functional asplenia, administer 2 primary doses of either MCV4 at least 8 weeks apart.
    • For children with anatomic/functional asplenia, if MCV4-D (Menactra) is used, administer at a minimum age of 2 years and at least 4 weeks after completion of all PCV doses.
    • See *MMWR* 2011;60:72–6, available at http://www.cdc.gov/mmwr/pdf/wk/mm6003. pdf, and Vaccines for Children Program resolution No. 6/11-1, available at http://www. cdc.gov/vaccines/programs/vfc/downloads/resolutions/06-11mening-mcv.pdf, and *MMWR* 2011;60:1391–2, available at http://www.cdc.gov/mmwr/pdf/wk/mm6040. pdf, for further guidance, including revaccination guidelines.

Courtesy of the Centers for Disease Control and Prevention

This schedule is approved by the Advisory Committee on Immunization Practices (http://www.cdc.gov/vaccines/recs/acip), the American Academy of Pediatrics (http://www.aap.org), and the American Academy of Family Physicians (http://www.aafp.org).
Department of Health and Human Services • Centers for Disease Control and Prevention

Figure 27-2   The recommended schedule for persons ages 0–6 years is approved by the Advisory Committee on Immunization Practices (http://www.cdc.gov/vaccines/recs/acip), the American Academy of Pediatrics (http://www.aap.org), and the American Academy of Family Physicians (http://www.aafp.org).

Recommended immunization schedule for persons aged 7 through 18 years—United States, 2012 (for those who fall behind or start late, see the schedule below and the catch-up schedule

Vaccine ▼ Age ►	7–10 years	11–12 years	13–18 years	
Tetanus, diphtheria, pertussis[1]	1 dose (if indicated)	1 dose	1 dose (if indicated)	Range of recommended ages for all children
Human papillomavirus[2]	see footnote[2]	3 doses	Complete 3-dose series	
Meningococcal[3]	See footnote[3]	Dose 1	Booster at 16 years old	
Influenza[4]	Influenza (yearly)			Range of recommended ages for catch-up immunization
Pneumococcal[5]	See footnote 5			
Hepatitis A[6]	Complete 2-dose series			
Hepatitis B[7]	Complete 3-dose series			Range of recommended ages for certain high-risk groups
Inactivated poliovirus[8]	Complete 3-dose series			
Measles, mumps, rubella[9]	Complete 2-dose series			
Varicella[10]	Complete 2-dose series			

This schedule includes recommendations in effect as of December 23, 2011. Any dose not administered at the recommended age should be administered at a subsequent visit, when indicated and feasible. The use of a combination vaccine generally is preferred over separate injections of its equivalent component vaccines. Vaccination providers should consult the relevant Advisory Committee on Immunization Practices (ACIP) statement for detailed recommendations, available online at http://www.cdc.gov/vaccines/pubs/acip-list.htm. Clinically significant adverse events that follow vaccination should be reported to the Vaccine Adverse Event Reporting System (VAERS) online (http://www.vaers.hhs.gov) or by telephone (800-822-7967).

1. **Tetanus and diphtheria toxoids and acellular pertussis (Tdap) vaccine.** (Minimum age: 10 years for Boostrix and 11 years for Adacel)
   - Persons aged 11 through 18 years who have not received Tdap vaccine should receive a dose followed by tetanus and diphtheria toxoids (Td) booster doses every 10 years thereafter.
   - Tdap vaccine should be substituted for a single dose of Td in the catch-up series for children aged 7 through 10 years. Refer to the catch-up schedule if additional doses of tetanus and diphtheria toxoid–containing vaccine are needed.
   - Tdap vaccine can be administered regardless of the interval since the last tetanus and diphtheria toxoid–containing vaccine.

2. **Human papillomavirus (HPV) vaccines (HPV4 [Gardasil] and HPV2 [Cervarix]).** (Minimum age: 9 years)
   - Either HPV4 or HPV2 is recommended in a 3-dose series for females aged 11 or 12 years. HPV4 is recommended in a 3-dose series for males aged 11 or 12 years.
   - The vaccine series can be started beginning at age 9 years.
   - Administer the second dose 1 to 2 months after the first dose and the third dose 6 months after the first dose (at least 24 weeks after the first dose).
   - See MMWR 2010;59:626–32, available at http://www.cdc.gov/mmwr/pdf/wk/mm5920.pdf.

3. **Meningococcal conjugate vaccines, quadrivalent (MCV4).**
   - Administer MCV4 at age 11 through 12 years with a booster dose at age 16 years.
   - Administer MCV4 at age 13 through 18 years if patient is not previously vaccinated.
   - If the first dose is administered at age 13 through 15 years, a booster dose should be administered at age 16 through 18 years with a minimum interval of at least 8 weeks after the preceding dose.
   - If the first dose is administered at age 16 years or older, a booster dose is not needed.
   - Administer 2 primary doses at least 8 weeks apart to previously unvaccinated persons with persistent complement component deficiency or anatomic/functional asplenia, and 1 dose every 5 years thereafter.
   - Adolescents aged 11 through 18 years with human immunodeficiency virus (HIV) infection should receive a 2-dose primary series of MCV4, at least 8 weeks apart.
   - See MMWR 2011;60:72–76, available at http://www.cdc.gov/mmwr/pdf/wk/mm6003.pdf, and Vaccines for Children Program resolution No. 6/11-1, available at http://www.cdc.gov/vaccines/programs/vfc/downloads/resolutions/06-11mening-mcv.pdf, for further guidelines.

4. **Influenza vaccines (trivalent inactivated influenza vaccine [TIV] and live, attenuated influenza vaccine [LAIV]).**
   - For most healthy, nonpregnant persons, either LAIV or TIV may be used, except LAIV should not be used for some persons, including those with asthma or any other underlying medical conditions that predispose them to influenza complications. For all other contraindications to use of LAIV, see MMWR 2010;59(No.RR-8), available at http://www.cdc.gov/mmwr/pdf/rr/rr5908.pdf.
   - Administer 1 dose to persons aged 9 years and older.

   - For children aged 6 months through 8 years:
     — For the 2011–12 season, administer 2 doses (separated by at least 4 weeks) to those who did not receive at least 1 dose of the 2010–11 vaccine. Those who received at least 1 dose of the 2010–11 vaccine require 1 dose for the 2011–12 season.
     — For the 2012–13 season, follow dosing guidelines in the 2012 ACIP influenza vaccine recommendations.

5. **Pneumococcal vaccines (pneumococcal conjugate vaccine [PCV] and pneumococcal polysaccharide vaccine [PPSV]).**
   - A single dose of PCV may be administered to children aged 6 through 18 years who have anatomic/functional asplenia, HIV infection or other immunocompromising condition, cochlear implant, or cerebral spinal fluid leak. See MMWR 2010:59(No. RR-11), available at http://www.cdc.gov/mmwr/pdf/rr/rr5911.pdf.
   - Administer PPSV at least 8 weeks after the last dose of PCV to children aged 2 years or older with certain underlying medical conditions, including a cochlear implant. A single revaccination should be administered after 5 years to children with anatomic/functional asplenia or an immunocompromising condition.

6. **Hepatitis A (HepA) vaccine.**
   - HepA vaccine is recommended for children older than 23 months who live in areas where vaccination programs target older children, who are at increased risk for infection, or for whom immunity against hepatitis A virus infection is desired. See MMWR 2006;55(No. RR-7), available at http://www.cdc.gov/mmwr/pdf/rr/rr5507.pdf.
   - Administer 2 doses at least 6 months apart to unvaccinated persons.

7. **Hepatitis B (HepB) vaccine.**
   - Administer the 3-dose series to those not previously vaccinated.
   - For those with incomplete vaccination, follow the catch-up recommendations (Figure 3).
   - A 2-dose series (doses separated by at least 4 months) of adult formulation Recombivax HB is licensed for use in children aged 11 through 15 years.

8. **Inactivated poliovirus vaccine (IPV).**
   - The final dose in the series should be administered at least 6 months after the previous dose.
   - If both OPV and IPV were administered as part of a series, a total of 4 doses should be administered, regardless of the child's current age.
   - IPV is not routinely recommended for U.S. residents aged 18 years or older.

9. **Measles, mumps, and rubella (MMR) vaccine.**
   - The minimum interval between the 2 doses of MMR vaccine is 4 weeks.

10. **Varicella (VAR) vaccine.**
   - For persons without evidence of immunity (see MMWR 2007;56[No. RR-4], available at http://www.cdc.gov/mmwr/pdf/rr/rr5604.pdf), administer 2 doses if not previously vaccinated or the second dose if only 1 dose has been administered.
   - For persons aged 7 through 12 years, the recommended minimum interval between doses is 3 months. However, if the second dose was administered at least 4 weeks after the first dose, it can be accepted as valid.
   - For persons aged 13 years and older, the minimum interval between doses is 4 weeks.

Courtesy of the Centers for Disease Control and Prevention

This schedule is approved by the Advisory Committee on Immunization Practices (http://www.cdc.gov/vaccines/recs/acip), the American Academy of Pediatrics (http://www.aap.org), and the American Academy of Family Physicians (http://www.aafp.org). Department of Health and Human Services • Centers for Disease Control and Prevention

Figure 27-3 The recommended schedule for persons ages 7–18 years is approved by the Advisory Committee on Immunization Practices (http://www.cdc.gov/vaccines/recs/acip), the American Academy of Pediatrics (http://www.aap.org), and the American Academy of Family Physicians (http://www.aafp.org).

Catch-up immunization schedule for persons aged 4 months through 18 years who start late or who are more than 1 month behind —United States • 2012

The figure below provides catch-up schedules and minimum intervals between doses for children whose vaccinations have been delayed. A vaccine series does not need to be restarted, regardless of the time that has elapsed between doses. Use the section appropriate for the child's age. **Always use this table in conjunction with the accompanying childhood and adolescent immunization schedules and their respective footnotes.**

Vaccine	Minimum Age for Dose 1	Minimum Interval Between Doses			
		Dose 1 to dose 2	Dose 2 to dose 3	Dose 3 to dose 4	Dose 4 to dose 5
Persons aged 4 months through 6 years					
Hepatitis B	Birth	4 weeks	8 weeks and at least 16 weeks after first dose; minimum age for the final dose is 24 weeks		
Rotavirus[1]	6 weeks	4 weeks	4 weeks[1]		
Diphtheria, tetanus, pertussis[2]	6 weeks	4 weeks	4 weeks	6 months	6 months[2]
Haemophilus influenzae type b[3]	6 weeks	4 weeks if first dose administered at younger than age 12 months / 8 weeks (as final dose) if first dose administered at age 12–14 months / No further doses needed if first dose administered at age 15 months or older	4 weeks[3] if current age is younger than 12 months / 8 weeks (as final dose)[3] if current age is 12 months or older and first dose administered at younger than age 12 months and second dose administered at younger than 15 months / No further doses needed if previous dose administered at age 15 months or older	8 weeks (as final dose) This dose only necessary for children aged 12 months through 59 months who received 3 doses before age 12 months	
Pneumococcal[4]	6 weeks	4 weeks if first dose administered at younger than age 12 months / 8 weeks (as final dose for healthy children) if first dose administered at age 12 months or older or current age 24 through 59 months / No further doses needed for healthy children if first dose administered at age 24 months or older	4 weeks if current age is younger than 12 months / 8 weeks (as final dose for healthy children) if current age is 12 months or older / No further doses needed for healthy children if previous dose administered at age 24 months or older	8 weeks (as final dose) This dose only necessary for children aged 12 months through 59 months who received 3 doses before age 12 months or for children at high risk who received 3 doses at any age	
Inactivated poliovirus[5]	6 weeks	4 weeks	4 weeks	6 months[5] minimum age 4 years for final dose	
Meningococcal[6]	9 months	8 weeks[6]			
Measles, mumps, rubella[7]	12 months	4 weeks			
Varicella[8]	12 months	3 months			
Hepatitis A	12 months	6 months			
Persons aged 7 through 18 years					
Tetanus, diphtheria/ tetanus, diphtheria, pertussis[9]	7 years[9]	4 weeks	4 weeks if first dose administered at younger than age 12 months / 6 months if first dose administered at 12 months or older	6 months if first dose administered at younger than age 12 months	
Human papillomavirus[10]	9 years	Routine dosing intervals are recommended[10]			
Hepatitis A	12 months	6 months			
Hepatitis B	Birth	4 weeks	8 weeks (and at least 16 weeks after first dose)		
Inactivated poliovirus[5]	6 weeks	4 weeks	4 weeks[5]	6 months[5]	
Meningococcal[6]	9 months	8 weeks[6]			
Measles, mumps, rubella[7]	12 months	4 weeks			
Varicella[8]	12 months	3 months if person is younger than age 13 years / 4 weeks if person is aged 13 years or older			

1. **Rotavirus (RV) vaccines (RV-1 [Rotarix] and RV-5 [Rota Teq]).**
   - The maximum age for the first dose in the series is 14 weeks, 6 days; and 8 months, 0 days for the final dose in the series. Vaccination should not be initiated for infants aged 15 weeks, 0 days or older.
   - If RV-1 was administered for the first and second doses, a third dose is not indicated.
2. **Diphtheria and tetanus toxoids and acellular pertussis (DTaP) vaccine.**
   - The fifth dose is not necessary if the fourth dose was administered at age 4 years or older.
3. **Haemophilus influenzae type b (Hib) conjugate vaccine.**
   - Hib vaccine should be considered for unvaccinated persons aged 5 years or older who have sickle cell disease, leukemia, human immunodeficiency virus (HIV) infection, or anatomic/functional asplenia.
   - If the first 2 doses were PRP-OMP (PedvaxHIB or Comvax) and were administered at age 11 months or younger, the third (and final) dose should be administered at age 12 through 15 months and at least 8 weeks after the second dose.
   - If the first dose was administered at age 7 through 11 months, administer the second dose at least 4 weeks later and a final dose at age 12 through 15 months.
4. **Pneumococcal vaccines.** (Minimum age: 6 weeks for pneumococcal conjugate vaccine [PCV]; 2 years for pneumococcal polysaccharide vaccine [PPSV])
   - For children aged 24 through 71 months with underlying medical conditions, administer 1 dose of PCV if 3 doses of PCV were received previously, or administer 2 doses of PCV at least 8 weeks apart if fewer than 3 doses of PCV were received previously.
   - A single dose of PCV may be administered to certain children aged 6 through 18 years with underlying medical conditions. See age-specific schedules for details.
   - Administer PPSV to children aged 2 years or older with certain underlying medical conditions. See MMWR 2010:59(No. RR-11), available at http://www.cdc.gov/mmwr/pdf/rr/rr5911.pdf.

5. **Inactivated poliovirus vaccine (IPV).**
   - A fourth dose is not necessary if the third dose was administered at age 4 years or older and at least 6 months after the previous dose.
   - In the first 6 months of life, minimum age and minimum intervals are only recommended if the person is at risk for imminent exposure to circulating poliovirus (i.e., travel to a polio-endemic region or during an outbreak).
   - IPV is not routinely recommended for U.S. residents aged 18 years or older.
6. **Meningococcal conjugate vaccines, quadrivalent (MCV4).** (Minimum age: 9 months for Menactra [MCV4-D]; 2 years for Menveo [MCV4-CRM])
   - See Figure 1 ("Recommended immunization schedule for persons aged 0 through 6 years") and Figure 2 ("Recommended immunization schedule for persons aged 7 through 18 years") for further guidance.
7. **Measles, mumps, and rubella (MMR) vaccine.**
   - Administer the second dose routinely at age 4 through 6 years.
8. **Varicella (VAR) vaccine.**
   - Administer the second dose routinely at age 4 through 6 years. If the second dose was administered at least 4 weeks after the first dose, it can be accepted as valid.
9. **Tetanus and diphtheria toxoids (Td) and tetanus and diphtheria toxoids and acellular pertussis (Tdap) vaccines.**
   - For children aged 7 through 10 years who are not fully immunized with the childhood DTaP vaccine series, Tdap vaccine should be substituted for a single dose of Td vaccine in the catch-up series; if additional doses are needed, use Td vaccine. For these children, an adolescent Tdap vaccine dose should not be given.
   - An inadvertent dose of DTaP vaccine administered to children aged 7 through 10 years can count as part of the catch-up series. This dose can count as the adolescent Tdap dose, or the child can later receive a Tdap booster dose at age 11–12 years.
10. **Human papillomavirus (HPV) vaccines (HPV4 [Gardasil] and HPV2 [Cervarix]).**
    - Administer the vaccine series to females (either HPV2 or HPV4) and males (HPV4) at age 13 through 18 years if patient is not previously vaccinated.
    - Use recommended routine dosing intervals for vaccine series catch-up; see Figure 2 ("Recommended immunization schedule for persons aged 7 through 18 years").

Clinically significant adverse events that follow vaccination should be reported to the Vaccine Adverse Event Reporting System (VAERS) online (http://www.vaers.hhs.gov) or by telephone (800-822-7967). Suspected cases of vaccine-preventable diseases should be reported to the state or local health department. Additional information, including precautions and contraindications for vaccination, is available from CDC online (http://www.cdc.gov/vaccines) or by telephone (800-CDC-INFO [800-232-4636]).

Courtesy of the Centers for Disease Control and Prevention

Figure 27-4 Catch-up immunization schedule for persons aged 4 months–18 years who start late or who are more than one month behind.

scheduled according to the recommended vaccination schedule to promote and facilitate maintenance of the schedule.

Vaccine storage should follow specific manufacturer's guidelines. Some vaccine preparations require refrigeration or protection from light.

Vaccines have trade names, and manufacturers have been tested for safety. The package insert of each vaccine describes the vaccine including its route of administration, purpose, contraindications, and possible side effects (see Table 27-1). Because some vaccines are grown in

Table 27-1 Vaccine Administration Guidelines

Vaccine	Disease	About the Disease	Precautions and Contraindications	Side Effects and Adverse Reactions	Vaccine Schedule	Dose and Route of Administration
DTaP, DT, Td	Diphtheria, tetanus, pertussis	Diphtheria can cause breathing problems, paralysis, heart failure, and death; tetanus causes paralysis of the jaw—cannot open mouth or swallow; pertussis (whooping cough) causes severe coughing so infants have difficulty eating, drinking, or breathing or causes brain damage/death	Moderate to severe acute illness, neurologic disorder, allergic reaction to prior dose	Local reactions, fussiness, seizures, fever, allergic reaction	2 months, 4 months, 6 months, 15–18 months, 4–6 years; not given at 7 years or older	0.5 mL IM
Inactive poliovirus (IPV) *	Poliomyelitis	Causes paralysis of skeletal muscles and diaphragm so that infants cannot breathe on their own	Allergic reaction to prior dose or to neomycin, streptomycin, or polymixin B; moderate to severe acute illness; pregnancy	Local reactions, allergic reaction	2 months, 4 months, 16–18 months, 4–6 years (booster)	0.5 mL IM or SQ
Haemophilus influenzae type B (Hib)	Meningitis, pneumonia, epiglottitis, pericarditis	Causes bacterial meningitis, pneumonia, epiglottitis, septicemia, death	Moderate to severe acute illness, allergic reaction to prior dose	Fever, swelling, redness and/or pain; allergic reaction	2 months, 4 months, 6 months, 12–15 months (booster); children younger than 6 weeks old should not get vaccine	0.5 mL IM

continues

Table 27-1   Vaccine Administration Guidelines (*Continued*)

Vaccine	Disease	About the Disease	Precautions and Contraindications	Side Effects and Adverse Reactions	Vaccine Schedule	Dose and Route of Administration
Combination vaccines containing Hib • DTaP_Hib (TriHIBit) • Hepatitis B-Hib (Comvax)	Diphtheria, tetanus, pertussis, *Haemophilus influenzae*, hepatitis B and *Haemophilus influenzae*		Moderate to severe acute illness	Local reaction, allergic reaction	Cannot be used at 2 months, 4 months, or 6 months; may be used as booster 2 months, 4 months, 12–15 months; not given to infants younger than 6 weeks old	0.5 mL IM
Hepatitis A (HAV)	Hepatitis A	Anorexia, fatigue, itching, low-grade fever, nausea and vomiting, jaundice, death	Known allergies, pregnancy, decreased immune function	Redness, pain or swelling at the injection site, fever, loss of appetite, nausea and vomiting	Two doses given over a 6–18 month period beginning between the ages of 1 and 2 years	Less than or equal to 18 years old 0.5 mL IM
Hepatitis B (HBV)	Hepatitis B	Anorexia, fatigue, diarrhea, vomiting, liver damage, cancer, death	Pregnancy, moderate to severe acute illness, allergic reaction to baker's yeast	Mild systemic effects, soreness, fever, allergic reaction	Within 12 hours of birth, 1–2 months, 6 months (3 doses needed)	Less than or equal to 19 years of age 0.5 mL IM
Pediatrix, DTap, HepV, IPV	Diphtheria, tetanus, pertussis, *Haemophilus influenzae*, hepatitis B, inactive poliovirus		Moderate to severe acute illness	Mild systemic effects, local reaction, allergic reaction	2 months, 4 months, 6 months	0.5 mL IM
Td	Tetanus, diphtheria		Moderate to severe acute illness, severe allergic reaction to prior dose	Soreness; swelling; severe allergic reaction; deep, aching pain in muscles of upper arm(s)	7 years or older then every 10 years for life	0.5 mL IM

Table 27-1 Vaccine Administration Guidelines (*Continued*)

Vaccine	Disease	About the Disease	Precautions and Contraindications	Side Effects and Adverse Reactions	Vaccine Schedule	Dose and Route of Administration
MMR	Measles, mumps, rubella	Measles can cause otitis media, pneumonia, seizures, brain damage, death; mumps can cause fever, swollen glands, deafness, meningitis, swelling of testicles or ovaries, death; rubella can cause pregnant women to have miscarriages or babies born with severe anomalies	Do not give if allergic to gelatin or the antibiotic neomycin, moderate to severe acute illness, breastfeeding, pregnancy, immunosuppressed individuals	Fever, mild rash, swelling of glands in cheeks and neck, seizures, temporary pain in joints, severe allergic reaction	Two doses: 12–15 months and 4–6 years (or any age if longer than 28 days from first dose)	0.5 mL SQ
Varicella	Chickenpox	Severe skin infection, pneumonia, brain damage, death; shingles (herpes zoster) may occur years later	Do not give if allergic to gelatin or the antibiotic neomycin, moderate to severe acute illness	Soreness and swelling at site, fever, mild rash, seizures, pneumonia	12–18 months or any age if never had chickenpox	0.5 mL SQ
Influenza inactivated (IM) Live, intranasal (IN) Ages 5–49	Influenza (flu)	Fever, cough, chills, aches, death	Do not give to pregnant women, egg allergy, history of Guillain-Barré syndrome	Soreness, redness, fever, aches, allergic reaction	All children 6–23 months	6–35 months: 0.25 mL ≥ 3 years: 0.5 mL IM
Pneumococcal conjugate	Pneumonia, bacterial meningitis	Meningitis, septicemia, otitis media, pneumonia, deafness, brain damage	Moderate to severe illness, allergic reaction to prior dose	Redness, swelling at site, fever, drowsiness	2 months, 4 months, 6 months, 12–15 months	0.5 mL IM
Meningococcal conjugate	Meningitis	Infection of the brain and coverings of the spinal cord, septicemia, mental retardation, seizures, stroke, death	Severe allergic reaction to prior dose	Allergic reaction, redness or pain at site, fever	Not for children younger than 2 years (two doses needed 3 months apart)	0.5 mL IM

continues

Table 27-1 Vaccine Administration Guidelines (*Continued*)

Vaccine	Disease	About the Disease	Precautions and Contraindications	Side Effects and Adverse Reactions	Vaccine Schedule	Dose and Route of Administration
Rotavirus (ROTA)	Kawasaki disease	Severe diarrhea, vomiting, fever, dehydration; cause unknown; serious in children; inflammation of small and medium-sized arteries, including coronary arteries; no test to diagnose disease (signs and symptoms used to help diagnose)	Serious allergic reaction from previous vaccine dose, serious allergic reaction to vaccine component		2 months, 4 months, 6 months	2.0 mL oral

© Cengage Learning 2014

bird eggs weakened by addition of chemicals or are made from animals, it is essential to know what allergies a child has. For example, a child who is allergic to eggs cannot receive an MMR (measles, mumps, rubella), varicella, or influenza vaccine because of the possibility of the child being allergic to the egg protein that is used in the manufacturing of the vaccine. Symptoms of side effects, contraindications, and allergies must be known by the medical assistant, who will ensure that the parents are informed and have given written consent before the vaccines are given. After administration of vaccines (see Procedure 27-1), the medical assistant is responsible for documentation of the types of vaccines, site of administration, manufacturer's lot number, and side effects, if any have been reported by the parents (Figure 27-5). The provider will report any clinically significant adverse reactions to the Vaccine Adverse Event Reporting System (VAERS) and will file a VAERS Events Form for the National Immunization Program. Vaccine records can be kept electronically. All children must have a personal immunization record as part of their permanent medical record. It is mandated that the following information be included in the patient's electronic medical record with each immunization:

- Month, day, and year of administration
- Vaccine given
- Vaccine information sheet (VIS) given to a parent or guardian
- Manufacturer name
- Lot number and expiration date
- Site and route of administration
- Name, address, and title of health care provider giving the vaccine
- Source of vaccine: federal (F), state (S), private (P)

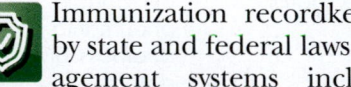 Immunization recordkeeping is mandated by state and federal laws. Total practice management systems include immunization recordkeeping as part of clinical care. Procedure 27-2 gives more information about maintaining immunization records.

Vaccines stimulate the immune system to produce antibodies against pathogens (see Chapter 22). Some patients may have conditions or preexisting conditions that would contraindicate vaccine administration. Safe vaccine administration requires assessment and recognition of conditions that would contraindicate vaccine administration at any specific time. When any vaccine is not given because of an existing contraindication, careful documentation and notification of the provider are required.

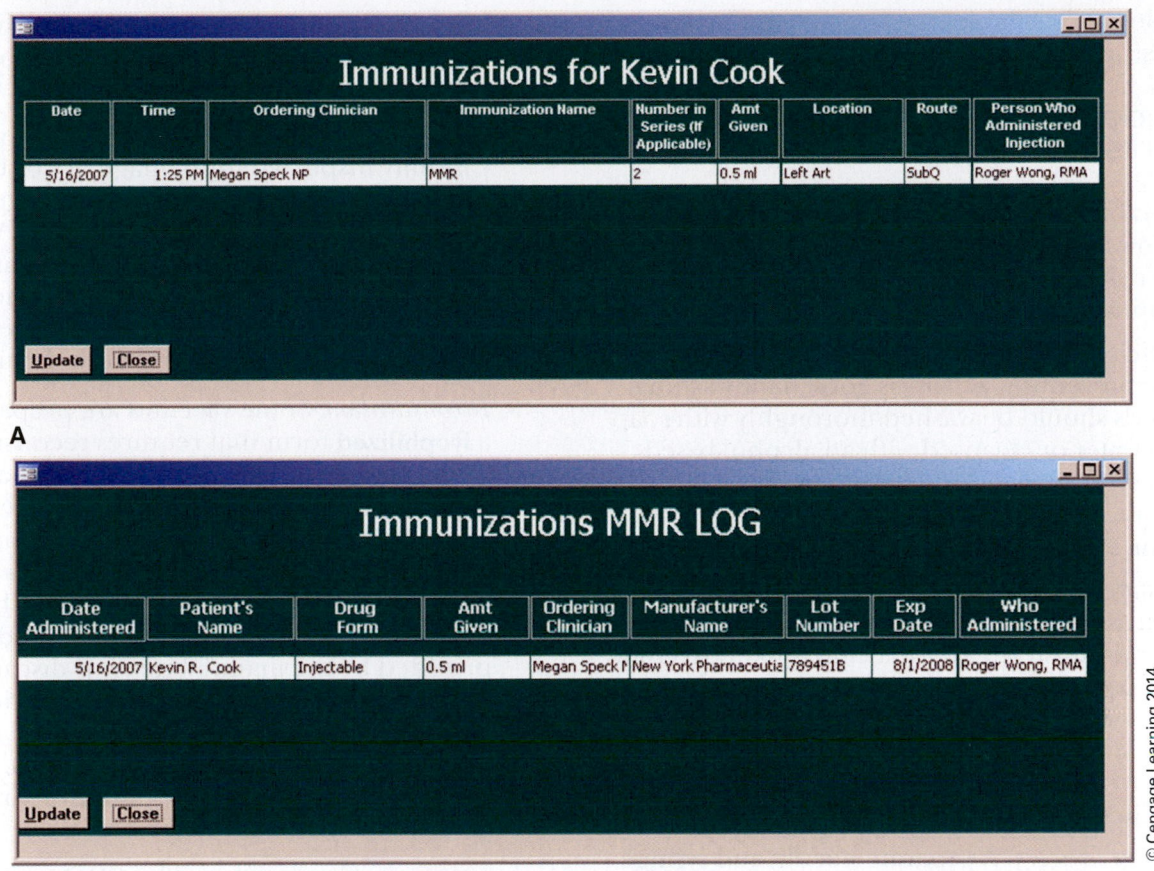

Date	Time	Ordering Clinician	Immunization Name	Number in Series (If Applicable)	Amt Given	Location	Route	Person Who Administered Injection
5/16/2007	1:25 PM	Megan Speck NP	MMR	2	0.5 ml	Left Art	SubQ	Roger Wong, RMA

A

Immunizations MMR LOG

Date Administered	Patient's Name	Drug Form	Amt Given	Ordering Clinician	Manufacturer's Name	Lot Number	Exp Date	Who Administered
5/16/2007	Kevin R. Cook	Injectable	0.5 ml	Megan Speck N	New York Pharmaceutic	789451B	8/1/2008	Roger Wong, RMA

B

© Cengage Learning 2014

Figure 27-5 Immunizations recorded in (A) a patient's electronic medical record and (B) in the practice's global immunization log for that vaccine.

Recommended Vaccination Schedule

The recommended vaccination schedule for infants and children is based on the premise that repeated doses of several vaccines are required and vaccine manufacturers recommend administering only compatible vaccines at any one visit to avoid drug interactions. If no contraindications are present at the various ages, vaccines should be administered according to the schedule to ensure complete vaccination by the age of 15 to 18 months, with

booster vaccines on school entry and again every 10 years throughout adult life. Should any vaccine be missed for any reason, vaccine "catch-up" schedules are available to ensure adequate vaccine administration (see Figure 27-4).

Considerations for Vaccine Administration

- *Infection control.* Health care providers should follow Standard Precautions to minimize the risks of spreading disease during vaccine administration.

- *Handwashing.* The single most effective disease prevention activity is good handwashing. Hands should be washed thoroughly with soap and water or cleansed with an alcohol-based waterless antiseptic between patients, before vaccine preparation, or any time hands become soiled (e.g., diapering, cleaning excreta).

- *Gloving.* Gloves are not required to be worn when administering vaccines unless the person administering the vaccine is likely to come into contact with potentially infectious body fluids or has open lesions on the hands. Clinic policy may require gloves be worn. It is important to remember that gloves cannot prevent needlestick injuries.

- *Syringe selection.* A separate needle and syringe should be used for each injection. A parenteral vaccine can be delivered in either a 1-mL or 3-mL syringe as long as the prescribed dosage is delivered. Syringe devices with engineered sharps injury protection are available, recommended by the Occupational Safety and Health Administration (OSHA), and required in many states to reduce the incidence of needlestick injuries and potential disease transmission. Personnel should be involved in evaluation and selection of these products. Staff should receive training with these devices before using them in the clinical area (see Table 27-2).

- *Needle selection.* Vaccine must reach the desired tissue site for optimal immune response. Therefore, needle selection should be based on the prescribed route, size of the individual, volume and viscosity of the vaccine, and injection technique. Typically, vaccines are not highly viscous; therefore, a fine-gauge needle (22–25 gauge) can be used (see Table 27-2).

- *Needle-free injection.* A new generation of needle-free vaccine delivery devices has been developed in an effort to decrease the risks of needlestick injuries to health care workers and to prevent improper reuse of syringes and needles. For more information on needle-free injection technology, see the Centers for Disease Control and Prevention (CDC) website: http://www.cdc.gov/nip/dev/jetinject.htm.

- *Inspecting vaccine.* Each vaccine vial should be carefully inspected for damage or contamination prior to use. The expiration date printed on the vial or box should be checked. Vaccine can be used up to and including the last day of the month indicated by the expiration date unless otherwise stated on the package labeling. Expired vaccine should never be used.

- *Reconstitution.* Some vaccines are prepared in a **lyophilized** form that requires reconstitution, which should be done according to manufacturer guidelines. Read package instructions carefully. Diluent solutions vary; use only the specific diluent supplied for the vaccine. Once reconstituted, the vaccine must be either administered within the time guidelines provided by the manufacturer or discarded. Changing the needle after reconstitution of the vaccine is not necessary unless the needle has become contaminated or bent. Continue with standard medication preparation guidelines.

- *Prefilling syringes.* The CDC strongly discourages filling syringes in advance because of the increased risk of administration errors. Once the vaccine is in the syringe, it is difficult to identify the type or brand of vaccine. Other problems associated with this practice are vaccine wastage and possible bacterial growth in vaccines that do not contain a preservative. Furthermore, medication administration guidelines state that the individual who administers a medication should be the one to draw up and prepare it. An alternative to prefilling syringes is to use filled syringes supplied by the vaccine manufacturer. Syringes other than those filled by the manufacturer are designed for immediate administration, not for vaccine storage. In certain circumstances, such as in large influenza clinics, more than one syringe can be filled. One person should prefill only a few syringes at a time, and the same person should administer them. Any syringes left at the end of the clinic day should be discarded. Under no circumstances should measles, mumps, and rubella (MMR), varicella, or zoster vaccines ever be reconstituted and drawn prior to the immediate need for them. These live virus vaccines are unstable and begin to deteriorate as soon as they are reconstituted with the diluent.

- *Labeling.* Once a vaccine is drawn into a syringe, the content should be indicated on the syringe. There are a variety of methods for identifying or labeling syringes (e.g., keep syringes with the appropriate vaccine vials, place the syringes in a labeled partitioned tray, use color-coded labels or preprinted labels).

- *Multiple vaccinations.* When administering multiple vaccines, never mix vaccines in the same syringe unless approved for mixing by the Food and Drug Administration (FDA). If more than one vaccine must be administered in the same limb, the injection sites should be separated by 1 to 2 inches so that any local reactions can be differentiated. It is best practice to utilize widely varied injection sites. For example, utilize bilateral vastus lateralis sites instead of two injections into the same muscle.

Vaccine doses range from 0.2 to 1 mL. The recommended maximum volume of medication for an intramuscular (IM) site varies among references and depends on the muscle mass of the individual. However, administering two IM vaccines into the same muscle would not exceed any suggested volume ranges for either the vastus lateralis or the deltoid muscle in any age group. The option to also administer a subcutaneous vaccine into the same limb, if necessary, is acceptable because a different tissue site is involved. If a vaccine and an immune globulin preparation are administered simultaneously (e.g., Td/Tdap and tetanus immune globulin [TIG] or hepatitis B vaccine and hepatitis B immune globulin [HBIG]), a separate anatomic site should be used for each injection. The location of each injection should be documented in the patient's chart or electronic medical record (Figure 27-6).

- *Nonstandard administration.* Deviation from the recommended route, site, and dosage of vaccine is strongly discouraged and can result in inadequate protection.

- *Needle gauge.* Use a 22- to 25-gauge needle.

- *Needle length.* For all IM injections, the needle should be long enough to reach the muscle mass and prevent vaccine from seeping into subcutaneous tissue, but not so long as to involve underlying nerves, blood vessels, or bone. The vaccinator should be familiar with the anatomy of the area into which the vaccine will be injected. Decision on needle size and site of injections must be made for each patient based on the size of the muscle, the thickness of adipose tissue at the injection site, the volume of the material to be

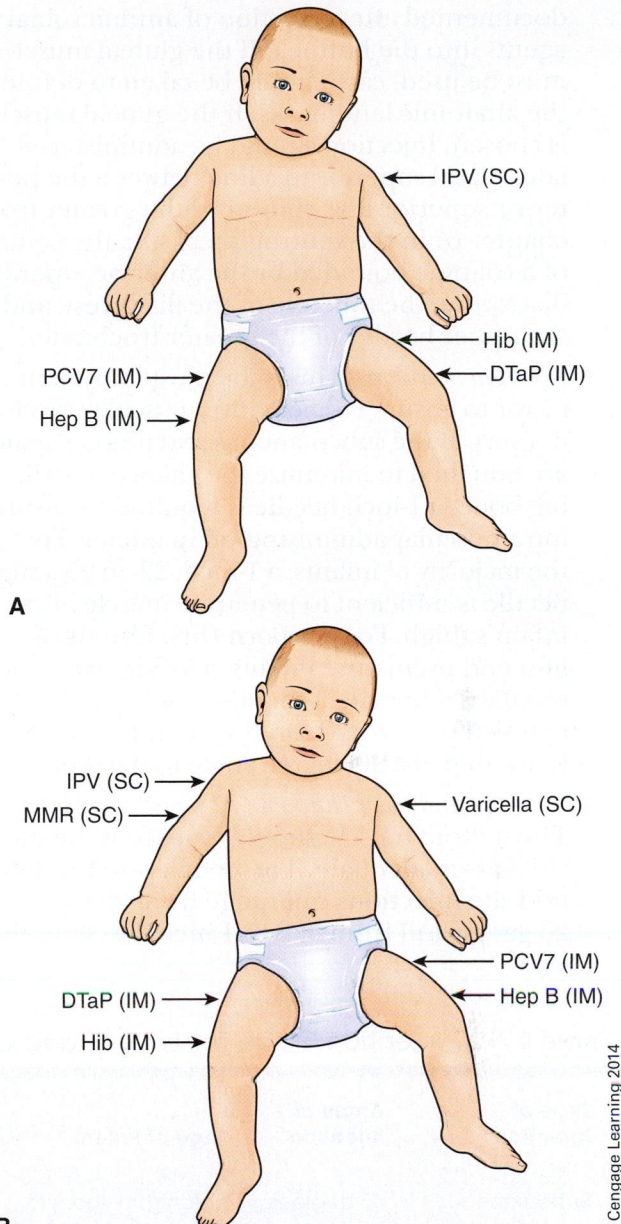

Figure 27-6 (A) An example of one way to give five doses at one visit. (B) An example of one way to give seven doses at one visit.

administered, the injection technique, and the depth below the muscle surface into which the material is to be injected (see Table 27-2).

- *Infants (younger than 12 months).* For the majority of infants, the anterolateral aspect of the thigh is the recommended site for injection because it provides a large muscle mass. The muscles of the buttock have not been used for administration of vaccines in infants and children because of concern about potential injury to the sciatic nerve, which is well documented after injection of antimicrobial agents into the buttock. If the gluteal muscle must be used, care should be taken to define the anatomic landmarks. If the gluteal muscle is chosen, injection should be administered lateral and superior to a line between the posterior superior iliac spine and the greater trochanter or in the ventrogluteal site, the center of a triangle bounded by the anterior superior iliac spine, the tubercle of the iliac crest, and the upper border of the greater trochanter.

- *Injection technique.* This is the most important factor to ensure efficient intramuscular vaccine delivery. If the subcutaneous and muscle tissue are bunched to minimize the chance of striking bone, a 1-inch needle is required to ensure intramuscular administration in infants. For the majority of infants, a 1-inch, 22- to 25-gauge needle is sufficient to penetrate muscle in an infant's thigh. For newborn (first 28 days of life) and premature infants, a 5/8-inch needle usually is adequate if the skin is stretched flat between thumb and forefinger and the needle is inserted at a 90-degree angle to the skin.

- *Toddlers and older children (12 months to 10 years).* The deltoid muscle should be used if the muscle mass is adequate. The needle size for deltoid site injections can range from 22 to 25 gauge and from 5/8 to 1 inch based on the

size of the muscle and the thickness of adipose tissue at the injection site. A 5/8-inch needle is adequate only for the deltoid muscle and only if the skin is stretched flat between thumb and forefinger and the needle is inserted at a 90-degree angle to the skin. For toddlers, the anterolateral thigh can be used, but the needle should be at least 1 inch long.

- *Adolescents and adults (11 years and older).* For adults and adolescents, the deltoid muscle is recommended for routine IM vaccinations. The anterolateral thigh can also be used. For men and women weighing less than 130 pounds (60 kg), a 5/8- to 1-inch needle is sufficient to ensure IM injection. For women weighing 130 to 200 pounds (60–90 kg) and men weighting 130 to 260 pounds (60–118 kg), a 1- to 1½-inch needle is needed. For women weighing more than 200 pounds (90 kg) or men weighing more than 260 pounds (118 kg), a 1½-inch needle is required.

Table 27-2 gives information on administering vaccines.

Giving Injections to Pediatric Patients

Infants and toddlers who have injections must be held in such a way that they cannot move. This is

Table 27-2 Injection Guide for Infants and Children

Type of Injection	Angle of Injection	Age of Patent	Needle Length	Needle Gauge	Injection Site
Subcutaneous	45 degrees	Infant (newborn to 12 months)	5/8"	23–25 gauge	Fatty subdermal tissue over anterolateral thigh muscle
	45 degrees	Children (12 months or older) adolescents and adults	5/8"	23–25 gauge	Fatty tissue over the triceps, abdomen, or anterior thigh over the quadriceps muscle
Intramuscular injection	90 degrees	Newborn (0 to 28 days)	5/8"	22–25 gauge	Vastus lateralis
	90 degrees	Infants (1 to 12 months)	1"	22–25 gauge	Vastus lateralis
	90 degrees	Toddlers (1 to 2 years)	5/8 to 1" / 1 to 1¼;"	22–25 gauge / 22–25 gauge	Deltoid muscle, vastus lateralis
	90 degrees	Children and teens (3 to 18 years)	5/8" to 1" / 1 to 1¼"	22–25 gauge / 22–25 gauge	Deltoid muscle, vastus lateralis

© Cengage Learning 2014

done for two reasons: to protect the child from injury and to provide access to an injection site. Parents must be informed of the procedure for administering injections. Their increased knowledge and understanding will allow the injection process to proceed with few complications.

For a child from birth to about 2 years of age, the vastus lateralis muscle is the preferred site. It is readily accessible when the infant is lying supine on the examination table.

Children who are 2 to about 4 years old are not emotionally developed enough to understand the need for cooperation. You will need help from the parent or another staff member to hold the child securely, thus avoiding injury. The deltoid is the preferred site for this age group. One method used to restrict the child's movement is to seat the child on the parent's lap. The parent wraps his or her legs around the child's legs to limit movement. The parent or staff member holds down the noninjection arm. The injection can be given once the child is securely immobilized.

Keep the syringe and needle out of the child's sight, because pediatric patients learn quickly that doctor clinic visits many times mean an injection, and with the injection comes some degree of fear and pain.

Do not tell the child that the injection will not hurt; rather, explain that it will sting for a short while, but it will help to keep him or her strong and healthy. A cartoon character adhesive strip applied to the site after the injection helps direct the child's attention away from the discomfort.

Although the vastus lateralis is the preferred site for intramuscular injections, the deltoid is used for subcutaneous pediatric injections (see Figures 27-7 and 27-8).

Clinical responsibilities for medical assistants during an immunization/well-baby visit include

How to Administer Intramuscular (IM) Vaccine Injections

Administer these vaccines by the intramuscular (IM) route: diphtheria-tetanus-pertussis (DTaP, Tdap); diphtheria-tetanus (DT, Td); *Haemophilus Influenzae* type b (Hib); hepatitis A (HepA); hepatitis B (HepB); human papillomavirus (HPV); inactivated influenza (TIV); quadrivalent meningococcal conjugate (MCV4); and pneumococcal conjugate (PCV). Administer inactivated polio (IPV) and pneumococcal polysaccharide (PPSV23) either IM or SC.

Patient age	Injection site	Needle size	Needle insertion
Newborn (0–28 days)	Anterolateral thigh muscle	⅝"* (22–25 gauge)	Use a needle long enough to reach deep into the muscle. Insert needle at a 90° angle to the skin with a quick thrust. (Before administering an injection of vaccine, it is not necessary to aspirate, i.e., to pull back on the syringe plunger after needle insertion.¶) Multiple injections given in the same extremity should be separated by a minimum of 1", if possible.
Infant (1–12 months)	Anterolateral thigh muscle	1"* (22–25 gauge)	
Toddler (1–2 years)	Anterolateral thigh muscle	1–1¼" (22–25 gauge)	
	Alternate site: Deltoid muscle of arm if muscle mass is adequate	⅝–1"* (22–25 gauge)	
Children (3–18 years)	Deltoid muscle (upper arm)	⅝–1"* (22–25 gauge)	
	Alternate site: Anterolateral thigh muscle	1–1¼" (22–25 gauge)	
Adults 19 years and older	Deltoid muscle (upper arm)	1–1½"*† (22–25 gauge)	
	Alternate site: Anterolateral thigh muscle	1–1½" (22–25 gauge)	

*A ⅝" needle usually is adequate for neonates (first 28 days of life) and preterm infants if the skin is stretched flat between the thumb and forefinger and the needle is inserted at a 90° angle to the skin.

†A ⅝" needle is sufficient in adults weighing less than 130 lbs (<60 kg) if the subcutaneous tissue is not bunched and the injection is made at a 90-degree angle; a 1" needle is sufficient in adults weighing 130–152 lbs (60–70 kg); a 1–1½" needle is recommended in women weighing 152–200 lbs (70–90 kg) and men weighing 152–260 lbs (70–118 kg); a 1½" needle is recommended in women weighing more than 200 lbs (>90 kg) or men weighing more than 260 lbs (>118 kg).

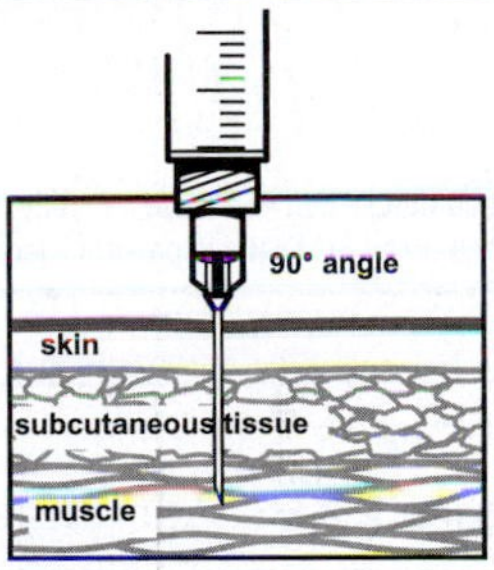

¶CDC. "ACIP General Recommendations on Immunization" at www.immunize.org/acip

90° angle

skin

subcutaneous tissue

muscle

IM site for infants and toddlers

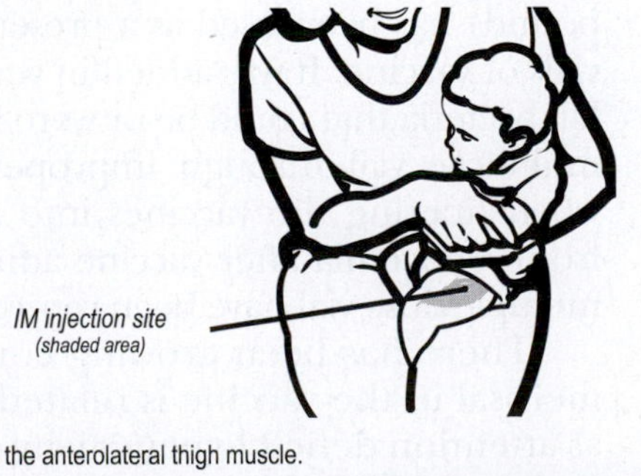

IM injection site (shaded area)

Insert needle at a 90° angle into the anterolateral thigh muscle.

IM site for children and adults

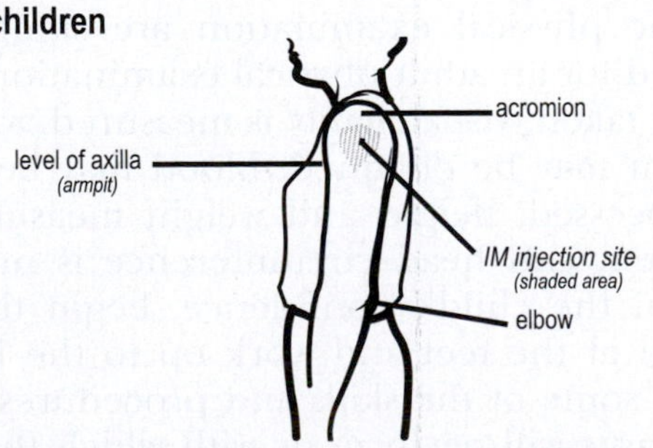

acromion

level of axilla (armpit)

IM injection site (shaded area)

elbow

Insert needle at a 90° angle into thickest portion of deltoid muscle — above the level of the axilla and below the acromion.

Technical content reviewed by the Centers for Disease Control and Prevention.

www.immunize.org/catg.d/p2020.pdf • Item #P2020 (8/12)

Immunization Action Coalition • 1573 Selby Ave. • St. Paul, MN 55104 • (651) 647-9009 • www.immunize.org • www.vaccineinformation.org • admin@immunize.org

From the Immunization Action Coalition, http://www.immunize.org

Figure 27-7 Administering intramuscular injections. The usual site for vaccine administration in infants is the vastus lateralis muscle of the upper thigh.

How to Administer Subcutaneous (SC) Vaccine Injections

Administer these vaccines by the subcutaneous (SC) route: measles, mumps, and rubella (MMR), varicella (VAR), meningococcal polysaccharide (MPSV4), and zoster (shingles [ZOS]). Administer inactivated polio (IPV) and pneumococcal polysaccharide (PPSV23) vaccines either SC or IM.

Patient age	Injection site	Needle size	Needle insertion
Birth to 12 mos.	Fatty tissue over the anterolateral thigh muscle	⅝" needle, 23–25 gauge	Pinch up on subcutaneous (SC) tissue to prevent injection into muscle. Insert needle at 45° angle to the skin. (Before administering an injection of vaccine, it is not necessary to aspirate, i.e., to pull back on the syringe plunger after needle insertion.*)
12 mos. and older	Fatty tissue over anterolateral thigh or fatty tissue over triceps	⅝" needle, 23–25 gauge	Multiple injections given in the same extremity should be separated by a minimum of 1". *CDC. "ACIP General Recommendations on Immunization" at www.immunize.org/acip

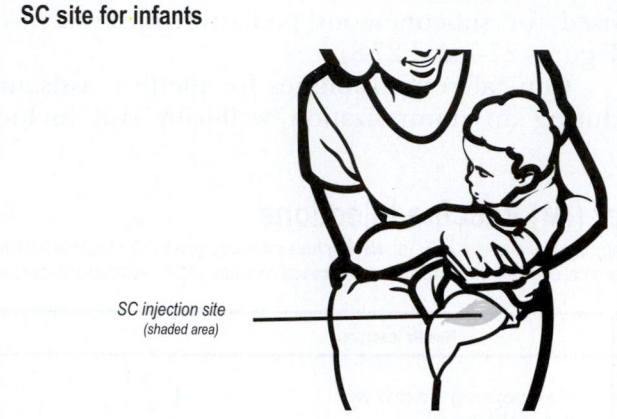

SC site for infants

SC injection site (shaded area)

Insert needle at a 45° angle into fatty tissue of the anterolateral thigh. Make sure you pinch up on SC tissue to prevent injection into the muscle.

SC site for children (after the 1st birthday) and adults

acromion

SC injection site (shaded area)

elbow

Insert needle at a 45° angle into the fatty tissue over the triceps muscle. Make sure you pinch up on the SC tissue to prevent injection into the muscle.

Technical content reviewed by the Centers for Disease Control and Prevention.

www.immunize.org/catg.d/p2020.pdf • Item #P2020 (8/12)

Immunization Action Coalition • 1573 Selby Ave. • St. Paul, MN 55104 • (651) 647-9009 • www.immunize.org • www.vaccineinformation.org • admin@immunize.org

From the Immunization Action Coalition, http://www.immunize.org

Figure 27-8 Administering subcutaneous injections. Subcutaneous tissue can be found all over the body. The usual sites for vaccine administration are the thigh (for infants) and the upper outer triceps of the arm (for children older than 12 months). If necessary, the upper outer triceps area can be used to administer subcutaneous injections to infants.

the same or similar procedures as the adult examination. The instruments used for the pediatric physical examination are similar to those used for an adult physical examination. Vital signs are taken, visual acuity is measured, a urine specimen may be obtained, blood may be drawn and processed, height and weight measurements are taken, and head circumference is measured. To gain the child's confidence, begin the examination at the feet and work up to the head. These are some of the skills and procedures medical assistants will perform or with which they will assist during the pediatric office or clinic visit.

It is important for the medical assistant to know that parents may ask about vaccine safety and preservatives. The following information is helpful; however, the provider is the best individual to answer specific questions parents may have.

Preservatives have been used in vaccines for more than 70 years. According to the CDC, thimerosol (an **organomercurial**, i.e., a mercury-containing compound) has been used as a preservative in multidose vials of vaccine. It was added in very small amounts to kill bacteria that could be or were introduced into the multidose vial through improper sterile technique when drawing the vaccines into a syringe. Fatalities from septicemia after vaccine administration using a multiple-dose vial have been reported.

There has been growing concern that the thimerosal in the vaccine is related to problems such as attention deficit hyperactivity disorder (ADHD), autism, and speech or language delays.

Many studies have been done over the last 30 years. The Institute of Medicine, the Immunization Safety Committee, the FDA, the CDC, and the National Institutes of Health (NIH) were involved throughout the studies. All have determined that there is no relationship between thimerosol and neurotoxicity from vaccine administration. The latest study in 2004 again investigated the situation and rejected the relationship between thimerosol and vaccines as a cause of neurotoxicity.

In 2000, the CDC, FDA, NIH, and the American Academy of Pediatrics (AAP) instructed the CDC to have thimerosol removed from all vaccines or to reduce it to trace amounts as soon as possible. There had been a movement by parents to remove all the preservatives. Parents still are involved in ongoing discussions about "reduced to trace amounts" in all routine vaccines for children 6 years and under. An exception, however, is inactivated flu vaccine. It contains thimerosol. A limited supply of preservative-free inactivated flu vaccine is available, but it is used for pregnant women, infants, and children. Perhaps over time all vaccines will be preservative-free. The CDC conducted a study in 2010 that indicated that exposure to thimerosol prenatally or as an infant does not increase the risk of autism spectrum disorder.

THEORIES OF GROWTH AND DEVELOPMENT

Before providing more in depth information about the various stages of growth and development in children, it is important to review the major theorists who contributed to understanding human growth and development.

There are at least eight or nine theories of human development put forth by Freud (psychosexual), Erickson (psychosocial), Sullivan (interpersonal), Piaget (cognitive), Kohlberg (moral), Bronfenbrenner (ecology), Pavlov, Skinner (behavioral), and Bandura (social learning). Each theory focuses on particular aspects of human development and its principles, strengths, and weaknesses.

No single theory can explain human development. The medical assistant can apply the theory or theories with relevance and understanding to each individual child or adult. This will allow for an inclusive approach to human development that is appropriate for children and families (Figure 27-9).

The following sections provide more information about growth and development at the various stages of a child's life (Figure 27-10).

Newborns

Even at a few days old, a newborn can imitate facial and manual gestures that adults make and can show a preference for certain colors (red, black, and white). The newborn can respond to auditory

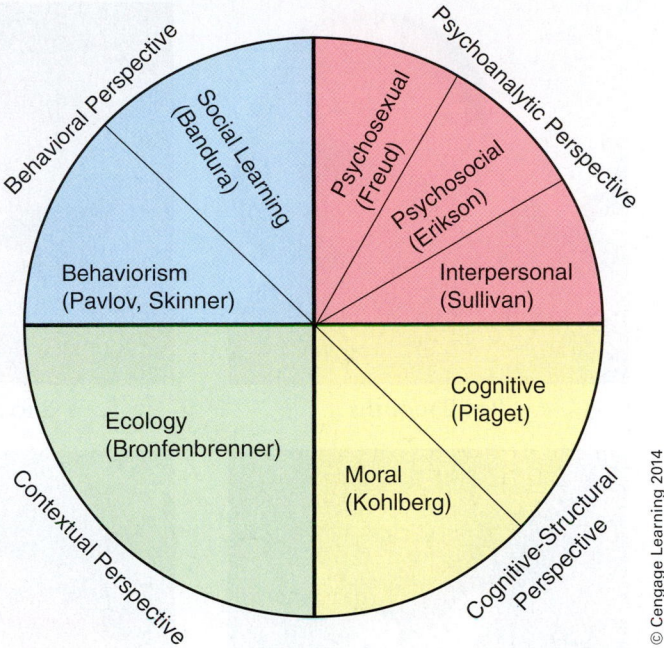

Figure 27-9 The eclectic nature of human development.

© Cengage Learning 2014

stimuli and is sensitive to being touched and handled. Respiratory rate is usually 30 to 60 breaths/minute; breaths are somewhat irregular in depth and rhythm, shallow and abdominal. The heart rate ranges from 110 to 130 beats/minute depending on whether the infant is awake or asleep. Urinary output is about 1 to 3 mL/hour or about 2 to 6 voidings a day.

Newborns can move and wiggle and can place themselves into dangerous or unsafe positions. One hand should always be kept on newborns whenever they are on top of any object because they can easily roll off. The safest place is in a crib with the sides raised.

It is important to note the vital signs at different ages will vary according to size, age, and gender. Comparisons can be made by finding values within the electronic medical record.

Infants

The infant stage is from 1 month to 1 year. Gross and fine motor skills develop starting at the head and moving toward the feet.

The infant usually doubles his or her birth weight during the first 6 months; by 12 months, birth weight has tripled. Height increases about 1 inch per month. By 12 months, the infant's height has slowed, and there can be a 50% increase from the birth length.

Head size changes quickly to accommodate fast brain growth. By 1 year old, the infant's brain

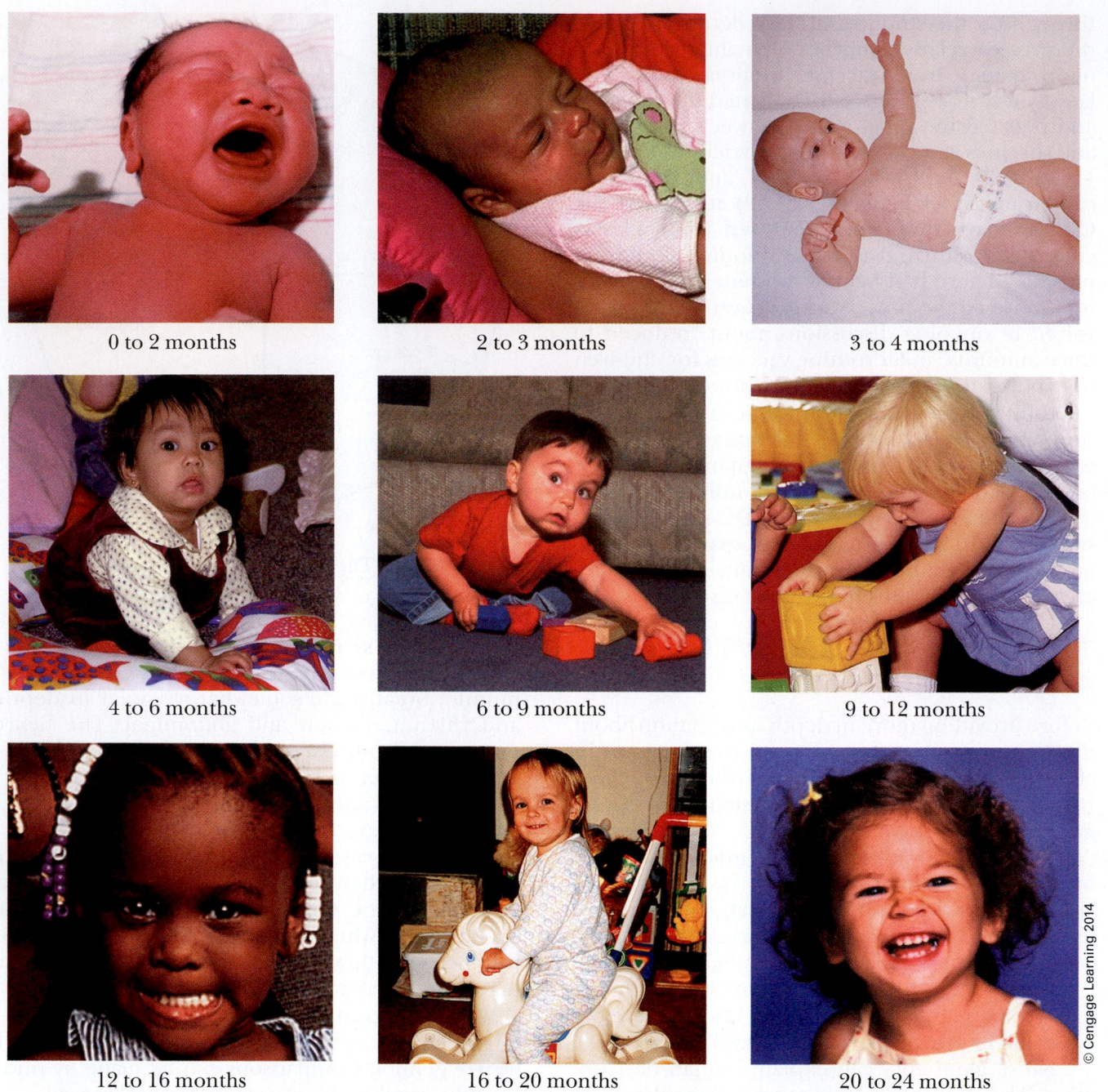

0 to 2 months   2 to 3 months   3 to 4 months

4 to 6 months   6 to 9 months   9 to 12 months

12 to 16 months   16 to 20 months   20 to 24 months

© Cengage Learning 2014

Figure 27-10 Growth and development stages of infants and toddlers.

is about 66% of the size of an adult brain, but growth does slow during the second 6 months of the first year. The **fontanels** (anterior and posterior) close by 2 months old (anterior) and 12 to 18 months old (posterior). The infant cannot control head movement until about 4 months old. This is known as "head lag," and the amount of head lag can be determined by pulling the infant by the arms from a supine to a sitting position. Because the infant cannot control the head, it will fall back until about 4 months old, at which time the infant has no head lag and can control the head while sitting.

Gross and fine motor development occurs quickly during the infant stage, but once developed, the infant can begin to walk, first with help, then alone. By 1 year old, in addition to being able to walk alone, the infant can feed himself or herself finger foods, grasp with his or her index finger and thumb, place and remove small objects from a container, and hold a crayon and make a mark with it.

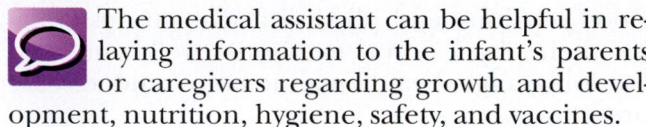 The medical assistant can be helpful in relaying information to the infant's parents or caregivers regarding growth and development, nutrition, hygiene, safety, and vaccines.

Toddlers

The toddler period covers 2 years in the child's life from about 1 to 3 years of age. During the toddler period, there is rapid change. The child is becoming more independent, is able to move about quickly, and is verbal and inquisitive. Environmental dangers are of utmost concern because of the toddler's rapid development of motor skills and lack of judgment. This is a time for discipline and guidelines but also for encouraging independence and natural curiosity. Most injuries and deaths occur as a result of airway obstruction, poisoning, drowning, falls, burns, and auto accidents.

During the 2 years that the toddler is developing, his or her physical growth slows. Height gain averages about 3 inches per year; weight gain is about 5 pounds per year. Most toddlers walk by 12 to 15 months old and climb stairs by 18 months old.

Bladder and bowel control usually occur during this period. Vital signs move closer to adult norms, respiration (25–30 breaths/minute awake) and pulse rates (96–105 beats/minute) slow, and blood pressure increases to greater than 90 mm Hg over 50 mm Hg. Serum lead levels are checked during this time.

It is during the toddler period that rapid onset of respiratory distress can occur, and there is an increase in tendency for airways to collapse. Otitis media, tonsillitis, and upper respiratory infections are common.

Often parents or caregivers are concerned their toddlers are eating little or they focus only on one particular food. Most toddlers eat when they are hungry and caregivers worry unnecessarily. The toddler is less interested in food because of his or her slowdown in growth, and thus fewer calories are needed.

Eating habits are established during the first 2 to 3 years of life, and good eating habits with children should start when they are toddlers. The early years are the time to teach lifelong healthy eating habits together with regular exercise. These two factors will significantly add years and quality of life because of disease prevention and maintenance of health. Many children in the United States are obese, perhaps because their parents are. A 2004 study reported in *Annals of Human Biology* found that almost half of children who were overweight at 1 year old were obese by 21 years old. The earlier that one can prevent obesity, the healthier one's children will be. Parents are their children's role models.

Preschoolers

The preschool years include ages 3 to 6 years. The child now has control over bowel and bladder, can dress and feed himself or herself, and can interact with others. During this period, preschoolers gain about 2 pounds of weight per year and 3 inches in height per year. Visual acuity rates decrease slightly.

The **Denver Developmental Screening Test** can be used to determine motor skills development levels. Running, jumping, skipping, jumping rope, and bike riding with training wheels usually occur in this time period. Preschoolers may begin to tie shoelaces.

Sexual curiosity is displayed, and questions about body parts, including genitalia, should be answered honestly. Children learn at this age that "private" body parts should not be touched by strangers.

Preschoolers learn through play and by imitating adult behaviors. It is now that children will play well with others and share. Preschoolers are creative and use their imaginations well.

During preschool years, a yearly physical examination should be done to note growth, vision, hearing, and blood pressure. Laboratory work includes a test for lead exposure, a tuberculosis test (once before beginning school), and a lipid profile. This age group suffers from otitis media, upper respiratory infections, and common stomach viruses. Teaching children the importance of good handwashing techniques and its significance in preventing illness is important.

Some preschoolers may refuse to eat for a few days or prefer one particular food every day. Parents and caregivers should avoid issues over these matters. Instead, spend mealtimes in a pleasant way.

Regular physical activity is beneficial because it helps develop lifetime habits of exercise, leading to disease prevention and health promotion. Sports are an ideal way to get preschoolers active and to have fun. Noncompetitive activities such as

CRITICAL THINKING

May Mobley has an appointment today for her 18-month checkup. She will be receiving her appropriate immunizations and the provider has asked that you perform a Denver Developmental Screening Test to assure that May is meeting her developmental benchmarks. After assessment, you see that May is delayed in several language activities. What is your best course of action?

dance, T-ball, karate, gymnastics, and bicycling also keep children active and healthy. Love of reading can be established now, especially when parents/caregivers read to their youngsters.

Playing near the road is an area of great concern for these children. They will listen to adults who set limits for their safety.

School-Aged Children

The school-aged group encompasses children from 6 to 12 years of age. A steady progression in children's rate of growth occurs during these years. Weight increases by about 5 pounds per year, and height increases about 2 inches per year. Muscle size increases, and the following motor skills continue to improve: climbing, running, jumping, throwing, catching, and balancing.

The circulatory and respiratory functions develop. The pulse and respiration rates slow. The pulse rate in this age group is about 90 beats/minute; the average respiration rate is about 20 breaths/minute. Both rates are while the children are at rest.

This period shows relatively few infectious diseases because of the immunity the children developed to microorganisms during their preschool years.

The last years of the school-aged period are known as prepuberty. Breast development, axillary and pubic hair, and body odor may appear as early as 9 or 10 years of age.

Peers begin to play a major role, and children seek support from their peers to begin gaining independence from their parents and family. Children have a sense of accomplishment when they focus their energy on sports, hobbies, and schoolwork and see themselves succeed in these activities.

Language is the way to communicate, and children use their language skills to socialize with their family and peers.

Usually school-aged children experience excellent health, and when they do become ill, it is usually a minor illness. The AAP recommends routine physical examinations about every 2 years, at ages 5, 6, 8, 10, 11, and 12 years. Height, weight, vital signs, physical examination, vision and hearing tests, review of nutrition, scoliosis screening, and tuberculosis testing are checked. Use of recreational drugs, tobacco, and alcohol is addressed.

Booster immunizations of DPT (diphtheria, pertussis, tetanus) and MMR (measles, mumps, rubella) are typically given between 4 and 6 years of age. Tetanus and diphtheria (Td) is usually repeated every 10 years.

Nutrition education is an ongoing process and children should be taught to eat breakfast daily and to make intelligent, healthy food choices.

Good nutrition and physical activity are essential for their physical and emotional well-being and for long-range health maintenance and disease prevention.

Accidents in this age group are the leading cause of death. The increased independence, need for their peer's approval, and increased involvement in physically challenging activities are some of the reasons. Most injuries are related to auto accidents and firearms. Violent crimes against children in this age group have increased dramatically in the last 20 years.

School-aged children comprehend rules about safety with regard to automobiles, bikes, swimming, and firearms, but they frequently resist these rules.

This group of children suffers from not looking the "same" as their peers, bullying, stress (peer pressure, divorce, drugs), and both parents/caregivers working and not being home when the children go home after school (latchkey children).

Adolescents

The adolescent period of growth and development is noticeable for its wide range of physiologic changes. It is the period between 11 and 21 years of age. During adolescence, there is a large growth spurt with gains in weight and height that occur rapidly. Boys can gain up to about 14 pounds and grow as much as 6 inches; girls gain up to about 10 pounds and grow up to 5 inches. Girls usually attain their adult height about 1 year before onset of menses; boys reach their adult height at about 13 years old, after axillary and pubic hair appear.

The average heart rate is about 60 to 70 beats/minute; average blood pressure is 100/50 to 120/70 mm Hg. Girls have a slightly higher pulse and body temperature than boys; girls' systolic blood pressure is a bit less. Respiration rates in both sexes average about 16 to 20 breaths/minute.

Adolescents direct their energy to nonfamily relationships and career goals. It is a time of conflict as adolescents try to become independent from their parents and establish their own identities.

The Department of Adolescent Health of the American Medical Association urges annual health screenings that focus not only on the physiologic and psychological health of the adolescent, but also on such matters as physical activity, birth control, recreational drugs, alcohol, depression, suicide ideation, injury prevention, and school accomplishments.

 Laboratory tests include human immunodeficiency virus (HIV) and other sexually transmitted diseases (gonorrhea, syphilis, chlamydia, and hepatitis B and C if sexually active). Tuberculosis testing is also recommended. The physical examination is comprehensive and includes vital signs, height and weight, vision and hearing testing, urinalysis, and complete blood count (CBC). At this time, the provider discusses issues of injury prevention (wearing seat belts, helmets for biking, no drinking and driving, contact sports, among others), violence prevention (gang memberships and anger management), nutrition (fast foods, high-sodium and fatty foods), how to avoid becoming overweight and obese, and regular physical activity. Motor vehicle accidents cause 50% of teenage deaths between ages 16 and 19 years, and they are common in drivers who use alcohol or other drugs.

 To be effective at all stages of growth and development, the medical assistant must understand the age and maturity level of pediatric patients, the psychological changes that occur, and the psychosocial aspects of the child at various ages.

   Communication with pediatric patients needs to be individualized, showing acceptance, empathy, honesty, and openness. Confidentiality must be maintained regardless of age. Parents and caregivers are involved with the care of their youngsters; therefore, they have the legal right to know the medical matters relating to their minor children. Adolescents may share information with the medical assistant that they do not want their parents or caregivers to know. It is important to stress that some matters may need to be shared with parents or caregivers, especially when adolescents are living at home (certain matters pertaining to birth control, abortion, pregnancy, and sexually transmitted diseases pose special problems). Some states allow minors to give their consent under these circumstances (see Chapter 7).

 Medical assistants can teach parents and caregivers in various ways. Handouts, demonstrations, videos, and one-on-one instruction are helpful in keeping children safe and healthy.

  The medical assistant must be caring, respectful, supportive, and nonjudgmental of all patients. The caregiver to pediatric patients must reflect these values. Family beliefs and values also must be taken into account. This will foster care for pediatric patients that is compliant and in the best interest of all.

GROWTH PATTERNS

Growth patterns provide valuable information to the pediatrician regarding the infant's physical progress. They are also used to calculate pediatric doses of medication. Height, weight, and head circumference are measured at each regularly scheduled appointment at the pediatric facility. The measurements are then plotted on a physical growth percentile chart that is part of the patient's permanent record (Figure 27-11). Careful measuring of the infant or child and monitoring of growth patterns are essential and should be done in a consistent and accurate manner.

Length and Weight Measurements

To record or plot length and weight measurements, you must first locate one growth value, either length or weight, in the vertical columns of the physical growth percentile chart shown in Figure 27-12. Find the child's age in months in the horizontal rows. Locate the area where the growth value lines intersect on the graph and plot the length and weight by marking with a dot. Connect dots from previous values with a ruler to provide a neat and accurate graphic recording. The date, age, measurements, and comments should also be indicated at the bottom of the chart.

The curved lines printed across the growth charts show the normal range of growth of infants and children in the United States. The numbers on the right side of the chart, in the vertical boxes between age 34 and 35 months, show the percentiles of other children the same age. To determine into which percentile the infant falls in relation to other infants of the same age, follow the line (percentile) upward to the percentage values along the edge of the graph. The National Center for Health Statistics (NCHS) growth charts become a permanent record of the child's development. These give the provider a quick way to check the child's growth in relation to that of other children the same age. Growth charts aid in the diagnosis of growth abnormalities and nutritional disorders and disease. Hereditary factors also influence growth patterns; therefore, having the family's history is important.

Infant Holds and Positions

Lifting and carrying infants must be done safely. The medical assistant should be especially careful of the infant's neck. It should be supported

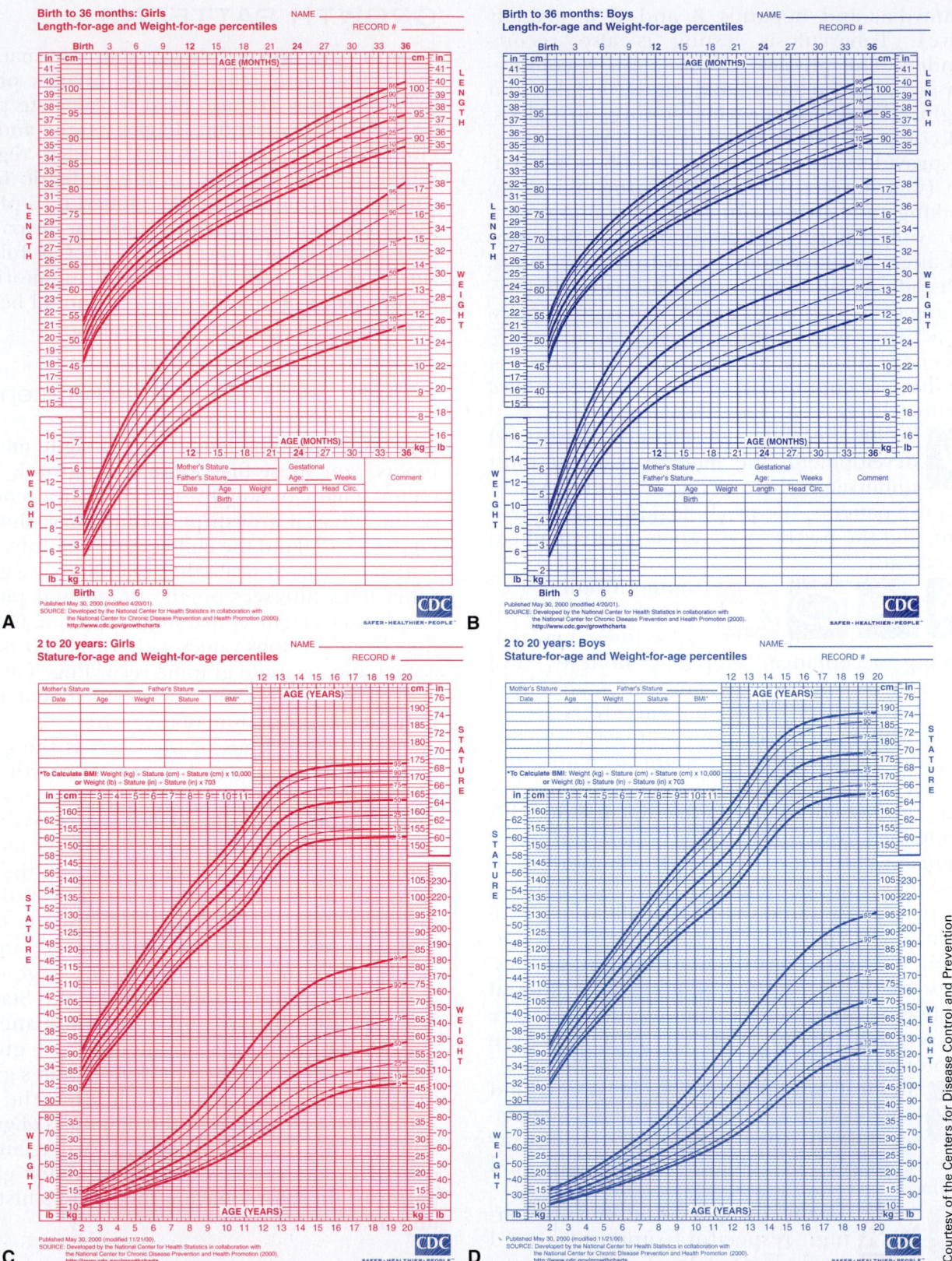

Figure 27-11 (A) Growth chart for girl's height and weight, age birth to 36 months. (B) Growth chart for boy's height and weight, age birth to 36 months. (C) Growth chart for girl's height and weight, age 2 to 20 years. (D) Growth chart for boy's height and weight, age 2 to 20 years. (Note that the growth charts shown in (A) and (B) provide space at bottom right of chart for date, age, weight, length and head circumference.)

Courtesy of the Centers for Disease Control and Prevention

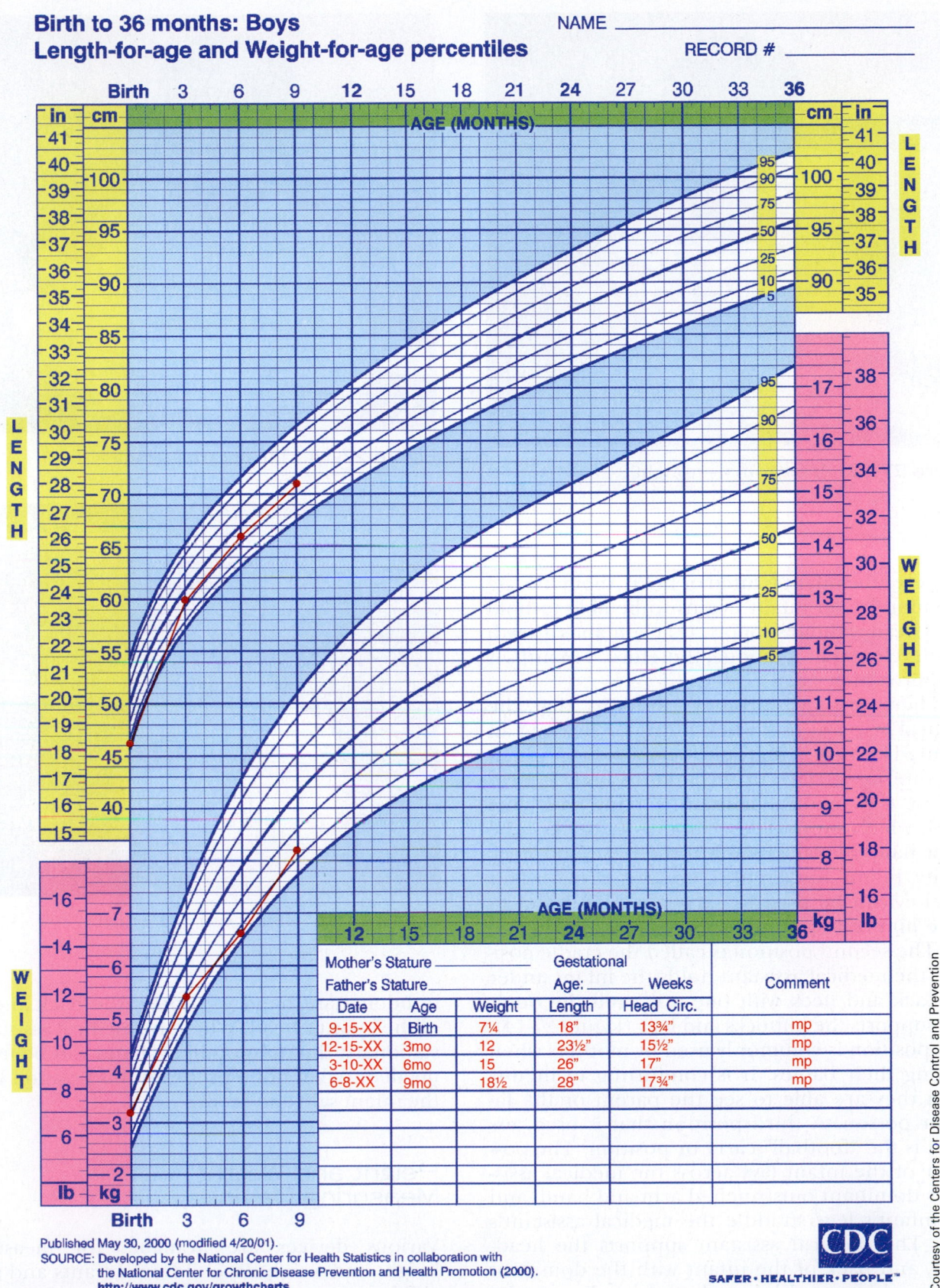

Birth to 36 months: Boys
Length-for-age and Weight-for-age percentiles

NAME _____

RECORD # _____

	Mother's Stature _____		Gestational			
	Father's Stature _____		Age: _____ Weeks			Comment
Date	Age	Weight	Length	Head Circ.		
9-15-XX	Birth	7¼	18"	13¾"		mp
12-15-XX	3mo	12	23½"	15½"		mp
3-10-XX	6mo	15	26"	17"		mp
6-8-XX	9mo	18½	28"	17¾"		mp

Published May 30, 2000 (modified 4/20/01).
SOURCE: Developed by the National Center for Health Statistics in collaboration with
the National Center for Chronic Disease Prevention and Health Promotion (2000).
http://www.cdc.gov/growthcharts

CDC
SAFER·HEALTHIER·PEOPLE™

Courtesy of the Centers for Disease Control and Prevention

Figure 27-12 Sample growth chart information plotted at birth, 3, 6, and 9 months. Sections in this figure are highlighted to help you locate the values: length (yellow), weight (pink), age (green), and percentiles (white).

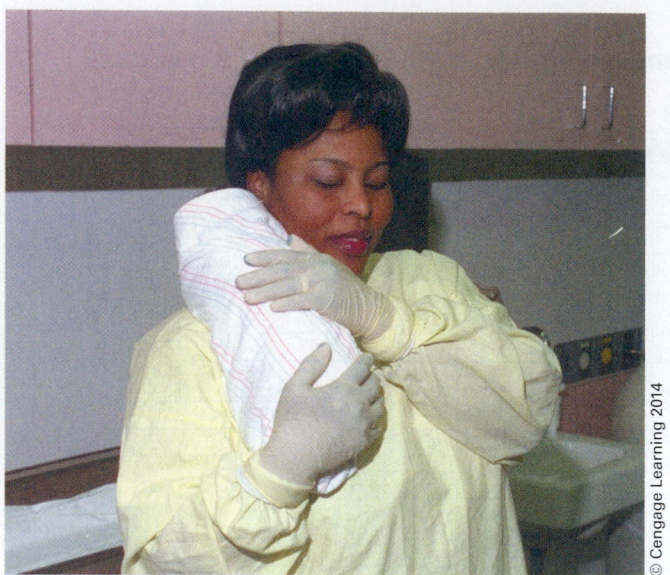

Figure 27-13 Infant carry—upright.

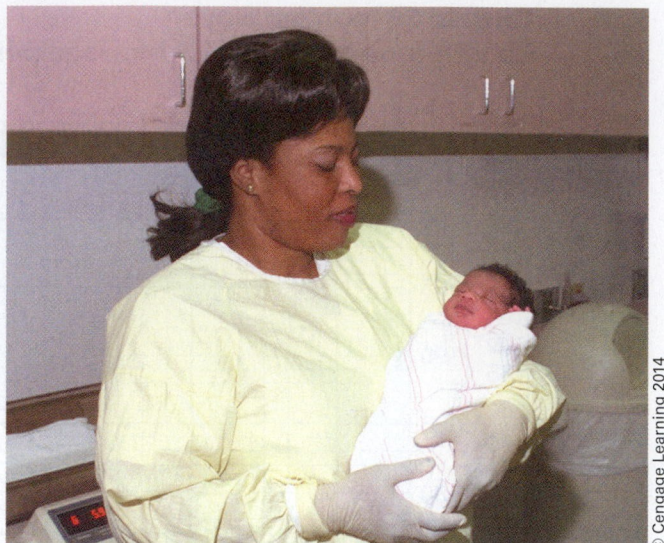

Figure 27-14 Infant carry—cradle.

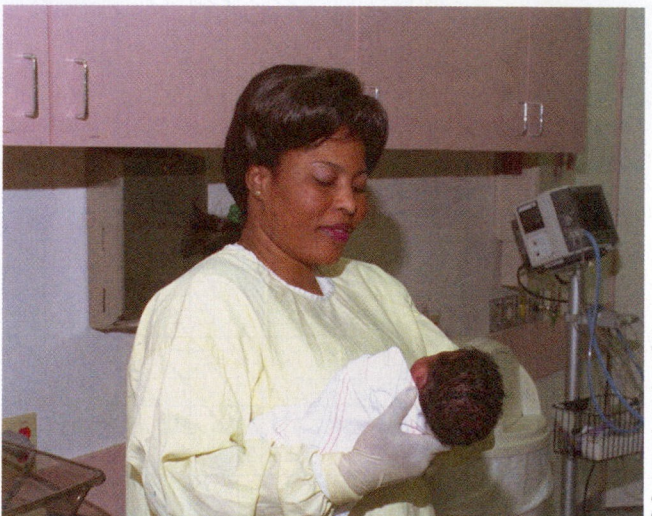

Figure 27-15 Infant carry—football.

whenever the infant is lifted or held. About the age of 4 months, an infant begins to be able to hold up its head without support. (Each infant's growth and development is unique; therefore, 4 months is an approximate age.)

There are two primary positions that the medical assistant uses when lifting or carrying an infant. The first is the upright position in which the anterior surface of the infant's body is held against the medical assistant's body with one hand, which supports the infant's buttocks. The other hand is placed behind the head and neck of the infant for support (Figure 27-13). This position can be used to carry the infant and to place him or her on the scale or examination table. The second position is called the cradle position; the medical assistant holds the infant under the back and neck with one arm, and the other arm supports the buttocks and legs (Figure 27-14). This position is commonly used by mothers when feeding their babies. It is comforting to infants when they are able to see the parent or the familiar person. A third position that is used less often is the "football" carry or position. The posterior of the infant lays across the medical assistant's dominant outstretched arm and hand, and the infant's legs straddle the medical assistant's arm. The medical assistant supports the head, neck, and back of the infant with the dominant hand and arm and keeps the infant close to the body (Figure 27-15). If transporting the infant in this position, the medical assistant uses the nondominant hand to protect the back and top of the infant's head. When the medical assistant is stationary, the nondominant hand can be used if needed. When done properly, this position keeps the infant safe and secure.

Height and Weight Measuring Devices

Various devices are available for measuring height and weight in children. Infants and small children are weighed on an infant platform scale, which provides a measurement in pounds and ounces and kilograms and grams (Figure 27-16).

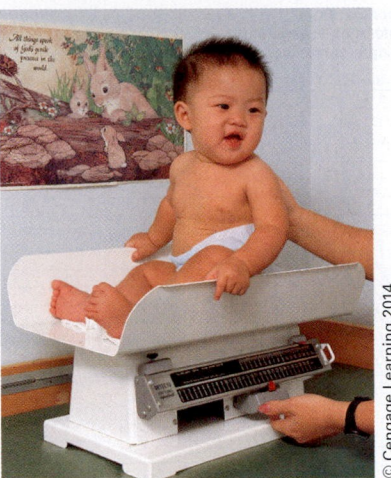

Figure 27-16 Infants who are able to sit and small children can be weighed on a platform scale.

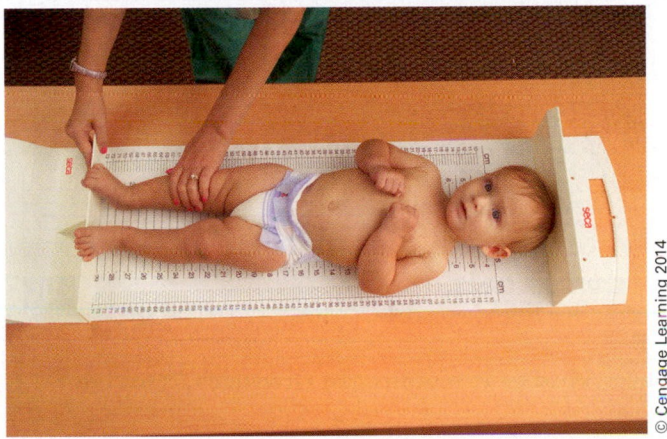

Figure 27-17 Measuring the recumbent length of an infant, from the vertex of the head to the heel.

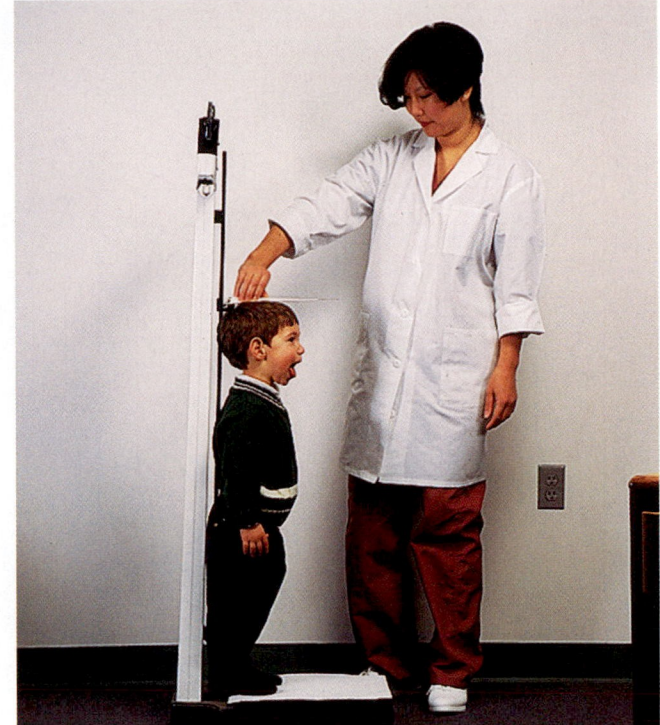

Figure 27-18 Measuring height in children.

The scale has a platform with curved sides in which the child may sit or lie. Weigh the infant or child in as few clothes as possible, removing the diaper and shoes or slippers. A small sheet, cloth diaper, or paper towel should be placed on the scale before weighing the infant or child, to avoid the transfer of microorganisms from bare skin. (The scale is sanitized and disinfected between patients.)

Infant length can be measured using an infant measuring board, which consists of a rigid headboard and movable footboard. Place the measuring board on a table and position the infant on his or her back on the board, with the head touching the headboard. Move the footboard up until it touches the bottom of the infant's feet (Figure 27-17).

An infant can also be measured on a pad by placing a pin into the pad or making a pencil mark at the top of the head and a second pin or mark at the heel of the extended leg. The length is the distance between the two pins. A tape measure can also be used. *NOTE:* 1 inch = 2.54 cm.

A stature-measuring device can be used to measure height once the child is able to stand erect without support. The device consists of a movable headpiece attached to a rigid measuring bar and platform (Figure 27-18). A paper towel should be placed on the platform before use to avoid the potential transmission of microorganisms from bare feet.

Measuring Head Circumference

Head circumference measurement is routinely recorded on an infant's chart to alert the provider to any abnormal development. This procedure should be performed during routine visits until the child is 36 months old. Thereafter, it should be measured on a yearly basis until the age of 6 years. Head circumference measurement requires a flexible paper or metal measuring tape. A cloth tape may stretch and give a false measurement. Head circumference is plotted similarly to height and

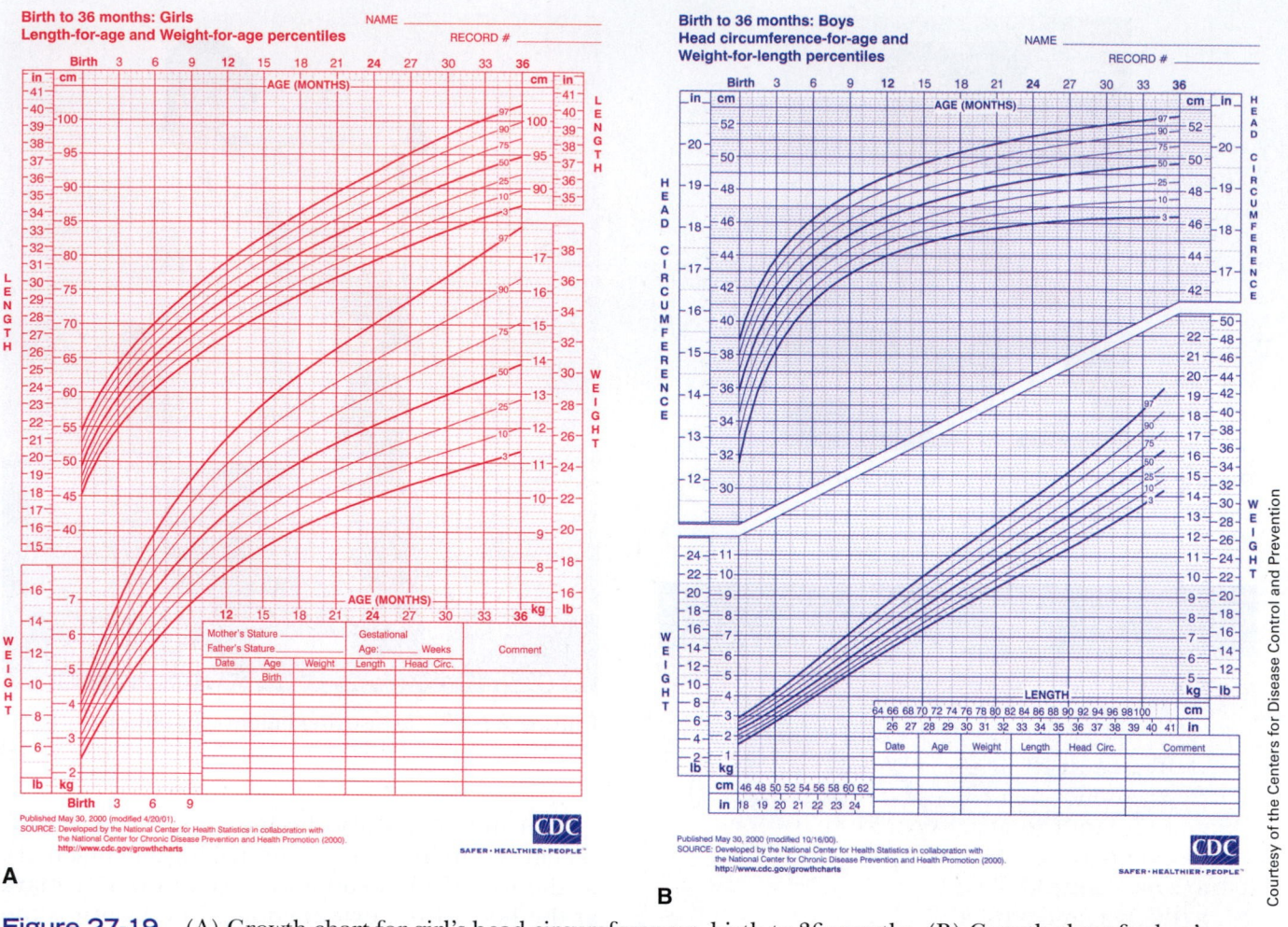

Figure 27-19   (A) Growth chart for girl's head circumferences, birth to 36 months. (B) Growth chart for boy's head circumferences, birth to 36 months.

weight but on separate growth percentile charts for head measurements (Figure 27-19). Generally, head and chest circumference are equal at about 1 to 2 years of age. Rapid growth above the normal percentile may indicate hydrocephalus, a disorder in which excessive fluid accumulates around the brain causing an increase in intracranial pressure and possible brain damage. This could lead to mental and physical problems. Conversely, the growth of the head that falls below the normal percentile may indicate microencephaly caused by a premature closure of the fontanels. In this instance, there is not enough room for the development of the brain, and mental retardation can result. Head circumference for a newborn should be between 12.5 and 14.5 inches or 31.75 and 36.83 cm.

Measuring Chest Circumference

Measuring the chest circumference of an infant is not normally performed during routine examinations. It may be performed and monitored when

there is a suspicion of overdevelopment or underdevelopment of the heart or lungs or calcification of rib cartilage. To measure the chest of an infant, snugly wrap the measuring tape around the chest at nipple level. It is preferable to read the measurement during the resting phase between respirations.

Occasionally it is necessary for the medical assistant to convert measurement results into inches or centimeters. To accomplish the task accurately, note that 1 inch equals 2.54 cm. (Procedure 27-3 gives steps for measuring infant chest and head circumference, weight, and height.)

Example: To convert inches to centimeters, multiply the number of inches by 2.54:

10 Inches × 2.54 = 25.4 Centimeters

Example: To convert centimeters to inches, divide the number of centimeters by 2.54:

10 Centimeters ÷ 2.54 = 25.4 Inches

Infant/Child Failure to Thrive

Sometimes an infant or child does not meet the expected standards of growth. The failure of an infant or a child to grow and thrive may have many organic and inorganic causes. There may be social and emotional causes. Many causes of an infant or a child failing to grow and thrive may be treated if found in time. The emotionally deprived infant needing affection will not grow because of lack of growth hormone production. Once this child is given physical and emotional warmth, the growth hormone is produced and the child will grow. Other reasons for an infant failing to thrive may be because the infant has a chronic disease; has a diet that is inadequate especially in calories and proteins; has a disorder of the heart, brain, or kidneys; or has been improperly fed. Adequate nutrition is especially critical in the first few years of life to assure physical growth and development.

PEDIATRIC VITAL SIGNS

As with older children and adults, pediatric vital signs are commonly taken by the medical assistant. The vital signs are more fully covered in Chapter 24 for adult patients; however, specific procedures for taking an infant's temperature, pulse, respiration, and blood pressure are explained here. These procedures are done differently for infants than for older children and adults.

Temperature

Body temperature may be measured in Fahrenheit (F) or Celsius (C) degrees through oral, rectal, axillary, or tympanic routes. Many types of thermometers are used. Mercury (glass) thermometers have been replaced in ambulatory care areas and clinics by digital thermometers, electronic thermometers, tympanic membrane sensors (aural), and temporal artery thermometers, which provide accurate temperature readings in less time. Broken mercury thermometers release vapors into the air that are toxic when inhaled and lead to mercury poisoning. They should not be used. Proper disposal of mercury is regulated by the health department and varies from state to state. Electronic and digital thermometers can display temperature within 15 to 60 seconds, depending on the model used. A read-ing can be obtained by infrared tympanic membrane and temporal artery sensor in a matter of seconds (see Procedure 27-4).

Oral Temperature. The oral route is used for children older than 5 years. Caution the child against biting down on the thermometer. Do not take an oral temperature if the child has a history of seizures.

Aural Temperature. The aural route uses the tympanic membrane thermometer. It is used on children older than 2 years because it is considered less accurate for children younger than 2 years. Otitis media and impacted cerumen are two other reasons why this route may not be selected. A reading can be obtained in a matter of seconds.

Rectal Temperature. Rectal temperatures may be taken with caution in infants and toddlers when other methods or routes are not advised. Place the child supine, with the knees flexed. An infant can also lie prone on a parent's lap. Do not force the thermometer. Rectal temperatures are not indicated for children who have had rectal surgery or for those who have diarrhea (see Procedure 27-4).

Axillary Temperature. Axillary temperatures are often preferable to rectal or oral temperatures for toddlers and preschoolers because they are safe and nonintrusive to take. Place the probe of the digital thermometer in the axillary space and have the child hold the arm close to the trunk. Leave in place until beep is heard. This route is not used if accuracy is critical.

Temporal Artery Temperature. Chapter 24 provides information and the procedure for taking a temperature using a temporal artery thermometer (TAT). Temporal artery thermometers a frequently used as a non-invasive method for obtaining temperature. It is especially useful with children as is the procedure is fast and gentle.

Pulse

The apical pulse is heard at the apex of the heart, located at the fifth intercostal space left side, midclavicular line, that is, between the fifth and sixth ribs in the middle of the clavicle (usually below the nipple), left of the sternum. A stethoscope is required to obtain an apical pulse. The apical pulse is generally preferred over pulses from other locations for infants and small children (younger than 5 years). Each "lub-dub" sound is counted as one heartbeat. The pulse is counted for 1 full minute (see Procedure 27-5).

The normal pulse rate varies with age, decreasing as the child grows older (Table 27-3). The heart rate may also vary considerably among children of the same age and size. The heart rate increases in

Table 27-3 Normal Heart Rate Ranges for Children

Age	Heart Rate Range (beats/minute)
Newborns	130–140
Infants to 2 years	110–130
2 to 6 years	96–115
6 to 10 years	70–110
10 to 16 years	60–100

© Cengage Learning 2014

Table 27-4 Normal Respiratory Rate Ranges for Children

Age	Respiratory Rate (breaths/minute)
Newborn	30–60
1 year	20–40
3 years	18–30
6 years	18–30
10 years	12–20
17 years	12–20

© Cengage Learning 2014

Table 27-5 Normal Blood Pressure Ranges for Children

Age	Systolic (mm Hg)	Diastolic (mm Hg)
3 years	110	65
6 years	110	65
10 years	118	75
17 years	118	75

© Cengage Learning 2014

response to exercise, excitement, anxiety, and fever and decreases to a resting rate when the child is still.

Listen to the heart rate, noting whether the heart rhythm is regular or irregular. Children often have a normal cycle of irregular rhythm associated with respiration called sinus arrhythmia. In sinus arrhythmia, the child's heart rate is faster on inspiration and slower on expiration. Record whether the pulse is normal, bounding, or thready.

Respirations

In older children and adolescents, respiratory rate is counted in the same way as in an adult. In infants and children younger than 6 years, however, the respiratory rate is assessed by observing the rise and fall of the abdomen. Inspiration, when the chest or abdomen rises, and expiration, when the chest or abdomen falls, are counted as one respiration. Because these movements are often irregular, they should be counted for 1 full minute for accuracy. Normal respiratory rate varies with the child's age (Table 27-4; see Procedure 27-6).

Blood Pressure

The blood pressure of an infant is not normally taken unless requested by the provider. In children 3 years of age and older, blood pressure should be measured annually as part of a routine vital sign assessment.

Blood pressure can be measured using electronic or aneroid equipment and a pediatric cuff. The size of the blood pressure cuff is determined by the size of the child's arm or leg. A general rule of thumb is that the width of the inflatable bladder should be 40% of the circumference of the extremity used. If the cuff is too small, pressure will be falsely high; if too large, falsely low. Sometimes it is difficult to hear the blood pressure in an infant or small child. Use a pediatric stethoscope over pulse sites if possible.

If the pulse still cannot be auscultated, the blood pressure can be measured by touch. Palpate for the pulse. Keeping your fingers on the pulse, pump up the cuff until the pulse is no longer felt. Slowly open the air valve, watching the dial, and note the number where the pulse is again palpated. This is called the palpated systolic blood pressure (Table 27-5).

COLLECTING A URINE SPECIMEN FROM AN INFANT

 Occasionally the medical assistant is required to obtain a urine specimen from an infant for laboratory testing. Special procedures

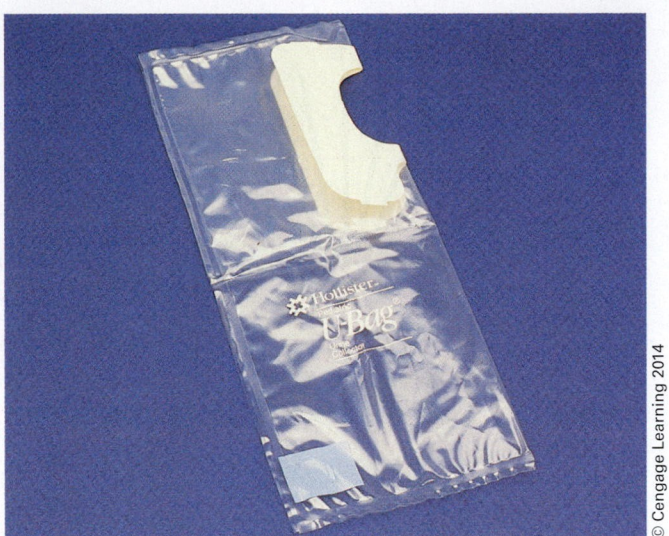

Figure 27-20 Pediatric urine collector. The collector is opened, and the paper backing is removed, exposing the adhesive surface. The collector is firmly attached over the child's cleansed genetalia to prevent leakage.

© Cengage Learning 2014

and equipment are required for this procedure. The collection bag is clear plastic with adhesive tabs (clean catch bag) for application to the perineum of the infant (Figure 27-20; see Procedure 27-7).

The clean catch bag has been a popular way to obtain a clean catch specimen for urinalysis in pediatric patients. The urinalysis is essential to the provider's workup of the patient. Not only is it time-consuming to wait for a child to void, but many times the bag is empty. There are risks of contamination of the specimen by the bag method. According to *The Internet Journal of Emergency Medicine,* a procedure known as direct urethral bladder catheterization is the preferred method for obtaining a sterile urine specimen. A very small catheter (5 French) is used. Using sterile technique, the catheter is inserted through the urethra into the bladder of the pediatric patient. The procedure used on an infant or child is the same as the procedures for performing a urinary catheterization on a male or female patient described in Chapter 30. Catheterization of a pediatric patient in order to obtain a sterile urine specimen is an invasive procedure performed by a licensed provider. A California study confirmed that catheterization is safe and effective particularly in the emergency department when a pediatric patient has a fever and symptoms of a urinary tract infection.

SCREENING INFANTS FOR HEARING IMPAIRMENT

In some hospitals, infants are screened for hearing impairment immediately after delivery. An automated system for checking hearing ability is used by some clinics. It is a more complex screening requiring the use of sensors. As the infant moves in response to sounds produced by the system, these responses are recorded by sensors attached to the infant. The procedure is a more definitive screening process. The medical assistant must maintain a quiet environment while these screening procedures are being performed because extraneous sounds may invalidate the results. For older children, a referral to an audiologist is indicated, especially if there is a delay in speech noted on developmental screening.

SCREENING INFANT AND CHILD VISUAL ACUITY

Measuring the visual acuity of an infant is difficult and is not usually performed unless visual impairment is suspected. Newborns will respond to light by tightly shutting their eyes and keeping them closed until the light is removed. Older infants will follow an object up and down when it is placed directly in front of the eyes. It is estimated that a newborn has the vision equivalent to 20/150, which will reach the adult level of 20/20 by the age of 6 months. The medical assistant will be required to maintain a nonstimulating environment while the provider is screening the infant, because any interference may invalidate results.

The kindergarten chart or Allen cards are used to test visual acuity in young children. It contains pictures in descending size, and the lines are labeled in the same manner as the Snellen chart. The child is asked to identify the picture as the medical assistant points to it (Figure 27-21).

The E chart is a series of Es pointing in different directions in descending size. The size and labeling are the same as the Snellen chart. This chart is used for older children. The child will be asked to point in the direction of the E as the medical assistant points to it (Figure 27-22).

Make a game out of measuring young children's visual acuity because their attention span is very limited.

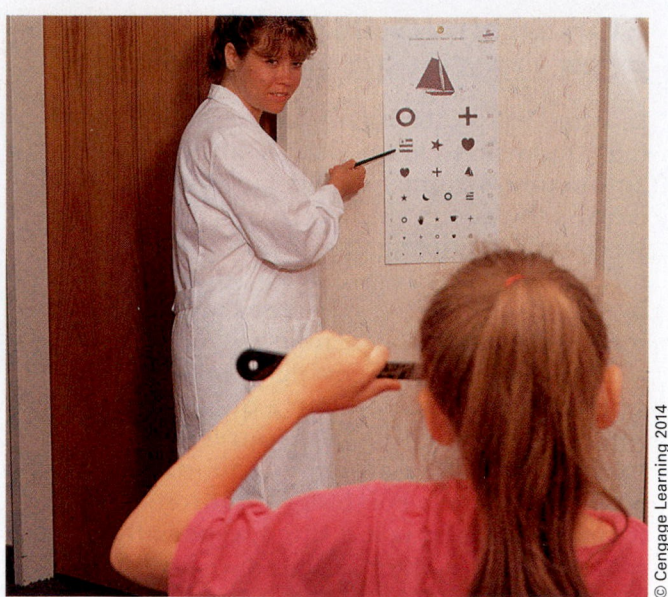

Figure 27-21 Measuring distance visual acuity of a child using a kindergarten vision screening chart.

COMMON DISORDERS AND DISEASES

Young children grow and physically change very quickly. Their immune systems develop normally when they are healthy infants and children. Immunizations, together with their own developing immune system, give them protection from dangerous childhood diseases. Many life-threatening illnesses have been controlled because of scheduled immunization, the child's own developing immune system, and the wise use of antibiotics for infections.

Otitis Media

Otitis media is a commonly occurring disorder in infants and young children. It is characterized by inflammation of the middle ear. Fluid accumulates behind the tympanic membrane, resulting in a degree of temporary hearing loss. It is commonly known as a middle ear infection. Because of the infant and young child's eustachian tubes' connection to the nose and throat, bacteria that cause throat and respiratory infections can easily access the inner ear via the eustachian tube. The fluid in the middle ear can become infected by the bacteria present in the nose and throat. The fluid turns to pus and is known as **suppurative** otitis media. Pain and loss of hearing are common symptoms. Many young children have eustachian tubes that are horizontal and narrow, which predisposes them to otitis media. As children develop physically, they can outgrow otitis media.

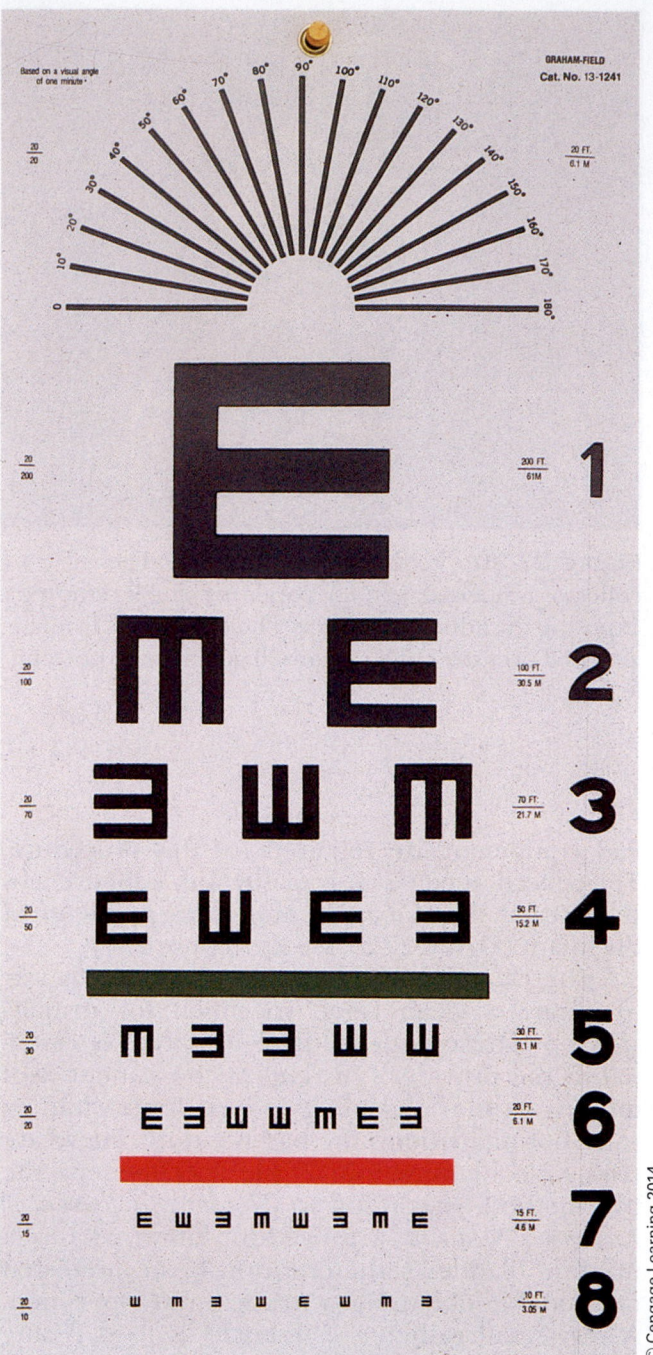

Figure 27-22 Snellen E or Big E chart for testing distance visual acuity of children.

The provider can diagnosis otitis media by visually examining the tympanic membrane with an otoscope. The membrane will be bulging and appear red and inflamed (Figure 27-23). If **exudates** or an oozing of pus is present, a culture and sensitivity test can be done. The treatment for otitis media is antibiotics. To prevent antibiotic overuse and pathogen resistance, providers attempt to

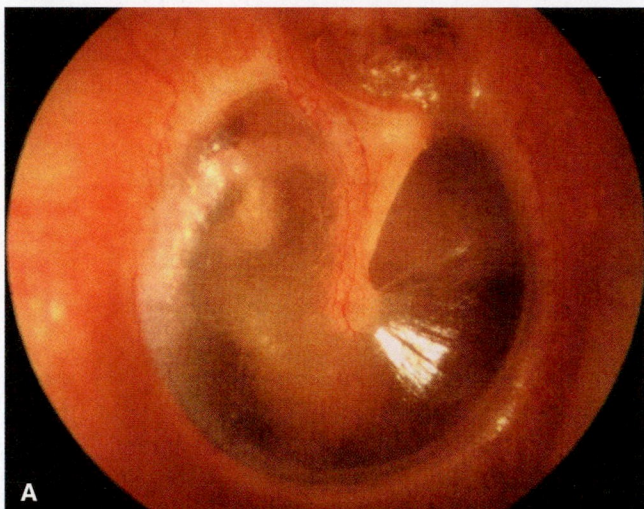

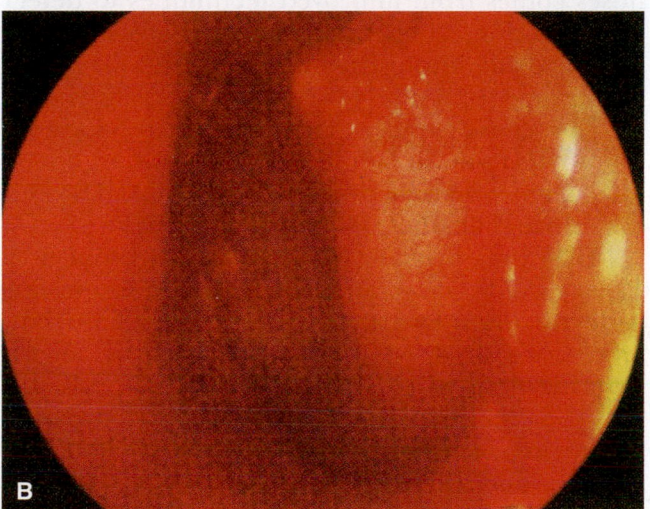

© Cengage Learning 2014

Figure 27-23 Comparison of (A) normal tympanic membrane and (B) acute otitis media.

prescribe antibiotic therapy only when necessary. Decongestants are helpful in some children. For chronic otitis media, a **myringotomy**, incision into the tympanic membrane, may be necessary to prevent rupture of the tympanic membrane and the scarring that results. Scarring can cause permanently impaired hearing ability.

Tympanostomy is a surgical procedure in which pediatric ear tubes are placed through the tympanic membrane to promote ongoing drainage. Chronic otitis media that is left untreated can result in permanent hearing loss.

Hearing loss causes serious major problems in a child's development. Treatment of hearing loss depends on its cause. Hearing aids may be helpful to amplify sounds if the loss is caused by sounds not being conducted to the inner ear. Sensorineural hearing loss does not improve with hearing aids. **Cochlear implantation**, approved by the FDA since 1990, is a procedure that can help children with bilateral **sensorineural** deafness.

The Common Cold

The common cold is aptly named because it is the most common and frequent disease that young children experience. Viruses are the usual microorganisms that cause a cold, and they are spread by direct contact and droplets through the air when children cough and sneeze. Some symptoms are inflammation of the nasopharynx, coughing, nasal discharge, sneezing, and fever. Treatment consists of getting sufficient rest, forcing fluids, and eating a well-balanced diet. Antibiotics are not helpful.

Tonsillitis

The tonsils are located in the back of the nose and throat. They aid in protecting the respiratory tract from infection but frequently become inflamed and infected while doing their job. The cause most often is group A beta-hemolytic streptococcus or a virus. Fever, cough, sore throat, and red, swollen tonsils are common symptoms. Diagnosis can be made by doing a culture and sensitivity test of tonsillar exudate. Antibiotics will rid the child of infection if it is bacterial, and must be taken as prescribed. Tonsillectomy is considered for older children who have chronic tonsillitis.

Pediculosis

Infestation with the head louse is known as pediculosis capitus and is common among school-aged children. The parasites suck blood from humans and are highly contagious. Diagnosis can be made by visual examination of the hair and scalp and observing the eggs (known as nits) on the hair. Special medications applied to the hair is an effective treatment. Care should be taken to launder bed linens and clothing every day. The louse is not a vector for disease.

Asthma

Asthma has increased dramatically in the general population but especially in children. The cause of asthma is not known, but it can be brought on by environmental substances, such as pollen, chemicals, cigarette smoke, mold, and dog and cat hair. Its symptoms include wheezing, coughing, and shortness of breath. It is a serious chronic respiratory disease. Spasms of the bronchi trap air and mucus in the lungs. The child will complain of a tight chest and will have shallow respirations and a nonproductive cough. The asthma attack may become an emergency situation. The pediatrician may refer the child to an allergy specialist who will test the child for various allergies. Respiratory therapy is helpful for some children. Airways can become damaged over time as a result of chronic inflammation.

Croup

The common viral condition croup has symptoms of a croupy or "barking"-type cough, a high-pitched sound on inspiration (stridor), and respiratory distress. The condition is often associated with an upper respiratory infection that leads to inflammation of the larynx, trachea, and bronchi. Respiratory obstruction can occur if severe, but children with croup generally are not seriously ill.

Pertussis (Whooping Cough)

Pertussis is a highly contagious respiratory tract infection caused by a bacterium. At the start, the disease appears to be a cold, but pertussis may become serious, especially in infants. Infected infants are at risk for pneumonia, seizures, brain diseases, and death. After about 2 weeks, the child has numerous rapid coughs that can last for months. Vaccines are available to prevent the disease. In recent years there have been outbreaks of pertussis in college-age individuals and adults. The thinking by providers is that these people have lost their immunity to pertussis and need to be revaccinated with a booster vaccine.

Respiratory Syncytial Virus

In most children, the virus causes mild cold-like symptoms. Death can occur in high-risk babies, such as premature infants, infants with a suppressed immune system, and infants with congestive heart failure. It is the most common cause of pneumonia in children under 1 year.

The virus spreads easily and rapidly through the air and can survive for 1 hour on hands and clothes and for several hours on toys, countertops, and other surfaces. There is no vaccine, but the infection can be treated with antiviral drugs such as ribavirin in **aerosolized** form. The drug inhibits the virus from replicating, so the sooner it is given, the better the results. This treatment is recommended only for severely ill and high-risk patients.

Attention Deficit Hyperactivity Disorder

Attention deficit hyperactivity disorder is a condition in which children have difficulties paying attention and focusing on the task at hand. Parents question whether the disorder is overdiagnosed. Many researchers believe that the increase in diagnoses comes from improved techniques to detect the condition. There are three types of symptoms: hyperactivity, impulsivity, and inattention. Symptoms range from mild to severe.

The cause is uncertain, but researchers note that ADHD runs in families, with a possible genetic link. There also may be a link between ADHD and tobacco and alcohol use during pregnancy.

Diagnosis is made when a child is about 6 to 12 years old. Observation of the child's behavior is documented by parents, teachers, pediatrician, family care provider, psychologist, and psychiatrist. Tests are done to identify other medical problems that can help explain the child's symptoms such as hearing or vision impairment, lead exposure, anemia, and thyroid disease. Symptoms can be controlled, but there is no cure. Stimulant medications (e.g., Adderall, Ritalin, Concerta) and behaviorial therapy help control the symptoms.

Child Abuse

 Child abuse has increased significantly in recent years. By law, health care professionals, including medical assistants, as well as others, must report suspected child abuse. The individual reporting the suspected abuse is protected against liability as a result of the reporting. If suspicion of abuse exists, the provider and health care professional should:

- Treat the child's injuries
- Send the child to the hospital if necessary
- Inform parents of the diagnosis
- Inform parents that the incident will be reported to the public and social service agency
- Notify child protective agency

- Document all information
- Provide court testimony if requested

Child abuse is any physical or mental injury, sexual abuse, negligence, or mistreatment of a child under 18 years of age. Some child abuse signs are:

- Bruises
- Broken bones
- Lacerations
- Burns (cigarette, rope, and burns from being immersed in scalding water)
- Poor hygiene
- Failure to thrive
- Malnutrition
- Head injuries
- Neglected well-baby appointments

The AAP recommends that parents be taught to monitor television, videos, DVDs, and other types of media to limit viewing time and exposure to violence. Children 2 years and younger should not be exposed to any of these media.

 The cultural background of the family should be taken into consideration, as should some folk medicine practices. Latin American and Russian cultures treat headaches or abdominal pain by placing a cup on the skin, creating a vacuum, and placing a small amount of burning material on the skin. These children may present with burns. To treat minor ailments, Southeast Asians rub a coin or spoon in hot oil and rub it onto the child's neck, spine, and ribs, and a burn may occur.

MALE CIRCUMCISION

Circumcision of the male is the surgical removal of the foreskin (prepuce) of the penis. Female circumcision includes a variety of surgical procedures performed on a female's genitalia (see Chapter 30).

Male circumcision is a religious rite in the Jewish and Muslim religions. It is performed on a majority of males in the United States for hygienic reasons. The belief is that male circumcision is a prophylaxis against urinary tract infections and sexually transmitted diseases, especially HIV.

Most circumcisions usually are performed in the hospital shortly after birth. Some consider the procedure to be "cultural" surgery. It has become a tradition, and the majority of male babies are circumcised. According to the CDC, it is the most commonly performed neonatal surgical procedure in the United States.

The practice of circumcision arose during the nineteenth century when circumcision was deemed necessary for male infants. The belief was that not being circumcised resulted in males who habitually masturbated or suffered from insanity.

Proponents of circumcision say it is important for male babies to have penises that resemble their fathers', for improved hygiene, and for males to conform socially with peers.

Although circumcision is generally safe, it is not harmless surgery. The infant is restrained in a specially designed device on a table, and the surgery is performed using sterile technique with analgesia. (In the nineteenth century it was advocated that no analgesic be given so that the male would feel pain, thus accomplishing a means of averting masturbation.) Scientists have shown that during circumcision, without analgesia, the infant's heart rate and blood pressure rise. There is a risk of hemorrhage, sepsis, and laceration.

Advocates for not circumcising male infants claim there is no medical reason to perform the procedure. Research has shown that urinary tract infections and sexually transmitted diseases are no more common in noncircumcised infants than in circumcised infants. Some view the surgery as a profit-driven surgery. According to the AAP about 80% of American male babies are circumcised yearly. At one time the AAP had a pro-circumcision stance, but in 1975 it reversed its position stating there is "no absolute medical indication for routine circumcision of newborns." If it is performed, the AAP recommended that pain relief be provided.

Some believe that elective circumcisions of males and females should not be accepted by conscientious health care providers. Furthermore, those who are averse to the surgery say that a child is normal when born and that circumcision results in loss of a body part, is unnecessary, leaves a scar, and removes a functioning body part in the name of custom or tradition. It is viewed as a nonessential, pathologic procedure and a violation of basic human rights because infants are too young and helpless to consent or refuse.

How can parents decide what to do? Circumcision or not? It is a choice they will make, and it will take courage. Deeply rooted cultural and traditional customs can be difficult to sort through. With courage, education, and research, parents can gain perspective about whether or not to circumcise their sons. The AAP has information available on its website (http://www.aap.org).

PROCEDURE 27-1
Administration of a Vaccine

STANDARD PRECAUTIONS:

PURPOSE:
To administer a vaccine.

EQUIPMENT/SUPPLIES:
Vaccines ordered by provider
Vaccine Information Statement (VIS)
Medication note
Appropriate syringe needles
Alcohol wipes
Gloves (if office/clinic policy)
Sharps container

PROCEDURE STEPS:

1. Review the provider's order. Write out a medication card. RATIONALE: Helps eliminate giving an incorrect medication or dose. Writing the vaccine order on the note prevents giving vaccine to the wrong patient.

2. Follow the six "rights" of medication administration (see Chapter 36).

3. Perform medical asepsis handwashing following OSHA guidelines.

4. Work in a well-lighted, quiet, clean area.

5. *Paying attention to detail,* assemble the appropriate equipment (see Table 27-2). RATIONALE: The appropriate size needle and syringe for the vaccine being given are important to prevent patient injury.

6. Give parents/guardians the Vaccine Information Statement (VIS) for the intended vaccine and *give them time to read the VIS and ask questions.*

7. Carefully select the appropriate vial of vaccine. *Pay attention to detail.* Check the label three times and check the medication note. RATIONALE: Safeguards patient from incorrect medication, dose, and route.

8. Check for expiration date on vial. RATIONALE: Expired medication is not safe to give.

9. Maintain sterile technique throughout. RATIONALE: Compromising the vaccine or syringe and needle by poor technique can introduce microorganisms into the patient or vaccine with serious consequences.

10. Select the correct needle and syringe for the type of injection and the size of the patient. (see Table 27-2).

11. Shake the vial or reconstitute powder medication using all of the diluents according to the manufacturer's instructions. RATIONALE: Ensures medication is mixed properly.

12. Invert the vial and withdraw the correct dose of vaccine. Recheck the label on the vial and the medicine note. RATIONALE: Ensures you have the correct vaccine.

13. Wash hands and, if clinic policy, don nonsterile gloves. RATIONALE: Gloves must be worn if the medical assistant has any openings in the skin or on the hands.

14. *Introduce yourself to the patient. Identify the patient.*

15. *Being courteous and respectful,* enlist the assistance of the parents to restrain the child. RATIONALE: Avoids injury to child.

16. *Speaking at the patient's level of understanding, explain the procedure. Allay the parent's and patient's fears regarding the procedure. Help them to feel safe and comfortable.*

17. Locate the appropriate site for administration. Cleanse the site with alcohol wipe and let dry. RATIONALE: The alcohol is an antiseptic and will lower the number of bacteria at the site. Letting the area dry lessens the sting when needle is inserted.

18. Inject the vaccine steadily at the appropriate angle. RATIONALE: Avoid rapid injection of the vaccine as it increases the discomfort to the child.

19. Withdraw needle and syringe at angle of insertion.

Procedure 27-1 (continued)

20. Immediately dispose of the needle and syringe in the appropriate biohazard container.

21. Apply gentle pressure to injection site. Rub gently. RATIONALE: Vaccine will be distributed evenly. This also encourages blood flow to the area to increase the absorption of the vaccine.

22. Remove gloves, if required by policy.

23. Wash hands.

24. Accurately record all of the information in the patient's chart or electronic medical record and on the vaccine administration record. Include lot number, manufacturer, site, VIS date, and your name and initials.

25. Update child's record of immunizations and remind parent or guardian to bring it to each visit.

26. Be aware of the location of the emergency drugs (epinephrine and others). RATIONALE: Medication must be readily available to counteract an allergic reaction.

PROCEDURE 27-2
Maintaining Immunization Records

STANDARD PRECAUTIONS:

PURPOSE:
To establish and maintain a record of preventive immunizations against childhood diseases for the provider and parent or legal guardian.

EQUIPMENT/SUPPLIES:
Vaccine Administration Record
Vial of vaccine as ordered

PROCEDURE STEPS:
1. Give the parent or legal guardian the most recent copy of the Vaccine Information Statement (VIS). The statements explain risks and benefits of vaccines for each dose of vaccine given.

2. After the administration of a scheduled vaccine for the child, accurately record all of the information in the patient's chart or electronic medical record and on the Vaccine Administration Record.

3. Using the medicine card and the vaccine vial, fill out the Vaccine Administration Record (Figure 27-24) according to which vaccine you administered. Note the headings, type of vaccine (use generic abbreviations, not the brand name), date given, month, day, year, dose, route, site, vaccine lot number and manufacturer, VIS; date on VIS, date given (VIS), and your initials as the individual who administered the vaccine.

4. The immunization record is kept by the provider and the parent or legal guardian. *NOTE:* Remind parent or legal guardian to keep immunization records safe and readily accessible for proof of immunization for daycare and school.

DOCUMENTATION:
5/2/20XX   DTaP 0.5 mL IM (R) vastus lateralis. Recorded on vaccine administration record. Parent given Vaccine Information Statement. S. Thomas, CMA (AAMA)————————

continues

Procedure 27-2 (continued)

Vaccine Administration Record for Children and Teens

(Page 1 of 2)

Patient name: _____

Birthdate: _____

Chart number: _____

Before administering any vaccines, give copies of all pertinent Vaccine Information Statements (VISs) to the child's parent or legal representative and make sure he/she understands the risks and benefits of the vaccine(s). Always provide or update the patient's personal record card.

Vaccine	Type of Vaccine[1]	Date given (mo/day/yr)	Funding Source (F,S,P)[2]	Site[3]	Vaccine		Vaccine Information Statement (VIS)		Vaccinator[5] (signature or initials & title)
					Lot #	Mfr.	Date on VIS[4]	Date given[4]	
Hepatitis B[6] (e.g., HepB, Hib-HepB, DTaP-HepB-IPV) Give IM.[7]									
Diphtheria, Tetanus, Pertussis[6] (e.g., DTaP, DTaP/Hib, DTaP-HepB-IPV, DT, DTaP-IPV/Hib, Tdap, DTaP-IPV, Td) Give IM.[7]									
***Haemophilus influenzae* type b**[6] (e.g., Hib, Hib-HepB, DTaP-IPV/Hib, DTaP/Hib) Give IM.[7]									
Polio[6] (e.g., IPV, DTaP-HepB-IPV, DTaP-IPV/Hib, DTaP-IPV) Give IPV SC or IM.[7] Give all others IM.[7]									
Pneumococcal (e.g., PCV7, PCV13, conjugate; PPSV23, polysaccharide) Give PCV IM.[7] Give PPSV SC or IM.[7]									
Rotavirus (RV1, RV5) Give orally (po).									

See page 2 to record measles-mumps-rubella, varicella, hepatitis A, meningococcal, HPV, influenza, and other vaccines (e.g., travel vaccines).

How to Complete This Record

1. Record the generic abbreviation (e.g., Tdap) or the trade name for each vaccine (see table at right).

2. Record the funding source of the vaccine given as either F (federal), S (state), or P (private).

3. Record the site where vaccine was administered as either RA (right arm), LA (left arm), RT (right thigh), LT (left thigh), or IN (intranasal).

4. Record the publication date of each VIS as well as the date the VIS is given to the patient.

5. To meet the space constraints of this form and federal requirements for documentation, a healthcare setting may want to keep a reference list of vaccinators that includes their initials and titles.

6. For combination vaccines, fill in a row for each antigen in the combination.

7. IM is the abbreviation for intramuscular; SC is the abbreviation for subcutaneous.

Abbreviation	Trade Name & Manufacturer
DTaP	Daptacel (sanofi); Infanrix (GlaxoSmithKline [GSK]); Tripedia (sanofi pasteur)
DT (pediatric)	Generic (sanofi pasteur)
DTaP-HepB-IPV	Pediarix (GSK)
DTaP/Hib	TriHIBit (sanofi pasteur)
DTaP-IPV/Hib	Pentacel (sanofi pasteur)
DTaP-IPV	Kinrix (GSK)
HepB	Engerix-B (GSK); Recombivax HB (Merck)
HepA-HepB	Twinrix (GSK); can be given to teens age 18 and older
Hib	ActHIB (sanofi pasteur); Hiberix (GSK); PedvaxHIB (Merck)
Hib-HepB	Comvax (Merck)
IPV	Ipol (sanofi pasteur)
PCV13	Prevnar 13 (Pfizer)
PPSV23	Pneumovax 23 (Merck)
RV1	Rotarix (GSK)
RV5	RotaTeq (Merck)
Tdap	Adacel (sanofi pasteur); Boostrix (GSK)
Td	Decavac (sanofi pasteur), Generic (MA Biological Labs)

Technical content reviewed by the Centers for Disease Control and Prevention, March 2011.

For additional copies, visit www.immunize.org/catg.d/p2022.pdf • Item #P2022 (3/11)

This form was created by the Immunization Action Coalition • www.immunize.org • www.vaccineinformation.org

Figure 27-24   Vaccination Administration Record.

PROCEDURE 27-3

Measuring the Infant: Weight, Length, and Head and Chest Circumference

STANDARD PRECAUTIONS:

PURPOSE:

To obtain an accurate measurement of an infant's weight, length, and head and chest circumference for medical records and to screen for growth abnormalities.

EQUIPMENT/SUPPLIES:

Infant scale
Pen
Paper protector
Ruler
Flexible measuring tape without elasticity
Biohazard waste container
Growth chart

PROCEDURE STEPS:

Measuring infant weight:

1. Wash hands.

2. *Introduce yourself to the parents. Identify patient.*

3. *Explain procedure to parent(s), speaking at the parent's level of understanding. Allay the parent's fears regarding the procedure.*

4. *Being courteous and respectful,* enlist the assistance of the parents to undress infant (including the diaper).

5. Place all weights to left of scale to check balance.

6. *Paying attention to detail.* Place a clean utility towel on scale and check balance scale for accuracy, being sure to compensate for the weight of the towel. RATIONALE: The protection that the paper utility towel affords helps to reduce transmission of microorganisms and provides warmth because the scale is cool.

7. Gently place small infant on her back on the scale. Larger infants can sit on the scale. Place your hand slightly above the infant's body to ensure safety (Figure 27-25). RATIONALE: This will safeguard the infant from falling.

8. Place the bottom weight to its highest measurement that will not cause the balance to drop to the bottom edge.

9. Slowly move upper weight until the balance bar rests in the center of the indicator. A balanced scale will provide an accurate weight. Read the infant's weight while he or she is lying still.

10. Return both weights to their resting position to the extreme left.

11. Gently remove infant and apply diaper. (Parent can help with diapering and holding infant.)

12. Discard used protective paper towel per OSHA guidelines.

13. Sanitize scale.

14. Wash hands.

15. Accurately record all information in patient's chart or electronic medical record or in growth chart and patient's booklet if available. Document results according to clinic policy (pounds and ounces or kilograms). Connect dot from previous examination with a ruler to complete graph.

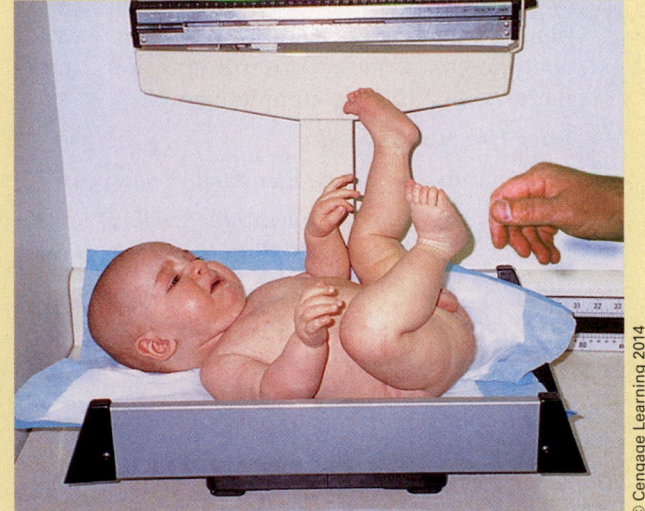

Figure 27-25 Infants who are unable to sit erect should be weighed on their back on the scale.

© Cengage Learning 2014

continues

Procedure 27-3 (continued)

Measuring infant length:

1. Wash hands and follow Standard Precautions.

2. ***Explain procedure to parent(s), speaking at the parent's level of understanding. Allay the parent's fears regarding the procedure.***

3. ***Being courteous and respectful,*** enlist the assistance of the parents to remove infant's shoes.

4. Gently place infant on his or her back on the examination table. If the pediatric table has a headboard, ask parent to hold infant's head against headboard (end) of table at zero mark of ruler while you place infant's heels against footboard. Gently straighten infant's back and legs to line up along ruler. If there is no footboard (to place infant's feet against), use your right hand as a guide (Figure 27-26). If necessary, gently place your left hand over the child's legs at the knees to secure the child in place and straighten the legs so you can read the recumbent length from the head to the heel. RATIONALE: Sometimes it is difficult to straighten the legs.

5. Read length on the measuring device in inches or centimeters.

6. ***Being courteous and respectful,*** enlist the assistance of the parents to dress the patient.

7. Wash hands.

8. Accurately record all information in patient's chart or electronic medical record or in growth chart and patient's booklet if available. Document according to clinic policy (inches or centimeters). Connect dot from previous examination with a ruler to complete graph.

Measuring Head Circumference:

1. Wash hands and follow Standard Precautions.

2. ***Explain procedure to parent(s), speaking at the parent's level of understanding. Allay the parent's fears regarding the procedure.***

3. ***Being courteous and respectful, talk to infant and parents to gain cooperation.*** Infant may be held by parent or lie on examination table for procedure. Older children of 2 or 3 years may stand or sit if they will remain still.

4. Place the measuring tape snugly around the head from the occipital protuberance to the supraorbital prominence. This is the largest part of the head (Figure 27-27).

5. Read the measurement, which will be in either inches (to nearest 1/2 inch) or centimeters (to nearest 0.01 cm).

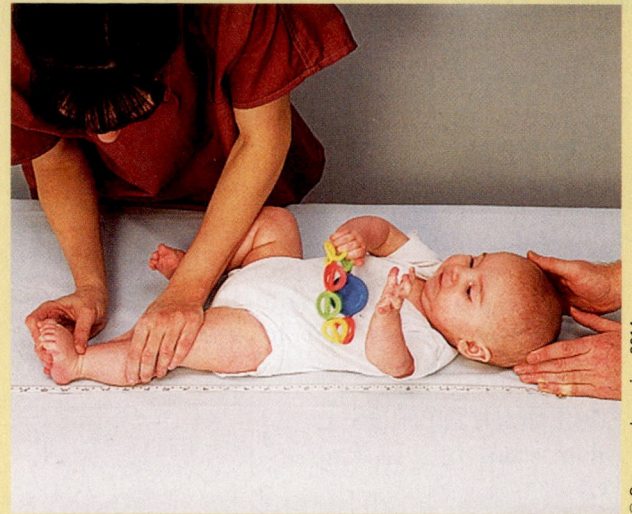

Figure 27-26   Measuring recumbent length of an infant.

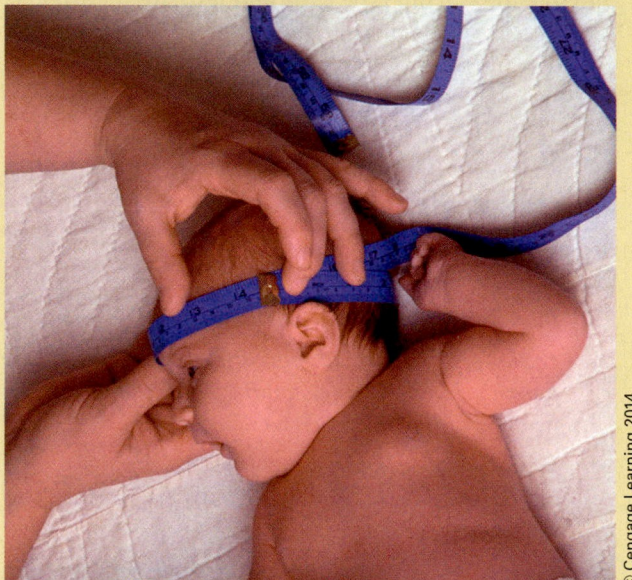

Figure 27-27   Measuring infant's head circumferences.

6. Wash hands.

7. Accurately record all information in patient's or electronic medical record, or in growth chart and parent's booklet if available. Connect dot from previous examination with a ruler to complete graph.

Measuring infant's chest circumference:

1. Wash hands and follow Standard Precautions.

2. ***Explain procedure to parent(s), speaking at the parent's level of understanding. Allay the parent's fears regarding the procedure.***

3. Use one thumb to hold tape measure with zero mark against the infant's chest at the midsternal area. With the other hand, bring the tape

Procedure 27-3 (continued)

around/under the back to meet the zero mark of the tape in front. Take the measurement of the chest just above the nipples with the tape fitting around the child's chest under the axillary region. If you need assistance in holding the child still, ask the parent or another assistant. The measurement should be taken when the child is breathing normally and during the resting phase between respirations (Figure 27-28).

4. Read measurement to the nearest 0.01 cm or one-eighth inch.

5. Wash hands.

6. Accurately record all information in patient's chart or electronic medical record or on growth chart and patient's booklet if available. Document according to office policy (inches or centimeters).

DOCUMENTATION:
3/10/20XX 4:00 PM   6 months of age, wt. 15 lb. Recorded on growth chart. A. Jarreau, RMA (AMT)

DOCUMENTATION:
3/10/20XX 4:00 PM   6 months of age, length 26 inches long. Recorded on growth chart. A. Jarreau, RMA (AMT)

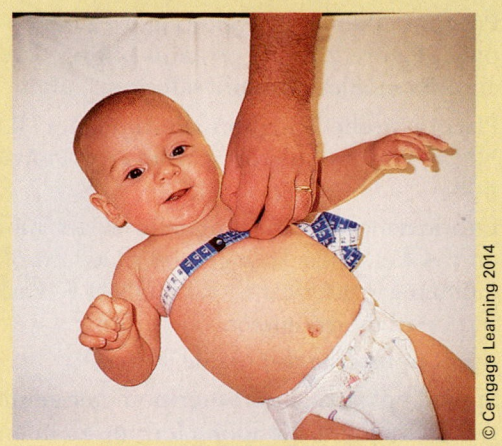

© Cengage Learning 2014

Figure 27-28   Measuring infant's chest circumferences.

DOCUMENTATION:
3/10/20XX 4:00 PM   6 months of age, head circumference 43 centimeters. Recorded on growth chart. C. McInnis, RMA (AMT)

DOCUMENTATION:
3/10/20XX 4:00 PM   6 months of age, chest circumference 30 centimeters. Recorded on growth chart. A. Jarreau, RMA (AMT)

PROCEDURE 27-4

Taking an Infant's Rectal Temperature with a Digital Thermometer

STANDARD PRECAUTIONS:

PURPOSE:
To obtain a rectal temperature using a digital thermometer.

EQUIPMENT/SUPPLIES:
Digital thermometer (red probe) and probe cover
Lubricating jelly
4 × 4 gauze sponges
Gloves
Biohazard waste container

PROCEDURE STEPS:
1. Wash hands and follow Standard Precautions.

2. *Introduce yourself to the parents. Identify patient.*

3. *Explain procedure to parent(s), speaking at the parent's level of understanding. Allay the parent's fears regarding the procedure.* RATIONALE: Gain cooperation and assistance in disrobing infant and positioning properly.

4. *Paying attention to detail,* assemble equipment.

5. *Being courteous and respectful,* enlist the parent's assistance to undress the infant (including the diaper).

continues

Procedure 27-4 (continued)

6. Position infant in a prone (Figure 27-29A) or supine (Figure 27-29B) position having parent or another medical assistant safeguard infant.

7. Place a probe cover on thermometer. RATIONALE: Prevents microorganism cross contamination.

8. Lubricate with lubricating jelly. (Place lubricant on a 4 × 4 gauze sponge and place tip of thermometer in lubricant.) RATIONALE: Easier insertion of thermometer.

9. Apply nonsterile disposable gloves.

10. Spread buttocks, insert thermometer gently into the rectum past the sphincter; for an infant this is 0.5 inch (Figure 27-29B).

11. Hold buttocks together while holding the thermometer. If necessary, restrain infant movement by placing your arm across infant's back. Parent can immobilize infant's legs. RATIONALE: Ensure infant's safety and comfort.

12. Hold in place until beep is heard. Do not let go of the thermometer. RATIONALE: Movement by infant can cause thermometer to move and injure the infant.

13. Remove from rectum.

14. Provide wipes to remove any additional lubricating jelly.

15. Have parent attend to infant.

16. Note temperature reading.

17. Remove probe cover by ejecting it into a biohazard container.

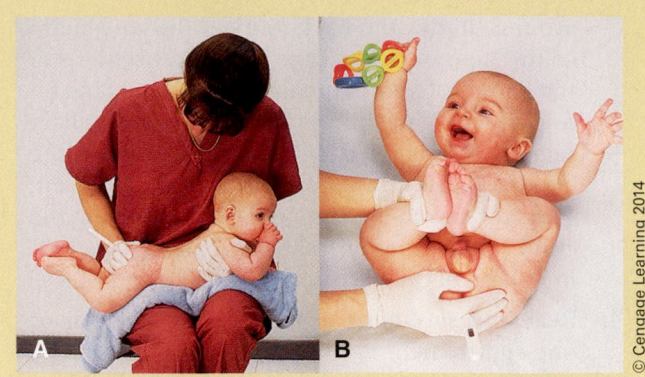

Figure 27-29 Taking the rectal temperature of an infant in (A) the prone position and (B) in the supine position.

© Cengage Learning 2014

18. Wipe probe with antiseptic wipe. Replace thermometer on holder.

19. Remove gloves, discard in biohazard waste container.

20. Wash hands.

21. *Being courteous and respectful,* enlist the parents in dressing the infant.

22. Accurately record all information in patient's chart or electronic medical record with the designation of (R) indicating rectal temperature.

DOCUMENTATION:
5/3/20XX 4:00 PM   T99.8 F (R). S. Thomas, CMA (AAMA)——

PROCEDURE 27-5
Taking an Apical Pulse on an Infant

STANDARD PRECAUTIONS:

PURPOSE:
To obtain an apical pulse rate.

EQUIPMENT/SUPPLIES:

Stethoscope
Watch with second hand
Alcohol wipes

PROCEDURE STEPS:

1. Wash hands and follow Standard Precautions.

2. *Paying attention to detail,* assemble equipment.

3. *Introduce yourself to the parents. Identify patient.*

4. *Explain procedure to parent, speaking at the parent's level of understanding. Allay the parent's fears regarding the procedure.* RATIONALE: Gain cooperation and assistance.

Procedure 27-5 (continued)

5. ***Being courteous and respectful,*** enlist the assistance of the parents to undress the infant (including the diaper).

6. Provide a drape for infant's warmth if necessary.

7. Gently position the infant in a supine position or sitting in the parent's lap. RATIONALE: The supine position may offer easier access to apex of heart if the child is calm.

8. Locate the fifth intercostal space, midclavicular line, left of sternum. RATIONALE: Location of apex of heart.

9. Place warmed stethoscope on the site and listen for the lub-dub sound of the heart.

10. Count the pulse for 1 minute; each lub-dub equals one heartbeat or pulse.

11. Wash hands.

12. Assist parents as needed to redress the infant.

13. Clean earpieces and diaphragm of stethoscope with alcohol wipes. RATIONALE: Prevents cross-contamination of microbes between patients.

14. Accurately record the pulse in the patient's chart or electronic medical record. Designate (AP) to indicate apical pulse. Note any arrhythmias.

DOCUMENTATION:
3/10/20XX 4:00 PM   Pulse 140 (AP). Regular. S. Thomas, CMA (AAMA)—————————————————————

PROCEDURE 27-6

Measuring Infant's Respiratory Rate

STANDARD PRECAUTIONS:

PURPOSE:
The respiratory rate is normally taken immediately before or after the pulse rate to obtain an accurate respiratory rate.

EQUIPMENT/SUPPLIES:
Watch with second hand

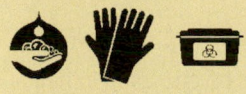

PROCEDURE STEPS:
1. Wash hands and follow Standard Precautions.

2. ***Identify the patient and explain the procedure to the parent, speaking at the parent's level of understanding.*** RATIONALE: To gain cooperation and assistance.

3. Position infant in a supine position.

4. Place hand on the chest to feel the rise and fall of the chest wall for 1 minute.

5. Note depth and rhythm while counting.

6. Wash hands.

7. Accurately record all information in patient's chart or electronic medical record. Note any irregularities in depth or rhythm.

DOCUMENTATION:
3/10/20XX 4:00 PM   Respirations 22. Regular. S. Thomas, CMA (AAMA)—————————————————————

PROCEDURE 27-7

Obtaining a Urine Specimen from an Infant or Young Child

STANDARD PRECAUTIONS:

PURPOSE:
To obtain a specimen of urine from an infant or young child.

continues

Procedure 27-7 (continued)

EQUIPMENT/SUPPLIES:
Urine collection bag
Urine cup
Laboratory request form
Biohazard transport bag
Gloves
Cleansing cloth
Towel
Biohazard waste container

PROCEDURE STEPS:
1. Wash hands and follow Standard Precautions.
2. ***Identify patient and explain procedure to parent(s), speaking at the parent's level of understanding.*** RATIONALE: To gain cooperation and assistance.
3. ***Paying attention to detail,*** assemble equipment.
4. ***Being courteous and respectful,*** enlist the assistance of the parents to disrobe patient and remove the diaper.
5. Wash and dry perineal area. RATIONALE: Cleaning area reduces microorganism level and provides better quality urine specimen.
6. Apply collection bag, secure with adhesive tabs (see Figure 27-19).
   a. Girls: spread perineum, place bag over labia.
   b. Boys: place bag over penis and scrotum.
7. Replace diaper carefully.
8. Frequently check bag for urine.
9. Once specimen has been collected, remove bag carefully.
10. Prepare specimen as required. Send to laboratory in an appropriate container with a requisition or process the specimen in the clinic laboratory.
11. Remove gloves and discard in biohazard waste container.
12. Wash hands.
13. Accurately record collection in patient's chart or electronic medical record.

DOCUMENTATION:
3/10/20XX 4:00 PM   Urine specimen collected via urine collection bag. Specimen sent to Bay Laboratory with requisition for routine urinalysis. J. Guerro, CMA (AAMA)———

CASE STUDY 27-1

Refer to the scenario at the beginning of the chapter.

CASE STUDY REVIEW

1. In what ways can Sarah learn about new vaccines that are required for pediatric patients?

2. Other than the provider giving information, describe two ways in which Sarah can stay current with vaccines and immunizations.

CASE STUDY 27-2

After examining Joey Little, Dr. King confirms the diagnosis of otitis media.

CASE STUDY REVIEW

1. Explain otitis media, the most common reason for its occurrence, and its treatment.

2. How can parents and caregivers be educated to help prevent otitis media?

SUMMARY

Caring for the health and well-being of infants and children throughout their various developmental stages and into adolescence is the responsibility of the pediatric practice.

Careful observation of the parent or caregiver and the child is helpful to the treatment and care given to the child. The medical assistant is responsible for reporting to the provider any suspicion of child abuse. Opportunities abound for educating parents about topics that will keep their children healthy throughout life and include nutrition, sleep, immunizations, and exercise. Pamphlets, videos, and demonstrations are available to share with parents and caregivers.

Children need respect and should be treated with empathy, love, and honesty; in doing so, a positive relationship can be developed with the child.

STUDY FOR SUCCESS

To reinforce your knowledge and skills of information presented in this chapter:

- Review the *Key Terms*
- Role-play with other students to apply attributes of professionalism pertinent to this chapter.
- Consider the *Case Studies* and discuss your conclusions
- Answer the questions in the *Certification Review*
- Apply your knowledge by completing the Activities in the *Study Guide* and the *Games and Quizzes* in the StudyWARE **StudyWARE** software on the *Premium Website*
- Perform the Procedures using the *Competency Assessment Checklists* in the *Competency Manual*
- Practice your problem-solving skills with the *Critical Thinking Challenge 3.0* on the *Premium Website*

Additional resources for this chapter include:

- Module 21 of the *Medical Assisting Learning Lab*
- *CourseMate for Delmar's Comprehensive Medical Assisting*
- *WebTutor for Delmar's Comprehensive Medical Assisting*

CERTIFICATION REVIEW

1. At what age should the first polio vaccine be given?
   a. birth
   b. 1 month
   c. 2 months
   d. 3 months
   e. 6 months
2. One procedure to treat otitis media is:
   a. suppuration
   b. tympanostomy
   c. ear irrigation
   d. otoscopy
   e. myringectomy
3. The pathogen usually responsible for causing tonsillitis is:
   a. *Staphylococcus aureus*
   b. meningococcus
   c. beta-hemolytic streptococcus group A
   d. beta-hemolytic streptococcus group B
4. Head circumference is measured on the child until what age?
   a. 12 months
   b. 24 months
   c. 36 months
   d. 72 months

5. An apical pulse is taken over which of the following sites?
   a. Third intercostal space on the left side
   b. Fourth intercostal space on the left side
   c. Fifth intercostal space on the left side
   d. Sixth intercostal space on the left side
6. The soft spot lying between the bones of the skull in a newborn and infant is called:
   a. frontal lobe
   b. fontanel
   c. foramen
   d. cranium
7. Most childhood immunizations are administered within what time period:
   a. the first 6 months of life
   b. the first 10 months of life
   c. the first 12 months of life
   d. the first 18 months of life
8. The measurement of chest circumference is important to determine:
   a. underdevelopment of the infant's heart and lungs
   b. overdevelopment of the infant's heart and lungs
   c. calcification of rib cartilage
   d. all of the above
9. When collecting a sterile urine specimen from an infant, it is important to use which method to assure no contamination:
   a. clean catch bag
   b. direct catheterization
   c. diaper extraction
   d. none of the above
10. The most definitive method for hearing testing of an infant is:
    a. automated system with the use of sensors
    b. manual system with the use of systems
    c. observation and exposure to loud noises
    d. extraneous sound monitoring

REFERENCES/BIBLIOGRAPHY

Ambroz, K. G., & Eilber, W. (2003). An enhanced method of pediatric urine collection. *The Internet Journal of Emergency Medicine 1*(1).

Clifton, J. C., 2nd. (2007). Mercury exposure and public health. In *Pediatric clinics of North America* (pp. 237–269). The National Library of Medicine and the National Institutes of Health. Retrieved July 2, 2008, from www.pubmed.gov

Hegner, B. R., Acello, B., & Caldwell, E. (2008). *Nursing assistant: A nursing process approach*. Clifton Park, NY: Delmar Cengage Learning.

Keir, L., Wise, B., Krebs, C., & Kelley-Arney, C. (2008). *Medical assisting: Administrative and clinical competencies* (6th ed). Clifton Park, NY: Delmar Cengage Learning.

Mandleco, B. L. (2004). *Growth and development handbook: Newborn through adolescent*. Clifton Park, NY: Delmar Cengage Learning.

Potts, N. L., & Mandleco, B. L. (2002). *Pediatric nursing: Caring for children and their families*. Clifton Park, NY: Delmar Cengage Learning.

Taber's cyclopedic medical dictionary (20th ed.). (2006). Philadelphia: F. A. Davis.

Tamparo, C., & Lewis, M. (2005). *Diseases of the human body* (4th ed.). Philadelphia: F. A. Davis.

Price, C. S., Thompson, W. W., & Goodson, B., et al. (Oct. 2010, pp. 656–664). Prenatal and infant exposure to thimerosal from vaccines and immunoglobins and risk of autism. *Pediatrics 126*(4).

OUTLINE

Anatomy of Male Reproductive System
  External Anatomy
  Internal Anatomy
Disorders of the Penis
  Priapism
  Erectile Dysfunction
  Penile Cancer
  Other Disorders of the Penis

Disorders of the Testes
  Testicular Trauma
  Testicular Torsion
  Testicular Cancer
  Epididymitis
  Hypogonadism
Disorders of the Prostate
  Prostatitis

Benign Prostatic Hyperplasia
Prostate Cancer
Other Disorders of the Male Reproductive System
  Sexually Transmitted Diseases
  Infertility
Assisting with the Male Reproductive Examination

LEARNING OUTCOMES

1. Define, spell, and pronounce the key terms as presented in the glossary.
2. Describe common disorders and diseases of the male reproductive system.
3. Discuss signs and symptoms of the various disorders and diseases of the male reproductive system.
4. Explain erectile dysfunction, its causes, and its treatments.
5. Describe the common diagnostic tests and procedures used in the male reproductive system.

6. Explain testicular self-examination to a male patient.
7. Prepare patient teaching materials for intravenous pyelogram and transurethral resection of the prostate.
8. Demonstrate compassion and empathy.
9. Analyze the professionalism questions and apply them to this chapter's content.

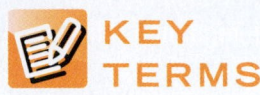

KEY TERMS

balanitis

benign prostatic hypertrophy (BPH)

bulbourethral glands

cryptorchidism

epididymitis

erectile dysfunction (ED)

hypogonadism

infertility

intravenous pyelogram (IVP)

libido

nocturia

orchiectomy

Peyronie's disease

phimosis

priapism

prostatectomy

prostatitis

retention

scrotum

spermatic cord

spermatogenesis

testicular torsion

testes

transurethral resection of the prostate (TURP)

vas deferens

ATTRIBUTES OF PROFESSIONALISM

Communication

- Did you introduce yourself? Did you identify the patient through name and birth date or other identifying feature?
- Did you listen to and acknowledge the patient?
- Did you speak at the patient's level of understanding?
- Did you display appropriate body language?
- Did you allay patient's fears regarding the procedure being performed and help them feel safe and comfortable?
- Did you demonstrate empathy in communicating with patients, family, and staff?

Presentation

- Did your actions attend to both the psychological and the physiologic aspects of the patient's illness or condition?
- Were you courteous, patient, and respectful to the patient?
- Did you display a calm, professional, and caring manner?

Competency

- Were you knowledgeable and accountable?
- Did you apply critical thinking skills in performing patient assessment and care?

Initiative

- Did you direct the patient to other resources when necessary or helpful, with the approval of the provider?

Integrity

- Did you demonstrate sensitivity to patient's rights?
- Did you protect personal boundaries?
- Were you respectful of others?
- Did you demonstrate respect for individual diversity?
- Did you demonstrate an appreciation for the patient's attitude toward his or her illness or condition?
- Did you protect and maintain confidentiality?

SCENARIO

Kimberly Sanchez, CMA (AAMA), has worked with Dr. Olani for the last 6 years. As the lead medical assistant in this busy urology practice, Ms. Sanchez interacts with patients in many settings. Mr. Range is seeing Dr. Olani today for evaluation of a testicular lump found on a self-examination. With the understanding that this is a stressful time for the patient, Ms. Sanchez introduces herself and begins collecting the patient's history. After Dr. Olani completes the physical examination and orders an ultrasound of the testicular mass, Mr. Range asks "What does all of this mean?" Ms. Sanchez stands near Mr. Range as he asks Dr. Olani to clarify all of the information that the provider had just delivered. Ms. Sanchez, with Dr. Olani's permission, gives Mr. Range a Patient Education Flyer from the National Institute for Health regarding Ultrasound of the Testicles.

INTRODUCTION

The male reproductive system is a specialized set of structures that serves the purpose of producing and delivering semen for sexual interaction and reproduction. It also has the important dual function of secreting male sex hormones that impact the growth and function of sexual organs and development of secondary sexual characteristics. This chapter will discuss the structure, function and disease processes of this system.

Diseases, disorders, conditions, diagnostic tests, procedures, and treatments common to the male reproductive system are listed in Table 28-1.

ANATOMY OF MALE REPRODUCTIVE SYSTEM

Males have a reproductive system that is both internal and external. The internal components are located near and interact closely with the urinary system and this must be kept in mind when considering the pathophysiology of this system.

External Anatomy

The penis is a biologic feature of male primary sexual characteristics. Its role in reproduction is to allow delivery of semen deep into the female reproductive tract via the vagina. The penis has several anatomic portions that include the glans (head), corpus cavernosum, corpus spongiosum, and the urethra. Features of the glans include a loose layer of skin called the foreskin and the opening of the urethra. The shaft of the penis is constructed of several internal chambers. These structures hold the blood involved in an erection and protect the urethra from compression during ejaculation. The urethra provides the route to the exterior of the body for semen.

SPOTLIGHT ON CERTIFICATION

RMA Content Outline

- Anatomy and physiology
- Medical terminology
- Principles of medical ethics and ethical conduct
- Patient relations
- Patient education
- Physical examination

CMA (AAMA) Content Outline

- Medical terminology
- Anatomy and physiology
- Developmental stages of the life cycle
- Professional communication and behavior
- Medicolegal guidelines and requirements
- Patient preparation and assisting the provider
- Collecting and processing specimens; diagnostic testing

CMAS Content Outline

- Medical terminology
- Anatomy and physiology
- Legal and ethical considerations
- Basic health history interview

Table 28-1   Male Reproductive System Diseases and Disorders

Disease/Disorder	Laboratory Diagnostics	Radiography and Technical Diagnostics	Medical/Surgical Diagnostics	Treatments
Prostatitis (inflammation of the prostate gland)	Complete blood count; urinalysis and culture; analysis of prostate secretion	Urodynamics (if not caused by a bacterium)	Digital rectal examination	Long-term treatment with antibiotics; increase fluid intake
Benign prostatic hypertrophy/enlargement of the prostate (BPH)	Prostate-specific antigen (PSA); urinalysis	Intravenous pyelogram (IVP); pelvic ultrasound	Digital rectal examination; cystoscopy; ultrasound, and biopsy	Medications; transurethral resection prostatectomy (TURP) is rare
Prostate cancer	PSA; urinalysis; acid phosphatase (blood)	IVP; pelvic ultrasound	Digital rectal examination; cystoscopy; ultrasound, and biopsy	Prostatectomy; hormone manipulation; chemotherapy, radiation, or both
Epididymitis (inflammation of the tubes on the testis)	Complete blood count; urinalysis (culture and sensitivity test); culture and sensitivity testing of urethral discharge	IVP; pelvic ultrasound	Physical examination	Antibiotics, scrotal support
Testicular cancer		Testicular ultrasound	Physical examination (palpation of testis); biopsy	Excision of the testis; radiation therapy; chemotherapy
Testicular torsion	Lab diagnostics			
Erectile dysfunction (ED) (inability of male to achieve erection)	Complete blood count; fasting blood sugar; lipid profile; testosterone level; urinalysis	Angiogram, rarely; magnetic resonance imaging of the brain, rarely	Physical examination; neurologic examination; psychological evaluation	Oral medications; localized injected medication; penile implant; penile pump
Balanitis (inflammation of the glans of the penis)	Culture, rarely		Physical examination; skin culture	Localized soaks and frequent cleansing; antibiotics
Sexually transmitted diseases (STDs):				
Nonspecific urethritis (NSU)	Rule out other STDs; culture and sensitivity testing of urethral discharge			Increase fluid intake; antibiotics; possibly test/treat partner
Chlamydia infection	Urinalysis; urethral smear			Patient education; antibiotics; test/treat partner
Genital herpes (type II herpes simplex)	Culture of lesion			Patient education; antiviral medications; test/treat partner
Gonorrhea	Urethral smear			Patient education; antibiotics; test/treat partner
Syphilis	Urinalysis with culture; Venereal Disease Research Laboratory (VDRL) studies; culture of the lesion			Patient education; antibiotics; test/treat partner

The testes are held within a soft tissue structure called the **scrotum**. The **testes** are divided into two sections by a ridge, and the left portion hangs lower as the spermatic cord is longer on the left. The exterior appearance varies depending on several factors. These factors include pathologic conditions, but more commonly, variations are due to the response to ambient temperature.

The scrotum is made up of two layers. The first is integumentary and the second is more muscular in nature. This structure protects the arteries, veins, lymphatics, nerves, and excretory duct of the testes. The largest bundle of these tissues is referred to as the **spermatic cord**.

Each smooth, oval testis is suspended in the scrotum by the spermatic cords. The testes serve important roles in the secretion of hormones and are responsible for **spermatogenesis**. The testes produce androgens, primarily testosterone, and follicle-stimulating hormone. These are required to support the process of spermatogenesis. Spermatogenesis is the formation and development of spermatozoa (mature, motile male sex cells).

The **epididymis** is a structure that is attached to the posterior aspect of each testicle. It is a tightly coiled tube-like structure that appears solid but is actually greater than 15 feet of convoluted tubules. Spermatozoa are produced in the testes and enter the epididymis for storage. They are immature gametes upon leaving the testis. While awaiting ejaculation, these spermatozoa mature and are then able to swim and are capable of fertilization when introduced to a mature ovum.

Attached to the epididymis is the **vas deferens**. The vas deferens connects the testes with the urethra. The vas deferens is a muscular tube that is approximately 30 to 35 cm long. Its function is to conduct the mature sperm to the penis during ejaculation. The muscles in this structure contract rhythmically to propel the sperm to the prostatic urethra.

Internal Anatomy

The vas deferens attaches to the urethra inside the body of the prostate. The prostate is a plum-sized gland that sits at the base of the urinary bladder. It performs multiple functions. As it relates to the male reproductive system, the prostate provides approximately one third of the fluid that composes semen. It is also thought to enhance pleasurable sensations during arousal and orgasm.

The fluid that is secreted by the cells of the lining of the prostate keep the semen in a liquid form, support and nourish the sperm, and provide a protective protein to shield the sperm from the acidity of the female vagina.

Also located behind the bladder are the seminal vesicles. These tube-like glands make 70% of the fluid portion of semen. Included in this fluid are vital nutrients to support the mature sperm including glucose and vitamins. This fluid is added to the ejaculate in the vas deferens. A vasectomy is the surgical interruption of this structure in order to disrupt the pathway of the sperm to the outside of the body, therefore rendering the male infertile (see Figure 28-1).

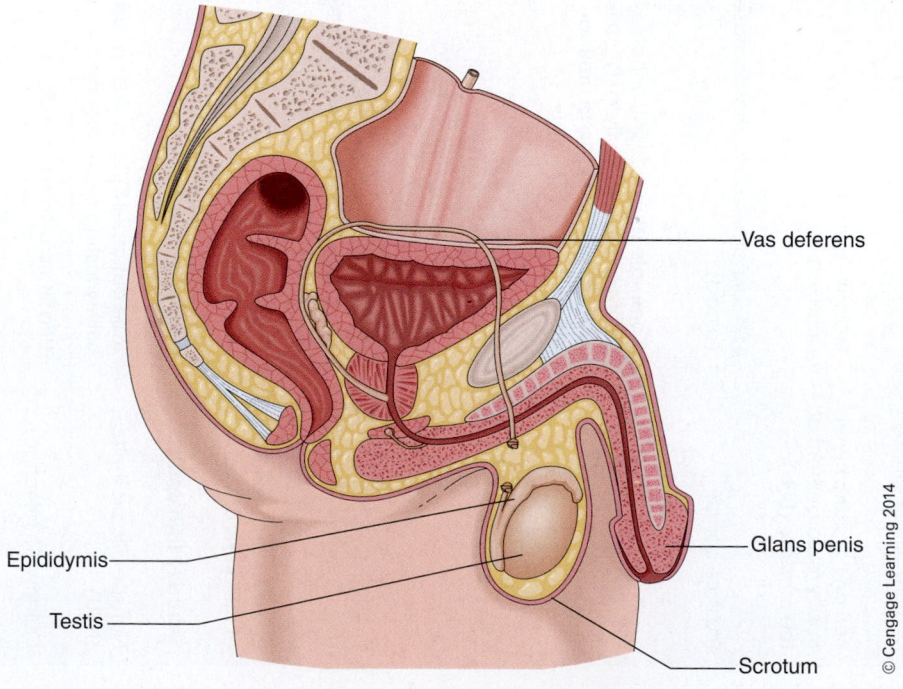

Vas deferens

Glans penis

Epididymis

Testis

Scrotum

© Cengage Learning 2014

Figure 28-1 Vasectomy (one side).

CRITICAL THINKING

What test will be done at the first postoperative clinic visit following a vasectomy?

The Cowper's or **bulbourethral glands** are also located internally at the base of the penis and are part of the male reproductive system. These glands are responsible for the manufacture and discharge of a clear viscous secretion known as pre-ejaculate. This fluid lubricates the urethra in preparation for ejaculation.

DISORDERS OF THE PENIS

Priapism

Priapism is defined as an erection lasting more than 4 hours and can occur with or without sexual stimulation. Priapism is the result of the filling of the erectile tissue in the penis that persists and interferes with the normal blood flow to the penile tissues. This interruption can result in tissue death and permanent erectile dysfunction. Predisposing factors are sickle cell disease and the use of pharmacologic agents to enhance sexual function.

The treatment for priapism includes the application of ice packs to the groin area and increased physical activity. If these measures do not relieve the symptoms, emergency medical treatment is indicated.

Erectile Dysfunction

Also called impotence, **erectile dysfunction (ED)** occurs when a man is unable to achieve or to sustain an erection of the penis during sexual intercourse. This condition or dysfunction is not normal at any age and is different from other issues that impede sexual intercourse, such as lack of **libido**.

Many men, at some point in their lives, can experience the inability to achieve an erection. This can happen on occasion from consuming too much alcohol or from extreme fatigue. This is not ED. The inability to achieve an erection more than 50% of the time is generally a reason for seeking treatment and is usually an indication of ED.

For an erection to occur, certain physiologic conditions must be present. There must be a stimulus from the brain and adequate circulation and nerve supply to the penis. If any of these conditions is impeded, an erection cannot be achieved. Some reasons why ED occurs include conditions or diseases that impair circulation (atherosclerosis) and nerve stimulation (nerve diseases) and psychological factors such as stress and depression. Medications such as those used to treat certain conditions such as hypertension can cause ED. Diabetes, multiple sclerosis, cerebral vascular accident (stroke), surgery on the prostate or bladder, and brain and spinal cord injuries are other causes of ED.

Treatment of the dysfunction is based on the cause. Referral to a urologist, psychologist, or both is made if appropriate. Blood and urine tests will be done after the provider examines the individual for medical problems. Medications the patient may be taking will be addressed. Some of the ways ED can be treated include oral medications (Viagra, Levitra, Cialis), penile injections (medication injected into the penis), sex therapy, surgery such as penile implants (device surgically implanted to overcome impotence), and vacuum pumps. A vacuum pump device is a pump put over the penis; air is pumped out of the cylinder, creating a vacuum. This vacuum causes blood to fill the penis, making it erect. Once the penis is erect, the pump can be removed.

Because of the very nature of ED, many men are embarrassed if they have the disorder, feeling they are somehow less "manly" than other men. It is of extreme importance to be conscientious and sensitive when assisting the provider with the care of these patients. Confidentiality on the telephone and during in-person conversations must be maintained. Protect your patient's privacy at all times. It is not only the law, but it is also an important attribute of a professional medical assistant.

Some experts say ED should be considered a possible risk factor for heart disease if atherosclerosis is present.

Penile Cancer

The incidence of penile cancer is greater in uncircumcised men. There is also an increased rate in men who smoke, have been infected with human papillomavirus, or have accumulations of smegma (the oily substance secreted by the skin of the penis and foreskin). The most common symptoms include lesions that do not heal on the penis as well as penile pain and bleeding.

Although penile cancer is fairly uncommon, it is a psychologically devastating disease.

Men commonly delay seeking medical treatment and physicians (especially male) delay intervention in preference for much less invasive treatment modalities such as topical steroids and antibiotics.

Usually a referral to a urologist is indicated, and the first step in treatment is a biopsy of the tissues. Treatment then depends on the severity of the lesion. Chemotherapy, radiation, and surgery are all components of the treatment regimen. A worst case scenario would be total removal of the penis, called a penectomy.

Other Disorders of the Penis

Peyronie's Disease. Curvature of the penis during erection is known as **Peyronie's disease**. It occurs due to fibrous tissue that is present subcutaneously on the shaft of the penis. This tissue can be scarring from penile trauma or is associated with other diseases that involve the formation of thickening and contracture of soft tissues.

Treatment includes the medical interventions of direct injections into the affected tissue, radiation therapy, and vitamin supplementation.

Balanitis. The swelling or inflammation of the glans penis is known as **balanitis**. If a male is uncircumcised, it is essential that the foreskin be retracted and the glans of the penis be cleansed as a part of daily hygiene. Also, care must be taken to remove any soap residue prior to returning the foreskin to its anatomic position. The exposure to soaps and other potentially irritating substances is the major cause of balanitis. Infection, diabetes, and some autoimmune disorders might also be the basis for this diagnosis.

Treatment is based on the cause of the balanitis. For example, infection may be treated with oral or topical antibiotics.

Phimosis. This condition is most common in children. **Phimosis** is the tightening of the foreskin that does not allow retraction. By the age of 3 years, an uncircumcised male should able to retract the foreskin from the tip of the penis.

The diagnosis of phimosis is usually made by a pediatrician, and the treatment involves steroid application, manual manipulation with lubrication, or a small incision to relieve the tension.

DISORDERS OF THE TESTES
Testicular Trauma

Even though the testicles are located on the exterior of the body, testicular trauma is less common than

one might expect. Owing to the mobility of the scrotum, the testes are protected from most impacts.

Testicular trauma is usually caused by a direct blow to the area, an object that penetrates the scrotum, or an injury that involves the removal of the protective integument. If the scrotum is intact and the testes have been spared, the treatment is scrotal support, methods to decrease inflammation (i.e., anti-inflammatory drugs and ice), and bed rest. If there has been interruption in the integrity of the skin or damage to the internal structures, emergency medical treatment must include surgical intervention.

Testicular Torsion

As previously discussed, each testicle is suspended in the scrotum by the spermatic cord. This cord consists of blood vessels, nerves, and other vital structures. A small percentage of males have a predisposition for a twisting of this cord, known as **testicular torsion** (see Figure 28-2). This creates an emergency situation if it is not resolved, with or without medical intervention. Testicular torsion is most common in males between the ages of 12 to 18 years. It can occur post-traumatically, after intense physical exercise, or without any evident reason.

A patient may see the practitioner complaining of sudden, severe pain in the scrotum with or without swelling. He might be nauseated, vomiting, and feel faint. To make the diagnosis, the practitioner will physically examine the testicles, looking for a palpable lump and visually evaluate whether one testicle is significantly higher than the other. Diagnosis might also include Doppler ultrasound to assess blood flow.

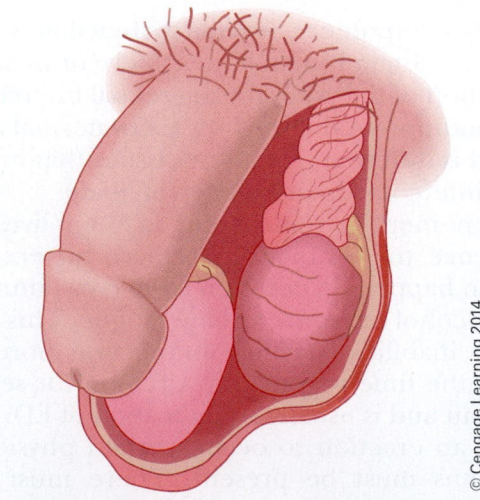

© Cengage Learning 2014

Figure 28-2   Testicular torsion.

Treatment can include manual distortion, but the most common intervention is emergency surgery to release the torsion and secure the testicle to the inner layers of the scrotum to prevent future events.

Testicular Cancer

This cancer affects young men between the ages of 15 and 40 most commonly. Those males at a higher risk have a family history of testicular cancer or other risk factors including abnormal testicular development, such as an undescended testicle (**cryptorchidism**, Figure 28-3) and Klinefelter syndrome. Exposure to industrial or farming chemicals and human immunodeficiency virus (HIV) also increases risk.

There are several types of testicular cancer. Seminoma arises in men between the ages of 30 and 40 most commonly. This type of cancer usually spreads via the lymph system. It can be deadly, but it responds well to radiation therapy. This cancer is highly curable if detected early. Monthly testicular self-examinations are recommended by the American Cancer Society and can be essential in early detection. It is the role of a medical assistant to integrate this important patient teaching topic, with the practitioner's approval,

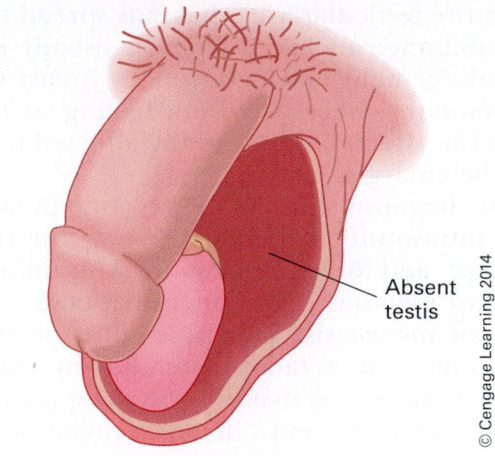

Figure 28-3   Cryptorchidism.

into the patient care plan. Figure 28-4 illustrates a testicular self-examination, and Procedure 28-1 outlines steps for instructions usually given to the patient by the medical assistant.

There is another classification of testicular tumors—nonseminoma. These tumors are the most common tumors that then translate into seminomas. The patient's symptoms will include

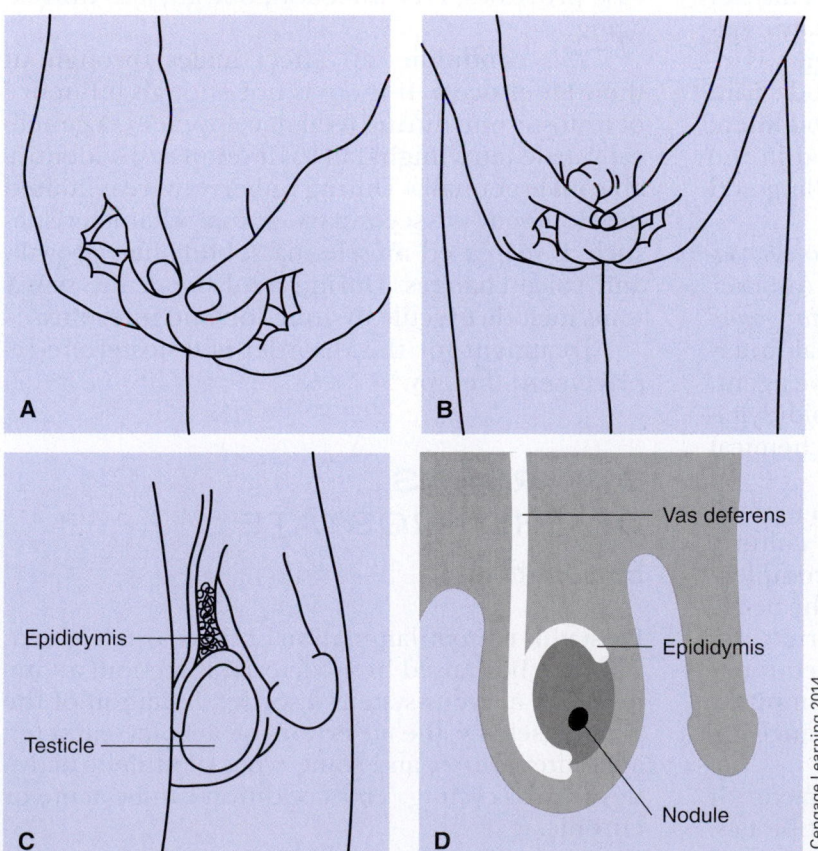

Figure 28-4   Testicular self-examination should be performed once a month after a warm bath or shower. The heat will relax the scrotum, making it easier to find abnormalities. (A) Stand in front of the mirror. Look for swelling on the skin of the scrotum. (B) Examine each testicle with both hands. Position your index and middle fingers under the testicle with the thumbs on top. Gently roll the testicle between your thumbs and fingers (having one testicle larger than the other is normal). (C) Find the epididymis (the soft tubelike structure at the back of the testicle). Do not mistake the epididymis for an abnormal lump. (D) If you find a lump, notify your provider immediately. Most lumps are found on the sides of the testicle, but some are located on the front. Testicular cancer is highly curable when detected early and treated promptly.

pain in the testicular area that may spread to the lower abdomen or back. There is usually testicular enlargement and occasionally breast tissue enlargement. There may be a feeling of heaviness in the affected side, and the affected testicle might be enlarged.

The diagnosis will include an abdominal and pelvic ultrasound, laboratory testing for tumor markings, and other testing to determine the degree of metastasis. Treatment depends on the extent of metastasis. The procedure of choice for treatment is a radical **orchiectomy** with biopsy of surrounding tissues for staging purposes. Postsurgical treatment includes radiation and chemotherapy.

It is important to provide patient teaching materials that cover what to expect postoperatively. Infertility is a certainty due to excision of the testis as well as the follow-up radiation and chemotherapy. There are also other associated risks to other organ systems from chemotherapy.

Epididymitis

Inflammation of the epididymis can be caused by various factors. Most commonly, the causative factor is a bacterial infection. A sexually transmitted disease is usually the causative organism. This can be a hallmark of sexual abuse in the pediatric setting and reporting to a child protective agency is indicated. Patients have symptoms that include pain in the groin, testicular area, flank, or abdomen; fever; discharge from the penis; and blood in the urine. There may be scrotal pain and swelling and pain upon urination.

The causative organism, *Chlamydia trachomatis*, is present in 50% to 60% of the cases. Another common infectious organism is *Neisseria gonorrhoeae*. For men who participate in anal intercourse, *Escherichia coli* might be the infective agent. There are other conditions that lead to epididymitis. Retrograde urine flow can cause a chemical epididymitis, as can some medications.

A diagnosis of epididymitis is based on a physical examination, urinalysis, and urine culture. Also, the white blood cell count on a complete blood count, and a urethral culture might be included in the evaluation. In order to rule out other causes for this type of pain, your practitioner might prescribe a testicular ultrasound, computed tomography (CT) scan, or magnetic resonance imaging (MRI) of the affected area.

Treatment is based on the causative factor. If bacterial, this condition is treated with antibiotics.

It is an important aspect of care, once the diagnosis is made, that the patient is counseled to inform all sexual partners of the causative organism, because they must be treated as well.

Hypogonadism

One of the functions of the testes is to produce testosterone. This hormone is responsible for the development of many male characteristics. In men, **hypogonadism** occurs when the testes produce little or no testosterone. Hypogonadism is often the result of a chromosomal abnormality, Klinefelter syndrome, which is a genetic disorder in which males have an additional X chromosome. Instead of XY, the chromosomal pattern is XXY. Not all males with this pattern demonstrate the symptoms of Klinefelter syndrome. The abnormality is so common that the National Institutes of Health estimate that 1 in 500 males has the extra X chromosome, but not all have the syndrome. Those males with symptoms are designated as XXY males.

Other causative factors for hypogonadism include cyrptorchisism, infection of the testicles from mumps, injury to the testicles, and cancer treatment. Some secondary causes are disorders of the hypothalamus or pituitary, inflammatory disease processes, HIV infection, obesity, and normal aging.

This condition can affect males throughout their life process. If there is not enough influence of testosterone during fetal development, a genetically male fetus might fail to develop easily identifiable male genitalia. During puberty there is limited development of secondary sexual characteristics such as increased muscle mass, body hair growth, and voice changes. During adulthood, the symptoms include erectile dysfunction and infertility.

Treatment for this disorder is testosterone replacement therapy.

DISORDERS OF THE PROSTATE
Prostatitis

Prostatitis is an inflammation of the prostate gland. This can be caused by a bacterial infection, an immune or nervous system disorder, irritation of the gland itself by the insertion of a Foley catheter, anal intercourse, and some types of athletic activities such as cycling. This condition can be acute or chronic.

Patients will present complaining of painful or difficult urination, nocturia, pain in the groin or lower back, pain in the testicular area, painful orgasms, or flu-like symptoms. In order to obtain an accurate diagnosis, your practitioner will do a thorough physical examination, order a blood culture, and might suggest a cystoscopy or urodynamic testing.

Prostatitis (called pelvic pain syndrome) may be either acute or chronic. The treatments include antibiotics, alpha blockers to assist in the relaxation of the bladder and aid in the flow of urine, pain relievers, and prostate massage.

Benign Prostatic Hyperplasia

Enlargement of the prostate gland that is not due to infection or cancer is known as **benign prostatic hyperplasia (BPH)**. This condition is common in men over the age of 50 and is of concern because an enlarged prostate gland blocks the flow of urine and does not allow complete emptying of the bladder.

The most common symptoms involve not being able to sleep through the night because of frequent urination. This symptom is known as **nocturia**. Your patient might also report a weak urine stream, dribbling at the end of the urine stream, or the feeling of being unable to completely empty the bladder.

Treatment is based on the severity of the symptoms. Treatment is indicated for complications such as sudden, painful inability to urinate, frequent urinary tract infections, or kidney damage caused by high pressure in the bladder due to urinary retention.

To determine the treatment after the detailed history, the practitioner will perform a thorough physical examination. Evaluation will include a laboratory workup to assess the prostate-specific antigen (PSA), rectal digital examination to palpate the prostate through the anterior wall of the rectum, and a urinalysis. It is important to note that the PSA needs to be drawn prior to the digital examination as this manipulation can cause a rise in the PSA. Diagnosis is also based on several procedures that measure the flow of urine from the bladder. These tests include:

- Urine flow studies are performed to determine the strength and amount of urine flow.
- Postvoiding residual urine studies to determine the amount of urine left in the bladder after voiding. This analysis can be conducted using an ultrasound or by accessing the bladder using a catheter to measure the amount of urine remaining.
- Ultrasound of the prostate is performed transrectally to measure the anatomy.

More invasive methods include:

- **Intravenous pyelogram (IVP)** using venous access and injecting a radiopaque medium that will allow the radiologist to observe the flow of urine through the urinary tract.
- Prostate biopsy to rule out prostatic cancer.
- Urodynamic studies to monitor pressures in the bladder, discover any urinary **retention** issues, and assess the function of the bladder muscles.

After a complete assessment, if treatment is needed, medications that relax the bladder neck or shrink the prostate are utilized. If the symptoms are severe, surgery may be indicated. A **transurethral resection of the prostate (TURP)** is a common procedure (see Figure 28-5). As the name indicates, a scope is inserted in the urethra and small tools are utilized to access the prostate and carve away enough to allow adequate urine flow. A more invasive surgery is the open prostatectomy. This is indicated if the prostate is very large and there are other complicating factors. There are many associated risks with this procedure and the recovery time is much longer.

Recently, there have been strides in surgical modalities that allow the patient to recover more rapidly. These methods include laser, microwave, and cryotherapy to reduce the size of the prostate.

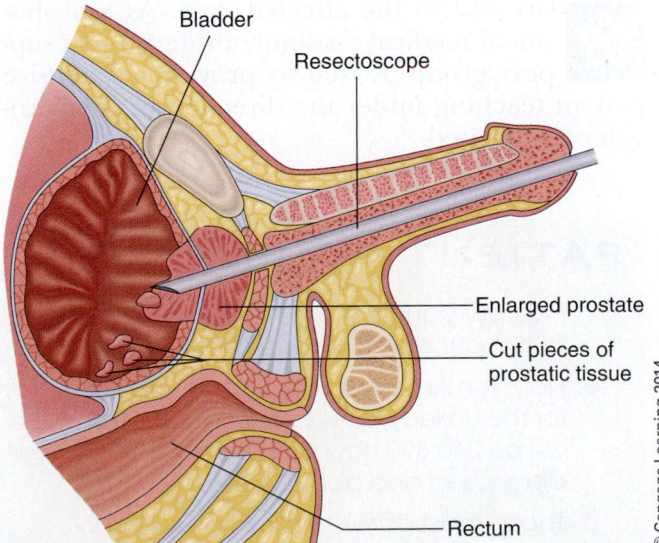

© Cengage Learning 2014

Figure 28-5   Transurethral resection of the prostate (TURP).

Prostate Cancer

Prostate cancer is the leading cause of cancer-related death in men 75 and older. With the availability of better screening tools, like the PSA test, early diagnosis is enabling earlier treatment for men with this form of cancer. Many times, this blood test indicates prostate cancer before there are symptoms. If symptoms are present, they are very similar to those associated with BPH (see above).

A prostate cancer screen also includes a digital rectal examination by the health practitioner. If transrectal examination shows are irregularities in the surface of the prostate, for further investigation is warranted. Transrectal ultrasonography and guided core needle biopsy are useful tools for diagnosis.

After a diagnosis of prostatic cancer, it must be staged to determine the patient's prognosis and most effective treatment plan. Prostate cancer is staged using a Gleason score. Dr. Donald Gleason invented this score in 1966. He biopsied more than 3000 patients with a diagnosis of prostate cancer and developed this method to relate the severity of the disease. A higher Gleason score indicates a greater aggressiveness of the cancer. This score serves as a guide to effective treatment.

Treatment most often includes a **prostatectomy** and can be followed by chemotherapy and radiation. There is often an added component of hormone therapy. The surgical prostatectomy can lead to many complications with the urinary system and with sexual function. This can be psychologically stressful to the affected man. As a professional medical assistant, a referral to a support group as well as providing extensive patient teaching under the direction of your provider is indicated.

OTHER DISORDERS OF THE MALE REPRODUCTIVE SYSTEM

Sexually Transmitted Diseases

STDs affect men and women; they can damage health and become life-threatening (Table 28-2). (See Chapter 26 for additional information regarding STDs.)

Table 28-2   Sexually Transmitted Diseases

Disease	Description
Chlamydial infection	Common in male and female individuals. A prevalent sexually transmitted disease that often coexists with gonorrhea.
Genital herpes	Painful viral disease that is dormant and recurs periodically. There is no cure. Characterized by blisters similar to chickenpox. Common in male and female individuals.
Gonorrhea	Caused by a bacterium. Infection can spread, producing a stricture of the urethra or the vas deferens. Sterility can result if both vas deferentia become involved.
Syphilis	Caused by a spirochete. Chancres develop and can subsequently heal. If untreated, the disease progresses to stages two and three. Severe damage to the cardiovascular system and brain and vision and hearing loss occur. General paralysis and death can result. Highly contagious.
Hepatitis B and C virus and HIV infections	All are caused by a virus and have no cure.

© Cengage Learning 2014

PATIENT EDUCATION

1. Prostate cancer is the most common cause of cancer death in men over the age of 75.

2. From the American Cancer Society estimates for the United States population in 2011, there will be 240,890 new cases of prostate cancer diagnosed and about 33,720 deaths.

3. Those most at risk for prostate cancer are men over the age of 60, and those with a family history of prostate cancer, with African-American men at a slightly higher risk.

4. A Gleason score is the manner of reporting the risk of metastasis. This score ranges from 1 to 10.

5. Survival depends on the staging.

6. The treatment for prostate cancer can impact sexual performance and urinary control.

Infertility

When couples regularly have unprotected sexual intercourse, the majority of them usually conceive within 1 year. The inability or diminished ability to conceive is known as **infertility**.

A provider who is treating couples for infertility might order a semen analysis as an early test to determine if the source of nonconception is related to an insufficiency in the sperm count. Sperm present in semen may not be of a sufficient number or quality to allow fertilization. A semen analysis includes a measure of the volume of the ejaculate, the time it takes for the semen to become liquid, and the number of mature, mobile sperm in the semen. The semen is tested to reveal the pH, presence of fructose, and white blood cells. All of these components assure the health of the sperm contained in the semen. If there is a determination of a low sperm count, treatment is based on the underlying cause. If there is venous congestion in the testicle (varicocele) surgery might be indicated to correct this issue. If an infection is the cause, antibiotics are indicated. Further investigation may prove that there are male hormone deficiencies and this can be treated with supplementation. Depending on a provider's specialty, he or she may chose to treat these conditions or refer the patient to a urologist or a specialist in the treatment of infertility.

Multiple causes of infertility are unrelated to a low sperm count. These causes include an infection in the genitourinary tract or the presence of an STD, either of which can block the tract and prohibit sperm from being fully ejaculated. An injury to the blood or nerve supply in the area, radiation exposure, stress, and hormonal imbalances are other factors that can promote infertility.

A complete physical examination and medical history (including childhood illnesses such as parotitis [mumps]), semen analysis for count and motility, and tests for endocrine disorders can help determine the cause of infertility.

Treatment of a male patient with infertility depends on the cause. Treatments include surgery to remove a blockage, antibiotics to treat an infection, use of artificial insemination, or use of pharmaceuticals to treat the infertility.

Prevention of the factors that may cause infertility is preferable because the percentage of couples treated for infertility who successfully become pregnant is relatively low.

ASSISTING WITH THE MALE REPRODUCTIVE EXAMINATION

  A female medical assistant usually is not required to assist the provider with the examination of the male reproductive system. However, it is within your professional responsibility to assist your provider as requested. Remember to conduct yourself in a respectful, appropriate manner, including nonverbal communication.

The provider examines the penis and the foreskin of the penis in an uncircumcised patient. In the United States, it is common for males to be circumcised shortly after birth. However, that is not the cultural expectation in many other countries.  Remember that cultural norms vary from country to country. There are many men who require health care that are from other nations and cultures. It is important to understand that diversity is acceptable. The penis and testes are examined for swelling, masses, or discomfort. The provider performs a digital rectal examination to check the size of the prostate and also checks for an inguinal hernia.

When working in a total practice management system, the provider completes the examination, orders tests and procedures, charts the findings, orders prescriptions as needed, and orders a follow-up appointment for the patient—right in the examination room (Figure 28-6).

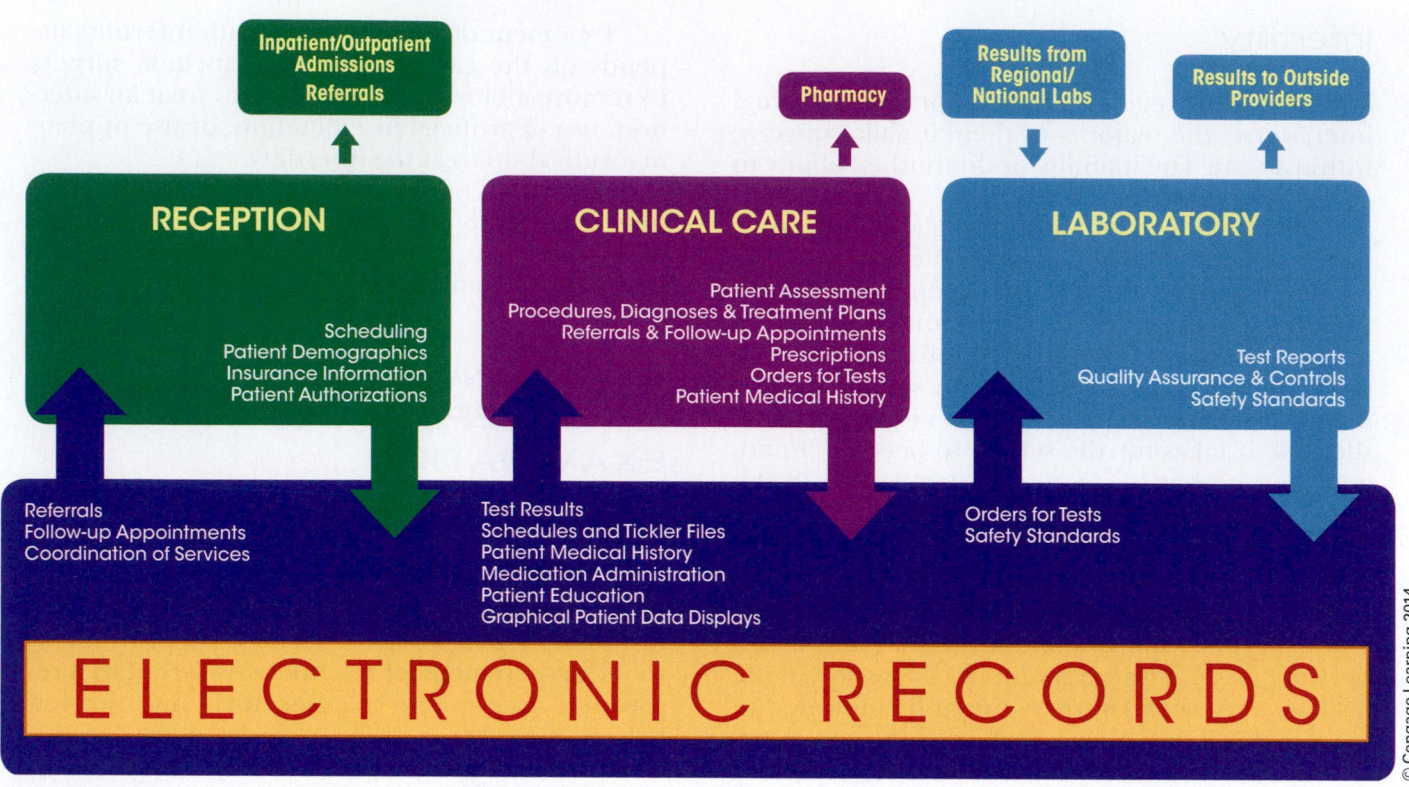

Figure 28-6 Clinical care, laboratory, and reception arms of a total practice management system.

PROCEDURE 28-1

Instructing Patient in Testicular Self-Examination

PURPOSE:

To provide a patient with information concerning testicular screening for the presence of a painless mass in the scrotum.

EQUIPMENT/SUPPLIES:

Testicular self-examination card
Anatomy illustration

PROCEDURE STEPS:

1. *Identify yourself and explain the procedure, speaking at the patient's level of understanding. Identify patient.*

2. *Being courteous and respectful,* instruct the patient to examine his testicles monthly in a warm shower. RATIONALE: The warmth causes the scrotal skin to relax.

3. Hold the penis out of the way and check one testicle at a time.

4. Examine each testicle separately with both hands.

5. Place the index and middle fingers underneath the testicle and the thumbs on top. Roll the testicle gently between the fingers.

6. Look and feel any hard lumps, any smooth rounded bumps, or change in size, shape or consistency of the testes.

7. Locate the epididymis. Provide a chart to the patient that illustrates the testes and epididymis. RATIONALE: A lump can be similar in size to the epididymis and needs to be distinguished from the epididymis.

8. Look for swelling or changes in the scrotal area.

9. Encourage the patient to report anything unusual to the provider.

10. Accurately record all information in patient's chart or electronic medical record.

DOCUMENTATION:

11/4/20XX   Patient instructed on how to perform testicular self-examination. Patient returned the demonstration and had no questions. K. Sanchez, CMA (AAMA)———————

CASE STUDY 28-1

Refer to the scenario at the beginning of the chapter.

After Dr. Olani has examined Mr. Range, he asks you to schedule a testicular ultrasound to assess the testicular mass that was discovered during a routine testicular self-examination.

CASE STUDY REVIEW

1. What can be determined from these tests?
2. What is the best method to deliver the results of this testing to Mr. Range?

CASE STUDY 28-2

Adam Desmond has an appointment today in the clinic for a physical examination. His chief complaint is that he has been having trouble sitting through ball games or movies without having to go to the bathroom to urinate several times.

CASE STUDY REVIEW

1. How can the provider make a diagnosis of benign prostatic hyperplasia?
2. What preliminary tests might the provider order for Mr. Desmond today?

CASE STUDY 28-3

Mr. Ranger called Dr. Olani's clinic to say that he discovered "something hard in his right testicle, like a marble."

CASE STUDY REVIEW

1. What will Dr. Olani's examination consist of?

SUMMARY

A thorough knowledge of the diseases and disorders of the male reproductive system and the diagnostic tests and procedures that are performed for this specialty will enhance the quality of care given by the medical assistant.

STUDY FOR SUCCESS

To reinforce your knowledge and skills of information presented in this chapter:

- Review the *Key Terms*
- Role-play with other students to apply attributes of professionalism pertinent to this chapter.
- Consider the *Case Studies* and discuss your conclusions
- Answer the questions in the *Certification Review*
- Apply your knowledge by completing the *Activities* in the Study Guide and the *Games and Quizzes* in the StudyWARE **StudyWARE** software on the *Premium Website*
- Perform the *Procedures* using the *Competency Assessment Checklists* in the *Competency Manual*
- Practice your problem-solving skills with the *Critical Thinking Challenge 3.0* on the *Premium Website*

Additional resources for this chapter include:

- Module 18 of the *Medical Assisting Learning Lab*
- *CourseMate for Delmar's Comprehensive Medical Assisting*
- *WebTutor for Delmar's Comprehensive Medical Assisting*

CERTIFICATION REVIEW

1. Cancer of the prostate may be detected early by which of the following?
   a. Prostate-specific antigen
   b. Transurethral resection of the prostate
   c. Semen analysis
   d. Urine culture
2. The best preventive measure for testicular cancer is which of the following?
   a. Yearly physical examination
   b. Yearly intravenous pyelogram
   c. Monthly self-examination
   d. Monthly urinalysis with cultures
3. Benign prostatic hypertrophy (BPH) is thought to be caused by:
   a. excessive consumption of alcohol
   b. aging and hormonal changes
   c. recurrent epididymitis
   d. chronic chlamydia infections
4. Which of the following is a symptom of prostatitis?
   a. Painful urination
   b. Low sperm count
   c. Eruptions on the scrotum
   d. High testosterone level
5. The most definitive way to diagnose cancer of the prostate is by which of the following?
   a. Ultrasonography
   b. Intravenous pyelogram
   c. Biopsy of the prostate
   d. Semen analysis
6. Erectile dysfunction is defined as:
   a. the inability to achieve an erection
   b. the inability to sustain an erection
   c. lack of libido
   d. both a and b
7. Important aspects of documentation of patient education regarding testicular examination are:
   a. patient questions
   b. return demonstration
   c. medical assistant name
   d. all of the above
8. The vas deferens attaches to what structure?
   a. Bladder
   b. Penis
   c. Urethra
   d. Prostrate
9. Prostate cancer is the leading cause of death in men from which age group?
   a. 45–55 years old
   b. 55–65 years old
   c. 65–75 years old
   d. 75 years and older
10. The incidence of penile cancer is greater in what population?
    a. Men over 75 years
    b. Men with a history of STDs
    c. Uncircumcised men
    d. Men who are infertile

REFERENCES/BIBLIOGRAPHY

Common male sexual problems—erectile dysfunction. Retrieved May 26, 2007, from http://www.webmd.com/sexual-conditions/guide/mens-sexual-problems

Taber's cyclopedic medical dictionary (20th ed.). (2005). Philadelphia: F. A. Davis.

Tamparo, C., & Lewis, M. (2005). *Diseases of the human body* (4th ed.). Philadelphia: F. A. Davis.

Warner, J. (ed.). (2007). *Erectile dysfunction.* Retrieved May 29, 2007, from http://www.webmd.com/sexual-conditions/guide/mens-sexual-problems

CHAPTER 29

Gerontology

OUTLINE

Societal Bias

Facts about Aging

Physiologic Changes

  Senses

  Integumentary System

  Nervous System

  Musculoskeletal System

  Respiratory System

  Cardiovascular System

Gastrointestinal System

Urinary System

Reproductive System

Prevention of Complications

Psychological Changes

The Medical Assistant and the Geriatric Patient

  Memory-Impaired Older Adults

Visually Impaired Older Adults

Hearing Impaired Older Adults

Elder Abuse

Healthy and Successful Aging

LEARNING OUTCOMES

1. Define, spell, and pronounce the key terms as presented in the glossary.
2. Identify expected physiologic changes that occur as part of the aging process.
3. List five common functional changes that can occur as part of the aging process.
4. Describe prevention techniques for complications arising from age-related disorders.
5. Explain two myths about aging.
6. Explain the importance of communication with older adults.
7. Identify several techniques or strategies to communicate with visually and hearing impaired older adults.
8. Describe strategies for healthy and successful aging.
9. Analyze the professionalism questions and apply them to this chapter's content.

KEY TERMS

andropause

arteriosclerosis

cognitive functioning

cystitis

dementia

dyspneic

empathize

geriatrics

gerontology

hyperthermia

hypothermia

incontinence

macular degeneration

menopause

nevus

osteoporosis

pernicious anemia

presbycusis

residual urine

senile

transient ischemic
attack (TIA)

ATTRIBUTES OF PROFESSIONALISM

Communication

- Did you listen to and acknowledge the patient?
- Did you speak at the patient's level of understanding?
- Did you provide appropriate responses/feedback?
- Did you display appropriate body language?
- Did you respond honestly and diplomatically to the patient's concerns?
- Did you demonstrate empathy in communicating with patients, family, and staff?
- Did you maintain eye contact with the patient during communication?
- Did you accurately and concisely update the provider on any aspect of the patient's care?
- Did you include the patient's support system as indicated?

Presentation

- Did your actions attend to both the psychological and the physiologic aspects of the patient's illness or condition?
- Did you attend to any special needs of the patient? Did you ask first if assistance was needed, rather than taking charge?
- Were you courteous, patient, and respectful to the patient?
- Did you display a calm, professional, and caring manner?

Competency

- Did you display sound judgment?
- Were you knowledgeable and accountable?
- Did you recognize the importance of local, state, and federal legislation and regulations in the practice setting?

Initiative

- Did you direct the patient to other resources when necessary or helpful, with the approval of the provider?

Integrity

- Did you demonstrate an appreciation for the patient's attitude toward illness or condition?
- Did you protect and maintain confidentiality?
- Did you report situations that were harmful or illegal?
- Did you maintain your moral and ethical standards?
- Did you do the "right thing" even when no one was observing?

SCENARIO

Mrs. Johnson is an 82-year-old patient of Dr. King, and she is scheduled for an appointment in the cardiac clinic. She is being evaluated for congestive heart disease and has had hypertension for many years. Her condition was difficult to control, but now she responds to medication.

She has become a volunteer at the gift shop at St. Louis Hospital. She is an example of an older adult with chronic illnesses who has changed some long-time behaviors that were harmful to her health.

INTRODUCTION

Gerontology is the scientific study of the problems associated with aging. *Geriatrics* is the branch of medicine that specializes in all aspects of aging: physiologic, pathologic, psychological, economic, and sociologic. The importance of studying gerontology is becoming more recognized because the expected life span is increasing. Thousands of people are living to be 100 years old or older. The aging population is growing rapidly, and according to the U.S. Census Bureau, by 2030, there will be 60 million people in the United States older than 65 years. The 80 and above age group is currently the fastest growing population group. As a medical assistant, you will be experiencing the impact on the health care system of this growing population of people.

  Through knowledge of the physical and psychological changes that occur as an individual ages, as a medical assistant you will be better able to recognize the special needs of this group of people. You will draw on and use effective communication skills and provide quality health care to geriatric patients.

SOCIETAL BIAS

In our culture, there is a deeply ingrained bias about aging. Older adults are stereotyped, and there is much discrimination because of age. Myths and stereotypes are common, and the medical assistant can be an advocate for older adults and can be sensitive to these myths and stereotypes. Accurate information and useful concepts about aging must be communicated to the general public. Older adults oftentimes are viewed as sick, frail, powerless, sexless, and burdensome. As a society, we are obsessed with the negative, rather than the positive, aspects of aging. The most popular myth is, "To be old is to be sick." Recent studies indicate that older adults in the United States are generally healthier than their counterparts of nearly a decade ago. Even in advanced old age, a majority of the older population has little functional disability. Years of research have debunked

CRITICAL THINKING

What do you consider common myths about older adults? What are your thoughts about these myths?

this myth. Because of better education about the practice of healthier lifestyles, to be old in the United States does not mean to be sick and frail. Thousands of people are living to be older than 100 years because of the recognition that healthy lifestyles are the most important factor in helping people to live long, healthy, productive lives. Such factors as good nutrition, regular exercise, stress reduction, yearly physical examinations, not smoking, and today's technology help forestall the aging process.

FACTS ABOUT AGING

Following are general facts about aging:

- Aging is a progressive, universal, and slow process.
- There are no diseases specific to aging.
- As people age, not all functional changes are related to disease. Interest, personal and financial resources, family structure, genetics, and attitude all play a part. The individual's lifestyle is a major factor. For example, smoking, misuse of chemicals such as alcohol or drugs, type of diet, and lack of exercise all play a part in how people age.
- There is a wider range of what is considered "normal" function among older adults than among younger people. There is a greater variability among older people in their physical

abilities, sizes, and characteristics than among younger groups (Figure 29-1).

- All older ages are not alike. People in their 60s, 70s, 80s, and 90s are all different.

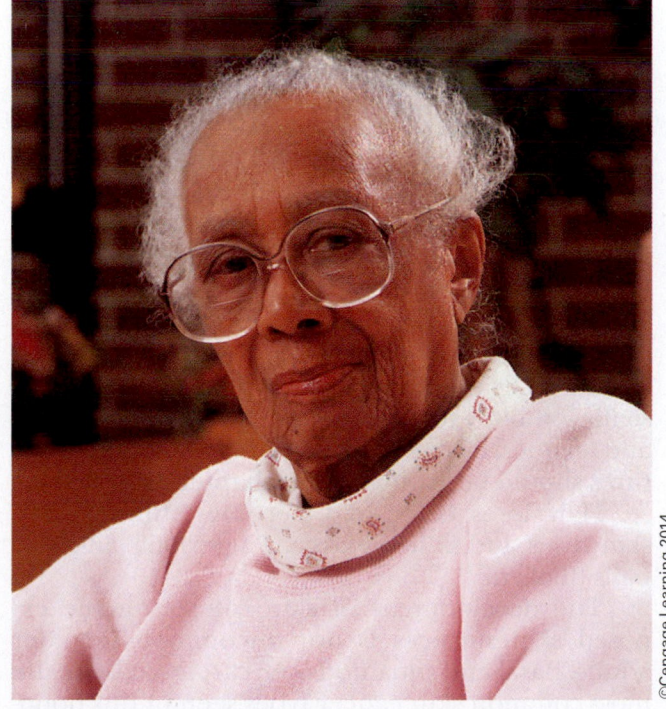

Figure 29-1   Note the many signs of aging.

©Cengage Learning 2014

PHYSIOLOGIC CHANGES

Although aging is a normal process, not all individuals age in the same way or at the same rate, because no two people have exactly the same genetic inheritance, personal lifestyle, or experiences in life. All of these factors strongly influence the ways in which we grow older. Some believe that the body endures wear and tear and stress during life and that because of this, eventually the body loses its ability to function as well as it had. Others believe that as people grow older, the body produces smaller and smaller amounts of various hormones and other chemicals that keep the body functioning. The fewer of these kinds of substances that are produced, the more susceptible an individual becomes to disease.

Every body system undergoes changes as we age. The changes are physiologic and psychological. As individuals move into their 60s and beyond, they will show physiologic changes that are part of the aging process. As people age, their body systems function less effectively, causing them to have difficulty performing their ordinary, everyday tasks of living. Also, as people grow older, they can become more susceptible to disorders and diseases. When taking the medical history of an older patient, it is evident that many have one or several chronic illnesses. Heart disease, diabetes, arthritis, hypertension, and vision and auditory impairments are common.

Although it is important to be knowledgeable about the physiologic changes that occur as part of aging, it is important to realize that the majority of older adults are free of serious, chronic health problems.

Senses

Vision. Many changes occur in the eye's ability to function. Pupil size diminishes, limiting the amount of light that can go through it to reach the retina. There is a diminished production of tears, so the eye may be dry, red, and irritated. The lens may become cloudy, and the cornea thickens. There is increased sensitivity to glare. Several problems can occur as a result of these changes. There is less ability to see clearly at any distance and to discern various shades of colors. Older people will need eyeglasses to help correct their vision loss, but reading small print can remain difficult (Figure 29-2). Glare can be minimized by incorporating a process known as polarization into corrective lenses.

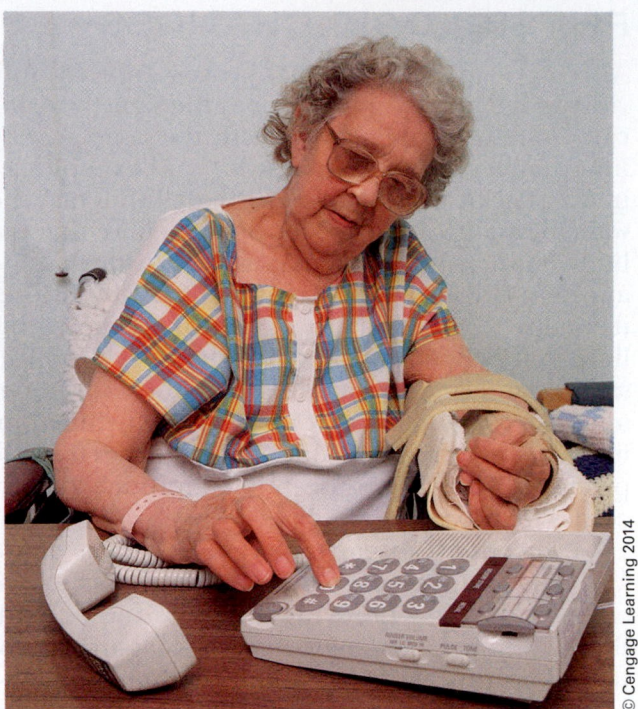

© Cengage Learning 2014

Figure 29-2　Good lighting and large numbers on a telephone can help improve vision.

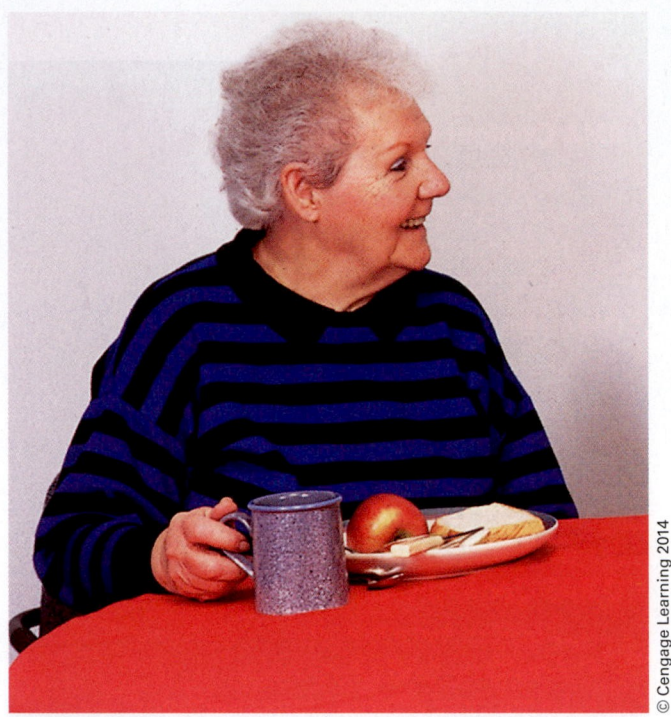

© Cengage Learning 2014

Figure 29-3　Older adults may add more salt and sugar to their food to compensate for their diminished sense of taste.

Cataracts, **macular degeneration**, and glaucoma are common findings in older adults. Cataracts can be surgically excised if they are large. Glaucoma can be treated medically or surgically but if left untreated can lead to blindness. Macular degeneration can lead to vision impairment. The macula of the retina is an important area in the visualization of fine details. Macular degeneration is the leading cause of visual impairment in adults older than 50 years, making it difficult to do fine work or such activities as threading a needle. Laser surgery may halt the progression of the degeneration.

Because of failing vision and impaired balance and coordination, older adults should be cautioned to use handrails whenever possible.

Hearing. Loss of hearing in the aging process is not uncommon. It usually occurs over a period of years, and the older person may not be aware of the loss. Loss of the ability to hear begins at about the third decade of life. Many times, individuals with hearing loss seem inattentive or confused and are thought to be mentally weak or **senile**. Presbyacusia or **presbycusis** is the progressive loss of hearing ability caused by the normal aging process.

Taste and Smell. Taste and smell diminish with age, making food less appealing because it no longer tastes as good as it once did (Figure 29-3). Taste buds decrease in size. Detecting odors becomes difficult and impaired, further lessening the desire for food. It is not unusual for older adults to lose weight and even to become malnourished because of the loss of the ability to taste and smell. Lacking the sense of smell can be dangerous because of the inability to smell smoke or gas and other dangerous fumes.

Integumentary System

Aging individuals' skin becomes more fragile with less subcutaneous and connective tissue. Exposure to sunlight is the major cause of wrinkled skin, liver spots, and leathery looking skin.

Sweat glands become smaller and the body becomes nonsensitive to heat and cold. **Hyperthermia**, an unusually high fever, and **hypothermia**, an unusually low body temperature, are serious problems, and exposure to excessive hot or cold temperatures should be avoided (see Chapter 33).

Hair loses color and becomes thinner. The skin dries and is less elastic. Fingernails and toenails thicken.

The development of skin cancer on the exposed skin surfaces is not uncommon in older adults. Basal and squamous cell carcinomas are the most common skin cancer types seen in this population. Both types of cancer can be serious if left untreated, but squamous cell cancer can metastasize. A complete skin assessment should be done on a yearly basis. Melanoma, a malignant tumor developing from a **nevus**, is the least common skin cancer, but it can be serious because it metastasizes readily. It is caused by exposure to the sun. Many older adults live in the Sunbelt areas of the United States and should be cautioned to wear sunscreen of SPF 15 or higher. People of all ages should protect their skin daily with a sunscreen of SPF 15 or higher, regardless of where they reside.

Nervous System

The brain shrinks in size as an individual ages because brain cells do not continue to divide throughout life as other cells do. Some loss of memory or delay in memory can be expected in many, but not all, aging people. Mental competence is the rule rather than the exception for older adults. Sudden loss of memory accompanied by confusion and inability to do tasks once able to be performed could be an indication of an organic problem, such as **transient ischemic attack (TIA)**, a temporary interference of the blood supply to the brain, or a brain lesion.

Problems with balance, temperature regulation, diminished pain sensation, and insomnia can occur as part of the physical changes of aging that affect the nervous system.

Chronic illnesses from which many older people suffer often require several different medications for control. Side effects of medication (over-the-counter, prescription, and herbals) can cause decreased mental capacity, as can malnutrition and substance abuse.

Loss of balance can be a problem for some older adults. Their coordination of muscles for movement may need more time for processing than it does with younger individuals. Older adults need to be reminded to be sure of their balance before starting to walk and to do so slowly. There is a general unsteadiness and lack of coordination not only because of the aging process, but also possibly because of medications the older adult takes (Figure 29-4). Older adults may need to use a cane to help steady their gait.

Musculoskeletal System

Musculoskeletal system changes are evident because older adults may have less muscle strength.

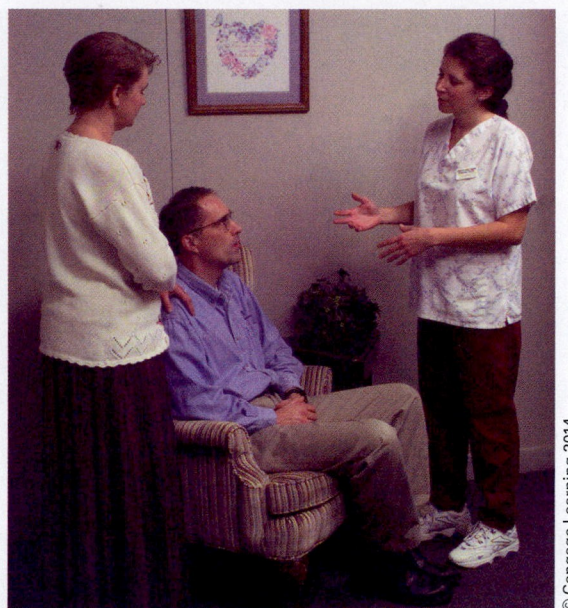
© Cengage Learning 2014

Figure 29-4   Older adults should be instructed to take their time when sitting, standing, and walking.

This results in loss of mobility, and the activities of daily living become more difficult. There is less flexibility and joints can stiffen. Loss of height and a stooped appearance can result. Arthritis and osteoporosis are not unusual, and older adults can suffer fractured bones more easily. Poor nutrition, malnourishment, and lack of exercise all contribute to these conditions and prolong healing time as well (see Chapters 33 and 34).

Osteoporosis—a thinning of the long bones, pelvic bones, and vertebrae—is a fairly common problem in the aging population, with more women than men affected. This thinning of bone makes these individuals more susceptible to pain and fractures in these and other bones. New medications (Fosamax, Actonel, Evista) plus 1500 mg of calcium daily helps to slow the progress of osteoporosis. Vitamin D is essential for utilization of calcium. A deficiency of vitamin D in older adults occurs either because it is insufficient in their diets or because of insufficient exposure to sunlight. Vitamin D is added to milk.

Physical activity and a nutritional diet, including dairy products, can stall the development of bone and muscle loss; therefore, older adults should be encouraged to keep active by walking, gardening, swimming, bicycling, golfing, and so on. The pace of these activities should be suited to the individual's level of ability (Figure 29-5).

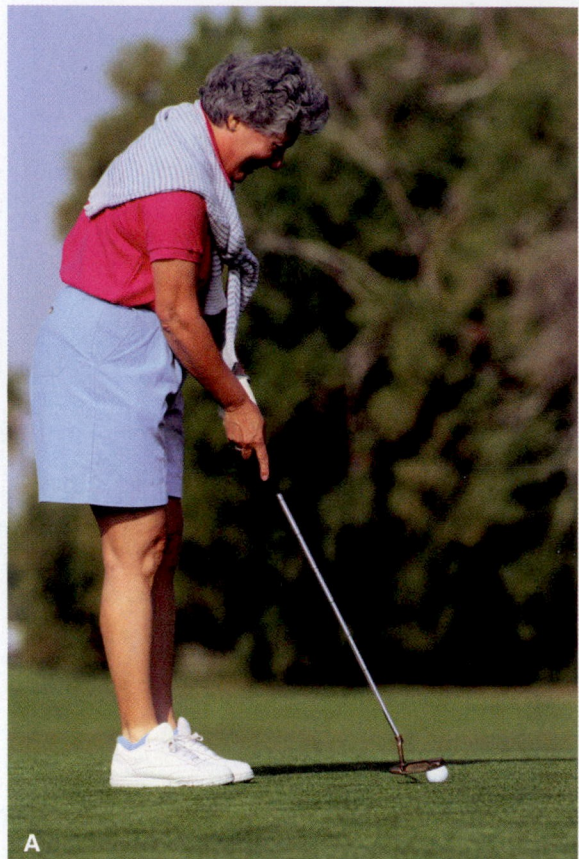

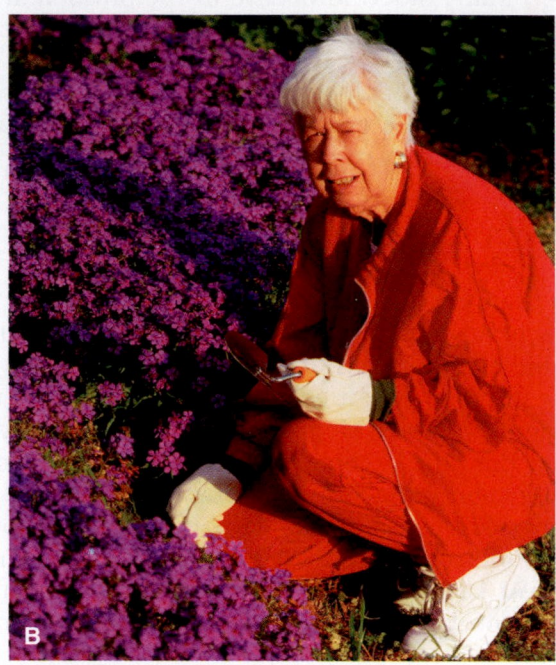

© Cengage Learning 2014

Figure 29-5   (A) A regular exercise program helps promote successful aging. (B) Gardening is a beneficial form of exercise.

Respiratory System

Breathing capacity diminishes with age, and oxygen and carbon dioxide exchange is lessened. The rib and chest muscles become smaller and less efficient. Lungs lose their elasticity, and the older adult may be **dyspneic**, short of breath (SOB), and more prone to pneumonia.

   As people age, there is a gradual decline in the muscle structure of the respiratory system, leading to a diminished ability to breathe deeply; thus, development of cough and pneumonia is not uncommon. Regular exercise can help to maintain the ability to breathe and cough effectively. In people who have been active throughout their lives, there is greater lung capacity.

Cardiovascular System

Heart disease and blood vessel disorders are the major cause of death in the United States. Lifestyle has been implicated as the most significant cause of cardiovascular disease. Blood vessels lose their elasticity, become narrower, and build up with plaque, and the arteries harden. This is known as **arteriosclerosis**. The myocardium loses some of its ability to pump effectively. This, together with narrowed and plaque-filled arteries, causes the heart to pump harder. Hypertension, or sustained high blood pressure, is a direct result of these factors. Hypertension can contribute to the accumulation of plaque in artery walls. Congestive heart failure is the inability of the heart to pump effectively to meet the body's demand for blood. Myocardial infarction, or heart attack, is another result of arteriosclerotic heart disease. Regular exercise and a healthy diet are the most beneficial activities for older adults in order to maintain adequate cardiac output throughout their life spans.

Gastrointestinal System

Stomach secretions and motility slow as part of aging. Peristalsis slows, and food moves through the gastrointestinal tract more slowly. **Pernicious anemia** is a disorder that can occur when cells of the stomach lining fail to secrete the intrinsic factor. Associated with the absence of hydrochloric acid, pernicious anemia affects the nervous system and red blood cell formation.

Fewer calories are needed during this time because metabolism slows. Many overeat if they are lonely, gain weight, and may become obese. Eating is a social as well as a physiologic event, and if they have no one to eat with, many older adults will not prepare a meal or eat properly to have good nutrition. Loss of vigor and vitality occur. Malnourishment is not uncommon.

Poor eating habits, poor nutrition, overeating, or undereating can lead to dental problems. Poor dental hygiene leads to gum disease and loss of teeth, many times making the chewing of food difficult and discouraging. Sometimes cardiac problems, such as endocarditis and myocardial infarction, occur from gum disease due to the invasion of pathogens and inflammation.

Urinary System

With aging, the kidneys decrease in size, resulting in less urine production and output. With cardiovascular arteriosclerosis, blood flow to the kidney is less. Filtering of waste products from the blood is impaired. Medications are not excreted as quickly as they are in a young, healthy person. Levels of medication may increase to a dangerous level with impaired kidney filtration. The bladder walls become more inelastic, and the ability to empty the bladder completely becomes difficult. **Residual urine** remains in the bladder, and microorganisms can cause an infection. **Cystitis** is infection and inflammation of the bladder. Urinary **incontinence**, the uncontrollable loss of urine, can be the result of many factors, such as relaxed muscles in the female pelvic floor, cystitis, hypertrophy of prostate gland, and diabetes.

Reproductive System

Women experience **menopause** at about age 55 years. Estrogen produced by the ovaries ceases, and changes in the female are noticeable with shrinking of vulva and genitalia. Hot flashes are not uncommon because of blood vessel dilation and contraction. Vaginal secretions diminish, the vagina becomes smaller, and infections are more likely. Estrogen replacement therapy helps to lessen symptoms but is used only for short-term therapy in women who experience severe menopausal symptoms. Long-term

use of estrogen and progesterone has been proved to increase the risk for heart disease and breast cancer (see Chapter 26 for more information regarding menopause and hormone therapy).

Men continue to produce sperm well after 50 years of age; however, testosterone levels diminish and midlife changes occur in men. This is known as **andropause**. It is about this time that many men older than 50 years experience benign hypertrophy of the prostate (see Chapter 28). Medication may help in some cases; otherwise, surgery, a prostatectomy, may be performed.

Aging men and women maintain their sexual desires, and many enjoy sexual intercourse more when children are no longer in the home. They have more privacy and time to relax.

PREVENTION OF COMPLICATIONS

Older adults are at risk for complications as a result of changes in the structure and function of their body systems.

Accidents can happen because of impaired vision or the inability to hear a warning sound, such as a fire alarm.

Malnutrition and anemia can develop because of poor nutrition or poor absorption of food. This can be caused by lack of interest in food because of lack of sense of taste or smell.

Older adults may have diminished sensitivity and lack the ability to feel pain as well as a younger person does. Heat and cold applications can injure an aging person if not watched carefully. Simple fractured bones may go unnoticed for some time. Loss of balance, disorientation, and confusion may be signs of impaired nervous system function.

Because many older adults suffer from osteoporosis, bones are more easily fractured. Falls are more common because of a loss of vision and balance.

Respiratory tract infections are not unusual. Pneumonia is a serious complication in this group of people. Encourage fluid intake and activity to keep the lungs healthy.

Urinary infections are more common. Adequate fluid intake (eight 8-ounce glasses of liquid per day) help keep infections at bay. Incontinence occurs when pelvic floor muscles are relaxed after childbirth.

Circulatory problems because of cardiovascular disease can cause poor circulation to the extremities, especially the legs. Fluid retention with noticeable edema is a common complication, together with hypertension and congestive heart failure.

Vaginitis is more common because of vaginal dryness and irritation caused by lack of estrogen. The prostate gland enlarges, making urination difficult for men.

It is especially important for older adults to alert and consult with their providers when consuming an alternative substance or when considering engaging in an alternative therapy. Many older adults take prescription drugs for a variety of health problems, and there could be harmful effects because of the interactions of the prescribed medications with the alternative substance. Tai chi, massage therapy, yoga, art therapy, music therapy, and meditation are examples of some alternative or complementary therapies in which as older adult patients can participate. Balance, mobility, strength, creativity, and stress reduction are some of the benefits for older adults who choose to add these alternatives to enhance their health and well-being.

PSYCHOLOGICAL CHANGES

There is a great deal of variation in the psychological functioning of older adults. Among the factors that contribute are the person's health; psychosocial history; race; sex; and environmental aspects, such as education, support system, and social class.

The level of decline in an older adult's intelligence can be affected by social factors. People who maintain their intelligence tend to be in better health, have had more education, are in a higher socioeconomic group, and are involved with others and in their community.

Dementia affects memory, personality, and **cognitive functioning** (awareness, reasoning, judgment, intuition) and is permanent. Alzheimer's disease is a common form of dementia. Some research has shown that there may be a genetic, as well as environmental, link to the cause of Alzheimer's disease.

People who have had a stroke, which interferes with blood circulation to brain cells, may suffer from dementia, impairing brain functioning. Other forms of dementia include Parkinson's disease, caused by a deficiency of dopamine, a chemical in the brain; syphilis, caused by a spirochete bacterium that causes brain damage (which manifests about 20 years after initial infection); and Huntington's disease, a genetic disease. When caring for patients  with dementia, protect them from injury, allow them to be independent if possible, and do not be critical or judgmental of their behaviors (it is unintentional) or what they say. Scientists have not determined what is in the minds of patients with dementia.

 Depression in older adults can occur from loss of a spouse, chronic illness, or financial problems. When caring for older adults, look for signs and symptoms of depression such as poor hygiene, insomnia or excessive sleep, crying, depressed mood (sad every day, most of the day), inability to concentrate, and increased alcohol consumption. Personality seems to help determine how individuals adapt to changes that they experience as they grow older.

THE MEDICAL ASSISTANT AND THE GERIATRIC PATIENT

Many older adults experience dementia, mental illness, depression, stress, boredom, fear of the unknown, loss of independence, feelings of rejection and worthlessness, low self-esteem, loneliness, dependence, failed expectations, and disappointments. All of these factors coupled with the physiologic changes that can occur offer a special challenge to the medical assistant caring for the health and needs of this group of patients.   Allow patients time to ventilate and express their concerns, allow for private and confidential discussion, and **empathize** with their situation by being aware of their feelings, emotions, and behavior. Good communication is essential for quality care of older adults. Do not talk to older adults as if they were children. Speak slowly and clearly. Face the individual while talking. Write instructions in addition to verbalizing them.

Memory-Impaired Older Adults

Geriatric care poses challenges when attempting to communicate with impaired older adults. The inability to communicate on a meaningful level can be frustrating and challenging, especially for the older person who is struggling to communicate but cannot find the right words. Following are some techniques that can be effective in improving verbal communication with older people experiencing memory impairment:

1. Talk to the person in a nondistracting place. It can be difficult for an older adult to concentrate or to sort things out when there are environmental distractions, such as other conversations, equipment noises, or people walking by.

2. Begin conversations with orienting information. Identify yourself, and call older adults by their preferred names. Explain the purpose of your visit.

3. Use short words and short, simple sentences using specific descriptive nouns rather than vague pronouns. For example, "Do you have difficulty using your walker?" instead of, "Do you have difficulty using it?".

4. Speak slowly and say individual words clearly.

5. Never "talk down" or be condescending. This is demeaning. Speak in an adult manner as you would to a coworker or friend. Provide the dignity and respect you wish to receive yourself.

6. Lower the tone (pitch) of your voice. A raised pitch is a signal that one is upset. A lower pitch is also easier for people with hearing impairments to understand.

7. Talk to the person in a warm and pleasant manner. Use nonverbal cues, such as facial expression, tone of voice, or touch, to show your feelings of affection and concern. Smiling, taking the older person's hand, or touching the person on the arm can vividly communicate that you are interested and really care.

8. When giving instructions, allow plenty of time for the information to be absorbed.

9. Give clear and simple instructions.

10. Ask the person to do one task at a time.

11. Listen actively. If you do not understand, apologize to the person by saying that you did not understand exactly what was said. It is extremely important to phrase responses in a way that does not damage the self-esteem of the older adult.

12. Avoid asking direct questions that require the person to remember a fact.

13. Focus on well behavior or things that you know the patient can still do.

14. Use humor when appropriate. If expressed naturally, humor brings much needed laughter, a dimension that is often lost in the health care setting.

15. Let the person know when you leave and if you are returning.

16. **HIPAA** When discussing a case with another staff member, do so in private to protect patient confidentiality.

Visually Impaired Older Adults

Visually impaired people need to know you are present, but do not approach the individual until you make your presence known. Help by explaining his or her location, and identify others who may also be present (Figure 29-6).

Hearing Impaired Older Adults

  For the hearing impaired older adult to communicate and understand instructions, there are some techniques the medical assistant should keep in mind. These strategies will be beneficial and will facilitate communication and understanding. These techniques include:

1. Face the hearing impaired person directly and on the same level when possible. (If he or she is standing, the medical assistant should stand; if the patient is seated, the medical assistant should be seated.)

2. Keep your hands away from your face while talking.

3. Reduce background noises when talking. Move to a quieter room away from extraneous sounds and activities.

4. Hearing impaired individuals hear and understand less when they are tired or sick.

5. Get the person's attention before beginning to speak and do not talk from another room.

6. Speak in a normal tone; do not shout.

7. Be sure that light is not shining in the eyes of the hearing impaired individual.

8. If the hearing impaired patient has trouble understanding, reword what you have said. Do not repeat the same words again and again.

9. Written instructions are useful, but the medical assistant must be certain that what is written is understood.

Elder Abuse

What is elder abuse? Massachusetts law defines elder abuse as the committing or omitting of an act

---

CRITICAL THINKING

Describe strategies for communicating with hearing impaired patients.

Making Contact

Introduce yourself. Ask the visually impaired patient if he would like assistance. If he does, offer your arm by saying so and by touching your hand or forearm against his.

Grip

The patient grips your arm just above the elbow. The grip must be firm but not so tight that it becomes uncomfortable.

Stance

The patient stands next to you, slightly behind. His arm is bent and held close to his side. Relax your arm and let it hang naturally at your side.

Pace

The pace should be comfortable for both of you. If the patient tightens his grip or pulls on your arm, slow down; your pace may be too fast or he may be anxious. You should alert the patient to obstacles such as curbs, stairs, doors, and thresholds. Be specific, but do not confuse him with too much information.

Stairs

When approaching stairs, tell the patient. Let him know whether you are going to go up or down. Be sure you approach the stairs directly, not at an angle. Have the patient stand next to the handrail if there is one.

Pause at the top (or bottom) of the stairs and describe anything unusual about them. The patient will find the handrail and reach forward with his foot to locate the edge of the first step. Start down (or up) the stairs, keeping yourself one step ahead. Keep a steady pace.

When you reach a landing, stop immediately. (Do not take an extra step.) Doing so lets the patient know that there are no more steps, and he can then match his stride with yours.

The same procedure should be used when approaching curbs. Point out any changes in the terrain, even small ones.

Sitting

When guiding someone to a chair, walk up to it and place your hand on the back of the chair. Let the patient trail your arm down to its back. Tell him which way the chair is facing, and he can then seat himself.

If the chair lacks a back or is very large, bring the patient up to the chair so that his legs are against the front of it. He can then reach down to locate the arms and seat of it before he sits.

If the chair is at a table, describe the relationship of the chair, the table and the patient. Place one of his hands on the chair and the other hand on the table.

Doors

When approaching a closed door, tell the patient its position when open. For example, "The door opens away and to the left." Or say, "Take the door with your left hand." After you open the door and begin to walk through, the patient will have his hand ready to help hold it open as you walk through together. The patient will move his arm across the front of his body to find the door with the palm of his hand. He should close it behind you if it is not a self-closing door. Use the narrow passage technique in addition to this technique if the doorway is narrow.

Narrow Passage Technique

When coming to a narrow passage, tell the patient. Move your guiding arm to the center of your back. Slow your pace. He will move behind you and extend his arm, placing you in a single-file position. Once you pass through the narrow passage, bring your arm forward and return to the normal stance.

Figure 29-6 Sighted guide techniques.

that results in serious physical or emotional injury to an older adult. All states have elder abuse laws. Abuse includes physical, emotional, and verbal abuse, and neglect. The law protects elders abused or neglected by caretakers.

  All persons 60 years and older living in the community are protected under the law. Who must report elder abuse? Providers, medical interns, dentists, medical assistants, nurses, family counselors, police officers, psychologists, home caregivers, licensed home health care aides, and many others may be required to report abuse. Agencies are also liable. Any person required to report abuse who fails to do so is subject to a fine. Anyone who has reasonable cause to believe an older adult has been abused may report it and has a moral obligation to protect older adults. In most states, the department responsible for elder affairs has established an elder abuse hotline to receive reports of abuse. Reports may also be made to the designated protective service agency in your community. Reporting is required for signs and symptoms of physical abuse, neglect, emotional or psychological abuse, financial abuse, exploitation or sexual abuse, and abandonment. Once reports are received by the elder protective services program, if appropriate, a caseworker will assess the

situation to determine the nature and extent of the abuse. If abuse is confirmed, services will be provided to eliminate or alleviate abuse. Many social services are usually available. Mental health, legal, home caregiver services, and alternative living arrangements may be provided (see Chapter 7).

The National Center for Elder Abuse (NCEA) is directed by the U.S. Administration on Aging. Their mission is to ensure that the elderly in America will live with dignity, integrity, and independence without abuse, neglect, or exploitation. This agency serves as a resource to local, state, and federal agencies for research, policy, and law as it affects the elderly. It serves as an excellent contact for information on the latest policies relating to elder care in the United States.

Some signs and symptoms of mistreatment or abuse include:

Psychological Signs and Symptoms	*Physical Signs and Symptoms*
• Increasing depression	• Lack of personal care
• Anxiety	• Lack of supervision
• Withdrawn/timid	• Bruises
• Hostile	• Welts
• Unresponsive	• Lack of food
• Confused	• Beatings
• New poverty	• Neglect
• Longing for death	• Unsatisfactory living conditions
• Vague health complaints	
• Anxious to please	

There are other signs and symptoms, and not all of those listed by themselves indicate mistreatment, neglect, or abuse. If any seem to increase in number or severity, it may indicate a problem. By observing closely, you may be able to initiate corrective action or reduce or prevent the situation from deteriorating. Careful documentation in the **EHR** patient's chart or electronic medical record over time can show continuous signs and symptoms of abuse. Usually the victim is frail (weak), physically or emotionally, and dependent on the abuser for basic survival needs. The victim may be afraid to speak out for fear of retaliation. Many times the abuser is the caregiver or a member of the patient's family.

For information, contact elder protective services programs in the Yellow Pages of your phone book, or contact the Eldercare Locator toll free at 1-800-677-1116 or via their website (http://www.eldercare.gov/public/resources/assessment.esp).

HEALTHY AND SUCCESSFUL AGING

Older adults are enjoying longer, healthier lives. Some reasons for healthy aging are the increase in the number of gerontologists (specialists who provide medical care only to older adult patients), greater awareness and involvement of older adults with their health care, improved nutrition, regular exercise, new medications, and advancing medical technology (Figure 29-7).

Some tips for healthy aging according to the National Institute on Aging of the National Institutes of Health are:

1. Eat a balanced diet.
2. Exercise regularly.
3. Get regular checkups.
4. Don't smoke.
5. Wear a seatbelt when in the car.
6. Practice safety to avoid falls and fractures.
7. Keep in contact with family and friends and stay active through work, community, and recreation.
8. Avoid overexposure to the sun and cold.
9. Drink alcohol in moderation. Don't drink and drive.

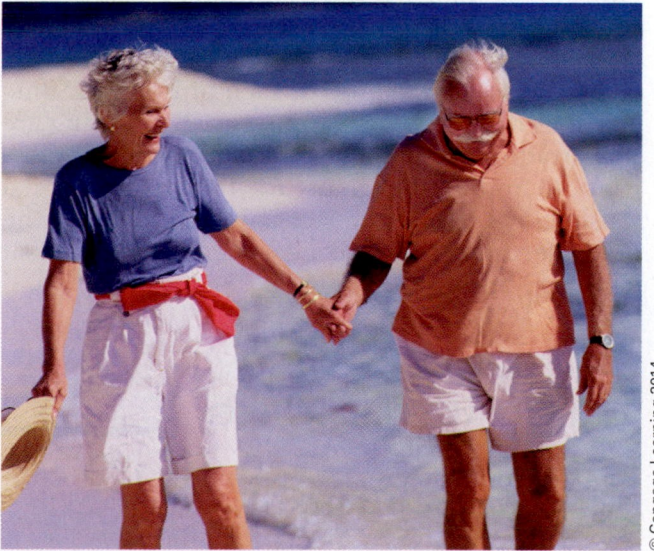

Figure 29-7 With improved geriatric care, older adults can look forward to longer, healthier lives.

© Cengage Learning 2014

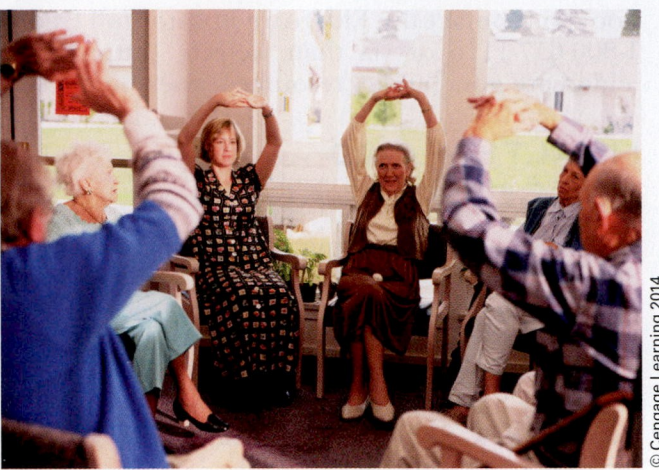

Figure 29-8 An exercise class in an assisted-living facility.

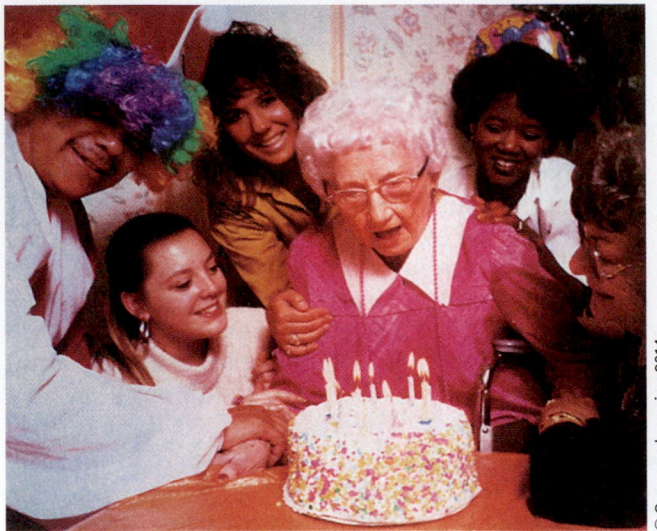

Figure 29-9 This woman is celebrating her 100th birthday and is surrounded by her family and friends.

10. Keep personal and financial records in order to simplify budgeting and investing. Plan for long-term financial needs and housing.

11. Keep a positive attitude toward life and engage in activities that make you happy.

12. Get vaccines: pneumonia, influenza, and herpes zoster (Zostavax). Zostavax is approved for people over age 60. It prevents herpes zoster (shingles).

Successful aging requires that healthy living and daily activities be combined. To age successfully, individuals need to be continually involved, must pursue what makes them happy, and make an effort to maintain a positive attitude. These actions of healthy habits should begin in childhood when they can be formed and encouraged. They become the responsibilities of each individual. Some activities that are important to successful aging are socialization with friends and family, intimacy, education, and employment (for income and social satisfaction). For successful aging to happen, the older person must make a commitment to work at it (Figure 29-8 through Figure 29-10).

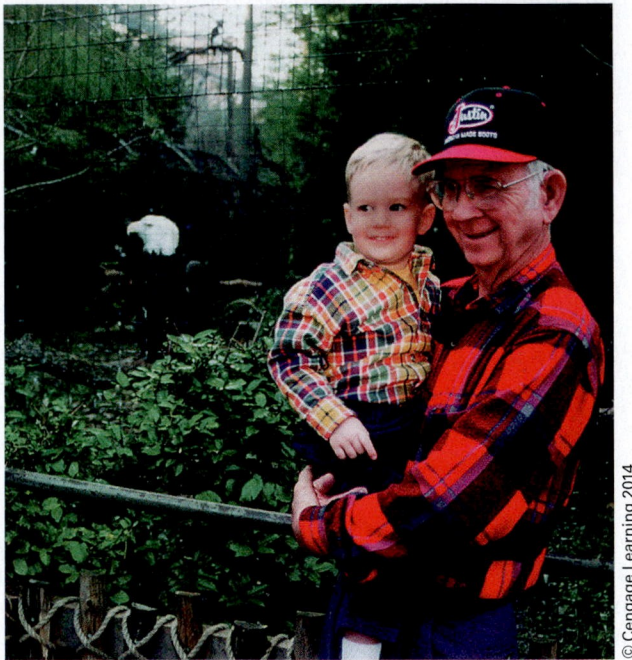

Figure 29-10 Caring for grandchildren is a very satisfying social relationship for many older adults.

CRITICAL THINKING

What are some strategies that older adults can do to keep mentally and physically stimulated?

CASE STUDY 29-1

Refer to the scenario at the beginning of the chapter.

CASE STUDY REVIEW

1. Describe five strategies older adults such as Mrs. Johnson can use to help slow the aging process.

CASE STUDY 29-2

Adelaide Robinson, 83 years old, has an appointment Thursday morning for a recheck of her most recent complaint. She tells you that she is moving slower than she did just 6 months ago, and she has noticed less flexibility as well.

CASE STUDY REVIEW

1. What are the possible causes of Mrs. Robinson's complaints?

2. What effect will these problems have on Mrs. Robinson's daily routine?

3. What might Dr. King suggest Mrs. Robinson do to help alleviate symptoms?

CASE STUDY 29-3

Sally Donovan, 92 years old, is in the gerontology clinic today. She currently lives with her 65-year-old son. You notice that she has lost 30 pounds since her last visit 2 months ago. Her demeanor is submissive and she looks to her son to answer any direct questions from the medical assistant and the provider. At checkout, her son opens her checkbook and writes the check for her co-payment, including signing her name on the signature line.

CASE STUDY REVIEW

1. What are the alarm signs for potential elder abuse with Ms. Donovan?

2. What are your next steps in reporting suspected elder abuse?

SUMMARY

Many aging people live well into their 80s, 90s, and even to 100 years of age. They remain physically and mentally stimulated. They learn a foreign language, learn to play a musical instrument, love to read, garden, and volunteer. Older people are more aware today than ever before of the importance of a healthy lifestyle and of its significant contribution to their long and healthy life span.

Other older adults, because of genetic inheritance, wear and tear, and stress, and loss of chemicals and hormones, seem to age quickly and have little control over these factors.

Many others practice poor health habits, some by choice and others by circumstance. These habits contribute to chronic diseases, disability, and a shorter and unhealthy life span.

Above all, dispel myths about older adults. Be patient, kind, consistent, and thoughtful.

STUDY FOR SUCCESS

To reinforce your knowledge and skills of information presented in this chapter:

- Review the *Key Terms*
- Role-play with other students to apply attributes of professionalism pertinent to this chapter.
- Consider the *Case Studies* and discuss your conclusions
- Answer the questions in the *Certification Review*
- Apply your knowledge by completing the *Activities* in the *Study Guide* and the *Games and Quizzes* in the StudyWARE **StudyWARE** software on the *Premium Website*
- Practice your problem-solving skills with the *Critical Thinking Challenge 3.0* on the *Premium Website*

Additional resources for this chapter include:

- *CourseMate for Delmar's Comprehensive Medical Assisting*
- *WebTutor for Delmar's Comprehensive Medical Assisting*

CERTIFICATION REVIEW

1. The most chronic condition associated with older adults is:
   a. arteriosclerotic heart disease
   b. cystitis
   c. presbycusis
   d. pernicious anemia

2. An eye disease common to older adults that is characterized by fluid pressure buildup is:
   a. macular degeneration
   b. presbyopia
   c. cataract
   d. glaucoma

3. Joints in older adults become worn because:
   a. cartilage erodes in the joints
   b. osteoporosis makes bones brittle
   c. muscle fibers decrease
   d. vertebrae become thinner

4. Inability to cough deeply and raise mucus makes older adults more susceptible to which of the following?
   a. Emphysema
   b. Asthma
   c. Pneumonia
   d. Bronchitis

5. Residual urine refers to:
   a. catheterized urine for urinalysis
   b. first-voided specimen
   c. amount of urine left in bladder after voiding
   d. total amount of urine in the bladder when full

6. Physiologic changes that are associated with age affect the following systems:
   a. integumentary
   b. musculoskeletal
   c. cardiovascular
   d. all of the above

7. With age, the damage to the retina that results in permanent loss of vision in the central visual field is:
   a. cataracts
   b. glaucoma
   c. macular degeneration
   d. none of the above

8. In order to prevent age-related disorders, these behaviors are indicated:
   a. eat a balanced diet
   b. include at least five alcoholic drinks a day
   c. increase exercise
   d. a and c

9. Patient education in a nondistracting environment, using short words and simple sentences, as well as speaking slowly and clearly demonstrates:
   a. good communication techniques
   b. professionalism
   c. adhering to medicolegal guidelines
   d. a and b

10. Thinning of the long bones, pelvis, and vertebrae is a symptom of:
    a. osteomalacia   c. osteoporosis
    b. osteoarthritis   d. osteochondroma

REFERENCES/BIBLIOGRAPHY

Cox, H. (2001). *Later life: The realities of aging* (5th ed.). Upper Saddle River, NJ: Prentice Hall.

Hegner, B. R., Accello, B., & Caldwell, E. (2008). *Nursing assistant: A nursing process approach* (20th ed.). Clifton Park, NY: Delmar Cengage Learning.

Hogstel, M. O. (2001). *Gerontology: Nursing care of the older adult.* Clifton Park, NY: Delmar Cengage Learning.

Lodge, H. S. (2007). You can stop "normal" aging. *Parade Magazine,* March 6, 2007.

Markson, E., & Hollis-Sawyer, G. (2000). *Readings in social gerontology.* Los Angeles, CA: Roxbury Publishing Co.

Perls, T. (2007). Simple steps may slow aging. *Consumer Reports on Health, 19,* 1–4.

Simmers, L. (2008). *Diversified health occupations* (7th ed.). Clifton Park, NY: Delmar Cengage Learning.

Taber's cyclopedic medical dictionary (21st ed.). (2003). Philadelphia: F. A. Davis.

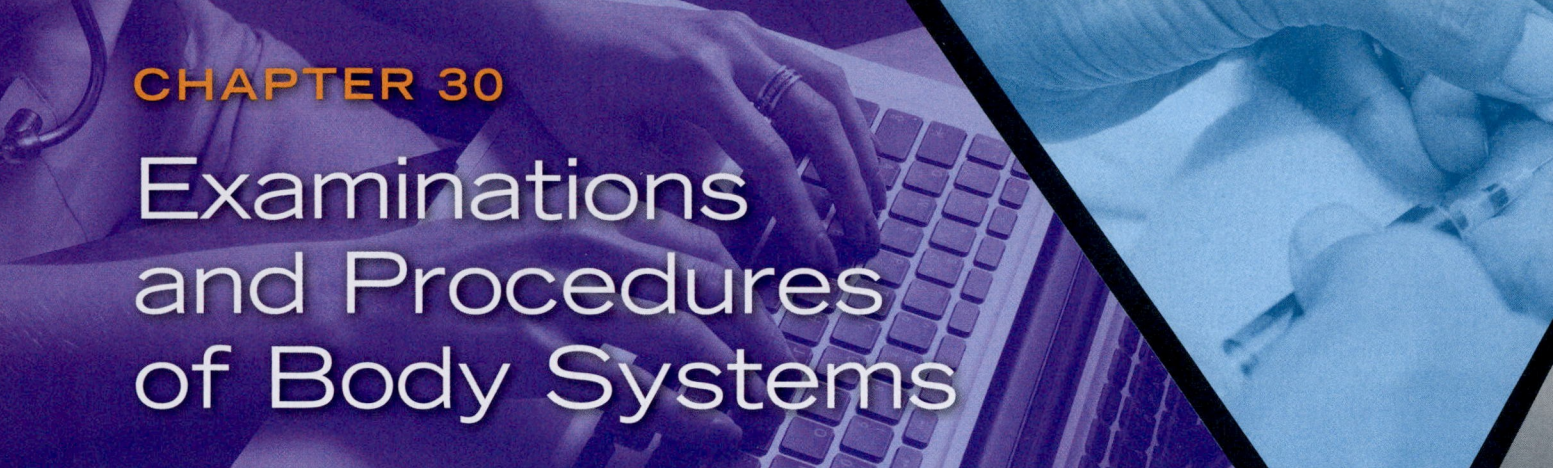

CHAPTER 30

Examinations and Procedures of Body Systems

OUTLINE

Integumentary System
    Allergy Skin Testing
Neurologic System
    Components of a Neurologic Screening
Sensory System
    The Eye
    The Ear
    The Nose
Respiratory System
    Signs and Symptoms of Respiratory Conditions and Disorders

Diagnostic Tests
Spirometry
Peak Expiratory Flow Rates
Pulse Oximetry
Inhalers
Circulatory System
Blood and Lymph System
Musculoskeletal System
    Fractures, Casting, and Cast Removal
Digestive System

Signs and Symptoms of Digestive Conditions and Disorders
Diagnostic Tests
Bariatrics
Urinary System
    Signs and Symptoms of Urinary Conditions and Disorders
Diagnostic Tests
Urinary Catheterization

LEARNING OUTCOMES

1. Define, spell, and pronounce the key terms as presented in the glossary.
2. List major organs in each body system.
3. Describe the normal function of each body system.
4. List basic integumentary assessment keys.
5. Define components of neurological examination.
6. List essentials of a sensory system examination.
7. Explain the value of each chart utilized in the eye exam.
8. Describe the proper use of a metered dose inhaler.
9. Briefly discuss the role of the medical assistant during spirometry and pulse oximetry.
10. Explain oxygen administration using a nasal cannula.
11. Identify patient education information for sputum collections.
12. Describe patient preparation for occult blood testing.
13. List items required by a provider for a neurologic examination and explain the medical assistant's role in the examination.
14. Discuss the different types of visual acuity charts and how to use them appropriately.
15. Differentiate between an instillation and irrigation.
16. Describe how to perform a nasal irrigation.
17. Explain the medical assistant's role when assisting with audiometry.
18. Describe how to perform a urinary catheterization.
19. Analyze the professionalism question and apply them to this chapter's content.

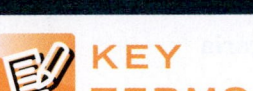

KEY TERMS

acute or adult
  respiratory distress
  syndrome (ARDS)
amblyopia
anorexia nervosa
aphasia
appendicular skeleton
auricle
axial skeleton
bariatrics
biopsy
bronchodilator
bulimia
carbuncle
cerebral vascular
  accident (CVA)
cerumen
colonoscopy
comedones
conjunctivitis
deep tendon
  reflexes (DTRs)
demyelination
dislocation
dysuria
endoscope
epistaxis
erythema
external respiration
fibromyalgia
frequency
furuncle
glaucoma
gout
hematuria
hemoptysis
hordeolum
hyperopia

(continues)

ATTRIBUTES OF PROFESSIONALISM

Communication

- Did you introduce yourself? Did you identify the patient through name and birth date or other identifying feature?
- Did you listen to and acknowledge the patient?
- Did you speak at the patient's level of understanding?
- Did you provide appropriate responses/feedback?
- Did you allay patients' fears regarding the procedure being performed and help them feel safe and comfortable?
- Did you respond honestly and diplomatically to the patient's concerns?
- Did you demonstrate empathy in communicating with patients, family, and staff?
- Did you accurately and concisely update the provider on any aspect of the patient's care?

Presentation

- Did your actions attend to both the psychological and the physiologic aspects of the patient's illness or condition?
- Did you attend to any special needs of the patient? Did you first ask if assistance was needed, rather than taking charge?
- Were you courteous, patient, and respectful to the patient?
- Did you display a calm, professional, and caring manner?

Competency

- Did you pay attention to detail?
- Were you knowledgeable and accountable?
- Did you apply critical thinking skills in performing patient assessment and care?

Initiative

- Did you seek out opportunities to expand your knowledge base?
- Did you direct the patient to other resources when necessary or helpful, with the approval of the provider?

Integrity

- Did you work within your scope of practice?
- Did you protect personal boundaries?
- Did you protect and maintain confidentiality?

KEY TERMS   *(continued)*

inhalers	morbid obesity	otoscope	salicylates
internal respiration	myasthenia gravis	oximetry	sigmoidoscopy
intravenous pyelogram (IVP)	myopia	polyp	Snellen chart
	nebulizer	presbyopia	spirometry
lesion	nocturia	proteinuria	strabismus
malabsorption	nystagmus	pruritus	tympanostomy
malaise	oliguria	pyuria	urgency
metered dose inhaler (MDI)	otitis media	rosacea	urticaria

SCENARIO

At Inner City Health Care, a number of specialty examinations are scheduled for Tuesday the eighth. Administrative medical assistant Jane O'Hara, who is office manager, is careful to schedule patients requiring specialty procedures so that times do not overlap; before she schedules, Jane makes certain examination rooms are available with an extra margin of time between patients. Clinical medical assistants Sam Tyler, CMA (AAMA), and Hannah Casey, RMA (AMT), take responsibility to ensure that all supplies and equipment are assembled, that both provider and patient are comfortable with the physical environment, and that all safety precautions are followed before, during, and after the examination or procedure.

INTRODUCTION

 New techniques and developments occur frequently in medicine, and medical assistants must refine existing skills and learn new ones to be knowledgeable and proficient and to provide the most current, up-to-date, quality care to patients. The medical assistant who works in a specialist's clinic or an ambulatory care setting that treats a variety of patient problems needs additional skills when providing specialty care to patients. Patients with conditions specific to a particular body system or body part need specialized care such as urinary catheterization or assisting with a lumbar puncture. The medical assistant assists the provider with a multitude of clinical procedures that are an integral part of each specialty examination.

This chapter covers specialty and body system examinations and the appropriate clinical procedures in urology; endoscopy; and the sensory, respiratory, musculoskeletal, neurologic, circulatory, blood and lymph, and integumentary systems.

Each specialty description includes tables that contain information on diseases, disorders, and diagnostic tests and procedures used to confirm diagnoses. Other diseases and disorders and procedures related to each specialty are addressed in the body of the chapter.

INTEGUMENTARY SYSTEM

The integumentary system consists of the skin and its associated structures, such as hair, nails, nerve endings, and the sebaceous (oil) and sudoriferous (sweat)

SPOTLIGHT ON CERTIFICATION

RMA Content Outline
- Anatomy and physiology
- Medical terminology
- Patient education
- Physical examinations

CMA (AAMA) Content Outline
- Medical terminology
- Anatomy and physiology
- Medicolegal guidelines and requirements
- Treatment area
- Patient preparation and assisting the provider
- Patient history and interview
- Nutrition

CMAS Content Outline
- Medical terminology
- Anatomy and physiology
- Basic charting
- Examination preparation

glands. This system provides protection for the body against invasion of microorganisms and trauma and helps regulate body temperature. Nerve endings sense pressure, touch, and pain. Structurally, the skin consists of two layers (Figure 30-1), which function differently from one another to perform specific activities.

- Epidermis is the outer layer of the skin that is composed of squamous epithelium and produces keratin and the pigment melanin.
- Dermis is the inner layer of the skin made up of connective tissue and contains blood vessels, nerve endings, and glands. This layer provides strength and elasticity.
- Subcutaneous connective tissue is the layer on which the skin and muscles lie and consists of elastic and fibrous connective tissue and adipose tissue. This layer guards against heat loss and provides insulation.

Skin disorders frequently produce a **lesion** unique to a specific skin disease, thus allowing for the diagnosis to be based on the appearance of the lesion, the patient's history, allergies, emotional well-being, and inherited diseases. If the lesion appears suspicious, the provider may perform a **biopsy** for tissue analysis. This procedure aids in the diagnosis and treatment of specific skin disorders.

Table 30-1 lists integumentary system diseases and diagnostic procedures. Table 30-2 describes skin disorders of the integumentary system.

Diagnostic procedures involving the skin range from the simple to the complex. Simple observations such as skin color, texture, size and shape of a lesion, and patient history can lead to a quick diagnosis. Confirmatory procedures such as clinical studies of urine and blood, culture of a purulent lesion, radiographs, and biopsies of the affected tissues can further delineate the disease.

The clinical procedures for the skin most commonly performed by the medical assistant are obtaining wound cultures, applying a sterile dressing to the wound site, and allergy skin testing.

Allergy Skin Testing

Medical assistants often perform allergy skin testing. When performing allergy skin tests, severe allergic reaction is a distinct possibility. Emergency treatment must be available immediately and consists of the following: (1) notify provider immediately; (2) have patient lie down; (3) have epinephrine, benadryl, and corticosteroid injections ready to be administered; and (4) check patient's vital signs.

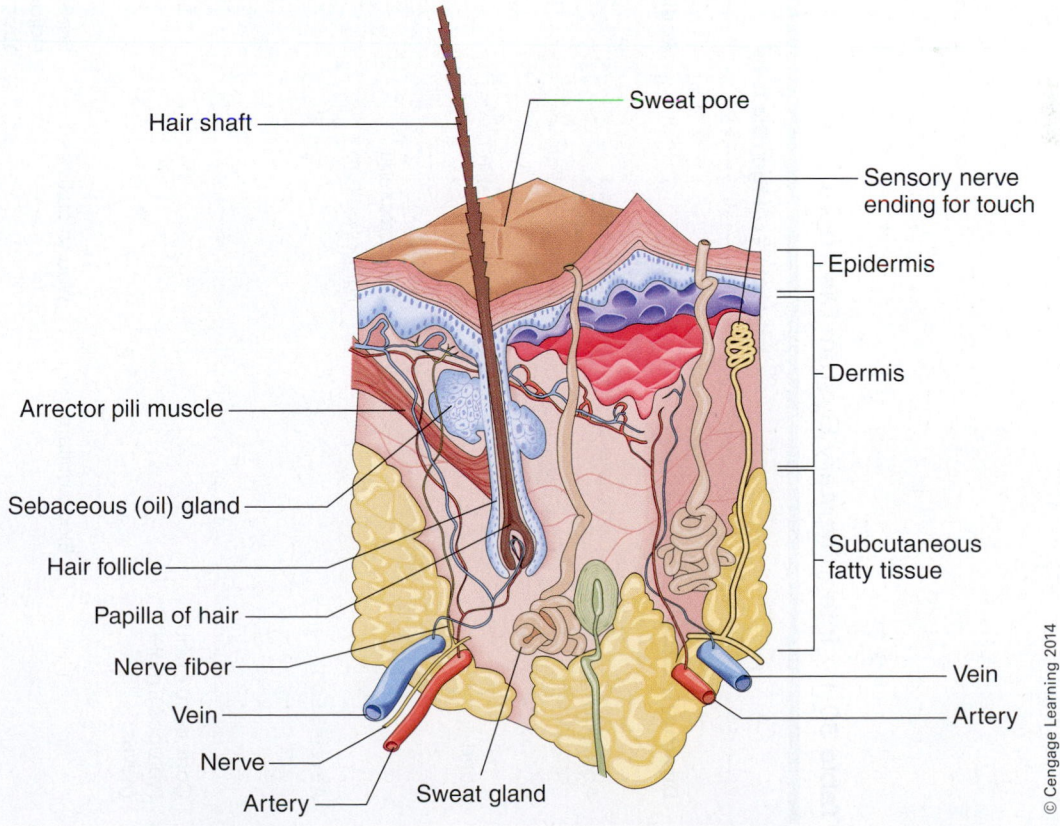

Hair shaft — Sweat pore — Sensory nerve ending for touch — Epidermis — Dermis — Arrector pili muscle — Sebaceous (oil) gland — Hair follicle — Papilla of hair — Nerve fiber — Vein — Nerve — Artery — Sweat gland — Subcutaneous fatty tissue — Vein — Artery

© Cengage Learning 2014

Figure 30-1   Cross-section of skin.

Table 30-1 Integumentary System Disorders

| Disease/Disorder | Laboratory/Diagnostic Tests | | | | Medical Tests or Procedures | Treatment |
	Blood	Other	Radiography	Surgery		
Abscess (furuncle, carbuncle)	Complete blood count Blood glucose	Culture and sensitivity of wound exudate		Incision and drainage		Antibiotics Incision and drainage
Acne		Culture of skin lesions				Antibiotics Steroids Retin-A
Athlete's Foot		Skin scrapings Fungal culture			Wood's lamp examination	Over-the-counter antifungal medications Prescription antifungal medications
Corn, callus, wart (verucca), mole (nevus)				Excisional biopsy Electrocautery		Surgical excision
Decubitus ulcers	Blood cultures	Wound cultures	Radiographs of adjoining bony structures	Rotational skin flap Débridement		Relieve pressure Antibiotics Nutritional supplementation Pain management Hyperbaric oxygen therapy

Condition						
Dermatitis	Serum IgE			Biopsy of lesion		Depends on cause
Dermatophytosis		Culture			Wood's rays (ultraviolet rays)	Antifungal medication
Impetigo	Complete blood count	Gram stain of discharge from lesion				Antibiotics
Melanoma			Chest radiograph	Biopsy of lesion		Surgical excision Chemotherapy
Psoriasis				Skin biopsy		Medication Light therapy
Scleroderma	Sedimentation rate Rheumatoid arthritis factor Antinuclear antibodies	Urinalysis Kidney function tests	Gastrointestinal radiograph Chest radiograph	Tissue biopsy		Medication
Skin cancer				Biopsy of lesion		Surgical excision Laser therapy Radiation therapy

Table 30-2   Description of Skin Disorders

Abscess. **Furuncle** ("boil"): Acute circumscribed infection of the subcutaneous tissues and surrounding tissues caused by staphylococci. **Carbuncle**: A circumscribed inflammation and infection of the skin and deeper tissues accompanied by fever, leukocytosis, and sometimes prostration. Caused by staphylococcus and common in patients with diabetes.

Acne. Chronic inflammatory disease caused by blocked sebaceous glands, characterized by **comedones** (blackheads), papules, and pustules.

Athlete's foot. Infection of the feet caused by fungus. It is also known as tinea pedis.

Corn and callus. Thickening and hyperplasia of the stratum corneum (outermost skin layer) caused by pressure or friction to the affected area.

Decubitus ulcers. Ulceration of skin layers due to pressure. The degree depends on the depth of tissue injury.

Dermatitis. Caused by a specific irritant characterized by **erythema** or redness, as in inflammation.

Dermatophytosis. A highly contagious infectious fungus infection of the skin. Common on hands and feet. When feet are infected, it is known as athlete's foot or tinea pedis.

Herpes zoster. An acute infectious disease caused by varicella-zoster virus. Characterized by inflammation of the ganglia of the spinal or cranial nerves. Painful, vesicular eruptions occur along the course of the nerves.

Impetigo. Contagious small pustules caused by a staphylococci or streptococci or a combination of both and spread by direct contact.

Melanoma. A malignant pigmented mole. Virulent and invasive. Can be caused by ultraviolet light exposure.

Nevus. A mole. Usually congenital.

Psoriasis. Chronic, genetically determined dermatitis, characterized by flat, reddened areas with silvery scales.

Scleroderma. Progressive thickening of the skin involving collagen tissue. Systemic involvement occurs. Cause is unknown.

Skin cancer. Malignant lesions on the skin surface caused by exposure to ultraviolet rays.

Verruca. A wart caused by a virus.

© Cengage Learning 2014

There can be a broad range of inflammatory responses to allergens. Some responses include **urticaria**, swelling at the injection site, **pruritus**, and redness. A response or reaction can be immediate, life-threatening, and systemic in nature. The allergen reaches the circulatory system triggering a massive release of substances (histamine) that can produce severe airway obstruction, vasodilation, hypotension, laryngeal edema, and anaphylactic shock. See Chapter 9.

Three Kinds of Skin Tests.
The scratch test, the patch test, and intradermal test are the three skin test procedures the provider can perform on patients to evaluate for allergies. Together with the patient's medical history, laboratory values, physical exam, and the skin test results, the provider compiles the data to determine the substances to which the patient is allergic.

Scratch Test. The back and arms are used for the scratch test. The skin surface is numbered in rows approximately 2 inches apart so that they can be identified. A small scratch is made on the surface of the skin and the allergen is placed on the scratch. As many as 50 allergens can be tested at one time. A reaction to the allergen usually occurs within one-half hour. If the patient is allergic to a substance, a wheal will develop at the scratch site. The site is compared with a scratch test with no allergens introduced into it, but just an allergy-free fluid. The provider reads the results, which are graded on a scale from 2 to 4. A number 2 reaction indicates a wheal larger than the control scratch reaction. A number 3 is given to

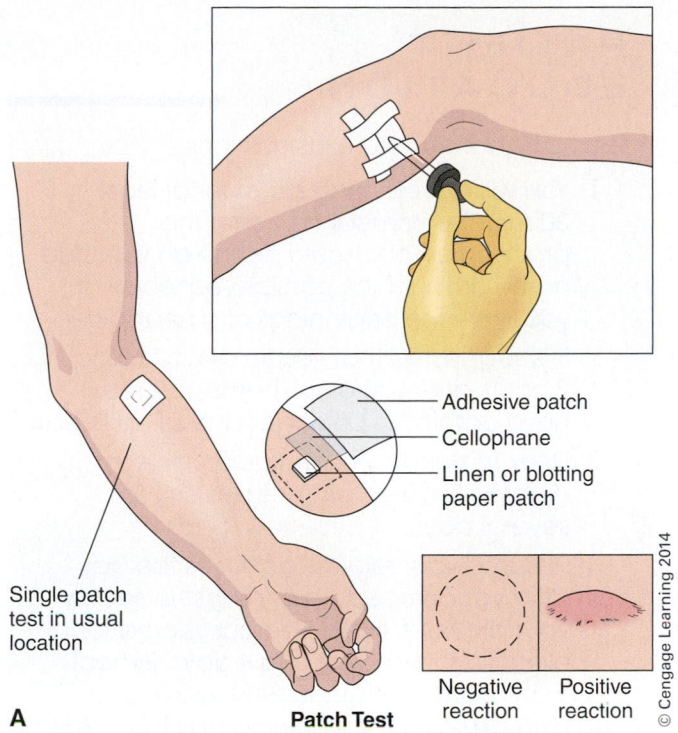

Single patch test in usual location

Adhesive patch
Cellophane
Linen or blotting paper patch

A   **Patch Test**

Negative reaction   Positive reaction

© Cengage Learning 2014

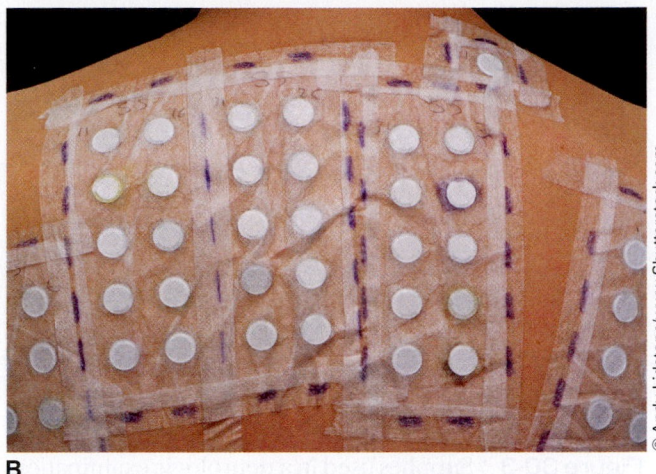

B

© Andy Lidstone/www.Shutterstock.com

Figure 30-2 (A) Patch test being applied. Tell the patient to keep the patch clean, dry, and covered until the provider reads the results. (B) Skin allergy patch test on back.

a larger reaction, and a 4 is given to a reaction in which the wheal extends beyond the usual circumscribed area of the injection. The allergen extract should be wiped away from the scratch area that is exhibiting a number 4 reaction (see Chapter 22).

Patch Test. The suspected allergen is placed on the skin and is covered with a square of cellophane and held in place by tape. As many as 25 tests can

be done at one time and results are read in 24 to 96 hours (Figure 30-2).

Intradermal Test. A dose of 0.1 mL of an allergen is injected intradermally into the forearm. Ten to fifteen tests can be done simultaneously on each arm, and the patient can experience a severe reaction more quickly. This test is always done on the patient's forearm.

PATIENT EDUCATION

Early detection of skin changes can make the difference in the overall health and prognosis of patients who have risk factors associated with skin cancer. The Cancer Research Institute recommends a simple ABCD method for identifying moles that might be malignant.

A – *Asymmetry.* Melanoma usually has an irregular shape, benign skin lesions usually have a smooth, rounded shape.

B – *Borders.* Like the shape, melanoma usually has wavy irregular borders, unlike benign moles, which have smooth borders.

C – *Colors.* Just like asymmetry and borders, the colors included in the melanoma lesion are irregular and contain shades

of brown and black; benign moles are usually one shade of brown.

D – *Diameter.* Melanoma lesions are usually larger (greater than ¼ inch or 6 mm in diameter); benign moles are usually smaller than that.

It is important to instruct your patients that melanoma might include pink or white in the coloration. They can grow slowly or quite rapidly. It is essential that a patient seek medical intervention to increase the chance of surviving this type of cancer. There are several types of treatment, including surgical excision, chemotherapy and radiation therapy, or immune therapy. Patients need to be aware that time is of the essence with this type of integumentary disease.

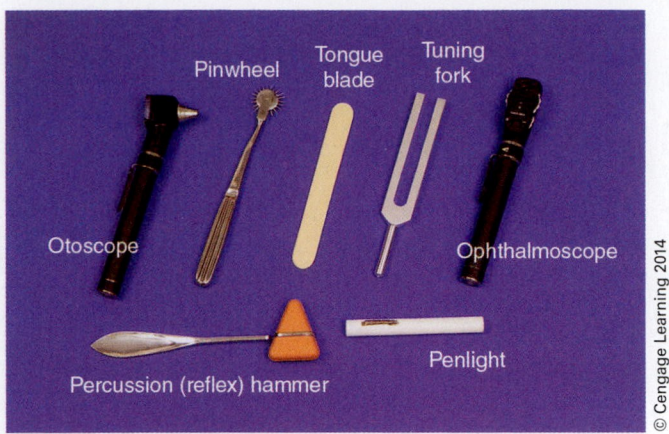

Figure 30-3   Supplies used in a neurologic examination.

NEUROLOGIC SYSTEM

The nervous system functions to coordinate the activities of body systems and allows for the body to adapt to its internal and external environments. Diagnosis and treatment of the brain, spinal cord, and peripheral nerve disorders are often difficult because of the interdependence of one part of the system on another.

The provider screens the patient during a physical examination for neurologic signs and symptoms. The medical assistant's role in a neurologic screening is to observe and evaluate the patient's mental status and to assist or perform other tests as directed by the provider. Most of the examination is performed in conjunction with the complete physical examination, but it can also be done when a patient is exhibiting specific signs and symptoms of a neurologic problem such as lack of sensation, seizures, confusion, paralysis, or **aphasia**, also known as the inability to speak.

The equipment and supplies used in a neurologic screening test the patient's reflexes, sense of touch, sense of smell, and degree of coordination, to name a few (Figure 30-3). The provider pays particular attention to symmetric strength and notes unequal weakness when comparing both sides of the body. A patient's sex and body build are considered when examining muscle mass and tone. Table 30-3 lists neurologic diagnostic procedures that are related to specific neurologic diseases. Table 30-4 describes common neurologic disorders.

Procedures performed to confirm a diagnosis of a neurologic problem or disease are limited to the use of various diagnostic imaging and electrical impulse studies. The medical assistant assists the providers during certain procedures. Patient teaching by the medical assistant before a procedure and active reinforcement during a procedure will promote patient cooperation. Procedure 30-1 outlines steps involved in removing cerebrospinal fluid from the lumbar area.

PATIENT EDUCATION

Post–Lumbar Puncture Instructions.

1. You will be kept lying down for at least 30 minutes immediately after the procedure. You should recline on your ride home as much as possible, especially if you have the beginnings of a headache.

2. It is suggested that you lie down for 6 to 8 hours after you arrive home. You may have bathroom privileges and sit up to eat.

3. Drink water and other liquids, at least eight to ten 8 oz. glasses per day for several days.

4. Resume your regular activities the day after your procedure or as instructed by your provider. Avoid rigorous recreational exercise for the next 3 to 4 days. Expect to be able to return to work and mild exercise the following day if no headache is present.

5. Notify your provider if you develop a headache after the procedure; headache is the most common complication of a lumbar puncture.

Components of a Neurologic Screening

 During the neurologic screening examination, various functions are observed. Procedure 30-2 outlines the steps involved in a neurologic screening examination:

- History
- Symptoms
- Duration of symptoms
- Important factors to note
  - *Changes in level of consciousness.* Periods of wakefulness, stupor, lethargy or history of coma
  - *Changes in mental function or mood.* Verifying the patient's orientation to person, place, and time, history of depression, dementia, or the inability to express thoughts or aphasia
  - *Headaches.* Frequency, location, severity, and duration, association with nausea or vomiting, aggravating and alleviating factors

Table 30-3   Neurologic System Disorders and Related Diagnostic Testing

| Disease/Disorder | Laboratory/Diagnostic Tests | | | | Medical Tests or Procedures | Treatment |
	Blood	Other	Radiography	Surgery		
Alzheimer's disease	Vitamin deficiency testing Thyroid profile		Magnetic resonance imaging (MRI) of the brain Positron emission tomography (PET) scan of the brain		Mental status and neuropsychologic tests	Cholinesterase inhibitor medications N-methyl-D-aspartate (NMDA) medications
Amyotropic lateral sclerosis (ALS)	Blood tests to rule out other conditions Genetic testing	Physical exam Patient history Pulmonary function tests	Computed tomography (CT) of the cervical spine and head MRI of the head	Gastrostomy for swallowing difficulty	Elecromyography Nerve conduction studies Swallowing studies Lumbar puncture (spinal tap)	Medications to control spasms Physical therapy Caloric supplementation Assistive ventilation devices
Bell's palsy	Complete blood count		MRI of brain			Warm moist heat Facial exercises Analgesics Eye patch if unable to close eye
Carpal tunnel syndrome		Physical exam	Wrist radiography		Electromyography (EMG) Nerve conduction velocity study	Support of the extremity Anti-inflammatory medications Surgery to relieve pressure on the median nerve
Cerebral vascular accident (CVA) (stroke)			Cerebral angiography CT MRI	To remove clots	Electroencephalography Lumbar puncture	Anticoagulant therapy Physical therapy Speech therapy Tissue-plasminogen activator (tPA)
Epilepsy			CT MRI		Electroencephalography	Antiepilepsy medication

continues

Table 30-3 Neurologic System Disorders and Related Diagnostic Testing (*Continued*)

Disease/Disorder	Laboratory/Diagnostic Tests				Medical Tests or Procedures	Treatment
	Blood	Other	Radiography	Surgery		
Herpes zoster	Varicella-zoster antibody				Culture of cell Scrapings from lesion	Analgesics Steroids Antiviral medication (acyclovir, Famvir) Zostavax vaccine
Multiple sclerosis			Bran scan CT MRI		Lumbar puncture	Steroids Medications: experimental Physical therapy Muscle relaxants Assistive devices
Parkinson's disease	Complete blood count				Medical history Neurologic exam	Dopamine-like medications Dopamine antigonists MAO-B inhibitors Catechol-O-methyltransferase inhibitors (COMT) Physical therapy Deep brain stimulator implant

© Cengage Learning 2014

Disease						Treatment
Rabies	Complete blood count Blood serum Reverse transcription Polymerase chain reaction (RT-PCR)	Saliva Cerebral spinal fluid for antibodies to rabies virus				Wash wound immediately with soap and water Antirabies injections Medication for convulsions
Reye's syndrome	Complete blood count Serum ammonia	Liver function studies		Liver biopsy Brain biopsy	Lumbar puncture Examination of cerebrospinal fluid	Supportive physical therapy Control of brain swelling
Sciatica	Blood serum		Myelogram CT MRI	Diskectomy (if caused by herniated disk)		Physical therapy Massage Exercise Analgesics Antiinflammatory drugs Surgery
Tic douloureux				Biopsy of trigeminal nerve		Analgesics Surgery to dissect the trigeminal nerve
West Nile virus	Complete blood count	Cerebral spinal fluid	MRI		Neurologic work-up	No specific treatment Supportive

Table 30-4 Description of Neurologic Disorders

- *Amytropic lateral sclerosis* (Lou Gehrig's disease). Disease of the nerve cells in brain and spinal cord that control voluntary movement.

- *Bell's palsy.* Paralysis of seventh cranial nerve caused by an acute inflammation. Usually characterized by unilateral facial paralysis and pain, but it can be bilateral.

- *Cerebral vascular accident (CVA).* Loss of blood supply to the brain (anoxia). May be caused by a ruptured or clogged blood vessel or clot in the brain. Symptoms include sudden loss of consciousness and paralysis. Also referred to as a stroke.

- *Epilepsy.* Episodes of seizures caused by changes in electrical brain potentials that result in disturbed brain impulses or function.

- *Headache.* Diffuse pain in different parts of the head. May be acute or chronic with varying degree of pain and may be caused by a variety of reasons.

- *Herpes zoster.* An acute infectious viral disease caused by varicella-zoster virus. Painful vesicular eruptions. Known as "shingles."

- *Meningitis.* Inflammation of the membranes of the spinal cord or brain. Symptoms include a stiff neck, headache, anorexia, and irregular fever. Caused by either a bacterium or a virus.

- *Multiple sclerosis.* Chronic progressive disease characterized by **demyelination** (destruction of nerve covering) of nerve fibers. The cause is unknown. First symptoms are visual disturbances and muscle weakness.

- *Parkinson's disease.* A slowly progressive disease, usually occurring in later life, caused by a degeneration of brain cells as a result of lack of dopamine in the brain. Muscle rigidity and akinesia are common symptoms.

- *Rabies.* Caused by a virus and transmitted to humans by scratches or bites from animals infected with the virus. The disease infects the brain and spinal cord and causes acute encephalitis. It can be fatal.

- *Reye's syndrome.* A neurologic illness usually seen in young children after a viral infection such as influenza, varicella, Epstein-Barr. There may be a connection between the viral infection and aspirin. Cause is unknown, but characteristic symptoms include vomiting, rash, lethargy and neurologic involvement, seizures, and coma.

- *Sciatica.* Severe pain in the leg along the course of the sciatic nerve felt at the back of the thigh and running down the inside of the leg. Caused by compression of the nerve by a ruptured intervertebral disk or osteoarthritis. Characterized by sharp, shooting pain running down back of thigh. Leg movement aggravates the pain.

- *Tic douloureux.* Degeneration of or pressure on the trigeminal (fifth cranial) nerve causing severe stabs of pain that radiate from the angle of the jaw along one of the branches. Pain may be felt in the eye, lip, nose, tongue. Pain may come and go for hours.

- *West Nile virus infection.* A potentially serious illness that affects the central nervous system. Symptoms may include headache, stupor, disorientation, tremors, convulsions, and coma. Spread by bite of infected mosquitoes.

© Cengage Learning 2014

- *Visual changes.* Double vision, nystagmus
- *Changes in hearing or tinnitus*
- *Dizziness/vertigo.* Related to position or movement, intermittent or constant, aggravating or alleviating factors
- *Abnormal sensation.* Numbness, tingling, burning
- *Weakness.* Location, duration, paralysis, localized or generalized
- *Pain.* Quality, quantity, description, continuous or intermittent
- *Gait.* Balanced, staggering, shuffling

- Level of consciousness
  - *Awake.* Eyes open wide spontaneously and immediately to minimal stimuli
  - *Alert.* Responds quickly and appropriately
  - *Drowsy.* Has the appearance of sleepiness, but responds to stimuli
  - *Lethargic.* Sleeps intermittently, awakens to stimuli, but may drift off to sleep again once the stimulus is removed
  - *Stuporous.* Can be awakened with more intense stimuli, can be disoriented when aroused, and returns to sleep once the stimulus is removed

- *Comatose.* No purposeful response even to painful stimuli, reflexes may be intact
- Memory (recall of past and present)
  - *Immediate.* Commonly a patient is given a verbal list of three objects and then asked to recite them correctly after 5 minutes
  - *Recent.* To check recent memory, the patient is asked about noteworthy current events
  - *Remote.* This test is recall of a patient's history such as birth date, name of children, first job, or hometown
- Cranial nerve function
  - *Cranial nerve I.* The olfactory nerve is responsible for the sense of smell. A patient is asked to identify the essence of coffee, peppermint, and vanilla using each nostril.
  - *Cranial nerve II.* The optic nerve is tested using an eye chart with a patient's glasses on. Peripheral vision is checked, and the provider will examine the interior of the eye and the retina.
  - *Cranial nerves III, IV, and VI.* The oculomotor, trochlear, and abducens nerves are tested together because they work in concert to control eye movement. Pupillary reaction and other extraocular movements are tested.
  - *Cranial nerve V.* The trigeminal nerve is responsible for corneal reflexes, facial sensation, and the opening and closing of the mouth.
  - *Cranial nerve VII.* The facial nerve controls the muscles of the face. The health of this nerve is determined by evaluation of facial expressions, especially smiling. The patient is examined for facial drooping and for the ability to tightly close the eyes.
  - *Cranial nerve VIII.* The vestibulocochlear nerve is responsible for hearing. The examination of this nerve involves a variety of hearing tests including air versus bone conduction using a tuning fork.
  - *Cranial nerves IX and X.* The glossopharyngeal and vagus nerves are evaluated together. The practitioner evaluates the quality of the voice, the ability to cough and swallow, and the gag reflex.
  - *Cranial nerve XI.* The accessory nerve controls the shoulders and the muscles of the neck. The functionality of this nerve is evaluated by observing the shoulders shrugging and the turning of the head against resistance.
- *Cranial nerve XII.* The hypoglossal nerve controls the movement of the tongue. To evaluate this nerve, a patient is asked to open the mouth so that the tongue can be examined for any abnormal movements, to thrust the tongue out of the mouth, and to speak in order to check articulation.

The provider continues with the neurologic examination by checking the patient for the following:

- Motor function

  Aspects of the motor function exam are focused on evaluation of the muscles of the body. Muscle groups are examined to determine muscle mass, tone, and strength. Any abnormalities such as tenderness and involuntary or abnormal muscle movement should be noted. The exam also evaluates the symmetry of the muscles of the body, comparing right to left. Muscle strength is evaluated by applying resistance to the extremities during flexion and extension. This strength is usually rated on a scale of 0 to 5.

- Sensory function

  It is important to evaluate the sensory as well as the motor function of the body to obtain a complete examination reflecting the status of the neurologic system. A number of tests can be used to test for appropriate sensory function. The aspects of sensation that are evaluated are pain, touch, joint position sense, and thermal perception. Pain is tested using a pin to gently prick the skin. Light touch is evaluated by touch with a cotton ball. Vibration is tested with the use of a tuning fork.

- Cerebellar function

  The cerebellum is a smaller brain structure than the cerebrum. However, it contains 50% of the total number of neurons in the brain. The cerebrum is a structure that controls motor movement and posture. To evaluate the functionality of the cerebellum, a patient is asked to perform several tests. They are described as follows:

  - *Finger-to-nose (FTN) testing.* The patient is asked to alternately point from his or her nose to the examiner's finger. The examiner moves his finger to different locations to assure the patient's ability to adapt.
  - *Romberg test.* The patient is asked to stand still with his or her feet together and the arms straight at the sides. It is a normal result if the patient does not lose his or her balance.

- *Heel-to-shin (HTS) test.* The patient is asked to run the heel of one foot along the shin of the opposite leg and to then alternate and repeat the procedure on the other side. There is an abnormal result if the patient cannot maintain coordination with rapid repeat of the exercise.
- Reflex function

    The evaluation of **deep tendon reflexes (DTRs)** examines the arc that sensation travels from the source to the spinal cord and back to the muscle tissue. The usual manner for testing DTRs is to utilize a reflex hammer to tap on tendons in the upper and lower extremities. When the tendon is tapped, it activates the stretch fibers in the muscle and causes contraction of the muscle. If there is damage or injury, the impulse is delayed and the reaction is slowed. One of the aspects of assessment is symmetry. Reflexes should be bilaterally equal. Babinski's sign is an assessment of upper motor neurons. With this test, the handle of the reflex hammer strokes from the toes to the heel on the plantar aspect of the foot. If the great toe extends downward, the upper neurons are intact. Reflexes are rated on a 0-4 scale with 0 indicating no response and 4+ indicating a hyperactive response. Normal is midscale at 2+.

- Gait and stance

    Specific neurologic disorders are identified by the rate, rhythm, and coordination of movement that represents gait. The observance of gait can be an indicator of a lack of integration of the peripheral and central nervous systems. It is the role of the medical assistant to be familiar with the components of a neurologic examination and to be able to accurately record the results of this exam at the direction of the provider (Procedure 30-2).

Additional tests:

- Angiography provides visualization of the circulation of the blood throughout the brain.
- Computed tomography (CT) helps to diagnose hemorrhage and tumors (see Chapter 32).
- Electroencephalography (EEG) records the electrical activity of the brain and helps to diagnose seizures and tumors.
- Magnetic resonance imaging (MRI) helps to diagnose tumors and hemorrhage (see Chapter 32).

- Lumbar puncture (LP) and the examination of cerebrospinal fluid (CSF) are used in many diagnoses related to the brain and spinal cord. These diagnoses include subarachnoid hemorrhage, meningitis, multiple sclerosis, and dementia.
- Positron emission tomography (PET) scans are tests of brain function as they assess chemical activity and metabolic rates within the brain. These scans are used to diagnose movement disorders, cerebral vascular disorders, epilepsy, tumors, dementia, and other disorders.
- Electromyography (EMG) is the assessment of the nerve and muscle interaction. EMG measures the electrical potential of muscles at rest and during contraction. The test diagnoses diseases that interrupt the electrical signal from the muscle to the spinal cord and back via the nerve-muscle junctions. Diseases of the peripheral nervous system are easily diagnosed using EMG.

SENSORY SYSTEM

The special senses of vision, hearing, equilibrium (balance), smell, touch, and taste permit the body to detect information about the environment. The eyes, ears, nose, taste buds, and skin are all sense organs that contain specialized receptor organs. Table 30-5 lists diseases and disorders of the sensory system and diagnostic tests and procedures for eyes and ears.

The Eye

The eye is the primary organ for sight and is one of the few organs of the body externally exposed. Its accessory structures—the eyelids, eyelashes, lacrimal ducts, and extrinsic muscles—provide protection for the eye. The anterior portion of the eyeball protrudes outward and the remainder is protected by the orbit.

The intraocular structures consist of some parts of the eye visible externally and parts visible only through an ophthalmoscope. The intraocular structures include the following:

- *Sclera.* White area covering the outside of the eye except over the pupil and iris
- *Cornea.* Clear tissue covering the pupil and iris
- *Iris.* Round disk of smooth and radial muscles giving the eye its color
- *Pupil.* Round opening in the iris that changes size as the iris reacts to light and dark

Table 30-5   Sensory System Disorders

| Disease/Disorder | Laboratory/Diagnostic Tests | | | | Medical Tests or Procedures | Treatment |
	Blood	Other	Radiography	Surgery		
Amblyopia					Ophthalmologic examination	Cover the normal eye to force weaker eye to function
Astigmatism					Ophthalmic exam	Corrective lenses
Cataract					Ophthalmologic examination Slit lamp	Phacoemulsification Surgical extraction
Chalazion				Excision		
Color blindness (achromatopia)					Ishihara color plates	
Conjunctivitis		Culture and sensitivity tests of eye discharge		Stained smears of conjunctival scrapings		Antibiotic drops or antibiotic ointment
Corneal abrasion					Fluorescein stain	Antibiotic ointment, dressing over affected eye
Diabetic retinopathy				Laser	Fluorescein agiography	Laser
Diplopia (double vision)					Ophthalmologic examination	Corrective lenses Treatment of underlying medical conditions
Epistaxis	Complete blood count			Nasal	Blood pressure	Electrocautery

continues

Table 30-5 Sensory System Disorders *(Continued)*

Disease/Disorder	Laboratory/Diagnostic Tests				Medical Tests or Procedures	Treatment
	Blood	Other	Radiography	Surgery		
External otitis	Complete blood count	Culture and sensitivity tests of exudate			Otologic examination	Antibiotic therapy Laser (if severe)
Glaucoma					Vision field testing Ophthalmologic examination including intraocular pressure Tonometry	Medicated eye drops Oral medication Laser surgery, conventional surgery, or a combination
Impacted cerumen					Otologic examination	Removal with curette Irrigation
Macular degeneration					Ophthalmologic examination Angiography Amsler grid	Laser Intraocular injections Intravenous medication Some cases are untreatable
Ménière's disease					Audiometry MRI Electrocochleography	Medication, surgery only if severe
Motion sickness						Medication
Myopia					Ophthalmologic examination	Radial keratotomy
Nystagmus					Opticokinetic drum test Neurologic examination	Directed at cause (inner ear or central nervous system)
Hyperopia					Astigmatoscopy	Corrective lenses

Condition	Complete blood count	Culture and sensitivity	Imaging	Procedure	Examination	Treatment
Presbyopia					Snellen chart	Corrective lenses
Nasal polyps				Biopsy of polyp (lesion)	Nasal examination	Electrosurgery
Otitis media	Complete blood count	Culture and sensitivity tests of exudate		Myringotomy Tympanostomy	Tympanography	Antibiotics Myringotomy
Otosclerosis					Audiometry Rinne test	Stapedectomy
Retinal detachment				Laser or surgery to reattach	Ophthalmologic examination	Laser
Retinoblastoma			CT of head MRI of head Ultrasound of the eye		Ophthalmologic examination Bone marrow biopsy CSF exam	Laser surgery Cryosurgery Radiation Chemotherapy
Sinusitis	Complete blood count	Culture and sensitivity tests of exudate	Sinus radiographs			Antibiotics for bacterial infection
Strabismus					Ophthalmologic examination Neurologic examination	Cover the normal eye to force weaker eye to function
Stye (hordeolum)		Culture and sensitivity tests if exudate present		Incision and drainage		Antibiotic ointment
Vestibular neuritis (labyrinthitis)			CT of head MRI of head		EEG Electrostagmography Audiology/audiometry Caloric stimulation of the inner ear	Antihistamines Medications for nausea and vomiting Sedatives Environmental management to reduce vertigo

- *Anterior chamber.* Space between cornea and iris/pupil filled with clear fluid called aqueous humor
- *Posterior chamber.* Space between the iris and lens that is filled with aqueous humor
- *Lens.* Clear fibers enclosed in a membrane that refract and focus light to the retina
- *Posterior cavity.* Space in the posterior part of the eyeball filled with thick, gelatinous material called vitreous humor
- *Posterior sclera.* White opaque layer covering the posterior part of the eyeball
- *Choroid layer.* Layer between the sclera and retina containing blood vessels
- *Retina.* Inside layer of the posterior part of the eye that receives the light rays (visual stimuli)

The mechanism of vision occurs after impulses leave the retina and travel through the optic nerves to the brain. At the optic chiasm, the nerve fibers cross and continue to the thalamus. These fibers synapse with other neurons that send the impulses to the right and left visual area of the occipital lobe of the brain. Because the tracts cross at the optic chasm, the stimuli coming from the right visual fields are translated in the visual area of the left occipital area, and the stimuli coming from the left visual fields are translated in the visual area of the right occipital lobe. Table 30-6 describes common eye disorders. Figure 30-4 illustrates the visual pathways of the eye.

Signs and symptoms that are common to eye diseases and disorders are conjunctivitis, **hordeolum**, or stye, decreased visual acuity, and any visual changes such as seeing sudden flashes of

Table 30-6   Description of Eye Disorders

Refraction and Other Disorders

- *Astigmatism.* Irregular lens curvature or cornea shape causing improper focusing of objects.

- *Cataract.* Lens loses its transparent nature caused by changes in its proteins. Usually brought on by aging or exposure to sunlight.

- *Color blindness.* Inability to distinguish among colors. Caused by an absence of a cone photopigment; a genetic disorder.

- **Conjunctivitis.** Caused by a bacterial infection or irritant resulting in irritated and reddened conjunctiva. If caused by bacteria, conjunctivitis is treated with the appropriate antibiotic ophthalmic ointment or drops.

- *Corneal abrasion.* Caused by an injury to the cornea by a foreign body resulting in pain, tearing, redness, and possible infection.

- *Diabetic retinopathy.* Diabetes mellitus causes damage to the retina because the disease causes vascular changes. This is the leading cause of blindness in the United States.

- **Glaucoma.** Condition caused by increased intraocular pressure due to a buildup of aqueous humor. This results in mild visual disturbances with little or no pain but can lead to severe visual impairment if untreated.

- *Nearsightedness (myopia).* Caused by an elongated (irregularly shaped) eyeball; the image is focused in the front of the retina, resulting in the inability to focus on objects at a distance.

- *Farsightedness (hyperopia).* Caused when the eyeball is irregularly shaped (shortened); the image is focused behind the retina, causing distance vision to be unclear.

- *Presbyopia.* Attributed to the aging process when the lens loses its elasticity and the ability to accommodate. Vision is hampered when items are close.

- *Retinal detachment.* Complete or partial separation of the retina from the choroid layer of the eye, leading to possible blindness.

- *Stye (hordeolum).* Inflamed sebaceous gland of the eyelid caused by bacterial infection. Erythema and tenderness at site are common symptoms.

© Cengage Learning 2014

LEFT VISUAL FIELD   RIGHT VISUAL FIELD

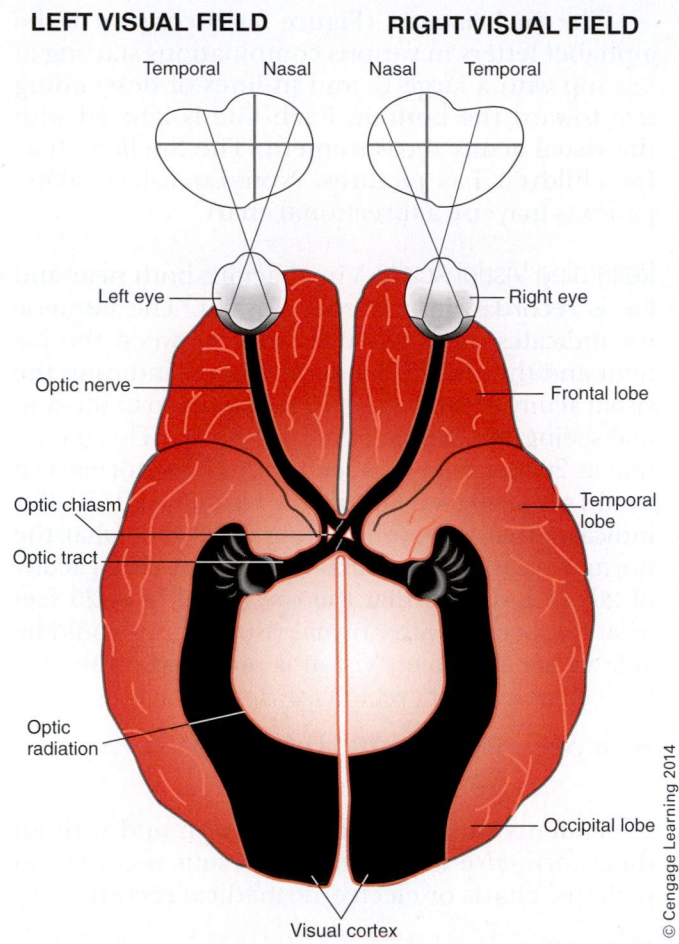

Figure 30-4 The visual pathways of the eye.

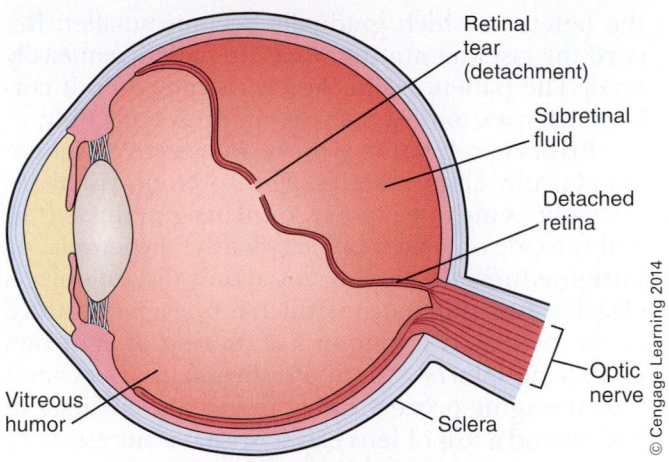

Figure 30-5 Detachment of the retina.

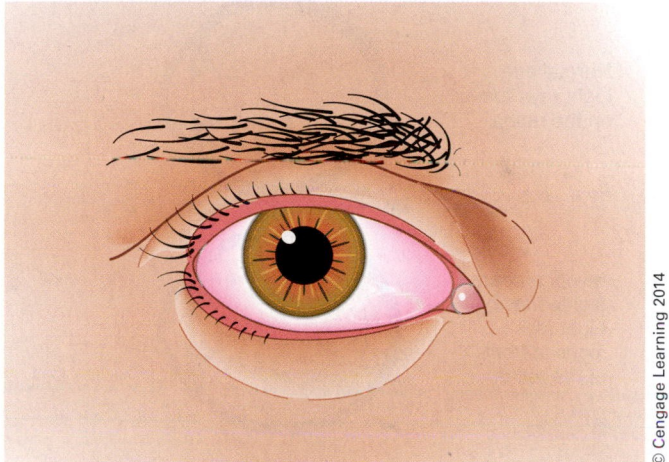

Figure 30-6 Conjunctivitis.

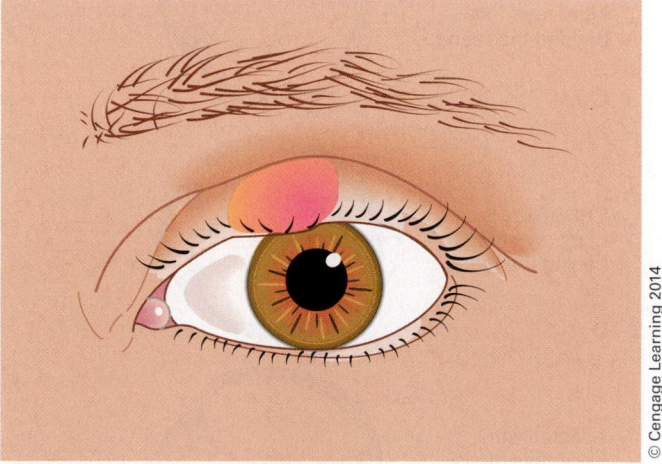

Figure 30-7 Stye (hordeolum).

light, which may indicate retinal detachment (see Figure 30-5 to Figure 30-7).

Measuring Visual Acuity. A procedure commonly performed by the medical assistant is the measuring of a patient's visual acuity. This is only a screening process used when errors in refraction are suspected. The procedure must be performed in a well-lit, quiet area. While performing the procedure, the medical assistant must observe the patient for any action that may indicate difficulty with vision. These actions include squinting, wiping of the eyes, or leaning toward the chart. In near-vision acuity, these actions include holding the card nearer or farther than the stated position. The commonly used chart for distance visual acuity is the Snellen chart for the adult. Near-vision is commonly checked by using the Jaeger card.

The Jaeger chart used for checking clear vision is a small card that the patient holds between 14 and 16 inches from the eye. The medical assistant measures the distance for accuracy. This is the distance from which a person with normal vision is able to read printed material such as a newspaper. The Jaeger test consists of a series of reading material, the letters of which gradually become smaller. Record the last line number that the patient can easily read. The patient is checked with and without corrective lenses, and each eye is checked separately.

Errors in refraction is the term used to designate visual acuity abnormalities. The common visual abnormalities include myopia, or nearsightedness (the ability to see only near objects clearly); **hyperopia,** or farsightedness (the ability to see only distant objects clearly); and astigmatism, which is uneven curvature of the cornea, resulting in a scattering of light rays producing blurry vision. **Presbyopia** is associated with the aging process and is an increase in farsightedness and a loss of lens elasticity that is necessary to accommodate for near vision (Figure 30-8).

The **Snellen chart** (Figure 30-9) consists of the alphabet letters in various combinations starting at the top with a large E, and in lines of descending size toward the bottom. Each line is labeled with the visual acuity measurement. The Snellen chart for children has pictures. Non–English-speaking patients may use a directional chart.

Recording Visual Acuity. Visual acuity, both near and far, is recorded in a fraction format. The numerator indicates the 20-foot distance between the patient and the chart. The denominator indicates the visual acuity of the patient in relationship to the normal seeing eye. Normal vision is 20/20. This means that at 20 feet the eye is seeing what the normal eye would see at 20 feet. Should the vision be 20/30, this indicates that the eye is seeing at 20 feet what the normal eye would see at 30 feet away. A visual acuity of 20/15 indicates that the eye is seeing at 20 feet what the person with normal visual acuity would be able to see at 15 feet. Vision is recorded on the patient chart as right eye, left eye, and both eyes.

Example: Right 20/20   Left 20/20
Both 20/20

Patients should be screened with and without their corrective lenses and the results recorded in patients' charts or electronic medical records.

Color Vision. Checking color vision is not part of a routine examination. This procedure is usually performed on people who must distinguish color

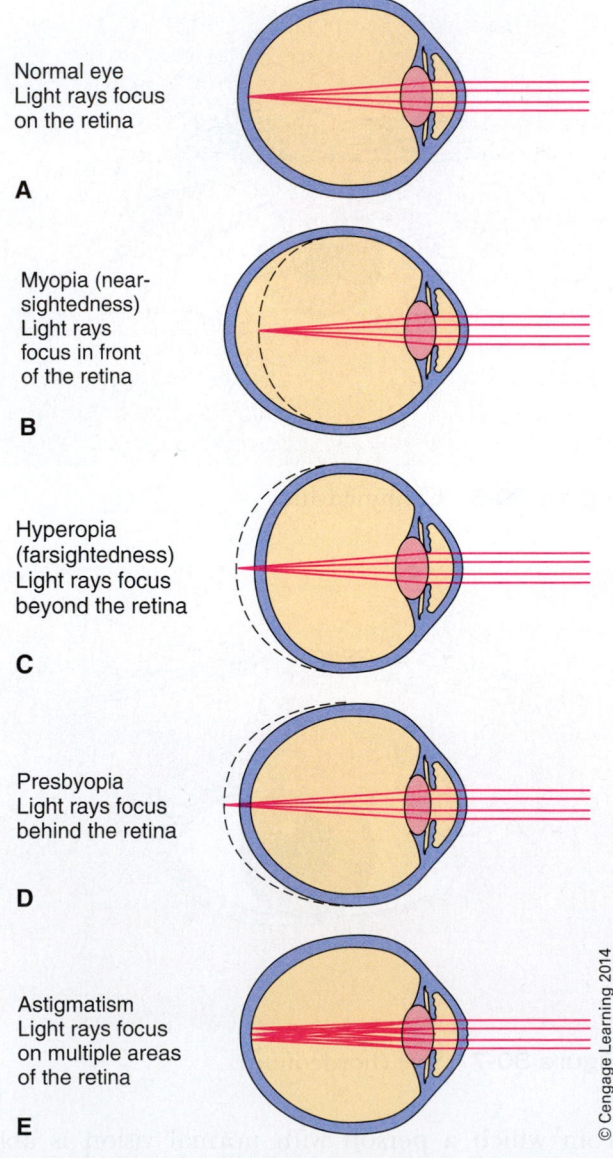

Figure 30-8 (A) Normal eye vision. (B) Myopia. (C) Hyperopia. (D) Presbyopia. (E) Astigmatism.

Normal eye
Light rays focus
on the retina

A

Myopia (near-
sightedness)
Light rays
focus in front
of the retina

B

Hyperopia
(farsightedness)
Light rays focus
beyond the retina

C

Presbyopia
Light rays focus
behind the retina

D

Astigmatism
Light rays focus
on multiple areas
of the retina

E

© Cengage Learning 2014

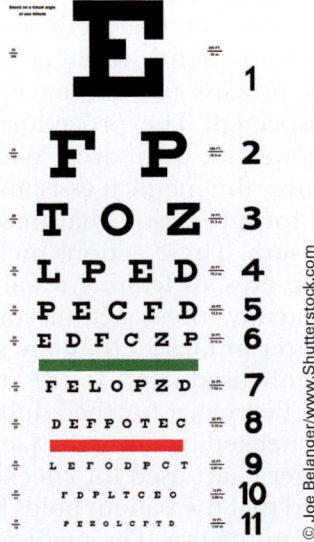

Figure 30-9 Snellen chart.

© Joe Belanger/www.Shutterstock.com

as part of their occupation (e.g., truck drivers, pilots, and salespeople). A commonly used color vision test is the Ishihara color graph. The Ishihara test chart book (Figure 30-10) contains pages composed of circles of varying sizes and colors. Inside the circles are numbers or lines that can be traced. The patient is seated for the procedure with the book held 14 to 16 inches away and is instructed to identify the numbers as the page is turned or is instructed to trace the line from the indicated starting point to the end. Inability to see the number or to follow the line may indicate color blindness. Should this occur, the medical assistant must inform the provider as to what number(s) could not be seen. The patient is referred to an ophthalmologist.

The medical assistant will be responsible for assisting the provider in ophthalmologic examinations and performing the tests for visual acuity. Diagnostic procedures for the special senses involve the use of specialized instruments. The use of the ophthalmoscope (lighted instrument used to view inside patient's eye; Figure 30-11) assists in identifying disease-related problems. The interior of the eye can be examined.

Procedures 30-3 through 30-8 list the steps for specialty procedures for the eye.

The Ear

The structures of hearing and equilibrium are divided into the external ear, the middle ear, and the inner ear. The external ear includes the pinna or **auricle** and the external auditory canal. The pinna is mostly cartilaginous tissue with a small amount of adipose tissue in the earlobe. The external auditory canal is about 1 inch in length and contains hair and wax-producing glands. Cerumen is the medical term for the wax that protects the ear canal. The external ear and middle ear are separated by the tympanic membrane, or eardrum.

The middle ear, also called the tympanic cavity, is a small space containing three bones—the malleus, incus, and stapes. Layman's terms for these three smallest bones in the human body are the hammer, the anvil, and the stirrup. Next to the stapes is the oval window that leads to the inner ear. The eustachian tube connects the middle ear to the throat.

The inner ear is the most sophisticated part of the ear. It is responsible for both hearing and

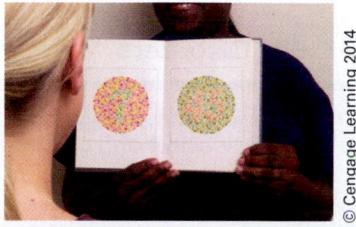

© Cengage Learning 2014

Figure 30-10   The patient's color vision acuity is tested using Ishihara plates.

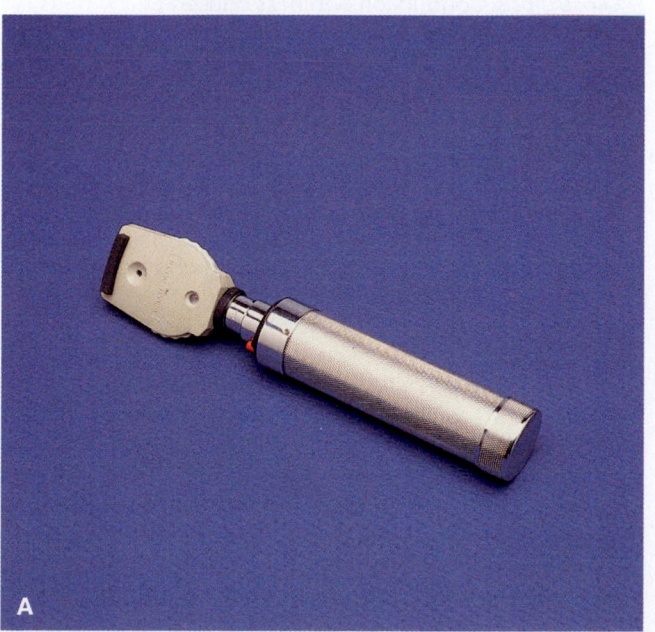

A

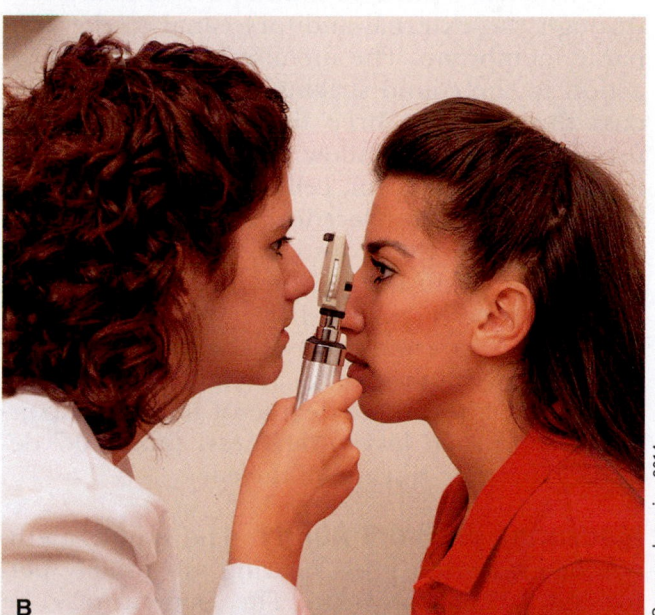

B

© Cengage Learning 2014

Figure 30-11   (A) The ophthalmoscope is used to identify eye disorders. (B) The provider uses the ophthalmoscope to view the interior of the patient's eye.

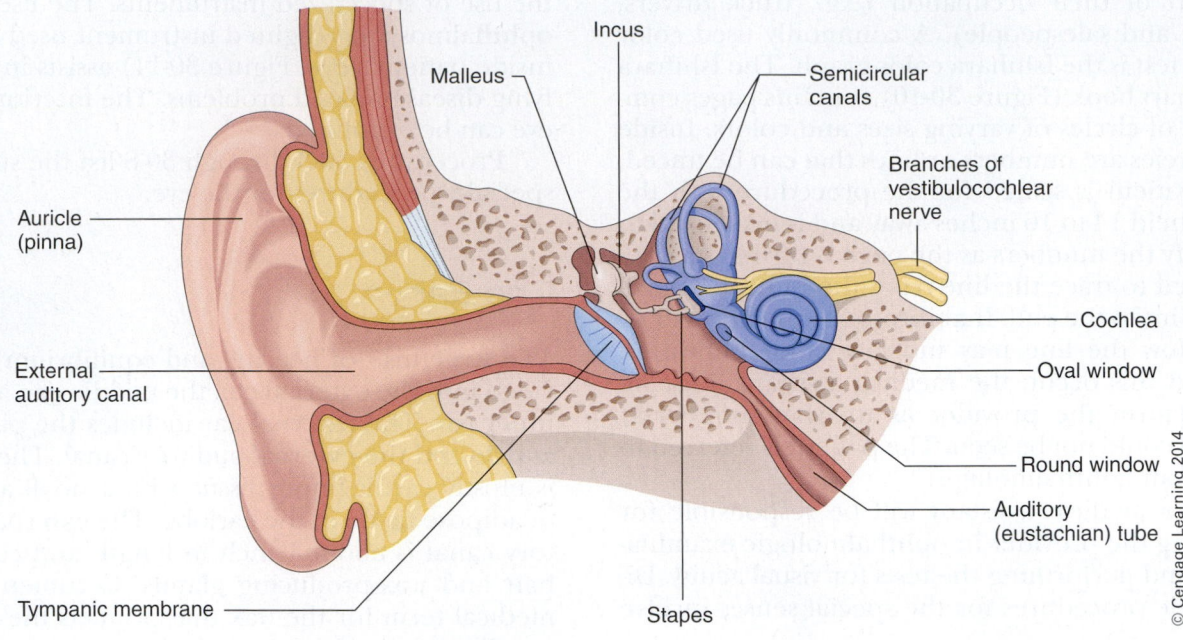

Figure 30-12   The ear.

© Cengage Learning 2014

equilibrium. The inner ear consists of a fluid-filled sterile space housing the vestibule, the semicircular canals, the round window, and the cochlea. The structures in the vestibule are responsible for maintaining equilibrium during movement of the head. The semicircular canals assist the body to adjust to changes in direction. The movement of fluid in this area can cause symptoms of dizziness. The cochlea is the organ of hearing.

The auricle picks up sound waves that are sent through the external auditory canal to the tympanic membrane. The membrane vibrates in reaction to the sound striking it. These vibrations pass through the three tiny middle ear bones through the oval window and into the fluid in the cochlea. Receptor cells respond and transfer the sounds into electrical impulses that travel to the brain via the acoustic nerve. The receiving area of the brain for auditory impulses is in the temporal lobe (Figure 30-12).

Diseases or conditions of the ear, if left untreated, can cause damage to nerves and tissues and can result in some degree of hearing impairment, from mild loss to deafness. Table 30-7 describes common diseases of the ear.

Measuring Auditory Ability.
The simple methods of measuring gross hearing are usually performed by the provider. The patient may be instructed to place a finger in one ear while the provider whispers one or two words in the other. The patient is then asked to repeat the words. A ticking watch may be placed by the patient's ear

Table 30-7   Ear Disorders

External otitis (swimmer's ear). Inflammation of ear canal. Symptoms are itchiness and crusting of ear canal.

Otitis media. Acute infection of the middle ear usually caused by bacteria. Symptoms are pain, fever, discharge, and decreased hearing acuity.

Otosclerosis. Conduction deafness caused by hardening of the stapes.

Ménière's disease. Characterized by deafness, vertigo, nausea, and tinnitus. Probable cause is edema of the labyrinth.

Impacted cerumen. Caused by accumulation of hardened cerumen that has built up against the tympanic membrane. Impaired hearing and tinnitus can result.

© Cengage Learning 2014

to ascertain hearing. A vibrating tuning fork may be placed on the mastoid process behind the ear and then on top of the head. The patient is asked if the sound vibrations could be heard or felt. This procedure will identify nerve or conduction deafness (Figure 30-13). Conduction deafness occurs when the sound wave is not transmitted to the middle ear. This type of deafness may be a result of the presence of impacted ear wax (cerumen) in the ear canal or a scarred tympanic membrane.

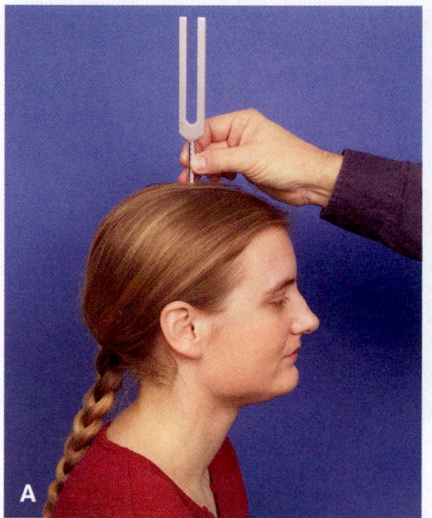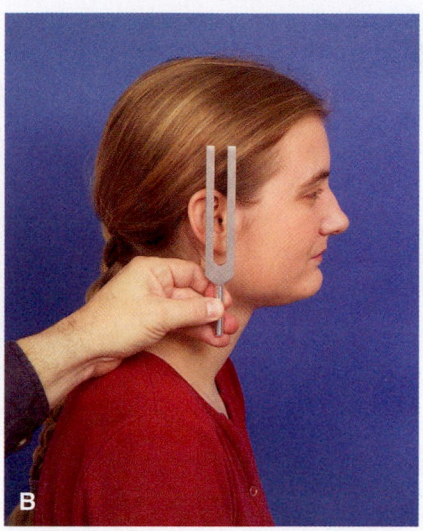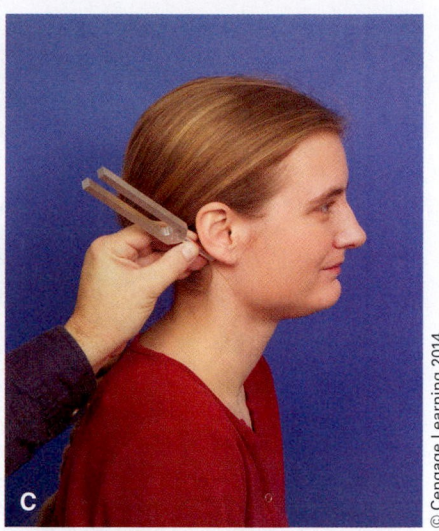

Figure 30-13 (A) The provider holds the tuning fork against the crown of the patient's head to determine which ear can hear the sound. (B) To check air conduction of sound, the provider holds the tuning fork 1 inch from the patient's auditory meatus. (C) The provider places the tuning fork on the bony prominence (mastoid bone) behind the patient's ear to check bone conduction of sound.

Cerumen is a substance secreted by glands at the outer third of the ear canal. In some individuals it can accumulate and block the canal and become impacted against the tympanic membrane. The sound waves cannot pass through the hardened cerumen to the middle ear, and conduction hearing loss results.

To remove impacted cerumen, the provider may use a curette. The patient may have had ear drops prescribed before the physical removal of the impacted cerumen. The drops are instilled in an effort to soften the cerumen to facilitate its removal. An ear irrigation may be performed by flushing the ear canal with warm water or a solution ordered by the provider. Commercial solutions are available for patients to use at home (see Procedure 30-9).

A tympanic membrane can become scarred from rupture or perforation. Scarring can occur from untreated acute otitis media or traumatic rupture. With acute otitis media, the tympanic membrane is red and bulges from accumulation of serous or purulent fluid behind it. The pressure of the fluid on the tympanic membrane may be so great that the membrane ruptures and drainage can be seen in the ear canal. The perforation or rupture will probably heal, but a small scar on the membrane will remain. Repeated ruptures from acute otitis media will cause repeated scarring and diminished hearing function, referred to as conduction hearing loss. A culture and sensitivity of any purulent or serous drainage will indicate the antibiotic to which the microorganism is sensitive.

A myringotomy is a surgical incision into the tympanic membrane made to remove accumulated fluid caused by infection. Because the procedure is surgical in nature, the tympanic membrane can be incised to allow the fluid to drain. Scarring is minimized because the incision is made with a scalpel in a controlled location and will heal with less scarring. Tubes may be placed in the opening made by the myringotomy, called a **tympanostomy**, to equalize pressure and prevent fluid from accumulating (see Chapter 27).

Nerve deafness is a result of injury or disease that affects the nerves leading from the inner ear to the auditory centers of the brain.

A more complex procedure for measuring hearing may be performed by the medical assistant but more often by an audiologist, using an audiometer. A quiet room with no distractions is required for the procedure to be accurate. The patient is seated facing away from the medical assistant and the audiometer, then ear phones are placed over the ears. The patient is instructed to raise a hand when a sound is heard. The audiometer has two dials, one for the various wavelengths and the other for wave intensity. Starting at the lowest pitch, the intensity is increased until the patient responds to the sound. The next pitch is then tested in the same manner. This process continues until the highest pitch sound is tested. The results are obtained by noting the number of intensity at which the sound was heard. When performing the procedure, the medical assistant must not develop a pattern that can be detected by the patient. The ears should be tested in an alternating fashion to ensure accuracy (see Procedure 30-10 and Figure 30-14).

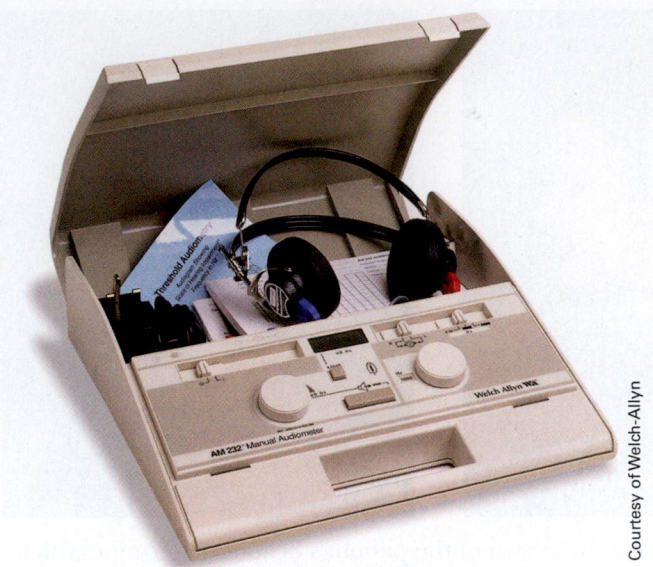

Courtesy of Welch-Allyn

Figure 30-14 Manual audiometer.

The medical assistant employed in an industrial medical facility may be required to monitor hearing of some employees. In this case, care must be taken to have the hearing test performed before the employee goes to work for the day. Hearing loss may result from the day's activities in some noisy facilities even when ear plugs are worn.

Tympanometry is a procedure used to ascertain the ability of the middle ear to transmit sound waves and is commonly performed on children to diagnose middle ear infections. A probe is inserted into the ear canal to measure the air pressure of the ear canal in relation to the air pressure found in the middle ear. Tympanogram is the recording produced by this procedure. The waves and peaks are measured, providing an indication of possible middle ear abnormalities (Figure 30-15).

The medical assistant or the provider may perform the audiometry test. Diagnostic procedures for the ear involve the use of specialized instruments, including the **otoscope** (lighted instrument to examine the tympanic membrane), which assists in identifying disease-related ear problems (Figure 30-16).

Procedures 30-9, 30-10, and 30-11 describe steps for audiometry, ear irrigation, and ear instillation.

The Nose

The provider inspects the exterior surface of the patient's nose for skin lesions such as **rosacea**, squamous or basal cell carcinoma, and other

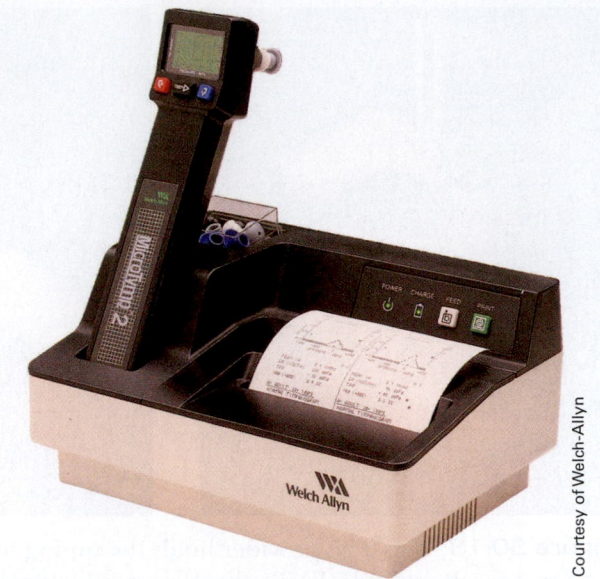

Courtesy of Welch-Allyn

Figure 30-15 A portable tympanometric instrument with charger. A printout of the tympanogram can be seen. Testing is done in 1 second and is useful for diagnosing otitis media and other middle ear conditions, such as patency of tympanostomy tubes and otosclerosis.

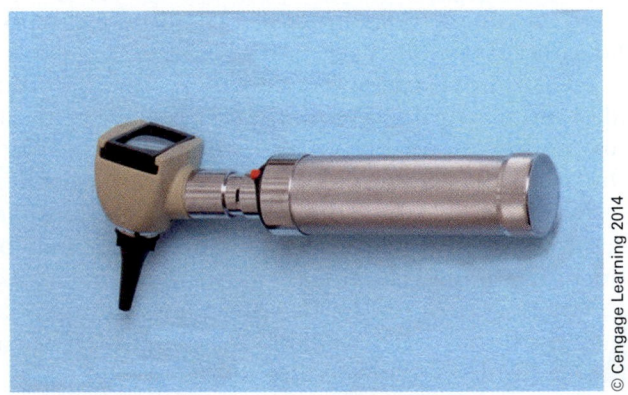

© Cengage Learning 2014

Figure 30-16 The otoscope is used to examine the patient's tympanic membrane.

dermatologic problems. The provider examines and palpates to determine if the nose is patent and the patient's ability to breathe in and out through each nostril. The mucous membrane is checked for polyps, superficial blood vessels, and foreign bodies. The septum is noted for deviation. Epistaxis is a common problem and can be treated with electrocautery or nasal packing. Procedures 30-12, 30-13, and 30-14 describe steps for specialized procedures and examinations for the nose.

RESPIRATORY SYSTEM

The respiratory process is all important to the life process. **External respiration** allows for the exchange of carbon dioxide and oxygen across the cell walls into the airspaces of the lungs. **Internal respiration** is the exchange of these gases at the cellular levels of the organs.

The respiratory process begins with air entering the nose or mouth, where it passes through the pharynx, down into the trachea, and into the bronchi, and then enters the lungs. Gas exchange takes place when the blood filters through the alveoli (Figure 30-17). Table 30-8 lists diagnostic procedures for respiratory diseases and disorders. Table 30-9 describes respiratory disorders.

Signs and Symptoms of Respiratory Conditions and Disorders

If a patient's chief complaint indicates a respiratory condition or disorder, medical attention is essential. Some signs and symptoms include:

- *Dyspnea.* Shortness of breath or air hunger
- *Chest pain.* Not only a symptom of cardiac disease
- *Fatigue.* Overall feeling of general tiredness or weakness due to decreased oxygen supply to the tissues
- *Hemoptysis.* Blood that is present in the sputum
- *Chills and fever.* Related to respiratory infection
- *Hoarseness.* Due to inflammation of the respiratory tract including the larynx
- *Wheezing.* A coarse whistling sound that arises from the lungs due to inflammatory or infectious narrowing of the respiratory passages
- *Cough, productive or nonproductive.* Productive cough results in bringing secretions up from the lower portions of the respiratory tract

Irrigations of the nose, collection of sputum specimens, and assisting with pulmonary tests are the roles of the medical assistant.

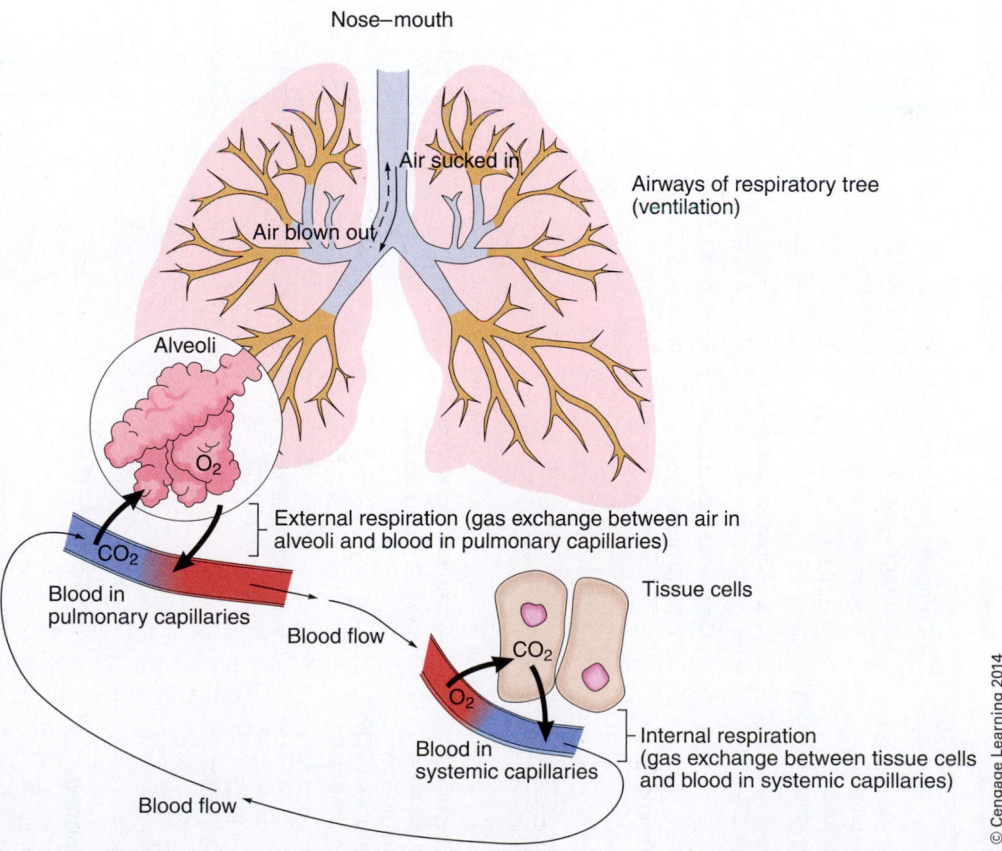

Figure 30-17   Gas exchange in the lungs and tissues.

Table 30-8   Respiratory System Disorders

Disease/ Disorder	Laboratory/Diagnostic Tests				Surgery	Medical Tests or Procedures	Treatment
	Blood	Other	Radiography				
Acute or adult respiratory distress syndrome (ARDS)	Complete blood count Blood chemistry Prothrombin time Partial thromboplastin time Arterial blood gases	Electro-cardiography Urinalysis	Chest radiograph (CXR)		Tracheotomy	Thoracentesis	Antibiotics Ventilator Oxygen
Asthma	Complete blood count Arterial blood gases	Sputum analysis Peak expiratory flow rate	Chest radiograph (CXR)			Pulmonary function tests Skin testing for allergies	Medication (bronchodilators) Metered-dose inhaler Treatment of hypersensitivity
Bronchitis	Complete blood count	Sputum culture and analysis	Chest radiograph (CXR)			Bronchoscopy	Antibiotics if secondary bacterial infection occurs
Chronic obstructive pulmonary disease (COPD) Emphysema	Complete blood count Arterial blood gases	Spirometry	Chest radiograph (CXR)			Pulmonary function tests Pulse oximetry	Bronchodilators
Cystic fibrosis	Immunoreactive trypsinogen (IRT)	Sweat chloride test Fecal fat test	Chest radiograph (CXR) CT scan			Pulmonary function testing	Antibiotics Inhalation treatments Enzyme therapy Lung transplant Oxygen therapy
Epistaxis	Complete blood count			Nasal cauterization		Blood pressure	Packing of nose, cautery
Influenza	Complete blood count		Chest radiograph (CXR)				Symptomatic Antibiotics if secondary bacterial infection occurs
Laryngitis	Complete blood count	Throat culture Rapid strep test				Laryngoscopy	Throat lozenges Analgesics

Condition						
Lung cancer	Complete blood count	Sputum cytology	Chest radiograph (CXR), CT scan	Biopsy of lung tissue	Bronchoscopy	Surgery, Chemotherapy, Radiation
Nasal polyps	Complete blood count			Biopsy of lesions	Nasal examination	Surgical excision
Pharyngitis	Complete blood count	Throat culture, Rapid strep test				Lozenges, Gargling
Pleurisy	Complete blood count		Chest radiograph (CXR)			Taping of chest, Antibiotics if bacterial, Analgesics
Pneumonia	Complete blood count	Blood culture, Sputum smear	Chest radiograph (CXR)			Antibiotics if bacterial, Symptomatic treatment if viral
Pneumothorax	Arterial blood gases (ABGs)		Chest radiograph (CXR)	Insertion of a chest tube		Oxygen, Rest, Chest tube insertion, Pleurodesis
Pulmonary embolism (PE)	Arterial blood gases (ABGs), Complete blood count (CBC), D-dimer	Electrocardiogram	Chest radiography (CXR), CT angiography, Pulmonary angiography, Ventilation/perfusion scan		Venous Doppler studies	Oxygen, Anticoagulants, Thrombolytics
Severe acute respiratory syndrome (SARS)	Complete blood count, Blood chemistry, Serum antibodies of SARS	Throat or nasopharyngeal swab, Viral culture	Chest radiography (CXR)			Antiviral drugs, Steroids, Symptomatic treatment
Sinusitis	Complete blood count	Culture and sensitivity tests	Sinus radiographs		Nasal examination	Decongestants, Antibiotics
Tonsillitis	Complete blood count, Streptococcal antibody test	Throat culture		Tonsillectomy		Antibiotics
Tuberculosis	Complete blood count	Sputum culture, Acid-fast smear of sputum	Chest radiograph (CXR), Bronchoscopy	Biopsy of lung tissue	Tuberculin skin test: Mantoux intradermal test	Multiple anti-tuberculosis medications

Table 30-9   Description of Respiratory Disorders

Acute or adult respiratory distress syndrome (ARDS). A life-threatening condition that occurs when there is severe fluid buildup and hemorrhage in the lungs. ARDS is breathing failure that can occur in critically ill patients with underlying illnesses. There is a high mortality rate. Patients may be placed on isolation precautions (see Chapter 22).

Asthma. Inflammation and spasm of the smooth muscle of the bronchi brought on by an allergen or emotional upsets. Characterized by dyspnea and wheezing.

Bronchitis. Inflammation of the bronchi, caused by viral or bacterial infection with a dry, painful cough, progressing to a productive cough of greenish yellow sputum. Symptoms include cough, slight fever, chills, malaise, and soreness under the sternum.

Cystic fibrosis. A genetic disease that causes an abnormal thickness and increased mucous secretions. These secretions build up in the respiratory, gastrointestinal, and other systems of the body. This buildup causes lung infections that can be life-threatening, and intestinal digestive disorders.

Emphysema. Enlargement of the alveoli due to lost elasticity, usually brought on by a long-time irritant, such as cigarette smoking. Results in dyspnea, chronic cough, weight loss, and the appearance of a "barrel chest."

Epistaxis. A nosebleed. May be caused by trauma, chronic sinus irritation, drug abuse (caused by "snorting" drugs), hypertension, blood disorders, and high altitude.

Influenza. A viral infection of various strains of the upper respiratory tract. Sudden onset of chills, fever, cough, sore throat, gastrointestinal disorders are common. Can range from mild to life-threatening.

Laryngitis. Hoarseness, cough, aphonia caused by infections from nose or throat.

Lung cancer. Cancer that may appear in trachea, air sacs, bronchi, and other lung tissues and cells.

Nasal polyp. A tumor of the nose that can bleed easily. Should be removed surgically.

Pharyngitis. Inflammation of the pharynx caused by bacteria, virus, or an irritant. Difficulty in swallowing, pain, redness, and inflammation of the pharynx are some of the signs and symptoms. Streptococcus is the most common bacterial infection; influenza virus and the common cold virus are the most common viral agents involved. May be accompanied by fever, malaise, and headache.

Pleurisy. Inflammation of the pleurae caused by bacteria or viruses. Symptoms include pain, fever, cough, chills, and dyspnea.

Pneumonia. Inflammation of the lungs caused by bacteria, fungi, viruses, and chemical irritants. Usually has sudden onset and is characterized by chills, fever, chest pain, cough, and purulent sputum. Symptoms include sore throat, fever, and lymphadenopathy.

Pneumothorax. The collapse of a lung due to disease or trauma. This results in a collection of air in the space around the lungs. This interferes with the lungs' ability to expand during inspiration.

Pulmonary embolism. A pulmonary embolism is a sudden blockage in a lung artery. Usually the blockage is caused by a blood clot that originated in a vessel in a lower extremity. The blockage causes damage to the lung tissue due to a lack of blood flow and oxygen.

Severe acute respiratory syndrome (SARS). An acute viral respiratory illness that begins with fever, headache, body aches, general malaise, and diarrhea. There may be mild respiratory symptoms at the onset. Most patients will develop pneumonia. The virus is spread by close person-to-person contact (i.e., kissing, hugging, sharing eating or drinking utensils, talking to someone within 3 feet [respiratory droplets], and touching someone directly). The patient will be placed on isolation precautions (see Chapter 22).

Sinusitis. Inflammation and infection of a sinus or sinuses. May be caused by allergies, bacteria, viruses, or polyps.

Tonsillitis. Inflammation of the tonsils usually caused by streptococcus. Tonsils become red and enlarged causing severe pharyngitis and fever.

Tuberculosis. Inflammatory infiltrations, formation of tubercles, abscesses, fibrosis, and calcification. Can lead to infection of other body systems. Is highly infectious. Airborne precautions are necessary to prevent transmission of the disease.

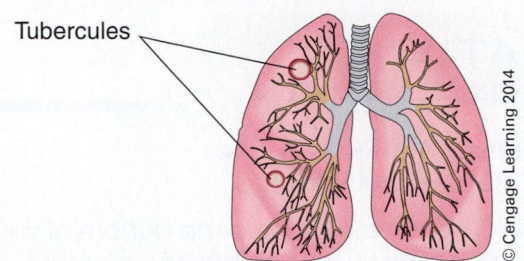

Figure 30-18 Tuberculosis.

Tubercules

© Cengage Learning 2014

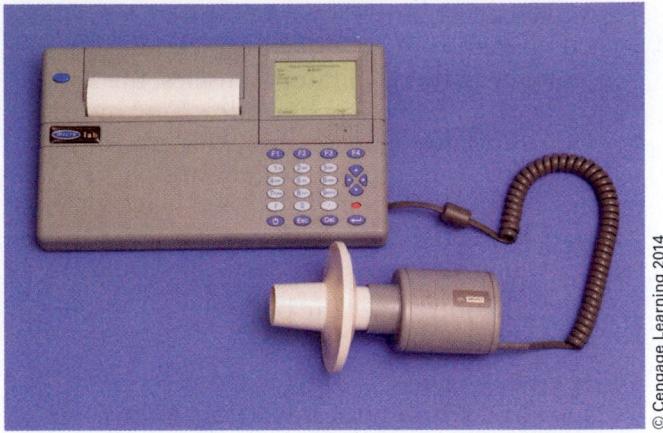

© Cengage Learning 2014

Figure 30-19 The spirometer is used to measure pulmonary function.

Diagnostic Tests

A fundamental test, auscultation of the chest, is used to check for abnormalities in breathing rate and quality. Lung function tests can be done. Chest x-ray studies are useful in helping to diagnose tuberculosis (Figure 30-18), lung lesions, pneumonia, and other respiratory conditions. Cultures of sputum can help diagnose infections in the respiratory tract. Bronchoscopy is used to take a sample of lung tissues (biopsy) for help in the determination of lung cancer and for culture of lung abscesses, washing, and irrigation. CT scanning allows very precise diagnosis of soft tissue disorders. This testing can be especially helpful in diagnosing diseases of the respiratory system.

Arterial blood gases (ABGs) measure the amount of oxygen and carbon dioxide in the arterial blood. ABGs also evaluate the mechanisms that help the body maintain a homeostatic pH. The quantities of oxygen and carbon dioxide found in the arterial blood indicate how well the process of internal respiration is functioning. This respiratory function requires that the lungs are functioning well to deliver oxygen to the alveoli and allow gas exchange across the capillary membrane, releasing carbon dioxide for exhalation. Higher amounts of carbon dioxide and lower amounts than normal of oxygen indicate poor lung function.

Multiple procedures and interventions relieve symptoms and treat various respiratory diseases. You will find the most common of these therapies in Procedures 30-15 through 30-17. These procedures provide detailed descriptions of the role of the medical assistant in common treatments and interventions.

Spirometry

The measurements of airflow, lung volume, and lung capacity are known as pulmonary function tests (PFTs). PFTs measure how well air moves in and out of the lungs and how well the lungs utilize the oxygen delivered. The patient's height, age, and sex are used in interpreting the PFT values. Many times the provider requests the PFT be performed before the administration of a **bronchodilator** and again after the bronchodilator is used. This is useful in evaluating the effectiveness of the medication (see Procedure 30-16).

A commonly used tool in the medical office or clinic, **spirometry** (test to measure lung capacity) assists the provider in the evaluation of signs and symptoms of pulmonary disease by measuring the air capacity (airflow and volume) of the lungs (Figure 30-19). Many components of lung functions are measured, including the following components:

1. Expiratory reserve volume (ERV) represents the maximum volume of air that can be exhaled from the lungs after normal expiration.

2. Forced vital capacity (FVC) represents the volume of air that can be forcibly exhaled from the lungs after taking the deepest breath possible.

3. Forced expiratory volume (FEV) is the volume of air that can be blown out in 1 second after full inspiration.

4. Forced expiratory flow (FEF) represents the speed of the air exiting the lungs in the middle of forced expiration.

5. Mean expiratory flow (MEF) is the measurement in liters per second of the peak of expiratory flow.

6. Tidal volume (VT) reflects the volume of air during either inspiration or exhalation during a single breath while resting.

7. Total lung capacity (TLC) is the maximum volume of air present in the lungs.

8. Maximum voluntary ventilation (MVV) is the value that is a good indicator of the health and strength of the respiratory muscles, the ability of the thorax to expand to allow lung movement, and airway resistance. This number is obtained by having the patient breathe in and out as fast as possible for 15 seconds. The result is reported in liters per second or per minute.

9. Residual volume (RV) measures the volume of air in the lung after the patient has exhaled all the air possible.

10. Total lung capacity (TLC) is the amount of air that the lungs can hold. It is about 6 L in humans.

Most spirometers are computerized, and thus automatically calculate the lung functions. Results are stored in the electronic health record and are readily accessible for comparison. This information is vital to determining the health of a patient's respiratory system.

Peak Expiratory Flow Rates

Peak expiratory flow rates (PEFRs) are measured using a peak flow meter (Figure 30-20). This is a fairly "low tech" device as compared to a computerized spirometer that is utilized for PFTs. A patient could utilize this tool at home to monitor asthma or other respiratory disorders. The PEFR measures the amount of air that can be pushed from the lungs. Utilizing a peak flow meter can indicate a worsening of conditions, such as asthma even before symptoms are noticeable. This allows early intervention to prevent serious episodes of illness.

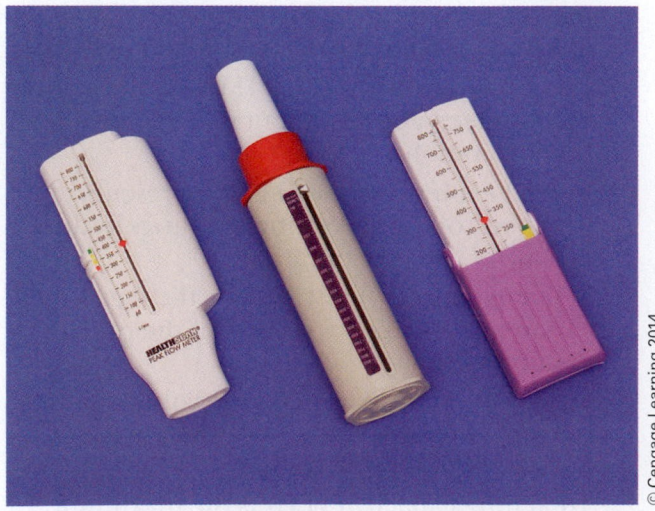

Figure 30-20   Examples of peak flow meters.

© Cengage Learning 2014

Pulse Oximetry

Pulse **oximetry** is a test that uses a small probe with an infrared light. The probe is placed on the earlobe, toe, finger, or bridge of the nose. It evaluates the amount of oxygen saturation in the blood. This test is helpful because cyanosis is not manifested until the saturation of oxygen is less than 85%. Pulse oximetry is useful in the diagnosis and evaluation of impaired respiratory and cardiac functions. A reading less than 95% indicates hypoxemia. It is not unusual for a patient being tested for sleep apnea to experience a pulse oximetry reading of under 75%.

The pulse oximeter sensor is placed on the fingertip or earlobe most commonly. One side of the sensor is an infrared light, and the other side is a photo detector. The infrared light passes through the tissues and blood vessels, and the detector measures the amount of light absorbed by hemoglobulin. This noninvasive procedure measures the amount of hemoglobin and can be performed on any patient, but is especially useful in those with impaired heart and lung function. Postoperative patients are attached to an oxygen pulse oximeter in the recovery room. The patient is likely to

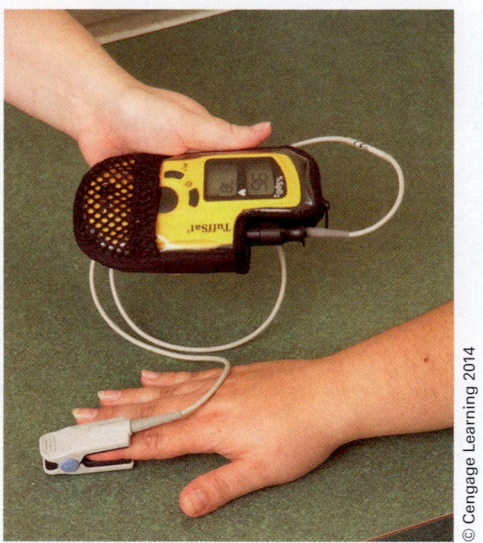

Figure 30-21   Apply the sensor to the selected site-in this case, the finger.

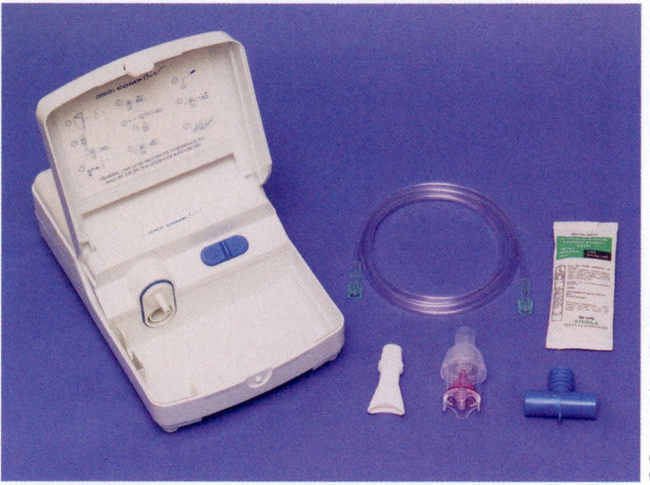

Figure 30-22   A nebulizer is used to administer breathing treatments.

have shallow, less effective respirations because of the anesthesia or narcotics. The patient must not be wearing nail polish (see Procedure 30-18 and Figure 30-21).

Inhalers

Inhalers are devices that are used to deliver medication into the lungs and are most often used to treat asthma. A number of different types of inhalers are available: **metered dose inhaler (MDI)**, metered dose inhaler with spacer (MDIS), dry powder inhaler (DPI), and nebulizer.

The MDIS is the preferred method. A tube that attaches to the inhaler and holds the medication until the patient can breathe it in is called the *spacer*. It makes the MDI easier to use and helps get the medication into the lungs better. A mask can be attached to the spacer for children or for an individual who has difficulty inhaling correctly with a conventional spacer. However, an MDI can be used without a spacer.

Some medications for asthma are in the form of a powder and can be taken with a handheld device known as a DPI. This device delivers medication to the lungs when the patient inhales through the device. However, some patients cannot inhale through the device with sufficient force to breathe in the medication well.

A **nebulizer** (Figure 30-22) is an apparatus that changes the medication for asthma from a liquid form into a mist for ease of inhaling the medication into the lungs. Nebulizers work well for infants and young children and for any person who is unable to use an MDIS. The different types of nebulizers all work in essentially the same way. The nebulizer hose is connected to an air compressor. The medicine cup is filled with the appropriate dose of liquid along with saline. For a single dose, the contents of the vial are squeezed into the medicine cup. The hose and mouthpiece are attached to the medicine cup. The patient puts the mouthpiece into the mouth and exhales, and then breathes through the mouth until all the medication is used, about 10 to 15 minutes. Alternatively, the nebulizer can be used with a mask. The mask must fit well to prevent medication from getting in the eyes. The medicine cup and mouthpiece are washed with water and allowed to air dry.

CIRCULATORY SYSTEM

The circulatory system is composed of the heart and a complex network of blood vessels. Their function is to pump and transport the blood to all parts of the body, thus supplying oxygen and removing waste products from body tissues. Table 30-10 lists circulatory system disorders and diagnostic procedures. Table 30-11 describes disorders of the circulatory system.

The variety of diagnostic procedures used to determine the patient's diagnosis is necessary because of the complexity of the cardiovascular system. The medical assistant assists with and performs some of the procedures used for clinical diagnosis. Electrocardiography (ECG) is explained in Chapter 37.

Table 30-10 Circulatory System Disorders

Disease/Disorder	Laboratory/Diagnostic Tests			Surgery	Medical Tests or Procedures	Treatment
	Blood	**Other**	**Radiography**			
Abdominal aortic aneurysm (Figure 30-23)			Abdominal radiography Abdominal ultrasound CT of abdomen Magnetic resonance angiography (MRA) MRI of abdomen		Abdominal ultrasound	Surgical repair
Angina pectoris			Ultrasonography Angiography Cardiac catheterization	Coronary artery bypass Angioplasty	Electrocardiography Stress test	Nitroglycerin and other medications Coronary artery bypass surgery Angioplasty with stent Lifestyle changes
Arteriosclerosis	Homocystine Fibrinogen Lipoprotein a Lipid profile C reactive protein		CT		Catheterization	Cardiology management Lifestyle changes Risk factor management Percutaneous angioplasty
Congestive heart failure	Chemistry panel		Chest radiograph	Removal of part of myocardium	Electrocardiography Venous pressure	Medication Heart transplant Lifestyle changes
Cardiomyopathy	B-type natriuretic peptide (BNP) Chemistry profile Complete blood count Thyroid panel		Chest radiograph Echocardiography MRI of heart		Electrocardiography Cardiac catheterization and biopsy	Beta blockers Digoxin Diuretics Pacemaker insertion Implantable cardioverter-defibrillator (ICD) insertion Heart transplant

Disorder	Laboratory tests (blood)	Laboratory tests (other)	Diagnostic examinations	Surgical procedures	Electrocardiography	Treatment
Coronary artery disease	Electrolytes Blood chemistry panel: low-density, high-density lipoprotein, cholesterol, triglycerides	High sensitivity C-reactive protein (hsCRP)	Angiography Thallium stress test Cardiac catheterization	Coronary artery bypass Angioplasty	Electrocardiography	Medication Coronary artery bypass surgery Lifestyle changes
Essential hypertension	Electrolytes Chemistry panel	Urinalysis Kidney function	Chest radiograph		Electrocardiography Blood pressure	Medication Lifestyle changes
Mitral valve stenosis			Ultrasonography Echocardiography Cardiac catheterization	Valvotomy	Electrocardiography	Valve replacement Medication
Myocardial infarction	Cardiac enzymes Complete blood count		Thallium stress test Cardiac catheterization Ultrasonography	Coronary artery bypass Angioplasty	Electrocardiography	Oxygen Medication Lifestyle changes
Pericarditis	Complete blood count Erythrocyte sedimentation rate Cardiac enzymes Bacterial antibodies	Urinalysis Blood culture	Chest radiograph		Electrocardiography	Medication Antibiotics Pericardiocentesis
Rheumatic fever	Complete blood count Streptococcal antibodies Erythrocyte sedimentation rate (ESR) Cardiac enzymes Kidney function Liver function	Throat culture	Echocardiography		Electrocardiography	Antibiotic therapy
Thrombophlebitis	Bleeding and clotting time Complete blood count	Urinalysis	Doppler ultrasonography Angiography Radioactive fibrinogen	Thrombectomy		Elevation of affected limb Medication (anticoagulant) Support hose
Varicose veins			Venography Doppler ultrasonography	Ligation and stripping Laser		Elastic stockings Sclerotherapy Ligation and stripping

Table 30-11   Description of Circulatory System Disorders

- *Angina pectoris.* Chest pain caused by lack of oxygen to the myocardium. Usual cause is coronary arteriosclerosis.

- *Congestive heart failure.* A syndrome characterized by the heart's inability to pump blood adequately to the body tissues. Characterized by congestion in the lungs, or edema of lower extremities, dyspnea on exertion, cough, and related edema.

- *Coronary artery disease.* Arteriosclerosis of the coronary arteries leading to impaired blood flow to the myocardium. Complete occlusion leads to myocardial infarction. May also be caused by thrombus in a coronary artery. Angina pectoris is the name of the chest pain caused by lack of oxygen to the myocardium.

- *Essential hypertension.* Consistently high blood pressure of unknown cause.

- *Mitral valve stenosis.* Narrowing of mitral valve obstructing flow from atrium to ventricle. Usual cause is a rheumatic heart disease as a result of a streptococcal infection (throat or scarlet fever). Thrombi can form. Atrial fibrillation possible.

- *Myocardial infarction.* Death of myocardial tissue caused by anoxia to the myocardium. Symptoms include dyspnea, chest pain, nausea, vomiting, and diaphoresis.

- *Pericarditis.* Inflammation of the pericardium. Caused by tuberculosis, pyogenic organisms, uremia, and myocardial infarction. Characterized by fever, dry cough, dyspnea, and palpitations.

- *Rheumatic fever.* A systemic disease affecting the heart, joints, and central nervous system after a group A beta-hemolytic streptococcal infection. May occur without symptoms. Symptoms include fever, migratory joint pain, pericarditis, and heart murmur.

- *Thrombophlebitis.* An inflammation of a vein with thrombus formation, may be caused by trauma. Symptoms include pain and swelling in affected vein.

- *Varicose veins.* Enlarged, twisted, and engorged veins, commonly occurring in the saphenous veins but may occur in any vein in the body. Caused by conditions that hamper venous return, such as pregnancy, standing for long periods of time, and obesity. Symptoms include pain in feet and ankles, swelling, and leg ulcers.

© Cengage Learning 2014

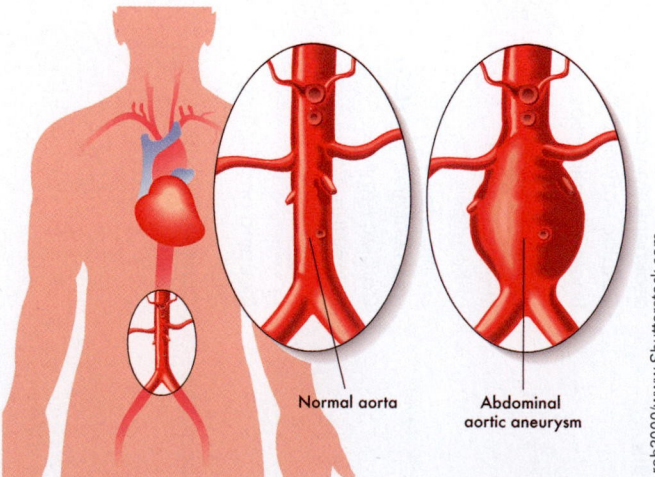

Normal aorta   Abdominal aortic aneurysm

© rob3000/www.Shutterstock.com

Figure 30-23   Abdominal aortic aneurysm.

BLOOD AND LYMPH SYSTEM

The blood and lymph are excellent indicators of many underlying diseases. As blood circulates through body tissues and organs, it deposits nutrients and removes wastes. Failure to accomplish this leaves the body in a disease state. Blood cells include erythrocytes, leukocytes, and platelets, and each has its own function. Studying the results of laboratory findings assists the provider in making a diagnosis.

Lymph is important because of its filtering properties. The body's immune system relies heavily on the fact that the lymph passes through the lymph glands and bacteria and other substances are filtered out. Table 30-12 describes diseases and disorders and the diagnostic procedures for the blood and lymphatic system; Table 30-13 describes certain blood and lymph system disorders.

Table 30-12 Blood and Lymph System Disorders

| Disease/Disorder | Laboratory/Diagnostic Tests | | | | | Medical Tests or Procedures | Treatment |
	Blood	Other	Radiography	Surgery			
Anemias	Ferritin Serum iron Complete blood count Red blood cell count Serum vitamin B_{12}	Gastric analysis	Ferrokinetic studies Radioactive vitamin B_{12}			Bone marrow	Depends on cause Increase dietary intake of iron or folic acid Vitamin B_{12} injections
Hemophilia	Complete blood count						Infusion of hormones or clotting factors based on the type of hemophilia
Hodgkin's disease	Complete blood count Liver function tests		Chest radiograph Lymphangiography	Lymph node biopsy		Bone marrow	Radiation Chemotherapy
Infectious mononucleosis	Complete blood count Monoscreen Heterophile antibody Epstein–Barr virus Liver function tests						Analgesics Rest
Leukemia	Complete blood count Liver function tests Platelet count Bleeding time			Bone marrow transplant		Bone marrow	Chemotherapy Bone marrow transplant
Lymphedema			Lymphangiography				Antibiotics Surgery Lymphedema therapy
Non-Hodgkin's lymphoma	Complete blood count		CT MRI PET scan	Lymph node biopsy		Bone marrow biopsy Lumbar puncture	Chemotherapy Radiation Radioimmunotherapy

Table 30-13 Description of Blood and Lymph System Disorders

Anemias. All anemias are manifested by a reduction in circulating red blood cells and the amount of hemoglobin, which is the volume of packed red blood cells per 100 mL blood. Symptoms include pallor of the skin, nailbeds, and mucous membranes; weakness; vertigo; headache; drowsiness; and general malaise.

- *Iron deficiency.* Lack of reserve iron in the body and in red blood cells that lack hemoglobin resulting from inadequate dietary intake of iron, iron **malabsorption** (poor absorption of nutrients), blood loss, or pregnancy.
- *Pernicious anemia.* Lack of intrinsic factor in the stomach secretions (hydrochloric acid). Vitamin B_{12} cannot be absorbed. Red blood cells cannot develop properly.
- *Sickle cell anemia.* A hereditary chronic anemia characterized by abnormal red blood cells causing lysis of the cells and the formation of clumps in the blood vessels, impairing circulation. Not curable.

Hodgkin's disease. An idiopathic malignancy of the lymphatic system causing enlargement of lymphatic tissue, spleen, and liver. Symptoms include fever and night sweats. Often curable.

Leukemia. Overproduction of abnormal and immature white blood cells. Cause is unknown. Symptoms include anemia, fatigue, fever, and joint pain.

Lymphedema. Abnormal accumulation of lymph in the extremities caused by obstruction of the lymphatics. Symptoms include edema in arms or legs.

Non-Hodgkin's lymphoma. A cancer of the immune system, specifically the lymphocytes.

© Cengage Learning 2014

Common laboratory and diagnostic procedures requested by the provider include some of the following:

- *Chemistry profile.* This test provides information on the functioning of several organ systems and can be an early diagnostic tool for many chronic illnesses such as diabetes, and kidney and liver disorders.
- *Coagulation studies.* Prothrombin time (PT), partial thromboplastin time (PTT), and international normalization ratio (INR) are all common lab tests that reflect the clotting time of blood.
- *Complete blood count (CBC).* This routine test includes a hemoglobin, hematocrit, and red and white blood cell count.
- *Differential.* The differential blood count distinguishes among the various types of white blood cells.
- *Erythrocyte sedimentation rate (ESR)* (sedimentation rate). This test is performed to time the speed of red blood cells settling to the bottom of a test tube.
- *Platelet count.* This test counts the number of platelets in a blood specimen.
- *Lipid profile.* High-density and low-density lipoproteins are measured as well as

triglycerides to determine the risk for vascular disease. The lipid profile is a good measure of risk factors that are predictors of coronary heart disease.

- *Liver function studies.* These tests measure coagulation factors, prothrombin, and fibrinogen necessary for blood coagulation.
- *Thyroid profile.* This measure of thyroid hormones circulating in the bloodstream accurately reflects the function of the thyroid gland.

Procedures to collect blood specimens and venipuncture are explained in Chapter 40; hematology is discussed in Chapter 41.

MUSCULOSKELETAL SYSTEM

The muscular and skeletal systems interact to coordinate the supporting framework and movements of the body. The musculoskeletal system includes bones, joints, muscles, and surrounding tissue. The skeletal system provides support; protects vital organs; and allows for the attachment of ligaments, tendons, and muscles. The muscular system gives the body form and shape and is responsible for the coordination of movement.

Bones of the skeletal system store minerals for later use by the body. They are classified according

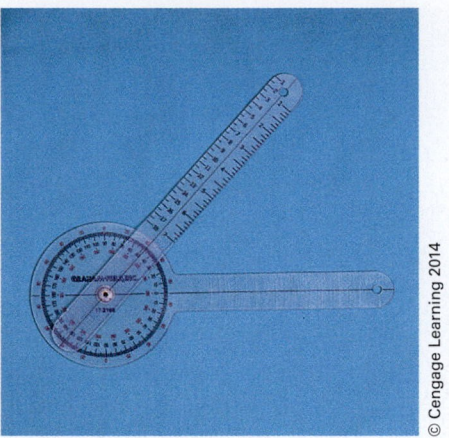

Figure 30-24 Goniometer.

© Cengage Learning 2014

to their shape. Bones provide for the attachment of muscles and joining of another bone, which allows for the passage of nerves and blood vessels. The skeletal system is divided into two parts: the **appendicular skeleton** (126 bones) and the **axial skeleton** (80 bones).

One of the top four reasons a patient visits a provider is back pain. During the visit, the provider evaluates the patient for contributory factors for the pain by assessing the patient for deformities, asymmetry, and signs of restricted motion. The provider performs a functional assessment by observing the patient's gait (manner of walking) for indications of decreased mobility and postural changes associated with aging or injury. Flexion tests with a goniometer (Figure 30-24) detect the degree of resistance applied to a given force, thus defining restricted motion and the amount of discomfort associated with movement. Supine straight-leg raising (SLR) tests detect the amount of hamstring flexibility and strength and can assess sciatic nerve damage.

There are more than 600 muscles in the body. Muscles are composed of bundles of muscle fibers, each with the ability to contract and relax. Any disease process that disrupts the balance between the muscular and skeletal systems severely hampers a person's ability to move effectively and painlessly (Tables 30-14, 30-15, and 30-16).

Diagnostic procedures involving the skeletal system involve the extensive use of various forms of radiographs and visual examination techniques. A bone biopsy may be ordered when additional diagnostic data are required.

Muscular system diseases and disorders can be treated by electromyostimulation (EMS). Electrical current directly stimulates motor nerves. A low frequency charge of electricity is given to muscle(s) through electrodes placed on the skin to elicit muscle contraction. The therapy improves muscle strength and is used to help strengthen atrophied muscles caused by surgery or injuries. EMS therapy can re-educate muscles that have become paralyzed. It can be used in sports training to improve muscle strength.

Therapeutic treatment of muscular system injuries caused by trauma is clinically handled by the use of cold and hot therapy and physical therapy including ultrasound therapy. These procedures are discussed in Chapter 33.

Fractures, Casting, and Cast Removal

Closed fractures of the wrist, forearm, fingers, lower legs, or upper arm are often treated in the ambulatory care setting. Table 30-17 lists types of fractures (see Chapter 9).

Types of casting materials used are the plaster cast, synthetic or plastic cast, and the air cast. Plaster casts are formed by wetting bandage rolls impregnated with calcium sulfate and molding them to the injured body part. Synthetic casts are formed by using tape embedded with a polyester/cotton combination, fiberglass, or plastic resin. Air casts are a type of inflatable immobilizer and are used for sprains and postcast support. The type of casting material used is dependent on provider preference and the body part to which a cast is being applied. Synthetic casts are lighter, stronger, and more water resistant, but they have less room for swelling.

- *Short arm cast (SAC).* Extends from the fingers to just below the elbow (fracture or dislocation of wrist and forearm).

- *Long arm cast (LAC).* Extends from the fingers to the axilla, with a bend at the elbow (fracture of the upper arm).

- *Long and short leg casts.* Extend from the thigh to the toes (LLC) or from below the knee to the toes (SLC) and usually include a walking heel.

The medical assistant's role in cast application and removal consists of setting up supplies and assisting the provider. Patient teaching of cast care is also a primary function of the medical assistant. Procedures 30-18 and 30-19 outline steps in applying a plaster cast and assisting in cast removal.

Table 30-14 Musculoskeletal System Disorders

Disease/Disorder	Laboratory/Diagnostic Tests			Surgery	Medical Tests or Procedures	Treatment
	Blood	Other	Radiography			
Avascular necrosis			MRI Radiograph Bone scan CT	Bone biopsy	Measurement of intraosseous pressure	Analgesics Corticosteroids Physical therapy Limited weight bearing Bone grafting Osteotomy Joint replacement
Bone cancer • Multiple myeloma • Osteosarcoma • Ewing's sarcoma • Chondrosarcoma	Complete blood count		Radiograph CT MRI	Needle biopsy Open biopsy		Surgical resection Amputation Radiation therapy Chemotherapy
Carpal tunnel syndrome	Erythrocyte sedimentation rate Uric acid Complete blood count			Surgical repair	Electromyography	Cortisone injection Physical therapy Antiinflammatory drugs Splinting Surgery
Dislocation			Radiograph of affected joint	Reduction		Reduction with anesthesia if necessary Surgical tightening of ligaments
Gout	Uric acid Complete blood count Erythrocyte sedimentation rate	Synovial fluid analysis Urinalysis	Skeletal radiographs			Bed rest when severe Ice to affected joint(s) Antiinflammatory agents Analgesics Corticosteroids Antigout drugs
Herniated disk			Myelogram CT MRI			Muscle relaxants Analgesics Brace for affected disk Epidural injection(s) of corticosteroids Surgical incision and release

Condition						Treatment
Myasthenia gravis	Acetylcholine receptor antibodies	Detailed history and neurologic examination	CT MRI		Electromyography (EMG)	Lifestyle changes Stress reduction Neostigmine Prednisone Plasmapheresis Surgical excision of the thymus gland
Osteoarthritis	Complete blood count Sedimentation rate		Skeletal radiographs including vertebrae CT scan MRI			Physical therapy Antiinflammatory drugs Analgesics Muscle relaxants Corticosteroid injection into affected joint Surgery to replace knee, hip, or shoulder
Osteoporosis	Serum calcium Alkaline phosphatase Estrogen level Total protein Creatinine	Urine calcium Urine creatinine	Bone scan	Bone biopsy		Calcium supplements Vitamin D supplements and sunshine Drug therapy Weight-bearing exercises
Rheumatoid arthritis	Rheumatoid factor Antinuclear antibody test Lupus erythematosus test Erythrocyte sedimentation rate Complete blood count	Synovial fluid analysis	Skeletal radiographs	To correct deformity		Antiinflammatory drugs Corticosteroids Immunosuppression drugs Splinting of affected joints Exercises Replacement of joint with artificial joint
Rickets	Serum phosphorus Vitamin D Creatinine	Urine calcium Urine phosphorus Urine creatinine	Skeletal bone scan	Bone biopsy		Vitamin D and calcium supplements Sunlight exposure
Spinal curvatures • Scoliosis • Lordosis • Kyphosis			Radiographs of spine			Exercise Brace Spinal fusion Body cast

Table 30-15   Muscular/Connective Tissue Disorders

Disease/ Disorder	Laboratory/Diagnostic Tests			Surgery	Medical Tests or Procedures	Treatment
	Blood	**Other**	**Radiography**	**Surgery**	**Medical Tests or Procedures**	**Treatment**
Back pain		Urinalysis	Radiograph of vertebrae	Surgery may be necessary	CT MRI	Treatment depends on diagnosis Analgesics Antiinflammatory medications Exercise Epidural corticosteroids Electronic stimulation device
Bursitis			MRI X-ray study of affected joint for calcium deposits	Excision of bursa wall		Moist heat Immobilization Antiinflammatory medications Local injection of corticosteroids
Fibromyalgia	Rheu- matoid arthritis antibody		Skeletal radiographs		Electromyography	Antiinflammatory medications may be useful Physical therapy Medication for sleep disturbances (antidepressants) Counseling Exercise
Strain, sprain			Radiographs of affected body part to rule out fracture	Surgery may be necessary		Cold wet packs to area for 24 hours; follow with warm packs Antiinflammatory medications Elevate and rest affected part Immobilization or movement of affected part (per provider's recommendation) Physical therapy*
Tendonitis			Arthrogram			Moist heat Antiinflammatory medications Local injection of corticosteroids Physical therapy*

© Cengage Learning 2014

*Physical therapy should be encouraged from the onset. Patient can prevent further damage. Provide patient education.

Table 30-16 Description of Skeletal and Muscular Disorders

Bone

Carpal tunnel syndrome. Causes pain and weakness of hand and fingers. May cause paresthesia of hand and fingers. Caused by compression of the median nerve against the carpal bones. Usually results from repetitive tasks (such as using computer keyboard or mouse or rolling hair).

Cleft palate. Congenital disorder caused by nonunion of the maxillary bones. Surgical repair needed to close palate.

Fractures. Break in a bone classified according to angle, usually caused by trauma or disease.

Herniated disk. A rupture of the cushioning mass between two intervertebral disks of the spine most often caused by injury or osteoarthritis. Causes back pain that may radiate into buttock(s) and down leg.

Osteoporosis. Diminished bone mass caused by lack of calcium deposits in the bone, predisposing patients to fracture.

Paget's disease. Chronic disease marked by a high rate of bone destruction and irregular bone repair. The new bone fractures easily. Cause unknown but may be hereditary.

Rickets. Abnormal bone softening caused by inadequate utilization of vitamin D, inadequate vitamin D intake, or loss of calcium. One symptom is night fever (known as osteomalacia in adults).

Spinal curvatures. Spinal defects with exaggerated curves caused by diseases of the spine, faulty posture, or congenital malformations.
- Scoliosis: right or left sideway curvature of the spine
- Lordosis: inward curvature of the lower spine (swayback)
- Kyphosis: outward curvature of the upper spine (hunchback)

Joints

Dislocation. A bone forcibly displaced from its joint; usually caused by trauma.

Gout. Form of arthritis caused by metabolic disturbances in purine metabolism resulting in uric acid crystal deposits in the joints. Causes periodic attacks of arthritis pain and joint inflammation.

Osteoarthritis. Common, chronic inflammatory process of the joints, with overgrowth of bone and spur formation. Accompanies aging. Causes swollen joints and pain.

Rheumatoid arthritis. More serious and crippling form of arthritis caused by inflammation of the synovial tissues of several joints; may be caused by antigen-antibody reaction. Systemic symptoms include fatigue, body temperature elevation of affected joint, sensory disturbances, pain, and joint deformities.

Muscle Disorders

Back pain. Localized discomfort usually in the lumbar area caused by stretching or straining of muscles.

Bursitis. Inflammation of the cavity found in connective tissue of a joint that is lined with synovial fluid usually caused by trauma.

Fibromyalgia. Discomfort of muscles, tendons, ligaments, and soft tissues brought on by trauma, strain, and emotional stress.

Spasm. Sudden involuntary muscle contraction; can cause pain.

Sprains. Caused by trauma to a joint with torn ligament if severe.

Strain. Trauma to a muscle from violent contraction.

Tendonitis. Inflammation of tendons and attachments caused by trauma such as strain.

Table 30-17   Types of Fractures

Fractures can be simple, or closed, so called because the bone is broken with no penetration of the skin; or they can be compound, or open, so called because the broken bone has protruded through the skin and there is an open wound in addition to the fracture.

Two of the most common fractures are both simple fractures: Colles' fracture and Pott's fracture. Colles' fracture is a fracture of the lower end of the radius. Pott's fracture is a fracture of the lower part of the fibula and the malleolus of the tibia.

Fractures are described by their characteristics:

Greenstick. The bone is bent on one side and fractured on the other.

Oblique. The bone is fractured and runs obliquely to the axis of the bone.

Transverse. The bone is fractured at a right angle to the axis of the bone.

Comminuted. The bone is splintered into fragments.

Impacted. The bone is fractured into fragments and the fragments have been driven into the interior of another bone. See Chapter 9.

© Cengage Learning 2014

PATIENT EDUCATION

Cast Care Guidelines

The medical assistant should instruct the patient on managing and caring for a cast.

- Allow the casting material to dry by exposing it to the air and keeping it uncovered, even during the night. Applying pressure to the cast before drying can result in tissue damage under the pressure area.

- Elevate the casted extremity to aid in reducing swelling and pain. This allows for a better fitting cast, and thus less discomfort.

- Observe the fingers or toes for changes in color; temperature changes; and decreased sensation, pain, or tingling. This is called nerve and circulation assessment, and changes could indicate the cast is too tight.

- Do not place objects into the cast to scratch irritated skin. A break in the skin will provide a breeding ground for bacteria. Do not use powder or creams.

- Do not get the cast wet. This could lead to malformation of the cast, resulting in misalignment of the extremity and breakdown of the skin. Cover with waterproof covering when bathing. If the cast gets wet, dry it with a hair dryer.

- Cleaning a cast can be accomplished by using a damp cloth.

- When decorating a cast, use only water-soluble paints or marking pens. This allows the cast to breathe, thus preventing tissue damage.

- Do not cut or trim the cast. Use masking tape if there is a sharp edge, or use a nail file to smooth a rough edge.

Notify the provider if any of the following occurs:

1. Fever.
2. A bad odor coming from the cast may indicate an infection.
3. Numbness, tingling, severe pain, difficulty moving, severe swelling, or cold fingers or toes may indicate that the cast is too tight.
4. A burning sensation over a bony area may indicate that the cast is too tight.
5. If there is bleeding or pink to red discoloration on the cast, there may be bleeding from a wound under the cast.

DIGESTIVE SYSTEM

The gastrointestinal (GI) system performs the following five functions:

1. Ingestion (taking in) of food and breaking it into smaller particles
2. Passage of food through the digestive system (peristalsis)
3. Digestion of food through secretions of digestive enzymes
4. Absorption of nutrients into the bloodstream
5. Elimination of the solid waste products of digestion (defecation)

When any of these functions is hindered, the digestive system malfunctions.

The digestive process begins in the mouth and concludes at the anus. As food passes through the alimentary canal, gastrointestinal tract, or digestive tract, it is mixed with gastric juices and enzymes, allowing it to break down into smaller nutrients, which allows absorption through the walls of the small intestine. Contents that have not been absorbed travel through the large intestine and are excreted through the anus. Tables 30-18 and 30-19 list common tests, procedures, disorders, and conditions of the digestive system. Figure 30-25 shows the major organs of the digestive system.

Signs and Symptoms of Digestive Conditions and Disorders

Common signs and symptoms of disorders and diseases of the digestive tract include nausea, vomiting, stomach cramping, diarrhea, heartburn, loss of appetite, weight loss, indigestion, fatigue, hematemesis or vomiting blood, melena or blood in feces, and hematochezia or bright red blood in feces.

Many disorders and diseases of the digestive tract can cause these signs and symptoms. Gastritis, a common ailment of the stomach, can be caused by caffeine, aspirin and other medications, spicy foods, and alcohol. It is characterized by epigastric pain, nausea, and vomiting of blood or hematemesis. Epigastric pain, chest pain, heartburn, and difficulty swallowing can also be caused by a pathologic condition known as a hiatal hernia. This pain occurs as a result of the upper portion of the stomach protruding through an enlarged opening in the diaphragm. This allows a backflow of gastric contents, including gastric acid, into the esophagus. The soft tissues of the esophagus cannot

withstand this exposure to stomach contents and erosion occurs.

Gastroenteritis, described as inflammation of the stomach and small intestine, is a common ailment that can be caused by infection or ingesting foods that have been contaminated with pathogens. It can be caused by infections from contaminated food or water, drug reactions, and allergic reactions to particular foods. Peptic ulcers found in the stomach are called gastric ulcers and can be caused by the action of pepsin, an enzyme. It is an erosion (eating away of tissue) of the mucous lining of the stomach. **Salicylates** (such as aspirin), alcohol, smoking, oversecretion of hydrochloric acid, and stress seem to be implicated in this disease.

It has been discovered in recent years that some gastric ulcers may be caused by the bacterium *Helicobacter pylori* and require antibiotic treatment. Ulcers found in the duodenum are called duodenal ulcers and are similar to gastric ulcers. A duodenal ulcer is an erosion of the mucous lining of the duodenum, a part of the small intestine. If the ulcer is determined to be caused by the bacteria, antibiotics will be prescribed. Both types of ulcers seem to run a chronic course. If they are not controlled, the ulcerated area can perforate, creating a hole caused by ulceration, and hemorrhage ensues. Contents of the stomach or intestine can spill out into the abdominal cavity and cause a serious complication called peritonitis. Peritonitis is caused by the introduction of infectious organisms into the abdominal cavity that is covered by the mucous membrane called the peritoneum. See Figures 30-27 and 30-28.

Diarrhea is characterized by frequent liquid bowel movements. Diarrhea and vomiting may have many causes such as allergic reactions, infections from food or water, or stress. Dehydration can become a problem if diarrhea continues for several days. Infants, children, and older adults are especially vulnerable to dehydration from vomiting and diarrhea.

Diagnostic Tests

Diagnostic tests for the digestive system commonly include radiography and endoscopy, which is defined as viewing within the body with a lighted scope. An upper gastrointestinal (GI) series (see Figure 30-30) or barium swallow is done to visualize the esophagus, stomach, and upper portion of the small intestine. A lower GI series (see Figure 30-29)

Table 30-18 Digestive Systems Disorder

| Disease/ Disorder | Laboratory/Diagnostic Tests | | | | Surgery | Medical Tests or Procedures | Treatment |
	Blood	Urine	Other	Radiography			
Anorexia nervosa	Complete blood count Electrolytes Blood glucose	Urinalysis				Electrocardiography	Replacement of fluids and electrolytes if needed Caloric supplementation Psychiatric care
Appendicitis	Complete blood count	Urinalysis Pregnancy test	Abdominal ultrasound		Appendectomy	Rectal examination	Appendectomy
Bulimia	Complete blood count Electrolytes	Urinalysis				Electrocardiography	Replacement fluids and electrolytes if needed Caloric supplementation Care of esophagus and teeth erosion Psychiatric care
Celiac disease	Albumin Alkaline phosphatase Clotting factors abnormalities Cholesterol Complete blood count Liver enzymes Prothrombin time Genetic testing					Endoscopy Duodenal biopsy	Gluten-free diet Vitamin and mineral supplementation Corticosteroids
Cholecystitis	Complete blood count Serum bilirubin	Urinalysis		Cholecystogram (oral or intravenous) Ultrasound of gallbladder			Cholecystectomy

Disease	Laboratory tests		Radiography	Biopsy	Endoscopy	Treatment
Cholelithiasis	Complete blood count Serum bilirubin		Radioisotope scan Ultrasound of gall bladder Intravenous cholangiogram			Cholecystectomy Asymptomatic—no treatment other than diet modification (low-fat diet)
Colon Cancer	Complete blood count Electrolytes	Fecal occult blood testing	Barium enema Abdominal ultrasound Computerized tomography (CT) scan of abdomen	Biopsy of colon	Sigmoidoscopy Colonoscopy	Colectomy Resection of the colon Endoscopic mucosal resection Chemotherapy Targeted drug therapy
Crohn's Disease	Complete blood count Electrolytes Sedimentation rate		CT of abdomen Abdominal ultrasound Abdominal radiograph	Biopsy of colon	Upper GI series Barium enema Colonoscopy Sigmoidoscopy Stool culture Pillcam	Nutritional support Antibiotics Antiinflammatories Resection of the affected area of the colon
Diverticulitis (Figure 30-28)	Complete blood count Erythrocyte Sedimentation rate		Abdominal radiography Barium enema		Sigmoidoscopy Colonoscopy	Antibiotics Colectomy in the case of perforation
Drug-induced ulcer	Complete blood count Electrolytes	Fecal occult blood testing	Upper gastro-intestinal series	Biopsy of stomach	Gastroscopy	Cessation of: • Aspirin • Antiinflammatory drugs (Ibuprofen, Naproxen, etc.) • Corticosteroids • Iron • Methotrexate treatments • Histamine H_2 blocking agents (Pepcid, Prilosec, Tagamet, Zantac)

continues

Table 30-18 Digestive Systems Disorder (*Continued*)

Disease/ Disorder	Laboratory/Diagnostic Tests					Surgery	Medical Tests or Procedures	Treatment
	Blood	Urine	Other	Radiography				
Duodenal ulcer	Complete blood count		Breath test H. pylori Occult blood test	Upper gastro-intestinal series		Biopsy duodenum	Upper endoscopy Esophagogastric duodenoscopy (EGD)	Medication: gastric secretion–blocking agent Antibiotics Lifestyle changes Small, frequent meals Gastrectomy if perforation
Enterobiasis	Complete blood count		Stool sample for ova and parasites				Perianal examination	Medication
Gastric ulcer	Complete blood count Serum albumin Transferrin		Guaiac test H. pylori Culture stomach secretions Breath test	Upper gastro-intestinal series Abdominal radiographs		Biopsy stomach lining	Upper endoscopy	Medication: gastric secretion–blocking agent Antibiotics Lifestyle changes Small, frequent meals Gastrectomy if perforation
Gastroenteritis	Complete blood count Electrolytes		Stool culture	Upper gastro-intestinal series			Upper endoscopy	Usually self-limiting Maintain electrolyte balance Antibiotics if indicated Infection control
Gastritis	Complete blood count		Samples of gastric content	Upper gastro-intestinal series		Biopsy of stomach	Gastroscopy	Antacid medications (Prilosec, Tagamet, Zantac) Antibiotics if needed
Gastro-esophageal reflux disease (GERD)				Esophageal ultrasonography Gastroscopy			Esophageal manometry	Medication Diet modification Weight loss

Hemorrhoids	Complete blood count				Hemorrhoid-ectomy	Physical examination Proctoscopy	Hemorrhoidectomy Ligation Cryosurgery
Hepatitis	Protein Bilirubin Liver functions Alkaline phosphatase Gammaglobulin	Urinalysis		Ultrasonography of liver	Liver biopsy	Liver scan	Hepatitis A • Immunoglobulin Hepatitis B • No specific treatment Hepatitis C • Medication (alpha-interferon; ribavirin)
Hiatal hernia (Figure 30-26)			pH studies of gastric secretions	Upper gastro-intestinal series Chest radiograph	Biopsy	Gastroscopy	Elevate head of bed for sleep Antacid medications (Prilo-sec, Tagamet, Zantac) Avoid foods that irritate stomach and esophagus Avoid overeating
Irritable Bowel Syndrome (IBS)		Testing to rule out celiac disease	Log of symptoms to include: • Abdominal discomfort lasting more than 12 weeks • Change in frequency or consistency of stools • Feeling of being unable to empty your rectum • Mucus in stool • Abdominal bloating Breath test for lactose intolerance	CT scan of abdomen		Sigmoidoscopy Colonoscopy	Fiber supplements Anti-diarrheal medications Dietary modification Anti-cholinergic drugs Antidepressants Antibiotics Stress management counseling

continues

Table 30-18 Digestive Systems Disorder (*Continued*)

Disease/Disorder	Laboratory/Diagnostic Tests					Medical Tests or Procedures	Treatment
	Blood	Urine	Other	Radiography	Surgery		
Pancreatic cancer	Complete blood count			Ultrasonography Computerized axial tomography scan Endoscopic retrograde cholangiopancreatography (ERCP)		Percutaneous needle aspiration biopsy	Surgical resection (if possible) Radiation therapy Chemotherapy
Pancreatitis	Serum amylase Complete blood count Erythrocyte sedimentation rate			Ultrasonography Computerized axial tomography scan Endoscopic retrograde cholangiopancreatography (ERCP)			Analgesics Diet modification
Rectal cancer	Complete blood count			CT scan of the abdomen DNA stool testing		Colonoscopy Sigmoidoscopy	Surgical resection Chemotherapy Radiation therapy
Stomach cancer	Complete blood count Chemistry profile Liver function studies		Fecal occult blood testing	CT scan of the abdomen Magnetic resonance imaging (MRI) PET imaging Chest radiography		Upper endoscopy Gastric biopsy	Laparoscopy

Table 30-19 Description of Digestive Disorders and Conditions

Anorexia nervosa. An eating disorder of psychological origin. Because of the need to avoid weight gain the individual does not eat and becomes emaciated (extremely thin) and malnourished.

Appendicitis. Acute inflammation of the appendix usually caused by infection or obstruction. Characterized by pain, nausea, vomiting, and fever.

Bulimia. A syndrome in which an individual binges on food and then purges by inducing vomiting. Laxative abuse is common. The reason individuals engage in this behavior is to avoid weight gain; it is of psychological origin.

Celiac disease. A genetic disease that damages the lining of the GI tract. This damage inhibits the ability to absorb nutrients in the small intestines. The ingestion of gluten causes an immune response that damages the villi in the small intestine that are important in the absorption of nutrients.

Cholecystitis. Inflammation of the gallbladder. Usual cause is gallstones, but other causes may be bacteria or chemical irritants.

Colon cancer. Common malignancy characterized by change in bowel habits, diarrhea or constipation, and abdominal discomfort as tumor grows.

Crohn's disease. Chronic disease that exhibits inflammation of the ileum resulting in diarrhea, right lower quadrant pain, and attacks of diarrhea and frequent blood in the stools.

Diverticulitis. Inflammation of diverticula usually caused by impacted feces or bacteria in the sacs. Pain, cramplike, usually in left side of abdomen. Obstruction can develop.

Diverticulosis. Diverticula in colon without symptoms (see Figure 30-28).

Drug-induced ulcers. Ulcers of the stomach or duodenum caused by taking salicylates (aspirin), corticosteroids, anti-inflammatory medications (ibuprofen, naproxen), iron, and methotrexate.

Duodenal ulcer. Lesion in the mucous membrane of the small intestine usually caused by hyperacidity or *Helicobacter pylori*.

Enterobiasis (pinworms). Intestinal parasites causing intestinal and rectal infection. Pruritus of the anus is a symptom.

Gastric ulcer. Caused by *Helicobacter pylori*, a bacterium, salicylates, smoking, and alcohol.

Gastritis. Inflammation of the stomach lining usually caused by an undefined irritant including alcohol, bacteria, or viruses. It can result in stomach discomfort, nausea, or vomiting.

Gastroenteritis. Inflammation of the stomach and intestinal tract. Causes nausea, vomiting, and diarrhea. May be caused by ingestion of pathogen.

Gastroesophageal reflux disease (GERD). A small valve in the lower esophagus (between the stomach and esophagus) leaks, allowing stomach acid to back up from the stomach into the esophagus. It causes frequent heartburn and discomfort behind the sternum.

Hepatitis. Inflammation of the liver caused by infection from a virus resulting in hepatomegaly, anorexia, and jaundice.
- *Hepatitis A.* Spread by fecal contamination of food or water.
- *Hepatitis B.* Spread by blood and body fluids contamination through sexual contact, contaminated needles, perinatal fluids, semen.
- *Hepatitis C.* Spread by blood (i.e., transfusion), contaminated needles, and sexual contact.
Refer to Chapter 22 for more information about hepatitis.

Hiatal hernia. Congenital or traumatic protrusion of stomach through the diaphragm into the chest cavity (Figure 30-26).

continues

Table 30-19   Description of Digestive Disorders and Conditions (Continued)

Irritable bowel syndrome (IBS). A disorder whose symptoms include bloating, diarrhea, cramping, constipation, and abdominal pain. There is no permanent harm to the digestive tract and IBS can be managed by diet, stress management, and medications.

Rectal cancer. Cancer of the mucous membranes in the portion of the large intestine called the rectum. This malignancy can spread to the adjacent structures in the pelvis. The current survival rate is approximately 50% with treatment.

Stomach cancer. Uncommon in the United States, the worldwide diagnosis of stomach or gastric cancer is declining. Risk factors include salty or smoked food intake, diet low in fruits and vegetables, and a family history of stomach cancer.

Pancreatic cancer. Cancer of the pancreas (usually the head). One of the leading causes of cancer deaths in the United States. Most commonly seen in the 60- to 70-year age group.

Pancreatitis (acute and chronic). Inflammation of the pancreas. Acute: can be a life-threatening event; pancreatic enzymes begin to digest the pancreas, causing necrosis and hemorrhage. Chronic: a slow, progressive destruction of the pancreas thought to be from enzymes digesting the pancreas as seen in acute pancreatitis. May be idiopathic or related to alcoholism. Diabetes can be a complication of pancreatitis.

© Cengage Learning 2014

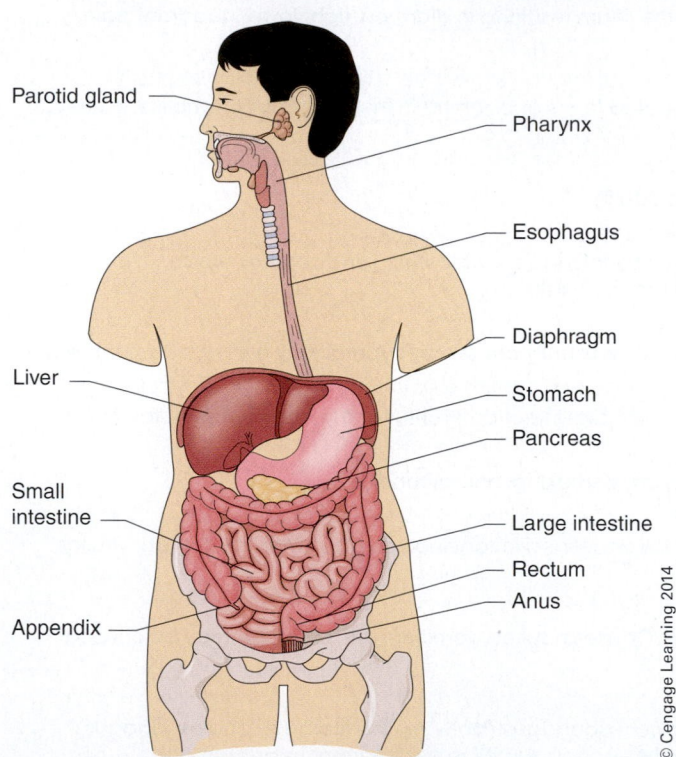

Figure 30-25   The digestive system.

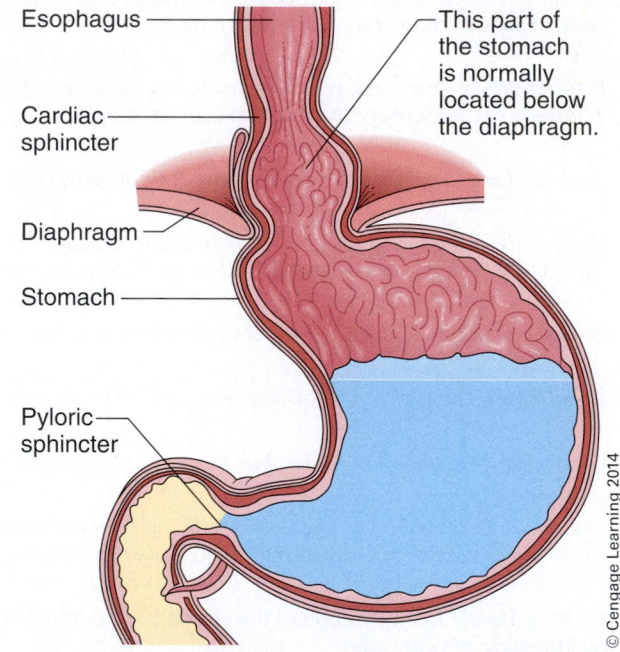

Figure 30-26   Hiatal hernia.

or barium enema visualizes the large intestine (see Figures 30-29 and 30-30 and Chapter 32).

Endoscopic Procedures.
An **endoscope** is an instrument or device that is used to observe the inside of a hollow organ or cavity. Using an endoscope, procedures can be done on many internal organs without surgical intervention. These are known as fiberoptic endoscopic procedures or endoscopy, and they can be performed through a natural body opening or a small incision. A fiberoptic endoscope permits the provider to observe within the body cavity for disorders such as polyps, tumors, cysts, stenoses, calculi, and malignancies. Biopsies and cultures can be taken during the procedure. Small lesions, such as polyps, can be totally removed during endoscopy. Photographs can be taken for documentation also.

PATIENT EDUCATION

With the provider's direction, you may discuss with your patients the following topics about their digestive health.

1. Remind them that laxatives and enemas should only be used by direction of the provider.

2. Constipation may be avoided/relieved by including fresh fruits and vegetables, cereals, and grains in the diet; drinking plenty of liquids (water); and getting regular exercise.

3. Instruct them that if they have any of the following symptoms persistently it could mean that a disease or an abnormal condition is present and consulting the provider is strongly advised: heartburn or indigestion, nausea or vomiting (especially if coffee grounds consistency), constipation or diarrhea, excessive gas or bloating, stool that is tarry (black), or other than a normal brown color.

4. Inform patients who are 40 years of age and older that they should routinely test their stool for occult blood every 2 years for screening of cancer of the colon, or more often if advised by the provider (if family history indicates). All patients older than 50 years should test annually for occult blood and have a colonoscopy.

5. Advise patients to include high-fiber foods in their diets, avoid fat (especially saturated fats) and cholesterol, and eat red meats sparingly.

6. Urge patients to eat a variety of foods (from Choosemyplate.gov) and to eat four to six small meals rather than one or two large meals daily to promote better utilization of nutrients and more energy.

7. Suggest to patients that they select snacks and beverages wisely such as fruits, vegetables, and juices over coffee/tea/soda and high-calorie sweets or salty chips.

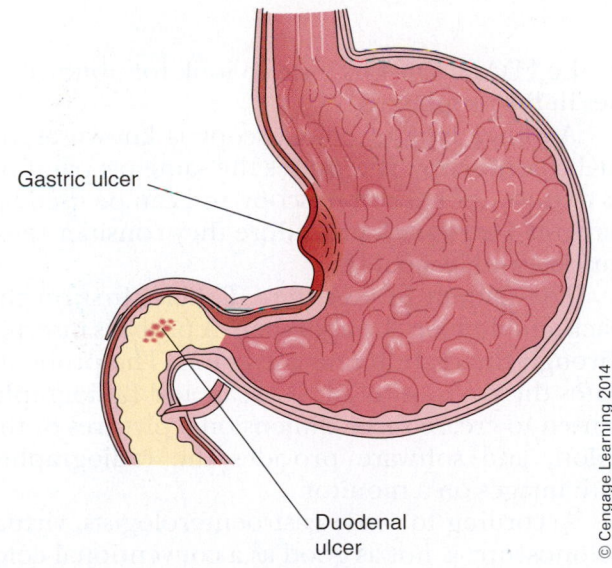

Figure 30-27 Peptic ulcers.

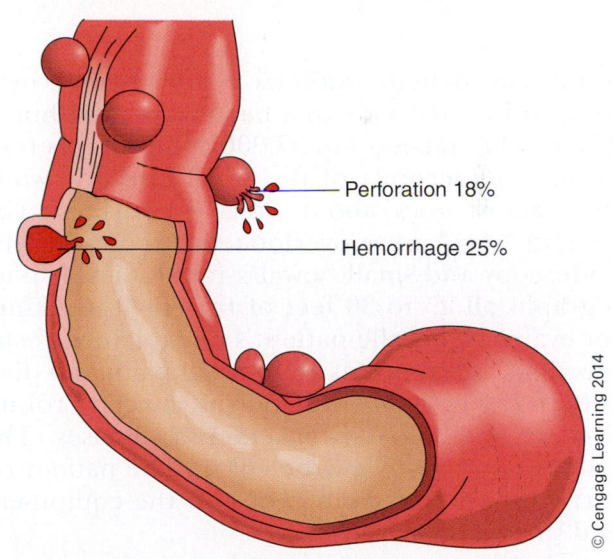

Perforation 18%

Hemorrhage 25%

Figure 30-28 Diverticulosis.

An endoscopic procedure known as capsule video endoscopy (CVE), wireless capsule endoscopy (WCE), or PillCam (all three are the same type of endoscopy) can be performed. The patient must fast for 10 hours before the procedure and needs a bowel preparation similar to that used for a colonoscopy preparation. When the patient arrives at 7:30 AM at the gastroenterology clinic, sensor-like wires are attached to the abdominal wall (they look similar to electrocardiogram sensors) and an 8-hour battery-operated data recording device is attached to the patient's

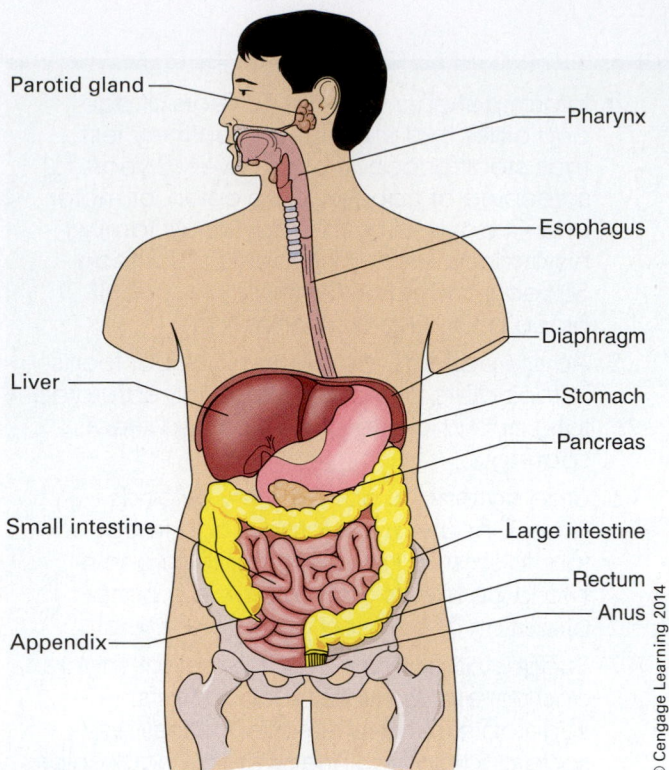

Figure 30-29 Lower gastrointestinal series; highlighted area is visualized.

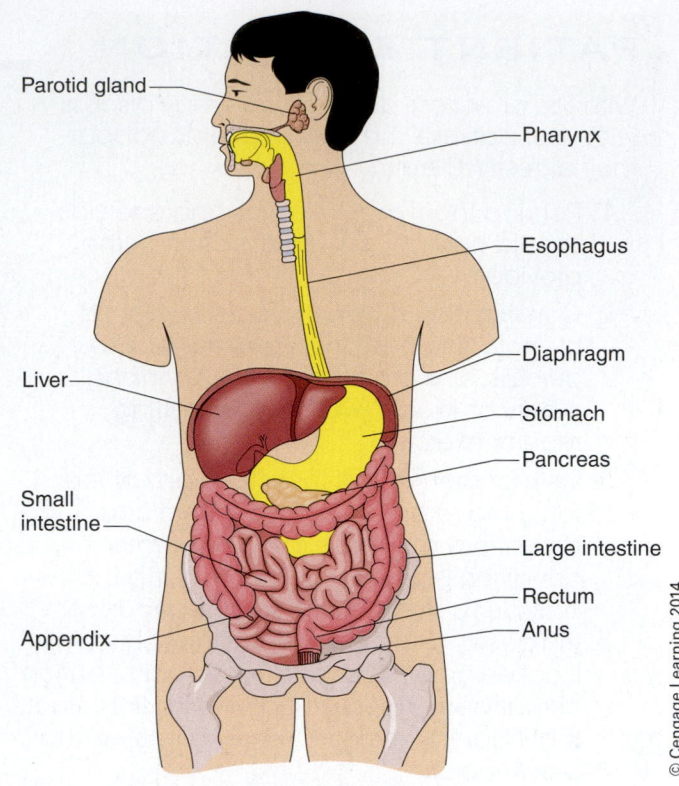

Figure 30-30 Upper gastrointestinal series; highlighted area is visualized.

waist. The patient swallows a pill about 1 inch long and ½ inch wide that has a camera within it. The camera takes up to 57,000 color images (two photos per second) of the small intestine while the patient goes about normal activities. The camera "sees" areas overlooked by conventional endoscopy and small bowel x-ray studies. It photographs all 25 to 30 feet of the small intestines for evaluation of the patient's unexplained rectal bleeding, intermittent abdominal pain, and diarrhea. It can help diagnose polyps, cancer, Crohn's disease, and other disorders and diseases. The PillCam does not view the colon. The patient returns after 8 hours and drops off the equipment and the data receiver.

The data from the recorder are downloaded onto a computer, and the photos are compressed into a video. The provider views the photographed images on a monitor.

The Food and Drug Administration (FDA) approved the capsule endoscopy (PillCam) in 2001. The FDA said the PillCam is safe and has few side effects. The patient excretes the camera in a bowel movement. A PillCam Colon is being used in Europe but has not been approved for use in the United States. A PillCam ESO, which was approved

by the FDA in 2004, is used to look for abnormalities in the esophagus.

Another type of colonoscopy is known as virtual colonoscopy. It requires the same preparation as a conventional colonoscopy and can be used for patients who want a procedure they consider to be quicker and less painful.

The patient lies on the CT table, first on the back and then on the abdomen. A probe is inserted through the rectum into the colon. The probe inflates the colon with air. CT scan and radiography is used to create three-dimensional pictures of the colon, and software provides the radiographer with images on a monitor.

According to some gastroenterologists, virtual colonoscopy is not as good as a conventional colonoscopy because of the lower quality of images of the colon.

The medical assistant must be certain that the patient has signed a consent form before the procedure and that the patient has followed the preparatory instructions. Table 30-20 lists endoscopic procedures, their importance in diagnosis, and patient preparation.

Endoscopy allows the provider to look directly into the digestive organs with a lighted scope.

Table 30-20   Endoscopic Procedures

Endoscopic Procedure	Importance in Diagnosis	Patient Preparation
Capsule video endoscopy	Helps diagnose Crohn's disease, polyps, and cancer of the small intestine	Laxative NPO (nothing by mouth) for 10 hours before procedure
Colonoscopy (views entire colon)	Detects polyps, tumors, bleeding, and malignancies Can take biopsies, photos, and cultures, and remove polyps	Clear liquids for 2 days before NPO after 10:00 PM the night before Night before bowel preparation: laxatives and enemas
Endoscopic retrograde cholangiopancreatography (ERCP) (examines the liver, gallbladder, bile ducts, and pancreas)	Helps diagnose problems in the liver, gallbladder, bile ducts, and pancreas, such as cholelithiasis, stenoses, and malignancies of these organs and structures	NPO after 10:00 PM the night before
Esophagogastroduodenoscopy (EGD) (examines esophagus, stomach, and duodenum)	Detects abnormalities in the esophagus, stomach, and duodenum, such as hiatal hernia, stenoses, tumors, ulcers, erosion Performs biopsies, brushings, photos	NPO after 10:00 PM the night before
Gastroduodenoscopy	Examines stomach and duodenum for lesions, such as tumors, polyps, strictures, and ulcers	NPO after 10:00 PM the night before
Laparoscopy (examines the peritoneal cavity, abdomen, and pelvis)	Camera photographs entire small intestine with 57,000 colored images, two photos per second Can photograph areas overlooked by conventional endoscopy and small bowel radiographs	Laxative and enemas
PillCam	Evaluates unexplained rectal bleeding, intermittent abdominal pain, and diarrhea	Laxative NPO for 10 hours before procedure
Proctosigmoidoscopy (views sigmoid colon and rectum)	Detects polyps, rectal abscesses, tumors, fissures, and fistulas	Bowel preparation: 3-day special diet
Wireless capsule endoscopy	Evaluates unexplained rectal bleeding, intermittent abdominal pain, and diarrhea	NPO after midnight the night prior

© Cengage Learning 2014

Some examples of endoscopies used in the digestive tract are named by the organ being scoped:

Stomach: gastroscopy

Colon: colonoscopy

Sigmoid colon: sigmoidoscopy

Entire upper GI area: esophagogastroduodenoscopy (EGD); see Figure 30-31

Biopsies can be taken during an endoscopic procedure.

Sigmoidoscopy. **Sigmoidoscopy** is a diagnostic examination of the interior of the sigmoid colon. It is a useful aid in the diagnosis of cancer of the colon, ulcerations, polyps, tumors, bleeding, and other lower intestinal disorders. The sigmoidoscope is a flexible instrument with a light source and a magnifying lens, which permits visualization of the mucous membrane of the sigmoid colon.

Providers commonly use the flexible sigmoidoscope. Because it is flexible, it can be inserted

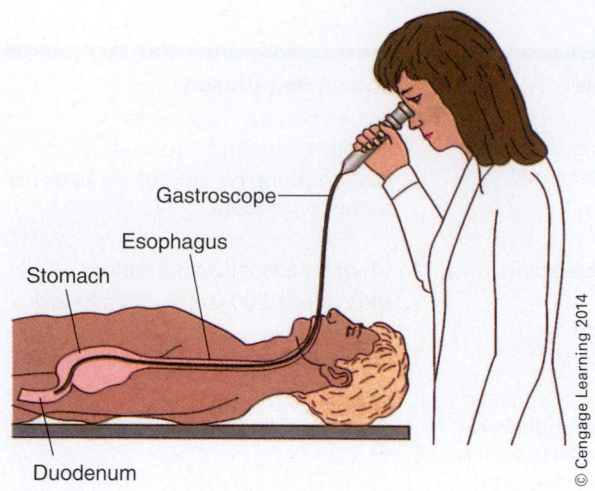

Stomach
Esophagus
Gastroscope
Duodenum

© Cengage Learning 2014

Figure 30-31 Esophagogastroduodenoscopy (EGD) procedure.

farther into the colon, making it possible to view more of the mucous membranes of the intestines (Figure 30-32).

As with any examination of the pelvic or abdominal cavity, you should advise the patient to empty the bladder and evacuate the bowel before the procedure begins. This will make the examination easier for both patient and examiner. During the procedure the patient should be instructed to breathe through the mouth deeply and slowly to relax abdominal muscles. Patients may feel the urge to defecate during a colon examination because of the stretching of the intestinal wall from the instrument passing through and air being introduced with it. If patients use the breathing technique mentioned, this discomfort can be relieved. Pain relievers and sedation are not usually necessary because of the short duration of the

procedure. The procedure should last only a few minutes, especially if patients have followed preparation instructions.

Air is sometimes introduced into the sigmoid colon (by the examiner's use of the inflation bulb attached to the scope with tubing) to distend the wall of the colon for easier placement of the lumen of the endoscope. Patients find this to be uncomfortable and sometimes painful. The provider may need to use suction to remove mucus, blood, or fecal material that is obstructing the view of the sigmoid colon.

During these examinations, the medical assistant's roles are to hand necessary items to the provider and to give support to the patient.

Most often it is the medical assistant who teaches the patient how to prepare for the sigmoidoscopy and explains how the test is performed. For successful examination, proper preparation is essential. Have patients restrict dairy products, raw fruits and vegetables, and grains and cereals from their diet, and encourage them to drink plenty of clear liquids and eat lightly the day before the scheduled appointment for the sigmoid colon examination. A plain commercial enema should be self-administered at home approximately 2 hours before the examinations. The provider may vary the instructions according to the patient's condition. If patients are not completely informed about preparations and the examination is attempted with unsatisfactory results, the examination will have to be repeated, which is both costly and inconvenient. Satisfactory results are obtained by giving patients both oral and written instructions.

There are occasions when, during an appointment for which the patient was "worked in" to the

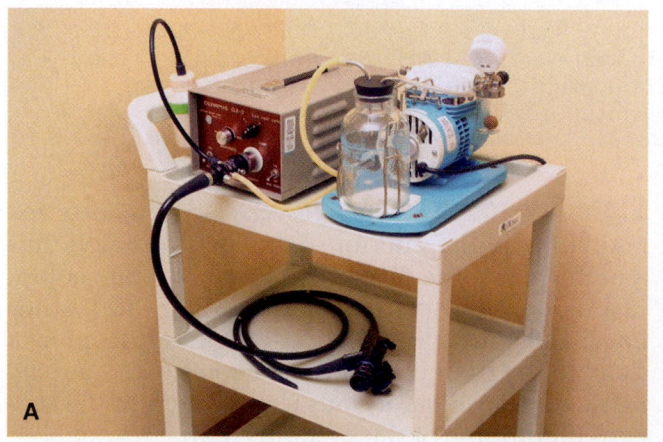

A

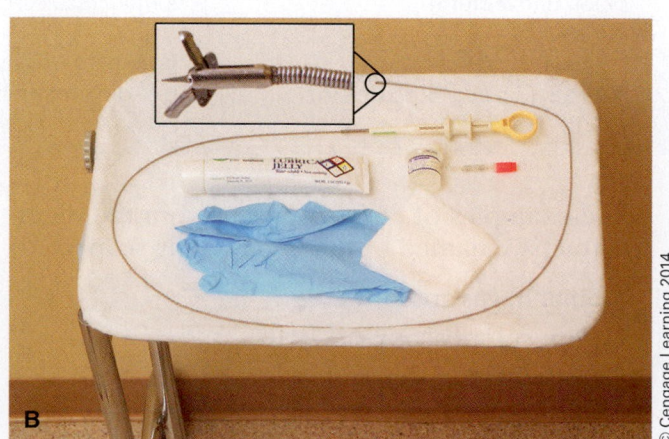

B

© Cengage Learning 2014

Figure 30-32 (A) Setup for a proctosigmoidoscopy with a flexible sigmoidoscope. (B) Control head of proctosigmoidoscopy.

schedules, the provider believes that the patient's condition warrants examination of the sigmoid colon. In this case, the provider will order an enema to be given to the patient in the clinic.

Administering an enema to a patient in the medical office or clinic is not a common procedure, but it is sometimes necessary for the successful completion of a sigmoidoscopy or other rectal examination. Even though a patient may have received proper instructions and carried them out before the scheduled appointment, there is no guarantee that the patient achieved success. In the event that the patient comes in for the appointment and the colon is not sufficiently evacuated of feces for a sigmoidoscopy, the provider may order a cleansing enema so that the examination can be completed. It is generally best to proceed with the planned procedure, even with the delay of the enema. Usually this works out well for patient and staff, because rescheduling presents difficulties for everyone.

Often the patient did follow the list of instructions but was not able to retain the enema solution long enough to get satisfactory results. You will more likely be able to encourage the patient to retain the contents of the enema longer. You may want to explain that the longer the contents are retained, the more successful the results will be. Otherwise, it may have to be repeated, or the examination rescheduled. Be certain that you use an examination room that is close to the rest room for the patient's convenience when you administer an enema. Your patience and understanding are needed, because many patients are embarrassed to have an enema administered to them.

Some examinations, such as diagnostic sigmoidoscopy and x-ray studies, require the use of laxatives by the patient the day before or the morning of the examination. This may present a problem in the patient's personal or employment schedule if instructions are not made clear before the appointment is made. Most patients are fearful of what the diagnostic examination will disclose. Helping them choose a convenient appointment time and explaining the reasons for the preparations they must undergo is usually appreciated.

Proper positioning of the patient during the sigmoidoscopy is important for both the provider's viewing of the rectum and sigmoid colon and the patient's comfort. Proctology tables are designed especially for this procedure (refer back to Figure 25-11). They provide support of the patient's chest and head with the arm resting against the headboard as the table is tilted to the knee-chest position. Patients who cannot tolerate this position are assisted into Sims' position for the examination. Many providers find this acceptable and it is more comfortable for the patient. You should ask about the provider's preference for patient position because there are many variations.

The provider may wish to view the intestinal mucosa after a normal bowel movement. More often, the patient is instructed to eat a light diet containing plenty of clear liquids and avoiding dairy products for 24 hours before the examination, and to have a plain cleansing enema the morning of, or 2 hours before, the examination. Still other providers may wish patients to use laxatives the day before and an enema the night before and also the morning of the examination.

When making a diagnosis of hemorrhoids, fissures, and ulcerations, the provider usually begins investigative procedures by examining the anus and the interior of the rectum with a proctoscope. During the sigmoidoscopy, the provider may want to take a biopsy of questionable tissue from the sigmoid colon to aid in confirming the diagnosis. It is a good rule to have all possible necessary items available. When the patient has been prepared and the provider is ready to begin the examination, the medical assistant hands the necessary instruments and supplies to the provider as needed. Remember to advise patients to report any problems, such as bleeding, discharge, swelling, or any other unusual discomfort, after the procedure. A biopsy laboratory request form must be completed and accompany the tissue to the laboratory. Containers for biopsy specimens have a formaldehyde solution to preserve the tissue until the analysis is done.

Whereas the proctosigmoidoscope examines the rectum and sigmoid colon with a flexible scope, a procedure known as a **colonoscopy** (viewing the colon with a lighted scope) can be scheduled in the outpatient department of the hospital or endoscopy center or performed in the office or clinic. A flexible fiberoptic colonoscope is used, and the entire length of the large intestine (colon) can be examined for lesions such as tumors, polyps, fissures, and masses. Biopsies that consist of small tissue pieces can be removed with a snare-type instrument inserted through the colonoscope. The tissue is microscopically examined by a pathologist to determine whether a malignancy (cancer) is present in the colon (Figure 30-33). The patient may receive a muscle relaxant/tranquilizer to facilitate the examination. (See "Endoscopic Procedures" later in this chapter.)

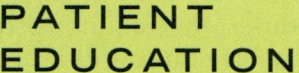

Transverse colon 5%

Hepatic flexure 3%

Cecum 9%

Splenic flexure 3%

Descending colon 5%

Sigmoid colon 21%

Rectum 54%

© Cengage Learning 2014

Figure 30-33 Incidence of colorectal cancer by site.

PATIENT EDUCATION

An important aspect of your role as a medical assistant is to provide patient education. Your provider may have created teaching materials specifically for patients or there might be preprinted educational materials in the clinic for this purpose. After a sigmoidoscopy, it is important that the patient follow instructions to avoid any complications after the procedure.

After sigmoidoscopy, patients should drink plenty of clear fluids to help relieve the abdominal discomfort and flatulence. Prevention of constipation is essential. High-fiber foods and exercise will assist in re-establishing resumption of regular bowel habits. Patients may also find relief in lying in a prone position with a pillow across the midabdominal area to aid in the passage of gas.

Fecal Occult Blood Test. Patients may be instructed to obtain three stool specimens at home for examination of a fecal sample for occult (hidden) blood. The patient will be given occult blood slides, applicators, and envelopes to take home (Figure 30-34). The patient will need to obtain two small stool samples from each of three separate bowel movements. Three separate samples are used to allow detection of blood from GI lesions that exhibit intermittent bleeding. The medical assistant's role is to instruct the patient about how to properly collect the stool specimens on the test

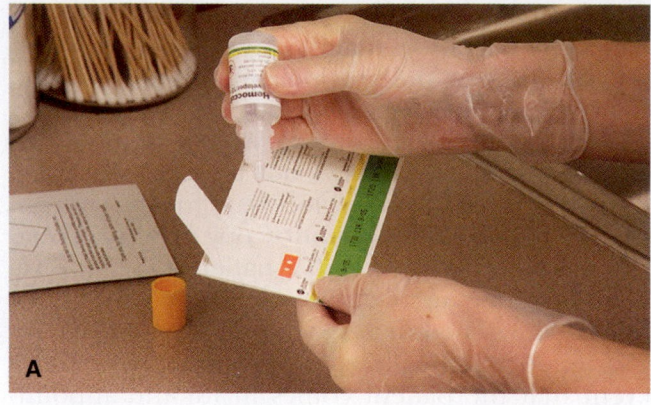

A

READING AND INTERPRETING THE HEMOCCULT® TEST

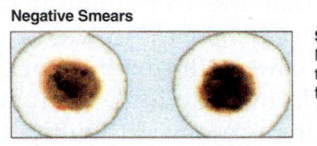

Negative Smears

Sample report: negative
No detectable blue on or at the edge of the smears indicates the test is negative for occult blood.

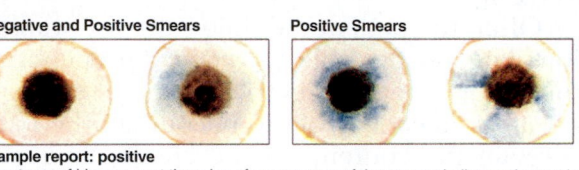

Negative and Positive Smears

Positive Smears

Sample report: positive
Any trace of blue on or at the edge of one or more of the smears indicates the test is positive for occult blood.

B

© Cengage Learning 2014

Figure 30-34 (A) Place the required number of drops of developing solution on the exposed guiac paper. (B) A change in color indicates the blood may be present in the stool.

slides, and then how to care for and store the slides until they are returned to the clinic by the patient (see Procedure 30-21). Biohazardous material (feces) cannot be sent through the U.S. Postal Service.

For patients who have daily bowel movements, this will not be a problem. For patients who have difficulty with daily elimination, collecting the samples may take several days. Patients should not use laxatives unless directed by the provider.

Positive tests for occult blood require further testing, because occult blood testing is a screening tool only. Sigmoidoscopy and colonoscopy help to identify the source of bleeding. If a lesion is found in either the rectum or colon, a biopsy can be performed and the sample sent to the laboratory for examination of cells for malignancy (see Procedure 30-21).

Radiographic Studies of the Digestive System.

Endoscopic procedures are done routinely but have not replaced the need for radiographic studies of the gastrointestinal tract. There

PATIENT EDUCATION

Your provider has ordered fecal occult blood testing to rule out colon cancer. It is important to instruct your patient on obtaining, handling, and storing the specimen until it can be returned to the clinic. The instructions for a successful and accurate test are provided here. First, always follow specific package instructions. These steps should be followed 2 days before the fecal occult blood test and continued until three slides have been prepared:

1. Avoid red meats, processed meats, and liver. These foods release hemoglobin, which can produce a false-positive result.
2. Avoid turnips, broccoli, cauliflower, and melons. These foods may contain a substance, peroxidase, that will cause a false-positive result.
3. Avoid aspirin, iron supplements, and large doses of vitamin C for 7 days before the test. These substances may cause gastric bleeding that can mask bleeding from a lesion.
4. Consume a high-fiber diet. Fiber provides roughage to promote bowel movement and encourage bleeding from any lesion that may be present.
5. Do not begin the test during menses, for 3 days after menses, or if bleeding from hemorrhoids.
6. Drink plenty of fluids to help prevent constipation.
7. Store slides at room temperature and protect from heat, sun, and fluorescent lights.

CRITICAL THINKING

Phyllis Lomeli, a new patient of Dr. Reynolds, has been experiencing gastrointestinal problems. Dr. Reynolds has ordered fecal occult blood tests for the patient. What diet instructions does the medical assistant give to the patient? What directions and supplies does the medical assistant give to the patient? When the guaiac slides are returned by the patient, how does the medical assistant develop and interpret them?

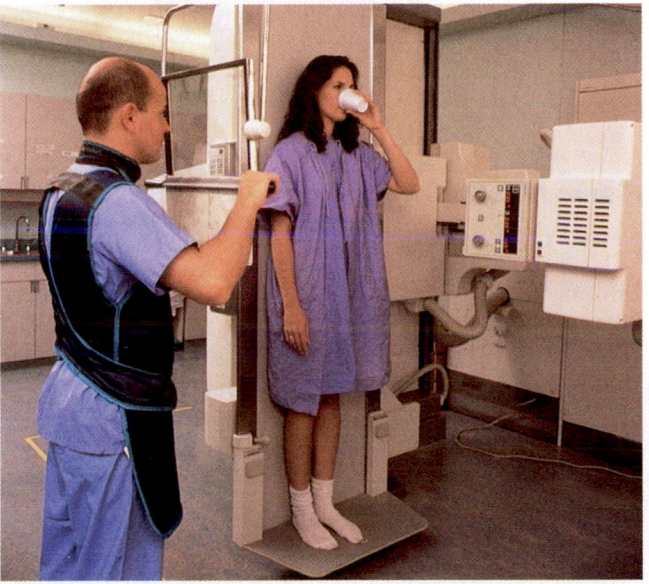

© Cengage Learning 2014

Figure 30-35 In a barium swallow test, barium sulfate is swallowed and radiographs are taken of the esophagus, stomach, and small intestine. This is also known as an upper gastrointestinal series.

are several diagnostic radiographic studies can be performed in order to study digestive structures and functions looking for disease. They include the upper GI series or barium swallow (Figure 30-35), lower GI series or barium enema, and the cholecystogram. Table 30-21 lists the purpose, patient preparation, and procedures for each of these three studies.

Bariatrics

Millions of people in the United States are obese and are ill with or at serious risk for diabetes, heart disease, hypertension, certain cancers, stroke, sleep apnea, and many other conditions. Obesity affects every body system in a negative way.

Emotional problems such as depression, rejection, low self-esteem, isolation, and chemical substance abuse are common. **Bariatrics** is the field of medicine that treats obesity and conditions associated with obesity.

Some obese patients decide, with their provider's recommendation, to undergo bariatric surgery

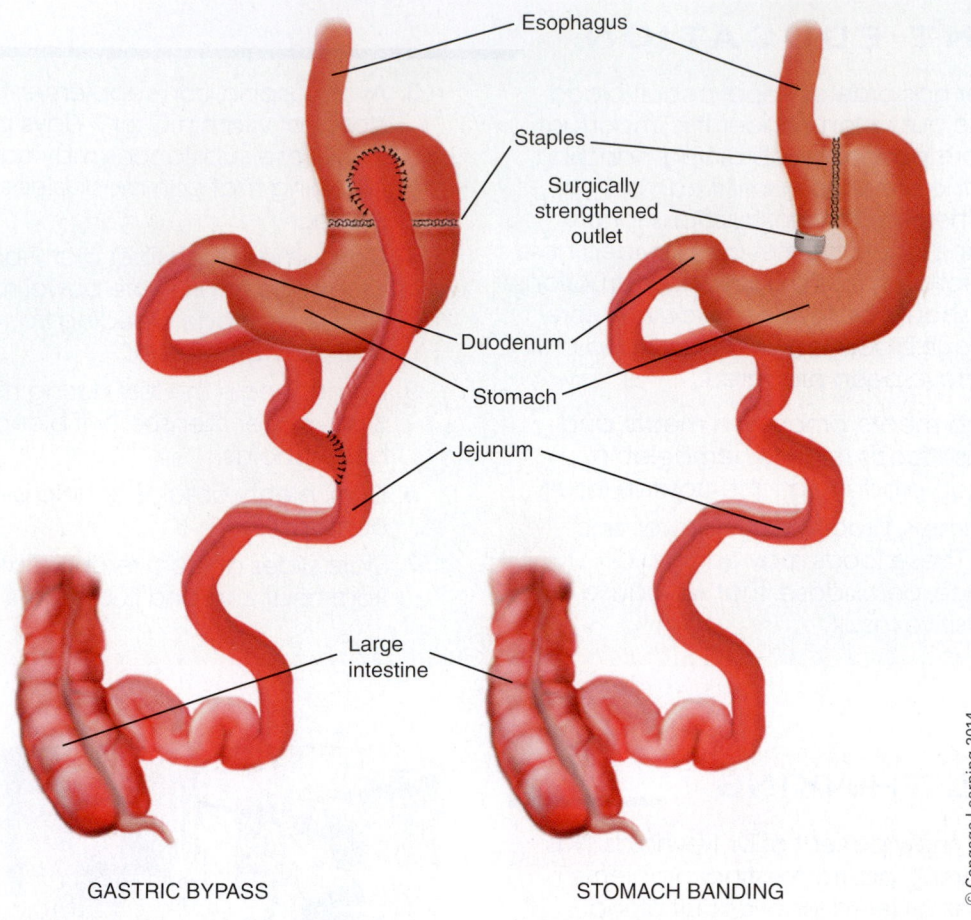

© Cengage Learning 2014

GASTRIC BYPASS   STOMACH BANDING

Figure 30-36   Gastric bypass and stomach banding are bariatric surgical procedures.

because of the physical and emotional problems caused by their obesity. Prior to surgery, patients must participate with their provider to bring their existing medical problems, such as uncontrolled diabetes, severe hypertension, hyperlipidemia, and gallbladder disease, under control. Stabilization is important to prevent serious complications before, during, and after surgery.

Bariatric surgery is performed to treat obesity and to help the patient lose weight. It can be accomplished with a standard abdominal incision or laparoscope. Two procedures that can be performed are "banding" or "stapling" and gastric bypass surgery (Figure 30-36). With banding or stapling, the bottom of the esophagus (where it enters the stomach) is banded or stapled, thus shrinking the stomach. An adjustable port in the abdomen controls the tightness of the band or staples. In gastric bypass surgery, the surgeon creates a pouch out of a small portion of the stomach and attaches it directly to the small intestine, thereby passing the stomach and duodenum. As a result, absorption, which occurs in the small

intestine, is reduced. Before surgery, patients are counseled about possible side effects, such as malabsorption, anemia, vomiting, diarrhea, hernias, and blood clots.

Bariatric surgery is considered for patients with **morbid obesity** who have tried numerous weight loss and exercise regimens without results and are at serious risk for heart disease, stroke, cancer, and other conditions. Body mass index (BMI) is another factor considered when providers evaluate patients for surgery. A BMI around 30 to 40 (a general guideline) is one of the criteria used to determine which patients are candidates for the surgery (normal BMI is 18.5–24.9). The presence of other diseases is also a factor in the evaluation.

  Caring for bariatric patients is challenging. Their emotional health is important. Being nonjudgmental and showing empathy for these patients are very important. They suffer from discrimination, prejudice, and isolation. Obesity is a chronic illness that requires patience and understanding.

Table 30-21 Patient Preparation and Procedure for Radiographic Studies of the Digestive System

Test	Purpose	Patient Prep	Procedure	Time
Barium swallow (upper gastrointestinal [GI] series)	To study the esophagus, stomach, duodenum of the small intestine for disease (ulcers, tumors, hiatal hernia, esophageal varices)	Day before radiograph: 1. Light evening meal 2. NPO after midnight Day of test: 1. NPO Postprocedural: 1. Increase fluid intake 2. Take laxative as prescribed	1. The patient is asked to drink a flavored barium mixture while standing in front of fluoroscope 2. The radiologist observes the passage down the digestive tract 3. The patient is turned to various positions to allow good visualization of the intestine 4. Radiographs are taken	1 hour
Barium enema (lower GI series)	To study the colon for disease (polyps, tumors, lesions)	Clear liquid 1 day prior (allowed: non-carbonated beverages, clear gelatin, clear broth, coffee and tea with sugar) No milk or milk products 8 oz water every hour until bedtime Prep kit: to include bottle of magnesium citrate, Dulcolax tab(s) Day before radiograph: 1. Late afternoon drink bottle of magnesium citrate 2. Early evening take Dulcolax tab(s) as prescribed 3. Light evening meal. NPO except water, after dinner Morning of procedure: 1. NPO 2. Cleansing enema Postprocedural instructions: 1. Increase fluid intake and dietary fiber 2. Report to provider if no bowel movement within 24 hours of test	1. The colon is filled with a barium sulfate mixture 2. The patient is turned in various positions to allow the barium to fill the colon. Air is injected to move the barium along the colon 3. When the colon is full, radiographs are taken	1–2 hours
Cholecystogram	To study the gall bladder for disease (stones, duct obstruction), inflammation	1. Evening before test fat-free dinner 2. Take dye tablets with 8 oz water 3. Cathartic or cleansing enemas may be prescribed 4. NPO after dinner and tablets	1. A series of radiographs is taken 2. A fatty meal may be given to stimulate the gall bladder to empty 3. Other radiographs can then be taken to check gall bladder function	1 hour

URINARY SYSTEM

The urinary system includes the kidneys, ureters, and bladder. The main function of the kidneys is to form and excrete urine, which contains waste products harmful to body tissues. The kidneys also regulate water balance in the body and help maintain the acid–base balance of body fluids.

Collecting and processing urine for laboratory analysis is covered in Chapter 42. Several other clinical and diagnostic procedures of the urinary system are covered in this section, including urinary catheterization and an overview of performing a urine drug screen and a diagnostic x-ray study known as an intravenous pyelogram (IVP) or excretory urography used to diagnose disorders of the urinary tract.

Diagnostic tests, procedures, disorders, and conditions common to the urinary system are given in Tables 30-22 and 30-23.

Signs and Symptoms of Urinary Conditions and Disorders

Signs and symptoms of urinary tract diseases include any abnormality in urine or in the ability to urinate. Some common signs and symptoms are **dysuria** or painful urination, **proteinuria** or protein in the urine, **hematuria** or blood in the urine, **pyuria** or pus in the urine, **frequency**, **urgency**, **oliguria** or absence of urine production, and **nocturia** or excessive urination at night. Patients may report flank or low back pain or experience fever, nausea, vomiting, general **malaise**, known as general discomfort, and fatigue.

Urinary tract infection (UTI) is the most common disorder of the urinary system, and it manifests itself with many of the above signs and symptoms. UTI is a broad diagnosis covering any infection of the urinary tract including the urethra, ureters, bladder, and kidneys. UTIs may be caused by virus or fungus, but by far the most common infection is caused by bacteria. The most common area is the bladder. The medical term for inflammation of the bladder is cystitis.

Bacteria may reach the urinary tract through the blood, called a hematogenous infection, or enter the tract through the urethra, known as an ascending infection. Hematogenous infection is less common and is usually the result of septicemia. In this case, the urinary tract is a site of secondary infection. Primary infection of septicemia may begin in the respiratory or gastrointestinal tract and is carried to the urinary tract through the blood.

Diagnostic Tests

The most commonly performed test to diagnose urinary system disorders is a urinalysis. Many different disorders of the urinary system can be identified, making this test extremely valuable. A specimen of urine can be analyzed for many components such as pH, specific gravity, protein, glucose, leukocytes, and blood. The specimen can be further analyzed by examination under the microscope to look for bacteria, white and red blood cells, crystals, and casts.

Urine culture and sensitivity can be performed and will indicate if a UTI is present so the appropriate antibiotic can be prescribed by the provider. To obtain a urine specimen for culture, there are two ways to collect the specimen: clean catch or by catheterization (insertion of sterile tube into urinary bladder; see Procedures 30-21 and 30-22 and Chapter 42).

Blood tests can be done to determine whether waste products are being adequately filtered out of the circulatory system. A test for kidney function confirms the status of glomeruli function.

Two nitrogenous waste products normally filtered from the blood are urea and creatinine. A blood urea nitrogen (BUN) test checks the levels

Table 30-22   Urinary System Disorders

Disease/ Disorder	Laboratory/Diagnostic Tests			Surgery	Medical Tests or Procedures	Treatment
	Blood	Urine	Radiography			
Cancer of urinary bladder	Complete blood count	Urinalysis Culture and sensitivity of urine	Intravenous pyelogram Pelvic ultrasound Computed tomography scan	Cystoscopy with biopsy of the bladder		Resection of cancer (transurethral resection of a bladder tumor [TURBT]) Cystectomy Radium implants Chemotherapy
Cystitis	Complete blood count	Urinalysis including microscopic examination Culture and sensitivity of urine	Intravenous pyelogram		Cystoscopy	Appropriate antibiotic therapy
Glomerulo-nephritis	Blood urea nitrogen Creatinine Blood culture Sedimentation rate Electrolytes	Urinalysis Culture and sensitivity of urine	Intravenous pyelogram Ultrasound of kidneys X-ray of kidneys, ureters, and bladder	Kidney transplant	Biopsy of kidney(s)	Diuretics Antihypertensives Dialysis (if necessary)
Polycystic kidneys	Blood urea nitrogen Creatinine Electrolytes	Urinalysis	Intravenous pyelogram Ultrasound of kidneys Computerized tomography scan	Kidney transplant		Dialysis

continues

Table 30-22   Urinary System Disorders (*Continued*)

Disease/Disorder	Laboratory/Diagnostic Tests				Surgery	Medical Tests or Procedures	Treatment
	Blood	Urine	Radiography				
Pyelonephritis	Blood urea nitrogen Creatinine Blood culture Electrolytes	Urinalysis	Intravenous pyelogram Ultrasound of kidneys				Appropriate antibiotics
Renal calculi	Complete blood count Uric acid	Urinalysis	X-ray of kidneys, ureters, and bladder (KUB) Ultrasound of kidneys, ureters, and bladder Intravenous pyelogram		Cystoscopy	Lithotripsy (crushing of a kidney stone) Surgery (nephrolithotomy)
Urinary tract infection	Complete blood count	Urinalysis Culture and sensitivity of urine			Cystoscopy	Appropriate antibiotics

Table 30-23 Description of Urinary Disorders and Conditions

Cancer of urinary bladder. Linked to cigarette smoking, industrial chemicals, and ingested toxins. Microscopic hematuria is one of the first signs.

Cystitis. Inflammation of the urinary bladder. More common in female patients due to the short length of the urethra. *Escherichia coli* may travel from the rectum to the bladder. Infectious organisms can invade the bladder during sexual intercourse. Frequency, burning, dysuria, and urgency are common symptoms.

Glomerulonephritis. Seen in children and young adults after streptococcal infection; strep throat, scarlet fever. Causes degenerative inflammation of glomeruli. Chills, fever, weakness are common symptoms. Edema and albumin in urine are common. Hypertension occurs.

Polycystic kidneys. A congenital anomaly. Kidneys contain multiple cysts and greatly dilated tubules do not open into renal pelvis. Hypertension, kidney failure, and death can result.

Pyelonephritis. Caused by pyogenic bacteria such as *E. coli*, streptococci, staphylococci, pregnancy, or calculi. May originate in the bladder and ascend to the kidneys. Pyuria, chills, fever, and sudden back pain are symptoms. Dysuria is common. Tenderness in suprapubic area.

Renal calculi. May be present with or without symptoms. Cause intense pain when they lodge in the ureter(s). Formed by certain salts (perhaps calcium). Urinary urgency, nausea and vomiting, fever.

© Cengage Learning 2014

of these two wastes. High levels of waste products can result in uremia (waste products in the blood), a toxic condition of the blood that, if not reversed, leads to death (see Chapter 42).

An IVP, kidney-ureter-bladder (KUB) radiograph, and cystogram are radiologic examinations of the urinary tract.

Intravenous Pyelogram.
An **intravenous pyelogram (IVP)** is used to examine the urinary tract for blockage, narrowing, growths, and calculi. This urinary tract diagnostic radiograph is also used to diagnose disorders such as lesions, hydronephrosis, a collection of urine in renal pelvis, and kidneys with many cysts, known as polycystic kidneys.

Patient Preparation for IVP. In studies of the urinary system, the IVP requires that the patient prepare with laxatives, enemas, and fasting (Table 30-24). The IVP consists of an intravenous injection of an iodine-based contrast medium that is used to define the structures of the urinary system. A retrograde pyelogram is a study of the urinary tract done by inserting a sterile catheter into the urinary meatus. Radiopaque contrast medium then flows upward into the kidneys. This diagnostic test is usually done in conjunction with cystoscopy. Patients should have iodine-sensitivity tests before the examination to determine the possibility of an allergic reaction. If there is an iodine and shellfish allergy, the patient will be required to be premedicated.

A voiding cystogram may be ordered in conjunction with an IVP. In this case, the contrast medium is instilled into the bladder by catheter and no special patient preparation is needed (see Chapter 32).

Cystoscopy.
Cystoscopy is a sterile procedure that uses a lighted cystoscope to view the urethra and bladder. Inflammation, bladder calculi, **polyps**, and tumors can be seen using a cystoscope. A biopsy of the bladder can be done while performing a cystoscopy (Figure 30-37).

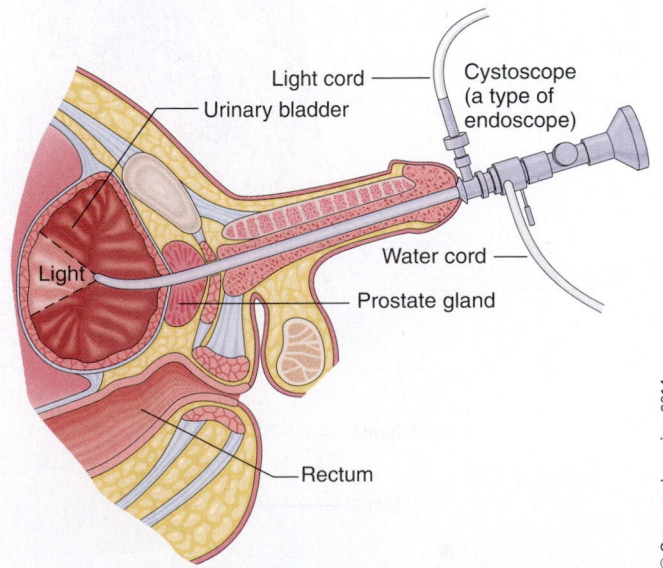

Figure 30-37 Cystoscopy.

© Cengage Learning 2014

Table 30-24   Intravenous Pyelogram Procedure and Precautions

Purpose	Patient Education	Precautions
To examine the urinary tract—kidneys, ureters, bladder—for blockage, narrowing, growths, and calculi	1. Only clear liquids the day prior to the procedure 2. Laxatives as ordered 3. NPO after midnight the evening before the IVP 4. Cleansing enema(s) the morning of the procedure	Contrast medium of iodine used for visualization (check with patient regarding seafood or iodine allergies) Warn patients of possible warm flushed sensation when dye is injected and that they may experience a metallic taste

© Cengage Learning 2014

Biopsy of the Kidney. Biopsies of the kidney will help confirm a diagnosis. Using radiology and ultrasonography, a fine-gauge needle is inserted through the flank to remove a piece of kidney tissue for analysis and determination of possible malignancy.

Urinary Catheterization

In some states medical assistants can either perform or assist with urinary bladder catheterization, which is the introduction of a sterile catheter through the urethra into the bladder for withdrawal of urine. Figure 30-38 shows male and female anatomy for catheterization. There are basically four reasons to catheterize patients:

1. To obtain a sterile urine specimen for analysis
2. To relieve urinary retention
3. To instill medication into the bladder, after the bladder is emptied
4. To measure the amount of postvoid residual urine

In some cases, this procedure is done by a urologist; however, some providers in obstetrics/gynecology and general and family practice perform or have the medical assistant perform the catheterization. The provider may order a culture

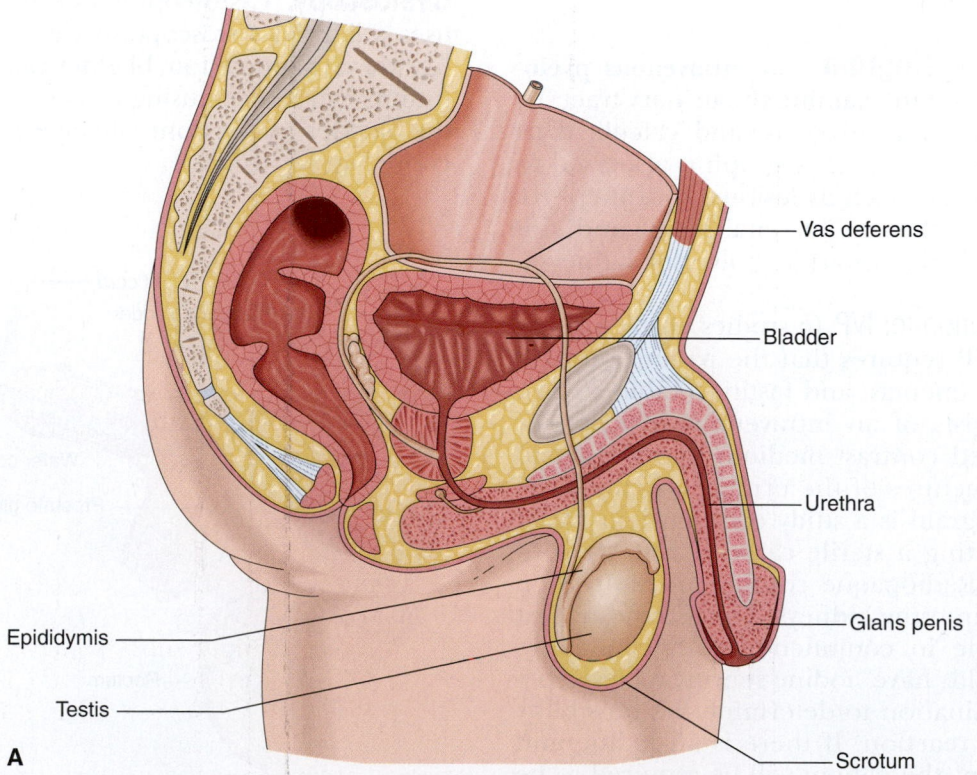

A

Figure 30-38   (A) Cross-sectional view of male anatomy showing urethra and bladder for catheterization.

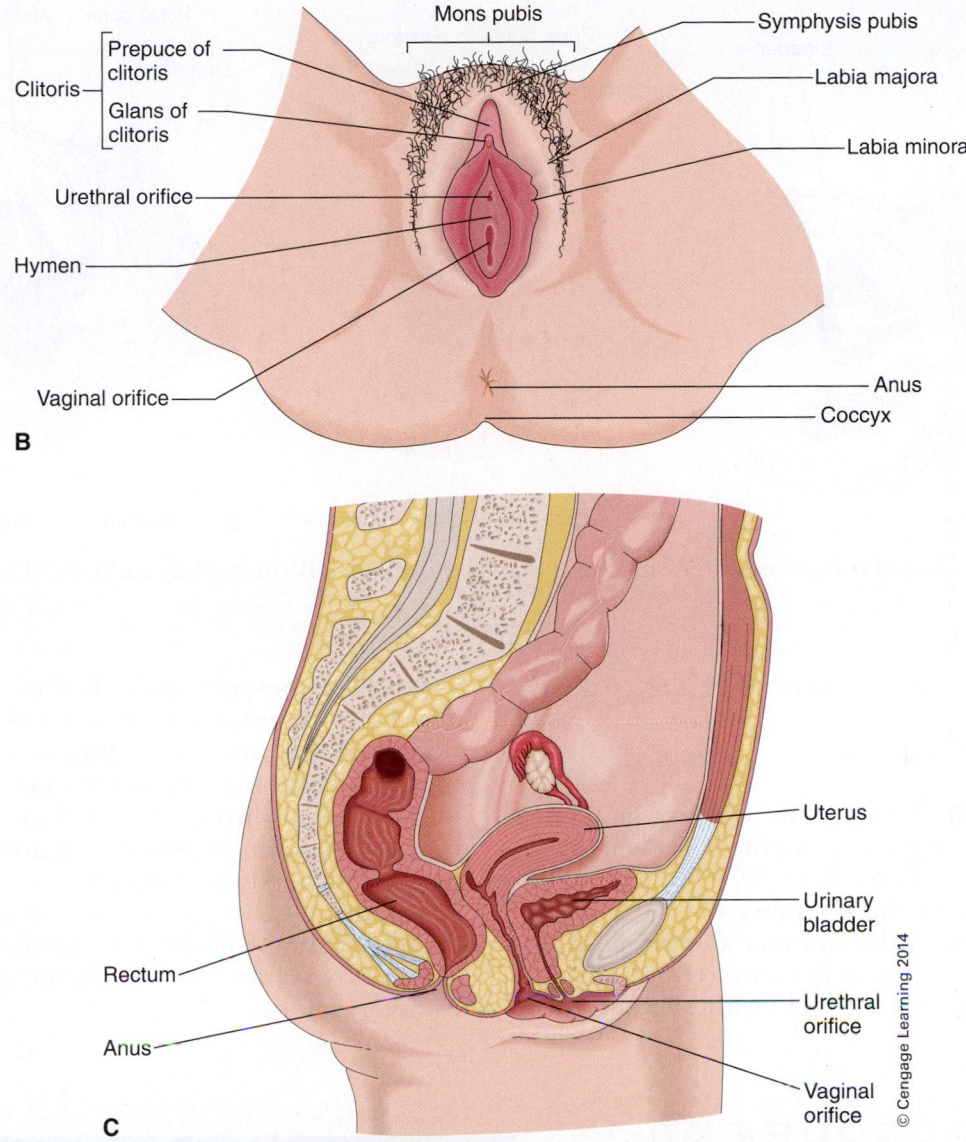

Figure 30-38 (*Continued*) (B) External genitalia of the female. (C) Cross-sectional view of female anatomy showing urethra and bladder for catheterization.

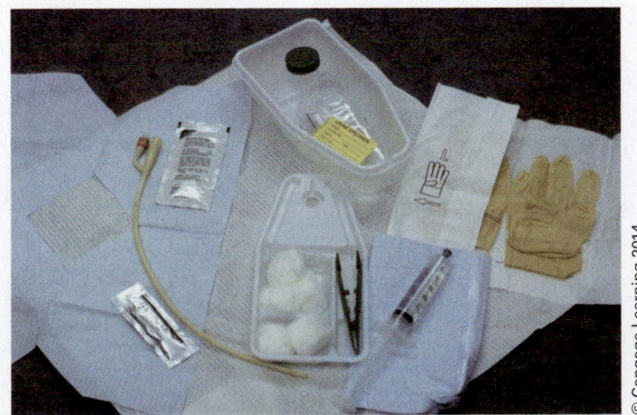

Figure 30-39 Catheterization kit.

and sensitivity test of the urine obtained from catheterization if the patient is experiencing dysuria, frequency, hematura, and urgency. This is done to determine if microorganisms are present and, if so, what the causative microorganism is and which medication would irradicate it, in order to prescribe the appropriate antibiotics.

Sterile technique must be maintained throughout the catheterization. Contamination of any items during the procedure requires discarding the items and obtaining new sterile equipment before continuing the procedure (Figure 30-39). Procedure 30-22 gives steps for performing a

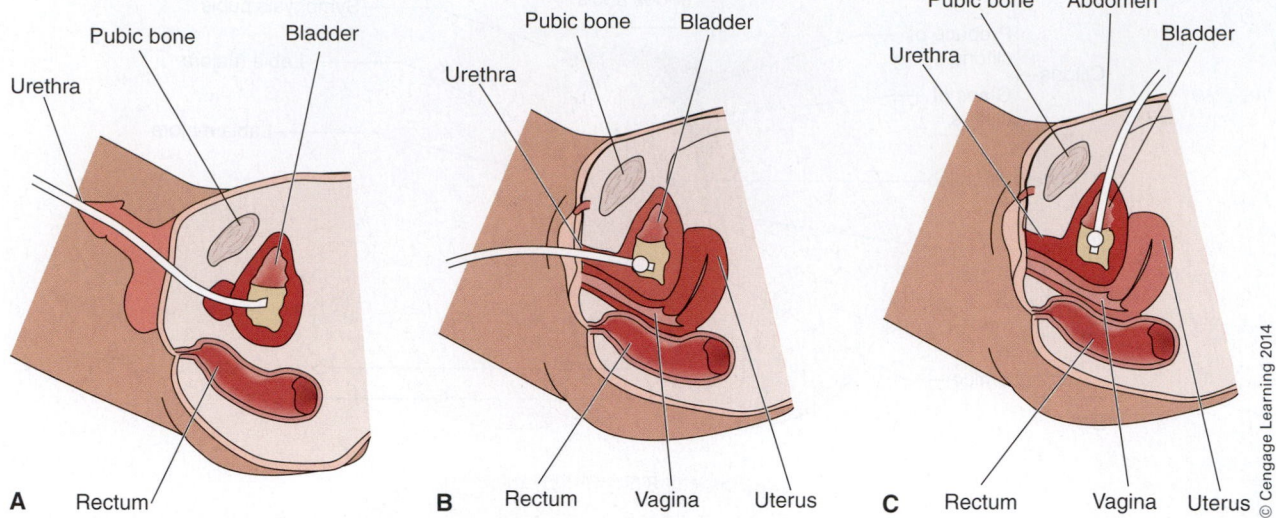

Figure 30-40   Types of urinary catheterizations: (A) Straight catheter. (B) Indwelling catheter. (C) Suprapubic catheter.

 urinary catheterization of a male patient, and Procedure 30-23 gives these steps for a female patient.

Catheterization Equipment. Urinary catheters are sized according to a system of French sizes. A common size catheter is Fr 12. The higher the number, the larger the diameter of the catheter. The provider orders the catheter size when ordering the catheterization procedure. Urethral catheters, sometimes called straight catheters, are used when the catheter is removed after the procedure. The Foley catheter is used when the catheter will remain in the urinary bladder (indwelling catheter). A suprapubic catheter (indwelling) is placed in the bladder during a surgical procedure. An incision is made in the suprapubic area. The bladder empties through the catheter.

Sterile, disposable catheterization kits are available that contain all necessary items to perform the procedure. Figure 30-40 shows the types of urinary catheterizations.

 PROCEDURE 30-1

Assisting the Provider during a Lumbar Puncture or Cerebrospinal Fluid Aspiration

STANDARD PRECAUTIONS:

PURPOSE:
To assemble supplies and position the patient for removal of cerebrospinal fluid from the lumbar area, which will be sent to the laboratory for analysis.

EQUIPMENT/SUPPLIES:
Gown
Sheet or blanket
Waterproof drape

Local anesthetic per provider's order (Xylocaine 1 or 2%)
Appropriately sized syringe and needle length and gauge for administration of anesthetic
Sterile gloves for provider and the medical assistant
Sterile water
Surgical prep kit that contains:
    Antiseptic soap
    Sponges
Disposable sterile lumbar puncture tray that includes:
    Skin antiseptic (providone-iodine) with applicator
    Adhesive bandage

Procedure 30-1 (continued)

Spinal needle
Three to four vials for cerebral spinal fluid collection
Fenestrated drape
Manometer
Laboratory requisition
Examination light
Gauze sponges

PROCEDURE STEPS:

1. Wash hands.

2. *Paying attention to detail,* gather appropriate equipment and supplies.

3. *Introduce yourself and identfy patient.*

4. *Reinforce provider's explanation of the procedure and answer questions, speaking at the patient's level of understanding.*

5. Verify the patient's signature on the informed consent. If the patient has questions, notify the provider that the patient requires further information.

6. *If needed, assist the patient* to the restroom to empty bladder and bowel. RATIONALE: Patient cannot move during the procedure.

7. Wash hands.

8. Using a mayo stand as a base, open the sterile lumbar puncture tray in a manner that maintains sterility of contents and establishes a sterile field for the provider.

9. *Allay the patient's fears and help him feel safe and comfortable* while positioning him in a lateral recumbent position with his back at the edge of the examination table. Provide a small pillow for comfort under his head. RATIONALE: Patient's alignment of the spine is best achieved in a horizontal position.

10. Drape the patient for warmth and privacy, *protecting the patient's personal boundaries.*

11. *Attending to any special needs of the patient,* instruct and then assist him to draw his knees up to his abdomen and to grasp the knees to hold them in place. His chin should be angled toward his chest and the back should be arched toward the edge of the exam table. RATIONALE: Position allows for easier needle insertion into the subarachnoid space of the spinal cord because this position widens the spaces between the lumbar vertebrae. Procedure is performed at the fourth intervertebral space of the lumbar region (Figure 30-41).

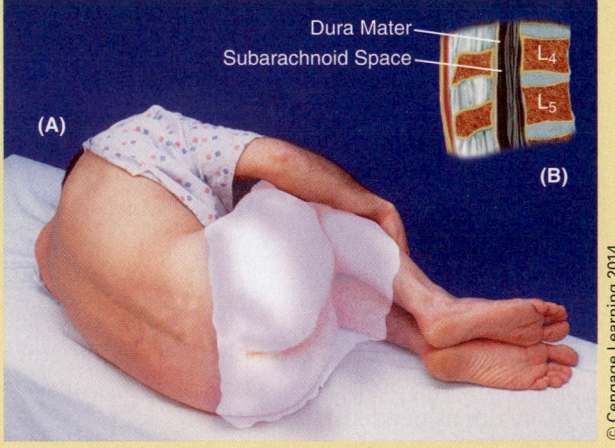

Figure 30-41 (A) Have the patient draw up the knees to the abdomen and grasp knees. Chin should flex on chest. (B) The site for the lumbar puncture.

12. Instruct the patient that during the procedure, he must remember to breathe slowly and evenly and refrain from talking.

13. Tuck a waterproof drape under the patient's side in the area to be prepped.

14. Open the surgical prep tray and pour sterile water into the provided area. Be careful to avoid splashing.

15. Don sterile gloves.

16. Prep the puncture site with antiseptic soap solution beginning at puncture location and prepping in a circular manner to a diameter of at least 6 inches. Discard the prep swab and repeat × 3 or per provider's orders. Rinse if required per provider's orders or manufacturer's instructions. Dry with sterile toweling.

17. Remove sterile gloves and dispose of appropriately.

18. Assist the provider as needed to swab the puncture site with the providine-iodine solution.

19. Assist the provider as needed to drape the puncture site with the sterile fenestrated drape.

20. Assist the provider to draw up the anesthetic solution by inverting the vial and holding it stable to be accessed.

21. Encourage and assist the patient to maintain the knee-chest position until the spinal needle is inserted and a free flow of cerebrospinal fluid (CSF) is obtained. RATIONALE: Movement by the patient could produce trauma to the spinal cord area.

22. When the manometer is attached and measurements are being taken, remind the patient to

continues

Procedure 30-1 (continued)

breathe slowly and evenly and refrain from talking so that an accurate pressure measurement can be obtained.

23. At the direction of the provider, have the patient straighten his legs. RATIONALE: Muscle tension can give false pressure reading. The provider reads manometer to determine the pressure of the spinal fluid.

24. Assist the provider as needed with the vials of CSF.

25. A sterile dressing will be applied to the puncture site once the procedure is completed. Assist the provider as needed.

26. Assist the patient to a supine position and instruct him that he must remain in this position for 2–4 hours or per the provider's orders. RATIONALE: Helps prevent the possibility of cerebrospinal fluid from leaking through the puncture site.

27. Monitor vital signs per office policy or provider's orders.

28. Provide comfort measures and medicate per provider's orders.

29. At the conclusion of the procedure, don sterile gloves and cap CSF specimens tightly.

30. Remove gloves and dispose of appropriately.

31. Wash hands.

32. Appropriately label the CSF vials with the date, patient's name, and order of collection (i.e., CSF #1, CSF #2, CSF #3). Place in biohazard specimen bag for transport.

33. *Paying attention to detail*, complete the laboratory requisition and following policy, send samples to the selected laboratory.

34. Don non-sterile disposable gloves.

35. Dispose of equipment per OSHA guidelines, including disposing of all sharps in approved sharps container.

36. Follow office policy or provider's orders to provide written instructions for after care.

37. Accurately record procedure per provider's instruction in the patient's medical record or EMR. Be sure to include patient education, any medications given, the patient's tolerance of the procedure, any pressure measurements obtained, and the disposition of the CSF samples.

DOCUMENTATION:
6/12/20XX 3:10 PM   Lumbar puncture performed by Dr. King. Three samples of cerebrospinal fluid obtained. Labeled #1, #2, #3. Taken to laboratory. Pt appeared to tolerate procedure. BP 142/82, P 88. Instructed to remain flat for 3 hours and to drink increased amounts of fluids. S. Tyler, CMA (AAMA)———

PROCEDURE 30-2
Assisting the Provider with a Neurologic Screening Examination

STANDARD PRECAUTIONS:

PURPOSE:
To determine a patient's neurologic status.

EQUIPMENT/SUPPLIES:
Percussion hammer
Safety pin or sensory wheel
Peppermint or alcohol prep for odor identification
Cotton ball
Solid objects such as keys, coins, paper clips

Tuning fork
Flash light or pen light
Tongue blade

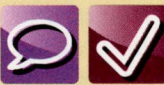

PROCEDURE STEPS:
1. Wash hands.

2. *Paying attention to detail,* gather appropriate equipment and supplies.

3. *Introduce yourself and identify patient.*

Procedure 30-2 (continued)

4. *Speaking at the level of the patient's understanding, explain the procedure and expectations to the patient.*

5. While taking the patient's medical history, observe the following:
   - Orientation to person, place, and time
   - Memory
   - Mood
   - Cognition
   - Appropriate behaviors

6. Assist the provider as requested when testing reflexes with a percussion hammer.

7. Assist the provider by assuring the smooth flow of assessment during the neuro exam by providing the following when requested:

   - Safety pin or sensory wheel and cotton ball
   - Solid objects such as keys, paper clips, coins
   - Peppermint or alcohol prep
   - Tuning fork
   - Flash light or pen light
   - Tongue blade

8. Accurately record findings of neurological exam per provider's instruction in the patient's medical record or EMR.

DOCUMENTATION:

8/22/20XX 3:20 PM   Assisted Dr. Woo with neurologic screening examination. Made appointment for patient to see Dr. Sullivan, neurologist, on 9/4/XX at 3:00 PM. J. Backus, RMA (AMT)

PROCEDURE 30-3

Performing Visual Acuity Testing Using a Snellen Chart

STANDARD PRECAUTIONS:

PURPOSE:

To perform a visual screening test to determine a patient's distance visual acuity.

EQUIPMENT/SUPPLIES:

Snellen eye chart placed at eye level (appropriate for age and reading ability of the patient)
Pointer
Occluder
Alcohol wipes

PROCEDURE STEPS:

1. Wash hands.
2. Assemble equipment and supplies, *paying attention to detail.*

3. Prepare a well-lit room, free from distractions and with a distance mark 20 feet from the eye chart. Be certain there is no glare on the chart.

4. *Speaking at the level of the patient's understanding, explain the procedures to the patient.*

5. Patients should be tested with glasses or contact lenses, unless otherwise indicated by the provider.

6. Instruct the patient to stand behind the mark and cover the right eye with the occluder (Figure 30-42). RATIONALE: Closing of the eye not being tested may cause the person to squint when reading the chart.

7. Instruct the patient to keep the left eye open under the occluder and not to apply pressure to the eyeball.

8. Stand next to the chart, point to row 3, and instruct the patient to read each letter with the left eye, verbally identifying each letter read (Figure 30-43). If unable to read line 3, go to line 2 or 1. RATIONALE: Pointing to each row

continues

Procedure 30-3 (continued)

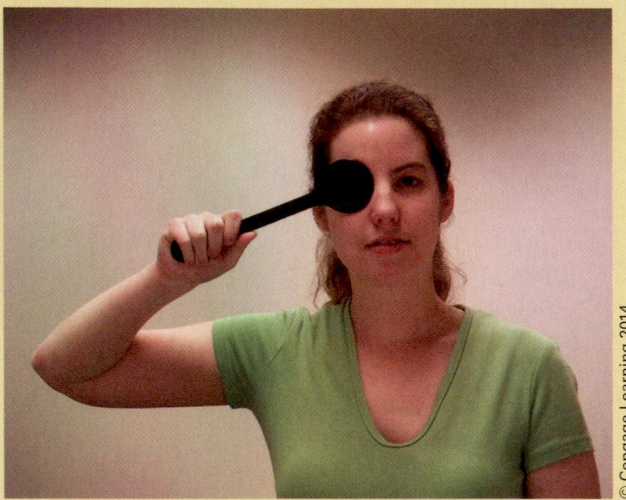

Figure 30-42 The patient covers the right eye with the occluder, keeping the eye open under the occluder.

helps the patient to focus on one row of letters at a time. Beginning at row 3 saves time.

9. Accurately record the results at the smallest line the patient can read with two or fewer errors. Vision is recorded as right eye, left eye, or both eyes.

   Example: Right eye 20/25; Left eye 20/20; Both eyes 20/20

   RATIONALE: Visual acuity is recorded as a fraction. The number above the line on the chart is the distance the patient is standing from the chart. The number below the line on the chart is the distance from which a person with normal vision can read that row of letters.

10. Record the patient's reaction during the test. RATIONALE: Leaning forward, squinting or straining, or tearing from the eye may indicate eye problems.

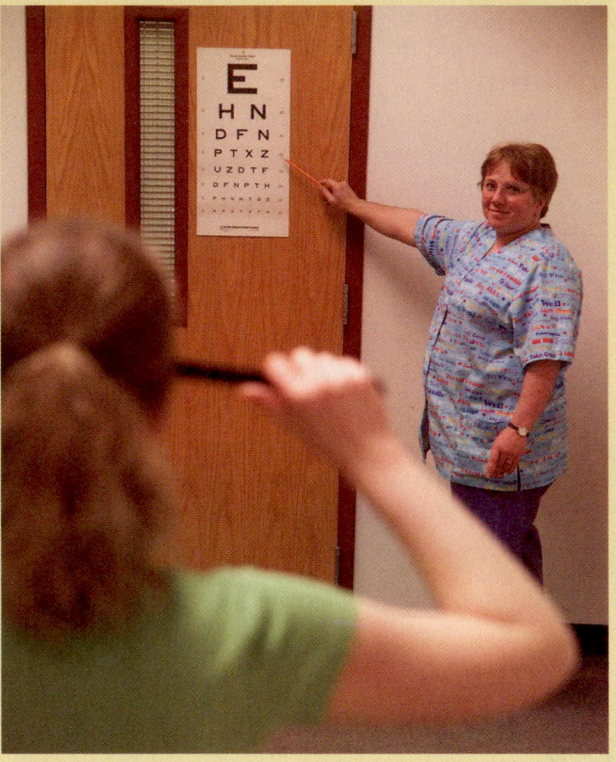

Figure 30-43 The patient uses the left eye to read the letters on the chart. The patient is instructed to start with row 3. Here she is reading row 4.

11. Repeat the procedure with the right eye.

12. Disinfect the occluder with alcohol wipes.

13. Wash hands.

14. Accurately record the results in the patient's chart or electronic medical record.

DOCUMENTATION:

4/14/20XX 1:15 PM   Visual acuity checked using Snellen chart. Results: right 20/30; left 20/20; both 20/20. H. Casey, RMA (AMT)

PROCEDURE 30-4
Measuring Near Visual Acuity

STANDARD PRECAUTIONS:

PURPOSE:
To measure the near vision of the patient.

EQUIPMENT/SUPPLIES:
Appropriate near vision chart (Jaegar)
Occluder
Measuring tape
Alcohol wipes

PROCEDURE STEPS:
1. Wash hands.
2. *Paying attention to detail*, assemble equipment and supplies.
3. Prepare a well-lit room, free from distractions.
4. *Identify patient. Speaking at the level of the patient's understanding, explain the procedures to the patient.* RATIONALE: To obtain patient cooperation.
5. Patients who wear corrective lenses should be tested wearing glasses or contact lenses, unless otherwise indicated by the provider.
6. Position the near visual acuity card 14 inches from the patient by measuring with a measuring tape. RATIONALE: To obtain accurate results.

7. Cover the left eye for right eye measurement. Instruct the patient to keep the left eye open under the occluder and not to apply pressure to the eyeball. RATIONALE: Pressure will cause blurring of the other eye.
8. *Demonstrating respect for individual diversity,* provide language appropriate paragraphs printed on a card.
9. Once patient has reached a line where more than two mistakes are made, note the visual acuity for that line for that eye (allow the patient to repeat the line to verify acuity).
10. Repeat the process to measure the left eye.
11. Repeat the process with both eyes open.
12. Record the patient's reaction during the test.
13. Disinfect the occluder with alcohol wipes. RATIONALE: To prevent microorganism cross contamination.
14. Wash hands.
15. Accurately record the results. Vision is recorded as right eye, left eye, or both eyes. Normal vision using this method is recorded as 14/14.

DOCUMENTATION:
7/22/20XX 4:00 PM   Near visual acuity checked. Results: 14/14. S. Tyler, CMA (AAMA)————————

PROCEDURE 30-5
Testing Color Vision Using the Ishihara Plates

STANDARD PRECAUTIONS:

PURPOSE:
To assess a patient's ability to distinguish between the colors red and green.

Patient education:
1. Explain that the purpose of the test is to determine if the patient has a color vision deficiency.
2. Show patient plate number 12 as an example of the test process.

EQUIPMENT/SUPPLIES:
Ishihara Plates (1-2) (Figure 30-44)
Measuring tape

PROCEDURE STEPS:
1. Wash hands.
2. *Paying attention to detail,* assemble equipment and supplies.
3. Assure that the plates have been stored covered and protected from sunlight to ensure that no

continues

Procedure 30-5 (continued)

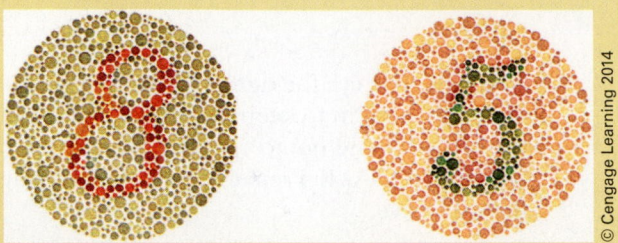

© Cengage Learning 2014

Figure 30-44   Ishihara plates are used to assess the patient's ability to distinguish between the colors red and green.

fading of the colors on the plates has occurred. This would invalidate the test.

4. Prepare a room lit by daylight, free from distractions. RATIONALE: Direct sunlight or electric light may produce errors in the results because of an alteration in the appearance of shades of color.

5. *Speaking at the level of the patient's understanding, explain the procedures to the patient.*

6. Hold each plate 30 inches from the patient and tilted so that the plane of the plate is at a right angle to the line of the patient's vision.

7. Record the number given by the patient on each plate.

8. Assess the patient's readings. RATIONALE: If 10 or more plates are read correctly, the color vision is regarded as normal.

9. *Concisely update the provider with the test results.*

10. Accurately record the results in the patient's chart or electronic medical record.

   Source for error: Test plates should be kept covered when not in use. Undue exposure to sunlight causes a fading of the color plates, thus leading to inaccurate test interpretation.

DOCUMENTATION:

3/12/20XX 11:00 AM   *Color vision test performed using Ishihara plates. Twelve plates read correctly. H. Casey, RMA (AMT)*

PROCEDURE 30-6
Performing Eye Instillation

STANDARD PRECAUTIONS:

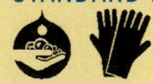

PURPOSE:
To treat eye infections, soothe irritation, anesthetize, and dilate pupils. Ophthalmic medication is supplied in liquid or ointment form. Use separate medication for each eye, if both are affected. Medication is sterile.

EQUIPMENT/SUPPLIES:
Sterile eye dropper for single use
Medication as ordered by provider
Nonsterile disposable gloves
Tissues

PROCEDURE STEPS:
1. Wash hands.

2. *Paying attention to detail,* assemble supplies using sterile technique.

3. Verify the provider's order and prepare a medication card.

4. Follow the "Six Rights" of medication administration.

5. Work in a well-lighted, quiet, clean area.

6. *Paying attention to detail,* review the medication card. Select the correct medication from the medication area.

7. Compare the medication label with the medication card (first check).

8. If unfamiliar with the medication, consult the PDR or other reputable reference. Familiarize yourself with:
   - Drug name (commercial and generic)
   - Mechanism of action
   - Routes of administration
   - Common side effects

9. Check the expiration date. RATIONALE: Verifies correct medication and ensures medication has not expired.

Procedure 30-6 (continued)

10. Compare the medication label with the medication card (second check).

11. Carefully transport the medication to the patient exam room. Bring the medication card.

12. Check the medication and medication card at the patient's bedside (third check).

13. ***Introduce yourself and identify patient.***

14. ***Speaking at the level of the patient's understanding, explain the procedure and expectations to the patient.*** State the name of the medication and the purpose of the injection.

15. ***Allay the patient's fears regarding the procedure being performed and help them feel safe and comfortable.***

16. Ask the patient about medication allergies.

17. Position the patient in a sitting or lying position.

18. Don gloves.

19. Open the bottle and remove the cap without allowing anything to touch the dropper tip of the medication bottle.

20. Have the patient look up at the ceiling and expose the lower conjunctival sac of the affected eye by gently pulling downward on the lower lid (Figure 30-45).

21. Place the dropper lid as close to the eye as possible (without touching the eye or the lid). Brace the remaining fingers on the nose.

22. Gently squeeze the bottle and administer one drop or appropriate amount of ointment (or as directed by the provider's order) into the pouch formed by the lower lid.

23. Instruct the patient to close eye gently and keep closed for at least 60 to 90 seconds to allow the medication to bathe the eye. RATIONALE: Movement distributes the medication evenly.

24. With the patient's eye closed, gently place your finger on the lower lid at the nasal corner to occlude the tear duct. This will inhibit the drops and any additional tearing that the eye drops

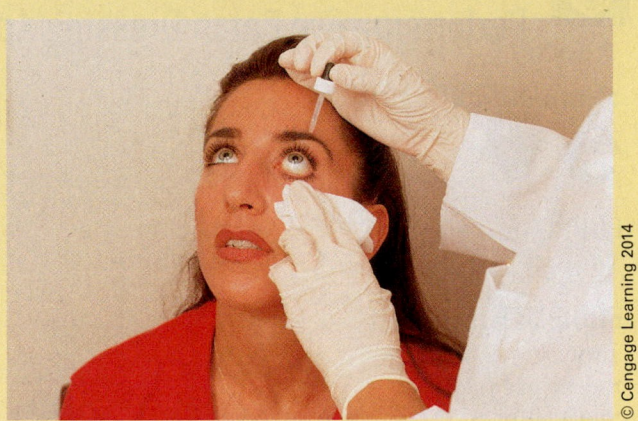

Figure 30-45 When medication is being instilled into the patient's eye, the patient should look up to the ceiling and the medical assistant should pull down on the lower lid. Contact with the eyeball should be avoided.

© Cengage Learning 2014

might cause from flowing into the tear drainage system.

25. Blot excess medication and tears from the patient's face with tissues. RATIONALE: Wipe from cleaner to dirtier.

26. Dispose of supplies in appropriate biohazard container.

27. Wash hands.

28. If the patient is to continue with medications at home, instruct regarding continued administration of eye preparation.

29. Accurately record the administration of medication to include name of medication, dose, route, date, time and initials. Also document patient teaching.

DOCUMENTATION:

9/12/20XX 11:30 AM   Ophthalmic drops (2) instilled in right eye. Eye red and swollen. No exudate noted. H. Casey, RMA (AMT)

PROCEDURE 30-7

Performing Eye Patch Dressing Application

STANDARD PRECAUTIONS:

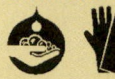

PURPOSE:
To apply a sterile eye patch.

EQUIPMENT/SUPPLIES:
Tape
Sterile eye patch
Sterile gloves

PROCEDURE STEPS:

1. Wash hands.

2. *Paying attention to detail,* gather appropriate equipment and supplies.

3. *Introduce yourself and identify patient.*

4. *Speaking at the level of the patient's understanding, explain the procedure and expectations to the patient.* Assure that the patient has a ride home. RATIONALE: Monovision is misleading, and the patient cannot see well enough to drive.

5. Position the patient in a sitting or supine position.

6. Instruct the patient to close both eyes during the application of the eye patch.

7. Open package containing the sterile eye patch, observing sterile technique.

8. Don sterile gloves.

9. Place the patch over the affected eye.

10. Secure the patch with three to four strips of transparent tape diagonally from mid-forehead to below the ear.

11. Remove gloves and dispose of in appropriate biohazard waste container.

12. Instruct patient regarding length of time to wear patch and return visit to provider.

13. Accurately record the application of a sterile eye patch and patient education in the patient's chart or electronic medical record.

DOCUMENTATION:
8/1/20XX 2:30 PM   Sterile eye patch applied to right eye. Eye appeared red. No exudate seen. Patient instructed not to drive with eye patch on. Wife to drive patient home. H. Casey, RMA (AMT)

PROCEDURE 30-8

Performing Eye Irrigation

STANDARD PRECAUTIONS:

PURPOSE:
To irrigate the patient's affected eye.
a. To cleanse debris
b. To cleanse discharge
c. To remove chemicals
d. To apply antiseptic
e. To apply warmth for comfort

EQUIPMENT/SUPPLIES:
Sterile irrigation solution as ordered by the provider
Sterile bulb syringe
Kidney-shaped basin
Sterile basin
Sterile gauze 2 × 2s
Sterile gloves in the appropriate size
Towel

Procedure 30-8 (continued)

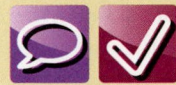

PROCEDURE STEPS:

1. Wash hands.
2. *Paying attention to detail*, gather appropriate equipment and supplies. *NOTE:* If both eyes need to be irrigated, use separate equipment for each eye. RATIONALE: Prevents cross contamination.
3. *Introduce yourself and identify patient.*
4. *Speaking at the level of the patient's understanding, explain the procedure and expectations to the patient.*
5. Position the patient in the supine position.
6. Check the solution and the provider's order (first check).
7. Warm the solution to body temperature. Check the expiration date on the solution. RATIONALE: More comfortable for patient.
8. Check the label with the provider's order (second check).
9. Have the patient turn her head to the side of the affected eye. RATIONALE: Avoid cross contamination of unaffected eye by allowing the solution to flow from the affected eye into the kidney basin and away from unaffected eye.
10. Place a towel over that shoulder to absorb any fluid that splashes.
11. Place the kidney basin along the affected side of the face to catch the irrigation solution. RATIONALE: Allows for the solution to drain into a catch receptacle.
12. Open the sterile basin using sterile technique.
13. Open the sterile bulb syringe and flip into the sterile basin.
14. Open and flip 3 packages of sterile 2 × 2 gauze sponges onto the sterile field.
15. Check the label of the irrigation solution against the provider's order (third check).
16. Carefully pour the sterile solution into the sterile basin.
17. Don sterile gloves.
18. Moisten two or three gauze sponges in the sterile saline.

19. If indicated, clean the eyelid and eyelashes of the affected eye from the nasal side to the outer aspect of the eyelid. Discard the sponge after each wipe. RATIONALE: Wipe from cleaner to dirtier.
20. Expose the lower conjunctiva by separating the eyelids with the index finger and the thumb of your non-dominant hand. RATIONALE: To facilitate flowing of solution.
21. Instruct the patient to stare at a fixed spot during the procedure.
22. Fill the bulb syringe with the sterile irrigation.
23. Irrigate the affected eye with sterile solution by resting the sterile bulb syringe on the bridge of the patient's nose, being careful not to touch the eye or conjunctival sac with the syringe tip. RATIONALE: Prevents a flow of solution into the unaffected eye causing cross contamination.
24. Gently squeeze the bulb syringe to allow the flow of irrigation from the inner corner to the outer corner of the eye.

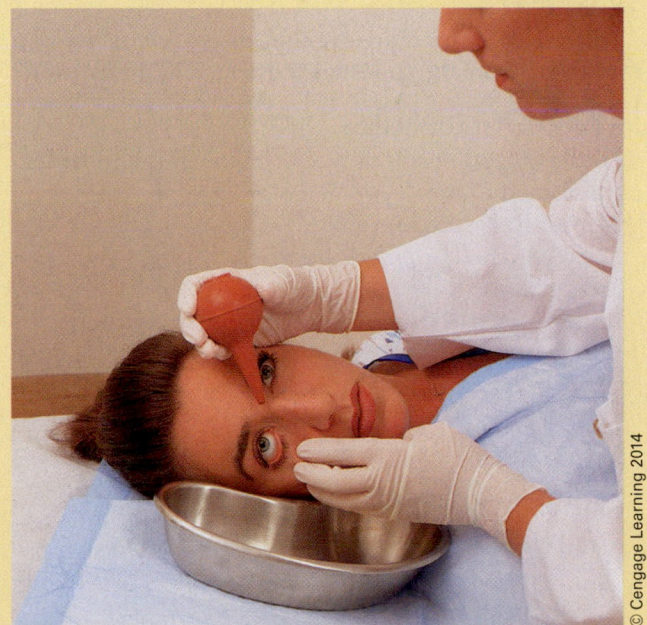

Figure 30-46   The medical assistant irrigates the patient's eye. Note that the solution will go from inner to outer canthus. The patient is turned toward the affected eye.

© Cengage Learning 2014

continues

Procedure 30-8 (continued)

25. Repeat several times until the debris is dislodged.

26. After irrigation, dry the eyelid and eyelashes with a sterile gauze sponge.

27. Before disposing of the setup, consult the provider. If needed, there may be a stain added to the irrigation to detect corneal abrasions.

28. Assist the provider as needed.

29. Discard the supplies as indicated in biohazard waste containers.

30. Remove and discard gloves appropriately.

31. Wash hands.

32. Accurately record the irrigation process in the patient's paper chart or electronic medical record.

DOCUMENTATION:

11/26/20XX 10:00 AM   Right eye irrigated with 100 mL sterile normal saline (100°F). Eye appears slightly red. No exudate noted. Fluorescein stain (stain strip used for diagnosis and detecting foreign bodies or lesions on the cornea) instilled into right eye by Dr. Woo. Patient seemed to tolerate procedure well. Says she has "no discomfort." H. Casey, RMA (AMT)———

PROCEDURE 30-9

Performing Ear Irrigation

STANDARD PRECAUTIONS:

PURPOSE:
To remove impacted cerumen, discharge, or foreign materials from the ear canal as directed by the provider.

EQUIPMENT/SUPPLIES:
Sterile irrigation solution as ordered by the provider, warmed to 98.6°–103°F
Nonsterile disposable gloves
Kidney-shaped or emesis basin
Sterile basin
Impervious pad to protect the patient's clothing
Bulb syringe

PROCEDURE STEPS:
1. Wash hands.

2. *Paying attention to detail,* gather appropriate equipment and supplies.

3. *Introduce yourself and identify patient.*

4. *Speaking at the level of the patient's understanding, explain the procedure and expectations to the patient.* Include the information that the patient might feel a bit of discomfort and that dizziness is not unusual as the fluid comes in contact with the tympanic membrane. RATIONALE: Ensures irrigation needed.

5. Assist the patient into a comfortable sitting position.

6. Check the label on the sterile solution and the provider's order (first check).

7. Check the expiration date.

8. Place the impervious drape on the patient's shoulder to protect her clothing.

9. Pour the warmed, sterile irrigation into the sterile basin. Check the label and the provider's order (second check).

10. Instruct the patient to tilt her head toward the affected side.

11. Check the label and the provider's order (third check).

12. Don gloves.

13. Tilt the patient's head slightly forward and toward the affected side (Figure 30-47). RATIONALE: This position allows the solution to flow into the basin by gravity.

14. Place the kidney basin (or emesis basin) under the affected ear and ask the patient to assist by holding it steady.

15. Fill the bulb syringe with the warmed solution.

16. With the non-dominant hand, gently pull the auricle upward and back to straighten the ear canal (for adults). RATIONALE: Allows better access to external ear canal.

17. Instruct the patient to immediately inform you of any severe discomfort or pain. If reported, stop immediately and report the findings to the provider.

Procedure 30-9 (continued)

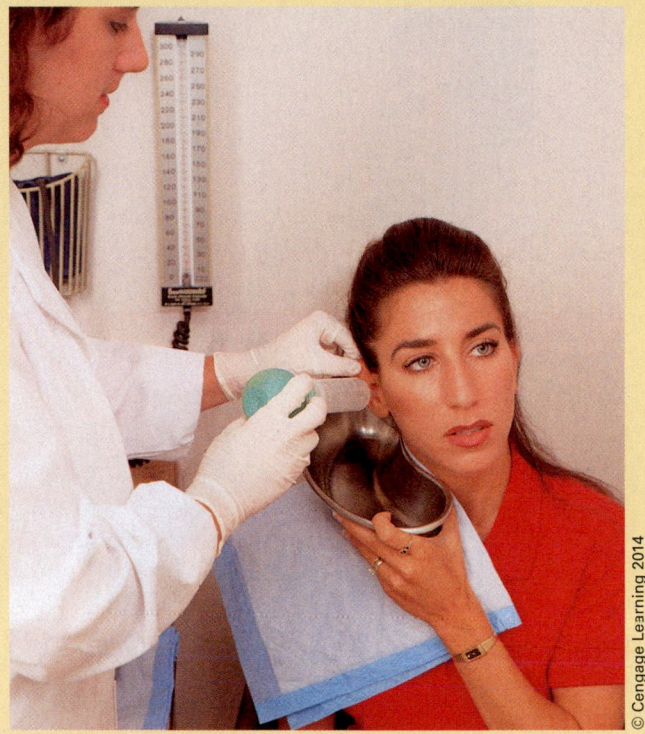

© Cengage Learning 2014

Figure 30-47   When irrigating the patient's ear, tip the affected ear to facilitate the flow of solution. The tip of the syringe does not occlude the opening to the external auditory canal.

18. Expel air from the syringe, leaving the warmed solution filling the bulb and the neck of the syringe.

19. Carefully and gently, insert the syringe tip into the affected ear. Do not insert the tip too deeply. Do not occlude the external auditory canal. RATIONALE: Avoids injury to the tympanic membrane and prevents occlusion of external auditory canal, allowing solution to drain out.

20. Very gently, squeeze the bulb syringe to deliver a slow, steady stream of warmed fluid in an upward direction into the ear canal.

21. Allow the fluid and debris to drain out into the kidney basin.

22. Repeat Steps 18 to 21 as ordered by the provider.

23. Blot the outer ear dry.

24. Notify the provider to re-examine the ear to assure that the procedure is completed.

25. If procedure is complete, remove the kidney basin. Discard the contents as indicated per OSHA guidelines.

26. Instruct the patient to lie on the affected side with a towel under her head to allow complete drainage of the ear.

    a. Report any pain or dizziness to the provider.

    b. Do not insert any foreign object (i.e., cotton applicator) into the ear canal.

27. Appropriately dispose of any remaining supplies.

28. Remove gloves.

29. Wash hands.

30. Accurately record the type and amount of irrigation utilized. Describe any cerumen noted in irrigation in the patient's paper chart or electronic medical record. Record any complaints of pain or dizziness and provider notification.

DOCUMENTATION:

6/4/20XX 3:30 PM   Left ear irrigated with normal saline (100°F). Three pieces (size of pencil eraser) of cerumen in solution returns. No complaints of pain or dizziness. Inner ear and tympanic membrane appear clear. Dr. King notified of results. Examined by Dr. King. S. Tyler, CMA (AAMA)———

PROCEDURE 30-10
Assisting with Audiometry

STANDARD PRECAUTIONS:

PURPOSE:
To assist in testing patient for hearing loss.

Patient education:

1. Explain the use and purpose of the audiometer and that the test measures frequency of sound waves and ability of patient to hear various frequencies of sound waves (one frequency at a time).

continues

Procedure 30-10 (continued)

2. When the patient hears a new frequency, signal the tester.

EQUIPMENT/SUPPLIES:
Audiometer with headphones
Quiet room

PROCEDURE STEPS:

1. Wash hands.
2. *Paying attention to detail,* gather appropriate equipment and supplies.
3. *Introduce yourself and identify patient.*
4. *Speaking at the level of the patient's understanding, explain the procedure and expectations to the patient.* Reinforce the instruction to patient to raise her hand when a new frequency is heard.
5. Assure that the room is quiet without extraneous noises. RATIONALE: Outside interference may cause inaccurate test results, especially in the lower frequencies, which are more difficult to hear.
6. Assist the patient into a comfortable sitting position.
7. Assist the patient to apply the earphones and adjust for fit and comfort. RATIONALE: To test each ear for hearing loss.
8. If the medical assistant has been trained to perform the procedure, the provider may authorize the medical assistant to perform the audiometry (Figure 30-48).
9. Begin the audiometry with the audiometer set at the lowest frequency.
10. The patient will indicate when the first sound is heard and the medical assistant will plot this information on the appropriate graph (the audiogram).

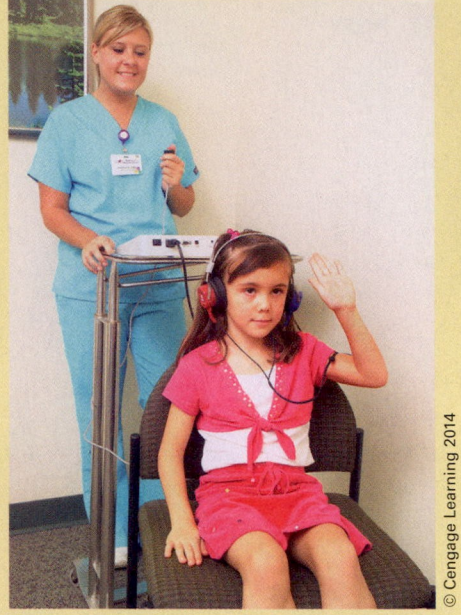

Figure 30-48   The patient raises her hand each time she hears a sound.

11. The frequency is gradually increased and information plotted until the exam is completed.
12. The other ear is checked in the same manner.
13. *Accurately and concisely provide the information to the provider* for interpretation.
14. Clean the equipment as indicated by manufacturer's instructions.
15. Wash hands.
16. Accurately record the procedure in the patient's paper chart or electronic medical record.

DOCUMENTATION:
4/12/20XX 2:00 PM   Audiometry performed. Results given to Dr. Woo. H. Casey, RMA (AMT)—————————

PROCEDURE 30-11
Performing Ear Instillation

STANDARD PRECAUTIONS:

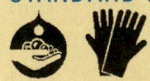

PURPOSE:
To soften impacted cerumen, fight infection with antibiotics, or relieve pain.

EQUIPMENT/SUPPLIES:
Otic medication as prescribed by the provider
Sterile ear dropper
Cotton balls
Gloves

Procedure 30-11 (continued)

PROCEDURE STEPS:

1. Wash hands.
2. *Paying attention to detail,* gather appropriate equipment and supplies.
3. *Introduce yourself and identify patient.*
4. *Explain procedure to the patient, speaking at the patient's level of understanding.*
5. Ask patient either to lie on unaffected side or to sit with head tilted toward unaffected ear. RATIONALE: Facilitates flow of medication.
6. *Paying attention to detail,* check otic medication three times against the provider's order and check expiration date of the medication. RATIONALE: Only otic medication can be used in the ear. Checking the medication three times minimizes medication error.
7. Draw up the prescribed amount of medication.
8. Gently pull the top of the ear upward and back (adult) or pull earlobe downward and backward (child) (Figure 30-49).
9. Instill prescribed dose of medication (number of drops) by squeezing rubber bulb on dropper into the affected ear.
10. Have the patient maintain the position for about 5 minutes to retain medication.
11. When instructed by the provider, insert moistened cotton ball into external ear canal for

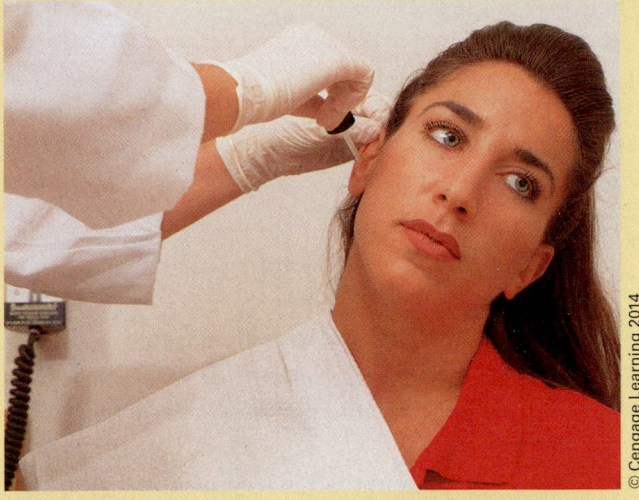

Figure 30-49 When instilling drops into patient's ear, have the patient tilt head so that the affected ear is uppermost.

15 minutes. RATIONALE: Moistened cotton ball will not absorb medication and will help retain medication in ear.

12. Dispose of supplies.
13. Wash hands.
14. Document procedure in patient's chart or electronic medical record.

DOCUMENTATION:

12/10/20XX 4:00 PM   Otic solution (4 drops) instilled into patient's right ear. Moistened cotton ball inserted in ear. No exudate noted. S. Tyler, CMA (AAMA)—————————

 PROCEDURE 30-12

Assisting with Nasal Examination

STANDARD PRECAUTIONS:

PURPOSE:

To assist the provider with the nasal examination when looking for polyps and engorged superficial blood vessels, and to assist in the possible removal of a foreign body.

Patient education:
When a foreign object is involved, instruct the patient not to blow the nose or to attempt to remove the object because this could cause tissue damage or push the object deeper into the nasal passage.

EQUIPMENT/SUPPLIES:

Nasal speculum
Light source
Disposable, nonsterile gloves

continues

Procedure 30-12 (continued)

Bayonet forceps
Kidney basin

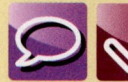

PROCEDURE STEPS:

1. Wash hands.
2. *Paying attention to detail,* gather appropriate equipment and supplies.
3. *Introduce yourself and identify patient.*
4. *Speaking at the level of the patient's understanding, explain the procedure and expectations to the patient.*
5. Assist the patient to sit in a comfortable position.
6. *Allay the patient's fears regarding the procedure being performed and help him feel safe and comfortable.*

7. Assist the provider by handing the equipment and supplies as needed/requested.
8. Appropriately discard disposable supplies according to OSHA guidelines.
9. Sanitize non-disposable instruments following office procedures.
10. Remove gloves and dispose of appropriately.
11. Wash hands.
12. Accurately document procedure in patient's chart or electronic medical record, noting foreign object if applicable.

DOCUMENTATION:

2/4/20XX 4:30 PM   Nasal examination done by Dr. Woo. Small polyp noted in left nostril. Arrangements made with Bayside Surgery for polyp removal on 2/10. H. Casey, RMA (AMT)

PROCEDURE 30-13
Cautery Treatment of Epistaxis

STANDARD PRECAUTIONS:

PURPOSE:

Patient education:
Depending on the location and severity of the nosebleed, the provider will either pack the nasal canal or chemically cauterize the vessel. Generally, chemical cautery is attempted first; if that fails, nasal packing or a nasal balloon is inserted. If cauterization is performed, the patient should be instructed to not blow the nose or otherwise irritate/disturb the scab that will form. Cautery will sting, and the patient should be appropriately prepared.

EQUIPMENT/SUPPLIES:

Patient gown and drapes
Appropriate syringe and needles
Kidney basin
Tissues
Vienna nasal speculum
Hands free light source
Electrocautery

Non-sterile, disposable gloves
PPE as required based on severity of bleeding
Bayonet forceps
Medications as ordered by provider (Xylocaine with epinephrine or cocaine 4%)
Silver nitrate sticks
Cotton balls or 2 × 2 gauze sponges
Nasal packing or nasal tampons
Absorbable packing (Gelfoam or Surigcel)
Medicine cups
Local anesthesia as ordered by provider
Antibiotic/antiseptic ointment

PROCEDURE STEPS:

1. Wash hands.
2. *Paying attention to detail,* gather appropriate equipment and supplies.
3. Provide kidney basin and tissues to allow the patient to manage bleeding until provider can intervene.

Procedure 30-13 (continued)

4. Instruct the patient to pinch all the soft structures of the nose between the thumb and index finger and press against the bones of the face. Have the patient lean forward with his head tilted forward until the provider can intervene.

5. *Introduce yourself and identify patient.*

6. *Speaking at the level of the patient's understanding, explain the procedure and expectations to the patient.*

7. *Allay the patient's fears regarding the procedure being performed and help them feel safe and comfortable.*

8. Assist the patient into a comfortable sitting position.

9. Monitor patient to assure maintenance of airway and breathing.

10. Don non-sterile, disposable gloves.

11. Assist the provider by handing the equipment and supplies as needed/requested.

12. If instructed by the provider, use a syringe and needle to withdraw the prescribed amount of anesthetic (Xylocaine or lidocaine with epinephrine for example) and inject it carefully into a medicine cup being careful to avoid splashing.

13. Soak cotton balls or gauze sponges in the anesthetic agent.

14. As instructed by provider, hand instruments and medication soaked packing as needed.

15. Remain with patient as anesthesia takes effect.

16. Assist the provider as needed to apply vasoconstrictive medication (epinephrine or cocaine) on cotton balls or 2 × 2s to the site of the bleeding.

17. Apply pressure to the external aspect of the nose if instructed by the provider.

18. If the bleeding is controlled, skip to Step 20. If the bleeding is not controlled, prepare electrocautery or silver nitrate sticks per provider preference.

19. If bleeding is controlled, skip to Step 20. If the bleeding continues, prepare nasal packing or nasal tampons per provider preference.

20. *Speaking at the level of the patient's understanding and including the patient's support system,* instruct patient per provider's orders regarding post-epistaxis care. For example:

- Nasal packing should remain in place for 24 to 48 hours
- A follow-up appointment must be made with an otolaryngologist for further treatment
- Avoid aspirin or anti-inflammatory medications

21. Gather and dispose of equipment per OSHA guidelines.

22. Sanitize non-disposable instruments following office procedures.

23. Remove gloves and dispose of appropriately.

24. Wash hands.

25. Accurately document the procedure in the patient's chart or electronic medical record. Include medications, dose, route, time and date, and initials. Document patient education.

DOCUMENTATION:

8/6/20XX 2:45 PM Patient treated for epistaxis with epinephrine and pressure on the exterior of nose and silver nitrate cautery was also used. Bleeding finally controlled with a nasal packing. Instructions given to avoid blowing nose or otherwise irritate/disturb the scab and to call/ return immediately if nose begins to bleed again. S. Tyler, CMA (AAMA)

PATIENT EDUCATION

Nasal Irrigation

Advise the patient that commercial nasal irrigation kits are available at the pharmacy or department store, or the patient can make his own solution of salt and warm water (½ teaspoon salt to a pint of water). Use a bulb-type syringe for irrigation. Instruct patient not to blow nose for 5 minutes after the irrigation. This could force the solution into the sinuses or ears and possibly cause an infection in either or both.

PROCEDURE 30-14
Performing Nasal Instillation

STANDARD PRECAUTIONS:

PURPOSE:
To provide medication to the nasal membranes as ordered by the provider.

Patient education:

1. Instruct the patient to keep the head tilted back slightly during the procedure to allow the medication to cover the nasal tissues.

2. Do not blow nose immediately after treatment. Medication could be forced out of nose.

EQUIPMENT/SUPPLIES:
Nasal medication as prescribed by provider
Sterile dropper (if required)
Tissues
Nonsterile disposable gloves

PROCEDURE STEPS:

1. Wash hands.

2. *Paying attention to detail,* gather appropriate equipment and supplies.

3. *Introduce yourself and identify patient.*

4. *Speaking at the level of the patient's understanding, explain the procedure and expectations to the patient.*

5. Assist the patient to sit comfortably with the head tilted back slightly.

6. *Paying attention to detail,* compare the nasal medication to the provider's order (first check).

7. Check the expiration date.

8. If the medication is not a single-user, self-contained dropper, calculate the medication.

9. Compare the medication and the provider's order (second check).

10. Don nonsterile disposable gloves if indicated.

11. Compare the medication and the provider's order (third check).

12. Utilize the sterile dropper or the self-contained dropper with the medication ready into the center of the nostril. Take care not to touch the inside of the nasal passage. RATIONALE: Touching the inside of the nostril will lead to contamination of the dropper.

13. Instruct the patient to inhale during the instillation of the nasal drops.

14. Instill the prescribed dose (correct number of drops).

15. Repeat the procedure for the other nostril if ordered.

16. Provide tissues to the patient for management of any drainage.

17. *Speaking at the level of the patient's understanding,* instruct the patient not to blow nose after treatment in order to keep the medication in contact with the mucous membranes of the nasal passages. RATIONALE: Allow time for medication to be absorbed by the nasal membranes.

18. If utilizing a dropper, dispose of properly per OSHA guidelines. If non-disposable, follow office procedure for sanitization and sterilization. If utilizing a self-contained medication, recap using sterile technique.

19. Remove gloves and dispose of appropriately.

20. Wash hands.

21. Accurately record the administration of medication to include name of medication, dose, route, date, time and initials.

DOCUMENTATION:
4/13/20XX 6:00 PM   Neosynephrine nasal drops (3 drops) instilled into each nostril. S. Tyler, CMA (AAMA)————————

PROCEDURE 30-15

Administer Oxygen by Nasal Cannula for Minor Respiratory Distress

STANDARD PRECAUTIONS:

PURPOSE:

To provide a low dose of concentrated oxygen to a patient during periods of respiratory distress (e.g., chronic obstructive pulmonary disease).

Patient education:

1. Demonstrate the position of the nasal prongs of the cannula into the nose. They face upward and the tab rests above the upper lip.

2. Describe how to clear the oxygen cylinder valve by turning it counterclockwise.

3. Oxygen supports combustion and a fire can start with oxygen in use. Friction, static electricity, a spark, or a lighted cigarette or cigar can cause ignition.

EQUIPMENT/SUPPLIES:

Portable D cylinder oxygen tank with stand
Disposable nasal cannula with 6 ft tubing
Flowmeter with Christmas tree adapter
Pressure regulator with gauge

PROCEDURE STEPS:

1. Wash hands.

2. *Paying attention to detail,* gather appropriate equipment and supplies.

3. *Introduce yourself and identify patient.*

4. *Speaking at the level of the patient's understanding, explain the procedure and expectations to the patient.*

5. *Allay the patient's fears regarding the procedure and help her feel safe and comfortable.*

6. Open the cylinder with one full turn in a counterclockwise direction.

7. Check the pressure gauge to assure that oxygen is present in the tank. RATIONALE: This will determine the amount of pressure in the cylinder.

8. Attach the nasal cannula and tubing to the Christmas tree adapter on the flowmeter.

9. Adjust the flow rate according to the provider's order (first check).

10. Check the nasal cannula to assure that oxygen is flowing.

11. Check the flow rate and the provider's order (second check).

12. Carefully place the nasal cannula into the nares of the patient with the tips curving inward to follow the curve of the nasal passage and the tab resting below the nose (Figure 30-50). Check with patient for comfort. Compare the flow rate and the provider's order (third check).

13. Adjust the tubing around the patient's ears and adjust slide for comfort under the chin (Figure 30-51).

14. Instruct the patient to breathe slowly through her nose in order to achieve the maximum benefit from oxygen therapy.

15. Oxygen is flammable. Instruct the patient and family members that smoking is not allowed near the patient.

16. Wash hands.

17. Accurately document the procedure in patient's chart or electronic medical record to include name of medication, dose, route, date, time and initials.

NOTE: Oxygen is usually humidified to prevent drying of respiratory mucosa (Figure 30-52).

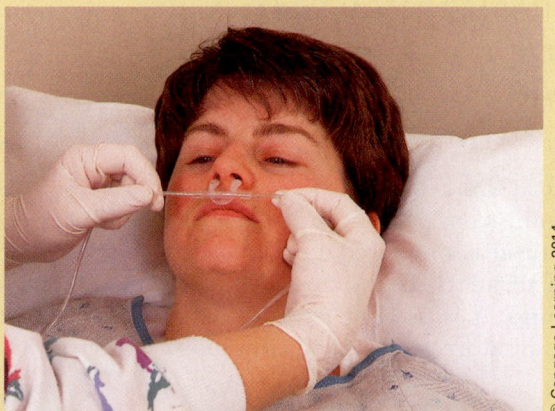

© Cengage Learning 2014

Figure 30-50 Insert cannula prong into nostrils.

continues

Procedure 30-15 (continued)

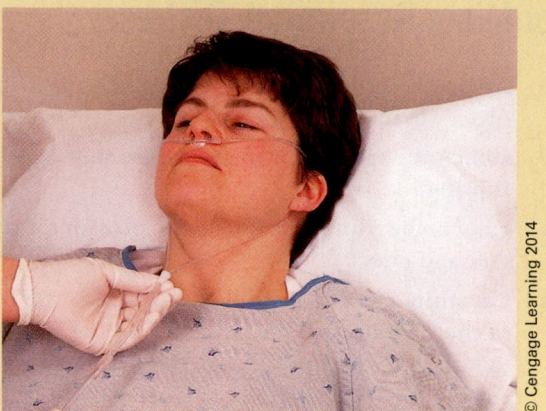

Figure 30-51 Adjust tubing.

DOCUMENTATION:

4/19/20XX 2:45 PM   Oxygen 3 L/minute by nasal cannula.
Color slightly improved. Less cyanosis. S. Tyler, CMA (AAMA)——

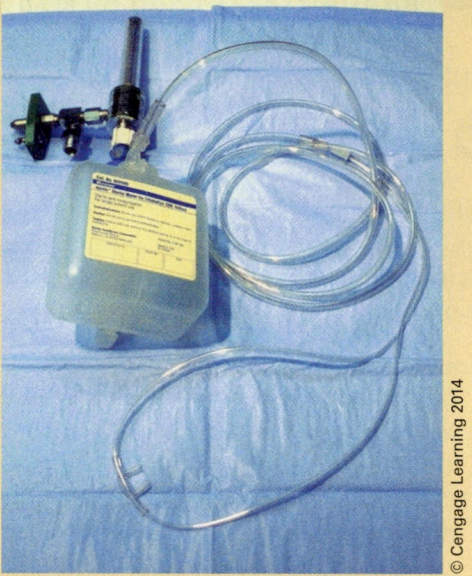

Figure 30-52 Nasal cannula and oxygen tubing attached to a humidifier.

PROCEDURE 30-16

Instructing Patient in the Use of a Metered Dose Inhaler With and Without a Spacer

STANDARD PRECAUTIONS:

PURPOSE:

To instruct patient on the use of a handheld device known as a metered dose inhaler. The device delivers medication to the respiratory tract including the lungs. It is used to treat asthma, COPD, and other respiratory diseases and conditions.

Patient education:
1. Remind the patient to inhale slowly.
2. Close the mouth and lips around the mouthpiece.

3. Clean the inhaler by rinsing the mouthpiece in warm water.
4. Adhere to prescribed dose.

EQUIPMENT/SUPPLIES:
Handheld inhaler with mouth piece
Spacer
Medication as ordered by practitioner

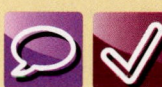

PROCEDURE STEPS:
1. Wash hands.
2. ***Paying attention to detail,*** gather appropriate equipment and supplies (see Figure 30-53).

Procedure 30-16 (continued)

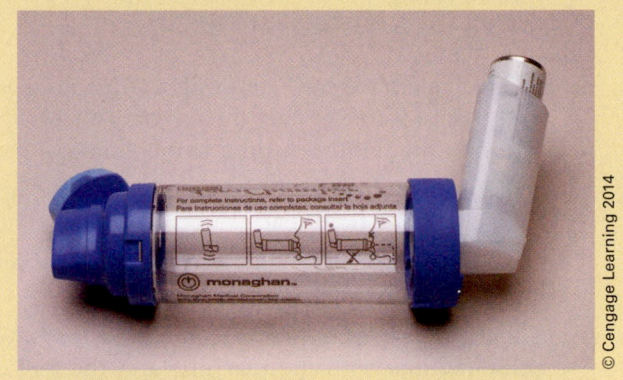

Figure 30-53   Metered dose inhaler and spacer.

3. Check the medication and the provider's order (first check).

4. *Introduce yourself and identify patient.*

5. *Speaking at the level of the patient's understanding, explain the procedure and expectations to the patient.*

6. Check the medication and the provider's order (second check).

7. Instruct the patient regarding:

   A. The purpose of using the medication via the metered dose inhaler as it relates to the diagnosis

   B. The dose and frequency of the medication

   C. Breathing out completely prior to administering the dose

   D. Shaking the inhaler to mobilize the medication

   E. Inserting the mouthpiece between the teeth and closing the lips to create a seal

   F. Breathing in slowly while simultaneously pressing the top of the inhaler once. RATIONALE: Releases medication.

   G. Removing the inhaler from the mouth

   H. Holding breath for at least 10 seconds. RATIONALE: Medication can enter into lungs well.

   I. Breathing out completely

   J. Waiting 30 seconds if an additional dose is required

   K. Shaking the inhaler again and repeating steps C–I. RATIONALE: To mix medication thoroughly.

   L. Rinsing the mouth, especially if the inhaled medication contains a steroid. RATIONALE: Prevents dry mouth, hoarseness, and micro-organism growth.

8. Check the medication and the provider's order (third check).

9. If a spacer is to be used, skip to Step 14.

10. Review and simulate the use of the metered dose inhaler (MDI) and then have the patient return the demonstration.

11. After administration of the dose, note any patient condition changes or comments. Record in the patient record.

12. Replace the cap on the MDI when finished.

13. Instruct the patient on the care of the MDI to include:

    • Storing at room temperature

    • After use, removing the metal canister from the plastic mouth piece and spacer (if utilized) and cleaning with mild soap and water and leaving to dry overnight

    • Never using water on the metal canister

    • Reassembling the MDI

    • Reloading the MDI by spraying a puff into the air prior to the next dose

14. If a spacer is to be used, instruct the patient on assembly:

    • Remove the cap on the MDI

    • Insert the MDI into the appropriate end of the spacer

15. Follow Step 7 to 12 above.

16. Accurately document in patient's chart or electronic medical record the administration of medication to include name of medication, dose, route, date, time and initials. Document patient education.

DOCUMENTATION:

4/19/20XX 2:45 PM   Instructed patient on use of handheld metered dose inhaler. Patient encouraged to cough following procedure. Performed procedure well. No adverse reactions noted. W. Slawson, CMA (AAMA)—

© Cengage Learning 2014

PROCEDURE 30-17

Spirometry

STANDARD PRECAUTIONS:

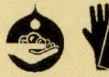

PURPOSE:

To prepare a patient for a spirometry to obtain optimum test results. To assist with diagnosis of asthma and chronic obstructive pulmonary disease (COPD).

Patient education:

1. Reinforce the importance of good posture during the process. RATIONALE: Good posture expands lungs more fully.

2. When blowing into the mouthpiece, the lips must seal tightly around it.

3. Explain the parameters needed for successful completion of the test.

Parameters:

1. Patient must refrain from the use of bronchodilators and tobacco for 24 hours before test.

2. Explain to the patient that maximum effort is required for accurate test results.

3. Patient must inhale deeply and quickly and exhale quickly and forcibly until no air can be expelled.

EQUIPMENT/SUPPLIES:

Spirometer
Disposable mouthpiece

PROCEDURE STEPS:

1. Wash hands.

2. *Paying attention to detail,* gather appropriate equipment and supplies.

3. *Introduce yourself and identify patient.*

4. *Speaking at the level of the patient's understanding, explain the procedure and expectations to the patient.*

5. *Allay the patient's fears regarding the procedure and help him feel safe and comfortable.*

6. Include the following in the patient education:

   • The patient should not have eaten a large meal before the test.

   • The use of tobacco products must have been avoided for 4–6 hours prior to the spirometry.

   • The patient will have received instructions from the provider regarding the use of bronchodilators or other inhalers prior to the testing.

   • When exhaling into the mouthpiece, the lips must form a tight seal.

   • Maximum effort is required for accurate test results.

7. Allow the patient to practice several times to become familiar with the machine and the feel of the testing.

8. Enter patient demographic data as required by the spirometry program. This will include the patient's height and weight.

9. Place the nose clip on the patient's nose to assure that all exhalation occurs via the oral airway.

10. Place the disposable mouthpiece on the spirometer.

11. Instruct the patient that several readings may be needed to assure accurate test results for interpretation by the provider.

12. Remind the patient to exhale forcibly and rapidly until unable to exhale any more air. RATIONALE: Provides more accurate results.

13. Coach the patient during the inhalation and exhalation in order to achieve maximum results. Instruct the patient that he must continue to exhale until instructed to stop.

14. Remind the patient to remain upright during the exhalation. RATIONALE: Helps patient take as large an inhalation and exhalation as possible.

15. *Be supportive and encouraging throughout the test. Attend to any special needs of the patients.*

16. At the conclusion of the procedure, discard the disposable mouth piece into a biohazard container. Disinfect and sanitize the equipment per policy.

17. Wash hands.

18. *Concisely update the provider* with the results of the spirometry for interpretation.

19. Accurately record the procedure, the patient's tolerance of the procedure, and patient education. Affix the record of the spirometry in the patient's chart or scan into the medical record.

DOCUMENTATION:

12/22/20XX 4:00 PM   Spirometry performed. Results given to Dr. Woo. H. Casey, RMA (AMT)

PROCEDURE 30-18

Pulse Oximetry

STANDARD PRECAUTIONS:

PURPOSE:

To measure arterial oxyhemoglobin saturation within seconds by using an external sensor.

EQUIPMENT/SUPPLIES:

Pulse oximeter
Sensor
Soap and water or alcohol wipe
Nail polish remover, if needed

PROCEDURE STEPS:

1. Wash hands.

2. *Paying attention to detail,* gather appropriate equipment and supplies.

3. *Introduce yourself and identify patient.*

4. *Speaking at the level of the patient's understanding, explain the procedure and expectations to the patient.*

5. Select a site for the sensor. A finger is usually chosen, but other sensors are available for the forehead or the earlobe. Adequate circulation is required for an accurate reading, so move to other sites if fingers are cold or peripheral vascular disease limits circulation to the hands.

6. Make sure the site is clean. If fingers are to be utilized, have the patient wash hands with soap and water. If fingernail polish is present, remove. If a site other than the hands is to be utilized, clean with an alcohol prep pad. **RATIONALE:**

Fingernail polish inhibits infrared light from passing through the oximeter.

7. Secure the sensor to the cable. Assure a tight connection between the cable and the pulse oximeter (see Figure 30-21).

8. Apply the sensor to the selected site. If applied to a finger, insert the finger into the sensor clip. For an earlobe, insert as much of the earlobe as possible into the specialized sensor. If a forehead is to be utilized, apply the appropriate sensor and secure with adhesive strip provided.

9. Turn the pulse oximeter on. A tone can be heard and a pulse fluxuation can be seen on the digital readout. Adjust the volume.

10. Review the alarm parameters.

11. Palpate the patient's pulse and compare to the digital representation of the pulse to assure an accurate reading.

12. Refer to manufacturer's information if troubleshooting is required.

13. *Accurately and concisely update the provider* with results.

14. Accurately document procedure in patient's chart or electronic medical record, noting type of sensor used, site of application, and results.

15. Plug in oximeter for recharging when not in use so that the battery does not get low. *NOTE:* When measuring, cover the sensor with a towel to eliminate sensor's exposure to light. It could interfere with the sensor and give incorrect results.

DOCUMENTATION:

3/16/20XX 4:00 PM   Pulse oximetry 98%. S. Thomas, CMA (AAMA)—————————————————————

PROCEDURE 30-19

Assisting with Plaster Cast Application

STANDARD PRECAUTIONS:

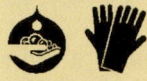

PURPOSE:
To assist provider in cast application.

EQUIPMENT/SUPPLIES:
Cast material:
Plaster or fiberglass casting material
Container or warm water with liner
Stockinette (diameter based on limb to be immobilized)
Webril or similar rolled padding material
Bandage scissors
Casting gloves
Waterproof pad

PROCEDURE STEPS:

1. Wash hands.

2. *Paying attention to detail,* gather appropriate equipment and supplies.

3. *Introduce yourself and identify patient.*

4. *Speaking at the level of the patient's understanding, explain the procedure and expectations to the patient.*

5. *Allay the patient's fears and help him feel safe and comfortable.*

6. Remove clothing that could interfere with cast application and provide a gown, sheet, and warm blanket to the patient.

7. *Attending to any special needs of the patient,* assist him into position per provider's orders for comfort and ease of cast application. RATIONALE: Proper alignment ensures fracture heals properly.

8. Medicate per provider's orders.

9. Drape the area of cast application, including applying a waterproof pad under the extremity to be casted.

10. Don non-sterile disposable casting gloves.

11. Cleanse the area to be casted per provider's orders.

12. Dry the area completely.

13. Accurately document any areas of skin lesions, soft-tissue injuries and neurovascular status as indicated per provider in the patient's chart or electronic medical record. RATIONALE: Appropriate documentation of skin condition is needed to assist in evaluation of the extremity at a later time.

14. Select the appropriate diameter of stockinette for the extremity to be casted. If too tight, it can cause neurovascular impairment. It too large, it can wrinkle and contribute to skin breakdown.

15. Measure stockinette to a length long enough to cover the area to be casted. Add 2 to 3 inches to each end of the measurement to allow for stockinette to fold back over the casting material and provide a smooth finish and padded edge. RATIONALE: A stockinette that is too large will form creases, thus allowing for injury to tissues.

16. Assist the provider with the correct width of Webril or other padded roll material. RATIONALE: Webril (soft cotton bandage) provides protection to the patient's skin, preventing pressure sores. Folds in the padding could lead to irritation of the skin.

17. Assist the provider with the alignment and immobilization of the extremity while applying the stockinette and padding. This will provide comfort for the patient. RATIONALE: Protects from pressure.

18. When instructed by the provider, immerse the chosen casting material in water per manufacturer's instructions.

19. Upon removal from the water bath, gently squeeze the cast material roll to remove excess water. Do not wring.

20. Assist with the application of casting material per provider's request/instruction.

21. *Reassure patient as needed.*

22. After completion of cast material application, support the extremity in a manner that will not distort the molding of the cast material.

23. Clean the area. Remove any plaster from the patient's exposed skin.

24. Evaluate the neurovascular status of the affected area. Document in the patient's chart or electronic medical record. *Notify the provider immediately* of any abnormal findings. RATIONALE: Reviewing possible complications with the patient enhances the immediate reporting of circulatory impairment and infection.

Procedure 30-19 (continued)

25. Per office policy or provider order, furnish and review written cast care and after care instructions with the patient, ***including the patient's support system.***

26. Discard the water bath in the sink or hopper using extreme care not to allow any casting material to enter the drain.

27. Discard the liner containing the plaster or other residue in the trash receptacle.

28. Remove gloves and dispose of appropriately.

29. Wash hands.

30. Schedule follow up appointment for cast check.

31. Accurately record the casting procedure, the neurovascular status of the affected limb, all patient education, and the date for follow up in the patient's chart or electronic medical record.

DOCUMENTATION:

12/14/20XX 2:00 PM   Plaster cast applied to left arm by Dr. King. Fingers warm to touch. Patient says there is no tingling or numbness in her fingers. Instructed about cast care, exercises, and reporting of circulatory impairment and infection. Sling applied. Next appointment 12/28/20XX. H. Casey, RMA (AMT)————

PROCEDURE 30-20

Assisting with Cast Removal

STANDARD PRECAUTIONS:

PURPOSE:

To assist the provider with removal of a cast.

EQUIPMENT/SUPPLIES:

Cast cutter
Cast spreader
Bandage scissors
Bag for disposing of cast materials
Drape

PROCEDURE STEPS:

1. Wash hands.

2. ***Paying attention to detail,*** gather appropriate equipment and supplies.

3. ***Introduce yourself and identify patient.***

4. ***Speaking at the level of the patient's understanding, explain the procedure and expectations to the patient.***

5. Drape the area of cast removal, taking care to protect the patient's clothing.

6. ***Allay the patient's fears and help them feel safe and comfortable.*** Explain that the cast cutter will not damage soft tissue as it vibrates, it does not spin. RATIONALE: Explaining the procedure reduces apprehension and fears about being cut with the blade.

7. Explain that there may be a sensation of warmth and some pressure during the cutting of the cast.

8. Assist the provider by handing instruments and supplies as requested.

9. Once the cast has been removed, cleanse the area under the cast of excess skin and dry completely.

10. Reassure the patient that muscle tone will return with physical therapy.

11. Remove gloves and dispose of appropriately.

12. Wash hands.

13. Follow office policy or provider's orders to provide written instructions for after care.

14. ***Follow up with collateral allied health professionals to optimize the patient's plan of care*** by arranging physical therapy follow up.

15. Accurately record removal of the cast. Be sure to document skin, neurovascular, and bony assessment per provider's orders. Document patient teaching. RATIONALE: Condition of the patient's arm size, skin appearance, and color are important factors to note for future evaluation.

DOCUMENTATION:

6/12/20XX 2:45 PM   Cast removed from left arm by Dr. King. Arm seems slightly atrophied. Skin color good, circulation seems good. Patient given skin care instructions. Appointment for physical therapy scheduled for 6/14/XX at 3:00 PM. S. Tyler, CMA (AAMA)————

PROCEDURE 30-21

Fecal Occult Blood Test

STANDARD PRECAUTIONS:

PURPOSE:

To test feces for occult blood.

EQUIPMENT/SUPPLIES:

Three occult slide test kits containing three slides, applicators, and envelope

PROCEDURE STEPS:

1. *Paying attention to detail,* check the expiration dates on the slides. RATIONALE: Outdated slides can give an inaccurate reading.

2. *Introduce yourself and identify patient.*

3. Complete the information on the front flap of all three slide packages (Figure 30-54).

4. *Explain the procedure, speaking at the patient's level of understanding* as follows:

   • Keep slides at room temperature.

   • Obtain a stool specimen in a clean, dry container.

   • Write date of collection on the front flap and then open the packet.

   • Use one end of the wooden applicator to apply a thin smear of the stool sample from the container to Box "A" on the slide. *NOTE: Do not collect during menstrual cycle or if hemorrhoids are present.*

   • Repeat the procedure using the other end of the applicator, obtaining a sample from a different area of the stool specimen and applying a thin smear to Box "B." RATIONALE: Occult blood may be distributed differently throughout a bowel movement.

   • Dispose of the applicator appropriately.

   • Close the cover after air drying overnight.

   • Repeat the process with the next two bowel movements, on subsequent days.

5. Provide the patient with an envelope to return the slides to the provider's office. Review with the patient instructions on diet and medication (Figure 30-55). RATIONALE: Slides are considered biohazardous material.

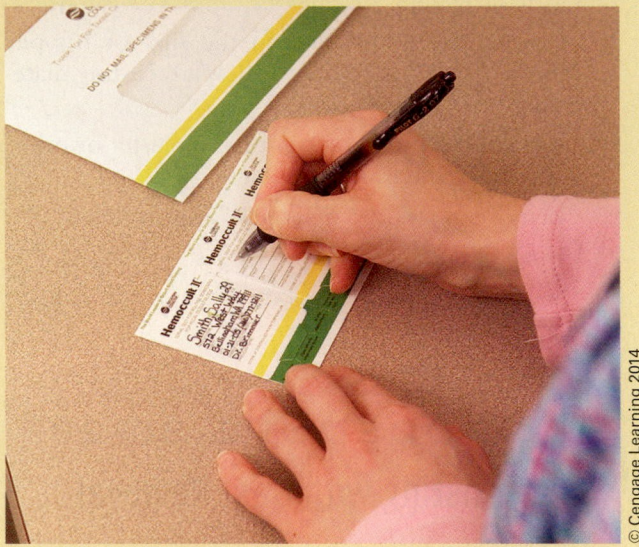

© Cengage Learning 2014

Figure 30-54 The medical assistant writes the patient's name, the date, and the specimen number on each occult slide.

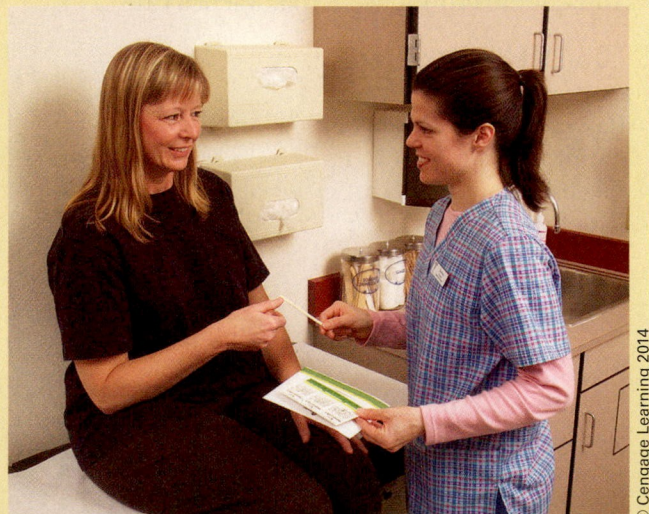

© Cengage Learning 2014

Figure 30-55 The medical assistant explains the process to the patient.

6. Instruct the patient NOT to mail the slides to the provider's office.

7. Accurately record all information regarding instructions and provision of test kits in patient's chart or electronic medical record.

Procedure 30-21 (continued)

Developing the Fecal Occult Slide

When the patient returns the fecal occult samples to the clinic, the medical assistant is responsible for developing the slides. Although most slides can be stored for up to 14 days before developing, the medical assistant should develop them as soon as possible because the patient may have already stored them for several days. Test results are important to ensure prompt treatment should a problem be discovered.

EQUIPMENT/SUPPLIES:

Prepared fecal slides from patient
Occult blood developer
Reference card that accompanies kit
Nonsterile disposable gloves
Clock or watch with a second hand

PROCEDURE STEPS:

1. Wash hands and check the expiration date on the label of the developer, *paying attention to detail.*

2. Don nonsterile disposable gloves.

3. Establish a work area in a well-lit environment by covering a flat, dry surface with surface protections such as paper towels.

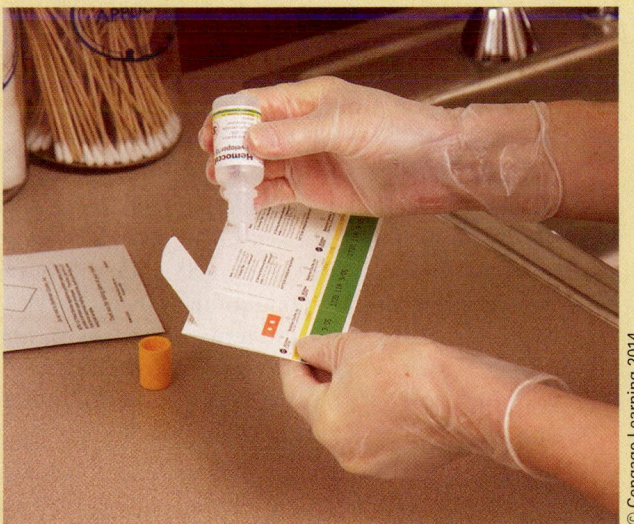

© Cengage Learning 2014

Figure 30-56   The medical assistant places developing solution on the slides.

4. Refer to package directions if unsure of the procedure.

5. Open the window flap on the back of the slide packet.

6. Apply two drops of the developer to each Box, "A" and "B," directly over each smear (Figure 30-56). RATIONALE: Paper contains the chemical guaiac, which will help identify occult blood.

7. Using a watch with a second hand, interpret the results within 30 to 60 seconds or per manufacturer's instructions.

8. A positive reaction consists of a blue halo appearing around the perimeter of the specimen. Any blue color is positive.

9. Perform the quality-control procedure by processing the positive and negative monitor strip on each slide to confirm the test system is functional. RATIONALE: Failure of the positive strip to turn blue or of the negative strip to remain neutral indicates faulty supplies. Recheck expiration dates on slide and developer. Repeat test if necessary.

10. Dispose of all supplies according to OSHA guidelines.

11. Remove gloves and dispose in appropriate biohazard waste container.

12. Wash hands.

13. Accurately, record all information in patient's chart or electronic medical record.

DOCUMENTATION:

1/14/20XX 2:00 PM   Given 3 occult slides, 3 wooden applicators, and an envelope with instructions. Instructed patient on dietary restrictions, collection of the stool specimens, and need to keep the slides at room temperature, away from sunlight. Patient instructed to bring specimens to clinic. S. Tyler, CMA (AAMA)——————

5/12/20XX 3:00 PM   Three hemoccult slides returned. Results: all three slides negative. Reported to Dr. Woo. Dr. Woo wants patient notified of results and to remind patient to make an appointment with her gastroenterologist for a colonoscopy. Spoke to patient. Understands slides were negative for hidden blood in the stool. She will make an appointment for a colonoscopy. S. Tyler, CMA (AAMA)——————

PROCEDURE 30-22
Urinary Catheterization of a Male Patient

STANDARD PRECAUTIONS:

PURPOSE:

To obtain a sterile urine specimen for analysis or to relieve urinary retention.

EQUIPMENT/SUPPLIES:

Catheterization kit (commercially available) containing:
- Sterile gloves
- Betadine® solution or swabs
- Lubricant
- Sterile fenestrated drape
- Sterile cotton balls
- Sterile urine container with label
- Sterile 2 × 2 gauze sponges
- Forceps (sterile)
- Sterile absorbent plastic pad

Additional supplies needed:
- Sterile catheter (size and type as ordered by provider)
- Biohazard waste container

PROCEDURE STEPS:

1. Wash hands and follow Standard Precautions.
2. *Introduce yourself and identify patient.*
3. *Explain the procedure, speaking at the patient's level of understanding. Allay the patient's fears and help him to feel safe and comfortable.*
4. Wash hands.
5. *Paying attention to detail,* assemble equipment.
6. Place unopened catheter kit on Mayo stand near the patent.
7. Provide good lighting.
8. *Being courteous and respectful,* have the patient disrobe below the waist and provide a drape, *respecting patient's personal boundaries.* Cover from umbilical area to pubic hairline.
9. *Attending to any special needs of the patient,* assist the patient into position lying on his back with knees slightly bent and legs separated on the examination table. RATIONALE: This allows for access to the urinary meatus.
10. Drape patient with sheet exposing only the external genitalia.
11. Wash hands.
12. Open outer wrapping of the sterile kit. This becomes the sterile field (Figure 30-57A). RATIONALE: Provides sterile field.
13. Utilizing sterile principles, place sterile absorbent plastic pad under patient's buttocks. Touching only the corners, empty contents of tray onto sterile field. Drape perineal area with fenestrated drape. Add sterile catheter to field.
14. This will place the sterile catheter tray between the patient's legs. Open catheter using sterile technique and place on the sterile field.
15. Ask patient to keep knees apart.
16. Apply sterile gloves.
17. Open fenestrated drape and, being careful not to contaminate drape or gloves, position drape opening over penis (Figure 30-57B).
18. Pour Betadine® over three cotton balls in appropriate compartment of the kit or open Betadine® swabs.
19. Open urine specimen container.
20. Apply sterile lubricant to a gauze sponge and place tip of catheter in lubricant.
21. Instruct patient to breathe slowly and deeply during procedure.
22. With nondominant hand, hold the penis just below the glans. In uncircumcised males, the glans must be pulled back to expose the meatus. This must be done entirely with the nondominant hand. RATIONALE: The dominant hand remains sterile so as not to contaminate remaining sterile equipment.
23. With the dominant hand, taking the Betadine® swabs or sterile forceps and a cotton ball that has been saturated with Betadine®, cleanse the meatus in a circular motion from the center to the outside of the glans. Use all three cotton balls or swabs (Figure 30-58). RATIONALE: Ensures that as many microorganisms as possible will be removed from the meatus and surrounding areas before insertion of sterile catheter.
24. Using the dominant, sterile gloved hand, pick up the catheter. While holding the head of the

Procedure 30-22 (continued)

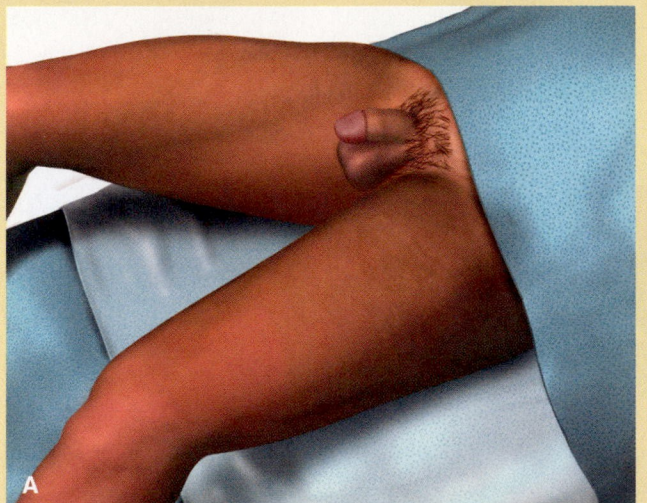

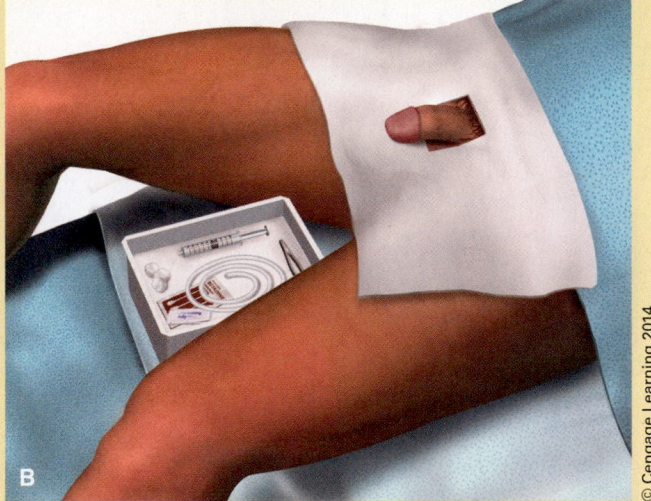

Figure 30-57 (A) First, have patient bend knees and separate legs. Then, place sterile underpad between patient's legs. (B) Open fenestrated drape. Be careful not to contaminate sterile underpad or drape. Place over penis.

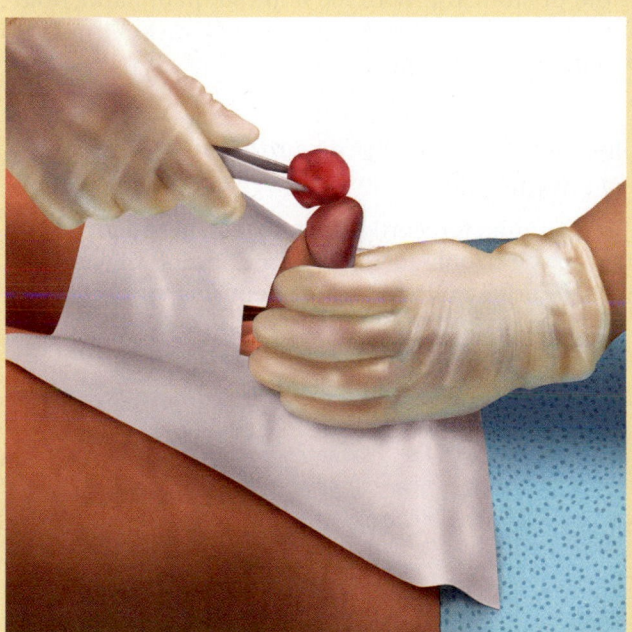

Figure 30-58 With dominant hand, take the sterile forceps and a cotton ball dipped in Betadine solution and cleanse around the urinary meatus moving from the center toward the outside. Use all three cotton balls and Betadine.

penis upright and straight with the nondominant hand, insert the catheter slowly approximately 6 inches until the urine begins to flow (Figure 30-59). RATIONALE: Holding the penis by the glans so that the penis will be upright and straight facilitates insertion of the catheter. CAUTION: Do not force the catheter. If problems arise attempting insertion, do not continue the procedure and notify the provider.

25. Interrupt urine flow by clamping or pinching off.

26. Position end of catheter into urine specimen container.

27. Collect specimen by releasing clamp and collecting approximately 60 mL of urine.

28. Allow remaining urine to flow into basin until flow ceases. Pinch catheter closed.

29. Remove catheter gently and slowly.

30. Clean Betadine® from penis with remaining cotton balls.

31. Tighten lid on the urine specimen container.

32. Remove procedure items and dispose of appropriately in biohazard waste container.

33. Remove sterile gloves and discard appropriately in biohazard waste container.

34. Position patient for comfort.

35. *Attending to any special needs,* assist the patient to sit on the edge of the table or relaxing in a horizontal recumbent position.

36. Offer tissues for cleanup of lubricant.

37. When patient is ready for sitting up, assess patient's color and pulse. Take blood pressure if indicated.

38. Don nonsterile disposable gloves.

Procedure 30-22 (continued)

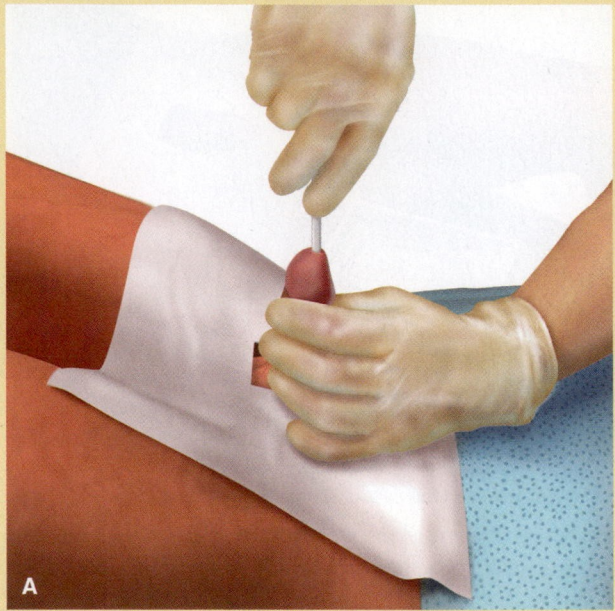
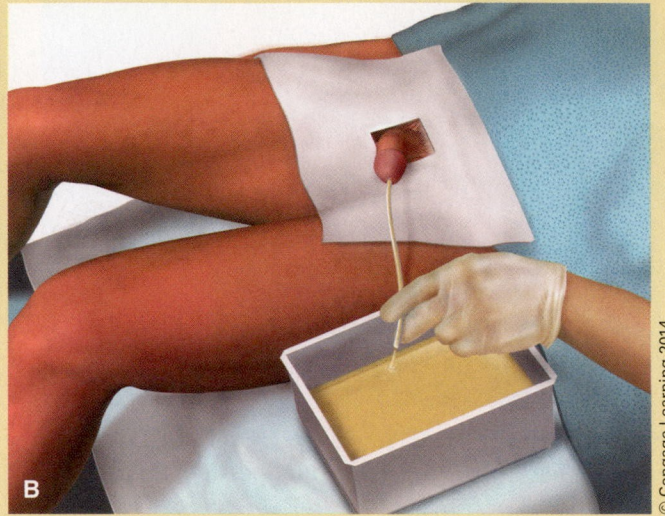

© Cengage Learning 2014

Figure 30-59   (A) With the dominant hand, take catheter out of lubricant. With the nondominant hand, hold the head of the penis so that the penis is an upright, straight position. Insert the catheter about 6 inches until urine flows into the sterile kit. (B) Obtain a specimen if ordered.

39. Dispose of items utilized per Occupational Safety and Health Administration (OSHA) guidelines.

40. If collecting urine specimen for analysis, label specimen container and attach to completed laboratory requisition form. Place in biohazard transportation bag.

41. Remove gloves and dispose of appropriately.

42. Wash hands.

43. Assist patient from examination table.

44. Don nonsterile disposable gloves.

45. Clean room and table.

46. Remove gloves and discard appropriately.

47. Wash hands.

48. Accurately record all information in patient's chart or electronic medical record, noting the amount of urine collected. Document that specimen was sent to outside laboratory (if appropriate).

DOCUMENTATION:

9/07/20XX 10:15 AM   Catheterized with straight catheter to relieve urinary retention. 700 mL clear urine obtained. S. Tyler, CMA (AAMA)

PROCEDURE 30-23

Urinary Catheterization of a Female Patient

STANDARD PRECAUTIONS:

PURPOSE:
To obtain a sterile urine specimen for analysis or to relieve urinary retention.

EQUIPMENT/SUPPLIES:
Catheterization kit (commercially available) containing:
   Sterile gloves
   Betadine® solution or swabs
   Lubricant
   Sterile fenestrated drape

Procedure 30-23 (continued)

Sterile cotton balls
Sterile urine container with label
Sterile 2 × 2 gauze sponges
Forceps (sterile)
Sterile absorbent plastic pad
Additional supplies needed:
Sterile catheter (size and type as ordered by provider)
Biohazard waste container

PROCEDURE STEPS:

1. Wash hands and follow Standard Precautions.
2. *Introduce yourself and identify patient.*
3. *Explain the procedure, speaking at the patient's level of understanding.*
4. Wash hands.
5. *Paying attention to detail,* assemble equipment.
6. Place unopened catheter kit on Mayo stand near the patient.
7. Provide good lighting.
8. *Being courteous and respectful,* have the patient disrobe below the waist and provide a drape, *protecting the patient's personal boundaries.*
9. *Attending to the special needs of the patient,* assist the patient into the dorsal lithotomy position on the examination table. RATIONALE: This allows for access to the urinary meatus.
10. Drape patient with sheet exposing only the external genitalia.
11. Wash hands.
12. Open outer wrapping of the sterile kit. This becomes the sterile field.
13. Utilizing sterile principles, place sterile absorbent plastic pad under patient's buttocks. Touching only the corners, empty contents of tray onto sterile field. Drape perineal area with fenestrated drape. Add sterile catheter to field.
14. This will place the sterile catheter trap between the patient's legs. Open catheter using sterile technique and place on the sterile field.
15. Ask patient to keep knees apart. RATIONALE: This position provides good visualization of the urinary meatus.
16. Apply sterile gloves.
17. Pour Betadine® over three cotton balls in appropriate compartment of the kit or open Betadine® swabs.

18. Open urine specimen container.
19. Apply sterile lubricant to a gauze sponge and place tip of catheter in lubricant.
20. Instruct patient to breathe slowly and deeply during procedure. RATIONALE: This helps the patient relax the abdominal and pelvic muscles and facilitates easier insertion of the catheter.
21. Spread labia with nondominant hand. Dominant hand remains sterile. With dominant hand and sterile forceps, wipe genitalia with each of three antiseptic soaked cotton balls or Betadine® swabs with a front to back motion. First wipe the right labia using a front to back motion. Discard cotton ball or swab into biohazard waste container. Second, wipe the left labia with cotton ball or swab and discard. Lastly, wipe down the center with the cotton ball or swab, discarding after each wipe. Discard forceps if used. Continue to hold labia apart until catheter is inserted. RATIONALE: Holding labia open will keep urinary meatus from becoming contaminated while inserting catheter.
22. Using sterile gloved hand, pick up the catheter and hold it 3 to 4 inches from lubricated end. The other end of the catheter should remain in the sterile tray.
23. Gently insert lubricated tip of the catheter into the urinary meatus approximately 6 inches or until urine begins to flow.
24. Interrupt urine flow by clamping or pinching off. RATIONALE: Stop flow of urine while specimen container is positioned.
25. Position end of catheter into urine specimen container.
26. If urinalysis is required, wait until catheterization is complete and pour urine into sterile container.
27. Collect specimen by releasing clamp and collecting approximately 60 mL of urine.
28. Allow remaining urine to flow into basin until flow ceases. Pinch catheter closed.
29. Remove catheter gently and slowly.
30. Clean Betadine® from perineum with remaining cotton balls.
31. Tighten lid on the urine specimen container.
32. Remove procedure items and dispose of appropriately in biohazard waste containers.
33. Remove sterile gloves and discard appropriately in biohazard waste container.

continues

Procedure 30-23 (continued)

34. Position patient for comfort.

35. *Attending to any special needs,* assist the patient to sit on the edge of the table or relax in a horizontal recumbent position.

36. Offer tissues for cleanup of lubricant.

37. When patient is ready for sitting up, assess patient's color and pulse. Take blood pressure if indicated.

38. Don nonsterile disposable gloves.

39. Dispose of items utilized per Occupational Safety and Health Administration (OSHA) guidelines.

40. If collecting urine specimen for analysis, label specimen container and attach to completed laboratory requisition form. Place in biohazard transportation bag.

41. Remove gloves and dispose of appropriately.

42. Wash hands.

43. Assist patient from examination table.

44. Don nonsterile disposable gloves.

45. Clean room and table.

46. Remove gloves and discard appropriately.

47. Wash hands.

48. Accurately record all information in patient's chart or electronic medical record, noting the amount of urine collected. Document that specimen was sent to outside laboratory (if appropriate).

DOCUMENTATION:

9/07/20XX 10:15 AM   Catheterized with straight catheter to relieve urinary retention and to obtain specimen for urinalysis. 700 mL clear urine obtained. Urine specimen sent to laboratory with requisition for urinalysis. S. Tyler, CMA (AAMA)—————————————————

CASE STUDY 30-1

Refer to the scenario at the beginning of the chapter.

Both medical assistants are responsible for ensuring that the supplies and equipment needed for the specialty examinations are available and that safety precautions are followed before, during, and after the examination.

CASE STUDY REVIEW

1. Determine what supplies and equipment should be assembled for the following specialty examinations: fecal occult blood testing, performing an eye instillation, performing an ear irrigation, and performing color vision testing.

2. Explain four safety precautions that must be in place when allergy skin testing is being performed.

CASE STUDY 30-2

Corey Bayer is a 15-year-old patient at Inner City Health Care. He sustained an injury to his right wrist today during soccer practice. Dr. Rice examined him and ordered a radiograph of the right forearm. The results show that Corey has sustained a Colles' fracture of the right wrist. Dr. Rice asks you to prepare the equipment to apply a cast.

CASE STUDY REVIEW

1. Describe cast application. What are the medical assistant's responsibilities?

2. After Corey's cast application, describe the cast care instructions that will be given to him and his mother.

CASE STUDY 30-3

Dr. Rice has scheduled Anita Blanchette for a spirometry test and wants you to telephone her the day before the test to prepare her so that optimal results are obtained.

CASE STUDY REVIEW

1. What information do you give to Anita before her spirometry so that the best test results can be obtained?

SUMMARY

 Medical assistants are a vital link in the health care team. A thorough knowledge and understanding of the various body system examinations and clinical procedures routinely performed as part of patient care will enhance the quality of care given.

Some of the specialty procedures are performed on a routine basis in the ambulatory care setting; others are performed occasionally and perhaps only in larger settings that offer specialized and primary care.

Sometimes, to feel comfortable assisting with the less common procedures, medical assistants may need to broaden their base of knowledge by conducting independent research. Medical assistants who are willing to constantly expand their clinical understanding will not only fine-tune their professional skills but will derive greater satisfaction from their job performance.

STUDY FOR SUCCESS

To reinforce your knowledge and skills of information presented in this chapter:

- Review the *Key Terms*

- Role-play with other students to apply attributes of professionalism pertinent to this chapter.

- Consider the *Case Studies* and discuss your conclusions

- Answer the questions in the *Certification Review*

- Apply your knowledge by completing the *Activities* in the *Study Guide* and the *Games and Quizzes* in the StudyWARE **Study**WARE software on the *Premium Website*

- Perform the *Procedures* using the *Competency Assessment Checklists* in the *Competency Manual*

- Practice your problem-solving skills with the *Critical Thinking Challenge 3.0* on the Premium Website

Additional resources for this chapter include:

- Modules 13-18 of the *Medical Assisting Learning Lab*

- *CourseMate for Delmar's Comprehensive Medical Assisting*

- *WebTutor for Delmar's Comprehensive Medical Assisting*

CERTIFICATION REVIEW

1. What is the name of the elevated skin lesions affecting the epidermis caused by the papillomaviruses?
   a. Scleroderma
   b. Moles
   c. Calluses
   d. Warts

2. What is the disorder that is characterized by discomfort of the muscles, tendons, ligaments, and soft tissues brought on by trauma, strain, and emotional stress?
   a. Carpal tunnel syndrome
   b. Bursitis
   c. Gout
   d. Fibromyalgia

3. What type of fracture has its bone fragments driven into each other?
   a. Greenstick
   b. Impacted
   c. Oblique
   d. Comminuted

4. What disease is caused by a degeneration of brain cells caused by lack of dopamine, bringing about muscle rigidity and akinesia?
   a. Multiple sclerosis
   b. Bell's palsy
   c. Parkinson's disease
   d. Tic douloureux

5. An acute circumscribed infection of the subcutaneous tissues caused by staphylococcus is a:
   a. comedone
   b. carbuncle
   c. verruca
   d. psoriasis

6. A device that provides a specific amount of medication per puff of medication is:
   a. a ventilator to increase lung volume
   b. a spacer that contains medication
   c. a specific dose of medication
   d. none of the above

7. A reflex hammer, alcohol swab, and cotton ball are supplies for which system assessment?
   a. Integumentary
   b. Musculoskeletal
   c. Neurologic
   d. None of the above

8. Scratch, patch, and intradermal testing are part of which system testing?
   a. Integumentary
   b. Immune
   c. Respiratory
   d. Neurologic

9. Occult blood is a test of which body fluid?
   a. Blood
   b. Gastrointestinal
   c. Cardiovascular
   d. None of the above

10. Pulse oximetry measures:
    a. pulse rate
    b. respiratory rate
    c. oxygen saturation
    d. all of the above

REFERENCES/BIBLIOGRAPHY

Altman, G. B. (2004). *Delmar's fundamental and advanced nursing skills* (2nd ed.). Clifton Park, NY: Delmar Cengage Learning.

American Cancer Society. (2011). *Stomach cancer.* Retrieved June 30, 2012, from www.cancer.org/Cancer/StomachCancer/DetailedGuide/stomach-cancer-diagnosis

Asthma guide, overview and facts, treatment and self-care. Retrieved from www.webmd.com

Borowitz, D., Robinson, K. A., Rosenfeld, M., et al. (2009). Cystic Fibrosis Foundation evidence-based guidelines for management of infants with cystic fibrosis. *Journal of Pediatrics, 155*(6 Suppl), S73–93.

Cancer Research Institute. (2009). *Conquering melanoma: prevent it, spot it, treat it.* Retrieved July 15, 2012, from www.cancerresearch.org/resources/conquering-melanoma/p2.html

Chernecky, C. C., & Berger, B. J. (2008). *Laboratory tests and diagnostic procedures* (5th ed.). Philadelphia, PA: Saunders Elsevier.

Chronic obstructive pulmonary disease overview and treatment overview. Retrieved October 4, 2008, from www.copdfoundation.org

Delaune, S. C., & Ladner, P. K. (2002). *Fundamentals of nursing standards and practice* (2nd ed.). Clifton Park, NY: Delmar Cengage Learning.

Donohoe Dennison, R. (2000). *Pass CCRN!* (2nd ed.). St. Louis, MO: Mosby.

Examinations and tests for COPD. Retrieved September 7, 2007, from www.webmd.com

Farley, A., & McLafferty, E. (2008). Lumbar puncture. *Nursing Standards, 22* (22), 46–48.

Feldman, E. L. (2007). Amyotrophic lateral sclerosis and other motor neuron diseases. In: Goldman, L., & Ausiello, D., eds. *Cecil textbook of medicine* (23rd ed.). Philadelphia, PA: Saunders Elsevier; chap. 435.

Gallager, C. (2009). Parkinson's disease. In: Rakel, D., ed. *Integrative medicine* (2nd ed.). Philadelphia, PA: Saunders Elsevier.

Goldberg, S. (2004). *The four-minute neurologic exam.* Miami, FL: MedMaster Publishing Co.

Green, P. H., & Cellier, C. (2007). Celiac disease. *New England Journal of Medicine, 357*:1731–1743.

Kahn, S., & Chang, L. (2010). Diagnosis and management of IBS. *Nature Reviews Gastroenterology and Hepatology, 7*(565).

Kline, J. A., & Runyon, M. S. Pulmonary embolism and deep venous thrombosis. In: Marx, J. A., Hockenberger, R. S., & Walls, R. M., eds. *Rosen's emergency medicine concepts and clinical practice* (Vol 2. 6th ed.). 1368–1382.

Metered dose inhalers and how to use them correctly. Retrieved October 11, 2008, from www.aafp.org/afp/20010815/603.html

Middleton, F. A., & Tillery, S. I. H. (2003). Cerebellum. In: Nadel, L., ed. *The encyclopedia of cognitive science.* London: Macmillan, pp. 467–475.

National Heart, Lung, and Blood Institute. (2011). *What is cardiomyopathy?* Retrieved December 7, 2011, from www.nhlbi.nih.gov/health/health-topics/topics/cm/

Neighbors, M., & Tannehill-Jones, R. (2006). *Human diseases*. Clifton Park, NY: Delmar Cengage Learning.

O'Toole, M. T., ed.. (1997). *Miller-Keane encyclopedia and dictionary of medicine, nursing and allied health* (5th ed.). Philadelphia: W. B. Saunders.

Robinson, P. D., Cooper, P., & Ranganathan, S. C. (September 2009). Evidence-based management of paediatric primary spontaneous pneumothorax. *Paediatric Respiratory Reviews 10*(3), 110–117.

Roe, S. (2003). *Delmar's clinical nursing skills and concepts*. Clifton Park, NY: Delmar Cengage Learning.

Section 4, Managing asthma long term overview. (2007). Retrieved October 11, 2008, from www.nhlbl.gov/idex.htm (pp. 277–280).

Spotlight on John McGuire, mobile spirometry unit. (2008). Retrieved October 11, 2008, from www.copdfoundation.org. 2(2).

Taber's cyclopedic medical dictionary. (2003). (22nd ed.). Philadelphia, PA: F. A. Davis.

Tamparo, C., & Lewis, M. (2005). *Diseases of the human body* (3rd ed.). Philadelphia, PA: F.A. Davis.

U.S. Department of Health and Human Services, National Institutes of Health. (2010). *Alzheimer's disease medication fact sheets*. Retrieved July 2, 2012, from www.nia.nih.gov/alzheimers/publication/alzheimers-disease-medications-fact-sheet

U.S. National Library of Medicine, PubMed Health. (2011). *Myasthenia gravis*. Retrieved March 29, 2012, from www.ncbi.nlm.nih.gov/pubmedhealth/PMH0001731/

CHAPTER 31
Assisting with Office/Ambulatory Surgery 886

CHAPTER 32
Diagnostic Imaging 954

CHAPTER 33
Rehabilitation and Therapeutic Modalities 972

CHAPTER 34
Nutrition in Health and Disease 1006

CHAPTER 35
Basic Pharmacology 1040

CHAPTER 36
Calculation of Medication Dosage
and Medication Administration 1078

CHAPTER 37
Electrocardiography 1140

Assisting with Office/Ambulatory Surgery

OUTLINE

Surgical Asepsis and Sterilization
    Hand Cleansing (Hand Hygiene) for Medical and Surgical Asepsis
Sterile Principles
Methods of Sterilization
    Gas Sterilization
    Dry Heat Sterilization
    Chemical ("Cold") Sterilization
    Steam Sterilization (Autoclave)
Common Surgical Procedures Performed in Providers' Offices and Clinics
Additional Surgical Methods
    Electrosurgery
    Cryosurgery

Laser Surgery
Suture Materials and Supplies
    Suture/Ligature
    Suture Needles
    Staples
    Staple Removal
Instruments
    Structural Features
    Categories and Uses
    Care of Instruments
Supplies and Equipment
    Drapes
    Sponges and Wicks
    Solutions/Creams/Ointments
    Dressings and Bandages
    Anesthetics

Patient Care and Preparation
    Patient Preparation and Education
    Informed Consent
    Medical Assisting Considerations
    Postoperative Instructions
    Wounds, Wound Care, and the Healing Process
Basic Surgery Setup
    Basic Rules and Concepts for Setup of Surgical Trays
Surgery Process
Preparation for Surgery
    Using Dry Sterile Transfer Forceps

LEARNING OUTCOMES

1. Define, spell, and pronounce the key terms as presented in the glossary.
2. Define surgical asepsis and differentiate between surgical asepsis and medical asepsis.
3. List eight basic rules to follow to protect sterile areas.
4. State four methods of sterilization.
5. List supplies and equipment necessary to achieve surgical asepsis when using an autoclave.
6. Explain competent wrapping and operation of the autoclave.
7. State storage measures and expiration periods for autoclaved materials.
8. Explain the sizing standards of suture material and the criteria used to select the most appropriate type and size.
9. Given a variety of surgical instruments, be able to identify each and describe its intended use.
10. Demonstrate the ability to select the most appropriate type of dressings for a given situation.

11. State advantages and disadvantages of Betadine®, Hibiclens®, isopropyl alcohol, and hydrogen peroxide when each is used as a skin antiseptic.
12. Define anesthesia, and explain the advantages and disadvantages of epinephrine as an additive to injectable anesthetics.
13. List five preoperative concerns to be addressed in patient preparation and education.
14. List five postoperative concerns to be addressed with the patient and the caregiver.
15. Demonstrate applying sterile gloves.
16. Demonstrate setting up a surgical tray, including laying the field, applying supplies and instruments, pouring a sterile solution, using transfer forceps, and covering the sterile tray.
17. Explain what is meant by alternative surgical methods.
18. Analyze the professionalism questions and apply them to this chapter's content.

Communication

- Did you introduce yourself? Did you identify the patient through name and birth date or other identifying feature?
- Did you listen to and acknowledge the patient?
- Did you speak at the patient's level of understanding?
- Did you provide appropriate responses/feedback?
- Did you allay the patient's fears regarding the procedure being performed and help them feel safe and comfortable?
- Did you respond honestly and diplomatically to the patient's concerns?
- Did you demonstrate empathy in communicating with patients, family, and staff?
- Does your knowledge allow you to speak easily with all members of the health care team?
- Did you maintain eye contact with the patient during communication?
- Did you accurately and concisely update the provider on any aspect of the patient's care?
- Did you include the patient's support system as indicated?

Presentation

- Did you do something to bond with the patient?
- Did you attend to any special needs of the patient? Did you first ask if assistance was needed, rather than taking charge?
- Were you courteous, patient, and respectful to the patient?
- Did you display a calm, professional, and caring manner?

Competency

- Did you pay attention to detail?
- Did you ask questions if you were out of your comfort zone or did not have the experience to carry out tasks?
- Were you knowledgeable and accountable?

Initiative

- Did you show initiative?
- Were you flexible and dependable?
- Did you direct the patient to other resources when necessary or helpful, with the approval of the provider?
- Did you assist coworkers when appropriate?

Integrity

- Did you work within your scope of practice?
- Did you protect personal boundaries?
- Did you immediately report any error you had made?

KEY TERMS

anesthesia
approximate
autoclave
avascularized
Betadine
caustic
cautery
contamination
electrosurgery
epinephrine
exudate
fenestrated
friable
Hibiclens
infection
inflammation
informed consent
isopropyl alcohol
ligature
Mayo stand/
  instrument tray
preference cards
ratchets
sitz bath
steam sterilization
sterile field
strictures
suppurant
surgical asepsis
suture
swaged
volatile

SCENARIO

Dr. Mark Beahm is a solo practitioner and runs a busy cosmetic surgery practice. He frequently performs smaller surgical procedures in his clinic. Today, Ms. Raquel Grindley is in the clinic to have a suspicious skin lesion removed from her left forearm. This lesion is suspected basal cell carcinoma. Jessica Goodwin, RMA (AMT), is Dr. Beahm's lead medical assistant. It is her responsibility to set the room up for the procedure and to care for the instruments and the specimen afterwards. Ms. Goodwin pulls Dr. Beahm's preference card and begins to collect the supplies needed for this procedure.

INTRODUCTION

Office/ambulatory surgery differs from hospital surgery not only in complexity, but in the supplies, equipment, instruments, and personnel needed. Some office/ambulatory surgery is performed by the provider alone; some surgeries require the assistance of the medical assistant. Most ambulatory care settings do not need a large variety of surgical instruments but often need more than one of the more frequently used instruments. As a personal preference, special instruments may be purchased and maintained for a specific provider to use during a particular surgical procedure. These particular instruments are generally not used by the other providers.

The equipment and supplies used in office/ambulatory surgery are usually portable and easily maintained. Larger practices that perform many office/ambulatory surgeries generally can afford the space and expense of maintaining a special room just for that purpose. Often patient examination rooms serve as small surgical suites with portable Mayo stands/instrument trays, supplies, and equipment brought into the room for the procedure.

Whether assisting with office/ambulatory surgery is a routine or an infrequent event for the medical assistant, it is nonetheless important to be knowledgeable about sterile technique, the use and care of instruments and the room, as well as patient preparation for the surgery. Medical assistants should understand the preferences of each provider on staff to make the surgical procedure comfortable and effective for both patient and provider.

SURGICAL ASEPSIS AND STERILIZATION

Surgical asepsis means all microbial life (pathogens and nonpathogens) is destroyed before an invasive procedure is performed. Therefore, all equipment to be used is sterile. The terms *surgical asepsis* and *sterile technique* often are used interchangeably.

Regardless of the number and complexity of surgical procedures performed in the clinic or ambulatory care center, surgical asepsis must be strictly maintained. Surgical asepsis uses practices known as sterile techniques and these techniques are always used during an invasive procedure. Some examples of invasive procedures include creating an opening in the skin such as a surgical incision, suturing a wound such as a laceration, giving

SPOTLIGHT ON CERTIFICATION

RMA Content Outline

- Medical ethics
- Patient relations
- Patient education
- Asepsis
- Sterilization
- Instruments
- Minor surgery

CMA (AAMA) Content Outline

- Anatomy and Physiology
- Medicolegal guidelines and requirements
- Principles of infection control
- Patient preparation and assisting the physician
- Collecting and processing specimens; diagnostic testing

CMAS Content Outline

- Basic clinical medical office assisting
- Asepsis in the medical office

an injection, or inserting a sterile catheter into a sterile body cavity such as the urinary bladder.

Because microorganisms are on virtually every surface, such as skin, instruments, surgical instrument trays, clothing, and even in the air, it is necessary to destroy as many as possible before performing any surgical procedure. Surgical asepsis or sterile technique prevents microorganism entry into the body during an invasive procedure and, therefore, helps to protect the patient from infection. Once the items and areas are sterilized, every precaution must be taken to prevent **contamination** of the sterile items or areas either by a nonsterile item or surface or from airborne contamination. In this context, to contaminate means to make impure; for example, by introducing microorganisms or infectious material into or onto sterile goods or areas. The cardinal rule for maintaining surgical asepsis is "If in doubt, throw it out." There is no room for error when protecting a patient from the introduction of pathogens into the body during an invasive procedure. It is the responsibility of the medical assistant to scrupulously maintain sterility of all instruments, sutures, and other items utilized during a procedure.

 Living tissue surfaces such as skin cannot be sterilized but can be made as free of pathogens as possible before the use of a sterile covering. One example of this concept is the use of the surgical hand cleansing technique before applying sterile gloves (see Procedure 31-1). Another example of surgical asepsis is preparing the patient's skin with a surgical scrub solution before applying sterile drapes around the intended surgical site.

Refer to Chapter 22 for more complete information on the concepts of asepsis and aseptic techniques, including hand cleansing for medical asepsis.

The differences between hand cleansing for medical asepsis as discussed in Chapter 22 (see Procedure 22-1) and hand cleansing for surgical asepsis are addressed in the following section (Table 31-1).

Table 31-1   Differences between Medical and Surgical Hand Cleansing (Hygiene)

Medical Hand Cleansing (Hygiene)	Surgical Hand Cleansing (Hygiene)
Liquid soap and water sufficient for most routine clinical activities.	Performed before any invasive procedure.
One-minute duration.	Three to six-minute duration.
Wash hands and wrists.	Wash hands, wrists, and forearms to the elbows. Brush may be used.
Hands should be held down during rinsing.	Hands should be held up during washing and rinsing.
Scrub nails with brush and clean under nails with cuticle stick.	Scrub nails with brush and clean under each nail with cuticle stick.
Alcohol-based preparations are practical alternatives to soap and water on visibly clean hands.	Alcohol-based applications have no role in surgical asepsis.
Apply lotion.*	Do not apply lotion.*
Utilize Universal Precautions.	Glove for sterility.
	Higher level of decontamination.

© Cengage Learning 2014

*The use of lotions is encouraged to help prevent chafing of the skin, especially with frequent hand cleansings. Nevertheless, studies have determined that lotions containing petroleum or mineral oil can break down latex and should be avoided if latex gloves are going to be worn within 1 hour after applying the lotion. If lotions are applied immediately before gloving, the use of water-based lotions is recommended. Of special interest to persons with latex sensitivities (see Chapter 22) is the fact that using lotions and creams containing petroleum products actually increases the amount of latex protein that is transferred from the gloves into the skin, thereby increasing the symptoms of latex sensitivity.

Hand Cleansing (Hand Hygiene) for Medical and Surgical Asepsis

Hand cleansing (hygiene) for medical asepsis is defined as removing pathogenic microorganisms from the hands after they become contaminated. Medical hand cleansing is used many times throughout the day to cleanse the skin after removing contaminated gloves, assisting with patient care, and touching unclean surfaces.

Preparation for an invasive procedure requires a surgical hand scrub to achieve surgical asepsis for all health care personnel who will participate in any invasive procedure during an episode of patient care. This is a crucial step in preventing Healthcare Associated Infections (HAI). A major risk factor for HAI is the behavior of health care professionals regarding decontamination, hand hygiene/asepsis, and compliance with universal precautions.

The beginning steps of the surgical scrub involve antimicrobial soap; warm water; and vigorous scrubbing of hands, wrists, and forearms. This process begins with removing any jewelry. The scrub includes cleaning under the nails, applying the soap, and scrubbing the hands for at least three minutes. The first two minutes are focused on the fingers, palms, and the posterior aspect of the hands. Next, scrub the wrist area and the arms to at least a few inches above the elbows for an additional minute. Care should be taken to keep the hands above the elbows during the entire scrub process to avoid contamination from the bacteria-laden soap running across the already clean areas of skin. Always maintain the hands above the elbows while rinsing hands and arms, and avoid contact with any of the surfaces of the sink.

After a thorough drying of the hands and then the arms, it is appropriate to don sterile gloves and prepare for the procedure.

Proper protocol when assisting with surgery requires the use of surgical hand cleansing at the beginning of each workday, as well as before every sterile technique, with the complementary use of medical hand cleansing before leaving the clinic and when returning and between patients and procedures. Any opening in the medical assistant's skin should be covered with a sterile adhesive dressing, and gloves are worn during any direct patient contact. See Chapter 22 for information on medical asepsis and Standard Precautions.

STERILE PRINCIPLES

Sterile principles are a set of guidelines designed to designate what items and areas are considered sterile and what actions cause contamination. Some areas are logical and clear, some are subtle and less clear. Some surfaces, such as skin, cannot be sterilized. Large items such as instrument stands and their trays cannot fit into an autoclave for sterilization. To create sterile areas and surfaces where sterility is not possible, sterile barriers should be used; for example, sterile gloves can be worn over the hands. Sterile drapes can be applied to trays once they have been washed, rinsed, dried, and disinfected.

Guidelines to protect sterile items and areas include:

- A sterile object may not touch a nonsterile object.

- Sterile objects must not be wet. Moisture can draw microorganisms into or onto the sterile object.

- An acceptable border between a sterile area and a nonsterile area is 1 inch. The portion of a drape that hangs over the edge is considered nonsterile, no matter what its size. Sterile articles should be placed in the center of the **sterile field** and away from the edge as much as possible.

- Do not turn your back on a sterile field. If you cannot see the field, you cannot be aware of what touched it.

- Anything below the waist is considered contaminated. In support of this principle, all surgery trays should be positioned above the waist. All articles are to be held above the waist.

- All sterile objects (such as gloved hands) must be held in front and away from the body and above waist level.

- Do not cough, sneeze, or talk over a sterile field. Airborne particles may fall onto the sterile area and contaminate it.

- Do not reach over the sterile area. Contaminants may fall onto the area and clothing may touch, thereby contaminating the area. Spend as little time as possible reaching into the sterile area.

- Do not pass contaminated dressings or instruments over the sterile field.

- Arrange for the provider to place contaminated instruments into a separate container or area.

- Always be aware of your actions and the actions of others to determine whether the sterile field has been contaminated. When in doubt, err on the side of safety.

- When opening sterile packages, the outer wrapper is contaminated. It should be opened without touching the inner contents, and the contents are then dropped onto the sterile field. Double wrapping can be used (see Procedure 31-3).

- Sterile solutions in bottles should be poured into sterile basins or cups on the sterile field without touching the rim of the bottle and without splashing solution onto the sterile field. If the sterile field is not polylined and becomes wet, it is considered contaminated because a field that is wet acts as a wick and draws microorganisms into the article. Using polylined drapes as sterile fields protects against contamination.

METHODS OF STERILIZATION

There are four methods of sterilization:

1. Gas sterilization
2. Dry heat sterilization
3. Chemical ("cold") sterilization
4. Steam sterilization (autoclave)

Gas Sterilization

Gas sterilization is considered low-temperature chemical sterilization. Toxic gases permeate and destroy organisms on heat- or moisture-sensitive equipment. This process takes 16–18 hours to complete and the temperature range is 50°F–60°F. This method is best utilized when there are large loads of sensitive equipment to be sterilized and is best suited for large organizations such as hospitals. Ethylene oxide, or EtO, is the gas most utilized and it presents a risk to health care workers. There is a prolonged aeration time needed to make items safe for handling by providers and for patient use.

Dry Heat Sterilization

Dry heat sterilization requires higher temperatures than steam sterilization and requires longer exposure times as well (320°F to 356°F for 90 minutes to 3 hours). This method can be used for instruments that easily corrode, such as sharp cutting instruments. Powders, oils, ointments, rubber goods, and plastic tubing can be sterilized using the dry heat method. Procedures for wrapping are the same as when wrapping for steam sterilization (see Procedure 31-3). Dry heat is seldom used in today's medical office or clinic.

Chemical ("Cold") Sterilization

Chemical sterilization, or cold sterilization, may use the same chemical agents used to chemically disinfect instruments or fomites. However, the exposure time for chemical sterilization is achieved through prolonged immersion. Items must be sanitized first. The handling of instruments after chemical sterilization differs from handling procedures for instruments that are steam sterilized in that chemically sterilized instruments must be handled with sterile gloves, rinsed with sterile water, and dried with sterile towels before placement on a sterile surface.

The position of the Food and Drug Administration is that sterilization with liquid chemicals is different from sterilization with heat, moisture, or low-temperature gas. It is the position of the CDC that utilization of liquid sterilants is actually high level disinfection and does not convey the same sterility assurances as the aforementioned methods.

Chemical sterilization is a method used in many medical clinics when the object being sterilized is too large or too heat sensitive for autoclaving (see following section for information on autoclaving). Fiber-optic endoscopes are one of the most common items sterilized with the use of chemicals. These items are delicate and unable to withstand the high heat of an autoclave. The necessary equipment for chemical sterilization is a container or basin of adequate size for the intended item (which should be maintained for that purpose only) with a well-fitting lid and the chemical of choice. A vent hood is required for safety. Two of the most popular brands of chemicals available through medical supply sources are Wavicide and Cidex. Both have advantages and disadvantages. Clinics must make individual choices based on convenience, expense, and other personnel preferences.

The effectiveness of any of these products depends greatly on the strength of the solution. If the specified strength is a 1:1 ratio of water to chemical, effectiveness will be lost if the solution is not mixed according to that dilution. Any attempt to cut cost by mixing a weaker solution will greatly compromise the effectiveness. The item will not be sterile. Sometimes solutions are weakened unintentionally by placing wet items into them, thereby adding more water than is intended. For this reason, wet items must be carefully dried before chemical sterilization. A well-fitting tight lid is essential to prevent evaporation, which also interferes with the strength of the solution. The lid also lessens the chance of dust and airborne microbes falling into the solution.

Another factor influencing the effectiveness of the sterilizing chemicals is exposure time. The manufacturers provide specific time charts for each purpose. Manufacturers' directions also include a time frame for replacing the solution. The ability of the solution to kill pathogens is directly related to its freshness or shelf life. Regardless of the chemical used for sterilization, ventilation is important.

 When using commercial chemicals, make certain that the lid is placed on the soak basin at all times except when placing or removing items. Care must be taken to avoid contact with skin, eyes, and mucous membranes. Wear protective gloves, goggles, and apron. The effects on skin can range from slight irritation to serious caustic burns.

Before any chemically sterilized item is used for patient contact, the chemicals must be thoroughly rinsed off using either sterile gloves or sterile transfer forceps to remove the item from the container. To maintain sterility, sterile water must be used for the rinsing process. Then dry with a sterile towel, and place onto a sterile field. This process is performed just before use of the item (see Procedure 31-2).

Steam Sterilization (Autoclave)

Steam sterilization is the most widely used method of sterilization used in the medical clinic. An **autoclave**, basically a pressure cooker, is used to achieve sterilization. The autoclave uses steam under pressure to obtain higher temperatures than can be achieved with boiling (Figure 31-1). Water reaches a maximum temperature of 212°F through boiling. When under pressure, water is converted to steam and is then able to reach a temperature of 270°F and higher. Exposing items to this extremely high heat and at least 15 pounds of pressure for a specific amount of time ensures that all microorganisms and their spores are killed. The autoclave is an inner sterilizing chamber surrounded by a metal jacket. This creates a middle steam chamber between the inner sterilizing chamber and the jacket. Inside the jacket is a reservoir for water. When water is poured into the reservoir, the autoclave door closed and secured, and the autoclave turned on, several processes occur. The water in the reservoir heats until vapor is produced. The vapor enters the middle steam

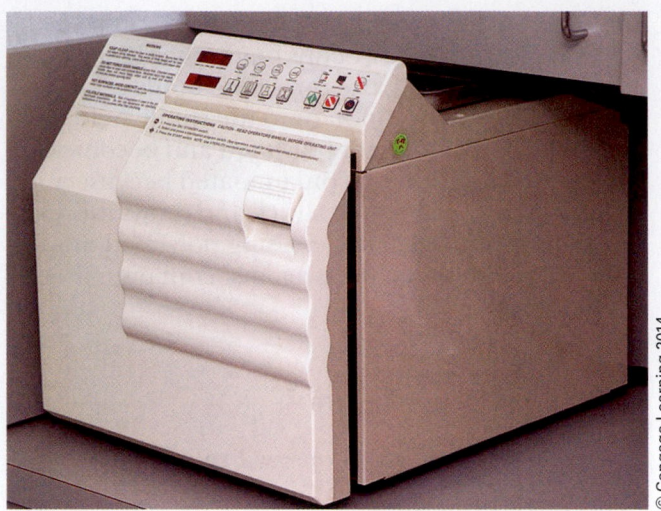

Figure 31-1 Commonly found in providers' offices, autoclaves are used for sterilization by steam pressure, usually at 270°F (118°C) for a specified length of time.

chamber inside the jacket. The air in the steam chamber is pushed out and replaced with steam. Because the air has been pushed out, the pressure increases. The increase of pressure causes the steam to then enter the inner sterilizing chamber (where the items and instruments for sterilization are placed), which pushes out the air. With the air being displaced with steam, the pressure increases in the inner chamber. The steam under pressure is able to reach a much higher temperature than boiling water. When the steam is able to reach all surfaces of the items placed in the autoclave and exposure is maintained for adequate amounts of time, sterility of those items is ensured.

The recommended temperature for effective sterilization in an autoclave is 270°F. Unwrapped items should be sterilized for 20 minutes, loosely wrapped items for 30 minutes, and tightly packed items for at least 40 minutes. When uncertain about the proper amount of time necessary, the medical assistant should refer to the manufacturer's recommendations. The overall effectiveness of the autoclave in sterilizing contents is totally dependent on the medical assistant following proper operating procedure.

In order to prevent mineral buildup in the machine, only distilled water should be used. Before every use, check the water level and add distilled water to the fill line, if necessary. Distilled water is inexpensive and readily available.

How to Load Packages. It is of extreme importance that instruments and materials be positioned

CRITICAL THINKING

What is the purpose of OSHA's Bloodborne Pathogen Standard and whom does it cover?

GENERAL RULES TO ENSURE PROPER STERILIZATION USING AN AUTOCLAVE

- Articles placed into the autoclave must have been sanitized, rinsed, and dried.
- The articles are wrapped and placed to allow adequate exposure of all surfaces (see Figure 31-2). Instruments inside packages should have hinges open and serrations exposed.
- To prevent formation of trapped air pockets, containers should be placed on their sides with lids loosely in place.
- Any wrapping material used must be approved for autoclave use.
- Timing should not start until the gauges read 15 pounds of pressure and 270°F.
- When the cycle is complete, the door must be opened slightly to allow steam to escape. The sterile wrapped articles will be hot and damp and should be left in the autoclave to cool and dry. Microorganisms can contaminate the sterile articles through the damp wrapping if the door is opened too wide or if articles are handled while damp.

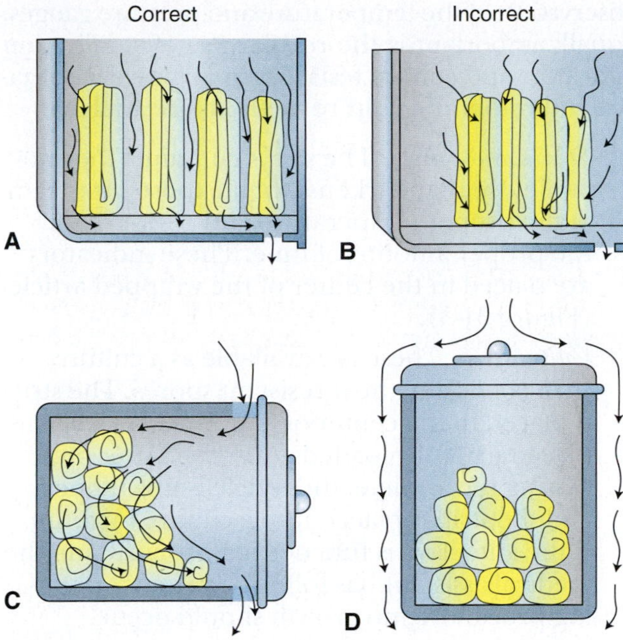

Courtesy of Steris Corporation, Mentor, OH

Figure 31-2 (A) Proper placement of packages in the autoclave allows steam to circulate and penetrate from all sides. (B) Packages incorrectly loaded in autoclave. (C) When placed correctly, the jar should lie on its side with the cover loosely in place to allow steam to freely circulate through the jar and properly sterilize the dressings. (D) Incorrect method.

properly in the autoclave for the steam to circulate through and between packs and penetrate them. Do not overload the autoclave. Place items as loosely as possible inside the chamber. Leave a 1- to 3-inch space between packs and the walls of the autoclave. Correct positioning and spacing allows sterilization to take place provided the medical assistant adheres to proper temperature, pressure, and time requirements (Figure 31-2).

Autoclave Maintenance and Cleaning. The autoclave, like any piece of equipment in the medical clinic, needs regular cleaning and maintenance. Frequency of cleaning the autoclave depends somewhat on its usage. If the autoclave is used every day, the inner chamber should be washed with a mild detergent and cloth, rinsed, and dried on a daily basis. The outer jacket should be wiped clean of dust and soil. Follow the manufacturer's instructions and recommendations for cleansers. Omni® Cleaner XL s a well-known brand of autoclave cleanser.

At least once a week or following the manufacturer's instructions, the autoclave should be drained of water and cleaned thoroughly. Cleaning

the autoclave requires that it be drained, filled with cleaning solution, run through a 20-minute heated cycle, drained of solution, filled with distilled rinse water, run through another 20-minute heated cycle, drained of rinse solution, and then filled with distilled water again. Then the inner shelves are removed and scrubbed, and the inner chamber is wiped clean. Because this process is fairly time-consuming and puts the autoclave out of use for a while, consideration should be given to scheduling the weekly cleaning at a time when personnel can devote the time and when the autoclave is not in demand for sterilization processes.

During the cleaning process, attention should be given to inspecting the rubber seal for cracks or wear. An extra replacement rubber seal should always be kept on hand. The seals are available through medical supply sources. Refer to the manufacturer's instructions for regularly scheduled replacement of the rubber seal and other recommended maintenance procedures.

Quality Control and Assurance for Autoclave.
Quality control when using an autoclave consists of proper maintenance, proper operation, and

observation of the temperature and pressure gauges. Equally important is the regular use of sterilization indicators and culture tests. Several types of sterilization indicators and culture methods are available:

- *Sterilization strips.* The strips contain a thermolabile dye that darkens when exposed to steam at the proper temperature and pressure for the proper amount of time. These indicators are placed in the center of the wrapped article (Figure 31-3).

- *Culture tests.* These are available as a culture strip containing heat-resistant spores. The strip is placed in the center of a wrapped article and placed in a fully loaded autoclave. After processing is complete, the article is unwrapped and the strip is placed into a culture medium. If the autoclave is functioning properly and the medical assistant has followed proper operating procedure, no growth should occur.

- *Biological indicators.* Also available through Becton-Dickinson Microbiology Systems is an ampule called the Kilit Ampule. These biological indicators are ampules that contain spores of the thermophile *Bacillus stearothermophilus*. After being processed through the autoclave, the Kilit Ampule is sent to a cooperating laboratory for a week-long observation for survival of the bacilli spores. A written report of the results is generated by the laboratory and sent to the clinic for its records. The CDC recommends biological indicators.

Autoclave Wrapping Material and Packaging Supplies.
Wrapping or otherwise packaging surgical instruments and other surgical and medical articles before placing them in the autoclave will extend their shelf life. Before these articles are wrapped, they must first be sanitized, rinsed, and dried. Several materials are available for wrapping. Cost, convenience, visibility, time, space, and ease of use will help determine which to use. Many clinics use a combination of materials.

- Muslin is a cloth wrap available in several sizes and colors. Even with the cost of the initial purchasing, occasional replacements, autoclave tape, and laundering, muslin is still an economical option. Besides these cost-effective advantages, many surgical instruments can be wrapped together in muslin, making up a convenient surgery/procedure set. One of the main disadvantages of muslin is the inability to view the contents. Another disadvantage is the need for constant examination for holes, tears, and wearing out of the cloth. Patching is not a reasonable option because iron-on patches impede penetration of steam and sewn-on patches create their own set of perforations. A defective muslin cloth should be discarded. Wrapping space and training of personnel are necessary when using cloth. Special autoclave tape is required to seal the package.

- Paper sterilization wrapping squares are available in many different sizes and types. This disposable type of material requires that a new paper be used each time items are sterilized, but it eliminates the need for laundering. Similar to cloth wrapping, paper wraps also lend themselves to larger sets of articles being wrapped together for surgery or procedural packs. As with muslin cloth, wrapping space and some personnel training are necessary. Paper wraps are opaque, making viewing of the contents impossible. Autoclave tape is required to seal the package.

- Sterilization pouches or bags may be plastic, paper, or a combination (Figure 31-4). They

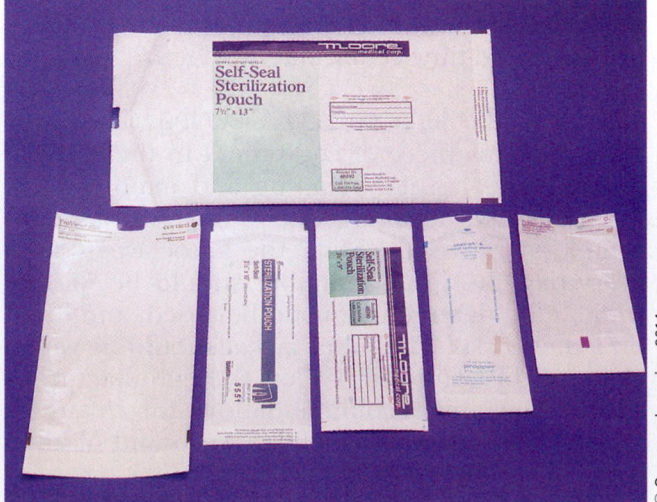

Figure 31-4 Various types and sizes of self-sealing bags for sterilization.

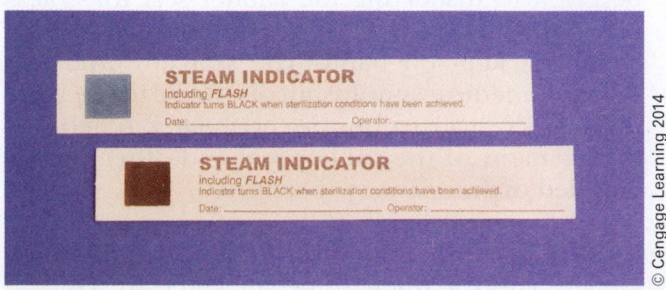

Figure 31-3 Types of sterilization indicators.

are fairly inexpensive and very easy to use. Because no wrapping is involved, additional work space is not required. Another advantage of bags is the visibility of the items inside. Some pouches are packaged on a continuous roll and are available in a variety of widths. This allows the medical assistant to cut the bag to fit the article. Because both ends must be taped closed, it is difficult to remove the article while maintaining its sterility. Probably the best bag-type option is individual bags with the top end open for instrument placement and the bottom end factory closed with a peel-apart seal. The article is inserted into the top opening, the bag is taped closed, and the package is sterilized (Figure 31-5). When needed, the sterile article is removed through the factory-sealed bottom end in a peel-apart sterile fashion. These individual bags need to be purchased in several sizes and are expensive, but they have the advantages of ease of use and item visibility and are probably the preferred method for most medical clinics today.

Autoclave Tape.

Autoclave tape is chemically treated to appear "striped" when exposed to heat. The striped pattern indicates exposure to high temperature but does not measure pounds of pressure or duration of exposure. Because of these limitations, autoclave tape does not assure that the wrapped package is sterile, only that it has been in a heated autoclave. The tape is placed on the outside of the package, so it does not assure that steam has penetrated to the inner article. It does help to determine if a package has been in the autoclave (Figure 31-6).

Labeling Packages for Autoclave.

Surgical packages should be labeled clearly. Clear bags usually have a designated place for labeling, and muslin- or paper-wrapped packages may be labeled across the autoclave tape. Proper labeling should include the name(s) of the articles in the pack, the date of sterilization, and the initials of the medical assistant responsible for the wrapping. The name of the instrument or article should be as specific as possible, especially when using the opaque cloth or paper wraps. If many instruments have been wrapped together for a specific surgery or for a specific provider, the label should clearly state which surgery or surgeon. For example, a "laceration repair set" could contain all the necessary instruments for repairing a laceration. "Dr. Peterson's vasectomy set" would contain all the instruments Dr. Peterson needs to perform a vasectomy, including, perhaps, personal preference instruments. The date of sterilization helps determine the expiration of sterility and a "pull date" for resterilizing. Initialing the package allows for accountability, if necessary. Labels should always be written with a permanent marker. Ballpoint pen should never be used because the ink will smear when wet. Caution should be taken to avoid puncturing through the package during labeling.

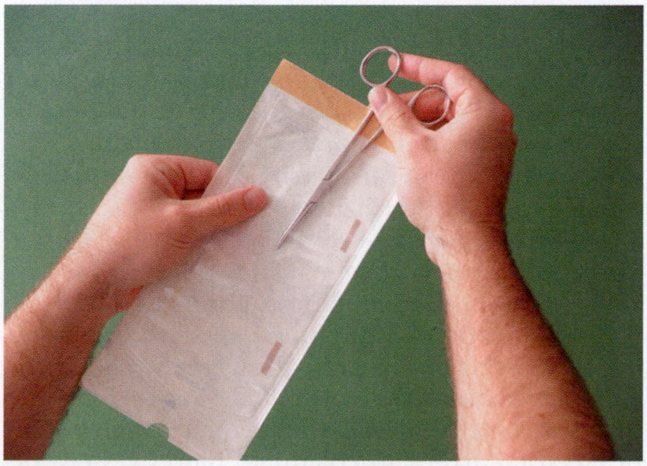

Figure 31-5 The medical assistant is placing a sanitized instrument into a sterilization bag for autoclaving by inserting the tips of the instrument in first.

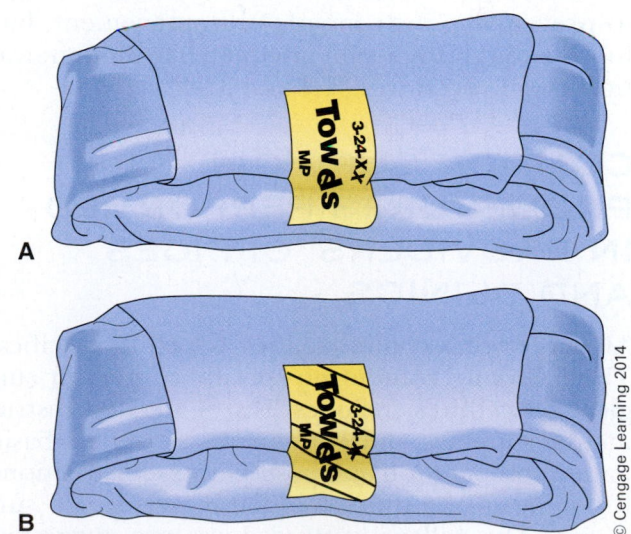

Figure 31-6 Package of towels (A) before and (B) after autoclaving. Note that the autoclave tape has a striped pattern indicating that the package was exposed to a high temperature. However, this does not assure sterility.

CRITICAL THINKING

You have removed a double-wrapped instrument pack from the autoclave and notice a small tear in the outermost wrap. The innermost wrap appears to be intact. What would your action be? Why?

Wrapping Techniques. Articles must be wrapped in a specific way to ensure they remain sterile when opened. Wrapped surgical instruments need to be double wrapped. Some methods advocate placing both layers of wrapping material together and double wrapping the pack in one process. A much more useful method is the "wrapping twice" technique (see Procedure 31-3). The wrapping twice technique allows for additional options at the time of opening. Wrapping twice allows for a completely wrapped inner sterile package to be applied to the surgical tray. This wrapping twice technique eliminates struggling to control multiple instruments during the unwrapping process; and, if the outer package becomes contaminated during the unwrapping, the medical assistant has the additional option of unwrapping the inner package using the same technique without having to discard the instruments and begin again with another sterile package. All packs should be neatly and securely wrapped—firm enough to prevent the instruments from movement, but loose enough to permit adequate steam penetration (see Procedures 31-3 and 31-4).

COMMON SURGICAL PROCEDURES PERFORMED IN PROVIDERS' OFFICES AND CLINICS

All surgery has commonalities as well as specifics. The following content on specific surgery or surgical procedures includes lists of needed instruments, supplies, and equipment, as well as basic patient preparation and postoperative instructions for some of the more frequently performed surgeries. The following procedures are suggested protocol only because providers will have preferences and techniques unique to them and their practices.

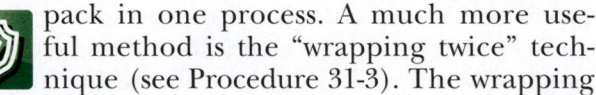

This section includes a general procedure for assisting with surgery and is followed by specific office/ambulatory surgical procedures, including:

- Assisting with Office/Ambulatory Surgery (Procedure 31-8)
- Dressing Change (Procedure 31-9)
- Wound Irrigation (Procedure 31-10)
- Preparation of Patient's Skin before Surgery (Procedure 31-11)
- Suturing of Laceration or Incision Repair (Procedure 31-12)
- Sebaceous Cyst Excision (Procedure 31-13)
- Incision and Drainage of Localized Infection (Procedure 31-14)
- Aspiration of Joint Fluid (Procedure 31-15)
- Hemorrhoid Thrombectomy (Procedure 31-16)
- Suture/Staple Removal (Procedure 31-17)
- Application of Sterile Adhesive Skin Closure Strips (Steri-Strips) (Procedure 31-18)

ADDITIONAL SURGICAL METHODS

Additional surgical methods are those methods not requiring the use of a surgical knife or scalpel but using other methods of cutting or destroying, such as electric current, heat, freezing, chemicals, or laser beam. The method used is determined by the provider's preference.

Electrosurgery

Electrosurgery uses an electric current in a concentrated area to either cut or destroy tissue whenever pathologic examination is not required. The equipment for electrosurgery consists of a power source, usually a small boxed unit, and a detachable handheld applicator with removable tips. The tips are available in various sizes and are removable for cleaning and sterilizing.

Electrosurgery is useful in removing benign skin tags and warts. The main advantage of electrosurgery is that the bleeding is controlled through the cauterization of the blood vessels as the electric current is applied. The terms *electrocoagulation, electrofulguration, electrodessication, electroscission, electrosection,* and *eletrocautery* all refer to various uses of electric current to coagulate blood vessels, destroy tissue either with a spark or by drying, or cut tissue. Disposable battery-operated units designed for one-time use are available.

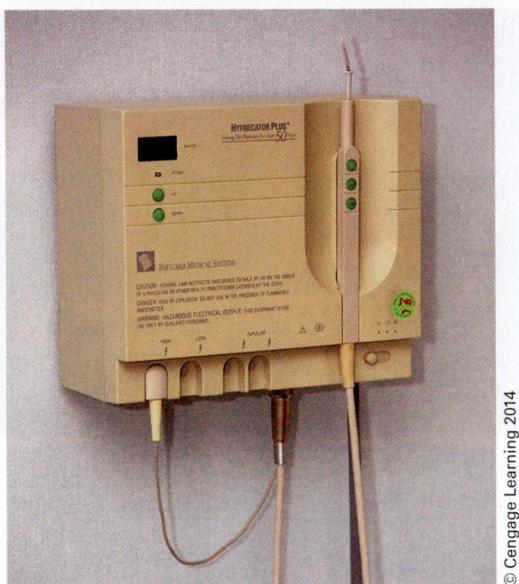

Figure 31-7   Electrosurgical equipment is used to destroy tissue, such as warts, or to coagulate blood vessels to decrease bleeding during surgery.

Cautery. The word **cautery** comes from the term *caustic* and means the application of a **caustic** chemical or destructive heat. Electrosurgery, cautery, and electrocautery are often used interchangeably. The burning of tissue, either chemically or electrically, is known as cauterization. Sometimes during surgical procedures unnecessary bleeding can be controlled by use of electrosurgical equipment (Figure 31-7). Tissues that do not need to be pathologically examined, such as benign skin tags, can be destroyed using cauterization. Some common chemicals used to destroy tissue and stop bleeding are silver nitrate, liquid nitrogen, and sodium hydroxide.

Chemical Tissue Destruction. Silver nitrate is available in a solid form, impregnated on the end of a wooden applicator stick. Silver nitrate is especially useful inside the nose to cauterize **friable**, easily broken, blood vessels in the treatment of epistaxis (nosebleed).

Liquid chemical caustic agents such as sodium hydroxide are used to permanently destroy the growth plates of toenails whenever total and permanent removal of the toenail is necessary.

Cryosurgery

Cryosurgery refers to the destruction of tissue by freezing. Some types of tissues react differently to heat than to cold in the rate of healing and level of scarring. The cryogenic substance most often used to destructively freeze tissue is liquid nitrogen. Liquid nitrogen, often incorrectly referred to as "dry ice," is extremely **volatile** (easily evaporated) and must be kept in a covered insulated canister. Liquid nitrogen is obtained when nitrogen gas is compressed under cold temperatures into a liquid. It is most often used to destructively "freeze" warts. Liquid nitrogen can be applied to cervical erosions to facilitate healing and growth of normal tissue; to remove lesions on the anus; and for cataract extraction, retinal detachment, prostate gland destruction, and removal of superficial lesions in the nose and throat. Some units are single purpose use. There is less trauma, more control of bleeding, and less pain with cryosurgery.

Many patients experience pain with liquid nitrogen because it is colder than other chemical cryosurgery options. Liquid nitrogen is usually kept in a large canister in a central location in the clinic and is carefully transferred to a small thermos for transport into the treatment room. The medical assistant must take care to keep the canister and thermos covered because of the volatile properties (evaporation rate) of the liquid nitrogen.

The cryogenic properties of solid liquid nitrogen make it useful for freezing warts and nevi. Nitrous oxide is another chemical used in cryosurgery. Nitrous oxide requires a gas cylinder, a regulator, a pressure gauge, and a cryogun with assorted tips. Nitrous oxide is applied in a more direct and controlled pattern because of the precision of the probes, and nitrous oxide does not evaporate as readily as liquid nitrogen. The tank, probes, and other supplies can be expensive. Nitrous oxide is not as cold as liquid nitrogen; therefore, although it is not so uncomfortable for the patient, it is not as destructive. It is not appropriate for use with cancerous lesions, which must be completely destroyed. Because nitrous oxide is a carcinogen, the Occupational Safety and Health Administration (OSHA) requires that all nitrous oxide systems have outside venting. It is not practical for most ambulatory clinics.

All volatile gases are dangerous to inhale, and appropriate ventilation must be used. Refer to the Material Safety Data Sheet (MSDS) information (available in printed form or on the manufacturers' Web sites) for specific cautions.

Laser Surgery

Laser is an acronym for Light Amplification by Stimulated Emission of Radiation. The laser instrument converts light into an intense beam. By focusing the laser beam onto the target, the application can be extremely precise without damaging surrounding tissue. Over the past two decades, laser surgery has become less expensive, more readily available, and consequently much more widespread as a treatment of choice for surgery in dermatology, ophthalmology, nerve surgery, vascular surgery, plastic surgery, and others. Most specialty surgery uses laser technology in various ways. Because many providers use laser technology in the ambulatory care setting, medical assistants must be familiar with the dangers involved with laser surgery, and safety precautions must be implemented. Attending a laser education and safety workshop is recommended for all personnel intending to work with lasers.

 The following precautions are designed to heighten awareness and serve as a safety guide:

- When the laser beam is focused on the target tissue, the cells explode and vaporize. Care should be taken not to inhale the vapors.

- Whenever high levels of electricity are used, care should be taken to avoid burns and to ensure that the equipment is always in good working order.

- Safety glasses should be worn by the provider, the medical assistant, and the patient.

- If the patient's skin has been prepared with flammable products such as alcohol-based antiseptics, the skin must be dry with no pooling of liquid. Read the product label for alcohol and other flammable substances.

- Sterile water should be readily available to extinguish any fire if the laser beam accidently ignites cloth or paper in the area.

SUTURE MATERIALS AND SUPPLIES

Suture/Ligature

The word **suture** can be used as a verb to describe the motion of sewing or as a noun to describe the material used to sew. Suturing, or sewing, a wound is a common procedure in provider's clinics. The purpose is to **approximate**, or bring together, the edges of a wound. Suturing hastens healing and lessens scarring. Whether the wound is an accidental laceration or a surgical incision, the suturing process is basically the same. When suture material

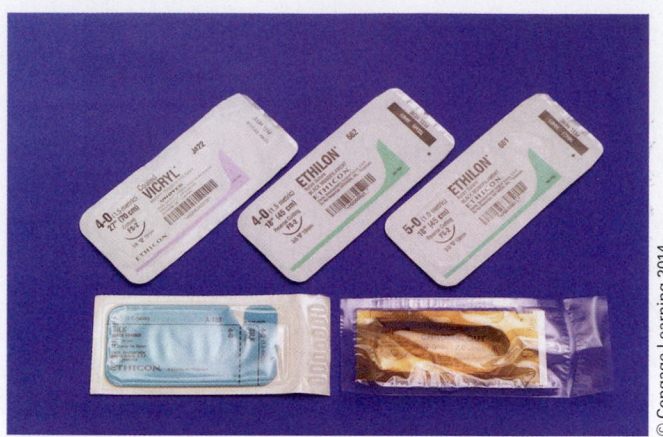

Figure 31-8 A variety of prepackaged suture materials with needles of various sizes and shapes.

© Cengage Learning 2014

is used for tying off the ends of tubular structures during surgery, it is termed **ligature**. The terms *suture* and *ligature* both refer to suture material, but they are named according to their uses.

Most suture material used in office/ambulatory surgical procedures comes already fused, or **swaged**, to a needle and packaged in various lengths (Figure 31-8). These are also called atraumatic needles. Eighteen inches is a preferred length because it is short enough to be manageable yet long enough to complete most suturing procedures. Combinations of sizes and types of suture materials and sizes and shapes of needles are endless, but most providers use a select few. Selection from among the many different suture materials and needles is based on the needs of the tissue and tissue healing. Suture ranges in size on a scale from the smallest gauge below 0 (aught) to the largest gauge above 0. The scale from 6–0 to 4 includes all sizes from the smallest to the largest:

6–0, 5–0, 4–0, 3–0, 2–0, 0, 1, 2, 3, 4

Sometimes 2–0 is labeled 00, 3–0 labeled 000, 4–0 labeled 0000, and so on. Ambulatory care settings use sizes 6–0 to 3–0.

If the tissue being sutured is delicate, as on the face or neck, smaller suture material such as 6–0 is used; the finer the stitch, the less scarring. Some sutures are made from materials that dissolve when they come in contact with the tissue enzymes. These are referred to as absorbable sutures. The original absorbable suture was called surgical gut or "cat gut." It was made from sheep intestinal tissue. Left "natural" or uncoated, it is called plain gut suture. It dissolves or is absorbed in about 1 to 2 weeks. If more time is needed to heal, surgical gut may be coated with chromic salts and is called chromic gut. It allows for a longer period of healing before dissolving. Absorbable gut suture is used for underlying tissues where removal is not reasonable and areas where suture removal is inconvenient. Individual body chemistries influence the exact absorption rate of both plain and treated gut suture. Surgical gut is rarely used now, having been replaced by manmade absorbable suture (such as Vicryl® and PDS* II®). Suture is also made of nonabsorbable materials such as stainless steel, silk, cotton, nylon, and Dacron. Some are natural (cotton, silk) and some are synthetic/manmade (Dacron®, Ethilon®, Prolene®). Each type of suture material comes in a variety of options such as different colors for ease of visualization, braiding for additional elasticity and strength, and coatings for lubrications and to lessen irritability to tissues.

Suture Needles

The atraumatic needles swaged to the suture material are also varied (see Figure 31-8). For office/ambulatory surgery, the needles are usually curved. They are categorized according to size, shape, radius of curve, and type of point. Needles may be termed *cutting needles, round taper point needles,* or *blunt point needles.*

Staples

Many surgical incisions can be approximated using staples (made of stainless steel or titanium) and a stapler made for this purpose (Figure 31-9). The length, width, and number of staples depend on the tissue. They are safe to use, reduce blood loss, and reduce the length of time of the surgery. Wound healing is quicker, and there is less trauma. Staplers are made for specific types of tissues (e.g., blood vessels, skin, gastrointestinal tract, and so forth). It is more difficult to remedy incorrectly placed staples than it is for manually placed sutures.

Staple Removal

 Staple removal (see Procedure 31-17) is done wearing sterile gloves and using sterile instruments. The staples are removed using a sterile prepackaged staple remover

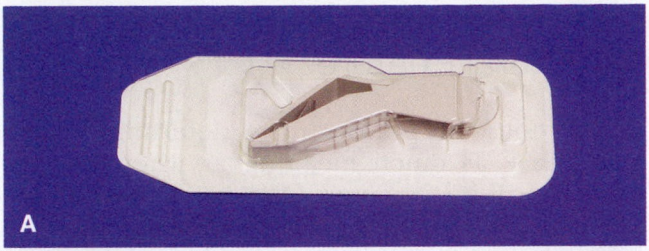

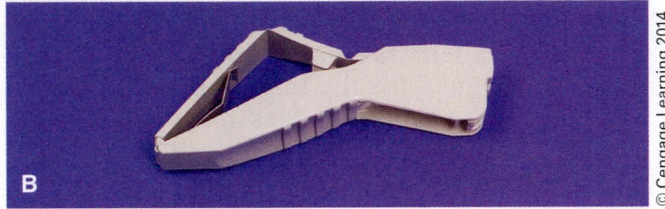

Figure 31-9 Disposable prepackaged skin stapler (A) in package and (B) out of package.

© Cengage Learning 2014

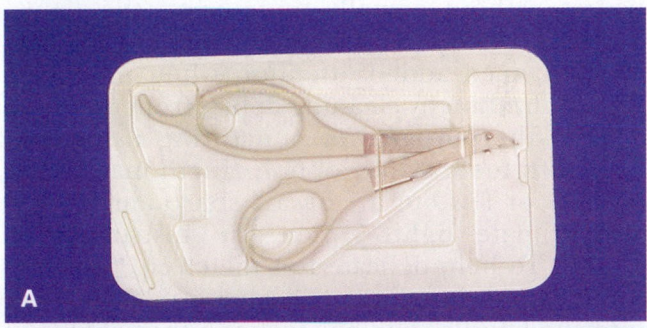

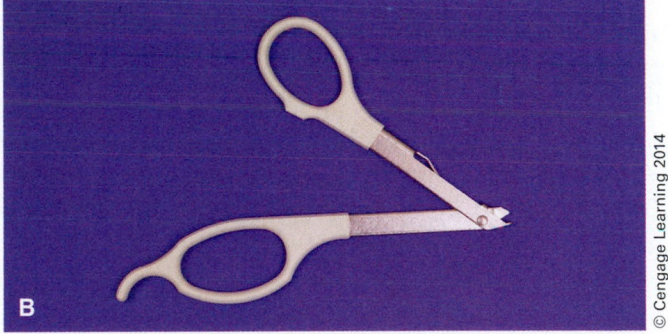

Figure 31-10 Disposable staple remover (A) in package and (B) out of package.

© Cengage Learning 2014

(Figure 31-10). The staple remover is carefully positioned under the staple and, when the handle is squeezed, the staple flattens out and it can be carefully lifted out. Cleanse with an antiseptic solution such as Betadine® and pat dry. Be certain all staples have been removed by verifying that the number that were inserted matches with the number you have removed.

INSTRUMENTS

Structural Features

Rarely does the phrase "form determines function" have as much meaning as when discussing surgical instruments. One can almost always correctly imagine function simply by close examination of the instrument's design. Handles designed to be squeezed between the thumb and finger are called "thumb" handles. "Ring" handles are designed for the insertion of the thumb and finger into rings. **Ratchets** are locking mechanisms located between the rings of the handles and are used for locking the instrument closed. Ratchets are designed to close in varying degrees of tightness. Serrations are the crevices etched into the surfaces of the jaws of hemostats, some forceps, and needle holders. The serrations provide a more secure grip during use with slippery tissues without actually puncturing the tissue. These serrated surfaces hold onto tissue and fluids and need added attention when preparing for sterilization by cleaning debris from this area.

For the purposes of puncturing tissue, forceps with teeth are an option. Teeth may be numerous or few but are always sharp and should approximate tightly when the instrument is closed. To help delicate tips match up properly, some thumb instruments have a guide pin built into the handle. The box-lock is a special type of hinge found on most ring-handled instruments, especially grasping instruments such as hemostats, forceps, and needle holders. This is also an area that requires special attention prior to sterilization. Because the box-lock provides strength and aids in the prevention of warping, most instruments with ratchets also need the box-lock hinge. Other features include prongs, hooks, and loops (Figure 31-11).

Categories and Uses

Several companies publish and distribute large pictorial catalogs of well over 30,000 medical-surgical instruments. A glance through these references shows the many choices available. For ease of discussion, learning, and cataloging, most surgical instruments are placed according to their uses into three basic categories.

Instruments designed for specific purposes within medical specialties often do not readily fit into any one group and are called specialty instruments. This group includes long-handled

CATEGORIES OF INSTRUMENTS

Cutting	Scissors and scalpels
Grasping/Clamping	Hemostats, forceps, clamps, and needle holders
Dilating/Probing	Specula, scopes, probes, retractors, and dilators

gynecologic instruments, as well as other instruments designed to meet specific needs within specialty practices.

Scissors and Scalpels. Most of the cutting instruments are scissors. Scissors have ring handles and two blades and vary in size, shape, and function. Because scissors have two blades, the word *scissors* is always plural. Bandage scissors have one rounded tip to allow insertion under a bandage without causing injury to the patient. Bandage scissors do not have to be sterile to use. The two most common styles are the Lister bandage scissors and the finer Knowles finger bandage scissors (Figure 31-12).

Operating scissors are used to cut tissues and generally have very sharp blades. The blades may be curved or straight, and the tips may be sharp, blunt, or a combination of each. They are described as sharp/sharp (s/s), blunt/blunt (b/b), or sharp/blunt (s/b) (Figure 31-13). A special type of scissors, the Mayo dissecting scissors, may be straight or curved, with curved more often used, but are never described as sharp or blunt because the tips are specifically designed to be neither but have a beveled edge with slightly rounded points (Figure 31-14). Iris scissors are useful, delicately bladed scissors, originally named for their usefulness in eye surgery but now widely used in many procedures. Iris scissors may be either curved or straight (Figure 31-15). Suture scissors, also called stitch or stitch removal scissors, have a distinctively notched blade to facilitate the insertion of one tip under a suture (Figure 31-16). All of these scissors must be sterilized before use.

The scalpel is the knife used to cut the skin. The scalpel is actually a blade secured to a handle that, when combined, becomes a surgical knife or scalpel. Disposable one-piece units with a protective retractable blade are available. The most common blade sizes are #10, #11, and #15, with #11 often referred to as a "stab blade" because of its

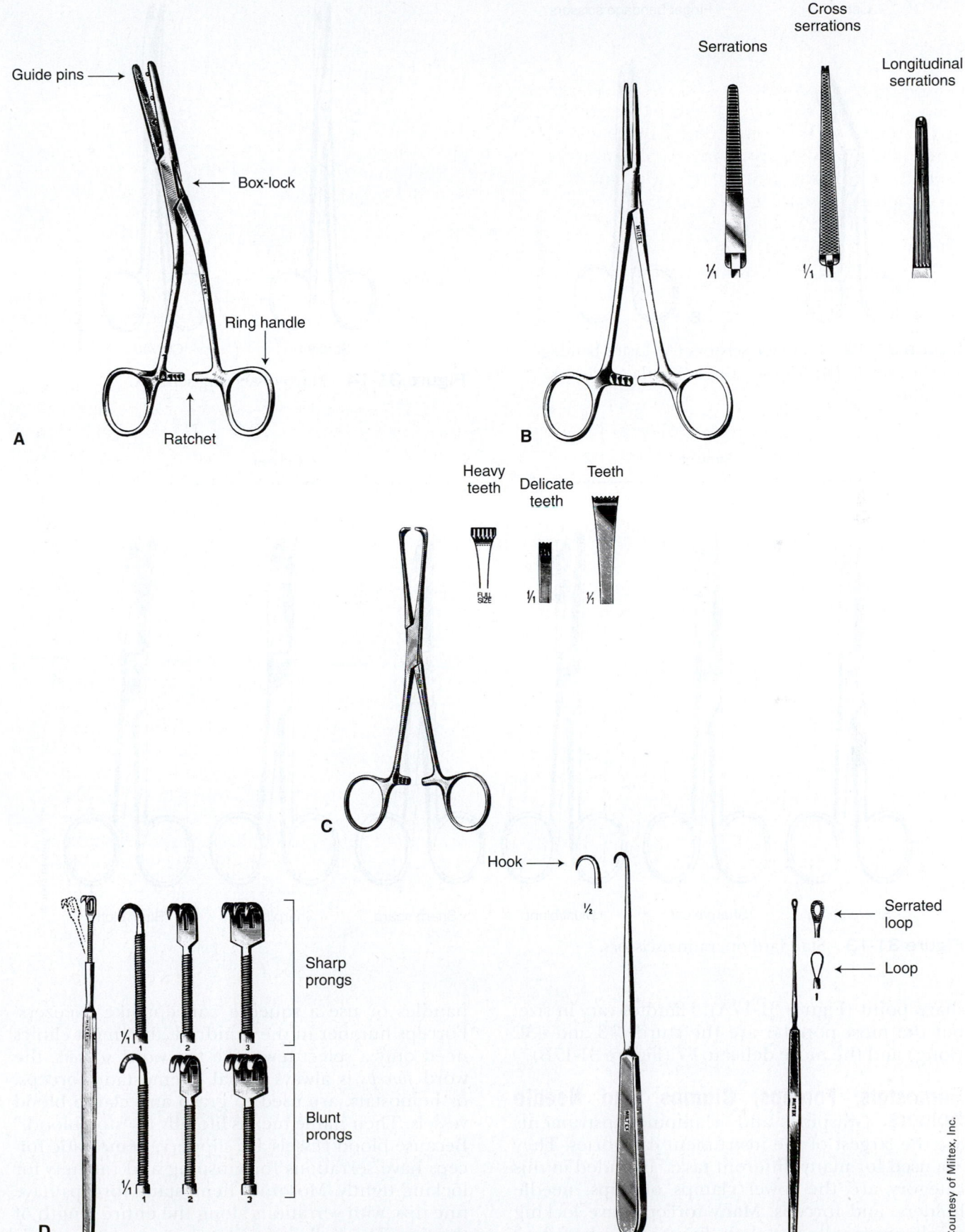

Serrations

Cross serrations

Longitudinal serrations

Guide pins

Box-lock

Ring handle

Ratchet

A

B

Heavy teeth

Delicate teeth

Teeth

C

Hook

Serrated loop

Loop

Sharp prongs

Blunt prongs

D

Courtesy of Miltex, Inc.

Figure 31-11 Structural features of instruments include (A) ratchets, box-locks, pins, and ring handle; (B) serrations; (C) teeth; and (D) prongs, hooks, and loops.

Lister   Finger bandage scissors

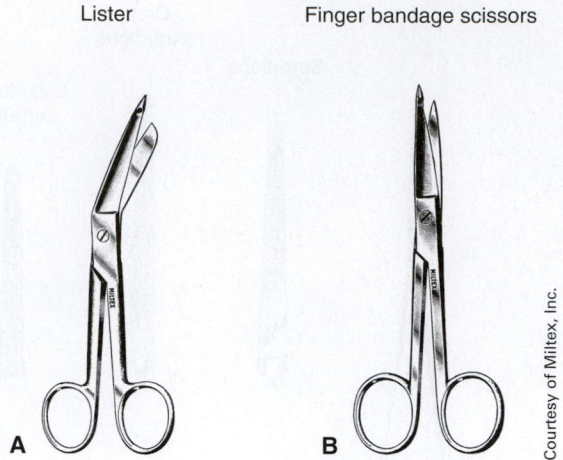

Courtesy of Miltex, Inc.

Figure 31-12   Bandage scissors (A) Lister bandage scissors, small; (B) Knowles finger bandage scissors, straight.

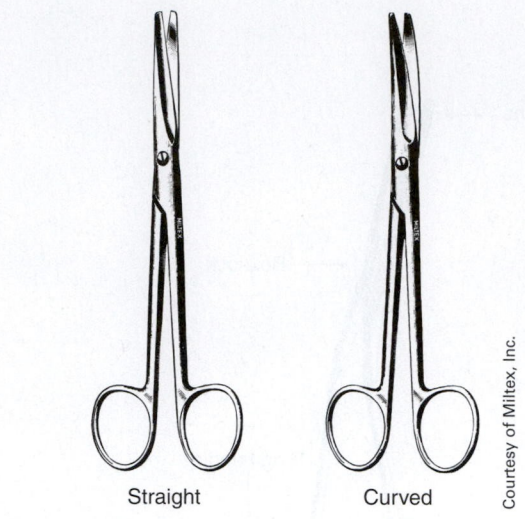

Straight   Curved

Courtesy of Miltex, Inc.

Figure 31-14   Mayo dissecting scissors.

Straight   Curved

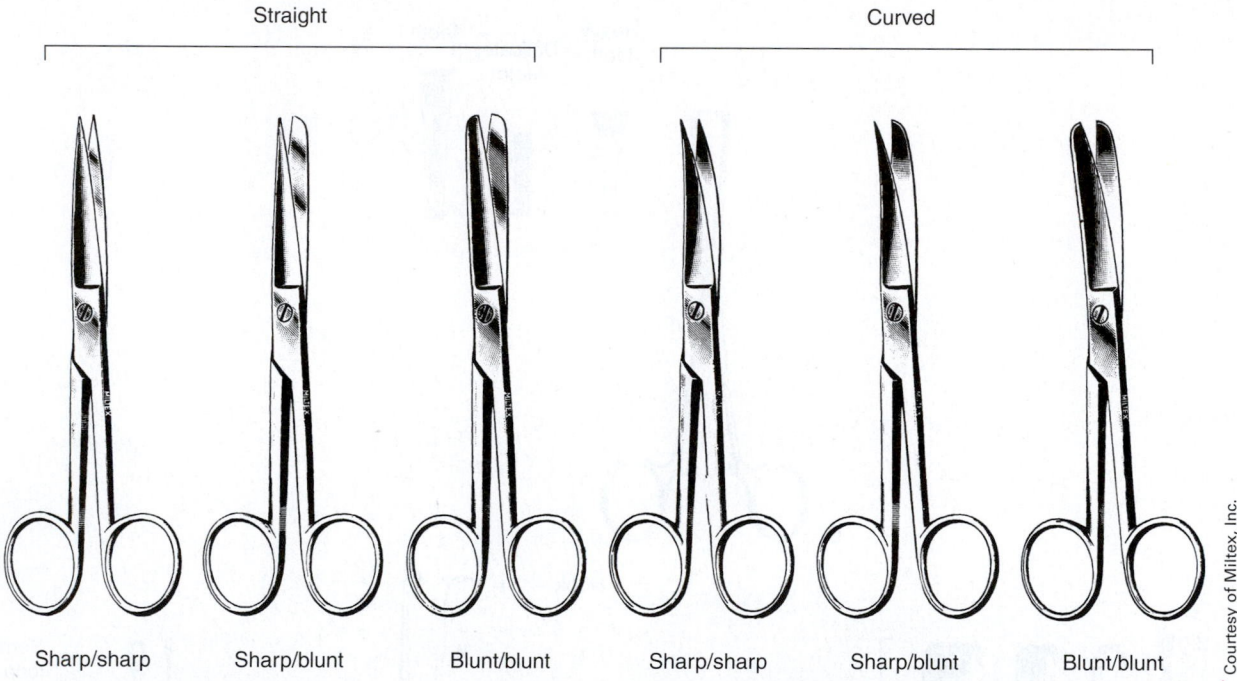

Sharp/sharp   Sharp/blunt   Blunt/blunt   Sharp/sharp   Sharp/blunt   Blunt/blunt

Courtesy of Miltex, Inc.

Figure 31-13   Standard operating scissors.

sharp point (Figure 31-17A). Handles vary in size, but the most popular are the sturdy #3 and #3L (long) and the more delicate #7 (Figure 31-17B).

Hemostats, Forceps, Clamps, and Needle Holders.

Grasping and clamping instruments are the largest of the instrument categories. They are used for many different tasks. Included in this category are the towel clamps or clips, needle holders, and forceps. Many forceps have locking mechanisms called ratchets. Forceps may have ring handles or use a squeeze concept like tweezers. Forceps number in the hundreds, but most clinics need only a select few. Like the word *scissors*, the word *forceps* is always plural. Hemostatic forceps, or hemostats, are used to grasp and clamp blood vessels. Their name means literally to "stop blood." Because blood vessels are slippery, hemostatic forceps have serrations for grasping and ratchets for locking tightly. Mosquito hemostatic forceps have fine tips, with serrations along the entire length of the tips. The Kelly hemostats have serrations only

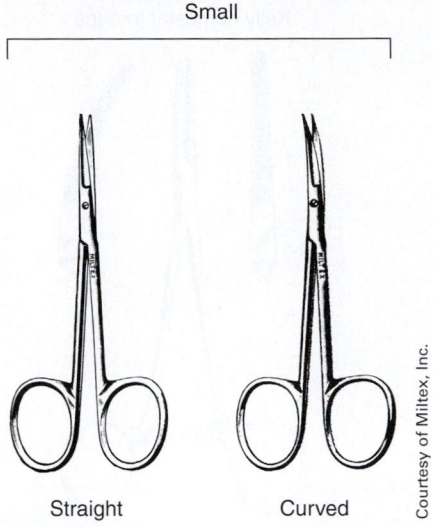

Small

Straight   Curved

Courtesy of Miltex, Inc.

Figure 31-15   Iris scissors.

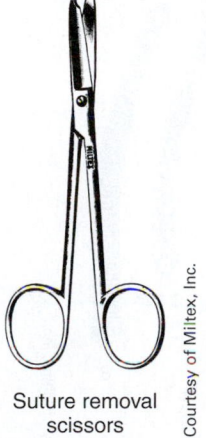

Suture removal
scissors

Courtesy of Miltex, Inc.

Figure 31-16   Suture or stitch removal scissors.

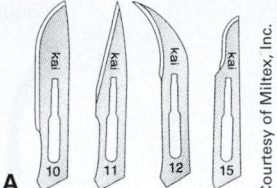

A

Courtesy of Miltex, Inc.

Figure 31-17A   Surgical blades: #10, #11, #12, #15.

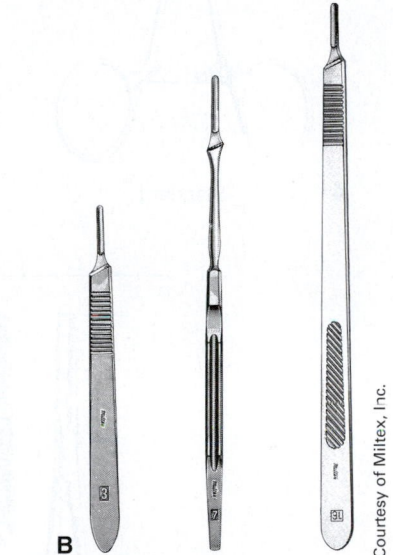

B

Courtesy of Miltex, Inc.

Figure 31-17B   Scalpel handles: #3, #7, #3L.

along partial length of the tips. The Kelly hemostatic forceps are sturdier, and some hemostatic forceps have teeth. All types may be straight or curved (Figure 31-18).

Allis tissue forceps are of a similar design to hemostatic forceps but have unique angular jaws with teeth. Thumb forceps are another type of grasping instrument, sometimes referred to as "pickups." Thumb forceps do not have ring handles or ratchets but are more like the common tweezers. Thumb forceps with teeth are called tissue forceps because of their ability to grasp tissue. Dressing forceps (plain) do not have teeth and are useful for dressing wounds and applying sterile skin closure strips. Dressing forceps are also used to insert sterile gauze packing strips into wounds to facilitate drainage. The Adson, a special type of thumb

forceps, is easily differentiated by its shape. Adsons may have teeth or be plain and have a finer tip.

The Lucae bayonet-type forceps, used in nose and ear procedures, have a thumb handle and are curved to allow the simultaneous use of other instruments and scopes and to facilitate viewing. In contrast, the Hartman ear forceps, duckbill ear alligator-type forceps, and the Hartman nasal dressing forceps have ring handles but also are bent for ease in ear and nose procedures. Figure 31-19 shows examples of each.

Splinter forceps do not have teeth and are used for pulling splinters. Many splinter forceps such as the plain splinter forceps and the Walter splinter forceps are of the thumb-handled style, but the physician's splinter forceps have ring handles and the Virtus splinter forceps have a spring-type handle (Figure 31-20).

Sponge forceps such as the Foerster may have rings on the tips and, as the name implies, are used to hold surgical gauze sponges. Sponge forceps may have long handles, making them useful for gynecologic procedures, and are called uterine sponge forceps. Many medical clinics use uterine

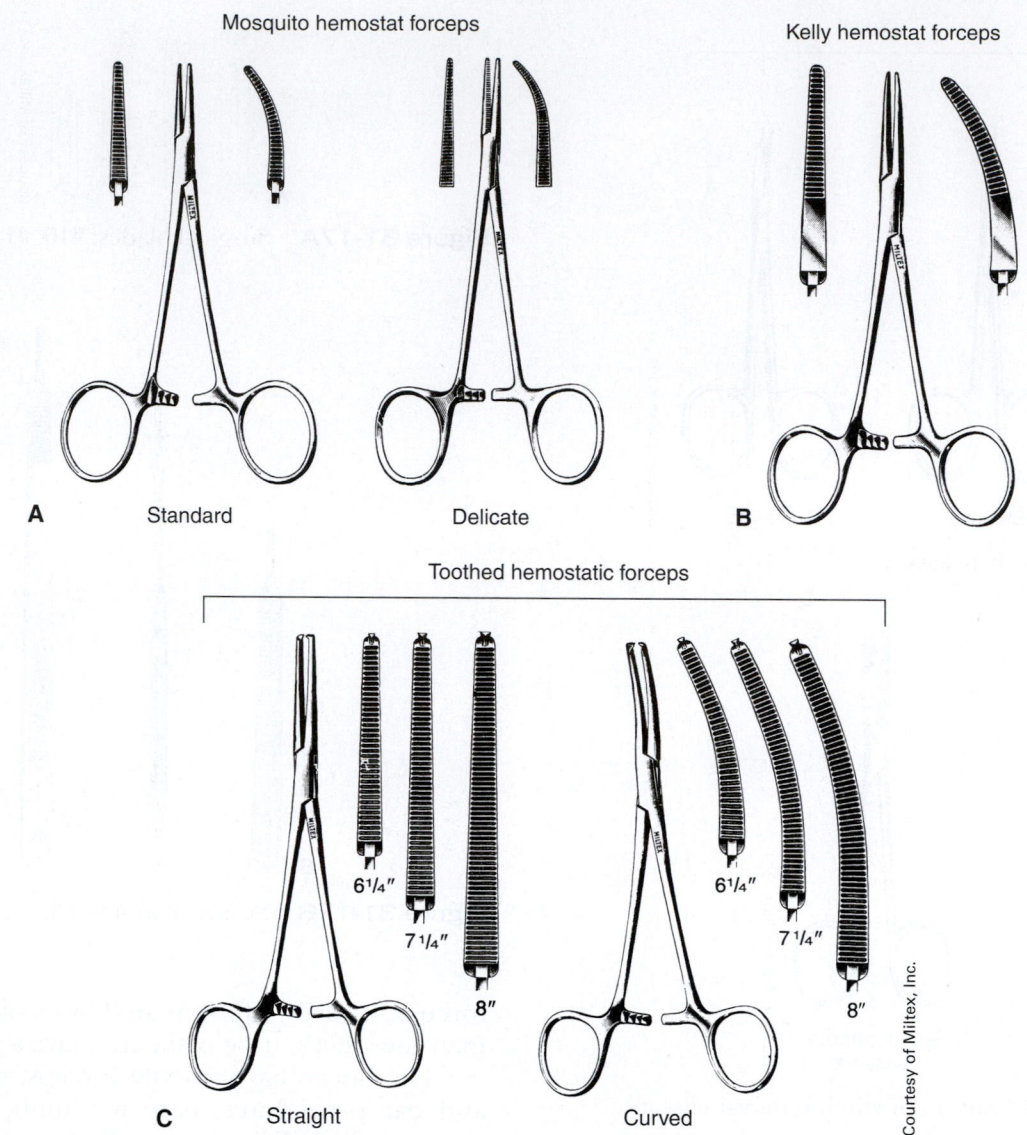

Mosquito hemostat forceps

Kelly hemostat forceps

A Standard   Delicate

B

Toothed hemostatic forceps

6¹/₄″
7¹/₄″
8″

6¹/₄″
7¹/₄″
8″

C Straight   Curved

Courtesy of Miltex, Inc.

Figure 31-18 Hemostatic forceps include (A) mosquito hemostat forceps; (B) Kelly hemostat forceps; and (C) toothed hemostatic forceps.

sponge forceps as transfer forceps (Figure 31-21). (See Basic Surgery Setup later in this chapter.)

Towel clamps are used to attach surgical field drapes to each other and in some situations, such as when bisecting the vas deferens in a vasectomy, to clamp onto dissected tissue. In the case of a vasectomy, the Backhaus towel clamp is used to hold the dissected section of the vas deferens (Figure 31-22).

Needle holders are ratcheted instruments similar to hemostats but with a wider and more stout jaw. Often called needle drivers, they are designed to hold the needle firmly without crushing it while suturing. Most needle holders have a

vertical ditch in the center of the jaw to disperse tension and help prevent slipping of the needle. Needle holders such as the Crile-Wood may have a special groove in which to place the needle during suturing. Some needle holders come in various sizes and some are equipped with a cutting edge that eliminates the need for a separate scissors to cut the suture material (Figure 31-23).

Specula, Scopes, Probes, Retractors, and Dilators. The category of dilators and probes includes specula that are designed for enlarging and exploring body orifices (Figure 31-24). The vaginal speculum is available in various lengths and

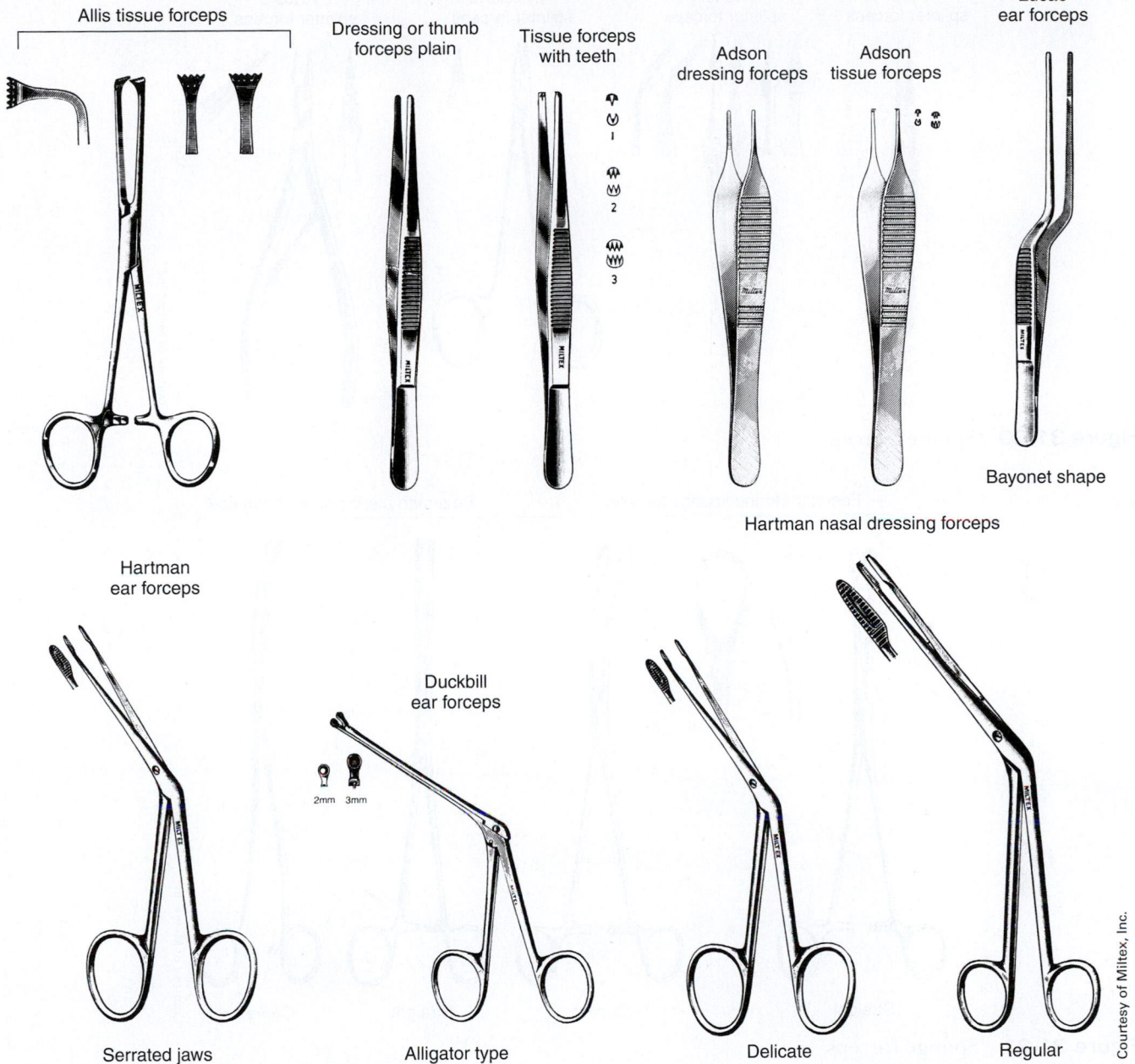

Figure 31-19 Tissue and dressing forceps.

widths and may be made of metal or disposable plastic. The most common instrument for enlarging the nostril is the Vienna nasal speculum. This instrument is used with the Lucae bayonet forceps to perform procedures within the nose.

Scopes are lighted instruments used for viewing. The otoscope, used to visualize the ear canal and eardrum, has a small light aimed into an ear speculum. Ear specula may be disposable or reusable. If reused, they are sanitized, chemically disinfected, rinsed, and dried between uses. Proctoscopes, anoscopes

(Figure 31-25), and rigid sigmoidoscopes are used for viewing the rectum, anus, and the sigmoid portion of the large intestine and have guides called obturators to ease insertion. The light source for the proctoscopes and anoscopes is usually a separate lamp. Although the light sources cannot be sterilized, they can be meticulously disinfected. The speculum portion that is inserted into the rectum may be made of disposable plastic or metal. Both the metal speculum and its obturator can be sanitized and sterilized in the autoclave.

Plain
splinter forceps

Walter
splinter forceps

Physician's
splinter forceps

Virtus
splinter forceps

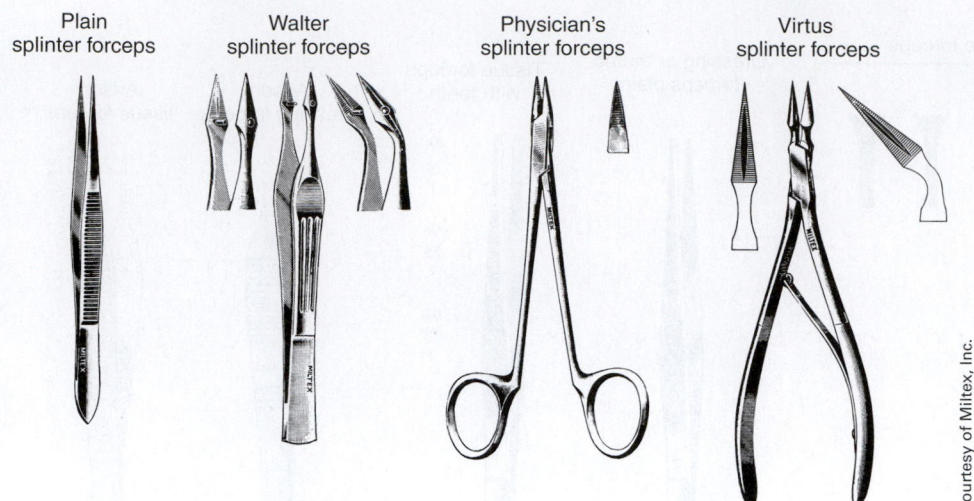

Courtesy of Miltex, Inc.

Figure 31-20 Splinter forceps.

Foerster uterine sponge forceps

Bozeman uterine sponge forceps

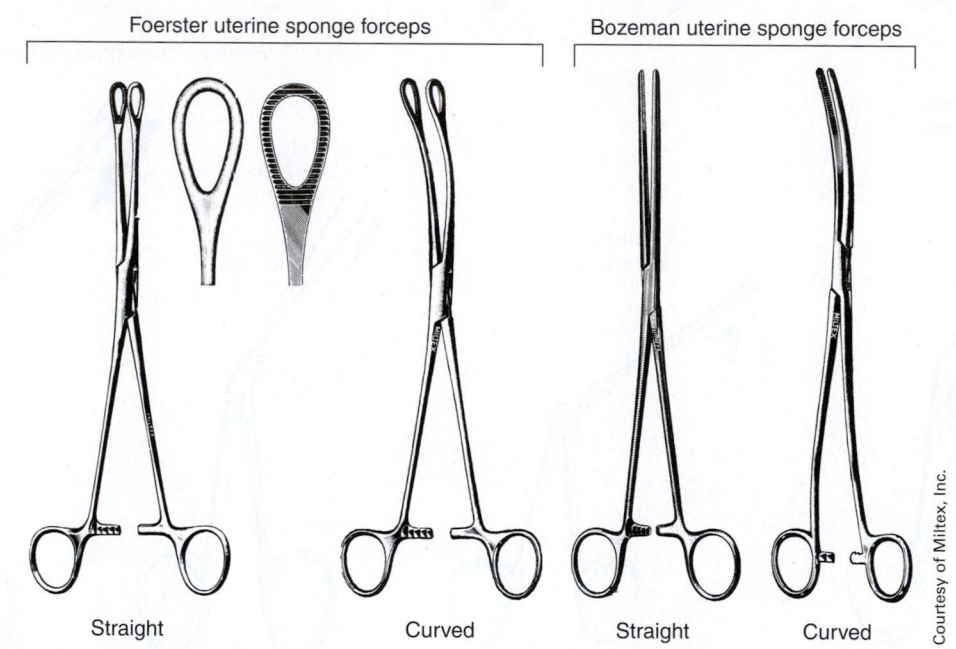

Straight

Curved

Straight

Curved

Courtesy of Miltex, Inc.

Figure 31-21 Sponge forceps.

Jones
towel clamp

Backhaus
towel clamp

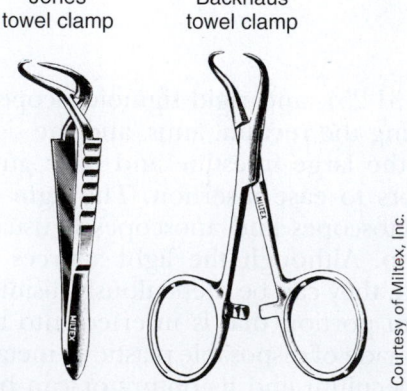

Courtesy of Miltex, Inc.

Figure 31-22 Towel clamps.

Another group of scopes are long, flexible, and much more complex and use fiber-optic light sources. Fiber-optic scopes are considered medical equipment rather than surgical instruments. Although considered to be medical equipment, these flexible scopes are inserted into body cavities and must be sanitized and sterilized between uses.

Probes are slender instruments used to probe into a hidden area, body cavity, or wound. Sounds are long, slender probing instruments used to determine the size and shape of the area being probed or to detect the presence of an unseen foreign body. Sounds may be calibrated in centimeters or inches (Figure 31-26).

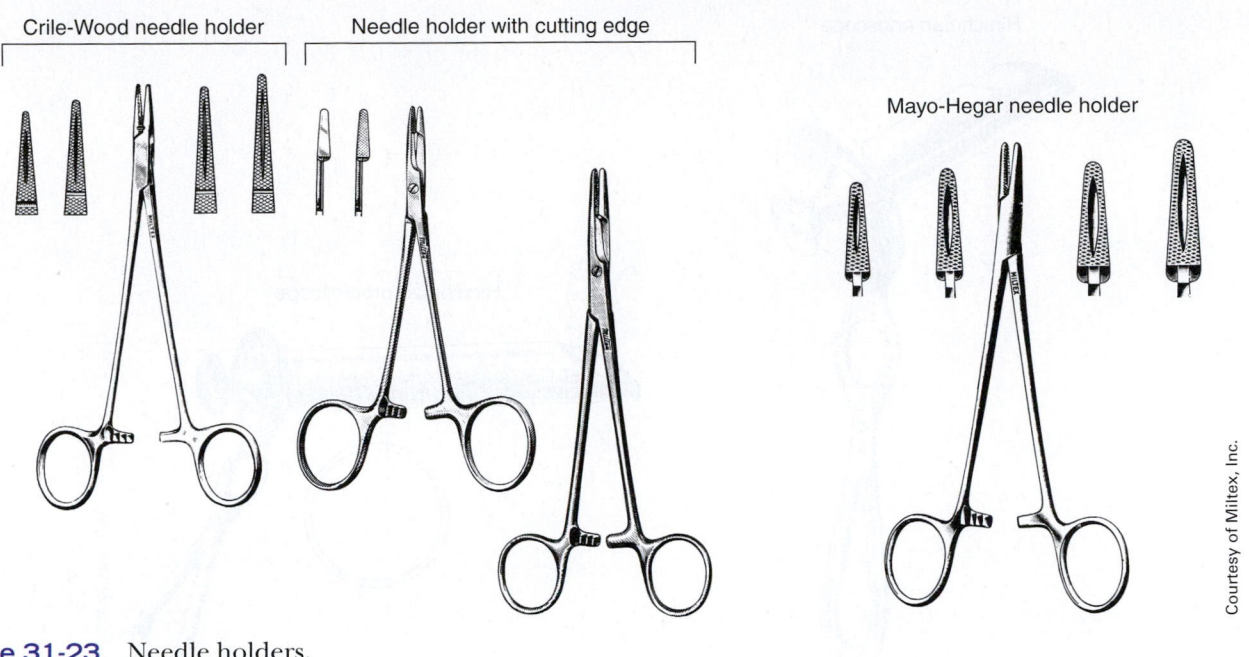

Crile-Wood needle holder   Needle holder with cutting edge

Mayo-Hegar needle holder

Courtesy of Miltex, Inc.

Figure 31-23   Needle holders.

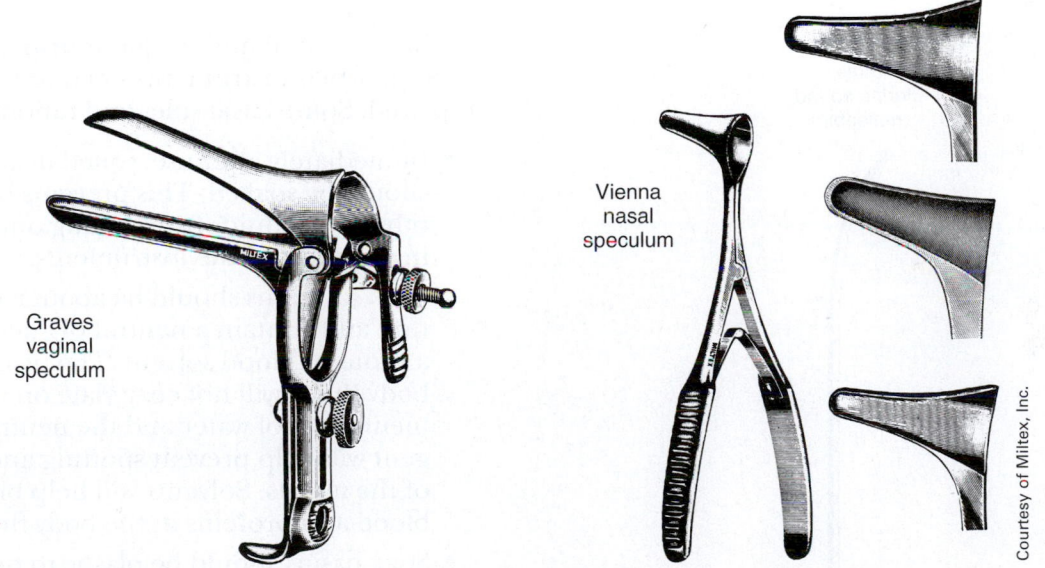

Graves
vaginal
speculum

Vienna
nasal
speculum

Courtesy of Miltex, Inc.

Figure 31-24   Specula and scopes are used to explore body openings by widening for better viewing.

Retractors used in office/ambulatory surgery are often called skin hooks and are used to hook onto and retract the edges of a wound to facilitate better viewing. Skin hooks are fine-tipped and delicate. As with all of the finer surgical instruments, special care should be taken to avoid damaging the delicate tips (Figure 31-27).

Dilators are double-ended metal rods with smooth, rounded tips, ranging in calibrated sizes from small to large. Dilators are inserted into narrowed or constricted ducts and tubes for the purpose of gradually dilating or enlarging the opening. Hegar uterine dilators are used to dilate the cervix to gain access to the inside of the uterus. Esophageal dilators are used to relieve **strictures**, or narrowing, of the esophagus. Urethral dilators are used to relieve strictures of the urethra (Figure 31-28).

Care of Instruments

Medical/surgical instruments require special care to prevent excessive wear and tear and unnecessary

Hirschman anoscope

Hirschman proctoscope

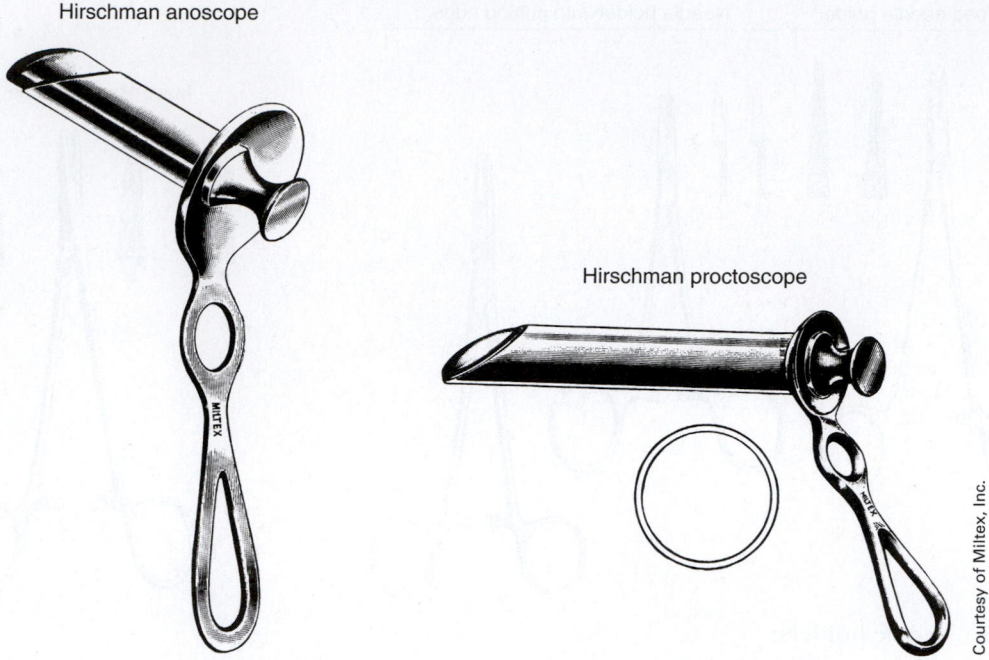

Courtesy of Miltex, Inc.

Figure 31-25   Scopes and specula are used to expose body orifices by opening for better viewing.

Sims
uterine sound
(maleable)

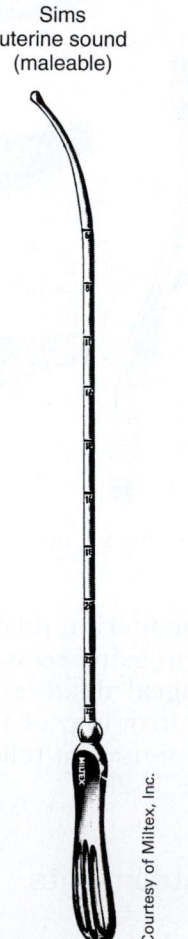

Courtesy of Miltex, Inc.

Figure 31-26   Uterine sound.

damage. Careful and frequent inspections will determine when instruments need to be replaced or repaired. Some basic rules and rationales include:

- Immediately after use, soiled instruments should be soaked. This prevents blood and other body fluids from drying onto the working surfaces of the instruments.

- Soak solutions should be about room temperature and contain a neutral pH detergent with a protein/blood solvent. The proteins in the body fluids will not coagulate on the instruments in cool water and the neutral pH detergent will help prevent spotting and corrosion of the metals. Solvents will help break up the blood and proteins in the body fluids.

- Soak basins should be plastic to prevent damaging points and edges. If a metal soak basin is used, placing a towel on the bottom as padding will help prevent damage to the instruments.

- Heavy-duty rubber gloves should be worn when cleaning instruments to lessen the likelihood of being stuck or cut with the sharp points and edges.

- Goggles should be worn to protect eyes from splashes.

- Delicate instruments should be separated from heavier instruments to prevent the delicate instruments from being bent or otherwise damaged.

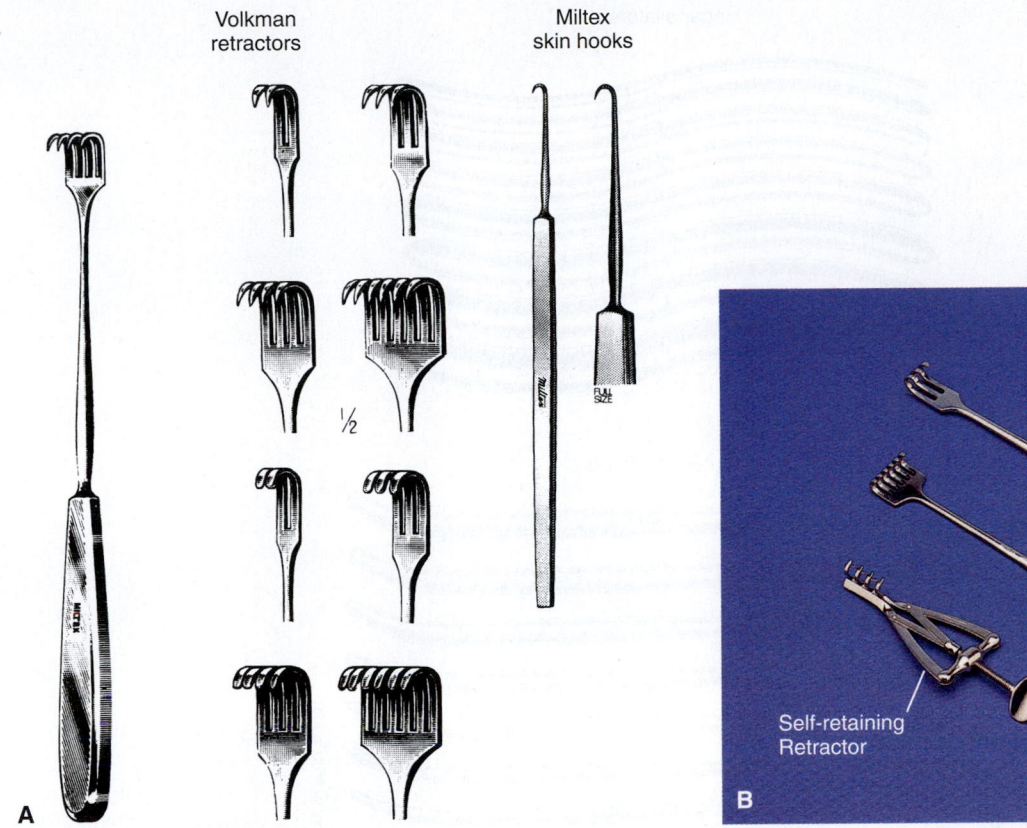

Volkman
retractors

Miltex
skin hooks

½

FULL
SIZE

A

B

Volkman
Rake Retractor
Hand Held

Volkman
Rake Retractor

Self-retaining
Retractor

Courtesy of Miltex, Inc.

Figure 31-27   Various types of retractors (sharp and blunt).

- Sharp instruments should be carefully separated from the other instruments and washed with extreme caution. The danger of being cut or punctured by sharp instruments is greater when cleaning them than at most other times, and the sharp instruments are usually the most contaminated.

- A soft bristle brush should be used to scrub hinges, ratchets, and serrations. The brush should be firm enough to clean crevices thoroughly yet soft enough to prevent scratching instruments. Instruments with multiple parts must be taken completely apart.

- Immediately after sanitization, instruments should be thoroughly rinsed and dried to prevent spotting and water damage.

- Carefully inspect all surfaces, edges, and points. Check for nicks, dulling, and warping. Test blades for sharpness. Be sure the instrument is not bent or pitted. Handles should also be checked for nicks that may snag and tear surgical gloves, thus disrupting the protective barrier and causing contamination.

- Damaged or malfunctioning instruments should be repaired or replaced.

Ultrasonic Cleaning. Surgical instruments can be sanitized by using an ultrasonic cleaner. Instruments are placed into an ultrasonic container with special cleaning solution. Sound waves vibrate to loosen debris and contaminants. Place instruments with ratchets or hinges into the cleaner in an open position. The articles, when finished, are rinsed well, dried, and wrapped for sterilization. The process of sanitizing contaminated instruments by ultrasound is safe for all instruments including delicate instruments. It is preferred for endoscopes. Follow manufacturer's directions for use and care of the ultrasonic cleaner (see Chapter 22).

Sanitization by use of an ultrasonic cleaner eliminates cleaning instruments by hand, thereby reducing the risk for contamination to the medical assistant.

- Instruments should be processed in the cleaner for the full recommended cycle time, usually 5 to 10 minutes.

- Place instruments in open position into the ultrasonic cleaner. Make sure that sharp blades and points do not touch other instruments.

Hegar dilators

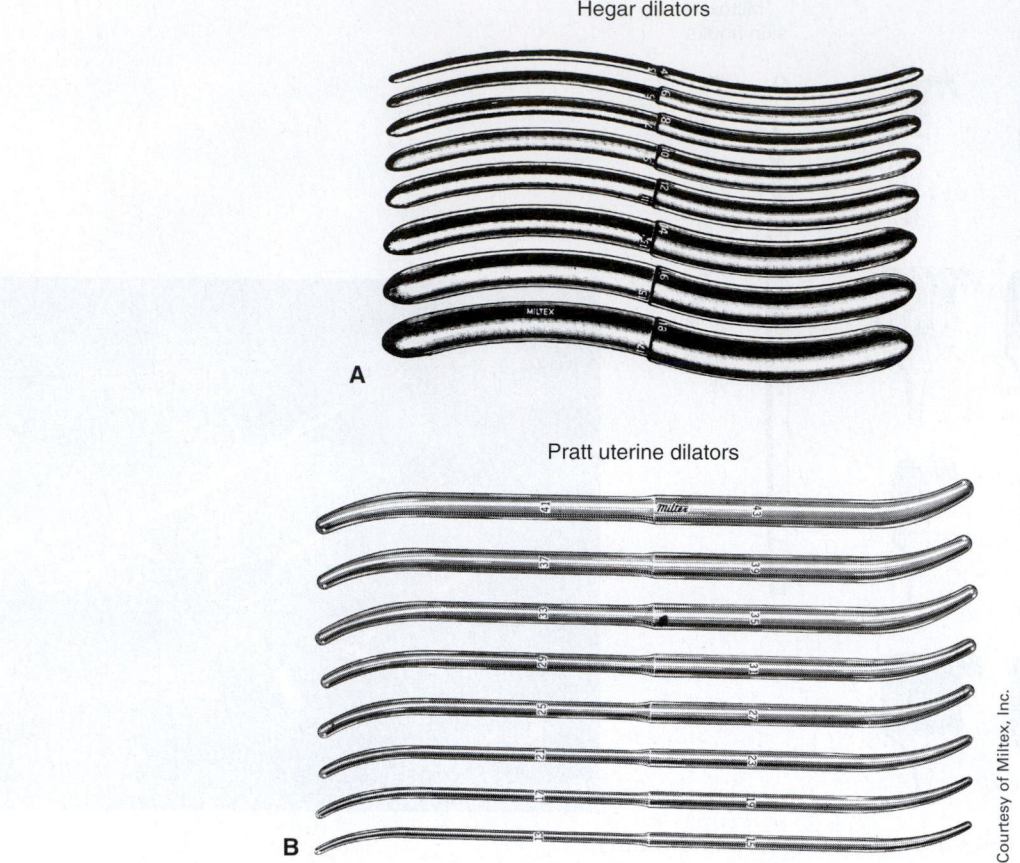

A

Pratt uterine dilators

B

Courtesy of Miltex, Inc.

Figure 31-28   Two types of dilators. Hegar dilators arranged smallest to largest. Pratt dilators arranged largest to smallest.

- All instruments must be fully submerged.
- Do not place dissimilar metals (stainless steel, copper, chrome plated) in the same cleaning cycle.
- Change solution frequently—at least as often as the manufacturer recommends.
- Rinse instruments thoroughly with distilled water after ultrasonic cleaning to remove ultrasonic cleaning solution.

Chemical "Cold" Sterilization. This type of sterilization is sometimes referred to as "cold" sterilization, which indicates that heat-sensitive items such as fiber-optic endoscopes and delicate cutting instruments can be immersed in a chemical solution. The chemicals used are reliable and capable of destroying bacteria and their spores and, when used in strict accordance with the manufacturer's instructions regarding length of immersion time, can ensure sterility. Procedure 31-2 gives steps for chemical ("cold") sterilization.

SUPPLIES AND EQUIPMENT

The supplies necessary for office/ambulatory surgery are often disposable and should be replenished as needed. Most medical/surgical supply companies have catalogs and Web sites available for ordering, and many companies have sales representatives who make regular stops or are available by telephone or email to assist in the ordering process. Sales representatives are familiar with the products marketed by their company and are extremely useful as a resource. Samples of new products are often available for trial, and optional choices are always offered. Medical/surgical supply companies frequently offer special prices for larger quantity purchases. If a medical/surgical supply item is being used frequently and storage space is available, buying in larger quantities might be more cost-effective. If a product currently being used is not meeting expectations, requesting optional trial products is usually the first step toward finding a better product. Following are some of the more commonly used supplies associated with office/ambulatory surgery.

Drapes

There are a variety of surgical drapes available for use in an ambulatory care setting. Drapes are used during surgery to create a sterile field over and around the surgical site. There are many types of drapes and the most appropriate should be selected to provide the best protection for the patient. Your provider will select the type of drape based on the type and complexity of the procedure. The drape may be impermeable, adherent, conformable, natural fiber, or antimicrobial. Natural fiber drapes are reusable after laundering and sterilization. Most adherent, conformable, and antimicrobial drapes are disposable. Care must be taken to appropriately manage these drapes after use. Disposable drape material must be placed in a biohazard container for disposal. Those drapes that are reusable must be managed utilizing Universal Precautions in the handling of materials contaminated with blood or body fluids.

Specialized drapes that are specific to a surgical site are referred to as **fenestrated** drapes. This specialized drape, being of either a reusable or disposable variety, has an opening large enough to accommodate the surgical field. This means that the area that needs to have the practitioner's attention, and no more, is exposed.

Sponges and Wicks

Surgical sponges are prepackaged squares of folded gauze used in surgery. In the provider's clinic, sponges are most often referred to by their size. A gauze square measuring 4 inches by 4 inches is called a "4 × 4" (Figure 31-29). The other most common sizes are 3 × 3 and 2 × 2. The gauze sponges are packaged in individual peel-apart packages of two or may be purchased in nonsterile bulk packages of two hundred. The individual packages are convenient, sterile, and useful for most purposes but cost more per sponge than the nonsterile bulk packages. For larger surgical needs, the medical assistant may wrap several bulk sponges together and autoclave them for later use. Most sponges are simply folded gauze, but some have cotton, rayon pads, or radiopaque fibers embedded in them to increase their absorption ability; to create a softer texture; and, in larger wounds, to be visible upon X-ray if left in the wound.

The provider using the sponge has a preference among the different types and uses. Gauze sponges are used in wound cleansing, in skin preparation, as absorbable sponges during surgery, as dressings and coverings, and for padding. The

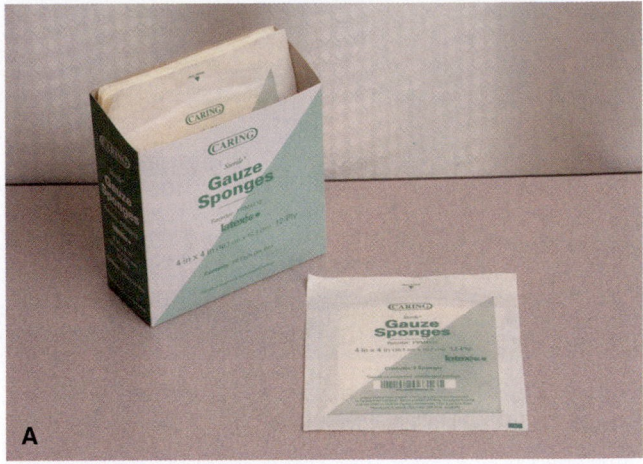

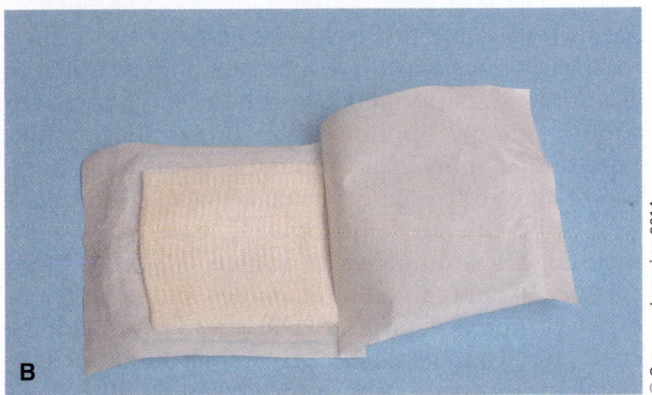

Figure 31-29 (A) Box of sterile gauze sponges. These are also referred to as 4 × 4s or, in surgery, as surgical sponges. (B) Peel-apart sterile open package of 4 × 4 gauze.

© Cengage Learning 2014

ambulatory care setting may prefer to have different sizes and types in stock to meet different needs.

Sterile surgical wicks or wound packing strips are used when an infected wound must remain open for drainage. The sterile wicking material is made of narrow strips of gauze packaged in long lengths in opaque glass bottles (Figure 31-30). The most recognizable product name is iodoform. The iodoform is sterile and packaged in multiple-use bottles. Extreme care should be taken to prevent contamination during removal of individual lengths. The bottle is opened using sterile technique, sterile dressing forceps are inserted into the bottle, the strip is cut to the desired length using sterile scissors, and the lid is applied without compromising the sterility of the remaining wicking material in the bottle.

Solutions/Creams/Ointments

Many different soaps and solutions are available and effective as skin cleansers, preoperative scrubs,

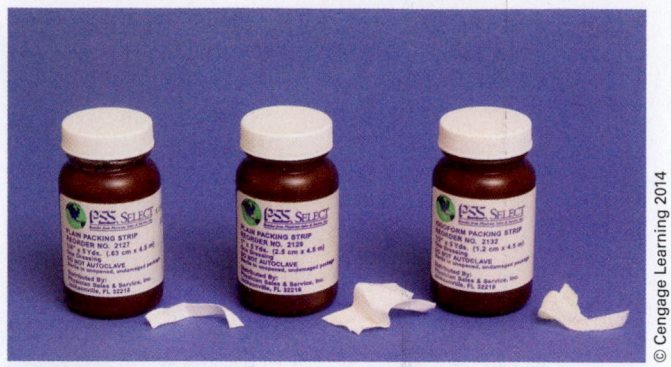

Figure 31-30 Various sizes of iodoform gauze: ¼ inch, ½ inch, 1 inch, 2 inches.

© Cengage Learning 2014

paints, soaks, and antiseptics. **Betadine**® (povidone-iodine) is a well-known antiseptic and is available as a surgical soap called a "scrub" and as a nonsoap solution for preoperative skin preparation/paint. Betadine® comes in multiple-use bottles, in single use, and in individually packaged swabs. **Hibiclens**® is another effective antiseptic that does not have the staining tendencies of iodine. Medical/surgical supply companies have names and samples of other products. Consideration should be made to cost, effectiveness, ease of use, shelf life, and personal preferences. **Isopropyl alcohol**, a 70% alcohol solution, is of limited medical/surgical use, although because of its rapid volatility rate and its ability to dissolve oils, it is still preferred for skin preparation before injections and venipuncture. Isopropyl alcohol is available in bottles for use with cotton/rayon balls or in convenient individually packaged pledgets. Isopropyl alcohol can be irritating and is not effective as a preoperative skin preparation. Hydrogen peroxide is a noncaustic mildly effective skin antiseptic. It bubbles on contact with mucous membranes and other moist skin surfaces, dissolving blood and proteins, and has a mechanical cleansing action. Hydrogen peroxide is ineffective as a skin prep before surgery but is useful for cleaning after surgery. Many providers do not recommend using hydrogen peroxide on surgical wounds because of its abrasive "scrubbing action," which can cause increased scarring and irritations. Do not use or recommend the use of hydrogen peroxide without consulting your provider.

Antibacterial creams and ointments are sometimes applied topically on wounds to aid healing. Antibacterial creams are usually white, water-based, and nongreasy. Antibacterial ointments are usually clear and oil based. If a wound requires thorough cleaning between dressing changes, an antibacterial cream is preferred because of the ease of removal.

Some examples of sterile solutions are sterile saline, sterile distilled water, and Betadine® solution.

Silvadene® is the brand name of a sterile cream used on burns and other abrasion wounds. It is an excellent antibacterial cream but must be applied ⅛- to ¼-inch thick to help ensure that the dressing does not absorb all the cream, thus drying out the wound. Sterile tongue blades are handy to apply the Silvadene® cream to large area burns. Silvadene should be thoroughly removed and reapplied fresh with each dressing change. Silvadene® is available by prescription only and comes in small tubes for individual use as well as larger jars for multiple uses. Silvadene® is fairly expensive. When using a multiple-use jar, as with any multiple-use container, extreme caution must be taken to avoid contamination of the product.

Dressings and Bandages

Dressings are the sterile material applied directly onto the surface of a wound or surgical site. Bandages are the supportive material applied over the top of dressings and are not sterile. A dressing, being sterile, should be handled with care to avoid contamination of the wound. Often a sterile nonstick pad or topical medication is applied to the wound to prevent the dressing from adhering to the wound.

Dressings are usually made of gauze and need to completely cover the wound. The dressings chosen should be adequately absorbent for any wound drainage.

Bandages are used to keep dressings in place, to provide padding and protection, and to immobilize. Bandaging may consist of rolled gauze wrapped around the wound area with an additional sturdier wrap applied overall. An elastic bandage may provide additional support, and a triangular bandage, sling, brace, or splint provides even more. A unique type of bandage is the tubular gauze bandage. Tubular gauze bandages are used to cover appendages such as fingers, arms, toes, and legs and come in various sizes according to the size of the body part being covered. Chapter 9 provides information about wounds and bandages. Figure 31-31 illustrates various bandage-wrapping techniques.

Anesthetics

The word **anesthesia** means the loss of feeling or sensation. An anesthetic is any mechanism that causes this loss of feeling. The application of extreme cold can be an anesthetic because it causes numbness to nerve endings and thus the loss of feeling. Anesthetics may be inhaled, topically applied, or sprayed, or injected directly into a vein

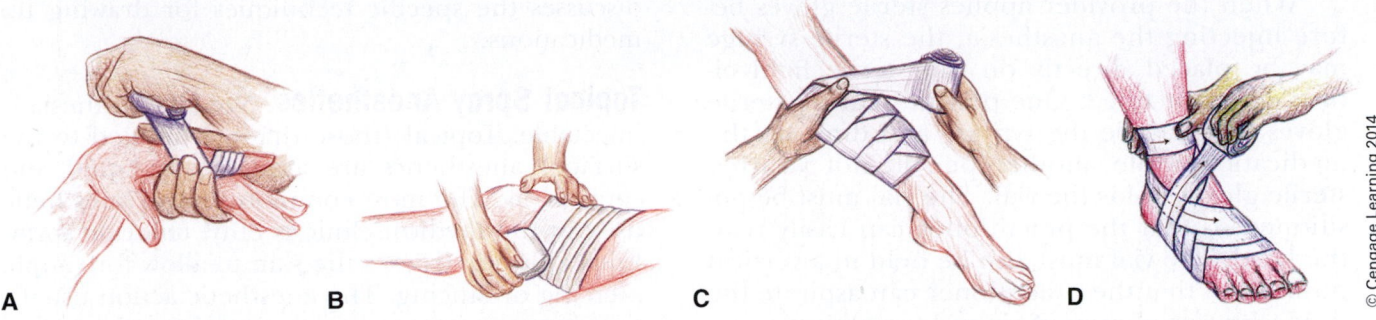

A   **B**   **C**   **D**

© Cengage Learning 2014

Figure 31-31   Bandage-wrapping techniques illustrating the circular, spiral, and figure-eight turns. (A) Circular turns are wrapped around a body part several times to anchor a bandage or to supply support. (B) Spiral turns begin with one or two circular turns, then proceed up the body part, with each turn covering two-thirds the width of the previous turn. (C) Reverse spiral turns begin with a circular turn. Then the bandage is reversed or twisted once each turn to accommodate a limb that gets larger as the bandaging progresses. (D) Figure-eight turns crisscross in the shape of a figure-eight and are used on a joint that requires movement.

(intravenously), the spinal column (intrathecally), or locally (subcutaneously) into the tissues at the site of the surgical procedure.

Injectable Anesthetics. Most anesthetics used in office/ambulatory surgery are administered locally through injection into the subcutaneous tissues. The nerves exposed to the anesthetic become temporarily unable to conduct sensations and feelings to the brain, thereby causing a lack of pain sensation in the area during the surgery. All synthetic local anesthetics have names that end in *-caine*. Some of the most common are Xylocaine (lidocaine), Novocaine (procaine), Marcaine, and Carbocaine. Local anesthetics are available in single-dose vials or ampules of 10 mL, but most medical clinics prefer the cost-effectiveness of multiple-dose vials containing 30 to 50 mL. Local anesthetics are also available in varying strengths such as 0.5%, 1%, and 2%. The local anesthetic is chosen based on the mechanism of action. These decisions include the duration of anesthesia, and whether or not there are additives that constrict the local vasculature to reduce bleeding at the site.

Injectable anesthetics may contain an additive called **epinephrine**. It has a red label. Epinephrine causes vasoconstriction and is used when reduced blood flow to the area is desired. The medical assistant is often delegated the responsibility of filling the syringe with the prescribed amount and strength of the ordered anesthesia or may assist the provider in drawing up the medication. Be sure to identify the drug and dose for the provider. The professional medical assistant must make the practitioner aware that a patient has hypertension if an anesthetic with epinephrine is used. Epinephrine can increase blood pressure.

Any time the medical assistant draws up a medication for the provider or pours a solution into a prep basin on the sterile tray, the original vial or bottle that the medication or solution comes from should be brought into the procedure room with the surgical/procedure tray and other supplies. It is the responsibility of the medical assistant to check the expiration date prior to providing the medication for the practitioner's use. The provider should check the vial and container before using the medication or solution to be sure it is exactly what has been ordered. A good practice is to set the vial or container on the counter within plain view for the provider to see. Often the provider verbally confirms what medication is in the syringe or what solution is in the prep basin before using them. An alternative is to use a sterile marker, while wearing sterile gloves, to label the syringe or container that the practitioner will utilize.

Anesthetics with epinephrine should not be used on fingers, toes, noses, or earlobes because of their vasoconstriction. Patients with circulatory complications may have even more restrictions/cautions on the use of epinephrine. This is one reason why it is important to bring the vial into the procedure room with the patient.

Drawing Techniques. If the provider plans to inject the anesthesia before applying sterile gloves, either the medical assistant or the provider may draw up the medication. The filled syringe is then placed on the side, rather than directly on the sterile field. This allows the provider to anesthetize the patient before beginning the sterile procedure. After the anesthesia has taken effect, the provider performs a surgical hand cleansing, applies sterile gloves, and begins the surgery.

When the provider applies sterile gloves before injecting the anesthesia, the sterile syringe may be placed directly on the sterile field either empty or filled. One person wearing sterile gloves may handle the syringe and draw up the medication while another person not wearing sterile gloves holds the vial. The vial must be positioned so that the practitioner can easily read the label. The vial must also be held in a vertical position so that the practitioner can aspirate the fluid with a minimum of air and maintain the sterility of the syringe.

This method requires that the syringe and needle either be applied directly to the sterile tray or be handed directly to a "sterile" person. The medical assistant may draw up the anesthesia under sterile process when the sterile tray is set up. As stated previously, if the tray contains a filled syringe, the vial from which it was drawn should accompany the tray into the procedure room and be set on the counter for the provider to verify. Chapter 36 discusses the specific techniques for drawing up medications.

Topical Spray Anesthetics.

Not all anesthesia is injectable. Topical (those that are applied to the surface) anesthetics are available in liquid and spray form. The most common topical anesthetic used in the medical clinic is ethyl chloride spray. Ethyl chloride freezes the skin to allow for simple piercing or lancing. The anesthetic action usually only lasts for a few seconds; therefore, the procedure must be performed quickly. It is highly flammable. One example for the use of ethyl chloride spray is to briefly numb an area before an injection. A lesion that is infected is extremely painful to inject with a local anesthetic; however, by using ethyl chloride spray before the injection, the patient is able to remain still. Ethyl chloride spray may also be used before installing intravenous lines.

Table 31-2 summarizes supplies and equipment commonly used in minor surgery.

Table 31-2   Supplies and Equipment Commonly Used in Minor Surgery

Item	Use/Description
Anesthetics	A mechanism used to cause the loss of feeling. May be inhaled, topically applied, sprayed, or injected directly into a vein, the spinal column, or locally into the tissues at the site of the surgical procedure.
Bandages	Nonsterile supportive materials applied over dressings to keep the dressing in place. May be rolled gauze, elastic bandage, or tubular gauze bandage.
Creams and ointments	Antibacterial. May be used topically on wounds to promote healing. Creams are water-based; ointments are oil-based.
Drapes	Used to create a sterile field over and around the operation site. They are made in various sizes and different materials. A fenestrated drape is commonly used in surgery.
Dressings	Sterile material applied directly onto surface of a wound or surgical site. Usually made of natural or synthetic fibers. Must be adequately absorbent and must completely cover the wound.
Solutions	Used as skin cleansers, preoperative scrubs, paints, soaks, and antiseptics. Most common are Betadine®, an antiseptic often used in soap form as a scrub; Hibiclens®, an effective antiseptic without iodine's staining properties; isopropyl alcohol, a 70% alcohol solution favored for skin preparation before injections and venipuncture but not effective as a preoperative skin preparation; and hydrogen peroxide, a mildly effective abrasive skin antiseptic.
Sponges	Used in wound cleansing, skin preparation, as absorbable sponges during surgery, as dressings and coverings, and for padding. Also called 4 × 4s. Typically made of folded gauze, though some have cotton or rayon pads embedded in them to increase absorption.
Wicks	Used when an infected wound needs to remain open for drainage. Wicking material is made of narrow strips of gauze packaged in long lengths in opaque glass bottles, which should be opened using sterile technique (see Figure 31-30).

PATIENT CARE AND PREPARATION

Patient Preparation and Education

For the patient who will undergo a planned surgical procedure, there is time for patient preparation. Patients may need to modify their diet, adjust medication, acquire special supplies, adjust their personal home and work situations, obtain prior approval from their insurance, and prepare for the postoperative period. For the patient undergoing an unplanned procedure, such as a laceration repair, there is less time for preparation. In either case, the medical assistant needs to follow an established protocol about wound care, patient education, patient health consideration, and consent. In the case of an accidental wound, the medical assistant needs to determine the cause of the wound and the date of the last tetanus injection. Chapters 22 and 35 provide specific information about tetanus and immunization schedules. The medical assistant must also check to determine whether the patient has allergies or sensitivities of any kind, particularly to medication and medically related substances.

Diet modifications include an absence of eating and drinking for several hours before the surgical procedure, as well as restricting the types and amounts of certain foods or liquids consumed before and directly after the procedure. When patients are aware of special dietary needs after surgery, they can shop early and be prepared. An example of a medication treatment includes prescribing an antibiotic to be taken as a precaution against acquiring an infection after surgery or adjusting anticoagulant medications to prevent excessive bleeding during surgery. Each clinic, provider, procedure, and patient has individual requirements and preferences. The patient might be required to obtain special supplies for the convalescent period. For instance, immediately after a vasectomy a scrotal support is usually recommended. Crutches or special foot coverings might be necessary after foot or leg surgery. Specific wound dressing and bandages might need to be purchased before the surgery in anticipation of the postoperative need. Having another person accompany the patient to the clinic for the surgery is required for the safe return home. Knowing the planned period for recovery allows the patient to make the necessary arrangements for work, child care, and other personal situations.

Informed Consent

Before a surgical procedure, the patient's written consent must be obtained. For many medical and all surgical procedures, an **informed consent** form must be signed. An informed consent is a document that may be created specifically for a particular procedure or that may be an established document available for duplication. An informed consent document informs the patient of the medical or surgical procedure to be performed, describes the actual procedure in lay terms, cites alternative treatments, and lists the possible undesirable outcome and risks involved in the procedure. Chapter 7 provides additional information about informed consent and a model consent farm.

The cost of the procedure is important information. Some insurances companies and Medicare require patients to sign an Advanced Beneficiary Notice (ABN) if their out-of-pocket expenses will go above a certain amount. It is always a good idea to discuss financial arrangements with all patients before an elective procedure or surgery. In some clinics, the bookkeeper or office manager comes into the examination room, sits down with the patient, and goes over the forms and financial arrangements. Any questions the patient has about the surgery should be answered completely by the provider, and an assessment should be made that the patient understands the answers. Even in the best of circumstances, results cannot be guaranteed. Most of the difficult situations between providers' practices and patients come from misunderstandings about unexpected outcomes. If patients are informed completely, even unplanned results are better tolerated.

Medical Assisting Considerations

The general health and condition of the patient before surgery is important when planning the recovery. A frail, weak man living alone may need home health care after even a simple surgical procedure. Some people may not be able to follow standard preoperative or postoperative instructions. The recovery may depend on the availability of supplies beyond what the patient can financially afford. If difficult circumstances can be identified before the surgery, arrangements can be made with home health care services, community assistance services, or friends and family. As a professional medical assistant, your role is to be a patient advocate. You must utilize the principles that you have learned in your training to provide holistic patient care. Understanding the health care benefits that your patient has access to beyond the care provided in the clinic could dictate the successful outcome of any intervention. It is the responsibility of the professional medical assistant to collaborate with the provider, the insurer, and the family to ensure that the best interest and the care of the patient are assured.

This can help avoid complications. Prior medical history should also be established and questions should be asked regarding allergies and sensitivities to medications and medical substances. A patient who has received a general anesthetic must be watched carefully for cardiopulmonary problems that can arise from the anesthesia. An elderly, weak patient who received a general anesthetic (inhalation or intravenous) may experience hypotension or hypoxia. A pulse oximeter is applied to the patient to monitor blood oxygen percentage (see Chapter 30). Vital signs are watched carefully. The policy and procedure of the clinic or ambulatory surgery center will establish the guidelines for the safe discharge of the patient post-procedure.

Postoperative Instructions

Postoperative instructions should be written and clearly understood by the patient or their designee. If the patient has a caregiver at home, the postoperative instructions should be clearly understood by the caregiver as well. The telephone number of the clinic and an after-hours number should be written on the postoperative instructions and brought to the attention of the patient and caregiver. It is good practice to plan to call patients within the first postoperative day to check on their condition.

Wounds, Wound Care, and the Healing Process

There are many different types of wounds based on the type of injury incurred. Wounds may be classified as open or closed, accidental, or intentional (surgical).

Lacerations, incisions, avulsions, and punctures are all examples of open wounds (Figure 31-32).

Ecchymosis, contusion, and hematoma are examples of closed wounds. They are caused by a blunt trauma that damages underlying tissues but leaves the skin intact (Figure 31-33).

Wounds are classified as superficial if the injury does not extend deeper than the subcutaneous tissues. Deep wounds extend beyond the subcutaneous layer. The size, location, and depth of the wound are important descriptors both for the medical record and for proper insurance reimbursement. A typical description of a patient wound that is an intermediate laceration might be, "patient sustained a deep 3.5-cm laceration to the anterior surface of the right knee caused by a fall onto a rock." A puncture wound might be described as, "patient presents with a 2-cm deep puncture wound on the plantar surface of the left foot obtained from stepping on a rusty nail." Both statements describe not only the size, depth, location, and type of wound, but also the causative factor.

PATIENT EDUCATION

The basic signs of inflammation are redness, heat, swelling, pain, and loss of function. Any one or more of these may be present in varying intensities during an inflammatory process. Most wounds will have a mild inflammation described as slightly red or pink, mild warmth, slightly tender to the touch, and mildly swollen. The symptoms are caused by increased blood supply to the traumatized area and the infiltration of white blood cells in reaction to the trauma. Patients should be taught to watch for an increase in the intensity of redness, pain, swelling, and heat or any drainage, fever, or lymph gland swelling, which can indicate an **infection** from invading pathogens. Patients should be given instructions as to what actions to take if these symptoms of infection are noticed. They should also be instructed to take their temperature twice a day and phone the provider if their temp reaches 101°F or higher.

The instructions should include a name and telephone numbers to call during the day or night. The medical assistant should reassure the patient not to hesitate to contact the center or provider if infection is suspected.

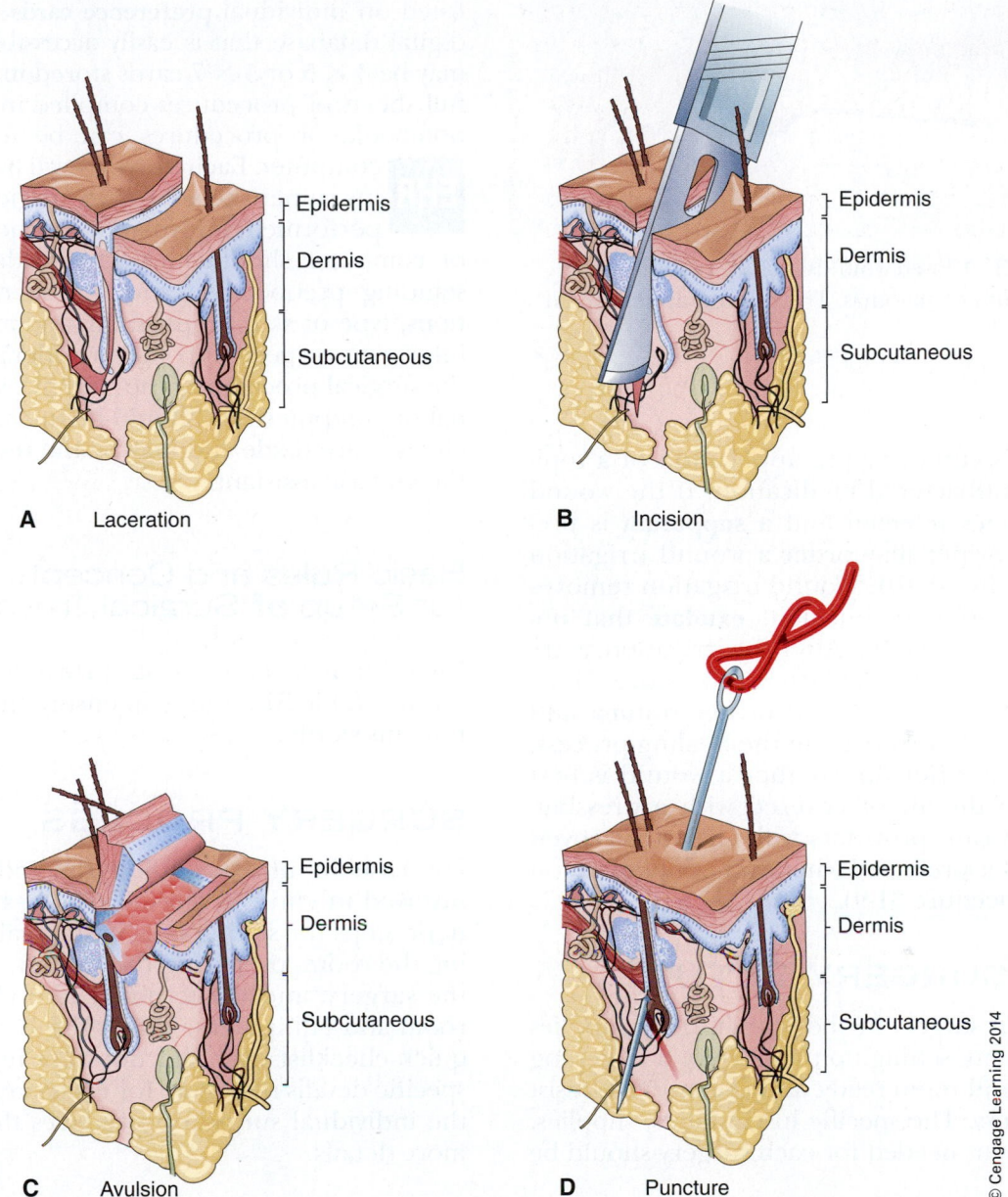

Figure 31-32 Open wounds. (A) Lacerations are accidental tearing of the body tissue usually made by sharp objects. The torn flesh may be smooth or jagged and often is difficult to clean and suture properly. There may be extensive bleeding. A cut from a sharp knife is an example of a laceration. (B) Incisions are intentional cuts typically made with a scalpel for surgical procedures. (C) Avulsions are accidental tearing away of a part or structures of the skin. (D) Punctures are holes or wounds made by a pointed object and can be either accidental or intentional. Puncture wounds have little bleeding because the point of entry is small. These wounds typically are not much larger than the instrument entering the skin. A puncture wound may also be the result of stepping on a nail.

Inflammation is the body's natural reaction to trauma. Inflammation is also a normal process of wound healing. Occasionally, inflamed tissue will become infected if the trauma is caused by a pathogen. Although a certain degree of inflammation is expected, prevention of infection is a primary goal (see Chapter 22).

Chapter 9 describes wounds and emergency care of wounds.

The best treatment of infection is prevention. Instructing the patient about proper wound care is extremely important. Encourage the patient to keep the wound clean and dry. In certain circumstances, the provider may prescribe a warm

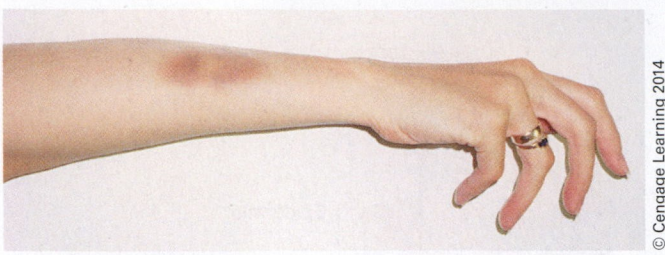

Figure 31-33 Closed wounds include contusions, ecchymoses, and hematomas. This photograph shows an ecchymosis.

soak solution or the application of a topical antibacterial medication. If the wound becomes infected and a **suppurant** is present, the provider may order a wound irrigation (see Procedure 31-10). Wound irrigation removes the accumulation of purulent **exudate** that impairs and delays healing. After the irrigation, a dry sterile dressing is applied (see Procedure 31-9). Protecting the wound from further trauma and contamination will also aid in the healing process. Opinions will differ on whether a wound is best left open to the air or covered with a dressing. Most health care providers will agree that covering a wound is preferred whenever contamination is likely (Procedure 31-9).

BASIC SURGERY SETUP

Preparing for surgery includes assembling supplies and equipment, setting up the surgery tray, getting the patient and room ready, and preparing to assist during surgery. The specific instruments, supplies, and equipment needed for each surgery should be listed on individual **preference cards** or listed in a digital database that is easily accessible. The cards may be 3 × 5 or 5 × 7 cards stored in a card file or full sheets of procedures compiled in a manual or notebook, or procedures can be found on the computer. Each provider will have individual instrument sets for each surgical procedure performed. Information on the surgery card or computer should include provider glove size, standing preoperative and postoperative instructions, type of skin preparation, and any additional information specific to the provider's needs or to the surgical procedure. The card file, whether manual or computerized, should be updated whenever changes are made and may be the responsibility of the medical assistant.

Basic Rules and Concepts for Setup of Surgical Trays

In addition to basic sterile principles, the guidelines in Table 31-3 will help ensure the sterile field remains sterile.

SURGERY PROCESS

For ease in understanding the individual tasks involved in clinic surgery, Table 31-4 provides generic steps for setting up the surgical tray, preparing the room, preparing the patient, assisting with the surgery, and the terminal care process of the room and equipment. Table 31-4 is intended as a quick checklist only and does not include all the specific details necessary for each surgery. Refer to the individual surgical procedures that follow for more details.

Table 31-3   Guidelines for Sterile Tray Setups

Set up the sterile surgery tray just before the surgery to minimize the chance of accidental contamination.

If a tray is to be set up prior to a procedure or in another location, after the tray is set up, cover it with a sterile drape immediately.

Once the tray is prepared and covered, move it directly into the surgery area rather than leaving it in a common area.

Inform the patient and others in the surgery room that the tray is sterile and should not be touched. Patients are often curious about instruments and may attempt to look under the cover if not cautioned against it.

If the medical assistant is interrupted while preparing the tray and it becomes necessary to leave the tray unattended, cover the tray and move it out of traffic paths to prevent it from being bumped.

© Cengage Learning 2014

Table 31-4   Preparations for Office/Ambulatory Surgery

Tray Setup

1. Wash hands.
2. Reference surgery card, manual, or computer.
3. Gather equipment and supplies.
4. Sanitize and disinfect Mayo instrument tray.
5. Wash hands.
6. Set up sterile field.
7. Place sterile instruments and supplies on the sterile field.
8. Apply sterile gloves or use sterile transfer forceps.
9. Arrange instruments and supplies in an organized and logical manner.
10. Medication may be drawn up with assistance (optional) (Figure 31-34).
11. Recheck tray for accuracy and completeness.
12. Remove gloves.
13. Cover and transport tray.
14. Add sterile solution (skin antiseptic) to tray if required.

Room Preparation

In preparing a room for a surgical procedure, all equipment should be clean and in good working order. Be certain to have spare parts such as light bulbs and filters readily available. Turn on equipment before the procedure to make sure all is working properly.

1. Check room equipment (light, stool, equipment, examination table, waste receptacle).
2. Check room supplies (tissue, extra gloves, and so on).
3. Arrange accessory supplies on the side counter in a logical order (pathology specimen bottle containing preservative, laboratory requisition, sterile glove package, dressings/bandages, postoperative medications, and instructions).

Patient Preparation

1. Wash hands.
2. Greet patient and ensure identity.
3. Escort the patient to the procedure room and offer restroom facilities.
4. Discuss the patient's compliance to preoperative instructions.
5. Explain the procedure again and address any questions.
6. Review postoperative instructions.
7. Check for signed informed consent form and financial forms.
8. Have the patient remove appropriate clothing and position the patient on the examination table. Offer a drape, gown, pillow, and blanket for comfort.
9. Prepare the skin for the surgical procedure (see Procedure 31-11).

Assisting with the Surgery

1. Remove the sterile cover, using appropriate technique, from the surgical tray while the provider applies sterile gloves.
2. Assist the provider with stool and lamp adjustment as needed.
3. If the medical assistant did not perform the skin preparation, assist the provider as needed during skin preparation and draping. The equipment and supplies for skin preparation are separate from the surgery tray and equipment (see Procedure 31-11).
4. Adjust the instrument tray and equipment around the provider.
5. Assist with drawing up local anesthetic or other medication as needed.
6. Apply clean gloves for protection or sterile gloves to assist.
7. Surgery begins.
8. The medical assistant either assists with sterile procedure or supports the patient as needed.
9. After surgery, assist with or perform dressing of wound.
10. Clean patient.
11. Label any specimens obtained with the patient's name, date of birth, patient number (if available), date and time of procedure, and type of specimen.
12. Prepare lab requisition to accompany specimen.
13. Apply formalin or refrigerate as needed based on type of specimen and pathology testing to be preformed.
14. Dispose of biohazardous waste materials.
15. Remove contaminated gloves; wash hands.
16. Assist the patient after surgery.

(continues)

Table 31-4   Preparations for Office/Ambulatory Surgery (*Continued*)

Assisting the Patient after Surgery

1. Check patient vital signs.
2. Remain with patient to ensure patient safety. Allow patient to rest if necessary.
3. Assist patient off examination table and assist with clothing as necessary.
4. Review written postoperative instructions with patient and caregiver. Dressing should be kept clean and dry. Patient should report any signs of infection.
5. Clarify any medication orders with patient and caregiver.
6. If not previously arranged, schedule follow-up appointment.
7. Document postoperative instructions in patient chart or electronic medical record.

Terminal Care of the Room and Equipment

1. Apply barrier gloves, gown, and goggles (if appropriate).
2. Dispose of drapes, table cover, pillowcase, and so on. Use biohazardous waste receptacle whenever appropriate.
3. Transfer contaminated surgical tray to cleanup area.
4. Using forceps, isolate sharps from surgical tray and dispose of them into designated sharps container.
5. Place instruments into a soak solution.
6. Sanitize Mayo instrument tray and all surfaces (examination table, stool, counter, lamp, machinery, and equipment).
7. Dispose of contaminated barrier gloves and apply protective gloves.
8. Disinfect all surfaces (examination table, stool, counter, lamp, machinery, and equipment).
9. Allow to air dry.
10. Sanitize, dry, wrap, and sterilize instruments.
11. It is the medical assistant's responsibility to make certain there are enough of each instrument and surgical set.

© Cengage Learning 2014

NOTE: During most surgical procedures, if tissue is excised, it is placed in a biopsy specimen jar containing formalin (a preservative) and sent to the pathology laboratory with an appropriately completed requisition (Figure 31-35).

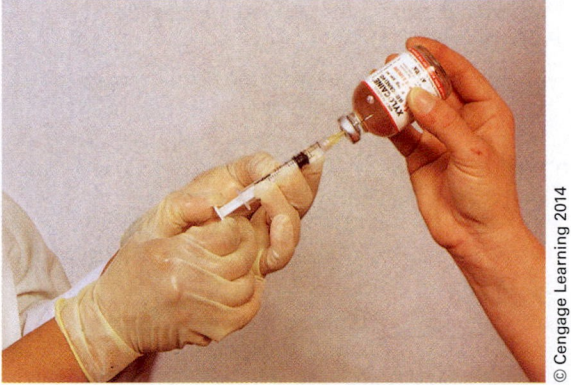

Figure 31-34   Hold the anesthetic solution in a convenient position so that the provider can fill the syringe without contaminating the needle.

PREPARATION FOR SURGERY

    The following procedures are used in preparation for minor surgery:

- Applying Sterile Gloves (Procedure 31-1)
- Setting Up and Covering a Sterile Field (Procedure 31-5)

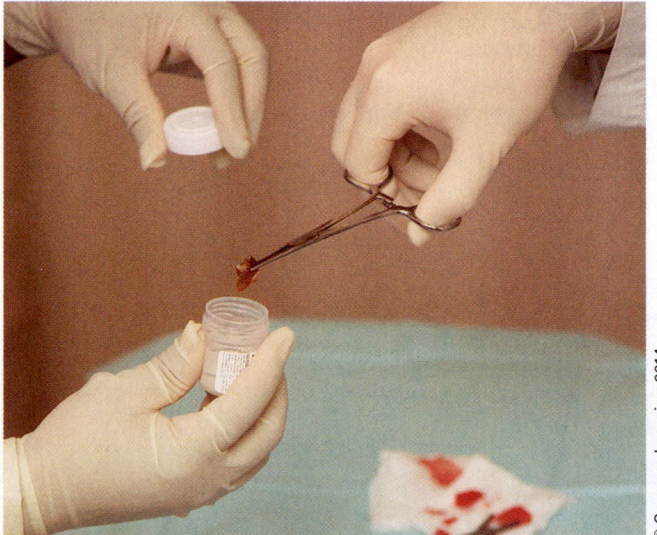

Figure 31-35   The provider places biopsy tissue into specimen jar. The specimen will be sent to the pathology laboratory for examination.

- Opening Sterile Packages of Instruments and Supplies and Applying Them to a Sterile Field (Procedure 31-6)

CRITICAL THINKING

Dr. Woo asks you to assist him in repairing the laceration on Jaime Carrera's hand. Though you are unsure, you think you may have noticed a tiny hole in the palm of your left glove. What is your next step?

CRITICAL THINKING

You are setting up a sterile surgical tray and have already applied your sterile gloves before you realize you forgot to place the suture package on the tray. You have several options. What are they, and what are the advantages and disadvantages of each?

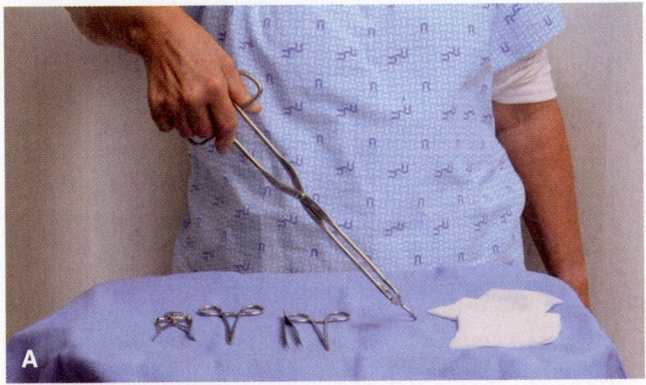

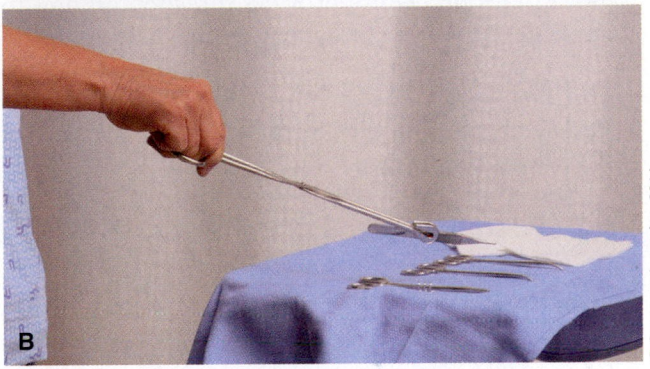

Figure 31-36 (A) If sterile gloves have been removed, use dry sterile transfer forceps to apply or rearrange sterile items on the Mayo stand. (B) Instruments and supplies can be moved around using dry sterile transfer forceps if necessary.

- Pouring a Sterile Solution into a Cup on a Sterile Field (Procedure 31-7)
- Preparation of Patient's Skin before Surgery (Procedure 31-11)

Setting up surgical trays for specific surgeries is addressed in the procedures of this chapter.

Using Dry Sterile Transfer Forceps

Occasionally after a sterile tray has been set up and sterile gloves removed, an additional item needs to be applied to or removed from the tray. The use of dry sterile transfer forceps allows sterile items to be applied or sterile items on the tray to be rearranged without the application of another pair of sterile gloves (Figure 31-36). The practice of using wet sterile transfer forceps is no longer recommended. Instead, when the use of sterile transfer forceps is needed, dry sterile transfer forceps are unwrapped, used only once, and then reprocessed for sterilization and subsequent use.

PROCEDURE 31-1

Applying Sterile Gloves

STANDARD PRECAUTIONS:

PURPOSE:

Because hands cannot be sterilized, everyone performing sterile procedures must wear sterile gloves. This procedure provides direction on how to apply sterile gloves without compromising sterility.

EQUIPMENT/SUPPLIES:

Packaged pair of sterile gloves of appropriate size
Flat, clean, dry surface

PROCEDURE STEPS:

1. Remove rings and watch.

2. Wash hands using surgical asepsis. RATIONALE: Rings and watches can snag and tear gloves, and therefore interfere with barrier protection.

3. Inspect glove package for tears or stains (Figure 31-37A). RATIONALE: Tears and stains indicate that the gloves are no longer considered sterile and must be disposed of or used for a nonsterile purpose.

4. Place the glove package on a clean, dry, flat surface above waist level. RATIONALE: Using a contaminated surface could compromise the sterility of the sterile package.

5. *Paying attention to detail,* peel open the package taking care not to touch the sterile inner surface of the package. Do not allow the gloves to slide beyond the sterile inner border (Figure 31-37B). RATIONALE: Care must be taken to maintain the sterility of the gloves.

6. The gloves should be opened with the cuffs toward you, the palms up, and the thumbs pointing outward. If the gloves are not positioned properly, turn the package around, being careful not to reach over the sterile area or touch the inner surface or the gloves. RATIONALE: Sterile gloves are packaged in this position for ease in application.

7. With the index finger and thumb of the nondominant hand, grasp the *inner* cuffed edge of the opposite glove. The glove should be picked straight up off the package surface without dragging or dangling the fingers over any nonsterile area. RATIONALE: Picking up the glove by grasping the inner cuff prevents the outer glove from becoming contaminated. Strict adherence must be made to the sterile principles listed in the beginning of this chapter.

8. With the palm up on the dominant hand, carefully slide the hand into the glove. Do not allow the outside of the glove to come in contact with anything and stand away from sterile package. Always hold the hands above the waist and away from the body with palms up (Figure 31-37C). RATIONALE: Keeping the palm up allows the glove to remain sterile in the palm area if it rolls slightly on the back of the hand.

9. With the gloved hand, pick up the glove for the remaining hand by slipping four fingers under the outside of the cuff. Lift the second glove up, keeping it held above the waist and away from the body. Do not allow the glove to drag across the package or touch nonsterile surfaces (Figure 31-37D). RATIONALE: The outside of the second glove is sterile and may only be touched by another sterile surface.

10. With the palm up, slip the second hand into the glove. Do not allow the outside of the gloves to touch nonsterile skin and be especially mindful of the thumb (Figure 31-37E).

11. Adjust the gloves on the hands as needed, but avoid touching the wrist area. Keep gloved hands above the waist and away from the body. Do not touch nonsterile surfaces with the gloved hands (Figure 31-37F and G).

Procedure 31-1 (continued)

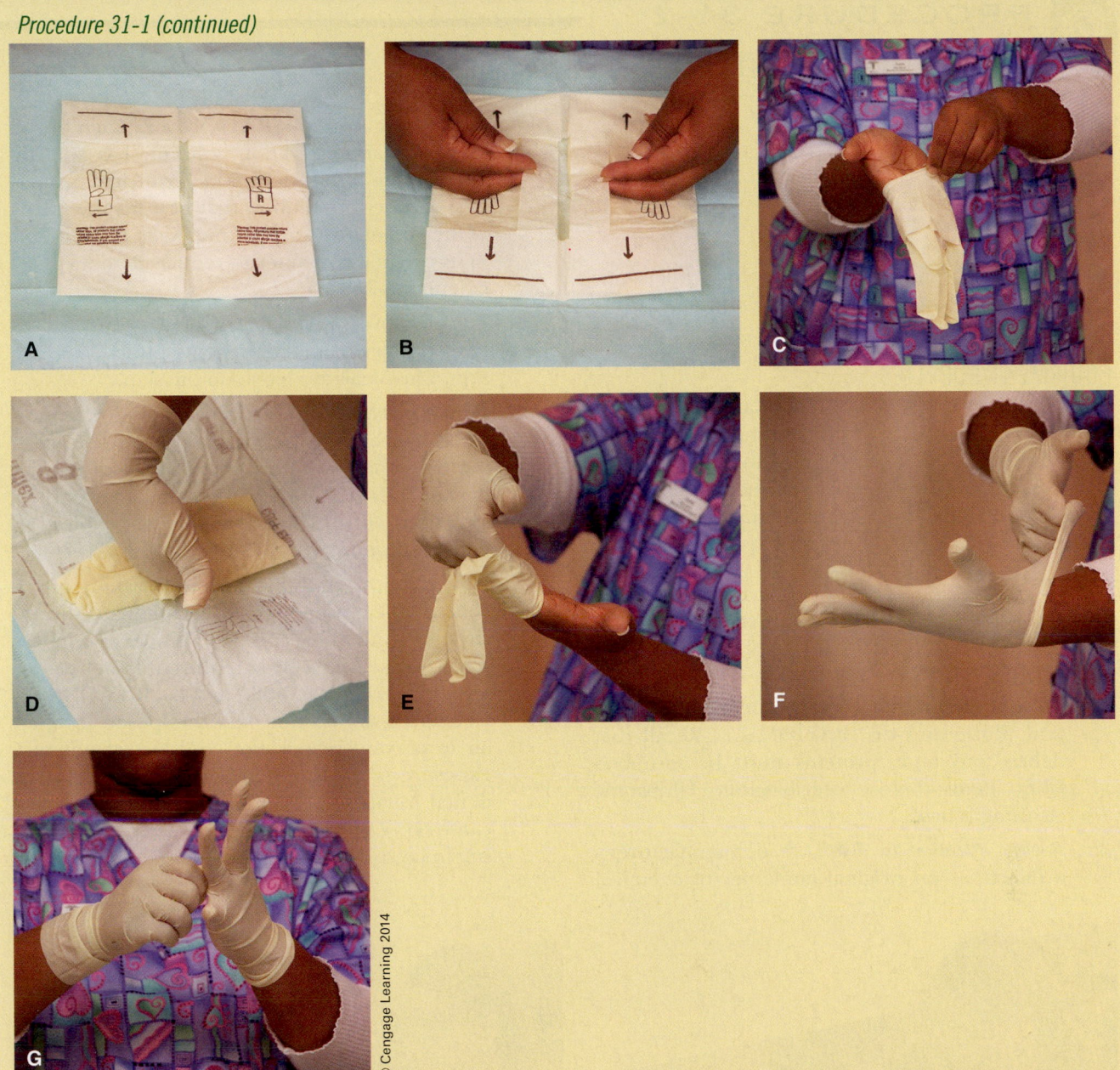

© Cengage Learning 2014

Figure 31-37 (A) Sterile gloves often are packaged with right and left clearly marked. (B) Using only the fingertips, reach in from each side and grasp the edges of the paper. Pull out and lay paper flat without touching any area except the very edges. (C) With the nondominant hand, grasp the inner cuffed edge of the opposite glove. Pick the glove up and step away from the sterile area, keeping your hands above your waste and away from your body. With palm up on the dominant hand, slide the hand into the glove. (D) Step back to the sterile area. With the gloved hand, pick up the glove for the remaining hand by slipping four fingers under the outside of the cuff. (E) With palm up, slip the second hand into the glove. Keep the gloved thumb in a "hitchhiking" position. (F) Keeping hands above the waist and away from the body, pull on the second glove. (G) Adjust gloves if desired, staying away from the wrist area. Keep gloved hands above the waist and away from the body.

PROCEDURE 31-2

Chemical "Cold" Sterilization of Endoscopes

STANDARD PRECAUTIONS:

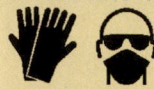

PURPOSE:

To sterilize heat-sensitive items such as fiber-optic endoscopes and delicate cutting instruments using appropriate chemical solutions.

EQUIPMENT/SUPPLIES:

Chemical solution such as Cidex Steris System® (peracetic acid)	Sterile water Gloves (heavy-duty) Sterile towel
Airtight container	Plastic-lined sterile drapes
Timer	Sterile transfer forceps Sterile basin

PROCEDURE STEPS:

1. Sanitize items that require chemical sterilization. Rinse and dry. RATIONALE: Recall that debris and body proteins must be scrubbed from items before sterilization. Ultrasonic cleaning is best.

2. *Paying attention to detail,* read manufacturer's instructions on original container of chemical sterilization solution. RATIONALE: Each brand of chemical sterilization solution has specific preparation instructions and germicidal properties; choose the solution that best fits the needs of the ambulatory care setting. Keep the solution in its original container to reduce chances of accidental poisoning.

3. Put on gloves. RATIONALE: Heavy-duty gloves help protect from sharp items puncturing the skin. Chemicals are harsh on the skin.

4. *Paying attention to detail,* prepare solution as indicated by manufacturer; place the date of opening or preparation on the container and initial it. RATIONALE: Following manufacturer's instructions ensures sterility. Note the expiration date of solution.

5. Pour solution carefully to avoid splashing into a container large enough to accomodate the instrument and allow complete immersion in the sterilizing solution. Be sure the container has an airtight lid (Figure 31-38A and B). RATIONALE: Chemicals should not be left exposed to open air to prevent evaporation and loss of potency, exposure to environmental contaminants, accidental inhalation, or poisoning. Splashing may cause skin or mucous membrane contact and result in injury.

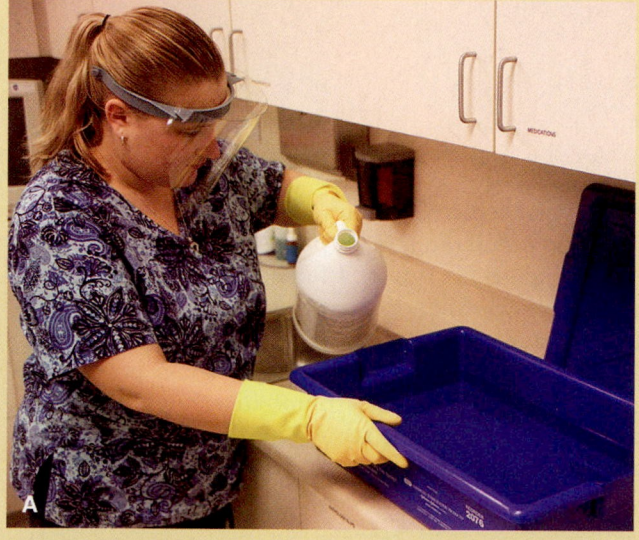
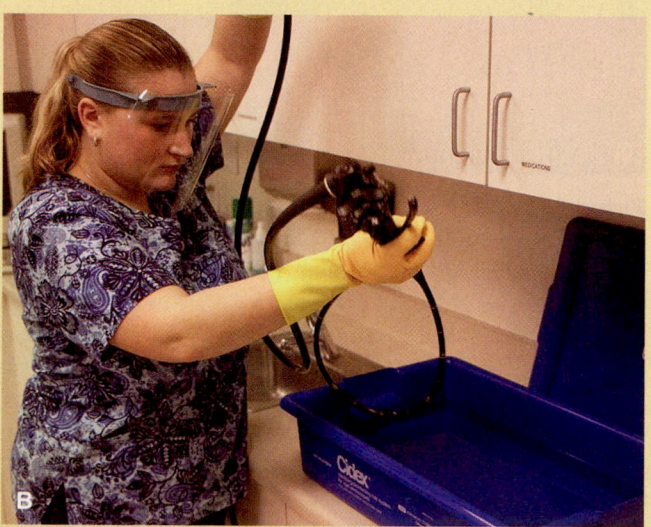

Figure 31-38 (A) Medical assistant pours chemical sterilization solution into a large soaking container. Note the use of heavy-duty gloves and face shield. (B) Medical assistant adds the endoscope to the chemical sterilization solution in the container.

Procedure 31-2 (continued)

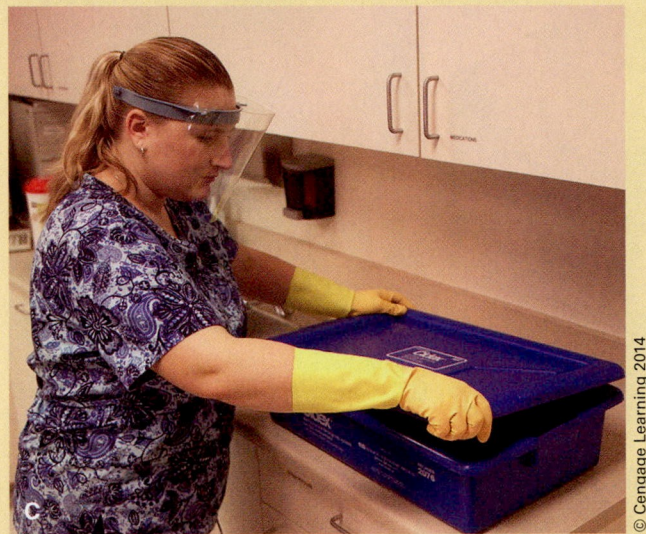

© Cengage Learning 2014

Figure 31-38 (*continued*) (C) Medical assistant secures lid tightly, then records the date, time of day, and her initials.

6. Place sanitized and dried items into the solution, completely submerging item(s). Avoid splashing when placing items into airtight container. RATIONALE: Total immersion is necessary for sterility to be achieved.

7. Close lid of container, label with name of solution, date, and time required per manufacturer, and initial (Figure 31-38C). RATIONALE: Exposure time is the required time indicated by the manufacturer to achieve sterility. Initialing work ensures accountability and responsibility.

8. Do not open lid or add additional items during the processing time. RATIONALE: Adding to the container interrupts the sterilization process and limits the effectiveness of the chemical.

9. Following the recommended processing time, lift item(s) from the container using sterile gloved hands or sterile transfer forceps. Carefully hold item above sterile basin and pour copious amounts of sterile water over it and through it (endoscopes) until adequately rinsed of chemical solution. RATIONALE: Item(s) once processed are sterile and must be handled appropriately. Using sterile gloved hands or sterile transfer forceps ensures sterile-to-sterile contact and no contamination of the item(s). Sterile water is poured through the inner channels of endoscopes to rinse chemicals from the inside, as well as the outside.

10. Hold item(s) upright for a few seconds to allow excess sterile water to drip off.

11. Place the sterile item on a sterile towel (which has been placed on a sterile field) and dry it with another sterile towel. The towel used for drying is removed from the sterile field. The use of sterile drapes that have a plastic polylined barrier layer between two layers of paper is recommended for the sterile field. RATIONALE: Plastic-lined sterile drapes create a barrier to prevent moisture from drawing contaminants from the metal surgical instrument tray or countertop up into the sterile area.

PROCEDURE 31-3

Preparing Instruments for Sterilization in Autoclave

PURPOSE:
To properly wrap sanitized instruments for sterilization in an autoclave.

EQUIPMENT/SUPPLIES:
Sanitized instruments
Wrapping material (muslin or disposable wrapping paper)
Sterilization indicator
2 × 2 gauze or cotton balls (if instrument has hinges)
Autoclave wrapping tape
Permanent marker or felt-tip pen (Figure 31-39A)

PROCEDURE STEPS:
1. *Paying attention to detail,* prepare a clean, dry, flat surface of adequate size to lay the wrapping material. RATIONALE: A clean area reduces risk for contamination. Adequate space is required for proper wrapping.

2. Select two wraps of adequate size in which to wrap instruments.

3. Place one square of wrapping material at an angle in front of you on the dry surface with one corner pointed directly toward you.

continues

Procedure 31-3 (continued)

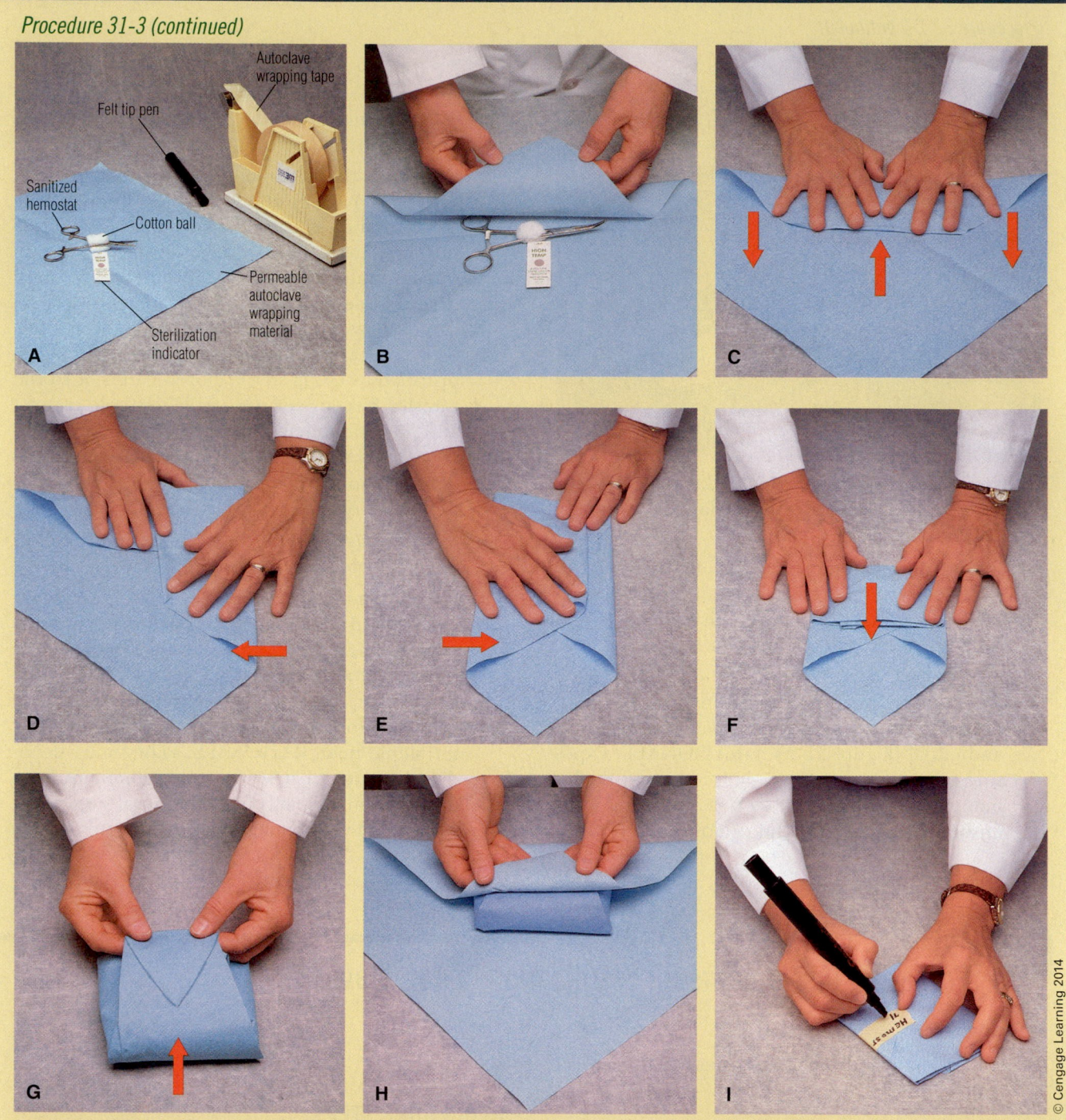

Figure 31-39   (A) Equipment needed to wrap surgical instruments or equipment for sterilization in an autoclave. (B) Place a cotton ball between the hinge joints of instruments to keep them open. Do not ratchet instruments closed. Pad the tips of sharp instruments. Put a sterilization indicator in with the instruments to be wrapped. (C) The wrapping paper is folded toward center. A small corner is turned back on itself. (D) Fold one side toward center, leaving small corner turned back on itself. (E) Fold other side toward center, leaving small corner turned back on itself. (F) The package is folded up from the bottom and secured. (G) Fold corner back on itself. (H) Wrap first package in another wrap. Double wrapping allows more control of multiple instruments when setting up a surgical tray. (I) Wrapped package is secured with heat-sensitive autoclave tape and labeled with the date, contents, and medical assistant's initials.

© Cengage Learning 2014

Procedure 31-3 (continued)

4. Place the sanitized instrument or articles to be placed in the autoclave just below the center of the wrap. Open instruments with hinges as wide as possible and place a 2 × 2 gauze or cotton ball in the opening (Figure 31-39B). RATIONALE: Instruments with hinged parts that are not spread open before autoclaving may not be properly sterilized.

5. Place one sterilization indicator with the instrument. RATIONALE: Sterilization indicators inside packages ascertain sterilization of each individual package. Indicators change colors when the required temperature has been reached, documenting the effectiveness of the sterilization. *NOTE:* Quality control for autoclave operation can be evaluated with sterilization indicators.

6. Bring the corner of the wrap closest to you up and over the article toward the center. Bring the tip of the same corner back toward you until it reaches the folded edge, creating a fan-fold effect. Smooth the edges of the fold. The article should remain completely covered (Figure 31-39C).

7. Fold one side edge toward the center line; fan-fold back to side, and crease (Figure 31-39D).

8. Repeat step 7 for the other side edge (Figure 31-39E).

9. Fold the package up from the bottom (Figure 31-39F).

10. Fold the top edge down and over the entire package (Figure 31-39G). RATIONALE: Final edge should wrap entire package for assurance of adequate coverage and protection once contents are sterilized. If wrap does not cover adequately, unwrap and start over with larger wrapping material.

11. To "wrap twice," place this package into the center of a second wrap (Figure 31-39H). Repeat Steps 7 through 10. RATIONALE: Double wrapping allows more control of multiple instruments when setting up a surgical tray.

12. Tape with autoclave tape across the point left exposed. RATIONALE: Autoclave tape indicates whether the package has been through the autoclave; it is not a form of sterilization indicator or quality control.

13. Label the tape with the name of the instrument or type of pack (i.e., laceration repair pack), date of sterilization, and your initials (Figure 31-39I). RATIONALE: Proper instrument labeling is required to identify wrapped sterilized instruments. Instruments wrapped and sterilized in paper or cloth wrappers are considered sterile for four weeks from the date of sterilization. Initialing packages ensures accountability and responsibility.

14. Place wrapped instruments in autoclave. RATIONALE: If wrapped instruments are not to be immediately autoclaved, do NOT date the package. Leave the package on a clean, dry surface and date the package just before autoclaving.

PROCEDURE 31-4

Sterilization of Instruments (Autoclave)

PURPOSE:
To rid items for use in invasive procedures of all forms of microbial life (microorganisms).

EQUIPMENT/SUPPLIES:
Steam sterilizer (autoclave)
Autoclave manufacturer's instructions
Wrapped sanitized instrument package(s) with sterilization indicatorsplaced inside package (or unwrapped item if removed with sterile transfer forceps)

PROCEDURE STEPS:
1. *Paying attention to detail,* check water level in the autoclave reservoir and add distilled water to fill line if necessary. RATIONALE: Not enough or too much water will impair the efficiency of the autoclave. Distilled water will not leave deposits (tap water leaves deposits) inside the autoclave. Deposits can impair the efficiency of the autoclave.

2. Depending on your autoclave, turn the knob to "fill" line and allow water into the chamber until it reaches the "fill" line. Turn the knob to the next position. This stops water from continuing to enter the chamber.

3. Load packages into autoclave tray; allow room for steam to circulate (Figure 31-40). RATIONALE: Steam circulates in predictable patterns in an autoclave. When packages are loaded too

continues

Procedure 31-4 (continued)

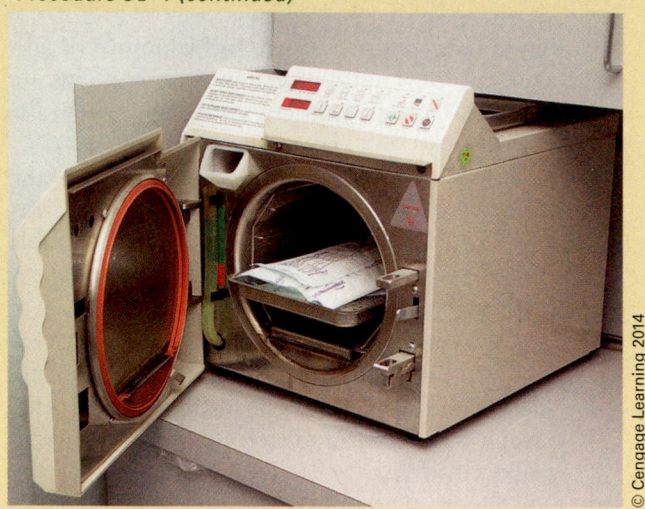

© Cengage Learning 2014

Figure 31-40 Load packages into the autoclave so that steam is able to reach all surfaces, allowing for proper sterilization.

closely or improperly, proper sterilization will not occur in individual packages.

   a. Load jars of dressings or cups on their sides, with tops ajar or loosely in place. RATIONALE: Steam is trapped within a jar when it is right side up; containers and goods will not be sterilized if loaded sitting up vertically.

   b. Load unwrapped instruments flat with handles opened, exposing all surfaces. RATIONALE: Steam must reach all surfaces.

4. Close autoclave door and seal. RATIONALE: Pressure cannot be achieved without a proper seal.

5. Turn on autoclave. When the temperature dial indicates 270°F (118°C) and 15 pounds of pressure has been achieved inside the autoclave, begin necessary exposure time by setting timer. RATIONALE: Proper heat, pressure levels, and exposure time must be achieved to kill all microorganisms within the autoclave. Careful note should be given to setting exposure time only after the proper temperature and pressure settings have been achieved.

Item	Required Exposure Time
Wrapped instrument packages or trays	30 minutes
Unwrapped items	15 minutes
Unwrapped items covered with cloth	20 minutes

6. After completion of the autoclave cycle, vent exhaust steam pressure from the autoclave by following the manufacturer's instructions. RATIONALE: Following the manufacturer's instructions carefully will ensure safe and proper use of the autoclave.

7. Open the door approximately 1 inch after the pressure gauge indicates zero (0) pressure and the temperature gauge indicates a decrease to at least 212°F. RATIONALE: You will not be able to open the door until the pressure is zero. Be aware that steam burns can occur when opening the door. Use caution.

8. Allow the contents to completely dry, approximately 30 to 45 minutes; do NOT touch contents until completely dry. RATIONALE: If packages are still wet or damp, microorganisms can enter a wrapped package, rendering it contaminated. Liquids travel along paper or cloth by capillary action and will be contaminated by microorganisms on countertops or from hands.

9. Remove wrapped contents with dry, clean hands and store in a clean, dry, closed cupboard or drawer. RATIONALE: Sterilized wrapped packages can be held with clean hands, because only the interior contents require maintenance of sterility. If the outer wrapper is required to remain sterile, remove with sterile transfer forceps and place on a sterile field or in sterile storage areas.

10. Remove unwrapped contents with sterile transfer forceps; resanitize and resterilize the transfer forceps following use. RATIONALE: Sterile transfer forceps must have been sterilized immediately prior to or along with the unwrapped item if they are to be used immediately in a sterile procedure. Place onto sterile surface.

11. Perform quality control on a regular basis, based on usage. RATIONALE: Quality control and maintenance of an autoclave are critical to assurance of proper operation. Accountability and responsibility to monitor quality control should be the responsibility of the medical assistant(s) most often responsible for sterilization.

   a. Monitor sterilization indicators with each use of sterilized instruments.

   b. On a weekly basis, perform quality control by documenting sterilization indicator outcome on a log; date and initial quality-control log entries.

12. Clean and service the autoclave regularly according to the manufacturer's guidelines. When

---

Procedure 31-4 (continued)

sterilization is not being achieved, take equipment out of service and contact a service agency for repair. RATIONALE: As a component of risk management, it is the responsibility of the

medical assistant to take out of service any equipment that is not operating properly.

13. Maintain a log of cleaning, services, and quality-control measures performed.

PROCEDURE 31-5

Setting Up and Covering a Sterile Field

STANDARD PRECAUTIONS:

PURPOSE:
Disposable sterile field drapes or sterile towels are used to isolate a sterile area or field, as well as to cover the sterile field for use in surgery and sterile procedures. They are available in convenient peel-apart packages, fanfolded for ease of use, and often are two-tone in color to aid in differentiating one side from the other. Cloth drapes may be packaged separately and sterilized fanfolded.

NOTE: A variety of materials, both disposable and nondisposable, can be used to set up and cover a sterile field. All material has certain criteria to be safe for use and all have advantages and disadvantages. For example, woven textile fabrics are moisture retardant and are effective barriers to microbial penetration. Polylined paper disposable drapes are excellent barriers against microorganisms and moisture. Many times medical clinic preference is determined by financial considerations.

EQUIPMENT/SUPPLIES:
Disposable sterile polylined field drapes (two) or
    reusable sterile towels (two) (muslin or linen with
    water-repellent finish)
Mayo instrument tray/stand positioned above the
    waist with stem to the right
Sterile transfer forceps (if needed)
Nonsterile disposable gloves

PROCEDURE STEPS:
1. Wash hands. Put on nonsterile disposable gloves.
2. Sanitize and disinfect a Mayo instrument tray. Adjust tray to above waist level and have the stem to the right.

3. Remove gloves and dispose of properly. Wash hands again.
4. Select an appropriate disposable sterile field drape and place the drape package on a clean, dry, flat surface.
5. Open the package exposing the fanfolded drape. Ensure that the cut corners of the drape are toward you; turn the package if necessary (Figure 31-41A). RATIONALE: Sterile field drapes are fanfolded and positioned within the package to facilitate ease of use.
6. With thumb and forefinger of one hand, carefully grasp the top cut corner without touching the rest of the drape or towel and pick the drape or towel up high enough to ensure that as it unfolds it does not drag across a nonsterile area (Figure 31-41B). RATIONALE: The drape or towel will naturally unfold as it is lifted, so care must be taken to ensure that it is lifted quickly and allowed to unfold without touching a nonsterile surface.
7. Holding the drape or towel above waist level and away from the body, grasp the opposing corner so that both corners along the long edge of the drape are being held (Figure 31-41C).
8. Keeping the drape or towel above waist level and away from the body, reach over the Mayo tray with the drape or towel. Take care that the lower edge of the drape or towel does not drag across the tray (Figure 31-41D). RATIONALE: Sterile principles state that sterile items should be kept above the waist and not touch other objects.
9. Gently pull the drape or towel toward you as it is laid onto the tray. If adjustment is needed to center the drape or towel, do not touch the center of the drape or towel, or reach over the sterile field. Walk around or reach underneath the tray to move it or make adjustments. RATIONALE: The

continues

Procedure 31-5 (continued)

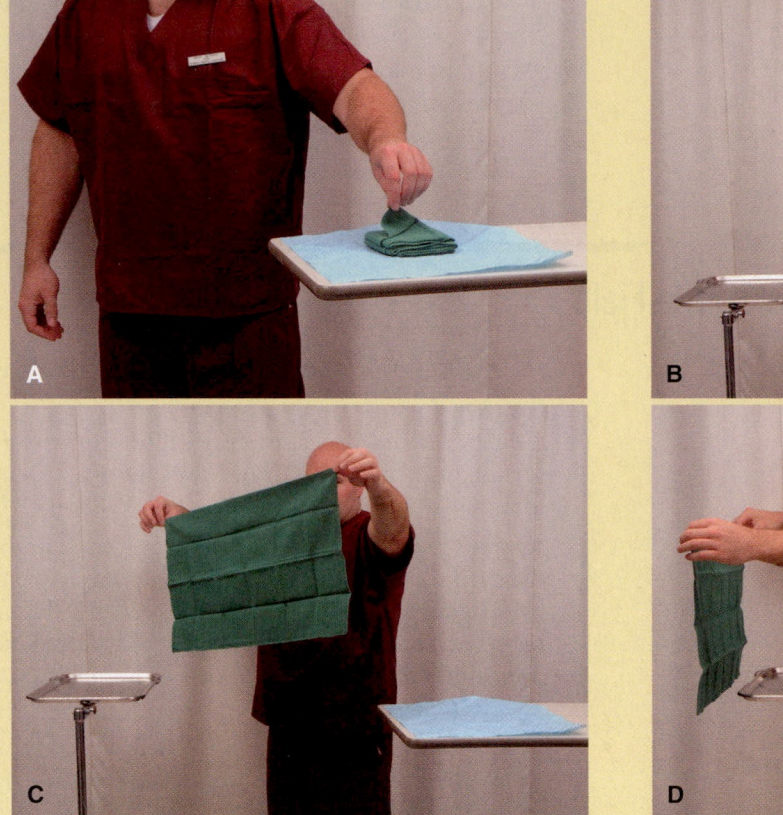
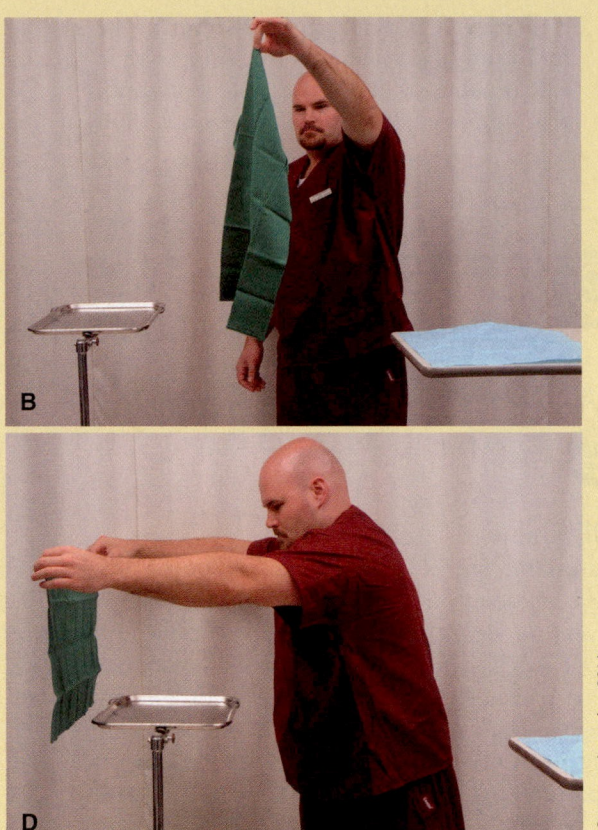

© Cengage Learning 2014

Figure 31-41 (A) Open the sterile drape package onto a flat, dry surface 90 degrees perpendicular to the Mayo tray. Grasp the corner of the sterile drape. (B) Pull the drape straight up, allowing it to unfold. Do not shake it out. (C) Carefully grasp another corner of the drape and apply the drape to the Mayo tray by pulling it toward you. Do not reach over the field; do not allow the "top" surface to touch anything. (D) Continue laying the drape as a sterile field.

corners/edges that hang over the tray are no longer considered sterile.

10. After setting the instruments and supplies on the tray, it must be covered.

11. To cover the sterile field with a second sterile drape or towel, follow Steps 4 through 7; then instead of pulling the drape or towel toward you (as described in Step 8), which would necessitate reaching over the sterile field, apply the covering drape or towel by holding it up in front of the field. Adjust the lower edge so it is even with the lower edge of the field drape or towel (see Figure 31-42H). With a forward motion, carefully lay the cover over the sterile field (see Figure 31-42I). RATIONALE: Reaching over the sterile field would contaminate the tray.

PROCEDURE 31-6

Opening Sterile Packages of Instruments and Supplies and Applying Them to a Sterile Field

STANDARD PRECAUTIONS:

NOTE: Sterile instruments and supplies are packaged in a manner that allows them to be opened and accessed without compromising sterility. Refer to other sections of this chapter for the specific steps of wrapping techniques, sterile gloving, and setting up sterile fields. The "wrapping twice" method of double wrapping was used in preparing the surgical packs for this procedure. Prepackaged items such as gauze squares should be in peel-apart packs.

PURPOSE:

To open sterile packages of surgical instruments and supplies and place them onto a sterile field using sterile technique.

EQUIPMENT/SUPPLIES:

Mayo instrument tray draped with sterile field
Sterile gloves
Wrapped-twice sterile surgical instruments
Prepackaged sterile surgical supplies

PROCEDURE STEPS:

1. *Paying attention to detail,* assemble supplies.

2. Wash hands and set up sterile field (see Procedure 31-5).

3. Position package of surgical instruments on palm of nondominant hand with outer envelope flap on top (Figure 31-42A). RATIONALE: This will facilitate opening the pack while protecting its sterile contents.

4. Grasping the taped end of the top flap, open the first flap away from you. Do not touch the inside of the flap (Figure 31-42B).

5. Grasping just the folded-back tips of the side flaps, pull the right-sided flap to the right. Then pull the left-sided flap to the left, taking care not

to reach over the package (Figure 31-42C). RATIONALE: Pulling the tips of the flaps toward each side allows the inner portion of the package to be exposed without contamination.

6. Pull the last flap toward you by grasping the folded-back tip, taking care not to touch the inner contents of the package (Figure 31-42D). RATIONALE: Pulling the last tip toward you allows you to avoid reaching over the inner contents of the package.

7. Gather all of the loose edges together to obtain a snug covering over your nondominant hand. Close your covered hand over the inner package and carefully apply the inner package to the sterile field (Figure 31-42E). RATIONALE: Gathering the loose edges prevents them from being dragged across the sterile field.

8. Open peel-apart packages using sterile technique by grasping both edges of the flaps and pulling them apart in a rolling down motion, keeping both hands together. The sterile item should be exposed gradually between the two peel-apart edges (Figure 31-42F). The sterile inner contents may then be offered to the sterile-gloved provider or applied to the sterile field using a flipping motion, or dropped as shown in Figure 31-42G, taking care not to contaminate either the package contents or the field.

9. Apply sterile gloves. Arrange instruments and supplies in an organized and logical manner according to the provider's preference. RATIONALE: Instruments should be arranged in the order of use. All handles should be pointed toward the user. Instruments should be separated as much as possible within the space of the field so entanglement of instruments is not a problem.

10. Apply the sterile field cover (Figure 31-42H, I, and J) (see Procedure 31-5). RATIONALE: A sterile cover will need to be applied if the surgical tray will not be used immediately, needs to be moved, or if the medical assistant leaves the tray unattended.

continues

Procedure 31-6 (continued)

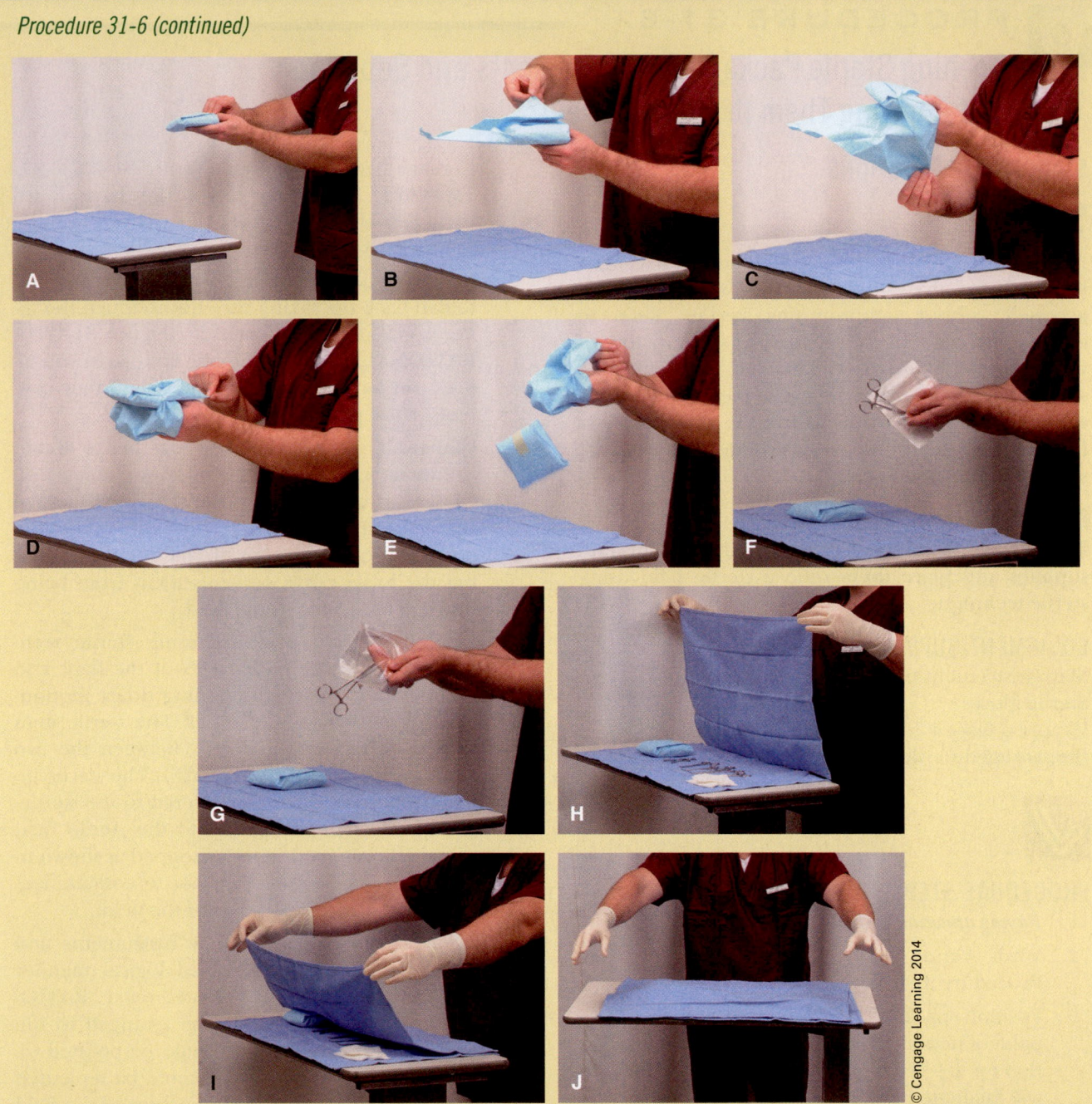

© Cengage Learning 2014

Figure 31-42 (A) To open a twice-wrapped pack, grasp the taped end of the top flap and open the first flap away from you. You should have the Mayo tray at or above waist height. Stand back from the sterile field. (B) Allow the pack to unroll on your hand. Do not touch the inside of the flap. Notice the medical assistant's thumb is under the flap, where he can securely grasp the inner pack. (C) Grasp just the folded back tips of the side flaps. First pull the right-sided tip to the right, then, reaching around or under, pull the left-sided tip to the left. Do not reach over the package. (D) Gather the loose edges together to form a snug covering over your nondominant hand. Securely grasping the wrapped inner pack, step toward your sterile field, and invert your hand. (E) Release (drop) the inner pack onto the center of the sterile field. Step back. (F) Open peel-apart packages using sterile technique, exposing sterile items slowly and gradually. Continue to peel back the sides of the package while securely holding onto the tip of the instrument. (G) Hold the sides of the package over your hand, step toward the Mayo tray, and apply the instrument, handle first, onto the sterile field. Apply other supplies as needed. Arrange instruments and supplies according to provider's preference using sterile gloves or sterile transfer forceps. (H) Apply the sterile drape cover to the surgical tray in a similar manner as the field was set up, except apply drape away from you. (I) Be sure the edges of the cover align with the edges of the field drape before letting go and applying the cover. (J) Do not adjust cover after it has been laid.

PROCEDURE 31-7

Pouring a Sterile Solution into a Cup on a Sterile Field

STANDARD PRECAUTIONS:

NOTE: Occasionally, sterile solutions need to be poured into a sterile cup that has been placed onto the sterile tray. The solution is sterile, but the outside of the container is not; therefore, special precautions need to be taken to pour the solution into the cup without contaminating the sterile field. The solution is always poured after the tray has been moved into the surgical area to avoid spilling during transport.

PURPOSE:
To pour a sterile solution into a cup on a sterile tray in a sterile manner.

EQUIPMENT/SUPPLIES:
Covered sterile surgical tray with a sterile cup in
   upper right corner
Container of sterile solution (as ordered)

PROCEDURE STEPS:
1. Wash hands.
2. ***Paying attention to detail,*** transport the surgical tray into the surgical area before pouring the solution; or, the surgical tray can be set up for immediate use in the surgical area. RATIONALE: The solution may tip and spill during transport.
3. Read the label of the solution container three times and check the expiration date. RATIONALE: To eliminate the possibility of pouring the wrong solution or an outdated solution.
4. Remove the cap from the solution container, taking care not to touch the inner surface of the cap. Place the cap upside down on a nonsterile surface to avoid touching the inner surface of the cap with a nonsterile surface. When the cap is held in the hand, hold it right side up. RATIONALE: Touching the inside of the cap with either your hand or a nonsterile surface will contaminate the inside of an otherwise sterile container.
5. ***Paying attention to detail,*** read the label again to ensure accuracy. Place palm over the label to protect the label from stains. Pour a small amount of the solution into a bowl, cup, or sink that is outside the sterile field. RATIONALE: This action will cleanse the lip of the container. *NOTE:* the surgical tray is set up in a surgical area, the solution can be poured before covering the surgical tray with a sterile drape or towel.
6. Carefully pull back the upper right corner of the tray cover to expose the cup. Take care to only touch the corner tip of the cover and not reach over the exposed field. RATIONALE: Touching the underside of the cover or reaching over the exposed sterile field will contaminate the sterile surgical tray.
7. Approaching from the corner of the tray and using the cleansed side of the lip of the container, pour the needed amount of solution into the sterile cup (Figure 31-43). Precaution should be taken to avoid splashing, spilling, reaching over the field, or touching any of the sterile surfaces. RATIONALE: Splashing or spilling of the solution would cause the sterile field drape to become wet, which may cause contaminants to "wick" from the metal tray into the sterile field. Use of a polylined sterile field drape will create a barrier to avoid wicking.
8. Replace the corner of the drape cover using sterile technique or cover with a sterile drape or towel.
9. Replace the cap of the solution container using sterile technique.
10. Read the label again, ***paying attention to detail.***

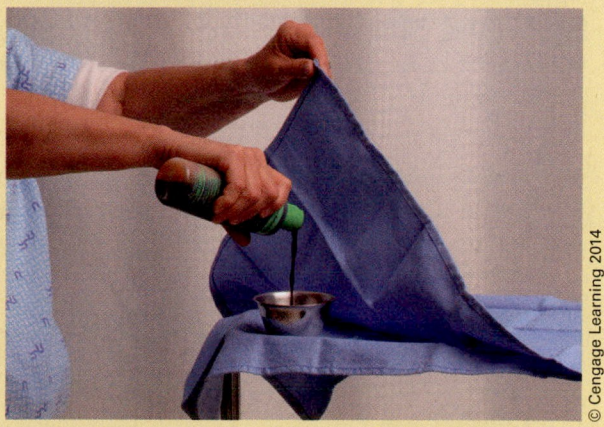

© Cengage Learning 2014

Figure 31-43 Approaching from the corner of the Mayo stand, pour the needed amount of solution into the sterile cup. Use the clean side of the container lip for pouring.

PROCEDURE 31-8

Assisting with Office/Ambulatory Surgery

STANDARD PRECAUTIONS:

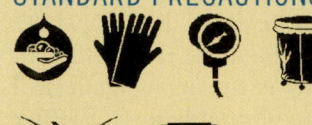

PURPOSE:

To maintain sterility during surgical procedures that require surgical excision.

EQUIPMENT/SUPPLIES:

Mayo stand:
Needles and syringe for anesthesia
Prep bowl/cup
Gauze sponges
Scalpel and blade
Operating scissors
Fenestrated drape
Hemostats (curved and straight)
Thumb dressing forceps
Thumb tissue forceps
Needle holder
Suture pack
Transfer forceps

Side table (unsterile field):
Sterile gloves (in package)
Labeled biopsy containers with formalin
Appropriate laboratory requisition
Anesthesia vial
Alcohol wipes
Dressing, tape, bandages
Biohazard container
Betadine® solution

PROCEDURE STEPS:

1. Check room and equipment for readiness and cleanliness.

2. Wash hands.

3. *Paying attention to detail,* set up side table of nonsterile items. RATIONALE: Nonsterile items cannot be placed onto a sterile field because they will contaminate it.

4. Perform surgical asepsis hand cleansing.

5. Set up sterile field on a sanitized and disinfected Mayo stand or on a clean, dry, flat surface (see Procedure 31-5).

6. *Paying attention to detail.* add sterile items (see Procedure 31-6).

7. Apply sterile gloves or use sterile transfer forceps (per Procedure 31-1).

8. Arrange instruments according to provider's instructions.

9. Remove sterile gloves and dispose of appropriately or remove forceps from area.

10. Wash hands.

11. Cover the sterile field with a sterile towel if not being used immediately.

12. *Introduce yourself. Identify the patient and explain the procedure at the patient's level of understanding.*

13. Prepare the patient based on the procedure to be performed and per provider's preference. Refer to Patient Preparation in Table 31-4.

14. Use appropriate skin prep.

15. *Paying attention to detail.* remove the sterile cover from the sterile setup as the provider applies sterile gloves. Lift the towel by grasping the tips of the corners farthest away from you and lifting toward you. Do not allow arms to pass over sterile field. RATIONALE: Avoids crossing over sterile field.

16. *Working within your scope of practice,* assist the provider as necessary, being certain to follow the principles of surgical asepsis.

   - Appropriately hold the vial of anesthetic agent with the provider withdraws the required dose.

   - The provider injects the local anesthetic, applies Betadine® or other antiseptic to the surgical site, applies sterile drapes, and begins the surgery. Apply sterile gloves to assist as requested.

   - Adjust the instrument tray and equipment around the provider.

   - Ensure a good light source.

   - *Allay the patient's fears regarding the procedure being performed and help them to feel safe and comfortable.*

17. Hand instruments to the provider and receive used instruments from the provider and place in a basin or container out of the patient's line of sight.

18. If necessary, hold biopsy container to receive specimen being excised. Do not contaminate the inside of the container. Assist with or apply sterile dressing to the operative site.

19. *Being courteous and respectful,* assist the patient as necessary. *Attend to any special needs of the patient.*

20. The specimen container must be tightly covered; labeled with the patient's name, date, type, and source of specimen; and sent to the laboratory accompanied by the appropriate laboratory requisition.

Procedure 31-8 (continued)

21. Wearing appropriate personal protective equipment (PPE), clean surgical or examination room.
    - Dispose of used gauze sponges in biohazard container and knife blades and other disposable sharps in puncture-proof sharps container.
    - Rinse used surgical instruments; soak, sanitize, and sterilize for reuse (see Chapter 22).
    - Remove gloves and other PPE and dispose of per Occupational Safety and Health Administration (OSHA) guidelines.

22. Wash hands.
23. Accurately document in patient's chart or electronic medical record that the specimen was sent to the laboratory.

DOCUMENTATION:

*8/12/20XX 2:30 PM   Skin tag from left axilla excised by
Dr. King. Biopsy specimen in its entirety sent to laboratory.
S. Tyler, CMA (AAMA)——————————————————————————*

PROCEDURE 31-9

Dressing Change

STANDARD PRECAUTIONS:

  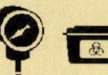

NOTE: After most surgical procedures have been completed, the wound is usually covered with a dry sterile dressing (DSD) that may need to be removed periodically so that the wound can be checked for healing or for suture removal. Another dry sterile dressing may then be applied. Burns require daily dressing changes.

PURPOSE:
To remove a wound dressing and apply a dry sterile dressing.

EQUIPMENT/SUPPLIES:
Sterile Field:

Several sterile gauze sponges and other dressing material as needed or prepackaged sterile dressing kit
Sterile bowl with Betadine® solution or prepared sterile Betadine® swab sticks
Sterile dressing forceps
Sponge forceps

Side Area (Unsterile Field):

Nonsterile gloves
Sterile gloves
Hydrogen peroxide
Container of sterile water
Cotton-tipped applicators
Adhesive strips
Antibacterial ointment/cream as ordered

Tape
Sponge forceps
Bandage scissors
Waterproof waste bag
Biohazard waste container

PROCEDURE STEPS:
1. Check provider's order.
2. Wash hands.
3. *Paying attention to detail,* prepare sterile field. Add gauze sponges, bowl with solution, and forceps.
4. Position a waterproof bag away from sterile area.
5. Pour Betadine® solution into sterile bowl or use Betadine swab sticks.
6. *Introduce yourself. Identify the patient and explain the procedure, speaking at the patient's level of understanding.*
7. *Allay the patient's fears regarding the procedure being performed and help them to feel safe and comfortable.*
8. Don nonsterile gloves or use forceps.
9. Loosen tape on dressing by pulling tape toward wound, or cut off bandage if necessary.
10. Carefully remove bandage; place in biohazard waste container. Do not pass over sterile field. RATIONALE: Passing dirty (used) bandage or dressing over sterile field contaminates it.

continues

Procedure 31-9 (continued)

11. Remove dressing, taking care not to cause stress on the wound.

    a. If the dressing is stuck to the wound, pour small amounts of sterile water or saline over the dressing; allow to soak for a short time. Remove dressing when loose enough to remove without resistance. Note type and amount of drainage.

12. Place used dressing in waterproof bag without touching inside or outside of bag. RATIONALE: Dirty (used) dressing can contaminate outside of bag.

13. Assess wound and note any drainage or signs of infection. Remove and discard gloves in waterproof bag.

14. Wash hands.

15. Don sterile gloves.

16. Clean the wound with antiseptic solution as ordered (Figure 31-44B). Gauze may be held with forceps, or use swabs.

17. Dispose of used gauze in waterproof bag.

18. Using sterile cotton-tipped applicators, apply cream/ointment as ordered. Using sterile forceps or sterile gloves, apply sterile gauze sponge(s) to wound (Figure 31-44C).

19. Remove gloves and dispose of appropriately. Wash hands.

20. Secure dressing with roller bandage and adhesive tape (Figure 31-44D and (Figure 31-44E) or elastic bandage.

21. Wash hands.

22. Accurately document procedure in patient's chart or electronic medical record, describing wound appearance (i.e., discharge, signs of infection, healing, and so on).

DOCUMENTATION:

11/24/20XX 10:30 AM   Dressing change to laceration left forearm. Small amount (dime-size) of serosanguinous discharge noted. No signs of redness or swelling in incisional area. DSD applied. Says she "feels fine and that my arm hurts very little." S. Tyler, CMA (AAMA) ————————

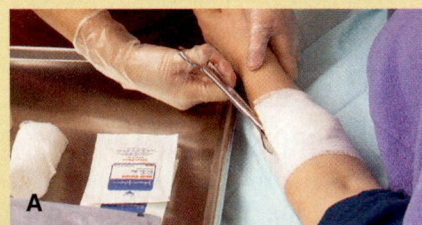
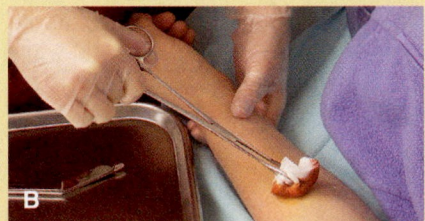
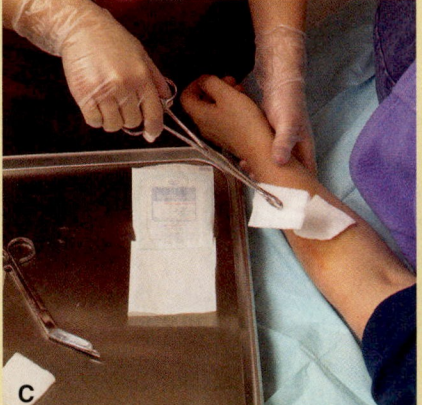
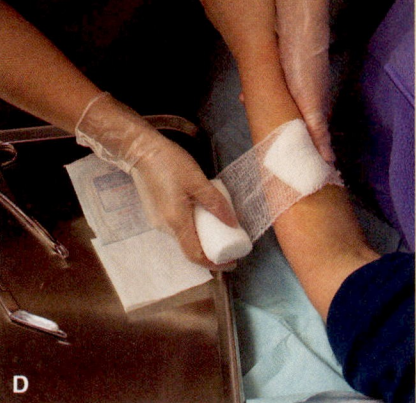
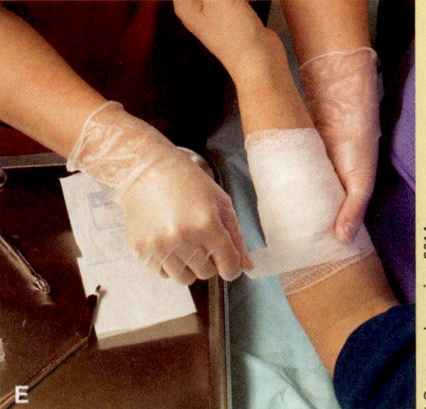

© Cengage Learning 2014

Figure 31-44 To change a dressing: (A) Gently remove dressing. Do not cause stress on wound. (B) Clean wound with Betadine® solution using sponge forceps. (C) Using dressing forceps, new sterile sponge forceps, and a hemostat or sterile gloves, apply sterile gauze sponge(s) to wound. (D, E) Secure dressing with elastic bandage and adhesive tape or roller bandage.

PROCEDURE 31-10

Wound Irrigation

STANDARD PRECAUTIONS:

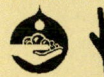

PURPOSE:

To irrigate a wound to remove the accumulation of exudate that impairs and delays healing.

EQUIPMENT/SUPPLIES:

On Mayo Tray:

Sterile gloves in package
Sterile irrigation kit (irrigating syringe, basin, and container for solution)
Sterile dressing material in package

Side Area/Unsterile Field:

Waterproof pad
Sterile solution for irrigation (per provider's order)
Nonsterile gloves
Waterproof waste bag

PROCEDURE STEPS:

1. Check the provider's order.
2. Select the correct solution and appropriate solution strength. It should be at least body temperature. (Solutions kept in warming closet.)
3. *Introduce yourself. Identify the patient and explain the procedure, speaking at the patient's level of understanding.*

4. *Allay the patient's fears regarding the procedure being performed and help him to feel safe and comfortable.*
5. Wash hands.
6. Place the waterproof pad under the body part that will be irrigated.
7. Position the patient in such a way that directs the flow of the solution into the wound. The basin catches the flow from the wound.
8. Don nonsterile gloves, remove the dressing, and dispose into waterproof waste bag.
9. Note the wound's appearance, color, amount of discharge, and odor to the discharge. RATIONALE: Allows ongoing assessment of the wound.
10. Remove and discard gloves into biohazard container.
11. Wash hands.
12. Maintaining sterile technique, open the sterile irrigation tray and the dressings. Use the inner kit wrapping as a sterile field.
13. Pour the irrigation solution into the sterile solution bowl or container. (Should be at least room temperature.) RATIONALE: Room temperature solution is more comfortable for the patient.
14. Don sterile gloves.
15. Place the sterile basin against the edge of the wound. RATIONALE: The basin will collect the irrigation solution.
16. Fill the irrigating syringe (or bulb syringe) with the solution and carefully wash out the wound with the flow of solution (Figure 31-45A and B).

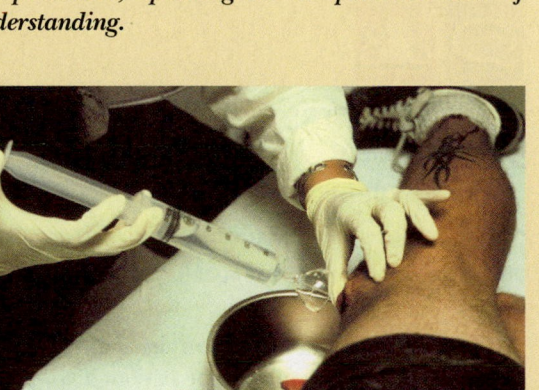

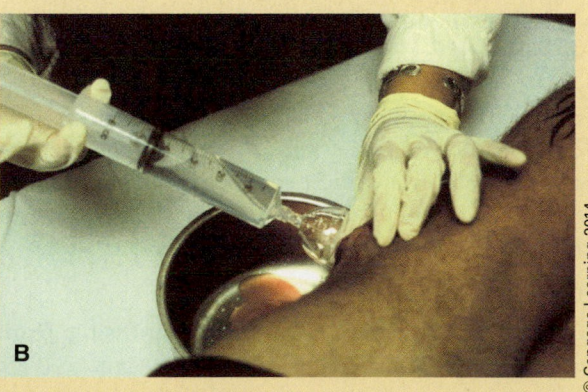

© Cengage Learning 2014

Figure 31-45   (A) Flush the wound gently. (B) Hold the syringe close to the wound, but do not touch the wound with the syringe.

continues

Procedure 31-10 (continued)

17. Continue to fill the syringe and continue to wash out the wound until the solution becomes clear and there is no drainage noted.
18. Dry the wound edge with sterile gauze.
19. Reassess the wound.
20. Apply a dry sterile dressing.
21. Remove gloves. Dispose in biohazard container.
22. Wash hands.
23. Accurately document in patient's chart or electronic medical record.

DOCUMENTATION:

8/6/20XX 2:30 PM   Dressing removed from abdominal wound. Wound red and filled with serosanguinous exudate. Irrigated with 500 mL sterile normal saline (fluid returns were clear). Wound slightly red and clean-appearing after irrigation. Wound dried with sterile 4 × 4s. Dry sterile dressing applied. Patient states, "I feel much better now that my wound has been cleaned out. That only hurt a little." Patient says she does not want anything for pain. S. Thomas CMA (AAMA)

PROCEDURE 31-11
Preparation of Patient's Skin before Surgery

STANDARD PRECAUTIONS:

NOTE: The skin and hair contain many microorganisms, and the patient's skin must be prepared before surgery to remove as many of the microorganisms as possible. Wound infection results when microorganisms enter the body. The patient may be told to scrub the site of the surgery using antimicrobial soap on the night before surgery. Because it is impossible to sterilize the skin, the operative site and an area surrounding it are scrubbed, shaved (hair harbors microorganisms), washed, and painted with an antiseptic such as Betadine® solution. A skin prep self-contained unit is a sponge applicator with a cylinder of antiseptic solution inside. One brand is known as DuraPrep. It contains iodophor and isopropyl alcohol. The medical assistant can use the unit with nonsterile gloves. The unit is compressed, the seal to the inner cylinder is broken, and the sponge end becomes the applicator. The mixture is thick and should be allowed to dry and not be blotted. Because it contains alcohol, which can be a fire hazard, the site must be dry before draping. The chemical action decontaminates the patient's skin.

PURPOSE:
To remove as many microorganisms as possible from the patient's skin immediately before surgery.

EQUIPMENT/SUPPLIES:
Absorbent pads
Drape

Disposable prep kit (includes antiseptic solution, several sponges, razor, and a container for water, or self-contained skin prep unit)
Sterile water
Sterile bowl
Sterile gloves for medical assistant and provider (two pair)

If Kit is Unavailable, Equipment Needed Is:
Sterile bowls (two)
Antiseptic solution
Sterile gauze sponges
Sterile razor
Basin for soiled sponges
Sterile transfer forceps

PROCEDURE STEPS:
1. Wash hands.
2. Assemble equipment.
3. ***Introduce yourself. Identify patient.***
4. ***Explain procedure, speaking at the patient's level of understanding.***
5. ***Remaining courteous, patient, and respectful to the patient,*** provide privacy, and drape patient if appropriate.
6. Prior to prepping and draping for the procedure, verify the location of the procedure by asking the patient to state or indicate the surgical site. Some facilities require that the appropriate site be marked with an indelible ink pen to be certain that the correct site is identified.

Procedure 31-11 (continued)

7. Provide a good light source.

8. Position patient for comfort and exposure of site.

9. Wash hands.

10. Insert waterproof absorbent toweling under the patient in the area to be prepped.

11. Open kit or individual items required for prep.

12. Don sterile gloves or use sterile transfer forceps.

13. Apply Betadine® or other antiseptic to the sponges or gauze being careful to avoid splashing.

14. *Paying attention to detail,* beginning at the site that the incision is to be made, cleanse in an outward circular motion form the site of the incision. Do not return to the center with the same sponge.

15. Discard used sponges as necessary.

16. Hold skin taut to avoid nicks, shave hair away from the operative site, following the hair growth pattern. RATIONALE: Prevents accidental nicks. Nicked skin can cause infection.

17. When hair has been removed, scrub again in a circular fashion as in Step 14 for at least three minutes or according to the provider's order.

18. Rinse shaved area with sterile water and dry with a sterile 4 × 4 gauze sponge.

19. Remove and appropriately discard absorbent pad, 4 × 4 sponges, disposable prep kit, and gloves. RATIONALE: This removes used supplies and equipment from prepped skin area and prevents contamination.

20. Wash hands.

21. Don sterile gloves, place a sterile towel under the operative site taking care not to contaminate sterile hands. RATIONALE: Placing a sterile towel under the operative area keeps site free from contamination.

22. Instruct patient not to touch the area.

23. Pour antiseptic solution (Betadine®) into the sterile bowl. Avoid splashing.

24. If instructed by the provider, don sterile gloves and prep the area with antiseptic solution. Using the same approach as in Step 14, paint the operative site with antiseptic three times, discarding the sponge after creating a cleansed area much larger than the intended incisional area.

25. Allow the area to completely dry prior to proceeding.

26. The provider will cover the patient with the fenestrated drape and begin the surgical procedure.

27. Accurately document the skin prep in patient's chart or EMR if instructed by the provider.

PROCEDURE 31-12
Suturing of Laceration or Incision Repair

STANDARD PRECAUTIONS:

 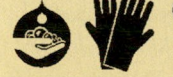
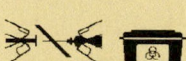

PURPOSE:

Suturing is recommended if a laceration or incision is gaping; is bleeding uncontrollably; is located on the face, neck, or a bend of a body part; or extends deep into underlying tissue. Suturing facilitates healing by approximating the edges of the wound. Suturing decreases scarring, helps decrease the likelihood of infection, and promotes healing. The wound and the surrounding area must be meticulously cleaned of any dirt and debris. Many providers have standard orders for wound cleaning, such as a 10-minute soak in Hibiclens® solution and sterile water, before

suture repair of either a laceration or incision-type wound.

EQUIPMENT/SUPPLIES:

Surgical Tray:

Appropriate size syringe and gauge of needle for administering anesthesia

Hemostats (curved)

Adson tissue forceps

Iris scissors (curved)

Suture material as ordered by provider

Needle holder

Gauze sponges

Sterile water or saline

Side Table (Unsterile Field):

Anesthetic as ordered by the provider

Dressings, bandages, and tape

Splint/brace/sling (optional)

Sterile gloves in package

continues

Procedure 31-12 (continued)

PROCEDURE STEPS:

1. Wash hands.

2. Assemble equipment.

3. *Introduce yourself. Identify the patient and explain the procedure, speaking at the patient's level of understanding.*

4. Obtain a signed consent for the procedure.

5. *Being courteous, patient, and respectful to the patient, provide privacy,* and drape patient if appropriate.

6. *Allay the patient's fears regarding the procedure being performed and help her to feel safe and comfortable.*

7. Assess cause of wound and its severity. *Accurately and concisely update the provider.*

   - Inquire regarding allergies and last tetnus shot. Document appropriately.

   - *Using active listening skills,* review health history to avoid possible complications. Share information with provider.

   - *Paying attention to any special needs of the patient,* assist her to a supine position

   - Soak wound in an antiseptic solution as ordered by provider.

   - Clean and dry wound.

8. Assist the provider as requested.

9. *Being courteous, patient, and respectful,* support the patient as needed.

Postoperative Care:

10. Don sterile gloves.

11. Using sterile water or saline and a 4 × 4 sponge, clean the area around the wound and dry with a 4 × 4 sponge or sterile towels.

12. Dress/bandage/splint wound following provider's preference.

13. Remove gloves and dispose of in biohazard waste container.

14. Wash hands.

15. Obtain vital signs to assess patient stability post–procedure. Document in the patient's chart or EMR.

16. Educate patient regarding care of the wound per provider's orders. *Include the patient's support system as indicated.* Provide written instructions that include the signs and symptoms of infection and an after-hours contact number.

17. *Demonstrating respect for individual diversity,* assist the patient with any questions or concerns.

18. Arrange for a follow-up appointment and post-operative medication as required.

19. Accurately document procedure in patient's chart or EMR.

20. Don PPE.

21. Dispose of supplies as per OSHA guidelines. Clean room, sanitize instruments, and sterilize for reuse.

22. Wash hands.

DOCUMENTATION:

11/17/20XX 10:15 AM   Patient sustained a 2 × 1.5 cm laceration on right elbow. Wound soaked in Hibiclens® solution and water for 10 minutes, and then dried. Dr. King sutured the laceration after injecting Xylocaine (1%) into area around laceration site. Ten nonabsorbable Ethicon sutures used to close wound. Dry sterile dressing applied to wound. Given a prescription by Dr. King for Percodan, 1 tab PO of 4-6h prn for pain, and Amoxicillin 500 mg PO of 6 h. Postoperative instructions reviewed and she appears to understand. Last tetanus 12 years ago. Tetanus injection given I.M. right deltoid (0.5 cc). S. Tyler, CMA (AAMA)—————————————

PROCEDURE 31-13

Sebaceous Cyst Excision

STANDARD PRECAUTIONS:

  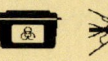 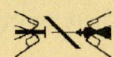

NOTE: A sebaceous cyst is a benign retention cyst, sometimes called a "wen." Sebaceous cysts are caused by an oil duct becoming "plugged," which causes the sebum (oil) to accumulate in the gland. Eventually the oil gland becomes distended. Sebaceous cysts that become inflamed or infected need to be removed. The patient may also elect to have a noninflamed sebaceous cyst removed if it is unsightly or located in a bothersome area. Incision and drainage of sebaceous cysts is usually not the treatment of choice because they tend to recur if the entire cyst is not completely excised. Ideally, the entire cyst sac is removed intact, but occasionally the sac ruptures during removal and large amounts of malodorous biohazardous sebum can be expelled. In preparation for this occurrence, extra gauze sponges, gloves, and goggles should be available.

PURPOSE:

To remove an inflamed or infected sebaceous cyst. To remove a sebaceous cyst that is not inflamed or infected but is located on an area of the body where the cyst is unsightly or where it may become irritated from rubbing.

EQUIPMENT/SUPPLIES:

Sterile Field:

Appropriate size syringe and gauge of needle for administering anesthesia
Iris scissors (curved)
Mosquito hemostat (curved)
Knife handle and blade
Suture material as ordered by provider
Needle holder
Tissue forceps (two)
Mayo scissors (curved)
Sterile 4 × 4 gauze sponges
Fenestrated drape
Antiseptic solution as per provider preference

Side Area (Unsterile Field):

Skin prep supplies
Anesthetic as ordered by the provider

Dressings, bandages, and tape
Splint/brace/sling as indicated
Prepackaged sterile gloves (appropriate sizes for medical assistant and provider)
Nonsterile disposable gloves
PPE
Alcohol pads
Tube for culture
Biohazard specimen transport bag
Appropriate lab requisitions

PROCEDURE STEPS:

1. Wash hands.

2. *Paying attention to detail,* assemble equipment.

3. *Introduce yourself. Identify the patient and explain the procedure, speaking at the patient's level of understanding.*

4. Obtain a signed consent for the procedure.

5. *Being courteous, patient, and respectful to the patient, provide privacy,* and drape patient if appropriate.

6. *Allay the patient's fears regarding the procedure being performed and help them to feel safe and comfortable.*

7. Inquire regarding allergies and last tetanus shot. Document appropriately.

8. *Using active listening skills,* review health history to avoid possible complications. Share information with provider.

9. *Paying attention to any special needs of the patient,* assist him to a supine position.

10. Don appropriate PPE, including goggles if indicated. RATIONALE: Purulent material may drain out of the wound and splash.

11. Don sterile gloves.

12. Perform skin prep as ordered by provider.

13. Remove gloves and dispose of in biohazard waste container.

14. Assist the provider to withdraw the ordered anesthetic by holding the vial in an inverted position.

15. Assist provider as needed during the procedure.

continues

Procedure 31-13 (continued)

Give Postoperative Care:

16. Don sterile gloves.

17. Using sterile water or saline and a 4 × 4 sponge, clean the area around the wound and dry with a 4 × 4 sponge or sterile towels.

18. Dress and bandage wound per provider's orders.

19. Dispose of items utilized during the procedure according to OSHA guidelines.

20. Remove gloves and dispose of in biohazard waste container.

21. Wash hands.

22. Obtain vital signs to assess patient stability post-procedure. Document in the patient's chart or EMR.

23. ***Explain wound care to the patient (and caregiver), speaking at the patient's level of understanding, and provide written instructions*** including symptoms of infection.

24. ***Demonstrating respect for individual diversity,*** assist the patient with any questions or concerns.

25. Arrange for a follow-up appointment and post-operative medication as required.

26. Document procedure in patient's chart or electronic medical record, noting that the culture specimen was sent to laboratory if appropriate.

27. Don PPE, including nonsterile disposable gloves.

28. Clean room, sanitize instruments, and sterilize for reuse.

29. Remove PPE and dispose of appropriately.

30. Wash hands.

DOCUMENTATION:

05/12/20XX 2:00 PM   Sebaceous cyst (0.5 × 0.5 cm) excised by Dr. King. Moderate amount of purulent exudate noted as cyst ruptured during removal. Specimen of exudate obtained and sent to the laboratory for culture and sensitivity. Five nonabsorbable sutures used to close the incision. Wound cleansed with Betadine®; dry sterile dressing applied. Patient given verbal and written instructions on caring for the dressing and for watching for signs of infection. BP 118/74, P 88. Skin color good. Will call clinic for results of culture and sensitivity and to discuss the need for antibiotic therapy. Will return on 5/22/20XX or sooner if necessary. S. Tyler, CMA (AAMA)————————————————

PROCEDURE 31-14

Incision and Drainage of Localized Infection

STANDARD PRECAUTIONS:

 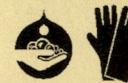

NOTE: An abscess is a localized accumulation of pus surrounded by inflamed tissue. The body attempts to isolate pus into a pocket or abscess as a means of protecting itself by walling off the pathogens and preventing them from spreading throughout the body. Incision and drainage is the procedure of cutting into an area (often an abscess) for the purposes of draining the fluid/material. A culture of the exudate can be done to identify microorganisms. Rather than suturing or otherwise closing the wound, the provider may place a gauze wick or a latex Penrose drain into the wound to facilitate continued drainage. The most commonly used type of wick is Iodoform. Iodoform is available in 5-yard lengths and widths of ¼, ½, 1, and 2 inches. Iodoform is packaged sterile in glass bottles under the Johnson & Johnson brand name of Nu Gauze (see Figure 31-31). Care must be taken when removing the desired length from the bottle to avoid contaminating the remaining gauze. To accomplish this, the medical assistant might hold the bottle and remove the lid to allow the provider to reach into the bottle with a sterile thumb dressing forceps and pull out the desired length. Sterile scissors are then used to cut the strip without contaminating the remaining wick. The Iodoform is packed into the wound with a short length exposed. After several hours or days of continued draining, the wick may be removed, and the wound allowed to heal without sutures. The patient may be prescribed an appropriate antibiotic.

Procedure 31-14 (continued)

The medical assistant should exercise caution by wearing appropriate PPE including goggles when assisting with this procedure because the exudate can be heavy and contains pathogenic microorganisms.

PURPOSE:

To incise and drain an abscess or other localized infection.

EQUIPMENT/SUPPLIES:

Surgical Tray:

Appropriate size syringe and gauge of needle for administering anesthesia

Iris scissors (curved)

Mosquito hemostat (curved)

Knife handle and blade

Suture material as ordered by provider

Needle holder

Tissue forceps (two)

Mayo scissors (curved)

Sterile 4 × 4 gauze sponges

Fenestrated drape

Antiseptic solution as per provider preference

Sterile culture swabs

Iodofom® gauze or Penrose drain

Side Area (Unsterile Field):

Skin prep supplies

Anesthetic as ordered by the provider

Dressings, bandages, and tape

Splint/brace/sling as indicated

Prepackaged sterile gloves (appropriate sizes for medical assistant and provider)

Nonsterile disposable gloves

PPE

Alcohol pads

Biohazard specimen transport bag

Appropriate lab requisitions

PROCEDURE STEPS:

1. Wash hands.
2. *Paying attention to detail,* assemble equipment.
3. *Introduce yourself. Identify the patient and explain the procedure, speaking at the patient's level of understanding.*
4. Obtain a signed consent for the procedure.
5. *Being courteous, patient, and respectful to the patient, provide privacy,* and drape patient if appropriate.
6. *Allay the patient's fears regarding the procedure being performed and help them to feel safe and comfortable.*
7. Inquire regarding allergies and last tetanus shot. Document appropriately.
8. *Using active listening skills,* review health history to avoid possible complications. Share information with provider.
9. *Paying attention to any special needs of the patient,* assist her to the appropriate position.
10. Don appropriate PPE, including goggles if indicated.
11. Don sterile gloves.
12. Perform skin prep as ordered by provider.
13. Remove gloves and dispose of in biohazard waste container.
14. Assist the provider as needed to inject the anesthesia by holding the vial while the appropriate amount is aspirated for injection. The provider incises the abscess and inserts either Iodoform gauze or a latex Penrose drain into the wound to encourage drainage. No sutures are used. Specimen taken for culture and sensitivity.
15. *Being courteous, patient, and respectful,* support the patient as needed.

Postoperative Care:

16. Don sterile gloves.
17. Using sterile water or saline and a 4 × 4 sponge, clean the area around the wound and dry with a 4 × 4 sponge or sterile towels.
18. Dress and bandage as directed. Several thicknesses of dressing material will be needed to absorb exudate, or the accumulated fluid in the cavity.
19. Dispose of items utilized during the procedure according to OSHA guidelines.
20. Remove gloves and dispose of in biohazard waste container.
21. Wash hands.
22. Obtain vital signs to assess patient stability post-procedure. Document in the patient's chart or EMR.
23. *Explain wound care to the patient (and caregiver), speaking at the patient's level of understanding* and provide written instructions such as to apply warm moist compresses to wound. Explain to watch for symptoms of infection. Stress caution when handling contaminated items.
24. *Demonstrating respect for individual diversity,* assist the patient with any questions or concerns.

continues

Procedure 31-14 (continued)

25. Arrange for a follow-up appointment and post-operative medication as required.

26. Accurately document procedure in patient's chart or electronic medical record.

27. Don PPE including nonsterile disposable gloves.

28. Clean room, sanitize instruments, and sterilize for reuse.

29. Remove PPE and dispose of appropriately.

30. Wash hands.

DOCUMENTATION:

6/20/20XX 10:00 AM   Incision and drainage of an abscess (2 × 1 cm) on the left buttock. Large amount purulent exudate noted. Wound packed with 1 inch iodoform gauze and DSD applied with large amount of 4 × 4s and abdominal dressings. Culture tube with specimen of exudate sent to laboratory with a requisition for C &S. BP 138/92, P 100. Postoperative wound care explained to patient and given written instructions as well. BP 142/72, P 88. S. Tyler, CMA (AAMA)————————

PROCEDURE 31-15
Aspiration of Joint Fluid

STANDARD PRECAUTIONS:

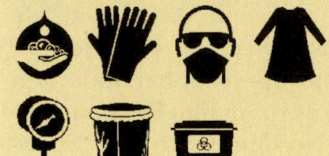

NOTE: The most common reason for aspirating fluid is to remove excess fluid from a joint, often the knee. A long, sterile, sturdy needle is inserted into the joint capsule and fluid is removed. Often a long-acting anesthetic and cortisone are injected at the same time. The aspirated fluid can be diagnostically examined for blood, pus, and fatty substances and also cultured for pathogens. After surgery the patient may be placed on anti-inflammatory medications to treat the inflammation and antibiotics if the culture is positive for pathogens.

PURPOSE:
To remove excess synovial fluid from a joint after injury.

EQUIPMENT/SUPPLIES:
Surgical Tray:

Appropriate size syringe and gauge of needle for administering anesthesia
Sterile basin for aspirated fluid
Appropriate size syringe and gauge of needle for joint aspiration per provider preference
Hemostat
Sterile 4 × 4 gauze sponges
Fenestrated drape
Antiseptic solution as per provider preference

Side Area (Unsterile Field):

Skin prep supplies
Anesthetic as ordered by the provider

Medication for joint injection per provider's orders
Dressings, bandages, and tape
Splint/brace/sling as indicated
Prepackaged sterile gloves (appropriate sizes for medical assistant and provider)
Nonsterile disposable gloves
PPE
Alcohol pads
Biohazard specimen transport bag
Supplies to obtain culture of joint fluid
Specimen container
Appropriate lab requisitions

PROCEDURE STEPS:

1. Wash hands.

2. *Paying attention to detail,* assemble equipment.

3. *Introduce yourself. Identify the patient and explain the procedure, speaking at the patient's level of understanding.*

4. Obtain a signed consent for the procedure.

5. *Being courteous, patient, and respectful to the patient, provide privacy,* and drape patient if appropriate.

6. *Allay the patient's fears regarding the procedure being performed and help them to feel safe and comfortable.*

7. Inquire regarding allergies and last tetanus shot. Document appropriately.

8. *Using active listening skills,* review health history to avoid possible complications. Share information with provider.

Procedure 31-15 (continued)

9. ***Paying attention to any special needs of the patient,*** assist him to the supine position.

10. Don appropriate PPE, including goggles if indicated.

11. Don sterile gloves.

12. Perform skin prep as ordered by provider.

13. Remove gloves and dispose of in biohazard waste container.

14. Assist the provider by holding the vial as anesthesia is aspirated. The provider injects anesthesia, inserts a long, sturdy needle into the synovial sac, and aspirates fluid with a large syringe. The aspirated fluid is put into a sterile bowl as the syringe fills with fluid. A hemostat is used to remove the syringe from the needle, leaving the needle in the joint. The syringe is reapplied to the needle, and the process continues until excess fluid is removed.

15. ***Being courteous, patient, and respectful,*** support the patient as needed.

Give Postoperative Care:

16. Don sterile gloves.

17. Using sterile water or saline and a 4 × 4 sponge, clean the area around the wound and dry with a 4 × 4 sponge or sterile towels.

18. Dress and bandage wound per provider's instructions. Dress to absorb exudates.

19. Dispose of items utilized during the procedure according to OSHA guidelines.

20. Remove gloves and dispose of in biohazard waste container.

21. Wash hands.

22. Obtain vital signs to assess patient stability post-procedure. Document in the patient's chart or EMR.

23. ***Explain wound care to the patient (and caregiver), speaking at the patient's level of understanding and provide written instructions*** including symptoms of infection.

24. ***Demonstrating respect for individual diversity,*** assist the patient with any questions or concerns.

25. Arrange for a follow-up appointment and post-operative medication as required.

26. Apply gloves and eye/mouth protection if sending specimen to laboratory. Place aspirated fluid into a sterile container and cover tightly.

27. Send labeled specimen container and requisition to the pathology laboratory after placing specimen in biohazard transport bag.

28. Accurately document the procedure in patient's chart or electronic medical record.

DOCUMENTATION:

10/12/20XX 11:30 AM   Left knee aspirated. 250 mL clear fluid withdrawn after injection of anesthetic. Sent to pathology department. Patient says she "feels better." Dressing applied to aspiration site. Postoperative verbal and written directions given. BP 118/64, P 72. Follow-up appointment made for discussion about results of analysis of fluid sent to laboratory. H. Casey, RMA (AMT)————————————

PROCEDURE 31-16
Hemorrhoid Thrombectomy

STANDARD PRECAUTIONS:

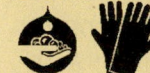 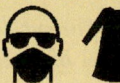

NOTE: Hemorrhoids are dilated or varicose veins in the rectum, either internal or external. Sometimes a blood clot can form in a protruding portion of the hemorrhoid and the vessel can become inflamed. The hemorrhoid is incised with a scalpel blade and the clot removed with a hemostat forceps. Suturing is not usually necessary. Soaking the area in a **sitz bath** aids in healing. Hemorrhoidectomy can be performed in much the same manner as a hemorrhoid thrombectomy, and the supplies and equipment are similar. The anal sphincter is dilated, the hemorrhoid pedicle is tied, and then each hemorrhoid is removed with either laser, electrosurgery, or cryosurgery. Another alternative is to ligate the internal hemorrhoids after visualizing the area with an anoscope. Two rubber bands are placed

continues

Procedure 31-16 (continued)

around the pedicle of each hemorrhoid. They will slough off after a week to 10 days because of the loss of blood supply to them (**avascularized** hemorrhoid).

PURPOSE:

To incise inflamed hemorrhoids and remove thrombus. To remove hemorrhoids with laser, electrosurgery, cryosurgery, or banding.

EQUIPMENT/SUPPLIES:

Surgical Tray:

Appropriate size syringe and gauge of needle for administering anesthesia

Sterile basin

Appropriate size syringe and gauge of needle for joint aspiration per provider preference

Mosquito hemostat (curved)

Sterile 4 × 4 gauze sponges

Fenestrated drape

Antiseptic solution as per provider preference

Rubber band

Side Area (Unsterile Field):

Skin prep supplies

Anesthetic as ordered by the provider

Medication for joint injection per provider's orders

Soft absorbent hold in place

Pad, similar to a sanitary napkin

T-bandage to hold in place

Prepackaged sterile gloves (appropriate sizes for medical assistant and provider)

Nonsterile disposable gloves

PPE

Biohazard specimen transport bag

Specimen container

Appropriate lab requisitions

PROCEDURE STEPS:

1. Wash hands.

2. *Paying attention to detail,* assemble equipment.

3. *Introduce yourself. Identify the patient and explain the procedure, speaking at the patient's level of understanding.*

4. Obtain a signed consent for the procedure.

5. *Allay the patient's fears regarding the procedure being performed and help them to feel safe and comfortable.*

6. Inquire regarding allergies and last tetanus shot. Document appropriately.

7. *Using active listening skills,* review health history to avoid possible complications. Share information with provider.

8. *Attending to any special needs of the patient,* position her per provider's preference (Sim's position).

9. *Being courteous, patient, and respectful to the patient, provide privacy,* and drape patient if appropriate, *being sure to protect the patient's personal boundaries.*

10. Don appropriate PPE, including goggles if indicated.

11. Don sterile gloves.

12. Perform skin prep as ordered by provider.

13. Remove gloves and dispose of in biohazard waste container.

14. Assist the provider to aspirate the appropriate amount of local anesthesia. After administering the anesthesia, the provider either bands or excises the hemorrhoids with a scalpel. Suturing is usually not necessary.

15. *Being courteous, patient, and respectful,* support the patient as needed.

Give Postoperative Care:

16. Don nonsterile disposable gloves.

17. Assist the provider in placing the soft absorbent pad against the wound. It may be held in place with the T-shaped bandage.

18. Dress and bandage wound per provider's instructions. Dress to absorb exudates.

19. Dispose of items utilized during the procedure according to OSHA guidelines.

20. Remove gloves and dispose of in biohazard waste container.

21. Wash hands.

22. Obtain vital signs to assess patient stability post-procedure. Document in the patient's chart or EMR.

23. *Explain wound care to the patient (and caregiver), speaking at the patient's level of understanding,* per provider. Sitting in a tub of warm water is soothing and aids healing. *Provide written instructions* including signs of complications such as excessive bleeding or pain.

24. *Demonstrating respect for individual diversity,* assist the patient with any questions or concerns.

25. Arrange for a follow-up appointment and postoperative medication as required.

Procedure 31-16 (continued)

26. ***Demonstrating respect for individual diversity,*** assist the patient with any questions or concerns.

27. Don PPE including nonsterile disposable gloves.

28. Clean room, sanitize instruments, and sterilize for reuse.

29. Remove PPE and dispose of appropriately.

30. Wash hands.

DOCUMENTATION:

3/17/20XX 1:00 PM   A. Thrombus removed from hemorrhoid. Perineal pad applied and secured with a T-binder. Patient seemed to tolerate the procedure well. BP 110/70, P 88. Postoperative instructions, verbal and written, given to patient. Prescription for Percodan, 1 tab PO q 4-6 h prn given to patient. Return appointment made for 4/4/20XX. S. Thomas, CMA (AAMA)———————————————————

B. Internal hemorrhoids removed with electrosurgical equipment. Very little bleeding noted. Perineal pad and T-binder applied. Patient seemed to tolerate the procedure well. BP 110/68, P 72. Postoperative instructions given to patient (verbal and written). Prescription for Percodan 1 tab. PO q 4-6 h prn given to patient. Return appointment made for 4/4/20XX. S. Thomas, CMA (AAMA)———————————————————

PROCEDURE 31-17
Suture/Staple Removal

STANDARD PRECAUTIONS:

  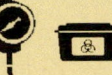

NOTE: Many minor surgical procedures require that suturing be done to approximate the skin edges to promote healing. Because these sutures or staples are nonabsorbable, they must be removed when the wound has healed. The patient returns to the office or clinic to have the sutures or staples removed. The medical assistant removes the dressing and checks the wound. The provider also checks the wound for degree of healing and determines that the sutures/staples can be removed.

PURPOSE:
To remove sutures from a healed surgical wound (as per provider).

EQUIPMENT/SUPPLIES:
(See Figure 31-46)
Gauze sponges
Bandage scissors
Biohazard waste container
Tape
Forceps
Suture removal kit (suture scissors or staple remover, thumb forceps, and 4 × 4s)
Sterile latex gloves
Antibiotic cream if ordered

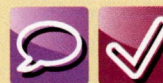

PROCEDURE STEPS:
1. Wash hands.
2. ***Paying attention to detail,*** assemble equipment.
3. ***Introduce yourself. Identify patient.***
4. ***Speaking at the level of the patient's understanding, explain the procedure.***
5. ***Allay the patient's fears regarding the procedure being performed and help them to feel safe and comfortable.***
6. Apply nonsterile gloves and remove bandage.
7. Dispose of bandage and gloves in biohazard waste container.
8. Wash hands.
9. Open suture or staple removal kit.
10. Apply sterile gloves.

    If removing sutures follow the steps below. If removing staples, jump to Step 17.

11. If the sutures are covered with dried fluids, don sterile gloves, soak a sterile 4 × 4 gauze sponge with sterile water or saline and gently place on the suture line to allow removal in order to visualize the sutures.

12. Using thumb forceps, gently pick up one knot of a suture. Gently pull upward toward suture line.

continues

Procedure 31-17 (continued)

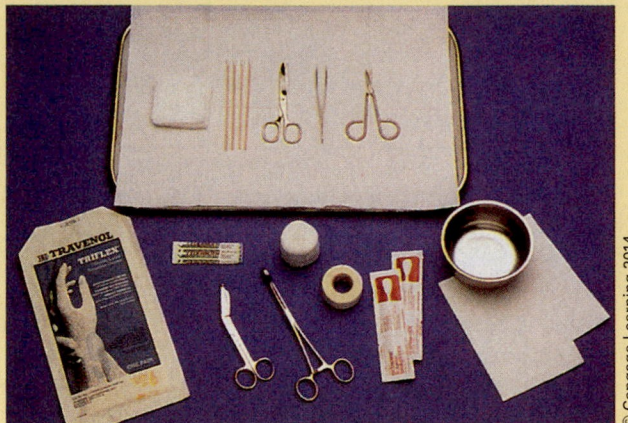

Figure 31-46 Equipment and supplies for suture removal.

> RATIONALE: Less pressure is exerted on suture line.

13. Using suture scissors, cut ONLY one side of the suture as close to the knot as possible. (Figure 31-47A).
    RATIONALE: Holding knot with forceps and cutting suture as close to skin as possible, the suture will be pulled out from under the skin, avoiding contamination of the wound.

14. Grasping the knot, pull slowly and continuously until the suture is free of the skin.

15. Repeat until all sutures are removed.

16. CAUTION: If suture line opens as sutures are removed, **STOP** and consult provider.

If removing staples, begin here:

17. If the staples are covered with dried fluids, don sterile gloves, soak a sterile 4 × 4 gauze sponge with sterile water or saline and gently place on the suture line to allow removal in order to visualize the staples.

18. Gently insert staple remover under the first staple with the two prongs positioned below the staple and the single prong on top of the staple.

19. With slow, continuous pressure, close the staple remover handles to remove the staple.

20. Repeat until all staples are removed.

21. CAUTION: If incision line opens as staples are removed, STOP and consult provider.

22. Apply antibiotic ointment/cream per provider's orders.

23. Place sterile dressing over wound per provider's orders.

24. Remove sterile gloves and dispose of in biohazard waste container.

25. Wash hands.

Postoperative Care:

26. Don nonsterile disposable gloves.

27. Dispose of items utilized during the procedure according to OSHA guidelines.

28. Remove gloves and dispose of in biohazard waste container.

29. Wash hands.

30. Obtain vital signs to assess patient stability postprocedure. Document in the patient's chart or EMR.

31. *Demonstrating respect for individual diversity,* assist the patient with any questions or concerns.

32. Arrange for a follow-up appointment and postoperative medication as required.

33. Accurately document procedure in patient's chart or electronic medical record.

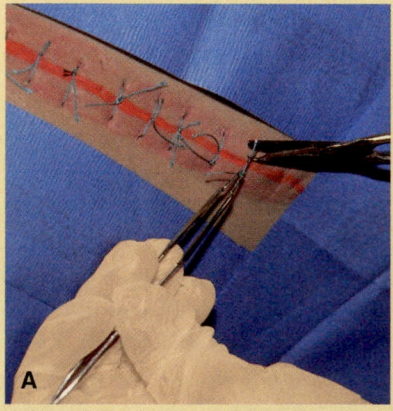
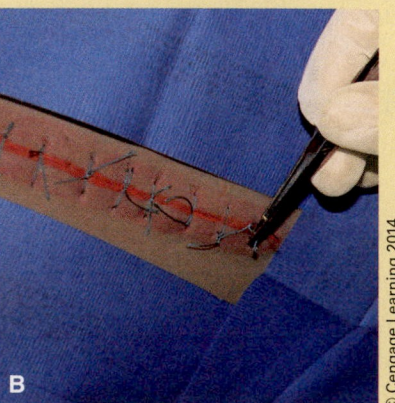

Figure 31-47 To remove sutures: (A) Grasp suture knot with thumb forceps. Place curved tip of suture removal scissors right next to the skin under the suture. Clip. (B) Gently pull the suture knot up and toward the incision with thumb forceps to remove.

Procedure 31-17 (continued)

DOCUMENTATION:

11/27/20XX 2:30 PM   Ten sutures removed from right forearm. Wound appears clean, well healed. No discharge seen. Edges of wound well approximated. H. Casey, RMA (AMT)————
OR

11/27/20XX 2:30 PM   Six staples removed from right forearm. Wound appears clean, well healed. No discharge seen. Edges of wound well approximated. H. Casey, RMA (AMT)————

PROCEDURE 31-18

Application of Sterile Adhesive Skin Closure Strips

STANDARD PRECAUTIONS:

NOTE: On occasion, a superficial wound does not require sutures. However, the edges of the wound can be drawn together and sterile strips of adhesive used to hold the edges of the wound together to facilitate healing.

PURPOSE:

To approximate the edges of a wound after the removal of sutures. Sometimes used in lieu of sutures or to give additional support along with sutures.

EQUIPMENT/SUPPLIES:

Sterile Field:

Suture removal instruments (if indicated)
Sterile adhesive skin closure devices
Iris scissors (straight)
Adson dressing forceps
Tincture of benzoin per provider's preference
Sterile cup
Sterile cotton-tipped applicators (for tincture of benzoin)
OR
Sterile prepackaged benzoin swabs

Side Area (Unsterile Field):

Prepackaged sterile gloves in the appropriate size
Dressings, bandages and tape
Waterproof bag

PROCEDURE STEPS:

1. Wash hands.
2. *Paying attention to detail,* assemble equipment.
3. *Introduce yourself. Identify patient.*
4. *Speaking at the level of the patient's understanding,* explain the procedure.
5. *Allay the patient's fears regarding the procedure being performed and help them to feel safe and comfortable.*
6. *Considering any special patient needs,* position patient comfortable.

If applying additional support to sutures at an incision line begin here. If placing strips post-suture or staple removal, skip to Step 19.

7. Using existing steril e field, open strips and drop onto sterile field.
8. Open sterile cup and cotton-tipped applicators (or use prepackaged swabs) and drop onto sterile field.
9. Carefully pour a small amount of tincture of benzoin into cup. (Skip step if using prepackaged swabs) RATIONALE: Tincture of benzoin Is applied to the periphery of the wound to prepare for the application of skin closure strips and to provide a better sticking surface and aid in easier removal with less skin irritation.
10. Don sterile gloves.
11. Clean and dry wound.
12. Apply tincture of benzoin to wound edges using sterile cotton-tipped applicator or swab stick. *DO NOT* allow benzoin to come into contact with the incison. Allow to dry.
13. Cut strips to size if needed.
14. Carefully peel strips from backing using thumb forceps.
15. Place the first strip at the center of the wound.

continues

Procedure 31-18 (continued)

16. Apply one end of the skin closure strip to one side of the wound and using slight tension, apply to the other side of the wound. *Do not pucker the skin.*

17. Secure the strip to the skin by pressing gently.

18. Apply the strips as needed to reinforce the suture line per provider's instructions.

If applying post-suture or staple removal, begin here:

Give Postoperative Care:

19. Dress and bandage if necessary.

20. Dispose of used items per OSHA guidelines.

21. Remove gloves and wash hands.

22. Check the patient's vital signs, if indicated.

23. ***Explain wound care to the patient (and caregiver), speaking at the patient's level of understanding, and provide written instructions*** including symptoms of infection.

24. ***Demonstrating respect for individual diversity,*** assist the patient with any questions or concerns.

25. Arrange for follow-up appointment and medication as ordered.

26. Document procedure in patient's chart or electronic medical record.

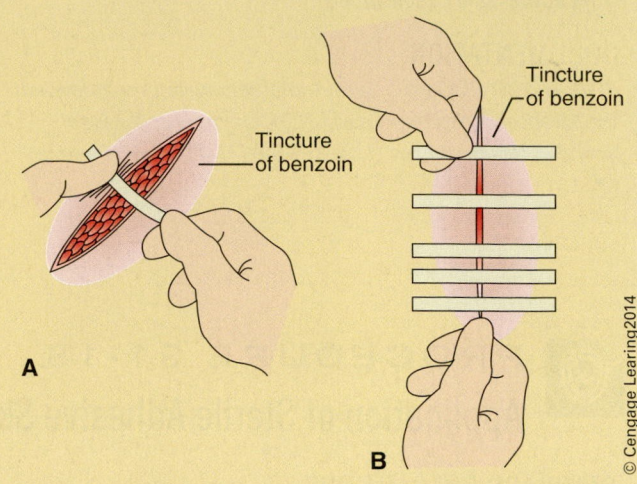

Figure 31-48 To apply skin closure strips: (A) Apply first strip in center of incision. (B) Apply closures to each side of center.

DOCUMENTATION:

3/17/20XX 4:00 PM   Nine skin closure strips applied to wound on shoulder after tincture of benzoin applied to skin around sutures. Suture line approximated well; no puckering of skin noted. Wound appears clean and to be healing. No redness or swelling. Patient says there is "very little discomfort." H.Casey, RMA (AMT)

CASE STUDY 31-1

Refer to the scenario at the beginning of the chapter. Distinguish between the types of surgery that would be performed in a high-volume patient practice and the surgery that would be performed in a smaller practice.

CASE STUDY REVIEW

1. Where would the medical assistant begin when preparing the equipment for Dr. Beahm and the procedure?

2. Describe the process for assuring that the specimen obtained during the biopsy is delivered to the pathology lab in a condition to allow a diagnosis.

CASE STUDY 31-2

Cele Little, an 84-year-old patient at Dr. Beahm's clinic, is having office surgery performed on Thursday morning. Her sister, Dottie Tate, also a patient and also in her 80s, will come with Cele. A friend from the local senior citizen center has offered to drive them to the center and home again. Dottie is more nervous about the procedure, the removal of a bothersome cyst, than Cele. After talking with the sisters about the procedure, clinical assistant Jessica Goodwin, RMA (AMT), MLT, realizes this and wants to reassure Dottie but also wants her to be prepared to be caregiver to Cele.

CASE STUDY REVIEW

1. Where should Jessica begin in her communication with the two sisters?

2. What specific advice should Jessica give Cele and Dottie before the procedure?

3. What instructions should Jessica give the sisters to follow after the procedure?

CASE STUDY 31-3

Letisha Brown has been scheduled to have a nevus excised from her upper back by Dr. Beahm.

CASE STUDY REVIEW

1. Explain how Jessica would prepare her for the surgery.

2. Explain how Jessica would care for her after the surgery.

3. What will become of the excised nevus? Explain your actions.

SUMMARY

In assisting with surgery in the ambulatory care setting, the medical assistant needs to know sterile principles and understand the difference between medical and surgical asepsis. Knowledge of suture materials, instruments, and other supplies such as dressings and bandages is also critical. In preparing for surgical procedures, the medical assistant's communication skills will be needed, because patients can be apprehensive and will require both reassurance and education. In addition to understanding the basic process and preparations for assisting with minor surgery, the medical assistant should be aware of the steps involved in some of the more common surgical procedures.

STUDY FOR SUCCESS

To reinforce your knowledge and skills of information presented in this chapter:

- Review the *Key Terms*
- Role-play with other students to apply attributes of professionalism pertinent to this chapter.
- Consider the *Case Studies* and discuss your conclusions
- Answer the questions in the *Certification Review*
- Apply your knowledge by completing the *Activities* in the *Study Guide* and the *Games and Quizzes* in the StudyWARE StudyWARE software on the *Premium Website*
- Perform the *Procedures* using the *Competency Assessment Checklists* in the *Competency Manual*
- Practice your problem-solving skills with the *Critical Thinking Challenge 3.0* on the *Premium Website*

Additional resources for this chapter include:

- Module 24 of the *Medical Assisting Learning Lab*
- *CourseMate for Delmar's Comprehensive Medical Assisting*
- *WebTutor for Delmar's Comprehensive Medical Assisting*

CERTIFICATION REVIEW

1. Which of the following describes the primary purpose of surgical asepsis?
   a. To prevent microorganisms from collecting on the Mayo stand
   b. To prevent microorganisms from causing inflammation
   c. To prevent microorganisms from entering the body during an invasive procedure
   d. To prevent microorganisms from multiplying

2. A basic rule to follow to protect sterile items is:
   a. a sterile object can touch a nonsterile object under certain circumstances
   b. it is safe to turn your back on the sterile field if you leave plenty of room between you and the field
   c. provide the provider a separate container for contaminated instruments
   d. gloved hands are held at the same height as the hip bone

3. Which of the following is the smallest size suture material?
   a. 0
   b. 2–0
   c. 4–0
   d. 1

4. Which of the following is an example of absorbable suture material?
   a. Vicryl
   b. Nylon
   c. Silk
   d. Cotton

5. What is the purpose of adding epinephrine to the local anesthetic?
   a. To prevent an allergic reaction
   b. To reduce blood flow in the operative site through vasoconstriction
   c. To reduce patient discomfort during the procedure
   d. To maintain patient vital signs

6. Which of the following actions might the provider take if a sebaceous cyst were infected?
   a. Remove the cyst
   b. Do a biopsy of the cyst
   c. Perform cryosurgery on the cyst
   d. Incise and drain the cyst

7. Key methods to protect a sterile object include the following:
   a. sterile objects must not touch unsterile objects
   b. never turn your back on a sterile field
   c. anything below the waist is considered unsterile
   d. all of the above

8. Which of the following is the gauge of the largest suture material?
   a. 0 silk
   b. 2–0 silk
   c. 3–0 silk
   d. 4–0 silk

9. Anesthesia is defined as:
   a. loss of sensation
   b. increased sensation
   c. localized sensation
   d. general sensation

10. Preference cards are used to:
    a. make setup for a procedure less difficult
    b. make sure that the practitioner has the instruments needed
    c. standardize procedures no matter which staff member sets up
    d. all of the above

REFERENCES/BIBLIOGRAPHY

Alguire, Patrick, MD, & Mathes, Barbara, MD (1998). Skin Biopsy Techniques for the Internist. *Journal of General Internal Medicine, 13*(1), 46–54. Retrieved April 5, 2012, from http://www.ncbi.nlm.nih.gov/pmc/articles/PMC1496896/

Association of Surgical Technologists, Inc. (2008). *Surgical technology for the surgical technologist.* Clifton Park, NY: Delmar Cengage Learning.

Phillips, N. (2004). *Barry and Kohn's operating room technique* (10th ed.). St. Louis, MO: Mosby.

Simmers, L. (2004). *Diversified health occupations.* (6th ed.). Clifton Park, NY: Delmar Cengage Learning.

Taber's cyclopedic medical dictionary (20th ed.). (2005). Philadelphia: F. A. Davis.

U.S. Department of Health and Human Services, Centers for Disease Control and Prevention (2011). *Guideline for Prevention of Surgical Site Infection, 1999.* Retrieved April 5, 2012, from http://www.cdc.gov/ncidod/dhqp/pdf/guidelines/SSI.pdf

U.S. Food and Drug Administration. (2011). *Liquid Chemical Sterilization.* Retrieved April 5, 2012, from http://www.fda.gov/MedicalDevices/ProductsandMedicalProcedures/GeneralHospitalDevicesandSupplies/ucm208018.htm

CHAPTER 32

Diagnostic Imaging

OUTLINE

Radiation Safety

Radiography Equipment

Contrast Media

Patient Preparation

Positioning the Patient

Fluoroscopy

Bone Densitometry

Diagnostic Imaging

Positron Emission
Tomography (PET)

Computerized Tomography
(CT)

Magnetic Resonance
Imaging (MRI)

X-Rays (Flat Plates)

Ultrasonography

Mammography

Filing Films and Reports

Radiation Therapy

Nuclear Medicine

LEARNING OUTCOMES

1. Define, spell, and pronounce the key terms as presented in the glossary.

2. Describe safety precautions for personnel and patients as they relate to ionizing radiation treatments.

3. Explain how fluoroscopy is used and explain its benefits.

4. Describe the various positions used during X-ray procedures.

5. Describe four X-ray procedures that require patient preparation.

6. Discuss the uses of ultrasonography, positron emission tomography, computerized tomography, magnetic resonance, and flat plates.

7. Discuss how radiographs are stored.

8. Explain the differences among radiology, radiation therapy, and nuclear medicine.

9. Recall four possible side effects of radiation.

10. Analyze the professionalism questions and apply them to this chapter's content.

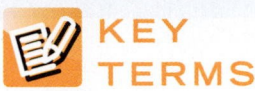

KEY TERMS

bone densitometry

cathode

claustrophobia

Doppler

dosimeter

echocardiogram

esophageal varices

fluoroscope

implantable cardioverter-defibrillator (ICD)

ionizing radiation

isotope

magnetic resonance imaging (MRI)

mammogram

oscilloscope

palliative

positron emission tomography (PET)

radioactive

radiograph

radiolucent

radionuclides

radiopaque

radiopharmaceuticals

stomatitis

transducer

ATTRIBUTES OF PROFESSIONALISM

Communication
- Did you speak at the patient's level of understanding?
- Did you allay patients' fears regarding the procedure being performed and help them feel safe and comfortable?
- Did you demonstrate empathy in communicating with patients, family, and staff?

Presentation
- Were you courteous, patient, and respectful to the patient?

Competency
- Were you knowledgeable and accountable?
- Did you recognize the importance of local, state, and federal legislation and regulations in the practice setting?

Initiative
- Did you seek out opportunities to expand your knowledge base?

Integrity
- Did you work within your scope of practice?

In the radiology department of Inner City Health Care, several patients are waiting to have their procedures performed. Wanda Slawson, CMA (AAMA), brings Don Waite to the department for an excretory urogram known as an intravenous pyelogram. She is careful to make certain that Mr. Waite has been properly prepared for the procedure. She does not want the procedure to have to be repeated because of the inconvenience and anxiety it may cause Mr. Waite, nor does she want there to be additional expense and time spent repeating the procedure.

INTRODUCTION

Radiology is a branch of medicine concerned with **radioactive** *substances, including* **radiographs,** *radioactive* **isotopes,** *and* **ionizing radiation.** *There are three specialties into which radiology can be classified: diagnostic radiology, radiation therapy, and nuclear medicine. Radiology can further be classified as imaging, interventional, and therapeutic. All the specialties are extremely valuable tools that can be used to diagnose and treat diseases.*

X-rays were named when a German physicist, Wilhelm Roentgen, discovered them in 1895. He received the first Nobel Prize in physics for his discovery. Roentgen noticed while working with a **cathode** *ray tube that the rays of energy emitted could pass through skin, paper, wood, and other solid materials. Because he didn't know what the rays were, he called them X-rays.*

Radiologic procedures are not often performed in an office setting; rather, they are performed in the radiology department of a hospital, clinic, or a freestanding facility outside of the hospital or clinic.

Some radiographs, such as those looking for a fractured bone, require no preparation, whereas others, such as an excretory urography (intravenous pyelogram [IVP]) or a computerized axial tomography (CAT) scan, require special preparation.

SPOTLIGHT ON CERTIFICATION

RMA Content Outline
- Anatomy and physiology
- Medical terminology
- Patient relations
- Patient education

CMA (AAMA) Content Outline
- Medical terminology
- Anatomy and physiology
- Medicolegal guidelines and legal requirements
- Patient preparation and assisting the provider with selected tests

CMAS Content Outline
- Medical Terminology
- Anatomy and physiology
- Legal and ethical considerations
- Examination preparation

RADIATION SAFETY

X-rays, though invisible to the human eye, are extremely powerful, and they can be beneficial or they can be dangerous and harmful. Exposure to radiation can destroy tissue and permanently damage the eyes, bone marrow, and skin. They are harmful to the developing embryo and fetus, causing severe anomalies and death.

One of the most important tasks of a medical assistant is to make sure that patients are adequately prepared for any radiologic procedure. Patient education is essential in preparing for many procedures. Without adequate patient education, the patient will not receive the desired outcome.

The benefit of X-rays is the ability to use the information obtained from them to diagnose and manage a patient's disease. The diagnostic benefits outweigh the risks that may result from X-ray exposure. Radiographers are educated to be certain that patients receive as low a dose of radiation as possible but still obtain a useful radiograph, and that they themselves and the patients are protected from exposure to radiation that is not necessary. Radiation is rarely used during pregnancy because of the danger it poses to the fetus and embryo. The first trimester is the most critical because severe congenital anomalies can be the result of the fetus's or embryo's exposure to radiation. Women

CRITICAL THINKING

What are the effects of radiation on a fetus or an embryo?

are routinely asked if there is a possibility of their being pregnant. X-rays of fertile women should be taken only when necessary and with a minimal exposure to the fetus or embryo. If a radiologic examination is necessary, a radiologic physicist calculates the dosage of radiation to estimate how little radiation to which the fetus or embryo should be exposed. The past guideline stated that X-rays of fertile women should not be taken until 10 days after the onset on their last menstrual period. The thinking was that women were unlikely to be pregnant during these 10 days. This guideline is now considered to be outdated because the ovum for the next menstrual cycle is most susceptible during this 10-day period.

 In some states, medical assistants and other health care professionals who are not licensed to take radiographs are not allowed by law to take or assist with radiologic procedures. Licensure in those states (about 35 states) is mandated because of the possibility of severe injury to an unlicensed individual and to patients. In some states, a limited license is required. The medical assistant must undergo additional training and is limited to "skeletal films" (arms, legs, and so forth). Education and training in radiologic techniques is of utmost importance for the safety of the patient and health care worker. Medical assistants must have a basic understanding of radiology and radiology safety to instruct patients in the correct preparation for procedures and to keep patients and themselves safe. They must protect themselves from radiation exposure by not participating in procedures for which they have not been adequately educated and trained.

 On August 5, 2010, a bill called the CARE bill (Consistency, Accuracy, Responsibility, and Excellence in Medical Imaging and Radiation Therapy) was introduced before the U.S. Congress. If passed, it would require all persons who perform medical imaging (including X-rays) and radiation therapy (excluding ultrasound) procedures to meet specific federal education and credentialing standards in order to participate in Medicare and Medicaid. Presently, the law in some states requires only voluntary basic training standards. This situation allows individuals without formal education to perform imaging procedures.

The AAMA supports the legislation that would require specific educational and certification standards for individuals performing medical imaging.

Personnel in the X-ray department and others who are exposed to X-rays must wear a **dosimeter**, a small badge-like device worn above the waist. The dosimeter contains a strip of film that measures the amount of X-rays to which a person is exposed. The dosimeter film is read on a regular basis, and radiation exposure is reported to a supervisor. Exposure can come from the X-ray beam itself or from scattered rays that are produced when going through the patient's body. Tracking of exposure to ionizing radiation is mandatory for health care professionals.

Patients must wear lead aprons over the reproductive organs, and technicians must shield themselves with lead aprons and gloves when they are assisting. However, shields are not necessary when technicians are standing behind the lead wall and working the control panel. In addition, walls in rooms where X-rays are taken are lead-lined to absorb scattering rays.

The World Health Organization held an international meeting in Geneva, Switzerland on March 1–3, 2010, to discuss "Referral Guidelines for Appropriate Use of Radiation Imaging." The meeting focused on standardizing an international evidence-based set of referral guidelines to limit unnecessary medical radiation exposure. As a result of this meeting, a guideline was developed in collaboration with experts and institutions to meet the goal of minimizing health risks while maximizing benefits to the patient.

RADIOGRAPHY EQUIPMENT

There are three main parts to an X-ray machine: the table, the X-ray tube, and the control panel. The tube is where the X-rays are produced and then come out as a beam of X-rays. Lead surrounds the tube except for the area where the beams of X-rays are sent out. The table on which the patient lies is movable in several directions, even upright or angled. The control panel is positioned behind a lead wall specially designed for shielding the

CRITICAL THINKING

What do some state laws require of personnel who take X-rays?

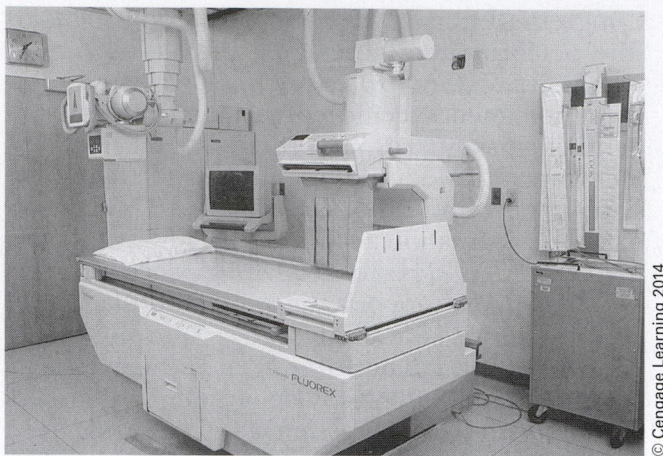

© Cengage Learning 2014

Figure 32-1 Radiography room prepared for procedure.

radiographer from X-rays when an X-ray is being taken (Figure 32-1).

Photographic film is placed beneath or behind the patient's body and a radiograph, or X-ray film, is produced by sending X-rays from the tube of the machine through the body and onto the film. After the film is processed, an image is created (see Figure 32-4A and Figure 32-4B). Bone is denser than skin and other soft tissues, and therefore can absorb more X-rays. The image of the hand bones on the X-ray film is white due to absorption of the X-rays.

EHR Radiologic procedures can be done without using X-ray film. The technique, known as computed radiography (CR), uses similar equipment. Computers and laser technology are used to obtain and process digital images. CR images can be recorded on an imaging plate that is put through a computer scanner, which reads and digitalizes the images.

The technique provides clear images that assist the provider in making a diagnosis. The CR images can be sent to other providers on the computer network for consultation or referral. Images are accessible in 3 minutes.

The process produces excellent images without film. It makes film storage unnecessary, thereby reducing costs. Transmission of patient data is quicker.

CR equipment is costly, and technologists who use the equipment require training on its operation.

CONTRAST MEDIA

Various body structures are of different densities. Bone is denser than skin and, therefore, can absorb more X-rays, leaving fewer to be picked up by the X-ray film. Thus, an X-ray film of bone will appear white. A lung is less dense, and the X-rays can penetrate lung tissue. The lung appears black on the radiograph. If X-rays do not penetrate a structure easily, it is termed **radiopaque**; if they penetrate readily, it is termed **radiolucent**. Contrast media are radiopaque and help to obtain a radiographic image of an internal organ or structure that ordinarily would be difficult to see, because the contrast media cause the organs or structures of the body to absorb more radiation (Figure 32-2A through Figure 32-2C).

Some commonly used contrast media are barium sulfate, iodine compounds, air, and carbon dioxide. Barium is a chalky compound and, when mixed with water, can be swallowed by the patient or administered as an enema by a radiologic technician. It is not absorbed by the body. It is used for upper and lower gastrointestinal (GI) series of X-rays (Figure 32-3A and Figure 32-3B). The patient is told to drink extra fluids to flush out the barium after the procedure. Iodine salts are radiopaque and are used for kidney, gall bladder, and thyroid examinations. Some individuals are allergic to the iodine salts used as contrast media. Patients are asked whether they have any allergies, particularly allergies to foods that contain iodine, such as fish.

Air and carbon dioxide are used to visualize the spinal cord and joints but have been replaced by use of the **magnetic resonance imaging (MRI)** machine.

Although contrast media is widely used, it is not without risk. The effects can range all the way from minor changes in homeostasis to life-threatening situations. Informed consent may be required by the facility that is performing the study. Risk factors for adverse reactions include specific allergies (as mentioned above), asthma, and renal insufficiency.

PATIENT PREPARATION

By law, without special education and training about X-rays, the medical assistant's role in X-ray procedures in most states is limited to giving patient preparation information and explanations about what the patient can anticipate.

 A thorough knowledge of the procedure ordered by the provider is essential, and the medical assistant must be certain that patients understand the preparation they are about to undergo. Verbal explanations should be followed up with written instructions. Many patients, fearful of what the ordered X-ray will show, are anxious and frightened and can easily forget verbal instructions. Proper preparation is essential for the best results on the radiographs. Having to repeat a procedure because of inadequate preparation results in increased patient anxiety, time, expense, and inconvenience (Table 32-1).

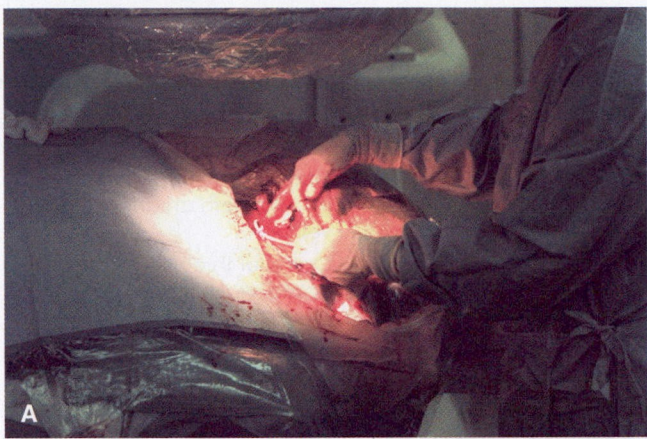

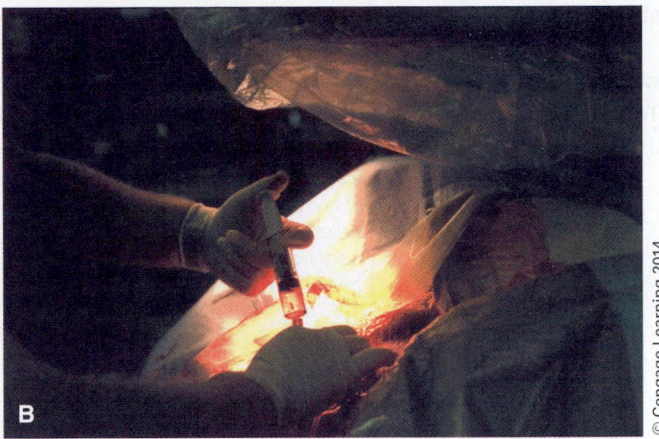

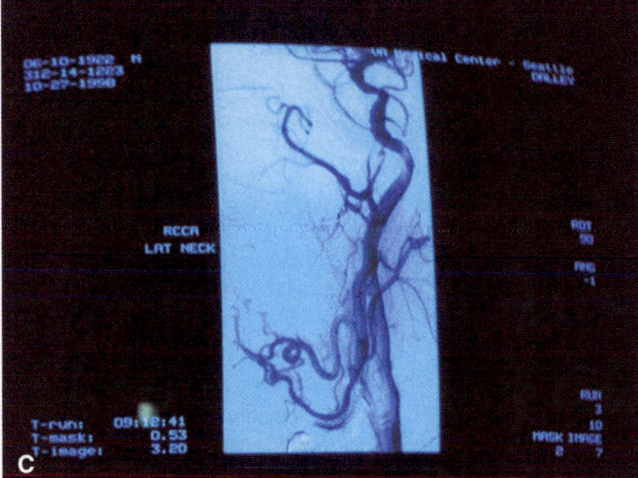

Figure 32-2 Angiography. (A) An intra-arterial catheter is inserted. (B) Radiopaque contrast material is injected. (C) The arteries are visualized. Note the many signs of aging.

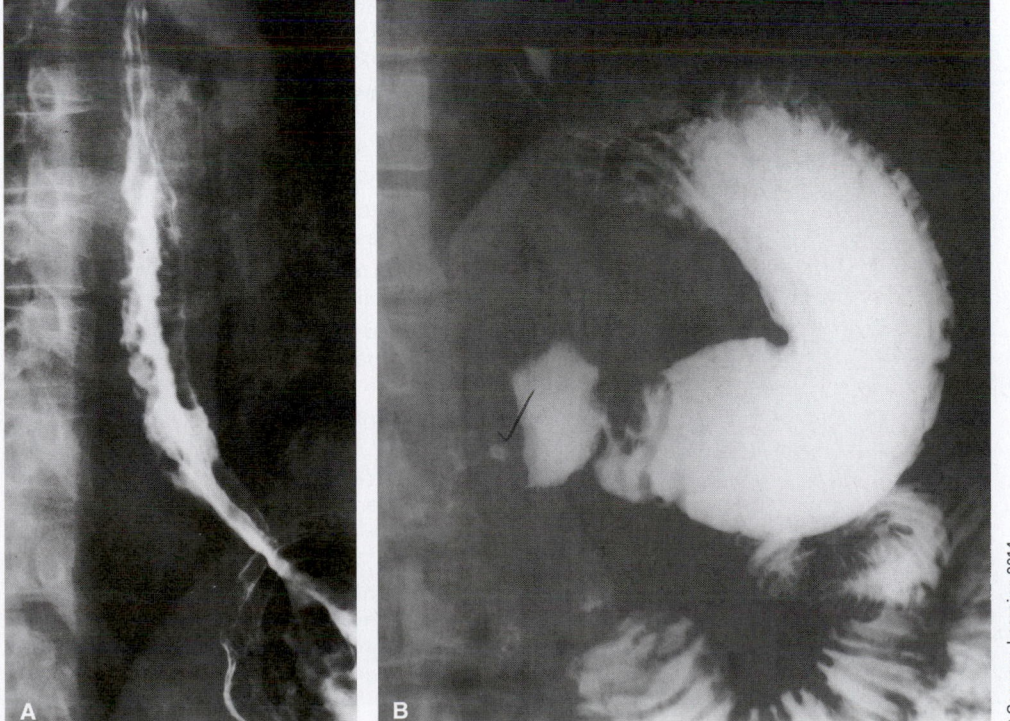

Figure 32-3 (A) Barium swallow showing esophageal varices. (B) Barium swallow showing duodenal ulcer.

Table 32-1   Examples of Diagnostic Procedures, their Purpose, Patient Preparation, and the Procedure

Test	Purpose	Patient Preparation	Procedure
Angiography	To visualize the inside of blood vessel walls. Helps to diagnose heart attacks, stroke, aneurysm (Figure 32-2).	NPO 6 to 8 hours before examination.	1. Contrast medium (iodine) injected into an artery or vein. 2. Catheter threaded to the appropriate site. 3. Digital angiography can be done and stored on computer disk.
Barium swallow (upper gastrointestinal [GI] series)	To study the esophagus, stomach, duodenum, and small intestine for disease (ulcers, tumors, hiatal hernia, esophageal varices) (see Figure 32-3).	Day prior: Light evening meal. NPO after midnight. Day of test: NPO. Postprocedural: Increase fluid intake. Take laxative as prescribed.	1. The patient is asked to drink a flavored barium mixture while standing in front of the fluoroscope. 2. The radiologist observes the passage down the digestive tract. 3. The patient is turned to various positions to allow good visualization of the intestines. 4. Radiographs are taken.
Barium enema (lower GI series)	To study the colon for disease (polyps, tumors, lesions).	Prep kit (usually supplied by provider's clinic), which includes bottle of magnesium citrate and Dulcolax tablet(s). Day prior: 1. Clear liquid allowed: carbonated beverages, clear gelatin, clear broth, coffee and tea with sugar. No milk or milk products. 2. 8 oz. of water every hour until bedtime. 3. Late afternoon, drink bottle of magnesium citrate. 4. Early evening, take Dulcolax tablet(s) as prescribed. 5. Liquid evening meal. NPO except water after dinner. Morning of procedure: NPO, cleansing enema Postprocedural: 1. Increase fluid intake and dietary fiber. 2. Report to provider if no bowel movement within 24 hours of test.	1. The colon is filled with a barium sulfate mixture. 2. The patient is turned in various positions to allow the barium to fill the colon. Air is injected to move the barium along the colon. 3. When the colon is full, radiographs are taken.
Cholangiography	To view the bile ducts for possible calculi or lesions.	May have cleansing enema 1 hour before examination. Meal preceding examination is withheld.	Contrast medium injected and radiograph of bile ducts is taken.

Table 32-1 Examples of Diagnostic Procedures, their Purpose, Patient Preparation, and the Procedure (*Continued*)

Test	Purpose	Patient Preparation	Procedure
Cholecystography	To study the gall bladder for disease (stones, duct obstruction), inflammation.	1. Evening before test, fat-free dinner. 2. Patient takes dye tablets with 8 oz. of water. 3. Cathartic or cleansing enemas may be prescribed. 4. NPO after dinner and tablets.	1. A series of radiographs is taken. 2. A fatty meal may be given to stimulate the gall bladder to empty. 3. Other radiographs can then be taken to check gall bladder function.
Cystography	To view the urinary bladder for lesions, calculi.	Day prior: Light evening meal. Laxative in evening. NPO after midnight.	Contrast medium injected and radiograph of the urinary bladder is taken.
Hysterosalpingography	To view the uterus and fallopian tubes for blockage and lesions. To check for pelvic masses.	Laxative evening before. Cleansing enema day of exam. Meal prior to examination is withheld.	Contrast medium injected and radiographs taken of uterus and fallopian tubes. Carbon dioxide may also be used.
Excretory urography (intravenous pyelogram) [IVP]	Visualization of kidneys, ureters, and bladder to detect kidney stones, lesions, strictures of urinary tract.	Eat a light evening meal and nothing after midnight. A laxative and enema are used to clean out the intestines to prevent a blocked view of the ureters behind the intestines.	A contrast medium of iodine salts is given intravenously after it has been determined that the patient is not allergic to iodine (see Chapter 30).
Mammography	To detect abnormalities in the breast, especially breast cancer.	Do not wear lotion, deodorant, or powders. Remove clothing from waist up. No contrast medium required.	Breast is positioned on the mammograph and compressed to flatten it. Two radiographs are taken of each breast, from the side and from above.
Retrograde pyelography	To view the kidneys and urinary tract for abnormalities.	Drink four to five glasses of water before examination unless sedated, then NPO.	Contrast medium injected and radiographs taken of the kidneys and urinary bladder.

© Cengage Learning 2014

POSITIONING THE PATIENT

The correct patient position is important for obtaining the best quality radiograph, and the type of examination that is necessary determines patient position. Some basic views are:

- *Anteroposterior view (AP)*. The anterior surface of the body faces the X-ray tube and X-rays are directed from the front toward the back of the body.
- *Posteroanterior view (PA)*. The posterior surface of the body faces the X-ray tube and X-rays are directed from back to front (Figure 32-4A and Figure 32-4B).
- *Lateral view*. X-rays pass through the body from one side to the opposite side.
- *Right lateral view (RL)*. X-rays are directed through the body from the left to the right side. The right side of the body is next to the film.
- *Left lateral view (LL)*. X-rays are directed through the body from the right to the left side. The left side of the body is next to the film.

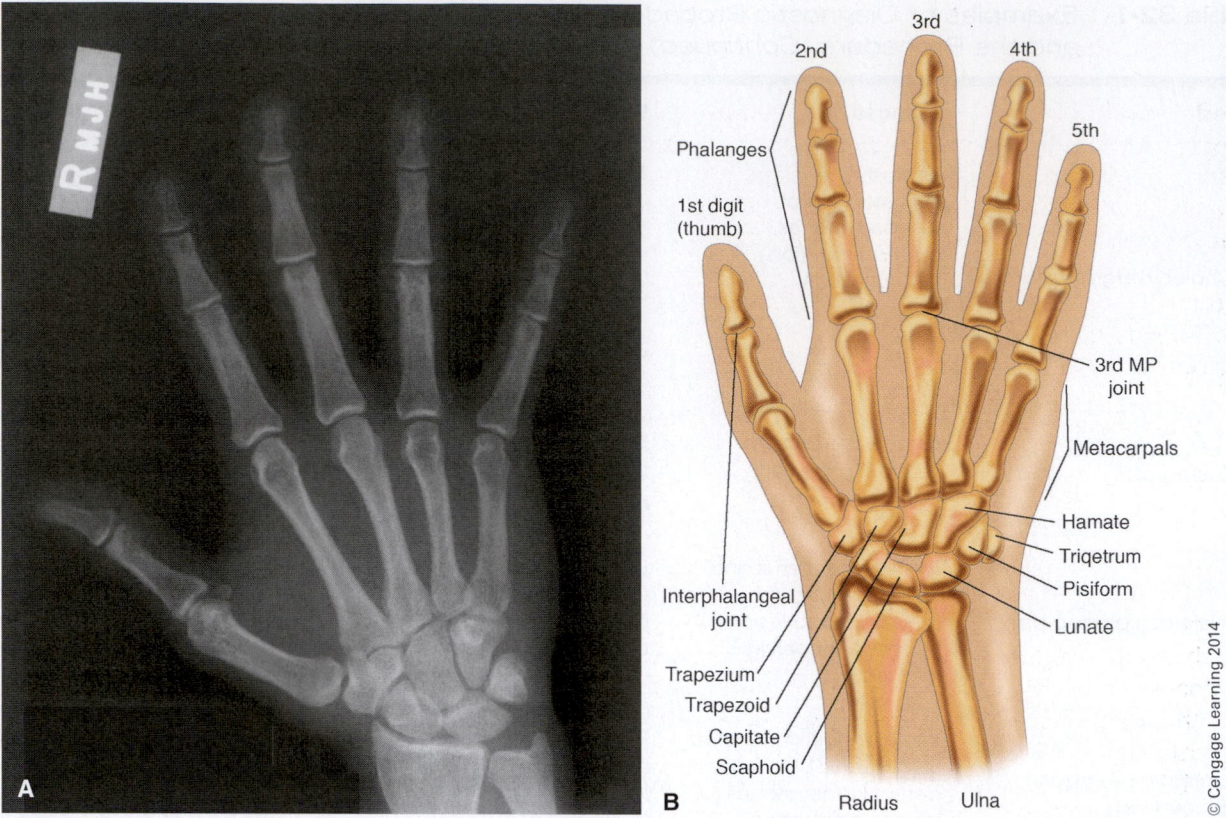

Figure 32-4 (A) Posteroanterior (PA) view of a hand. Note the dark spaces between the bones. This is because the bones (denser) pick up X-rays (absorb them) and appear white. The soft tissue (less dense) does not absorb X-rays and appears dark. (B) PA hand.

- *Oblique view.* The body is positioned at an angle.
- *Supine view.* The body is lying face up, on the back.
- *Prone view.* The body is lying face down, on the abdomen.

FLUOROSCOPY

Fluoroscopy is the process of using a **fluoroscope** to view internal organs and structures of the body so that they can be seen in motion immediately by the radiologist. The patient is usually given a contrast medium and placed between the X-ray tube and the fluoroscope. Fluoroscopy is used for procedures such as cardiac catheterization and for viewing the function of the stomach and intestinal structures to detect any abnormalities. A television screen and camera are available so that the radiographer can watch and take photos of the body system(s) in operation (Figure 32-5). Most fluoroscopes have radiographic properties and can be used for both fluoroscopy and X-rays. X-rays can be taken and recorded during fluoroscopy.

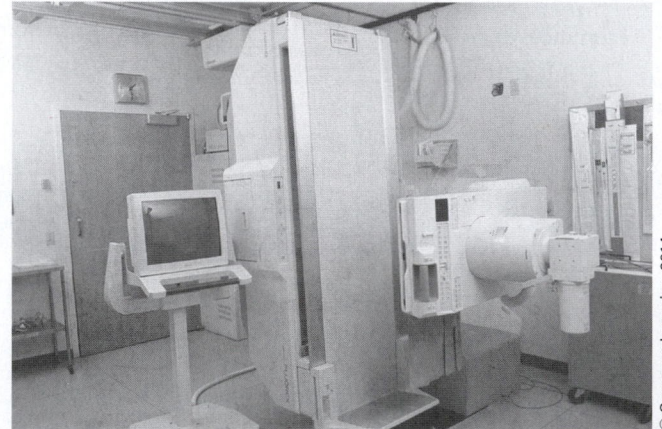

Figure 32-5 Fluoroscopy room ready for upper gastrointestinal study.

BONE DENSITOMETRY

An enhanced form of X-ray technology (low dose) is used during **bone densitometry**. X-rays check areas of the body (hip, hand, spine, foot) for signs of mineral loss and bone thinning. The test determines the density of bone and is used to diagnose osteoporosis, often found in women after menopause. It can occur in men as well. Bone densitometry can assess an individual's risk for fractures. It is a painless procedure.

The patient is told to refrain from taking calcium supplements for 24 hours prior to the examination, to wear loose clothing without metal zippers or buttons or a belt, and to remove jewelry and any metal objects. These items can interfere with the X-ray images.

Most machines have software that computes and displays the bone density on a computer monitor. The test takes from 10 to 30 minutes. The lower the density, the greater the risk for fractures.

DIAGNOSTIC IMAGING

Positron Emission Tomography (PET)

PET is a radiographic procedure that uses a computer and a radioactive substance. The radioactive substance is injected into the patient's body and gives off charged particles. They combine with particles in the patient's body to produce color images that reveal the amount of metabolic activity in an organ or structure.

PET is primarily a diagnostic medical imaging modality. It makes use of specialized, intravenously injected **radiopharmaceuticals** that emit positrons, which can be detected out of the body due to high-energy releases. Specialized detectors arranged around the patient sense the energy and map the location from which it originated inside the body. These radiopharmaceuticals can be chemically designed to localize in the heart, brain, or certain types of tumors (e.g., breast tumors) throughout the body. A clinical image is formed by the accumulation of positron emissions in a target organ. The patient's emission pattern forms a clinical image. This image is compared with the normal distribution by the nuclear medicine provider.

Generally, low-to-moderate doses are used to diagnose disease in patients. The PET scan can detect cancer and the effects of chemotherapy. Certain nuclear medicine treatment studies use specialized radiopharmaceuticals that isolate in the area to be treated. These agents emit their energy locally, irradiate tissue, and usually do not leave the body, unlike diagnostic radiopharmaceuticals. The properties and intent of diagnostic radiopharmaceuticals are different from therapeutic radiopharmaceuticals (Figure 32-6A through Figure 32-6C).

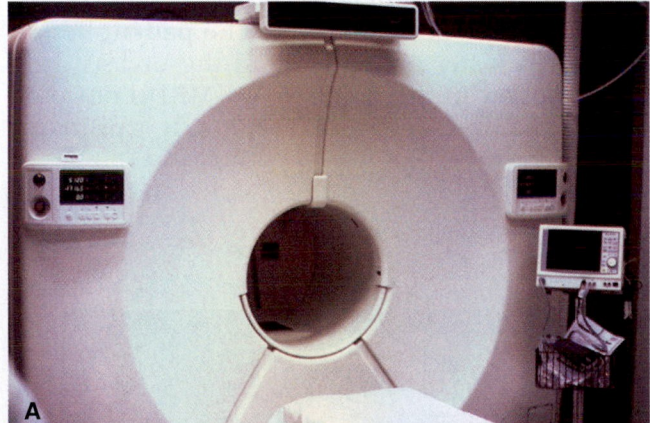

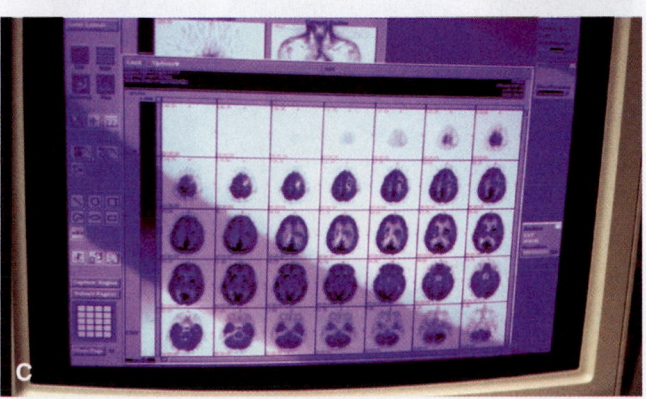

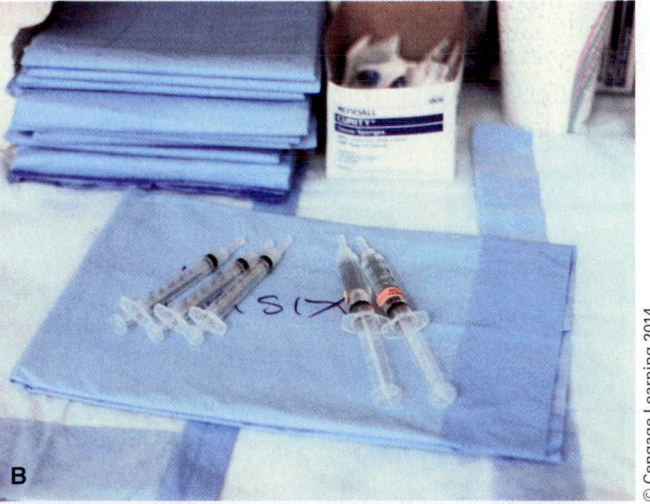

Figure 32-6 (A) Position Positronemission tomography (PET) scanner. (B) Medications ready for injection. (C) PET scan output images.

© Cengage Learning 2014

Computerized Tomography (CT)

CT uses a small amount of radiation. The beams penetrate body tissues to produce a series of cross-sectional images of the body part being examined. It allows images of structures that cannot be seen with regular X-rays. It is a noninvasive test that usually requires no preparation.

EHR The CT machine has software and hardware for storing and managing information. The images can be examined on a computer monitor, and hard copies of the images can be made. It rotates 360 degrees around the patient to obtain cross-sectional images that are processed by a computer and can be viewed on a monitor and on film. It can also be used to guide biopsies, plan surgery, and identify internal organ injury due to trauma. It is ideal for early detection of tissue tumors such as childhood cancers and abdominal tumors, and it helps in directing radiation therapy for tumor masses. The cardiac CT is more useful for diagnosing coronary artery disease than cardiac stress testing. On occasion, a contrast medium is injected for a better view of internal structures. If contrast medium is used, the patient must be NPO (have nothing by mouth) for 4 hours before being placed onto a motorized table that moves the body part to be examined into a scanner that surrounds that part of the patient. An entire body can be scanned in 15 to 20 minutes (Figure 32-7A and Figure 32-7B). Newer multislice CT scanners produce thinner slices in a shorter time with greater detail.

Magnetic Resonance Imaging (MRI)

EHR Images produced by MRI are of exceptionally high quality. No ionizing radiation is used, and it is a noninvasive, safe, and painless procedure that can produce computer-processed images. All body areas can be viewed by MRI, but it is especially helpful for soft tissues. It is good for the spine, pelvis, and joints and is superior for visualizing the brain and abdominal organs. It shows more detail than CT. The examiner can see through fluid-filled tissue with exceptional detail using an MRI machine. The computer forms the visual image.

Magnetic resonance angiography (MRA), a noninvasive test, evaluates arteries and veins throughout the body and is very useful for showing neck and brain blood flow. This technique uses a magnetic field and pulses of radio waves to image blood vessels inside the body. The computer converts the data into digital images of slices. No catheterization is needed, but a contrast medium may be given intravenously. The procedure helps diagnose blood vessel and heart disorders as well as strokes. Another imaging technique, functional MRI, measures split-second nerve cell activity of the brain.

Another application of the technology is breast imaging using an MRI that is linked to the computer. Hundreds of detailed pictures of the breast are taken from several angles. The patient lies on the table on her abdomen, and the breasts drop into a hollow in the table. Breast MRI is not used for routine breast cancer screening. It is primarily

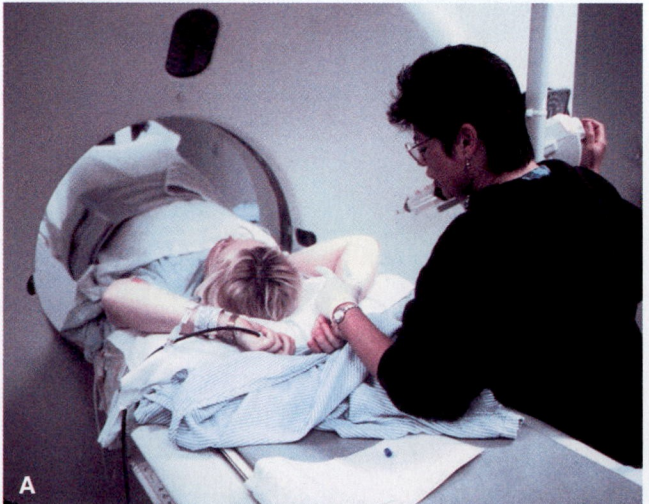
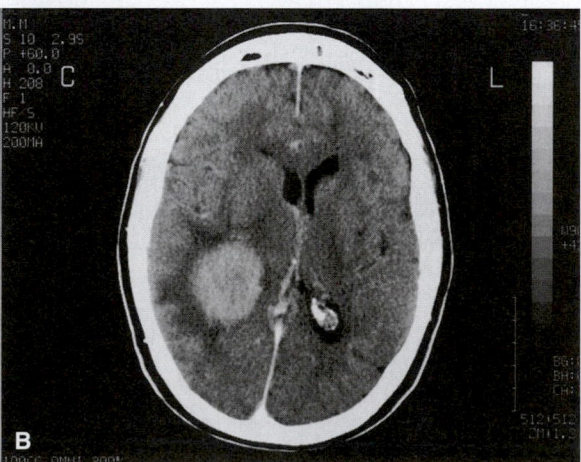

Figure 32-7   (A) Computed tomography (CT) scanning. Instruct patient to lie still. (B) This axial CT scan demonstrates a meningioma surrounded by edema.

© Cengage Learning 2014

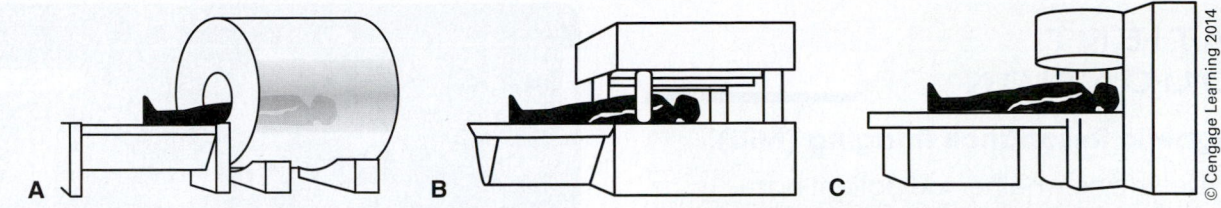

Figure 32-8   Three types of MRI machines: (A) closed MRI, (B) open-air MRI, and (C) open MRI.

used to evaluate breast implants for leaks and to assess abnormalities seen on a conventional mammogram. Breast MRI does not take the place of conventional mammography and ultrasonography and is not routinely used to diagnose breast cancer.

For MRI, the patient lies on a table. The machine has an electromagnet. Three types of MRI machines are available: closed MRI, open-air MRI, and open MRI (Figure 32-8).

The conventional closed MRI has high magnetic strength. According to Lexington Medical Center, nine of ten MRI machines used in hospitals and clinics are the closed MRI. It produces high-quality images.

The open-air type MRI has open sides and ends. Most open machines have low-strength magnets and are not as powerful as the closed MRI. Images are of lesser quality.

The open-type MRI is an advanced MRI machine that is completely open on all sides. It eliminates patient **claustrophobia** and can accommodate obese patients. It has a powerful magnet that is much stronger than the magnet used in open air–type MRIs. Greater image detail results in information providers need to make a diagnosis (Figure 32-9).

A drawback to MRI and CT is that they cannot be used in patients with a pacemaker; an **implantable cardioverter-defibrillator (ICD);** or metal clips, pins, or other permanent hardware left in place on an internal organ or structure as part of a surgical procedure. The metal may become damaged during testing. Controlled studies investigating whether patients with implantable devices such as a pacemaker and/or an ICD can undergo CT and/or MRI are inconclusive. The FDA has not approved either procedure for these patients. Some researchers found that newer CTs and MRIs did not cause difficulties for patients with implantable-devices compared with earlier models, which did cause minor difficulties in some patients. An MRI is not as useful as conventional radiographs or a CT scan for diagnosing fractured bones.

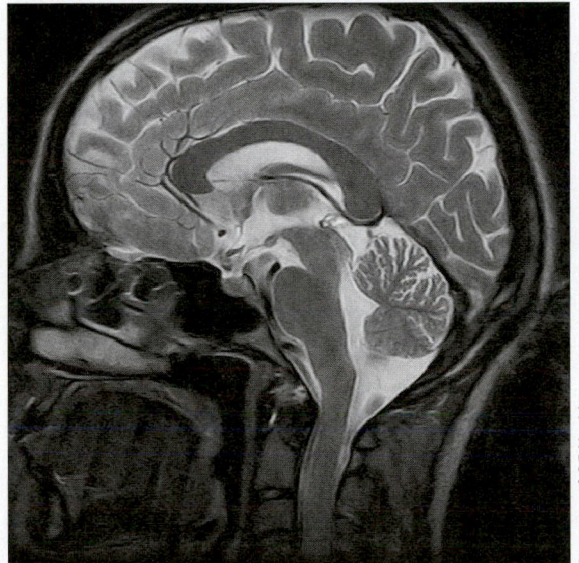

Figure 32-9   A sagittal MRI of the head.

Patients are asked to remove all objects that have metal (watches, belts, hairpins, rings, other metal jewelry) and credit cards because of the strong magnet in the MRI machine. Loose, comfortable clothing without zippers or snaps should be worn. The procedure takes about 45 minutes to an hour, during which time the patient must remain still. The technician, although not in the room with the patient, has a camera and microphone with which to communicate with the patient. An intermittent tapping sound can be heard throughout the procedure, and earphones are available if the patient wants them.

X-Rays (Flat Plates)

Flat plates are also known as "plain" films because they require no special technique or use of contrast medium. This type of X-ray is used on various parts of the body and is helpful in diagnosing problems in the skull, abdomen, chest, sinuses, and bone.

PATIENT EDUCATION

Magnetic Resonance Imaging (MRI)

1. Determine whether the patient has followed the preparation instructions, if there were any.

2. Explain the procedure and what the patient can expect.

3. Have patient remove all metal objects (jewelry, watch, and so on). The magnet in the MRI machine is strong, and metal can disrupt images.

4. Have patient empty bladder before the procedure because it takes about 45 minutes and patient cannot move during that time.

5. Explain to patient that machine makes humming and tapping noises.

6. Tell patient that the intravenous contrast medium may be slightly uncomfortable when injected into vein.

7. Remind patient to lie still and not to move.

8. Tell patient that there is a microphone for communication between the patient and technician.

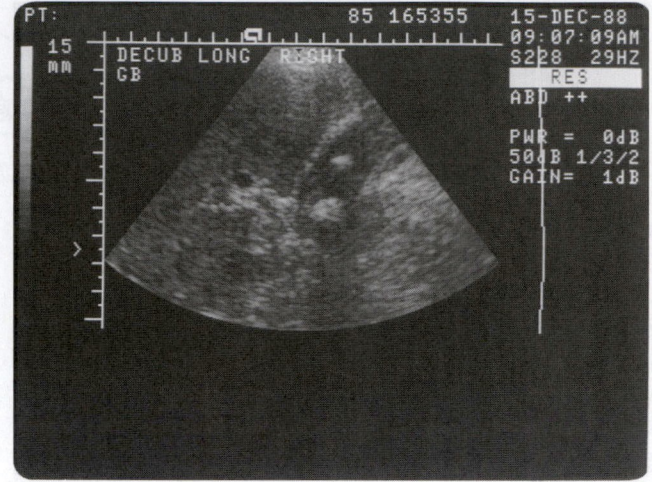

Figure 32-10 Sonogram of gall bladder with gallstones.

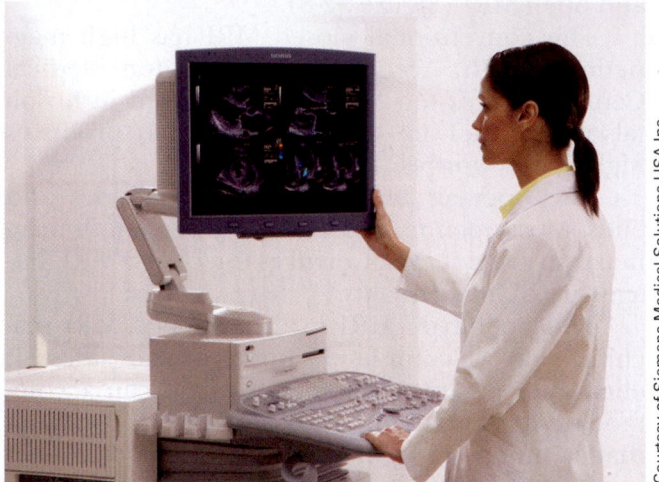

Figure 32-11 Electrocardiograph machine.

Ultrasonography

Ultrasonography, CT, and MRI allow for greater imaging detail than conventional radiographs. Ultrasonography, or ultrasound, has been available longer than the other technologies. High-frequency sound waves (inaudible to the human ear) are used to image internal soft tissues. It can be used to help diagnose problems in the abdominal organs, liver, gall bladder, uterus, ovaries, and spleen (Figure 32-10). It cannot be used for skeletal structures or the lungs.

Doppler ultrasonography is a noninvasive technique used to evaluate blood flow through the major arteries and veins of the neck, arms, and legs. It can reveal blockages such as plaque or thrombi (blood clots). An **echocardiogram**, an ultrasound of the heart, can view the heart and determine its size, shape, and position and the motion made by the valves opening and closing (Figure 32-11). Ultrasound has advantages over other methods of viewing internal organs and structures in that it

uses no X-rays and allows for continuous viewing while organs and structures are in motion.

During ultrasound, a **transducer** is used with a coupling agent, and sound waves are emitted from the head of the transducer. The transducer is placed firmly on the patient's body over the organ to be examined. The sound waves pass through the skin and bounce off the body's tissues and are reflected back to the transducer. These echoes are displayed on an **oscilloscope**, showing a visual pattern or picture. The image or record produced is known as a sonogram or echogram. A permanent film for the patient's record and videotape can also be made.

EHR Integration of ultrasonography with a computer stores data and then produces three-dimensional images. Ultrasonography can be used to guide the provider while performing a biopsy.

Ultrasonography, because it is noninvasive (i.e., the procedure does not puncture skin or enter the body), is widely accepted for obstetrical use. Gestational age can be determined, congenital anomalies detected, multiple fetuses noted, ectopic pregnancy diagnosed, and fetal size and position determined (see Chapter 26).

Ultrasound takes 15 to 45 minutes, and the preparation depends on the body part being examined. An obstetrical ultrasound may require the patient to have a full bladder to push aside the intestines. An ultrasound of the gallbladder and liver requires the patient to have had nothing to eat or drink for 8 to 12 hours before the examination. The patient must remain still unless requested to change positions. Therapeutic ultrasonography is discussed in Chapter 33.

Mammography

More than any other X-ray, the **mammogram** must be of the highest resolution and contrast. High resolution and contrast call for an increase in exposure to radiation, but mammography currently is safer than ever because of strong regulations (the only radiography examination fully regulated by the federal government) and improved technology. The machines used for mammography must meet stringent requirements. They are used with special screens, film, and cassettes. Currently, the equipment can produce high-resolution and extremely high-contrast images with exposures that are lower than ever. Digitalization helps improve images. Although some newer mammography equipment is digitalized, according to some experts, it produces images that are only slightly better than those produced by nondigitalized equipment. Imaging techniques help providers perform biopsies of the breast, especially of abnormal areas that cannot be felt but are seen by conventional mammography or with ultrasound. A type of needle biopsy, stereotactic-guided biopsy, involves the exact location of the abnormal area in three dimensions using conventional mammography. (Stereotactic refers to use of a computer and scanning devices to create three-dimensional images.) A sterile needle is inserted into the precise location, and tissue or cell samples can be obtained. The samples are examined by a pathologist who looks for cancer cells.

Computer-Aided Detection (CAD). Computer-aided detection uses the computer to bring suspicious areas on a mammogram to the radiologist's attention. The CAD scans the mammogram with a laser beam and converts it into a digital signal that is processed by the computer. The image is displayed on a video monitor, with the suspicious area highlighted. The radiologist can compare the digital image with the conventional mammogram to see if any of the highlighted areas were missed on the initial review and require further investigation. CAD technology may improve the accuracy of a screening mammogram. CAD provides a second set of eyes for the radiologist with the goal of increased analysis of suspicious areas. Researchers continue to seek ways to reduce the exposure of X-rays to the patient even further. Chapter 26 provides more information on mammography.

Filing Films and Reports

Because radiographs are part of the patient's permanent record, they must be safeguarded from the environment. Conditions such as heat, moisture, light, and radiation can damage them. Processed films are stored in special envelopes with the patient's name, date, and identification number marked on the outside. They are stored in a cool, dry place. The films are the property of the hospital or other facility where the films were taken and usually remain where they were taken. Storage on-site makes them accessible for future use for comparison purposes and eliminates the possibility of their being lost if they were allowed to be taken away from the facility where they were processed. Written reports of the findings are prepared by the radiologist and sent to the patient's provider(s) (Figure 32-12). Computed radiography eliminates the need for film storage (hard copy).

RADIATION THERAPY

Radiation therapy is generally used to treat tumors that cannot be surgically removed or that are inaccessible for surgical removal, and for treatment of a malignant tumor that was surgically excised but a portion of the tumor remains. It is a specialty within radiology. When used to treat inaccessible or inoperable tumors, the treatment is considered **palliative** treatment. The treatments shrink the tumor, thereby lessening the symptoms. The treatments can be either external, with direct radiation aimed through the surface of the skin to an area within the body, or internal, using various

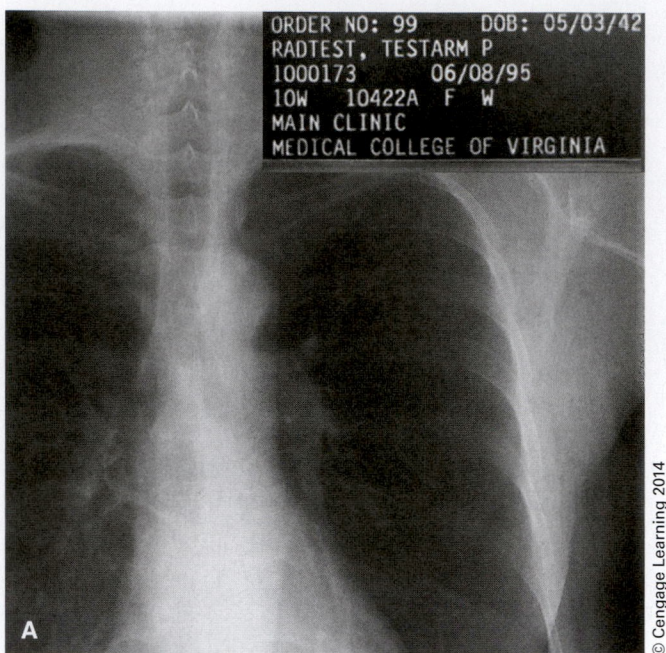

Figure 32-12A Radiograph showing patient identification information.

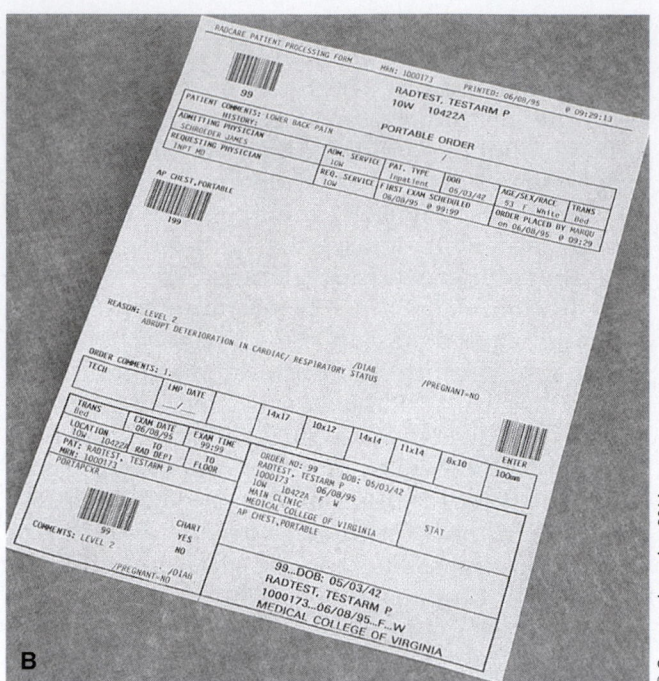

Figure 32-12B Sample requisition form.

applications of radioactivity such as seeds or beads that are planted inside the body and left there for a certain amount of time. The radiation is the same as X-rays, with doses carefully calculated. The aim of radiation therapy is to interfere with malignant cell growth and to disrupt the DNA. The object is to destroy as many of the malignant cells as possible without harming healthy cells surrounding the tumor. Possible side effects are nausea, vomiting, hair loss, anorexia, bone marrow suppression, and **stomatitis**.

NUCLEAR MEDICINE

Nuclear medicine is the branch of medicine involved with the use of radioactive (i.e., emitting rays or particles from the nucleus) substances for diagnosis, therapy, and research. Specific training is necessary for this specialty.

Radioactive substances are administered to the patient either by mouth or by injection. The radioactive compounds, known as **radionuclides**, travel to an organ or area in the body that attracts them and creates an image of that area. The gamma rays omitted are detected by camera.

If the radionuclide is in an area that is abnormal, such as a tumor, the area is referred to as "hot." If the radionuclide does not concentrate in the abnormality, but surrounds it instead, the area is referred to as "cold." Both hot and cold areas are suggestive of abnormalities.

EHR The provider may order a nuclear medicine scan for the following reasons: to analyze kidney function, image blood flow through the heart, scan lungs, measure thyroid function, identify bleeding into the colon, determine the spread of cancer, bone scan, brain scan, and others. Nuclear imaging techniques use a camera and a nearby computer to detect emissions of the rays, measure the amount of radioactivity, and provide a digitalized image of the organ (e.g., the thyroid gland).

Data gathered from all of these diagnostic imaging devices are stored electronically in a hospital information system (HIS). Picture archiving and communication systems (PACS) store all radiologic exam results and are available online to providers on demand. The level of access to the data can be defined by each system. The benefits of these systems are that the examination reports and images will not become lost and no time is spent waiting for a report.

CRITICAL THINKING

Describe how radiation therapy helps to destroy malignant neoplasms.

CASE STUDY 32-1

Refer to the scenario at the beginning of the chapter.

CASE STUDY REVIEW

1. What is the patient preparation for excretory urography (IVP)?

2. What should Wanda tell Mr. Waite about what to expect as he begins to have his procedure?

CASE STUDY 32-2

Gloria McDermott is scheduled to have a GI series of X-rays next week because of persistent episodes of stomach pain that is unrelieved by the medication Dr. King has prescribed for her.

CASE STUDY REVIEW

1. How will you explain to her the purpose of the test?
2. What will you tell her about how to prepare for the examination?

CASE STUDY 32-3

Raymond Brunnelle has had a series of X-rays, a GI series, a cholecystogram, and an MRI of his abdomen. He has scheduled an appointment with a gastroenterologist and asks you to get all of the films for him.

CASE STUDY REVIEW

1. What is your response to his request?
2. Explain why they should be kept on-site.

SUMMARY

Radiology and diagnostic imaging are helpful in the diagnosis and treatment of diseases and conditions because procedures can be done to visualize internal structures and their functions. Radiation is not without its risks to personnel and patients, but by following specific safety precautions, the health and safety of all involved can be safeguarded.

The three specialty areas are radiology, radiation therapy, and nuclear medicine.

STUDY FOR SUCCESS

To reinforce your knowledge and skills of information presented in this chapter:

- Review the *Key Terms*
- Role-play with other students to apply attributes of professionalism pertinent to this chapter.
- Consider the *Case Studies* and discuss your conclusions
- Answer the questions in the *Certification Review*
- Apply your knowledge by completing the *Activities* in the *Study Guide* and the *Games and Quizzes* in the StudyWARE **StudyWARE** software on the *Premium Website*
- Practice your problem-solving skills with the *Critical Thinking Challenge 3.0* on the *Premium Website*

continues

STUDY FOR SUCCESS (CONTINUED)

Additional resources for this chapter include:

- Module 23 of the *Medical Assisting Learning Lab*
- *CourseMate for Delmar's Comprehensive Medical Assisting*
- *WebTutor for Delmar's Comprehensive Medical Assisting*

CERTIFICATION REVIEW

1. Which of the following radiologic procedures does *not* require a contrast medium?
   a. Hysterosalpingogram
   b. Mammogram
   c. Cholecystogram
   d. Angiogram

2. A cholecystogram requires which type of contrast medium?
   a. Air
   b. Tablets
   c. Carbon dioxide
   d. Barium

3. A cholangiogram will examine:
   a. upper GI tract
   b. lower GI tract
   c. bile ducts
   d. kidneys and ureters

4. In which of the following positions does the posterior aspect of the body face the X-ray tube and the anterior face the film?
   a. Oblique
   b. Anteroposterior
   c. Posteroanterior
   d. Prone
   e. Supine

5. The radiologic procedure of choice for brain imaging is:
   a. computerized tomography
   b. positron emission tomography
   c. magnetic resonance imaging
   d. ultrasonography
   e. thermography

6. A key way to limit your exposure to radiation as an allied health provider is to:
   a. utilize a camera and microphone to communicate with patient during exam
   b. allow the practitioner to perform all radiographic procedures
   c. move quickly when in the room with the patient
   d. none of the above

7. With a right lateral view, the beam of radiation travels:
   a. through the body from the left to the right
   b. through the body from front to the back
   c. through the body from the right to the left
   d. through the body from the back to the front

8. The following is true of a CT scan:
   a. it uses a large amount of radiation
   b. it produces cross-sectional images of the body
   c. it allows imaging of structures that standard radiography cannot
   d. both b and c

9. The purpose of radiation therapy is:
   a. to diagnose medical conditions
   b. treatment of neoplasms that cannot be surgically removed
   c. to provide palliative therapy
   d. both b and c

10. Fluoroscopy can be described as:
    a. a form of x-ray that measures bone density
    b. using a computer and contrast media
    c. X-rays that are viewed in motion
    d. none of the above

REFERENCES/BIBLIOGRAPHY

Bone mineral density test. (n.d.). *MedlinePlus Medical Encyclopedia*. Retrieved February 18, 2008, from http://www.nlm.nih.gov/medlineplus/ency/article/007197.htm

Carlton, R. R., & Adler, A. M. (2001). *Principles of radiographic imaging: An art and a science* (3rd ed.). Clifton Park, NY: Delmar Cengage Learning.

Cornuelle, A., & Gronefeld, D. (1998). *Radiographic anatomy and positioning: An integrated approach.* Stanford, CT: Appleton and Lange.

Cowling, C. (1998). *Radiographic positioning procedures, Volume II: Advanced imaging procedures.* Clifton Park, NY: Delmar Cengage Learning.

Mettler, F. A., Jr., & Guiberteau, M. J. (2005). *Essentials of nuclear medicine imaging* (5th ed.). Philadelphia: W. B. Saunders.

Orenstein, B. W. (2006). Hot issues—MRI and implantable devices. *Radiology Today, 7*(4), 8.

Taber's cyclopedic medical dictionary. (22nd ed.). (2005). Philadelphia: F. A. Davis.

CHAPTER 33

Rehabilitation and Therapeutic Modalities

OUTLINE

The Role of the Medical Assistant in Rehabilitation

Principles of Body Mechanics
  Posture

Using the Body Safely and Effectively
  Lifting Techniques

Transferring Patients

Assisting Patients to Ambulate

Assistive Devices
  Walkers
  Crutches
  Canes
  Wheelchairs

Therapeutic Exercises
  Range of Motion
  Muscle Testing
  Types of Therapeutic Exercise

Electromyography

Electrostimulation of Muscle

Therapeutic Modalities
  Heat and Cold
  Moist and Dry Heat
  Moist and Dry Cold
  Ultrasound
  Massage Therapy

LEARNING OUTCOMES

1. Define, spell, and pronounce the key terms as presented in the glossary.
2. Define rehabilitation medicine and explain its importance in patient care.
3. Discuss the importance of correct posture and body mechanics, and demonstrate how to safely transfer patients and lift or move heavy objects using proper body mechanics.
4. Describe safety precautions and techniques used when helping a patient to ambulate and demonstrate how to assist the patient to safely stand and walk.
5. Demonstrate how to safely care for the falling patient.
6. Describe assistive devices and the importance of each in helping patients to ambulate.
7. Demonstrate how to measure patients for a walker, crutches, and a cane, and help them ambulate safely with each device.
8. Describe the ambulation gaits used with crutches.
9. Discuss the safety precautions and techniques used when pushing a wheelchair.
10. Explain the importance of joint range of motion and the method used to measure joint movement.
11. Explain the importance of therapeutic exercise and the types of therapeutic exercises used in patient rehabilitation.
12. Describe electromyography and its purpose.
13. Explain the purpose of the electrostimulation of muscle.
14. Explain the body's physiologic reactions to heat and cold therapeutic modalities.
15. Be able to identify and describe the various types of hot and cold modalities, and describe how ultrasound works.
16. Describe various conditions for which massage therapy is used.
17. Analyze the professionalism questions and apply them to this chapter's content.

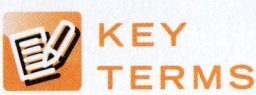

KEY TERMS

abduction

activities of daily living (ADL)

adduction

ambulation

assistive device

body mechanics

circumduction

contracture

diathermy

dorsiflexion

effleurage

eversion

extension

flexion

gait

gait belt

goniometer

goniometry

hemiplegia

hydrocollator

hyperextension

inversion

modalities

petrissage

plantar flexion

pronation

range of motion (ROM)

rehabilitative medicine

rotation

supination

thermotherapy

ultrasound

vasoconstriction

ATTRIBUTES OF PROFESSIONALISM

Communication

- Did you introduce yourself? Did you identify the patient through name and birth date or other identifying feature?
- Did you speak at the patient's level of understanding?
- Did you explain procedures and expectations to the patient?
- Did you allay patients' fears regarding the procedure being performed and help them feel safe and comfortable?

Presentation

- Did your actions attend to both the psychological and the physiological aspects of the patient's illness or condition?
- Did you attend to any special needs of the patient? Did you first ask if assistance was needed, rather than taking charge?
- Were you courteous, patient, and respectful to the patient?

Competency

- Were you knowledgeable and accountable?

Initiative

- Did you seek out opportunities to expand your knowledge base?
- Did you direct the patient to other resources when necessary or helpful, with the approval of the provider?
- Did you assist coworkers when appropriate?

Integrity

- Did you work within your scope of practice?

SCENARIO

In a large urgent care center such as Inner City Health Care, a team of therapists is responsible for providing patients with a high level of rehabilitative care. However, the clinical medical assistants at Inner City also are involved on a daily basis in the care of patients who have experienced injuries such as fractures or severe back pain. Clinical medical assistant Sam Tyler, CMA (AAMA), MLT, and clinical medical assistant Sarah Thomas, CMA (AAMA), are often responsible for transferring patients and getting them safely from the reception area to the examination room and from wheelchair to examination table. Although acutely aware of the needs and safety of the patient, Sam and Sarah also make sure they protect themselves by using proper body mechanics, by observing good posture, by using their arm and leg muscles and not their back muscles, and by always bending from the hips and knees, not the waist. Sam's and Sarah's observation of these important principles protects their health and ensures the safety of their patients.

INTRODUCTION

Physical disability affects millions of people in the United States, regardless of age, race, or socioeconomic status. Every year thousands of people survive strokes, head or spinal cord injury, or other debilitating illness or injury that leaves them unable to perform complete independent function. Some of these individuals recover completely. Others recover to their fullest ability, living the rest of their lives with some type of disability. Still other patients experience chronic conditions such as arthritis or severe back pain that incapacitates them to the extent they cannot work or completely care for themselves.

Rehabilitation medicine is a field of medical disciplines that uses physical and mechanical agents to aid in the diagnosis, treatment, and prevention of diseases or bodily injuries. Its goal is to aid in the restoration of those functions that have been affected by the patient's condition. For those who have experienced permanent loss of ability, it seeks to find practical substitutions for that loss, thereby assisting patients to make the most of their remaining abilities.

Most rehabilitation services are prescribed by the provider in charge of a patient's care and, depending on the patient's condition, can include a recommendation to one or several rehabilitation specialists. Most likely, that specialist will be a physical therapist, occupational therapist, speech therapist, or sports medicine specialist, although the field of rehabilitation medicine is certainly not limited to these four areas of specialty. Professional rehabilitation therapists, in whichever field they practice, are specifically trained and licensed in their field of expertise to assess, plan, and execute the patient's treatment in an overall effort to restore that patient to the highest level of physical and social independence possible. The medical assistant, as a member of an interdisciplinary health team, can use medical assisting skills to enable patients to regain normal or near-normal function after an illness or injury. Chapter 7 provides information on legal considerations and the Americans with Disabilities Act (ADA).

SPOTLIGHT ON CERTIFICATION

RMA Content Outline

- Anatomy and physiology
- Medical terminology
- Human relations
- Patient education
- Therapeutic modalities

CMA (AAMA) Content Outline

- Medical terminology
- Anatomy and physiology
- Medicolegal guidelines and requirements
- Treatment area
- Patient preparation and assisting the physician

CMAS Content Outline

- Medical terminology
- Basic anatomy and physiology

THE ROLE OF THE MEDICAL ASSISTANT IN REHABILITATION

As a medical assistant, you may find yourself working in one of the rehabilitation fields. Such opportunities might include an ambulatory care setting with a specialty in physical therapy or sports medicine, an orthopedic surgeon's practice, the occupational or speech therapy department of a large suburban hospital, or other outpatient clinic or medical clinic. For the more chronically ill, nursing homes and rehabilitation hospitals also focus on restoring patients to as much independence as possible.

Even if you do not work in the field of rehabilitation and therapeutic modalities, you may be referring patients for treatments and perhaps even performing insurance coding or rehabilitative and therapeutic **modalities**. Either way, a good working knowledge of the field is important for a well-rounded understanding of today's medical treatments.

Whatever the rehabilitation setting, you will most likely find that you are a member of an interdisciplinary team of health care professionals who bring a broad knowledge base to patient care (Table 33-1). However, the provider is responsible for prescribing any type of **rehabilitative medicine**.

It is important to remember that patients seeking rehabilitation treatment may have sub-stained a tremendous loss of physical ability, leaving them vulnerable to feelings of helplessness. They may be able to perform only limited **activities of daily living (ADL)** or normal daily self-care such as brushing their teeth, getting dressed, and eating. Perhaps they cannot even do the simple tasks we take for granted every day, leaving them completely dependent on another person for help.

Understanding and encouragement are vital to the recovery process of these patients. While working with disabled persons, remember that certain tasks may be challenging to them. More than

likely they are acutely aware of their impairment and feel frustrated at their loss of function and discouraged about the future. Some patients may suffer some speech impairment, making communication difficult or impossible. Respect for their dignity will build their self-esteem and have a positive effect on their treatment.

Patients' safety is essential. Many have a loss of ability to move and are vulnerable to falls.

PRINCIPLES OF BODY MECHANICS

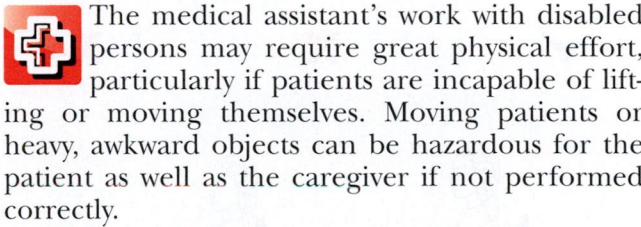The medical assistant's work with disabled persons may require great physical effort, particularly if patients are incapable of lifting or moving themselves. Moving patients or heavy, awkward objects can be hazardous for the patient as well as the caregiver if not performed correctly.

Body mechanics is the practice of using certain key muscle groups together with good body alignment and proper body positioning to reduce the risk for injury to both patient and caregiver. Always be conscious of using proper body mechanics, not just on the job, but in everything that requires moving, lifting, pushing, or pulling heavy or awkward objects.

Posture

Practicing good body mechanics starts with good posture. Good posture protects the entire body, particularly the back, whether standing, sitting, or lying down. Following the principles of good posture allows all of the structural components of the body to work together to perform at a peak level and to avoid injury.

The central idea of good posture is body alignment. When standing, the body should be balanced. Keep your head in the midline and your earlobes equally distant from the shoulders. Hold your chest high while keeping your shoulders back and relaxed. Keep your abdominal muscles tight and pull in your buttocks. Balance your weight evenly on both feet and keep your knees relaxed.

Good posture when sitting includes keeping the spine in a neutral position. Sit with your buttocks against the back of the chair and rest your back on the chair back. Feet should be resting on the floor with knees level with hips. Keep your head and neck straight with your shoulders relaxed, not rounded, elevated, or pulled back.

Table 33-1   Some of the Specialized Fields of Rehabilitative Medicine

Physical Therapy/ Physiotherapy	The treatment of disorders with physical and mechanical agents and methods to restore normal function after injury or illness.
Occupational Therapy	The use of activities to help restore independent functioning after an injury or illness.
Speech Therapy	The diagnosis and treatment of speech disorders.
Sports Medicine	A branch of medicine that specializes in the treatment and prevention of injuries caused by athletic participation.

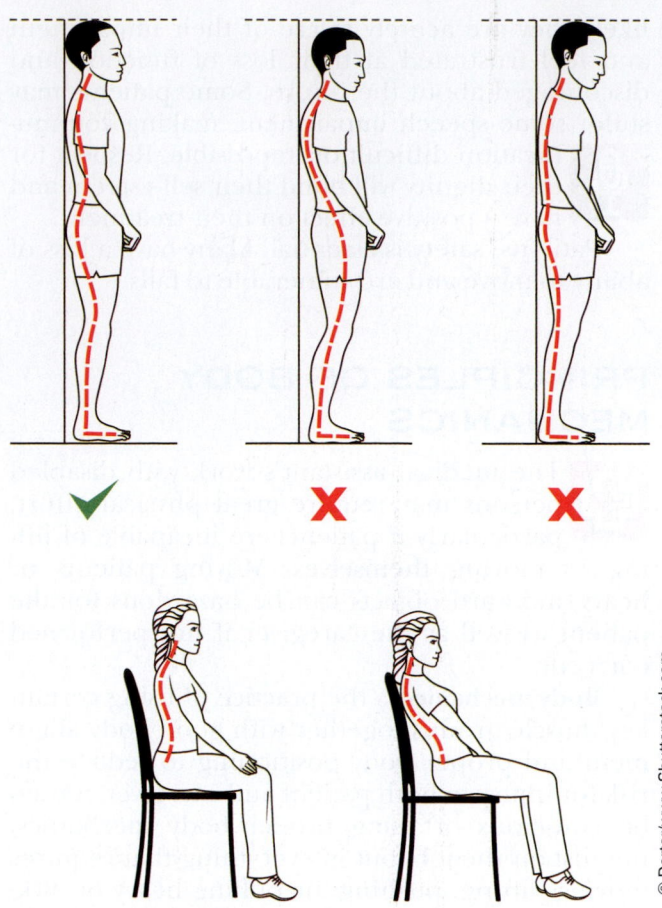

Figure 33-1   The correct position of the spine while standing or sitting.

Good posture when lying down includes maintaining your spine in a neutral position. A firm mattress for support is essential. When lying on your side, use a pillow between your knees to maintain proper alignment. If lying on your back, place the pillow under both knees to maintain proper positioning.

Refer to Figure 33-1 as a guide for proper posture when standing or sitting.

USING THE BODY SAFELY AND EFFECTIVELY

The spine is a flexible rod, designed to bend in many directions and hold the back steady. However, the muscles of the back are small and not meant for lifting heavy loads. They can be easily damaged if called on to work beyond their natural ability. The muscles in the arms and legs, however, are large and were designed for heavy work. Rely on these muscles when lifting and carrying heavy objects, bending over or bending down, or moving patients.

It is important to keep several basic rules in mind whenever performing any task:

- Keep the back as straight as possible and feet shoulder-width apart to provide a good base of support (Figure 33-2).
- Always bend from the hips and knees, enabling the largest muscles of the legs to do the hard work, but *never* bend from the waist.
- Pivot the entire body instead of twisting it.
- Use the body's weight to push or pull any heavy object.
- Obtain help if unable to move a patient or object that is too heavy.
- Hold heavy objects close to the body.
- Make sure the path is clear and the area to receive the object is ready before lifting or moving it.
- Get into the habit of wearing a body support if a job includes much lifting.

Lifting Techniques

There is great risk for back injuries when dealing with immobile or partially immobile patients. The greatest risk occurs when attempting to assist a person to a sitting position from a reclining position, transferring a person from a bed to a chair, or when leaning over a person for a long period of time.

When lifting patients or moving or lifting heavy objects, certain techniques should be used to prevent back injury:

- Get as close as possible to the object or person being lifted, because this allows the center of gravity to be maintained over the base of support.
- Keep the feet apart, one slightly in front of the other, and knees slightly bent.
- Use the large muscles of the legs and arms to lift, not back muscles.
- Keep the back straight to transfer the workload to larger arm and leg muscles. Avoid twisting movements.
- Bend from the hips and knees, squat down, and push up with leg muscles.

TRANSFERRING PATIENTS

It may be necessary to transfer patients if they cannot walk or lift themselves. Such patients may have a wide variety of disabilities, ranging from severe

© Derter/www.Shutterstock.com

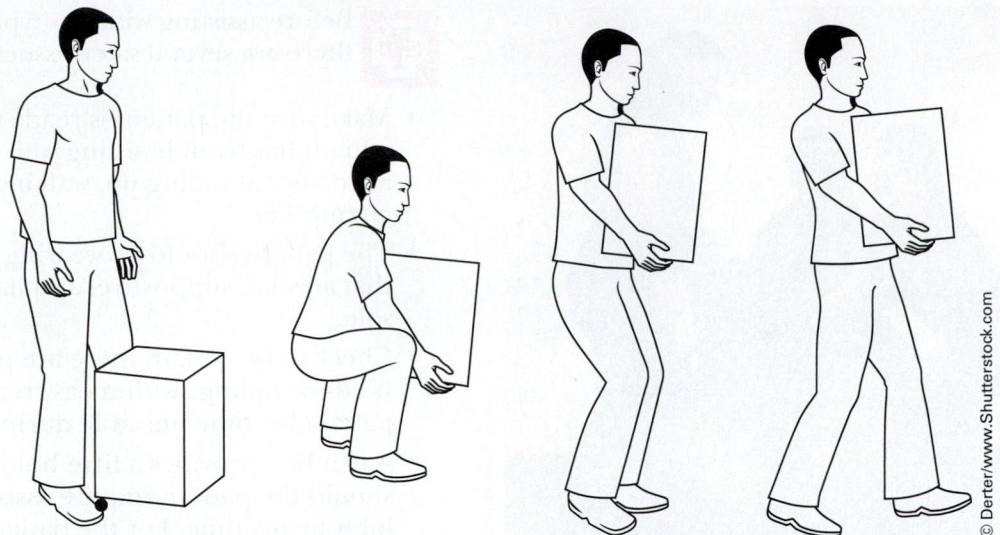

Figure 33-2   Provide a good base of support by keeping the back straight and feet apart.

back pain to **hemiplegia**, or paralysis of one side of the body resulting from a stroke, accident, or other condition. Frail older adults also require particular care when being transferred, because they are more prone to bruising and broken bones, and they may be unsteady on their feet.

As a safety precaution, it is important to remember good body mechanics when transferring patients. The act of lifting and moving someone can throw off one's center of gravity and therefore the base of support. Provide a wider base of support by moving the feet farther apart and bending slightly, using strong arm and leg muscles to lift.

Before beginning any transfer, observe certain precautions:

- Make sure the equipment is stable and firm. Lock the brakes of the wheelchair and make sure the examination table or other surface will not move during the transfer.

- Check that there are no obstructions to trip over when making the transfer.

- Take small shuffling steps, and avoid crossing the feet.

- It is best if the transfer surfaces being used are close to the same height. If possible, lower the examination table or bed to the height of the wheelchair.

- Position the equipment according to the patient's physical limitations or disability. If the patient is stronger on one side, make sure that is the side on which the transfer will take place. It not only makes the transfer easier, it gives the patient more confidence.

- Always use a **gait belt**, a safety belt worn around the patient's waist, when transferring a patient. Lift the patient by grasping the belt from underneath and lifting up. The utilization of a gait belt provides balance assistance during transfers and ambulation. This reduces the risk that either the patient or the staff will be injured. Never lift a patient by the arms, or under the armpits, because this could cause injury to you and the patient.

- Take advantage of any assistance the patient can provide in lifting and moving.

- Never have patients put their arms around your neck or on your shoulders, because it could cause you to be injured.

- Make sure both you and the patient are wearing footwear that will not slip or hinder the transfer process in any way. If a prosthesis or brace is involved, make sure it is secure and will not present a problem.

- Thoroughly explain to the patient what you intend to do, and make sure the patient understands what to expect during the transfer. Instructions need to be simple and repeated when necessary.

- Practice good body mechanics. Get close enough to the patient so you can lift with your legs (Figure 33-3). Always bend at the hips instead of the waist.

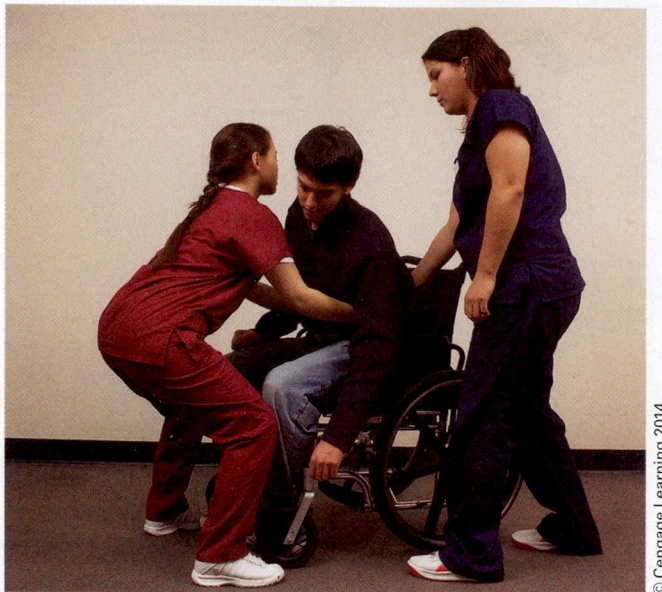

Figure 33-3 When a patient or object is too heavy, get help if necessary. Consider wearing a body support to protect the back if a job requires frequent lifting.

- Ascertain beforehand whether assistance will be needed with the transfer.
- Finally, take sufficient time when completing each step. Many patients will want to help themselves. Respect their courage and determination, but remember that safety is of the utmost importance.

 Procedure 33-1 gives the proper steps for transferring patients from a wheelchair to an examination table. Procedure 33-2 outlines steps for transfer from examination table to wheelchair.

ASSISTING PATIENTS TO AMBULATE

Despite great strides that have been made in providing access for disabled persons, **ambulation**, or walking, is a functional activity that still provides the ultimate level of independence and freedom. For many patients, being able to ambulate again gives them tremendous satisfaction, because the act of walking more than anything else signifies their return to wellness. Some patients take months to walk again by undergoing exercises and treatment designed to strengthen specific muscles. They may still need help while in your clinic or in a clinic specializing in orthopedics or sports medicine.

 Before assisting with any type of ambulation, there are several safety issues to remember:

- Make sure the patient is ready to walk. If a patient has trouble sitting well or cannot balance once standing up, walking should not be attempted.
- The patient should be wearing good shoes that are flat, supportive, and have a rubber sole.
- Check to be certain there are plenty of handholds or railings within easy reach should the patient become unstable during walking.
- A gait belt provides a firm hold on the patient should the patient require assistance with stability at any time. For the patient just starting to walk, this device should be used and held by the caregiver throughout the session.
- Monitor the patient when standing and throughout the ambulation session for signs of fatigue and vertigo.
- Ambulate only as long as the patient has strength. Never push the patient beyond endurance.
- Never hurry a patient.
- Be ready should a patient start to fall. Generally, patients will fall toward their weaker side, but sometimes their legs lose stability and they go straight down.

 Procedures 33-3 and 33-4 detail the steps involved in assisting patients to stand and walk and in caring for a falling patient.

ASSISTIVE DEVICES

For some patients, the extent of their physical disability may determine that ambulation is only possible with the help of an **assistive device**, or walking aid such as a walker, crutches, or cane. For others, their physical disability is such that mobility is not possible at all without the use of a wheelchair.

Some assistive devices provide stability and support, whereas others require more coordination. Depending on the patient's condition, one assistive device may be used until the patient has gained enough strength and coordination to move on to another type of assistive device, with the ultimate goal of walking unaided. The device a patient needs depends both on the disability and the patient's recuperation curve, and is prescribed after careful evaluation by the attending provider or other health professional (Table 33-2).

Table 33-2 Types of Assistive Devices

Assistive Device	Features	Patient Requirements
Walkers		
Standard	• Adjustable • Rubber tips	• Requires upper body strength • Provides maximum stability and support • Excellent for older adults
Rolling	• Legs have wheels • Otherwise same as regular walker	• Good for patients who need walker only for balance and not support
Crutches		
Axillary	• Wooden or steel • Worn under axillae	• Requires good upper body strength and balance • Not recommended for older adults • Best for younger persons with lower extremity or hip fractures that will heal in a short time • Provides greatest range of ambulation
Forearm (Lofstrand or Canadian)	• Shorter than axillary crutches • Has metal cuff worn around forearm	• Less stable than axillary crutches • Best for long-term crutch use • Reduces stress on axillary vessels and nerves • Requires upper body strength and more stability and coordination • Provides most maneuverability of all crutches
Platform	• Platform affixed to a crutch • Patient bears weight on forearm	• Best for patients with severe arthritis or poor use of hands • Does not require as much upper body strength • Requires good balance
Canes		
Standard	• Single leg • Curved handle • Rubber tip	• Good for patients with only one good arm, lateral instability, or balance conditions
Quad (four-point)	• Single cane resting on a platform with four legs • Rubber tips on legs	• Better for patients with more severe conditions • Does not require as much coordination, but still requires balance and upper body strength in one arm
Walkcane or Hemiwalker	• Has four legs that come all the way up to a handlebar • Rubber tips on all legs	• Provides most stability of all canes • Best for hemiplegic patients who require extra support on one side

© Cengage Learning 2014

Whatever device a patient will be using, medical assistants may be called on to measure the patient for the correct size and to provide instruction in its proper use and care. Once the patient has become proficient on level surfaces, provide instruction on sitting; standing; turning around; and negotiating stairs, curbs, ramps, doors, and other obstacles. In addition, patients should be taught how to protect themselves should they fall while alone and how to get back up.

Walkers

Walkers are best used for patients who require maximum assistance with balance and coordination, because walkers provide stability and support when patients are standing or walking. They provide patients with the ability to ambulate independently with confidence. To use one, patients must be strong enough to be able to hold themselves upright while leaning on the walker.

Various styles of walkers are available. The two most widely used walkers are those that have rubber tips on the legs (stationary walkers), and those with wheels on the bottom of the legs (rolling walkers). Walkers that have wheels can be easily pushed ahead by the patient while walking and are best for patients who primarily need a walker for balance.

Most walkers are made of aluminum and are lightweight; most can be easily folded for storage or transport. The major disadvantage is that they must be used on level ground and cannot be used on stairs. Walkers are also difficult to use when attempting to go through doorways and in small areas around the house.

Fitting a Walker. Most walkers can be adjusted for a proper fit. The height of the handgrip should be adjusted to the individual patient just below the patient's waist, or at the top of the femur, so the elbow can be bent at a 30-degree angle when the patient is standing with hands on the handgrip (Figure 33-4).

 Procedure 33-5 provides steps for assisting a patient to ambulate with a walker.

Crutches

Crutches provide the ambulating patient with a great deal more mobility and flexibility. They provide good stability and support, therefore allowing for a broad range of gait patterns and ambulating speeds.

Three basic types of crutches are prescribed, depending on the patient's physical limitations and abilities: axillary crutches, forearm crutches (also called Lofstrand or Canadian crutches), and platform crutches (Figure 33-5).

Axillary crutches are made of wood or aluminum and are used primarily for individuals who need crutches temporarily while a lower extremity heals. Axillary crutches are ideal for stronger patients and pediatric patients who have minor injuries; they are not recommended for frail older adults because upper body strength and balance are required to use them (Figure 33-6). These crutches are easily transported and can be used to maneuver on stairs or in tight places.

Forearm crutches, also known as Lofstrand or Canadian crutches, are shorter and provide less stability than axillary crutches. Forearm crutches are fixed with a metal or hard plastic cuff that fits around the patient's forearm. The weight is borne

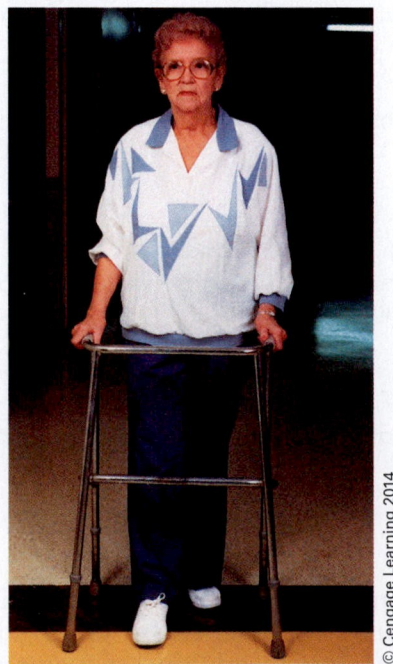

Figure 33-4   Proper fit for a walker. Note the patient's elbows are flexed at a 30-degree angle.

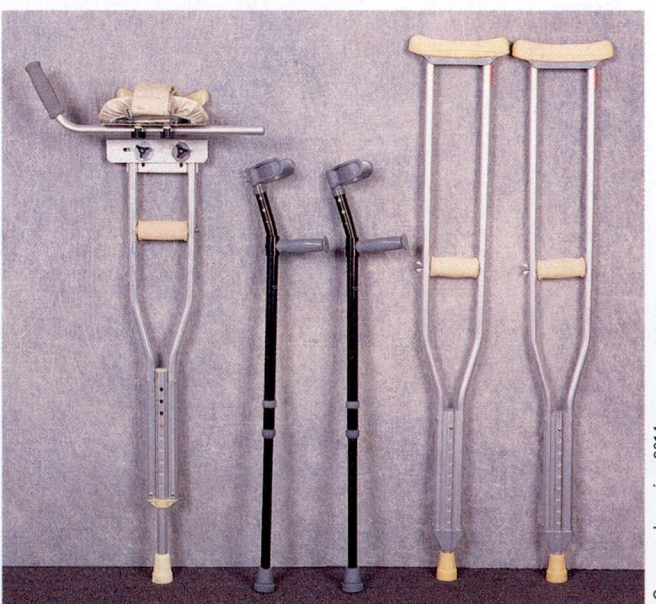

Figure 33-5   Types of crutches, from left to right: platform, forearm (or Lofstrand), and axillary.

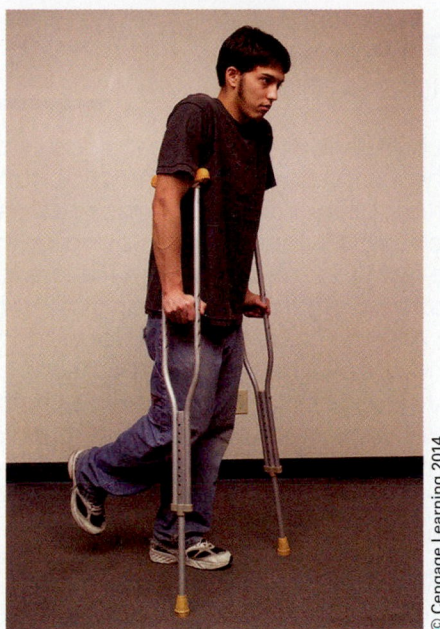

Figure 33-6 Patient using axillary crutches.

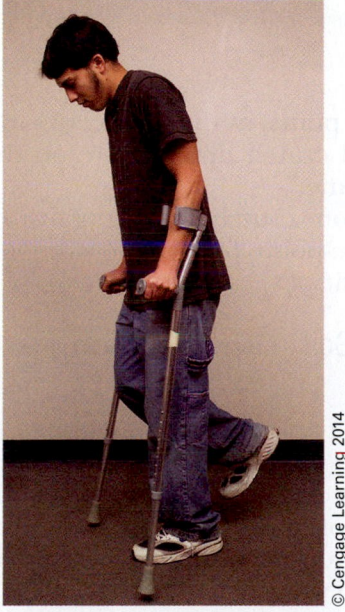

Figure 33-7 Patient using Lofstrand or forearm crutches.

almost exclusively on the hand grip, requiring a great deal of upper body strength and coordination to use. This type of crutch is generally recommended for patients who will need crutches permanently or for a long period because they do not put any pressure on the axillary vessels and nerves (Figure 33-7).

The *platform crutch* is a third type of crutch that is recommended for patients who cannot

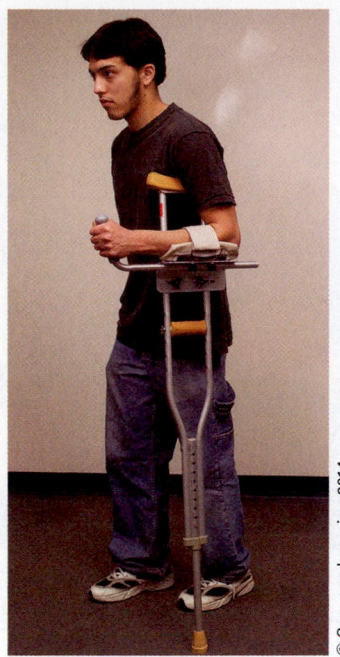

Figure 33-8 Patient using a platform crutch. This crutch is an ideal substitute for a cane if the patient cannot bear weight in his upper arm or on his hand.

grip the handles of other types of crutches or bear weight through their wrists or hands. The crutch has a platform attached to the top that includes a hand grip. It is high enough for the patient to use with the elbow bent at a right angle. The patient bears his or her weight completely on the forearm, which requires stability, strength, and coordination. The platform crutch is an ideal substitute for a cane when a patient only requires minimal weight transfer but cannot bear weight on or grip with the hands (Figure 33-8).

Measuring a Patient for Axillary Crutches.
To determine the right height of the crutches, the patient should stand tall. Be sure the patient is wearing good walking shoes. Adjust the height of the crutch so it is about two to three fingers, or 2 inches, below the patient's axillae, or armpits (Figure 33-9). Adjust the hand grips so the patient's elbows are bent at about a 20- to 30-degree angle. Position the crutch tips about 2 inches lateral and 6 inches anterior to the foot. When the patient is standing correctly, the crutch tips and patient's feet should form a triangle (Figure 33-10).

Procedure 33-6 gives steps for teaching patients to ambulate with axillary crutches.

Crutch-Walking Gaits.
The type of **gait**, or walk, a patient uses depends on the patient's injury and condition and is determined by the provider or

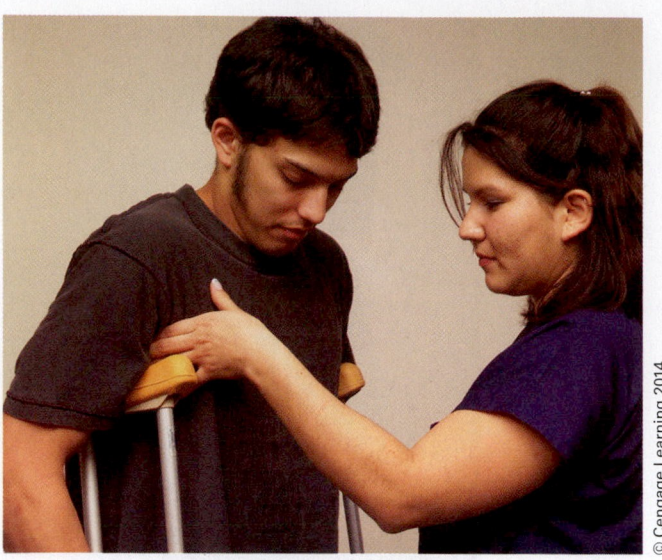

Figure 33-9 Measuring for axillary crutches. Note the height is about two to three fingers below the patient's axillae.

© Cengage Learning 2014

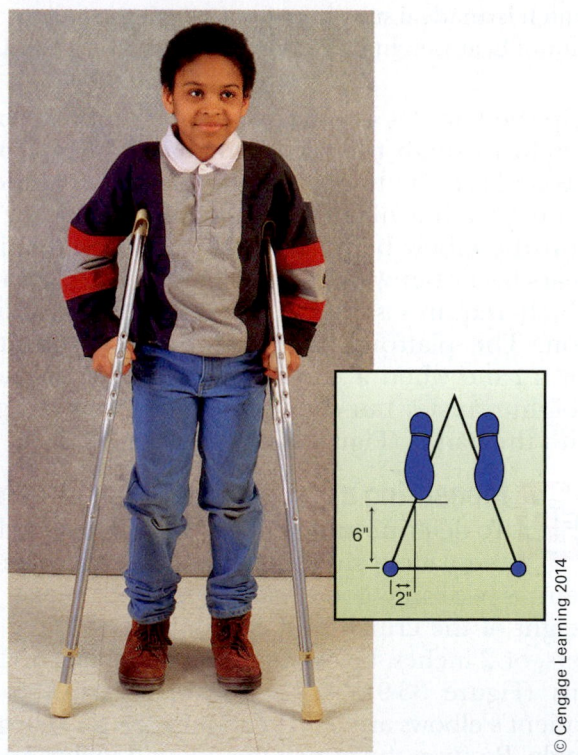

Figure 33-10 The distal end of the crutch should be 2 inches lateral and 6 inches anterior to the foot to form a triangle.

© Cengage Learning 2014

licensed therapist. In crutch-walking gaits, each time the patient's foot or crutch touches the ground it is called a *point*. There are five gaits that are commonly used in crutch ambulation. The

When instructing patients in the use of axillary crutches, impress on them the importance of putting all their weight on their hands, not on the axillae. Many patients using crutches for the first time mistakenly put the pressure on their axillae, which can damage the axillary nerve. Also reinforce the need for wearing flat, nonskid shoes when using crutches.

Throw rugs and other obstacles in the home or work area are a danger to patients on crutches. Remind them to have such hazards removed. Teach patients to examine crutches daily for the following:

- Check that the wing nuts that adjust the crutches are tight.
- Check the crutch tips for wear and tear.
- Check the foam pads of the hand grips and axilla rests for tears.

number of points in the gait relates to the number of feet and crutch tips that are on the ground at the same time.

Common crutch-walking gaits include two-point, three-point, four-point, swing-to, and swing-through gaits.

Two-Point Gait. There are two types of two-point gaits:

1. The first type is a non-weight-bearing gait. Patients place the crutch tips about 18 inches in front of them. They push off, taking the weight off their body and transferring it to their hands, and then bring their strong leg forward past the crutches.

2. The second gait, called the two-point alternating gait, is used when the patient can bear weight on both legs. The opposite foot and crutch are advanced forward at the same time (Figure 33-11). This gait is a more advanced gait and is used after the four-point gait has been mastered.

Three-Point Gait. This gait is used when the patient can only bear partial weight on one leg, or just touch that foot to the floor. Both the crutches and the weak leg are advanced at the same time. The body weight is then transferred forward to the crutches, and the stronger leg is advanced and placed slightly in front of the crutches (Figure 33-12).

Four-Point Alternating Gait.
This is a slower gait that is used for patients who can bear weight on both legs and move each leg separately. The patient moves one crutch forward, then the opposite foot.

The patient then moves the other crutch forward, then the opposite foot (Figure 33-13).

Swing-To Gait.
Patients start with the crutches at their side. They move both crutches forward, transfer their weight forward, and swing both feet together up to the crutches.

Swing-Through Gait.
Start with the crutches at the side. Move both crutches forward. Transfer the weight and swing both feet through the crutches, stopping slightly in front of the crutches.

Sitting.
The patient backs into a straight chair with armrests until the seat of the chair touches the back of the legs. Crutches are held in the hand on the strong side and opposite the weak leg. With the other hand the patient can grasp the armrest of the chair and lower slowly into the chair.

Standing.
The patient holds both crutches in the hand on the strong side, moves forward in the chair, grasps the armrest with the hand on the weaker side, then pushes up to a standing position.

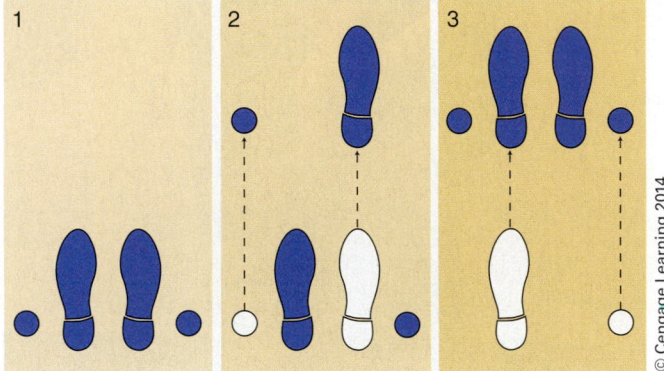

Figure 33-11 Two-point gait. The patient is bearing weight on both legs.

© Cengage Learning 2014

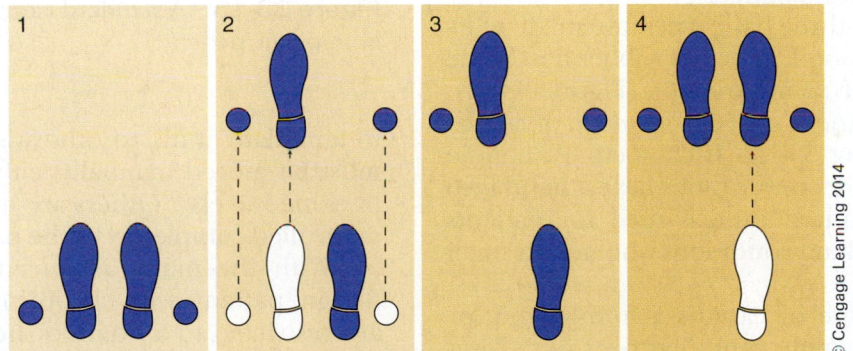

Figure 33-12 Three-point gait. The left leg is the weaker leg and bears no weight.

© Cengage Learning 2014

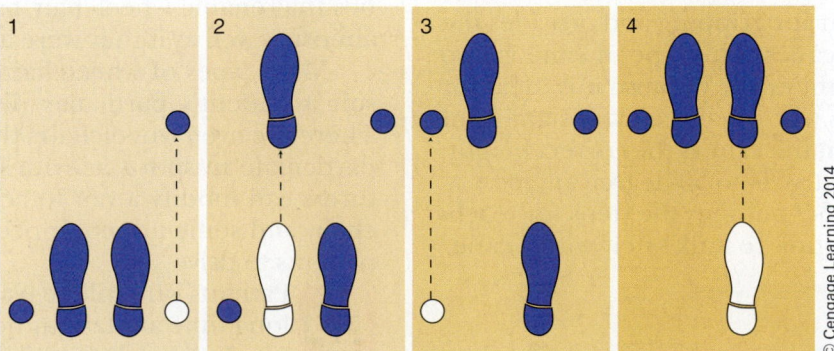

Figure 33-13 Four-point gait. The patient is bearing weight on both legs.

© Cengage Learning 2014

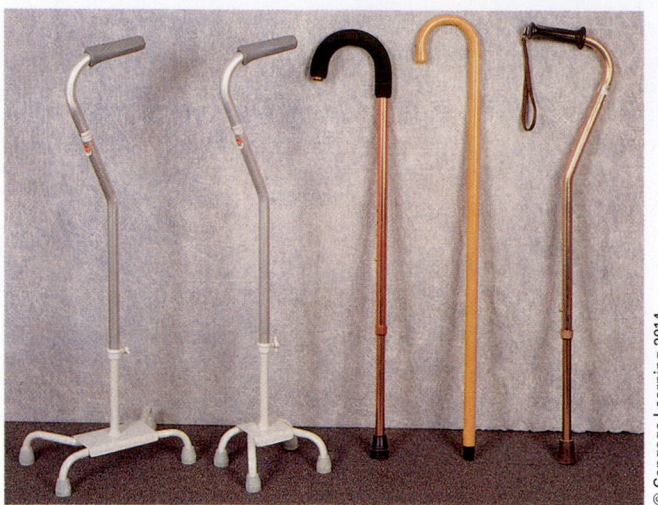

© Cengage Learning 2014

Figure 33-14 Types of standard canes: quad canes and single-tip canes.

Canes

A cane is used when the patient has one weak side and will need this assistive device for a longer period than crutches. It is also useful for patients who have a general but minor weakness on one side or those who have poor balance.

Canes come in three basic types, are made of either aluminum or wood, and have rubber tips. Some are adjustable and some are not (Figure 33-14). The first type of cane is called a *standard,* or single-tipped, cane (Figure 33-15). It has a curved handle for gripping, and the newer canes have a hand grip attached. The standard cane is used for patients with less severe walking conditions who need a small amount of support.

The second type of cane is a four-legged, or *quad,* cane. It is a single cane that rests on a four-legged platform, provides stability and a wide base of support, and is for patients with more severe walking difficulties.

The third type of cane is a *walkcane.* It has four legs and a handlebar for gripping and provides the best support of all canes. This type of cane is also referred to as a Hemiwalker because it is ideal for hemiplegic patients who need the extra stability of this wide base. When the cane is the correct height, the elbow is flexed at a 20- to 30-degree angle.

 Procedure 33-7 outlines the steps for teaching a patient how to walk safely with a cane.

Wheelchairs

Wheelchairs are mobile chairs that enable patients with severe ambulation conditions, or no ability

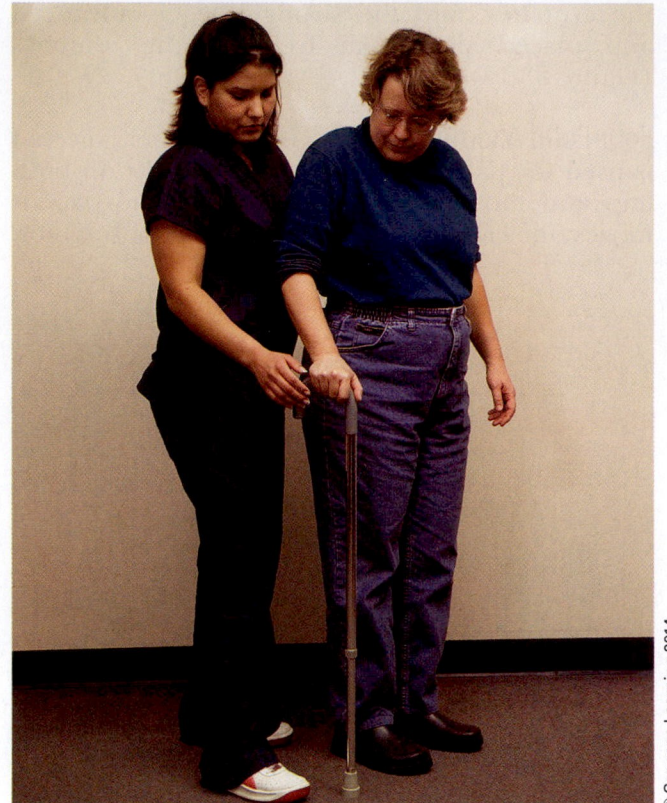

© Cengage Learning 2014

Figure 33-15 A standard cane being used by a hemiplegic patient.

to ambulate at all, to otherwise get around. Some must be moved manually, either by the patient or by someone else. Others are motorized and can be controlled completely by the patient (Figure 33-16).

With the many advancements in wheelchair design, patients with chronic conditions no longer are restricted to a home or hospital environment. Today, all public buildings and many private ones have handicapped access ramps as an alternative to stairs, remote-controlled doors, elevators that can accommodate a wheelchair, and other amenities that enable wheelchair patients to get around almost as well as if they were ambulating.

Many types of wheelchairs can be modified to suit a patient's particular disability and lifestyle. There are even wheelchairs that enable patients to participate in sports activities. Many car manufacturers can modify a van to accommodate a wheelchair, and some are equipped to allow wheelchair patients to drive.

Patients who will be using a wheelchair for a long time are taught how to maintain it. Depending on their abilities, they check it regularly to make sure all the parts are working correctly, and, if they are able, to make any

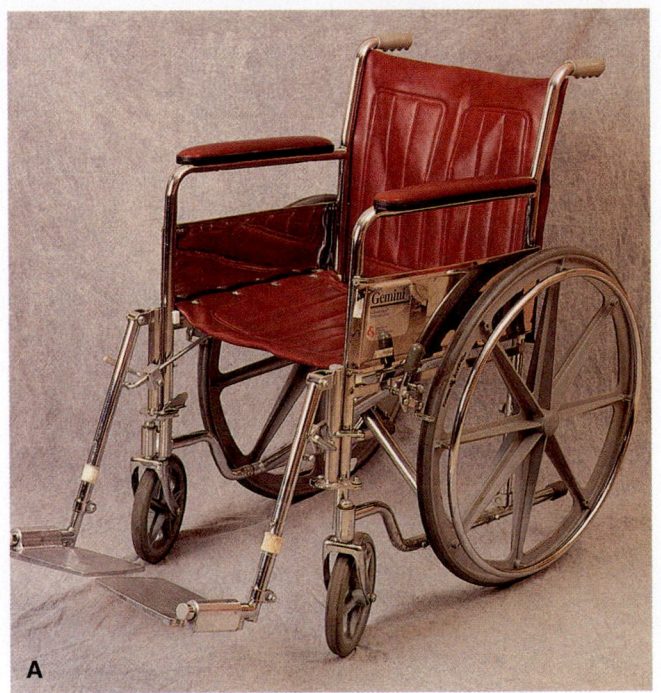

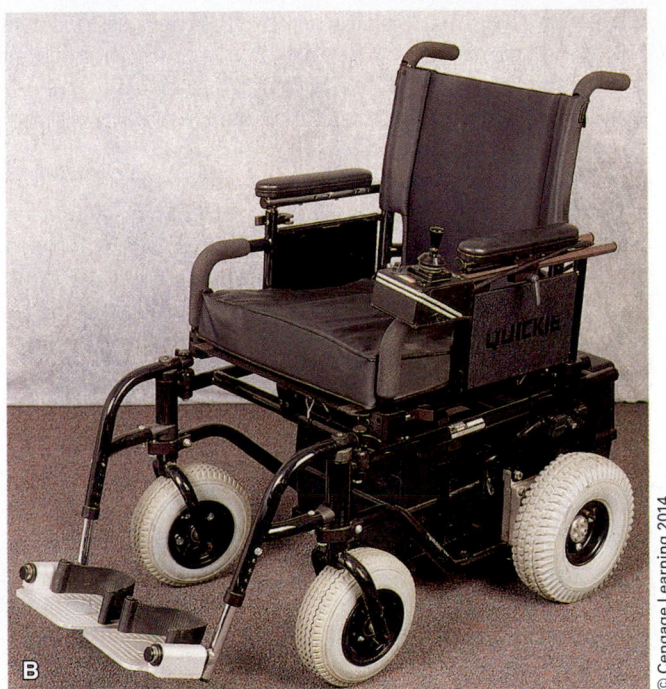

Figure 33-16 (A) A manual wheelchair. (B) A motorized wheelchair.

necessary repairs. Patients are taught to use the wheelchair safely and how to maneuver into and out of difficult spaces.

If a patient is being pushed by someone else, that individual must learn basic safety rules for transporting a patient:

- Make sure that the brakes are locked when transferring a patient into and out of a wheelchair; and if a patient must be left alone in the wheelchair for any length of time, lock the brakes (Figure 33-17).
- Make sure the patient's feet are placed on the footrests when the wheelchair is in use.
- Be certain the patient feels safe.
- Always back into and out of elevators.
- Stay to the right in corridors.
- Back down slanted ramps.

THERAPEUTIC EXERCISES

Range of Motion

The musculoskeletal system is a complex joining of bones, joints, ligaments, and tendons. Not only does it give structure to the body and protect the body's vital organs but also it allows for movement so we can carry out a multitude of activities.

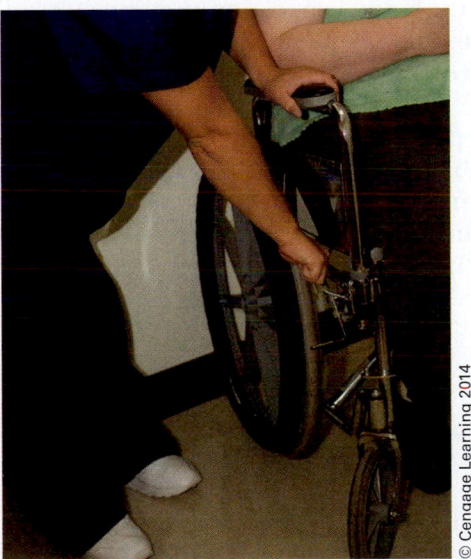

Figure 33-17 The patient's wheelchair should be locked when transferring a patient in and out of it, or when the patient is left alone in the wheelchair for any length of time.

The bones of almost all the joints of the body are designed to move as well. Each joint has its own **range of motion (ROM)**, the amount of movement that is present in a joint.

Normal ROM varies among people and depends on several factors, such as age, sex, and whether the motion being performed is passive (assisted motion) or active (voluntary motion). There is a standard ROM for all movable joints, and it is this standard that is used when evaluating the joint movement of a particular patient.

The measurement of joint motion is called **goniometry**. Joint movement is measured with an instrument called a **goniometer** and is always expressed in degrees. For example, the average person lying flat with arms to the sides can move the elbows from a 20-degree hyperextension (extending the arm beyond its normal limits) to 0-degree extension, through to 150 degrees of flexion, or bending (Figure 33-18).

ROM evaluation is one of several tools used when developing a therapeutic program for a patient.

As a medical assistant, you need to be familiar with ROM exercises (Figure 33-19). ROM exercises are designed to maintain joint mobility and are performed either passively (someone else does the movement) or actively (the patient does the movement).

The importance of maintaining ROM is the prevention of contractures. **Contractures** occur when the body is in a non-moving state. The usually flexible connective tissues become stiffened and are replaced with fiber-like tissues. This restricts movement and the immobility can become permanent. To avoid this complication of immobility, joints must be passively or actively in motion.

Joint movement has a special vocabulary, and it is helpful to learn the terms and their definitions (Table 33-3).

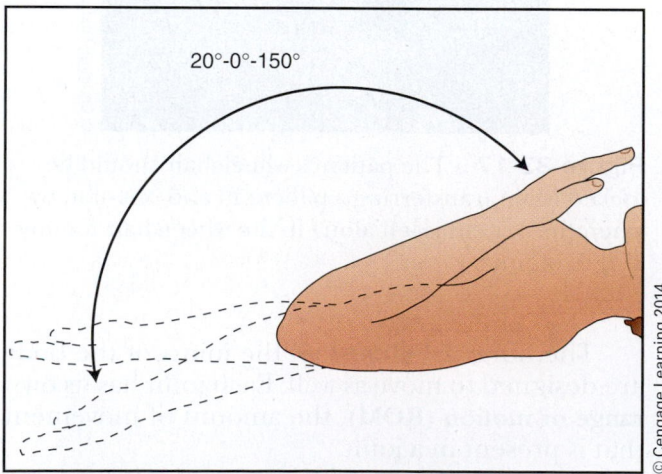

Figure 33-18 Joint mobility is measured against standard ranges of motion and is always expressed in degrees.

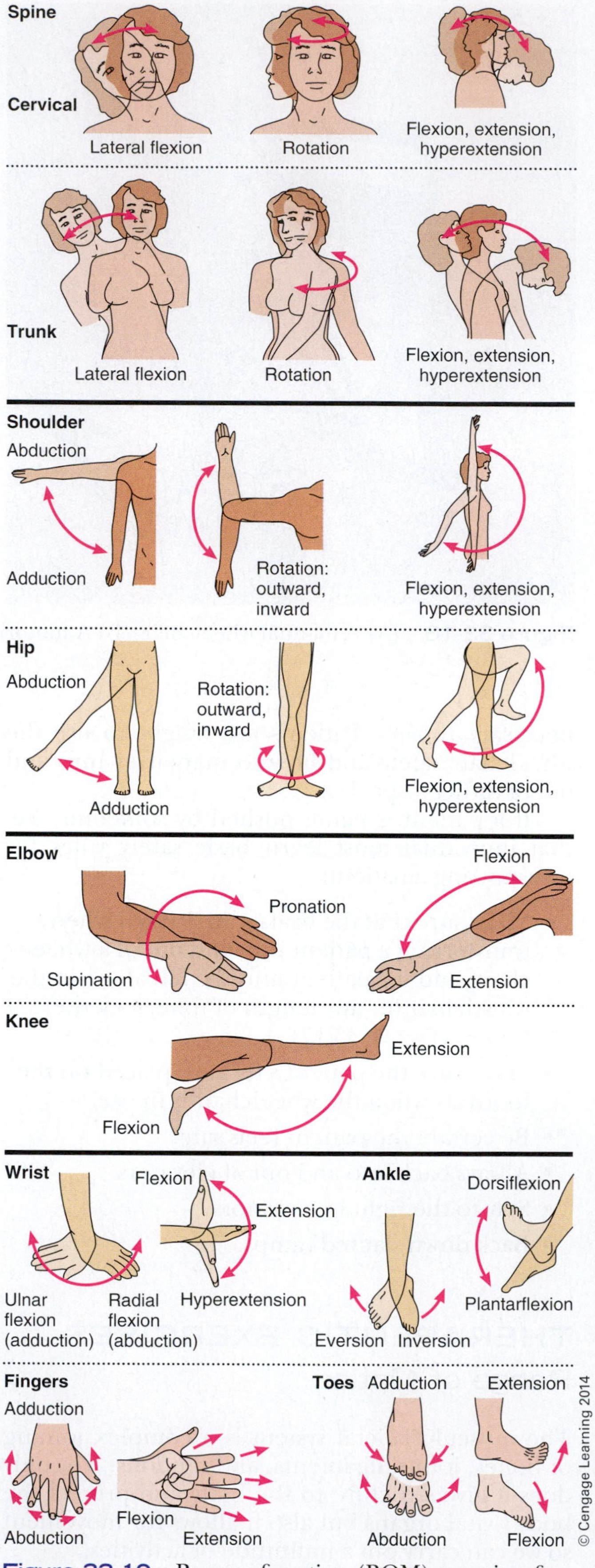

Figure 33-19 Range of motion (ROM) exercises for specific joints.

Table 33-3 Terminology of Joint Movement

Abduction	Motion away from the midline of the body
Adduction	Motion toward the midline of the body
Circumduction	Circular motion of a body part
Dorsiflexion	Moving the foot upward at the ankle joint
Eversion	Moving a body part outward
Extension	Straightening of a body part
Flexion	Bending of a body part
Hyperextension	A position of maximum extension, or extending a body part beyond its normal limits
Inversion	Moving a body part inward
Plantar flexion	Moving the foot downward at the ankle
Pronation	Moving the arm so the palm is down
Rotation	Turning a body part around its axis
Supination	Moving the arm so the palm is up

© Cengage Learning 2014

Before performing ROM exercises on a patient, the caregiver will need to observe some general precautions:

- Always move the patient's limbs gently, within pain tolerance and within the flexibility of the limb.
- Use slow, careful movements that allow the muscles time to adjust to the movement.
- Always support the limb above and below the joint.
- It is best to perform passive ROM with the patient in the supine position.
- ROM should never cause pain. If the patient reports pain at any time, the ROM exercises should be discontinued until the provider or other health care professional can determine the source of pain.
- Repeat each movement several times or as prescribed by the provider.
- Provide for patient privacy.

Muscle Testing

The other tool used for evaluating the movement abilities of a patient is muscle testing. Whereas goniometry focuses on joint movement, muscle testing evaluates the motion, strength, and task potential of a given muscle. *ROM* testing for muscles determines how flexible and resilient a muscle may be. *Strength testing* shows how hard a muscle can work. *Task potential* of a muscle means how well a muscle can aid in accomplishing a given activity. As a medical assistant, you may assist with testing the patient for joint mobility, posture, and strength of muscles.

Types of Therapeutic Exercise

Without constant exercise, the musculoskeletal system would deteriorate. Joints would become stiff and contractures, or deformities, could develop. Muscles would atrophy, or shrink and lose strength. Bones would lose vital minerals such as calcium and phosphorus. The body's overall circulation would decrease, which in turn would create a separate set of unhealthy conditions. Like drugs, exercise has a powerful and systemic effect on the body. It involves the function of joints, bones, muscles, nerves, tendons, and ligaments, as well as the circulatory and respiratory systems. Therapeutic exercises are prescribed after careful evaluation by a trained specialist and are tailored to each patient depending on that patient's individual condition and rehabilitation goals. It is the role of the medical assistant to understand the goals and objectives of the therapeutic exercise program to better support and encourage patients to complete their program.

Whereas an athlete uses exercise to build strength and endurance to attain a certain level of performance, therapeutic exercises are prescribed for a variety of therapeutic and preventive effects. They are used most commonly for therapeutic reasons to correct or prevent deformities, regain body movement after an accident or disease, restore joint motion after immobility, improve neuromuscular coordination, and improve or develop ADLs.

Exercise is also used for another important reason: It can prevent many common problems brought on by inactivity, such as those associated with respiration and circulation.

A variety of exercise programs are used for therapeutic or preventive purposes:

1. *Active exercises,* which are self-directed and performed by the patient without assistance
2. *Passive exercises,* which are performed by another person with no voluntary participation from the patient

3. *Assisted exercises,* which help the patient voluntarily move weakened muscles with the use of an assistive device, such as a therapy pool

4. *Active resistance exercises,* which provide voluntary movement against various types of manual or mechanical pressure to increase muscle strength

Electromyography

Electrical activity of muscles can be recorded on a graph or film to help determine how well muscles contract. An electromyograph is the instrument used to test the electrical activity of a muscle. An electrode (using a small gauge needle) is inserted through skin into the muscle, and measurements of muscle strength are made.

Electrostimulation of Muscle

An electric current of low voltage can help stimulate muscles to exercise by stimulating the sensory and motor nerves for that muscle. It is helpful for a patient who has nerve damage to the muscle and cannot voluntarily move the muscle. The purpose is to prevent atrophy of the muscle and help restore muscle function.

The low current of electricity passing through the patient's muscle acts similarly to the patient's own nerves, causing the muscle to contract and relax. The stimulation is helpful to retrain a patient after experiencing an injury to a muscle or muscle group. Disposable gel electrodes are applied, and low-voltage current stimulates the muscles to prevent atrophy.

A method of using electric current to stimulate nerves is known as *transcutaneous electric nerve stimulation* (TENS). It is used for patients who have severe pain, for example, chronic lower back pain from an injury. In this method, electrodes are attached to the patient's skin over a painful area. This causes interference with the transmission of painful stimuli, thus reducing the patient's pain sensation. Many patients with chronic severe pain need narcotics to ease the pain. However, TENS can control the pain and lesson the need for addictive drugs. TENS can be used by patients at home.

THERAPEUTIC MODALITIES

Sometimes, therapeutic exercise is not the best or only way to restore injured or painful joints and tissues. A patient's condition may respond equally well to certain physical agents, called modalities, which take advantage of the properties of heat, cold, electricity, light, and water to improve circulation, minimize pain, and correct or alleviate muscular and joint malfunction.

Many modalities have been around for centuries, and some can easily be performed by the patient or caregiver at home. Modalities can be used locally to treat a small area at a time or systemically to alter a patient's temperature or soothe many groups of painful muscles or joints. The patient's condition and rehabilitation program both influence the modality or combination of modalities used.

A provider order is required for any therapeutic modality.

Heat and Cold

Heat, or **thermotherapy**, acts on the body by causing vasodilation (dilation of the blood vessels). The effect of heat increases circulation to an area and acts to speed up the repair process. Heat can be used to:

- Relax muscle spasms
- Relieve pain in a strained muscle or sprained joint
- Relieve localized congestion and swelling
- Increase drainage from an infected area
- Increase tissue metabolism and repair
- Combat local infection
- Increase circulation
- Improve mobility before exercise

However, because heat dilates the blood vessels and increases circulation, it also acts to speed up the inflammatory process, which can lead to more serious problems, such as increased bleeding and swelling. Heat should not be used longer than its prescribed length of time.

Cold applications, or cryotherapy, are used to constrict blood vessels and slow or stop the flow of blood to an area. This process, also called **vasoconstriction**, slows down the inflammatory process, which can reduce or prevent swelling of inflamed tissues, reduce bleeding, numb the pain sensation by acting as a topical anesthetic, and reduce drainage to an area.

By understanding how heat and cold affect the body, it is easier to observe whether they are having the desired therapeutic effect. Because heat and cold modalities can be extremely effective, they are widely used for treating certain physical conditions. However, the effects of heat and cold modalities depend on several conditions: the type of modality used, the length of time it is applied, the patient's condition, and the area or areas being treated.

Precautions for Heat and Cold Applications.

When applying either heat or cold modalities, you need to take certain precautions to avoid injury. If misused, any therapeutic modality can actually cause more damage to the site it is trying to heal. Before starting any treatment, keep the following precautions in mind:

- Infants and patients who cannot report a burning sensation should be watched carefully. Infants and older adults are particularly susceptible to burns.
- Heat and cold sensitivity varies with patients; check patients frequently and never leave them alone.
- Never have a patient lie on a heating pad because severe burning can result. Place a rubber cover over the heating pad if using with moist dressings.
- Always wrap appliances, whether warm or cold, with cloth before applying them to the skin.
- Only soak or immerse patients in water between 104°F and 113°F (40°C–45°C). Temperatures of 116°F (47°C) or greater can cause burning.
- Never use heat within the first 48 hours of an acute inflammatory process and never apply heat to newly burned skin.
- Watch carefully persons with impaired circulation; cardiovascular, renal, sensorineural, or respiratory conditions; or osteoporosis. Tell patient to report pain or numbness.
- Excessive cold can damage tissues.
- Lack of sensation to a therapy may mean impaired circulation to an area, and the patient may be unable to report a burning sensation.
- Heat concentrates in metal materials, so have patients remove all jewelry and other metal objects, and administer the treatment on nonmetal tables and chairs.
- **EHR** Document in the patient's chart or electronic medical record the type of modality, length of time applied, color of patient's skin, and any discomfort.

Moist and Dry Heat

Moist Heat Therapies.
Moist heat refers to heat modalities that feel moist against the skin. Moist heat penetrates better than dry heat and aids in improving circulation, relaxation, and mobility.

Warm Soaks. Warm soaks are generally used for soaking the extremities and can be administered easily at home by the patient or caregiver. The patient's body part is gradually immersed in plain or medicated water no hotter than 110°F (44°C) for a short time, usually no more than about 15 minutes. The patient should be positioned to be comfortable. Observe the patient's skin for excessive redness and, if noticed, remove the limb at once. Always dry the skin carefully by patting, not rubbing, it.

Total body immersion in water 104°F–113°F can be administered in a whirlpool bath or special Hubbard tank. This treatment is often prescribed to promote relaxation, circulation, and movement of limbs in preparation for exercise. The mechanical action of agitating water moving over the body in a whirlpool is called hydromassage and can both relax muscles and stimulate circulation. The Hubbard tank is a bit larger and provides room for limited body exercise without the effects of gravity.

Sitz Bath. A sitz bath is a bath of warm water in which only the hips and buttocks (perineum) are immersed for relief of pain and discomfort from conditions such as rectal surgery and episiotomy. It is therapeutic and cleansing and will help relieve discomfort by reducing swelling and will improve healing by stimulating blood flow.

Warm Wet Compresses and Packs. A warm wet compress is usually applied to a small area. It is prepared by soaking and wringing out either a square of gauze or other absorbent material (such as a clean washcloth) and applying it for a limited time to the affected area (Figure 33-20). Warm compresses can be administered easily at home. A warm pack is used for a larger area and generally involves the use of a professional warm pack (**hydrocollator**) administered in the clinical setting. This type of warm pack is soaked in water 150°F–170°F, removed with tongs and drained, and placed over larger areas such as the back or shoulders. Check color of patient's skin frequently.

Paraffin Wax Bath. This type of treatment is most often used for chronic joint disease, such as rheumatoid arthritis. The bath mixture of seven parts

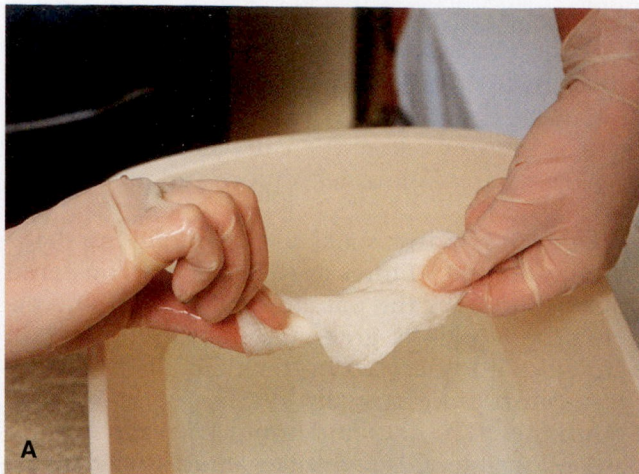

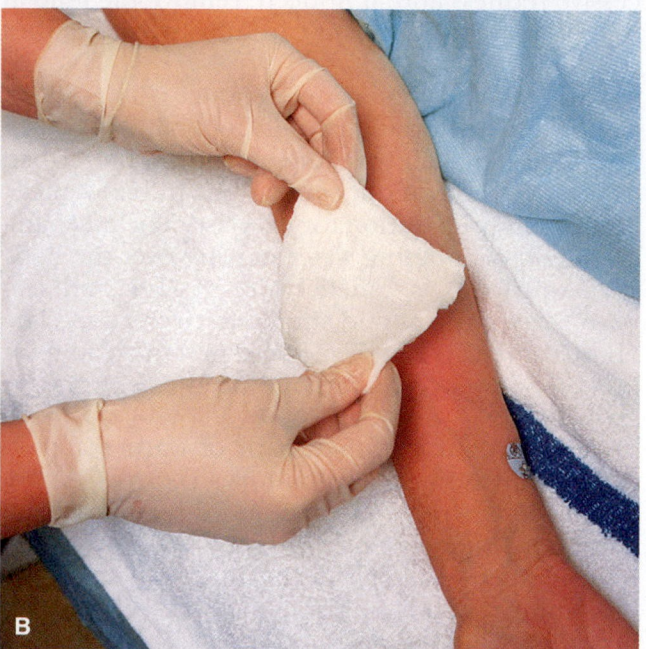

Figure 33-20   (A) Dip warm compresses frequently into a basin of warm water to keep them warm. (B) Apply compresses directly to the skin. *NOTE:* Limb will be wrapped in a towel that will then be covered with a blue plastic wrap. This helps keep the compresses warm.

paraffin to one part mineral oil is heated to melting (about 127°F) and the body part is dipped in the mixture several times until a thick coat of wax builds up. The body part is then wrapped in foil, cloth, or plastic wrap to help insulate the heat, then left on for 30 minutes or less. Once peeled off, the circulatory effects of this treatment can last up to several hours. It is an excellent modality for warming up joints before ROM or other exercises. This modality, ordered by the provider, will be carried out in the physical therapy department by a professional therapist (Figure 33-21).

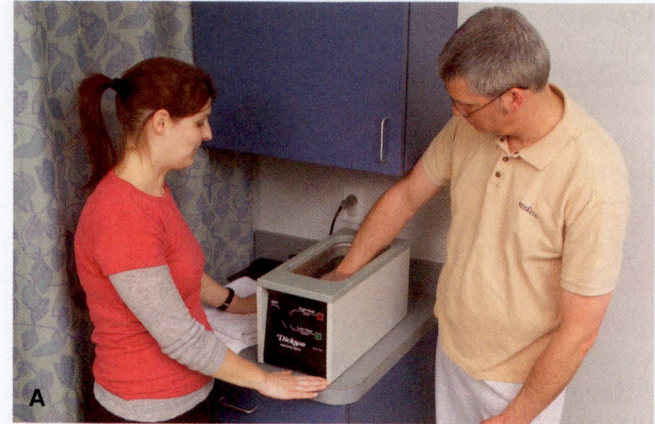

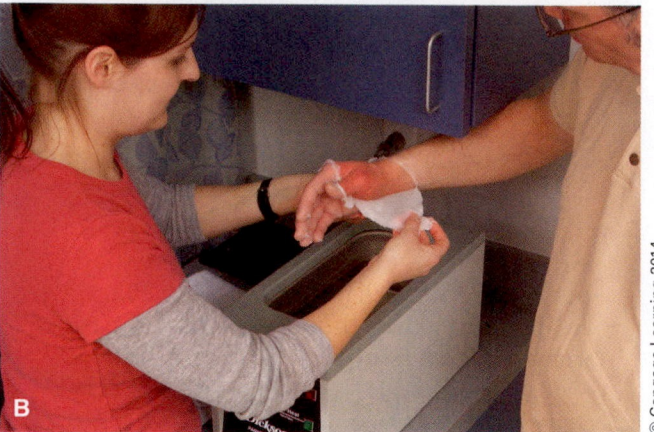

Figure 33-21   (A) A body part is dipped into the paraffin bath three or four times to create a layer of warm wax on the skin. (B) After the wax has been placed for 20 to 30 minutes, it is peeled off and discarded.

Dry Heat Therapies. Dry heat applications feel dry against the skin and do not penetrate like moist heat. They are used more to improve circulation for the purposes of relieving swelling and healing wounds, as well as to relax muscles and reduce muscle spasms. Most dry heat modalities can be performed easily by the patient or caregiver at home.

Heating Pads and Packs. Heating pads and commercially prepared packs are used for smaller areas and should always be covered with a cloth before applying against the skin. Never let a patient lie directly on a heating pad because burns can result. Set the switch on the heating pad to a low or medium setting and observe the proper time of exposure.

An Aquamatic K-Pad® is a commercial pad that is safer to use than a heating pad or commercially prepared pack because you can maintain a constant temperature and regulate that temperature more carefully. It is a pad with tubes that are filled with distilled water and heated by a control unit. The pad must be covered and left on the patient for no more than about 30 minutes. The temperature usually is set between 95 and 100°F.

Moist and Dry Cold

Moist Cold Therapies. Moist cold therapies refer to cold modalities that feel moist against the skin. Moist cold, as with moist heat, penetrates better than dry cold and is used to prevent swelling or edema, relieve pain or tenderness, and reduce body temperature. Most cold therapies can be performed easily at home by the patient or caregiver.

Cold Compresses and Packs. Cold compresses are used for smaller areas, and cold packs are used for larger areas. For a cold compress, immerse the cold cloth, gauze, or other clean material in a basin filled with ice and cold water or solution prescribed. Wring out the cloth and apply it to the affected area. Keep the cloth cold by immersing it several times throughout the treatment or use a syringe to add cold water to the compress. Cold or ice packs are administered in the same manner. Check patient's skin frequently.

Dry Cold Therapies. Dry cold treatments are used for the same reasons as moist cold treatments but are better for bleeding and acute injuries. Dry cold is also an excellent therapy for sprains, strains, burns, or bruises.

The temperature used depends on the area being treated and the method used, as well as the patient's tolerance for cold temperatures. In general, the colder the temperature, the shorter the duration of exposure.

Ice Packs. Dry cold treatments include ice packs and commercially prepared chemical ice packs or cold packs. Always cover the pack with cloth before applying it to the skin (Figure 33-22). Generally, ice packs can be kept on the body longer than heat packs, about 30 minutes. Check color of patient's

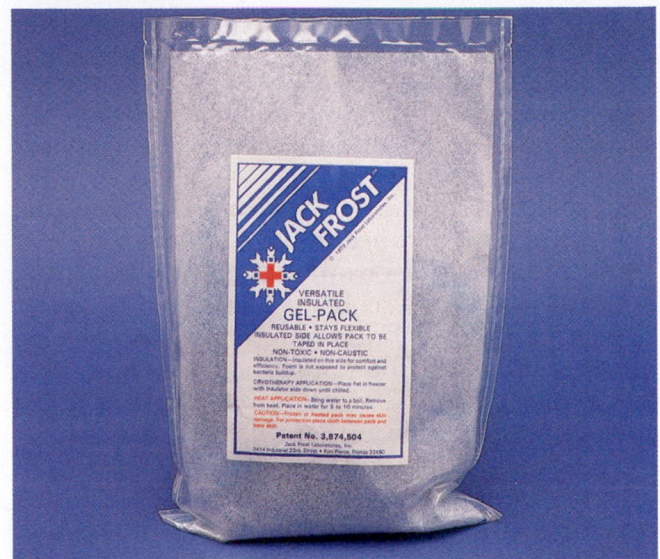

© Cengage Learning 2014

Figure 33-22   A chemical ice pack. These should be covered with a cloth before applying to the skin.

PATIENT EDUCATION

Neither heat nor cold applications should be left on the skin for prolonged periods, because both can have counterproductive effects if not monitored carefully. When applying heat or cold, periodically check the skin for signs of paleness or redness. If the patient experiences any numbness or tingling reaction, discontinue the application. Report the observations, and document.

skin frequently (see Chapter 9). A commercial ice pack can be used for smaller areas and can usually be chilled in the freezer. Because they do not freeze and become solid, these ice packs are pliable, making them ideal for contouring to the body part being treated. The cold packs are usually single-use. They must be activated by a blow to the pack before applying or by squeezing the pack.

Ultrasound

Ultrasound is a high-frequency acoustic vibration that is part of the electromagnetic spectrum, and its frequencies are beyond the perception of the human ear. This type of treatment uses high-frequency sound waves that are converted to heat in the deeper tissues.

CRITICAL THINKING

How do heat and cold affect the body's physiology and for what conditions should each be used?

Ultrasound is an effective form of treatment for chronic pain or acute injuries such as sprains or strains. It relaxes muscle spasms, increases the elasticity of tissue such as tendons and ligaments, and stimulates circulation, which, in turn, speeds up the healing process.

Ultrasound waves travel best in tissue that has a high concentration of water, such as muscles. They cannot penetrate and move through tissue such as bone that has a low water content. In fact, ultrasound treatment must be used carefully near bones, particularly those near the surface, because their waves are capable of concentrating in one area and causing damage.

Because ultrasound waves cannot be conducted through air, a special gel is applied to the skin surface that acts as a conduit. The sound waves are generated through an applicator that is rubbed over the gel. This applicator must be kept moving to prevent any internal damage caused by too high a concentration of sound waves. The duration of treatment lasts anywhere from 5 to 15 minutes, depending on the condition being treated and the recommendation of the physician or other health care provider. It is important to note that, because of its potential dangers, ultrasound treatment should only be administered if the medical assistant or other caregiver is specially trained in its safe and effective use.

Massage Therapy

Massage therapy has become recognized as a modality that is basic to physical therapy. The majority of states require a massage therapist to be licensed in order to practice the profession.

History shows massage therapy is one of the earliest practices for helping the body restore healthy functioning. It is used to relieve minor aches and pains, thus helping patients feel relaxed and refreshed. Massage therapy is safe and advantageous for most individuals, from infants to older adults.

Some physiologic benefits include increased metabolism, promotion of healing, soothing of muscles, relief of discomfort and pain, and improved circulation. Massage therapy can be used to manage the pain associated with conditions such as whiplash injury, muscle spasm, sciatic nerve pain, arthritis, and many other health problems.

Therapists use their hands to handle or touch the soft tissues of the patients' body. The movements stimulate the patients' circulation, help relieve discomfort, improve range of motion, and relax muscles. Some of the movements include percussion (tapping), rubbing, pressing, **petrissage** (kneading), and **effleurage** (stroking) of the soft tissue (Figure 33-23).

Massage therapy is inappropriate for patients with open wounds, neuropathies, shock, severe upper respiratory illnesses, varicose veins, phlebitis, high blood pressure, and often patients with osteoporosis (bones can easily break).

There are psychological benefits as well. Massage therapy relieves stress and tension; refreshes the patient, thereby lessening fatigue; and regenerates energy.

Massage therapy has been accepted and recognized by the medical community and the community-at-large as a complementary or alternative form of medicine.

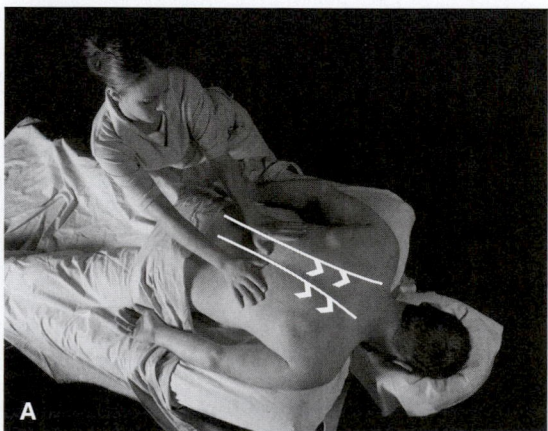
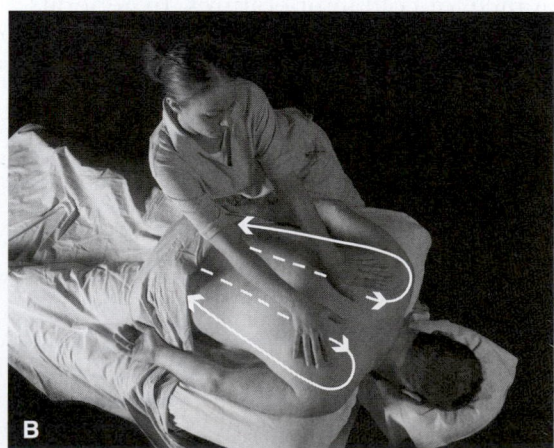

Figure 33-23 (A) The therapist applies long strokes up along the muscles on each side of the spine. (B) Effleurage strokes are used up the back and over the shoulders. Effleurage or gliding strokes are applied in the direction of venous blood and lymph flow.

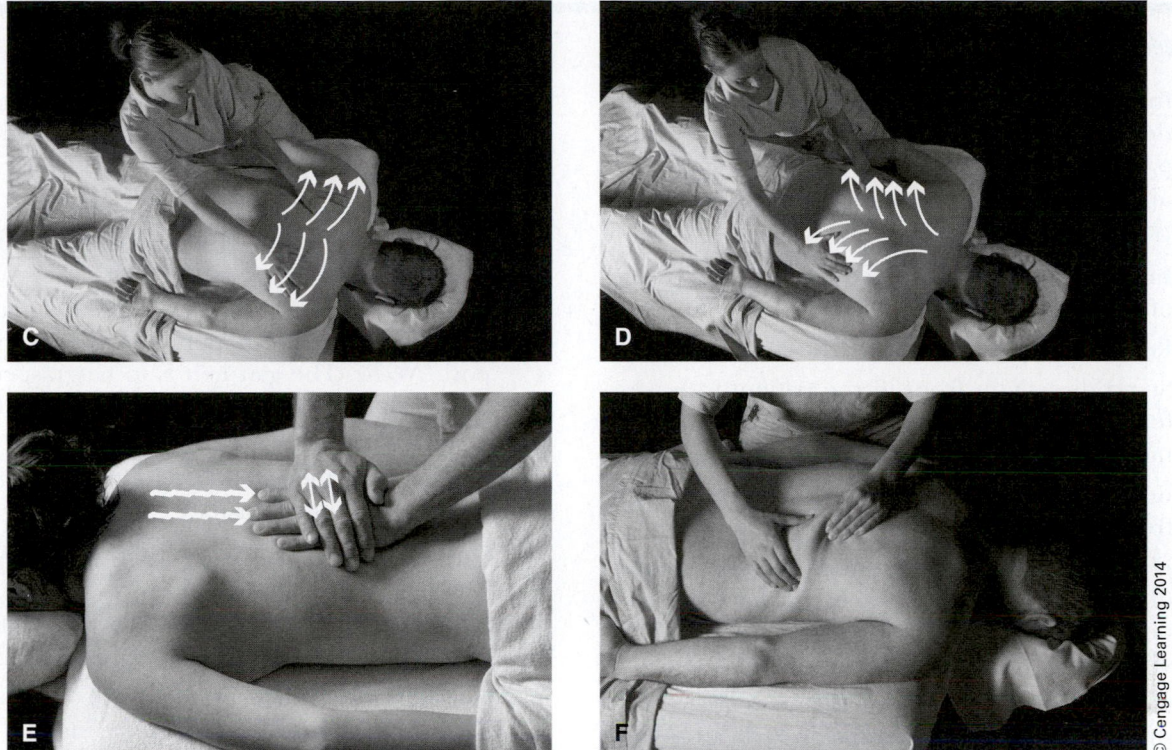

© Cengage Learning 2014

Figure 33-23   (continued) (C) The muscles of the back are stroked outward. (D) Fan stroking is applied to the back. (E) Vibration movements are applied to the vertebrae, and vibrations go back and forth as the therapist moves down along the spine. (F) Petrissage is applied to the entire side opposite the therapist.

PROCEDURE 33-1

Transferring Patient from Wheelchair to Examination Table

STANDARD PRECAUTIONS:

PURPOSE:
To move a patient safely from a wheelchair to the examination table.

EQUIPMENT/SUPPLIES:
Footstool with hand rail and non-skid
    rubber tips
Gait belt

PROCEDURE STEPS:
1. Wash hands.
2. *Introduce yourself and identify patient.*

3. *Speaking at the level of the patient's understanding, explain the process of transfer* so that the patient is able to assist as much as possible.

4. Place the wheelchair next to the examination table and lock the brakes. CAUTION: The side nearest the examination table should be the patient's stronger side to allow the patient to balance on that leg during the transfer.

5. Assure that the wheelchair is parked with the patient's strongest side near the exam table. The patient can balance on this leg during the transfer.

6. Place the gait belt snugly around the patient's waist and tuck the excess belting under the belt to avoid tripping or entanglement (Figure 33-24A).

7. Move the wheelchair's footrests up and out of the way. If the footrests are removable, that is preferred.

continues

Procedure 33-1 (continued)

8. Instruct the patient to place their feet flat on the floor. Assist him if needed.

9. Position stool in front of the examination table and as close to the wheelchair as possible (Figure 33-24B).

10. Instruct the patient to move forward to the edge of the wheelchair.

11. Remind the patient of instructions and signal.

12. Stand directly in front of the patient with your feet slightly apart. Remember to use good body mechanics (Figure 33-24C).

13. Bend at the hips and knees. Grasp the gait belt from underneath.

14. Have the patient place his hands on the armrests of the wheelchair. At your signal, have your patient push on the armrests to assist in lifting himself to a standing position.

15. Steady the patient momentarily and observe for strength, balance, and skin color. If there are any changes or as indicated by patient statements ('I'm dizzy'), carefully lower the patient to a sitting position in the wheelchair and check vital signs.

16. If the patient appears steady, stable and is balanced, proceed by standing slightly behind and on the weakest side of the patient.

17. Grasp the gait belt with one hand and place the other hand on the patient's bent arm for support. *NOTE:* The gait belt is to be grasped with fingers under the belt, palm facing upwards, and elbow bent.

18. Still grasping the gait belt, have the patient grasp the handle of the footstool.

19. Instruct the patient to carefully step up on the footstool.

20. Assist the patient to pivot so that his back is toward the examination table (Figure 33-24D).

21. The buttocks should be slightly above the edge of the bed. Steady the patient.

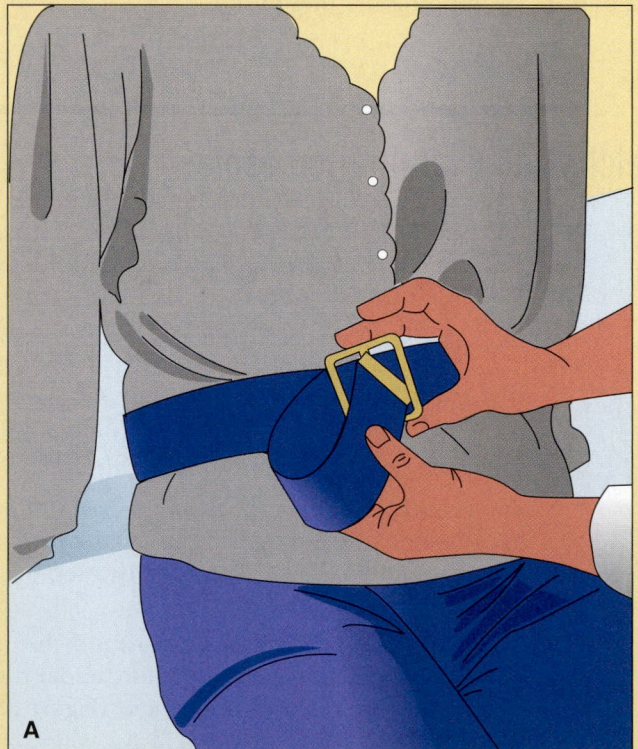

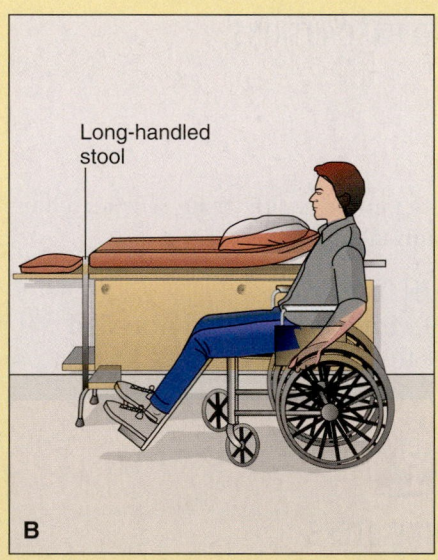

Long-handled stool

Figure 33-24 (A) The gait belt is always applied snugly around the patient's waist before attempting to move or ambulate with the patient. (B) Position the long-handled stool in front of the examination table and as close to the wheelchair as possible.

Procedure 33-1 (continued)

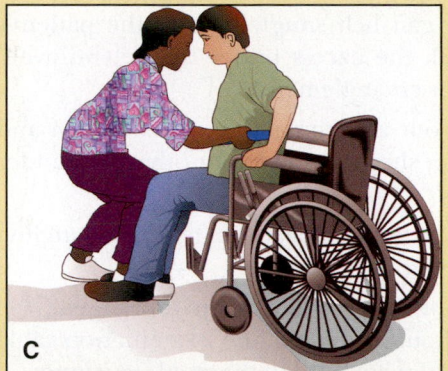

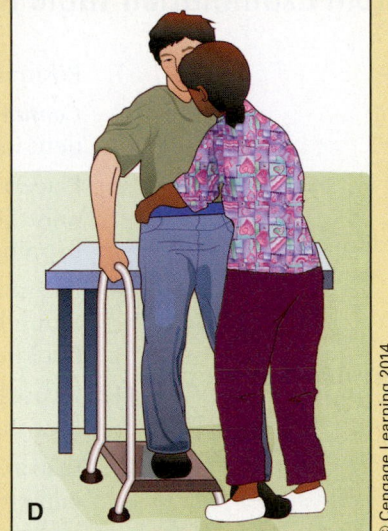

Figure 33-24 (continued) (C) Before lifting, observe proper body mechanics to avoid injuring yourself or the patient. (D) Check that the patient's foot is firmly placed on the stool before completing the transfer.

Figure 33-25 A two-person transfer is used when the patient does not have the upper body strength to help move himself or herself.

22. Instruct the patient to place one hand on the safety handle of the footstool and one hand on the examination table.

23. ***Considering any special patient needs,*** gently ease the patient onto the examination table.

24. Position the examination table as necessary.

25. Move the wheelchair and footstool out of the way.

Modification: Two-Person Transfer

1. Follow Steps 1 to 7 above.

2. Position one staff member in front of the patient and one on the patient's weakest side.

3. Both persons should grasp the gait belt from underneath.

4. Remind the patient and your assistant of your instructions and have the patient place his hands on the armrests of the wheelchair. At your signal, have your patient push on the armrests to assist in lifting himself to a standing position (Figure 33-25).

5. Upon your signal, coordinate the upward motion gripping the gait belt.

6. The person nearest the examination table should move the wheelchair out of the way.

7. The other person should assist the patient to pivot.

8. Have the patient grasp the handle of the footstool. Instruct and assist the patient to place the foot on his strongest side upon the footstool.

9. On your signal, both persons lift the patient onto the examination table.

10. ***Considering any special needs of the patient,*** position the patient on the examination table as necessary.

PROCEDURE 33-2
Transferring Patient from Examination Table to Wheelchair

STANDARD PRECAUTIONS:

PURPOSE:
To move a patient safely from the examination table to a wheelchair.

EQUIPMENT/SUPPLIES:
Safety handrail footstool with non-slip rubber tips
Gait belt

PROCEDURE STEPS:
1. Wash hands.
2. *Introduce yourself and identify patient.*
3. *Speaking at the level of the patient's understanding, explain the procedure.*
4. *Allay the patient's fears regarding the procedure being performed and help her to feel safe and comfortable.*
5. Position the wheelchair next to the examination table and lock the brakes. *NOTE:* Place the wheelchair so it is closest to the patient's stronger side so the patient can transfer weight onto the stronger foot as he or she gets down.
6. Park the wheelchair so that it is closest to the patient's strongest side. This will allow the transfer of weight onto the strongest leg when descending from the examination table.

7. Position the stool next to the wheelchair.
8. *Considering any special patient needs,* assist the patient into a sitting position.
9. Place the gait belt snugly around the patient's waist. Tuck the excess under the belt to avoid tripping or entanglement.
10. Position your arm under the patient's arm and around her shoulders and your other arm under her knees.
11. Pivot the patient so that her legs are dangling over the edge of the table.
12. Instruct the patient that upon your signal, the patient should push off the examination table and grasp the handrail of the stool for support.
13. Give the signal and pull the patient slightly toward you so that her feet land squarely on the footstool.
14. Still grasping the gait belt, instruct and then assist the patient to step to the floor with the strongest leg and pivot at the same time so that she is facing away from the wheelchair.
15. Instruct and assist the patient to swing her hands backwards and grasp the armrests of the wheelchair.
16. Bending from your knees and hips, gently lower the patient into the wheelchair controlling her rate of descent with the gait belt.
17. Assist her to attain comfort in the seated position.
18. Lower or replace the footrests. Assist the patient to comfortably place her feet on the footrests.

PROCEDURE 33-3
Assisting the Patient to Stand and Walk

STANDARD PRECAUTIONS:

PURPOSE:
To help a patient ambulate safely.

EQUIPMENT/SUPPLIES:
Gait belt

PROCEDURE STEPS:
1. Wash hands.
2. *Introduce yourself and identify patient.*
3. *Speaking at the level of the patient's understanding, explain the procedure.*

Procedure 33-3 (continued)

4. Lock the brakes on the wheelchair, if the patient is using one.

5. ***Considering any special patient needs,*** place the patient's feet on the floor and move the foot plates out of the way.

6. Instruct and/or assist the patient to slide forward to the edge of the wheelchair.

7. Place the gait belt snugly around the patient's waist. Tuck the excess under the belt to avoid tripping or entanglement.

8. Remembering the principles of good body mechanics, stand directly in front of the patient.

9. Bend at the hips and knees. Grasp the gait belt from underneath (Figure 33-26).

10. Have the patient place his hands on the armrests of the wheelchair. At your signal, have your patient push on the armrests to assist in lifting himself to a standing position.

11. Steady the patient momentarily and observe for strength, balance, and skin color. If there are any changes or as indicated by patient statements ('I'm dizzy'), carefully lower the patient to a sitting position in the wheelchair and check vital signs.

12. If the patient appears steady, stable, and is balanced, proceed by standing slightly behind and on the weakest side of the patient.

13. Grasp the gait belt with one hand and place the other hand on the patient's bent arm for support. *NOTE:* The gait belt is to be grasped with fingers under the belt, palm facing upwards, and elbow bent.

14. Indicate when you are ready to begin ambulation. Step forward with the same leg as the patient and remain in step.

15. Accurately document the procedure in the patient's chart or electronic medical record, including date, time, duration of ambulation, any gait disturbances, response of patient, and instructions given.

Modification: Two-Person Assist with Ambulation

1. Perform the preceding Steps 1 through 7.

2. Position a person on each side of the patient.

3. Utilizing good body mechanics, bending at hips and knees, grasp the gait belt from underneath with one hand and place the other hand on the patient's back for support.

4. During ambulation each person should remain on either side and slightly behind the patient (Figure 33-27).

5. Both people must retain a grip on the gait belt throughout the ambulation.

6. Accurately document in the patient's chart or electronic medical record indicating date, time, duration of ambulation, and any gait disturbances noted, response of patient, vital signs if taken, and patient education.

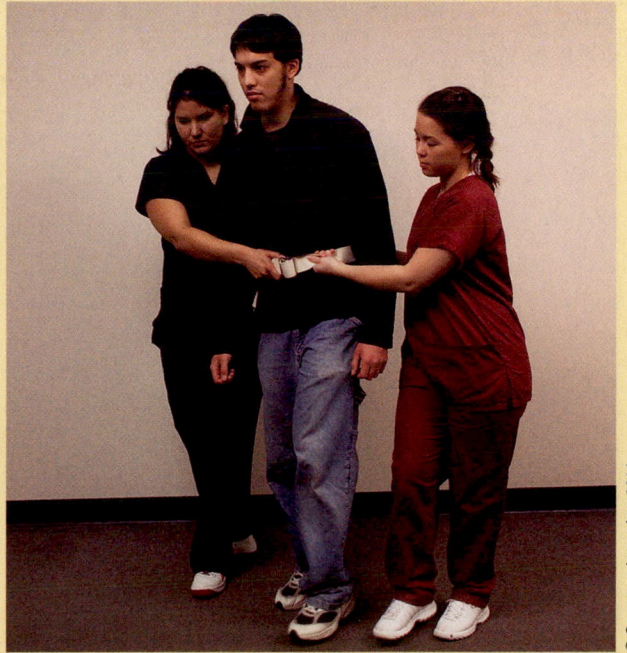

Figure 33-27 When two persons are assisting with ambulation, they should stand on either side of the patient.

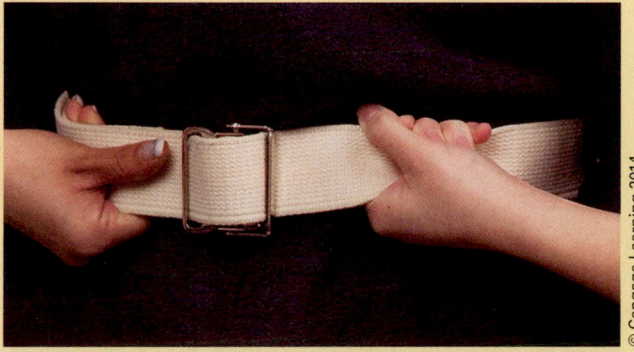

Figure 33-26 Firmly grasp the gait belt from underneath, with the palm up and elbow bent.

Procedure 33-3 (continued)

DOCUMENTATION:

7/14/20XX 2:30 PM   Patient states she has been doing "fairly well" in physical therapy. She says she walks short distances, about 10 feet. Assisted with ambulation. Seems steady on her feet. Says she feels "very good." S. Tyler, CMA (AAMA)——————————————

DOCUMENTATION:

7/14/20XX 2:30 PM   Patient has been to physical therapy a total of 15 times. Dr. Woo wants patient to ambulate to see her progress. Assisted patient to ambulate with another person assisting. Did very well. Walked about 100 feet. Color remained good. P 100. H. Casey, RMA (AMT)——————————

PROCEDURE 33-4
Care of the Falling Patient

PURPOSE:
To help the patient fall safely to prevent injury.

EQUIPMENT/SUPPLIES:
Gait belt (should already be on patient)

PROCEDURE STEPS:
1. Firmly grip the gait belt. Never grab clothing as it can shift and become unstable.

2. If the patient falls backwards, widen your stance to become a more stable base of support to accept the patient's weight(Figure 33-28).

3. Gently guide the patient to the floor, call for assistance, and assess vital signs.

4. If the patient falls to either side, attempt to assist the patient back to center of gravity by moving your foot in the direction of the fall.

5. Assess the patient to determine whether to terminate the ambulation session.

6. Call for assistance if needed.

7. Assess vital signs.

8. If the patient falls forward, provide support by utilizing a firm grip on the gait belt (Figure 33-29).

9. Gently lower patient to the floor.

10. Call for assistance.

11. Assess vital signs.

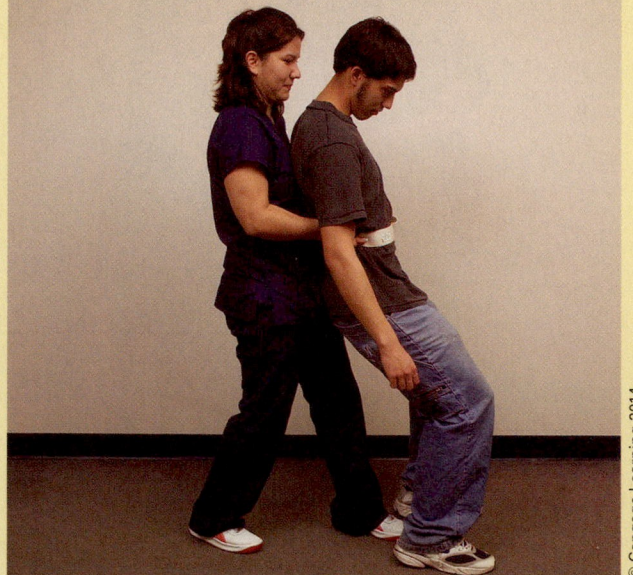

Figure 33-28   Support a falling patient with a wide base of support.

© Cengage Learning 2014

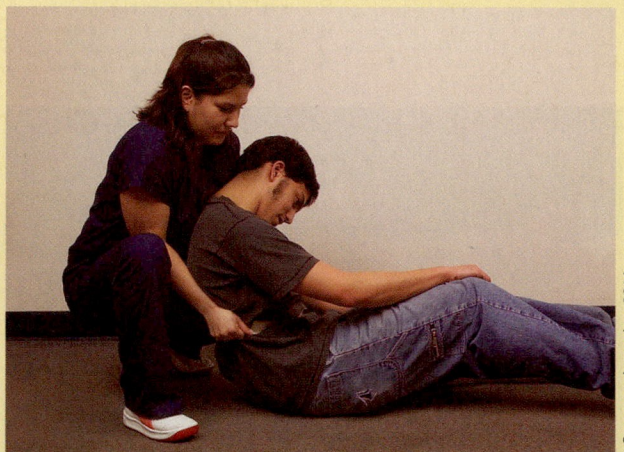

Figure 33-29   Ease the falling patient to the floor and try to protect the head.

© Cengage Learning 2014

Procedure 33-4 (continued)

12. Notify the provider of the need for assessment prior to moving patient.

13. Accurately document in the patient's chart or electronic medical record indicating date, time, factual description of the event, response of patient, vital signs if taken, and any injuries noted by provider.

14. Complete occurrence report if required.

DOCUMENTATION:

1/21/20XX 11:30 AM   While walking to exam room with assistance the patient suddenly began to fall forward with knees buckling. Says she feels "faint." Eased to the floor gently. Did not strike any body parts during fall. BP 110/60, P 108 (lying on floor). BP and pulse rechecked when patient placed in wheelchair. 11:35 am BP 120/78, P 92. Dr. King notified. H. Casey, RMA (AMT)

PROCEDURE 33-5

Assisting a Patient to Ambulate with a Walker

STANDARD PRECAUTIONS:

PURPOSE:

To allow a patient to ambulate independently and safely with a walker.

EQUIPMENT/SUPPLIES:

Walker
Gait belt

PROCEDURE STEPS:

1. Wash hands.

2. ***Introduce yourself and identify patient. Explain to the patient what you are going to do, speaking at the patient's level of understanding.***

3. Notify the provider of the need for assessment prior to moving patient.

4. Place the gait belt snugly around the patient's waist and tuck the excess belting under the belt to avoid tripping or entanglement.

5. Check the walker to be sure the rubber suction tips are secure on all legs.

6. Check the handles for rough and damaged edges that could injure the patient.

7. Assure that the walker is locked in the open position.

8. Check the height of the walker. The hand rests should be level with the patient's hip joint. When placing hands on the hand rest, the elbows should be bent at an approximately 30° angle.

9. Check the patient's footwear. It must be sturdy with a flat, non-slip sole.

10. Have the patient step into the walker and have her hold onto the hand rests.

11. Instruct the patient to keep the walker out in front of her as she begins to ambulate.

12. Position yourself behind and slightly to the side of the patient. (If one side is weaker, choose that side for your placement.)

13. Instruct the patient to lift the walker and place all four legs of the walker in front of herself. The back legs of the walker should be even with the patient's toes.

14. The patient should then lean forward placing hands on the hand rest. Have the patient utilize her arms to transfer some of the weight to the walker.

15. Have the patient step into the walker using the stronger leg, then the weaker leg. Ensure that the patient's stronger leg is within the embrace of the walker.

16. Steady the patient momentarily and observe for strength, balance, and skin color. If there are any changes, or as indicated by patient statements ('I'm dizzy'), rest and make a decision about continuing to ambulate.

17. If the walker has rollers, the patient simply rolls the walker ahead a comfortable distance, then walks

continues

Procedure 33-5 (continued)

into it. The patient can also walk normally with a rolling walker by simply rolling it in front and leaning into the gait, using the walker for support.

18. Accurately document in the patient's chart or electronic medical record indicating date, time, duration of ambulation, response of patient, vital signs if taken, and any injuries noted by provider.

DOCUMENTATION:

2/12/20XX 1:35 PM   Patient assisted with ambulation using a walker for the first time. Walked approximately 50 feet. Did well. Walked to reception desk and back. No change in color. P 100. S. Thomas, CMA (AAMA)————————

PROCEDURE 33-6

Teaching the Patient to Ambulate with Crutches

STANDARD PRECAUTIONS:

PURPOSE:
To teach the patient how to ambulate safely using crutches.

EQUIPMENT/SUPPLIES:
Crutches
Gait belt

PROCEDURE STEPS:

1. Wash hands.
2. *Introduce yourself and identify patient. Explain to the patient what you are going to do, speaking at the patient's level of understanding.*
3. Assemble the crutches and be sure they are in good working order.
4. Check the rubber, non-slip tips on the end of each crutch.
5. Check the bar and hand rest to be sure they are covered with padding. If the padding is cracked or worn, replace them.
6. Assure that the wing nuts are tightened appropriately.
7. Measure for crutches. Place tape in the axillary area. Measure from there to a spot 2 inches before and 6 inches to the side of the foot. Adjust crutches to this measurement.
8. Place the gait belt snugly around the patient's waist and tuck the excess belting under the belt to avoid tripping or entanglement.
9. *Speaking at the level of the patient's understanding,* instruct the patient to bear the weight of the body using the hands on the hand rests. Do not bear weight on the axillary area.
10. Place both crutches at a comfortable distance in front of the patient's feet.
11. Stand tall, looking forward rather than down at your feet.
12. Move the affected leg up even with crutches.
13. Transfer weight via the hands onto the crutches.
14. Repeat the same sequence for the next step.
15. Accurately document in the patient's chart or electronic medical record indicating date, time, duration of ambulation, patient instruction, response of patient, vital signs if taken.

DOCUMENTATION:

3/24/20XX 4:45 PM   Crutches adjusted to patient's height. Three-point gait used. Tolerated well. S. Tyler, CMA (AAMA)————————————

PROCEDURE 33-7

Assisting a Patient to Ambulate with a Cane

STANDARD PRECAUTIONS:

PURPOSE:

To teach patients how to walk safely with a cane.

EQUIPMENT/SUPPLIES:

Appropriate cane for patient
Gait belt

PROCEDURE STEPS:

1. Wash hands.

2. *Introduce yourself and identify patient.*

3. Select the appropriate cane per the providers orders.

4. Examine the tip of the cane to assure that the rubber is not worn. If a quad cane or walk cane is to be used, be sure that all legs have rubber tips.

5. Assemble cane and gait belt.

6. Place the gait belt snugly around the patient's waist and tuck the excess belting under the belt to avoid tripping or entanglement.

7. Place the cane relatively close to the body to the side of the foot of the strong leg (Figure 33-30).

8. Adjust the cane so that the handle is level with the hip joint.

9. During weight bearing, the patient's elbow should be flexed 20 to 30°.

10. The cane and the involved leg are advanced simultaneously.

11. Have the patient move the weak leg forward while transferring the weight to the cane.

12. Have the patient step forward with the unaffected leg past the cane.

13. Repeat the procedure for the next step.

14. Support the patient by grasping the gait belt in the back while standing slightly behind the patient.

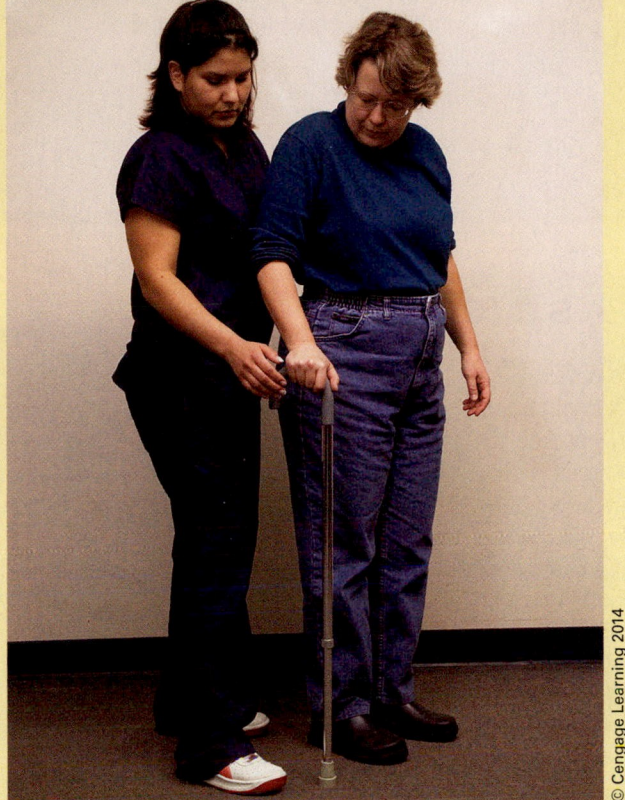

Figure 33-30 When placing the cane, be sure the handle comes to the top of the patient's hip and elbow is flexed 20 to 30 degrees.

© Cengage Learning 2014

15. Follow along behind and on the patient's affected side.

16. Wash hands.

17. Accurately document in the patient's chart or electronic medical record indicating date, time, duration of ambulation, patient instruction, response of patient, vital signs if taken.

DOCUMENTATION:

4/17/20XX 10:30 AM Standard cane adjusted to patient's hip joint. Ambulated about 100 yards and seemed to tolerate it well. S. Tyler, CMA (AAMA)

CASE STUDY 33-1

Refer to the scenario at the beginning of the chapter.

Mrs. Williams comes to Inner City Health Care because she fell when she tripped on a scatter rug at home. Her son helped her to the clinic. Her left ankle is swollen and painful.

CASE STUDY REVIEW

1. What action(s) should you take immediately to help Mrs. Williams?
2. After X-rays, Dr. King determined that Mrs. Williams has an ankle fracture, and he applied a cast to it. He wants you to fit Mrs. Williams to crutches and teach her how to use them. What gait will Dr. Cox have you teach the patient? Why?

CASE STUDY 33-2

It is a mild summer afternoon in River City, the home of Inner City Health Care. The softball season is in full swing, and Inner City has treated its share of players and spectators who have had minor injuries. On this particular Tuesday, Bill Schwarz, a regular patient, comes in late in the day in obvious pain. Sam Tyler, the clinical medical assistant on duty, quickly gets the patient into a wheelchair. From the patient's description of the situation and the pain, Sam suspects a sprained ankle. Dr. Woo is on call and is available to examine the patient immediately. Dr. Woo asks Sam to transfer Bill from the wheelchair to the examination table.

CASE STUDY REVIEW

1. What are some of the general principles the medical assistant should observe during any transfer?
2. Summarize the steps involved in transferring the patient from the wheelchair to the examination table.
3. What are possible treatment choices Dr. Woo may use?

CASE STUDY 33-3

After diagnosing Mr. Schwarz with a sprained left ankle, Dr. Woo has prescribed an Ace bandage to the ankle, crutches, and an ice pack to be applied to the ankle. He has also given Mr. Schwarz a prescription for pain relievers and has recommended that Mr. Schwarz stay off his feet as much as possible. He is to keep the leg elevated with an ice pack on it.

CASE STUDY REVIEW

1. Explain what you would tell Mr. Schwarz about applying the ice pack to his ankle at home.
2. What patient education can be used in this situation?

SUMMARY

Rehabilitation medicine is a field of medical disciplines that specializes in both preventing disease or injury and restoring physical function. It uses a combination of physical and mechanical agents to aid in the diagnosis, treatment, and prevention of diseases or bodily injury, including exercise and a variety of treatment modalities.

Much of what a medical assistant might do on the job in this field involves some form of lifting or moving of heavy objects. It is important to remember to use good body mechanics to prevent back or other injury. When transferring patients, good body mechanics ensures the safety of both caregiver and patient. If necessary, get someone to help with the transfer.

Helping patients to ambulate safely after a period of sedentary recuperation is an important part of a rehabilitation program. If they are not able to ambulate on their own, patients can be fitted for a variety of assistive walking devices, including walkers, crutches, and canes. Crutch walking, by far the most common use of an assistive device, can be done using one of several walking patterns, or gaits, depending on the patient's condition, strength, and stability. Whatever assistive device is used, it is important that the patient be measured correctly for that device and taught how to periodically check it for safety.

In addition to ambulation, there are a number of other types of therapeutic exercises. Depending on the patient's condition, an exercise program can be prescribed after evaluating the patient's joint ROM and muscle strength. Joints and muscles must be exercised regularly to prevent muscle atrophy or joint contractures, as well as to improve circulation and maintain or improve overall health. ROM and other exercises can be performed by the caregiver, the patient, or a combination of the two.

In addition to exercise, a variety of therapeutic modalities might be used as part of the patient's rehabilitation program. The various properties of heat, cold, light, electricity, and water act on the body to improve circulation, minimize pain, or correct or alleviate joint and muscle malfunction. Heat dilates the blood vessels, thereby increasing circulation to an area and speeding up the repair process. Cold constricts the blood vessels, slowing circulation and therefore the inflammatory process. Ultrasound and other electrical **diathermies** use an electrical current to create heat in the deeper tissues of the body. It is important to understand how each modality affects the physiologic functioning of the body and to observe certain safety precautions to avoid injuring the patient.

STUDY FOR SUCCESS

To reinforce your knowledge and skills of information presented in this chapter:

- Review the *Key Terms*

- Role-play with other students to apply attributes of professionalism pertinent to this chapter.

- Consider the *Case Studies,* and discuss your conclusions

- Answer the questions in the *Certification Review*

- Apply your knowledge by completing the *Activities* in the *Study Guide* and the *Games and Quizzes* in the StudyWARE *StudyWARE* software on the *Premium Website*

- Perform the *Procedures* using the *Competency Assessment Checklists* in the *Competency Manual*

- Practice your problem-solving skills with the *Critical Thinking Challenge 3.0* on the *Premium Website*

Additional resources for this chapter include:

- Module 27 of the *Medical Assisting Learning Lab*

- *CourseMate for Delmar's Comprehensive Medical Assisting*

- *WebTutor for Delmar's Comprehensive Medical Assisting*

CERTIFICATION REVIEW

1. Brushing teeth, getting dressed, and eating are referred to as:
   a. rehabilitation medicine
   b. activities of daily living
   c. assistive behaviors
   d. occupational therapy

2. Hemiplegia is defined as:
   a. inability of the patient to ambulate properly
   b. severe back pain
   c. paralysis of one side of the body
   d. confinement to a wheelchair

3. Ambulatory assistive devices include:
   a. gait belts
   b. walkers, canes, and crutches
   c. wheelchairs
   d. stools with handholds
4. Motion away from the midline of the body is called:
   a. adduction
   b. pronation
   c. extension
   d. abduction
5. Supination involves:
   a. placing the patient in the supine position
   b. moving the arm so the palm is up
   c. bending a body part
   d. straightening a body part
6. The use of a gait belt serves which function(s)?
   a. Assists in fall prevention
   b. Protects staff from accidental back injury
   c. Teaching patients proper gait
   d. Both a and b
7. The purpose of electrostimulation of a muscle is:
   a. stimulation of the sensory and motor nerves in a muscle
   b. preventing atrophy
   c. restoring muscle function
   d. all of the above

8. Massage therapy is sometimes utilized in combination with physical therapy. The benefits include:
   a. increased circulation
   b. healing of bones
   c. walker training
   d. none of the above
9. To provide maximum assistance for a person with mobility problems, the most appropriate assistive device is:
   a. a cane
   b. crutches
   c. a walker
   d. none of the above
10. Which of the following is **not** an effect of ultrasound as a therapeutic modality?
   a. Provides heat to deeper tissues
   b. Decreases circulation
   c. Assists with management of chronic pain
   d. Decreases muscle spasms

REFERENCES/BIBLIOGRAPHY

Beck, F. (2006). *Theory and practice of therapeutic massage* (4th ed.). Clifton Park, NY: Delmar Cengage Learning.

Hegner, B., & Caldwell, E. (2008). *Nursing assistant: A nursing process approach* (10th ed.). Clifton Park, NY: Delmar Cengage Learning.

O'Sullivan, S. B., & Schmitz, T. (2000). *Physical rehabilitation: Assessment and treatment* (4th ed.). Philadelphia: F. A. Davis.

Taber's cyclopedic medical dictionary. (22nd ed.). (2003). Philadelphia: F. A. Davis.

Weiss, R. C. (1999). *The physical therapy aide: A work text.* Clifton Park, NY: Delmar Cengage Learning.

CHAPTER 34

Nutrition in Health and Disease

OUTLINE

Nutrition and Digestion

Types of Nutrients

Energy Nutrients (Organic)

Other Nutrients (Inorganic)

Reading Food Labels

Items on the Nutrition Label

Comparing Labels

Nutrition at Various Stages of Life

Pregnancy and Lactation

Breast-Feeding

Infancy

Childhood

Adolescence

Older Adults

Therapeutic Diets

Weight Control

Diabetes Mellitus

Cardiovascular Disease

Cancer

Diet and Culture

LEARNING OUTCOMES

1. Define, spell, and pronounce the key terms as presented in the glossary.
2. Describe the relation of nutrition to the functioning of the digestive system.
3. Identify the seven basic nutrient types.
4. Explain the relationship and balance among the three energy nutrients.
5. Distinguish between water-soluble and fat-soluble vitamins.
6. Discuss herbal supplements.

7. Explain the reason for nutrition labels on food packaging.
8. Read and interpret nutrition facts and ingredients on three food packages.
9. Discuss various therapeutic diets, and explain how each can help to control a particular disease state or accommodate a change in the life cycle.
10. Analyze the professionalism questions and apply them to this chapter's content.

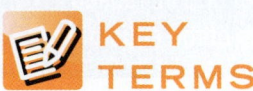

KEY TERMS

amino acid
antioxidant
ascorbic acid
basal metabolic rate (BMR)
beriberi
bulimia
cachectic
calorie
carotene
catalyst
cellulose
cheilosis
cholecalciferol
cobalamin
coenzyme
digestion
diuretic
electrolytes
extracellular
fat-soluble
folic acid
glycogen
homeostasis
macrobiotic
major mineral
metabolism
niacin
nutrient
nutrition
oxidation
preservative
processed food

pyridoxine
riboflavin
saturated fat

scurvy
thiamin
tocopherol

trace mineral
water-soluble
xerophthalmia

ATTRIBUTES OF PROFESSIONALISM

Communication

- Did you introduce yourself? Did you identify the patient through name and birth date or other identifying feature?
- Did you listen to and acknowledge the patient?
- Did you speak at the patient's level of understanding?
- Did you respond honestly and diplomatically to the patient's concerns?
- Did you refrain from sharing your personal experiences?
- Did you include the patient's support system as indicated?

Presentation

- Did your actions attend to both the psychological and the physiological aspects of the patient's illness or condition?
- Were you courteous, patient, and respectful to the patient?
- Did you display a positive attitude?
- Did you display a calm, professional, and caring manner?

Competency

- Were you knowledgeable and accountable?

Initiative

- Did you direct the patient to other resources when necessary or helpful, with the approval of the provider?

Integrity

- Were you respectful of others?
- Did you demonstrate respect for individual diversity?

SCENARIO

Becky Slack, RMA (AMT) works with Dr. Hannah, a pediatrician in a small rural setting. She initiated a discussion with Dr. Hannah about the recent increase in childhood obesity. Knowing that the percentage of children aged 6–11 years in the United States who were obese increased from 7% in 1980 to nearly 20% in 2008, and realizing the impact on their patient population, Ms. Slack wanted to know what solutions the practice might offer to these patients and their families. Dr. Hannah has agreed to collaborate with Ms. Slack to begin a nutritional education class that will be held at the clinic once a week. This class will include children and their parents who are concerned about weight. As treatment includes changes in diet and increased physical activity, this will be the focus of the education.

INTRODUCTION

The human body is in a constant state of fluctuation. The outside environment is constantly changing, and the body requires homeostasis, *or a continual internal environment, which, in turn, gives us a requirement for nutrients. The nutrients we take into our bodies replenish the materials we have used. In this way, homeostasis is maintained, and our bodies have a relatively balanced internal environment.* Nutrition *is the study of the taking of nutrients into the body and how the body uses them.*

The normal healthy individual will consume and use close to what the body needs to stay healthy. However, some individuals either do not consume enough nutrients or consume too much of a particular type of nutrient. These are poor diets that can cause particular disease states, and these diets must be modified to return the patients to good health. In addition, specific disease states, such as diabetes mellitus, warrant a change from a normal diet to control the progress of the disease. The human body also goes through many changes in a lifetime and with these changes come new nutritional needs. Protecting health requires paying attention to strategies to prevent disease. The choices made regarding foods consumed and the quality of nutritional intake have a significant impact on the quality and longevity of life. Healthy food choices contribute to living longer and preventing major health issues.

This chapter explores the balance of nutrients required for good health and examines therapeutic modifications to the diet that should take place at various life stages or in the presence of disease. The astute medical assistant will recognize the role of nutrition in maintaining health and will use a knowledge of nutritional principles to encourage patients to adopt a healthy lifestyle.

NUTRITION AND DIGESTION

Nutrition includes ingestion, digestion, absorption, and metabolism of food. Good nutrition results in longer life spans and healthier individuals

SPOTLIGHT ON CERTIFICATION

RMA Content Outline
- Disorders and diseases
- Medical terminology
- Human relations
- Patient education

CMA (AAMA) Content Outline
- Medical terminology
- Medicolegal guidelines and requirements
- Patient preparation and assisting the physician
- Nutrition

CMAS Content Outline
- Medical terminology
- Anatomy and physiology

through the control of preventable diseases. The food eaten by an individual is used to build and repair cells and tissues of the body. Therefore, it is important to have knowledge and information about nutrition and to make appropriate food choices for optimum health. A well-nourished individual is less susceptible to infection and disease.  Patient education is important especially when the normal diet must be modified to treat the patient's illness. The medical assistant can answer patient questions only through a knowledge of both good nutrition and what constitutes the therapeutic diets prescribed by the provider.

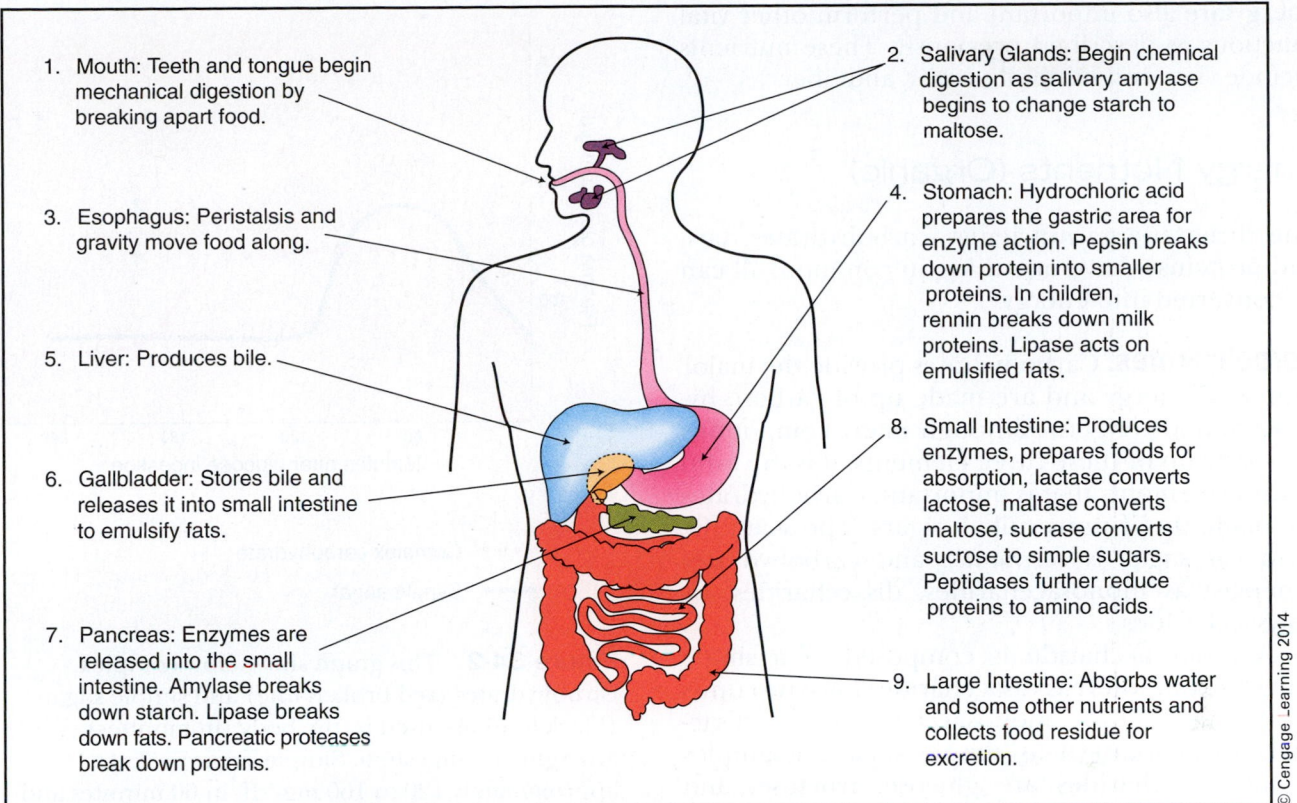

1. Mouth: Teeth and tongue begin mechanical digestion by breaking apart food.

2. Salivary Glands: Begin chemical digestion as salivary amylase begins to change starch to maltose.

3. Esophagus: Peristalsis and gravity move food along.

4. Stomach: Hydrochloric acid prepares the gastric area for enzyme action. Pepsin breaks down protein into smaller proteins. In children, rennin breaks down milk proteins. Lipase acts on emulsified fats.

5. Liver: Produces bile.

6. Gallbladder: Stores bile and releases it into small intestine to emulsify fats.

8. Small Intestine: Produces enzymes, prepares foods for absorption, lactase converts lactase, maltase converts maltose, sucrase converts sucrose to simple sugars. Peptidases further reduce proteins to amino acids.

7. Pancreas: Enzymes are released into the small intestine. Amylase breaks down starch. Lipase breaks down fats. Pancreatic proteases break down proteins.

9. Large Intestine: Absorbs water and some other nutrients and collects food residue for excretion.

© Cengage Learning 2014

Figure 34-1   The digestive system.

Digestion involves the physical and chemical changes to food that the body makes to make it absorbable. Absorption is the transfer of the nutrients from the gastrointestinal tract into the bloodstream. Without absorption, the body would not receive the nutrients. Figure 34-1 shows the digestive system and its basic functions.

TYPES OF NUTRIENTS

Nutrients serve many purposes in the body. Some nutrients provide energy for the body to perform activities such as the pumping of the heart, the division of cells, or the contraction of muscles. Nutrients also provide building blocks so that proteins or phospholipids can be made within the body, or they can act as catalysts to help processes such as the clotting mechanism proceed at a faster rate. Essentially, ingested substances that help the body stay in its homeostatic state can be called **nutrients**.

Nutrients can be divided into two groups: those that provide energy and those that do not. Both groups are necessary for good health. Table 34-1 lists examples of each of these two groups. Those that provide energy are composed of three types: carbohydrates, fats (lipids), and proteins. Each of

these three substances is used in ways other than making energy, but it is important to remember that these are the only substances from which the body can derive energy. Nutrients that do not provide

Table 34-1   Types of Nutrients

Energy Nutrients (Organic)	Function
Carbohydrates (CHO)	Provide energy
Fats (lipids)	Provide energy
Proteins	Build and repair tissues
Other Nutrients	**Function**
Vitamins	Regulate body processes
Minerals	Regulate body processes
Water	Regulate body processes
Fiber	Regulate body processes

© Cengage Learning 2014

energy are also important and perform other vital functions as described previously. These nutrients include vitamins, minerals, water, and fiber.

Energy Nutrients (Organic)

The three energy nutrients—carbohydrates, fats, and proteins—have one thing in common: all can be converted into energy.

Carbohydrates. Carbohydrates provide the major source of energy and are made up of carbon, hydrogen, and oxygen. Although many compounds are made up of these three elements, it is the ratio of these elements that is important. Carbohydrates are made up of units called sugars. The scientific term for sugar is *saccharide,* and carbohydrates can exist as monosaccharides, disaccharides, or polysaccharides.

A monosaccharide is composed of a single unit of sugar, whereas disaccharides have two units of sugar. Together, monosaccharides and disaccharides are known as simple sugars. Examples of monosaccharides are glucose, fructose, and galactose. Glucose is the sugar that the body uses most efficiently, thus most ingested sugar is broken down in the intestines and converted to glucose in the liver. Fructose is found largely in fruits, whereas galactose is a product of lactose digestion. Examples of disaccharides are lactose, maltose, and sucrose. Lactose is found primarily in milk or milk products. Maltose is a product of starch breakdown. Sucrose is one of the sweetest sugars and is what we commonly refer to as table sugar. It occurs naturally in many fruits and vegetables, as well as sugar cane and the sugar beet, which are commercial sources of refined sugar.

Polysaccharides are also known as complex carbohydrates. They are made up of many units of sugar connected together. The most common polysaccharides are starches, glycogen, and fiber. Starches are the most important dietary complex carbohydrate. **Glycogen** is only ingested in small quantities, but is an important carbohydrate form for storage of glucose in the body. Fiber is a special polysaccharide because it cannot be digested.

Because the simple sugars are composed of only one or two units of sugar, their digestion takes little time, and absorption occurs soon after ingestion. The body initially experiences a large increase in sugar concentration in the blood, which is brought down to within a normal range by the release of insulin. The complex carbohydrates require more time to digest, and as a result there is

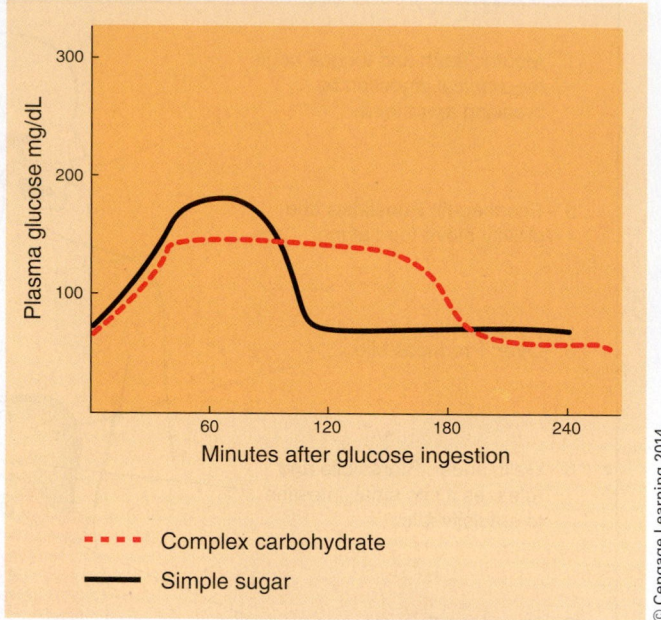

Figure 34-2 This graph shows how complex carbohydrates (red broken line) and simple sugar (black line) are used by the body (in minutes) after glucose ingestion. Simple sugar peaks to approximately 120 to 160 mg/dL in 60 minutes and returns to a normal level within 120 minutes. Complex carbohydrates (red broken line) never increase to more than approximately 130 to 140 mg/dL during a 60-minute period; that level is maintained for the next 180 minutes and then returns to normal.

a slow absorption of the single-carbohydrate units as the larger starch molecule is broken down. This is demonstrated in Figure 34-2. In this case, there would be a moderate increase in the sugar levels in the blood, and this would continue for a longer period. A continuous level of sugar in the bloodstream is necessary for a constant energy supply. The principle sources of carbohydrates are fruits, vegetables, cereal grains, and sugar. It is important to limit the amount of added sugar as an additional source of carbohydrates. One gram of carbohydrate contains 4 calories.

Fats. Fats, also called lipids, are also composed of carbon, hydrogen, and oxygen, but in a ratio different from carbohydrates. They exist as triglycerides in the body. A triglyceride has three fatty acids attached to a glycerol molecule (Figure 34-3). The fatty acid component of a triglyceride has several important characteristics. The first is whether it is essential to the diet. The only true essential fatty acid in the human diet is linoleic acid, and all

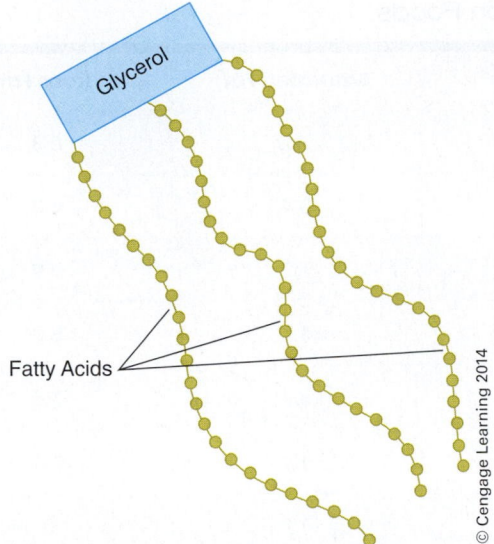

Figure 34-3   A triglyceride has three fatty acids attached to a glycerol molecule.

other fatty acids the body requires can be derived from this. Another important characteristic of fatty acids is saturation. When a fatty acid is saturated, every carbon molecule on the fatty acid holds as many hydrogens as possible. If it does not hold all the hydrogens possible, it is called unsaturated. The more unsaturated the fatty acid, the more liquid the fat. For example, lard has saturated fatty acids and a thick consistency compared with corn oil, which has relatively unsaturated fatty acids and a thin consistency. If an unsaturated fat is hydrogenated, combined with hydrogen, it becomes more saturated. **Saturated fats** are more common in foods from animal sources than from plant sources. Generally, saturated fatty acids tend to increase the level of fats and cholesterol in the blood. It is important to know that fats contain the most condensed caloric values. One gram of fat contains nine calories.

Trans unsaturated fatty acids (trans fats) are unhealthy fats because they increase low-density lipoproteins (LDL), bad cholesterol, and decrease high-density lipoproteins (HDL), good cholesterol.

Trans fats are produced by a process known as hydrogenation. Vegetable oil (liquid) is heated and hydrogen is added to it. This makes the product solid at room temperature. It gives certain foods a longer shelf life (stay fresh longer) and a better taste. The process, however, turns healthy fat (vegetable oil) into unhealthy fat, trans fats.

Trans fats are found in meat and dairy products, as well as in stick margarine, solid shortening, and many commercially prepared foods. Foods that are considered convenience foods such as snacks, potato chips, cookies, crackers, and cakes are high in trans fats. Margarine, fast foods, cereal, doughnuts, and French fries are also examples. Experts recommend that the daily amount of trans fats be as close to zero as possible. The FDA requires that all food packaging labels show the amount of trans fats per serving in the product. Table 34-2 lists some common foods and their grams of total fat and trans fat per serving.

Proteins. Although protein is also composed of carbon, hydrogen, and oxygen, it contains one more important element: nitrogen. The basic structural unit of protein is the **amino acid**. There are 22 amino acids in proteins. Eight of these are needed in the diet for the body to function normally. One more, histidine, is essential only during childhood. The rest of the amino acids can be synthesized from the eight, provided that they are present in adequate quantities. A complete

PATIENT EDUCATION

Trans Unsaturated Fatty Acids

- Use a margarine that is soft at room temperature; it is lower in trans fat. Some margarines are available that are entirely trans fat free.
- Olive oil is a wise choice for salads and for dipping bread, and butter is a better option than margarine.
- Olive oil and canola oil are best for sautéing and frying.

- Make foods from scratch to avoid trans fats. Foods such as breads, dips, salad dressings, cereals, and soups can be made without hydrogenated fats.

If a food label lists hydrogenated oil or shortening as one of its main ingredients (usually one of the first listed ingredients), it has a large amount of trans fats in it. Avoid the product altogether, or eat only small amounts.

Table 34-2 Grams of Fat per Serving of Some Common Foods

Product	Serving Size	Total Fat	Saturated Fat	Trans Fat
Butter	1 tbsp	10.8	7.2	0.3
Cake (pound)	1 slice	16.4	3.4	4.3
Cookies (filled with cream)	3	6.1	1.2	1.9
Doughnut	1	18.2	4.7	5.0
French fries (fast food)	Medium	26.9	6.7	7.8
Granola bar	1 bar	7.1	4.4	0.4
Ground beef (75% lean)	4 oz.	28	12	0
Margarine (stick)	1 tbsp	11.0	2.1	2.8
Margarine (tub container)	1 tbsp	6.7	1.2	0.6
Mayonnaise	1 tbsp	10.8	1.6	0.0
Milk (whole)	1 cup	6.6	4.3	0.2
Peanut Butter	1 oz.	14	3	0
Potato chips	Small bag	11.2	1.9	3.2
Ramen noodle soup	42 g	7.2	3.2	0.9
Shortening (solid)	1 tbsp	13.0	3.4	4.2
Wheat crackers	50 g	10.0	2.0	4.0
Yogurt (low fat)	1 cup	4	2	0

Source: Food and Drug Administration Center for Food Safety and Applied Nutrition; U.S. Department of Agriculture National Nutritional Database.

protein is so named because it has all eight of the essential amino acids. An incomplete protein does not contain all of these. The best sources for complete proteins are meats and animal products such as milk and eggs. Most plants provide only incomplete proteins and must be combined with complementary incomplete proteins to obtain all eight amino acids (Figure 34-4).

Although protein is described as an energy nutrient, its main function is not to provide energy but to provide amino acids to be used as building components of body proteins, which can be used as enzymes, hormones, and as the basic structural unit in all body

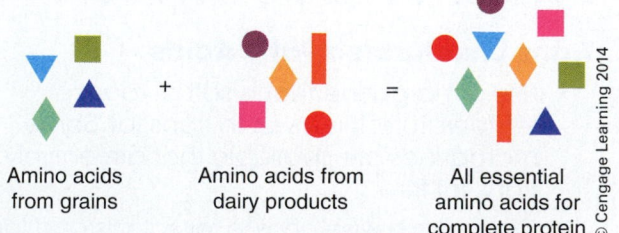

Amino acids from grains + Amino acids from dairy products = All essential amino acids for complete protein

© Cengage Learning 2014

Figure 34-4 Some foods, such as grains and dairy products, may not have all the essential amino acids when considered separately. Combined, however, these form a complete protein and therefore are considered complementary.

tissues and cells. The body uses carbohydrates and fats as its primary energy sources; however, when these are in short supply, the body diverts its use of protein for structural purposes to use it as an energy source. This has detrimental effects on the body.

Protein contains 4 calories per gram.

Deficiencies in protein usually occur together with deficiencies in total calories. Foods high in protein are more expensive than those high in carbohydrates and fats. This leads to dietary choices that are based on economics for some families. Failure to thrive is caused by a lack of protein in infants and young children.

Energy Balance. Although all of the energy nutrients are capable of supplying energy to the body, they do so in different ways and in varying amounts. The amount of energy that a substance is able to supply can be measured in large **calories**. Nutrition is discussed in terms of the large calorie, which is always capitalized to distinguish it from the small calorie. The large calorie (abbreviation: C or Cal) is also expressed as a kilocalorie (abbreviation: kcal). One thousand small calories equal one large calorie or one kilocalorie.

Carbohydrates and proteins both give four calories for each respective gram. So, if 10 g pure carbohydrate were ingested, it would yield 40 calories.

$$\frac{10 \text{ g}}{\text{carbohydrate}} \times \frac{4 \text{ calories}}{1 \text{ gram of carbohydrate}} = 40 \text{ calories}$$

Similarly, if 10 g protein were used for energy, it would yield 40 calories.

$$\frac{10 \text{ g}}{\text{protein}} \times \frac{4 \text{ calories}}{1 \text{ gram of protein}} = 40 \text{ calories}$$

Fats, in comparison, yield nine calories for every gram of fat. Fats, therefore, are a more energy-rich food source than carbohydrates or proteins because they give more calories for every gram used. If 10 g fat were used, it would yield 90 calories.

$$\frac{10 \text{ g}}{\text{fat}} \times \frac{9 \text{ calories}}{1 \text{ gram of fat}} = 90 \text{ calories}$$

The total of all changes, chemical and physical, that take place in the body is called **metabolism**. The metabolic rate concerns itself with the changes in the body with respect to energy. It is the balance between the energy that is brought into the body and the energy used by the body. Energy is used during every action of the body, including voluntary activities such as walking or riding a bicycle and involuntary activities such as breathing and cellular repair.

The level of energy required for activities that occur when the body is at rest is called basal metabolism. The **basal metabolic rate (BMR)** varies according to several factors. For example, the BMR is higher in individuals with leaner body mass (muscle) because more energy is needed to fuel the muscles than to store fat. BMR also is higher in individuals during periods of high growth rate, such as in children and pregnant women.

Ideally, an individual will take in as many calories as the body will use each day. When a person takes in more calories than will be used, the body will store the excess energy in the form of fat. When a person uses more energy than is brought into the body, the body breaks down these stores. When the stores of fat are depleted, the body will start to break down its protein structures.

For an optimal energy balance in the body, the largest percentage of calories in the diet should come from carbohydrates. Ideally, the percentage should be 45% to 65% of total calories consumed. The percentage of calories attributable to fat should not be greater than 35%, with a percentage closer to 20% being preferred. Proteins should make up 10% to 35% of calories in the diet.

Take note that these values are the percentage of the total calories derived from each energy nutrient—not the percentage of grams. This distinction is important because of the difference in calories derived from each energy nutrient. Figure 34-5 gives an example of these calculations. Note the percentages of fat, carbohydrate, and protein found in the "mystery" food. All fall outside of the recommended percentages for each.

In many cultures outside of the United States, rice, bread, and noodles are the basis of the diet. In the United States, we have available great amounts of food from the dairy and meat groups. Unfortunately, dairy products and meats, although containing many good nutrients, also contain a great deal of fat. Studies have shown that many Americans are obese (defined as their weight being at least 20% greater than what their ideal weight should be). The U.S. diet is too high in fat, has too many calories, has too much salt and cholesterol, and has insufficient amounts of complex carbohydrates and fiber. As a result, many illnesses and diseases occur, such as heart disease, high blood pressure, diabetes, and cancer.

Because obesity in the United States has become such a serious problem, there has been much interest in modifying the Food Guide Pyramid developed by the U.S. Department of Agriculture for maintaining ideal weight. Health experts believe that the emphasis on 6 to 11 daily

Label for Mystery Food:	Amount Per Serving
Calories	149
Total Fat	9g
Total Carbohydrate	14g
Total Protein	3g

The first calculation to make is one that converts grams to calories.

$$9 \text{ grams of fat} \times \frac{9 \text{ calories}}{\text{gram}} = 81 \text{ calories due to fat}$$

$$14 \text{ grams of carbohydrate} \times \frac{4 \text{ calories}}{\text{gram}} = 56 \text{ calories due to carbohydrate}$$

$$3 \text{ grams of protein} \times \frac{4 \text{ calories}}{\text{gram}} = 12 \text{ calories due to protein}$$

The next calculation is to find the percentage of total calories due to each of the energy nutrients.

$$\frac{81 \text{ calories due to fat}}{149 \text{ total calories}} = 54\%$$

$$\frac{56 \text{ calories due to carbohydrate}}{149 \text{ total calories}} = 38\%$$

$$\frac{12 \text{ calories due to protein}}{149 \text{ total calories}} = 8\%$$

© Cengage Learning 2014

Figure 34-5 Calculations of percentages of total calories from fat, carbohydrate, and protein.

servings from the bread, cereal, rice, and pasta groups (carbohydrates) is a contributing factor to obesity. Ongoing studies and research has led to redesign of the pyramid with less emphasis on the carbohydrate group and more emphasis placed on the fruits, vegetables, whole grains, legumes, and nuts. This research was instrumental in developing the MyPlate Food Guidance System (Figure 34-6).

The new food guide has specific information about portions and calories. It can help individuals get individualized nutrition and exercise advice.

Each color on the MyPlate guide represents a food group:

- *Orange* represents grains, which are divided into two groups: whole grains and refined grains. The recommendation is to eat 5 to 8 ounces of grain per day, half of which should be from whole grain breads, pasta, rice, cereal, or crackers.

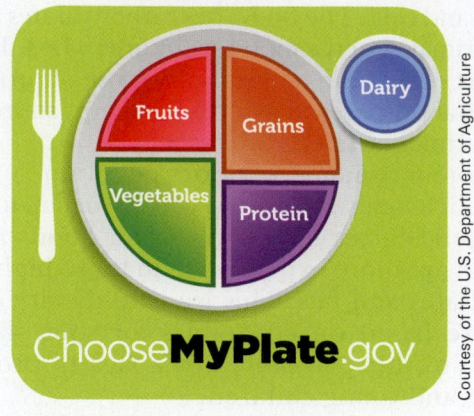

Courtesy of the U.S. Department of Agriculture

Figure 34-6 MyPlate is the "new generation" food icon to prompt consumers to think differently about their food choices.

- *Green* represents vegetables. For a low calorie per day intake, 2½ cups of vegetables should come from all five vegetable groups several times a week.
- *Red* represents fruits. 1½ to 2 cups daily is the recommended intake.
- *Blue* represents dairy products. Three cups per day of fat-free or low-fat milk or milk products is recommended.
- *Purple* represents protein. The recommendation is to eat 5 to 6½ ounces of protein per day, choosing from lean meat, poultry, fish, eggs, processed soy products, beans, nuts, seeds, and peas.

The new government Web site (http://www.choosemyplate.gov) allows individuals to input their age, gender, and activity level. By doing so, they get a recommendation about their personal daily calorie intake and physical activity level (Figure 34-7). Download the ChooseMyPlate.gov brochure at http://www.choosemyplate.gov/print-materials-ordering/dietary-guidelines.html.

Other Nutrients (Inorganic)

Many other nutrients are essential to maintaining good health. Although they do not provide the body with energy, they perform a variety of necessary functions. They include vitamins, antioxidants, herbal supplements, minerals, water, and fiber.

Vitamins. Vitamins are a class of nutrients in which each specific vitamin has a function entirely its own. They are complex molecules and are required by the body in minute quantities. Vitamins

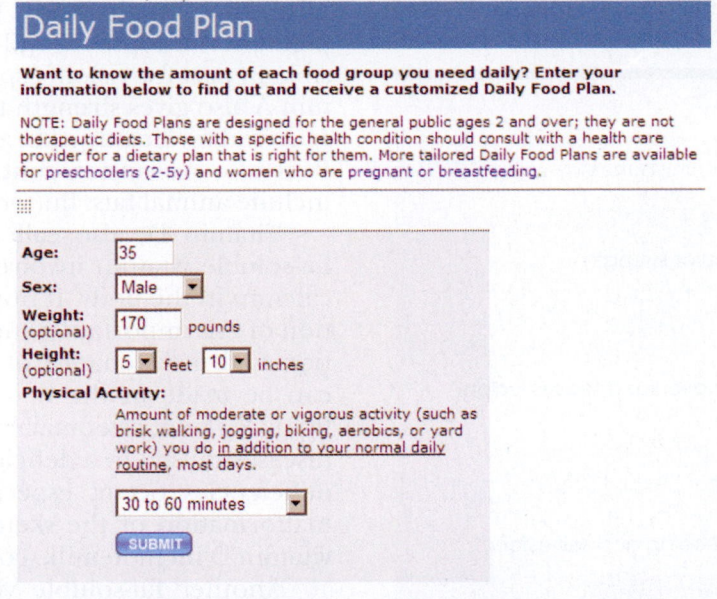

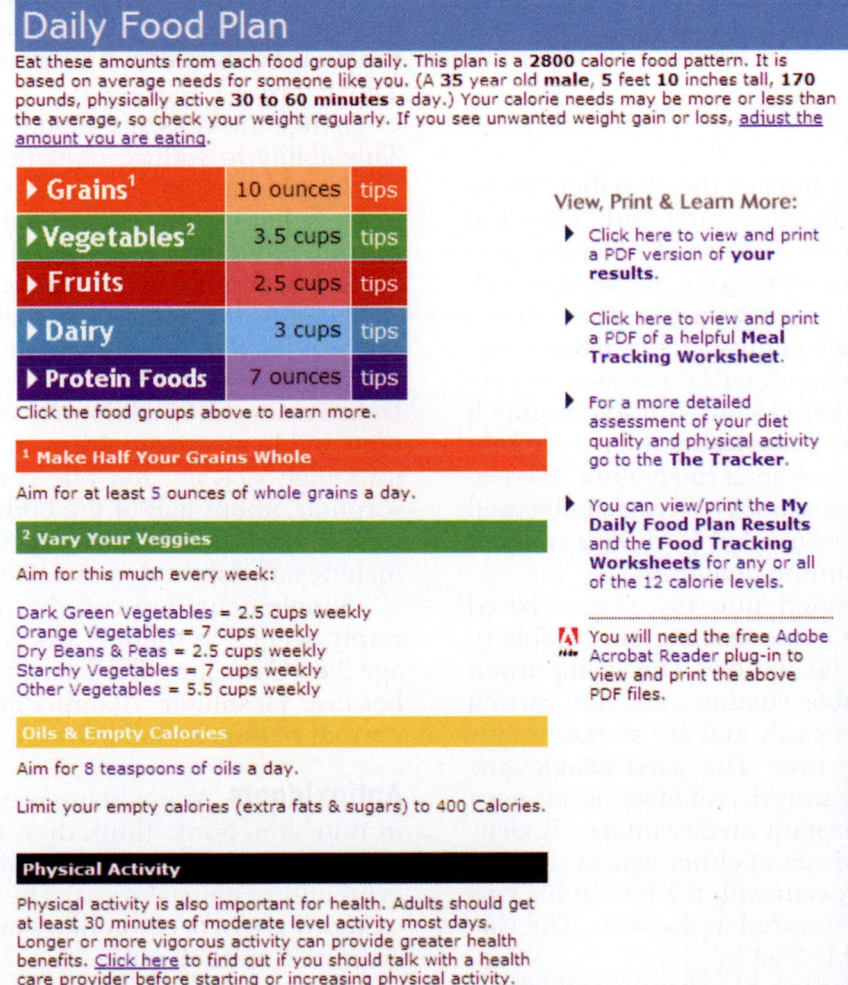

Figure 34-7 Daily food plan screens on www.ChooseMyPlate.gov: (A) You can enter your individual information. (B) The results of your information input.

Table 34-3 Health Benefits of Regular Physical Activity

Increase physical fitness
Helps build and maintain healthy bones, muscles, and joints
Builds endurance and muscular strength
Helps manage weight
Lowers risk factors for cardiovascular diseases, colon cancer, and type 2 diabetes
Helps control blood pressure
Promotes psychological well-being and self-esteem
Reduces feelings of depression and anxiety

Source: Nutrition and Your Health: Dietary Guidelines for Americans (6th ed.), 2005.

were first named as letters of the alphabet. These names have been supplemented with chemical names and both should be learned. Vitamins generally have one of two functions: to facilitate cellular metabolism by acting as a coenzyme with a catalyst, and to act as a component of tissue structure. A **catalyst** allows a chemical reaction to proceed at a much quicker rate and without as much energy input, and the **coenzyme** is the nonprotein part that acts with it. Neither a catalyst nor its coenzyme is used in the reaction, thus each can be used again and again. Vitamins that work with catalysts are only needed in minute quantities.

Vitamins are divided into two classes based on solubility. The vitamins that are not soluble in water are said to be fat soluble. This is important because the **fat-soluble** vitamins are not carried into the bloodstream easily and are stored in fatty tissue, especially the liver. The **water-soluble** vitamins are not so easily stored, and blood levels must be maintained by constant dietary intake. Toxicity can occur with high doses of either type of vitamin, but is more likely to occur with the fat-soluble vitamins because they are stored in the body. The vitamins are listed in Table 34-4.

There are four fat-soluble vitamins, which include vitamins A, D, E, and K. The first one, vitamin A, has two forms. The form that is used by the body is retinol, which is found in animal foods. The form found in plants is carotene. **Carotene** is converted

into retinol in the body. Vitamin A is part of the pigment rhodopsin found in the eye and is responsible in part for vision, especially night vision. Vitamin A also gives strength to epithelial tissue and is required for healthy skin and mucous membranes. It is also an antioxidant. Sources of vitamin A include animal fats, butter, and cheese.

Vitamin D, also called **cholecalciferol**, is the fat-soluble vitamin involved in the metabolism of calcium in the body. It not only helps with absorption of this important mineral, but also with formation and maintenance of bone tissue. Vitamin D can be made in the body with exposure to sunlight. Rickets, osteomalacia, and osteoporosis are diseases caused by a deficiency in vitamin D. When deficiencies occur, especially during childhood, malformation of the skeleton is seen. Sources of vitamin D include milk, cod liver oil, and egg yolk.

Another fat-soluble vitamin is vitamin E, or **tocopherol**. It too is an **antioxidant**, possibly reducing the likelihood of **oxidation** of substances. As the body breaks down nutrients, oxidation occurs. This is process releases free radicals that can kill or change the cells of the body and create disease. This ability to reduce oxidation has recently led to suggestions that vitamin E may slow the aging process, but its true effectiveness is yet to be demonstrated. Vitamin E is found in lettuce and other green leafy vegetables, wheat germ, and rice.

Vitamin K is a fat-soluble vitamin required for the production of prothrombin. Prothrombin is one agent responsible for the clotting of blood. Deficiencies can result in prolonged blood clotting time and hemorrhage. Vitamin K is synthesized by intestinal bacteria, and bile is required for its absorption. About half of the body's requirement for vitamin K is fulfilled in this way. Sources of vitamin K include fats, fishmeal, oats, alfalfa, wheat, and rye.

Supplementation of fat-soluble vitamins is rarely needed as there is a rich supply in the average diet. Care must be taken with supplementation because fat-soluble vitamins are stored for long periods of time and toxicity is a possibility.

Antioxidants. Antioxidants are an important topic in nutrition. Some think they are as important as the discussion about fats. Antioxidants are powerful and beneficial to us. The four primary antioxidants are beta-carotene (vitamin A), vitamin C, vitamin E, and selenium.

When our bodies use oxygen to burn (oxidize) food for energy, the process results in the formation of free radicals. Most times our bodies take care of the free radicals by producing enzymes to fight them.

Table 34-4   Vitamin Sources and Functions

Name	Food Sources	Functions	Deficiency/Toxicity
Fat-Soluble Vitamins			

Vitamin A (carotene or retinol)	Animal
	  Liver
	  Whole milk
	  Butter
	  Cream
	  Cod liver oil
	Plants
	  Dark green leafy vegetables
	  Deep yellow or orange fruit
	  Fortified margarine
		Antioxidant
		Dim light vision
		Maintenance of mucous membranes
		Growth and development of bones
			Deficiency
			  Night blindness
			  Xerophthalmia
			  Respiratory infections
			  Bone growth ceases
			Toxicity
			  Cessation of menstruation
			  Joint pain
			  Stunted growth
			  Enlargement of liver

Vitamin D (cholecalciferol)	Animal
	  Eggs
	  Liver
	  Fortified milk
	Plants
	  None
		Bone growth	Deficiency
			  Rickets
			  Osteomalacia
			  Osteoporosis
			  Poorly developed teeth
			  Muscle spasms
			Toxicity
			  Kidney stones
			  Calcification of soft tissues

Vitamin E (alpha-tocopherol, beta-tocopherol, delta-tocopherol, gamma-tocopherol)	Animal
	  None
	Plant
	  Wheat germ
	  Margarines
	  Salad dressing
	  Nuts
		Antioxidant	Deficiency
			  Neurologic defects
			  Destruction of red blood cells (RBCs)
			Toxicity
			  Hypertension

Vitamin K (phytonadione)	Animal
	  Egg yolk
	  Liver
	  Milk
	Plant
	  Green leafy vegetables
	  Cabbage
		Blood clotting	Deficiency
			  Prolonged blood clotting
			Toxicity
			  Hemolytic anemia
			  Jaundice

Water-Soluble Vitamins			

Thiamin (vitamin B_1)	Animal
	  Liver
	  Eggs
	  Fish
	  Pork
	  Beef
	Plants
	  Whole and enriched grains
	  Legumes
		Coenzyme in oxidation of glucose	Deficiency
			  Beriberi
			  Gastrointestinal tract, nervous and cardiovascular system problems
			Toxicity
			  None

continues

Table 34-4   Vitamin Sources and Functions (*Continued*)

Name	Food Sources	Functions	Deficiency/Toxicity

Thiamin	Animal
	  Pork
	  Beef
	  Liver
	  Eggs
	  Fish
	Plants
	  Whole and enriched grains
	  Legumes
	  Brewer's yeast
		Metabolism of carbohydrates
		Maintains normal appetite and nervous system function
			Deficiency
			  Cardiovascular system, nervous system and gastrointestinal system disorders
			Toxicity
			  None

Riboflavin (vitamin B$_2$)	Animal
	  Poultry
	  Milk
	  Fish
	Plants
	  Green vegetables
	  Cereals
	  Enriched bread
		Aids release of energy from food	Deficiency
			  Cheilosis
			  Glossitis
			  Photophobia
			Toxicity
			  None

Pyridoxine (vitamin B$_6$)	Animal
	  Pork
	  Milk
	  Eggs
	Plants
	  Whole grain cereals
	  Legumes
		Synthesis of nonessential amino acids
		Conversion of tryptophan to niacin
		Antibody production
			Deficiency
			  Irritability
			  Depression
			  Dermatitis
			Toxicity
			  Liver disease
			  Rare

Vitamin B$_{12}$ (cobalamin)	Animal
	  Seafood
	  Meat
	  Eggs
	  Milk
	Plants
	  None
		Synthesis of RBCs
		Maintenance of myelin sheaths
			Deficiency
			  Degeneration of myelin sheaths
			  Pernicious anemia
			Toxicity
			  None

Niacin (vitamin B$_3$, nicotinic acid)	Animal
	  Milk
	  Eggs
	  Fish
	  Poultry
		Transfers hydrogen atoms for synthesis of adenosine triphosphate	Deficiency
			  Pellagra
			Toxicity
			  Vasodilation of blood vessels

Folate (folic acid)	Animal
	  Liver
	Plants
	  Spinach
	  Asparagus
	  Broccoli
	  Kidney beans
		DNA synthesis
		Synthesis of RBCs
		Protein metabolism
			Deficiency
			  Anemia
			  Glossitis
			  Macrocytic anemia
			  Neural tube defects
			Toxicity
			  None

Table 34-4   Vitamin Sources and Functions (*Continued*)

Name	Food Sources	Functions	Deficiency/Toxicity

Biotin	Animal
	  Milk
	  Liver
	Plants
	  Legumes
	  Mushrooms
		Coenzyme in carbohydrate and amino acid metabolism
		Niacin synthesis from tryptophan
			Deficiency
			  None
			Toxicity
			  None

Pantothenic acid (vitamin B_5)	Animal
	  Eggs
	  Liver
	  Salmon
	Plants
	  Mushrooms
	  Cauliflower
	  Peanuts
	  Yeast
		Metabolism of carbohydrates, lipids, and proteins
		Synthesis of acetylcholine
			Deficiency
			  None
			Toxicity
			  None

Vitamin C (ascorbic acid)	Fruits
	  All citrus
	Plants
	  Broccoli
	  Tomatoes
	  Brussels sprouts
	  Potatoes
		Prevention of scurvy
		Formation of collagen
		Healing of wounds
		Release of stress hormones
		Absorption of iron
		Antioxidant
			Deficiency
			  Scurvy
			  Muscle cramps
			  Ulcerated gums
			Toxicity
			  Increase uric acid level
			  Hemolytic anemia
			  Kidney stones

Vitamins are divided into two classes based on water solubility: fat-soluble and water-soluble vitamins.

If free radicals are excessive, health can be seriously impaired. Evidence has shown that excess free radicals cannot be fought successfully and the body cannot get rid of them.

The radicals attack the cells' DNA and blood vessel cells, contributing to cardiovascular disease, strokes, arthritis, cataracts, and other diseases that may be degenerative in nature. These are seen in older adults.

Free radicals are not only a by-product of oxidation, they form with exposure to environmental influences such as water and air pollution, cigarette smoke, and certain foods, such as fried foods.

Antioxidants fight free radicals through those enzymes already in our bodies, those we ingest in food, and those we take as supplements. Vitamins A (as beta-carotene), C, and E and selenium provide powerful benefits because they fight against oxidation that produces free radicals.

Vitamin C, or **ascorbic acid**, is a water-soluble vitamin. Vitamin C is a constituent of connective tissue and acts to hold cells together. A deficiency of vitamin C causes **scurvy**, in which the walls of the capillaries become so weakened that they burst. Vitamin C also helps with wound healing and with the absorption of iron. Sources include most fresh fruits (especially citrus fruits) and vegetables (especially tomatoes).

The last group of water-soluble vitamins are the B-complex vitamins. It is important to remember that each vitamin in the B-complex is a separate vitamin with distinct functions. Vitamin B_1, or **thiamin**, helps in the conversion of glucose to energy. The disease **beriberi** is caused by thiamin deficiency and is characterized by neuritis, edema, and cardiovascular changes. Sources of thiamin include whole grain cereals, peas, beans, vegetables, and brewer's yeast. Vitamin B_2, or **riboflavin**, is also involved in energy production. It is important in the production of proteins and is necessary for normal growth. Sources include eggs, liver, milk, brewer's yeast, and green vegetables. A third

B-complex vitamin, **niacin**, works with both thiamin and riboflavin in the production of energy. Lack of niacin results in gastrointestinal and central nervous system disturbances. All three of these vitamins are important throughout the body.

Vitamin B_6, or **pyridoxine**, has an important role in protein metabolism, especially the synthesis of proteins. It is also important in the metabolism of fats and carbohydrates. Vitamin B_6 is found in rice, beans, and yeast. Another B-complex vitamin, **folic acid**, is involved in the formation of DNA and the formation of red blood cells. Folic acid is found in liver, yeast, and green leafy vegetables. Vitamin B_{12}, or **cobalamin**, is another vitamin important to the functioning of red blood cells. This vitamin is responsible for the synthesis of the heme portion of hemoglobin, and deficiencies in vitamin B_{12} result in the disease pernicious anemia. Because vitamin B_{12} is only found in animal foods such as liver, kidney, and dairy products, pernicious anemia may be a problem for some vegetarians. Pernicious anemia may also occur when there is decreased production of a factor within the stomach that is required for vitamin B_{12} absorption. Other B-complex vitamins, pantothenic acid, vitamin B_5, and biotin, are generally responsible for energy metabolism.

Multivitamin supplements may help reduce the risk for certain diseases, especially in individuals who do not eat nutritionally sound diets. Individuals who may be more likely to suffer vitamin deficiencies because of poor nutrition include the elderly, mentally challenged individuals, young children without proper care, alcoholics, and patients with chronic diseases such as Crohn's disease, cystic fibrosis, and celiac disease. Some studies show a reduced risk for coronary artery disease in patients who take a multivitamin coupled with antioxidants. Researchers believe that B vitamins and antioxidants may help keep plaque from forming in arteries.

Most patients who are healthy and eat a nutritious diet do not need a supplement in the form of a multivitamin. A balanced diet is the best overall source of nutrients. Some people may need a supplement because they are at risk for disease such as cancer and heart disease. Examples of people at high risk are patients who have a chronic illness such as AIDS or cancer; patients who have gastrointestinal problems that impair digestion or absorption; patients who are dieting; patients who are vegans or vegetarians; pregnant and breastfeeding women; and patients older than 50 years (many adults older than 50 years have difficulty absorbing B vitamins from food, and their level of vitamin D may be low because of lack of sunshine and eating poorly).

Patients should check with their provider before beginning to take multivitamin supplements.

Herbal Supplements. Herbs are medicinal plants and are also known as botanicals or phytomedicines. Many have been used as far back as Roman times and are used as traditional herbal medicine.

Many patients use herbs for the treatment of illnesses and diseases and to maintain health. It is part of a movement toward alternative or complementary therapies. Herbal supplements can be found in health food stores, pharmacies, supermarkets, large outlet stores, through the mail, and on the Internet.

Herbs are made from dried plants and plant juices. Herbal teas are made by placing the herb into boiling water. Natural hormones can be found in soy products.

Some supplements are helpful; other supplements are harmful and are banned in several countries but may be available in the United States. The Food and Drug Administration (FDA) is exempt from having authority over dietary supplements, although under the Dietary Supplement Health and Education Act of 1994, the FDA must prove a product is unsafe before it can order its removal from store shelves. An example of a potentially unsafe herbal supplement that the FDA removed from the shelves in 2004 is ephedra. It was used as an anorectic and as a bronchodilator, it acts as a stimulant, and it can increase blood pressure and pulse to dangerous levels. In 2005, a federal judge struck down the FDA's year-long ban on ephedra and supplements containing ephedra. A Utah supplement company had challenged the ban, which prompted the judge's ruling. In 2006, the ruling was appealed to the U.S. Court of Appeals for the Tenth Circuit in Denver, Colorado, and the court of appeals upheld the FDA's ban on ephedra. The sale of ephedra or supplements containing ephedra is illegal in the United States. Although ephedra is an illegal and banned substance, it is widely used by athletes.

Be sure to ask patients about all substances or remedies they may be using, including herbs, vitamins, teas, or others. Most patients do not consider supplements to be medicines and may not think to mention them when asked what medications they are taking. Herbs can interact unfavorably with certain prescription, over-the-counter medications, and anesthetics.

Minerals. Minerals differ from vitamins in two distinct ways. Whereas vitamins are complex molecules, minerals are singular elements. Another way that minerals differ from vitamins is that, although vitamins are only required in minute quantities, some minerals are required in larger amounts. The foundation of the classification of minerals falls into two groups: major and trace minerals. No matter how small the quantity required of either a mineral or vitamin, all are vital to a healthy body. Some minerals are considered **electrolytes**, in that they become ionized and carry a positive or negative charge. The levels of these minerals in the bloodstream must be carefully balanced for the body to function in a healthy state.

There are seven **major minerals** (Table 34-5). They are calcium, phosphorus, sodium, potassium, magnesium, chloride, and sulfur.

Calcium (Ca) is the mineral present in the largest quantity in the body because of its involvement in the structure of bone and teeth. It is also important in blood clotting, muscle contraction, and nerve conduction. Its levels in the blood must

Table 34-5   The Seven Major Minerals and Their Food Sources

Name	Food Sources	Functions	Deficiency/Toxicity

Calcium (Ca)	Milk exchanges
	  Milk, cheese
	Meat exchanges
	  Sardines
	  Salmon
	Vegetable exchanges
	  Green vegetables
		Development of bones and teeth
		Permeability of cell membranes
		Transmission of nerve impulses
		Blood clotting
		Normal heart action
			Deficiency
			  Osteoporosis
			  Osteomalacia
			  Rickets
			  Poor bone and teeth formation

Phosphorus (P)	Milk exchanges
	  Milk, cheese
	Meat exchanges
	  Lean meat
		Development of bones and teeth
		Transfer of energy
		Component of phospholipids
		Buffer system
			Deficiency
			  (Same as calcium)
			  Anorexia
			  Weakness

Potassium (K)	Fruit exchanges
	  Oranges, bananas
	  Dried fruits
	  Legumes
		Contraction of muscles
		Maintaining water balance
		Transmission of nerve impulses
		Carbohydrate and protein metabolism
			Deficiency
			  Hypokalemia
			Toxicity
			  Hyperkalemia

Sodium (Na)	Table salt
	Meat exchanges
	  Beef, eggs
	Milk exchanges
	  Milk, cheese
		Maintaining fluid balance in blood
		Transmission of nerve impulses
			Toxicity
			  Increase in blood pressure

Chloride (Cl)	Table salt
	Meat exchanges
	Eggs
		Gastric acidity
		Regulation of osmotic pressure
		Activation of salivary amylase
			Deficiency
			  Imbalance in gastric acidity
			  Imbalance in blood pH

Magnesium (Mg)	Vegetable exchanges
	  Green vegetables
	Bread exchanges
	  Whole grains
		Synthesis of adenosine triphosphate
		Transmission of nerve impulses
		Activator of metabolic enzymes
		Relaxation of skeletal muscles
			Unknown, perhaps mental and emotional disorders

Sulfur (S)	Meat exchanges Eggs, poultry, fish	Maintaining protein structure Formation of high-energy compounds	Unknown

© Cengage Learning 2014

be kept within narrow limits to ensure that the nervous and muscular tissues can function. This is especially important for the beating heart tissue. When there is a deficiency of calcium in the diet, calcium is taken from the bones to keep the blood calcium levels constant. The resulting deficient peak bone mass may put a person at risk for osteoporosis. This condition develops when there is not enough calcium in the bones and the bones become porous and easily broken.

Women older than 60 years are at greater risk for osteoporosis than are men. There are no symptoms of the disease, and the first indication for the patient is when he or she sustains a fracture caused by weakened bones.

Most adults in the United States older than 60 years do not consume enough calcium in their diets and risk development of osteoporosis. Dairy products contain high amounts of calcium, as do sardines, figs, oranges, almonds, greens, and beans.

Supplemental estrogen for menopausal women was once a common preventative for bone loss. Since 2002, estrogen has not been given as a preventive measure because a large study by the Women's Health Initiative showed an increased risk for heart disease, stroke, cancer, and breast cancer in postmenopausal women who took estrogen.

Phosphorus (P) is another mineral important in bone formation. Phosphorus also is involved in numerous activities associated with energy metabolism, as well as maintaining a proper pH balance in the blood.

Sodium (Na) and potassium (K) are two minerals that act as electrolytes. Together they work to maintain proper water balance. They also help in maintenance of proper pH balance and are involved in nerve and muscular conduction and excitability. In addition, potassium is involved in protein synthesis and release of insulin from the pancreas. Most importantly, potassium plays a role in cardiac function and in skeletal and smooth muscle contraction.

Magnesium (Mg) is another mineral that is involved with energy metabolism. It also functions in nerve and muscle excitability and is stored in bone. Magnesium is critical to more than 300 enzyme-driven biochemical reactions in the body. It is critical to glucose and fat breakdown, and creation of DNA and RNA.

Chloride (Cl) is important in pH balance and is the major **extracellular** (outside the cell) anion. It is also a major component of gastric secretions in the form of hydrochloric acid. Chloride is present in white cells as hypochlorite and is a part of the immune response.

The last major mineral is sulfur (S). It is a component of one of the amino acids, and therefore is found in protein. It is also involved in energy metabolism. It is essential in the production of collagen as well.

The **trace minerals** are required in smaller quantities but are as important as the major minerals. Some of the more important trace minerals include iron, copper, chromium, molybdenum, selenium, manganese, iodine, zinc, cobalt, and fluorine.

Iron is vital to life because of its role in the heme molecule, which carries oxygen to every cell in the body. Iron-deficiency anemia results when the diet is low in iron and is characterized by small, pale red blood cells. Iron is also part of the molecule myoglobin, found in muscle cells, and is involved in a number of metabolic reactions.

Copper, chromium, molybdenum, selenium, and manganese are trace minerals important as factors in a number of metabolic reactions. Selenium acts as an antioxidant and has been receiving much of the recent publicity that vitamin E has. Iodine is also involved in metabolism but is unique in that the only place that iodine is found is in the thyroid hormone produced by the thyroid gland. Without it, the thyroid gland would be unable to regulate the overall metabolism of the body.

Zinc is an important constituent of many parts of the body but most notable is its involvement with the immune system and growth of tissues. Deficiencies lead to decreased ability to heal and reduced immune resistance. Cobalt is part of vitamin B_{12} and is therefore important for the functioning of red blood cells. Fluorine is involved in calcified tissues. Its involvement in strengthening teeth has led to the fluoridation of most public water supplies. Its role in the prevention of osteoporosis has been suggested but is still under investigation.

Water. Water is an important nutrient. The human body can go far longer without food than it can without water. Water has a multitude of functions in the body. It is the major solvent of the body and is the medium in which most biochemical reactions of the body take place. As a solvent, water is essential for the removal of toxic waste from the body. In addition, it is an important component of many structures; the body is composed of 50% to 60% water. Being the major component of blood, water serves as a transporter. Another function of water is its lubricating role, especially in joints and in the digestive system. In addition, water helps control temperature within the body by eliminating excess heat through the evaporation of water secreted in the form of perspiration.

Because the body cannot efficiently store water, water that is lost daily must continually be replenished. Water is lost through perspiration, feces, urine, and respiration. Water can be replenished in part from foods that are ingested, but additional water should also be consumed. It is suggested that six to eight glasses of water be taken in per day. Although other beverages are important sources of water, it should be considered that caffeine and alcohol are **diuretics** and may cause the body to lose water through increased urinary output.

Fiber. Although most fiber is carbohydrate in composition, it is included in its own section because of its special characteristics. Fiber comes only from plant sources. An adequate supply of fruits, vegetables, and grains is necessary to ensure enough fiber in the diet. Fiber cannot be digested and therefore is not absorbed into the body. Although fiber is not digested, it is important for the proper functioning of the gastrointestinal tract because it adds bulk to feces as it is passed through the intestines; therefore, it gives the muscles of the tract something against which to work. Lack of fiber in the diet has been implicated in such gastrointestinal disorders as diverticulitis, constipation, and colorectal cancer.

There are several types of fiber. Most are carbohydrates and include **cellulose**, gums, mucilages, algal polysaccharides, pectins, and hemicellulose. Another important fiber, lignin, is not a carbohydrate. It is recommended that the diet contain 20 to 35 g of fiber per day. The U.S. diet tends to be far below this recommendation (approximately 11 g), in part because of the consumption of processed foods. During processing, fiber is often removed. Fiber levels should be increased gradually to prevent gastrointestinal distress, which can include diarrhea or flatulence.

READING FOOD LABELS

When assisting patients in changing or modifying their diets, the medical assistant must be knowledgeable not only about types of nutrients, but also about how these nutrients are expressed in the foods we eat. The nutritional analysis presented on a package's food label is a helpful guide to understanding levels of fat, cholesterol, sodium, carbohydrate, protein, and vitamins contained in a particular food.

Many of the foods we eat are **processed foods** which are cooked or packaged with parts removed or ingredients added. We rely on the labels on the cans, bottles, and boxes to tell us what nutrients

are inside. The government wants to make it easier for people to understand the labels.

The government also wants to prevent food companies from fooling people into thinking something has good nutrition when it really does not. Food companies often put words on their labels to make people believe a product is healthy. Words such as "healthy" and "light" or "lite" are not adequately descriptive. To discover what is in the package and whether it is healthy, it is important to read the nutrition label (Figure 34-8).

Items on the Nutrition Label

Serving Size. The nutrition information given is for one serving of the food. In this case, one serving is one-half cup of the food. The package contains four servings.

Calories. The label lists the number of calories per serving, as well as the number of calories from fat per serving. This number should be less than 30% of the total calories. For example, if the total calories amount is 100, the calories from fat should be 30 or less.

The Percentage (%) Daily Value. The percentage (%) daily value is the amount of a nutrient obtained by eating one serving of the product. The amount is given in a percentage based on a diet of 2,000 calories a day. For example, if the packaged food has 3 g fat, the total fat from eating

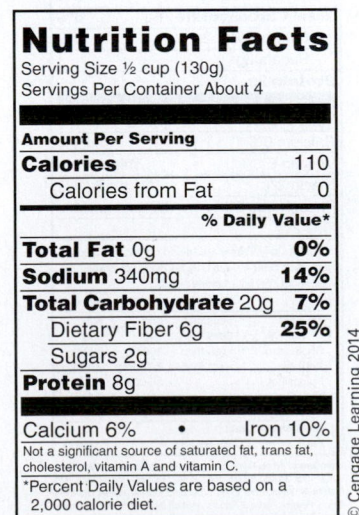

Figure 34-8 Labels on food packages give facts about the ingredients and nutrition of the food in the package.

one serving is 5% of the total fat that should be ingested in an entire day.

Fat and Cholesterol. Because it is important to eat a low-fat diet, nutrition labels list both the total amount of fat and the amount of saturated fat and trans fat per serving. Saturated fat comes from an animal source and contains more cholesterol than unsaturated fats, which come from vegetable sources. The cholesterol content is also listed.

Sodium. The amount of sodium per serving is listed. This category is especially important for patients on a sodium-restricted diet, such as those with cardiac disease and hypertension.

Carbohydrates. The total amount of carbohydrates per serving is listed together with the amount of carbohydrates that come from simple sugar. These two types of carbohydrates are separated for individuals who are trying to eat more complex carbohydrates and less simple sugar.

Other Information. The amounts of fiber, protein, and some vitamins and minerals are listed.

Ingredients. The ingredients contained in a packaged food are listed on the label. The item that is in the largest quantity is listed first. For example, if a product lists flour first and water second, there is more flour than water in the product. **Preservatives**, or chemicals added to food to keep it fresh longer, and artificial flavors and colors are often added to processed foods.

Comparing Labels

Look at some labels from snack foods that people eat when they want something crunchy and salty. Figure 34-9 shows labels from potato chips, pretzels, and snack crackers. When comparing products, compare equal amounts. These products list the serving as 30 or 28g. That is close enough to compare the labels.

A

Nutrition Facts
Serving Size 1 oz. (28g/About 15 chips)
Servings Per Container About 12

Amount Per Serving	
Calories 140	Calories from Fat 60
	% Daily Value*
Total Fat 6g	**10%**
Saturated Fat 1g	**5%**
Polyunsaturated Fat 2g	
Monounsaturated Fat 3.5g	
Trans Fat 0g	
Cholesterol 0mg	**0%**
Sodium 130mg	**5%**
Potassium 75mg	**2%**
Total Carbohydrate 18g	**6%**
Dietary Fiber 2g	**9%**
Sugars 3g	
Protein 2g	

Vitamin A 0%	Vitamin C 0%
Calcium 0%	Iron 2%
Vitamin E 8%	Thiamin 2%
Niacin 2%	Vitamin B_6 4%
Phosphorus 6%	Magnesium 4%
Zinc 2%	

*Percent Daily Values are based on a 2,000 calorie diet. Your Daily Values may be higher or lower depending on your calorie needs:

	Calories:	2,000	2,500
Total Fat	Less than	65g	80g
Sat Fat	Less than	20g	25g
Cholesterol	Less than	300mg	300mg
Sodium	Less than	2,400mg	2,400mg
Potassium		3,500mg	3,500mg
Total Carbohydrate		300g	375g
Dietary Fiber		25g	30g

Calories per gram:
Fat 9 • Carbohydrate 4 • Protein 4

Ingredients: Whole Corn, Sunflower Oil, Whole Wheat, Rice Flour, Whole Oat Flour, Sugar, Salt, Whey Protein Concentrate, Dry Buttermilk, Whey, Sour Cream (Cultured Cream, Nonfat Dry Milk), Onion Powder, Natural Flavors, Hydrolyzed Soy Protein, Cultured Whey, Corn Starch, Autolyzed Yeast Extract, Mozzarella Cheese (Pasteurized Part Skim Milk, Cheese Cultures, Salt, Enzymes), Citric Acid, Garlic Powder, Gum Arabic, Glycerol, Disodium Phosphate, Spice, and Artificial Color (Including Red 40, Blue 1).
CONTAINS WHEAT, MILK, AND SOY INGREDIENTS.

B

Nutrition Facts
Serving Size 6 Crackers (15g)
Servings Per Container About 24

Amount Per Serving	
Calories 60	Calories from Fat 15
	% Daily Value*
Total Fat 1.5g	**2%**
Saturated Fat 0.5g	**3%**
Trans Fat 0g	
Polyunsaturated Fat 0.5g	
Monounsaturated Fat 0.5g	
Cholesterol 0mg	**0%**
Sodium 160mg	**7%**
Total Carbohydrate 11g	**4%**
Dietary Fiber less than 1g	**1%**
Sugars 1g	
Protein 1g	

Vitamin A 0%	Vitamin C 0%
Calcium 0%	Iron 2%

*Percent Daily Values are based on a 2,000 calorie diet. Your Daily Values may be higher or lower depending on your calorie needs:

	Calories:	2,000	2,500
Total Fat	Less than	65g	80g
Sat. Fat	Less than	20g	25g
Cholesterol	Less than	300mg	300mg
Sodium	Less than	2,400mg	2,400mg
Total Carbohydrate		300g	375g
Dietary Fiber		25g	30g

Ingredients: Enriched flour (wheat flour, niacin, reduced iron, thiamin mononitrate [vitamin B_1], riboflavin [vitamin B_2], folic acid), partially hydrogenated soybean and/or cottonseed oil† with TBHQ for freshness, sugar, contains two percent or less of salt, leavening (baking soda, sodium acid pyrophosphate, monocalcium phosphate), corn syrup, high fructose corn syrup, sodium stearoyl lactylate, sodium sulfite, soy lecithin.
†Less than 0.5g *trans* fat per serving
CONTAINS WHEAT, AND SOY INGREDIENTS.

C

Nutrition Facts
Serving Size 18 Pretzels (30g)
Servings Per Container about 8

Amount Per Serving	
Calories 120	Calories from Fat 0
	% Daily Value*
Total Fat 0g	**0%**
Saturated Fat 0g	**0%**
Trans Fat 0g	
Cholesterol 0mg	**0%**
Sodium 320mg	**13%**
Total Carbohydrate 25g	**8%**
Dietary Fiber 2g	**8%**
Sugars 3g	
Protein 3g	

Vitamin A 0%	Vitamin C 0%
Calcium 0%	Iron 2%

*Percent Daily Values are based on a 2,000 calorie diet. Your Daily Values may be higher or lower depending on your calorie needs:

	Calories:	2,000	2,500
Total Fat	Less than	65g	80g
Sat Fat	Less than	20g	25g
Cholesterol	Less than	300mg	300mg
Sodium	Less than	2,400mg	2,400mg
Total Carbohydrate		300g	375g
Dietary Fiber		25g	30g

Calories per gram:
Fat 9 • Carbohydrate 4 • Protein 4

Ingredients: Organic wheat flour, water, organic oat flour and oat bran, organic evaporated cane juice, salt, yeast, sodium bicarbonate.
Allergy information: Produced in a facility that handles peanut butter.

Figure 34-9 Examples of food labels from (A) potato chips, (B) wheat crackers, and (C) pretzels.

In reviewing these labels, note the amount of fat and saturated fat in each item. It might be assumed that potato chips, which are fried, would be high in fat. It may be surprising that the snack crackers have high fat content. Pretzels are the clear winner for a low-fat snack.

Although the labels show total fat and saturated fat, the amount of trans-fatty acids (TFA) is not listed. Previously, food labels included trans fats within the total fat amount. The FDA now requires the amount of TFAs be listed in the label. All three snack items contain TFAs. These snacks should be avoided or used sparingly.

In terms of sodium, calories, and sugar, pretzels have the most sodium, but all three are high in sodium.

All three are low in sugar. Their calories are nearly the same as are the amounts of fiber and protein. The pretzels have the most carbohydrates, and the crackers have the most artificial flavors, colors, and preservatives.

NUTRITION AT VARIOUS STAGES OF LIFE

For the nutrients discussed in the preceding sections, ranges of suggested normal requirements were given. These ranges should be used as a guide,

remembering that each individual is unique, and requirements will vary.

Pregnancy and Lactation

Pregnancy and lactation both cause marked changes in a woman's body and both require an increase in various nutrients. During pregnancy, not only does the growth of the fetus require additional nutrients, but the growth of the placenta, the increase in adipose tissue in the mother, the increased volume of blood, and the growth of breast tissue also require additional nutrients.

The increased demand for nutrients is not just a demand for calories, but also for other specific nutrients to be increased, most notably protein. Protein requirements are nearly double during pregnancy. Because of the role vitamins play in metabolism and structure, they are needed in greater quantities than usual. In addition, calcium, phosphorus, and iron are needed in such high amounts that usually a vitamin supplement is prescribed. It is important that diet modifications are not simply an increase in calories but include quality foods high in minerals, vitamins, and protein.

Pregnancy is an important time for both fetus and mother. It is normal and healthy for the mother to gain weight. Her provider will determine the appropriate amount of weight gain based on the individual. A general rule of thumb is 25 to 35 pounds. During lactation, the requirement for higher levels of nutrients continues; however, overall, it is not as high as during pregnancy. A baby is more likely to be healthy and develop normally if the mother has good nutritional habits during pregnancy and breast-feeding. A baby born to a mother who is malnourished may suffer from mental retardation and be of lower birth weight. Lower birth weight babies (less than 5.5 pounds) have a greater mortality rate than do babies of normal weight.

Breast-Feeding

There are several reasons why breast-feeding is encouraged. The nutrition the infant receives from breast milk is a perfect combination of water, lactose (sugar), fat, and protein. There are more than 100 ingredients in breast milk that are not found in formula milk. There are no allergic reactions to mother's milk. (On occasion, if the mother eats a particular food, the infant may react by being fussy.) Breast-feeding is nutritionally sound, economical, and sterile. Breast milk is easily digested and does not easily cause gastrointestinal upsets. Breast-fed babies receive temporary antibodies to many diseases from their mothers. Mother and infant bond during breast-feeding. Breast-feeding helps contract the uterus and bring it back to its nonpregnant state, thus helping to control postpartum bleeding.

While breast-feeding, the mother will continue to require nutritious foods taken from the MyPlate guidelines and will need to increase her intake of calories. If she consumes inadequate calories, the amount of milk produced will be decreased. When the mother terminates the period of breast-feeding (6 months is recommended for the greatest benefit to the infant), caloric intake should be reduced to avoid gaining weight.

CRITICAL THINKING

Write a response to a teenage girl who refuses to gain weight during her pregnancy.

Infancy

Infancy is a time of continuous growth, and many of the mother's nutritional requirements during pregnancy are still required by the baby after birth. In the first year of life, the baby will triple birth weight. The infant will need two to three times more calories per kilogram (kg) of body weight than the normal adult. This is true for protein as well, and most of the vitamins and minerals are required at greater levels per kilogram. Most of these can be furnished with breast milk or formula; however, once iron stores have been used up, usually in 3 to 6 months, the infant will require an iron supplement, which is why pediatricians prescribe an infant liquid iron supplement. Because of the high rate of growth, especially of the nervous system, infancy is an important time to be sure nutritional requirements are met. However, according to some pediatricians, overfeeding in infancy might lead to childhood obesity.

Childhood

Good eating habits develop during childhood. One way parents who have good eating habits can teach their children how to eat healthfully is by example. Family eating habits, physical activity, and lifestyle help children to adopt healthy habits. Poor habits are established during childhood and are often difficult to alter. This can lead to lifelong health problems, such as obesity, diabetes, and cardiovascular diseases. The effects of poor nutrition are not only physical but can also be emotional as well. When an obese child is "picked on" in school, anxiety, low self-esteem, depression, and irritability can result.

Childhood obesity is a serious problem, leading to type 2 diabetes because the disease is related to being overweight and having a poor diet. Obese children have a greatly increased chance of becoming obese as adults if they are obese before becoming a preteen (around age 11 years). Osteoporosis and cardiovascular diseases are other problems obesity can cause.

The availability of electronic devices, such as computers, video games, and television, contribute greatly to a child's reluctance to be active. Bike riding, jumping rope, swimming, and running are activities that most children enjoy if encouraged to engage in them.

Fast foods and carbonated sodas contribute to obesity because of their high fat and calorie content. They are even banned from some schools because they are consumed readily and are poor choices at any age.

Clearly, parental education (and therefore education of their children) about exercise and good nutrition is an excellent way to stop childhood obesity and type 2 diabetes. By following *ChooseMyPlate,* as recommended by the USDA, parents and children can learn to be active every day and to make healthy food choices. The government Web site (http://www.ChooseMyPlate .gov) gives ideas on how everyone in the family can eat better and exercise more.

Adolescence

During adolescence, individuals experience the greatest levels of growth. The period of growth varies from person to person but generally begins sooner with girls. Except for times of pregnancy and lactation, the need for total nutrients is greatest at this stage of growth. At the end of the growth spurt, nutrient requirements decrease, and young adults must then also decrease the amount of food they consume and must exercise regularly.

Two particular nutrients that especially need to be altered during adolescence are iron and calcium. Iron requirements increase for the female individual as she begins menstruation. Calcium requirements increase for both male and female individuals as bone development is occurring at a rapid rate.

Bulimia and Anorexia Nervosa. Two eating disorders that may occur at any age are **bulimia** and anorexia nervosa, and they are serious in all individuals. Girls are more likely than boys to suffer from these problems, although eating disorders are on the rise among the male population. The diets of adolescent girls in general are deficient in calories, vitamins, protein, and, as previously mentioned, iron and calcium. Many girls have concerns about their weight coupled with poor eating habits; when taken to extremes, these can result in bulimia or anorexia nervosa. When a patient is diagnosed with bulimia or anorexia nervosa, the provider monitors the patient's weight gain or loss, orders laboratory tests at each clinic visit, and makes an appropriate treatment plan.

EHR These tasks are facilitated in a total practice management system, as the patient's weight pattern can be viewed graphically and test results can be easily accessed (Figure 34-10).

Bulimia. Bulimia can be life threatening because it can result in an electrolyte imbalance. Dental caries, malnutrition, dehydration, and eroded mouth and esophagus are other problems related to the continuous exposure to stomach and digestive juices. Individuals with bulimia binge on food and then purge (vomit). Use of laxatives is common. Girls fear becoming overweight and usually binge on high-calorie dessert-type foods, then self-induce vomiting. Psychological therapy may help.

Anorexia Nervosa. Anorexia nervosa can be life threatening. It is characterized by the individual severely restricting caloric intake and exercising excessively. Problems that occur are low blood pressure, alopecia, altered metabolism, amenorrhea, brain damage, and death.

Both bulimia and anorexia nervosa seem to have some basis in U.S. culture, with teenagers (mostly women) wanting to look like the slim supermodels and fashion models (with distorted body images) seen in movies and in magazines.

These eating disorders are serious, and relapses are not unusual. Sometimes they become a lifelong struggle, and repeated therapy sessions are needed. Anorexia and bulimia are some of the most life-threatening disorders among the mental health disorders.

Older Adults

Aging is a natural process of the body. Although aging occurs in different stages and at different rates for each individual, some generalities can be made. As we age, our cellular metabolism tends to slow and, coupled with a general decline in physical activity, results in a decreased requirement for calories. At the same time, there may be an increase in nutrient requirement in special circumstances. There is always an increased requirement for nutrients, vitamins, and protein in particular during illness, especially the prolonged illnesses that may occur in older adults. With aging, there may be increased breakdown of cells; as a result, there is an increased requirement for nutrients that repair and build cells and tissues. There is also a need to ingest more nutrients because of decreased absorption within the digestive tract. Thus, although there is less need for calories, there is more need for nutrient-rich foods. Less need for calories along with less physical activity may lead to weight gain if calorie intake is not reduced.

This may become difficult for older adults for several reasons. One reason may be an individual's psychological state. Loneliness and depression affect many older adults, especially after the loss of a spouse. Older adults may not like the idea of

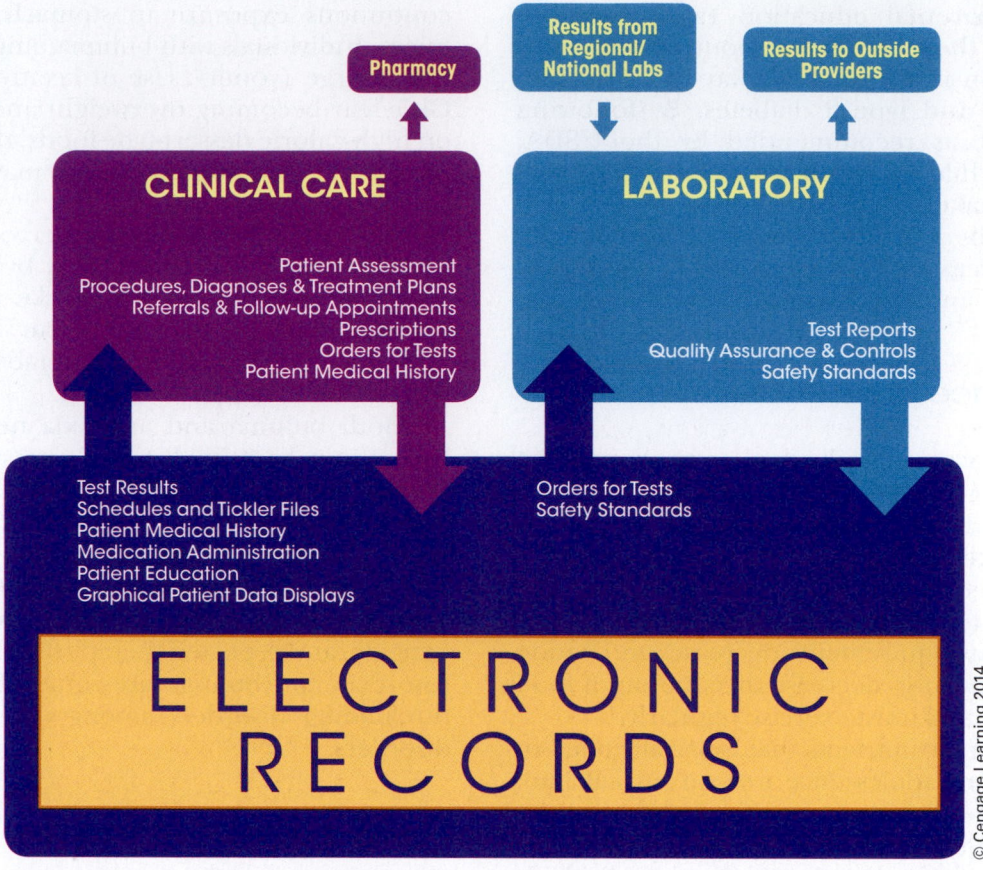

Figure 34-10   The clinical care and laboratory arms of the total practice management system (TPMS). Laboratory tests results and mensurations are tracked in the patient's electronic medical record and are accessible to providers when determining an appropriate treatment plan.

eating alone. The economic status of the individual also may present problems, as after retirement income generally decreases. Physiologically, taste tends to diminish with age and interest in food may decrease. In addition, problems with teeth and a decrease in salivary gland secretions may make eating painful. Many medications cause a decrease in saliva production. Also, decreased motility in the gastrointestinal tract may lead to constipation, making eating uncomfortable. All these factors, as well as a general unwillingness to break old habits, may make it difficult to change the diet to keep up with the body's aging process.

THERAPEUTIC DIETS

Thus far this chapter has examined the nutrient requirements of the body under normal conditions. There are times, however, when the body becomes diseased and nutrient requirements change. These changes may be necessitated by disease states such as diabetes mellitus or conditions resulting from a poor diet such as obesity. Therapeutic diets are designed to overcome or control these conditions.

The diet can be modified in a number of ways. The number of overall calories can be adjusted, or one type of nutrient can be restricted or encouraged. The consistency, texture, and spiciness of food can be varied. The frequency of eating can be increased or decreased. When counseling patients, remember that habits are hard to change. The medical assistant should be supportive and encouraging.

Weight Control

Overweight and underweight are both weight disorders. The problem in defining overweight or underweight stems from the fact that there is no ideal weight for an entire population. There is only an ideal weight for the individual. Ideal weight can depend on many factors including age, sex, lean muscle mass, bone structure, and physical activity.

Obesity is generally considered being more than 20% overweight. Underweight is weight 10% to 15% below average. Height-weight tables now generally give ranges that vary more than 20 pounds. The ratio of fat tissue to lean muscle mass is a better indicator than a specific weight of whether individuals are at their ideal weight.

Individuals will gain weight if they consume more calories than they need. Conversely, individuals will lose weight if they use more calories than they ingest. In either case, the individual must bring the amount of calories ingested into balance with the amount used. For the overweight individual, this means either decreasing calorie consumption or increasing calorie usage, or both. For the underweight individual, it usually means focusing entirely on increasing calorie consumption.

Weight loss has become a big business. However, individuals do not need to spend tremendous amounts of money to lose weight; patient education about low-calorie, low-salt foods and a moderate exercise program are basic starting points for weight loss. Because losing more than 1 to 2 pounds a week can put an individual into nutritional deficiency, goals should not be set higher than this. Modifications made to the diet should then be maintained even after the weight is lost and should be continued throughout life. Losing weight takes much effort, and the patient needs constant encouragement and support from medical personnel and family.

Obesity has become a serious health problem. It is defined as being severely overweight and having a body mass index (BMI) of 30 or above. BMI uses height and weight to calculate an individual's total amount of body fat. Go to http://www.nhlbisupport.com/bmi/ to calculate your own BMI.

Genetics may play a role in obesity. Several genes affect the rate at which the body burns calories. Playing a major role in obesity are family eating habits, other lifestyle habits, physical activity levels, and psychological factors such as stress and depression. Major causes of obesity are lack of physical exercise, oversized portions of high-fat foods, and the accessibility of fast foods. Many people eat more food than their bodies need.

Obesity causes increased risk for hypertension, heart and lung disease, hip and knee problems, certain cancers, and diabetes, and it shortens the life span.

Parents can be role models and teach their children to eat nutritious foods and not to consume more calories than their bodies need. Parents should provide nourishing foods, limit inactivity such as television and computer time,

engage the entire family in regular exercise, eat at regular mealtimes at the table, and encourage the family to drink plenty (six to eight glasses) of water daily. By parents setting good examples when their children are young, the children will learn that healthy eating habits and regular exercise will improve the quality of life (fewer illnesses) and prolong the length of life.

The American Heart Association and the American Cancer Society are community resources available with information about reducing the risk for heart disease and cancer. Keeping weight under control and regular exercise helps prevent heart attacks, hypertension, and certain cancers.

Because there has been a great deal of media attention given to the problem of obesity and the diseases it can cause, many people are looking for a quick fix to lose weight. There are many claims that people can lose weight without exercising or eating healthy foods. Most claims about weight loss products are deceptive or false.

Individuals who want to lose weight must strive to eat a healthful diet over time. A healthful diet together with regular exercise can reduce their risk for hypertension, coronary artery disease, and certain cancers (colon and breast).

Diabetes Mellitus

Diabetes mellitus is a disease in which there is either reduced or no production of insulin, or in which there is reduced or no response to insulin. Approximately 5% of the population has diabetes mellitus (type 1 or type 2) in some form. Most patients with this disease (type 2 diabetes) are not dependent on insulin and can control their condition by monitoring diet, exercise, and weight.

Normally, after a meal, the body secretes the hormone insulin, which makes its way to all cells of the body. Insulin signals the cells that the glucose is available and should be brought in so that it can be converted to energy. If the cells do not receive this signal, or do not respond to it, their ability to use glucose is markedly reduced. Because the body uses glucose as its main energy source, the ramifications of this affect almost every tissue of the body. In addition, the high level of glucose that remains in the bloodstream puts a tremendous strain on the kidneys and other major body organs, causing problems such as myocardial infarction, vascular diseases, neuropathy, and infections.

The effects of diabetes mellitus can be controlled with a general goal of maintaining a regular level of glucose in the bloodstream, avoiding large fluctuations between high and low levels. There are several ways suggested to accomplish this. Total calories need not be altered, unless the diabetic patient is overweight. However, the ratio of carbohydrate, fat, and protein must be closely monitored. Total carbohydrates should be increased, but simple sugars should be avoided. Because of the slower rate of digestion and absorption of complex carbohydrates, these will be released over a longer period and will prevent a sudden high level of glucose in the bloodstream; thus, these are the type of carbohydrates diabetics need. Increasing fiber content also increases the time of absorption and decreases the likelihood of sudden increases in glucose levels in the bloodstream. Regular snacks may be added between meals to maintain levels of glucose. The trend is for patients to take charge of their own care. The role of educator for the medical assistant will be an important one to facilitate patient self-management.

Type 2 Diabetes and Obesity.
Obesity has become epidemic in the last 10 years and is the most significant factor in the increase in diabetes. Children and young people who are obese are being diagnosed with type 2 diabetes at an extremely high rate. The longer individuals have diabetes, the greater their risk for development of the complications of the disease, including heart disease, stroke, kidney disease, blindness, and infections. Diabetes is a major cause of death.

Prevention of type 2 diabetes is of utmost importance. Changes in lifestyle such as weight loss, regular exercise, and a nutritious diet can prevent type 2 diabetes. If a patient has type 2 diabetes, it can be controlled by diet and exercise and by medication (see Chapter 36 for more information about diabetes and insulin).

Cardiovascular Disease

Cardiovascular disease is currently the leading cause of death in the United States. The unfortunate aspect of this is that much of it is preventable. Cardiovascular disease encompasses a variety of problems. Two of these problems, hypertension and atherosclerosis, often work hand in hand to perpetuate one another until a myocardial infarction occurs. It is important to remember that the conditions leading up to a myocardial infarction do not occur overnight. They have been developing slowly over many years, often asymptomatically. These conditions can be reduced or prevented with lifestyle modifications such as a healthy diet, moderate exercise, cessation of smoking, and weight management. This section focuses on a healthy diet to prevent cardiovascular disease.

Hypertension, or increased blood pressure, is often of unknown cause. Sometimes it has a familial connection. When the blood pressure is only moderately increased, certain diet modifications can be used to reduce it. If it is severe, drug therapy may be used in conjunction with diet therapy. One of the largest diet factors in controlling increased blood pressure is restricting sodium, because it can play such an important role in maintenance of water levels in the body. Some individuals are salt sensitive. An increased volume of blood and water will increase the pressure on the blood vessel walls. Eliminating sodium includes more than simply eliminating use of table salt. Foods that are particularly high in sodium include smoked meats, luncheon meats, olives, pickles, chips, crackers, catsup, and cheese. In some cases, eliminating foods with only moderate salt levels may be indicated. These may include certain meats, breads containing baking powder or baking soda, shellfish, and some vegetables.

Atherosclerosis is another condition that can lead to a myocardial infarction. Atherosclerosis is narrowing of the arteries because of deposits of fatty substance. It should not be confused with arteriosclerosis, which is a narrowing of the arteries because of loss of the elasticity of the arterial wall. Atherosclerosis leads to arteriosclerosis, which generally occurs because of a lack of exercise and increased blood cholesterol levels. The elasticity can be regained by increasing activity, although it should be started slowly and under a provider's guidance. Atherosclerosis and arteriosclerosis often occur together. Smoking and hypertension will increase the likelihood of development of both of these conditions.

The conditions of atherosclerosis and arteriosclerosis facilitate each other. The fatty deposits associated with atherosclerosis tend to occur at points of damage to the inner walls of the artery. One of the causes of this damage is high pressure at points where there may be narrowing because of deposits that are already there, or because of the constriction of blood vessels due to nicotine. Carbon monoxide brought into the bloodstream during smoking also causes damage to the arterial walls. The deposits and hardening increase the blood pressure, which, in turn, causes more damage and more deposits. It is a cycle that is difficult to stop. The best solution is prevention.

Fats and cholesterol in the diet have been strongly implicated in atherosclerosis. It is not only total fat that is important, but also the types of fat ingested. The effect of high levels of fats and cholesterol in the diet will vary among individuals, and the key factor in atherosclerosis is the level of these substances in the bloodstream. Some individuals are able to ingest high amounts of fat and cholesterol without the body maintaining high levels in the blood. Unfortunately, this is not the case for everyone, and fat and cholesterol levels in the bloodstream must be closely monitored. Fat levels are measured by looking at triglycerides and lipoproteins. Lipoproteins are a complex structure made of fatty acids and proteins and are used to carry fat and cholesterol in the bloodstream. LDLs are used by the body to transport fats and cholesterol to the body tissues. These are the lipoproteins more likely to deposit cholesterol and fat into the arterial wall. HDLs carry fats and cholesterol to the liver to be broken down and used. These lipoproteins are more likely to remove fats and cholesterol from the deposits in the arterial walls. HDL levels can be increased by exercise.

The Nurses' Health Study, conducted by Harvard University, showed an association between the intake of hydrogenated fats (trans fats) and heart disease. The women who consumed high levels of foods that contained hydrogenated fats experienced a much greater risk for having a heart attack than did the women who consumed few hydrogenated fats. Harvard School of Public Health researchers have found that hydrogenated fats are responsible for the thousands of premature heart disease deaths in the United States every year. Trans fats have also been implicated in increasing the risk for type 2 diabetes.

If total serum cholesterol and LDL levels are found to be increased, the individual must modify the diet, and, if severe enough, drug therapy may be indicated. The percentage of calories from fat should be kept to less than 20% to 30% of total daily dietary intake, with less than a third of these coming from saturated fats. Cholesterol consumption should be less than 200 mg per day.

If a person experiences a myocardial infarction, it is important that the heart muscle be allowed to rest to facilitate proper healing. This includes bed rest initially, with a gradual progression to limited activity over about a 2-week period. Depending on severity of damage from the MI and overall health, the recovery period is individualized. Rehabilitation consists of cessation of smoking; control of hypertension; weight reduction through a low-fat, low-calorie diet; and a program of exercise. All help to improve myocardial function.

Cancer

Some substances ingested or inhaled are thought to be carcinogenic. For example, nitrites that are found in foods such as smoked ham or bacon are thought to cause cancer of the stomach and esophagus. Smoking tobacco, although not a food, has been implicated in cancers of the mouth, larynx, esophagus, and lungs. High fat in the diet has been shown to be associated with cancer of the breast, uterus, and colon.

High fiber in the diet may protect from colon cancer. Foods with vitamins A and C protect from cancer of the stomach, lung, and bladder. Fruits and vegetables, legumes, and foods with soy may protect from certain cancers.

Wise choices of foods from MyPlate, avoiding foods with known carcinogens, keeping weight under control, and practicing a healthy lifestyle will improve the quality and length of life.

Cancer is a disease that comes in a variety of forms. It generally means that the normal regulatory mechanisms within a cell have broken down. The result is that cells continue to grow in an unrestrained manner, diverting energy and nutrients from the patient's body to the cells' uncontrolled growth. There are many stages through which these cells may go, and they will go through them at varying rates. The ramifications of this new growth will vary depending on what types of cells are affected.

For these reasons, each cancer patient will have varying nutritional requirements. However, there are some generalities that can be made. First, there is definitely a need for increased calories. Because the new cancerous growth has the ability to divert nutrients to itself, the result is that the body receives fewer nutrients. It will then break down its own tissue. In addition, there is an increased need for nutrient intake to supply the immune system with the energy and nutrients it needs in its attempt to destroy the cancerous cells.

The patient who is receiving chemotherapy or radiation treatment has an even greater need for increased nutrients. These therapies are directed at killing cells that are rapidly dividing. Affected cells include not only the cancerous cell but also healthy cells such as those of the lining of the gastrointestinal tract and hair follicles. Increased nutrients are needed for repair and replacement of the lost cells, and protein levels in particular should be increased. Because of the disturbance of the gastrointestinal lining, digestion and absorption may also be decreased. It is important that the patient maintain as healthy a nutritional status as is possible rather than having to make up for nutritional deficiencies.

The patient may experience loss of appetite, as well as nausea and vomiting. There are several ways to cope with this. First, food should be made as appealing as possible. If the patient has difficulty swallowing, food can be liquefied in a food processor. Generally, food will be better tolerated if it is slightly chilled; extremes of temperature should be avoided. Several smaller meals may be easier to eat than three large meals.

If patients lose large amounts of weight because of worry or concern or as a result of chemotherapy and/or radiation, they may become cachectic. In such cases, a tube is passed into the patient's stomach or duodenum through the nose, or directly into the jejunum, and liquid feedings are given through the tube. This is referred to a parenteral nutrition or tube feeding. Another method for providing nutrition to a patient who is unable to take in necessary amounts of food is through an intravenous catheter inserted into the subclavian vein to the superior vena cava, known as total parenteral nutrition (TPN). Feedings via the catheter provide very good nutrition and can be given for prolonged periods.

DIET AND CULTURE

Medical assistants are likely to come into contact with patients from many different ethnic groups. Many of these patients will have diets based on traditional cultures, and some of the foods they eat, or the ways they combine foods, may be unfamiliar to the medical assistant.

Often, diets in other cultures are sensible, with foods chosen or combined to make up a complete protein. The medical assistant who has some knowledge of ethnic food choices can help reassure patients that the dietary changes they need to make are within the parameters of their own cultures. Table 34-6 presents some highlights of the food choices of different ethnic groups.

Vegetarian diets are fairly common around the globe, including in the United States. With a good variety of grains, vegetables, fruits, and dairy products, a vegetarian diet can supply an individual with all the required nutrients. Pernicious anemia, a disease caused by lack of cobalamin (vitamin B_{12}), is sometimes associated with vegetarian diets that do not contain enough animal proteins (see the section on vitamins in this chapter). One type of vegetarian, the vegan, does not eat any product associated with animals, including milk or eggs. This type of diet is particularly susceptible to nutritional deficiencies. Patients who are vegan or vegetarian need additional dietary discussion to assure that they are ingesting an adequate amount of amino acids and in the right combination to provide complete proteins. These complete proteins are necessary for cellular repair and maintenance of health.

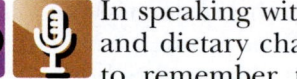In speaking with patients about diet and dietary changes, it is important to remember that patients choose their diets for a variety of reasons, including cultural, religious, or ethical beliefs. The medical assistant should respect the patient's reasons for following a certain diet while encouraging any modifications.

Table 34-6   Sample Food Choices of Various Cultural, Religious, and Ethnic Groups

Culture/Region/Group	Diet and Food Choices
Native American	It is thought that approximately half of the edible plants commonly eaten in the United States today originated with the Native Americans. Examples are corn, potatoes, squash, cranberries, pumpkins, peppers, beans, wild rice, and cocoa beans. In addition, they used wild fruits, game, and fish. Foods were commonly prepared as soups and stews, and also dried. The original Native American diets were probably more nutritionally adequate than their current diets, which frequently consist of too high a proportion of sweet and salty, snack-type, empty calorie foods. Native American diets today may be deficient in calcium, vitamins A and C, and riboflavin.
U.S. Southern	Hot breads such as corn bread and baking powder biscuits are common in the U.S. South because the wheat grown in the area does not make good quality yeast breads. Grits and rice are also popular carbohydrate foods. Favorite vegetables include sweet potatoes, squash, green beans, and lima beans. Green beans cooked with pork are commonly served. Watermelon, oranges, and peaches are popular fruits. Fried fish is served often, as are barbecued and stewed meats and poultry. There is a great deal of carbohydrate and fat in these diets and limited amounts of protein in some cases. Iron, calcium, and vitamins A and C may sometimes be deficient.

Table 34-6   Sample Food Choices of Various Cultural, Religious, and Ethnic Groups (*Continued*)

Culture/Region/Group	Diet and Food Choices
Mexican	Mexican food is a combination of Spanish and Native American foods. Beans, rice, chili peppers, tomatoes, and corn meal are favorites. Meat is often cooked with the vegetables as in chili con carne. Corn meal is used in a variety of ways to make tortillas and tamales, which serve as bread. The combination of beans and corn makes a complete protein. Although tortillas filled with cheese (called enchiladas) provide some calcium, the use of milk should be encouraged. Additional green and yellow vegetables and vitamin C–rich foods would also improve these diets.
Puerto Rican	Rice is the basic carbohydrate food in Puerto Rican diets. Vegetables commonly used include beans, plantains, tomatoes, and peppers. Bananas, pineapple, mangoes, and papayas are popular fruits. Favorite meats are chicken, beef, and pork. Milk is not used as much as would be desirable from the nutritional point of view.
Italian	Pastas with various tomato or fish sauces and cheese are popular Italian foods. Fish and highly seasoned foods are common to Southern Italian cuisine, whereas meat and root vegetables are common to northern Italy. The eggs, cheese, tomatoes, green vegetables, and fruits common to Italian diets provide excellent sources of many nutrients, but additional milk and meat would improve the diet.
Northern and Western European	Northern and Western European diets are similar to those of the U.S. Midwest, but with a greater use of dark breads, potatoes, and fish, and fewer green vegetable salads. Beef and pork are popular, as are various cooked vegetables, breads, cakes, and dairy products.
Central European	Citizens of Central Europe obtain the greatest portion of their calories from potatoes and grain, especially rye and buck wheat. Pork is a popular meat. Cabbage cooked in many ways is a popular vegetable, as are carrots, onions, and turnips. Eggs and dairy products are used abundantly.
Middle Eastern	Grains, wheat, and rice provide energy in these diets. Chickpeas in the form of hummus are popular. Lamb and yogurt are commonly used, as are cabbage, grape leaves, eggplant, tomatoes, dates, olives, and figs. Black, very sweet (Turkish) coffee is a popular beverage.
Chinese	The Chinese diet is varied. Rice is the primary energy food and is used in place of bread. Foods are generally cut into small pieces. Vegetables are lightly cooked, and the cooking water is saved for future use. Soybeans are used in many ways, and eggs and pork are commonly served. Soy sauce is extensively used, but it is salty and could present a problem with patients on low-salt diets. Tea is a common beverage, but milk is not. This diet may be low in fat.
Japanese	Japanese diets include rice, soybean paste and curd, vegetables, fruits, and fish. Food is frequently served tempura style, which means fried. Soy sauce (shoyu) and tea are commonly used. Current Japanese diets have been greatly influenced by Western culture.
Southeast Asian	Many Indians are vegetarians who use eggs and dairy products. Rice, peas, and beans are frequently served. Spices, especially curry, are popular. Indian meals are not typically served in courses as Western meals are. They generally consist of one course with many dishes.
Thai, Vietnamese, Laotian, and Cambodian	Rice, curries, vegetables, and fruit are popular in Thailand, Vietnam, Laos, and Cambodia. Meat, chicken, and fish are used in small amounts. The wok (a deep, round fry pan) is used for sautéing many foods. A salty sauce made from fermented fish is commonly used.

continues

Table 34-6   Sample Food Choices of Various Cultural, Religious, and Ethnic Groups (*Continued*)

Culture/Region/Group	Diet and Food Choices
Jewish	Interpretations of the Jewish dietary laws vary. Those who adhere to the Orthodox view consider tradition important and always observe the dietary laws. Foods prepared according to these laws are called kosher. Conservative Jews are inclined to observe the rules only at home. Reform Jews consider their dietary laws to be essentially ceremonial and thus minimize their significance. Essentially the laws require the following: • Slaughtering must be done by a qualified person, in a prescribed manner. The meat or poultry must be drained of blood, first by severing the jugular vein and carotid artery, then by soaking in brine before cooking. • Meat or meat products may not be prepared with milk or milk products. • The dishes used in the preparation and serving of meat dishes must be kept separate from those used for dairy foods. • A specified time, 6 hours, must elapse between consumption of meat and milk. • The mouth must be rinsed after eating fish and before eating meat. • There are prescribed fast days—Passover Week, Yom Kippur, and Feast of Purim. • No cooking is done on the Sabbath—from sundown Friday to sundown Saturday. These laws forbid the eating of: • The flesh of animals without cloven (split) hooves or that do not chew their cud • Hind quarters of any animal • Shellfish or fish without scales or fins • Fowl that are birds of prey • Creeping things and insects • Leavened (contains ingredients that cause it to rise) bread during the Passover Generally, the food served is rich. Fresh smoked and salted fish and chicken are popular, as are noodles, egg, and flour dishes. These diets can be deficient in fresh vegetables and milk.
Roman Catholic	Although the dietary restrictions of the Roman Catholic religion have been liberalized, meat is not allowed its adherents on Ash Wednesday and Fridays during Lent.
Eastern Orthodox	Followers of this religion include Christians from the Middle East, Russia, and Greece. Although interpretations of the dietary laws vary, meat, poultry, fish, and dairy products are restricted on Wednesdays and Fridays and during Lent and Advent.
Seventh Day Adventist	Generally, Seventh Day Adventists are ovo-lacto vegetarians, meaning they use milk products and eggs, but no meat, fish, or poultry. They may also use nuts, legumes, and meat analogues (substitutes) made from soybeans. They consider coffee, tea, and alcohol to be harmful.
Mormon (Latter Day Saints)	The only dietary restriction observed by Mormons is the prohibition of coffee, tea, and alcoholic beverages.
Islamic	Adherents of Islam are called Muslims. Their dietary laws prohibit the use of pork and alcohol, and other meats must be slaughtered according to specific laws. During the month of Ramadan, Muslims do not eat or drink during daylight hours.
Hindu	To the Hindus, all life is sacred, and small animals contain the souls of ancestors. Consequently, Hindus are usually vegetarians. They do not use eggs because they represent life.
Vegetarians	There are several vegetarian diets. The common factor among them is that they do not include red meat. Some include eggs, some fish, some milk, and some even poultry. When carefully planned, these diets can be nutritious. They can contribute to a reduction of obesity, high blood pressure, heart disease, some cancers, and possibly diabetes. They must be carefully planned so they include all needed nutrients. Ovo-lacto vegetarians use dairy products and eggs but no meat, poultry, or fish. Lacto-vegetarians use dairy products but no meat, poultry, or eggs.

Table 34-6   Sample Food Choices of Various Cultural, Religious, and Ethnic Groups (*Continued*)

Culture/Region/Group	Diet and Food Choices
Vegans	Vegans avoid all animal foods. They use soybeans, chickpeas, and meat analogues made from soybeans. It is important that their meals be carefully planned to include appropriate combinations of the nonessential amino acids to provide the needed amino acids. For example, beans served with corn or rice, or peanuts eaten with wheat, are better in such combinations than any of them would be if eaten alone. Vegans can show deficiencies of calcium; zinc; vitamins A, D, and B_{12}; and, of course, proteins.
Zen macrobiotic diets	The macrobiotic diet is a system of 10 diet plans developed from Zen Buddhism. Adherents progress from the lower number diet to the higher, gradually giving up foods in the following order: desserts, salads, fruits, animal foods, soups, and ultimately vegetables, until only cereals—usually brown rice—are consumed. Beverages are kept to a minimum, and only organic foods are used. Foods are grouped as Yang (male) or Yin (female). A ratio of 5:1 Yang to Yin is considered important. Most macrobiotic diets are nutritionally inadequate. As the adherents give up foods according to plans, their diets become increasingly inadequate. These diets can be especially dangerous because avid adherents promise medical cures from the diets that cannot be attained, and thus medical treatment may be delayed when needed.

© Cengage Learning 2014

PROCEDURE 34-1
Provide Instruction for Health Maintenance and Disease Prevention

PURPOSE:

To instruct patients about how to exercise more responsibility for and take control of their health in order to extend their lives and enjoy healthy years.

With the provider's permission, medical assistants have many opportunities on a daily basis to educate patients about ways to stay healthy and reduce the risk of disease. Patient education boxes throughout the textbook relate specific behaviors patients can adopt to prevent diseases and measures they can take to preserve health.

EQUIPMENT/SUPPLIES

Discussion
DVDs
Videos
Print material
Authentic Web-based interactive information
Community resources directories
Seminars
Classes (self-directed and self-paced)

PROCEDURE STEPS:

1. *Introduce yourself and identify patient.*
2. Gather materials to be utilized during the educational session for health maintenance and disease prevention.
3. Select a quiet and private are to begin the instruction.
4. Assess the patient's learning style and preference. *Involve the patient's support system.* RATIONALE: The patient's age, physical limitations, and learning preferences need to be taken into consideration by the medical assistant. The patient's family will learn along with the patient and provide instruction and encouragement to the patient at home.
5. *Speaking at the patient's level of understanding,* provide information to the patient regarding a specific illness, medical management, health maintenance, and/or disease prevention. Instruct patient to:
   - Schedule regular screenings for illness as is age appropriate (i.e., yearly examinations, Pap smear, mammogram, occult blood testing, colonoscopy, urinalysis, EKG, CXR, anemia testing, chemistry profiles, hearing and vision testing)
   - Avoid tobacco
   - Exercise at least 30 minutes a day most days of the week
   - Maintain a balanced diet (www.choosemyplate.gov)
   - Practice safety to prevent injuries (make sure smoke detectors work, wear seat belts, do not drink and drive)
   - Control weight, blood pressure, and cholesterol

continues

Procedure 34-1 (continued)

- Watch sun exposure and use sun block factor of at least SPF 30 all year
- Keep vaccine immunization current
- Practice food safety by preparing food with clean hands and on clean surfaces

6. Educate patients who do not have a home computer regarding access at the public library. With the prevalence of smart phones, and other electronics and wifi widely available, there are many ways to access the internet for information on health maintenance.

7. Some examples of websites that could be useful are:

- General health: http://www.healthfinder.com
- Cancer: http://www.cancer.org

- Osteoporosis: http://www.osteo.org
- Nutrition: http://www.usda.gov or http://www.fda.gov
- Alcohol and drug abuse: http://niaa.nih.gov
- Depression: http://nimh.nih.gov/health/topics/depression/index/html
- Heart and lung health: http://www.nhlbi.nih.gov
- Product safety: http://cpsc.gov

8. Accurately document in the patient's chart or electronic medical record indicating date, time, topic of education, demonstration of patient understanding and planned follow-up.

CASE STUDY 34-1

Refer to the scenario at the beginning of the chapter.

CASE STUDY REVIEW

1. What aspects of nutrition must be considered when Becky Slack, RMA (AMT), is considering the nutritional needs of an adolescent?

2. What are key ways that Becky can include parents in the educational process?

3. What guidelines should Becky follow when encouraging adolescents to incorporate exercise in their nutritional plans?

CASE STUDY 34-2

Anita Ferguson is a new patient at Inner City Health Care. She is a 16-year-old girl who is 4 months pregnant and came to the urgent care center only a couple of weeks ago. After Wanda Slawson, CMA (AAMA), took Anita's medical history, and after Anita was examined by the provider, Wanda set aside time to answer any questions Anita might have about her pregnancy. Anita is obviously scared; she wants the baby, but she does not want her life to change. According to the history, Anita has lost a few pounds in the last 2 weeks.

CASE STUDY REVIEW

1. What patient education can Wanda provide to alert Anita to the importance of diet and weight gain during pregnancy?

2. What foods should Wanda encourage Anita to eat?

3. If Anita resists Wanda's suggestions and has not gained any weight by the next visit, how should Wanda proceed?

CASE STUDY 34-3

Dr. Lewis prescribed an 1800-calorie ADA diet for Mrs. Johnson.

CASE STUDY REVIEW

1. Describe what is included in an 1800-calorie ADA diet.

2. Describe the patient education you would use to help Mrs. Johnson understand the diet and to help her reach her goal of improved health.

SUMMARY

Seven types of nutrients are required by the body for maintenance of good health. Carbohydrates, fats, and proteins provide energy for the body. Vitamins, minerals, fiber, and water cannot provide energy but are responsible for many vital processes within the body.

Some individuals take herbal supplements. Making the provider aware of which supplements are being taken is an important responsibility of the medical assistant.

Nutritional needs change at various points in the life cycle. During pregnancy, lack of nutrients can be detrimental to the development of the fetus and the health of the expectant mother. The need for nutrients is great during infancy and childhood, with the greatest need for total nutrients occurring during adolescence. During adulthood, the requirement for calories decreases. With the decrease in basal metabolism that occurs with aging, the requirement for calories decreases even more.

At times of disease, the diet of the individual must be modified to help relieve stress put on the body by the disease, to give energy to fight the disease, and, in cases where the disease is diet related, to decrease the severity of the disease.

It is important to have adequate nutritional intake during every stage of life. The healthier one is, the better one feels and enjoys a good quality of life. Nutritional status should be examined and adjustments made if necessary with the goal of helping patients maintain a healthy body.

STUDY FOR SUCCESS

To reinforce your knowledge and skills of information presented in this chapter:

- Review the *Key Terms*
- Role-play with other students to apply attributes of professionalism pertinent to this chapter.
- Consider the *Case Studies* and discuss your conclusions
- Answer the questions in the *Certification Review*
- Apply your knowledge by completing the *Activities* in the *Study Guide* and the *Games and Quizzes* in the StudyWARE [StudyWARE] software on the *Premium Website*
- Perform the *Procedure* using the *Competency Assessment Checklist* in the *Competency Manual*
- Practice your problem-solving skills with the *Critical Thinking Challenge 3.0* on the *Premium Website*

Additional resources for this chapter include:

- Module 27 of the *Medical Assisting Learning Lab*
- *CourseMate for Delmar's Comprehensive Medical Assisting*
- *WebTutor for Delmar's Comprehensive Medical Assisting*

CERTIFICATION

1. The transfer of nutrients from the gastrointestinal tract into the bloodstream is:
   a. ingestion
   b. digestion
   c. absorption
   d. elimination
2. Fats are considered a(n):
   a. mineral
   b. vitamin
   c. energy nutrient
   d. fiber
3. The total of all chemical and physical changes that take place in the body is called:
   a. homeostasis
   b. metabolism
   c. catalyst
   d. an antioxidant
4. What is the significance for the provider in determining the patient's use of herbal supplements?
   a. The FDA has authority over these dietary supplements, therefore they are safe.
   b. They are unsafe if bought in a supermarket.
   c. They may interact with over-the-counter and prescription medications.
   d. They are not considered medicines. It is not significant to inform the provider.
5. Another name for vitamin C is:
   a. tocopherol
   b. carotene
   c. biotin
   d. ascorbic acid

6. There are three energy nutrients. They are:
   a. vitamins, minerals, and herbal supplements
   b. fat, carbohydrates, and protein
   c. cholesterol, starch, and vitamins
   d. sugar, starch, and fats
7. Fat-soluble vitamins include:
   a. A, D, E, and K
   b. C, B, and Calcium
   c. A, C, and B
   d. none of the above
8. Nutrition labels provide the following information:
   a. vitamin content
   b. protein content
   c. fat content
   d. all of the above
9. An antioxidant serves to:
   a. reduce the amount of fat in our diet
   b. remove free radicals from our bodies
   c. increase the amount of energy produced
   d. impair overall health
10. During which phase of life do humans triple their body weight?
   a. Infancy
   b. Childhood
   c. Adolescence
   d. Adulthood

REFERENCES/BIBLIOGRAPHY

Centers for Disease Control and Prevention. (2007). *Overweight and obesity*. Retrieved May 24, 2007, from http://www.cdc.gov

Centers for Disease Control and Prevention. (n.d.). *Childhood Obesity Facts*. Retrieved April 8, 2012, from http://www.cdc.gov/healthyyouth/obesity/facts.htm

Ephedra. (2007). Retrieved May 25, 2007, from http://www.wikipedia.org/wiki/ephedra

Harrison, J. E., & Schultz, J. (1976). Studies on the chlorinating activity of myeloperoxidase. *Journal of Biological Chemistry, 251,* 1371–1374.

Mayo Clinic Staff. (n.d.). Healthy diet: End the guesswork with these nutrition guidelines. Retrieved April 8, 2012, from http://www.mayoclinic.com/health/healthy-diet/NU00200

Parcell, S. (2002). Sulfur in human nutrition and applications in medicine. *Alternative Medicine Review, 7*(1), 22–44.

Richardson, M. (2004). Calcium absorption in post-menopausal women. *Harvard Women's Health Watch, 5,* 1–3.

Roth, R. A. (2007). *Nutrition and diet therapy.* (9th ed.). Clifton Park, NY: Delmar Cengage Learning.

Spratto, G. R., & Woods, A. L. (2004). *PDR nurse's drug handbook.* Clifton Park, NY: Delmar Cengage Learning.

Taber's cyclopedic medical dictionary. (20th ed.). (2006). Philadelphia: F. A. Davis.

CHAPTER 35

Basic Pharmacology

OUTLINE

Uses of Medications

Research and Development

Drug Names

History and Sources of Drugs
- Plant Sources
- Animal Sources
- Mineral Sources
- Herbal Supplements
- Synthetic Drugs
- Genetically Engineered Pharmaceuticals

Drug Regulations and Legal Classifications of Drugs
- Controlled Substance Act of 1970

Prescription Drugs

Nonprescription Drugs

Proper Disposal of Drugs

Administer, Prescribe, Dispense

Drug References and Standards
- How to Use the PDR
- Other Reference Sources

Classification of Drugs

Principal Actions of Drugs
- Factors That Affect Drug Action
- Undesirable Actions of Drugs

Drug Routes

Forms of Drugs
- Liquid Preparations
- Solid and Semisolid Preparations
- Other Drug Delivery Systems

Storage and Handling of Medications

Emergency Medications and Supplies
- Bioterrorism

Drug Abuse

LEARNING OUTCOMES

1. Define, spell, and pronounce the key terms as presented in the glossary.
2. Recall five medical uses for drugs.
3. Describe three types of drug names and give an example, for one drug, of all three names.
4. List five sources of drugs.
5. Describe the federal Food, Drug, and Cosmetic Act and the Controlled Substances Act of 1970.
6. Name the five controlled substance schedules and describe appropriate storage of the substances.
7. Define the law in terms of administering, prescribing, and dispensing drugs.
8. Describe how to use the four most commonly used sections of the *Physician's Desk Reference* (PDR).
9. Describe the principal actions of drugs and three undesirable reactions.
10. Identify the classifications of medications.
11. Describe routes of drug administration and drug forms.
12. Describe handling and storing of drugs.
13. List emergency drugs and supplies.
14. Recall commonly abused drugs and describe their physical and emotional effects.
15. Critique the legal role and responsibilities of the medical assistant.
16. Analyze the professionalism questions and apply them to this chapter's content.

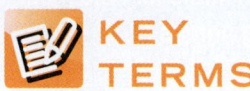

KEY TERMS

absorption

abuse

administer

anaphylaxis

bioequivalent

biopharmaceuticals

biotransformation

contraindication

controlled substances

dispense

distribution

elimination

pharmacogenomics

pharmacology

pharmazooticals

prescribe

pruritus

transdermal

urticaria

ATTRIBUTES OF PROFESSIONALISM

Communication
- Did you speak at the patient's level of understanding?

Presentation
- Did your actions attend to both the psychological and the physiological aspects of the patient's illness or condition?

Competency
- Did you pay attention to detail?
- Were you knowledgeable and accountable?
- Did you recognize the importance of local, state, and federal legislation and regulations in the practice setting?

Initiative
- Did you seek out opportunities to expand your knowledge base?
- Did you direct the patient to other resources when necessary or helpful, with the approval of the provider?

Integrity
- Did you work within your scope of practice?
- Did you immediately report any error you had made?
- Did you report situations that were harmful or illegal?
- Did you maintain your moral and ethical standards?
- Did you do "the right thing" even when no one was observing?

SCENARIO

Claire Bloom, CMA (AAMA), is the lead Medical Assistant for Dr. Jim Hoback, a busy cardiologist. Due to the many look-alike and sound-alike drugs, Ms. Bloom knows that it is very important to have patients bring in their prescription bottles in order to obtain an accurate medication history. She has been assigned the responsibility of developing a Policy and Procedure to be approved by the provider outlining the appropriate steps for all staff members when taking a medication history. This need for a procedure was identified after a patient reported that he was taking the medication amiloride when in fact the medication that was prescribed was amlodipine. This is an example of one of the drugs on the Institute for Safe Medication Practices list of confused drug names.

INTRODUCTION

Pharmacology is the study of drugs, the science that is concerned with the history, origin, sources, physical and chemical properties, uses, and effects of drugs on living organisms. Medical assistants in the ambulatory care setting need to understand basic pharmacology, including the uses, sources, forms, and delivery routes of drugs; they must know and be able to implement the intent of the law regarding controlled substances and other medications; and they must have a knowledge of drug classifications and actions to be able to caution patients who are taking prescription or nonprescription drugs. In addition, the medical assistant must be able to educate patients about a drug's intended purpose and the correct way to take the drug for maximum effectiveness.

This chapter provides an overview of pharmacology; it is considered a review for medical assistants who have had a formal course in the subject. Information on dosage, calculation, and medication administration can be found in Chapter 36.

USES OF MEDICATIONS

A drug is defined as a medicinal substance that may alter or modify the functions of a living organism. There are five medical uses for drugs:

- *Therapeutic.* Used in the treatment of a condition to relieve symptoms. An example is an antihistamine that may be used in the treatment of an allergy.
- *Diagnostic.* Used in conjunction with radiology and other diagnostic imaging procedures to allow the provider to pinpoint the location of a disease process. An example is dye tablets used in the X-ray study of the gallbladder.
- *Curative.* Used to kill or remove the causative agent of a disease. An example is an antibiotic.

- *Replacement.* Used to replace substances normally found in the body. Hormones and vitamins are examples of replacement drugs.

- *Preventive or Prophylactic.* Used to ward off or lessen the severity of a disease. Examples are immunizing agents such as vaccines.

RESEARCH AND DEVELOPMENT

It can take up to 15 years for a drug to make it to market. The process begins with scientists researching an illness to begin to understand the mechanics of the disease. The goal is to understand the process of change from health to illness from the level of the cellular components. These identified areas are referred to as targets. From this information, the next step is to begin to design chemical compounds and **biopharmaceuticals** that will interrupt the disease process at the selected target.

The average cost to research and develop an effective drug is between $800 million and $1 billion. Five to ten thousand compounds may enter the pipeline for one successful drug to enter the market. For up to 20 years, the new drug is protected by a drug patent. This patent will not allow any other company to make or market the drug. Delaying the transition to generic production allows the originating pharmaceutical company to recoup the investment in research and development to develop the drug.

In 2003, the Human Genome Project was completed. In a joint effort, the U.S. Department of Energy and the National Institutes of Health identified 20,000–25,000 genes in human DNA. The sequences in the 3 billion base pairs were also determined. This information was stored in databases that could allow access to these technologies by the private sector, such as pharmaceutical companies. By discovering the pharmacogenomics, drug companies can focus on the creation of drugs specifically for genome targets.

Pharmacogenomics is the study of the response of the body to various chemical compounds based on an individual's genetic inheritance. This knowledge could allow medications to be tailored to each individual and his or her disease process in the future. There is also potential for the creation of more effective medications. An added benefit is that the provider could prescribe the right drug the first time for a patient. Dosing could be customized more appropriately than the current weight-based method.

Utilizing **pharmacogenomics**, pharmaceutical companies could reduce the number of potential chemical compounds that are researched and get

an effective drug to market more rapidly and at less cost. Pharmacogenomics is in limited use today. However, the field is rapidly advancing.

DRUG NAMES

Most drugs have three types of names: chemical, generic, and trade or brand name.

- *The chemical name* describes the drug's molecular structure and identifies its chemical structure.
- *The generic name* is the drug's official name and is assigned to the drug by the United States Adopted Names Council. A generic drug can be manufactured by more than one pharmaceutical company. When this is the case, each company markets the drug under its own unique trade or brand name. Generic names begin with a lowercase letter.
- *A trade* or *brand name* is registered by the U.S. Patent and Trademark Office and is approved by the U.S. Food and Drug Administration (FDA). The ® symbol following a drug's trade or brand name indicates that the name is registered and protected for 17 years. No other manufacturer can make or sell the drug during that time. Once the patent expires, any manufacturer can sell the drug under its generic name or a new trade name. The original trade name cannot be reused. The brand name begins with a capital letter.

Example:

Chemical name: 1, 4:3, 6-dian hydrosorbitol-2, 5 dinitrate
Generic name: isosorbide dinitrate
Trade/Brand name: Sorbitrate®

When providers prescribe a drug, they may use either the generic or trade name. It is not uncommon for providers to prescribe the generic form of a drug because it is usually less costly for the patient. To reduce costs, some insurance companies pay for only generic brands. Sometimes, providers specify drugs by their trade names. Some states allow patients to request that their pharmacist dispense the generic drug equivalent unless the provider has specified that the drug be dispensed by its trade name.

The U.S. Food and Drug Administration (FDA) maintains strict regulations regarding generic drugs. In order for a copy of a brand-name drug to be allowed to enter the market, generic drugs must have the same high quality, strength, purity, and stability as the innovator drug. Generics must be **bioequivalent** to the original. In some states, a pharmacist may select a generic form of a drug if not specifically directed otherwise by the provider. Generic and trade name drugs have the same chemical composition and must adhere to identical FDA standards; therefore, according to most state laws, they can be used interchangeably. The drug label reflects the drug products dispensed.

HISTORY AND SOURCES OF DRUGS

 Drugs prepared from roots, herbs, bark, and other forms of plant life are among the earliest known pharmaceuticals. Their origin can be traced back to primitive cultures, where they were first used to evoke magical powers and to drive out evil spirits. Having discovered that certain plants were pharmacologically useful, a search was started for sources of drugs.

Today this search continues. In addition to plants, drugs are derived from animals and minerals and are produced in laboratories using chemical, biochemical, and biotechnologic processes.

Plant Sources

The leaves, roots, stems, or fruit of certain plants may contain medicinal properties. For example, the dried leaf of the foxglove plant (*Digitalis purpurea*) is a source of digitalis, a cardiac glycoside used in the treatment of certain heart conditions.

Herbals fit into this plant source category. The disadvantage of many natural herbals on the market today is that some drugs derived from plants may not be standardized. In any given crop, there may be plants that are more or less potent than their neighboring plants. This lack of consistency is related to the amount of sunshine and water a particular plant receives, as well as the nutrients in the soil. Another disadvantage of natural plant drugs is the pesticides that may be present. These may be man-made pesticides applied to the plants or taken up by the plant through the environment (soil, water, and air); they may also be natural pesticides originating from the plant itself to defend itself from molds, insects, and other threats. These pesticides all pose biologic threats to our chemical and biologic functions. These foreign chemicals can be interpreted by our bodies as irritants, free radicals, antigens, and antagonists. For these reasons, patients should be cautioned to purchase only reputable, standardized, natural herbal products.

Animal Sources

A few drugs are obtained from tissues such as the adrenal glands of animals. Drugs of this type are referred to as **pharmazooticals**. Examples of drugs obtained from animals are adrenaline and cortisone, extracted from the adrenal glands of animals. Adrenaline is used for allergic reactions and cortisone is an anti-inflammatory. Premarin® is another example. It is derived from urine produced by pregnant mares. It is used for treating menopausal symptoms in some women.

Some drugs are derived from unusual animal sources. Captopril®, an ACE inhibitor that is widely utilized to treat hypertension, is derived from a chemical substance found in the Brazilian arrowhead viper. ARC, a potent drug used to treat leukemia, is derived from the Caribbean sponge.

Mineral Sources

Some naturally occurring mineral substances are used in medicine in a highly purified form. One such mineral is sulfur, which has been used as a key ingredient in certain bacteriostatic drugs. It is now prepared synthetically and used in the treatment of urinary and intestinal tract infections.

Lithium is used to treat episodes of mania associated with a diagnosis of bipolar disease. Lithium is a mineral that is present in some rocks and in the sea.

Herbal Supplements

With the increased interest in alternative or complementary medicine, many patients and some practitioners use herbal products for treatment, prophylaxis, and maintenance of health and care of disease. *Phytomedicine* is the term used to describe the use of plants to promote optimum health.

Native cultures since ancient times had great respect for their medicine men and women because they knew about plants and herbs for medicinal purposes. Such diseases and conditions as cardiac arrhythmia, pain, blood thinning, digestive upsets, and increased urinary output (diuresis) have been successfully treated with herbal medicine.

European providers use herbal medicines routinely in their practices and have had classes on the topic throughout medical school. In the United States, it was not until 1974 that the FDA passed an act known as the Dietary Supplement Health and Education Act (DSHEA). Under the act the FDA examines any dietary supplement, such as an herbal product, and may remove it from the market if it presents a significant or unreasonable risk for illness or injury when used according to its labeling or under ordinary conditions of use.

In accordance with DSHEA, the FDA gathers and thoroughly reviews evidence about the pharmacology of a product, uses peer-review scientific literature on safety and effectiveness, examines adverse event reports, and includes public comments for information about associated health risks.

There is no efficacy, or proof of claim, oversight of herbal supplements by the FDA. Herbal supplements do not have to obtain the approval of the FDA prior to marketing. They are classified as dietary supplements. However, the FDA does monitor the quality of manufacturing to ensure that these compounds meet quality standards and do not include harmful substances such as pesticides.

Self-medication with herbal products is less in the United States than worldwide, but sales in the United States have been increasing yearly. There has been an abundance of interest by the public in herbal products because of the media attention given to them and their benefits.

Many providers combine herbal products (together with nutrition) in their practice(s), and certain herbal treatments have become part of the practitioner's treatment regimen.

Some examples of herbs and their uses are as follows: cascara—laxative; feverfew—headaches; garlic—antibacterial; licorice—gastritis, cough, menopause; St. John's wort—depression and anxiety; and saw palmetto—prostate health.

There are risks associated with self-medication with herbal products. Patients need to be informed that taking certain medications together with herbal products can produce dangerous interactions. It is important for you as the medical assistant to gather information about all medications, prescriptions, over-the-counter medications, and herbals. Pregnant patients should inform their provider about what they are taking and should be cautioned about possible harm to the fetus (see Chapter 26). It is important to remember that any medication and any herb can cause an allergic reaction and have side effects.

The dietary supplement ephedra, also known as ma huang, has been prohibited from being sold since April 2004 because, according to the DSHEA of 1994, ephedra presented an unreasonable risk for illness and injury. The herbal supplement had been promoted for use in weight loss and control and for enhancing performance in sports activities. Evidence showed modest effectiveness for weight loss with no clear health benefit. However, it was confirmed that, in many instances, the substance increased blood pressure and caused tachycardia, chest pain, myocardial infarction (MI), cerebral vascular accidents (CVA), seizures, psychosis, and death.

Once a dietary supplement is on the market and proves to be hazardous to the health of Americans, the FDA can file a claim against the manufacturer and issue a warning or have the supplement removed from the market. In 2005, the ban on ephedra was lifted because it had been challenged in court, and the judge ruled for the company that manufactures ephedra. During 2005 and 2006, ephedra was sold again. In August 2006, the FDA's ban on all ephedra and ephedra-like drugs was upheld. It now is illegal in the United States. In October 2006, the manufacturing company filed

PATIENT EDUCATION

If you want to use herbal therapy, you should find a qualified herbalist and work with him or her and your practitioner. Herbal products are not regulated or standardized by an agency or organization (see previous section for information about DSHEA). Report at once any symptoms that seem unusual. Herbal products should be used for the shortest amount of time needed to obtain results. Keeping track of herbs taken, for what purpose they are being taken, and the effect on symptom control is important and provides information about those products that are helpful and those that are not. Journals, newsletters, and the Internet can provide information about herbal medicine. These publications can be explored for information and are a valuable resource. Relevant publications include *HerbalGram, Phytomedicine, Alternative Medicine Alert,* and the *Journal of Alternative and Complementary Medicine.*

a petition for a rehearing on the issue. Ephedra remains illegal and is likely to remain so. Congress is rewriting laws so it will be easier for the FDA to take action and ban substances it believes are harmful. In 2007, the United States Supreme Court declined a rehearing of this ban.

Synthetic Drugs

Synthetic drugs are artificially prepared in pharmaceutical laboratories. By combining various chemicals, scientists can produce compounds that are identical to a natural drug or create entirely new substances. An advantage of synthetic drugs over natural is the ability to standardize doses. Thousands of drugs are now produced synthetically. Examples are Motrin® (ibuprofen), Feldene® (piroxicam), and Prilosec® (omeprazole).

Genetically Engineered Pharmaceuticals

Scientists are now capable of creating new strains of bacteria using a technique known as gene splicing. Through this process, hybrid forms of life have been created that benefit human beings by providing an alternative source of drugs, such as Humulin® (insulin) for the diabetic patient and interferon for use in the treatment of cancer. These drugs can be manufactured in large quantities; thus, they are less expensive than natural substances.

DRUG REGULATIONS AND LEGAL CLASSIFICATIONS OF DRUGS

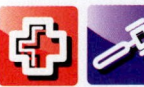 Qualified medical practitioners who prescribe, dispense, or administer drugs must comply with federal and state laws. The laws govern the manufacture, sale, possession, administration, dispensing, and prescribing of drugs. All drugs available for legal use are controlled by the federal Food, Drug, and Cosmetic Act. The law protects the public by ensuring the purity, strength, and composition of foods, drugs, and cosmetics. It also prohibits the movement in interstate commerce of altered and misbranded food, drugs, devices, and cosmetics. Enforcement of the act is the responsibility of the FDA, which is part of the Department of Health and Human Services (DHHS).

Controlled Substance Act of 1970

One category of drugs—those with potential for abuse or addiction—is regulated by the Controlled Substance Act of 1970. It controls the manufacture, importation, compounding, selling, dealing in, and giving away of drugs that have the potential for abuse and addiction. The drugs are known as controlled substances and include heroin and cocaine and their derivatives, other narcotics, stimulants, and depressants. The Drug Enforcement Agency (DEA) of the U.S. Justice Department monitors and enforces the act, which is also known as the Comprehensive Drug Abuse Prevention and Control Act. Under federal law, providers who prescribe, administer, or dispense controlled substances must register with the DEA and renew their registration as required by state law (Form DEA 224).

Applications for registration are available online (http://www.deadiversion.usdoj.gov). A licensed provider is issued a registration that must be renewed at regular intervals. The renewal form is sent approximately 2 months before the expiration date.

Controlled Substances Schedules. Controlled substances are classified according to five schedules:

- *Schedule I* specifies drugs that have a high potential for abuse and are not accepted for medical use within the United States. Examples are heroin, lysergic acid diethylamide (LSD), and marijuana.

- *Schedule II* drugs include those that also have a high abuse potential but have an accepted medical use within the United States. Examples are amphetamines and cocaine. Because of their high potential for abuse, a special DEA form must be used to order these drugs. The form is not necessary for Schedule III and Schedule IV drugs. A written prescription is required for Schedule II drugs and the prescription cannot be renewed. Examples of Schedule II drugs are morphine, codeine, Ritalin, and Percocet.

- *Schedule III* drugs have a low-to-moderate potential for physical dependence, yet have a high potential for psychological dependency. Some examples are barbiturates and various drug combinations containing codeine and paregoric. Prescriptions for Schedule III drugs can be either written or oral. They can be refilled, but only five times within 6 months. Schedule III drugs are accepted for medical use in the United States.

- *Schedule IV* drugs have a lower potential for abuse and have an accepted use in the United States. Examples of these drugs include chloral hydrate and diazepam. Prescriptions for Schedule IV drugs may include refills, but refills are limited to five times within 6 months.

- *Schedule V* drugs have the lowest abuse potential of controlled substances. Some examples from this schedule are Lomotil® and Donnagel®. Some drugs from Schedule V may include refills, but refills are limited to five times within 6 months.

On occasion, the DEA will reclassify drugs and move them from one schedule to another.

So that they can be readily identified, controlled substances are labeled with a large C with a Roman numeral inside it to indicate from which schedule the drug has come; for example, C_{II} represents a Schedule II drug.

The provider's DEA number must appear on each prescription for controlled substances.

A copy of the federal law and a complete list of controlled substances and their schedules are available from any DEA office or online.

Storage of Controlled Substances.
Federal law requires that all controlled substances be kept separate from other drugs. They must be stored in a well-constructed metal box or compartment that has a double lock. Controlled substances must be protected from possible misuse and abuse, and persons who administer controlled substances must record them in a separate record book. The record must be maintained on a daily basis and kept for a minimum of 2 to 3 years, depending on state laws. Patient name, address, date of administration of the controlled substance, drug name, dose, and route and method of administration must be included in the record.

EHR Record keeping applies only to persons who administer or dispense controlled substances. Record-keeping data can be stored electronically.

Controlled substances (Schedule II) stored and used on the premises must be counted at the end of each workday, verified by two individuals for accuracy of count, and recorded on an audit sheet. An inventory record of Schedule II drugs must be submitted to the DEA every 2 years.

Because of the increase in clinic drug theft and substance abuse, as well as the stringent federal laws that apply to storing, dispensing, and administration of controlled substances, many clinics do not keep controlled substances on the premises. However, agencies that do have controlled substances on the premises must comply with the DEA disposal policy.

Controlled Substance Disposal Policy (per DEA).
The DEA Disposal Policy for Controlled Substances requires that controlled substances be accounted for when they are disposed of. There are a variety of companies that contact with the DEA and will dispose of expired or unused controlled substances. Certain forms (DEA Form 41) must be completed, and the provider must have a current certificate of registration (DEA Form 222) with the DEA. Records of disposed controlled substances must be kept for 2 years. Application forms are completed and signed by the provider. A copy of the provider's DEA certificate of registration is included and sent to Universal Solutions (controlled substances are not sent at this time). Shipping instructions from Universal Solutions will be sent along with a label. Follow the instructions provided and ship to Universal Solutions. The company will confirm receipt of the material and its eventual destruction. Copies of application and confirmation of destruction must be sent to the DEA. Applications for forms for disposal of controlled substances are available from the nearest DEA office or online (http://www.usdoj.gov/dea).

Medical Assistant Role and Responsibilities.
 Medical assistants are required to know the legalities that surround controlled substances. Medical assistant responsibilities may include:

1. Monitor the provider's DEA registration renewal date.

2. **EHR** Maintain legally designated records and inventories of all drugs (Figure 35-1), including samples. This can be done electronically.

3. Provide security for all drugs, in particular controlled substances (Schedule II).

4. Provide security for prescription pads.

5. Properly destroy expired drugs and document.

6. Know and understand federal and state laws that regulate drugs, including all controlled substances and samples.

7. In some states, medical assistants are allowed, under the supervision of the provider, to call in routine refills of medications that are exact and have no change in dosage.

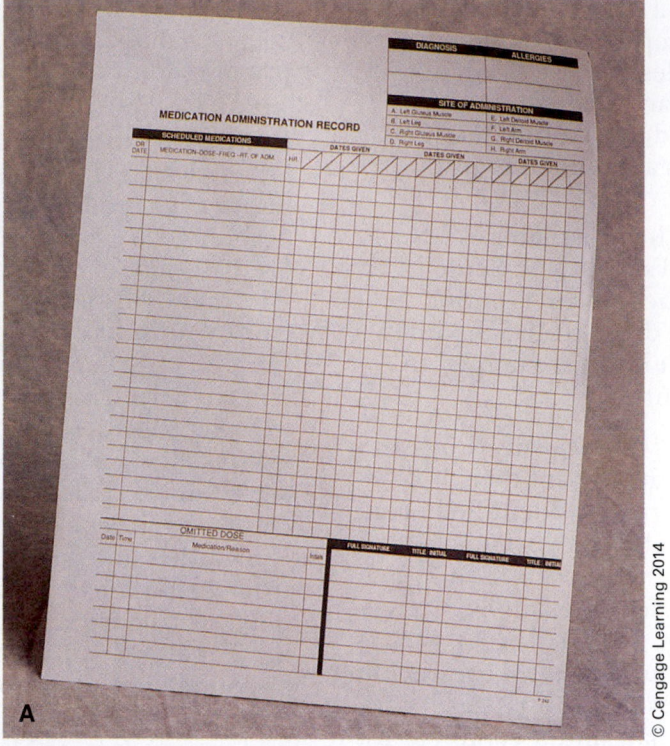

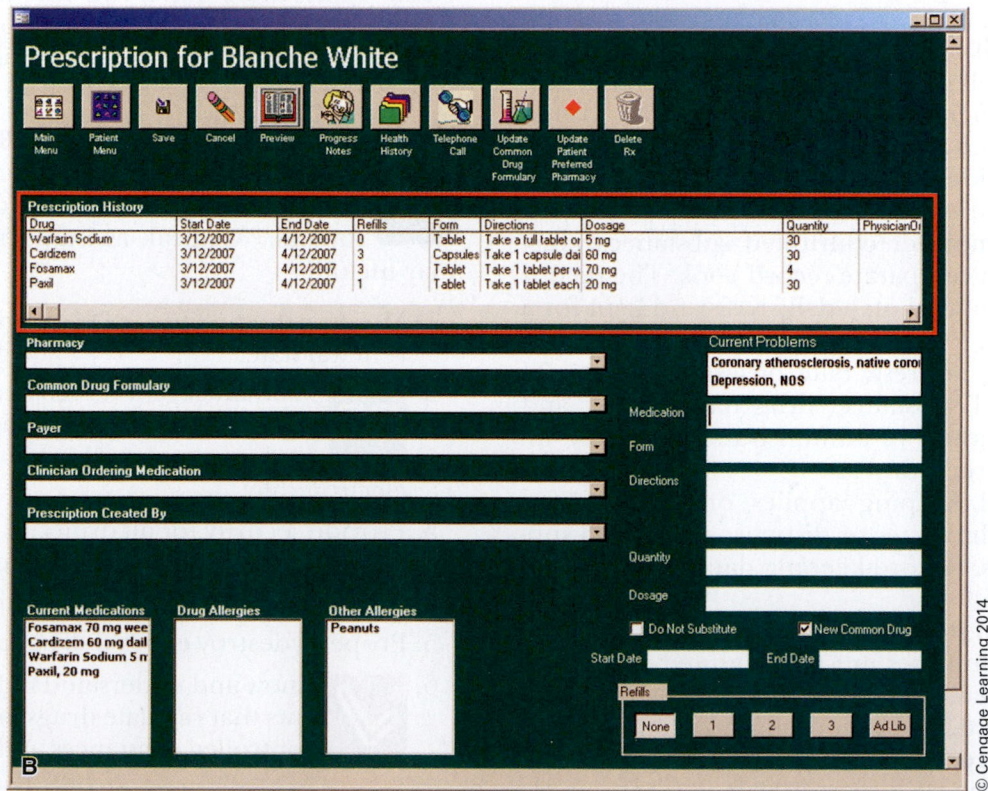

Figure 35-1 It is important to maintain patient medication records both for the safety of the patient and to protect the practice. (A) A paper-based patient medication record. (B) The patient medication record as part of the patient's electronic medical record.

The computer and its software have the capability of storing information regarding the due date for the provider's DEA registration renewal, maintaining legal records and inventories on all drugs including samples, keeping track of expiration dates of drugs and when they are destroyed, accessing the latest information regarding new DEA laws, and e-prescribing.

Since 2006, the DEA has been reluctant to approve regulations covering e-prescribing of controlled substances. This reluctance and the lack of DEA policies have been a hurdle to widespread adoption of e-prescribing. Presently, some providers can e-prescribe medications other than controlled substances (which require handwritten and signed prescriptions). This requires two separate systems, e-prescribing and handwritten prescriptions, and providers object, viewing this as time-consuming.

On March 24, 2010, the DEA issued its 334-page *Interim Final Rule on Electronic Prescriptions for Controlled Substances*. In brief, it states:

> The regulations provide pharmacies, hospitals, and practitioners with the ability to use modern technology for controlled substance prescriptions while maintaining the closed system of controls on controlled substances dispensing.... Additionally, the regulations will reduce paperwork for DEA registrants who dispense controlled substances and have the potential to reduce prescription forgery.
>
> Source: *FCW* (http://s.tt/1agIw).

This rule also states that e-prescribing has the potential to reduce errors and allow hospitals, doctors, and pharmacies to integrate their records.

E-prescribing of medications is safe, efficient, and effective. It can improve patient safety. The next section on Prescription Drugs discusses how e-prescribing is beneficial to providers and patients.

Prescription Drugs

State laws require that licensed practitioners who prescribe drugs must write and sign an order for the dispensing of drugs. This process is known as writing a prescription. Some examples of drugs that require a prescription are all of the controlled substances, except for Schedule I, which is not accepted for medical use in the United States, and other categories such as digoxin, a cardiac drug, and epinephrine, a vasoconstrictor.

Medical assistants need to advise patients after the provider prescribes a drug. Patients should also read warning labels on medication containers

(Figure 35-2). Prescription drugs are also called legend drugs.

The July 20, 2007, issue of *Medical Economics*, a periodical for providers and other medical professionals, reported the results of a survey they conducted that showed providers ranked computer systems high on timely access to records, better quality of care, and better documentation. E-prescribing is a feature many providers appreciate. Providers have instantaneous and remote access to records, in addition to many other capabilities. Some are:

- Automatically alerts to allergies and drug interactions
- Automatically calculates doses of medication according to the patient's age and weight
- Recommends brand and/or generic drug substitutions
- Prints prescriptions and faxes them to the patient's pharmacy

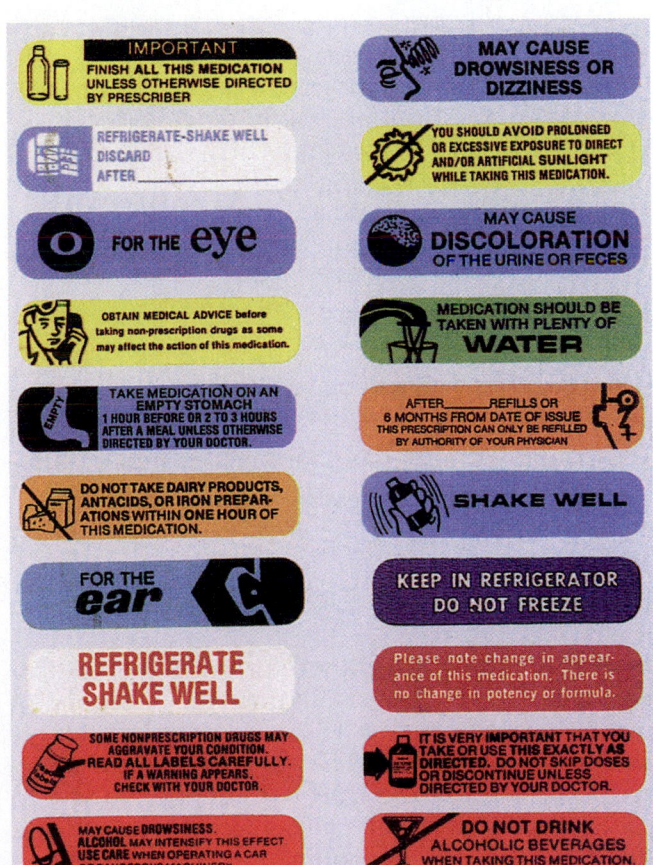

© Cengage Learning 2014

Figure 35-2 Warning labels are placed on prescription medication containers, and patients should be advised to read and adhere to the precautions or instructions.

PATIENT EDUCATION

Guidelines for patients who take prescription medications include:

1. Take exactly as directed.
2. Inform the provider or the medical assistant of unusual or adverse reactions.
3. Continue to take the medication for the duration of the prescribed number of days, weeks, and so on.
4. If you want to discontinue the medication, inform your provider or the medical assistant.
5. Do not take other medications or herbs concurrently without checking with your provider or medical assistant.
6. Do not take someone else's prescribed medication.
7. Store all medications away from children.
8. Discard unused medication properly. Many states require that unused medications be turned in to a community's biohazard waste collection. Medication substances have been found in some water supplies.
9. Heed warning labels on medication containers.

- Integrates with a drug reference such as the *Physician's Desk Reference* (PDR)
- Contains and updates patients' demographics
- Automatically processes renewals or refills

Nonprescription Drugs

Drugs that are frequently referred to as over-the-counter (OTC) drugs fall into the category of nonprescription drugs. These drugs are readily accessible to the public. They do not require a prescription because the FDA considers them safe to use without a provider's advice. Examples of OTC drugs are aspirin, ibuprofen, and vitamins such as vitamin C. Although OTC drugs are considered safe, it is useful for the medical assistant to offer patients some guidelines (Figure 35-3).

Prescription drugs can be reclassified to OTC if they meet the following criteria:

 Because patients are more aware and better informed about their health care needs, they are becoming more involved in making choices and decisions about their health care. When they choose to take over-the-counter (OTC) drugs, they need information and guidance. Over the past few years, some previous prescription drugs have been changed to OTC drugs. The safety of these drugs can only be ensured if patients take them as directed.

Patients need to realize that OTC medications:

1. Can interact with other drugs (either prescribed, herbal, or other OTCs) and cause undesirable or adverse reactions or complications
2. May be used in lieu of seeking professional help and thereby interfere with the need for medical care
3. Can mask symptoms and exacerbate an existing condition
4. May have several active ingredients, which may be found to be undesirable
5. Have a safe minimum dose, which may not have the desired therapeutic effect

© Cengage Learning 2014

Figure 35-3 Guidelines for patients when taking non-prescription (over-the-counter) medications.

- The indication or indications of use for OTC must be similar to the prescription indication and must permit easy diagnosis and monitoring by the patient.
- There must be a low incidence of adverse reactions and drug interactions.
- The drug must not have properties that need additional monitoring or a very narrow margin for therapeutic effect.

In 1972, the FDA launched the OTC Drug Review to ensure the safety, effectiveness, and appropriate labeling of over-the-counter products. As a result of this review, only 33% of OTC drugs were found to be safe and effective. 33% were found to be ineffective, and many more were found to be unsafe.

Proper Disposal of Drugs

 All drug labels contain an expiration date (Figure 35-4). When that date has been reached, the drug must be removed from the shelf and destroyed (see Procedure 35-1).

An expired drug cannot be dispensed or administered because it could be harmful.

When disposing of expired drugs, it is no longer recommended that expired and unused medications, whether prescription or over-the-counter, be released into the sewage system. Various

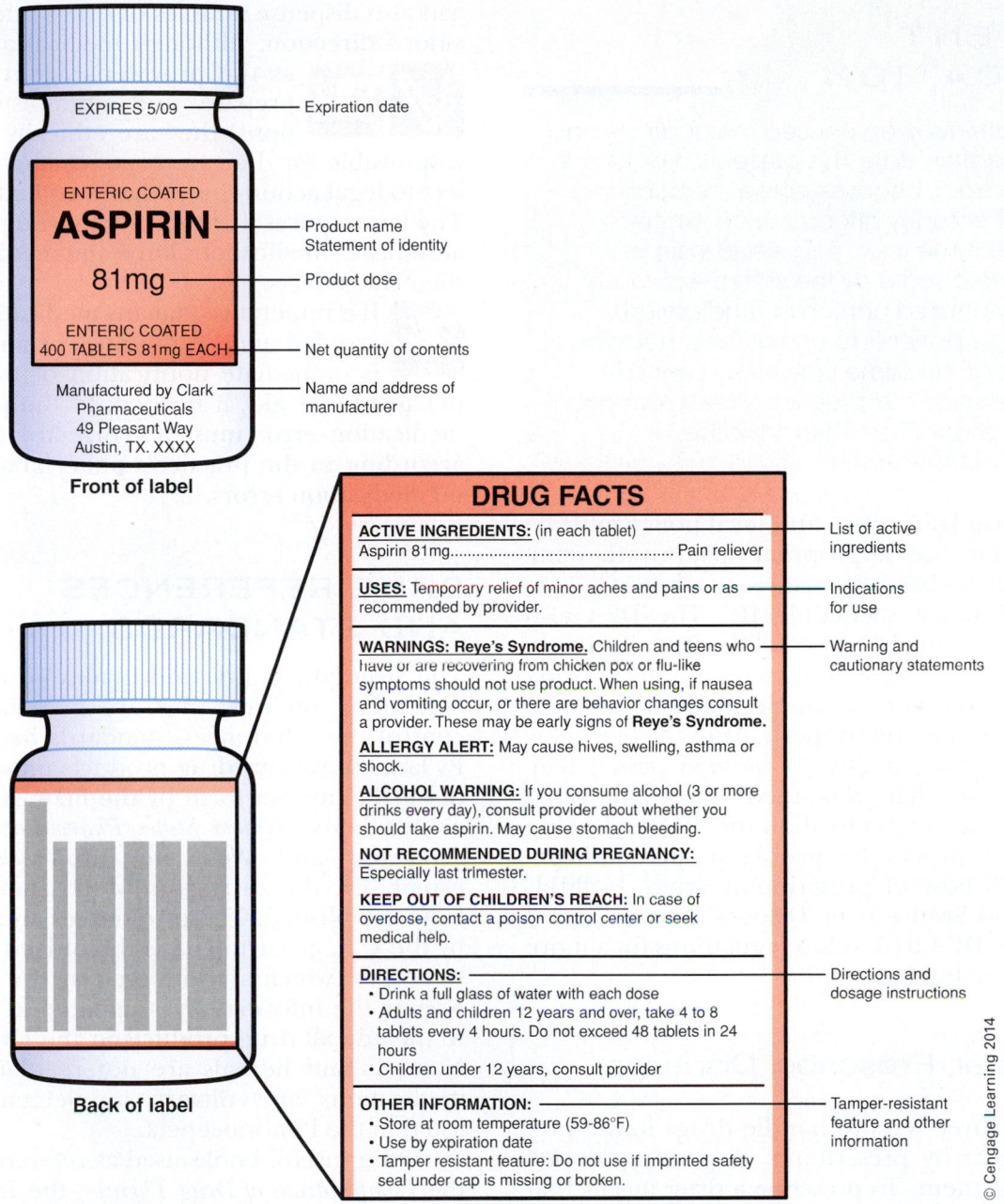

Figure 35-4   Medication labels contain valuable information essential to the safe and effective use of the drug.

antibiotics and hormones have been discovered in the water supplies. Pharmacists have been asked to allow patients to take their expired and unused medications to their pharmacies. Pharmacists can arrange to have the medications incinerated. Some communities have one day a year set aside for disposal of biohazard substances, including these medications.

If a medication is removed from its original container, it should not be used (for example, the patient refused the medication); do not replace it in the container. Dispose of it as outlined earlier.

Outdated and expired controlled substances (Schedule II) are handled differently. They must be returned to the pharmacy (as required by law). If a controlled substance (Schedule II) has been either dropped onto the floor (and is thus unfit to be given to a patient) or has spilled (if in liquid form), a witness should verify the incident and proper documentation must take place.

The local DEA office and local police must be notified and the appropriate paperwork completed if there has been a loss or theft of a controlled substance (Schedule II). The DEA also sponsors an annual National Take-Back Initiative. This is an opportunity for the community to bring in their expired and unwanted medications to be disposed of safely and properly. After the first Take-Back Day in 2010, Congress passed legislation that amended the Controlled Substances Act to allow the FDA to develop a permanent process for people to safely and conveniently dispose of prescription drugs. In 2011, the Safe and Secure Drug Disposal Act was signed to allow the DEA to develop regulations for a more permanent solution.

Administer, Prescribe, Dispense

There are three ways to handle drugs in the provider's clinic: by prescribing, dispensing, or administering them. To **prescribe** a drug means that the licensed practitioner with prescriptive authority (provider, physician assistant, or nurse practitioner) gives a written order to be taken to the pharmacist to be filled. To **dispense** a drug means to provide the medication as ordered by the provider to the patient to be taken at another time. To **administer** a drug means to give it to the patient by mouth or injection or any other method of administration as ordered by the provider.

Although state laws vary, some states allow certain professionals, including medical assistants, to prepare and administer medications under the licensed practitioner's supervision. Usually, it is the provider and pharmacist who dispense medications. However, medical assistants

can also dispense samples of drugs under the provider's direction. Although medical assistants act as the provider's agent when they prepare and administer medications, they are ethically and legally responsible for their own actions and can be subject to legal action should harm come to a patient. The law requires that individuals who prepare and administer medications know the medications and their side effects.

It is imperative that any medication error be avoided and, if one does occur, that there is immediate notification of the practitioner to render aid, if needed, to the patient. Any medication error must be correctly documented according to the practice's policy and procedure on medication errors.

DRUG REFERENCES AND STANDARDS

The strength, purity, and quality of drugs differ depending on how they are manufactured. To control the differences, standards have been set. By law, the various drug products must meet standards that are set forth by the FDA. A special reference book, *United States Pharmacopeia/National Formulary,* and Web site http://www.usp.org/usp-nf, list the drugs for which standards have been established. These resources are recognized by the U.S. government as the official list of drug standards, which are enforced by the FDA. Every 5 years the information is updated in an attempt to include all drug products in the United States. Naturals and herbals are not regulated. Herbal medications and dietary supplements are not listed in the Pharmocepeia.

Other useful books used as references include the *Compendium of Drug Therapy,* the *Desk Reference for Nonprescription Drugs,* and the *Physician's Desk Reference* (PDR). When using the PDR, it is helpful to understand that each medication is described using the manufacturer's package insert. The format for each medication is similar, but not uniform, as is often found in other references. Also, there are color photographs of each medication included for easy recognition. The PDR is published annually and supplements to the PDR are available two times a year. The supplements contain the newest drugs that were not yet available when the PDR was printed; thus, the supplements contain the most current information. The supplements are organized in the same way as the PDR. The PDR is available in print, on the Web, and for PDAs. The PDR

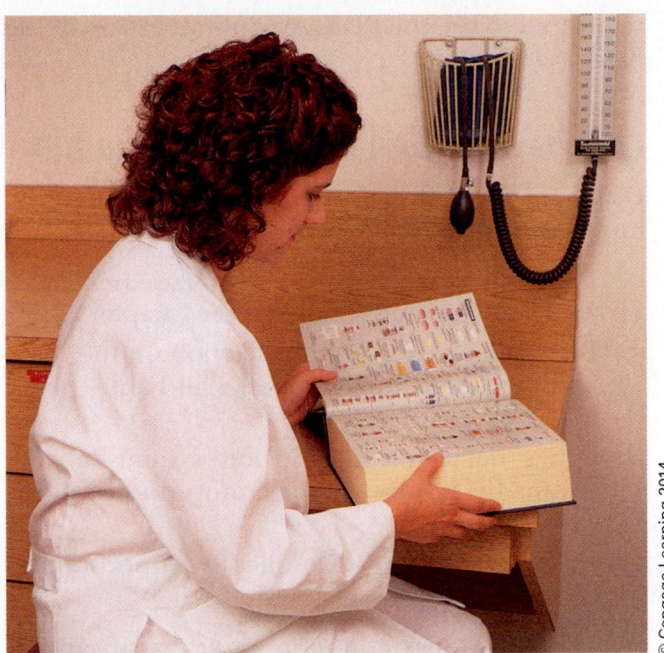

Figure 35-5 The Physician's Desk Reference (PDR) is a valuable resource for the medical assistant who wishes to obtain information about a specific medication.

© Cengage Learning 2014

is one of the most widely used reference books and is found in most offices and clinics. It is divided into sections of drug information, which are followed by other useful drug information such as a list of products, poison control 1-800 toll-free telephone numbers, conversion tables, and a guide to management of drug overdose (Figure 35-5).

Providers use electronic technology to assist them when they need references to drugs, their interactions, brand and generic names, and doses according to patient's needs. Some providers use personal digital assistants (PDAs), hand-held electronic devices that give them the information they need. The PDR comes with a CD-ROM, and an individual can register online to access medications information (http://www.PDR.net).

How to Use the PDR

The five most commonly used sections of the PDR list drugs according to:

- Brand name and generic name index (Section 2)
- Classification or category (Section 3)
- Product identification guide (Section 4)
- Product information and alphabetical arrangement by manufacturers (Section 5)

Section 2 of the PDR is the alphabetized section used for finding the page numbers for generic and brand name drugs. Each drug, whether generic or brand, has a page number listed to enable you to locate a specific drug. Each time a brand name appears, it is followed by the manufacturer's name and page number to check for more information. When more than one page number appears, the first number refers to the photo section, Section 4 (Product Identification Guide); the last number refers to the prescribing category, Section 3 (Product Category Index). Generic named drugs are underlined; brand names are not.

The PDR has many other sections within it, such as the Key to Controlled Substances category, the U.S. Food and Drug Administration telephone directory, telephone numbers for poison control centers, and herb and drug interactions.

The following guidelines will assist you as you learn to use the PDR:

1. If you know the brand or generic name of the drug, turn to Section 2 and locate the drug in the alphabetical listing. The manufacturer's name will be in parentheses, followed by a page number or two page numbers. The first number is the product identification page number, Section 4. The second number is the product information, Section 5.

Example:

Look up Zithromax® capsules in a current PDR.

Zithromax (Pfizer)
Note all the information provided for a drug.

- *Description.* Gives the origin and chemical composition of the drug.
- *Clinical Pharmacology.* Indicates the effect of the drug on the body and the process by which the drug exerts this effect.
- *Indications and Uses.* States the various conditions, diseases, types of microorganisms, and so on, for which the drug is used.
- *Contraindications.* States when the drug should not be given to a specified person.
- *Warnings.* Gives the potential dangers of the drug.
- *Precautions.* States the possible unfavorable effects that the drug may have on a patient.
- *Adverse Reactions.* Lists the undesired side effects or toxicity of the drug.

- *Dosage and Administration.* States the amount (usual daily dose for adults and children) and time sequence of administration.

- *How Supplied.* Lists the various forms of the drug and their dosages.

2. If you know the classification of the drug, turn to Section 3 and locate the category of the drug.

Example:

Antibiotics
Macrolide
Zithromax® capsules (Pfizer)

NOTE: All controlled substances listed in the PDR are indicated with the symbol C with the Roman numeral II, III, IV, or V printed inside the C to designate the schedule in which the substance is classified.

Example:

Duramorph® C$_{II}$, morphine sulfate USP

Other Reference Sources

On occasion, you may not find the drug that you are looking for listed in the PDR. When this happens:

- Refer to another drug reference book
- Research medications online, making sure your source is reliable
- Ask a pharmacist about the drug
- Refer to the packet insert that comes in the drug package

The package insert that most manufacturers provide with their products is an important source of information about a particular drug. This is a brief description of the drug, including its clinical pharmacology, indications and usage, **contraindications** (any symptom or circumstance that indicates that the use of a particular drug is inappropriate when it would otherwise be advisable), warnings, precautions, drug interactions, adverse reactions, overdose, dosage, and administration. The package insert can be a valuable source of information about drugs that might not be listed elsewhere, or if a PDR is unavailable.

Information about some older medications, such as digoxin, can be found in the package insert because they may have been deleted from the current PDR. You or your employer can become

registered to use the PDR. An online version of the PDR is available.

CLASSIFICATION OF DRUGS

Drugs can be classified (arranged in groups) in a number of ways. Some examples are:

- Drugs used to treat or prevent disease (examples are hormones and vaccines) (see Chapter 22)
- Drugs that have a principal action on the body (examples are analgesics and anti-inflammatory drugs)
- Drugs that act on specific body systems or organs (examples are respiratory and cardiovascular drugs)
- Drug preparation (examples are suppository, liquid)

Table 35-1 lists common drug classifications. See Appendix B for the 200 top prescribed brand name medications, or visit the following Web site: http://www.pharmacytimes.com/publications/issue/2011/May2011/Top-200-Drugs-of-2010.

PRINCIPAL ACTIONS OF DRUGS

In general, drugs can be grouped as follows: those that act directly on one or more tissues of the body; those that act on microorganisms; and those that replace body chemicals.

Certain drugs have selective action, such as stimulants, which increase cell activity, and depressants, which decrease cell activity.

Other drugs may have what is known as:

- *Local action.* The drug acts on the area to which it is administered.
- *Remote action.* A drug affects a part of the body that is distant from the site of administration.
- *Systemic action.* The drug is carried via the bloodstream throughout the body.
- *Synergistic action.* One drug increases or counteracts the action of another.

Factors That Affect Drug Action

The four principal factors that affect drug action are: absorption, distribution, biotransformation, and elimination. These factors depend

Table 35-1 Common Classifications of Drugs and Their Actions

Classification (with Phonetic Spelling)	Action	Examples of Drugs Commonly Used in Ambulatory Care Setting	Side Effects
Analgesic (an"al-je'sik)	An agent that relieves pain without causing loss of consciousness	Acetaminophen (Tylenol), acetylsalicylic acid (aspirin), ibuprofen (Advil, Motrin)	**Common:** GI changes **Severe:** Allergic reaction (rash, hives, tissue swelling, respiratory difficulty, chest tightness)
Anesthetic (an"es-thet'ik)	An agent that produces numbness May be local or general depending on the type and how administered	lidocaine HCl (Xylocaine) procaine HCl (Novacaine) } Both are local anesthetics	**Common:** Irritation, redness, changes in sensation, drowsiness, irregular heartbeat (based on route of administration) **Severe:** Allergic reaction (rash, hives, tissue swelling, respiratory difficulty, chest tightness)
Antacid (ant-as'id)	An agent that neutralizes acid	Amphojel, Gelusil, Mylanta, Milk of Magnesia	**Common:** Constipation, loss of appetite, urinary changes, muscle weakness, increased thirst
Antianemic (an"ti-an-em'ic)	An agent that replaces iron	Iron, ferrous sulfate	**Common:** Stomach upset, abdominal pain, nausea, constipation, diarrhea, or vomiting
Antianxiety (an"ti-ang-zi'e-te)	An agent that relieves anxiety and muscle tension	Benzodiazepines: diazepam (Valium), chlordiazepoxide HCl (Librium), alprazolam (Xanax)	**Common:** Drowsiness, incoordination, muscle weakness **Severe:** Allergic reaction (rash, hives, tissue swelling, respiratory difficulty, chest tightness); slurred speech; tremor; mood changes
Antiarrhythmic (an"te-a-rith'mik)	An agent that controls cardiac arrhythmias	Lidocaine HCl (Xylocaine), propranolol HCl (Inderal)	**Common:** Dizziness, nausea and vomiting, vision changes, decreased sexual ability **Severe:** Allergic reaction (rash, hives, tissue swelling, respiratory difficulty, chest tightness); slowed heart beat
Antibiotic (an"ti-bi-ot'ik)	An agent that is destructive to or inhibits growth of microorganisms	Penicillins (Pentids, Duracillin, Polycillin, Pipracil, Augmentin) and others	**Common:** Upset stomach, diarrhea, vomiting **Severe:** Allergic reaction (rash, hives, tissue swelling, respiratory difficulty, chest tightness)

continues

Table 35-1   Common Classifications of Drugs and Their Actions (*Continued*)

Classification (with Phonetic Spelling)	Action	Examples of Drugs Commonly Used in Ambulatory Care Setting	Side Effects
Anticholesterol or antihyperlipidemic (an"ti-ko"less-ter-ol)	An agent that reduces cholesterol	Zocor, Lipitor, Crestor, Mevacor	**Common:** Muscle pain or weakness, change in amount of urine produced **Severe:** Allergic reaction (rash, hives, tissue swelling, respiratory difficulty, chest tightness); renal changes/failure; liver damage
Anticholinergic (an"ti-ko"lin-er'jik)	An agent that blocks parasympathetic nerve impulses	Atropine, scopolamine, trihexyphenidyl HCl (Artane)	**Common:** Dilated pupils, blurred vision, dizziness, constipation **Severe:** Allergic reaction (rash, hives, tissue swelling, respiratory difficulty, chest tightness); renal changes/failure; liver damage
Anticoagulant (an"ti-ko-ag'u-lant)	An agent that prevents or delays blood clotting	Heparin sodium, dicumarol, warfarin sodium (Coumadin)	**Common:** Irritation at the site of injection **Severe:** Allergic reaction (rash, hives, tissue swelling, respiratory difficulty, chest tightness); bleeding gums; hematuria; gastric bleeding; shortness of breath; slurred speech
Anticonvulsant (an"ti-kon-vul'sant)	An agent that prevents or relieves convulsions	Carbamazepine (Tegretol), phenytoin (Dilantin), ethosuximide (Zarontin)	**Common:** Constipation, dizziness, headache, nausea, vomiting **Severe:** Allergic reaction (rash, hives, tissue swelling, respiratory difficulty, chest tightness)
Antidepressant (an"ti-dep-res'ant)	An agent that prevents or relieves the symptoms of depression	Monoamine oxidase (MAO) inhibitors: isocarboxazid (Marplan), phenelzine sulfate (Nardil); tricyclic: amitriptyline HCl (Elavil), imipramine HCl (Tofranil), sertraline HCl (Zoloft), paroxetine HCl (Paxil), trazodone (Desyrel), fluoxentine (Prozac)	**Common:** Anxiety, constipation, diarrhea, dizziness, drowsiness, GI symptoms **Severe:** Allergic reaction (rash, hives, tissue swelling, respiratory difficulty, chest tightness); bizarre behavior, severe mental status and mood changes; fast or irregular heartbeat; suicidal thoughts or attempts

Table 35-1   Common Classifications of Drugs and Their Actions (*Continued*)

Classification (with Phonetic Spelling)	Action	Examples of Drugs Commonly Used in Ambulatory Care Setting	Side Effects
Antidiarrheal (an"ti-di-a-re'al)	An agent that prevents or relieves diarrhea	Pepto-Bismol, Kaopectate, diphenoxylate HCl (Lomotil)	**Common:** Darkening of stools or tongue **Severe:** Persistent vomiting or diarrhea; dizziness; abdominal pain; allergic reaction (rash, hives, tissue swelling, respiratory difficulty, chest tightness)
Antidote (an-ti'dot)	An agent that counteracts poisons and their effects	Naloxone (Narcan)	**Severe:** Hypo- or hypertension, arrhythmias, pulmonary edema, cardiac arrest, coma
Antiemetic (an"ti-e-met'ik)	An agent that prevents or relieves nausea and vomiting	Tigan, Dramamine, Phenergan, Reglan, Marinol, Compazine	**Common:** Dry mouth, vomiting, dizziness, drowsiness, weakness **Severe:** Allergic reaction (rash, hives, tissue swelling, respiratory difficulty, chest tightness); blurred vision; irritation at injection site; hallucinations; loss of coordination; confusion; shortness of breath; twitching of face or tongue
Antihistamine (an"ti-his'ta-min)	An agent that counteracts histamine	Dimetane, Benadryl, Seldane, Allegra	**Common:** Constipation, diarrhea, dizziness, dry mouth, excitability, loss of appetite, nausea and vomiting **Severe:** Allergic reaction (rash, hives, tissue swelling, respiratory difficulty, chest tightness); blurred vision; chest pain; loss of coordination; irregular heartbeat; drowsiness
Antihypertensive (an"ti-hi"per-ten'siv)	An agent that prevents or controls high blood pressure	Methyldopa (Aldomet), clonidine HCl (Catapres), metoprolol tartrate (Lopressor)	**Common:** Anxiety, confusion, constipation, dizziness, weakness, ringing in ears, sweating **Severe:** Allergic reaction (rash, hives, tissue swelling, respiratory difficulty, chest tightness); chest pain; fainting; cardiac arrhythmias; hallucination; shortness of breath

continues

Table 35-1 Common Classifications of Drugs and Their Actions (*Continued*)

Classification (with Phonetic Spelling)	Action	Examples of Drugs Commonly Used in Ambulatory Care Setting	Side Effects
Anti inflammatory (an"ti-in-flam'a-to-re)	An agent that counteracts inflammation	Naproxen (Naprosyn), aspirin, ibuprofen (Advil, Motrin)	**Common:** GI changes **Severe:** Allergic reaction (rash, hives, tissue swelling, respiratory difficulty, chest tightness)
Antimanic (an"ti-man'ik)	An agent used for the treatment of the manic episode of manic-depressive disorder	Lithium	**Common:** Drying and thinning of hair, hand tremor, loss of appetite, nausea, tiredness **Severe:** Allergic reaction (rash, hives, tissue swelling, respiratory difficulty, chest tightness); abnormal eye movements; confusion; diarrhea; dizziness; muscle weakness; increased urination; blurred vision
Antineoplastic (an"ti-ne"o-plas'tik)	An agent that kills or destroys malignant cells	Busulfan (Myleran), cyclophosphamide (Cytoxan)	**Common:** Loss of appetite, diarrhea, changes in skin color, hair loss, nausea, vomiting, weakness **Severe:** Allergic reaction (rash, hives, tissue swelling, respiratory difficulty, chest tightness); hematuria; tarry stools; fever; chills; hallucinations; infections; mouth sores; unusual bleeding or bruising
Antipsychotic	An agent that helps in schizophrenia and chronic brain syndrome	Haloperidol (Haldol), chlorpromazine (Thorazine)	**Common:** Constipation, diarrhea, drowsiness, dry mouth, headache, nausea, restlessness **Severe:** Allergic reaction (rash, hives, tissue swelling, respiratory difficulty, chest tightness); chest pain; confusion; renal changes; difficulty swallowing; arrhythmias; mood changes
Antipyretic (an"ti-pi-ret'ik)	An agent that reduces fever	Aspirin, acetaminophen (Tylenol)	**Common:** GI changes **Severe:** Allergic reaction (rash, hives, tissue swelling, respiratory difficulty, chest tightness)

Table 35-1 Common Classifications of Drugs and Their Actions (*Continued*)

Classification (with Phonetic Spelling)	Action	Examples of Drugs Commonly Used in Ambulatory Care Setting	Side Effects
Antitussive (an"ti-tus'iv)	An agent that prevents or relieves cough	Codeine, dextromethorphan (Pertussin, Romilar)	**Common:** Blurred vision, constipation, dizziness, drowsiness, nausea and vomiting **Severe:** Allergic reaction (rash, hives, tissue swelling, respiratory difficulty, chest tightness); breathing changes, especially slowed breathing; arrhythmias
Antiulcer (an"ti-ul'ser) (H₂ blockers)	An agent that relieves and heals ulcers by blocking hydrochloric acid	Cimetidine (Tagamet), ranitidine (Zantac), omeprazole (Prilosec)	**Common:** Drowsiness, dizziness, headache **Severe:** Allergic reaction (rash, hives, tissue swelling, respiratory difficulty, chest tightness); agitation; anxiety; confusion; hair loss; joint or muscle pain
Antiviral (an"ti-viral)	An agent that fights a specific virus	Zovirax, Retrovir, Denavir	**Common:** Nausea, diarrhea, fever, headache, pain, aggressive behavior **Severe:** Allergic reaction (rash, hives, tissue swelling, respiratory difficulty, chest tightness); delirium; anemia; coma; psychosis; hepatitis; renal failure
Bronchodilator (brong"ko-dil-a'tor)	An agent that dilates the bronchi	Isoproterenol HCl (Isuprel), albuterol (Proventil)	**Common:** Flushing, headache, dizziness, tremors, nausea, sweating, weakness **Severe:** Allergic reaction (rash, hives, tissue swelling, respiratory difficulty, chest tightness); blurred vision; arrhythmias; chest pain
Contraceptive (kon"tra-sep'tiv)	Any device, method, or agent that prevents conception	LoEstrin 1.5/30, Ortho-Novum 7/7/7; 1/35, Triphasil-21, Ovral 28, Alesse, Levlen	**Common:** Breast tenderness, bleeding between periods, headache, nervousness, nausea, vomiting, cramping, vaginal infection **Severe:** Allergic reaction (rash, hives, tissue swelling, respiratory difficulty, chest tightness); chest pain; depression; loss of hair; severe headache; loss of vision

continues

Table 35-1   Common Classifications of Drugs and Their Actions (*Continued*)

Classification (with Phonetic Spelling)	Action	Examples of Drugs Commonly Used in Ambulatory Care Setting	Side Effects
COX-2 Inhibitor (kox-2 in-hib-it-or)	An agent that inhibits COX-2 (an enzyme) found in joints or other body parts that are inflamed	Celebrex	**Common:** Headache, constipation, diarrhea, gastrointestinal symptoms **Severe:** Allergic reaction (rash, hives, tissue swelling, respiratory difficulty, chest tightness); bloody, black, or tarry stools; chest pain; confusion; depression; seizures; headache; dizziness; gastrointestinal symptoms
Decongestant (de"con-gest'ant)	An agent that reduces nasal congestion or swelling	Oxymetazoline (Afrin), phenylephrine HCl (Neo-Synephrine), pseudoephedrine HCl (Sudafed)	**Common:** Increased nasal discharge, sneezing, stinging, burning **Severe:** Allergic reaction (rash, hives, tissue swelling, respiratory difficulty, chest tightness)
Diuretic (di"u-ret'ik)	An agent that increases the excretion of urine	Chlorothiazide (Diuril), furosemide (Lasix), mannitol (Osmitrol)	**Common:** Blurred vision, dizziness, headache **Severe:** Allergic reaction (rash, hives, tissue swelling, respiratory difficulty, chest tightness); confusion; drowsiness; arrhythmia; muscle pain; nausea and vomiting
Expectorant (ek-spek'to-rant)	An agent that facilitates removal of secretion from the bronchopulmonary mucous membrane	Gualifenesin (Robitussin)	**Common:** Dizziness, excitability, headache, weakness **Severe:** Allergic reaction (rash, hives, tissue swelling, respiratory difficulty, chest tightness); dysuria; hallucinations; arrhythmias; headache; tremor
Hemostatic (he"mo-stat'ik)	An agent that controls or stops bleeding	Humafac, Amicar, vitamin K	**Common:** Confusion, decreased vision, muscle aches, headaches, gastrointestinal symptoms **Severe:** Allergic reaction (rash, hives, tissue swelling, respiratory difficulty, chest tightness); muscle pain; arrhythmias; stroke; unusual bleeding

Table 35-1   Common Classifications of Drugs and Their Actions (*Continued*)

Classification (with Phonetic Spelling)	Action	Examples of Drugs Commonly Used in Ambulatory Care Setting	Side Effects
Hypnotic (hip-not'ik)	An agent that produces sleep or hypnosis	Secobarbital (Seconal), chloral hydrate, ethchlorvynol (Placidyl)	**Common:** Clumsiness, dizziness, lightheadedness **Severe:** Allergic reaction (rash, hives, tissue swelling, respiratory difficulty, chest tightness); confusion; hallucinations; fainting; depressed respirations
Hypoglycemic (hi"po-gli-se'mik)	An agent that reduces blood glucose level	Insulin, chlorpropamide (Diabinese), tolbutamide (Orinase)	**Common:** Scarring at injection site, enlargement of the skin at the site, depression in the skin **Severe:** Allergic reaction (rash, hives, tissue swelling, respiratory difficulty, chest tightness); confusion; dizziness; loss of consciousness; muscle weakness; shortness of breath; slurred speech; unusual sweating and hunger
Laxative (lak'sa-tiv)	An agent that loosens and promotes normal bowel elimination	Metamucil powder, Dulcolax, Docusate sodium (Colace)	**Common:** Abdominal bloating or fullness **Severe:** Allergic reaction (rash, hives, tissue swelling, respiratory difficulty, chest tightness); difficulty swallowing; dyspnea
Muscle relaxant (mus'el re-lak'sant)	An agent that produces relaxation of skeletal muscle	Robaxin, Norflex, Paraflex, Skelaxin, Valium	**Common:** Blurred vision, confusion, dizziness, nasal stuffiness, nausea and vomiting **Severe:** Allergic reaction (rash, hives, tissue swelling, respiratory difficulty, chest tightness); memory loss; seizures; bradycardia
Nonsteroidal anti-inflammatory drug (NSAID)	An agent that relieves mild to moderate pain due to headache, toothache, dysmenorrhea, backache	Aspirin (Bufferin, Ecotrin), ibuprofen (Advil, Excedrin, Motrin), naproxen (Aleve, Anaprox, Naprosyn), ketoprofen (Orudis)	**Common:** GI changes **Severe:** Allergic reaction (rash, hives, tissue swelling, respiratory difficulty, chest tightness)

continues

Table 35-1   Common Classifications of Drugs and Their Actions (*Continued*)

Classification (with Phonetic Spelling)	Action	Examples of Drugs Commonly Used in Ambulatory Care Setting	Side Effects
Proton-pump inhibitor (prōtōn pump in-hib-it-or)	An agent that suppresses gastric acid (GERD) ulcers	Aciphex, Nexium, Protonix	**Common:** Allergic reaction (rash, hives, tissue swelling, respiratory difficulty, chest tightness); bone pain; chest pain; arrhythmia; liver dysfunction; unusual bleeding; vision changes
Sedative (sed'a-tiv)	An agent that produces a calming effect without causing sleep	Amobarbital (Amytal), butabarbital sodium (Buticaps), phenobarbital	**Common:** Drowsiness, dizziness, nightmares, gastrointestinal symptoms **Severe:** Allergic reaction (rash, hives, tissue swelling, respiratory difficulty, chest tightness); depression; overexcitement; hepatitis; hallucinations; blood disorders
Tranquilizer (tran"kwi-liz'er)	An agent that reduces mental tension and anxiety	Diazepam (Valium), alprazolam (Xanax), chlordiazepoxide (Librium)	**Common:** Drowsiness, incoordination, muscle weakness **Severe:** Allergic reaction (rash, hives, tissue swelling, respiratory difficulty, chest tightness); slurred speech; tremor; mood changes
Vasodilator (vas"o-di-la'tor)	An agent that produces relaxation of blood vessels; reduces blood pressure	Isosorbide dinitrate (Isordil), atenolol (Tenormin), nitroglycerin, diltiazem (Cardizem)	**Common:** Dizziness, flushing of face and neck, headache, lightheadedness **Severe:** Allergic reaction (rash, hives, tissue swelling, respiratory difficulty, chest tightness); fainting; chest pain; arrhythmias; nausea and vomiting
Vasopressor (vas"o-pres'or)	An agent that produces contraction of muscles of capillaries and arteries; increases blood pressure	Metaraminol (Aramine), norepinephrine (Levophed)	**Common:** Anxiety, headache, irritation at the injection site **Severe:** Allergic reaction (rash, hives, tissue swelling, respiratory difficulty, chest tightness); arrhythmia; severe hypertension; photophobia; chest pain

on the individual patient, the form and chemical composition of the drug, and the method of administration.

1. *Absorption* is the process whereby the drug passes into the body fluids and tissues.
2. *Distribution* is the process whereby the drug is transported from the blood to the intended site of action, site of biotransformation, site of storage, and site of elimination.
3. *Biotransformation* is the chemical alteration that a drug undergoes in the body, usually in the liver.
4. *Elimination* is the process whereby the drug is excreted from the body. Elimination occurs via the gastrointestinal tract, respiratory tract, skin, mucous membranes, and mammary glands.

Undesirable Actions of Drugs

Most drugs have the potential for causing an action other than their intended action. For example:

1. *Side effect.* An undesirable action of the drug that may limit the usefulness of the drug.
2. *Drug interaction.* Occurs when one drug potentiates, i.e., increases or diminishes the action of another drug. These actions may be desirable or undesirable. Drugs may also interact with various foods, alcohol, tobacco, and other substances.
3. *Adverse reaction.* An unfavorable or harmful unintended action of a drug, such as an allergic reaction.

A patient may experience an allergic reaction to a drug after administration. It is often mild and may exhibit itself in the form of a rash, **urticaria**, or **pruritus**. On occasion, a severe reaction or **anaphylaxis** can occur, which is hypersensitivity to a drug or other foreign protein. It is the least common allergic reaction but can become severe quickly and result in dyspnea and shock. Loss of consciousness and death can result. To help prevent an allergic reaction or minimize its risk, the medical assistant should attempt to ascertain before administration of every drug whether the patient has any known allergies. The medical assistant should be aware of signs and symptoms of allergic reaction and notify the provider immediately so that appropriate emergency treatment can be given. One or two injections of epinephrine usually reverses the life-threatening symptoms of anaphylaxis, and is followed by administration of an antihistamine and/or H1 and H2 blockers such as Benadryl®, Tagamet®, or Zantac®. The patient needs to be immediately placed in the Trendelenburg position and supplemental oxygen applied. In severe cases that do not respond to this treatment, oxygen and immediate transfer to the emergency department is necessary.

DRUG ROUTES

Drugs are manufactured in a variety of forms and for various purposes. The route of a drug refers to how it is administered to the patient, and thereby transported into the patient's body. Certain medications can be administered by more than one route, whereas others must be administered via a specific route.

The route of administration is determined by a number of factors. One factor is the action of the medication on the body, either local or systemic. Intravenous medication reaches the systemic circulation rapidly via the bloodstream and quickly becomes effective. Injections of medications and medications absorbed through mucous membranes, such as suppositories and sublingual nitroglycerine, are absorbed quickly. Oral medications take longer to act because they first must be digested by the stomach and then must be absorbed into the bloodstream.

Another factor in route selection is the physical and emotional state of the patient. The patient's consciousness level, emotional status, and physical restrictions are considered when selecting a route to administer medication.

A third factor to consider is the characteristics of the drug. An example is insulin. Insulin is destroyed by digestive enzymes; therefore, the route of administration must be by injection.

The most frequently used routes of administering medication to the patient are oral and parenteral routes: oral medications are taken by mouth, parenteral generally by injection. Other routes of administration include:

- Direct application to the skin, i.e., topical (lotions, creams, liniments, ointments, transdermal [patch] systems)
- Sublingual (tablets, liquid, drops)
- Buccal (tablets)
- Rectal (suppositories, ointments)
- Vaginal (suppositories, creams, applications)
- Inhalation (sprays, aerosols)
- Instillation (liquid, drops)

FORMS OF DRUGS

Drugs are compounded in three basic types of preparations: liquids, solids, and semisolids. The ease with which a drug's ingredients can be dissolved largely determines the variety of forms manufactured. Some drug agents are soluble in water, others in alcohol, and others in a mixture of several solvents.

The method for administering a drug depends on its form, its properties, and the effects desired. When given orally, a drug may be in the form of a liquid, powder, tablet, capsule, or caplet. If it is to be injected, it must be in the form of a liquid. For topical use, the drug may be in the form of a liquid, powder, or semisolid. Oral and injectable medications are examples of preparations designed for internal use.

Liquid Preparations

Liquid preparations contain a drug that has been dissolved or suspended. Depending on the solvent used, the drug may be further classified as an aqueous (water) or alcohol preparation or as an aerosol or mist. When prescribed for internal use, liquid preparations other than emulsions are rapidly absorbed through the stomach, intestinal walls, or lungs.

Solid and Semisolid Preparations

Tablets, capsules, caplets, troches or lozenges, suppositories, and ointments are examples of solid and semisolid preparations. These products offer great flexibility as a means of dispensing different dosages of drugs. Figure 35-6 shows types of tablets and capsules.

Other Drug Delivery Systems

Technologic advances have introduced new ways by which drugs can be introduced into the patient. In addition to the conventional preparations, the following therapeutic systems offer special delivery of medication to targeted areas.

Transdermal System. The **transdermal** system of medication delivery consists of a small adhesive patch that may be applied to intact skin near the treatment site. For example, Transderm Scop®, used for preventing motion sickness, may be applied behind the ear; Nitro-Dur® (Figure 35-7), used for preventing angina pectoris, may be

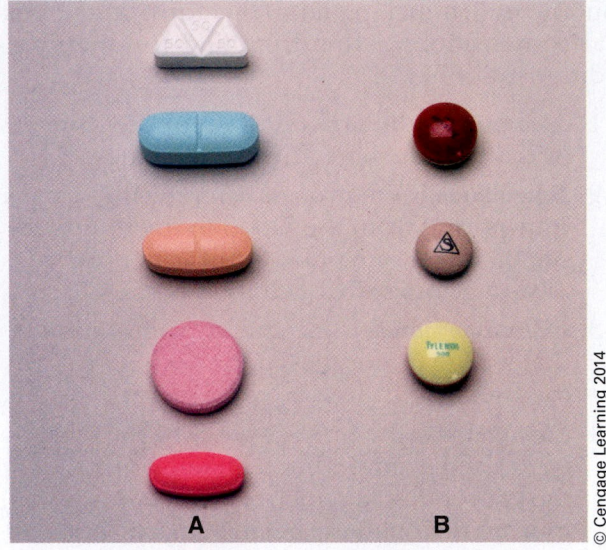

© Cengage Learning 2014

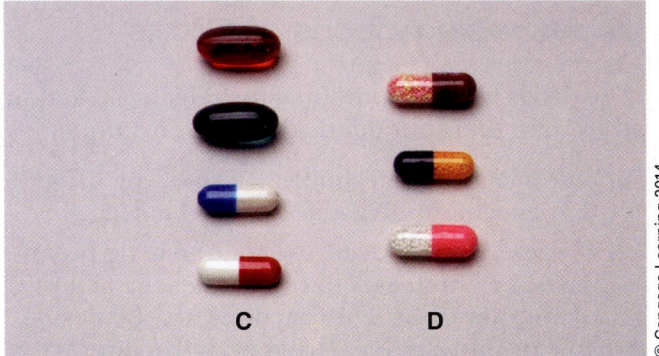

© Cengage Learning 2014

Figure 35-6 Drugs are manufactured in various forms, including solid preparations such as tablets and capsules. (A) Tablets, scored and unscored. (B) Enteric-coated tablets. (C) Capsules and gelatin-coated capsules. (D) Timed-release capsules.

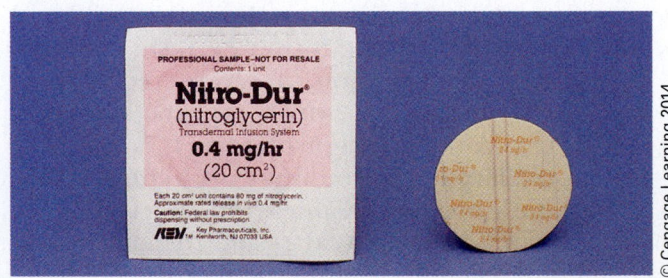

© Cengage Learning 2014

Figure 35-7 Nitro-Dur® is a transdermal system of delivering medication used for prevention and for long-term management of angina pectoris. It can be applied to the chest.

applied to the chest; Estraderm®, used to treat menopausal symptoms, may be applied to the trunk; and Nicoderm®, used to relieve the body's craving for nicotine, may be applied to any area above the waist. A transdermal system generally consists of four layers (Figure 35-8):

1. An impermeable backing that keeps the drug from leaking out of the system
2. A reservoir containing the drug
3. A membrane with tiny holes that controls the rate of drug release
4. An adhesive layer or gel that keeps the device in place

Inhalation Medications. Medication for respiratory diseases and conditions such as asthma, bronchiectasis (permanent dilation of one or more bronchi), bronchitis, and others may require treatment with inhalation medication from an aerosolized inhaler or a nebulizer. Some of the commonly prescribed

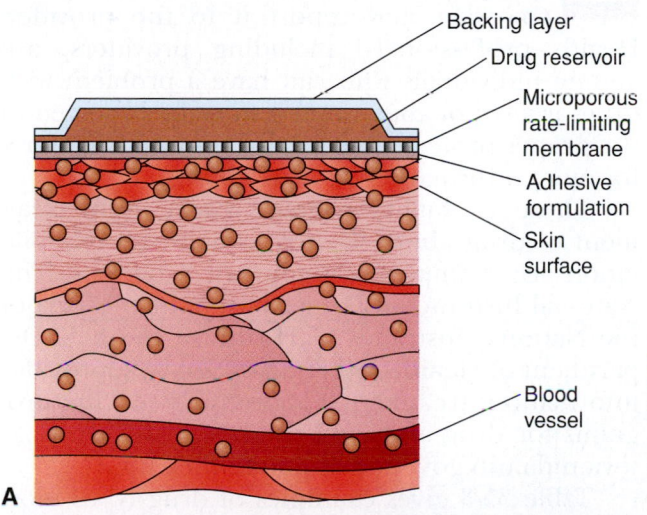

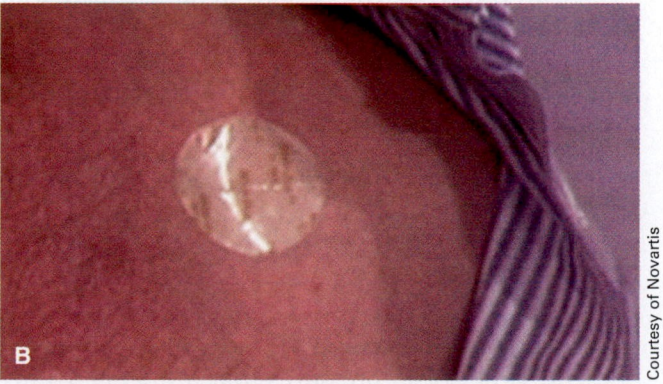

Courtesy of Novartis

Figure 35-8 (A) The multilayer unit comprising TransdermNitro® delivers nitroglycerin into the bloodstream in a consistent, controlled manner for 24 hours. The thin unit contains a backing layer, a reservoir of nitroglycerin, a unique rate-limiting membrane, and an adhesive layer that has a priming dose of nitroglycerin. (B) The patch is applied to the skin.

medications are bronchodilators such as aminophylline, albuterol, Isuprel, epinephrine, and cortisone-type medications. Oxygen may be prescribed for hypoxia caused by respiratory diseases. Oxygen may be prescribed for cardiovascular collapse, congestive heart failure, and pneumonia, among other examples. (See Chapter 30 for information about nebulizers, inhalers, and oxygen administration.)

Eye-Curing Lens. Another innovative drug delivery system is one in which a drug, contained between two ultrathin plastic membranes, is placed inside the lower eyelid. It appears to cause little or no discomfort and provides a controlled release of the medication for an extended period. Pilocarpine, a miotic that causes contraction of the pupils, is being used in this method for the treatment of glaucoma.

Implantable Devices. Implantable devices are available in several shapes and sizes and are positioned just beneath the skin near blood vessels that lead directly to the area to be medicated. For example, an infusion pump that is about the size of a hockey puck can be implanted below the skin near the waist to provide continuous delivery of chemotherapy to patients with liver cancer, insulin to a diabetic, or narcotics to a chronic pain patient. This device, which has a refillable drug reservoir, is connected by an outlet catheter to the patient's blood vessel or directly into the spinal fluid. In addition to providing a continuous supply of medication, these devices have the advantage of delivering greater doses with fewer side effects than can be realized through the systemic route.

STORAGE AND HANDLING OF MEDICATIONS

Certain precautions should be followed if the ambulatory care setting keeps medications on the premises. The goal should be to store all medications in their original containers in a separate room in a locked cabinet. Many medications require storage in a certain manner, such as a dark area or in a dark container (to keep light away from them) or in the refrigerator. Some must be kept in glass containers only because plastic may react with the medication's chemical composition. The drug label indicates proper storage and handling for each medication.

Keep medications that are for internal use separated from those intended for external use.

Access to medications is simplified if they are organized in the storage area either according to their classification (diuretic, hormones) or according to the alphabet. Always check expiration dates.

Labels on figure: Backing layer, Drug reservoir, Microporous rate-limiting membrane, Adhesive formulation, Skin surface, Blood vessel. A. B.

EMERGENCY MEDICATIONS AND SUPPLIES

The ambulatory care setting should maintain a tray, box, cabinet, or crash cart (see Chapter 9 for contents of crash cart) especially and solely for drugs and supplies needed in an emergency such as anaphylaxis or other form of shock. The drugs listed in Table 35-2 are a sample of some general drugs to keep readily available for emergencies.

Other supplies and equipment to keep together with the drugs on the emergency cart include:

- Intravenous (IV) materials such as IV fluids, needles, tubing, syringes, alcohol, swabs, constriction band, and tape
- Sphygmomanometer
- Stethoscope
- Oxygen and mask
- Airways
- Defibrillator
- Suction equipment (nasopharyngeal)
- Personal protective equipment

Check the tray on a regular basis (weekly or monthly, depending on use) according to need. Check the oxygen tank and gauge. Replace items that have been used as soon as possible, and discard drugs and supplies that have reached their expiration dates. Document that the tray has been checked and updated. (See Chapter 9 for more information about emergencies and emergency drugs used in the office and other ambulatory areas.)

Bioterrorism

Bioterrorism is the name given to the use of biologic weapons (pathogenic microorganisms) to create fear in people. There are many biologic agents that can be used in an attempt to cause serious diseases. Most diseases can be treated with pharmaceutical agents such as antibiotics and antitoxoids.

The most dangerous disease threats are anthrax, botulism, pneumonic/bubonic plague, smallpox, and tularemia.

Anthrax, pneumonic/bubonic plague, and tularemia can all be treated with antibiotics. Botulism is treated with botulism antioxides supplied by public health authorities. Smallpox is treated by early vaccination (within four days). The Centers for Disease Control and Prevention has the vaccine.

 Education plays a vital role in raising awareness and increasing the knowledge of health care professionals to aid them in being better prepared for threats to the public health. The World Health Organization, the Centers for Disease Control and Prevention, and state and local public health departments are excellent resources for more information about bioterrorism. (See Chapter 9 for information about emergencies, Chapter 22 for infectious diseases)

DRUG ABUSE

  There has been an enormous increase in the **abuse**, or misuse, of legal and illegal drugs. Any drug can be abused, whether it is penicillin, alcohol, or a controlled substance such as cocaine. Medical assistants, while caring for patients, may unexpectedly come in contact with patients who abuse or misuse drugs.

 Medical assistants must be able to recognize the symptoms of drug abuse in a patient or coworker and report it to the provider. Health professionals, including providers, are among individuals who can have a problem with drug or alcohol abuse, and it must be reported to the proper professional association (see Chapter 7 for more information on drug abuse).

There are many programs available for treatment of drug abuse. Detoxification and rehabilitation are examples of treatment programs. The National Institute on Drug Abuse, which is part of the National Institutes of Health of the U.S. Department of Health and Human Services, provides information, treatment options, and specific programs for drug abuse on their Web site (http://www.nida.nih.gov/podat/podatindex.html).

Table 35-3 gives examples of drug types most commonly abused.

In addition to the drugs of abuse listed in Table 35-3, another drug of abuse is dextromethorphan. It is an antitussive (cough suppressant) that has been an over-the-counter medication for more than 30 years and is a component of several cough medications. One of the drugs is Coricidin HBP (cough and cold tablets), also known as "ccc," "robo," or "red devils." Primarily it is used by youths as a recreational drug for its euphoric effects, but an overdose can result in coma and death. The cough and cold medications are easily available and often are shoplifted by persons who abuse them.

The same social pressures that influence young people to try alcohol are responsible for introducing people of all ages to the previously mentioned drugs and other chemical substances. Because it is easier to prevent drug abuse than it is to break an established habit, most efforts to combat drug abuse are directed at the young. However, people of all ages, including older people, may be or become abusers.

Table 35-2 Examples of Common Emergency Drugs

Drug	Description
Activate charcoal	A charcoal suspension. Used to treat poisoning.
Adrenaline (a-dren'a-lin) or **epinephrine** (ep-i-nef-rin)	A vasoconstrictor. Relieves anaphylactic shock.
Albuterol (al-bú-ter-ol)	A bronchodilator. Relaxes smooth muscle of the respiratory tract.
Atropine (a-fro-peen)	Helps restore heart rate.
Benadryl (ben'a-dril)	An antihistamine that relieves allergic symptoms.
Compazine (com-pa'zeen)	An antiemetic. Relieves symptoms of nausea and vomiting.
Dextrose (deks'trose) 50%	Used for hypoglycemia to counteract hyperinsulinism.
Diazepam (dī-i-az'-e-pam)	Helps control seizures. Antianxiety.
Digoxin (di-jox'in)	Cardiac drug. Used for congestive heart failure, arrhythmias. Slows and strengthens heartbeat.
Diuril (di'ur-il)	Promotes excretion of urine.
Hydrocortisone (hi"dro-cort'i-zon)	An anti inflammatory. Used to suppress swelling and shock.
Insulin (in'sah-lin)	Diabetic coma.
Isuprel (īcé-ū-prel)	Heart block.
Lasix (lā-siks, -ziks)	Pulmonary edema.
Lidocaine (lī'-dō-kāne)	Controls ventricular arrhythmia.
Morphine (mawr-feen)	Narcotic analgesic.
Narcan (nar'can)	Antidote. Used in narcotic overdose.
Nitroglycerin (ni"tro-glis'er-in)	Vasodilator. Dilates coronary arteries. Used in treatment of angina pectoris.
Valium (val'e-um)	Antianxiety, muscle relaxant. Used to calm anxious patients and to relax muscles. Valium is a Schedule IV drug, and therefore must be kept in a locked cabinet.
Verapamil (ver-ap'a-mil)	For cardiac arrhythmia, stable and unstable angina.

NOTE: Ipecac syrup, no longer used to induce vomiting, has proven to be cardiotoxic, and several cases of aspiration have occurred.

Table 35-3 Drugs of Abuse—Uses and Effects

Drugs	Controlled Substance Schedule	Trade or Other Names	Medical Uses	Dependence	
				Physical	Psychological
Narcotics					
Heroin	Substance I	Diamorphine, Horse, Smack, Black tar, *Chiva, Negra (black tar)*	None in United States, analgesic, antitussive	High	High
Morphine	Substance II	MS-Contin, Roxanol, Oramorph SR, MSIR	Analgesic	High	High
Hydrocodone	Substance II, Product III, V	Hydrocodone with acetaminophen, Vicodin, Vicoprofen, Tussionex, Lortab	Analgesic, antitussive	High	High
Hydromorphone	Substance II	Dilaudid	Analgesic	High	High
Oxycodone	Substance II	Roxicet, Oxycodone with acetaminophen, OxyContin, Endocet, Percocet, Percodan	Analgesic	High	High
Codeine	Substance II, Product III, V	Acetaminophen, Guaifenesin or Promethazine with Codeine, Fiorinal, Fioricet or Tylenol with Codeine	Analgesic, antitussive	Moderate	Moderate
Other Narcotics	Substance II, III, IV	Fentanyl, Demerol, Methadone, Darvon, Stadol, Talwin, Paregoric, Buprenex	Analgesic, antidiarrheal, antitussive	High-Low	High-Low
Depressants					
Gamma Hydroxybutyric Acid	Substance I, Product III	GHB, Liquid Ecstasy, Liquid X, Sodium Oxybate, Xyrem®	None in United States, anesthetic	Moderate	Moderate
Benzodiazepines	Substance IV	Valium, Xanax, Halcion, Ativan, Restoril, Rohypnol (Roofies, R-2), Klonopin	Antianxiety, sedative, anticonvulsant, hypnotic, muscle relaxant	Moderate	Moderate

Tolerance	Duration (hours)	Usual Method	Possible Effects	Effects of Overdose	Withdrawal Syndrome
Yes	3–4	Injected, snorted, smoked	Euphoria, drowsiness, respiratory depression, constricted pupils, nausea	Slow and shallow breathing, clammy skin, convulsions, coma, possible death	Watery eyes, runny nose, yawning, loss of appetite, irritability, tremors, panic, cramps, nausea, chills, sweating
Yes	3–12	Oral, injected	Same as above	Same as above	Same as above
Yes	3–6	Oral	Same as above	Same as above	Same as above
Yes	3–4	Oral, injected	Same as above	Same as above	Same as above
Yes	3–12	Oral	Same as above	Same as above	Same as above
Yes	3–4	Oral, injected	Same as above	Same as above	Same as above
Yes	Variable	Oral, injected, snorted, smoked	Same as above	Same as above	Same as above
Yes	3–6	Oral	Slurred speech, disorientation, drunken behavior without odor of alcohol, impaired memory of events, interacts with alcohol	Shallow respiration, clammy skin, dilated pupils, weak and rapid pulse, coma, possible death	Anxiety, insomnia, tremors, delirium, convulsions, possible death
Yes	1–8	Oral, injected	Same as above	Same as above	Same as above

continues

Table 35-3 Drugs of Abuse—Uses and Effects (*Continued*)

Drugs	Controlled Substance Schedule	Trade or Other Names	Medical Uses	Dependence Physical	Psychological
Other Depressants	Substance I, II, III, IV	Ambien, Sonata, Meprobamate, Chloral Hydrate, Barbiturates, Methaqualone (Quaalude)	Antianxiety, sedative, hypnotic	Moderate	Moderate
Stimulants					
Cocaine	Substance II	Coke, Flake, Snow, Crack, *Coca, Blanca, Perico, Nieve, Soda*	Local anesthetic	Possible	High
Amphetamine/ Methamphetamine	Substance II	Crank, Ice, Cristal, Krystal Meth, Speed, Adderall, Dexedrine, Desoxyn	Attention deficit/ hyperactivity disorder, narcolepsy, weight control	Possible	High
Methylphenidate	Substance II	Ritalin, Concerta, Focalin, Metadate	Attention deficit/ hyperactivity disorder	Possible	High
Other Stimulants	Substance III, IV	Adipex P, Ionamin, Prelu-2, Didrex, Provigil	Vasoconstriction	Possible	Moderate
Hallucinogens					
MDMA and Analogs	Substance I	(Ecstasy, XTC, Adam), MDA (Love Drug), MDEA (Eve), MBDB	None	None	Moderate
LSD	Substance I	Acid, Microdot, Sunshine, Boomers	None	None	Unknown
Phencyclidine and Analogs	Substance I, II, III	PCP, Angel Dust, Hog, Loveboat, Ketamine (Special K), PCE, PCPy, TCP	Anesthetic (ketamine)	Possible	High
Other Hallucinogens	Substance I	Psilocybe mushrooms, Mescaline, Peyote Cactus, Ayahausca, DMT, Dextromethorphan (DXM)	None	None	None

*Not regulated

Tolerance	Duration (hours)	Usual Method	Possible Effects	Effects of Overdose	Withdrawal Syndrome
Yes	2–6	Oral	Slurred speech, disorientation, drunken behavior without odor of alcohol, impaired memory of events, interacts with alcohol	Shallow respiration, clammy skin, dilated pupils, weak and rapid pulse, coma, possible death	Anxiety, insomnia, tremors, delirium, convulsions, possible death
Yes	1–2	Snorted, smoked, injected	Increased alertness, excitation, euphoria, increased pulse rate and blood pressure, insomnia, loss of appetite	Agitation, increased body temperature, hallucinations, convulsions, possible death	Apathy, long periods of sleep, irritability, depression, disorientation
Yes	2–4	Oral, injected, smoked	Same as above	Same as above	Same as above
Yes	2–4	Oral, injected, snorted, smoked	Same as above	Same as above	Same as above
Yes	2–4	Oral	Same as above	Same as above	Same as above
Yes	4–6	Oral, snorted, smoked	Heightened senses, teeth grinding, dehydration	Increased body temperature, electrolyte imbalance, cardiac arrest	Muscle aches, drowsiness, depression, acne
Yes	8–12	Oral	Illusions and hallucinations, altered perception of time and distance	Longer, more intense "trip" episodes	None
Yes	1–12	Smoked, oral, injected, snorted	Illusions and hallucinations, altered perception of time and distance	Unable to direct movement, feel pain, remember	Drug-seeking behavior*
Possible	4–8	Oral	Illusions and hallucinations, altered perception of time and distance	Unable to direct movement, feel pain, remember	Drug-seeking behavior*

continues

Table 35-3 Drugs of Abuse—Uses and Effects (*Continued*)

Drugs	Controlled Substance Schedule	Trade or Other Names	Medical Uses	Dependence Physical	Dependence Psychological
Cannibis					
Marijuana	Substance I	Pot, Grass, Sinsemilla, Blunts, *Mota, Yerba, Grifa*	None	Unknown	Moderate
Tetrahydrocanna-binol	Substance I, Product III	THC, Marinol	Antinauseant, appetite stimulant	Yes	Moderate
Hashish and Hashish Oil	Substance I	Hash, Hash oil	None	Unknown	Moderate
Anabolic Steroids					
Testosterone	Substance III	Depo Testosterone, Sustanon, Sten, Cypt	Hypogonadism	Unknown	Unknown
Other Anabolic Steroids	Substance III	Parabolan, Winstrol, Equipoise, Anadrol, Dianabol, Primabolin-Depo, D-Ball	Anemia, breast cancer	Unknown	Yes
Inhalants					
Amyl and Butyl Nitrite		Pearls, Poppers, Rush, Locker Room	Angina (amyl)	Unknown	Unknown
Nitrous Oxide		Laughing gas, balloons, Whippets	Anesthetic	Unknown	Low
Other Inhalants		Adhesives, spray paint, hair spray, dry cleaning fluid, spot remover, lighter fluid	None	Unknown	High
Alcohol					
Alcohol		Beer, wine, liquor	None	High	High

Tolerance	Duration (hours)	Usual Method	Possible Effects	Effects of Overdose	Withdrawal Syndrome
Yes	2–4	Smoked, oral	Euphoria, relaxed inhibitions, increased appetite, disorientation	Fatigue, paranoia, possible psychosis	Occasional reports of insomnia, hyperactivity, decreased appetite
Yes	2–4	Smoked, oral	Same as above	Same as above	Same as above
Unknown	14–28 days	Injected	Virilization, edema, testicular atrophy, gynecomastia, acne, aggressive behavior	Unknown	Possible depression
Unknown	Variable	Oral, injected	Same as above	Same as above	Same as above
No	1	Inhaled	Flushing, hypotension, headache	Methemoglobinemia	Agitation
No	0.5	Inhaled	Impaired memory, slurred speech, drunken behavior, slow-onset vitamin deficiency, organ damage	Vomiting, respiratory depression, loss of consciousness, possible death	Trembling, anxiety, insomnia, vitamin deficiency, confusion, hallucinations, convulsions
No	0.5–2	Inhaled	Impaired memory, slurred speech, drunken behavior, slow-onset vitamin deficiency, organ damage	Vomiting, respiratory depression, loss of consciousness, possible death	Trembling, anxiety, insomnia, vitamin deficiency, confusion, hallucinations, convulsions
Yes	1–3	Oral	Impaired judgments, uncoordinated movements, slurred speech, blurred vision	Motor vehicle accidents, gastritis, liver damage, brain damage, domestic violence	Anxiety, shakiness, depression, hallucinations, sweats, increased blood pressure, seizures

PROCEDURE 35-1
Proper Disposal of Drugs

STANDARD PRECAUTIONS:

PURPOSE:

To properly dispose of drugs that have reached their expiration dates.

EQUIPMENT/SUPPLIES:

Drugs (oral and parenteral) that have reached their expiration dates

PROCEDURE STEPS:

1. Consult practice policy for disposal of expired medications.

2. Access the drug closet or narcotics cabinet and evaluate the expiration date on all medications.

3. Gather expired drugs, either prescription or over-the-counter. RATIONALE: Expired drugs cannot be dispensed nor administered because they can be harmful to patients.

4. Medicine take-back programs for disposal are a good way to remove expired medications. Contact your city or county government's household trash and recycling service to learn about any special rules regarding which medicines can be taken back. Explain this process.

5. For safety reasons, FDA recommends that a few, select medicines be disposed of by flushing down the sink or toilet. *Pay attention to detail.* Only after checking the label or package insert for the medication should this method be utilized. RATIONALE: Disposal of drugs into the sewage system, either by flushing down the toilet or down the sink, is discouraged everywhere and is prohibited in some states (medication substances have been found in some municipal water supplies).

6. Wash hands.

7. Accurately document instructions in the medication log book or in the appropriate data collection area that medications with expired dates were disposed of. Be sure to document the method of disposal. Have a co-worker co-sign the entry.

DOCUMENTATION:

2/17/XX   Drugs from the crash cart, drugs in the medication closet, and drug samples all checked for expiration dates. Expired medications were removed and returned to the pharmacy for incineration. Drugs inventoried and restocked with new replacements. C. McInnis, RMA (AMT)——————

CASE STUDY 35-1

Refer to the scenario at the beginning of the chapter.
Mrs. Maynard has an appointment to see Dr. Hoback this morning. She brings in her bag with all of her prescription medications. When Claire Bloom, CMA (AAMA), is updating Mrs. Maynard's electronic medical record, she becomes aware that there is a mistake in the record of Mrs. Maynard's medication history. The prescription bottle states "Zantac 150 mg by mouth twice a day." The electronic record reveals that the medication prescribed was "Zyrtec 10 mg by mouth once a day."

CASE STUDY REVIEW

1. What are the first steps that Ms. Bloom should take to clarify this issue?

2. What kind of questions would Ms. Bloom need to ask Mrs. Maynard about the medications?

CASE STUDY 35-2

Maria Jover reports vaginal discharge and discomfort. Dr. King confirms the diagnosis of a yeast infection by performing a smear and identifying the microorganism. Dr. King prescribes over-the-counter vaginal suppositories. After asking Maria if she has any questions, clinical medical assistant Audrey Jones, RMA (AMT) proceeds to help Maria understand the self-administration of this particular medication.

CASE STUDY REVIEW

1. The patient, Maria, asks Audrey Jones whether she can use some vaginal suppositories she bought last year. How should Audrey respond?

2. Maria tells Audrey that the last time she had a vaginal yeast infection she only used part of the recommended number of suppositories because the infection cleared up. How should Audrey respond?

3. Maria does not really like using suppositories. Should Audrey ask Dr. King to prescribe another form of medication for the yeast infection? What other forms might be available?

CASE STUDY 35-3

Dr. Lewis keeps a small quantity of various controlled substances on the premises for use in an emergency situation.

CASE STUDY REVIEW

1. What are the legalities surrounding controlled substances that concern Joe Guerrero, CMA (AAMA), the clinical medical assistant?

2. What are his responsibilities?

SUMMARY

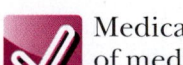 Medical assistants must know state and federal laws that govern the distribution and administration of medications and must understand their role and responsibilities in light of these laws. Knowledge of drug regulations; the legal classifications of drugs, including controlled substances; and prescribing, administering, and dispensing of drugs is essential to ensure compliance with the law.

Available resources and reference books will provide valuable information about pharmaceutical products, their classifications, routes, forms, storage and handling, and side effects.

Emergency drugs and supplies should be available on a crash cart or a tray or cabinet for the sole use in an office emergency.

 With the increase of drug abuse and misuse, it is important for medical assistants to recognize the signs of drug abuse in patients and coworkers and to report abuse to the provider or supervisor.

STUDY FOR SUCCESS

To reinforce your knowledge and skills of information presented in this chapter:

- 📝 Review the *Key Terms*
- Role-play with other students to apply attributes of professionalism pertinent to this chapter.
- Consider the *Case Studies* and discuss your conclusions
- Answer the questions in the *Certification Review*
- Apply your knowledge by completing the *Activities* in the *Study Guide* and the *Games and Quizzes* in the StudyWARE StudyWARE software on the *Premium Website*
- 🛡 Perform the *Procedure* using the *Competency Assessment Checklists* in the *Competency Manual*
- Practice your problem-solving skills with the *Critical Thinking Challenge 3.0* on the *Premium Website*

Additional resources for this chapter include:

- Module 25 of the *Medical Assisting Learning Lab*
- *CourseMate for Delmar's Comprehensive Medical Assisting*
- *WebTutor for Delmar's Comprehensive Medical Assisting*

CERTIFICATION REVIEW

1. Which of the following drugs is commonly used in an emergency such as anaphylactic shock?
   a. Lomotil
   b. Interferon
   c. Cytoxan
   d. Epinephrine
2. Which of the following types of drugs do providers prescribe most frequently?
   a. Generic
   b. Official
   c. Chemical
   d. Brand
3. An example of a drug that can be obtained from an animal is:
   a. digitalis
   b. cortisone
   c. imferon
   d. sulfur
4. Which of the following is an example of a controlled substance?
   a. Nembutal
   b. Keflin
   c. Inderal
   d. Aldomet

5. After you have poured a medication and taken it to the patient, he refuses to take it. You should:
   a. give it to another patient who has the same medication prescribed
   b. return the refused medication to its original container
   c. save it for the next time the patient is due for another dose
   d. dispose of it by returning it to the pharmacist to dispose of. Document.
6. The substances that have the highest potential for abuse are designated as which schedule?
   a. Schedule I
   b. Schedule II
   c. Schedule III
   d. Schedule IV
7. Sources of drugs include:
   a. plants
   b. animals
   c. minerals
   d. all of the above

8. Which of the following are considered medical uses for drugs?
   a. Therapeutic, diagnostic, curative
   b. Diagnostic, curative, recreational
   c. Preventative, curative, holistic
   d. Replacement, prophylactic, research
9. Which of the following is a commonly abused drug?
   a. Aspirin
   b. Oxycodone
   c. Fentanyl
   d. Both b and c

10. Which of the following is a category of drug names?
    a. Brand name
    b. Generic
    c. Chemical
    d. All of the above

REFERENCES/BIBLIOGRAPHY

Broderick, M. (2003, September). Spotting drug abuse. *RN Magazine, 66*(9), pp. 48–53.

Centers for Disease Control and Prevention. (2007). *Public emergency preparedness and response.* Retrieved September 11, 2007, from http://www.bt.cdc.gov

Facts & figures. (2007). Retrieved October 15, 2008, from http://drugtopics.modernmedicine.com

Human Genome Project Information. (2011). *Pharmacogenomics.* Retrieved April 27, 2012, from http://www.ornl.gov/sci/techresources/Human_Genome/medicine/pharma.shtml

The Medical Board of California, Department of Consumer Affairs. (2010). *Medical Assistants – Frequently Asked Questions.* Retrieved April 29, 2012, from http://www.mbc.ca.gov/allied/medical_assistants_questions.html

MedicineNet.com. (2005). *Wonder Drugs Using Pharmazooticals.* Retrieved April 28, 2012, from http://www.medicinenet.com/script/main/art.asp?articlekey=52324

Rice, J. (2006). *Principles of pharmacology for medical assisting* (4th ed.). Clifton Park, NY: Delmar Cengage Learning.

Spratto, G. R., & Woods, A. L. (2007). *Physician's desk reference—Nurse's drug handbook.* Clifton Park, NY: Delmar Cengage Learning.

Taber's cyclopedic medical dictionary (22nd ed.). (2003). Philadelphia: F. A. Davis.

United States Drug Enforcement Agency (DEA). (2007). *Drugs of abuse publication chart.* Retrieved February 16, 2008, from http://www.justice.gov/dea/docs/drugs_of_abuse_2011.pdf

U.S. Food and Drug Administration, Department of Health and Human Services. (2004, February 6). *FDA issues regulations prohibiting sale of dietary supplements containing ephedrine alkaloids and reiterates—it advises that consumers stop using these products.*

WebMD Health. (2006). *Crash carts and their typical contents and indications.* Retrieved October 15, 2008, from http://ucdmc.ucdavis.edu/cne/resources/clinical_skills_refresher/crash_cart/index.html

Wooten, J. M. (2003, April). Medicine cabinet staples are not without risks. *RN Magazine, 66* (4), 96.

World Health Organization. (n.d.). *Health aspects of biological and chemical weapons.* Retrieved September 10, 2007, from http://www.who.int

OUTLINE

Legal and Ethical Implications of Medication Administration
Ethical Considerations
The Medication Order
The Prescription
Drug Dosage
Age
Weight
Sex
Other Factors
Pediatric Considerations
The Medication Label
Calculation of Drug Dosages
Understanding Ratio
Understanding Proportion
Weights and Measures
Medications Measured in Units
How to Calculate Unit Dosages

Insulin
Diabetes
Calculating Adult Dosages
The Proportional Method
Understanding the Formula Method
Calculating Children's Dosages
Body Surface Area
Kilogram of Body Weight
Administration of Medications
The "Six Rights" of Proper Drug Administration
Medication Errors
Patient Assessment
Administration of Oral Medications
Equipment and Supplies for Oral Medications
Administration of Parenteral Medications

Hazards Associated with Parenteral Medications
Reasons for Parenteral Route Selection
Parenteral Equipment and Supplies
Principles of Intravenous Therapy
Site Selection and Injection Angle
Marking the Correct Site for Intramuscular Injection
Basic Guidelines for Administration of Injections
Z-Track Method of Intramuscular Injection
Administration of Allergenic Extracts
Administration of Inhaled Medications
Implications for Patient Care
Administration of Oxygen

LEARNING OUTCOMES

1. Define, spell, and pronounce the key terms as presented in the glossary.
2. Discuss the legal and ethical implications of medication administration.
3. Describe the medication order.
4. Identify abbreviations and symbols used in calculating medication dosage.
5. Describe the parts of a prescription.
6. Define drug dosage.
7. State what information is found on a medication label.

8. Understand ratio and proportion.
9. Use the metric, household, and apothecary systems of measurement and convert between the metric and apothecary systems.
10. Understand units of medication dosage.
11. Correctly calculate dosages for adults and children.
12. List the guidelines to follow when preparing and administering medications.
13. Administer oral medications.
14. Select proper sites for administering parenteral medication.

ATTRIBUTES OF PROFESSIONALISM

Communication
- Did you introduce yourself? Did you identify the patient through name and birth date or other identifying feature?
- Did you explain procedures and expectations to the patient?
- Did you speak at the patient's level of understanding?
- Did you allay patients' fears and help them feel safe and comfortable?

Presentation
- Were you courteous, patient and respectful to the patient?

Competency
- Did you pay attention to detail?
- Did you ask questions if you were out of your comfort zone or did not have the experience to carry out tasks?
- Did you display sound judgment?
- Did you apply critical thinking skills in performing patient assessment and care?
- Did you recognize the importance of local, state, and federal legislation and regulations in the practice setting?

Integrity
- Did you work within your scope of practice?
- Did you protect and maintain confidentiality?
- Did you immediately report any error you had made?
- Did you report situations that were harmful or illegal?
- Did you do "the right thing" even when no one was observing?

KEY TERMS

administering

apnea

body surface area (BSA)

compounding

dispensing

hypoxemia

meniscus

nomogram

parenteral

pharmacokinetics

phytomedicines

port

precipitate

retrolental fibroplasia

status asthmaticus

unit dose

LEARNING OUTCOMES (*continued*)

15. Describe safe disposal of syringes, needles, and biohazard materials.
16. Understand intravenous therapy.
17. Describe site selection for administration of injections.
18. Understand allergenic extracts.
19. Describe inhalation medication and its administration.
20. Analyze the professionalism questions and apply them to this chapter's content.

INTRODUCTION

Despite the fact that many ambulatory care centers use what is known as the "unit dose" type of medication preparation, there remains a responsibility for medical assistants to know and understand how to calculate dosages of medication and to safely administer them to patients.

This chapter addresses calculation of adult and pediatric dosages of medication using the metric and household systems. It also emphasizes the legal aspects of medication administration and discusses oral and parenteral medication administration.

LEGAL AND ETHICAL IMPLICATIONS OF MEDICATION ADMINISTRATION

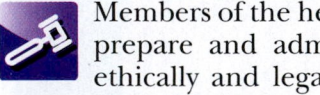 Members of the health care profession who prepare and administer medications are ethically and legally responsible for their own actions. Under law, these individuals are required to be licensed, registered, or otherwise authorized by a provider.

Each state has enacted laws governing the practice of medicine, nursing, and pharmacy. These laws vary from state to state; therefore, it is essential that medical assistants become familiar with the laws of the state in which they are employed before administering any medication. In some states, the only health professional authorized to give injections, other than a physician, is a registered nurse. In other states, legislation gives physicians broad authority to delegate responsibility for administering medication to other health care workers such as medical assistants. Laws have been passed in some states specifying which qualified and properly educated and trained persons may perform certain medical acts.

Regardless of the differences in state authorization laws, the courts will not permit the careless action of health care workers to go unpunished,

1. Drug name (generic and brand)
2. Action
3. Uses
4. Contraindications
5. Warnings when indicated
6. Adverse reactions
7. Dosage and route
8. Implications for patient care
9. Patient teaching
10. Special considerations

© Cengage Learning 2014

Figure 36-1 Medical assistants should have a thorough knowledge of any medication they administer to a patient and should consult references such as the Physician's Desk Reference (PDR).

especially when such actions result in harm or death to the patient. Under the law, those administering medications are expected to be knowledgeable about the drugs that they administer and the effects the drug(s) may or will have on the patient. Many states have uniform disciplinary acts. Never administer a medication without thorough knowledge of the drug. It is the medical assistant's responsibility to know the information about a medication listed in Figure 36-1 before administering it to a patient. You are an agent of the provider and accountable for your actions.

Ethical Considerations

Anyone who has access to medications may be tempted to use them for personal benefit. To do so not only is unethical, but also is considered to be illegal. The conversion to personal use of medications intended for another is unethical and may cause harm to the patient. It is also unethical and illegal to take any medication that belongs to your employer, even aspirin or drug samples, without proper authorization.

It is essential that attention is focused on the administration of medications. However, mistakes are sometimes made. If there has been a medication error, it is the responsibility of the professional medical assistant to demonstrate integrity and report this error immediately.

The Medication Order

The medication order is given by the provider. It is for a specific patient and denotes the drug to be given, the dosage, the form of the drug, the time for or frequency of administration, and the route by which the drug is to be given.

The Prescription

The prescription is a written legal document that gives directions for **compounding**, **dispensing**, and **administering** a medication to a patient. There are eight parts to a prescription (Figure 36-2).

The purpose of a prescription is to control the sale and use of drugs that can be safely and effectively used only under the supervision of a licensed provider. Federal law divides medicines into two main classes: prescription or legend medicines and over-the-counter (OTC) medicines. The prescription is written by the provider and signed with an ink pen or e-prescribed. The pharmacist fills the prescription according to the provider's order. Once the prescription has been filled, the assigned prescription number and all other information can be entered into a computer. The hard copy of the prescription is filed and kept for a minimum of 7 years. There are state and federal laws, as well as Drug Enforcement Agency guidelines that are applied to the prescribing provider and the pharmacy regarding controlled substances. Some examples are:

- There is a limit placed on the amount of time that a prescription is valid after the provider writes it and it is presented at the pharmacy to be filled.
- The number of day's supply is limited.
- The refilling of a prescription for a controlled substance listed in Schedule II is prohibited.
- A prescription for controlled substances in Schedules III, IV, and V issued by a practitioner, may be communicated either orally, in writing, or by facsimile to the pharmacist, and may be refilled if so authorized on the prescription or by call-in.
- Schedule III and IV controlled substances may be refilled if authorized on the prescription.

There are different guidelines for the management of the prescription once it is filled. These guidelines can be found in the DEA Pharmacist's Manual.

HIPAA. E-prescribing is the process of electronically accessing the patient's medical history, prescribing a medication, and selecting a pharmacy.

Parts of a Prescription

1. The physician's name, address, telephone and fax numbers, and DEA registration number. [1]
2. The patient's name, date of birth, address, and the date on which the prescription is written. [2]
3. The superscription that includes the symbol Rx ("take thou"). [3]
4. The inscription that states the names and quantities of ingredients to be included in the medication. [4]
5. The subscription that gives directions to the pharmacist for filling the prescription. [5]
6. The signature (Sig) that gives the directions for the patient. [6]
7. The physician's signature blanks. Where signed, indicates if a generic substitute is allowed or if the medication is to be dispensed as written. [7]
8. REFILL 0 1 2 3 p.r.n. This is where the physician indicates whether or not the prescription can be refilled. [8]

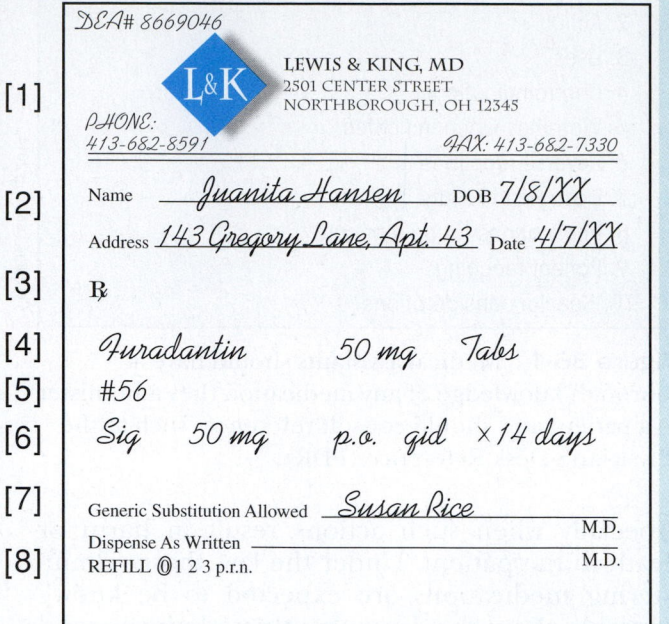

© Cengage Learning 2014

Figure 36-2 Prescriptions are written legal documents that give directions for compounding, dispensing, and administering a medication. Prescriptions have eight distinct elements.

EHR The Medicare Prescription Drug, Improvement, and Modernization Act (MMA) of 2003 and the Health Insurance Portability and Accountability Act (HIPAA) of 1996 have recommended e-prescribing standards. Medications handled electronically have reduced the problem of medication errors. Patients enjoy the ease of e-prescriptions because they do not have to drop off the prescription and then return to pick it up. Some states already have e-prescriptions in patients' electronic medical records. However, the possibility of a breach in confidentiality exists whenever electronic medical records are used.

Prescriptions for Controlled Substances.
Federal laws require that the provider follows specific procedures when prescribing controlled substances (Table 36-1).

All prescriptions for controlled substances must be dated and signed on the date issued, bearing the full name and address of the patient and the name, address, and Drug Enforcement Administration (DEA) number (see Chapter 35) of the provider. The prescription must be written in ink or typewritten and signed by the provider's own hand.

Prescription Abbreviations and Symbols.
It is important to be knowledgeable of the most common abbreviations used by the provider when an

Table 36-1 Requirements for Prescriptions for Controlled Substances

	Verbal Order or Prescription	Written Prescription	Refills
Schedule I	NOT FOR MEDICINAL USE		
Schedule II	No	Yes	No
Schedule III	Yes	Yes	5 × within 6 months
Schedule IV	Yes	Yes	5 × within 6 months
Schedule V	Yes	Yes	5 × within 6 months

© Cengage Learning 2014

order for a prescription drug is given. The abbreviations are a clear and concise means of writing orders. This medical shorthand is an international language used by professional and nonprofessional people involved with patient care. Medical assistants should memorize all abbreviations in Table 36-2 so that they can prepare medications safely and accurately for administration.

Table 36-2   Common Prescription Abbreviations and Symbols

Abbreviation or Symbol	Meaning	Abbreviation or Symbol	Meaning
aa	of each	non rep	do not repeat
ac	before meals	$\bar{p}$	after
ad lib	as desired	pc	after meals
aq	water	per	by or with
bid	twice a day	po	by mouth
$\bar{c}$	with	prn	as needed
cap	capsule	pt	patient
dil	dilute	q	every
elix	elixir	qh	every hour
g	gram	q (2, 3, 4) h	every (2, 3, 4) hours
gr	grain	qid	four times a day
gt or gtt	drop (drops)	qs	of sufficient quantity
h	hour	Rx	take
IM	intramuscular	$\bar{s}$	without
IV	intravenous	sol	solution
kg	kilogram	ss	one-half
L	liter	stat	at once
liq	liquid	tab	tablet
m or min	minim	Tbs	tablespoon
mg	milligram	tsp	teaspoon
mL	milliliter	tid	three times a day
mm	millimeter	tr	tincture
NPO	nothing by mouth	ung	ointment

© Cengage Learning 2014

The Joint Commission requires that facilities comply with the Joint Commission's minimum requirement for the banning of certain abbreviations, acronyms, symbols listed in their "*Do Not Use*" list. This ban, as part of the Joint Commission's 2004 patient safety goals, has been applied to protect patients from errors during documentation. The ban was reaffirmed in 2005 by the Joint

Table 36-3 Dangerous Abbreviations No Longer Allowed

Do Not Use	Possible Misinterpretation	How to Avoid Problem
U (for unit)	Mistaken for a four (4), zero (0), or cc	Write out the word "unit"
IU (for international unit)	Mistaken for IV or ten (10)	Write out "international unit"
Q.D., every day; Q.O.D, (every other day)	Mistaken for one another	Write "daily" Write "every other day"
Trailing zero (X.0 mg) Lack of preceding zero (.X mg)	Decimal point is missed and dose is either too much or not enough	Do not write a zero by itself after the decimal point (X mg) Always use zero before a decimal point (0.X mg)
mS mSO₄ MgSO₄	Can be interpreted to mean morphine sulfate or magnesium sulfate	Write out "morphine sulfate" Write out "magnesium sulfate"

© Cengage Learning 2014

Table 36-4 Additional Abbreviations, Acronyms, and Symbols That May Be Misinterpreted (for Possible Future Inclusion in the Official "Do Not Use" List)

Do Not Use	Possible Misinterpretation	How to Avoid Problem
> (greater than) < (less than)	Can be misinterpreted as number seven (7) or the letter "L" Confused for one another	Write out "greater than" and "less than"
Apothecary units	Unfamiliar to many practitioners Confused with metric units	Use metric units
@	Mistaken for number two (2)	Write "at"
cc	Mistaken for U (units) when written poorly	Write out "mL" or "milliliters"
μg	Mistaken for mg (milligrams) causing 1,000 × overdose	Write out "mcg" or micrograms

© Cengage Learning 2014

Commission. In 2010, the "Do Not Use" list was integrated into the Information Management standards to improve medication administration safety. This standard relates to documentation, both electronic and manual. The standard states that unapproved abbreviations cannot be used in any type or medication-related documentation. Table 36-3 lists abbreviations no longer allowed by the Joint Commission. Table 36-4 lists abbreviations and symbols that can be misinterpreted and are under consideration for possible inclusion on the "Do Not Use" list in the future.

Patients should be inquisitive when at the provider's office, clinic, pharmacy, or hospital and should ask questions about the medications they are prescribed or being given (see Patient Education box).

Many medications sound alike and look alike, which can cause confusion and errors. The Joint Commission recommends that pharmaceutical manufacturers examine their practices in naming

their medications and make changes to alleviate confusion and errors. Table 36-5 lists a few sound-alike, look-alike medications. The United States Pharmacopeia regularly updates a complete list of sound-alike, look-alike medications on their Web site (http://www.usp.org).

DRUG DOSAGE

The dosage or dose is the amount of medicine that is prescribed for administration. It is determined by the provider or qualified practitioner, who considers the following important factors: age, weight, sex, and other factors as well.

Age

The usual adult dose is generally suitable for the 20- to 60-year age group. Infants, young children, adolescents, and older adults require an individualized dosage regimen.

Table 36-5 Sound-alike, Look-alike Medications

Accupril (hypertension)	Aciphex (heartburn, ulcers)
Rimantadine (flu)	Ranitidine (heartburn)
Oxycontin (pain)	Oxybutynin (urinary incontinence)
Paxil (depression)	Plavix (prevent heart attack and stroke)
Pravachol (high cholesterol)	Propranolol (hypertension)
Singulair (asthma)	Sinequan (depression, anxiety)
Clonazepam (anticonvulsant)	Chlorazepate (anti-anxiety)
Darvon (analgesic)	Diovan (hypertension)
Clonazepam (anticonvulsant)	Lorazepam (anti-anxiety)

© Cengage Learning 2014

Weight

The average adult dosage is based on 150 pounds (about 68 kilograms). Individuals who weigh less or more than this should have the dosage based on **body surface area (BSA)** or kilograms of body weight.

Sex

Many medications are contraindicated during pregnancy and breast-feeding. It is important that these two factors be known before any dose of medication is prescribed.

Other Factors

Other factors that determine the dosage of a medication include the following:

1. Physical and emotional condition of patient
2. Disease process, especially kidney disease because of impaired excretion
3. Presence of more than one disease process

4. Causative microorganism(s) and the severity of the infection
5. Patient's medical history, allergies, and idiosyncrasies
6. Safest method, route, time, and amount to effect the desired maximum result

Pediatric Considerations

The term **pharmacokinetics** refers to the way a drug is handled by the body. For pediatric patients, it means that drugs are administered in smaller but more frequent doses. Dosages are weight-based in milligrams, micrograms, or milliequivalents per kilogram, which allows for much safer drug administration. Remember that those children 16 years of age and younger are considered pediatric patients. At age 16, it is generally accepted that the pharmacokinetics are similar to that of adults.

Only about one quarter of the drugs approved by the FDA are indicated for pediatric use. There is extensive testing required prior to approval to assure safety in the less mature body systems of pediatric patients.

As reported by the U.S. Pharmacopeia, there is an increased rate of medication errors in the pediatric population of almost three times the adult population rate of medication errors. There can be significant and life-altering results that are associated with these errors. Therefore, it is considered a best practice to always have a peer review the order, the calculation, and the medication prior to administering a drug to a pediatric patient.

THE MEDICATION LABEL

The medication label can be a source of valuable information to the medical assistant and the patient. Regardless of whether administering a prescription drug or taking a nonprescription product, an understanding of the information provided on the label is essential to the safe and effective use of any medicine. In addition to the name and address of the manufacturer, other important items of information on a medication label include:

- The trade or brand name for the medication
- The generic name (or listing of active and inactive ingredients)
- The National Drug Code (NDC) numbers that can be used to identify the manufacturer, the product, and the size of the container
- The dosage strength in a given amount of the medication

PATIENT EDUCATION

Patients should:

1. Question the provider, pharmacist, and staff administering the drug about the drug and its possible side effects.

2. Be sure the prescription has been written legibly. Many drugs sound alike (e.g., Ambien® for insomnia and Amen® for menstrual cycle control; Xanax® for anxiety and Zantac® for heartburn and ulcers; Fosamax® for osteoporosis and Flomax® for enlarged prostate).

3. Always check the label at the pharmacy to make sure it is clearly written.

4. Always check your medication at the pharmacy to be certain that the medication and directions are what you expect.

5. Have the provider or pharmacist explain the name and purpose of each new medication that is being prescribed. Be sure you understand.

6. Keep an updated list of all medications, prescriptions, OTC vitamins, minerals, and **phytomedicines**.

7. Take medications as directed, and do not discontinue use until the appropriate date as indicated by the provider.

8. Store medicines away from heat and humidity in their original containers.

9. Ask the provider or pharmacist what you should do if you miss a dose.

- The usual dosage and frequency of administration
- The route of administration
- Precautions and warnings
- The expiration date for the medication

Other information that may be on a medication label includes directions for storage and directions for mixing or reconstituting a powdered form of the drug (Figure 35-4).

CALCULATION OF DRUG DOSAGES

 The preparation and administration of medications is one of the most important and critical tasks that medical assistants perform. Today, drugs are more potent and more likely to cause physiologic changes in the body; therefore, anyone who administers medications must do so with extreme care.

 Incorrectly calculated or measured dosages are the leading cause of error in the administration of medications. A drug error is a violation of a patient's rights. It is important that medical assistants develop a working knowledge of mathematics to calculate or accurately measure a medication that is to be administered to a patient.

 According to the Institute of Medicine (IOM), each year medications kill several thousand hospital patients and injure another 1.5 million. About half of these deaths and injuries result from side effects; the other half result from errors. Because the majority of prescriptions are written in providers' clinics, the figures are likely to be proportionately higher. E-prescribing will reduce the number of errors. Hospital prescriptions and all OTC medications, vaccines, and blood will require standardized and universal bar codes to help prevent medication errors. Reading the bar code with a scanner can correlate the medication bar code with a patient identification bar code.

The IOM states that only a small percentage of health care agencies use a bar code medication system. However, studies have shown that use of bar codes (bar code on medication matches bar code on patient's wrist) results in far fewer errors.

 A study in 1999 by the IOM determined that many medical mistakes were made that were avoidable, including medication errors. Patient safety then became a primary concern. As a result, computer-based provider order-entry systems have been implemented in hospitals, outpatient centers, and non–acute care settings. These systems enable providers to enter prescriptions and other orders for patient care electronically. This reduces the errors that are caused by legibility and completeness problems, and improves the communication between the provider and the pharmacist. Patient records are also readily available and this improves patient safety and prevents medical errors and adverse drug events by checking allergies, previous medications, and dosages.

Additionally, the IOM recommended to the FDA that they lessen the confusion about sound-alike medications and simplify look-alike labels and packaging.

The Centers for Medicare and Medicaid Services (www.cms.gov) have initiated an EHR Incentive Program. As a part of this program, CMS has established 15 core measures to provide incentive payments to eligible providers, in- and outpatient clinics, urgent care, surgery centers, and hospitals as they adopt, implement, upgrade, or demonstrate meaningful use of certified EHR technology. The fourth core measure addresses e-prescribing.

The objective of this core measure is to generate and transmit permissible prescriptions electronically. Achievement of this objective is measured by proving that 40% of all permissible prescriptions written by the eligible professional are transmitted electronically using certified EHR technology. "Permissible prescriptions" refers to the current restrictions by the Department of Justice on the electronic prescribing of Schedules II–V controlled substances.

Understanding Ratio

Ratio is a method of expressing the relationship of a number, quantity, substance, or degree between two similar components. For example, the relationship of one to five is written 1:5. Note that numbers are side by side and separated by a colon.

In mathematics, a ratio may be expressed as a quotient, a fraction, or a decimal.

Ratio Expressed as a Quotient.
A quotient is the number found when one number is divided by another number. The ratio one to five written as a quotient is $1 \div 5$.

Ratio Expressed as a Fraction.
A fraction is the process of dividing or breaking a whole number into parts. The ratio one to five written as a fraction is $\frac{1}{5}$ or $\frac{1}{5}$.

Ratio Expressed as a Decimal.
A decimal is a linear array of numbers based on 10 or any multiple of 10. To express the ratio one to five as a decimal, divide the denominator (5) into the numerator (1).

$$\text{(denominator) } 5\overline{)1.0}^{\,0.2} \text{ (numerator)}$$

The ratio may be expressed as:

A quotient	A fraction	A decimal
$1 \div 5$	$\frac{1}{5}$ $\left(\frac{1}{5}\right)$	0.2

Understanding Proportion

Proportion is a process of expressing the comparative relationship between a part, share, or portion with regard to size, amount, or number. In mathematics, a proportion expresses the relationship between two ratios. In setting up a proportion, the ratios are separated by a colon (:) or an equal sign (=) sign. In this text, the equal sign (=) is used to separate ratios.

Example:

$6 : 4 = 3 : 2$

Read:

Six is to four equals three is to two.

The four terms of a proportion are given special names. The *means* are the inner numbers or the second and third terms of the proportion.

Example:

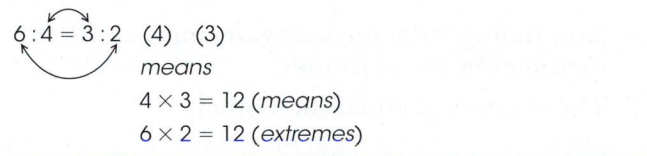

$6 : 4 = 3 : 2$ (4)   (3)
means
$4 \times 3 = 12$ (*means*)
$6 \times 2 = 12$ (*extremes*)

The *extremes* are the outer numbers or the first and fourth terms of the proportion.

Example:

$6 : 4 = 3 : 2$ (6)   (2)
extremes

In a true proportion, the product of the means equals the product of the extremes.

Example:

means   (16)   (1)
$8 : 16 = 1 : 2$
extremes   (8)   (2)
$16 \times 1 = 16$ (*means*)
$8 \times 2 = 16$ (*extremes*)

Solving for x.
The proportion is a useful mathematical tool. When a part, share, or portion of the problem is unknown, then x represents the unknown factor. You can determine the unknown

by solving for *x*. The unknown factor *x* may appear any place in the proportion.

Now solve for *x* in the problem: $3 : 4 = x : 12$.

1. Multiply the term that contains the *x* and place the product ($4x$) to the left of the equal sign.
2. Multiply the other terms and place the product (36) to the right of the equal sign.
3. To find *x*, divide the multiplier of *x* into the product of the other terms.

$$4x = 36$$
$$x = \frac{36}{4} \text{ or } 36 \div 4$$
$$x = 9$$

After finding the unknown factor, check your mathematical skills by determining if you have a true proportion. This technique is called proof or proving your answer. To prove your answer:

1. Place the answer you found for *x* back into the formula where *x* was.

$$3 : 4 = 9 : 12$$

2. Now multiply the means by the means, and the extremes by the extremes.
3. The results will equal each other.

Formula: $3:4 = x:12$

Proof: $3:4 = 9:12$

$$4 \times 9 = 36$$
$$3 \times 12 = 36$$

Weights and Measures

Two systems of measurement are used in pharmacology to calculate dosages: metric and household. The metric system is used throughout the world as the official language of communication in scientific and technical fields. It is based on the decimal system: the number 10 or multiples of 10.

Metric System Guidelines. The following guidelines are helpful when learning basic facts about the metric system:

1. Arabic numbers are used to designate whole numbers, e.g., 1, 250, 500, 1,000.
2. Decimal fractions are used for quantities less than one, e.g., 0.1, 0.01, 0.001, 0.0001.
3. To ensure accuracy, place a zero before the decimal point, e.g., 0.1, 0.001, 0.0001.
4. The Arabic number precedes the metric unit of measurement, e.g., 10 grams, 2 millimeters, 5 liters.
5. The abbreviation for gram should be capitalized (Gm) or written as (g) to distinguish it from grain (gr).
6. The abbreviation for liter is capitalized (L).
7. Prefixes are written in lowercase letters, e.g., milli, centi, deci, deka.
8. Capitalize the measurement and symbol when it is named after a person, e.g., Celsius (C).
9. Periods are no longer used with most abbreviations or symbols.
10. Abbreviations for units are the same for singular and plural. An *s* is not added to an abbreviation to indicate a plural.

The Seven Common Metric Prefixes. It is important to know common metric prefixes to have a solid foundation for determining metric equivalents. When a metric prefix is combined with a root of physical quantity, you arrive at multiples or submultiples of the metric system.

Example:

- **milli** (prefix): one-thousandth of a unit
  meter (root): a measure of length
  millimeter: one-thousandth of a meter
- **kilo** (prefix): one thousand units
  liter (root): a measure of volume
  kiloliter: one thousand liters
- **micro** (prefix): one-millionth of a unit
  gram (root): a measure of mass and/or weight
  microgram: one-millionth of a gram

Prefixes:

micro (mi'kro) = one millionth of a unit, written as 0.000001

milli (mil'i) = one-thousandth of a unit, written as 0.001

centi (sen'ti) = one-hundredth of a unit, written as 0.01

deci (des'i) = one-tenth of a unit, written as 0.1

deka (dek'a) = ten units, written as 10

hecto (hek'to) = one hundred units, written as 100

kilo (kil'o) = one thousand units, written as 1,000

Fundamental Units:
Following are the fundamental units of the metric system:

meter (m)	length
liter (L)	volume
gram (Gm, g)	mass and/or weight

The meter is the fundamental unit of length in the metric system and originally formed the foundation for the entire system. A meter is equal to 39.37 inches, which is slightly more than a yard, or 3.28 feet.

A millimeter is about the width of the head of a pin. It takes approximately 2½ centimeters to make an inch; a decimeter is approximately 4 inches.

Meter (m)		Length
1 millimeter (mm)	=	0.001 meter
1 centimeter (cm)	=	0.01 meter
1 decimeter (dm)	=	0.1 meter
1 meter (m)	=	1 meter
1 dekameter (dam)	=	10 meters
1 hectometer (hm)	=	100 meters
1 kilometer (km)	=	1,000 meters

The liter is the metric unit of volume. A liter is equal to 1.056 quarts, which is 0.26 gallon or 2.1 pints.

A milliliter is equivalent to one cubic centimeter (cc), because the amount of space occupied by a milliliter is equal to one cubic centimeter. The weight of one milliliter of water equals approximately one gram. It takes approximately 15 milliliters to make 1 tablespoon. It takes 15 or 16 minims to make one milliliter.

Liter (L)		Volume
1 milliliter (mL)	=	0.001 liter
1 centiliter (cL)	=	0.01 liter
1 deciliter (dL)	=	0.1 liter
1 liter (L)	=	1 liter
1 dekaliter (daL)	=	10 liters
1 hectoliter (hL)	=	100 liters
1 kiloliter (kL)	=	1,000 liters

The gram is the metric unit of mass and weight. It equals approximately the weight of 1 cubic centimeter or 1 milliliter of water. A gram is equal to approximately 15 grains or 0.035 ounce.

Gram (Gm, g)		Mass and Weight
1 microgram (mcg)	=	0.000001 gram
1 milligram (mg)	=	0.001 gram
1 centigram (cg)	=	0.01 gram
1 decigram (dg)	=	0.1 gram
1 gram (Gm, g)	=	1 gram
1 dekagram (dag)	=	10 grams
1 hectogram (hg)	=	100 grams
1 kilogram (kg)	=	1,000 grams

The metric equivalents most frequently used in the medical field are:

Length

2½ centimeters (cm)	=	1 inch

Volume

1,000 milliliters (mL)	=	1 liter (L)

Weight

1,000 micrograms (mcg)	=	1 milligram (mg)
1000 milligrams (mg)	=	1 gram (Gm, g)
1000 grams (g)	=	1 kilogram (kg)
1 kilogram	=	2.2 pounds (lb)

Household Measurements. Household measurements are approximate measurements. They are more frequently used in the home than in the medical field, but the medical assistant should be familiar with the common household measurements listed in Table 36-6.

Because medications can be prescribed in either metric or household measurements, it is important to know equivalents between both to calculate the dose of prescribed medication (Table 36-7).

Metric System Conversion. The process of changing into another form, state, substance, or product is known as *conversion*. In the metric system, changing from one unit to another involves multiplying or dividing by 10, 100, 1,000, and so forth. This can be done by the proportional method or by moving the decimal in the correct direction.

Table 36-6 Common Household Measures

60 drops (gtt)	is equal to:	1 teaspoon (t or tsp)
3 teaspoons (tsp)	is equal to:	1 tablespoon (T or tbsp)
2 tablespoons (tbsp)	is equal to:	1 ounce (oz)
8 ounces (oz)	is equal to:	1 measuring cup (c)
16 tablespoons or 8 ounces	is equal to:	1 measuring cup (c)
2 cups (c)	is equal to:	1 pint (pt)
2 pints (pt)	is equal to:	1 quart (qt)
4 quarts (qt)	is equal to:	1 gallon (gal)

© Cengage Learning 2014

Drop (gt) = approximate liquid measure depending on kind of liquid measured and the size of the opening from which it is dropped.

Table 36-7   Approximate Equivalents Among Metric and Household Systems

Metric	Household
DRY	
1 Gm	¼ tsp
15 Gm	1 tbsp (3 tsp)
30 Gm	1 oz (2 tbsp)
1 kg	2.2 lb
LIQUID	
	1 gt
1 mL	15 gtt
5 mL	1 tsp
15 mL	1 tbsp (3 tsp)
30 mL	1 fl oz (2 tbs)
500 mL	1 pt or 2 cups
1,000 mL	4 cups (1 qt)
LENGTH	
2.5 cm	1 in
1 m	39.37 in

© Cengage Learning 2014

Proportional Method for Converting Metric Equivalents. There are six basic steps in the proportional method, plus an additional step to prove the answer. The following example will serve as a model for future applications of the proportional method of converting metric equivalents.

Example:

Convert 1,500 milligrams to grams.

$$1,500 \text{ mg} = \_\_\_\_\_ \text{ g}$$

Step 1.

Because the unknown factor in the given formula is the number of grams contained in 1,500 milligrams, substitute the symbol x for grams in the equation.

Step 2.

Setting up the proportion requires that you know metric equivalents. For example, in this problem you have to know that 1,000 milligrams (mg) = 1 gram (g).

Step 3.

Since you know that 1,000 mg is equal to 1 g, you can create one-half of the equation. Write the equivalent and place it on the left of the equal sign.

$$1,000 \text{ mg} : 1 \text{ g} =$$

Step 4.

Now that you have the left side of the equation, set up the right side by using the designated metric value 1,500 mg : x g. Always write the smallest equivalent as to the largest equivalent, for example, mg : g. By being consistent, it is less likely errors will occur.

$$1,000 \text{ mg} : 1 \text{ g} = 1,500 \text{ mg} : x \text{ g}$$

Step 5.

Note that you have an equal equation:

$$\text{mg} : \text{g} = \text{mg} : \text{g}$$

The first values on either side of the equal sign are milligrams, and the second values on either side are grams.

Step 6.

Now solve for the unknown (x) by multiplication and division. Multiply the means by the means and the extremes by the extremes. *NOTE:* Once the proportion is correctly set up, simply use the numbers as you multiply and divide.

$$1,000 : 1 = 1,500 : x$$

$$
\begin{aligned}
1,000x &= 1,500 \\
x &= 1,500 \div 1,000 \\
x &= 1.5
\end{aligned}
$$

$$
\begin{array}{r}
1.5 \\
1,000\overline{)1,500.0} \\
\underline{1,000} \\
500.0 \\
\underline{500}
\end{array}
$$

Step 7.

To make sure the answer is correct, prove the work: Place the answer 1.5 g into the formula where x once was. Now multiply the means by the means and the extremes by the extremes.

$$
\begin{aligned}
1,000 \text{ mg} : 1 \text{ g} &= 1,500 \text{ mg} : 1.5 \text{ g} \\
1,500 &= 1,500
\end{aligned}
$$

MEDICATIONS MEASURED IN UNITS

Medications such as insulin, heparin, some antibiotics, hormones, vitamins, and vaccines are measured in units. These medications are standardized in units based on their strengths. The strength varies from one medicine to another, depending on the source, condition, and method by which it is obtained.

How to Calculate Unit Dosages

When calculating medications that are ordered in units, use either the proportional method or the formula method.

The Proportional Method.

Example:

The provider orders 4,000 USP units of heparin given deep subcutaneously. On hand is heparin 5,000 USP units per milliliter.

Step 1.

Use the following proportion to calculate the dose:

Known unit on hand	:	Known dosage form	=	Dose ordered	:	Unknown amount to be given
5,000 Units:		1 mL	=	4,000 Units:		x mL
		5,000x	=	4,000		
		x	=	$\frac{4}{5} = \frac{4}{5}$ mL or 0.8 mL		

Use a tuberculin syringe to draw up 0.8 mL, or convert ⅘ mL to minims.

Step 2.

Convert ⅘ mL to minims. *NOTE:* There are 15 or 16 minims per milliliter.

Multiply:

$$\frac{4}{\not{5}_1} \times \frac{\not{15}^{3}}{1} = \frac{4}{1} \times \frac{3}{1} = 12 \text{ minims}$$

Administer 12 minims (of 5,000 Units/mL for correct dose of 4,000 Units) to the patient.

The Formula Method.

Example:

The provider orders 450,000 Units of Bicillin 1M. On hand is Bicillin 600,000 Units per milliliter.

Step 1.

Use the following formula to calculate the dose:

$$\frac{\text{Dose ordered (desired)}}{\text{Dose on hand}} \times \text{Quantity (per mL)} = \text{Amount to give}$$

$$\frac{450{,}000 \text{ units}}{600{,}000 \text{ units}} \times 1 \text{ mL} = \frac{450{,}\not{000} \text{ units}}{600{,}\not{000} \text{ units}} = \frac{45}{60} = \frac{3}{4}$$

$$\frac{3}{4} \times 1 \text{ mL} = \frac{3}{4} \text{ mL}$$

Step 2.

You may convert to minims. If you do, multiply ¾ by 16.

$$\frac{3}{\not{4}_1} \times \frac{\not{16}^{4}}{1} = 12 \text{ minims}$$

The patient will receive 12 minims of Bicillin 600,000 Units for the ordered dose of 450,000 Units.

Insulin

Insulin is a chemical substance (hormone) secreted by the beta cells of the islets of Langerhans in the pancreas. Insulin is necessary for the proper metabolism of blood glucose and maintenance of the correct blood sugar level. Inadequate secretion or no secretion of insulin, as in the disease diabetes mellitus, results in hyperglycemia and subsequent excessive production of ketone bodies. Eventual coma can occur.

Patients' needs are individualized according to the severity of their disease; treatment includes taking insulin, controlling diet, and exercise. The diet is well-balanced and consists of the correct number of calories distributed among carbohydrates, fats, and proteins. Patients are taught to monitor blood and urine glucose levels at home throughout the day, because the dosage of insulin taken depends on the amounts of glucose detected. Uncontrolled diabetes mellitus can result in serious complications such as circulatory problems, especially in the feet and legs; kidney disease; loss of vision; bedsores; infection; and gangrene. Special care of the feet is essential. The mouth and teeth require excellent oral hygiene.

Diabetes

The National Diabetes Data Group of the National Institutes of Health organized the various forms of diabetes into the following categories:

Type 1	Insulin-dependent diabetes mellitus (IDDM)
Type 2	Noninsulin-dependent diabetes mellitus (NIDDM)
Type 3	Women who developed glucose intolerance in association with pregnancy (gestational)
Type 4	Other types of diabetes associated with pancreatic disease, hormonal changes, adverse effects of drugs, or genetic or other anomalies

Individuals with type 1 diabetes (IDDM) must take insulin on a regular basis to maintain life. Other insulin delivery devices besides the syringe and the needle can be used for injection. With an insulin pen, the patient can turn a dial on the top until the correct dose of insulin is displayed through a small window. Once the correct dose is chosen, the dial "locks" itself to prevent the pen from losing insulin or from the dial moving forward to give an unintended larger dose. The pen has a needle similar to the insulin syringe, and the patient presses the plunger and the dose of insulin is delivered under the skin.

Another delivery device is a jet injector. High-pressure air sends a fine mist of insulin through the skin. No needles are required. This device may be suitable for patients who dislike needles.

The insulin pump is a small device outside of the body that pumps insulin through flexible tubing that is connected to a catheter that is under the skin of the abdomen, thigh, or buttocks. The pump is programmed to deliver a steady flow of the correct dose of insulin 24 hours a day. The pump can allow the patient to add insulin in a short time if needed. Although it is convenient and helps keep the patient's blood glucose under control, the pump can be damaged if the patient engages in certain physical activities. Patients still must regularly monitor their blood glucose levels.

Other devices not yet approved but being worked on for approval are an insulin patch and a dry powder that is inhaled into the lungs through the mouth, then is absorbed from the lungs into the bloodstream. The dosage of insulin is expressed in units and is individualized by the provider for each patient. The amount of insulin that a person must take is based on blood and urine glucose levels, diet, exercise, and the individual's needs (Table 36-8).

It is *extremely important that the exact dosage of insulin be given to the patient.* Too little or too much insulin can cause serious problems ranging from a blood sugar level too low or too high, to coma, and even death. It may be the medical assistant's responsibility to administer insulin and to teach patients or their families how to administer insulin.

When administering insulin, the U-100 syringe (1 mL) is preferred. U-100 means there are 100 units of insulin per milliliter. Insulin dosage should always be expressed in units rather than in milliliters. For example, if the provider orders 30 units of U-100 NPH insulin, use a U-100 syringe and draw up 30 units of U-100 NPH insulin.

Table 36-8   Insulin Preparation Units 100

Type of Insulin	Onset	Appearance
Rapid-acting: Humalog Lispro	5 minutes after injection Peaks in 1 hour Works for 2–4 hours	Clear, colorless
Regular or short-acting: Humulin R Novolin Actrapid	30 minutes after injection Peaks in 2–3 hours Works for 3–6 hours	Clear, colorless
Intermediate: Lente L Humulin NPH	2–4 hours after injection Peaks in 4–12 hours Effective 12–18 hours	Cloudy
Long-lasting: Lantus	6–10 hours after injection Effective 20–24 hours	Clear, colorless
Premixed: Humalog Mix 75/25	5 minutes after injection Duration 1–24 hours	Clear, colorless
Humulin 70/30	1–2.5 hours after injection Peak 7–15 hours Duration 24 hours	Clear, colorless
Humulin 50/50	15–20 minutes after injection Peak 1–4 hours Duration 1–24 hours	Clear, colorless

© Cengage Learning 2014

Precautions to Observe When Administering Insulin.

The following precautions must be observed when administering insulin:

- Be sure to use the proper insulin, the one ordered by the provider. Refer to Table 36-8 for various insulin preparations.
- Do not substitute one insulin for another.
- Use the correct syringe, U-100.
- Dosage of insulin is always measured in units and is individualized for each patient.
- Check the label for the name and type of insulin, strength, and expiration date.

Encourage patients with diabetes to enroll in diabetic education classes, which are offered at most local hospitals. Patients also need to realize that treatment of diabetes is a lifelong commitment and that they must abide by everything that the hospital teaches.

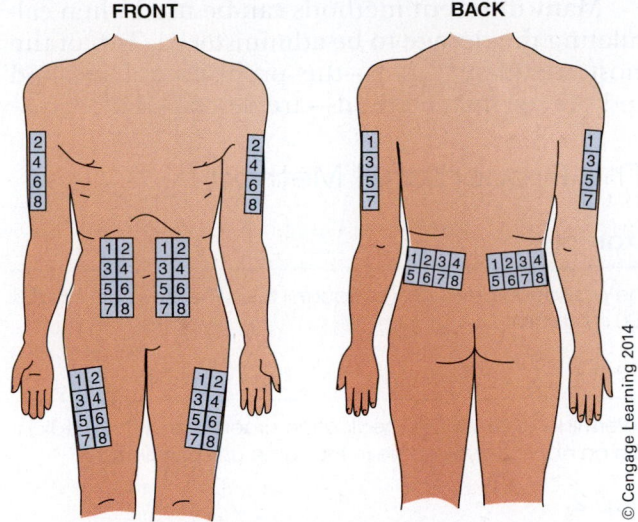

Figure 36 -3   Sites and rotation for insulin administration.

- Make sure the insulin has the proper appearance. Refer to Table 36-8 for the proper appearance of various insulins.
- When insulin is not in use, store it in a cool place and avoid freezing.
- When mixing insulins in one syringe, be certain they are compatible. NPH and Regular are compatible. Regular and Lente are not compatible.
- Avoid shaking the insulin bottle. Roll gently in palms of hand to mix. This method prevents bubbles in the medication.
- Use a subcutaneous needle, but inject at a 90-degree angle.
- Insulin pens are available prefilled with 300 units of insulin.
- Use a site rotation system and select an appropriate site. Insulin injection sites must be rotated to prevent tissue damage. Record site used (Figure 36-3).
- Do not massage after injection.
- Always follow the provider's order and clinic policy when mixing insulins.

Oral Hypoglycemic Medication. Persons with type 2 diabetes mellitus are known to have noninsulin-dependent diabetes mellitus (NIDDM). Type 2 diabetes has a gradual onset, usually seen in adults over 40 years of age. With the obesity epidemic in the United States, individuals are contracting type 2 diabetes at earlier ages (obesity contributes to and can cause type 2 diabetes). The pancreas in patients with type 1 diabetes secretes no insulin; in type 2, the pancreas has some ability to secrete insulin. Most individuals with type 2 diabetes do not have to inject insulin, although a few do. Exercise and diet management may be sufficient for type 2 diabetics to lose enough weight and not require oral hypoglycemic medication. For the majority, however, exercise and diet are not enough to bring the blood sugar to an acceptable level. Medication works by stimulating the pancreas to secrete more insulin, by making cells more receptive to insulin, and by slowing the body's carbohydrate absorption. Some oral hypoglycemics are Orinase, Tolinase, Micronase, Glucotrol, Glucophage, and Starlix.

CALCULATING ADULT DOSAGES

Two measures, weight and volume, are used to determine the amount of medication that is to be administered. The weight of a medication may be expressed as any of the following:

- milliequivalent (mEq)
- microgram (mcg)
- milligram (mg)
- gram (Gm, g)
- unit

The volume of a medication may be expressed as a:

- milliliter (mL)
- minim (m)
- dram (dr)
- ounce (oz)
- variety of household measures, such as the teaspoon (tsp)

Many different methods can be used when calculating the dosage to be administered. Two of the most useful methods—the proportional method and the formula method—are described next.

The Proportional Method

Example:

The provider orders 0.2 g of Equanil tabs. The dose on hand is 400 mg tabs.

Step 1.

Determine whether the medication ordered and the medication on hand are available in the same unit of measure.

Step 2.

If the medication ordered and the medication on hand are not in the same unit of measure, convert so that both measures are expressed using the same unit of measure.

Conversion: To change 0.2 g to mg

$$1,000 \text{ mg} : 1 \text{ g} = x \text{ mg} : 0.2 \text{ g}$$
$$x = 200 \text{ mg}$$

or

multiply $0.2 \times 1,000 = 200$

Step 3.

Now use the following proportion to calculate the dosage. Remember that 0.2 g was converted to 200 mg.

Known unit on hand	:	Known dosage form	=	Dose ordered	:	Unknown amount to be given
400 mg	:	1 tab	=	200 mg	:	x tab

$$400 : 1 = 200 : x$$

$$400x = 200$$

$$x = \frac{\overset{1}{\cancel{200}}}{\underset{2}{\cancel{400}}} \quad \text{(Reduce fraction to lowest terms)}$$

$$x = \tfrac{1}{2} \text{ tab of 400 mg}$$

Step 4.

Prove your answer. Place your answer in the original formula in the x position.

$$400 \text{ mg} : 1 \text{ tab} = 200 \text{ mg} : \tfrac{1}{2} \text{ tab}$$
$$200 = \tfrac{1}{2} \text{ of } 400$$
$$200 = 200$$

Understanding the Formula Method

One of the simplest methods for calculating dosages is the formula method. It is necessary to know what is needed or ordered, what is available or the concentration, and the vehicle in which the medication will be delivered: tablet, mL, or capsule.

The formula looks like this:

$$\frac{\text{Needed}}{\text{Available}} \times \text{Vehicle} = \text{Dose}$$

Example:

Your provider orders 250 mg of Cephalexin po now to be given to Ms. Jones for her diagnosis of cystitis. The bottle of Cephalexin in the drug cabinet holds capsules that contain 250 mg.

Step 1.

Identify each part of the formula:

Needed or ordered = 250 mg

Available = 250 mg

Vehicle = 1 capsule

Step 2.

The formula would be set up as follows:

$$\frac{\text{(Needed) 250 mg}}{\text{(Available) 250 mg}} \times \text{(Vehicle) 1 capsule} = \text{Dose}$$

Step 3.

Determine whether the medication ordered and the medication on hand are in the same unit of measure.

As the needed dose is in mg and the available dose is in mg, there is no further need to address the concentration, and the mg aspect of the equation disappears. We will explore the management of differing concentrations a little later.

You equation now looks like this:

$$\frac{250}{250} \times 1 \text{ capsule} = \text{Dose}$$

Step 4.

Do the math:

$$\frac{250}{250} \text{ is equal to 1}$$

Now multiple by the vehicle of 1 capsule:

$$1 \times 1 = 1 \text{ capsule}$$

The dose to be administered is 1 capsule.

Example:

The provider orders 5 mg of morphine to be given IM now. A check of the narcotics cabinet reveals that injectable morphine is available in 10 mg per 2 mL.

Step 1.

Identify each part of the formula.

Needed or ordered: 5 mg; available: 10 mg

Vehicle: 2 mL

Step 2.

The formula would be set up as follows:

$$\frac{\text{(Needed) 5mg}}{\text{(Available) 10mg}} \times \text{(Vehicle) 2 mL} = \text{Dose}$$

$$\frac{5 \text{ mg}}{10 \text{ mg}} \times 2 \text{ mL} = \text{Dose}$$

Step 3.

Determine whether the medication ordered and the medication on hand are in the same unit of measure.

As the needed dose is in mg and the available dose is in mg, there is no further need to address the concentration, and the mg aspect of the equation disappears.

Step 4.

Do the math:

$$\frac{5}{10} = 0.5$$

Now multiply by the vehicle of 2 mL:

$$0.5 \times 2 \text{ mL} - \text{Dose}$$

$$0.5 \times 2 \text{ mL} = 1 \text{ mL. 1 mL is the dose to be administered.}$$

1 mL of morphine will be administered using the appropriate needle gauge and length in the appropriate volume syringe IM.

If the concentration of the needed medication differs from the concentration of the available medication, this must be resolved.

Example:

Your provider prescribes 500 mg cefadroxil po now. The medication available in the drug cabinet is 1 Gm cefadroxil in scored tablets.

Step 1.

Identify each part of the formula:

Needed or ordered: 500 mg

Available: 1 Gm

Vehicle: 1 tablet

Step 2.

The equation would be set up as follows:

$$\frac{\text{(Needed) 500 mg}}{\text{(Available) 1 Gm}} \times 1 \text{ tablet} = \text{Dose}$$

Step 3.

Determine whether the medication ordered and the medication on hand are in the same unit of measure. As the concentrations of the needed medication and the available medication differ, we must apply the principles discussed earlier in the chapter. The concentrations must be the same in order to determine the dose.

To accomplish this, multiply 1 Gm × 1000 to convert Gms to mg. This results in 1000 mg. Insert this into the equation. It now looks like this:

$$\frac{500 \text{ mg}}{1000 \text{ mg}} \times 1 \text{ tablet} = \text{Dose}$$

Step 4.

Do the math. As the needed and available doses are now in the same unit of measure, the mg portion of the equation disappears:

$$\frac{500}{1000} = 0.5$$

Now multiply by the vehicle:

0.5×1 tablet $= 0.5$ tablet. 0.5 tablet is the dose to be administered.

This formula can also be expanded to accommodate weight-based dosing.

Example:

Your provider orders amoxicillin suspension of 40 mg/kg/day BID for a pediatric patient. The amoxicillin that is available is in a concentration of 400 mg/5 mL. The child weighs 22 lbs.

Step 1.

The order is based on kilograms and the weight is noted in lbs; therefore, you must convert:

2.2 kg = 1 lb

lbs divided by 2.2 = weight in kgs

22 lbs divided by 2.2 = 10 kgs

Step 2.

Next we need to calculate the dose that we are to administer at this time.

40 mg/kg can be calculated for the child as 40 mg × 10 kg = 400 mg. Further, the dosage is to be divided into two times a day.

400 mg divided by 2 = 200 mg

The single dose that you are preparing right now is 200 mg.

Step 3.

Now that we have calculated the dose based on weight and taken the dosing interval into twice a day dosing, we can identify each part of the formula.

Needed or ordered: 200 mg

Available: 400 mg

Vehicle: 5mL

Step 4.

The equation would be set up as follows:

$$\frac{200 \text{ mg}}{400 \text{ mg}} \times 5 \text{ mL} = \text{Dose}$$

Step 5.

Do the math. As the needed and available doses are now in the same unit of measure, the mg portion of the equation disappears:

$$\frac{200}{400} = 0.5$$

Now multiply by the vehicle:

$$0.5 \times 5 \text{ mL} = \text{Dose}$$

$$0.5 \times 5 \text{ mL} = 2.5 \text{ mL}. \quad 2.5 \text{ mL is the dose to be administered.}$$

CALCULATING CHILDREN'S DOSAGES

Each child is an individual differing from other children in age, size, and weight. In the past, formulas such as Young's, Clark's, and Fried's rules were used to calculate pediatric dosages. These formulas determined what fraction of an adult dose was appropriate for a child. Because each child does not develop in the same way during a given time span, these formulas have been replaced by more exact methods of determining the correct dosage of medication for a child.

Today, there are two basic methods used to calculate children's dosages:

- According to kilogram of body weight
- According to body surface area (BSA)

The body weight method is generally the method of choice, because most medications are ordered in this way and it is easier to calculate. The BSA is an exact method, but one must use a formula and a **nomogram** (a device-graph that shows a relation among numeric values) to determine a correct dosage (Figure 36-4).

Body Surface Area

The BSA is considered to be one of the most accurate methods of calculating medication dosages for infants and children up to 12 years of age. This method requires the use of a nomogram that estimates the BSA of the patient according to height and weight.

The body surface area is determined by drawing a straight line from the patient's height to the patient's weight. Intersection of the line with the surface area column is the estimated BSA. This figure is then placed in the following formula:

$$\frac{\text{BSA of child } (\text{m}^2)}{1.7 \ (\text{m}^2)} \times \text{adult dose} = \text{child dose}$$

This formula is based on the average adult who weighs 140 pounds and has a body surface area of 1.7 square meters (1.7 m^2).

Example:

Marion Carrera is a 4-year-old child who is 40 inches tall and weighs 38 pounds (BSA 0.7). The provider has ordered Demerol for pain. The average adult dose of Demerol is 50 mg per mL. What dosage will be given to Marion according to the BSA method?

$$\frac{0.7 \ (\text{m}^2)}{1.7 \ (\text{m}^2)} \times \frac{50 \text{ mg}}{1} = \text{child's dose}$$

$$\frac{0.7 \ (\text{m}^2)}{1.7 \ (\text{m}^2)} \times \frac{50}{1} = \frac{35}{1.7} = 20.5 \text{ mg} = 20.5 \text{ or } 21 \text{ mg}$$

Now use the formula $\dfrac{\text{Desired}}{\text{Have}} \times \text{Quantity}$ to convert mg to mL.

$$\frac{21 \text{ mg}}{50 \text{ mg}} \times 1 \text{ mL} = x \text{ mL}$$

$$\frac{21}{50} = 0.42 \text{ mL administered in a tuberculin syringe}$$

Kilogram of Body Weight

It may be the responsibility of the medical assistant to calculate the amount of dosage ordered by the provider according to the patient's body weight. Today, many medications are ordered in this manner; therefore, it is essential that you learn how to calculate dosage according to this method. The following example will guide you step by step through the mathematical process of calculating dosage according to kilogram of body weight.

There are 2.2 pounds in 1 kg.

Example:

The provider ordered the antiepileptic agent Depakene (valproic acid) 15 mg/kg/day capsules for Clark Kipperley, who weighs 110 pounds. The medication is to be given in three divided doses.

Step 1.

To express pounds in kilograms, divide the weight in pounds by 2.2. Convert the patient's weight to kilograms:

$$110 \div 2.2 = 50 \text{ kilograms}$$

Step 2.

Now, calculate the prescribed dosage by placing 50 in the appropriate place:

$$15 \text{ mg}/50/\text{day}$$

$$15 \times 50 = 750 \text{ mg/day}$$

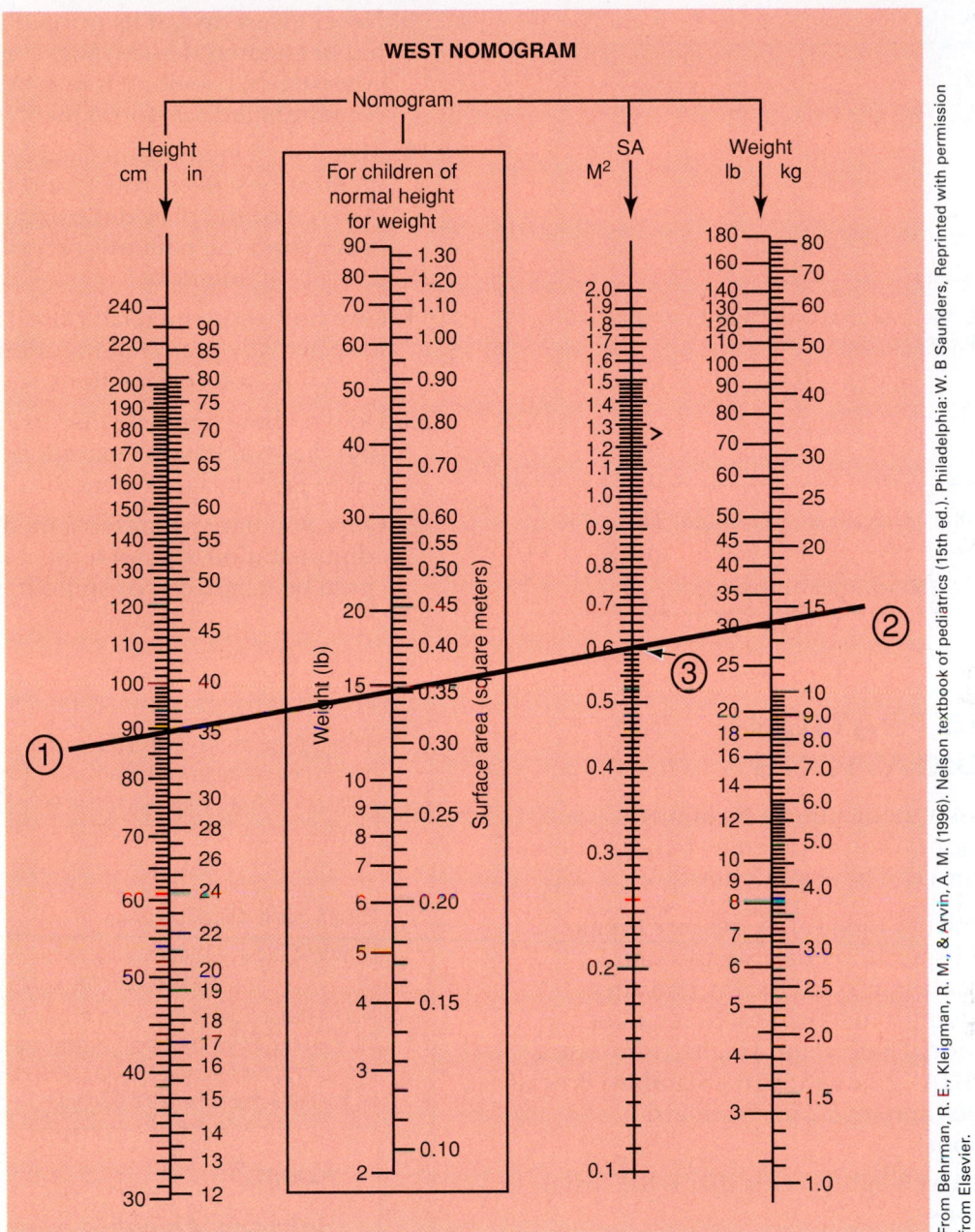

WEST NOMOGRAM

Nomogram

Height
cm   in

For children of
normal height
for weight

SA
M²

Weight
lb   kg

Weight (lb)

Surface area (square meters)

From Behrman, R. E., Kleigman, R. M., & Arvin, A. M. (1996). Nelson textbook of pediatrics (15th ed.). Philadelphia: W. B Saunders. Reprinted with permission from Elsevier.

Figure 36-4 Body surface area (BSA) is determined by drawing a straight line from the patient's height (1) in the far left column to his or her weight (2) in the far right column. Intersection of the line with BSA column (3) is the estimated BSA (m²). For infants and children of normal height and weight, BSA may be estimated from weight alone by referring to the enclosed area.

Step 3.

To determine the amount of each dose, divide 750 by 3 (divided doses).

$$750 \text{ mg} \div 3 = 250 \text{ mg}$$

Depakene is available in 250-mg capsules and 250-mg/5 mL syrup. The provider ordered the medication in capsules, so Clark will receive a 250-mg capsule every 8 hours for a total of 3 doses a day.

In the same example, use the proportional method to calculate kilogram of body weight.

Step 1.

To convert 110 pounds to kilograms, set up the proportion as follows:

$$2.2 \text{ lb} : 1 \text{ kg} = 110 \text{ lb} : x \text{ kg}$$

Step 2.

Now, solve for *x*.

$$2.2 : 1 = 110 : x$$
$$2.2x = 110$$
$$x = 50$$

Step 3.

Now, calculate the prescribed dosage by placing 50 in the appropriate place: mg/50 kg/day.

$$15 \times 50 = 750 \text{ mg/day}$$

Step 4.

To determine the amount of each dose, divide 750 by 3 (divided doses).

$$750 \div 3 = 250 \text{ mg per dose}$$

ADMINISTRATION OF MEDICATIONS

Regardless of a medication's form or the route by which it is administered, certain basic guidelines must be followed. These guidelines are:

1. Practice medical asepsis (see Chapter 22 for specific medical asepsis rules). Wash your hands before and after administering a medication. Remember Occupational Safety and Health Administration (OSHA) guidelines and Standard Precautions (see Chapter 22 for Standard Precautions).

2. Work in a well-lighted area that is free from distractions.

3. Follow the "Six Rights" of proper drug administration (see following section).

4. Always check for allergies before administering any medication.

5. Give only drugs ordered by a licensed practitioner who is authorized to prescribe medications.

6. Never give a medication if there is any question about the order.

7. Be completely familiar with the drug that you are administering before giving it to the patient. Look it up in the PDR or online.

8. Always check the expiration date on the medication label.

9. Never give a drug if its normal appearance has been altered in any way (color, structure, consistency, or odor); it may be outdated, contaminated, or stored incorrectly.

10. Make out a medication card (Figure 36-5) for medications, dose, route, and time exactly as ordered by the provider using the provider's order from the patient's record as a guide. Do not rely on memory.

11. Give only those medications that you yourself have actually prepared for administration. Trust only your own actions.

12. Do not allow someone else to give a medication that you have prepared. Depend on yourself to give the correct medication.

13. Once you have prepared a medication for administration, do not leave it unattended; it could be misplaced or spilled.

A medication card is written out prior to administration of any medication to the patient in the ambulatory care setting. The information is taken directly from the provider's order sheet of the patient's record. An example follows.

Information needed:

Patient name: Abigail Johnson

Provider's order: Cardizem (diltiazem hydrochloride) 180 mg po stat. Winston Lewis, MD.

The medicine card is then used to be certain you have the correct patient, and to document the information on Mrs. Johnson's record. Following documentation, tear up the medication card and discard.

> Room 3
>
> Johnson, Abigail
>
> Cardizem
>
> 180 mg
>
> po
>
> stat
>
> 10/24/XX – 10 A.M.

Figure 36-5 A medication card is used to prepare, administer, and record medications, dose, route, and time as ordered by the provider.

14. Be careful in transporting the medication to the patient. Do not spill or drop.

15. When administering oral medications, stay with the patient until you are certain that the medication has been taken to be sure patient swallowed the medication.

16. Shake (to mix) all liquid medications that contain a **precipitate** before pouring. A precipitate is a substance that separates from a solution if allowed to stand. This mixes the liquid for the proper medication.

17. When pouring a liquid medication, hold the measuring device at eye level or place it on a flat surface and squat down so you can observe it at eye level. Read the correct amount at the lowest level of the **meniscus**, which is the top surface of the column of liquid.

18. Do not contaminate the cap of a bottle while pouring a medication. Place the cap with the rim pointed upward to prevent contamination of that portion of the cap that comes into contact with the medication.

19. Keep all drugs not being administered in a safe storage place.

20. Carefully follow the procedural steps for the type of medication that you are giving or the type of procedure you are performing.

21. Always keep safety precautions in mind. The United States Department of Health and Human Services, Public Health Service, and Centers for Disease Control and Prevention recommend following Standard Precautions for prevention of hepatitis B and C viruses, human immunodeficiency virus, and other bloodborne diseases (see Chapter 22 for specifics about Standard Precautions).

The "Six Rights" of Proper Drug Administration

The "Six Rights" have been developed as a checklist of activities to be followed by those who give medications. This easy-to-remember list should always be followed to ensure the proper administration of any drug:

1. *Right drug.* To be sure that the correct drug has been selected, compare the medication order with the label on the medication bottle. A frequent check of the medication label is a good way to avoid a medication error. One should make a practice of reading the label on each of the following three occasions:

First:	When the medication is taken from the storage area.
Second:	Just before removing it from its container.
Third:	On returning the medication container to storage or before discarding the empty container.

2. *Right dose.* It is essential that the patient receive the right dose. If the dose ordered and the dose on hand are *not the same*, carefully determine the correct dose through mathematical calculation. When calculating dosage, it is advisable to have another qualified person verify the accuracy of your calculations before the medication is administered.

3. *Right route.* Check the medication order to be sure that you have the right route of administration (Figure 36-6A).

4. *Right time.* You are responsible for medicating the patient at the proper time. Check the medication order to ensure that a drug is administered according to the time interval prescribed. For a drug to be maintained at the proper blood level, care must be taken to administer it at the right time (Figure 36-6B).

5. *Right patient.* Before administering any medication, always be sure that you have the right patient. A good safety practice is to correctly identify the patient on each occasion when you administer a medication. In a hospital, the patient's identification bracelet is always checked. In the ambulatory care facility, call the patient by name or ask the patient to state his or her name (Figure 36-6C).

6. **EHR** *Right documentation.* The recording process is the vital link between provider, patient, and medical assistant. It is an account of the essential data that are collected and preserved. The patient's chart is a legal document; therefore, all data should be recorded in ink or entered into the computer. The data should be accurate and clearly stated. It is important that certain data about

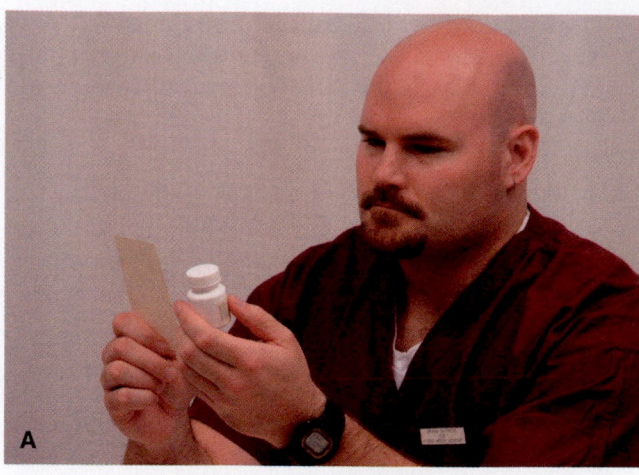

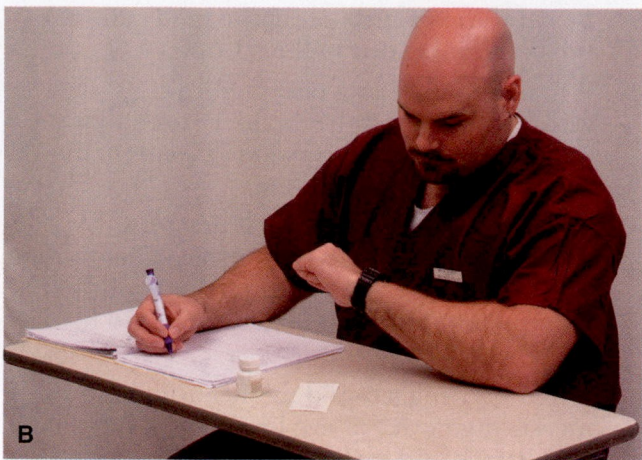

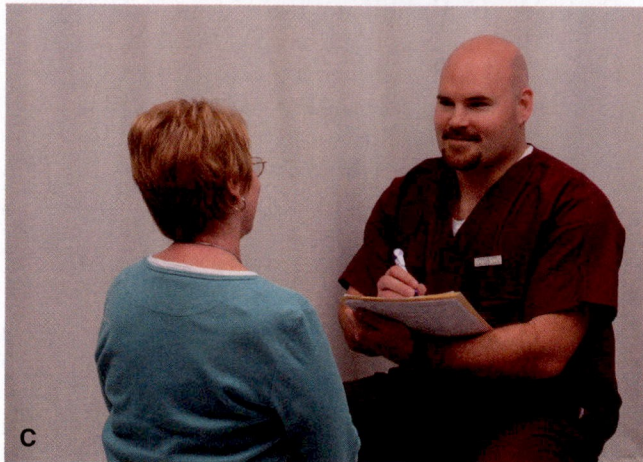

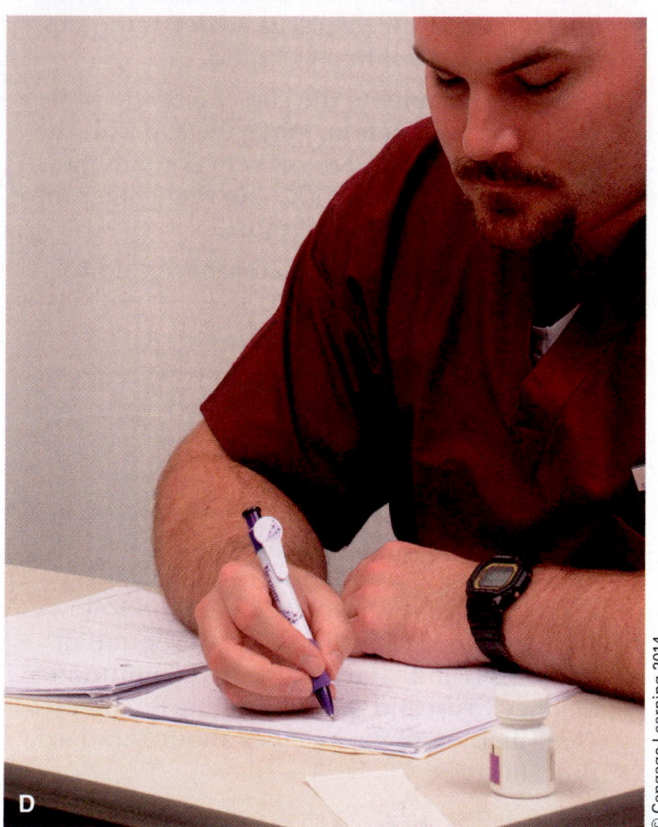

Figure 36-6   (A) Medical assistant checks for the right drug, the right route, and the right dose of medication to administer. (B) Medical assistant checks for the right time to administer medication to the patient. (C) Medical assistant assesses patient before administering the medication. The medical assistant ascertains he has the right patient and asks the patient if she has any allergies. (D) Medical assistant documents administration of medication in patient's chart.

© Cengage Learning 2014

drug administration be entered into the patient's chart (Figure 36-6D):

- Patient's name
- Date and time of administration
- Name of the medication and the amount (dosage) administered
- Route by which the medication was administered
- Any unusual reactions experienced by the patient

- Any complications in administering the drug (patient refusing to take the medication, difficulty in swallowing)
- If the medication was *not* given, state why and dispose of the medication according to agency policy and federal and state laws
- Patient data, such as blood pressure, pulse, respirations, when appropriate
- Your name or initials and title

WHEN A MEDICATION ERROR OCCURS, FOLLOW STANDARD PROCEDURE:

a. Recognize that an error has been made.

b.  Stay calm. Assess the patient's condition and reactions to the medication.

c.  Report the error immediately to the provider. Give the details of the mistake and the patient's reactions.

d. Follow the provider's orders for correcting the error.

e. Document the error in the patient's chart or electronic medical record or the facility's record form:

- Describe the type of error.
- Describe the patient's reactions.
- Describe the steps taken to correct the error.
- State date, time, and your name.

Medication Errors

Medication errors should not happen when personnel follow the "Six Rights" of proper drug administration and the essential medication guidelines; however, honest mistakes will be made periodically. A medication error occurs when any of the following happen:

1. A drug is given to the wrong patient
2. The incorrect drug is given
3. The drug is given via an incorrect route
4. The drug is given at the incorrect time
5. The incorrect dose is administered
6. Incorrect data are entered on the patient's chart or electronic medical record

Patient Assessment

Before administering any medication, carefully assess the patient's condition. An assessment should include, but is not limited to, the following conditions:

1. *Age.* Is the medication and route suitable for the patient at a particular stage in life? The stages of life include infancy, childhood, adolescence, adulthood, and old age. During infancy, early childhood, and old age, a smaller dose of medication may be required than would be appropriate for the other stages in life.

2. *Physical conditions.* Potential problems associated with the patient's physical condition must be considered. Female patients should not be given certain medications during pregnancy or while breast-feeding because they may be contraindicated.

3. *Body size.* The amount of medication given and size of the needle used are directly related to the size of the patient. Pediatric and geriatric patients usually have less subcutaneous and muscular tissue per BSA than the average adult (see Figure 36-4). Small, thin patients usually require less medication, and a shorter needle may be used to reach the appropriate tissue level. On the other hand, the large or obese patient may or may not require more medication than the average adult and a longer needle to reach the appropriate tissue level.

4. *Sex.* Consider differences that are related to the sex of the patient.

5. *Build.* Muscular patients generally have more muscular tissue. Obese patients have more adipose tissue. Always inspect and palpate muscle tissue with this in mind when determining the appropriate needle length to reach muscle tissue.

6. *Skin texture.* Some patients have tougher skin than others. A young person's skin might have more tone than that of an older adult. Slightly more force is required to penetrate skin that is tough or lacking in tone.

7. *Injection site.* Always inspect and palpate the skin before administering an injection. The following body areas should be avoided when choosing the site for an injection:

- Any type of skin lesion
- Burned areas
- Inflamed areas
- Previous injection sites
- Any traumatized area
- Scar tissue (vaccination, keloid)
- Moles, warts, birthmarks, tumors, lumps, hard nodules
- Nerves, large blood vessels, bones
- Cyanotic areas
- Edematous areas
- Paralyzed areas
- Arm on same side as mastectomy, or other lymphatic compromise

Correct injection sites are illustrated later in this chapter.

ADMINISTRATION OF ORAL MEDICATIONS

Oral medications are easily and economically administered. There are, however, several disadvantages associated with the oral route. For instance, the drug may:

- Have an objectionable odor/taste
- Cause discoloration of the teeth, mouth, and tongue
- Irritate the gastric mucosa
- Be altered by digestive enzymes
- Be poorly absorbed from the digestive system because of illness or nature of the medication
- Not be taken by the patient
- Have less predictable effects on the body when given orally than when given by the parenteral route (by injection)
- Not be able to be swallowed if in tablet, capsule, or caplet form

Equipment and Supplies for Oral Medications

Three measuring devices commonly used in the administration of oral medications are the medicine cup, the water cup, and the medicine dropper. The medicine cup (Figure 36-7) comes in various sizes and shapes, depending on its manufacturer and its intended use. Cups may be calibrated in fluid ounces, fluidrams, milliliters (mL), and tablespoons.

The water cup is a small plastic or paper cup that is disposable. The average water cup holds three ounces of liquid.

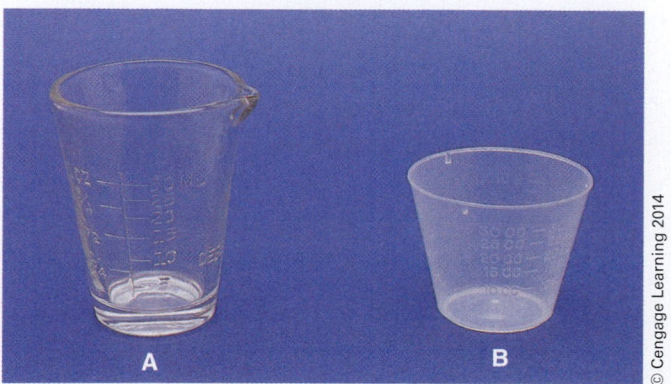

Figure 36-7 Medicine cups: (A) glass; (B) plastic.

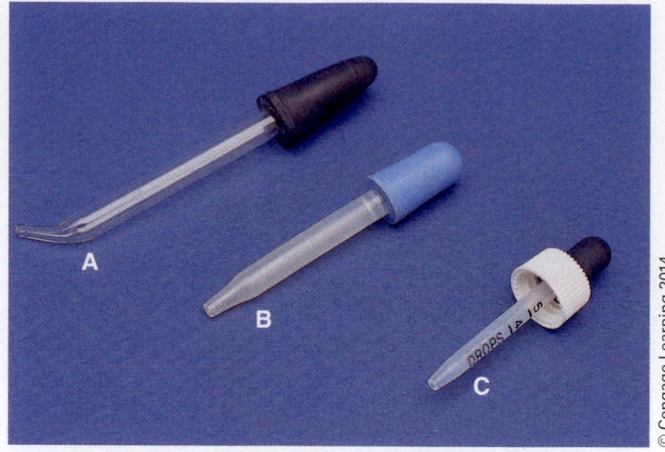

Figure 36-8 Various types of medicine droppers: (A) glass; (B) plastic; (C) plastic calibrated.

The medicine dropper (Figure 36-8) may be calibrated in milliliters, minims, or drops. Medicine droppers are often included with the bottle of medication. Uncalibrated droppers may be provided when the medicine is administered only in drops. The size of the drop varies with the size of the dropper opening, the angle at which it is held, the force exerted on the rubber bulb, and the viscosity of the medication.

It is important that the appropriate measuring device is selected for a medication and that the prescribed dosage is accurately measured. The selection of the measuring device depends on the physical structure of the medication (solid or liquid), the amount of medication prescribed, the size of the measuring device, and the calibrations on the container.

 Procedure 36-1 gives steps for administration of oral medications.

ADMINISTRATION OF PARENTERAL MEDICATIONS

The term **parenteral** is used to describe the injection of a substance into the body via a route other than the alimentary canal/digestive system. The most frequently used parenteral routes are:

- *Subcutaneous.* Just below the surface of the skin. A subcutaneous injection is usually given at a 45-degree angle.
- *Intramuscular.* Within the muscle. An intramuscular injection is given at a 90-degree angle, passing through the skin and subcutaneous tissue, and penetrating deep into muscle tissue.

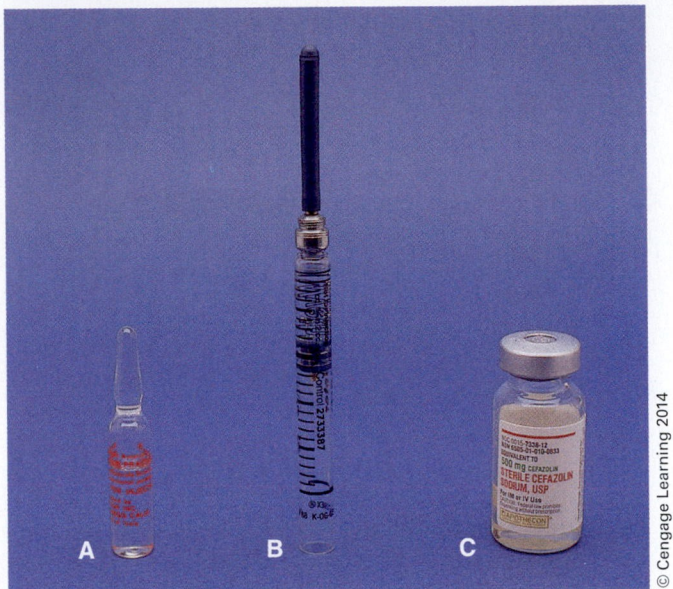

Figure 36-9 Medications given parenterally: (A) Ampule. (B) Sterile cartridge with premeasured medication. (C) Vial of powder for reconstitution.

- *Intradermal.* Within the dermal layer of the skin. An intradermal injection is given at an angle between 10 and 15 degrees.
- *Intravenous.* Within or into a vein.

Medications that have been prepared for use by injection are available in multiple-dose form (vials) and in unit dose form (ampules and cartridge-needle units) (Figure 36-9). **Unit dose** forms are premeasured amounts, packaged on a per-dose basis.

- *Ampule.* A small, sterile, prefilled glass container that usually holds a single dose of a hypodermic solution.
- *Cartridge-needle unit.* A disposable sterile cartridge containing a premeasured amount of medication. This unit is designed for use in a nondisposable cartridge-holder syringe such as the Tubex® or Carpuject®.
- *Vial.* A small, sterile, prefilled glass bottle with rubber stopper containing a hypodermic solution.

Hazards Associated with Parenteral Medications

Injections of medications must be done with extreme care. Sterile technique must be used because the needle and medication are being introduced into the patient's body

and microorganisms must not be transmitted. Appropriate site selection and proper technique ensure effectiveness of the medication.

Additional dangers to be aware of when administering medications parenterally (by injection) include:

- Allergic reaction (if present) will be swift
- Injury to bone, nerve, or blood vessel
- Breaking of needle in tissue (rare)
- Injecting into a blood vessel instead of tissue (this is avoided by checking for blood return, on aspiration)

Reasons for Parenteral Route Selection

The parenteral route is selected because of:

- Rapid response time to medication
- Accuracy of dosage
- Need to concentrate medication in a specific body part or area (into a joint or local anesthetic)
- Inability to administer orally because the medication is destroyed by gastric juices, or the patient is incapable of taking medication orally

Because parenteral medications are intended for use by injection, they must be injected as liquids. Some medications are supplied in powder form and must be reconstituted to a liquid form for injection (see Procedure 36-8).

Because they must be in liquid form, the amount of parenteral medications is expressed in terms of volume (milliliters, minims, or ounces). The strength of the drug contained in the liquid is usually expressed in terms of its weight (milliequivalents, micrograms, milligrams, grams, or units). Therefore, medications ordered for parenteral use are often ordered by both weight and volume.

The parenteral route of drug administration offers an effective mode of delivering medication to a patient when a rapid and direct result is desired. The effect of a parenteral medication is faster than one given by the oral route; however, the accuracy of dosage calculation for both is important.

Parenteral Equipment and Supplies

Syringes. Syringes are classified as disposable, nondisposable, or a combination of these two types. Most syringes used are plastic. They also may be classified according to their intended use. In addition to the standard hypodermic syringes that are in general use, there are special-purpose syringes for irrigations or oral feedings, tuberculin syringes, and insulin syringes.

Disposable Syringes.

Disposable syringes are those that are sterilized, prepackaged, nontoxic, nonpyrogenic, and ready for use. They are available as a syringe-needle unit and are generally enclosed in individual peel-apart packages of durable paper or clear plastic. They are available in sizes from 1 to 60 milliliters. The 1-, 3-, and 5-mL syringes are the ones most often used when parenteral medications are administered.

 A disposable syringe-needle unit consists of a syringe with an attached needle. The needle is covered by a hard plastic sheath to prevent it from accidentally penetrating the package or sticking the user. The unit may be sealed within a peel-apart package or encased in a rigid plastic container that has been heat sealed to ensure sterility. Labeling usually includes the manufacturer's name, type and size of the syringe, gauge and length of the needle, and a reorder number. Packages are usually color coded for ease of identification. Always read the label. Disposable syringes are generally preferred for the administration of parenteral medications because they ensure sterility and sharp needles. Also, disposable syringes eliminate the need for resterilization, which is costly, time-consuming, and possibly unsafe if not done properly.

Nondisposable Syringes.

Nondisposable syringes are usually made of specially strengthened glass resistant to thermal shock. These units, consisting of round glass barrels with individually fitted plungers, are manufactured to exacting specifications.

Nondisposable glass and plastic syringes are available in sizes from 1 to 50 milliliters. They may be used by providers to perform special procedures such as paracentesis, thoracentesis, thoracotomy, and tracheotomy.

Combination Disposable/Nondisposable Cartridge-Injection Syringes.

A cartridge-injection system, such as the plastic Carpuject® (Figure 36-10) or the metal Tubex®, consists of a disposable cartridge-needle unit and a nondisposable cartridge-holder syringe. The cartridge-needle unit is factory sealed and sterile and contains a precisely measured unit

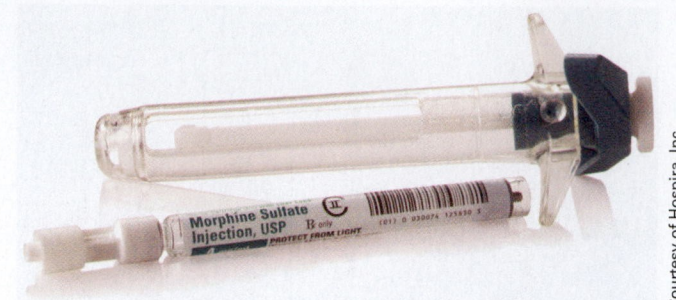

Courtesy of Hospira, Inc.

Figure 36-10 The Carpuject® is a type of cartridge-injection system with a click-lock mechanism for safety.

dose of medicine. The cartridge-holder syringe may be made of durable chrome-plated brass or of plastic. These reusable syringes are designed for quick and safe loading and unloading of cartridge-needle units, which are manufactured in various sizes and dosage capacities and contain a wide range of medications (Figure 36-11).

The combination of a disposable/nondisposable syringe system is easy to use and convenient. When using this system, be careful to read the label and compare the medication order with the label. For example, the provider may order Demerol® 25 mg and the cartridge is 50 mg/mL. Give ½ mL and properly discard the other ½ mL according to clinic policy. Another person must witness the disposal of the Demerol®, which is a controlled substance.

Parts of a Syringe.

The component parts of a syringe consist of a barrel, plunger, flange, tip (Figure 36-12), and safety shield on a safety syringe.

- The *barrel* is the part that holds the medication and has graduated markings (calibrations) on its surface for use in measuring medications.

- The *plunger* is a movable cylinder designed for insertion within the barrel; it provides the mechanism by which a medication (or other substance) is drawn into or pushed out of the barrel.

- The *flange* is at the end of the barrel where the plunger is inserted. It forms a rim around the end of the barrel where the plunger is inserted and has appendages against which one places the index and middle fingers when drawing up solution for injection. The flange also prevents the syringe from rolling when laid on a flat surface.

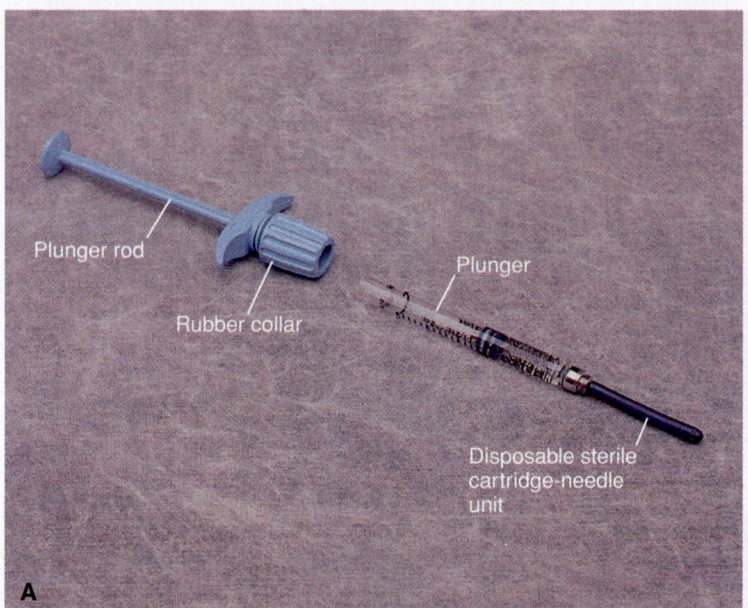

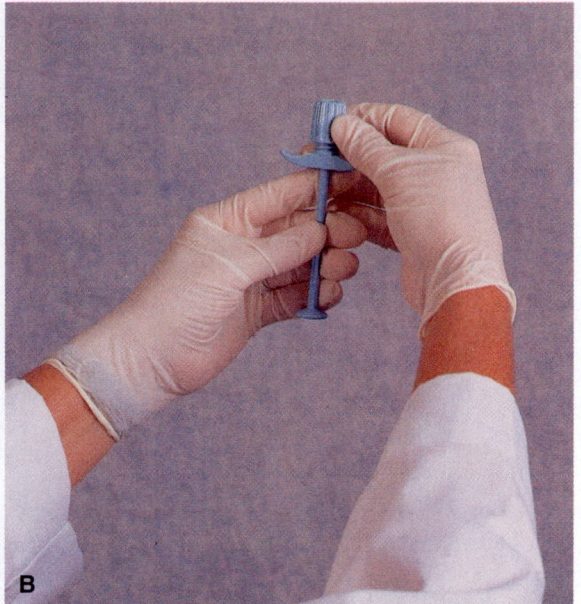

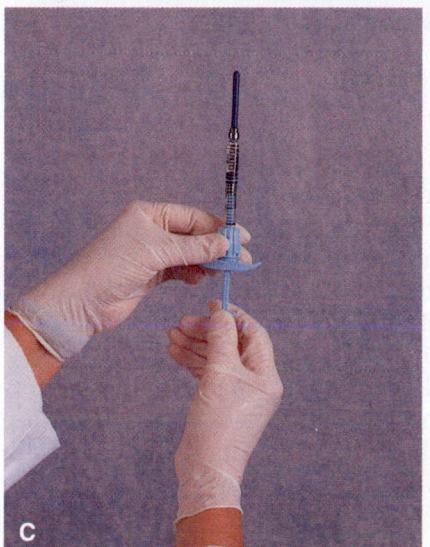

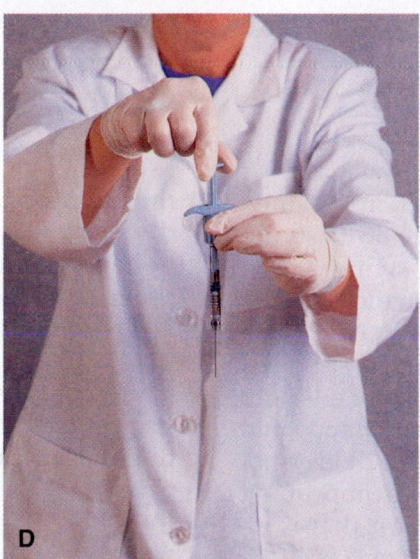

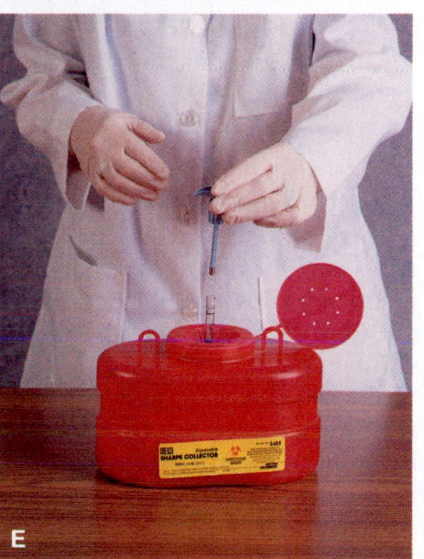

© Cengage Learning 2014

Figure 36-11 (A) Reusable cartridge holder with disposable sterile cartridge needle unit. (B) Turn ribbed collar to open position. (C) Insert the sterile cartridge-needle unit into the open end of the injector. The ribbed collar is firmly tightened. The plunger of the injector and the plunger of the cartridge-needle units are tightened and ready for use. (D) The medical assistant prepares to dispose of the cartridge-needle unit. The needle is not recapped. The plunger rod is disengaged by unscrewing. The ribbed collar is loosened. (E) The medical assistant holds the cartridge-needle unit over a sharps container, and the unit drops into the container.

- The *tip* is at the end of the barrel where the needle is attached.
- The safety shield is pulled over the needle while withdrawing it. Safety needles have a mechanism to either sheath the needle, retract it, or blunt it.

The parts of a syringe that must remain sterile during the preparation and administration of a parenteral medication are the inside of the barrel, the section of the plunger that fits inside the barrel, and the syringe tip to which the needle is to be attached.

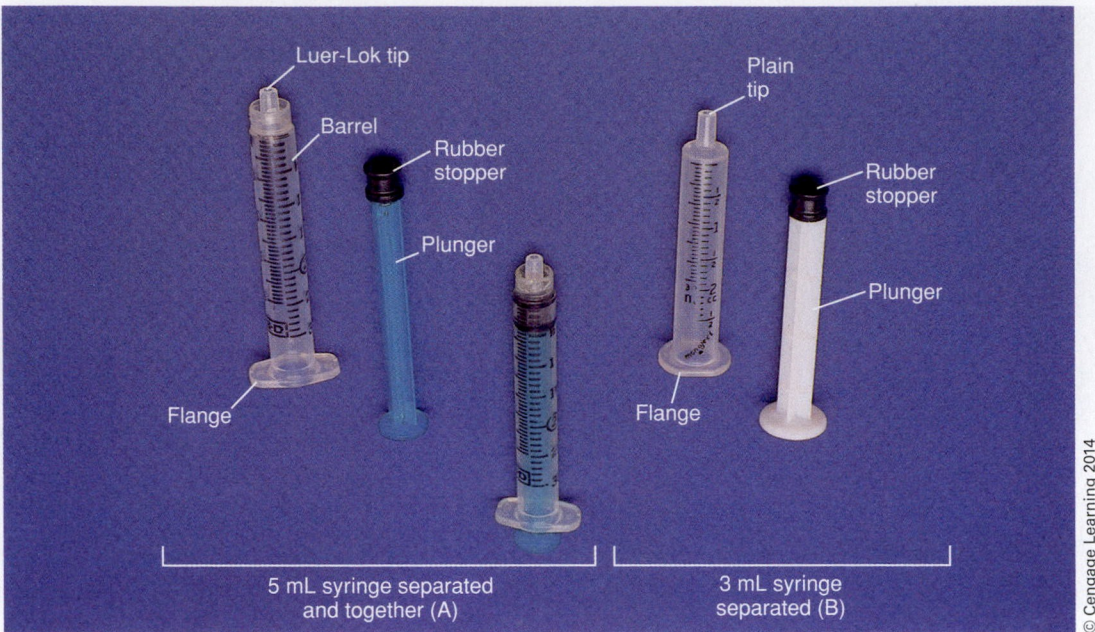

Figure 36-12 Parts of a syringe. (A) A 5-mL syringe separated and unseparated with Luer-Lok® tip. (B) A 3-mL syringe separated with plain tip.

Types of Syringes and Uses. Syringes are named according to their sizes and uses. Table 36-9 lists the types, sizes, calibrations, and uses of syringes used in the administration of parenteral medications.

One should always choose a needle with sufficient length to reach the desired tissue level (Table 36-10). A large person may require a longer needle to reach the correct body tissue than would be required for a smaller person. The delivery of medication to the proper tissue level is important. A concentrated or irritating medication that is intended for deep intramuscular injection could be delivered instead into the subcutaneous tissue of an obese patient if one selects a needle that is too short. Such an inappropriate injection may cause a sterile abscess and necrosis. This unnecessary complication can be avoided by considering the size of the patient when choosing the length of the needle.

Needles. Both disposable and nondisposable needles are available for use with syringes. Of these, the most frequently used are disposable needles, which are individually packaged in sterile paper or plastic containers. Disposable needles and syringe-needle units are available with a color-coded sheath. The sheath protects the needle and identifies its gauge and length. Common needle gauges (G) range from 16 to 32, and

their lengths vary from $\frac{3}{8}$ to 2 inches. The needle's gauge is determined by the diameter of the lumen or opening at its beveled tip. The larger the gauge, the smaller the diameter of its lumen. For example, a 32 gauge needle is much smaller than a 16-gauge needle.

Nondisposable needles are made of high-quality stainless steel. They are equipped with a mounting hub that has a cylindrical opening designed to slip over the lock onto the tip of a syringe, such as a Luer-Lok®. See Figure 36-13 for various sizes and types of needles.

Parts of a Needle. Figure 36-14 shows the parts of a needle used to administer parenteral medications.

- The *point* is the sharpened end of the needle. The point is formed when the end of the shaft is ground away to form a flat, slanted surface called the *bevel*.
- The *lumen,* the hollow core of the needle, forms an oval-shaped opening when exposed at the beveled point.
- The hollow steel tube through which the medication passes is the *shaft.*
- The other end of the shaft attaches to the *hub,* which is part of the needle unit that is designed to mount onto the syringe.

Table 36-9 The Most Frequently Used Syringes for Parenteral Medications

Type of Syringes	Size and Calibration	Typical Uses
Hypodermic	3 milliliter Calibrated 0.1 15/16 minims/milliliters	Intramuscular and subcutaneous injections
Hypodermic	5 milliliter Calibrated 0.2	Venipuncture and intramuscular Injections
Hypodermic	Larger sizes (10, 30, and 60 milliliter)	Medical/surgical treatments, aspirations, irrigations, venipuncture, gavage (tube-to-stomach) feedings
Tuberculin	1 milliliter Calibrated 0.1 and 0.01 16 minims/milliliters	To inject minute amounts for intradermal injections, allergy testing, allergy injections
Insulin	U-100 (0.5 milliliter) U-100 (1 milliliter)	Lo-Dose® administration of insulin Insulin administration

© Cengage Learning 2014

Table 36-10 Syringe-Needle Combinations for Various Parenteral Routes

Subcutaneous Injection	Intramuscular Injection	Intradermal Injection
3-mL syringe/ 25G, ⅝-inch needle	3-mL syringe/ 23G, 1-inch needle	1-mL syringe/25G, ⅝ -inch needle
3-mL syringe/ 26G, ⅜-inch needle	3-mL syringe/ 22G, 1½-inch needle	1-mL syringe/26G, ⅜ -inch needle
3-mL syringe/ 27G, ½-inch needle	3-mL syringe/ 21G, 1½- to 2-inch needle	1-mL syringe/27G, ½-inch needle
U-100 (1 mL)/ 26G, ½-inch needle for insulin		

© Cengage Learning 2014

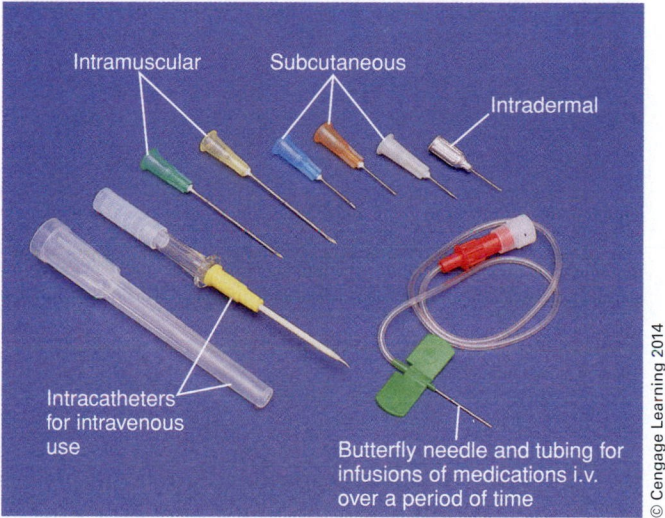

Figure 36-13 Various sizes and types of needles. Different colored hubs denote needle gauges.

- The point at which the shaft attaches to the hub is called the *hilt.*

Safety Syringes.
There are multiple manufacturers of safety syringes and multiple designs for the protection of the health care worker. Some safety syringes have covers that snap or slide over the used needle. There are other designs that have a needle that retracts into the plunger.

The Safe Disposal of Needles and Syringes.
The careless disposal of used needles and syringes may present a health risk to any person coming into contact with the used equipment. An accidental stick by a contaminated needle could transmit diseases such as hepatitis B, hepatitis C, syphilis, Rocky Mountain spotted fever,

tuberculosis, malaria, varicella zoster, and human immunodeficiency virus (HIV). Used needles and syringes should be discarded in a rigid, puncture-proof container (Figure 36-15). Never recap a needle after giving an injection. Do engage safety feature. Most needlesticks occur while recapping. Refer to Chapter 22 for OSHA regulations.

Most sharps-related injuries (needlesticks) occur in the hospital with inpatients. However, any health care worker who administers parenteral medications is at risk for an injury. Other types of sharps-related injuries besides disposable needles

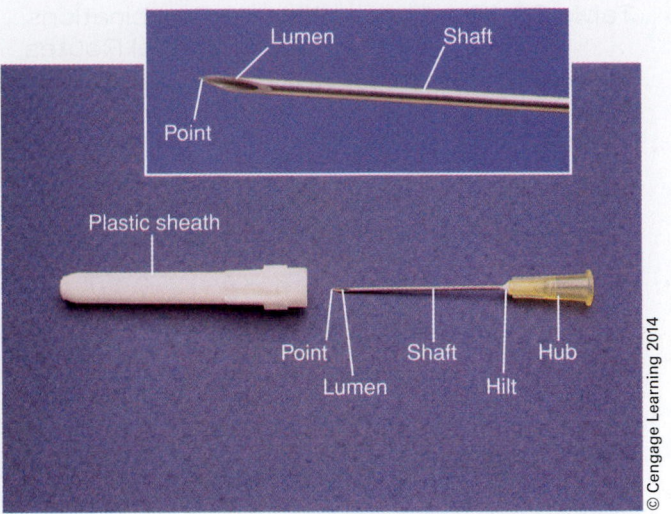

Figure 36-14 Parts of a needle and needle sheath. Inset shows point, lumen, and shaft.

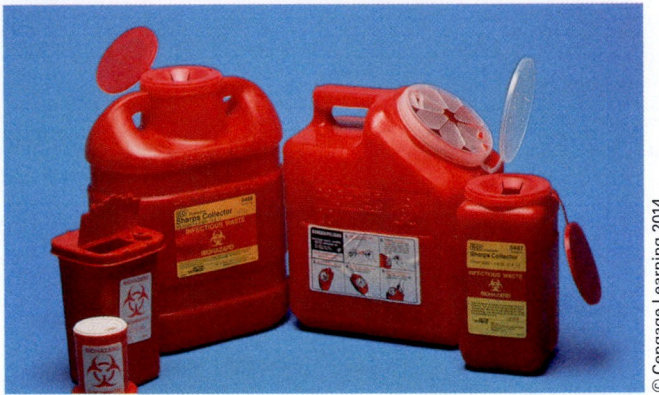

Figure 36-15 Place used needles, point down, in puncture-proof sharps containers.

include suture needles, butterfly needles, scalpel blades, phlebotomy needles, and IV catheter stylets.

A number of pathogens can enter the body during a sharps-related injury, but of greatest concern are hepatitis B and C viruses and HIV (see Chapter 22 for details about these and other bloodborne pathogens).

The National Alliance for the Primary Prevention of Sharps Injuries (NAPPSI) consists of medical device makers, health organizations, and health care providers whose goal is the prevention of sharps-related injuries. Besides safety needles (see information on retractable needles in Chapter 22), laser scalpels, and needleless drug delivery systems such as patches and inhaled medications, a needleless injection system is available (fluid under pressure). There are glues and adhesives available to approximate surgical incisions.

These alternative methods are helpful in reducing sharps-related injuries; however, phlebotomy and IV therapy still require a needle. Legal regulations (CDC and OSHA) require use of the safest needle available.

Proper use and disposal of sharps is of the utmost importance to health care workers and others. Avoid needles if there are other methods available, and never recap used needles. Engage the safety mechanism and dispose of needles and syringes immediately after use.

Sharps Collectors. Sharps collector systems eliminate the need to reshield the needle, thereby reducing the risk for an accidental needlestick.

Needles are placed into the container as a whole unit after safety mechanisms are engaged. Sharps containers need to be within reach any time injections are given.

PRINCIPLES OF INTRAVENOUS THERAPY

Patients who are unconscious, uncooperative, experiencing severe nausea and vomiting, have had severe burns, or have a significant amount of blood loss may need an intravenous infusion. All of these situations result in the patient losing body fluids, resulting in loss of homeostasis. The provider will order the fluids to be replaced by intravenous infusion according to the patient's condition or disease. The fluids will be specific for the needs of a particular patient. Some infusions maintain the patient's water (fluids) and electrolyte needs. For example, some elderly people who live alone and do not feel well, and perhaps have pneumonia, may not eat well or drink enough liquid to maintain the body's balance of fluids and electrolytes. If the situation goes on for a few days, during which time the patient becomes dehydrated, the patient will need IV fluids. Symptoms of dehydration are dry mouth, dark urine, and lightheadedness. It can lead to changes in the body's chemistry and become life-threatening.

Severe nausea and vomiting can quickly dehydrate an individual and eventually can lead to kidney failure. The patient needs replacement of fluids and electrolytes through an intravenous infusion. (If a patient is vomiting, any attempt at taking in fluids orally is not likely to be successful.)

When a patient is prescribed intravenous fluids, the provider takes into consideration the patient's age, weight, height, and clinical laboratory results.

When patients are receiving an intravenous infusion, they must be watched carefully. The flow rate is ordered by the provider. Blood pressure should be monitored. Breathing and chest tightness should be reported. Excessive volume (too much fluid too quickly) can result in overhydration and possible serious adverse cardiac and pulmonary consequences.

Inserting a needle or cannula into a vein for purposes of an infusion is an invasive procedure, and the possibility exists for microorganisms to enter the patient's body. Everything must be sterile because microorganisms can enter the bloodstream and cause serious problems. Infection at the site of needle entry is possible. Phlebitis (inflammation of the vein) can occur from the patient moving about and causing the needle to irritate the vein. The IV fluid can infiltrate the tissues around the needle site, causing pain, swelling, and possibly tissue damage. The IV must be terminated and a new site used to restart it. Monitor the skin around the injection site for swelling and redness. Standard Precautions must be used to avoid exposure to the patient's blood and/or body fluids. The fluid is infused into the patient drop by drop. The flow of the solution is carefully monitored. The rate of the IV flow is crucial, and the number of drops per minute must be accurate. Other essential factors for IV infusion are that both the prescribed fluid amount and the amount of time required for the infusion to finish are correct, and that the drop factor is calculated using a mathematical formula.

Electronic devices for IV infusion are battery operated, electrically operated, or a combination of both. The devices are safe and accurate and can be programmed to a specific drop-per-minute rate. The device has an alarm that signals if there is a problem and signals when the infusion is finished.

Equipment for an IV comes in a sterile kit. Within the kit are the needle and cannula for entering the vein, the tubing to attach to the needle and cannula (shielded), and a plastic (usually) or glass container of the prescribed fluid. This equipment constitutes a "basic" administrating set and is what is generally seen in ambulatory care (Figure 36-16). The tubing has a roller-type clamp for adjusting the drop rate. Some tubing is made with a **port** that gives ready access for addition of other fluids by using another infusion set simultaneously. The tubing can become kinked and slow down the flow of fluid. If the needle is not securely attached to the tubing, the fluid may leak out at the attachment site.

IV therapy or infusion is ordered by the provider for a variety of patient conditions. It provides for medication to be given for a rapid response, replaces fluids and electrolytes, helps to raise blood

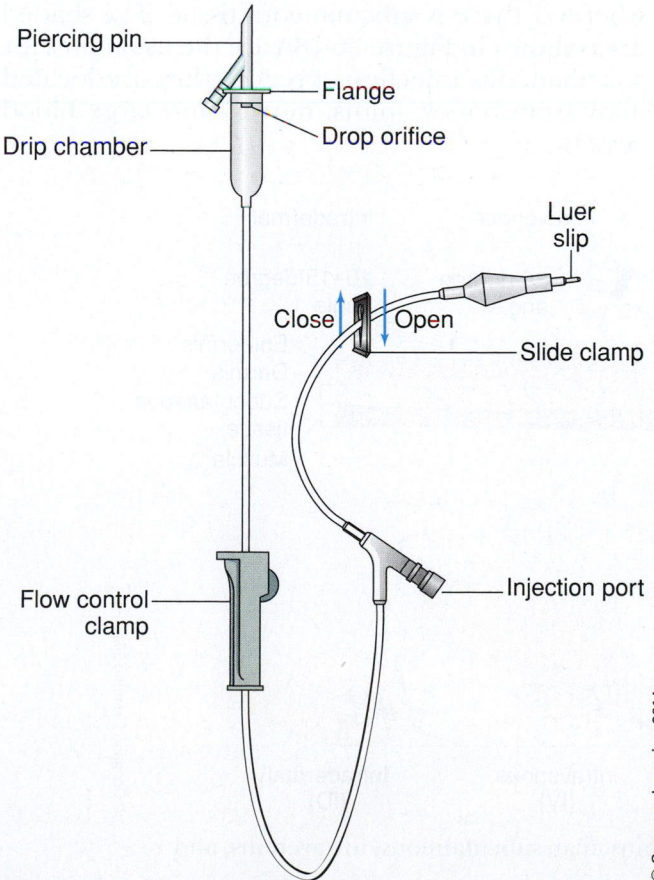

Figure 36-16A Basic IV administration set.

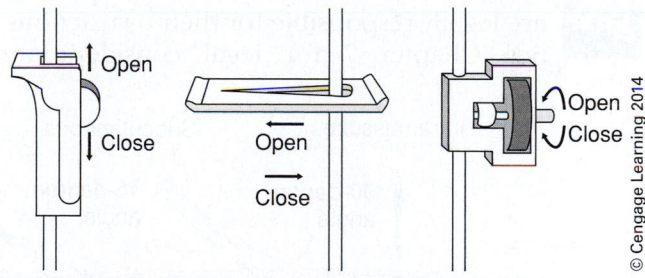

Figure 36-16B Administration set tubing clamps.

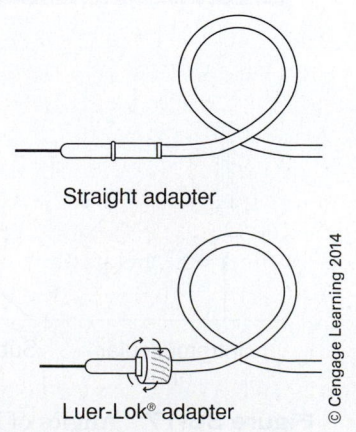

Figure 36-16C Straight and Luer-Lok® cannula hub adapters.

pressure when the patient suffers from shock due to blood or fluid loss, and can be used for nutritional supplements. Access to a vein when needed will have a systemic effect in a short period of time. The vein is accessible for emergencies. The route is useful for unconscious patients and provides a rapid route for countering poisonous substances or inappropriate medication response.

Veins may "collapse" (become very difficult to find) as a result of the patient's condition (dehydration, hypotension, blood loss), and locating an accessible vein may be difficult. The provider may order that the vein be kept opened (by continuous IV infusion). This is abbreviated KVO (keep vein open) or TKO (to be kept open) for immediate accessibility.

Some IV solutions commonly used for infusions in ambulatory settings are:

- 5% dextrose in water
- Saline solutions
- Dextrose in normal saline
- Lactated Ringer's solution

Although IV therapy is not a procedure medical assistants perform, they must be knowledgeable about the procedure, understand the purpose for IV infusions, recognize the precautions concerning this invasive procedure, and realize that state laws vary regarding IV infusion.

 All persons providing health care to patients are legally responsible for their own actions. See Chapter 7 for legal considerations

and Chapter 40 for information regarding phlebotomy.

It is important to realize that IV infusion is an invasive procedure much like the phlebotomy procedure. The veins for IV infusion are similar to those used for venipuncture in the hands and arms.

The AAMA excludes the preparation and administration of intravenous medications from their list of Clinical Competencies for the medical assistant. It is important to understand the scope of practice for the medical assistant in the state in which you are employed. Questions regarding scope of practice can be directed to the American Association of Medical Assistants.

SITE SELECTION AND INJECTION ANGLE

The selection of a proper site for a subcutaneous, intramuscular, or intradermal injection and the correct angle of insertion for each will ensure that the medication is delivered to the correct tissue type (Figure 36-17).

A subcutaneous injection is given at an angle of 45 degrees just below the surface of the skin wherever there is subcutaneous tissue. The shaded areas shown in Figure 36-18A are the usual sites for subcutaneous injections because they are located away from bones, joints, nerves, and large blood vessels.

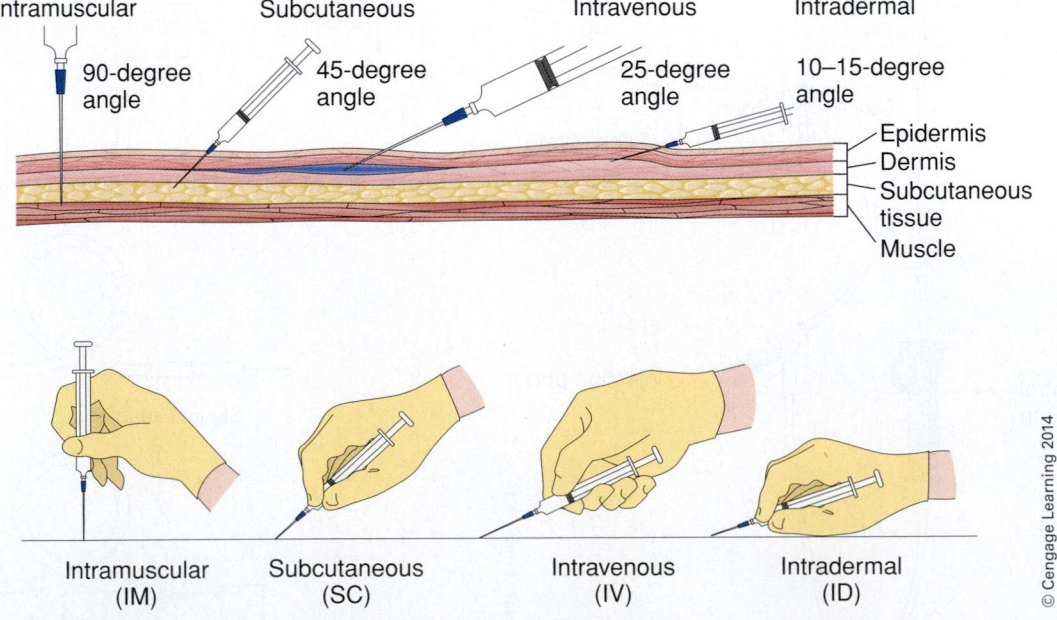

Figure 36-17 Angles of injection for intramuscular, subcutaneous, intravenous, and intradermal injections.

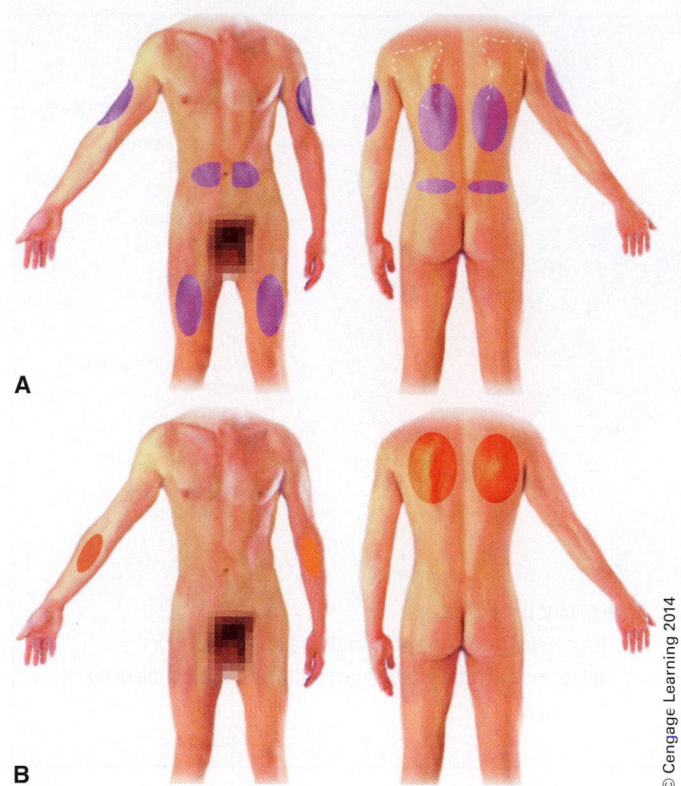

A

B

© Cengage Learning 2014

Figure 36-18   Injection sites: (A) subcutaneous; (B) intradermal.

An intramuscular injection is given at a 90-degree angle, passing through the skin and subcutaneous tissue and penetrating deep into muscle tissue. Body areas normally used for intramuscular injections are the dorsogluteal area, ventrogluteal area, deltoid muscle, and vastus lateralis.

After locating an appropriate vein, an IV injection is given at a 25-degree angle penetrating the skin and introducing the needle into the vein. The antecubital, median cephalic, median basilic, and median cubital veins are common sites appropriate for IV injections (see Chapter 40 for more information about vein selection).

Intradermal injections are given at an angle between 10 and 15 degrees into the dermal layer of the skin. The body areas used for intradermal injections are the inner forearm and the middle of the back (Figure 36-18B). These two sites are used because the skin in these areas is thin and contains little hair.

Marking the Correct Site for Intramuscular Injection

To give a safe injection, it is necessary to become familiar with the anatomic structures associated with the injection site. With knowledge of where such structures are located, it is easier to mark injection sites that avoid bones, nerves, and large blood vessels.

Dorsogluteal Site. The dorsogluteal site is the traditional location for giving most (adult) deep intramuscular injections (Figure 36-19A). Commonly referred to as the "upper outer quadrant of the buttocks," this description can be easily misinterpreted and result in an injection into the inappropriate area. To locate the correct site for a dorsogluteal injection, locate the superior posterior iliac spine and place a small *x* on this spot. Then locate the greater trochanter of the femur and mark this spot. Draw (or imagine) a diagonal line between the two locations. The area above and outside this line and about 3 inches below the iliac crest is the correct location of the dorsogluteal site.

Extreme caution should be used when giving intramuscular injections in the dorsogluteal area. Improper site selection can result in damage to the sciatic nerve or injection into the superior gluteal artery or vein. This site is contraindicated for infants and is used only as a site of last resort in children because of less muscle development. This muscle mass may be degenerated in older adults, the nonwalking, or the emaciated patient.

Ventrogluteal Site. The ventrogluteal site (gluteus medius muscle) can generally accommodate the majority of medications ordered for intramuscular injection. It may be used for individuals from infancy to adulthood. The ventrogluteal site is relatively free of major nerves and vessels, thereby making it a choice site for intramuscular injections. To locate the ventrogluteal injection site, palpate to find the greater trochanter, the anterior superior iliac spine, and the bony ridge of the iliac crest (Figure 36-19B). With these three locations identified, place the palm of your hand against the greater trochanter with the tip of your index finger on the anterior superior iliac spine. Then spread your middle finger as far from the index finger as possible. Place an *x* in the center of the triangle formed by the middle and index fingers to mark the correct injection site.

Deltoid Muscle. The deltoid muscle is a small but adequate site for certain intramuscular injections. These intramuscular preparations include vaccines, narcotics, sedatives, and vitamin preparations. The site should not be used for an infant. To

- Volume of drug administered:
  Usual   1.0 mL to 2.0 mL
- Needle sizes frequently used:
  20G to 23G. 1 inch to 1½ inches
  (greater length needed for very obese
  individuals)
- Acceptable patient position:
  Prone
- Angle of injection:
  90° angle to flat surface upon which prone patient is
  lying
- Advantages of site:
  Large muscle mass accommodates deep IM/Z-track
  injections.
  Injection not visible to patient.
- Disadvantages of site:
  Boundaries of the upper, outer quadrant are often arbi-
  trarily selected and may exceed margin of safety.
  Danger of injury to major nerves and vascular structures
  if incorrect site or technique is used.
  Subcutaneous fat in area is often very thick; an injection
  intended for muscle may in fact be subcutaneous.

- Additional considerations:
  IM injection using the dorsogluteal site requires strict
  adherence to proper anatomical site location and injection
  technique.

Iliac crest
Gluteus medius muscle
Posterior superior
iliac spine
Gluteus minimus
muscle
Greater trochanter of
femur
Sciatic nerve
Gluteus maximus
muscle
Iliotibial tract

© Cengage Learning 2014

Figure 36-19A Injection technique for dorsogluteal site, adult and pediatric (2 years and older).

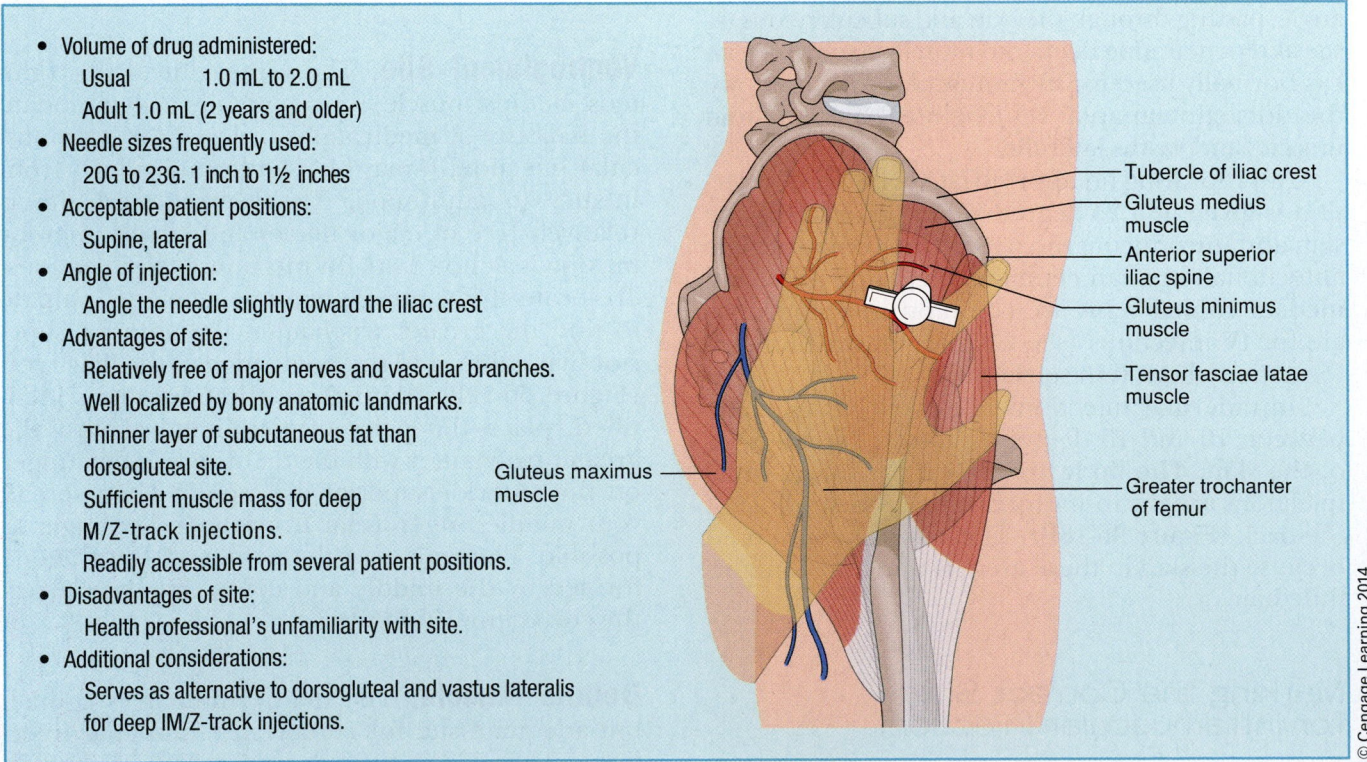

- Volume of drug administered:
  Usual   1.0 mL to 2.0 mL
  Adult 1.0 mL (2 years and older)
- Needle sizes frequently used:
  20G to 23G. 1 inch to 1½ inches
- Acceptable patient positions:
  Supine, lateral
- Angle of injection:
  Angle the needle slightly toward the iliac crest
- Advantages of site:
  Relatively free of major nerves and vascular branches.
  Well localized by bony anatomic landmarks.
  Thinner layer of subcutaneous fat than
  dorsogluteal site.
  Sufficient muscle mass for deep
  M/Z-track injections.
  Readily accessible from several patient positions.
- Disadvantages of site:
  Health professional's unfamiliarity with site.
- Additional considerations:
  Serves as alternative to dorsogluteal and vastus lateralis
  for deep IM/Z-track injections.

Tubercle of iliac crest
Gluteus medius
muscle
Anterior superior
iliac spine
Gluteus minimus
muscle
Tensor fasciae latae
muscle
Gluteus maximus
muscle
Greater trochanter
of femur

© Cengage Learning 2014

Figure 36-19B Injection technique for ventrogluteal site, adult and pediatric (2 years and older).

locate the deltoid injection site, place your fingers on the shoulder and find the acromion (lateral triangular projection of the spine of the scapula forming the point of the shoulder) and the deltoid tuberosity that lies lateral to the side of the arm, opposite the axilla (Figure 36-19C). The correct injection site is 1 to 2 inches (about the width of three fingers) below the acromion.

CAUTION: Do not inject medicine into the upper and lower aspects of the deltoid muscle.

Care should be taken to avoid brachial and axillary nerves and blood vessels, the radial nerve, acromion, and the humerus.

Vastus Lateralis Site.

The vastus lateralis is the preferred site for intramuscular injections in infants and children. It is also used for intramuscular injections in adults (Figure 36-19D). This site generally accommodates the majority of intramuscular injections ordered and is a relatively safe

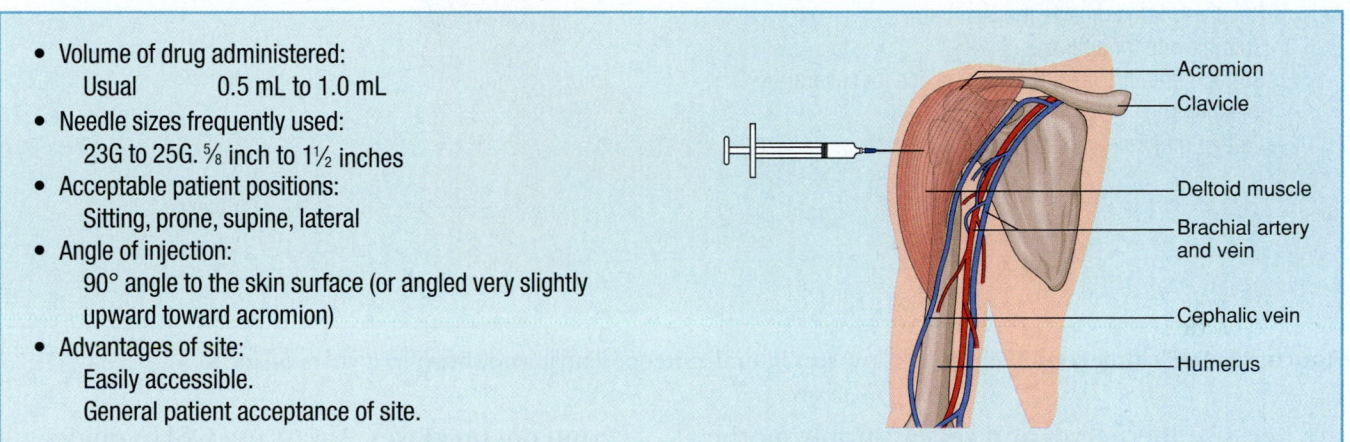

- Volume of drug administered:
  Usual   0.5 mL to 1.0 mL
- Needle sizes frequently used:
  23G to 25G. ⅝ inch to 1½ inches
- Acceptable patient positions:
  Sitting, prone, supine, lateral
- Angle of injection:
  90° angle to the skin surface (or angled very slightly upward toward acromion)
- Advantages of site:
  Easily accessible.
  General patient acceptance of site.

Acromion
Clavicle
Deltoid muscle
Brachial artery and vein
Cephalic vein
Humerus

© Cengage Learning 2014

Figure 36-19C Injection technique for deltoid site, adult and pediatric (15 months and older).

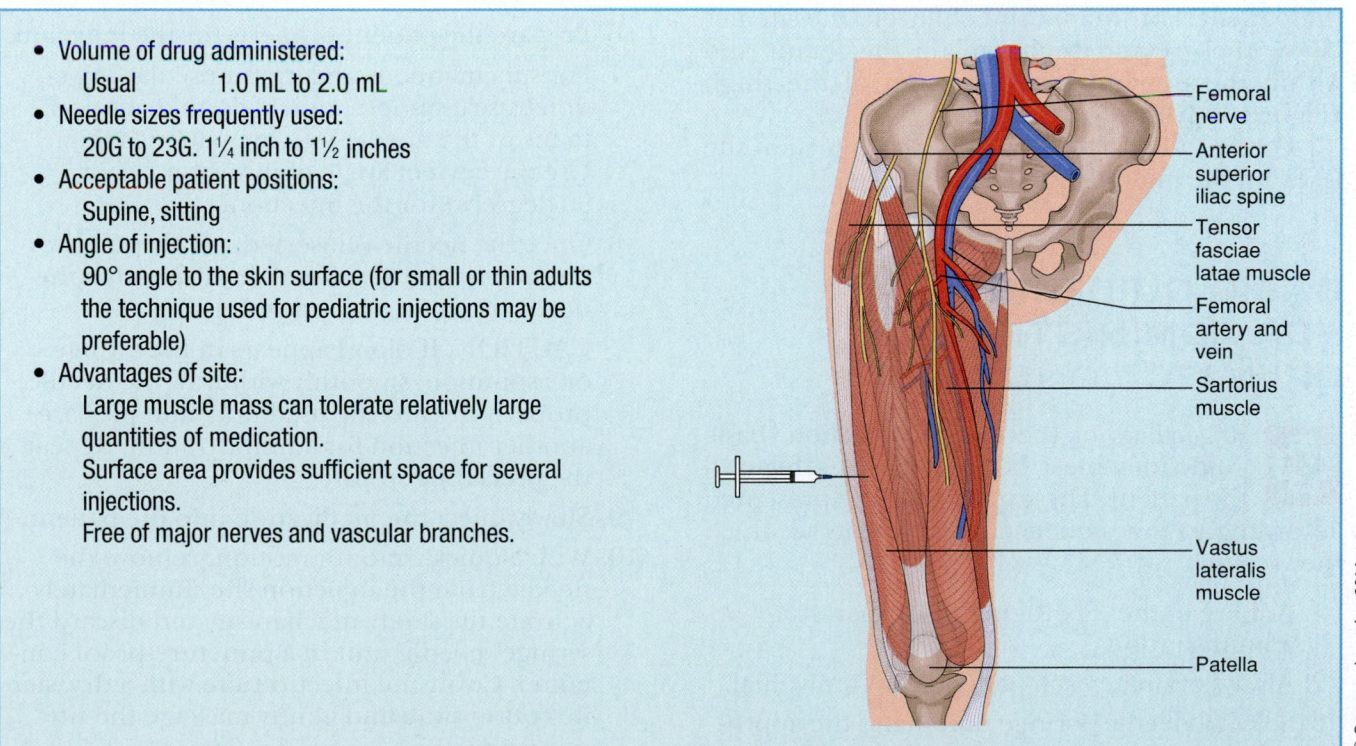

- Volume of drug administered:
  Usual   1.0 mL to 2.0 mL
- Needle sizes frequently used:
  20G to 23G. 1¼ inch to 1½ inches
- Acceptable patient positions:
  Supine, sitting
- Angle of injection:
  90° angle to the skin surface (for small or thin adults the technique used for pediatric injections may be preferable)
- Advantages of site:
  Large muscle mass can tolerate relatively large quantities of medication.
  Surface area provides sufficient space for several injections.
  Free of major nerves and vascular branches.

Femoral nerve
Anterior superior iliac spine
Tensor fasciae latae muscle
Femoral artery and vein
Sartorius muscle
Vastus lateralis muscle
Patella

© Cengage Learning 2014

Figure 36-19D Injection technique for vastus lateralis site, adult and pediatric (2 years and older).

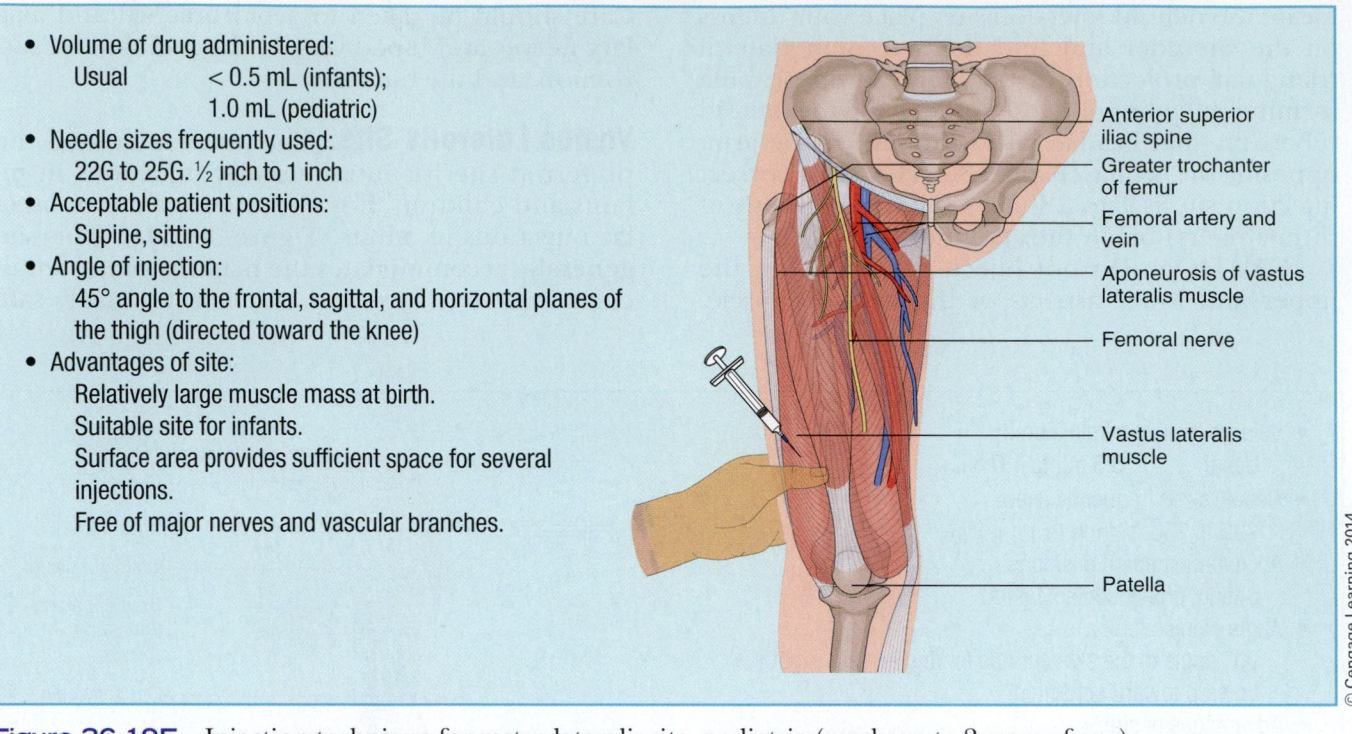

- Volume of drug administered:
  Usual   < 0.5 mL (infants);
           1.0 mL (pediatric)
- Needle sizes frequently used:
  22G to 25G. ½ inch to 1 inch
- Acceptable patient positions:
  Supine, sitting
- Angle of injection:
  45° angle to the frontal, sagittal, and horizontal planes of the thigh (directed toward the knee)
- Advantages of site:
  Relatively large muscle mass at birth.
  Suitable site for infants.
  Surface area provides sufficient space for several injections.
  Free of major nerves and vascular branches.

Labels: Anterior superior iliac spine; Greater trochanter of femur; Femoral artery and vein; Aponeurosis of vastus lateralis muscle; Femoral nerve; Vastus lateralis muscle; Patella

© Cengage Learning 2014

Figure 36-19E   Injection technique for vastus lateralis site, pediatric (newborn to 2 years of age).

site because the nerves and vessels supplying the area are not generally endangered. The vastus lateralis is a part of the quadriceps femoris. The muscle is located on the anterolateral aspect of the patient. For infants and children, the site lies below the greater trochanter of the femur and within the upper lateral quadrant of the thigh (Figure 36-19E).

For the adult patient, the correct injection site is within the middle third of the muscle.

BASIC GUIDELINES FOR ADMINISTRATION OF INJECTIONS

Regardless of the type of injection, basic guidelines must be followed to safeguard the patient. These guidelines are presented according to the sequence of the events to which they relate:

1. Adhere to the "Six Rights" of proper drug administration.
2. Always evaluate each patient as an individual.
3. Select a needle–syringe unit that is the appropriate size for the proper administration of a parenteral medication.
4. Correctly prepare the appropriate parenteral equipment and supplies for use. Wash hands

and put on gloves. Always use OSHA guidelines and follow Standard Precautions.

5. Select the correct site for the intended injection.
6. Prepare the patient properly for the injection.
7. For subcutaneous and intramuscular injections, use a smooth, quick, dartlike motion to insert the needle into the patient's skin. Use the correct angle of insertion (45 or 90 degrees) for the injection.
8. Once the needle is inserted, gently pull back on the plunger (aspirate) to ensure that the needle is not in a blood vessel.

CAUTION: If blood appears in the syringe on aspiration, smoothly withdraw the needle, properly discard the used unit, and prepare another injection for administration. Repeat the preceding steps.

9. Slowly inject the medication into the patient.
10. With a quick, smooth motion, remove the needle from the injection site. Immediately activate the safety mechanism and discard the syringe–needle unit in a puncture-proof container. Cover the injection site with a dry, sterile cotton swab and gently massage the site.

CAUTION: Do not massage the site when administering insulin, Imferon, or heparin.

11. Remove the cotton swab and check for bleeding. If bleeding occurs after applying pressure

for 30 seconds, apply a sterile adhesive strip to the injection site.

12. Remove gloves.

13. Observe the patient for any signs of hypersensitivity. Take precautions to ensure the patient's safety.

14. Properly and immediately discard the used equipment and supplies.

15. Wash hands.

16. Follow documentation procedures in patient's chart or electronic medical record, noting administration of the medication.

17. Before releasing the patient, wait the appropriate amount of time and make sure the patient is given proper instructions and is not experiencing any unusual effects.

18. Return medications to shelf/storage.

 Procedures 36-1 through 36-9 provide steps as follows:

- Procedure 36-1: Administration of Oral Medications
- Procedure 36-2: Withdrawing Medication from a Vial
- Procedure 36-3: Withdrawing Medication from an Ampule
- Procedure 36-4: Administration of Subcutaneous, Intramuscular, and Intradermal Injections
- Procedure 36-5: Administering a Subcutaneous Injection
- Procedure 36-6: Administering an Intramuscular Injection
- Procedure 36-7: Administering an Intradermal Injection of Purified Protein Derivative (PPD)
- Procedure 36-8: Reconstituting a Powder Medication for Administration
- Procedure 36-9: Z-Track Intramuscular Injection Technique

Z-TRACK METHOD OF INTRAMUSCULAR INJECTION

Imferon is an example of a medication that is administered using the Z-track method. This medication and others that are irritating to the subcutaneous tissues and may discolor the skin are given in this manner. (The *Physician's Desk Reference* [PDR] is a good reference source for help in determining the correct route technique for injections.)

The Z-track technique is similar to an intramuscular injection, except that the skin is pulled to the side before needle insertion. This causes a displacement of the tissues and the medication enters in a manner that will not allow it to seep back into the subcutaneous tissues and up to the skin's surface. Because the medications are irritating, for the comfort of the patient, change the needle on the syringe after aspirating the medication from the ampule or vial before injecting the patient with the medication (see Procedure 36-9).

ADMINISTRATION OF ALLERGENIC EXTRACTS

It may be the responsibility of the medical assistant to administer allergenic extracts. It is important to observe the following:

- Allergic extracts are *always* given in subcutaneous tissue, *never* in the muscle.
- Use a tuberculin syringe with a 25G, $^5/_8$-inch needle; 26G, $^3/_8$-inch needle; or 27G, ½-inch needle or 1-mL allergist syringe (Figure 36-20).
- Use a site rotation system for each injected extract.
- Correctly document the procedure and dosage.
- Allergenic extracts should be refrigerated; they should retain potency for 10 to 12 weeks.
- Adverse reactions such as itching, swelling, and redness should be reported immediately to the provider.
- Severe reactions such as anaphylactic shock have occurred; therefore, emergency

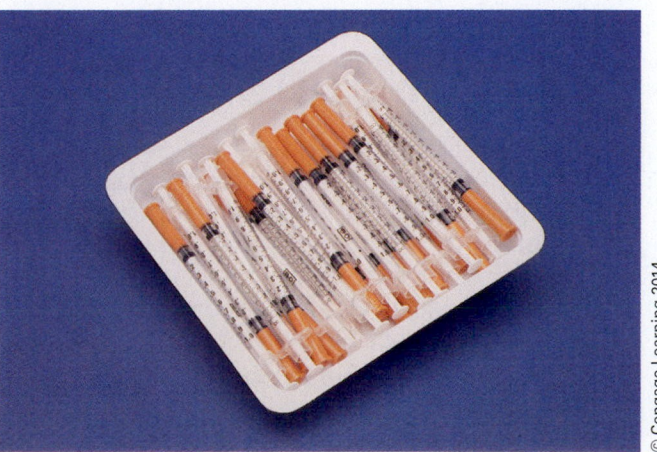

Figure 36-20 Allergist syringes.

equipment and supplies must be available for use. Epinephrine and Benadryl must be readily accessible. (See Chapters 9 and 35 for emergency supplies.)

- Allergy testing is done when the provider is present.
- Patient must wait 20 to 30 minutes after injection to be certain there has been no reaction.

Example:

Patient's Name:

Date	Dose	Site
6/24/XX	1st 0.01 mL SC	Lt. arm
6/27/XX	2nd 0.02 mL SC	Rt. arm
6/30/XX	3rd 0.03 mL SC	Lt. arm

 The patient should be observed for 20 to 30 minutes after the injection of an allergenic extract.

Susceptible individuals can experience development of allergic reactions to many foreign substances. It is wise for the patient with allergies to be aware of those substances and others that are known allergens.

ADMINISTRATION OF INHALED MEDICATIONS

The act of drawing breath, vapor, or gas into the lungs is known as *inhalation*. Inhalation therapy may involve the administration of medicines; water vapor; and such gases as oxygen, carbon dioxide, and helium.

An inhaler may be used to deliver medications to the lungs. Medications that use an inhaler include bronchodilators, mucolytic agents, and steroids. Inhalers are useful in the delivery of treatment for chronic obstructive pulmonary disease (COPD) and reversible obstructive airway disease. An inhaler is a small, handheld apparatus, usually an aerosol unit, that contains a microcrystalline suspension of medication. When activated, it produces a fine mist or spray containing the medication. This suspension is then drawn into the respiratory tract, settling deep into the lungs and alveoli. See Chapter 30 for information about pulmonary diseases and procedures.

Implications for Patient Care

Patients should be instructed to follow the prescribed medication regimen. The prescribed medicine and the type of inhaler to be used will determine the method of administration. A handheld inhaler may be used for oral or nasal inhalation, depending on the type ordered by the provider.

Inhalation therapy may be contraindicated in patients with delicate fluid balance, cardiac arrhythmias, **status asthmaticus**, and hypersensitivity to the medication. As with any medication, the provider will determine the treatment regimen for each patient. See Chapter 30 for information about pulmonary diseases and procedures.

Administration of Oxygen

Oxygen is a colorless, odorless, tasteless gas that is essential for life. When the body does not have an adequate supply of oxygen, a state of **hypoxemia** (lack of oxygen in the blood) develops, and irreversible damage to vital organs is possible. When a lack of oxygen threatens a person's survival, supplemental oxygen must be prescribed and administered immediately, and arterial blood gas analysis

PATIENT EDUCATION

- Patients should be advised to avoid overuse of the inhaler. Tolerance, rebound bronchospasm, and adverse cardiac effects can occur from overuse. Instruct the patient to notify the provider should the prescribed dose of medication fail to produce the desired effect.
- Instruct the patient to perform good oral hygiene, including rinsing of the mouth and mouthpiece of equipment, after the inhalation treatment (to prevent the possible growth of fungi).
- Caution the patient against the continued use of a metered-dose canister after the prescribed number of actuations. If the medication contains adrenaline, fatalities can occur if heart rate and blood pressure increase significantly.

will be necessary after oxygen administration has been started. If the situation is not an emergency or life threatening, arterial blood gas analysis can be performed before the provider prescribes the dosage and method of administration. The normal range for oxygen in the arterial blood is 80 to 100 mm Hg (millimeters mercury). Oxygen is supplied in tanks (Figure 36-21) for use in the ambulatory care setting, but in a hospital setting, oxygen is piped in through a wall pipe system.

Dosage.

When oxygen is to be administered, dosage is based on individual needs. Because oxygen is a drug, the provider will prescribe the flow rate, concentration, method of delivery, and length of time for administration. Oxygen is ordered as liters per minute (LPM) or L/min and as percentage of oxygen concentration (%).

It is the medical assistant's responsibility to follow provider orders and adhere to the guidelines for proper drug administration. Always assess the patient as an individual, explain the procedure, and carefully observe the patient for signs of improvement or symptoms of oxygen toxicity.

A noninvasive technology that monitors the safety and efficacy of oxygen administration is the pulse oximeter. O_2 liter flow per minute can be titrated based on the results obtained from the pulse oximeter (see Chapter 30).

CAUTION: Oxygen toxicity may develop when 100% oxygen is breathed for a prolonged period. As with any other drug, toxicity depends on dose, time, and the patient's response. The higher the dose, the shorter the time required to develop toxicity. Symptoms of oxygen toxicity are substernal pain, nausea, vomiting, malaise, fatigue, numbness, and a tingling of the extremities.

High concentrations of inhaled oxygen cause alveolar collapse, intra-alveolar hemorrhage, hyaline membrane formation, disturbance of the central nervous system, and **retrolental fibroplasia** in newborns.

NOTE: **Apnea** (absence of breathing) can result when giving oxygen at a flow rate greater than 2 liters per minute to patients with COPD, especially those with emphysema.

Methods of Oxygen Delivery.

Many methods are available today for the delivery of oxygen. The more commonly prescribed methods include the use of nasal cannulas, nasal catheters, and masks. Other methods of delivery involve the use of isolettes, hoods, and tents.

Nasal Cannula.

When a low concentration of oxygen is desired, the nasal cannula (Figure 36-22) is the simplest and most convenient method for the administration of oxygen. Made of plastic, the nasal cannula consists of two hollow prongs through which oxygen passes, and a strap or other device

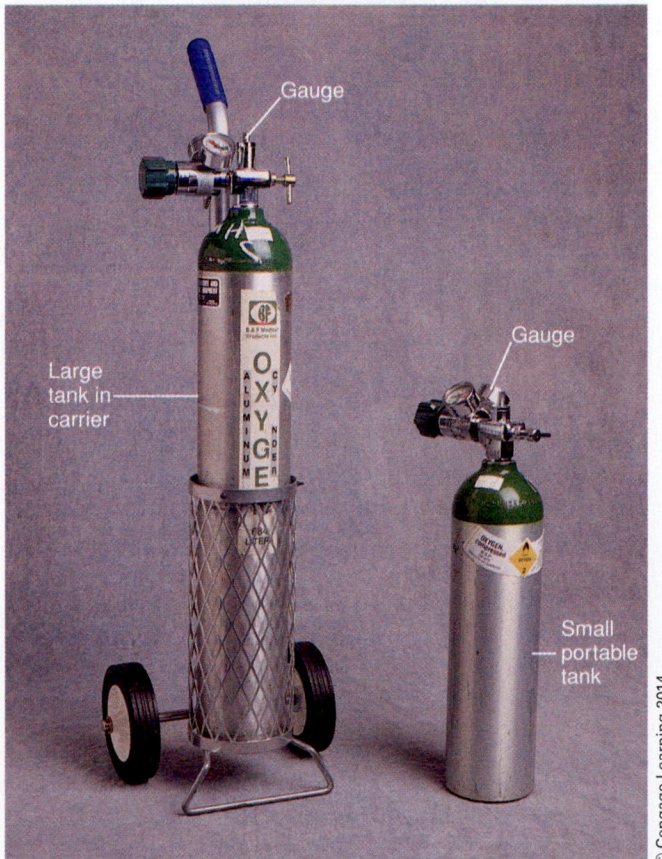

Figure 36-21 Oxygen tanks. Note gauge at top of tanks.

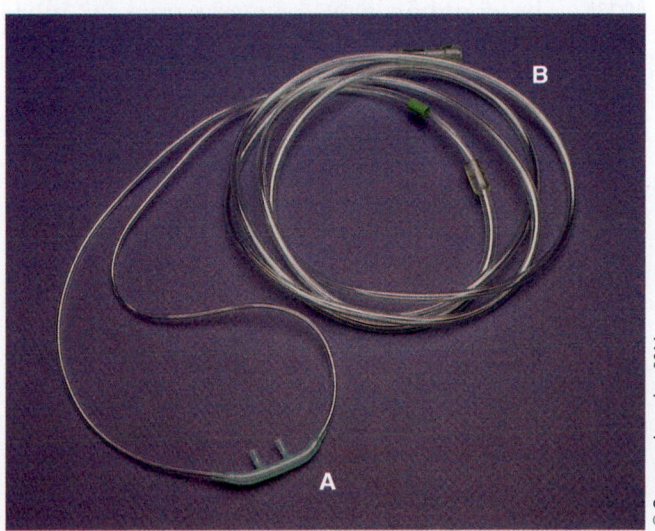

Figure 36-22 (A) Oxygen cannula. (B) Tubing.

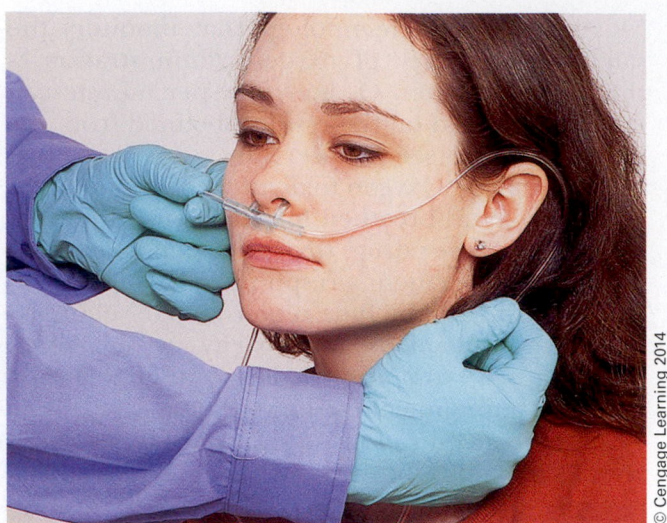

Figure 36-23 Medical assistant adjusts nasal cannula around patient's ears for oxygen administration.

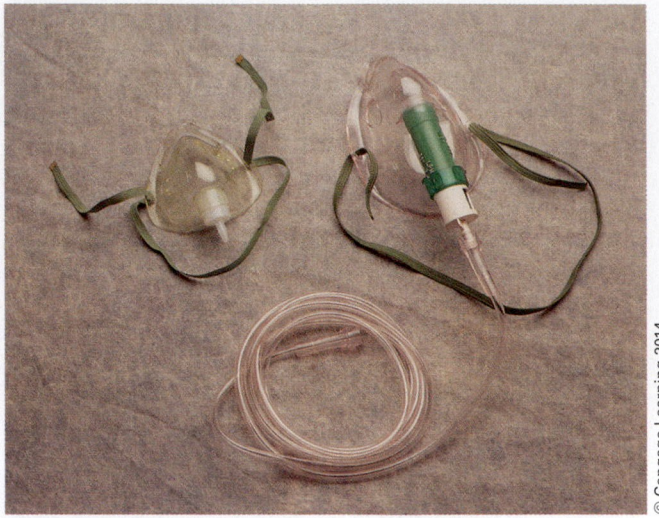

Figure 36-24 Oxygen masks: (A) without tubing; (B) with tubing.

to secure it to the patient's head (Figure 36-23). Do not place the direct flow of oxygen against the patient's nasal mucosa, because this causes tissue dehydration. Flow rates greater than 2 to 4 L/min require humidification.

Nasal Catheter. The nasal catheter is a disposable plastic tube that has small holes at the inserted end. These holes diffuse the flow of oxygen for better distribution to lung tissue with minimum dehydration. The nasal catheter is rarely used today because it causes mucous membrane irritation and has to be changed every 8 hours. Because of the discomfort caused to the patient by the catheter, the nasal cannula is the preferred method for the delivery of oxygen.

Mask. The common types of masks used for inhalation therapy include plastic disposable, partial rebreather, nonrebreather, and Venturi (Figure 36-24). These devices are used when the patient requires high humidity and a precise amount of oxygen. To be effective, the mask must be fitted snugly to the patient (Figure 36-25).

CAUTION: Oxygen must be humidified before delivery to the patient to prevent drying of the respiratory mucosa.

Oxygen Safety Precautions. Oxygen supports combustion; thus, there is the danger of a fire being started when oxygen is in use. Extreme caution should be exercised when oxygen is being administered because ignition can be caused by friction, static electricity, or a lighted cigar or cigarette. In the provider's clinic, oxygen is generally stored in tanks. These tanks

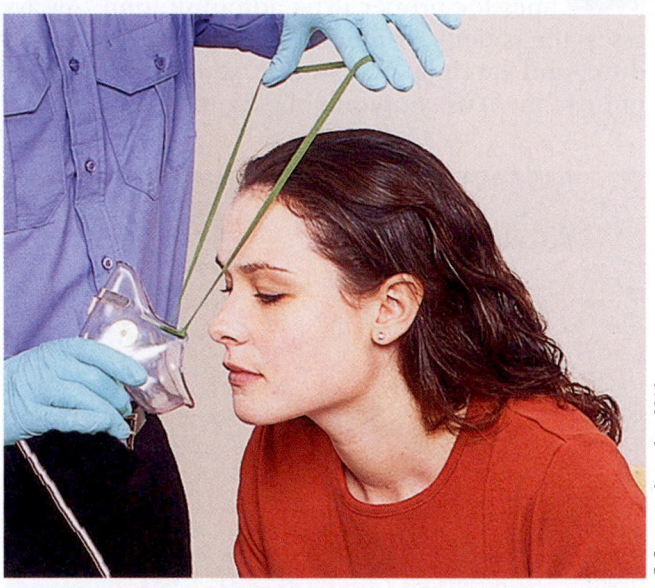

Figure 36-25 Medical assistant adjusts oxygen mask around patient's head.

must be checked on a regular basis and replaced as necessary. See Chapter 30 for information about pulmonary diseases and procedures.

PATIENT EDUCATION

Explain safety measures to the patient who uses oxygen at home. Cigarettes, lighters, candles, and other smoking materials should not be used in the room where oxygen is used. Instruct the patient to wear non–static producing clothing, such as cotton.

PROCEDURE 36-1

Administration of Oral Medications

STANDARD PRECAUTIONS:

PURPOSE:

Correctly administer an oral medication after receiving the provider's order and assembling the necessary equipment and supplies.

EQUIPMENT/SUPPLIES:

Medication order per provider
Medication card
Correct medication
Medicine cup
Fluid for swallowing the medication (water, juice, or milk)

PROCEDURE STEPS:

1. Perform medical asepsis handwashing procedure. Adhere to OSHA guidelines.

2. Verify the provider's order and prepare a medication card.

3. Follow the "Six Rights" of medication administration (Figure 36-26A).

4. Work in a well-lighted, quiet, clean area.

5. *Paying attention to detail,* gather appropriate equipment and supplies. RATIONALE: A well-lighted area for preparing medications is important because you must be able to see well to accurately pour medications. A quiet area is free from distractions, and medical asepsis helps fight transmission of microorganisms.

6. Review the medication card. Select the correct medication from the medication area.

7. Compare the medication label with the medication card (first check). RATIONALE: Reading from a medication card helps prevent errors while pouring the medication.

8. If unfamiliar with the medication, consult the PDR or other reputable reference. Familiarize yourself with:
   - Drug name (commercial and generic)
   - Mechanism of action
   - Routes of administration
   - Common side effects

9. Check the expiration date. RATIONALE: Outdated medication may be deteriorated or altered in some way and may be harmful to the patient.

10. Carefully calculate the dosage based on medication order and medication available.

11. Correctly prepare (a, b, or c) (Figure 36-26B and Figure 36-26C).
    a. Multiple-dose solid medication
    b. Unit dose medication
    c. Liquid medication

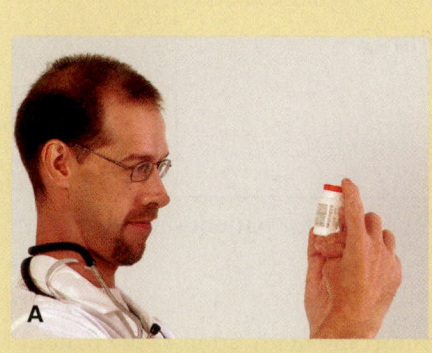 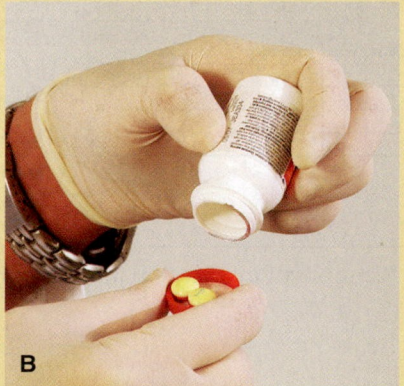 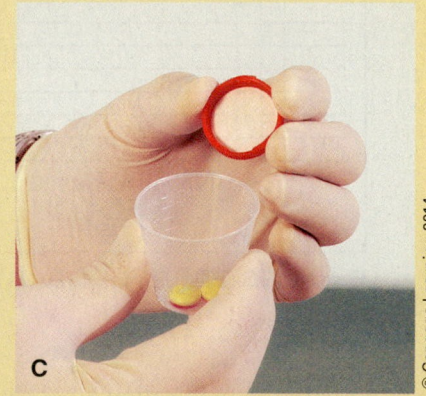

© Cengage Learning 2014

Figure 36-26   (A) Medical assistant checks for right drug, right dose, right route, and expiration date before pouring medication. (B) Medical assistant pours capsules from the cover of the medicine container into a medicine cup before administering medicine to patient. The medication is poured into cover to avoid contamination of medicine. (C) Medical assistant administers the medication, being certain that patient takes the medicine.

continues

Procedure 36-1 (continued)

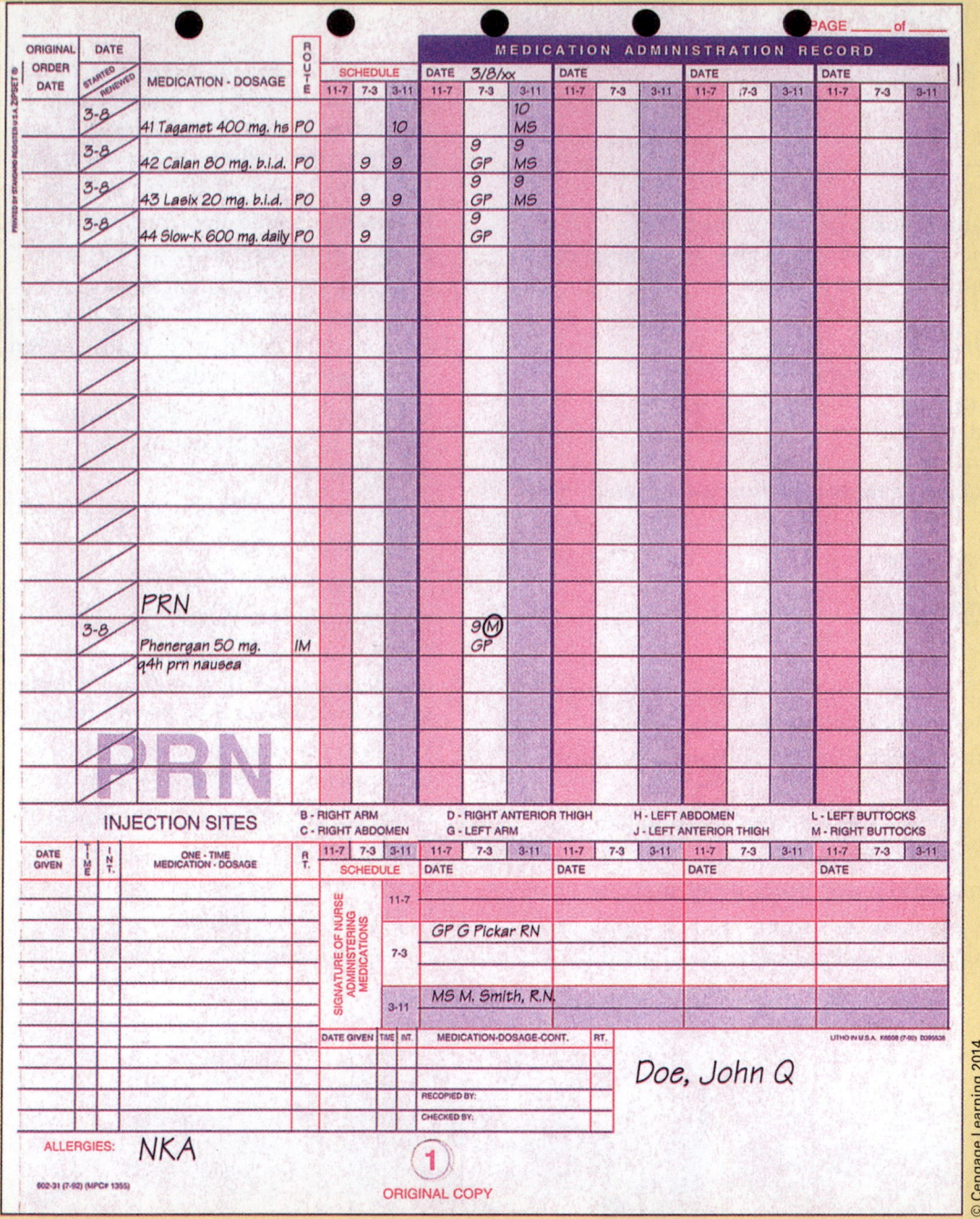

Figure 36-26   *(continued)* (D) Example of medication administration record for patient's chart.

12. Compare the medication label with the medication card (second check).

13. Discard any refuse generated during the preparation.

14. Carefully transport the medication to the patient exam room. Bring the medication container with the prepared medication.

15. ***Introduce yourself and identify patient.***

Procedure 36-1 (continued)

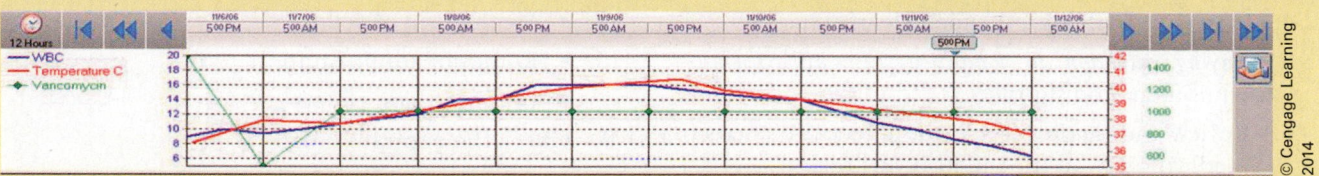

© Cengage Learning 2014

Figure 36-26 *(continued)* (E) The computer makes a graph when the appropriate patient data is input. The patient's white blood cell count (WBC), temperature (in Celsius), and antibiotic (Vancomycin) are shown. The patient has an infection, and the computer-generated graphic shows the patient's response to the antibiotic. The WBC and temperature climb over a period of 4 days, and then begin to drop in response to the antibiotic. The provider has access to the information on demand.

16. *Speaking at the level of the patient's understanding, explain the procedure and expectations to the patient.* State the name of the medication and the purpose of the dose.

17. Ask the patient about medication allergies.

18. Assess the patient. Take vital signs if indicated (i.e., apical pulse prior to administration of digoxin). RATIONALE: Always assess the patient for body size, physical condition, age, and gender to be certain the dose and route are appropriate prior to administration of certain medications. BP or pulse may need to be taken to ascertain if the vital signs are within normal limits.

19. Assure the patient is in a comfortable, upright position.

20. Review the medication card and the medication (third check).

21. Administer the medication. Provide an adequate amount of fluid to assure ease of swallowing.

RATIONALE: Some patients, for various reasons, may deliberately not swallow their medication.

22. Have the patient open his mouth and move his tongue around to assure that the patient has swallowed the medication.

23. If it is the first time that the patient has received the medication, have the patient remain in the office setting per the provider's preference.

24. *Being courteous, patient, and respectful,* assess the patient every 5 minutes for signs of reaction.

25. *Paying attention to detail,* return the medication container to the appropriate place in the medication area.

26. Accurately document in the patient's chart or electronic medical record the medication, dose, route, site of injection, and patient reaction. Sign and add date and time (Figure 36-26D and Figure 36-26E).

PROCEDURE 36-2
Withdrawing Medication from a Vial

STANDARD PRECAUTIONS:

PURPOSE:
Medication is supplied in a variety of packaging. Medication from a vial must be drawn into a syringe for parenteral injection.

EQUIPMENT/SUPPLIES:

Medication order per provider	Alcohol wipes
Medication card	Disposable nonsterile gloves
	Sharps container

Correct medication
Appropriately sized syringe and needle of the correct gauge and length

PROCEDURE STEPS:
1. Perform medical asepsis handwashing procedure. Adhere to OSHA guidelines.

2. Verify the provider's order and prepare a medication card.

3. Follow the "Six Rights" of medication administration.

continues

Procedure 36-2 (continued)

4. Work in a well-lighted, quiet, clean area.

5. ***Paying attention to detail,*** gather appropriate equipment and supplies.

6. Review the medication card. Select the correct medication from the medication area.

7. Compare the medication label with the medication card (first check).

8. If unfamiliar with the medication, consult the PDR or other reputable reference. Familiarize yourself with:

   - Drug name (commercial and generic)

   - Mechanism of action
   - Routes of administration
   - Common side effects

9. Check the expiration date.

10. Carefully calculate the dosage based on medication order and medication available.

11. Compare the medication label with the medication card (second check).

12. Remove the metal or plastic cap from the vial. Clean the vial stopped with an alcohol wipe using a circular motion (Figure 36-27A).

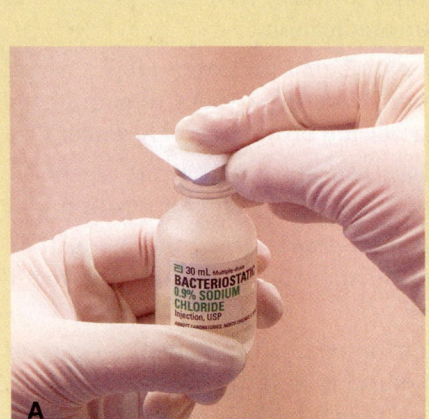

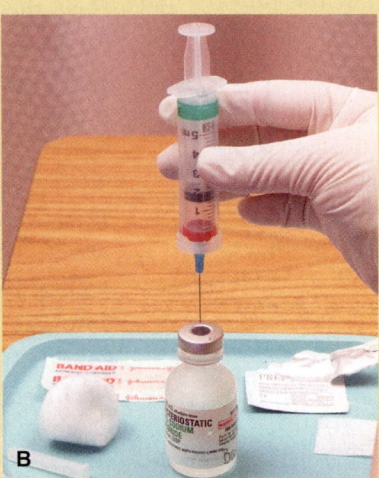

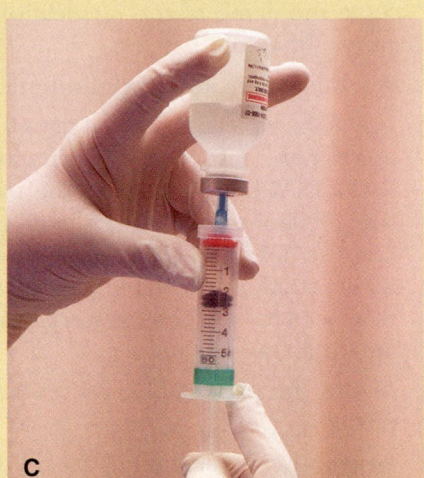

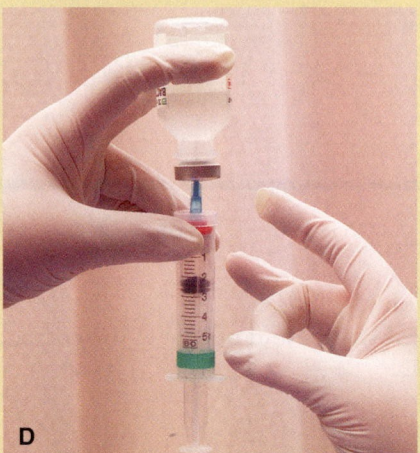

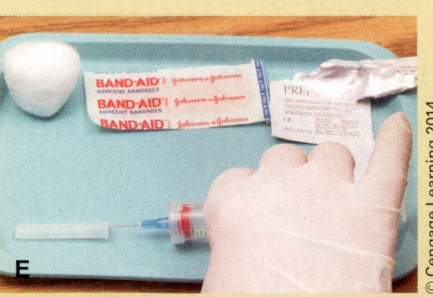

© Cengage Learning 2014

Figure 36-27   (A) Disinfect the rubber stopper on the medication vial with an alcohol wipe. (B) Keeping the bevel of the needle above the fluid level, inject an amount of air equal to medication quantity to be withdrawn. (C) Hold syringe pointed upward at eye level and with the bevel of the needle in the medication. Pull back plunger and aspirate the quantity to be withdrawn. (D) Tap syringe to eliminate air bubbles. Hand should hold syringe while tapping it. (E) After the correct dose has been withdrawn, recover the sterile needle using "scoop" method. Place medicine on a tray with medication card, the medication vial, and an alcohol wipe and safely transport to the patient.

Procedure 36-2 (continued)

13. Carefully remove the needle cover. Inject air into the vial as follows:

    - Hold the syringe pointed upward at eye level. Pull the plunger back to the level of the expected amount of medication to be withdrawn.
    - Leave vial on tabletop/countertop.
    - Insert the needle through the center of the rubber stopper of the vial.
    - Inject the air by pushing the plunger slowly (Figure 36-27B).

14. Invert the vial. Hold the vial and the syringe steady.

15. Carefully and slowly pull back on the plunger to withdraw the correct amount of medication.

16. Measure accurately. Keep the tip of the needle below the surface of the liquid; otherwise, air will enter the syringe. Keep the syringe at eye level (Figure 36-27C).

17. Check the syringe for air bubbles. Remove them by tapping sharply on the syringe. Push the air bubbles back into the vial (Figure 36-27D).

18. Check the measurement for accuracy, and draw out more medication if necessary.

19. Remove the needle from the vial.

20. Replace the sterile needle cover (Figure 36-27E) using the "scoop" technique. RATIONALE: The needle cover can be replaced because it is sterile and has not been used on a patient.

21. Check the label on the vial with the medication card (third check).

22. If the medication is a tissue irritant, change the needle utilized to withdraw the medication. RATIONALE: Tissue irritants can cause tissue necrosis.

23. Carefully carry the syringe and medication vial to the patient's bedside.

24. Refer to the appropriate procedure (subcutaneous, intradermal, or intramuscular injection).

25. Activate the safety mechanism to cover the needle. Immediately dispose of the needle and syringe in the sharps container.

26. Remove gloves (if utilized) and dispose of according to OSHA guidelines.

27. Wash hands.

28. ***Paying attention to detail,*** return the medication container to the appropriate place in the medication area.

29. Accurately document in the patient's chart or electronic medical record the medication, dose, route, site of injection, and patient reaction. Sign and add date and time.

30. Following office procedure, return the vial to the medication cabinet. Destroy the medication card.

DOCUMENTATION:

8/9/20XX 2:30 PM   Vitamin B$_{12}$ (Cyanocobalamin)
100 mcg IM (R) deltoid area. W. Slawson, CMA (AAMA)——

PROCEDURE 36-3

Withdrawing Medication from an Ampule

STANDARD PRECAUTIONS:

PURPOSE:

Medication is supplied in a variety of packaging. An ampule is a sterile, glass, single-dose container of liquid medication. It is aspirated into a syringe for injection.

EQUIPMENT/SUPPLIES:

Medication order per provider
Medication card
Ampule of correct medication
Appropriately sized syringe and needle of the correct gauge and length

Sterile gauze sponges
Sterile filter needle
Alcohol wipes
Disposable nonsterile gloves

PROCEDURE STEPS:

1. Perform medical asepsis handwashing procedure. Adhere to OSHA guidelines.

2. Verify the provider's order and prepare a medication card.

3. Follow the "Six Rights" of medication administration.

continues

Procedure 36-3 (continued)

4. Work in a well-lighted, quiet, clean area.

5. *Paying attention to detail,* gather appropriate equipment and supplies.

6. Review the medication card. Select the correct medication from the medication area.

7. Compare the medication label with the medication card (first check).

8. If unfamiliar with the medication, consult the PDR or other reputable reference. Familiarize yourself with:

   • Drug name (commercial and generic)

   • Mechanism of action

   • Routes of administration

   • Common side effects

9. Check the expiration date.

10. Carefully calculate the dosage based on medication order and medication available.

11. Compare the medication label with the medication card (second check).

12. Don nonsterile disposable gloves.

13. Grasp the ampule of medication. The medication will often get "trapped" in the neck of the ampule. To return it to the body of the ampule, swirl the ampule in a circular motion by holding onto the upper end above the neck. The medication will return to the body of the vial. (Figure 36-28A). RATIONALE: This is important

to ensure all medication is available in the body of the ampule to calculate the correct dose. If some of the medication remains trapped above the neck in the top of the ampule, some medication will not be available for use and it is possible to give an incorrect dose, especially if the patient is to receive the entire contents of the ampule.

14. Thoroughly disinfect the neck of the ampule by wiping with an alcohol wipe. RATIONALE: The needle will enter the opening of the ampule and wiping the neck of the ampule before removal of the top ensures disinfection of the neck on opening of the ampule.

15. With a sterile gauze, wipe dry the neck of the ampule.

16. Completely surround the ampule with the gauze and forcefully snap off the top of the ampule by pulling the top toward you (Figure 36-28B). RATIONALE: Ensures medical assistant safety from possible injury from broken glass. Discard top in sharps container.

17. *Paying attention to detail,* carefully place the open ampule on the countertop.

18. Check the provider's order, medication card and label on ampule (third check).

19. With a sterile syringe and a filter needle (sometimes included with the medication), aspirate the required dose into the syringe (Figure 36-28C). Cover needle with sheath using scoop method

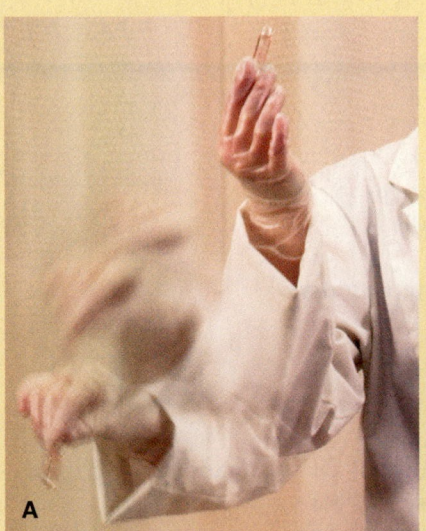 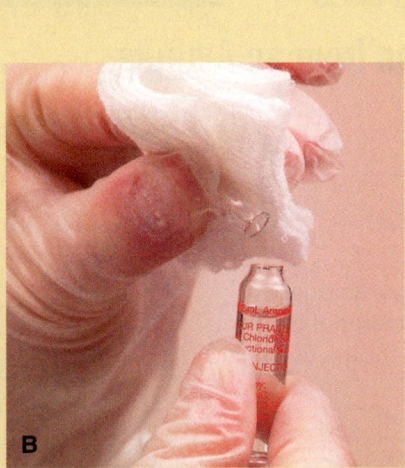 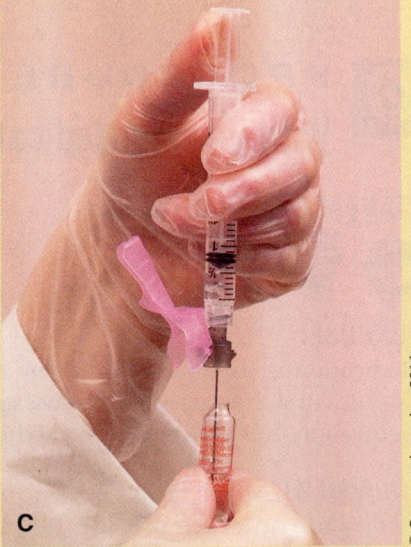

© Cengage Learning 2014

Figure 36-28   (A) Hold ampule by the top and force all the medication into the bottom of the ampule by a snap of the arm and wrist. (B) Remove top from ampule. Snap away from you by pulling top toward you. (C) Draw the required dose into syringe.

Procedure 36-3 (continued)

and transport it with medication ampule to patient on the medicine tray. **RATIONALE:** Filtered needles prevent glass particles from being aspirated with medication.

There is an alternate method for withdrawing the medication. The needle with the syringe attached can be inserted into the open ampule and then inverted. The medication will not flow out due to the force of surface tension. Then withdraw the appropriate amount of medication.

20. Cover the filter needle with the cap using the "scoop" method.

21. Remove the filter needle from the syringe and immediately discard in an appropriate sharps container. **RATIONALE:** The filter needle may contain glass particles.

22. Select the appropriate needle gauge and length for the injection.

23. Place the new needle, using sterile technique, on the syringe with the medication.

24. Follow the steps for appropriate administration of subcutaneous, intradermal, or intramuscular injection.

DOCUMENTATION:

5/12/20XX 11:20 AM   Phenergan 25 mg IM (R) dorsogluteal area. B. Abbott, RMA (AMT)———————————

PROCEDURE 36-4

Administration of Subcutaneous, Intramuscular, and Intradermal Injections

STANDARD PRECAUTIONS:

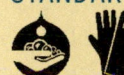

PURPOSE:
To properly administer subcutaneous, intramuscular, and intradermal injections.

EQUIPMENT/SUPPLIES:
Medication order per provider
Medication card
Ampule of correct medication
Appropriately sized syringe and needle of the correct gauge and length
Alcohol wipes
Disposable nonsterile gloves

PROCEDURE STEPS:
1. Perform medical asepsis handwashing procedure. Adhere to OSHA guidelines.

2. Verify the provider's order and prepare a medication card.

3. Follow the "Six Rights" of medication administration.

4. Work in a well-lighted, quiet, clean area.

5. *Paying attention to detail*, gather appropriate equipment and supplies.

6. Review the medication card. Select the correct medication from the medication area.

7. Compare the medication label with the medication card (first check).

8. If unfamiliar with the medication, consult the PDR or other reputable reference. Familiarize yourself with:
   - Drug name (commercial and generic)
   - Mechanism of action
   - Routes of administration
   - Common side effects

9. Check the expiration date.

10. Carefully calculate the dosage based on medication order and medication available.

11. Compare the medication label with the medication card (second check).

12. Don nonsterile disposable gloves.

continues

Procedure 36-4 (continued)

13. Withdraw medication from vial using correct syringe and needle (Figure 36-29A to Figure 36-29D).

14. Check the provider's order, medication card, and label on ampule (third check).

15. Keeping the syringe, medication, alcohol swab and medication card together (some practices use a medication tray), transport to the patient's bedside.

16. *Introduce yourself and identify patient.*

17. *Speaking at the level of the patient's understanding, explain the procedure and expectations to the patient.* State the name of the medication and the purpose of the injection.

18. *Allay the patient's fears regarding the procedure being performed and help her feel safe and comfortable.*

19. Ask the patient about medication allergies.

20. *If you are beyond your comfort zone or experience, ask a more knowledgeable peer or the provider to assist you. Remember to work within your scope of practice.*

21. Assess the patient to determine the most appropriate site to administer an injection. Rotate sites if appropriate.

22. Don nonsterile disposable gloves (if mandated by clinic policy and procedures).

23. Prepare the patient for injection (position, provide privacy, drape).

24. Cleanse the injection site that has been chosen. Use an alcohol wipe using a circular motion, beginning at the site of injection and circling outward to a diameter of 2 inches.

25. Allow the skin to dry.

26. Carefully, remove the needle cover.

27. Using the correct angle of injection, insert the needle into the proper anatomical area.

28. Aspirate by holding the syringe steady and gently pulling back on the syringe plunger. Check for blood in the syringe.

   • If blood is evident, remove the needle from the skin

   • Discard syringe appropriately in hazardous waste needle box

   • Notify provider

29. Remove the needle in the direction that it was inserted.

30. Activate the safety mechanism to cover the needle.

31. If indicated, massage the site using the alcohol wipe.

32. Cover the site if indicated with an adhesive bandage.

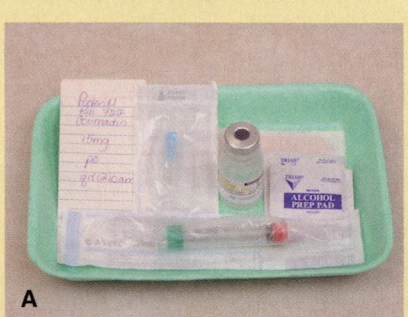
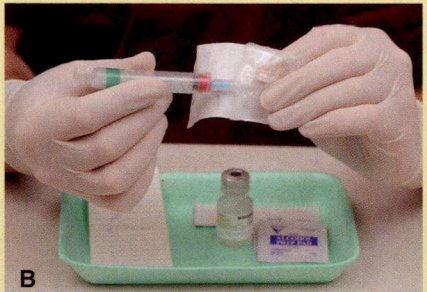
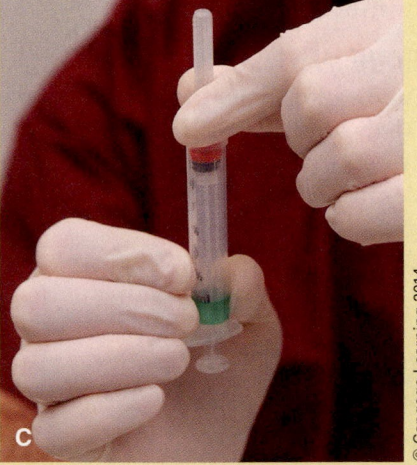

© Cengage Learning 2014

Figure 36-29   Preparing syringe-needle unit for use. (A) Assemble the equipment and supplies needed to draw up medication from a vial. (B) Open the sterile syringe and needle from packages. (C) Secure the needle by twisting it clockwise.

Procedure 36-4 (continued)

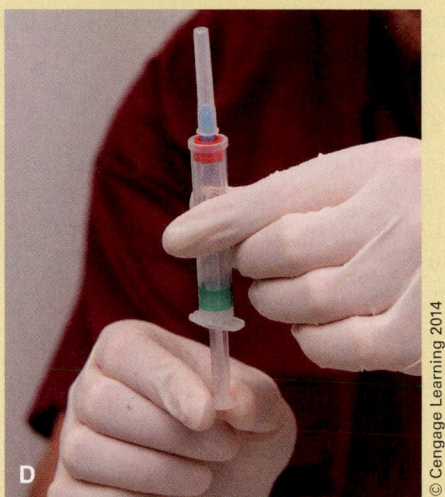

© Cengage Learning 2014

Figure 36-29 (*continued*) (D) Pull the plunger to check for ease of gliding operation.

33. Remove gloves (if utilized) and dispose of according to OSHA guidelines.

34. Wash hands.

35. If it is the first time that the patient has received the medication, she must remain in the exam room for 20 minutes to assure there is no reaction.

36. *Being courteous, patient, and respectful,* assess the patient every 5 minutes for signs of reaction.

37. *Paying attention to detail,* return the medication container to the appropriate place in the medication area.

38. Discard the medication card.

39. Accurately document in the patient's chart or electronic medical record the medication, dose, route, site of injection, and patient reaction. Sign and add date and time.

  Procedure to follow should the medical assistant sustain an accidental needlestick after the injection:

- Thoroughly wash the site where the needle stick occurred.

- Cleanse the skin with antiseptic.

- Report the incident to the supervisor and/or provider.

- Document the incident using an occurrence form. Retain a copy for your records.

- Follow the policy and procedure to access medical attention. Testing for Hep B and C and HIV are indicated.

- Complete an OSHA 300 form.

 ## PROCEDURE 36-5
Administering a Subcutaneous Injection

STANDARD PRECAUTIONS:

PURPOSE:
Correctly administer a subcutaneous injection after checking the provider's order and assembling the necessary equipment and supplies.

EQUIPMENT/SUPPLIES:
Medication order per provider
Medication card
Appropriate syringe size and needle gauge and length
Alcohol wipes
Nonsterile disposable gloves

Sharps container
Adhesive bandage

PROCEDURE STEPS:

1. Perform medical asepsis handwashing procedure. Adhere to OSHA guidelines.

2. Verify the provider's order and prepare a medication card.

3. Follow the "Six Rights" of medication administration.

4. Work in a well-lighted, quiet, clean area.

5. *Paying attention to detail,* gather appropriate equipment and supplies.

continues

Procedure 36-5 (continued)

6. Review the medication card. Select the correct medication from the medication area.

7. Select the correct medication.

8. Compare the medication label with the medication card (first check).

9. If unfamiliar with the medication, consult the PDR or other reputable reference. Familiarize yourself with:

   - Drug name (commercial and generic)
   - Mechanism of action
   - Routes of administration
   - Common side effects

10. Check the expiration date.

11. Carefully calculate the dosage based on medication order and medication available.

12. *Displaying sound judgment,* correctly prepare the parenteral medication.

13. Compare the medication label with the medication card (second check).

14. Withdraw the medication from the vial using proper technique.

15. Discard any refuse generated during the preparation.

16. Carefully, transport the medication to the patient exam room. Bring the medication container (vial) with the prepared medication.

17. *Introduce yourself and identify patient.*

18. *Speaking at the level of the patient's understanding, explain the procedure and expectations to the patient.* State the name of the medication and the purpose of the injection.

19. *Allay the patient's fears regarding the procedure being performed and help him feel safe and comfortable.*

20. Ask the patient about medication allergies.

21. *If you are beyond your comfort zone or experience, ask a more knowledgeable peer or the provider to assist you. Remember to work within your scope of practice.*

22. Assess the patient to determine the most appropriate site to administer an intramuscular injection.

23. Don gloves (if required by practice policy and procedure).

24. Prepare the patient for injection (position, provide privacy, drape).

25. Review the medication card and the medication (third check).

26. Cleanse the injection site that has been chosen. Use an alcohol wipe using a circular motion, beginning at the site of injection and circling outward to a diameter of 2 inches.

27. Allow the skin to dry.

28. Carefully remove the needle cover.

29. Using your non-dominant hand, grasp the skin and pinch upward to form a 1 inch fold.

30. Instruct the patient to take a deep breath and slowly release it.

31. Insert the needle quickly at a 45° angle (Figure 36-30).

32. Aspirate by holding the syringe steady and gently pulling back on the syringe plunger. Check for blood in the syringe.

   - If blood is evident, remove the needle from the skin

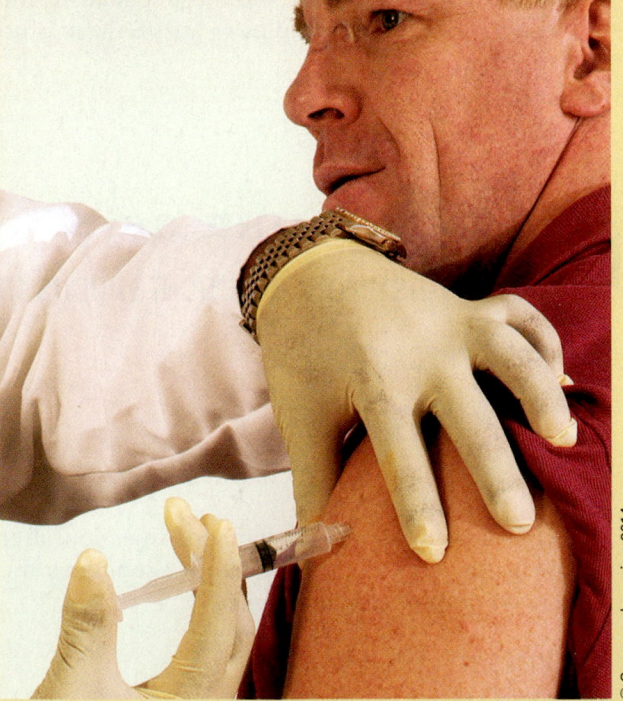

© Cengage Learning 2014

Figure 36-30 Insert needle at 45-degree angle into upper arm.

Procedure 36-5 (continued)

- Discard syringe appropriately in hazardous waste needle box
- Notify provider

33. Slowly and steadily inject the medication.

34. Remove the needle in the direction that it was inserted.

35. Activate the safety mechanism to cover the needle. Immediately dispose of the needle and syringe in the sharps container.

36. If indicated, massage the site using the alcohol wipe.

37. Cover the site, if indicated, with an adhesive bandage.

38. Remove gloves (if utilized) and dispose of according to OSHA guidelines.

39. Wash hands.

40. If it is the first time that the patient has received the medication, he must remain in the exam room for 20 minutes to assure there is no reaction.

41. ***Being courteous, patient, and respectful,*** assess the patient every 5 minutes for signs of reaction.

42. ***Paying attention to detail,*** return the medication container to the appropriate place in the medication area.

43. Accurately document in the patient's chart or electronic medical record the medication, dose, route, site of injection, and patient reaction. Sign and add date and time.

DOCUMENTATION:

12/16/20XX 10:00 AM   Sandostatin 100 mcg subcutaneously (L) deltoid. S. Jones, CMA (AAMA)——————

PROCEDURE 36-6
Administering an Intramuscular Injection

STANDARD PRECAUTIONS:

PURPOSE:

Correctly administer an intramuscular injection after receiving a provider's order and assembling the necessary equipment and supplies.

EQUIPMENT/SUPPLIES:

Medication order per provider
Medication card
Appropriate syringe size and needle gauge and length
Alcohol wipes
Nonsterile disposable gloves
Sharps container
Adhesive bandage

PROCEDURE STEPS:

1. Perform medical asepsis handwashing procedure. Adhere to OSHA guidelines.

2. Verify the provider's order and prepare a medication card.

3. Follow the "Six Rights" of medication administration.

4. Work in a well-lighted, quiet, clean area.

5. ***Paying attention to detail,*** gather appropriate equipment and supplies.

6. Review the medication card. Select the correct medication from the medication area.

7. Compare the medication label with the medication card (first check).

8. If unfamiliar with the medication, consult the PDR or other reputable reference. Familiarize yourself with:

- Drug name (commercial and generic)
- Mechanism of action
- Routes of administration
- Common side effects

9. Check the expiration date.

10. Carefully calculate the dosage based on medication order and medication available.

continues

Procedure 36-6 (continued)

11. ***Displaying sound judgment,*** correctly prepare the parenteral medication.

12. Compare the medication label with the medication card (second check).

13. Withdraw the medication from the vial using proper technique.

14. Discard any refuse generated during the preparation.

15. Carefully transport the medication to the patient exam room. Bring the medication container (vial) with the prepared medication.

16. ***Introduce yourself and identify patient.***

17. ***Speaking at the level of the patient's understanding, explain the procedure and expectations to the patient.*** State the name of the medication and the purpose of the injection.

18. ***Allay the patient's fears regarding the procedure being performed and help him feel safe and comfortable.***

19. Ask the patient about medication allergies.

20. ***If you are beyond your comfort zone or experience, ask a more knowledgeable peer or the provider to assist you. Remember to work within your scope of practice.***

21. Assess the patient to determine the most appropriate site to administer an intramuscular injection.

22. Don gloves (if required by practice policy and procedure).

23. Prepare the patient for injection (position, provide privacy, drape).

24. Review the medication card and the medication (third check).

25. Cleanse the injection site that has been chosen. Use an alcohol wipe using a circular motion, beginning at the site of injection and circling outward to a diameter of 2 inches.

26. Allow the skin to dry.

27. Carefully remove the needle cover.

28. Using your non-dominant hand, stretch the skin taut in the area that has been cleansed and is dry.

29. Instruct the patient to take a deep breath and slowly release it.

30. Using a dart-like motion, insert the needle at a 90° angle (Figure 36-31).

31. Release the skin.

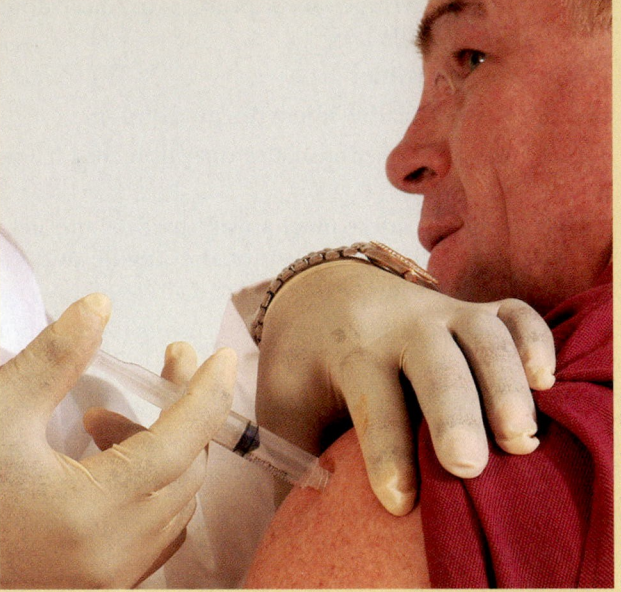

Figure 36-31 Using deltoid muscle, insert needle to the hub at a 90-degree angle.

32. Aspirate by holding the syringe steady and gently pulling back on the syringe plunger. Check for blood in the syringe.
    - If blood is evident, remove the needle from the skin
    - Discard syringe appropriately in hazardous waste needle box
    - Notify provider

33. Slowly and steadily inject the medication.

34. Remove the needle in the direction that it was inserted.

35. Activate the safety mechanism to cover the needle. Immediately dispose of the needle and syringe in the sharps container.

36. If indicated, massage the site using the alcohol wipe.

37. Cover the site if indicated with an adhesive bandage.

38. Remove gloves (if utilized) and dispose of according to OSHA guidelines.

39. Wash hands.

40. If it is the first time that the patient has received the medication, he must remain in the exam room for 20 minutes to assure there is no reaction.

Procedure 36-6 (continued)

41. ***Being courteous, patient, and respectful,*** assess the patient every 5 minutes for signs of reaction.

42. ***Paying attention to detail,*** return the medication container to the appropriate place in the medication area.

43. Accurately document in the patient's chart or electronic medical record the medication, dose, route, site of injection and patient reaction. Sign and add date and time.

DOCUMENTATION:

12/16/20XX 10:00 AM   Demerol 75 mg IM (L) deltoid.
S. Jones, CMA (AAMA)

PROCEDURE 36-7

Administering an Intradermal Injection of Purified Protein Derivative (PPD)

STANDARD PRECAUTIONS:

PURPOSE:
Correctly administer an intradermal injection of PPD after receiving a provider's order and assembling the necessary equipment and supplies.

EQUIPMENT/SUPPLIES:
Medication order per provider
Medication card
Appropriate syringe and needle gauge and length
Alcohol wipes
Nonsterile disposable gloves
Sharps container
Adhesive bandage

PROCEDURE STEPS:
1. Perform medical asepsis handwashing procedure. Adhere to OSHA guidelines.

2. Verify the provider's order and prepare a medication card.

3. Follow the "Six Rights" of medication administration.

4. Work in a well-lighted, quiet, clean area.

5. ***Paying attention to detail,*** gather appropriate equipment and supplies.

6. Review the medication card. Select the correct medication from the medication area.

7. Compare the medication label with the medication card (first check).

8. If unfamiliar with the medication, consult the PDR or other reputable reference. Familiarize yourself with:
   • Drug name (commercial and generic)
   • Mechanism of action
   • Routes of administration
   • Common side effects

9. Check the expiration date.

10. Carefully calculate the dosage based on the medication order and available medication.

11. ***Displaying sound judgment,*** correctly prepare the parenteral medication.

12. Compare the medication label with the medication card (second check).

13. Withdraw the medication from the vial using proper technique.

14. Discard any refuse generated during the preparation.

15. Carefully transport the medication to the patient exam room. Bring the medication (vial/container) with the prepared medication.

16. ***Introduce yourself and identify the patient.***

17. ***Speaking at the level of the patient's understanding, explain the procedure and expectations to the patient.***

continues

Procedure 36-7 (continued)

18. *Allay the patient's fears regarding the procedure being performed and help her feel safe and comfortable.*

19. Ask the patient about medication allergies.

20. *If you are beyond your comfort zone or experience, ask a more knowledgeable peer or the provider to assist you. Remember to work within your scope of practice.*

21. Assess the patient to determine the most appropriate site to administer an intradermal injection (Figure 36-17B).

22. Don gloves (if required by practice policy and procedure).

23. Prepare the patient for injection (position for injection, provide privacy, drape).

24. Review the medication card and the medication (third check).

25. Cleanse the injection site that has been chosen. Use an alcohol wipe in a circular motion, starting at the injection site and circling outward to a diameter of 2 inches (Figure 36-32A).

26. Allow the skin to dry.

27. Carefully remove the needle cover.

28. Using your nondominant hand, pull the skin taut.

29. Instruct the patient to take a deep breath and slowly release it.

30. Carefully, insert the needle at a 10–15° angle, bevel upward, to a depth of $\frac{1}{8}$ inch (Figure 36-32B).

31. Do not aspirate.

32. Release skin.

33. Steadily inject PPD to form a wheal or bleb (Figure 36-32C).

34. Carefully remove the needle in the direction that it was inserted. RATIONALE: Minimizes leakage.

35. Activate the safety mechanism to cover the needle.

36. Immediately dispose of the needle and syringe in the sharps container.

37. Blot site of injection. Do not massage.

38. Instruct the patient not to rub wheal.

39. Remove gloves (if utilized) and discard in appropriate waste container.

40. Wash hands.

41. If this is the first time that the patient has received a PPD injection, the patient must be observed for 20 minutes to assure no reaction.

42. *Being courteous, patient, and respectful,* assess the patient every 5 minutes for signs of reaction.

43. *Paying attention to detail,* return the medication vial to the appropriate area for storage.

44. Discard the medication card.

45. Accurately document in the patient's chart or electronic medical record indicating the medication, dose, route, site of injection, and any patient reaction. Sign and date.

DOCUMENTATION:

10/14/20XX 10:00 AM   0.1 mL PPD intradermally (L) forearm. Pt given appointment to return 10/16/20XX to have PPT read. S. Jones, CMA (AAMA)——————————

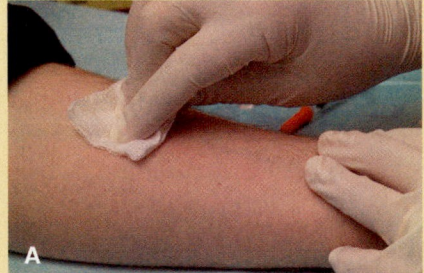
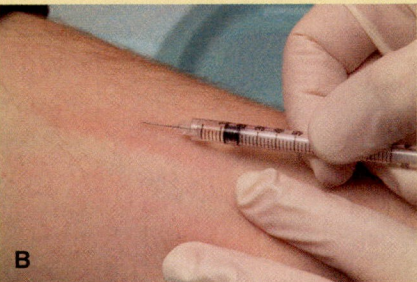
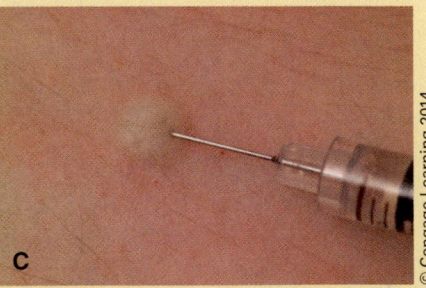

© Cengage Learning 2014

Figure 36-32   (A) Cleanse the injection site with alcohol and allow area to air-dry. (B) Insert the needle at a 10- to 15-degree angle, bevel upward at $\frac{1}{8}$ inch. (C) Steadily inject the medicine, allowing a wheal to form.

PROCEDURE 36-8

Reconstituting a Powder Medication for Administration

STANDARD PRECAUTIONS:

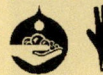

PURPOSE:

Drugs for injection may be supplied in a powdered (dry) form and must be reconstituted to a liquid for injection. A diluent (usually sterile water) is added to the powder, mixed well, and the appropriate dose is drawn up to be administered.

EQUIPMENT/SUPPLIES:

Medication order per provider
Powdered medication
Diluent
Medication card
Appropriate syringe and needle gauge and length
Alcohol wipes
Nonsterile disposable gloves
Sharps container

PROCEDURE STEPS:

1. Perform medical asepsis handwashing procedure. Adhere to OSHA guidelines.
2. Verify the provider's order and prepare a medication cart.
3. Follow the "Six Rights" of medication administration.
4. Work in a well-lighted, quiet, clean area.
5. ***Paying attention to detail,*** gather appropriate equipment and supplies.

   If unfamiliar with the medication, consult the PDR or other reputable reference. Familiarize yourself with:
   - Drug name (commercial and generic)
   - Mechanism of action
   - Routes of administration
   - Common side effects
6. Check the expiration date.
7. Prepare needle-syringe unit in preparation for reconstituting powdered medication.
8. Remove tops from diluents and powdered medication containers and wipe with alcohol swabs (Figure 36-33A).
9. Fill the syringe with air equal to the amount of diluent that is to be added to the medication.
10. Carefully insert the needle through the rubber stopper on the vial of diluent (Figure 36-33B).
11. Withdraw the appropriate amount of diluents to be added to the powdered medication (Figure 36-33C).
12. Inject the diluents slowly and carefully into the powdered medication (Figure 36-33D).

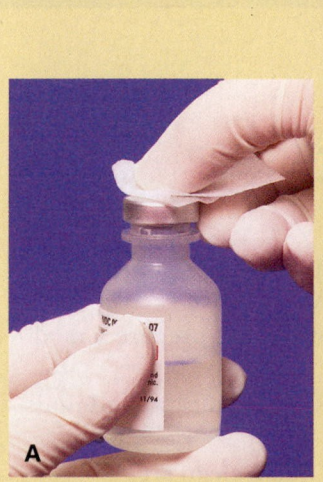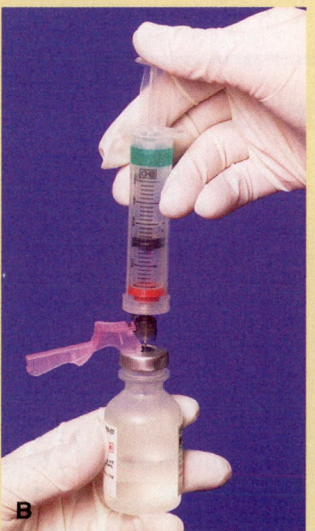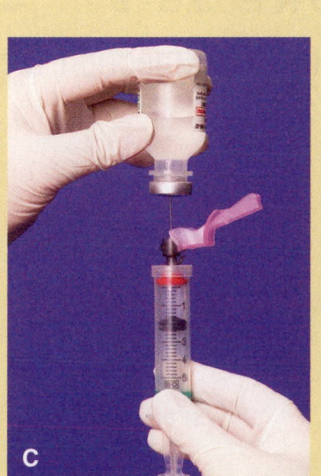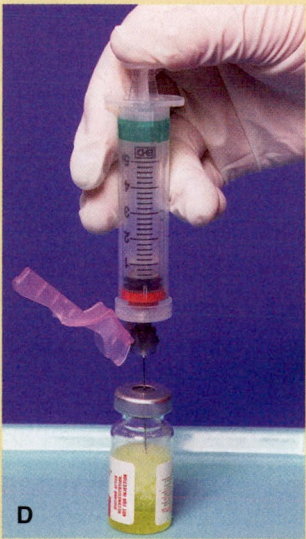

Figure 36-33   (A) Remove top from diluent and powdered medication. Wipe top of each with an alcohol wipe. (B) Inject air in an equal amount to diluent being removed from the vial. (C) Prepare to remove the needle from the vial after withdrawing diluent. (D) Inject diluent into vial containing powdered medication.

continues

Procedure 36-8 (continued)

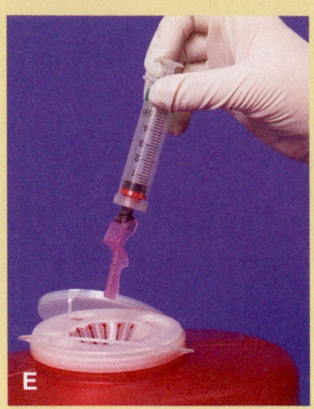
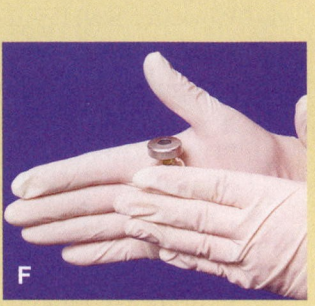
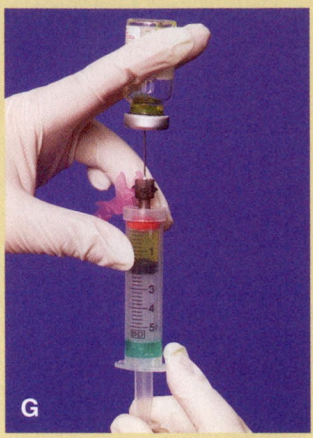
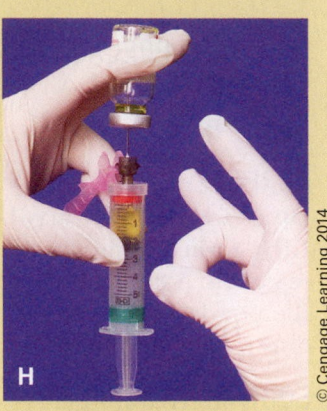

© Cengage Learning 2014

Figure 36-33 (*continued*) (E) Discard safety needle—syringe unit. (F) Roll vial of solution medication between palms of hands to mix well. Label vial with date, amount of diluent added, strength of dilution, time mixed, and your initials. (G) Use a second sterile needle—syringe unit to draw the prescribed dose of medication ordered by the provider. (H) Flick away any air bubbles that cling to the side of the syringe. Withdraw more medication if needed. Labeled, reconstituted medication will be taken to the room with the syringe and placed on the shelf or in the refrigerator according to the manufacturer's instructions after the injection is given.

13. Remove the needle and syringe appropriately in a biohazard sharps container (Figure 36-33E).

14. ***DO NOT SHAKE THE VIAL.*** Roll the vial between the palms of the hands to completely mix together the powder and the diluents (Figure 36-33F).

15. If the medication is contained in a multidose vial, label the vial with the name of the medication and the strength after dilution, the date and time, your initials, and the expiration date.

16. With a second sterile needle and syringe, withdraw the desired amount of medication (Figure 36-33G).

17. Flick away any air bubbles that cling to side of syringe (Figure 36-33H).

18. The medicine tray with reconstituted medication and medication card are ready for transport to patient.

19. Proceed as in Steps 12 to 43 of Procedure 36-6, Administering an Intramuscular Injection.

PROCEDURE 36-9
Z-Track Intramuscular Injection Technique

STANDARD PRECAUTIONS:

PURPOSE:
Correctly administer a Z-track intramuscular injection after receiving a provider's order and assembling the necessary equipment and supplies.

EQUIPMENT/SUPPLIES:
Medication order per provider
Medication card
Appropriately sized syringe and needle with correct gauge and length
Alcohol wipes
Disposable nonsterile gloves
Adhesive bandage

PROCEDURE STEPS:
1. Perform medical asepsis handwashing procedure. Adhere to OSHA guidelines.

2. Verify the provider's order and prepare a medication card.

3. Follow the "Six Rights" of medication administration.

4. Work in a well-lighted, quiet, clean area.

5. ***Paying attention to detail,*** gather appropriate equipment and supplies.

6. Select the correct medication from the medication storage area.

7. Check the expiration date.

Procedure 36-9 (continued)

8. Compare label information to provider's order (first check).

9. If unfamiliar with the medication, consult the PDR or other reputable reference. Familiarize yourself with:
   - Drug name (commercial and generic)
   - Mechanism of action
   - Routes of administration
   - Common side effects

10. Calculate the correct dose based on provider's order and medication on hand.

11. *Displaying sound judgment,* correctly prepare the parenteral medication.

12. Compare the medication label with the medication card (second check).

13. Withdraw the medication from the vial using proper technique.

14. Change the needle after aspirating the medication from the vial to avoid irritation of the tissues.

15. Discard any refuse generated during the preparation.

16. Carefully transport the medication to the patient exam room. Bring the medication container (vial) with the prepared medication.

17. *Introduce yourself and identify patient.*

18. *Speaking at the level of the patient's understanding, explain the procedure and expectations to the patient.* State the name of the medication and the purpose of the injection.

19. *Allay the patient's fears regarding the procedure being performed and help him feel safe and comfortable.*

20. Ask the patient about medication allergies.

21. *If you are beyond your comfort zone or experience, ask a more knowledgeable peer or the provider to assist you. Remember to work within your scope of practice.*

22. Assess the patient to determine the most appropriate site to administer an intramuscular injection.

23. Don gloves (if required by practice policy and procedure).

24. Prepare the patient for injection (position, provide privacy, drape).

25. Review the medication card and the medication (third check).

26. Cleanse the injection site that has been chosen. Use an alcohol wipe using a circular motion, beginning at the site of injection and circling outward to a diameter of 3–4 inches.

27. Allow the skin to dry.

28. Carefully remove the needle cover.

29. Using your nondominant hand, and placing fingers outside of the prepped area, gently pull the skin laterally about 1½ inches away from the chosen injection site. RATIONALE: Prevents medication from leaking.

30. Instruct the patient to take a deep breath and slowly release it.

31. Keeping the skin pulled laterally and using a dart-like motion, insert the needle at a 90° angle (Figure 36-34).

32. Aspirate by holding the syringe steady and gently pulling back on the syringe plunger. Check for blood in the syringe.
   - If blood is evident, remove the needle from the skin
   - Discard syringe appropriately in hazardous waste needle box
   - Notify provider

33. Slowly and steadily inject the medication.

34. Remove the needle in the direction that it was inserted.

35. Immediately release the traction of the Z position to seal off the needle track.

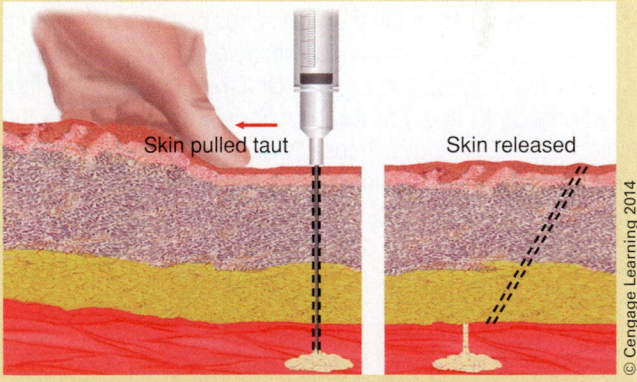

Skin pulled taut   Skin released

© Cengage Learning 2014

Figure 36-34   With patient supine, grasp and pull the muscle laterally before injecting medication. Inject medication. Keep skin pulled taut for 10 seconds. Quickly withdraw the needle and release the skin to seal the site.

continues

Procedure 36-9 (continued)

36. Activate the safety mechanism to cover the needle. Immediately dispose of the needle and syringe in the sharps container.

37. Cover the site. DO NOT MASSAGE.

38. Cover the site if indicated with an adhesive bandage.

39. Remove gloves (if utilized) and dispose of according to OSHA guidelines.

40. Wash hands.

41. ***Being courteous, patient, and respectful,*** assess the patient every 5 minutes for signs of reaction.

42. ***Paying attention to detail,*** return the medication container to the appropriate place in the medication area.

43. Accurately document in the patient's chart or electronic medical record the medication, dose, route, site of injection, and patient reaction. Sign and add date and time.

DOCUMENTATION:

12/01/20XX 2:00 PM　Interferon 1,000,000 International units IM (R) Dorsogluteal muscle using Z-track technique. J. Guerrero, CMA (AAMA)

CASE STUDY 36-1

Refer to the scenario at the beginning of the chapter.

CASE STUDY REVIEW

1. Explain the consequences of preparing and administering a medication without a medicine card.

2. Is it possible under normal circumstances to commit to memory the medication, dose, route, patient, and documentation?

CASE STUDY 36-2

Abigail Johnson, a patient of Dr. Lewis, has been unable to keep her type 2 non–insulin dependent diabetes mellitus under control with oral hypoglycemics, and Dr. Lewis has decided that Abigail needs to begin to take insulin injections. Today in the clinic, her fasting blood glucose level is 190 mg/mL. Dr. Lewis prescribes Humulin® insulin 10 units subcutaneously stat.

CASE STUDY REVIEW

1. What size insulin syringe should be used?

2. What does the medication label state are the number of units per milliliter? Show how to calculate the correct dosage.

3. Discuss the route of administration and the specifics regarding insulin administration that require it to be given slightly differently from other subcutaneous injections.

4. Describe several topics of discussion in which you would engage Abigail to help her learn how to better control her disease.

CASE STUDY 36-3

Alice Chambers weighs 28 pounds. Her pediatrician orders erythromycin 50 mg/kg/day po TID.

CASE STUDY REVIEW

1. Calculate Alice's weight in kg.
2. Calculate the dose of erythromycin Alice needs.

3. How much will Alice receive at each dosing?
4. If the erythromycin is available as erythromycin 400 mg per 5 mL, calculate the dose to be given TID.

SUMMARY

Administering medications is one of the most important and essential responsibilities that the medical assistant performs. This chapter reviewed of some of the fundamental elements of pharmacology, dosage calculations, and medication administration.

 Each state has enacted laws governing the practice of medicine, nursing, and pharmacy. These laws vary from state to state; therefore, it is essential that medical assistants become familiar with the laws of the state in which they are employed before administering any medication.

Under the law, those administering medications are expected to be knowledgeable about the drugs that they administer and the effects the drug may or will have on the patient. They are responsible for their own actions.

STUDY FOR SUCCESS

To reinforce your knowledge and skills of information presented in this chapter:

- Review the *Key Terms*
- Role-play with other students to apply attributes of professionalism pertinent to this chapter.
- Consider the *Case Studies* and discuss your conclusions
- Answer the questions in the *Certification Review*
- Apply your knowledge by completing the *Activities* in the *Study Guide* and the *Games and Quizzes* in the StudyWARE (StudyWARE) software on the *Premium Website*
- Perform the *Procedures* using the *Competency Assessment Checklists* in the *Competency Manual*
- Practice your problem-solving skills with the *Critical Thinking Challenge 3.0* on the *Premium Website*

Additional resources for this chapter include:

- Module 25 of the *Medical Assisting Learning Lab*
- *CourseMate for Delmar's Comprehensive Medical Assisting*
- *WebTutor for Delmar's Comprehensive Medical Assisting*

CERTIFICATION REVIEW

1. A written legal document that gives directions for compounding, dispensing, and administering medication to a patient is a:
   a. medication card
   b. prescription
   c. medication order
   d. subscription

2. An abbreviation symbol that means "nothing by mouth" is:
   a. non rep
   b. NPO
   c. IM
   d. mm

3. Insulin-dependent diabetes mellitus is:
   a. Type 1
   b. Type 2
   c. Type 3
   d. Type 4

4. Body surface area is used:
   a. when calculating children's dosages
   b. when calculating adult dosages
   c. when determining an injection site
   d. when selecting an appropriately sized needle

5. An injection given just below the surface of the skin at a 15-degree angle is called a(n):
   a. intramuscular injection
   b. intradermal injection
   c. subcutaneous injection
   d. parenteral injection

6. Methods for calculating dosage include:
   a. formula
   b. ratio and proportion
   c. body surface area
   d. a and b

7. Pediatric dosages must be carefully calculated based on:
   a. weight in kg
   b. body surface area
   c. divided dosing
   d. all of the above

8. Which of the following is a part of the "Six Rights" of proper medication administration?
   a. Right patient
   b. Right medication
   c. Right time
   d. All of the above

9. When a medication error occurs, the first step in standard procedure is to:
   a. tell the patient that an error has occurred.
   b. inform the provider that an error has occurred.
   c. recognize that an error has occurred.
   d. assess the patient's condition

10. Site selection for administering medications is based on:
    a. anatomic structures
    b. provider preference
    c. treating each patient in exactly the same manner
    d. knowledge of the Z-track method

REFERENCES/BIBLIOGRAPHY

Balasa, D. A. (2008). New roles for the certified medical assistant to enhance quality and effectiveness of care. *Journal of Medical Practice Management.* Retrieved May 10, 2012, from www.aama-ntl.org/resources/library/JMPM_New_Roles_CMAs.pdf

Centers for Disease Control and Prevention, Division of Health Care Quality Promotion. (2004, February). *Workbook for designing, implementing, and evaluating a sharps injury prevention program.* Retrieved August 9, 2004, from http://cdc.gov/sharpsafety/wk_info.html

Centers for Disease Control and Prevention. (2006). *Health care workers and regulations regarding safety needles.* Retrieved October 15, 2008, from http://www.cdc.gov/medicationsafety/

Centers for Medicare and Medicaid Services. (2010). *Eligible professionals meaningful use core measures.* Retrieved July 15, 2012, from www.cms.gov/Regulations-and-Guidance/Legislation/EHRIncentivePrograms/downloads/4_e-prescribing.pdf

Josephson, D. (2004). *Intravenous infusion therapy for nurses: Principles and practice.* (2nd ed.). Clifton Park, NY: Delmar Cengage Learning.

Keir, L., Wise, B., Krebs, C., & Kelley-Arney, C. (2008). *Medical assisting administrative and clinical competencies* (6th ed.). Clifton Park, NY: Delmar Cengage Learning.

Open Clinical Knowledge Management for Medical Care. (2006). *CPOE: Computer physician order entry systems.* Retrieved May 20, 2012, from www.openclinical.org/cpoe.html

Prescription for drug safety. (2003, March). *Consumer Reports on Health, 15*(3), 1, 4–6.

Rice, J., (2006). *Principles of pharmacology for medical assisting* (4th ed.). Clifton Park, NY: Delmar Cengage Learning.

Spratto, G., & Woods, A. (2009). *Delmar nurse's drug handbook, 2009 edition.* Clifton Park, NY: Delmar Cengage Learning.

Taber's cyclopedic medical dictionary (22nd ed.). (2005). Philadelphia: F. A. Davis.

To the point. (2004, August 2). *Advance for nurses serving RN's in New England, 4*(17), 30–31.

OUTLINE

Anatomy of the Heart

Electrical Conduction System of the Heart

The Cardiac Cycle and the ECG Cycle

Calculation of Heart Rate on ECG Graph Paper

Types of Electrocardiographs

Single-Channel Electrocardiograph

Multichannel Electrocardiograph

Automatic Electrocardiograph Machines

Electrocardiograph Telephone Transmissions

Facsimile Electrocardiograph

Interpretive Electrocardiograph

ECG Equipment

Electrocardiograph Paper

Electrolyte

Sensors or Electrodes

Lead Wires

Electrocardiograph Machine

Care of Equipment

Lead Coding

The Electrocardiograph and Sensor Placement

Standard Limb or Bipolar Leads

Augmented Leads

Chest Leads or Precordial Leads

Standardization and Adjustment of the Electrocardiograph

Standard Resting Electrocardiography

Mounting the ECG Tracing

Interference or Artifacts

Somatic Tremor Artifacts

AC Interference

Wandering Baseline Artifacts

Interrupted Baseline Artifacts

Patients with Unique Problems

Myocardial Infarctions (Heart Attacks)

Cardiac Arrhythmias

Atrial Arrhythmias

Ventricular Arrhythmias

Defibrillation

Other Cardiac Diagnostic Tests

Holter Monitor (Portable Ambulatory Electrocardiograph)

Loop ECG

Treadmill Stress Test or Exercise Tolerance ECG

Thallium Stress Test

Echocardiography/ Ultrasonography

Coronary MRI and CT Imaging

Cardiac Procedures

Procedures for Heart Disease

Procedures for Arrhythmias

LEARNING OUTCOMES

1. Define, spell, and pronounce the key terms as presented in the glossary.

2. Follow the circulation of blood through the heart starting at the vena cavae.

3. Describe the electrical conduction system of the heart.

4. State three reasons why patients may need an electrocardiogram (ECG).

5. Identify the various positive and negative deflections and describe what each represents in the cardiac cycle.

6. Explain the purpose of standardization of the ECG.

7. Identify the 12 leads of an ECG and describe what area of the heart each lead represents.

8. State the function of ECG graph paper, electrodes (sensors), and electrolyte.

9. Describe various types of ECGs and their capabilities.

10. Explain each type of artifact and how each can be eliminated.

11. Name and describe the purposes of the various cardiac diagnostic tests and procedures as outlined in this chapter.

12. Identify the placement of Holter monitor electrodes.

(continues on page 1142)

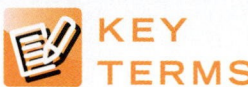

KEY TERMS

amplified
amplitude
angina pectoris
angiogram
arrhythmia
artifact
augment
baseline
bipolar
bradycardia, sinus
calibration
cardiac catheterization
cardiac cycle
cardioversion
countershock
defibrillation
defibrillator
deoxygenated
depolarization
diastole
electrocardiogram
electrocardiograph
electrocardiography
electrodes
electrolyte
galvanometer
Holter monitor
implantable
   cardioverter-
   defibrillator (ICD)
ischemia
isoelectric
lead wires
mounting
myocardial infarction
noninvasive
normal sinus rhythm
oscilloscope
percutaneous
   transluminal coronary
   angioplasty (PTCA)
precordial
repolarization
rhythm strip
sensor

sonographer
stylus
syncope
systole

tachycardia, sinus
test cable
thallium stress testing
tracing

transducer
ultrasonography
unipolar

ATTRIBUTES OF PROFESSIONALISM

Communication

- Did you introduce yourself? Did you identify the patient through name and birth date or other identifying feature?
- Did you speak at the patient's level of understanding?
- Did you allay patients' fears regarding the procedure being performed and help them feel safe and comfortable?
- Did you demonstrate empathy in communicating with patients, family, and staff?
- Did you accurately and concisely update the provider on any aspect of the patient's care?

Presentation

- Did you attend to any special needs of the patient? Did you ask first if assistance was needed, rather than taking charge?
- Were you courteous, patient, and respectful to the patient?
- Did you display a calm, professional, and caring manner?

Competency

- Did you pay attention to detail?
- Were you knowledgeable and accountable?
- Did you apply critical thinking skills in performing patient assessment and care?

Initiative

- Were you flexible and dependable?
- Did you direct the patient to other resources when necessary or helpful, with the approval of the provider?

Integrity

- Did you protect personal boundaries?
- Did you protect and maintain confidentiality?

LEARNING OUTCOMES   (*continued*)

13. Describe the reason for a patient activity diary during ambulatory electrocardiography.

14. Identify six arrhythmias and explain the cause of each.

15. Explain how to calculate heart rates from an ECG tracing.

16. Identify a common coding system used to code each lead on an ECG tracing.

17. Describe the procedure for mounting an ECG tracing.

18. Analyze the professionalism questions and apply them to this chapter's content.

SCENARIO

Wanda Slawson, CMA (AAMA), clinical medical assistant at Inner City Health Care, recently had her own physical examination that included her first electrocardiogram (ECG). This is now Wanda's baseline ECG, which provides a basis for future ECG readings to be compared. Because Wanda currently has no heart problems, future tests will indicate differences from her normal baseline ECG. It was different for Wanda to be the patient instead of the person performing the ECG. Having the test performed on her, Wanda can now relate to feelings many of her patients must have felt when having an ECG. These included feelings of fear that the test may be abnormal; a cold feeling because even though the room temperature was normal, she was partially uncovered and the pads were cold when applied; and anxiousness because she found it difficult to stay completely still through the entire tracing. Wanda could empathize more with her patients after she had the test than she did before her test. Wanda now makes a more concerted effort to allay patient fears and make patients comfortable during ECGs.

INTRODUCTION

Many providers include an **electrocardiogram** *(ECG or EKG) as part of a complete physical examination, especially for patients who are 40 years or older, for patients with a family history of cardiac disease, or for patients who have experienced chest pain. It is a noninvasive, safe, and painless procedure that can provide valuable information about the health of the patient's heart or suspected cardiac symptoms. A graphic representation of the heart's electrical activity, an ECG measures the amount of the electrical activity produced by the heart and the time necessary for the electrical impulses to travel through the heart during each heartbeat.*

Some reasons for **electrocardiography** *are to (1) detect myocardial ischemia, (2) estimate damage to the myocardium caused by a myocardial infarction, (3) detect and evaluate cardiac arrhythmia, (4) assess effects of cardiac medication on the heart, and (5) determine if electrolyte imbalance is present. An ECG cannot always detect impending heart disease or cardiovascular disease. The ECG is used in conjunction with other laboratory and diagnostic tests to assess total cardiac health. An ECG alone cannot diagnose disease. In a medical clinic or ambulatory care setting, it is the medical assistant who records the ECG; therefore, special knowledge and skills are necessary and include these aspects of the correct electrocardiography procedures: patient preparation; operation of the electrocardiograph; elimination of artifacts, mounting, and labeling the ECG; and maintenance and care of the instrument.*

ANATOMY OF THE HEART

The heart has four chambers: two upper chambers known as atria, and two lower chambers known as ventricles. **Deoxygenated** blood enters the right atrium from the superior and inferior vena cavae and passes through the tricuspid valve into the right ventricle. In a healthy heart, the blood between right and left sides cannot mix together. It then travels to

into the left atrium, through the mitral valve, into the left ventricle. The oxygenated blood then passes through the aortic valve into the aorta and from the aorta to all cells, tissues, and organs of the body (Figure 37-1). The cycle begins with each heartbeat.

On its external surface, the heart is surrounded by coronary arteries that supply the myocardium with its blood supply, from which oxygen and nutrients are obtained (see the section on the circulatory system in Chapter 30).

ELECTRICAL CONDUCTION SYSTEM OF THE HEART

There are basically two kinds of cardiac cells: electrical cardiac cells and myocardial cells. The electrical cells, which are located in distinct pathways around and through the heart, are sensitive to electrical impulses. Their pathways are referred to as the conduction system of the heart and have specific names.

The body's natural pacemaker, the sinoatrial (SA) node, is located in the upper part of the right atrium. The SA node is a bundle of specialized cardiac muscle cells that are self-excitatory or pacemaker cells. A healthy SA node "fires" at a rate of 60 to 70 times a minute in a resting heart. It sends out an electrical impulse that begins and regulates the heartbeat. When the electrical impulses are sent

the lungs via the pulmonary arteries. The deoxygenated blood gives off the carbon dioxide and picks up oxygen in the capillary bed of the lungs. Oxygenated blood is pumped through the pulmonary vein

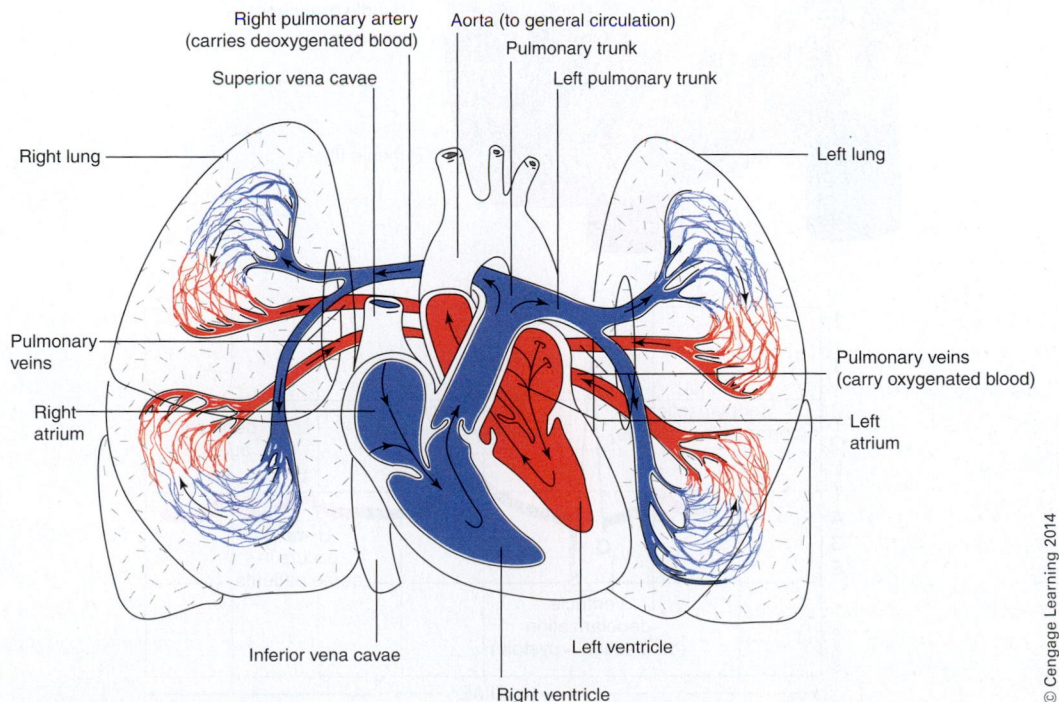

Figure 37-1   Oxygenated blood passing through the heart and then to the rest of the body.

along the pathways or conduction system of the heart (via the electrical cells), the myocardial cells contract, causing the heart muscle to pump the blood from chamber to chamber and through the lungs. The contraction of the cardiac cells is called **depolarization** (from the electrical "discharge"). The first chambers affected (contracted) by the electrical discharge from the SA node are the atria. From the atria, the electrical impulses travel along the conduction system toward the ventricles, to the atrioventricular (AV) node, located at the base of the right atrium. The AV node responds to signals from the SA node. However, if there is suppression of the SA node, the AV node can fire intrinsically at a rate of 40 to 60 times per minute. From here, the electrical impulses are transmitted to the bundle of His. The bundle of His divides into right and left bundle branches that continue the electrical impulses on to the Purkinje fibers. These fibers disperse the electrical impulses to the right and left

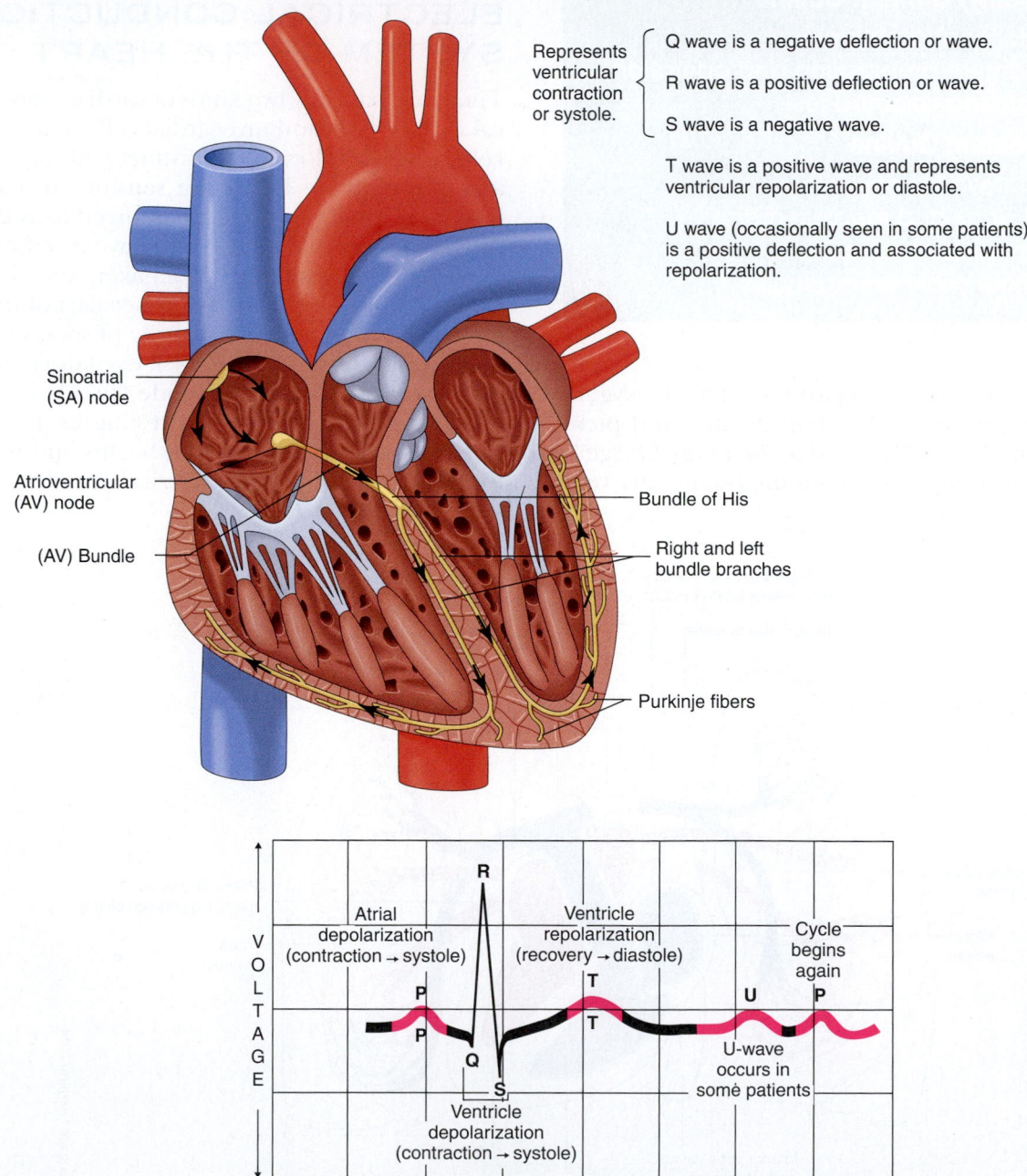

Represents ventricular contraction or systole.

Q wave is a negative deflection or wave.

R wave is a positive deflection or wave.

S wave is a negative wave.

T wave is a positive wave and represents ventricular repolarization or diastole.

U wave (occasionally seen in some patients) is a positive deflection and associated with repolarization.

Sinoatrial (SA) node

Atrioventricular (AV) node

(AV) Bundle

Bundle of His

Right and left bundle branches

Purkinje fibers

Atrial depolarization (contraction → systole)

Ventricle repolarization (recovery → diastole)

Cycle begins again

Ventricle depolarization (contraction → systole)

U-wave occurs in some patients

VOLTAGE

TIME

© Cengage Learning 2014

Figure 37-2 The heartbeat is controlled by electrical impulses that comprise the continuous cardiac cycle.

ventricles, causing them to contract. If there is an interruption in the electrical signals from the SA or the AV node, the Purkinje fibers can fire at a very slow and less effective rate of 15 to 40 times per minute. The heart recovers electrically **(repolarization)**, then relaxes briefly (polarization), and then a new impulse is begun by the SA node and the cycle begins again (Figure 37-2). This cycle is known as the **cardiac cycle** and it represents one heartbeat. The electrocardiograph records the electrical activity that causes the contraction **(systole)** and the relaxation **(diastole)** of the atria and ventricles. The ECG cycle is the recording or the graphic representation of the cardiac cycle. These electrical impulses can be recorded on special ECG paper or displayed on an **oscilloscope**.

THE CARDIAC CYCLE AND THE ECG CYCLE

The **baseline**, or **isoelectric**, line is the flat line that separates the various waves. It is present when there is no current flowing in the heart. The waves are either deflecting upward, known as positive deflection, or deflecting downward, known as negative deflection from the baseline.

The P, QRS, and T waves, recorded during the ECG, represent the depolarization (contraction) and repolarization (recovery) of the myocardial cells. They are recorded on specialized graph paper. This is accomplished by a heated **stylus** that moves on the heat-sensitive graph paper, recording the electrical impulses moving through the heart tissue. The P wave is initiated when the SA node fires and represents atrial depolarization. It is recorded as a positive deflection. The QRS complex is initiated when the AV node fires and represents ventricular depolarization. It is measured from the beginning of the first wave of the QRS complex to the end of the last wave of the QRS complex (see Figure 37-2). The T wave represents ventricular repolarization and is a positive deflection. The recovery of the atria is so slight that it is lost behind the QRS complex.

Each complete cardiac cycle takes about 0.8 second, with each wave taking an appropriate

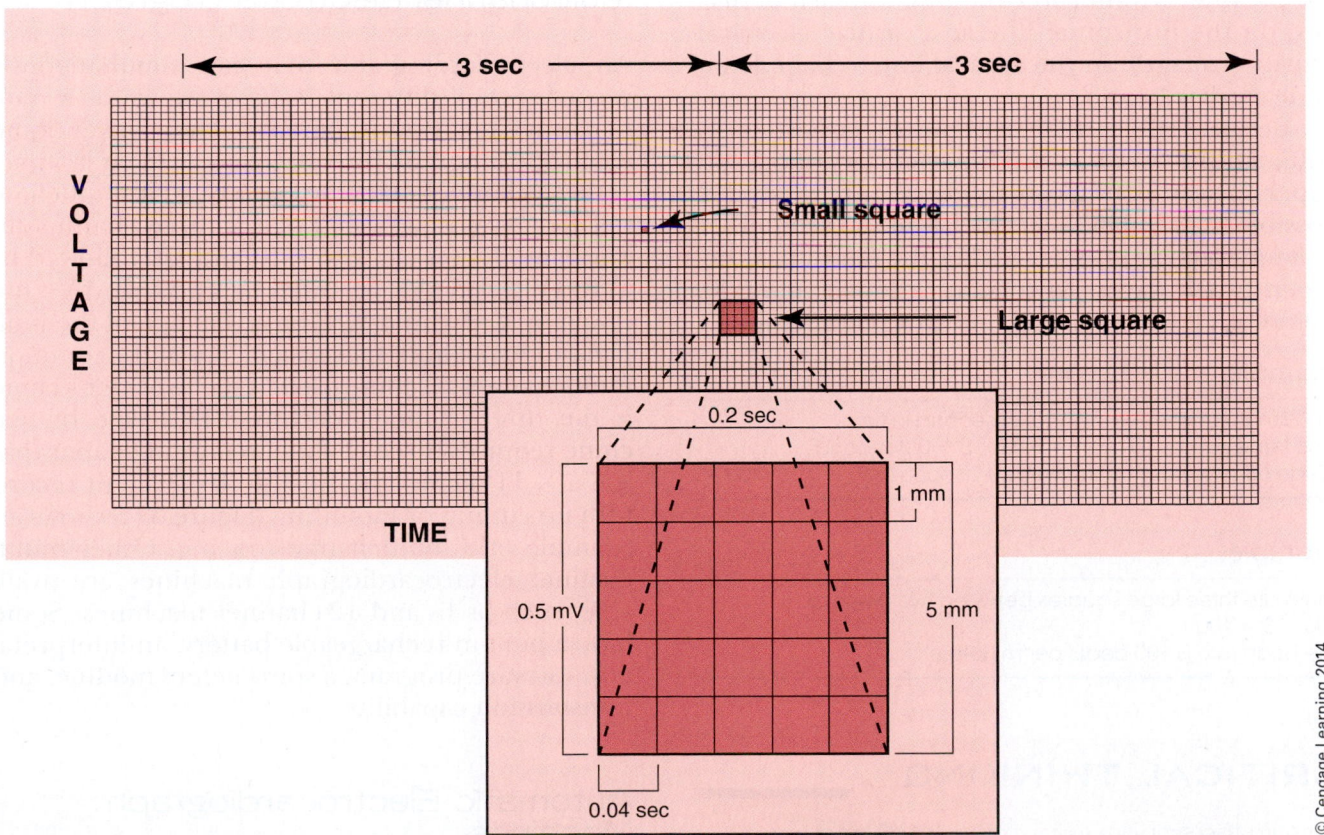

© Cengage Learning 2014

Figure 37-3 Electrocardiogram graph paper measurements allow medical professionals to determine the time and voltage of heartbeats. (A) The small square is 1 mm wide and 1 mm high. One small square = 0.04 second. (B) The large square consists of 25 small squares and measures 5 mm wide and 5 mm high. One large square = 0.04 second × 5, or 0.2 second.

amount of time if the heart is healthy. By observing and measuring the size, shape, and location of each wave on an ECG recording, the provider can analyze and interpret the conduction of electricity through the cardiac cells, the heart's rhythm and rate, and the health of the heart in general.

Calculation of Heart Rate on ECG Graph Paper

ECG graph paper is divided into 1-mm squares (small squares) and 5-mm squares (large squares). Each large square consists of 25 small squares and is 5 mm high and 5 mm wide. On the horizontal line, one small square represents 0.04 second. On the vertical line, one small square represents 1 mm of voltage. Because a large square is five small squares wide and five deep, each small square represents 0.2 second horizontal and 5 mm vertical. *Note:* Every fifth line, both horizontally and vertically, is darker than the other lines, making squares that are 5 × 5 mm (Figure 37-3). These measurements are accepted worldwide and enable the provider to interpret the time of each deflection on the horizontal line and cardiac electrical activity (voltage) on the vertical line to help determine cardiac health.

Because all cardiac complexes consist of P, QRS, and T waves, and the electrocardiograph paper measures time on the horizontal line, it is possible to calculate heart rate. Count the number of 5-mm boxes (number within the dark lines) between two R waves. Divide this number into 300. The result is the heart rate in beats per minute.

Example:

One small square (1 mm) = 0.04 second in time
One large square (5 mm) = 0.04 × 5 = 0.2 second
Divide 60 seconds (1 minute) by 0.2 second: 60 ÷ 0.2 = 300

Example:

There are three large squares between two R waves.
300 ÷ 3 = 100
The heart rate is 100 beats per minute.

CRITICAL THINKING

Explain the significance of the small and large boxes on ECG paper. There are 2.5 large boxes between each cardiac cycle. What is the heart rate in beats per minute?

TYPES OF ELECTROCARDIOGRAPHS

Single-Channel Electrocardiograph

A conventional 12-lead single-channel **electrocardiograph** can be used in either manual mode or automatic mode. When using automatic mode, the 12-lead ECG tracing is complete in less than 40 seconds. With a single-channel machine, only one lead can be recorded at a time. If not automatic, the single-channel ECG requires manually turning the lead selector on and off between each of the 12 leads. It may also require the leads to be coded so that they can be identified later and properly mounted. Lead coding and mounting are explained more fully later in this chapter. The ECG tracing from a single-channel machine will need to be cut and mounted onto special forms for filing into the patient record. Figure 37-4 shows a sample of a single-channel electrocardiograph machine and tracing.

Multichannel Electrocardiograph

An electrocardiograph that can simultaneously record several different leads is known as a multichannel electrocardiograph. The conventional electrocardiograph records one lead at a time. A three-channel machine, one type of multichannel electrocardiograph, records three channels at one time. It records lead I, II, and III, followed by aVR, aVL, and aVF, followed by V_1, V_2, and V_3, followed by V_4, V_5, and V_6. The advantage of the multichannel machine is its speed. The most common multichannel machine used in the provider's clinic is the three-channel machine. This type of machine requires three-channel recording paper that is 8½ × 11 inches and fits into the patient record with no cutting or mounting. Figure 37-5 shows an example of a multichannel tracing. Other multichannel electrocardiograph machines are available, such as 6- and 12-channel machines. Some have a built-in rechargeable battery, an interpretation software program, a spirometery module, and transmission capability.

Automatic Electrocardiograph Machines

When using an automatic electrocardiograph, the lead length and switching of leads are done automatically by the electrocardiograph and there is

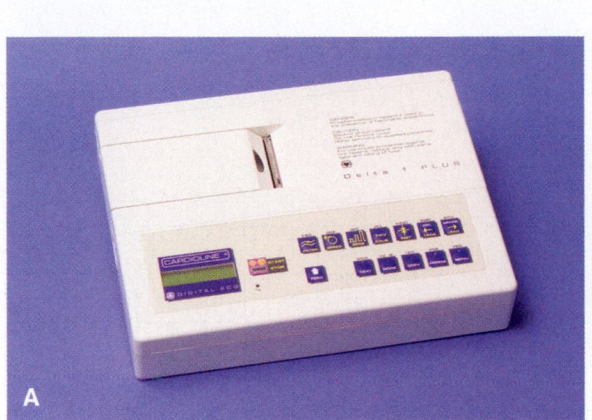

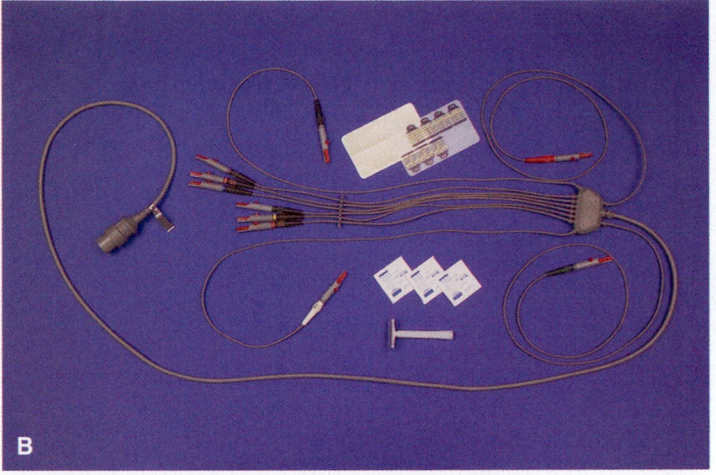

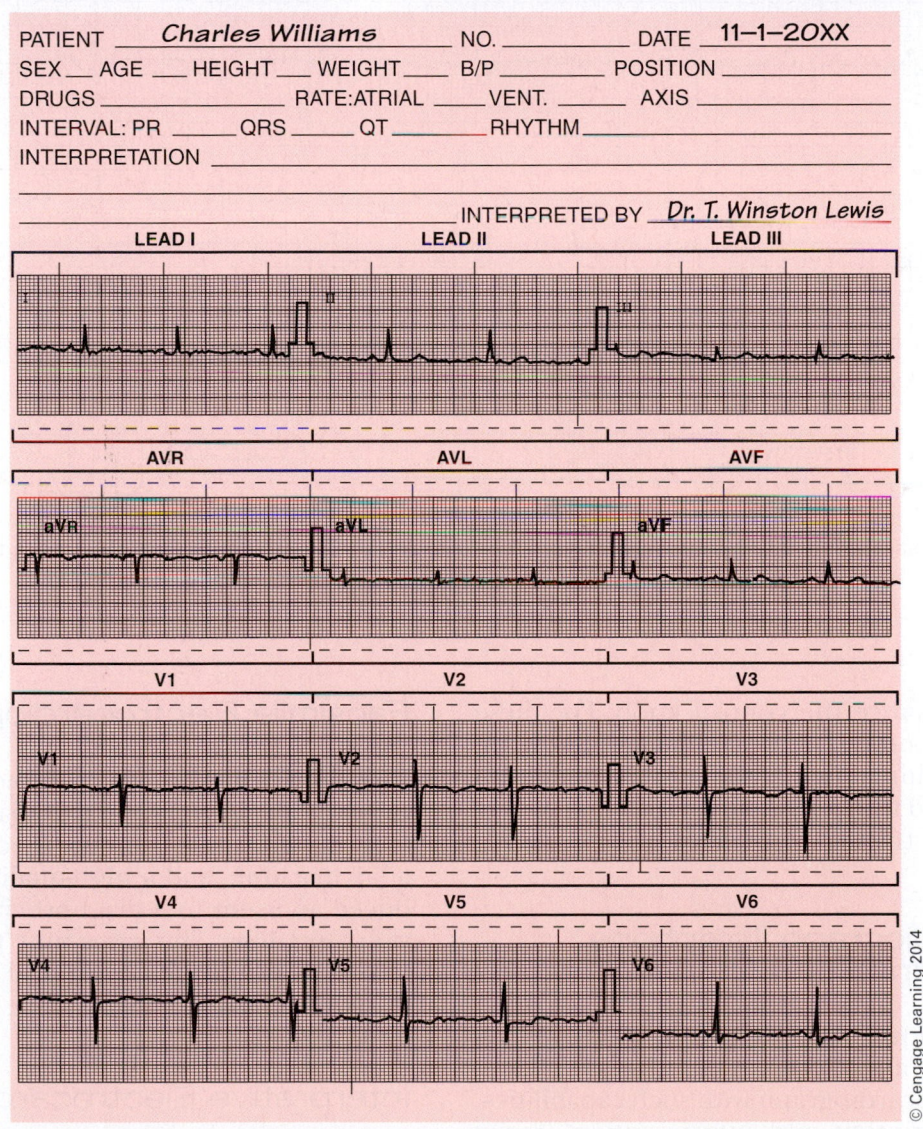

Figure 37-4 (A) Single-channel 12-lead electrocardiograph machine. (B) Supplies for single-channel 12 lead electrocardiograph. (C) Mounted single ECG tracing or recording.

© Cengage Learning 2014

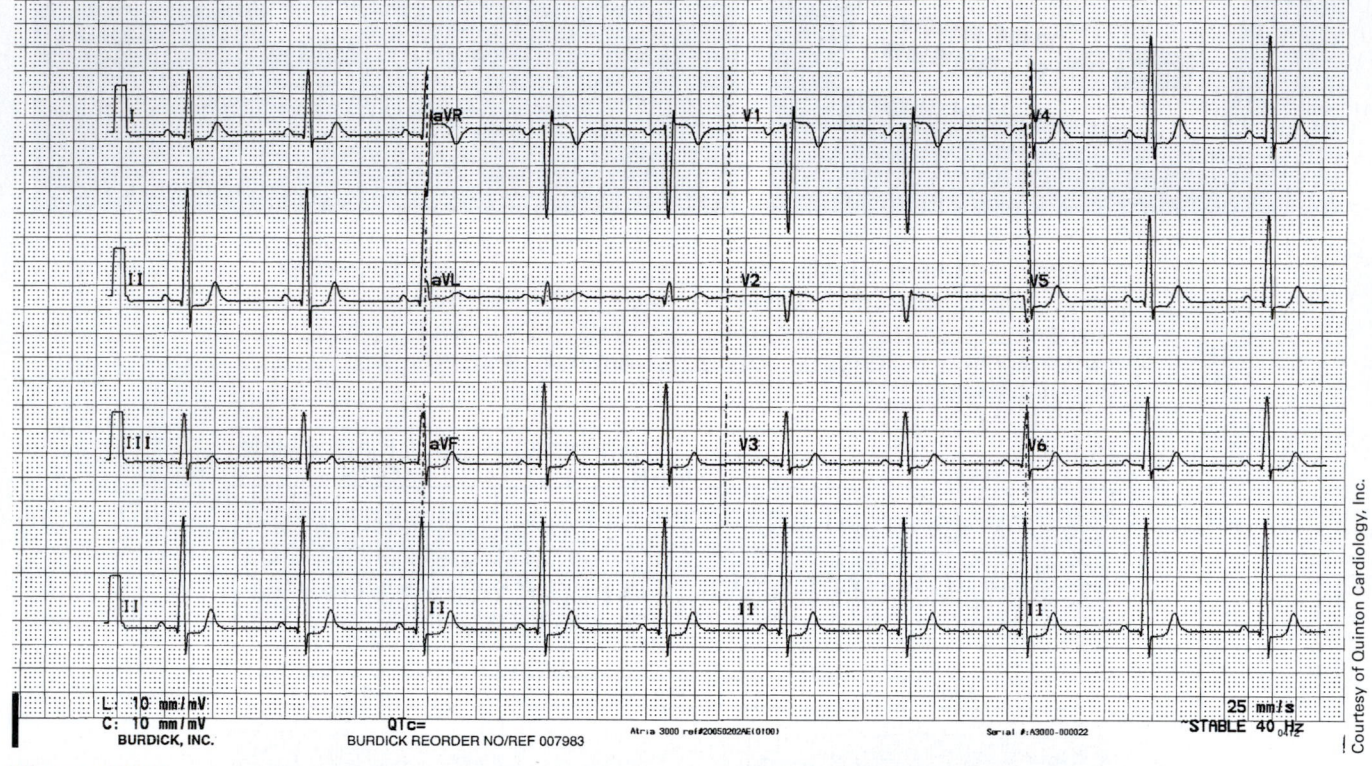

Figure 37-5 Example of three-channel electrocardiogram recording in which three leads are recorded simultaneously.

no need to advance the control knob. For these reasons, both time and paper can be saved with the automatic machine. The automatic machine also comes equipped with a manual control that can be used if a longer tracing is necessary.

Electrocardiograph Telephone Transmissions

An electrocardiogram can be transmitted via a telephone line to an ECG interpretation site when using an electrocardiograph with such capabilities. A recording printout and interpretation (many times interpretation is done by a cardiologist or by a computer) are transmitted automatically on the electrocardiograph. Results of the ECG can be transmitted verbally as well.

Facsimile Electrocardiograph

The provider may need a rapid, expert ECG interpretation from an off-site diagnostician. Direct ECG fax transmits from the electrocardiograph to a fax machine, and a high-quality facsimile is produced and sent to a diagnostician, who calls back with a reading. This saves time by eliminating the step of copying the report and sending it via the traditional fax machine.

Interpretive Electrocardiograph

The interpretive electrocardiograph has a built-in computer program that interprets the ECG tracing while it is being recorded, allowing for faster diagnosis and treatment. The provider in charge will review the tracing before a diagnosis is confirmed and treatment is begun.

ECG EQUIPMENT

Electrocardiograph Paper

ECG paper can be either black or dark blue and is wax- or plastic-coated with a white or pink background and color lines. The paper is heat and pressure sensitive. As the heated stylus of the electrocardiograph moves across the paper, the background coating is melted away, revealing the black or blue color of the paper, and the ECG cycles are recorded or traced. The heat of the stylus can be adjusted to obtain a sharp, clear recording, or **tracing**. Medical assistants should learn how to adjust the proper control using the specific manual or instructions that accompany the electrocardiograph in their facility.

Electrolyte

Because the skin is a poor conductor of electricity, there are various types of conductive **electrolyte** substances applied with each electrode to pick up the electrical current. The impulses are transmitted to the electrocardiograph by metal tips on the patient lead wires or cables that are attached to the sensors. Because electrolyte substances must contain moisture to properly conduct impulses, they are manufactured in the forms of gels, lotions, pastes, presaturated pads or, more commonly, are contained within adhesive sensors. For our purposes here, we use the disposable self-adhesive electropads/sensors.

Sensors or Electrodes

There are various types of **sensors** or **electrodes** made of metal or other conductive material. The sensors detect the electrical impulses on the body surface and relay them through cables, or lead, wires to the ECG machine.

Disposable Electrodes. Disposable sensors (electrodes) contain a layer of electrolyte gel on their adhesive surface and can be used on both the limbs and chest. They do not require additional electrolytes. These sensors are applied to the skin of the limbs and chest and held in place by the adhesive. The self-adhesive electrodes are discarded after use. They should be kept in an airtight bag because they dry out and will not stick well. Skin preparation is essential for an accurate tracing. In order to

provide the most conductive surface, it is recommended that the hair be cut or shaved from the area of electrode application. Then the dry, dead layer of the epidermis must be removed using soap and water, an alcohol prep pad, or a 4 × 4 gauze pad. Vigorously dry the skin to improve capillary circulation. Some providers encourage the use of an ECG prep pad that is similar to fine sand paper for the final step in preparation.

Lead Wires

Once the self-adhesive sensors are placed, a series of lead wires coming from the machine will be connected to them. Small clips, sometimes referred to as alligator clips, will grasp the tabs on the sensors (Figure 37-6). This completes the circuit from the patient to the machine.

Electrocardiograph Machine

Because the electrical activity that comes from the body is small, it is made larger, or **amplified**, by the amplifier of the electrocardiograph machine. The voltage is changed into a mechanical motion by the **galvanometer** and recorded on the paper by the heated stylus.

Care of Equipment

Once the ECG tracing is complete, remove the lead wires from the sensors, then remove the sensors from the patient. Dispose of the sensors. Check supplies on machine so it is ready for next use. Neatly and loosely place the lead wires on top of or beside the machine. Change the ECG paper when necessary according to manufacturer's suggestions.

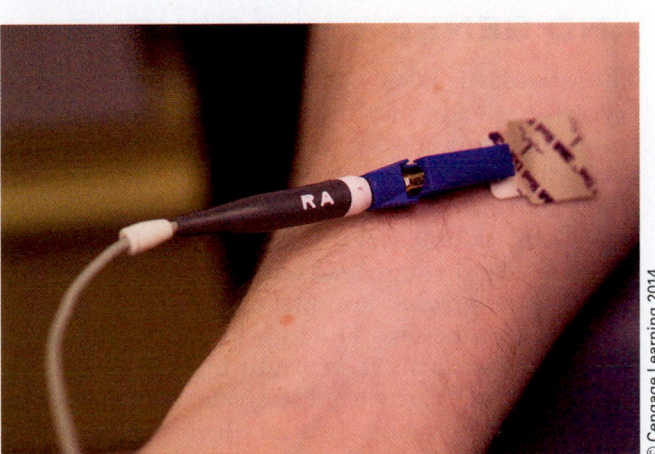

Figure 37-6 Alligator clip and disposable sensor.

© Cengage Learning 2014

THE PROCESS OF RECORDING CARDIAC ELECTRICITY

Skin—Poor conductor

Electrolyte—Must contain moisture to conduct current

Electrodes—Must contain metal to conduct current

Metal clips or tips—To connect the electrodes to the lead wires

Lead wires—To conduct the current from the patient to the machine

Amplifier in the machine—To amplify the electricity enough to measure it

Stylus—An instrument to record the electrical pattern

ECG paper—On which the stylus can record the pattern

Older electrocardiographs may have plain lead wire tips for use with the older metal plates and suction cups. They can easily and inexpensively be converted to use the current self-adhesive sensor electrodes. The only conversion equipment necessary is a set of "alligator" clips that will fit over the end of the lead wire tips. Contact the manufacturer or a medical supplier for conversion sets.

LEAD CODING

There are a number of codes used to identify each lead recorded on the ECG reading. There are 12 leads recorded using the 10 lead wires. These codes are necessary for later identification and for mounting purposes. Newer electrocardiographs automatically mark (code) each lead in the upper margin of the ECG paper during the recording. Older electrocardiographs must be manually coded by depressing the lead marker button. Figure 37-7 shows an example of a common coding system.

THE ELECTROCARDIOGRAPH AND SENSOR PLACEMENT

The standard ECG consists of 10 sensors that record 12 leads of the heart's electrical activity from different angles, allowing for a thorough three-dimensional interpretation of its activity. The electrical impulses given off by the heart are picked up by the electrodes and conducted into the machine through **lead wires**.

The electrodes are placed on the patient's four limbs and chest. The four limb leads are right arm (RA), left arm (LA), right leg (RL), and left leg (LL). The right leg electrode is not used as part of the recording. It is an electrical reference point only. The limb leads are placed on the fleshy, nonmuscular area of upper arms and lower legs. The chest leads are known as precordial leads, V leads, or C leads, and use an electrode for each of six areas on the chest wall or one electrode that is moved to six different positions on the chest wall. (This depends on the type of electrocardiograph being used.)

Standard Limb or Bipolar Leads

The first three leads that are recorded on a standard ECG are called leads I, II, and III (Figure 37-8A). These are known as **bipolar** leads because each of them uses two limb electrodes that record simultaneously. Lead I records electrical activity between the right arm (RA) and left arm (LA); lead II records electrical activity between the right arm (RA) and left leg (LL); and lead III records activity between the left arm (LA) and left leg (LL). Lead II is used as a **rhythm strip** because it portrays the heart's rhythm better than the other leads. The rhythm strip is usually a separate longer recording approximately 6 to 12 inches.

Augmented Leads

The next three leads are **augmented** (added to) leads and are designated aVR, aVL, and aVF (Figure 37-8B). The aV stands for augmented voltage; the R, L, and F stand for right, left, and foot (or leg). These are **unipolar** leads. Lead aVR records electrical activity from the midpoint between the left arm added to the left leg, directed to the right arm. Lead aVL records electrical activity from the midpoint between the right arm added to the left leg, directed to the left arm. Lead aVF records electrical activity from the midpoint between the right arm added to the left arm, directed to the left leg. Because these three leads produce such small electrical impulses, the electrocardiograph machine augments, or increases, their size to record

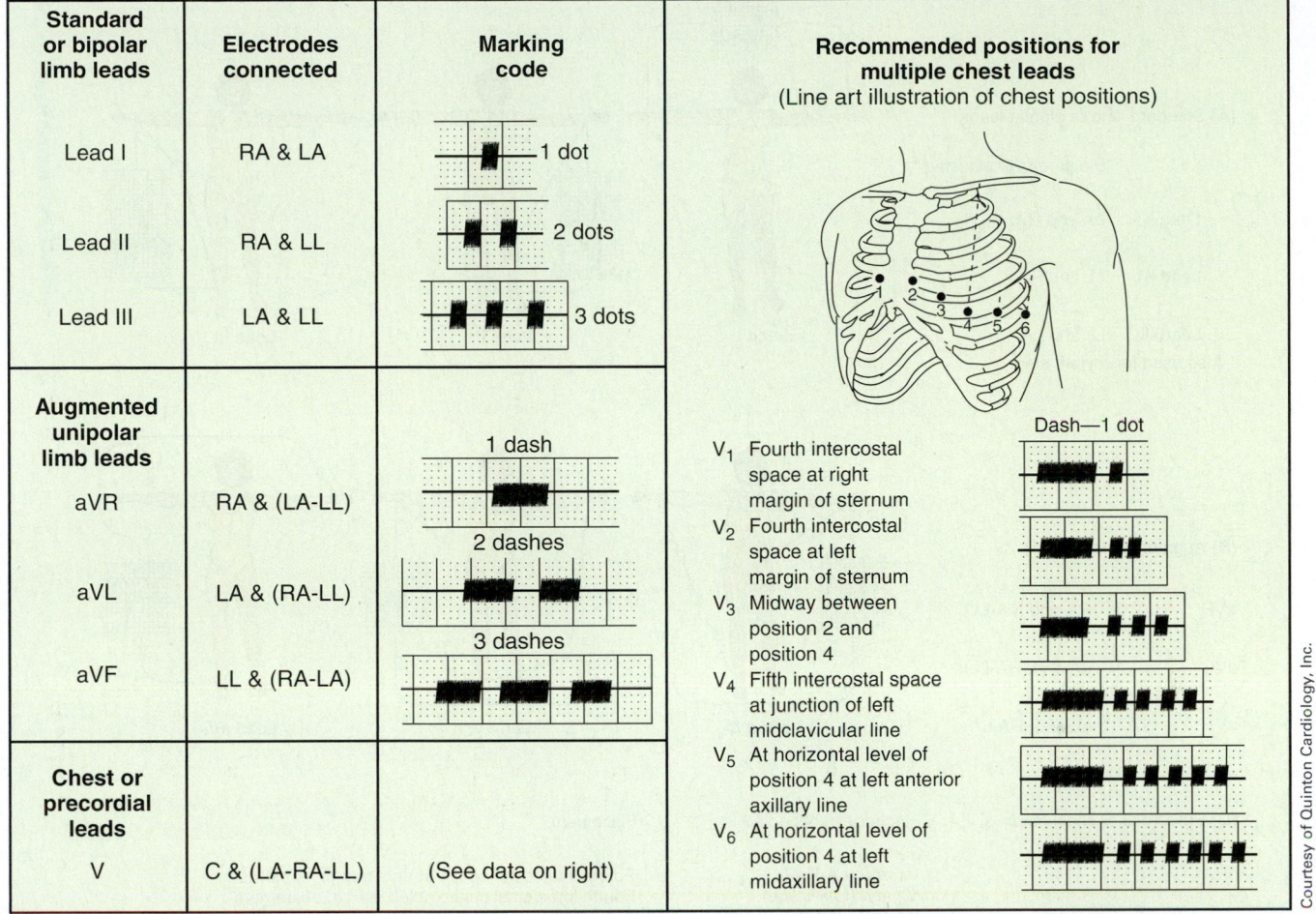

Standard or bipolar limb leads	Electrodes connected	Marking code	Recommended positions for multiple chest leads (Line art illustration of chest positions)
Lead I	RA & LA	1 dot	
Lead II	RA & LL	2 dots	
Lead III	LA & LL	3 dots	
Augmented unipolar limb leads			
aVR	RA & (LA-LL)	1 dash	V₁ Fourth intercostal space at right margin of sternum
aVL	LA & (RA-LL)	2 dashes	V₂ Fourth intercostal space at left margin of sternum
aVF	LL & (RA-LA)	3 dashes	V₃ Midway between position 2 and position 4
Chest or precordial leads			V₄ Fifth intercostal space at junction of left midclavicular line
V	C & (LA-RA-LL)	(See data on right)	V₅ At horizontal level of position 4 at left anterior axillary line
			V₆ At horizontal level of position 4 at left midaxillary line

Dash—1 dot

Courtesy of Quinton Cardiology, Inc.

Figure 37-7   Example of a common coding system for electrocardiogram leads that must be manually coded on older electrocardiographs. Accurate coding is accomplished by pressing the lead marker button appropriately.

them. Figure 37-8B will help you visualize the augmented process.

Chest Leads or Precordial Leads

The remaining six leads of the standard 12-lead ECG are the chest leads or **precordial** leads (Figure 37-8C). These are unipolar leads and are designated V₁, V₂, V₃, V₄, V₅, and V₆. These leads record the heart's electrical impulse from a central point within the heart to one of six predesignated positions on the chest wall where an electrode is attached. The correct position *must* be used for each lead recording.

The anatomic positions for placement of the chest or precordial leads are:

V₁: fourth intercostal space at right margin of sternum

V₂: fourth intercostal space at left margin of sternum

V₄: fifth intercostal space on left midclavicular line

V₃: midway between V₂ and V₄ (*Note:* This is correct order, V₃ after V₄.)

V₅: horizontal to V₄ at left anterior axillary line

V₆: horizontal to V₄ at left midaxillary line

When using an electrocardiograph with one chest wire, the chest electrode must be moved manually one by one to each of the six chest lead positions. This necessitates stopping the instrument between each chest lead to move the electrode to the next appropriate position on the chest wall. Some electrocardiographs have six lead wires allowing all six chest leads to be applied at one time; therefore, there is no interruption between chest lead recordings (see Figure 37-17C in Procedure 37-1).

(A) Standard limb or bipolar leads

Electrodes Connected

Lead I	LA and RA
Lead II*	LL and RA
Lead III	LL and LA

* Also used for rhythm strip

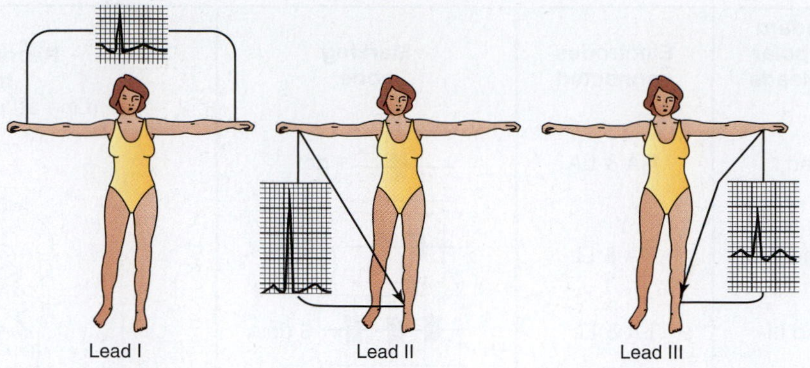

Lead I   Lead II   Lead III

(B) Augmented limb leads

aVR	RA and (LA-LL)
aVL	LA and (RA-LL)
aVF	LL and (RA-LA)

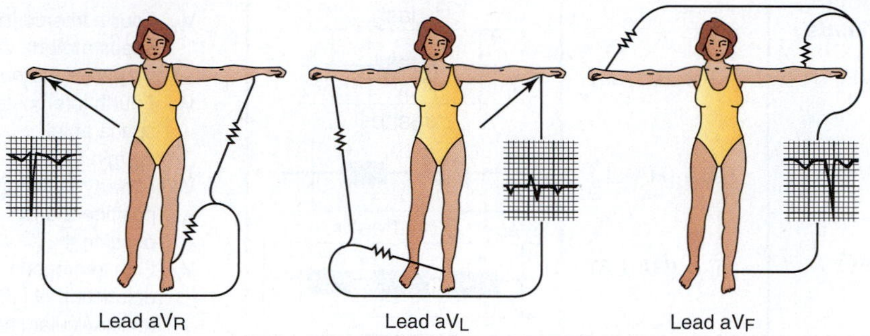

Lead aV$_R$ Lead aV$_L$ Lead aV$_F$

(C) Precordial or chest leads

	Electrodes connected	Placement
V$_1$	V$_1$ and (LA-RA-LL)	Fourth intercostal space at right margin of sternum
V$_2$	V$_2$ and (LA-RA-LL)	Fourth intercostal space at left margin of sternum
V$_4$	V$_4$ and (LA-RA-LL)	Fifth intercostal space at junction of left midclavicular line
V$_3$	V$_3$ and (LA-RA-LL)	Midway between position 2 and position 4
V$_5$	V$_5$ and (LA-RA-LL)	At horizontal level of position 4 at left anterior axillary line
V$_6$	V$_6$ and (LA-RA-LL)	At horizontal level of position 4 at left midaxillary line

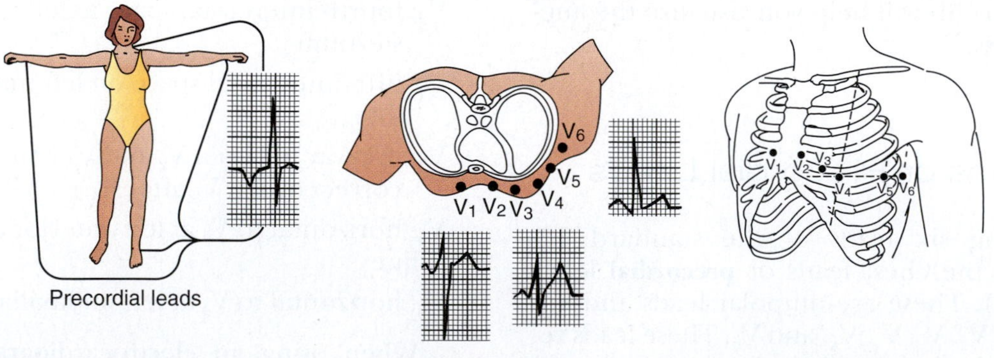

Precordial leads

Figure 37-8   Lead types, connections, and placement. (A) Standard limb or bipolar leads. (B) Augmented limb leads. (C) Precordial or chest leads.

© Cengage Learning 2014

STANDARDIZATION AND ADJUSTMENT OF THE ELECTROCARDIOGRAPH

The value of an ECG recording depends on it being performed accurately. To ensure a precise and reliable recording, you must standardize the ECG instrument before every ECG performed. The standardization of the machine is a quality-assurance check to determine if the machine is set and working properly. Standardization measurements have been adopted internationally as a means of accurate **calibration** according to universal measurements. The universal standard is that 1 mV (millivolt) of cardiac electrical activity will deflect the stylus exactly 10 mm high. This is the equivalent of 10 small squares on the ECG paper. Figure 37-9 shows an example of the 10-mm standardization at the beginning of each row.

On occasion, R waves may be large and go off the paper. Repositioning the stylus may not correct the situation. In such instances, the medical assistant can record the lead(s) in which the R wave is large at one-half sensitivity. This action will record all ECG cycles at half their normal **amplitude**.

Conversely, the waves of the ECG cycles may be small, making it difficult to interpret. In this circumstance, the medical assistant can record the ECG cycles at twice the normal standard. This action will record ECG cycles at twice their normal amplitude. Whenever a change is made from a normal standardization (10 mm high) to either a one-half standardization (5 mm high) or a double standardization (20 mm high), the medical assistant must include the adjusted standardization mark with that particular lead to alert the provider to the change in standard. The standard must be returned to normal to prevent accidentally running the next lead at a standard other than normal. The paper is usually run at a speed of 25 mm/second. If cycles are too close together, the paper speed can be adjusted to 50 mm/second. Make a note on the ECG paper if paper speed or amplitude is changed.

STANDARD RESTING ELECTROCARDIOGRAPHY

Regardless of the type of electrocardiograph used, the basic components of the standard electrocardiography procedure remain the same. Patient preparation, placement of limb and chest leads, attachment of lead wires, and elimination of

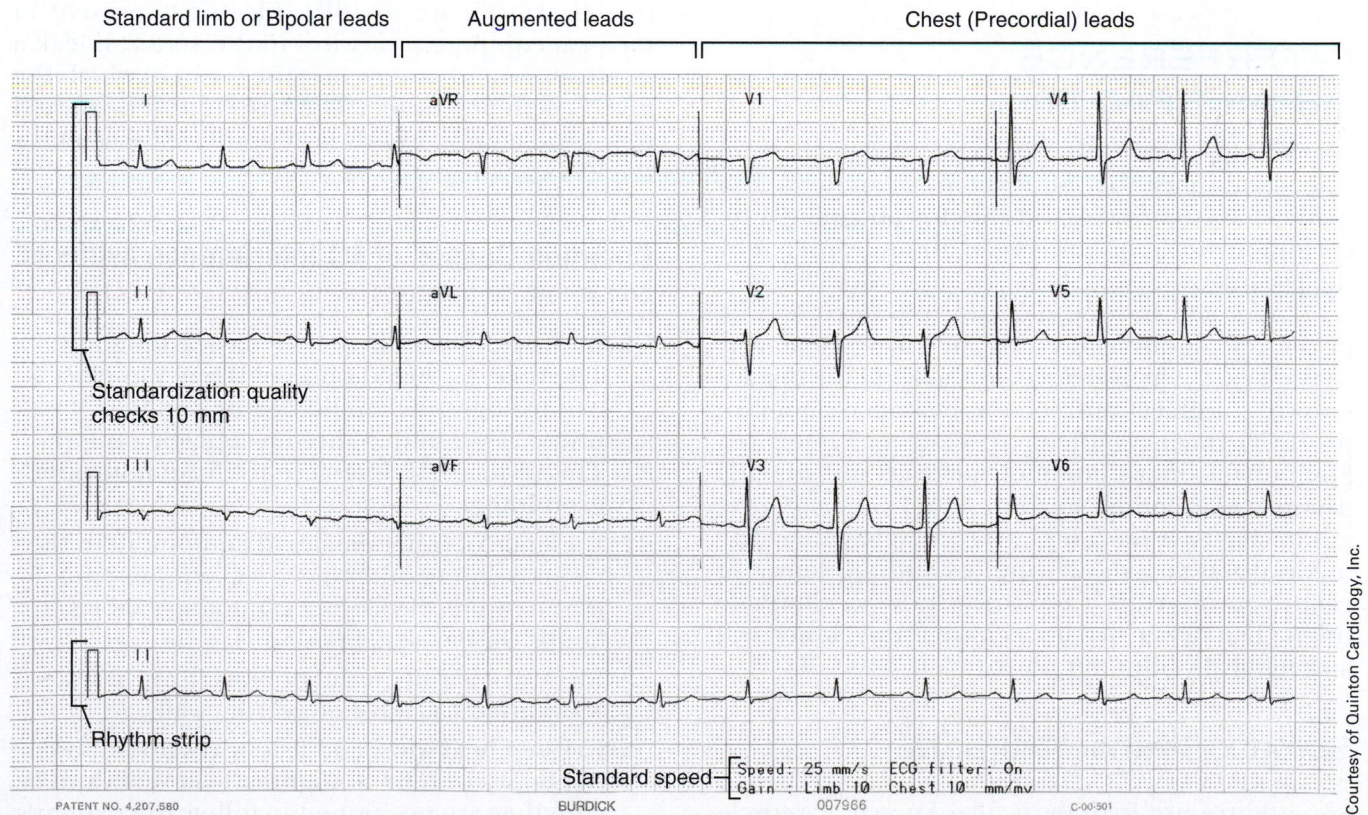

Standard limb or Bipolar leads   Augmented leads   Chest (Precordial) leads

I   aVR   V1   V4

II   aVL   V2   V5

Standardization quality checks 10 mm

III   aVF   V3   V6

II

Rhythm strip

Standard speed — Speed: 25 mm/s   ECG filter: On
Gain : Limb 10   Chest 10   mm/mv

PATENT NO. 4,207,580   BURDICK   007966   C-00-501

Courtesy of Quinton Cardiology, Inc.

Figure 37-9   An electrocardiogram showing all 12 leads recorded in minutes at one time with no interruption.

artifacts vary little from one electrocardiograph to another. Procedure 37-1 explains a 12-lead ECG using a multiple-lead channel electrocardiograph.

  Before performing the procedure, medical assistants must be familiar with the electrocardiograph machine in their facility and should thoroughly review the manufacturer's instruction manual that accompanies the machine. Knowledge of the basic procedures included here can be adapted for all other electrocardiographs.

MOUNTING THE ECG TRACING

Commercially prepared **mounting** forms are available, and the medical assistant should mount the completed tracing after the provider has reviewed the entire recording. The mounting of the ECG recording depends on the machine. Some machines produce a strip already printed on a durable paper record. Some machines produce a long strip that will need to be cut apart and adhered to a mounting paper or card. There are many options within these two varieties. Included with any ECG recording should be the patient's name, date, address, age, sex, blood pressure, height and weight, and cardiac medications on the mounting form.

INTERFERENCE OR ARTIFACTS

The ECG is a valuable diagnostic aid to the provider and must be performed accurately. The medical assistant is responsible for obtaining a recording that can be easily read and interpreted by the provider.

There can be unusual and unwanted activity in the tracing not caused by the electrical activity of the heart. These defects in the ECG tracing are known as **artifacts**, and their appearance can make the ECG tracing difficult to read and interpret. Four of the more common artifacts are somatic tremor, alternating current (AC) interference, wandering baseline, and interrupted baseline. The medical assistant should understand the causes of each type of artifact and know how to eliminate them. The newer machines have filters, which will automatically filter out the artifact.

Somatic Tremor Artifacts

Somatic tremor artifact is also known as muscle tremor. It is characterized by unnatural baseline deflections such as jagged peaks or irregularity of spacing and height. The tracing appears fuzzy (Figure 37-10A). Somatic tremor occurs when the patient is apprehensive or uncomfortable, resulting in involuntary muscle movement. Voluntary muscle movement occurs when the patient moves, talks, coughs, and so on. Parkinson's disease, a nervous system disorder, is an example of involuntary somatic tremor. It is not possible for the patient to control the muscle tremors. (Often, involuntary somatic tremor can be minimized somewhat by having the patient slide the hands under the buttocks during the recording.)

It is natural for the patient to feel apprehensive before and during the ECG tracing. Reassurance and an explanation of the procedure will allay apprehension and relax muscles. Be certain the patient is comfortable. Use pillows for the head and under the knees; be sure the temperature of the room is comfortable. These simple techniques will help to minimize somatic tremor.

AC Interference

The AC interference artifact is caused by electrical interference and appears as a series of small regular peaks (Figure 37-10B). Electricity present in medical equipment or wires in the area can leak a small amount of energy into the room in which the ECG is being recorded. The current can be picked up by the patient's body and it will be detected by the ECG tracing as an AC artifact.

Common Causes of AC Interference Artifacts.

Some common causes of AC interferences are:

1. Improper grounding of electrocardiograph. The three-pronged plugs in the newer electrocardiographs should be inserted into a properly grounded three-receptacle outlet. This reduces AC interference from improper grounding.

2. Presence of other electrical equipment in the room. Unplug other electrical equipment in the room (electrical examination tables, lamps, autoclaves, and so on).

3. Electrical wiring in the floor, ceiling, or walls. Move the ECG table away from walls.

4. Crossed lead wires and lead wires not following body contour. Straighten lead wires and be sure they are positioned to follow the patient's body contour.

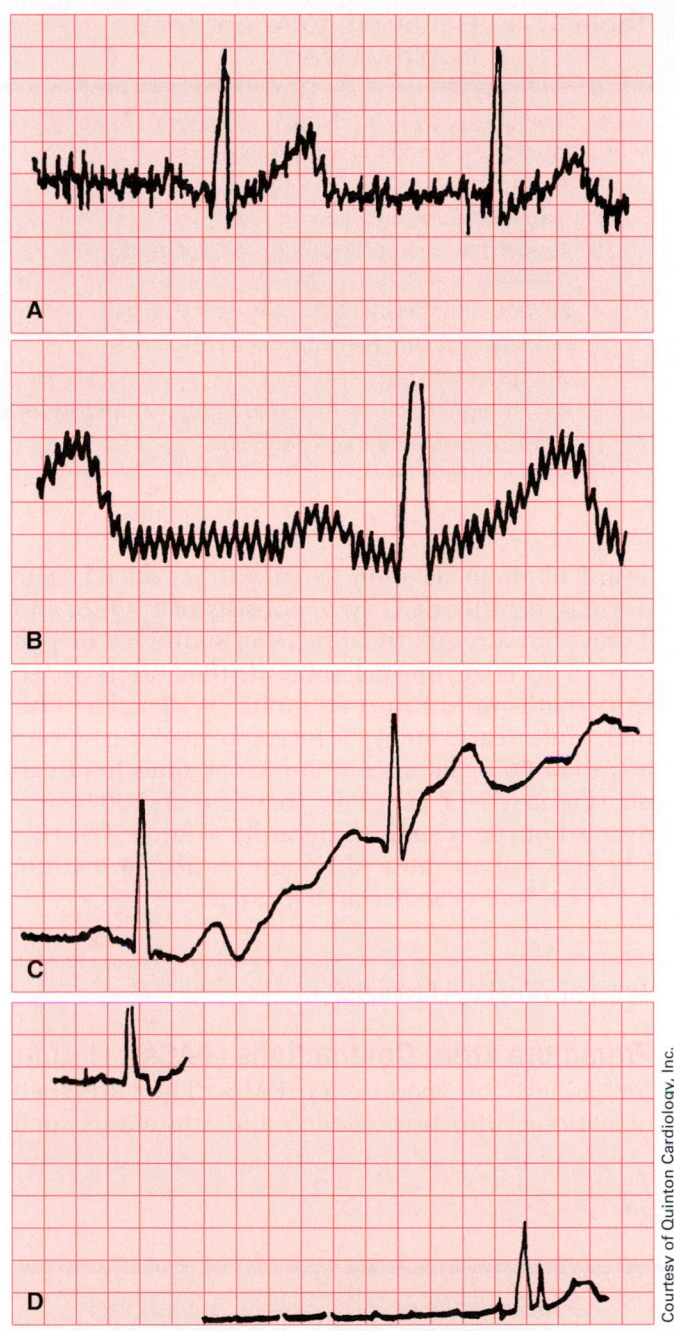

Figure 37-10   Electrocardiogram artifacts.
(A) Somatic tremor. (B) Alternating current.
(C) Wandering baseline. (D) Interrupted baseline.

Courtesy of Quinton Cardiology, Inc.

Wandering Baseline Artifacts

A wandering baseline occurs when the stylus moves from the center of the ECG paper, resulting in the complexes "wandering" across the ECG paper; for example, from the top of the paper to the bottom, or bottom to top (Figure 37-10C). This makes it difficult to follow the complexes when the provider reads and interprets the recording.

Common Causes of Wandering Baseline Artifacts.
Wandering baseline artifacts can be caused by the following conditions:

1. Electrodes applied too loosely or too tightly. There should be equal tension on all four limb leads, metal tips should be firmly attached to the electrodes, and the cable attached to patient should not have tension on it nor be dangling to cause pulling on the electrode.

2. Corroded or dirty electrodes or metal tips of the lead wires. Clean and rinse after each use.

3. Inappropriate amount or poor-quality electrolyte gel or paste. Each electrode should have the same amount of electrolyte gel or paste on it.

4. Lotions, oils, or creams on the patient's skin that interfere with the adhesive sticking well. Remove any of these substances before applying the electrode by cleansing the area with an alcohol wipe.

Wandering baseline artifacts are more often seen in older ECG machines that use metal electrodes and electrolyte. Newer machines use electrodes (sensors) that are disposable and self-adhesive, thereby eliminating the four causes of wandering baseline artifacts.

Interrupted Baseline Artifacts

On occasion, the baseline is interrupted and a break is seen between waves (Figure 37-10D). Possible causes are a broken cable, a lead wire that became detached from an electrode, or an electrode that came completely off.

Patients with Unique Problems

On occasion, the medical assistant performs an ECG on a patient who has unique medical problems. An obese patient, a woman with large breasts, or a patient with thick chest muscles will make it difficult to palpate the intercostal spaces. Place the chest leads on the chest as accurately as you can.

For a patient with a limb amputation or a cast, the medical assistant should apply the sensors as close to the preferred site as possible, higher on the limb. Place the sensor in a similar position on the other limb.

Do not place sensors on wounds, open areas, sutures, or staples. Try to situate the sensors as close as possible to the preferred site.

If the patient has dyspnea, the ECG can be taken with the patient in semi-Fowler's position (see Chapter 25 for positions).

CRITICAL THINKING

You have just performed an annual ECG on your patient, Ms. Cantrell. The tracing looks alarming. However, Ms. Cantrell is alert, oriented, and talking. What is your best course of action?

If you have difficulty performing an ECG on patients with certain medical problems or conditions, ask for assistance from your supervisor/delegator.

MYOCARDIAL INFARCTIONS (HEART ATTACKS)

Myocardial infarctions (heart attacks) are the number one cause of death in the United States today. With the approval of the employer–provider, medical assistants are in an excellent position to offer healthy tips and suggestions from which patients can benefit. For instance, they can offer patient health tips regarding diet and exercise while applying the ECG equipment and provide handouts and informational websites for patients to research (Table 37-1).

CARDIAC ARRHYTHMIAS

The medical assistant should recognize cardiac **arrhythmias** (anything other than normal sinus rhythm) that occur during the ECG recording and without alarming the patient make the provider

Table 37-1 Behaviors to Adopt for a Healthy Heart

The provider may want the medical assistant to remind patients of the following healthy behaviors:

1. Avoid tobacco
2. Take medications as prescribed
3. Report any unusual symptoms or problems to the provider
4. Eat a low-fat, low-cholesterol, low-sodium diet
5. Exercise regularly with provider's permission
6. Get adequate rest
7. Keep weight under control and at an acceptable level
8. Practice stress reduction behaviors

© Cengage Learning 2014

aware of them as soon as they are noticed. The normal, healthy ECG cycle consists of P, QRS, and T waves in a regularly appearing sequence or pattern. The term **normal sinus rhythm** refers to an ECG that is within normal limits (WNL). The normal adult heart rate is 60 to 100 beats/min. A rate less than 60 beats/min is known as **sinus bradycardia** (Figure 37-11A); a rate greater than 100 beats/min is known as **sinus tachycardia** (Figure 37-11B). These two heart rates, although regular in rhythm, are considered cardiac arrhythmias.

Atrial Arrhythmias

Premature Atrial Contractions (PACs). Healthy individuals can experience PACs. They are seen in patients who use tobacco and stimulants such

PATIENT EDUCATION

Atherosclerosis is the buildup of fatty deposits on the lining of coronary arteries causing narrowing and obstruction of the arteries. **Ischemia** or decreased blood flow to the heart muscle is diminished particularly when the heart is called on to work harder, for example, during increased physical activity, emotional stress, exposure to cold temperatures, and after a heavy meal. The heart's muscle tissue responds to these conditions by symptoms of pain or discomfort beneath the sternum, into the neck, jaw, left arm and shoulder, and throat. Rest usually relieves the pain. This condition is known as **angina pectoris**.

Treatment of angina consists of rest and medication. Nitroglycerin may be prescribed in tablet or patch form. Change in lifestyle and other suggestions (Table 37-1) may be recommended. Tests that the provider may order include a 12-lead ECG, a stress ECG (stress test), blood tests, chest radiograph, and coronary **angiogram**.

Pain that does not subside after rest may indicate a more serious condition such as a complete obstruction of the coronary arteries and no blood flow to the heart muscle, a myocardial infarction, or heart attack. Seek immediate medical attention if pain persists.

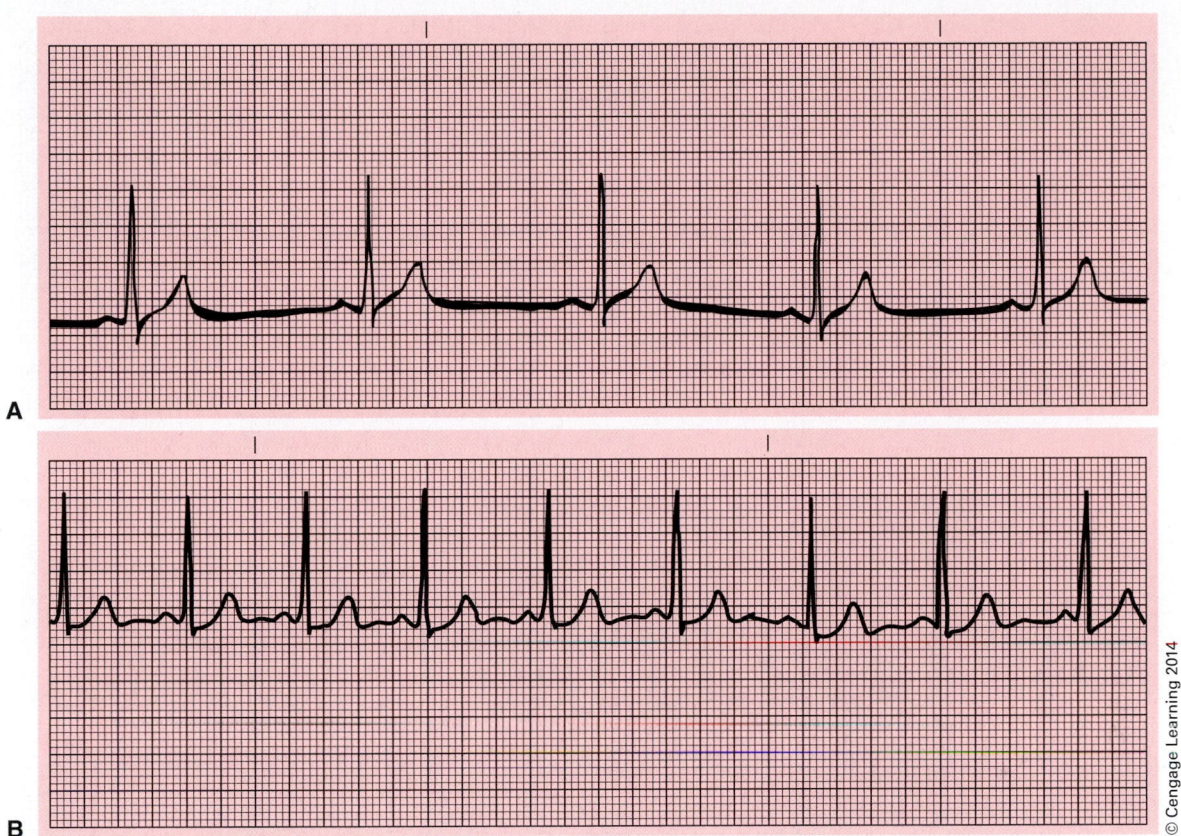

© Cengage Learning 2014

Figure 37-11   (A) Heart rate shown is 50 beats/min, known as sinus brachycardia because it is less than 60 beats/min. One large square = 0.2 second; 1 minute (60 seconds) ÷ 0.2 = 300. There are six large squares between R waves: 300 ÷ 6 = 50 beats/min. (B) Sinus tachycardia is a heart rate faster than 100 beats/min. There are three large squares between R waves: 300 ÷ 3 = 100 beats/min.

as caffeine, or even during exercise, but they can forewarn of more serious cardiac problems. This type of arrhythmia is characterized by a cardiac cycle that occurs before the next cycle is due. The P wave is shaped differently from the P wave of the normal cycle (Figure 37-12A).

Paroxysmal Atrial Tachycardia (PAT).

This arrhythmia can be seen in healthy individuals; and in persons with cardiac disease. PAT is characterized by its unprovoked sudden onset and abrupt termination. The heart rate is regular and ranges between 160 to 250 beats/min. The episode usually lasts only a few seconds; the heart rate then returns to its original rate (Figure 37-12B). The patient may describe a fluttering in the chest, apprehension, shortness of breath, and, on occasion, dizziness.

Atrial Fibrillation.

This arrhythmia can be seen in healthy individuals or in those with cardiac disease. In younger patients, common causes can be

congenital heart disease and mitral valve damage caused by rheumatic heart disease. In older patients, the arrhythmia can be caused by hypertension, coronary artery disease, or mitral valve prolapse. It is characterized by extremely rapid, incomplete contractions 400 to 500 beats/min of the atria resulting in irregular and uncoordinated contractions of the ventricles at a much slower rate. On an ECG tracing, this is seen as complexes that are difficult to measure accurately because the P waves cannot be distinguished and the ventricular rate is irregularly irregular (Figure 37-12C).

Ventricular Arrhythmias

Premature Ventricular Contractions (PVCs).

This arrhythmia can be seen in healthy individuals and in patients with hypertension, coronary artery disease, and lung disease. In healthy individuals, PVCs can be caused by tobacco, anxiety, alcohol, and medications that contain epinephrine

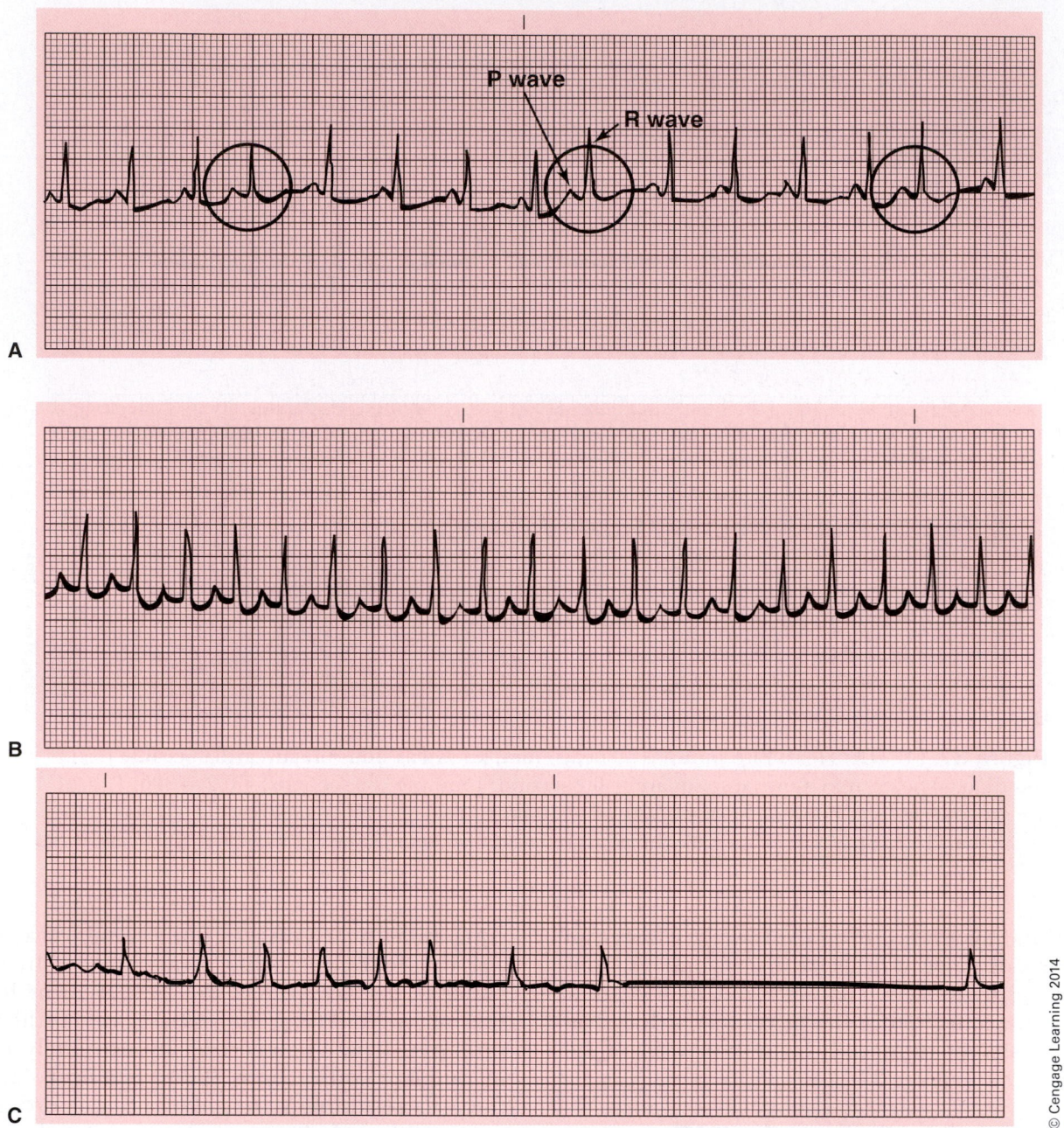

Figure 37-12   Atrial arrhythmias. (A) Premature atrial contractions. (B) Paroxysmal atrial tachycardia. (C) Atrial fibrillation.

(Figure 37-13A). PVCs are seen on ECG tracings fairly frequently and are considered common disturbances in the rhythm. They are characterized by a beat that comes early in the cycle, has no P wave, a wide QRS complex, and a different T wave. The PVC is followed by a pause before the occurrence of the next normal cycle. This rhythm is dangerous when there are pairs or groups of PVCs and they occur in an already compromised heart due to myocardial infarction, heart failure, or valvular disease. In this population, an increased number of PVCs per minute can indicate a progression into ventricular tachycardia (VT), a life-threatening condition.

Ventricular Tachycardia. This arrhythmia is seen in patients with cardiac disease, both acute and chronic. It is common in patients with coronary artery disease, and frequently the patient experiencing a myocardial infarction will have ventricular tachycardia as a result of the infarction (Figure 37-13B). The arrhythmia is manifested by a group or a

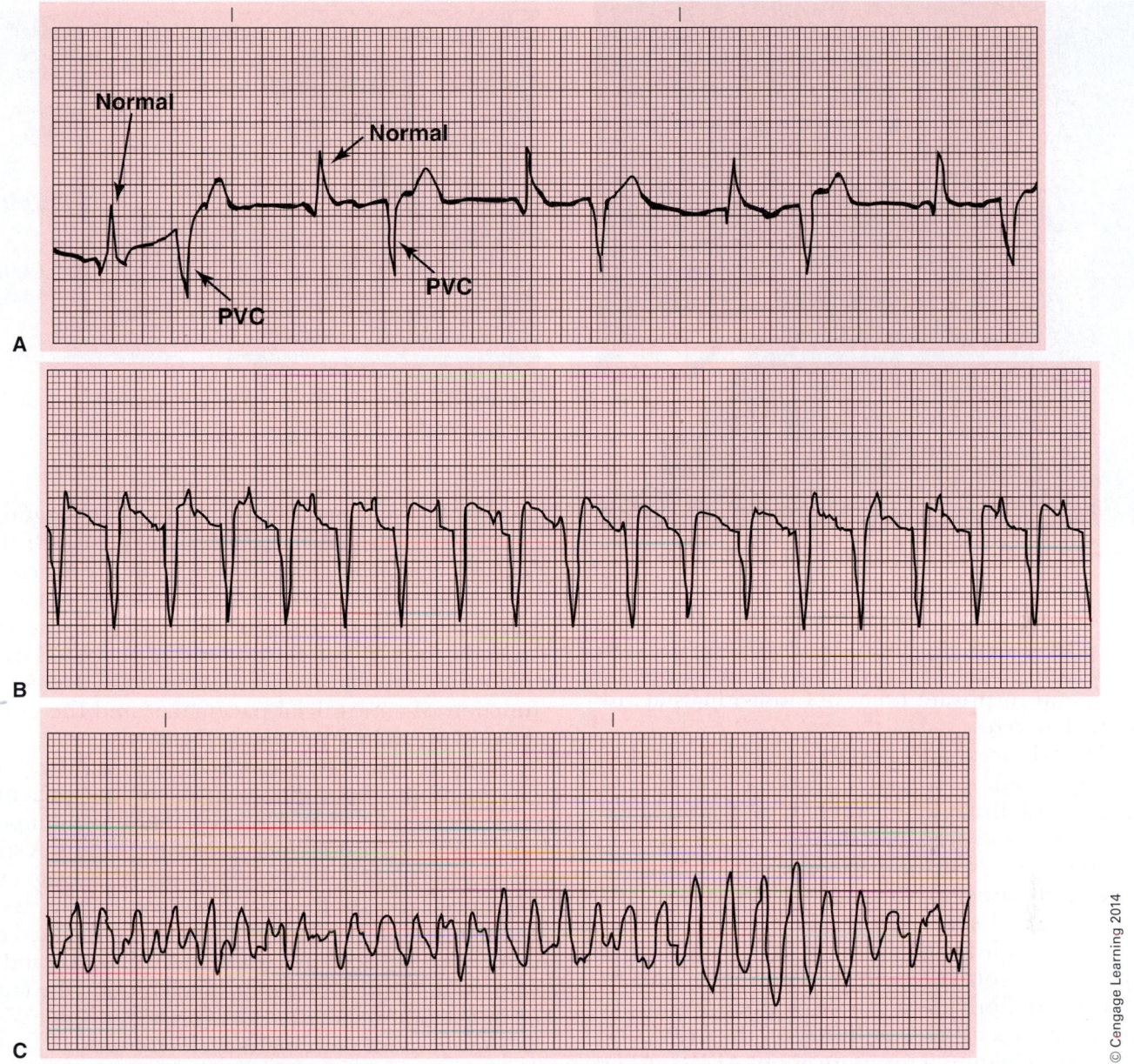

Figure 37-13   Ventricular arrhythmia. (A) Premature ventricular contractions (PVCs). (B) Ventricular tachycardia. (C) Ventricular fibrillation.

sustained run of PVCs that occur at a rate ranging from 150 to 250 beats/min. There are no P waves, and the QRS complexes are distorted. Ventricular tachycardia is life threatening and can rapidly deteriorate into fibrillation and cardiac standstill.

Ventricular Fibrillation. This arrhythmia is seen in patients experiencing a myocardial infarction or in patients with existing cardiac disease. It may be preceded by PVCs or ventricular tachycardia, or it may begin as ventricular fibrillation. It is a life-threatening arrhythmia (Figure 37-13C).

DEFIBRILLATION

A **defibrillator** is an electrical device that applies **countershocks** to the heart through electrodes or pads placed on the chest wall (Figure 37-14). The purpose is to convert cardiac arrhythmia into normal sinus rhythm. This is known as **defibrillation** or **cardioversion**. In most offices and clinics, a defibrillator is kept on a crash cart for quick access in emergency situations. The medical assistant should regularly check the equipment for proper operation and preparedness and assist the provider as needed.

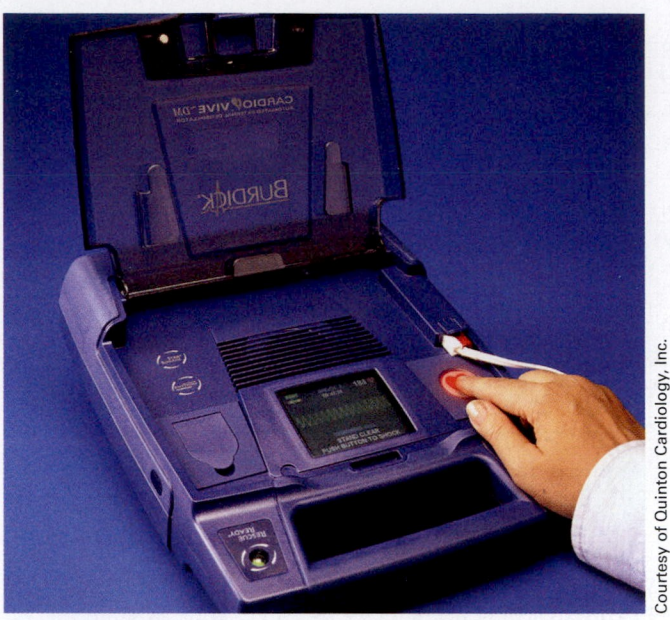

Courtesy of Quinton Cardiology, Inc.

Figure 37-14 The CardioVive DM AED.

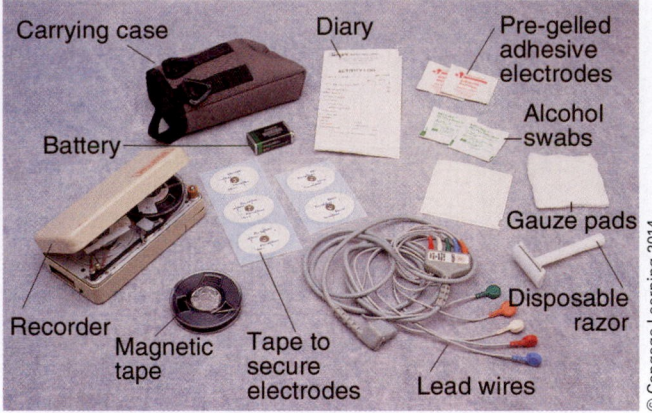

© Cengage Learning 2014

Figure 37-15 Holter monitor and supplies needed for application.

Automated external defibrillators (AEDs) are widely used and are found in places where many people congregate, such as airports and the workplace, and in private homes of individuals at risk for cardiac arrest.

The devices are portable, small, and battery operated. Emergency medical technicians, police, and firefighters trained in defibrillation techniques and who are the first to respond in an emergency were primarily the individuals who used these devices. Now, many citizens are certified to use AEDs (see Figure 37-14).

In an individual experiencing a myocardial infarction, ventricular fibrillation is not uncommon. If the fibrillation can be stopped within the first 5 minutes using a defibrillator, the life can be saved (see Chapter 9 for more about AEDs). AEDs are commonly found and come with very simple instructions about defibrillator pad placement. Once the unit is turned on, it uses a complex computer program to analyze the cardiac rhythm and provide audible instructions to the rescuer.

OTHER CARDIAC DIAGNOSTIC TESTS

Holter Monitor (Portable Ambulatory Electrocardiograph)

The Holter monitor is a portable continuous recording of cardiac activity for a 24-hour period (Figure 37-15). The patient is monitored while going about the usual daily activities with no restrictions. This **noninvasive** test helps to diagnose cardiac arrhythmias by correlating them with the patient's symptoms. Some symptoms are **syncope**, fatigue, chest pain, and vertigo. This type of monitoring is useful for patients whose arrhythmias are sporadic and are not found on a 12-lead ECG tracing. Also, ambulatory monitoring helps assess the function of an artificial pacemaker and the effectiveness of antiarrhythmic medications.

Special electrodes attached to lead wires are placed in the appropriate areas of the patient's chest. Remember that skin preparation is an important aspect of ensuring accurate information. A special portable tape recorder, either digital or magnetic continually records the heart's electrical activity for a 24-hour period. The monitor is a battery-operated recorder that is placed in a leather pouch or bag and is worn by the patient either on a belt around the waist or by a strap over the patient's shoulder. Table 37-2 lists locations for placement of electrodes.

One kind of digital **Holter monitor** is a three-channel (five-lead) ECG that has Windows-based software technology. A keypad is used to enter the patient's information, such as date of recording, patient identification number, etc. There is no need to check the effectiveness of the monitor by attaching it to a test cable and an ECG machine. Some monitors have a removable flash memory card and a flash card reader that can download information in 90 seconds. It can hold up to 48 hours of ECG information. The tracing is interpreted and sent back by computer. It can be accessed and printed. The electrode placement is the same for a digital Holter monitor as it is for a magnetic tape Holter monitor, but both digital and magnetic tape electrode placement is not the same as it is for a standard 12-lead resting ECG.

Table 37-2 Holter Monitor Electrode Placement

Electrode	Lead	Location
A (black)	mV_1	Fourth intercostal space at right of the sternal edge
B (white)	mV_5	Right clavicle, just lateral to sternum
C (brown)	mV_1	Left clavicle, just lateral to the sternum
D (red)	mV_5	Fifth intercostal space at left axillary line
E (green)	Ground	Lower right chest wall

© Cengage Learning 2014

PATIENT EDUCATION

When preparing patients to wear a 24-hour Holter monitor, instruct them in the following:

1. Keep a diary of daily activities, symptoms, and emotions, and note the time of occurrence.
2. Depress the event marker only briefly and only when experiencing a significant symptom. Overuse of the marker can mask the ECG tracing.
3. Do not shower, bathe, or swim while wearing the monitor because the recording could be interrupted or the monitor could be damaged.
4. Do not handle the electrodes. Doing so could cause artifacts.
5. Do not remove the recorder from its case.
6. Do not use an electric blanket. This can cause interference.

Other computerized continuous cardiac monitoring devices are available and are prescribed for patients according to the patient's symptoms and the practitioner's preference. The tracing can be read over the telephone or is computerized. Transtelephone monitor devices are frequently used by patients with a pacemaker and or **implantable cardioverter-defibrillator (ICD).** These patients have routine scheduled checks of their devices over the phone.

Some cardiac monitoring devices are sent directly to the patient from the supplier, complete with printed or telephone directions for the patient. When the specific time period has elapsed for the particular monitor being used, the patient is responsible for returning the device to the supplier.

Medical Assistant's Role. The medical assistant is responsible for preparing the patient, instructing the patient, checking and replacing the battery, and applying and removing the monitor.

Holter Monitor Electrode Placement. Special disposable electrodes, which are round plastic and have a strong adhesive backing, are available for the Holter monitor. These disposable electrodes contain an electrolyte gel. There may be either four or five electrodes depending on whether the monitor has a built-in ground. Notice that the leads for the Holter monitor are applied to different locations from the electrodes of a resting ECG. Table 37-2 lists the locations for lead placement.

Holter Monitor Attachment. Once the Holter monitor has been attached to the patient, the monitor should be checked for effectiveness by attaching the **test cable** to the monitor and the other end to an ECG instrument. A baseline strip can be recorded to verify the correct wave activity and lack of artifact. If there are inaccurate readings, the monitor may not have been applied properly. The medical assistant can reconnect the leads to the electrodes or reposition the electrodes and reconnect the leads (see Procedure 37-2). The skin should be cleansed with an alcohol wipe and rubbed with gauze to roughen it. Males should be shaved so that the electrodes adhere well. (See instruction for ECG lead placement.) It is essential that the leads be applied appropriately and secured with waterproof tape to allow the collection of clean, interpretable data from the Holter monitor.

Patient Activity Diary. The patient activity diary is an important component of the monitoring procedures. As noted in the Patient Education box, all activities and emotional states, and the time of their occurrence, should be noted during the 24-hour monitoring time. Symptoms such as chest pain, shortness of breath, dizziness, palpitations, and so on, and the time the event occurred should also be noted. Patient symptoms recorded while being monitored can be compared with the patient's

The following are examples of some of the daily activities that should be recorded by the patient in the patient activity diary:
- Eating meals
- Ascending and descending stairs
- Sexual activity
- Medications taken
- Times of sleep
- Smoking
- Bowel movements
- Physical exercise

notations in the activity diary and correlated to the heart's activity. Symptoms can be further noted by the patient briefly depressing an event marker button located at one end of the monitor. This places an electronic "tag" on the tape. This signal can alert the person interpreting the ECG to look for a significant event or abnormality on the tape.

Holter Monitor Removal. The patient is instructed to return to the clinic or ambulatory care center 24 hours later to have the monitor removed. Usually no appointment is necessary. The tape is analyzed by a Holter monitor scanner or by a computer. This is usually done in the ECG department of a nearby hospital. The provider can access the report from the computer with samples of any abnormalities that were picked up during the monitoring period. A follow-up appointment is scheduled with the provider to discuss the results.

Loop ECG

Another type of ambulatory electrocardiography is called *loop ECG*. It uses only two electrodes. It records a few minutes of the ECG at a time on a computer chip. It constantly records new information and discards the oldest information. Thus, the memory contains only the last few minutes of the ECG recording. When a patient has an "episode or event" (symptoms), the patient pushes the "record" button and the recording remains in the

device's memory. The recorded event is transmitted (played back) by telephone to the provider. The device then erases the event.

The recorder constantly refreshes its memory. It is suitable for capturing brief events and can be carried for long periods of time. Other types of recorders take a longer period of time, and if a patient is experiencing dizziness, it takes too long to apply a recorder. This may result in not being able to capture episodes associated with syncope.

Treadmill Stress Test or Exercise Tolerance ECG

On occasion patients have symptoms of cardiac problems that do not appear as abnormalities on a resting ECG. The provider may prescribe a treadmill stress test or exercise tolerance test to aid in the determination of the patient's diagnosis and prognosis. The test is done to diagnose heart disorders, to diagnose the probable cause of the patient's chest pain, and to assess the patient's cardiac ability after cardiac surgery. The treadmill stress test is a noninvasive ECG tracing taken under controlled conditions while the patient is closely monitored by the medical assistant and the provider. Frequent blood pressure readings are taken. The patient wears comfortable clothing and flat shoes such as sneakers with rubber soles and exercises on a treadmill at prescribed rates of speed (Figure 37-16). Electrodes are applied to the chest only.

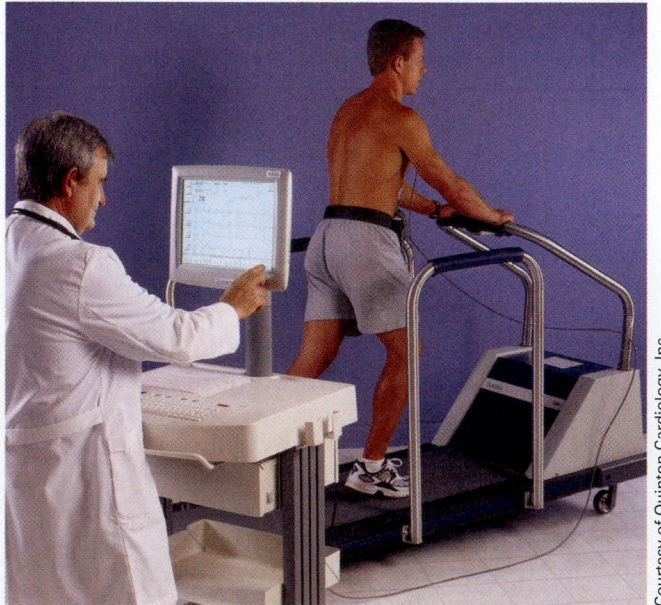

Figure 37-16 The Quest Exercise Stress System.

CRITICAL THINKING

State three purposes for using a Holter monitor and give the instructions that the patient will need to know while wearing the monitor.

As with the Holter monitor, the patient's skin should be cleansed with an alcohol wipe and rubbed with gauze to roughen it. Male patients should be shaved at the site of the electrodes to ensure electrode adherence.

The myocardium requires extra oxygen during exercise and in the presence of narrowed or obstructed coronary arteries; the additional workload on the myocardium will often be demonstrated as an abnormality on the ECG recording. The patient should have no pain, shortness of breath, or excess fatigue. If any of these or other unusual symptoms occur, the provider may terminate the test because this could indicate cardiac disease.

 At the conclusion of the test, the patient is told to rest. Monitoring continues until the vital signs and heart rate return to normal. Prior to the patient leaving the clinic, the patient should be instructed to rest, refrain from a hot bath or shower, avoid stimulants such as caffeine, and avoid extreme temperature changes for several hours.

Complications such as a myocardial infarction or a serious arrhythmia can occur during testing. Although these events are unusual, appropriate emergency equipment must be readily available, and the medical assistant should check them frequently for proper functioning. Some equipment to have available on a crash cart for cardiac emergencies include oxygen, antiarrhythmic drugs, an Ambu-bag, a defibrillator, an endotracheal tube, and a laryngoscope. The medical assistant is responsible for checking the supplies and plugging in the defibrillator.

Further diagnostic tests such as **cardiac catheterization** (angiogram) may be necessary to diagnose the extent of the atherosclerosis buildup and obstruction of the coronary arteries. A cardiac catheterization is an invasive procedure that is performed in an acute care setting on an outpatient basis. In order to visualize the coronary arteries and determine the extent of disease, if any, a large catheter is inserted into the femoral or brachial artery and threaded carefully to the origin of the coronary vessels via the vena cava. Once the specially shaped tip of the catheter is engaged in the coronary artery, radiopaque contrast medium is injected into the vessel and visualized using radiographic techniques. The course of intervention is determined at this point if disease is noted.

Thallium Stress Test

Thallium stress test is similar to a treadmill stress test in that the patient has an ECG tracing while exercising on the treadmill after having been given an injection of a radioactive substance such as thallium. The test shows how well blood flows to the heart muscle. It can help diagnose coronary artery blockage, the cause of a patient's chest pain, cardiac function, and status after myocardial infarction, and can check the level of exercise a patient can safely engage in.

The thallium is injected intravenously while the patient is being monitored on the treadmill and is exercising. After the stress test, the patient is "scanned" under a machine in the diagnostic imaging department. The patient leaves the department for 3 or 4 hours (rests), then returns, and another scan is done. Therefore, the patient has been "scanned" during exercise and after a rest period of a few hours.

The thallium intravenous injection mixes with blood in the bloodstream and in the arteries and enters the heart muscle cells. If a portion of the heart does not receive a normal blood supply, then a smaller amount of thallium will be present in those heart muscle cells. To the cardiologist this finding indicates a degree of block in the heart's blood supply. The patient most likely has ischemia of the heart muscle or an infarct of the heart muscle.

Patients who cannot tolerate an exercise stress test because of serious heart disease or patients with special needs, such as wheelchair-bound patients, can be given a vasodilator and undergo the ECG test seated in a chair or wheelchair. The medication will cause an increase in heart rate, thus simulating the stress of walking on a treadmill. The thallium stress test is performed in the outpatient department of the hospital or in a cardiology office or clinic.

Echocardiography/Ultrasonography

Echocardiography is a noninvasive, diagnostic test that uses ultrasound (ultrahigh-frequency sound waves) to image the internal structures of the heart. X-rays are not useful. General anatomy, myocardial function, valve function, and heart chamber size can be evaluated. Echocardiography may be performed in a cardiologist's office.

During **ultrasonography**, a handheld **transducer** acts as a transmitter and receiver of the high-frequency sound waves as it is held against the chest wall and moved over the heart area. As the sound waves go through the skin and hit internal structures, echoes are sent back to the transducer. A machine converts the images when the various structures provide different echoes. The images can then be examined by a computer and converted into photographs and films of structures and blood flow.

There is little patient preparation other than to have the patient lie on the examination table with the four-limb leads of a 12-lead electrocardiograph attached. The test is usually performed by a **sonographer**. The provider views the results later and informs the patient.

Coronary MRI and CT Imaging

Magnetic resonance imaging (MRI) is useful in identifying the location and thickness of cardiac muscle scars due to damage. Although neither MRI nor computed tomography (CT) has replaced x-ray angiography (XRA) as the clinical standard for the diagnosis of coronary stenosis, their use in determining if a vessel is open is increasing. Recently, 64-slice multidetector-row CT angiography (CTA) has shown potential as an alternative to x-ray angiography for the identification of coronary blockages.

CARDIAC PROCEDURES

The following section discusses cardiac procedures performed for heart disease and arrhythmias. Some cardiac procedures for diagnosing diseases of the heart are computerized, and the results are stored in the patient's electronic medical record. The data are accessible on demand.

Procedures for Heart Disease

Percutaneous transluminal coronary angioplasty (PTCA) is a procedure that widens a narrowed or blocked coronary artery. One type of PTCA is balloon angioplasty. A catheter with a deflated balloon is inserted into the patient's femoral artery and gently advanced to the coronary arteries via the inferior vena cava. Once the tip of the catheter is engaged in the correct coronary artery, a very thin and flexible wire is advanced through the catheter and down the course of the coronary artery, past or through any lesion that has been identified during the coronary angioplasty. An additional, smaller catheter that holds a compressed balloon in various lengths is advanced over the flexible wire and positioned at the site of the blockage. Very precise inflation pressures and times are applied by the cardiologist with the hope of opening the occluded artery and establishing blood flow downstream to the heart muscle.

For complicated lesions, it is sometimes necessary to utilize a coronary stent. Stents are small mesh tubes that are compressed around a balloon that is much like the angioplasty balloon. Using radiographic visualization, the stent is positioned within the area of blockage. As the balloon is slowly, carefully inflated, the stent is deployed against the wall of the vessel. Once the stent is deployed, all of the interventional catheters and wires are removed. Over time, the stent becomes a part of the vessel wall after the inner layer of cells or endothelium regrows over the area that was stented. Thus, a stent is a permanent intervention and there is a standard regimen of care to assure the best outcomes after insertion of a stent that includes the use of anticoagulant medications.

Other cardiac procedures that can be performed for heart disease are atherectomy and laser angioplasty. In atherectomy, the provider uses a very small device on the end of the catheter to cut away the blocked area inside the coronary artery. In laser angioplasty, the provider uses a laser beam to destroy the blockage in the artery.

Coronary artery bypass is a procedure in which a portion of a vein (typically the saphenous) is transplanted into one or more of the heart's coronary arteries. The transplanted vein circumvents or bypasses the blocked coronary artery, thus reestablishing blood supply to that portion of the heart. This is a major procedure and the recovery time is extended.

A catheter with a large balloon can be used to open a standard (normal) valve. The balloon is inflated and, as in the angioplasty, the valve can be loosened. The catheter with balloon is removed after the procedure.

A heart valve can be repaired or replaced. In a replacement procedure, a tissue or mechanical valve replaces the heart's damaged valve.

Procedures for Arrhythmias

A cardiac electrophysiologist is a specialist who provides care to patients with arrhythmias. After a study by the cardiac electrophysiologist determines the source of the patient's arrhythmia within the electrical conduction system of the heart, a catheter is inserted into the femoral artery and a special device with radio waves is "aimed" at the source of the abnormal heart rhythm. This is known as *cardiac ablation*. The tiny scar produced prevents the electrical conduction system from traveling through the scarred area, resulting in normal rhythm.

A permanent battery-operated pacemaker can be surgically implanted into the patient's chest wall for treatment of certain types of arrhythmias. Wires from the pacemaker are inserted into the heart to provide a steady, regular heartbeat.

An implantable cardioverter defibrillator (ICD) is a device surgically implanted into the patient's chest wall with wires leading into the heart. When the patient's heart rate is extremely low or the patient's heart stops beating, the defibrillator delivers a small electric shock to jar the heart back into a normal rhythm (works like the AED; see section on defibrillation and Chapter 9).

Two other diagnostic tools for cardiac disease are cardiac computed tomography (CCT) and cardiac magnetic resonance (CMR). Both are very useful tools, but they expose the patient to radiation and they are very expensive. Some cardiologists believe echocardiography (no radiation exposure) is just as useful in diagnosing heart disease.

PROCEDURE 37-1

Perform Single-Channel or Multichannel Electrocardiogram

STANDARD PRECAUTIONS:

PURPOSE:

To obtain an accurate, graphic, artifact-free reading of the electrical activity of the patient's heart to identify arrhythmias, estimate damage caused by myocardial infarction, assess effects of cardiac medication, determine if electrolyte imbalance is present, identify cardiac ischemia, and determine the effects of hypertension or other disorders on the heart.

EQUIPMENT/SUPPLIES:

Examination or ECG table with pillow and sheet or blanket
Patient gown (open in front)
Automated electrocardiograph with patient cable wires
Alligator clips
Electropads (sensors)
ECG paper
Alcohol wipes
Gauze squares
Mounting form/card
Razor

PROCEDURE STEPS:

1. Perform tracing in a quiet, warm, and comfortable room away from electrical equipment that may cause artifacts. RATIONALE: Patient is less apprehensive in a quiet atmosphere. AC interference is minimized when ECG is performed away from other electrical equipment.

2. Wash hands, gather equipment, *identify the patient, and explain the procedure to the patient, speaking at the patient's level of understanding.* RATIONALE: Following these universal steps minimizes transmission of microorganisms and reassures patient.

3. Have the patient remove clothing from the waist up and uncover lower legs; nylon stockings must be removed; socks can be worn. RATIONALE: Electropads must be placed on bare skin for optimum conductivity of electricity. Provide a sheet or blanket for privacy and warmth. Place the patient in supine position on the examination table with arms and legs supported. Pillows can be used under the knees and head. RATIONALE: All four limbs and chest must be uncovered for proper electrode placement.

4. Explain that the procedure is painless and why it is necessary not to move or talk during the procedure. RATIONALE: Patient cooperation ensures good quality tracing.

5. Place the electrocardiograph with the power cord pointing away from the patient. Do not allow the cable to go underneath the table. RATIONALE: Helps reduce AC interference.

6. Apply the limb electropads (sensors) first. Apply the sensors to the fleshy parts of the four limbs. If the sensor does not adhere well, use an alcohol wipe on the skin, let it dry, and apply a new sensor. Shave sites if necessary. RATIONALE: Skin oils can be removed by alcohol, thus improving

(continues)

Procedure 37-1 (continued)

the adherence of the sensor. By removing excess hair on the chest, the sensor will adhere better. Place sensors on a nonbony, nonmuscular (fleshy) area of the upper arms and lower legs. Arm sensors should have tab pointing down, leg sensors point upward. RATIONALE: Artifact can be reduced if sensors are placed on nonbony, nonmuscular areas of the limbs. Directing tabs properly reduces tension on the electrodes.

7. Place the sensors on the chest wall on the appropriate intercostal spaces with sensors pointing downward. Shave chest sites if necessary.

8. Attach lead wires from the ECG machine to each sensor using alligator clips, special clips applied to the ends of the lead wires (Figure 37-17 A–B). Be sure to connect lead wires to the correct sensors. Lead wires are labeled with abbreviations (RA, LA, RL, LL, and V or C) and are color-coded as follows: RA 5 white; LA 5 black; RL 5 green; LL 5 red, V or C 5 (chest) brown or multicolored depending on machine model. The lead wires should follow the patient's body contour (Figure 37-17 C–D). RATIONALE: Following body contour prevents sensors from being pulled off.

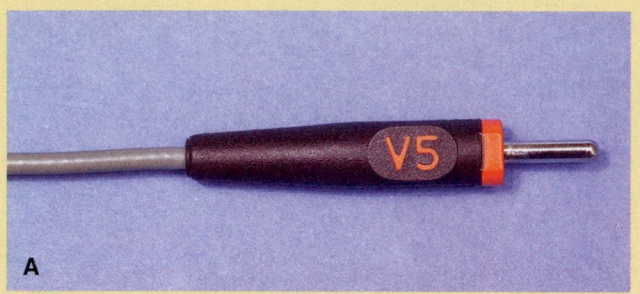

A

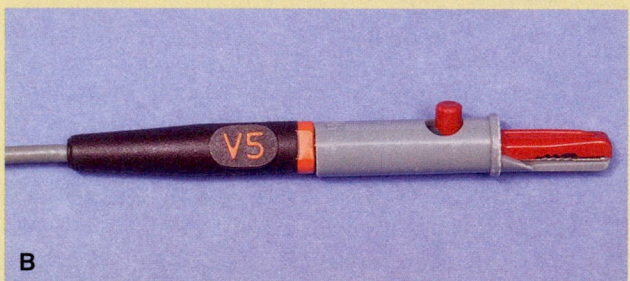

B

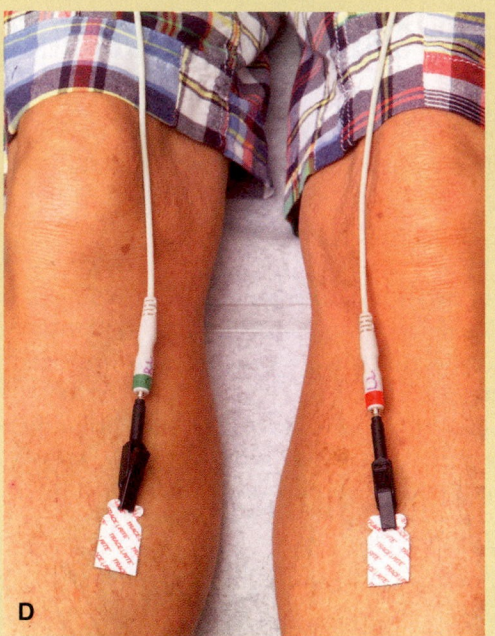

D

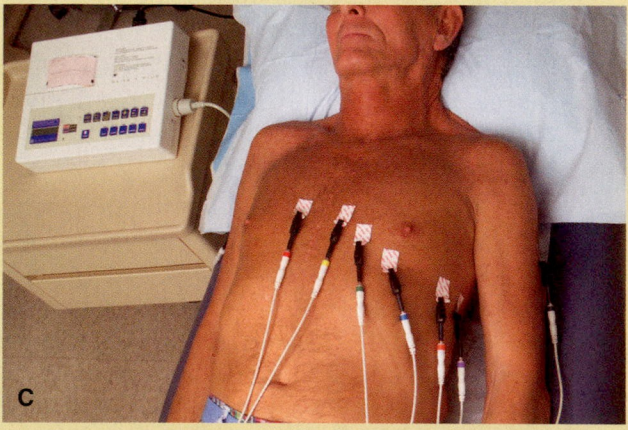

C

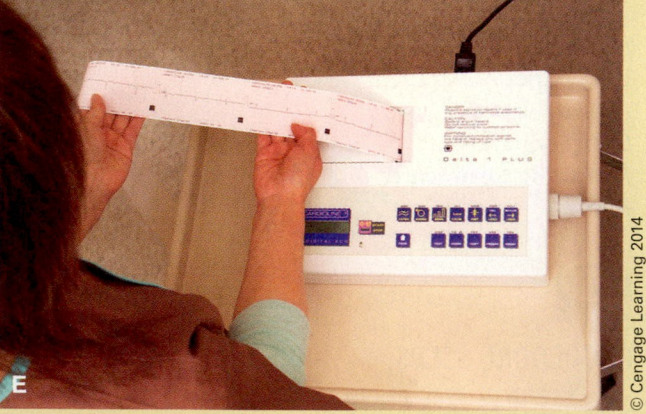

E

© Cengage Learning 2014

Figure 37-17 (A) Lead wires with nothing attached. (B) Alligator clip attached to top of lead wires. (C) Lead wires attached to the patient's chest and arms. (D) Lead wires attached to the patient's legs. (E) The machine prints each lead sequentially on a strip of ECG paper.

Procedure 37-1 (continued)

9. The patient cable is supported either on the table or on the patient's abdomen. Plug the patient cable into the electrocardiograph.

10. Turn the instrument to ON.

11. Enter information (patient name, date of birth, age, height, weight, sex, identification number, and cardiac medications the patient is presently taking). RATIONALE: The ECG machine automatically prints the information entered onto the ECG printout.

12. Remind the patient not to talk and to try not to move. (If the patient has a neuromuscular condition such as Parkinson's disease and cannot remain still, try having the patient slide his or her hands under the buttocks.) RATIONALE: Somatic tremor artifact may be lessened when the patient's hands are slid under the buttocks.

13. Press AUTO and the machine will automatically record and standardize the tracing. RATIONALE: Standardization ensures a dependable and accurate ECG.

14. The single-channel machine prints each lead sequentially on a strip of ECG paper (Figure 37-17E). A multichannel machine prints the tracing on an 8½ × 11-inch sheet of paper.

15. Check the quality of the tracing (artifacts, low voltage) before disconnecting lead wires. If it is necessary to repeat the tracing, first correct the problem that is causing a poor quality tracing. RATIONALE: Checking the tracing before removing the electropad sensors will save time if the ECG must be repeated.

16. Disconnect lead wires and remove the electropad sensor from the patient.

17. Assist patient as needed.

18. Be certain the patient information is on the tracing before giving it to the provider to read.

19. If the tracing is a single-channel tracing, cut and mount it, remembering to handle it carefully. Place in patient's record.

20. Document procedure in patient's chart or electronic medical record.

DOCUMENTATION:

4/19/20XX 2:00 PM   Twelve-lead ECG completed. Tracing given to Dr. Woo. Patient cooperative and seemed comfortable throughout procedure and says she "feels fine" after tracing. W. Slawson, CMA (AAMA)—————————

PROCEDURE 37-2
Holter Monitor Application (Cassette and Digital)

STANDARD PRECAUTIONS:

PURPOSE:
To detect sporadic cardiac arrhythmias, to determine correlation of symptoms with activity, and to evaluate chest pain and cardiac status after pacemaker implantation or after acute myocardial infarction.

EQUIPMENT/SUPPLIES:
Holter monitor
Patient activity diary
Blank magnetic tape or flash memory card
Disposable electrodes
Razor
Alcohol wipes
Gauze
Carrying case
Belt or shoulder strap

PROCEDURE STEPS:
1. Wash hands and assemble equipment.

2. Prepare the equipment by removing old (used) battery from the monitor and replacing it with a

(continues)

Procedure 37-2 (continued)

new battery. Insert a blank magnetic tape or flash card into the monitor. RATIONALE: Installing a new battery each 24-hour period will ensure the monitor will function because it will have sufficient power.

3. Wash hands.

4. *Identify the patient and explain the procedure, speaking at the patient's level of understanding.* RATIONALE: Adherence to patient guidelines helps ensure an accurate tracing.

5. Have patient remove clothing from the waist up.

6. Have patient sit on the examination table or chair. RATIONALE: This allows for patient comfort and relaxation and for the medical assistant to place the electrodes appropriately.

7. Locate the correct electrode placement sites. The skin must be prepared in the following way:

   a. Dry shave patient's chest at each electrode site if chest is hairy.

   b. Cleanse the shaved area with an alcohol wipe. Let area dry.

   c. Abrade the skin slightly with a dry 4 × 4 gauze. Areas should be red. RATIONALE: Shaved site and abraded skin help the electrodes to adhere better to the skin and facilitate easier removal.

8. Take the electrodes from the package and peel away the backing from one of them (electrode should be moist). Continue to remove electrodes one by one and attach as in Step 9.

9. Apply adhesive-backed electrode to the appropriate sites by applying firm pressure at the center of the electrode and moving outward toward the edges. Run your fingers along the outer rim to ensure firm attachment. Avoid moving from one side of electrode to the other. Gel could be forced out and could cause interference. RATIONALE: Firmly attached electrodes ensure a good quality tracing.

10. Attach the lead wires to the electrodes. Connect them to the patient cable.

11. Plug the monitor into the electrocardiograph with the test cable. Run a baseline tracing (not necessary with digital monitor). RATIONALE: Running a baseline tracing will validate proper setup of electrodes and confirm there is no malfunction of the leads or cable.

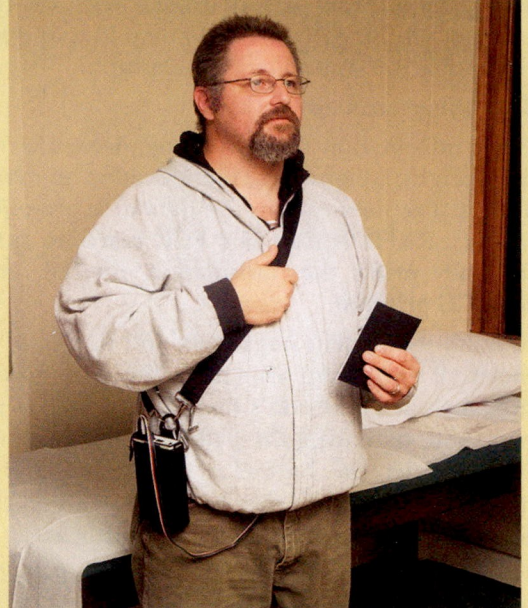

Figure 37-18 Correct placement of Holter monitor on patient.

12. Place the electrode cable so that it extends from between the buttons of the patient's shirt or from below the bottom of the shirt.

13. Place the recorder into its carrying case and either attach it to the patient's belt or over the patient's shoulder. Be certain there is no pulling on the lead wires (Figure 37-18). RATIONALE: Pulling on electrodes could cause them to become detached.

14. Plug the electrode cable into the monitor. Record the starting time in the patient activity log (diary). These data will already be recorded in a digital monitor. RATIONALE: The beginning time is noted to correlate cardiac activity with the patient activity log.

15. Help patient get dressed.

16. Give the activity log to the patient, being certain that the patient information is completed. RATIONALE: The activity log helps correlate cardiac activity with patient symptoms.

17. Inform patient what time the following day the monitor will be removed. Remind the patient to bring along the activity log/diary.

18. Wash hands.

© Cengage Learning 2014

Procedure 37-2 (continued)

19. Document procedure in patient's record or electronic medical record.

20. Upon the patient's return 24 hours later, take the patient's electrodes off, remove flash memory card, accept cassette, remove battery.

21. Document patient returned with equipment.

DOCUMENTATION:

3/2/20XX 10:00 AM   Holter monitor applied. Patient given complete written instructions and restrictions and seems to understand them well. Time and date noted on activity log. Patient reminded to return to cardiac clinic at the same time tomorrow (10:15 AM) to have monitor removed and also to bring the activity diary. Patient given after-hours number if he needs assistance. J. Guerro, CMA (AAMA) ——————————

3/3/20XX 10:00 AM   Holter monitor electrodes removed from patient. Cassette and activity log returned or flash memory card removed for later analysis on the computer analysis system. J. Guerro, CMA (AAMA) ——————————

CASE STUDY 37-1

Refer to the scenario at the beginning of the chapter.
   Wanda can empathize better with her patients now that she herself has had a baseline ECG.

CASE STUDY REVIEW

1. The feelings Wanda had while having her tracing are experienced by many patients. Explain what you can do for your patients to allay their fears when they are getting ready for an ECG and during the tracing.

CASE STUDY 37-2

Abigail Johnson, who is in her mid-70s, arrives at the urgent care center reporting chest pain. She has been seen on two other occasions for similar pain and has a history of diabetes, hypertension, arteriosclerotic heart disease, and angina pectoris. Medical assistant Wanda Slawson immediately alerts Dr. Rice of Mrs. Johnson's chest pain and then takes her into the cardiac examination and treatment room. Dr. Rice tells Wanda to have Mrs. Johnson take one of her nitroglycerin tablets and to perform an ECG on her. Mrs. Johnson is restless and anxious as Wanda prepares for the ECG and while the tracing is in progress. There is significant somatic tremor. Wanda attempts to allay Mrs. Johnson's apprehension to obtain a good quality ECG. The patient's pain subsides within a few minutes and she begins to feel better.

CASE STUDY REVIEW

1. What immediate action could Wanda have taken if Mrs. Johnson's pain had not subsided?

2. Mrs. Johnson tells Wanda that Dr. Rice explained arteriosclerotic heart disease and angina pectoris to her, but that she was nervous and understood little and that she is embarrassed to admit that to Dr. Rice. How can Wanda explain, in language that the patient can comprehend, what causes arteriosclerotic heart disease and angina, and what Mrs. Johnson experiences during an attack of angina? What strategies can Wanda teach Mrs. Johnson to promote healthier habits and prevent more serious heart problems?

3. Research community resources are available for persons with Mrs. Johnson's heart condition. Explain how Mrs. Johnson can locate them and how she could benefit from them.

CASE STUDY 37-3

George Matthews, a 79-year-old patient of Dr. Abbott, has a history of cardiovascular heart disease. He tells Dr. Abbott that today he has been experiencing "palpitations and slow and fast heartbeats and sometimes dizziness." Dr. Abbott orders a resting ECG that shows no evidence of arrhythmia and decides that a Holter monitor electrocardiograph for Mr. Matthews might be helpful in diagnosing a cardiac arrhythmia.

CASE STUDY REVIEW

1. Describe why Dr. Abbott ordered Holter monitor electro-cardiography for Mr. Matthews.
2. What instructions will you give to Mr. Matthews about wearing the monitor?
3. Mr. Matthews says he is not certain what activities should be recorded in the patient activity diary. Explain what they are and the reason for their importance.

SUMMARY

Electrocardiography is a noninvasive, painless procedure that is helpful in diagnosing heart arrhythmias, ischemia, and effects of cardiac medications. Wires with sensors are attached to the patient's arms, legs, and chest. The electrocardiograph amplifies the electrical currents generated by the electrical cells of the heart. A series of deflections (waves) is recorded on special ECG paper when a heated stylus on the electrocardiograph moves across the paper. The cardiac cycles that appear are then interpreted by the provider. The recording or tracing, known as an ECG, represents the heart's rate, rhythm, and other myocardial actions. Each of the 12 leads of the recording becomes part of the patient's permanent record.

In addition to a resting ECG, other types of electrocardiography can be done. Cardiac stress testing is done while the patient is physically challenged to perform increasingly strenuous exercises. The heart's tolerance to the increased demands placed on it during exercise can be observed and recorded while the patient is being closely monitored. This type of electrocardiography helps determine cardiac health and arrhythmias that would not be evident if a resting ECG were done.

Holter electrocardiography or ambulatory cardiac monitoring is an ECG test done as the patient goes about normal daily activities. The patient wears chest leads and carries a small recording device on a belt or on a strap over the shoulder for a period of 24 hours and documents activities in the patient activity diary. This type of electrocardiography helps diagnose cardiac arrhythmias that occur sporadically and may be difficult to capture on a resting ECG because of their unpredictability. Echocardiography is a diagnostic test that uses ultrasound to image the internal structures of the heart. Myocardial function, valvular function or defects, and chamber size can be determined.

In most cases, the medical assistant is responsible for patient preparation; patient education; operation of the electrocardiograph; elimination of artifacts; mounting, labeling, and placing ECG readings into the patient's file; and maintenance and care of the equipment. The diagnostic value of the test depends on the medical assistant's accuracy and skill.

STUDY FOR SUCCESS

To reinforce your knowledge and skills of information presented in this chapter:

- Review the *Key Terms*
- Role-play with other students to apply attributes of professionalism pertinent to this chapter.
- Consider the *Case Studies* and discuss your conclusions
- Answer the questions in the *Certification Review*

STUDY FOR SUCCESS (CONTINUED)

- Apply your knowledge by completing the Activities in the *Study Guide* and the *Games and Quizzes* in the StudyWARE (StudyWARE) software on the *Premium Website*

- 🛡 Perform the *Procedures* using the *Competency Assessment Checklists* in the *Competency Manual*.

- Practice your problem-solving skills with the *Critical Thinking Challenge 3.0* on the *Premium Website*.

Additional resources for this chapter include:

- Module 23 of the *Medical Assisting Learning Lab*

- *CourseMate for Delmar's Comprehensive Medical Assisting*

- *WebTutor for Delmar's Comprehensive Medical Assisting*

CERTIFICATION REVIEW

1. Which of the following is the most common type of artifact?
   a. Somatic tremor
   b. AC interference
   c. Wandering bascline
   d. Interrupted baseline

2. Which of the following may cause somatic tremor?
   a. Too much electrolyte
   b. Cable across patient's lap
   c. Corroded sensors
   d. Parkinson's disease

3. One cardiac cycle (heartbeat) takes approximately how long?
   a. 0.2 second
   b. 0.4 second
   c. 0.6 second
   d. 0.8 second

4. Which of the following indicates ventricular depolarization?
   a. QRS complex
   b. P wave
   c. T wave
   d. ST segment

5. Another name for V leads is:
   a. precordial
   b. augmented
   c. standard
   d. limb

6. An electrocardiograph is known as a 12-lead ECG. How many leads are placed on the patient?
   a. 6 leads
   b. 10 leads
   c. 12 leads
   d. 14 leads

7. Which of the following is a common cause of premature atrial contractions (PACs)?
   a. Coffee
   b. Tobacco
   c. Stress
   d. All of the above

8. Defibrillators are indicated to:
   a. deliver a countershock to restore normal heart rhythm
   b. deliver a countershock to keep respiratory rhythm
   c. deliver a countershock and work as a pacemaker
   d. deliver a countershock to synchronize pulse and respiration

9. A treadmill or stress test is used to diagnose cardiac problems. Prior to the test, a patient must:
   a. rest the day before
   b. avoid stimulants like coffee, caffeine, and tobacco
   c. remain NPO
   d. none of the above

10. When reading a patient's chart, the medical assistant sees a notation that the patient has had a PTCA. The professional medical assistant is aware that this means:
    a. partial transplant of coronary arteries
    b. percutaneous transition of coronary arteries
    c. percutaneous transluminal coronary angioplasty
    d. none of the above

REFERENCES/BIBLIOGRAPHY

Delaune, S. C., & Ladner, P. (2002). *Fundamentals of nursing standards and practice* (2nd ed.). Clifton Park, NY: Delmar Cengage Learning.

Fozzard, H. A., Haber, E., Jennings, R. B., et al. (Eds.) (1991). *The heart and cardiovascular system* (p. 2193). New York: Raven Press.

Heartsaver AED. Retrieved September 18, 2009, from http://www.americanheart.org

Passanisi, C. (2001). *Electrocardiology essentials.* Clifton Park, NY: Delmar Cengage Learning.

Pearlman, J. D., et al. (2011). *Imaging in coronary artery disease.* MedScape Reference: Drugs, Diseases & Procedures. Retrieved May 12, 2011, from http://emedicine.medscape.com/article/349040-overview

Taber's cyclopedic medical dictionary (20th ed., 2005). Philadelphia: F. A. Davis.

Van Belle, E., et al. (1998). Endothelial regrowth after arterial injury: from vascular repair to therapeutics. *Cardiovascular Research*, 38(1), 54–68, Retrieved May 11, 2002, from http://cardiovascres.oxfordjournals.org/content/38/1/54.full

UNIT IX
Laboratory Procedures

CHAPTER 38
Regulatory Guidelines in the Medical Laboratory 1174

CHAPTER 39
Introduction to the Medical Laboratory 1194

CHAPTER 40
Phlebotomy: Venipuncture and Capillary Puncture........ 1218

CHAPTER 41
Hematology 1266

CHAPTER 42
Urinalysis 1292

CHAPTER 43
Basic Microbiology 1326

CHAPTER 44
Specialty Laboratory Tests 1358

Regulatory Guidelines in the Medical Laboratory

OUTLINE

Clinical Laboratory Improvement Amendments of 1988

The Intention of CLIA '88

General Program Description

Categories of Testing

Contents of the Law

Criteria for PPMP

Criteria for CLIA Waived Tests

CLIA '88 Regulation for Quality Control in Automated Hematology

Aftermath of CLIA '88

Impact of CLIA on Medical Assistants

Where to Find More Information Regarding CLIA '88

OSHA Regulations

The Standard for Occupational Exposure to Hazardous Chemicals in the Laboratory

Chemical Hygiene Plan

OSHA Regulations and Students

Avoiding Exposure to Chemicals

Ergonomics and Cumulative Trauma Disorders

LEARNING OUTCOMES

1. Define, spell, and pronounce the key terms as presented in the glossary.
2. Identify and discuss the contents of the law of CLIA '88 and its importance to the medical assistant.
3. Describe how CLIA '88 regulates the use of quality control in automated hematology instruments.
4. Recall the categories of testing and list several from the waived category.
5. Describe CMS form 116 and explain its purpose.
6. Identify personal safety precautions as established by the Occupational Safety and Health Administration (OSHA).
7. Describe the importance of Material Safety Data Sheets (MSDS) in the health care setting.
8. Identify and comply with safety signs, symbols, and labels.
9. Evaluate the work environment to identify safe versus unsafe working conditions and safety techniques that can be used to prevent accidents and maintain a safe work environment.
10. Analyze the professionalism questions and apply them to this chapter's content.

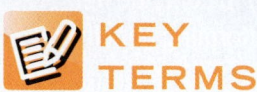

KEY TERMS

aegis

body fluid

calibration

certificate of
  waiver (COW)

communicable

excretion

fume hood

mandate

Material Safety Data
  Sheet (MSDS)

medical asepsis

proficiency testing

provider-performed
  microscopy
  procedure (PPMP)

quality assurance

quality control

reimbursement

requisition

secretion

waived

ATTRIBUTES OF PROFESSIONALISM

Competence
- Did you pay attention to detail?
- Were you knowledgeable and accountable?
- Did you recognize the importance of local, state, and federal legislation and regulations in the practice setting?

Initiative
- Did you seek out opportunities to expand your knowledge base?
- Did you develop a strategic plan to achieve your goals? Was your plan realistic?

Integrity
- Did you acknowledge the scope of practice of other health care professionals?
- Did you immediately report any error you had made?

SCENARIO

At Inner City Health Care, Dr. Susan Rice ordered a complete urinalysis for patient May Pankey. Dr. Rice's medical assistant, Wanda Slawson, CMA (AAMA), has obtained the specimen from the patient, has performed the physical examination and the chemical examination of the urine, and has documented her findings on the lab report form. She has also spun a test tube of urine in the centrifuge and has prepared a slide of the sediment for Dr. Rice to examine under the microscope. While Wanda is waiting for the doctor, she examines the slide to see if she can identify any abnormalities. She will compare her findings with Dr. Rice's findings to see how closely she comes to correctly identifying the cellular components in the urine sediment. This is one way for Wanda to continue her education on a daily basis while performing her clinical duties.

INTRODUCTION

Laboratory safety is a concern for all—management, staff, and patients. An unsafe work environment and work practices can threaten the emotional and physical health of the health care worker, as well as the patient. Injuries are costly on many levels: personally to the injured individual, lost work days, workers' compensation, medical treatment, potential legal action, and potential fines from regulatory agencies. These situations have a direct effect on the individuals involved, but they also have an indirect effect by lowering staff morale, ultimately resulting in less productivity. Management's response to safety is the key. Appropriate orientation, annual reviews, periodic drills, and consistent enforcement of staff adherence to policy are all part of a successful laboratory safety program.

All health care providers continually come into contact with patients who are ill. Some patients have **communicable** or contagious diseases; others may have a suppressed immune system that does not protect them from infection. In the course of performing your duties as a medical assistant, you will be in contact with blood and **body fluids** that may be highly infectious. It is of extreme importance that your health and safety, as well as the health and safety of your patients, be protected.

There are a number of infection control measures that can be used to reduce the transmission of bloodborne and other pathogens. **Medical asepsis**, also known as infection control, consists of procedures and practices that health care professionals use to prevent the spread of infection (see Chapter 22). State and federal agencies also have established policies, procedures, and guidelines for health care providers and employers to follow to reduce the risk for transmission of infectious diseases. This chapter, as well as Chapter 22, examines the major guidelines.

The Centers for Disease Control and Prevention (CDC) in Atlanta, Georgia, a division of the United States Public Health Service, is an agency that investigates various diseases in an attempt to control them and makes recommendations on how to prevent the spread of disease. The CDC issued the system of seven isolation categories for patients with infectious diseases and recommended the guidelines known as Universal Precautions. In 1996, the CDC released Standard Precautions, which represent the most current and comprehensive approach to infection control. The CDC Guidelines for Standard Precautions and Universal Precautions are covered thoroughly in Chapter 22. This chapter focuses on the federal regulations of the Clinical Laboratory Improvement Amendments of 1988 (CLIA '88) and the Occupational Safety and Health Administration (OSHA) in relation to the providers' office laboratory (POL).

CLIA '88 and OSHA, together with the CDC, regulate the safety of patients and health care workers. CLIA '88 comes under the **aegis**, or protection, of the Centers for Medicare & Medicaid Services (CMS), formerly known as the Health Care Financing Administration (HCFA) of the U.S. Department of Health and Human Services (DHHS) of the federal government. OSHA comes under the U.S. Department of Labor. Both agencies require that health care settings, including clinical laboratories, adhere to the strict regulations that they set forth.

The purpose of CLIA '88 is to safeguard the public by regulating all testing of specimens taken from the human body. The purpose of OSHA is to require employers to ensure employee safety in regard to occupational exposure to potentially harmful substances.

CLIA '88 and OSHA guidelines are discussed separately in this chapter. Keep in mind as you go through this chapter that CLIA '88 is designed to protect patients, and OSHA regulations are designed to protect workers. Table 38-1 summarizes the guidelines and purposes of CDC, CLIA '88, and OSHA.

Table 38-1 Federal Health and Safety Guidelines

Guidelines	Issuing Agency	Purpose
Standard Precautions	Centers for Disease Control and Prevention (CDC), U.S. Public Health Service	Issued in 1996 to augment and synthesize Universal Precautions and techniques known as body substance isolation (BSI). Standard Precautions contain measures intended to protect all health care providers, patients, and visitors from infectious diseases.
Transmission-Based Precautions	CDC	Designed to reduce the risk for airborne, droplet, and contact transmission of pathogens. These are used in addition to Standard Precautions and are intended for specific categories of patients.
Universal Blood and Body Fluid Precautions (Universal Precautions)	CDC	Released in 1985 to assist health care providers to greatly reduce the risk for contracting or transmitting infectious diseases, particularly AIDS and hepatitis B.
Clinical Laboratory Improvement Amendments of 1988 (CLIA '88)	Centers for Medicare & Medicaid Services (CMS), U.S. Department of Health and Human Services (DHHS)	Safeguards the public by regulating all testing of specimens taken from the body.
Occupational Safety and Health Administration (OSHA) Guidelines	OSHA, U.S. Department of Labor	Requires employers to ensure employee safety in regard to occupational exposure to potentially harmful substances.

© Cengage Learning 2014

SPOTLIGHT ON CERTIFICATION

RMA Content Outline
- Medical law
- Asepsis
- Laboratory procedures (safety)
- First aid

CMA (AAMA) Content Outline
- Medicolegal guidelines and requirements
- Principles of infection control
- Processing specimens
- Quality control
- Preplanned action

CMAS Content Outline
- Legal and ethical considerations
- Asepsis in the medical office
- Medical office emergencies
- Safety
- Supplies and equipment

CLINICAL LABORATORY IMPROVEMENT AMENDMENTS OF 1988

CLIA '88 was designed to set safety policies and procedures that protect patients.

In 1988, there was a public outcry as a result of articles published in the *Washington Post* and the *Wall Street Journal* and televised reports of deaths that were attributed to misread Pap smears. The public wanted action taken to ensure its safety, particularly in regard to laboratory testing. The outcry prompted the federal government to become more involved in regulating laboratories.

Although CLIA had been enacted into law in 1967, the issue of the misread Pap smears caused Congress to reexamine the regulations it had set forth in 1967. Thus, CLIA '88 was passed and included amendments to the original law. The amended regulations took effect on September 1, 1992.

States can seek exemptions from the CLIA standards if they have regulations that are comparable to those imposed by CLIA. If the federal government grants the state an exemption, laboratories in that state are under the control of state standards and applicable fees, not federal standards and fees.

The Intention of CLIA '88

The intent of CLIA '88 is to protect the public by regulating all laboratory tests performed on specimens taken from the human body, that is, tissue, blood, and body **secretions** and **excretions**, which are used in the diagnosis, treatment, and prevention of disease. Previous regulations (Medicare, Medicaid, and CLIA '67) were based on the site and scope of the laboratory testing. CLIA '88 regulates laboratory testing regardless of site, scope, volume, or frequency. As of May 2012, registered CLIA laboratories total more than 225,000, with POLs making up more than 50% of the total. The regulations require that all laboratories in the United States and its territories meet performance requirements that are based on how complex a test is and the risk factors that are associated with incorrect test results. Laboratories must comply with the requirements to be certified by the DHHS.

It is necessary to understand what the CLIA '88 regulations encompass and how they impact medical assistants and other health care workers who participate in testing human specimens. It is important because all laboratories, including POLs, must abide by the CLIA law.

CLIA '88 regulations are based on the complexity of tests performed and they affect all aspects of the laboratory. They specify the type of test performed, personnel involved in testing, and **quality control**.

General Program Description

Congress passed CLIA in 1988, establishing quality standards for all laboratory testing to ensure the accuracy, reliability, and timeliness of patient test results regardless of where the test was performed. A laboratory is defined as any facility that performs laboratory testing on specimens derived from humans for the purpose of providing information for the diagnosis, prevention, or treatment of disease, or impairment or assessment of health. CLIA is user-fee funded; therefore, all costs of administering the program must be covered by the regulated facilities.

Regulations were published based on the complexity of the test method; thus, the more complicated the test, the more stringent the

requirements. **Provider-performed microscopy procedure (PPMP)**; and high complexity. CLIA specifies quality standards for proficiency testing (PT), patient test management, quality control, personnel qualifications, and **quality assurance** as applicable. Because problems in cytology laboratories were the impetus for CLIA, there are also specific cytology requirements.

CMS is charged with the implementation of CLIA, including laboratory registration, fee collection, surveys, surveyor guidelines and training, enforcement, approvals of PT providers, accrediting organizations, and exempt states. The CDC is responsible for test categorization and CLIA studies.

To enroll in the CLIA program, laboratories must first register by completing an application, pay fees, be surveyed if applicable, and become certified. CLIA fees are based on the certificate requested by the laboratory (i.e., waived, PPMP, accreditation, or compliance) and the annual volume and types of testing performed. Waived and PPMP laboratories may apply directly for their certificate because they are not subject to routine inspections. Those laboratories that must be surveyed routinely—that is, those performing moderate- or high-complexity testing—can choose whether they wish to be surveyed by CMS or by a private accrediting organization. The CMS survey process is outcome-oriented and uses a quality assurance focus and an educational approach to assess compliance (Table 38-2).

Data indicate that CLIA has helped to improve the quality of testing in the United States. The total

Table 38-2 How to Tell What Level of CLIA Is Required

If these tests are performed	This type of certificate and/or survey is needed
Waived tests only	Certificate of Waiver (COW)
Provider-Performed Microscopy Procedure (PPMP)	Certificate of PPMP
Tests of moderate complexity	Certificate of Registration, CLIA survey, and Certificate of Compliance
Tests of high complexity	Certificate of Registration, survey by an accrediting agency, and Certificate of Accreditation

© Cengage Learning 2014

number of quality deficiencies has decreased significantly from the first laboratory survey to the second.

Work is currently in progress with the CDC and CMS to develop a final CLIA rule that will reflect all comments received and new technologies.

Categories of Testing

CLIA '88, under the aegis of the CMS of the DHHS, has designated three categories of testing and one subcategory:

1. Waived tests
2. Moderate-complexity tests, including Provider Performed Microscopy: PPM Procedures (also called PPMP)
3. High-complexity tests

Each of these categories has different requirements for personnel and quality control.

Waived tests are simple, are unvarying, and require a minimum of judgment and interpretation. Test error carries minimal hazard to the patient. Waived tests represent the lowest percentage of the total number of tests performed.

PPMP tests are moderate-complexity tests but represent a subcategory that was added at the request of providers.

The following criteria are used to categorize moderate- and high-complexity tests.

- The degree of operator intervention needed
- The necessary knowledge and experience the operator possesses
- The degree of maintenance and troubleshooting needed to perform the tests

Even though most of the tests medical assistants perform fall into the waived category, POLs will often perform moderate-complexity tests, including the PPMP tests. POLs are not limited to any category as long as they have sufficiently trained and credentialed personnel, equipment, and approval.

Manufacturers of self-contained test kits apply for and receive Food and Drug Administration (FDA) approval for their particular test to be on the CLIA waived list. To find out if your particular brand of self-contained test kit is on the CLIA waived list, access an up-to-date listing at the FDA website http://www.fda.gov and use the key search term "currently waived analytes" (be forewarned, though, the list is very long). You can obtain a list of categories and the complete CLIA '88 guidelines from the CDC website (http://www.cdc.gov and use key search term "CLIA").

Contents of the Law

1. All laboratories are required to register with CLIA '88 even if just one test is performed, regardless of whether there is Medicare and Medicaid **reimbursement** and regardless of the category in which the test is found.
2. The regulations apply to all laboratories.
3. The regulations are specific to the complexity of the test. The waived tests are the simplest with the fewest regulations. Standards become more stringent as the complexity of the test increases.
4. A laboratory must obtain a certificate to perform tests. An initial filing for a certificate is made on CMS form 116. One of five certificates can be obtained. (There can be a state exemption as previously mentioned.)
   a. *Certificate of Waiver (COW)*. This certificate is issued to a laboratory to perform only waived tests.
   b. *Certificate for PPMP*. This certificate is issued to a laboratory in which a provider, midlevel practitioner, or dentist performs no moderate-complexity tests other than the PPMP procedures (Table 38-3). This

Table 38-3 Examples of Provider-Performed Microscopy Procedures

All direct wet-mount preparations for the presence or absence of bacteria, fungi, parasites, and human cellular elements
All potassium hydroxide (KOH) preparations
Pinworm examinations
Fern tests
Postcoital direct, qualitative examinations of vaginal or cervical mucus
Urine sediment examinations
Nasal smears for granulocytes
Fecal leukocyte examinations
Qualitative semen analysis (limited to the presence or absence of sperm and detection of motility)

© Cengage Learning 2014

certificate permits the laboratory to also perform waived tests.

c. *Certificate of Registration.* This certificate enables the entity to conduct moderate- and high-complexity laboratory testing until the entity is determined by survey to be in compliance with CLIA regulations.

d. *Certificate of Compliance.* This certificate is issued to a laboratory after an inspection finds the laboratory to be in compliance with all applicable CLIA requirements.

e. *Certificate of Accreditation.* This is a certificate that is issued to a laboratory on the basis of the laboratory's accreditation by an organization approved by CMS.

5. All five certificates require renewal every 2 years.

6. After a laboratory has been certified, it must notify CMS within 6 months if it changes the type of tests it performs. Changing the tests performed may change the laboratory's classification.

7. Some examples of sanctions or penalties imposed by CMS for noncompliance with CLIA law are:

Infraction	*Penalty*
Failure to enroll with CMS	Denial or revocation of certificate
Nonparticipation in proficiency testing	A score of zero (a score of 80% is required)
Failure to return the proficiency testing result	A score of zero

In addition, Medicare and Medicaid payments may be suspended or terminated.

For CLIA '88 conditions other than proficiency testing, newly regulated laboratories will not be subjected to penalties during the first inspection cycle unless it is determined that the laboratories' inadequacies pose immediate patient danger.

8. The law **mandates** quality assurance for non-waived tests. Laboratories are required to establish policies and procedures through programs that assess test quality; identify problems and correct them; ensure precise, dependable, and punctual reporting of test results; and guarantee sufficient competent staff. In addition, laboratories must ensure that all quality-control data are studied, and if there is a complaint, an investigation must be

CMS FORM 116

CMS form 116 for the clinical laboratory collects information regarding a laboratory's operation and is needed to evaluate fees, to determine baseline data, to update existing data, and to fulfill legal requirements. The information obtained from the application will give the surveyor of the laboratory a perspective of the laboratory's operation and if it will be subject to an on-site inspection.

undertaken and appropriate action taken and recorded. It is a requirement that quality assurance records be maintained.

9. The law mandates quality control for non-waived tests. Laboratories are required to have an adequate supply of equipment to perform the number and types of tests that they offer. A procedures manual must be available in the testing area and must include complete testing instructions. Documentation of maintenance programs for instruments, equipment, and test systems must be evident.

10. The law establishes requirements for the correct collection, transportation, and storage of specimens and the reporting of results (see No. 16, Patient Test Management).

11. The law mandates maintenance of records, equipment, and facilities of laboratories performing nonwaived tests (see No. 17, Documentation).

12. The law mandates personnel standards. There are requirements for personnel who perform nonwaived tests and they spell out the necessary qualifications and responsibilities required of them. Each person who takes the tests must be licensed by the state if required, have a high school diploma or equivalent, have adequate training, and be able to demonstrate an understanding of laboratory procedures; **calibration**, or standardization of instruments; specimen collection; and quality control. Personnel must report test results accurately and with dependability. All high-complexity tests must be done by technologists and technicians except for cytology, which requires more stringent qualifications.

13. The law mandates **proficiency testing** for nonwaived tests. The procedures and tests found in the waived category are exempt from proficiency testing, regardless of the type of laboratory in which the tests are performed.

Moderate- and high-complexity test laboratories must enroll in proficiency testing programs that are approved by the DHHS. The proficiency testing samples are checked in the same manner as patient specimens. Unsatisfactory performance on a proficiency testing check can result in various penalties ranging from termination of the laboratory's license to operate to the termination of reimbursement from Medicare and Medicaid.

14. The law mandates unannounced on-site inspection. All laboratories in the moderate- and high-complexity categories are subject to unannounced inspections by DHHS or an agency assigned to the task by DHHS. Laboratories that perform only waived tests must prove that tests are being done according to the manufacturer's directions. Inspections can involve interviewing employees, observation of employees performing tests, analysis of data, and documentation of results. Violations of requirements by any laboratory can result in penalties. The cost of inspection will be billed to the laboratory.

15. The law mandates an annual listing of laboratories that have had action taken against them.

16. The law mandates patient test management. All laboratories must have a strategy for properly receiving and processing specimens and for the precise reporting of the results. Written instructions regarding collection, safeguarding of specimens, and labeling of specimens must be available for patients. There must be a specific procedure for the reporting of life-threatening results and a follow-through to the person requesting the test. Test records must be kept for 2 years after the reporting of results.

17. The law mandates documentation. The following documentation must be done and be available:

- Specimen
    Patient preparation
    Specimen collection procedure
    Proper labeling technique
    Preservation of specimen if applicable
- Proficiency testing
    Corrective action taken
- Quality control and quality assurance
    Any corrective action taken
- Problem and complaint log

- **Requisitions** or written requests
    Patient name
    Patient date of birth
    Patient identification number or record number
    Name and address of laboratory
    Date and time of collection
    Name of test requested
    Diagnosis
- Results
    Name and address of laboratory where test is done
    Test name
    Test results, including normal ranges listed on test results
    Disposition of unacceptable specimens must be released to authorized person
- Log of results
    Printouts from instruments report must be kept
    Identification of person performing test
    Patient identification number
    Specimen identification
    Date
    Time specimen is received in laboratory
    Specimen rejection log maintained
    Records and dates of all tests done

Criteria for PPMP

To be categorized as a PPMP, the procedure must meet the following criteria:

1. The examination must be personally performed by one of the following practitioners:
    a. A provider during the patient's visit on a specimen obtained from his or her own patient or from a patient of a group medical practice of which the provider is a member or an employee.
    b. A midlevel practitioner, under the supervision of the provider or in independent practice only if authorized by the state, during the patient's visit on a specimen obtained from his or her own patient or from a patient of a clinic, group medical practice, or other health care provider of which the midlevel practitioner is a member or an employee.
    c. A dentist during the patient's visit on a specimen obtained from his or her own

patient or from a patient of a group dental practice of which the dentist is a member or an employee.

2. The procedure must be categorized as moderately complex.

3. The primary instrument for performing the test is the microscope, limited to bright-field or phase-contrast microscopy.

4. The specimen is labile, or a delay in performing the test could compromise the accuracy of the test result.

5. Control materials are not available to monitor the entire testing process.

6. Limited specimen handling or processing is required.

Criteria for CLIA Waived Tests

To be categorized as a laboratory performing waived tests, the procedures must meet the following criteria:

1. The tests must be simple laboratory examinations and procedures that are cleared by the FDA for home use, use methods that are simple and accurate so errors are negligible, or pose no reasonable risk for harm to the patient if performed incorrectly.

2. The tests performed must be on CLIA's waived test list.

3. The manufacturer's instructions for performing the tests must be followed.

4. Minimal scientific and technical knowledge is required to perform the test, or knowledge required to perform the test may be obtained through on-the-job instruction.

5. Minimal training is required for preanalytic, analytic, and postanalytic phases of the testing process, or limited experience is required to perform the test.

6. Reagents and materials are generally stable and reliable, or reagents and materials are prepackaged; premeasured; or require no special handling, precautions, or storage conditions.

7. Operational steps are either automatically executed (such as pipetting, temperature monitoring, or timing of steps) or are easily controlled.

8. Calibration quality-control materials are stable and readily available, and external proficiency testing materials, when available, are stable.

9. Test system troubleshooting is automatic or self-correcting, clearly described, or requires minimal judgment, and equipment maintenance is provided by the manufacturer, is seldom needed, or can be performed easily.

10. Minimal interpretation and judgment are required to perform preanalytic, analytic, and postanalytic processes, and resolution of problems requires limited independent interpretation and judgment.

CLIA '88 Regulation for Quality Control in Automated Hematology

CLIA '88 regulations require that three different procedures be performed in the quality-control protocol for automated hematology instruments. The procedures are calibration, control sample testing, and proficiency testing. CLIA's regulations require that the automated hematology instrument be calibrated at regularly scheduled intervals with either a calibrator sample or a normal control sample testing. Many manufacturers of automated hematology instruments recommend or may require that the instrument be recalibrated at shorter intervals than are required by CLIA '88. CLIA '88 mandates that two levels of control samples be tested first each day on any parameter that will be performed on a patient's sample. These quality-control checks must be performed before the patient's sample is tested. The results for quality-control samples must fall within two standard deviations of the expected mean value for that sample.

In addition to calibrations and control sample testing, an ambulatory care setting that uses automated hematology instruments must enroll in a proficiency testing program with a reference laboratory that is CLIA '88 approved.

Aftermath of CLIA '88

There are many individuals who have serious concerns about whether CLIA has led to improved testing as was intended, or if the law has just produced an overload of paperwork and problems. Some question if the law will be fully implemented or even eliminated altogether.

Important developments help to put the law into perspective. CMS has postponed the date that Medicare payments would be

The findings of errors in processes at Certificate of Waiver (COW) laboratories and PPMP certificate laboratories are of concern. Both COW and PPMP laboratories currently have virtually no oversight. Results of studies indicate that, even though COW laboratories have the least amount of complexity to their tests, there are huge gaps in quality of the tests performed. It was discovered that POLs are lacking in the areas of following instructions, quality assurance, and quality control. PPMP laboratories were lacking in the areas of inappropriate certificates, not documenting personnel competency, and not evaluating test accuracy. Although these findings are of concern to the CLIA program, no patient harm has been documented as a result of these errors. Personnel performing the tests at COW laboratories surveyed were mostly nurses and physicians. The Centers for Medicare & Medicaid Services (CMS) confirmed that lack of routine oversight in COW and PPMP laboratories continues to be a significant challenge to ensuring quality testing. They recommend the following:

- Institute educational programs for COW and PPMP laboratories
- Validate the effectiveness of this educational program
- Survey a percentage of COW and PPMP laboratories annually
- Develop a self-assessment for PPMP laboratories
- Provide educational material as part of the CLIA enrollment process
- Have state survey agencies contact COW and PPMP laboratories to verify test menus

The law states that CLIA must be self supporting. However, far fewer laboratories registered than was originally anticipated, and the result is a significantly lower amount of revenue than had been expected.

It is interesting to note that the CDC has proposed easing CLIA regulations by adding another category of testing. It would fall between the waived tests and the moderately complex tests. The tests within this new category would be subject to minimal regulation. This proposal is under consideration. Many question whether CLIA will have any value if this event occurs.

Impact of CLIA on Medical Assistants

 CLIA '88 requires every facility that tests human specimens for diagnosis, treatment, and prevention of disease to meet specific federal requirements. The law applies to any facility that performs tests for the preceding purposes. This includes any POLs and ambulatory care setting, two typical areas where medical assistants are employed. The law covers all facilities even if only one test or a few basic tests are done and even if there is no charge for the testing.

 Medical assistants may be responsible not only for performing the tests but also for maintaining personnel records, including such information as workers' college diplomas, state licenses, national certifications, employees' continuing education, and recredentialing. Employee hepatitis B status must also be on file. Medical assistants may be involved with compiling a procedures manual on how to perform every test done; these must be reviewed every year. An instrument log must be available for each piece of equipment. Systems must be in place for calibration, quality control, quality assurance test recording, and proficiency testing (if higher than waived category tests are performed). Documentation by medical assistants is of utmost importance; for instance, a quality-control plan may be in action, but it may not be written down in detail.

Medical assistants are the only health care professionals trained specifically for the ambulatory setting, including the POL procedures. Lacking a medical laboratory technician or medical technologist in the POL, the burden of quality performance of the waived tests falls to the person specifically trained in that area, the medical assistant. Because laboratory training of the medical assistant focuses

cut off for failure to register. The deadline has been postponed at least three times. The American Medical Association (AMA) complained that unannounced inspections of POLs would disrupt patient office visits. As a result, the Secretary of DHHS declared that POL inspections would be announced.

The category of PPMP was added as another certificate and testing category because providers argued that the microscopic tests were essential to their practice. Already the PPMP has expanded to include midlevel practitioners such as nurse practitioners, nurse midwives, and physician assistants.

primarily on CLIA waived tests, it is of major concern that medical assisting programs offer the best training possible in the areas of quality assurance, quality control, and following manufacturer's instructions. Keep in mind that the medical assistant may be the only health care professional in the POL who has formal training in the performance of the waived laboratory tests. Add that to the received findings of errors in processes at COW and PPMP laboratories and medical assistants are definitely on the front lines of ensuring the best quality for test results performed in the POLs.

Because CMS has received only a fraction of the money that they expected to collect from application fees, there is little money to carry the CLIA '88 program forward. Medical assistants must realize that CLIA '88 is the law even though a number of laboratories have not seen inspectors nor felt any impact from the CLIA '88 regulations. Some laboratories are delaying concern about CLIA '88 rules and do not understand the law and, therefore, have not fully implemented the regulations. Medical assistants must know and comply with the law and be prepared for a CLIA inspection. Penalties are imposed on laboratories that are not in compliance with the law.

Medical assistants who perform clinical laboratory procedures must keep up with government changes.

Where to Find More Information Regarding CLIA '88

The original CLIA '88 guidelines and updates are available from the Federal Register for a fee. See the appendices for ordering information or visit the CMS website (http://www.cms.hhs.gov/CLIA).

OSHA REGULATIONS

OSHA regulations are intended to ensure employers have a safe and healthy work environment for their employees. This applies to all workers, not just health care workers. Some of the regulations include hard hats and steel-toed shoes for construction workers, safety switches for machinery, fire prevention equipment in restaurants, and, of course, safety equipment and supplies for health care workers. Two OSHA standards have the greatest impact: *The Occupational Exposure to Hazardous Chemicals* (revised from *The Hazard Communication Standard*) and *The Bloodborne Pathogen Standard*. *The Bloodborne Pathogen Standard* is reviewed in Chapter 22. This chapter discusses the standard

for *Occupational Exposure to Hazardous Chemicals*. It is important to note that states have their own worker safety standards. Those state standards are required to be as strict or greater than the federal OSHA standards.

The Standard for Occupational Exposure to Hazardous Chemicals in the Laboratory

In an effort to reduce the number of chemically related illnesses and injuries in the workplace, OSHA published its *Hazard Communications Standard* in 1983. This led many states to develop *right-to-know* laws. In 1992, OSHA expanded the *Hazard Communications Standard,* and published *The Occupational Exposure to Hazardous Chemicals in the Laboratory Standard,* which specifically addressed clinical laboratories.

The intention of this law is to heighten employee awareness of risks linked with chemical dangers. It serves to improve work practices through employee training and identification of hazardous chemicals that exist in the workplace. The use of protective equipment is utilized to protect employees from harmful chemicals.

Chemical Hygiene Plan

The Chemical Hygiene Plan (CHP) on hazardous chemicals is the core of the OSHA safety standard on hazardous chemicals. A written plan must specify the training and information requirements of the standard. Certain specific control measures such as **fume hoods** and glove boxes must be included in the plan. A designated employee is the chemical hygiene or safety officer. Provisions for housekeeping and maintenance of the facility are included. OSHA standards are not optional, and penalties are imposed for noncompliance with the standard. Employers must meet the requirements not only to be in compliance with the law but to protect employees as well.

 All laboratories and ambulatory care settings, including providers' offices, must comply with a chemical hygiene plan to

---

CRITICAL THINKING

Compare whom CLIA protects with whom OSHA protects. Do they have similar missions?

meet the OSHA regulations. The primary component of the OSHA standard is that a written chemical hygiene plan and program must be operational if chemicals are stored in a facility and handled by employees. Some examples of chemicals include, but are not limited to, stains, ethyl alcohol, sodium hypochlorite (household bleach), formaldehyde, fixatives, preservatives, injectables such as chemotherapeutic agents, and acetone. Many laboratory accidents result in chemical-related illnesses ranging from eye irritations to pulmonary edema.

There are three primary goals that an employer must accomplish to be in compliance with the OSHA standard for chemical exposure. The first is that there must be an inventory taken and a list compiled of all chemicals considered hazardous. The following information must be documented (Figure 38-1): the quantity of chemicals stored per month or year; whether the substance is gas, liquid, or solid; the manufacturer's name and address; and the chemical hazard classification.

Second, a **Material Safety Data Sheet (MSDS)** (Figure 38-2) manual must be assembled. The MSDS statements are provided by the manufacturer when the chemicals are purchased and give detailed information about the chemicals and whether they are a health hazard. The MSDS statements should be organized into a notebook for employee use and located in an area of immediate access by employees. Every employee who is exposed to or works with chemicals must read the

---

SAMPLE
CHEMICAL INVENTORY FORM

Office of _____

Date _____

Chemical Name	Catalog #	Quantity Stores L./gm. (monthly)	Physical State	Hazard Class				Manufacturer	Comments
				H	F	R	P		

(H) Health	**(F) Fire Hazard**	**(R) Reactivity**	**(P) Protection**
0 - Minimal	0 - Will not burn	0 - Stable is not reactive	A. - Goggles
1 - Slightly	1 - Slight	with water	B. - Goggles/Gloves
2 - Moderate	2 - Moderate	1 - Slight	C. - Goggles/Gloves/Apron
3 - Serious	3 - Serious	2 - Moderate	D. - Face Shield/Gloves/Apron
4 - Extreme	4 - Extreme	3 - Serious	E. - Goggles/Gloves/Mask
		4 - Extreme	F. - Goggles/Gloves/Apron/Mask
			X. - Gloves

Courtesy of POL Consultants, 2 Russ Farm Way, Delanco, NJ 08075, 856-824-0300

Figure 38-1   Sample chemical inventory form for listing chemicals on the premises, including quantity, physical state, hazard class, manufacturer, and comments.

MATERIAL SAFETY DATA SHEET

I – PRODUCT IDENTIFICATION

COMPANY NAME: We Wash Inc.

Tel No:	(314) 621-1818
Nights:	(314) 621-1399
CHEMTREC:	(800) 424-9343

ADDRESS: 5035 Manchester Avenue
Freedom, Texas 79430

PRODUCT NAME: Spotfree   Product No.: 2190

Synonyms: Warewashing Detergent

II – HAZARDOUS INGREDIENTS OF MIXTURES

MATERIAL: (CAS#)	% By Wt.	TLV	PEL
According to the OSHA Hazard Communication Standard, 29CFR 1910.1200, this product contains no hazardous ingredients.	N/A	N/A	N/A

III – PHYSICAL DATA

Vapor Pressure, mm Hg: N/A   Vapor Density (Air=1) 60–90F: N/A
Evaporation Rate (ether=1): N/A   % Volatile by wt: N/A
Solubility in H_2O: Complete   pH @ 1%   Solution 9.3–9.8
Freezing Point F: N/A   pH as Distributed: N/A
Boiling Point F: N/A   Appearance: Off-White granular powder
Specific Gravity H_2O=1 @25C: N/A   Odor: Mild Chemical Odor

IV – FIRE AND EXPLOSION

Flash Point F: N/AV   Flammable Limits: N/A

Extinguishing Media: The product is not flammable or combustible. Use media appropriate for the primary source of fire.

Special Fire Fighting Procedures: Use caution when fighting any fire involving chemicals. A self-contained breathing apparatus is essential.

Unusual Fire and Explosion Hazards: None Known

V – REACTIVITY DATA

Stability - Conditions to avoid: None Known

Incompatibility: Contact of carbonates or bicarbonates with acids can release large quantities of carbon dioxide and heat.

Hazardous Decomposition Products: In fire situations heat decomposition may result in the release of sulfur oxides.

Conditions Contributing to Hazardous Polymerization: N/A

Figure 38-2   Example of a Material Safety Data Sheet (MSDS) listing product name, hazardous ingredients, physical data, fire and explosion data, reactivity data, health hazard data, emergency and first aid procedures, spill or leak procedures, protection information/control measures, and special precautions.

Spotfree
VI – HEALTH HAZARD DATA

EFFECTS OF OVEREXPOSURE (Medical Conditions Aggravated/Target Organ Effects)
A. ACUTE (Primary Route of Exposure)   EYES: Product granules may cause mechanical irritation to eyes.
   SKIN (Primary Route of Exposure): Prolonged repeated contact with skin may result in drying of skin.
   INGESTION: Not expected to be toxic if swallowed, however, gastrointestinal discomfort may occur.
B. SUBCHRONIC, CHRONIC, OTHER: None known.

VII – EMERGENCY AND FIRST AID PROCEDURES

EYES: In case of contact, flush thoroughly with water for 15 minutes. Get medical attention if irritation persists.
SKIN: Flush any dry Spotfree from skin with flowing water. Always wash hands after use.
INGESTION: If swallowed, drink large quantities of water and call a physician.

VIII – SPILL OR LEAK PROCEDURES

Spill Management: Sweep up material and repackage if possible.
   Spill residue may be flushed to the sewer with water.

Waste Disposal Methods: Dispose of in accordance with federal, state and local regulations.

IX – PROTECTION INFORMATION/CONTROL MEASURES

Respiratory: None needed   Eye: Safety   Glove: Not
                                                                                  glasses   required

Other Clothing and Equipment: None required

Ventilation: Normal

X – SPECIAL PRECAUTIONS

Precautions to be taken in Handling and Storing: Avoid contact with eyes. Avoid prolonged or repeated contact with skin.
   Wash thoroughly after handling. Keep container closed when not in use.
Additional Information: Store away from acids.

Prepared by: D. Martinez   Revision Date: 04/11/XX

Seller makes no warranty, expressed or implied, concerning the use of this product other than indicated on the label. Buyer assumes all risk of use and/or handling of this material when such use and/or handling is contrary to label instructions.

While Seller believes that the information contained herein is accurate, such information is offered solely for its customers' consideration and verification under their specific use conditions. This information is not to be deemed a warranty or representation of any kind for which Seller assumes legal responsibility.

Courtesy of POL Consultants, 2 Russ Farm Way, Delanco, NJ 08075, 856-824-0800.

Figure 38-2   (*continued*)

MSDS about those chemicals and know where the manual is kept. The various chemicals are labeled using the National Fire Protection Association's color and number method (Figure 38-3). There are four colors, each signifying a warning to the person handling the chemical(s) (Figure 38-4). They are:

- Blue signifies a health hazard
- Red signifies a flammability hazard
- Yellow signifies reactivity or instability hazard
- White signifies a special hazard and the use of personal protective equipment (PPE)

The numbers 0 to 4 are used in conjunction with the colors to indicate the level of risk for each product and are assigned by the manufacturer using the rating system. The numbers can be found on the MSDS (Figure 38-5).

Third, the employer is required to provide a hazard communication educational program to the employee within 30 days of employment and before the employee handles any hazardous chemicals (Figure 38-6A). The training program should consist of the location and identification of hazardous chemicals, how to read and understand the labels on the chemicals, where the MSDS manual is kept, when to use PPE, and procedures to follow for chemical spills. The training sessions must be documented, signed by the employer, and permanently retained in the employee record (Figure 38-6B).

Requirements of Chemical Hygiene Plan (CHP).
The requirements for a CHP include:

- Employers must have an operational written plan (a manual) relevant to the safety and health of employees.
- Written instructions on the use of PPE must be available.
- Fume hoods or biohazard hoods must be checked regularly.

CHEMICAL WARNING LABEL DETERMINATION

The Hazard Communication Act contains specific labeling requirements. Labels must be on all hazardous chemicals that are shipped to and used in the workplace. Labels must not be removed. Material safety data sheets for all chemicals will be available to employees.

Manufacturer Requirements: Chemical manufacturers are required to evaluate chemicals, determine status as hazards, provide material safety data sheets (MSDS), and label all shipped chemicals properly. Manufacturer labels must never be removed. The best way to determine the hazards of the chemical is to read the MSDS, obtain an OSHA designated list or State Hazardous Substance list. For most mixed chemicals, it is necessary to contact the manufacturer for MSDS.

Office Chemicals: Search through your office and write down all chemicals you have in the office. Most pharmaceuticals and common household products do not come under this standard. Ingredients can then be compared to a list of regulated substances or MSDS sheets will provide necessary information.

Employer's Responsibility: Any hazardous chemical used in the workplace that is not in its original container must be labeled with the identity of the chemical and hazards. "Target Organ" chemical labels may be used. The label must include the chemical and common name, warnings about physical and health hazards, and the name and address of the manufacturer. The employer is to compile a chemical inventory list that is to be updated as needed. MSDS information should be located in a place where it is accessible to all employees. Label and MSDS information should be provided during the safety training program.

Identity: The term identity can refer to any chemical or common name designation for the individual chemical or mixture, as long as the term used is also used on the list of hazardous chemicals and the MSDS.

NOTE: If a chemical is poured into another container for immediate use, it does not need to be labeled.

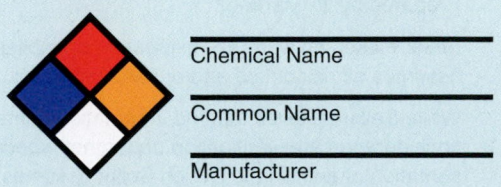

Courtesy of POL Consultants, 2 Russ Farm Way, Delanco, NJ 08075, 856-824-0800.

Figure 38-3   Chemical warning label determination indicates necessary information for labels, including manufacturer's requirements, office chemicals, employer's responsibility, and identity of chemical or its common name.

BLUE: HEALTH HAZARD

4 = Danger: May be fatal
3 = Warning: Corrosive or toxic
2 = Warning: Harmful if inhaled
1 = Caution: May cause irritation
0 = No unusual hazard

RED: FLAMMABILITY

4 = Danger: Flammable gas or extremely flammable liquid
3 = Warning: Flammable liquid
2 = Caution: Combustible liquid
1 = Caution: Combustible if heated
0 = Noncombustible

YELLOW: REACTIVITY/INSTABILITY

4 = Danger: Explosive at room temperature
3 = Danger: May be explosive if spark occurs or if heated under confinement
2 = Warning: Unstable or may react if mixed with water
1 = Caution: May react if heated or mixed with water
0 = Stable: Nonreactive when mixed with water

WHITE: SPECIAL HAZARD/PROTECTION

A   Goggles
B   Goggles, gloves
C   Goggles, gloves, apron
D   Face shields, gloves, apron
E   Goggles, gloves, mask
F   Goggles, gloves, apron, mask
X   Gloves

© Cengage Learning 2014

Figure 38-4   National Fire Protection Association's color and number method.

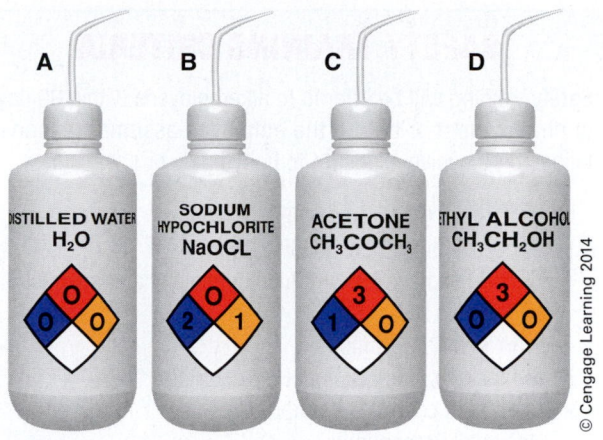

© Cengage Learning 2014

Figure 38-5   Four containers are marked using the National Fire Protection Association's color and number method for identifying and warning of chemical hazards. (A) Distilled water: Presents no health, flammability, or reactivity/instability hazard and requires no PPE when used (all areas are zero). (B) Sodium hypochlorite: Does not promote a flammability hazard (red is zero), is harmful if inhaled (blue is 2), and may react or become unstable if heated or mixed with water (yellow is 1). (C) Acetone: Flammable (red is 3), may cause irritation (blue is 1), and is stable/nonreactive when mixed with water (yellow is zero). (D) Ethyl alcohol: Flammable (red is 3), no unusual health hazards (blue is zero), and is stable/nonreactive when mixed with water (yellow is zero).

- Training sessions must be held for employees regarding their right to know what hazardous chemicals are in their work environment.
- It is the employer's legal responsibility to provide medical attention for an employee should an accidental chemical spill occur.
- The responsibility for executing training sessions, keeping manuals current, and documentation is designated to an employer.
- Instruction must be provided regarding disposal of hazardous waste produced in the workplace. (Usually a hazardous waste company is contracted by the employer.)
- Each employee's record must have a written statement, signed by the employer, stating the employer's responsibility to arrange for employee training and a safe work environment.

Importance of Chemical Standard to Medical Assistants. Meeting the requirements set forth by OSHA is not optional. All must comply or face penalties. All employees, including medical assistants, have the right to know and be given information and be educated regarding chemical hazards that they are exposed to in

CRITICAL THINKING

If you were to develop a chemical hazard training program for your clinic, what criteria would you determine to be vital for the safety of your coworkers?

SAFETY TRAINING CRITERIA

Safety training will be offered to all employees within 30 days of employment or before the employee assumes responsibilities that involve exposure to body fluids or chemicals.

Items to be covered in training session:

- General explanation of OSHA laws
- General explanation of the epidemiology and symptoms of HBV and HIV
- Who is at risk in office
- Modes of transmission of HBV and HIV
- Method of control in workplace
- Universal Precautions
- Handwashing
- Personal protective equipment
- How to clean up spills
- What to do after a needlestick injury
- Medical follow-up after an exposure
- Cleaning protocol for office
- Hazardous Communication Standard
- Types of chemical labels
- How to read MSDS and NFPA signs
- Warning signs
- How to get MSDS
- Location of MSDS
- How to store chemicals
- How to record chemical inventory
- Hazardous Waste laws
- How to comply with laws
- How to use and label bio-bins and sharps containers
- How to keep records
- Who keeps the records
- Medical consent forms
- HBV forms
- Safety training certificate
- Engineering control records

Courtesy of POL Consultants, 2 Russ Farm Way, Delanco, NJ 08075, 856-824-0800.

Figure 38-6A Safety Training Form lists the items to be covered by the employer during OSHA training sessions.

SAMPLE
CERTIFICATE OF TRAINING

_____

First Name　　　　Middle Initial　　　　Last Name

has completed the

OSHA HAZARD COMMUNICATION
INFORMATION TRAINING PROGRAM

This certificate indicates your successful participation in a program instructing you of your rights as a worker and the proper handling of hazardous substances in the workplace.

_____　　　_____
Date　　　　　　　　　　Employee Signature

　　　　　　　　　　　_____
　　　　　　　　　　　Instructor's Signature

　　　　　　　　　　　_____
　　　　　　　　　　　Employer's Signature

Courtesy of POL Consultants, 2 Russ Farm Way, Delanco, NJ 08075, 856-824-0800.

Figure 38-6B Sample Certificate of Training shows that the employee has completed an OSHA Hazard Communication Information Training Program.

 positions must use their knowledge and skills to provide a safe work environment for themselves and their staff.

OSHA REGULATIONS AND STUDENTS

With the passage of the OSHA laws, all students with potential exposure to chemicals and blood-borne pathogens should follow all safety procedures as outlined by OSHA. Because students are not considered employees of a health care facility and are attending an educational institution, they do not fall under the OSHA guidelines. They should, however, take precautions to avoid contact with potentially infectious materials and toxic chemicals wherever learning is taking place.

Avoiding Exposure to Chemicals

Students may come into contact with harmful chemicals when doing procedures that can cause

their place of employment. Medical assistants can be exposed to hazardous chemicals through skin contact, injection, or inhalation. Because many laboratory accidents result in chemical-related illnesses, it is important for medical assistants to understand how the law affects them, their place of employment, and their employer. Medical assistants and other health care providers should know what hazards they face, and know the proper technique for handling, storing, and disposing of hazardous chemicals. Medical assistants in administrative

such problems as burns to the skin and eyes. Students will be made aware of these through information packaged with kits and the MSDS. As a general rule, if the chemical comes in contact with the skin, it must be flushed with water immediately and continued for five minutes. Chemicals that get into the eye must be flushed for 15 minutes (unless contradicted on the label). Refer to the MSDS for specific post-exposure procotol. Eyewash stations and showers should be available in case of accidental exposure to hazardous chemicals with a follow-up in the emergency department.

Chemical spills should be carefully cleaned following the procedure for the particular chemical. The same chemical biohazard spill cleanup kits used in POLs can be used in school laboratories. Students should familiarize themselves with the contents of the kits and the instructions for use before an actual spill occurs.

Toxic fumes can occur with certain chemicals and certain tests can cause lung irritation and damage. This type of chemical should be handled under a fume hood that will take the fumes away by means of a ventilation mechanism.

A student safety laboratory manual outlining an exposure control plan with emphasis on Standard Precautions, PPE, work practice controls, lists of hazardous chemicals, and MSDS should be compiled and accessible. Students should be thoroughly familiar with its contents. In addition, students should be educated as to the location and identification of hazardous chemicals just as employees are.

It is of utmost importance that students learn about and understand the OSHA standards and comply with them. In so doing, they will safeguard themselves from harmful chemicals and blood-borne pathogens.

ERGONOMICS AND CUMULATIVE TRAUMA DISORDERS

OSHA has been focusing its attention on a new threat to the workplace: ergonomic hazards. Ergonomics is the study of the workplace. OSHA published its first standard, *Ergonomic Hazards,* in 1991. At the heart of these guidelines is the prevention of cumulative trauma disorders. Cumulative trauma disorders are injuries involving the musculoskeletal or nervous system, such as carpal tunnel syndrome and trigger finger. They are the result of long-term, repetitive work actions, such as gripping, keyboard use, pipetting, and microscopy. Limiting or preventing repetitive work actions is the key to minimizing cumulative trauma disorders. Use of ergonomically correct equipment and supplies, proper work site design, staff training, and job rotation are essential in creating an ergonomically sound workplace. See Chapter 11 for more specific ergonomics information.

CASE STUDY 38-1

Refer to the scenario at the beginning of the chapter. Wanda performs the microscopic examination of the urine slide even though the procedure is not a waived test. She compares her findings to Dr. Rice's assessment.

CASE STUDY REVIEW

1. Besides learning more about urine components and continuing her education, what benefit does Wanda obtain by putting forth this extra effort?
2. Do you think Dr. Rice will appreciate her extra effort?

CASE STUDY 38-2

Marie Tyndall is a student in the Jackson Heights Community College Medical Assisting Program. She and two other classmates have been assigned the project of creating a plan for cleaning up spills that might occur in the classroom laboratory and ensuring that all students using the laboratory have been trained in the proper procedure.

CASE STUDY REVIEW

1. What materials would her group need?
2. How would her group go about learning the proper steps in the clean-up process?
3. How would her group ensure that all other students in the laboratory also have the proper training?

SUMMARY

Infectious diseases and accidents occur through lack of education and carelessness. Medical assistants must understand the importance of the regulations and guidelines set forth by the federal government and follow through by helping employers implement them. In doing so, the health and safety of patients and health care workers will be protected, the spread of infectious diseases can be kept under control, and the risk for contracting an infectious disease such as AIDS or hepatitis B will be greatly minimized.

Every medical office and ambulatory care setting must, by law, have clearly written and readily available manuals containing information about Standard Precautions, CLIA '88, and OSHA for the safe handling, storage, and disposal of blood, body fluids, and chemicals.

Through consistent use of Standard Precautions and adherence to the CLIA and OSHA laws, health care providers can acquire the behaviors and techniques needed to safeguard themselves and their patients.

Because of frequent changes in the laws, it is necessary for medical assistants and all other health care providers to keep abreast of the government mandates.

STUDY FOR SUCCESS

To reinforce your knowledge and skills of information presented in this chapter:

- Review the *Key Terms*
- Role-play with other students to apply attributes of professionalism pertinent to this chapter.
- Consider the *Case Studies* and discuss your conclusions
- Answer the questions in the *Certification Review*
- Apply your knowledge by completing the *Activities* in the *Study Guide* and the *Games* and *Quizzes* in the StudyWARE (StudyWARE) software on the *Premium Website*
- Practice your problem-solving skills with the *Critical Thinking Challenge 3.0* on the *Premium Website*

Additional resources for this chapter include:

- *CourseMate for Delmar's Comprehensive Medical Assisting*
- *WebTutor for Delmar's Comprehensive Medical Assisting*

CERTIFICATION REVIEW

1. A major part of infection control is:
   a. medical asepsis
   b. communicable diseases
   c. state guidelines
   d. chemical hygiene
2. Standard Precautions were issued by:
   a. DHHS
   b. CDC
   c. CMS
   d. OSHA

3. CLIA '88 was made law to regulate:
   a. the disposal of infectious waste
   b. the use of chemicals in the workplace
   c. laboratory tests performed on specimens taken from the human body
   d. the transmission of the human immunodeficiency virus (HIV)

4. The core of the OSHA safety standard for chemical exposure is:
   a. the dipstick test
   b. the chemical hygiene plan
   c. the quantity of chemical stored per month
   d. the MSDS manual

5. The agency that requires employers to ensure employee safety concerning exposure to potentially harmful substances is:
   a. CDC
   b. U.S. Public Health Service
   c. CMS
   d. OSHA

6. Successful laboratory safety programs include:
   a. threats to the emotional and physical health of health care workers
   b. lost workdays and increased workers' compensation claims
   c. orientation, periodic drills, and consistent enforcement of policy
   d. potential fines from regulatory agencies

7. CLIA regulations specify all the following except:
   a. the type of test performed
   b. the personnel involved in testing
   c. quality control
   d. the methods used in testing

8. The agency charged with implementing CLIA is:
   a. CDC
   b. United States Public Health Service
   c. CMS
   d. OSHA

9. How many categories of testing are there in CLIA?
   a. 2
   b. 6
   c. More than 20
   d. 4

10. Which is not an approved provider for PPMP?
    a. A physician
    b. A nurse practitioner
    c. A dentist
    d. A medical assistant

11. MAs perform most of their tests in which CLIA category?
    a. Waived
    b. PPMP
    c. Moderately complex
    d. Highly complex

12. The standard published by OSHA to prevent cumulative trauma disorders is:
    a. *Workplace Standard*
    b. *Standard for Prevention of Cumulative Trauma*
    c. *Ergonomic Hazards*
    d. *Ergonomic Standard*

13. Material Safety Data Sheets do contain:
    a. flammability of the chemical
    b. cost of the chemical per use
    c. shelf life of the chemical
    d. other chemical options available

14. Reagents and materials used for waived testing generally:
    a. are prepackaged
    b. are premeasured
    c. require no special handling
    d. all of the above

REFERENCES/BIBLIOGRAPHY

Centers for Disease Control and Prevention. (2007). *Good laboratory practices for waived testing report.* Retrieved February 2012, from http://www.cdc.gov/mmwr

Centers for Medicare & Medicaid Services. Retrieved February 2012, from http://www.cms.hhs.gov

U.S. Food and Drug Administration. (2012). *CLIA—Clinical Laboratory Improvement Amendments.* Retrieved February 2012, from www.accessdata.fda.gov/scropts/cdrh/cfdocs/cfCLIA/clia.cfm

CHAPTER 39

Introduction to the Medical Laboratory

OUTLINE

The Laboratory
 Purposes of Laboratory
  Testing
 Types of Laboratories
 Laboratory Personnel
 Laboratory Departments
 Panels of Laboratory Tests
Billing for Laboratory
 Services

Quality Controls/Assurances
 in the Laboratory
 Control Tests
 Proficiency Testing
 Preventive Maintenance
 Instrument Validations
 The Medical Assistant's Role
Laboratory Requisitions
 and Reports

The Specimen
 Proper Procurement,
  Storage, and Handling
 Processing and Sending
  Specimens to a Laboratory
Microscopes
 Types of Microscopes
 How to Use a Microscope
 How to Care for a Microscope

LEARNING OUTCOMES

1. Define, spell, and pronounce the key terms as presented in the glossary.
2. Explain the reasons for performing laboratory testing.
3. Describe the main similarities and differences between an independent laboratory and a physicians' office laboratory (POL).
4. Explain the levels of laboratory personnel in relation to their education, skills, and duties, and where the medical assistant is placed in the hierarchy.
5. List eight different departments within the medical laboratory and list at least two types of testing performed within each of those departments.
6. Name nine of the most common laboratory panels and explain the body system or function being surveyed.

7. Explain the concepts of quality control and quality assurance in the medical laboratory.
8. Describe at least three methods of ensuring quality in the medical laboratory.
9. Demonstrate how to correctly complete a laboratory requisition.
10. Explain the rationale behind proper patient preparation before laboratory testing.
11. Explain where accurate and reliable information might be obtained about proper procurement, storage, and handling of laboratory specimens.
12. Demonstrate the proper use and care of a compound microscope.
13. Analyze the professionalism questions and apply them to this chapter's content.

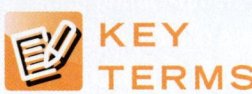

KEY TERMS

assay

baseline values

biopsy

clinical chemistry

clinical diagnosis

control test

culture and
  sensitivity (C&S)

cytology

diagnosis

differential diagnosis

DNA

electrolyte

glucose

hematology

histology

hospital-based
  laboratories

immunohematology

immunology

invasive

microbiology

mycology

panel

parasitology

patient service centers

peak

physician's office
  laboratory (POL)

qualitative test

quantitative test

reagent

reference laboratories

reference values

requisition

serum

therapeutic drug
  monitoring (TDM)

toxicology

trough

urinalysis

virology

ATTRIBUTES OF PROFESSIONALISM

Communication
- Did you speak at the patient's level of understanding?
- Did you explain procedures and expectations to the patient?

Competency
- Did you pay attention to detail?
- Were you knowledgeable and accountable?

Initiative
- Did you seek out opportunities to expand your knowledge base?

Integrity
- Did you work within your scope of practice?
- Did you acknowledge the scope of practice of other health care professionals?

SCENARIO

Dr. Susan Rice's patient, Annette Samuels, has come into the Inner City Health Care clinic complaining of lower abdominal cramps and burning when she urinates. After discussion of her symptoms and a brief examination, Dr. Rice's clinical diagnosis is urinary tract infection. She asks Wanda Slawson, CMA (AAMA), to obtain a urine sample for a urinalysis and culture with sensitivity. The urinalysis is to be performed in the physician's office laboratory (POL) within the Inner City Health Care clinic, and a portion of the sample will be sent to an outside independent lab for the culture and sensitivity testing. Wanda gives Annette specific instructions on how to prepare for the urine test and how to collect the urine. She asks Annette if she has questions and she has Annette repeat the instructions to be sure she understands them. When Annette returns with the specimen, Wanda

immediately labels it, transfers a portion of the urine into a labeled urine transport tube, places the tube into a bio-hazard transport bag, and completes a lab requisition for a culture and sensitivity test. The requisition and lab specimen are then ready to be sent to the outside lab for testing. Wanda performs a urinalysis on the remaining urine sample, and the test confirms Dr. Rice's clinical diagnosis of a urinary tract infection. Dr. Rice is able to prescribe an antibiotic for Annette while waiting for the culture results. The culture will determine what type of bacteria is in the urine, and the sensitivity will assure Dr. Rice that the proper antibiotic was prescribed. The culture will take 24 to 48 hours, so Wanda assures Annette that she will contact her the next day when the report is received. A return appointment is made for Annette for a follow-up check and urinalysis in about 10 days.

INTRODUCTION

Providers use laboratory tests to diagnose illnesses, assess patients' health, and manage chronic diseases such as diabetes and arthritis. Medical assistants in providers' offices, clinics, and laboratories may be responsible for patient preparation, obtaining specimens, and testing or sending specimens to an independent laboratory. It is important for medical assistants to be aware of laboratory procedures to ensure accurate testing.

THE LABORATORY

The current health care environment offers numerous options in the methods used to process laboratory tests.

- The specimen may be obtained and the test performed within the **physician's office laboratory (POL)**.
- The specimen may be procured and packaged for transport to a separate laboratory.
- The patient may be referred to a separate laboratory for collection and testing of the specimen.

Each laboratory setting has specific requirements for the training and qualifications of the health care personnel who work in that setting. The equipment, supplies, and paperwork, as well as the instructions given

SPOTLIGHT ON CERTIFICATION

RMA Content Outline
- Medical law
- Laboratory procedures

CMA (AAMA) Content Outline
- Medicolegal guidelines and requirements
- Principles of infection control
- Principles of operation
- Processing specimens
- Quality control

CMAS Content Outline
- Legal and ethical considerations
- Asepsis in the medical office
- Supplies and equipment

to the patient, are also determined by the type of laboratory. Whichever laboratory setting is selected, the focus should be on the safety of the public, the patient, and the health care personnel, while always maintaining quality testing to ensure accurate results.

Purposes of Laboratory Testing

Physicians depend on the ability of medical laboratories to help determine a patient's state of health or disease in some of the following ways.

To Record an Individual's State of Health. Blood tests may be performed periodically, usually during a routine physical examination, to be assured of healthy normal ranges, also known as **reference values**. Then in the future, if illness occurs, the **baseline values** are available for comparison.

To Satisfy Employment, Insurance, or Legal Requirements. If an accident occurs, quite often blood is tested for the presence of drugs and alcohol. Such a determination can prove a person guilty or innocent of a crime. Sometimes, places of employment or life insurance companies request laboratory tests to be assured that their employees or clients are free of illegal or dangerous drugs. Employment-required drug and alcohol testing is a classic example of this reason for testing.

To Gain Statistics for Research and Clinical Trials. Laboratory tests are sometimes a part of the data gathered for research and for clinical trials information. When we read about the relation between osteoporosis and hormone replacement therapy (HRT) the information is gathered through research. Clinical trials might address the efficacy of certain medications, vitamins, and minerals on osteoporosis in women receiving HRT.

To Detect Asymptomatic Conditions or Diseases. Occasionally, a patient has no complaints of illness and is asymptomatic—that is, exhibits no symptoms that might be associated with a disease process—but during routine screening or testing in another, perhaps unrelated, area, a disorder may be discovered. An example is a young man presenting at the office for an athletic physical. Routine urinalysis reveals he has a mild bladder infection.

To Confirm a Clinical Diagnosis. When a patient reports specific symptoms and describes a particular condition (subjective information), and data are compiled through a clinical examination (objective information), the provider may be able to determine a **diagnosis** without the aid of laboratory tests. This is referred to as a **clinical diagnosis**. To confirm a clinical diagnosis, the provider orders laboratory tests. For example, a child has symptoms of a strep throat infection such as sudden onset of sore throat, fever, headache, and upset stomach. On visual examination, the provider discovers small abscesses on the child's tonsils. The provider is almost certain that the diagnosis will be strep throat, but a quick and simple strep test is performed to confirm the clinical diagnosis.

To Differentiate between Two or More Diseases. Sometimes, a patient presents with a combination of symptoms that can be related to more than one condition. For the provider to diagnose accurately, a laboratory test is performed. In situations such as these, the provider chooses to perform the simplest and least **invasive** laboratory test to rule out a particular disease before requiring more extensive testing. This is known as a **differential diagnosis**. For example, if the child in the preceding case had a negative strep test but perhaps exhibited other more systemic symptoms, a blood test might confirm mononucleosis or another condition. The provider is then able to differentiate between the two diagnoses—strep throat and mononucleosis.

To Diagnose. If symptoms are vague, thereby making the clinical diagnosis difficult for the provider, a series of laboratory tests may be required. Sometimes a **panel**, or group of related tests, is ordered. This helps narrow the field for diagnosis. For example, a patient presents with reports of severe fatigue, but preliminary testing does not indicate a diagnosis. Further testing will eventually either lead the provider in a specific direction or at least eliminate a wide variety of conditions.

To Determine the Effectiveness of Treatments. After a patient has been diagnosed and has begun treatment, the provider monitors the patient's health to be sure that the treatment is therapeutic. For example, a patient diagnosed with epilepsy must take an effective amount of antiseizure medication. A blood test is used to check the level of medication in the patient's system. Sometimes the provider wants to know the highest and lowest ranges of medication in the patient's blood to determine if the levels are within a therapeutic range, called **therapeutic drug monitoring (TDM)**, and to check for drug toxicity (if the drug level is too high). To measure the highest level of medication in the patient's blood serum (called the **peak**), the specimen is taken about a half hour after the patient has taken his or her regular dose of medicine. To measure the lowest level (called the **trough**), the specimen is taken just before the patient takes his or her next scheduled dose of medicine. A periodic blood test can also be used to determine the effectiveness of dietary and lifestyle changes in reducing blood cholesterol levels.

To Prevent Diseases/Disorders. Protection of the public, families, and coworkers can warrant laboratory tests. An example is protecting an unborn child from contracting genital herpes through the birthing process. A culture of the mother's cervical and vaginal mucosa helps to determine if the child is at risk. If the culture is positive, performing a cesarean section is the treatment of choice to protect the newborn from contracting herpes. Because a newborn's immune system is not fully developed, contracting herpes can cause serious illness and even death.

To Prevent the Exacerbation of Diseases. Patients with chronic conditions require regular blood tests to prevent exacerbation of the disease. When the results of the blood test are obtained, the provider or patient determines whether it is necessary to adjust the diet or medication. For example, a patient with diabetes tests his or her blood regularly to measure the blood sugar, or **glucose**, level. If the blood sugar level is too high or too low, the patient may adjust the insulin dosage or have something to eat to return the blood sugar level to normal.

Types of Laboratories

There are many different types and locations of medical laboratories. They are identified by their size, capabilities, and affiliations. Independent laboratories may be located within medical centers or large clinics. They often have small satellite **patient service centers** located near more isolated medical facilities or in areas of convenience to patients. Satellite laboratories facilitate patients' specimens being obtained closer to their neighborhoods and ambulatory care settings. The specimens are usually couriered back to the independent central laboratory for processing.

Hospital-based laboratories perform most of the tests required by that hospital area, but even large hospitals use reference laboratories for specialized testing. **Reference laboratories** are independent, regionally located laboratories that service larger areas. Reference laboratories are used by hospitals and providers for complex, expensive, or specialized tests.

In a business sense, medical laboratories are quickly becoming more and more competitive. Growth and profitability depend on community relations and service, convenience, efficiency, cost, location, and even reputation. Competition often places the medical assistant and other medical personnel in a position of being asked to

recommend a particular medical laboratory over another. Unless the provider has a valid reason for using a particular laboratory or not referring to a particular laboratory, the patient should choose the laboratory. The patient's insurance plan may also be a factor in determining which laboratory is used. Many insurance plans require the patient to use a particular laboratory or to choose a laboratory from those participating in the plan to guarantee payment for the tests. The medical assistant is then a resource for options rather than a referral service. The law is clear that a provider may not have a financial interest in the laboratory to which he or she refers patients.

Point-of-Care Testing (POCT). POCT is sometimes referred to as near-patient testing or bedside testing, brings the laboratory services directly to the patient, wherever that may be. Medical conditions, location of the patient, and treatment methods often require laboratory results as quickly as possible so proper medical care can be administered without delay. POCT uses portable equipment and tests that provide rapid, accurate results when used correctly.

POLs. POLs are those laboratories physically set within the office. Some of the more commonly performed medical laboratory tests can easily and inexpensively be performed in the office by the medical assistant. With a simple fingerstick and a few readily available medical supplies, a patient's blood glucose levels can be determined. Another commonly performed test in the ambulatory care setting is **urinalysis**, in which urine is physically, chemically, and microscopically examined for irregularities. With the availability of the many varieties of self-contained kits, tests for strep throat, pregnancy, blood sugar (serum glucose) levels, and hidden (occult) blood in stool can be performed quickly. Other kits are being developed daily. Patients may use a kit that can be purchased without a prescription at home. Some of the home kits available to the general public are of the same quality as the kits used in medical offices. The major difference is that the person performing the test may not be trained, which may affect the accuracy of the test results. Consistent quality control measures might not be used by the nonmedical person (see Quality Control/Assurances in the Laboratory section). For example, a pregnancy test kit may be exposed to extreme temperatures while in the patient's care, on a grocer's shelf, or in the patient's home. These extreme temperatures may invalidate the chemical reaction in the test kit. More training, education, and credentialing are required as the complexity of the testing and equipment increases. (See CLIA'88 in Chapter 38 for specific testing parameters.) If the results are not within normal limits, the provider needs to be consulted for confirmation and diagnosis/treatment.

Laboratory Personnel

·All independent medical laboratories must be managed by a pathologist, a physician who specializes in disease processes. Additional staffing consists of clinical laboratory scientists, technicians, clinical laboratory assistants, phlebotomists, and medical assistants. Many agencies certify laboratory personnel. Table 39-1 gives specific information about laboratory personnel, their titles, training required, and duties performed within the clinical lab.

Laboratory Departments

Laboratories are usually divided into departments and may even be subdivided, depending on the size

Table 39-1 Laboratory Personnel

Credential/Title	Education Required	Duties Performed
Physician Pathologist (MD) or Scientist (PhD)	Board-certified medical doctor or PhD scientist (either must be CAP accredited).	Director of the lab. Manages the laboratory. Interprets biology results, Pap smears, and other cytology samples.
Clinical Laboratory Scientist (CLS) or Medical Technologist (MT) or Registered Medical Technologist (RMT) Clinical Laboratory Technologist (CLT)	Bachelor's degree in life sciences or medical technology, including 3 years of course work and 1 year of clinical experience. Must be certified by ASCP, AMT, DHHS, ISCLT, NCA, or NRM.	Qualified to perform analysis testing in all departments of the lab. Has leadership role; often trains, manages, and supervises other lab personnel. May perform routine lab tests as well as highly specialized lab tests. Troubleshoots problems with results, specimens, and/or instruments. Works directly with the lab director/manager. Performs quality control checks. Evaluates new instruments. Implements new test procedures. Often specializes in one area within the lab.
Medical Laboratory Technician (MLT) Clinical Laboratory Technician (CLT)	Usually has associate's degree or certificate from an accredited MLT/CLT program. May be certified by ASCP or NCA.	Performs routine tests. Performs microscopic exams and utilizes other lab equipment. May specialize in one area in the lab.
Phlebotomist/Phlebotomy Technician (PBT) ASCP Registered Phlebotomy Technician (RPT) AMT Certified Phlebotomy Technician (CPT) ASPT Clinical Laboratory Phlebotomist (CLP) AMT	High school and additional phlebotomy training through a certificate program or on-the-job training. May be certified through ASCP, AMT, ASPT, or NCA, and registered under state law.	Performs venipuncture and skin puncture. May perform CLIA waived testing. Collects specimens. Processes specimens for transport.
Certified Medical Assistant (CMA) AAMA Registered Medical Assistant (RMA) AMT	Generally an associate's degree or certificate from an ABHES- or CAAHEP-accredited program in a community college, technical school, or proprietary school. May be certified through AAMA or AMT. May be registered under state law.	May perform routine specimen procurement and waived testing as well as administrative duties, receptioning, computerized record keeping, and billing. Often works in POL.

© Cengage Learning 2014

Credentialing Associations: AAMA: American Association of Medical Assistants; ABHES: Accrediting Bureau of Health Education Schools; ASCP: American Society of Clinical Pathologists; ASPT: American Society for Phlebotomy Technicians; AMT: American Medical Technologists; CAAHEP: Commission on Accreditation of Allied Health Education Programs; CAP: College of American Pathologists; DHHS: Department of Health and Human Services; ISCLT: International Society of Clinical Laboratory Technology; NCA: National Credentialing Agency for Medical Laboratory Personnel; NRM: National Registry of Microbiologists.

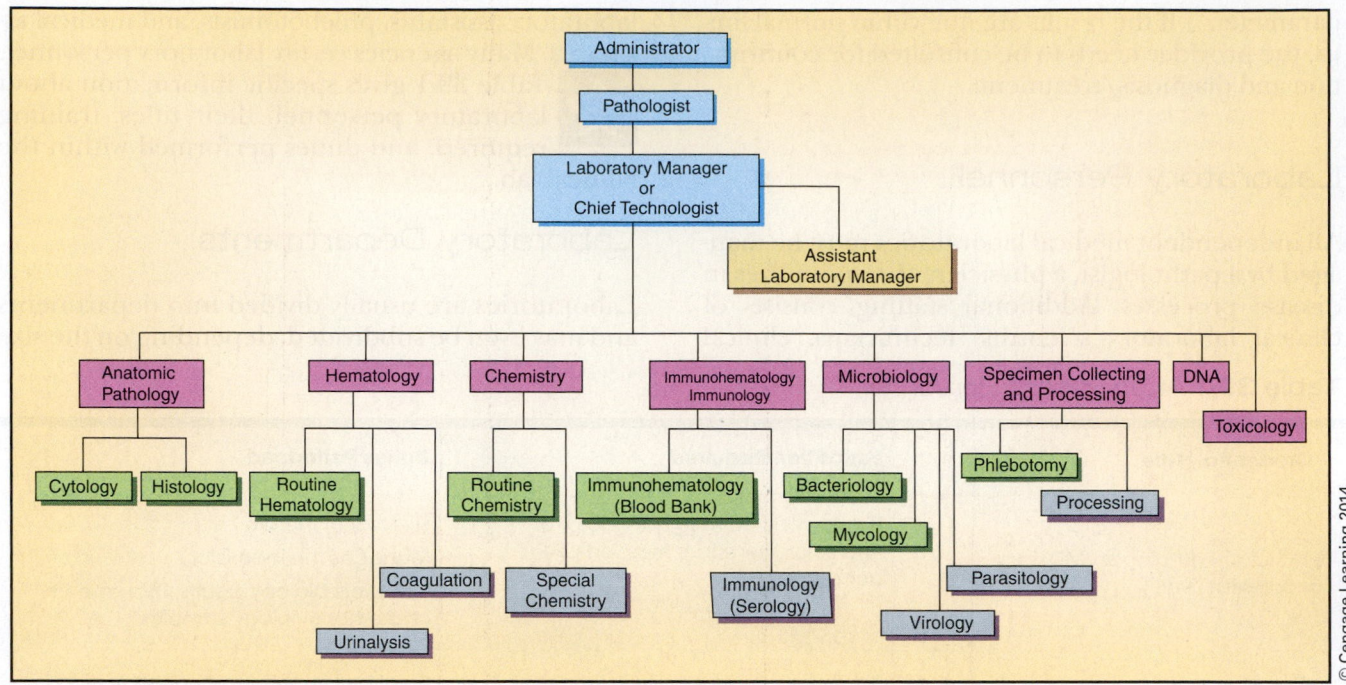

Figure 39-1　Departments of a typical medical laboratory.

and specialties within the laboratory (Figure 39-1). The various departments perform special tests categorized within their expertise (Table 39-2). Categorization becomes evident when test results are requested over the telephone or whenever there is a need to converse with laboratory personnel. Through knowledge of the various departments within the laboratory, information can be more readily obtained.

Hematology Department.
The **hematology** department tests the formed (cellular) elements of the blood. These tests may be quantitative (quantity) or qualitative (quality). The **quantitative tests** involve actual number counts such as counting the number of white blood cells (WBC), red blood cells (RBC), or platelets. The **qualitative tests** focus on the quality or characteristics of the components, such as the size, shape, and maturity of the cells. In addition, the hematology department tests the ability of the blood components to perform their individual tasks correctly. An example is testing the coagulation ability of clotting factors in blood.

Urinalysis Department.
Urinalysis is the physical, chemical, and microscopic examination of urine. Required cultures are sent to the microbiology or bacteriology department. In a large laboratory, the urinalysis department is often located under hematology because of the

microscopic examinations performed on urine (Figure 39-2).

Clinical Chemistry Department.
The **clinical chemistry** department analyzes the chemical composition of blood, cerebrospinal fluid, and joint fluid. Some of the procedures within this department include **assay** of enzymes in the **serum**, serum glucose, or **electrolyte** levels. Toxicology, including TDM and identification of drugs of abuse, is also performed in this department.

Immunohematology (Blood Bank) Department.
Immunohematology is a special area that deals with blood typing procedures, cross-matching, and the separation and storage of blood components for transfusion, as well as antibody-antigen reactions.

Serology (Immunology) Department.
The serology **(immunology)** department is the area of the laboratory that performs tests to evaluate the body's immune response, both production of antibodies and the cellular immune response. Procedures in this area include the detection of antibodies to bacteria and viruses, as well as antibodies produced against one's own body (autoimmune), as in rheumatic diseases such as rheumatoid arthritis and lupus erythematosus. Diseases such as AIDS have helped move laboratory evaluation of the cellular immune system out of the research setting

Table 39-2   Categories of Laboratory Tests

HEMATOLOGY

White blood cell (WBC) count	Hematocrit (Hct)
Red blood cell (RBC) count	Prothrombin time (PT)
Differential white blood cell count (Diff)	Erythrocyte sedimentation rate (ESR)
RBC indices	Platelet count
Hemoglobin (Hgb)	

CLINICAL CHEMISTRY

Glucose	Potassium
Blood urea nitrogen (BUN)	Bilirubin
Creatinine	Cholesterol
Total protein	Triglycerides
Albumin	Uric acid
Globulin	Lactate dehydrogenase, LD (LDH)
Calcium	Aspartate aminotransferase, AST (SGOT)
Inorganic phosphorus	Alanine aminotransferase, ALT (SGPT)
Chloride	Alkaline phosphatase
Sodium	Phospholipids

SEROLOGY (IMMUNOLOGY/IMMUNOHEMATOLOGY) AND BLOOD BANKING

Syphilis detection tests (VDRL, RPR)	Rheumatoid Arthritis factor (RA factor)
C-reactive protein test (CRP)	Mono test
ABO blood typing	Heterophil antibody titer test
Rh typing	Hepatitis tests
Rh antibody titer test	HIV tests: ELISA and Western blot
Cross-match	Antistreptolysin O (ASO) titer
Direct Coombs' test	Pregnancy tests
Cold agglutinins	

URINALYSIS

Physical analysis of urine:	Bilirubin
Color	Urobilinogen
Clarity	Nitrite
Specific gravity	Leukocyte esterase
Chemical analysis of urine:	Microscopic analysis of urine:
pH	Red blood cells
Glucose	White blood cells
Protein	Epithelial cells
Ketones	Casts
Blood	Crystals

continues

Table 39-2   Categories of Laboratory Tests (*Continued*)

MICROBIOLOGY

Candidiasis	Pneumonia
Chlamydia	Streptococcal sore throat
Diphtheria	Tetanus
Gonorrhea	Tonsillitis
Meningitis	Tuberculosis
Pertussis	Urinary tract infection
Pharyngitis	

PARASITOLOGY

Amebiasis	Scabies
Ascariasis	Tapeworm disease (cestodiasis)
Hookworm disease	Toxoplasmosis
Malaria	Trichinosis
Pinworm disease (enterobiasis)	Trichomoniasis

CYTOLOGY

Chromosome studies
Pap test

HISTOLOGY

Tissue analysis
Biopsy studies

DNA

DNA tests compare individuals according to their individual genotype

TOXICOLOGY

Tests for chemicals, specifically for drugs and other toxins in blood

and into the diagnostic setting of the medical laboratory. Molecular biology and flow cytometry are becoming commonplace in today's medical laboratory. Traditionally, serology has been an area within the microbiology department, but with the introduction of many new immunologic techniques, most medical laboratories now include a separate immunology department.

Toxicology. The **toxicology** department tests for toxic substances in a person's blood and monitors any drug usage, therapeutic levels of medication prescribed, or toxicity to the drugs being used. Medications commonly monitored for toxicity are digoxin, phenobarbital, lithium, and pain management drugs. Blood tests also determine levels of occupational exposure to metals and chemicals in the course of one's employment. Testing for drug usage/toxicity is now required in a growing number of pre-employment physical examinations. Toxicity levels for chemicals and metals include lead, zinc, iron, copper, arsenic, and carbon dioxide. The Department of Social and Health Services requires toxicology tests in child protection cases.

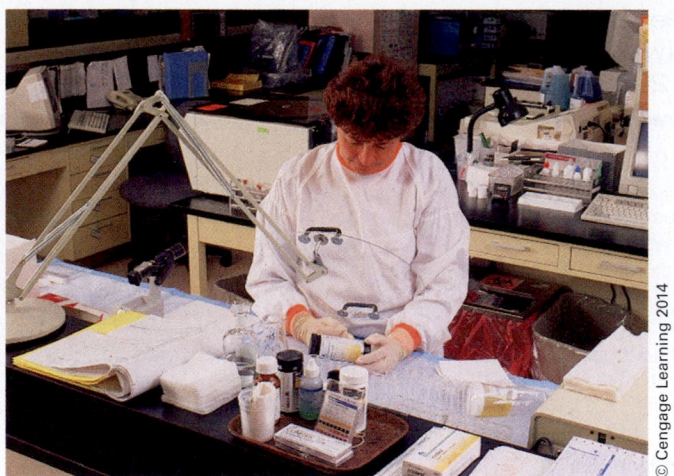

Figure 39-2 Clinical reference laboratories may have a separate urinalysis department where the laboratory professional tests urine for physical, chemical, and microbiologic properties.

Drug testing is often required for special assistance in low-income housing and other public financial assistance programs. The reasons for drug testing are wide and varied and are growing every year, making this department larger than in the past.

DNA. The second area within the medical laboratory growing larger each year is the DNA department. With the advent of **DNA** tests for proving paternity and maternity of children and the growing use of DNA testing for criminal cases, DNA testing is quickly becoming a major focus in many laboratories.

Microbiology Department. The **microbiology** department is the area in the laboratory where microorganisms such as bacteria and fungi are grown in an appropriate medium, cultured, and then identified. Sensitivity tests are then performed to identify which antibiotics can effectively eradicate the pathogenic organisms. The combination of culturing and identifying the best antibiotic is called **culture and sensitivity (C&S)**. **Mycology** is an area within the microbiology department where fungi are studied. **Virology** is an area within the microbiology department where viruses are studied.

Parasitology Department. **Parasitology** is a subdivision of the microbiology department where ova and parasite (O&P) tests are performed on specimens such as feces. The specimens are examined for the presence of parasites or their eggs.

Cytology Department. The **cytology** department is the area in which microscopic examinations of cells are performed to detect early signs of cancer and other diseases. The Papanicolaou test, known as the Pap smear, for irregular cervical cells is an example of a test performed in the cytology department.

Histology Department. **Histology** is the study of tissue sample biopsies for the determination of disease. Frozen samples or **biopsies** are sliced/stained and then microscopically examined for cancer and other anomalies.

Panels of Laboratory Tests

Laboratory tests are often categorized into related groups to provide information about a particular body system or related bodily function. The blood serum (the part of blood that doesn't contain cells) tests are usually referred to as panels, formerly called "profiles." In addition, requisition forms are organized into panels for ease of ordering. For a current list of CMS-approved organ- and disease-oriented panels, see Table 39-3.

Medicare requires that providers order tests under their approved panels. Providers may not refer to panels under other names such as the previously named Chem Screen, SMAC, Chem 7, and so on. The panels listed in Table 39-3 are the only panels allowed. If a provider would like a specific series or combinations of tests under a special panel, he or she must apply to the CMS for the approval to design their own panel.

BILLING FOR LABORATORY SERVICES

Providers must justify which lab tests are ordered by using the correct diagnosis code. For example, if the diagnosis is pneumonia, a urinalysis would not be justified and would not be covered. If a provider wants to order a test that probably will not be covered by insurance under CMS guidelines, the patient should sign a waiver. Medicare patients would sign an Advance Beneficiary Notice (ABN). The waiver/ABN notifies the patient that the test might not be covered and that the patient will have to pay for it. If the clinic fails to notify the patient, the patient does not have to pay for the test, and the provider is liable for the charges. Chapter 20 provides more information about insurances and billing practice.

Table 39-3 Centers for Medicare and Medicaid Services (CMS) Approved Organ- and Disease-Oriented Panels (with Current Procedural Terminology [CPT] Codes), Effective 2008

BASIC METABOLIC PANEL (CPT CODE 80048)

BUN (84520)	Creatinine (82565)
Calcium, total (82310)	Glucose (82947)
Carbon dioxide (82374)	Potassium (84132)
Chloride (82435)	Sodium (84295)

GENERAL HEALTH PANEL (CPT CODE 80050)

Comprehensive metabolic panel (CPT code 80053)	CBC w/manual differential (80054) or CBC w/automated differential (85025)
TSH (84443)	

ELECTROLYTE PANEL (CPT CODE 80051)

Carbon dioxide (82374)	Chloride (82435)
Potassium (84132)	Sodium (84295)

COMPREHENSIVE METABOLIC PANEL (CPT CODE 80053)

Albumin (82040)	Creatinine (82565)
Alkaline phosphatase (84075)	Glucose (82947)
Bilirubin, total (82247)	Potassium (84132)
BUN (84520)	Protein, total (84155)
Calcium, total (82310)	Sodium (84295)
Carbon dioxide (82374)	SGOT (AST) (84450)
Chloride (82435)	SGPT (ALT) (84460)

OBSTETRIC PANEL (CPT CODE 80055)

CBC w/manual differential (80054) or CBC w/automated differential (85025)	Syphilis test, qualitative (e.g., VDRL, RPR) (86592)
Hepatitis B surface antigen (87340)	Antibody screen, RBC (86850)
Rubella antibody (86762)	Blood typing, ABO (86900) and Rh (D) (86901)

LIPID PANEL (CPT CODE 80061)

Cholesterol (82465)	Triglyceride (84478)
HDL cholesterol (83718) and LDL cholesterol, calculated	

RENAL FUNCTION PANEL (CPT CODE 80069)

ALBUMIN (82040)	Creatinine (82565)
BUN (84520)	Glucose (82947)
Calcium, total (82310)	Phosphorus (84100)
Carbon dioxide (82374)	Potassium (2012)
Chloride (82435)	Sodium (84295)

ARTHRITIS PANEL (CPT CODE 80072)

Uric acid (84550)	Fluorescent noninfectious agent, screen (86255)
ESR, erythrocyte sedimentation rate (85651)	Rheumatoid factor, qualitative (86430)

ACUTE HEPATITIS PANEL (CPT CODE 80074)

Hepatitis A antibody, IgM (86709)	Hepatitis B surface antigen (87340)
Hepatitis B core antibody, IgM (86705)	Hepatitis C antibody (86803)

HEPATIC FUNCTION PANEL (CPT CODE 80076)

Albumin (82040)	Protein, total (84155)
Alkaline phosphatase (84075)	SGOT (AST) (84450)
Bilirubin, direct (82248)	SGPT (ALT) (84460)
Bilirubin, total (82247)	

TORCH ANTIBODY PANEL (CPT CODE 80090)

Cytomegalovirus antibody, IgG (86644)	Rubella antibody, IgG (86762)
Herpes simplex (1 & 2) antibody, IgG (86694/86695)	Toxoplasmosis antibody (86677)

QUALITY CONTROLS/ ASSURANCES IN THE LABORATORY

The accuracy of any laboratory test result depends on all safeguards being followed. These standards ensure the quality of the testing equipment, supplies, personnel, and the accuracy of the test results. Many factors can compromise the accuracy of laboratory test results. Among these factors are collection of specimen, temperature, amount or age of specimen, time limits of test, and using chemicals or reagents past their expiration dates. Even when laboratory guidelines are strictly followed, inaccurate results may be obtained by using test kits that have been exposed to extreme heat or cold, or using chemicals or reagents after their expiration. It is important to follow all laboratory guidelines, but the medical assistant must also confirm that the specimen, chemicals, and test kits are handled and processed properly.

Control Tests

To further ensure accurate test results, **control test** samples are tested together with the patient's sample. The control samples have a known value, negative or positive result, or abnormal or normal result, which is compared with the results of the patient's test. One of the purposes of this control measure is to minimize human error. By being able to compare a sample of known value or positive or negative test result with the patient's test, the health care worker performing the test can accurately determine the result. An error in the testing method may be discovered if the control sample does not test accurately.

Another purpose of the control test is to check the **reagents** or chemicals. If the control sample is not showing accurate results, it may be determined that the chemicals (reagents) are faulty or have expired. On receiving any test in the POL, the person responsible for quality assurance and quality control (probably the medical assistant performing the tests) should perform the calibration or control test provided by and as directed by the manufacturer. This ensures proper test function.

Proficiency Testing

CLIA '88 requires laboratories to participate in an accredited proficiency program for certain identified tests (see Chapter 38 for CLIA '88 requirements). Proficiency testing is similar to quality control in that "known" proficiency samples are tested the same as patient samples. The difference is an approved outside agency evaluates the accuracy of the testing and submits the performance records to CMS for CLIA '88 compliance.

Preventive Maintenance

Preventive maintenance helps identify potential problems before they actually occur. Procedures include manufacturer-recommended maintenance on equipment; daily temperature checks on refrigerators, freezers, and incubators; daily checks on expiration dates of reagents and supplies; and instrument log and centrifuge checks.

Instrument Validations

The quality of test results can be ensured by consistently checking the calibration and linear range of the instruments and machines. If the equipment is not maintained or is functioning improperly, accurate test results cannot be ensured.

The Medical Assistant's Role

 Medical assistants are educated to perform administrative office duties, prepare patients, collect specimens, and perform waived tests in such a manner that patients and health care personnel are safe from contamination, patients are not harmed, samples are reliable, and tests are accurate. These four aspects of quality laboratory testing are critical for accuracy. When the patient is prepared properly, the specimen is obtained as expertly as possible, the reagents and equipment are in the best condition and calibration possible, and the test is performed by a trained professional, the test results will be accurate. Professionals performing the lab tests should be able to explain the procedure to the patient, exactly follow the manufacturer's instruction, and follow proper protocol for labeling, handling and processing the specimen. Labeling should always occur in the presence of the patient.

LABORATORY REQUISITIONS AND REPORTS

A written **requisition** for laboratory work must be sent to the laboratory with the patient or with the specimen (Figure 39-3). These forms are preprinted with the most commonly requested tests separated into logical categories. Additional space is provided for writing special requests. The laboratories that patients use can provide your medical

Requested By

(1)

Courtesy Copy/Comments

Patient Information

Chart Number		Pre-Op? ☐ Y ☐ N	Surgery Date
Social Security Number		Sex	Date of Birth (required)
Patient Name	(2)		
Mailing Address		City	
State	Zip		Patient Phone

Insurance Information

| Insurance Company (Name/Billing Address) |
| |
| Guarantor (Responsible Party) |
| Insurance Number |
| Medicare Number |

(3)

REQUIRED REQUIRED

ICD.9 Diagnosis Code(s)

(4)

REQUIRED

Physician Notice: For reimbursement, Medicare **requires ABN signature** review (see reverse side) be made for the following tests in **bold,** that may NOT be covered under "Medical Necessity".

REQUIRED

☐ **STAT**   Phone Results ☐ # _____   Fasting _____   **Last Dose**   **Collected By**   Date
☐ **ASAP**   Medication _____
☐ **ROUTINE**   FAX Report ☐ # _____   hrs   Date/Time _____   ID _____   Time

Comments/Additional Tests

| SS = SST | L = LAV | B = BLUE | R = RED | G = GRAY | GN = GREEN | PK = PINK | U = URINE | C = CULTURE | S = SERUM | FROZEN | BIOPSY | SLIDES |

Alphabetical Test Listing	COLL CODE	Alphabetical Test Listing	COLL CODE	Alphabetical Test Listing	COLL CODE	Alphabetical Test Listing	COLL CODE	Microbiology
☐ ABO 50100 ☐ Rh 50200	R	☐ Creatinine 30570	S	☐ **Hepatitis Panel, Acute 40781**	S	☐ Prolactin 40450	S	Indicate Exact Specimen Source
☐ Albumin 30590	S	☐ Creatinine, Urine, 24hr 32100	U	• **Hep A Ab (IgM)** • **HBcAb (IgM)**		☐ Protein, Urine	U	
☐ Alkaline Phosphatase 30670	S	☐ Creatinine, Urine, Ran 32081	U	• **HBsAg** • **Hep C Ab**		☐ RAN 32180 ☐ 24hr 32200		☐ AFB Culture with Smear 64450
☐ **Alpha-fetoprotein 41150**	S	☐ Creatinine Clearance 32240	S,U	☐ **HIV-1 & -2 Antibody 42007**	S	☐ **PSA, Diagnostic 42158**	S	☐ C. difficile Toxin 68016
☐ ALT (SGPT) 30680	S	☐ C-Reactive Protein (CRP) 58200	S	☐ **HIV-1 RNA, PCR, Quant 42015**	L	☐ **PSA, Screen 41954**	S	☐ Chlamydia Only, Amplified 68361
☐ Amylase 31710	S	☐ CRP, Cardiac Risk 43575	S	☐ Homocysteine 43600	L	☐ **PSA Ratio, Free & Total 42147**	S	☐ Chlamydia/GC, Amplified 68395
☐ ANA (with Reflex) 69107	S	☐ **Digoxin 33060**	S	☐ Iron 30720	S	☐ **PT (Protime w/INR) 25000**	B	☐ Fungal Culture 64300
☐ Antibody Screen 50500	R	☐ Electrolytes 31310	S	☐ Iron, TRF Sat., (TIBC) 44210	S	☐ PTH (Whole Molecule) 40571	L	☐ Giardia Antigen 67031
☐ AST (SGOT) 30700	S	• Na • K • Cl • CO₂		☐ LDH 30710	S	☐ **PTT, Activated 25100**	B	☐ Gram Stain, Direct 60050
☐ **B₁₂ 41250**	S	☐ Electrophoresis, Serum 48010	S	☐ **LDL Direct 43571**	S	☐ **Reticulocyte Count 21150**	L	☐ Herpes simplex Virus Culture 68263
☐ B₁₂/Folate 41311	S	☐ Electrophoresis, Urine 48310	U	☐ LH 40500	S	☐ **Rheumatoid Factor 44480**	S	☐ Herpes/Varicella Virus Culture 68277
☐ Basic Metabolic Panel 31307	S	☐ **ESR (Sed Rate) 21050**	L	☐ Lipase 31740	S	☐ **RPR 58800**	S	☐ Influenza A & B, Direct Exam 65092
• Na • K • Cl • CO₂		☐ Estradiol 41600	S	☐ **Lipid Panel 1 43560**	S	☐ Rubella 58681	S	☐ KOH Prep 64200
• BUN • Creat • Gluc • Ca		☐ **Ferritin 41350**	S	• **Chol** • **HDL** • **Trig** • **LDL**		☐ Semen, Post Vasectomy 23540	Se	☐ Ova & Parasite 67002
☐ BNP 31379	L	☐ Folate 41300	S	• **Chol/HDL** • **LDL/HDL**		☐ T3, Free 40070	S	☐ Pinworm Prep 67200
☐ BUN 30560	S	☐ FSH 40400	S	☐ **Rflx Direct LDL, Trig> 400 43562**		☐ T3, Total 40200	S	☐ Polys (WBC's) 67455
☐ Bilirubin, Total 30640	S	☐ GGT 30690	S	☐ **Lithium 33320**	S	☐ **T4 (Thyroxine) 40000**	S	☐ Rapid Strep-A Antigen,
☐ Bilirubin, Direct 30650	S	☐ **Glucose 30550**	S	☐ Lymphocyte T-Cell Subsets 29100	LGN	☐ **T4, Free 40050**	S	Culture if Negative 65100
☐ **CA 125 41050**	S	☐ **Glucose Tolerance Test ___ hrs**	S	☐ Lymphocytes, T-Helper 29150	LGN	☐ **Free Thyroxine Index,**	S	☐ Rotavirus 68073
☐ **CA 19.9 42900**	S	☐ **Glucose 2hr PP 31820**	S	☐ **Magnesium 31280**	SS	☐ **FTI (T4 + TU) 40025**		☐ Trichomonas Wet Mount 60103
☐ **CA 27.29 41061**	S	☐ **hCG-beta, Quantitative 41100**	S	☐ Microalbumin, Urine	U	☐ Thyroid Peroxidase Ab 34720	S	**Culture, Bacterial**
☐ Calcium 30610	S	☐ **hCG-beta, Tumor Marker 41110**	S	☐ Ran 43980 ☐ 24hr 42101		☐ **Theophylline 33430**	S	☐ Anaerobic 61653
☐ Carbamazepine (Tegretol) 33050	S	☐ **HCV RNA, PCR, Quant 40738**	L	☐ Timed ___ hrs ___ min 42100		☐ Total Protein 30580	S	☐ Blood 60250
☐ Cardiolipin Abs, IgG, IgM 27500	S	☐ H. pylori, IgG 58322	S	☐ Microalbumin/Creat Ratio 43985	U	☐ **Triglycerides 30730**	S	☐ CSF 60450
☐ **CBC w/auto differential 20000**	L	☐ **Hemoglobin AIC (Glycol) 42550**	L	☐ Monotest 58550	S	☐ **Troponin I 31378**	S	☐ Catheter Tip 60420
☐ **Hemogram Only 20150**		☐ **Hepatic Function Panel 31306**	S	☐ **Occult Blood Screen 67100**	F	☐ **TSH 40250**	S	☐ E. coli – 0157, Only 61227
☐ **CEA 41000**	S	• **Alk Phos** • **Alb** • **DBil** • **TBil** • **TP**		☐ **Occult Blood Diagnostic 67105**	F	☐ **TSH with Reflex 40012**	S	☐ GC Only 60750
☐ **Cholesterol 30740**	S	• **ALT (SGPT)** • **AST (SGOT)**		☐ Phenytoin (Dilantin) 33360	S	☐ **Testosterone 40550**	S	☐ Genital, Full Culture 60800
☐ CK, Total 31350	S	☐ Hep A Ab, IgM 42114	S	☐ Phenytoin, Free & Total 87060	R	☐ Uric Acid 30630	S	☐ Group-B Strep Only, Genital 60217
☐ Comp Metabolic Panel 31305	S	☐ Hep B Core Ab, IgM 42141	S	☐ Phosphorus 30620	S	☐ **UA & Microscopic 24080**	U	☐ MRSA Screen, Nares 60867
• Na • K • Cl • CO₂ • Gluc		☐ Hep C Ab 40711	S	☐ **Potassium/NA 30510**	S	☐ **UA & Microscopic, Reflex**	U	☐ Sputum/Trach/Bronch 61100
• BUN • Creat • Ca • AST • ALT		☐ Hepatitis B Immunity Scrn 40770	S	☐ Prealbumin 44470	S	**with C&S if Indicated 11850**		☐ Stool, Full Culture 61150
• TP • Alb • A/G • Alk Phos • TBil		☐ HBsAg 42127	S	☐ Progesterone 41750	S			☐ Strep-A Screen, Throat 60207
								☐ Throat Culture 61350
								☐ **Urine Culture 61500**
								☐ Wound, 61657

(5)

Lab Use Only
Veni ☐ A 95370 ☐ C 95372
☐ NH 99561
Hfee ☐ 1 ☐ 2 ☐ 3

source:
_____

© Cengage Learning 2014

Many payors (including Medicare and Medicaid) have a necessity requirement for the diagnosis and treatment of the patient, therefore, only those tests which are medically necessary should be ordered.

Figure 39-3 Sample laboratory requisition form. 1. Physician information, 2. Patient information, 3. Billing information, 4. Specimen information, 5. Tests ordered.

agency with these forms. Laboratory requisition forms are computer generated, and the provider's name, address, and other information necessary for proper reporting and recordkeeping are often pre-printed on the forms. If the requisitions are not preprinted, spaces are provided for the information to be written in. The information must be complete, accurate, and clearly legible. A properly completed requisition contains the following data:

- *Provider's name, account number, address, and telephone number.* This information is necessary to contact the office for any clarification or further information and to report the results.

- *Patient's name, address, and telephone number.* Be sure the name is complete and spelled correctly. Avoid using alternate versions of the patient's name without also including the proper, legal name. Make certain to include apartment numbers and ZIP codes. This information will be used for billing purposes, as well as medical records. Social Security numbers and middle initials are helpful when it is necessary to differentiate between patients.

- *Patient's billing information, insurance, and identification number.* Because the patient is often not the person who is the subscriber to the insurance, the subscriber's name, address, telephone number, and insurance identification numbers are extremely important, especially if the patient does not live with the subscriber. Some patients have secondary insurance coverage. Be sure to include that data also. The laboratory would prefer to receive an additional sheet of information than to have incomplete insurance records in its business office.

- *Unique patient identifier.* This can be an identification number that is hospital or laboratory generated. In the outpatient setting, this can be the patient's Social Security number or date of birth.

- *Patient's age/date of birth and sex.* Age and sex both influence the results of some tests and should not be assumed.

- *Source of specimen.* This information is especially important when dealing with tests such as cultures and biopsies. In the case of cultures, knowing the source of the specimen aids the laboratory in determining whether the specimen contains normal flora or is abnormal for that area of the body.

- *Time and date of the specimen collection.* Some tests require that the specimen be tested fairly quickly after leaving the body; other tests must be performed after a certain period has elapsed. The time and date of the specimen collection are important because accuracy can be compromised if the specimen is not sent to the laboratory in a reasonable amount of time.

- *Test requested.* This is usually a matter of putting a check mark in the appropriate box on the requisition, but it is surprising how often laboratories receive specimens with nicely completed requisitions and no indication of the test desired.

- *Medications the patient is taking.* Because medication can influence some test results, it is important that the laboratory be provided this information. Patients are often asked to refrain from taking certain medications before testing. Be sure to consult with the provider to verify orders. If a medication is not discontinued before testing, the type of medication, the dosage amount, and the time of the last dose must be included on the requisition.

- *Clinical diagnosis.* The provider's tentative diagnosis is useful to the laboratory in helping to differentiate between diagnoses or confirm a diagnosis. The clinical diagnosis may also alert the laboratory personnel to any possible special considerations of which to be aware. For example, if diabetes is suspected, the laboratory will give special consideration to the glucose value. The diagnosis or preferably the ICD-9 code is also necessary for billing.

- *Urgency of results.* Sometimes the provider needs a test to be performed immediately (STAT) or would like a result as soon as possible (ASAP). The provider's orders need to be clearly stated on the requisition. Additional space is also provided for other special instructions if necessary.

- *Special collection/patient instructions.* Examples include fasting specimens, timed collections, and "do not collect from a specific area" instructions.

- If copies of the results are to be sent to a second provider, the medical assistant must include the provider's full name, address, and fax number. Be careful to print the fax number clearly so that the patient's results are not sent to the wrong place in error.

> Many offices copy both sides of the patient's insurance card and attach the copies to the laboratory requisition. This ensures the laboratory will have all the insurance information it needs to bill for its services.

```
Patient Name: FAKEY FAKERSON
Note: All result statuses are Final unless otherwise noted.

Tests (1) BASIC METABOLIC PANEL (31308)

    SODIUM                          [H]   155 mmol/L        136-145
    POTASSIUM                       [H]   5.7 mmol/L        3.5-5.1
    CHLORIDE                        [H]   115 mEq/L         96-108
    TOTAL CO2                             25 mmol/L         22-29
    GLUCOSE                         [H]   200 mg/dL         70-109
    UREA NITROGEN (BUN)                   15 mg/dL          5-20
    CREATININE                            1.1 mg/dL         0.6-1.3
    CALCIUM                         [H]   10.5 mg/dL        8.4-10.2


       Test Performed at Northwest Regional Laboratories

Note: An exclamation mark (!) indicates a result that was not dispersed into the flowsheet.
Document Creation Date: 09/18/2008 2:33 PM
_____

(1) Order result status: Final
Collection or observation date-time: 09/18/2008 14:12
Requested date-time: 09/18/2008 14:12
Receipt date-time: 09/18/2008 14:12
Reported date-time: 09/18/2008 14:16
Referring Physician:
Ordering Physician: MARK SMITH (17006)
Specimen Source:
Producer ID: SMSLIS
Filler Order Number: NZ80009408
Lab site:

Signed by: Mary L Ponder on 09/23/2008 at 10:14 AM
```

© Cengage Learning 2014

Figure 39-4   Sample computerized laboratory report.

The laboratory will send back a written report (Figure 39-4) that will contain the following information:

- Name, address, and telephone number of the laboratory
- Referring provider's name, address, and identification numbers
- Patient's name, identification number, age, and sex
- Date the specimen was received by the laboratory
- Date and time the specimen was collected
- Date the laboratory reported the results
- The test name, results, and normal reference ranges if applicable

EHR Lab requisitions may be electronically generated using an electronic health record (EHR) program and completed on screen and then either printed for the patient to take to the outside lab or sent electronically to the lab.

Occasionally a requisition will be faxed to a lab if the EHR is not available. Interestingly, today's medical clinic staff may perform a combination of electronic and manual communication with outside labs. Eventually the electronic format will replace all manual methods.

Reports are sent to the provider by fax (Figure 39-5), manually delivered to the clinic, or sent electronically using EHR software (Figures 39-4 and 39-5.)

Abnormal test results are always flagged in some way, either in a different color, a different column, or perhaps designated by a star or simply by *H* (for high) or *L* (for low). Critical values (results that may indicate serious medical conditions) are alerted to the provider by a phone call from the laboratory.

When the results are received, the medical assistant should attach them to the patient's chart for the provider to review and initial before filing them. The provider should be alerted to any abnormal test results as soon as possible. Laboratories

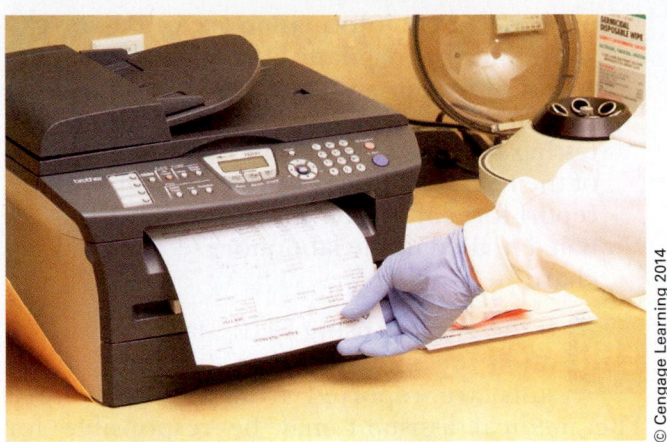

Figure 39-5 The computerized laboratory report is transmitted directly from the reference lab to the provider's office if the EHR is not available.

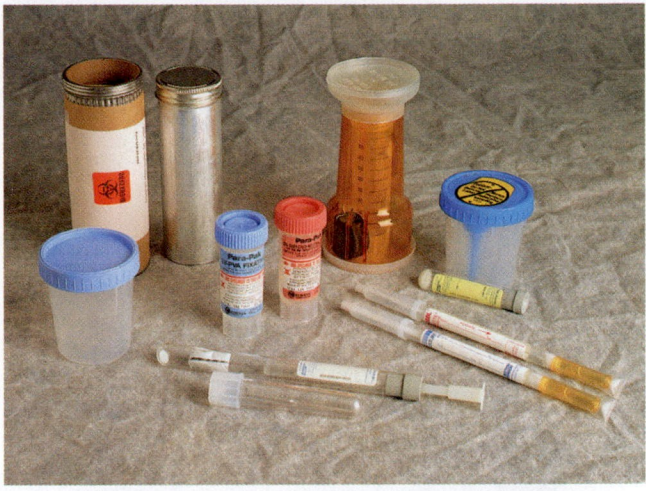

Figure 39-6 Various types of collection and transportation containers for laboratory specimens.

often send results via computer-generated reports directly to the provider's office or hospital.

THE SPECIMEN

Proper Procurement, Storage, and Handling

Instructions for procuring, storing, and handling and transporting laboratory specimens properly can be obtained from the independent laboratories. Most laboratories will provide the office/clinic with a step-by-step instruction manual, sometimes called a compendium, a laboratory manual, or a user manual and will also be available to answer any additional questions by telephone.

Obtaining the specimen in the proper manner and using the right equipment will ensure that a high-quality specimen is submitted to the laboratory. Some guidelines are as follows:

- Check the provider's orders and identify the patient.
- Refer to the laboratory instruction manual or consult the laboratory for specific collection instructions.
- Instruct the patient on any necessary dietary restriction (see Patient Education box).
- Instruct the patient to ingest special food or take other substances if required.
- Select or provide to the patient appropriate containers with the proper preservatives in them, if required.
- Be certain to label the specimen with the patient's name, identification number, date, type of specimen, time of collection, and

provider's name. Label the container, not the lid, because the lid will be removed during testing. Label the container, not the wrapping, because the wrapping will be separated from the container when testing is performed, for example, throat swabs.

- Obtain the specimen or instruct the patient to provide the specimen according to the directions given by the laboratory.
- Follow applicable OSHA bloodborne pathogens guidelines (see standard precautions in Chapter 22) when packaging the specimen for transport so it will not leak or contaminate the courier or other office staff and so that it will safely arrive at the laboratory without being damaged or destroyed (Figure 39-6).
- Place any biologic specimen to be sent to an outside laboratory into an approved biologic transport bag (Figure 39-7 A–C). These bags, which have the universal symbol for biohazard caution stamped on them, contain two sections: one for the specimen and one for the requisition. The requisition and specimen are placed in the proper areas within the transport bag, and the bag is sealed. When the testing laboratory receives the bag, the other end is torn open so that the specimen and requisitions can be removed without contaminating the receiver.
- Document in the patient's chart or electronic medical record the type of specimen collected, the tests ordered, which laboratory the specimen is being sent to (even if it is being tested in your POL), how the patient tolerated the procedure (including any complications), and

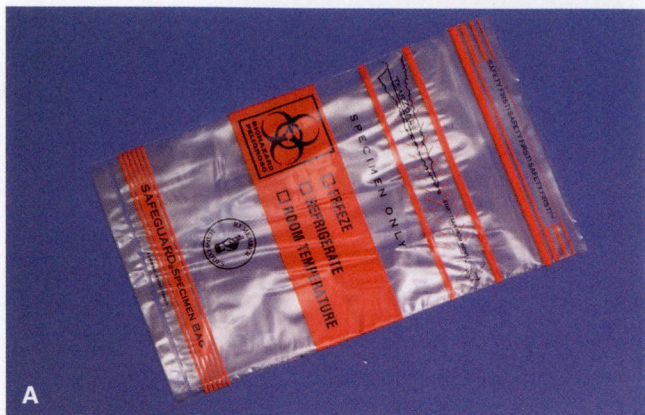

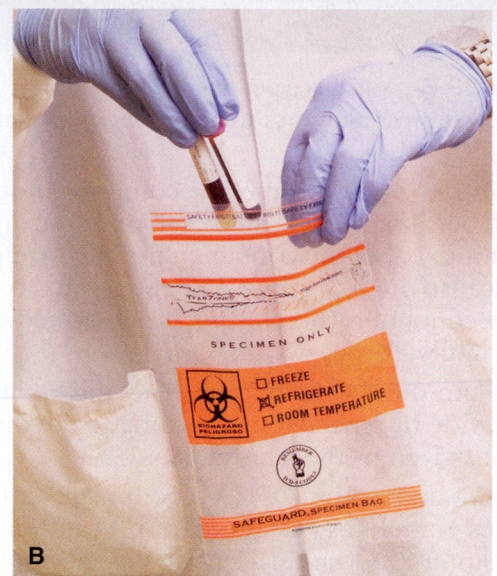

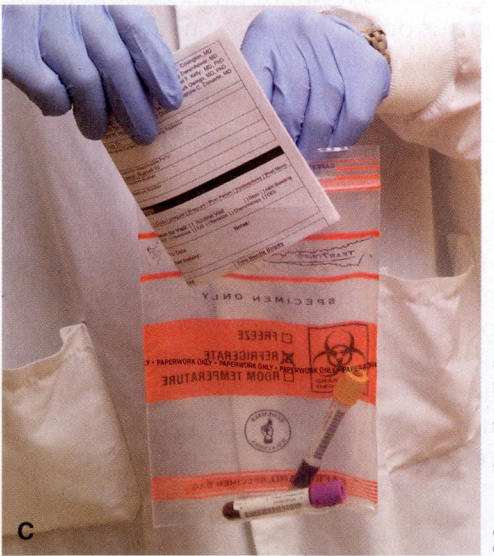

© Cengage Learning 2014

Figure 39-7 Preparing a biological specimen to be sent to an outside laboratory. (A) Laboratory specimen transport bag. (B) The medical assistant places the specimen into the transport bag and seals that part of the bag. (C) The medical assistant places the requisition into a separate compartment of the bag.

other pertinent information according to your office policy. Many offices also keep a copy of the laboratory requisition in the patient's chart for later reference. If the testing is performed in your POL, the results of the test should be recorded on a laboratory report form and, after the provider has initialed it, filed in the laboratory section of the chart.

EHR If the clinic is using EHRs, lab requisitions often stay in a "pending" file until the results are reported from the laboratory. The medical assistant may be responsible for tracking pending lab tests until the reports are received.

If the medical clinic and lab both are using EHRs, they may share an interface software program that allows the report to be imported onto the provider's desktop as an "unsigned" document. Many clinics have policies in place that require the provider to electronically "sign" lab reports within 36 or 48 hours of receipt.

Processing and Sending Specimens to a Laboratory

Specimens collected by the medical assistant are often sent from the office to a laboratory many miles away or are picked up by a courier representing the outside laboratory. These are often large commercial laboratories that are not associated with a local hospital laboratory. The patient's insurance often dictates the laboratory contracted to perform the patient's testing. It is not unusual for several different laboratories to pick up at one location. A situation could be that the blood work from patient Jones would go to laboratory A, the blood work from patient Smith would go to laboratory B, and a urine sample from patient Doe would be tested in the laboratory within the building. It sometimes can be confusing as to where to send the specimen.

All laboratory test results are dependent on the quality of the specimen submitted. The quality of the specimen depends on patient preparation, proper collection, correct patient identification, and transportation of the specimen. If there is any doubt or question regarding the type of specimen to be collected, it is imperative that the appropriate laboratory be called to clarify the specimen needed. There are often differences between laboratories; the type of specimen acceptable for one laboratory is not necessarily the acceptable specimen for another laboratory.

PATIENT EDUCATION

The patient will often need to be instructed on a specific preparation before a specimen is taken. Because food and medication can greatly influence test results, a patient may need to be instructed not to eat for several hours before having the specimen taken or drawn. Fasting means the patient may not have anything except water for the 12 hours before the test. NPO (Nothing by Mouth) means the patient may not have even water. The patient may need to refrain from taking a routine dosage of medication before the test is performed. Sometimes the patient preparation instructions will include a special diet for a few days. Regardless of how simple instructions may seem, it is important to give the patient clear, written directions. Take the time to go over any instructions with the patient (and sometimes other family members as authorized). Your patients will welcome the opportunity to ask questions and to have a written set of instructions to take home.

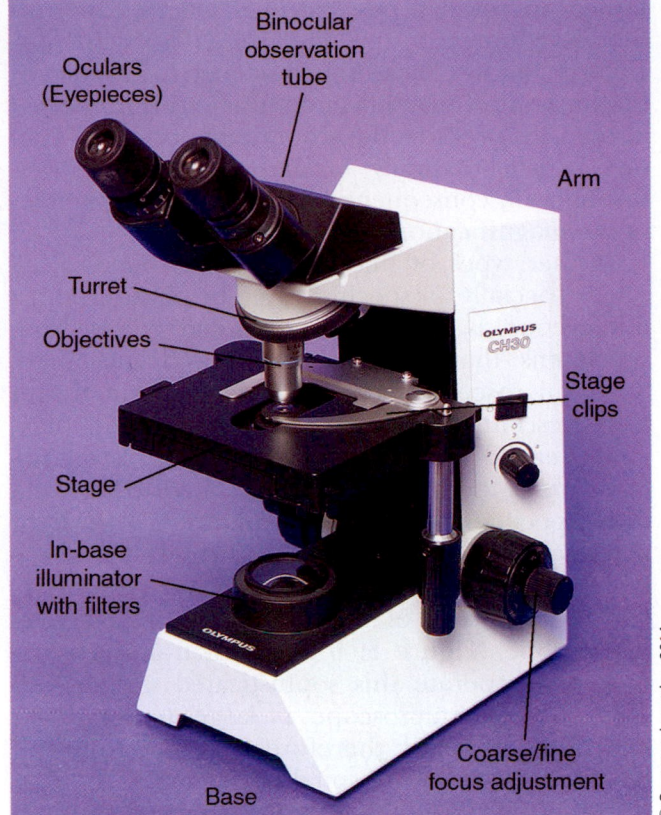

Figure 39-8   Basic compound microscope.

© Cengage Learning 2014

MICROSCOPES

One of the most used pieces of equipment in the medical laboratory is the microscope. Consisting of a light source, eyepieces, objectives, condenser and diaphragm, the microscope enables us to see bacteria and other microorganisms that are much too small to be seen without magnification.

Types of Microscopes

The most commonly used microscope in the clinic is the compound microscope (Figure 39-8). As the name indicates, the image is compounded by the use of two different lenses. One lens compounds or increases the magnification produced by the other lens. The first lens system is located in the objectives, and the second lens system is in the eyepiece (ocular). The light source is a bulb in the base. The light is directed up through the specimen on the slide and into the objective lenses. The light, or image, is then reflected by the condenser onto the specimen to the ocular lenses for visualization.

The eyepiece may have a single (monocular) lens, or there may be two (binocular) lenses. This lens is not adjustable or changeable. The magnification in the eyepiece is usually 10 times (10x) the normal size of the object being viewed.

The objective lenses are adjustable between low power, high power, and oil immersion. When viewing through the microscope under low power, more of the slide can be seen but with less detail than when using high power. When viewing under high power, a smaller portion of the field can be seen but with greater detail. The low-power objective lens allows the item being viewed to be magnified 10 times larger than life. This magnification combined with the 10 times magnification of the ocular lens gives the ability to see microscopically 100 times the normal size (10x × 10x = 100x).

Combining the 10-power (10x) ocular lens with the high-power objective lens, which has the magnification power of 40 times life (40x), increases magnification vision to 400 times the normal size (10x × 40x = 400x). This is enough magnification to see large microorganisms but is still not enough to see smaller organisms, such as bacteria, clearly. An oil-immersion lens is needed to view bacteria closely.

The oil-immersion lens gives the ability to multiply the ocular lens magnification (10x) by hundred

(100x) to reach a possible total magnification of thousand times normal life size (10x × 100x = 1,000x). Because more light is needed to actually see this amount of magnification, the lens is immersed in oil. This prevents the scattering and loss of light rays, which naturally occurs when light travels through air, consequently increasing the efficiency of the magnification.

Other types of microscopes have been developed especially for specific uses. The phase-contrast microscope is specifically designed for viewing specimens that are transparent and unstained. Some microscopic specimens must be stained with a fluorescent dye to be examined in detail (e.g., when detecting specific bacteria). A fluorescent microscope is the instrument best suited for viewing those specimens. In dark-field microscopy, the light is reflected from an angle, which causes the specimen to appear as a bright object on a dark field.

Another type of microscope is the electron microscope (Figure 39-9). Special training is required to operate this sophisticated instrument. The electron microscope is large (several feet tall) and expensive; therefore, it is only found in larger regional and hospital laboratories. An electronic beam, rather than light, is passed through the specimen. The image is projected onto a fluorescent screen and may then be photographed and enlarged. The electron microscope provides views of extremely small organisms, such as viruses, in great detail and in three dimensions. Figure 39-10 shows blood cells seen using an electron microscope.

How to Use a Microscope

Besides being able to adjust a microscope's magnification, it may be necessary to adjust focus. The microscope contains a coarse adjustment and a fine adjustment. The coarse adjustment is to be used with the low-power (short) objective only. The coarse adjustment is used to bring the object into view. The fine adjustment may then be used to sharpen the image. Depending on the individual microscope, the coarse and fine adjustments may raise and lower the nosepiece, which houses the objectives, or they may raise and lower the stage, or platform, on which the slide rests.

It is important always to remember to raise the platform of the lower objectives using the coarse adjustment and the low-power objective *while viewing the slide from the side.* This allows the lens to come close to the slide without actually touching it. If the slide is not viewed from the side for the coarse adjustment, there is the possibility of running the objective through the slide and seriously damaging the lens and the microscope, or of breaking the slide. After bringing the slide and objective together, the adjustments may be made through the ocular, always moving away from the slide. Once the item is in view, the fine adjustment may be used for clarity.

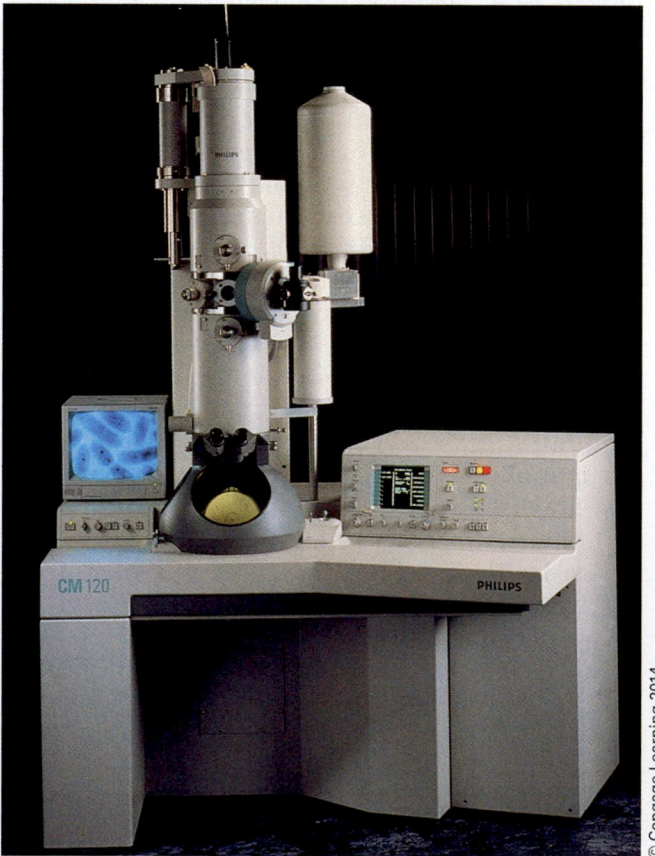

Figure 39-9   S440 scanning electron microscope.

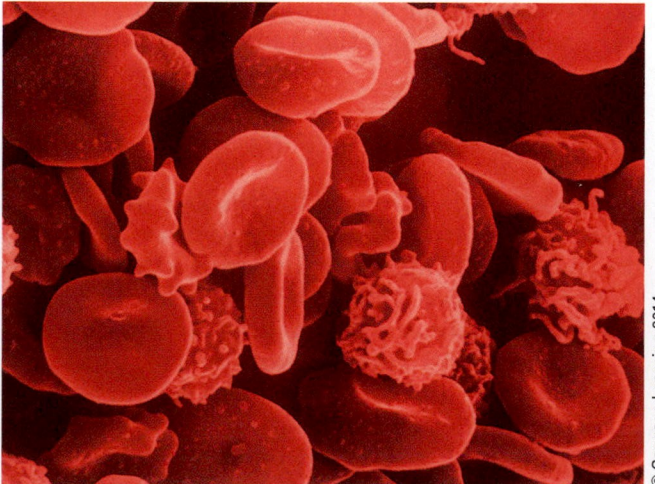

Figure 39-10   Blood cells as seen under an electron microscope.

The bulb in the base directs light through the slide. The light first goes through a condenser and then through an iris diaphragm. The condenser is used to control the intensity of the light, and the iris diaphragm may be adjusted to control the amount of light.

To use the oil-immersion lens, place a drop of cedar or mineral oil on top of the coverslip directly over the specimen on the slide. Then carefully lower the oil-immersion lens into the oil, making sure that the lens never actually touches the slide.

How to Care for a Microscope

Microscopes can be expensive and, like any precision instrument, should be treated with care. Some practices that will extend the life of a microscope and maintain the quality of its performance are:

- Always follow the manufacturer's and clinic's rules for the care and maintenance of the microscope.
- Carry the microscope with one hand securely supporting the base and the other hand holding the arm (Figure 39-11).
- Keep the microscope covered when it is not being used.
- Clean the lenses with special lens paper and lens cleaner after each use. Using standard tissue can scratch the lenses.

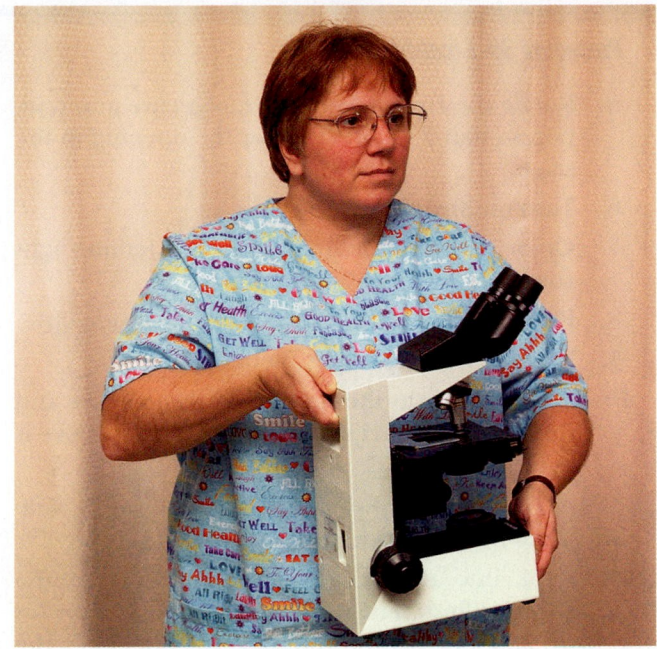

© Cengage Learning 2014

Figure 39-11 The proper way to carry a microscope.

- When looking through the eyepiece and focusing, always move the platform away from, never toward, the eyepiece to prevent the objective from coming into contact with the slide. If you are actually looking at the platform, then you can move it closer to the eyepiece without coming into contact with the slide.
- Use oil only with the oil-immersion lens.

PROCEDURE 39-1

Using the Microscope

STANDARD PRECAUTIONS:

PURPOSE:

To properly use a microscope to view microscopic organisms using the coarse and fine adjustments, as well as the low- and high-power and oil-immersion objectives.

EQUIPMENT/SUPPLIES:

Hand disinfectant
Microscope (monocular or binocular)
Manufacturer's manual
Lens paper
Lens cleaner

Prepared slides (commercially available)
Immersion oil
Solvent cleaner
Surface disinfectant

NOTE: Procedure will vary slightly according to microscope design. Consult the operating procedure in the microscope manual for specific instructions.

PROCEDURE STEPS:

1. Wash hands.
2. Assemble equipment and materials.
3. Clean the ocular(s) and objectives with lens paper.
4. Use the coarse adjustment to raise the eyepiece or lens unit.

continues

Procedure 39-1 (continued)

5. Rotate the 10x, or low-power, objective into position so that it is directly over the opening in the stage.

6. Turn on the microscope light.

7. Open the diaphragm until maximum light comes up through the condenser.

8. Place the slide on the stage (specimen side up).

9. Locate the coarse adjustment.

10. Look directly at the stage and 10x objective and turn the coarse adjustment until the objective is as close to the slide as it will go.

    NOTE: Do not lower any objective toward a slide while looking through the ocular(s).

11. Look into the ocular(s) and slowly turn the coarse adjustment in the opposite direction (as in Step 10) to raise the objective (or lower the stage) until the object on the slide comes into view.

12. Locate the fine adjustment.

13. Turn the fine adjustment to sharpen the image.

    NOTE: If a binocular microscope is used, the oculars must be adjusted for each individual's eyes

    a. Adjust the distance between the oculars so that one image is seen (as when using binoculars).

    b. Use the coarse and fine adjustments to bring the object into focus while looking through the right ocular with the right eye.

    c. Close the right eye, look into the left ocular with the left eye, and *use the knurled collar on the left ocular* to bring the object into sharp focus. (Do not turn the coarse or fine adjustment at this time.)

    d. Look into the oculars with both eyes to observe that the object is in clear focus. If it is not, repeat the procedure.

14. Scan the slide by either method:

    a. Use the stage knobs to move the slide left and right and backward and forward while looking through the ocular(s), or

    b. Move the slide with the fingers while looking through the ocular(s) (for microscope without movable stage).

15. Rotate the high-power (40x) objective into position while observing the objective and the slide to see that the objective does not strike the slide.

16. Look through the ocular(s) to view the object on the slide; it should be almost in focus.

17. Locate the fine adjustment.

18. Look through the ocular(s) and turn the fine adjustment until the object is in focus. Do not use the coarse adjustment.

19. Adjust the amount of light. This can be done by closing the diaphragm, lowering the condenser, or adjusting the light at the source.

20. Scan the slide as in Step 14, using the fine adjustment if necessary to keep the object in focus.

21. Rotate the oil-immersion objective to the side slightly (so that no objective is in position).

22. Place one drop of immersion oil on the portion of the slide that is directly over the condenser.

23. Rotate the oil-immersion objective into position, being careful not to rotate the 40x objective through the oil.

24. Look to see that the oil-immersion objective is touching the drop of oil.

25. Look through the ocular(s) and slowly turn the fine adjustment until the image is clear. Use only the fine adjustment to focus the oil-immersion objective.

26. Adjust the amount of light using the procedure in Step 19.

27. Scan the slide using the procedure in Step 14.

28. Rotate the 10x objective into position (do not allow the 40x objective to touch the oil).

29. Remove the slide from the microscope stage and gently clean the oil from the slide with lens paper. A copeland jar containing a solvent cleaner, such as xylene, can be used to remove excess oil from the slide.

30. Clean the oculars, 10x objective, and 40x objective with clean lens paper and lens cleaner.

31. Clean the 100x objective with lens paper and lens cleaner to remove all oil.

32. Clean any oil from the microscope stage and condenser.

33. Turn off the microscope light and disconnect.

34. Position the eyepiece in the lowest position using the coarse adjustment.

35. Center the stage so that it does not project from either side of the microscope.

36. Cover the microscope and return it to storage.

37. Clean the work area; return slides to storage.

38. Wash hands.

CASE STUDY 39-1

Refer to the scenario at the beginning of the chapter. Now imagine that Wanda sent Annette to the lab for the urinalysis rather than performing the test in the POL.

CASE STUDY REVIEW

1. What was the advantage of Wanda performing the urinalysis in the POL rather than sending Annette to the lab for the urinalysis?

2. What would have been an advantage of sending Annette to the outside lab for the urinalysis?

CASE STUDY 39-2

Edith Leonard came to Inner City Health Care because she was experiencing sight disturbances, constant thirst, and fainting spells. After examining Edith, Dr. Ray Reynolds ordered a glucose tolerance test. Certified medical assistant Wanda Slawson gave Edith a special diet that she was to follow for the 3 days preceding the test and instructions regarding fasting before the test.

Edith has returned to the clinic to have the test. "Did you follow the diet I gave you, Mrs. Leonard?" Wanda asks. "Yes, I did." "Did you have anything to eat this morning?" "No, but I did have a cup of coffee. I thought it would be all right because I drink it black. I can't start the day without my coffee."

CASE STUDY REVIEW

1. Should Wanda perform the test? Explain your answer.
2. How can Wanda emphasize the importance of following the diet, fasting, and test instructions?
3. What can Wanda do to try to ensure Edith's cooperation?

SUMMARY

If disease did not exist, we would have little need for clinical laboratories. If we were not susceptible to viral illnesses, if bacteria never infected our bodies, if our bodies always operated in their healthiest state regardless of what we did to them, and, perhaps most important of all, if we chose our parents wisely, there would be little that a clinical laboratory would be asked to do. The fact that our bodies are susceptible to disease necessitates the existence of clinical laboratories.

Together with clinical laboratory personnel, medical assistants play an important role in laboratory testing. They prepare patients for tests, obtain specimens, and perform simple, routine tests or send specimens to the appropriate laboratory. Medical assistants are educated to perform these tasks in a manner that ensures the accuracy of the test and safeguards the health of patients and health care personnel.

STUDY FOR SUCCESS

To reinforce your knowledge and skills of information presented in this chapter:

- Review the *Key Terms*
- Role-play with other students to apply attributes of professionalism pertinent to this chapter.
- Consider the *Case Studies* and discuss your conclusions
- Answer the questions in the *Certification Review*
- Apply your knowledge by completing the *Activities* in the *Study Guide* and the *Games and Quizzes* in the StudyWARE **StudyWARE** software on the *Premium Website*

continues

STUDY FOR SUCCESS (CONTINUED)

- Perform the *Procedure* using the *Competency Assessment Checklists* in the *Competency Manual*
- Practice your problem-solving skills with the *Critical Thinking Challenge 3.0* on the *Premium Website*

Additional resources for this chapter include:

- Module 22 of the *Medical Assisting Learning Lab*
- *CourseMate for Delmar's Comprehensive Medical Assisting*
- *WebTutor for Delmar's Comprehensive Medical Assisting*

CERTIFICATION REVIEW

1. All of the following statements concerning point-of-care testing are true *except:*
   a. performed at the patient's bedside
   b. must be performed by certified laboratory professionals
   c. provides for rapid, accurate results
   d. the medical laboratory's role includes training and management of quality control

2. Independent medical laboratories must be managed by a:
   a. clinical laboratory technologist
   b. pathologist
   c. clinical laboratory technician
   d. medical assistant

3. The hematology department of a laboratory:
   a. studies microorganisms and their activities
   b. studies blood and blood-forming tissues
   c. detects the presence of disease-producing human parasites or eggs present in specimens taken from the body
   d. detects the presence of abnormal tissues

4. The quality of patient test results is maintained by:
   a. instrument calibration procedures
   b. preventative maintenance procedures
   c. quality control testing
   d. all of the above

5. When a patient or specimen is sent to a laboratory for testing, the medical assistant also sends:
   a. a written requisition
   b. a report
   c. the patient's file
   d. an insurance form

6. The most commonly used microscope in the clinic is the:
   a. fluorescent microscope
   b. electron microscope
   c. phase-contrast microscope
   d. compound microscope

7. Testing a blood specimen for antibody-antigen reactions would be performed in which laboratory department:
   a. hematology
   b. chemistry
   c. toxicology
   d. immunohematology

8. Lab results that indicate a serious medical condition are labeled as:
   a. Provider Attention
   b. Critical Values
   c. Dangerous levels
   d. Urgent Results

9. A physician that specializes in disease processes is called a:
   a. physiatrist
   b. pathologist
   c. cytologist
   d. medical technologist

10. Qualitative testing determines all of the following factors of a specimen except:
    a. size
    b. shape
    c. number
    d. maturity

REFERENCES/BIBLIOGRAPHY

American Association for Clinical Chemistry. Retrieved February 2012, from http://www.aacc.org

American Society for Clinical Laboratory Science. Retrieved February 2012, from http://www.ascls.org

National Accrediting Agency for Clinical Laboratory Sciences. Retrieved February 2012, from http://www.naacls.org

Phlebotomy: Venipuncture and Capillary Puncture

OUTLINE

Why Collect Blood?

The Medical Assistant's Role in Phlebotomy

Anatomy and Physiology of the Circulatory System

Blood Collection

    Plasma and Whole-Blood Collection

    Collection of Blood Specimens

Venipuncture Equipment

    Syringes and Needles

    Safety Needles and Blood Collection Systems

    Vacuum Tubes and Adapters/ Holders

    Anticoagulants, Additives, and Gels

    Order of Draw

Tourniquets

Specimen Collection Trays

Venipuncture Technique

    Approaching the Patient

    Preparing Supplies and Greeting the Patient

    Patient and Specimen Identification

    Positioning the Patient

    Selecting the Appropriate Venipuncture Site

    Applying the Tourniquet

    Performing a Safe Venipuncture

Specimen Collection

    The Syringe Technique

    Vacuum Tube Specimen Collection

Butterfly Needle Collection System

Blood Cultures

Patient Reactions

The Unsuccessful Venipuncture

Criteria for Rejection of a Specimen

Factors Affecting Laboratory Values

Capillary Puncture

    Composition of Capillary Blood

    Capillary Puncture Sites

    Preparing the Capillary Puncture Site

    Performing the Puncture

    Collecting the Blood Sample

LEARNING OUTCOMES

1. Define, spell and pronounce the key terms as presented in the glossary.
2. Explain the medical assistant's responsibility to the patient in terms of quality of care and respect for the patient as a human being.
3. Explain why the medical assistant has a special responsibility to present a neat, pleasant, and competent demeanor.
4. Explain the supplies and equipment used in blood collections and demonstrate the ability to use them safely and comfortably.
5. Explain the importance of correct patient identification; complete specimen labeling; and proper handling, storage, and delivery.
6. Summarize the step-by-step procedure for drawing blood with a syringe, vacuum tube system, butterfly, or capillary puncture.
7. Explain how to handle the various reactions a patient might have to venipuncture.
8. Analyze the professionalism questions and apply them to this chapter's content.

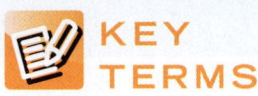

KEY TERMS

additive
aliquot
anticoagulant
buffy coat
cannula
centrifuge
edematous
erythrocyte
hematology
hematoma
hemoconcentration
hemolysis
hemolyzed
leukocyte
lipemia
palpate
phlebotomy
plasma
serum
thixotropic gel
thrombocyte
tourniquet
venipuncture
viscosity

ATTRIBUTES OF PROFESSIONALISM

Communication
- Did you introduce yourself? Did you identify the patient through name and birth date or other identifying feature?
- Did you listen to and acknowledge the patient?
- Did you speak at the patient's level of understanding?
- Did you provide appropriate responses/feedback?
- Did you explain procedures and expectations to the patient?
- Did you allay patients' fears regarding the procedure being performed and help them feel safe and comfortable?
- Did you respond honestly and diplomatically to the patient's concerns?

Presentation
- Were you dressed and groomed appropriately?
- Were you courteous, patient, and respectful to the patient?
- Did you display a positive attitude?
- Did you display a calm, professional, and caring manner?

Competency
- Did you pay attention to detail?
- Did you display sound judgment?
- Were you knowledgeable and accountable?
- Did you ask questions if you were out of your comfort zone or did not have the experience to carry out tasks?

Integrity
- Did you work within your scope of practice?
- Did you immediately report any error you had made?

SCENARIO

At Inner City Health Care, medical assistant Bruce Goldman often performs venipunctures. Bruce is personable and has an easy-going manner that makes patients feel comfortable with him. He takes time to talk to patients before performing a venipuncture to determine their feelings about the procedure and to learn about their previous experiences. Bruce is confident and professional in his interactions with patients. He is always well groomed, and he treats patients with respect. Using his social, technical, and administrative skills, Bruce is usually able to collect the necessary blood samples while providing a positive experience for patients.

INTRODUCTION

The task of collecting blood samples from patients for diagnostic testing is known as phlebotomy. The health care professional who performs this duty varies at each health care setting. The task of phlebotomy is not restricted to one individual. A variety of individuals are cross-trained to do phlebotomy and other tasks. Many health care settings do not have enough patients to justify having a phlebotomist available at all times. Therefore, the medical assistant may be designated to perform phlebotomy procedures.

WHY COLLECT BLOOD?

Hematology is the study of blood and its components, fluids, and cells. Hematology also includes the study of blood-forming organs and blood diseases.

Phlebotomy is the process of collecting blood for diagnostic purposes or bloodletting as a therapeutic measure. The history of bloodletting dates back to the early Egyptians and continues into modern times. Phlebotomy in the past was a method to cure individuals with "bad" blood. Blood was "let" (blood-letting) out of individuals as a treatment, thereby alleviating the patient's symptoms. Phlebotomy, also called **venipuncture**, is now used to help determine the disease process taking place and to determine the method of treatment. Testing blood samples gives the provider more tools for gathering diagnostic information.

THE MEDICAL ASSISTANT'S ROLE IN PHLEBOTOMY

A phlebotomist is a person trained to obtain blood specimens by venipuncture and capillary puncture techniques. The phlebotomist's primary role is to collect blood as efficiently as possible for accurate and reliable test results. How the medical assistant will be involved in phlebotomy will vary greatly from one health care environment to another. The medical assistant performing venipuncture will have direct contact with the patient and perform tasks that are critical to the patient's diagnosis and care. During the direct contact with the patient, the medical assistant will leave an impression with the patient. It can be positive or negative

SPOTLIGHT ON CERTIFICATION

RMA Content Outline

- Anatomy and physiology
- Human relations
- Asepsis
- Laboratory procedures

CMA (AAMA) Content Outline

- Systems, including structure, function related conditions, and diseases
- Maintaining confidentiality
- Medical records
- Principles of infection control
- Equipment preparation and operation
- Safety precautions
- Collecting and processing specimens; diagnostic testing
- Recognizing and responding to verbal and nonverbal communication
- Professional communication and behavior

CMAS Content Outline

- Anatomy and physiology
- Professionalism
- Asepsis in the medical office
- Communication

depending on the skill with which the medical assistant performs the venipuncture.

It is the medical assistant's responsibility to provide high-quality care to patients. The medical assistant must act professionally when working with patients. Professionalism is displayed by performing tasks in an efficient, competent manner; wearing clean, neat attire; and showing concern for patients and their feelings.

Patients will not tell family and friends that their blood was run through expensive state-of-the-art instruments but rather that the person drawing their blood sample was friendly and skilled. A smile and a kind word can allay a patient's fear and ensure a more satisfied and loyal patient.

ANATOMY AND PHYSIOLOGY OF THE CIRCULATORY SYSTEM

To be prepared to collect blood, the medical assistant must understand the system that carries the blood and the composition of the blood. The system in which the blood is transported is the circulatory system. Blood forms in the organs of the body. The bone marrow is the primary factory for production of blood cells. The lymph nodes, thymus, and spleen are also sites for the production of blood cells. The function of blood is to carry oxygen to body tissues and to remove the waste product, carbon dioxide. The blood also carries nutrients to all parts of the body and moves the waste products to the lungs, kidneys, liver, and skin for elimination.

The circulatory system consists of the heart, which pumps blood through the body by way of tubing called arteries, veins, and capillaries. When blood flows away from the heart, it flows in arteries; blood flowing back to the heart flows through the veins. Connecting most of the arteries and veins are the capillaries (Figure 40-1).

Arteries have a thick wall that helps them withstand the pressure of the pumping action of the heart. The arteries branch to form arterioles, which branch again to become capillaries. The capillaries then begin coming together to form venules, and the venules then become veins. As blood flows through the body, it follows this path of artery-arteriole-capillary-venule-vein. Oxygenated arterial blood, which contains a high level of oxygen, leaves the heart and carries the oxygen to the tissues by releasing the oxygen through the cell walls of the capillaries. At the same time, carbon

ARTERIES TO VEINS	
Arteries	**Veins**
1. Carry blood from the heart, carry oxygenated blood (except pulmonary artery)	1. Carry blood to the heart, carry deoxygenated blood (except pulmonary vein)
2. The blood is normally bright red	2. The blood is normally dark red
3. Elastic walls that expand with surge of blood	3. Thin walls/less elastic
4. No valves	4. Valves
5. Can feel a pulse	5. No pulse

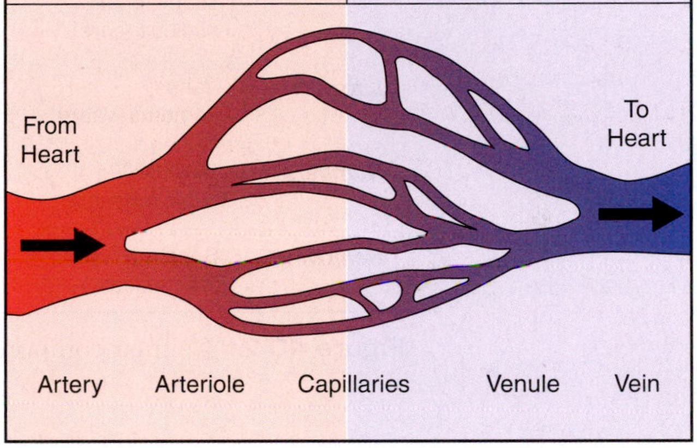

Figure 40-1 Blood flows from the heart through the larger arteries to arterioles to arterial capillary beds at the cellular level, then back to the heart through venous capillary beds into venules and finally larger veins.

dioxide is being absorbed by the blood, and then is transported to the lungs to be exhaled as a waste product. The flow of the blood also regulates body temperature. When the body gets warm, the capillaries in the extremities dilate and let off heat. This process then cools the body. If the body becomes cold, the capillaries constrict and less blood flows through, thereby conserving heat for the rest of the body.

The body contains approximately 6 liters (L) of blood, 45% of which is formed elements. The formed cellular elements consist of **erythrocytes**, **leukocytes**, and **thrombocytes** (Figure 40-2). The remaining 55% of the blood is liquid. Generally 2.5 milliliters (mL) of blood will yield about 1 mL of serum. The liquid portion of uncoagulated blood is known as plasma. **Plasma** is the fluid that provides a matrix for blood cells, electrolytes,

	White Blood Cell (Leukocyte)	Red Blood Cells (Erythrocytes)	Platelets (Thrombocytes)
Function	Body defense (extravascular)	Transport of oxygen and carbon dioxide (intravascular)	Blood clotting
Formation	Bone marrow, lymphatic tissue	Bone marrow	Bone marrow
Size/shape	9–16 micrometers; different size, shape, color, nucleus (core)	6–7 micrometers; bioconcave disc; normally no nucleus in circulatory blood	1–4 micrometers; fragments of megakaryocytes
Life cycle	Varies, 24 hours–years	100–120 days	9–12 days
Numbers	5–10,000/ cubic millimeter	4.5–5.5 million/ cubic millimeter	250–450,000/ cubic millimeter
Removal	Bone marrow, liver, spleen	Bone marrow, spleen	Spleen

© Cengage Learning 2014

Figure 40-2   Cellular components of blood.

proteins, and chemicals to travel throughout the body via the blood vessels. Blood flowing through the body contains a substance called fibrinogen. The clotting process converts the fibrinogen into fibrin. The fibrin is like a sticky spider web that traps the formed elements into the fibrin mass called a clot. The clot then contracts and the liquid **(serum)** portion is extracted. The serum is a clear, straw-colored liquid that is used for many of the tests done in the laboratory. The main difference between serum and plasma is that plasma contains fibrinogen, and serum does not.

The formed elements and the liquid portion of the blood are often separated for laboratory testing. To speed the removal of the serum from a tube of blood, an instrument called a **centrifuge** spins the blood. A carrier holds the tubes of blood, and when the centrifuge is activated, the carrier spins. The spinning action of the carrier pushes the blood cells to the bottom of the tube. The blood separates according to weight. The clot goes to the bottom of the tube and the serum goes to the top.

To produce a plasma specimen, the blood must be prevented from clotting by the use of a chemical anticoagulant. Blood collected in a tube containing an **anticoagulant** can be centrifuged to separate the formed elements (cells) from the plasma. The bottom layer will contain the erythrocytes, then there will be a thin layer called the **buffy coat**. The buffy coat contains a mixture of leukocytes and thrombocytes, which are lighter and less numerous than the red blood cells (RBCs). On top of all these layers is the plasma layer. The plasma will contain fibrinogen and usually is slightly hazy (Figure 40-3).

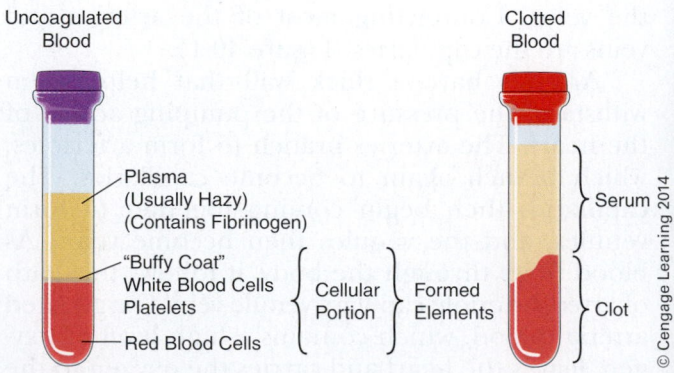

Figure 40-3   Vacuum collection tubes showing serum and plasma.

BLOOD COLLECTION

Most laboratory tests are performed on serum, plasma, or whole blood. Generally, when a serum sample is needed, a serum separator vacuum tube with **thixotropic gel** is used. The purpose of the thixotropic gel is to create a barrier between the clotted cells and the serum during centrifugation. This protects the serum from contamination from any **hemolyzed** (ruptured) RBCs. There will be certain restrictions in some cases; refer to the laboratory user manual to verify tube requirements. When a serum separator tube is used, several steps must be followed:

1. Perform venipuncture by the preferred method.
2. Invert the tube five times to activate the clotting.
3. Allow the specimen to clot with the tube in the upright position in a rack for at least 30 minutes but no longer than an hour.
4. Centrifuge the tube at 2,500 g for 15 minutes.
5. Store the tube upright or transfer the serum to a plastic transport vial for pickup by the laboratory. These are usually frozen specimens and require a stat pickup. Check the manual to see indications.

There will be different requirements for different laboratories. *NOTE:* Do not use serum separator tubes for therapeutic drug monitoring (TDM) or toxicology studies. The gel has a tendency to absorb the drugs, thereby decreasing the accuracy of the test results. Collect these samples in a plain red-top vacuum tube. Remove the serum immediately (if indicated in the test requirements) after centrifugation and place it in a plastic transport vial. Indicate if the specimen is a serum specimen or for type and cross-match.

Plasma and Whole-Blood Collection

Tubes containing anticoagulants are used to collect plasma and whole-blood samples. There are a variety of different anticoagulant tubes that can be used. The anticoagulant needed in the tube will be specified by the laboratory or testing requirements. Preparing the plasma specimen for transport or testing is similar to serum preparation:

1. Perform venipuncture by the preferred method.
2. Invert the tube 8 to 10 times to mix the blood with the anticoagulant.
3. Centrifuge the tube at 2,500 g for 10 minutes.
4. Transfer the plasma to a plastic transport vial for pickup by the laboratory. Do not allow any blood cells to mix with the plasma specimen. Indicate the specimen as a plasma specimen and what type of anticoagulant was used. There will be different requirements for different laboratories. Refer to your laboratory user manual for the appropriate test requirements.

To prepare whole-blood specimens for transport or testing:

1. Perform venipuncture by the preferred method.
2. Invert the tube 8 to 10 times to mix the blood with the anticoagulant.
3. Maintain the tube at room temperature unless otherwise instructed. Never freeze a whole-blood sample unless specifically instructed to do so.

Collection of Blood Specimens

The most commonly used method for blood collection is venipuncture. To obtain a blood sample, the medical assistant must locate a vein that is acceptable for blood collection. The preferred site for venipuncture is the antecubital space, which is located anterior to the elbow on the inside of the arm. The veins are near the surface and are large enough to give access to the blood (Figure 40-4). The median cubital vein is the vein that is used the majority of the time. When this vein is not available, any of the other veins that can be felt may be used. These veins include the basilic, cephalic, and median veins. When necessary, veins on the dorsal surface of the hand or wrist may be used for venipuncture, but they are more painful for the patient and may require a smaller needle or the use of a butterfly apparatus.

The veins of the feet are an alternative when the arms are not available. The provider's permission is needed before drawing blood from the veins of the legs and feet. The provider may not want the patient's leg or foot veins punctured because the act of drawing blood may cause clots to form. These clots then have the possibility of dislodging and causing a blockage elsewhere in the body. It would be extremely rare for a medical

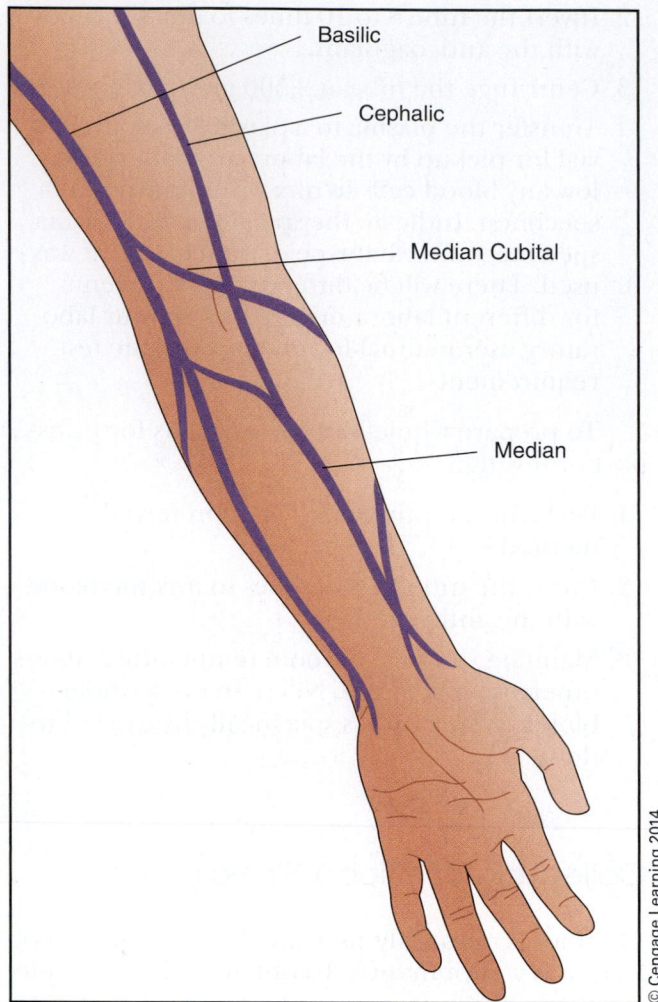

Figure 40-4   Superficial veins of the arm.

© Cengage Learning 2014

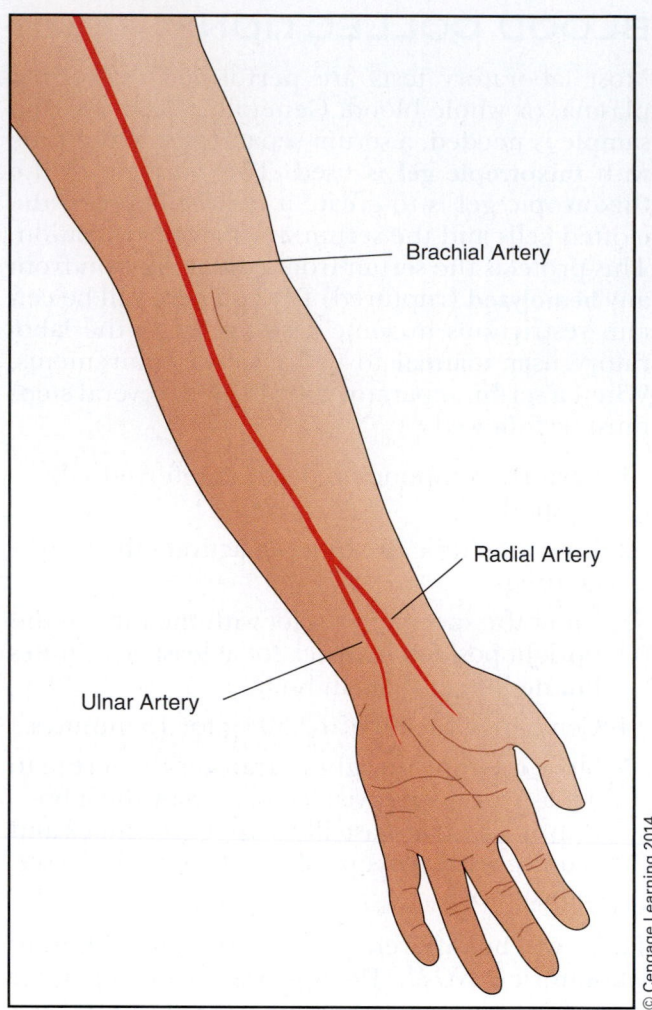

Figure 40-5   Arteries of the arm.

© Cengage Learning 2014

assistant to use this location. The provider should be consulted before a foot puncture is considered. The person performing a foot draw must be specially trained for that procedure.

The arteries in the arm consist of the brachial artery in the brachial region of the arm and the radial and ulnar arteries in the wrist (Figure 40-5). Special techniques are necessary to puncture arteries to obtain a blood specimen for the examination of gases absorbed by the blood. Arterial punctures and the techniques used to draw blood from these locations for blood gas testing are not generally done by a medical assistant. Refer to individual state laws for specific training and certification/registration requirements.

VENIPUNCTURE EQUIPMENT

All methods of venipuncture require the invasive procedure of puncturing into a vein to obtain a blood sample. The three methods used to perform venipuncture are the syringe method, the vacuum tube method, and the butterfly method. Each method has advantages and disadvantages (Table 40-1). It is important that the well-trained medical assistant have options when attempting to draw blood from a wide range of patients in a variety of situations. There will be times in one's career when one method will be preferred over another. Regardless of which method is chosen to perform the blood draw, the blood will probably be transferred into a vacuum tube eventually. This

Table 40-1   Comparison of Blood Collection Methods

Method	Indications for Use	Advantages	Disadvantages
Vacuum tube	Routine collection Multiple tubes are needed Whenever possible	Fast Relatively safe Best specimen quality Large collection amount possible	May not work well with: Small veins Fragile veins Difficult draws Small children Hand or feet draws
Butterfly assembly	Small or fragile veins Difficult draws Small children or older adult patients	Least likely to collapse vein Less painful to patient Can attach syringe Can attach vacuum tube adapter Least likely to pass through small veins Good specimen quality	Syringe not as safe because tube transfer is necessary Specimen may become hemolyzed Not recommended for large amounts of blood
Syringe	Children Infants Older adult patients Oncology patients Severely burned patients Obese patients Inaccessible veins Extremely fragile veins When specimen requires a drop of blood	Easier to perform Allows for smaller amount of specimen	Not recommended for dehydrated patients Not recommended for patient with poor circulation Cannot be used for: Blood cultures Erythrocyte sedimentation rate

Source: Courtesy of Sheri R. Greimes, CMA (AAMA), PBT (ASCP) RMA, RPT (AMT).

is because vacuum tubes contain the chemicals and substances necessary for the blood tests to be performed.

Syringes and Needles

Syringes used in venipuncture are usually made of plastic (Figure 40-6). They come in a variety of sizes. Each manufacturer has its own packaging and coloring, thus there is really no significance related to the color and design of syringes. Most syringes used in venipuncture will be 5 and 10 mL in size. Some syringes are designed with a Luer-Lok tip. This tip allows the needle to be securely twisted onto the syringe. The Luer-Lok tip may be preferred to the push-on tip for additional safety for the user.

Needles attached to syringes and used for venipuncture do not necessarily differ in function and design from needles used for injections (Figure 40-6). They come in a wide variety of lengths and gauges. Most common sizes for venipuncture are 20, 21, and 22 gauges and about 1 or 1.5 inches in length (Table 40-2). Sixteen-gauge needles are often used for blood banking procedures. Remember, the larger the number, the smaller the gauge.

Another type of needle used in venipuncture is the special needle, designed for use with the vacuum tube method. This needle has a double end—the longer needle to puncture the vein and the shorter needle to puncture into the vacuum tube (Figure 40-7). These needles also come in a variety of gauges and lengths; the most common is the same as the standard needle described

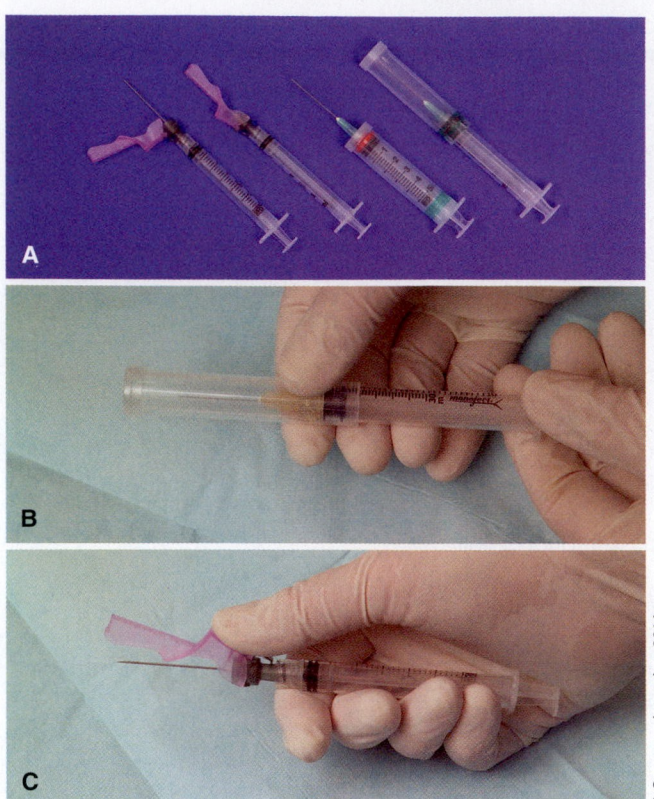

Table 40-2 Needle Gauges Used in Phlebotomy

Gauge Size	Comments
23	Often considered too small, can cause hemolysis of blood cells; used sometimes with butterfly system
22	Preferred for pediatric phlebotomy or very small veins of the hands or feet
21	Most common size used with vacuum tubes
20	Appropriate, but large for common phlebotomy
18	Not used for phlebotomy, but sometimes used in blood banking/donations
16	Most commonly used in blood banking/donations

© Cengage Learning 2014

Figure 40-6 (A) Safety syringes with needles, before and after safety mechanisms are engaged. (B) Pull entire casing over the needle to engage this type of safety mechanism. Once engaged, it is locked into place. (C) With the thumb and forefinger, press the safety mechanism over the needle; or, an even safer technique is to press it against a hard surface such as the edge of the counter. Be sure to listen for the click. Once engaged, the safety mechanism should be firmly locked in place.

previously: 20, 21, and 22 gauge, 1 to 1.5 inches in length. When selecting a double-ended needle for use with the vacuum tube, you will use a multidraw needle, which enables drawing of more than one tube of blood. The multidraw needles come with a

rubber sheath over the shorter needle, which goes into the vacuum tube. This rubber sheath prevents blood from leaking out of the needle during tube changes. Multidraw needles are sometimes referred to as multisample or multiple sample needles.

Another type of needle used in venipuncture is on a "winged" infusion set called the butterfly collection system (Figure 40-8). Because of the

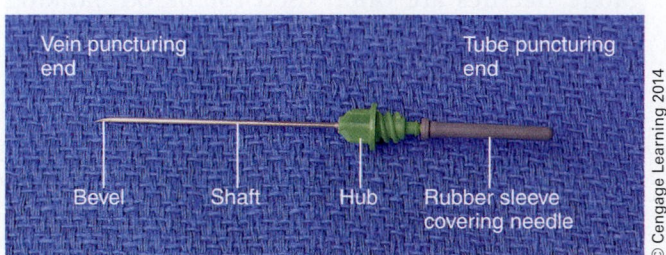

Figure 40-7 Multidraw needle for vacuum tube blood collection system.

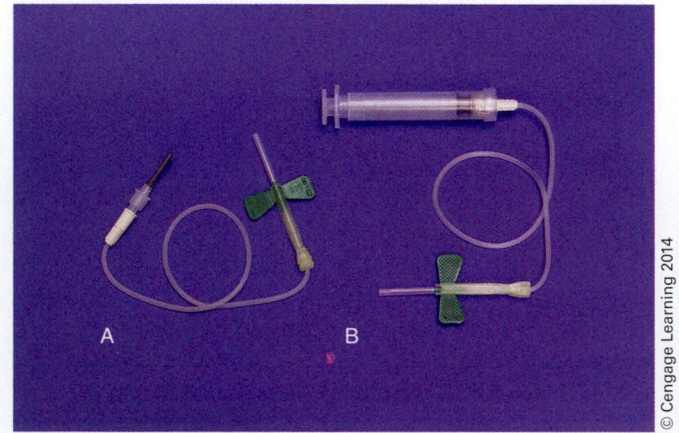

Figure 40-8 (A) Winged infusion set (butterfly) with safety needle. (B) Butterfly attached to syringe.

reasons for using the butterfly collection system, the needles are smaller, usually 21 or 23 gauge.

More details about each collection method are discussed later in this chapter.

Safety Needles and Blood Collection Systems

The Occupational Safety and Health Administration (OSHA) requires that safety needles be made available to employees to prevent on-the-job needle-stick injuries. The huge variety of safety needles and blood collection systems currently available greatly reduces the risks for accidental needlesticks. The main issue is deciding which to select for use in your clinic based on personal preferences. OSHA requires that employers make purchasing decisions based on formal feedback from front-line employees rather than costs and administrative contracts. This means that you have a great deal of choice about what systems you select to use. It is recommended that you examine a variety of safety systems on a regular basis to determine which one gives you the greatest protection from accidental needlestick injury. These systems are often referred to as needle-stick prevention devices (NPDs). Among the available systems are passive systems in which the needle is automatically covered when withdrawn and systems that require the medical assistant to activate a mechanism of covering the needle. Within each type are many options and brands. This chapter discusses and shows a few currently available options in no particular order. The first is the Plexus Puncture Guard system (Figure 40-9). Before withdrawing the needle from the patient's vein, a **cannula** is clicked into place. The cannula fills the inside of the needle, virtually blunting the tip. Another option is the Eclipse system by Becton-Dickinson (Figure 40-10), which requires the medical assistant to snap a cover over the needle after it is removed from the vein. A third option, called the Safety-Lok, also manufactured by Becton-Dickinson, requires the medical assistant to slide the cover over the needle until it locks into place. Whichever system you choose, always combine the safest equipment with the safest practices for the best all-around benefit for you, your coworkers, and your patients. Many accidents occur when we become distracted or hurried in our tasks.

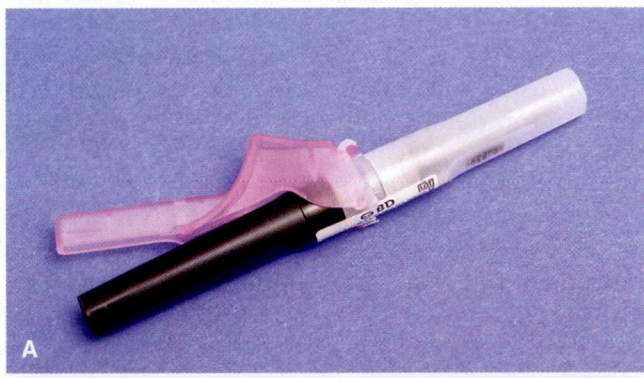
A

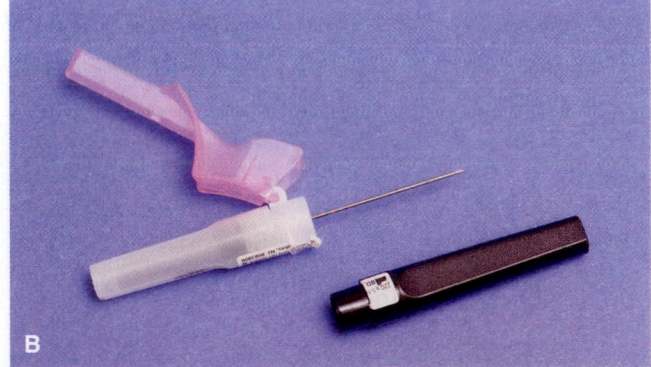
B

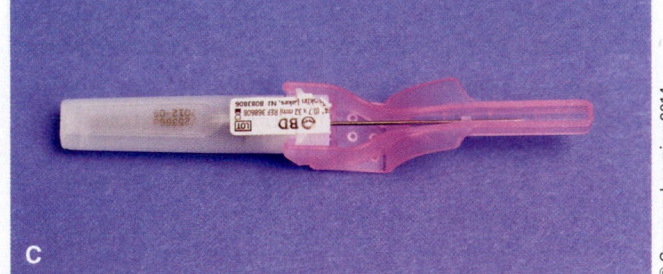
C

© Cengage Learning 2014

Figure 40-10 Three Eclipse safety needles for use with vacuum tubes. (A) Needle capped, safety mechanism not engaged. (B) Needle exposed, safety mechanism not engaged. (C) Safety mechanism engaged.

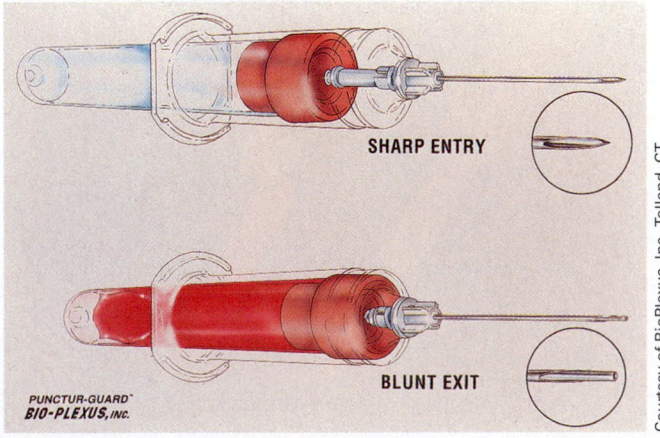

SHARP ENTRY

BLUNT EXIT

PUNCTUR-GUARD
BIO-PLEXUS, INC.

Courtesy of BioPlexus, Inc., Tolland, CT

Figure 40-9 Puncture Guard is one type of safety needle.

Vacuum Tubes and Adapters/ Holders

The vacuum tube system is often called the Vacutainer system. Vacutainer can be a misnomer because the term *Vacutainer*® is a brand name for the vacuum tube system manufactured by Becton-Dickinson. Medical personnel often say Vacutainer when they are using another company's product.

Vacuum tubes are vacuum-packed test tubes with rubber stoppers. The safest ones are made of plastic and have screw-on caps. They are available in a variety of sizes for a variety of uses (Figure 40-11). Vacuum tubes come plain or with added chemicals or substances necessary for the appropriate test to be run. The color of the rubber stopper designates the additive inside the tube. Although most colors are universal regardless of manufacturer, the shades may vary and can be confusing to beginners. It is always best to read the label to determine the additive if the shade is different.

Plastic holders or tube adapters (Figure 40-12) are used in conjunction with the vacuum tubes. Figure 40-13 shows safety holders developed to minimize the risk for accidental needle-sticks.

Some plastic holders are reusable, but there is much debate about the appropriateness of reusing them, even after disinfection. They are fairly inexpensive and the inner threads will eventually wear out, therefore replacing them frequently is always good practice. The holders with the safety mechanisms shown in Figure 40-13 are not reusable.

Anticoagulants, Additives, and Gels

Different tests require different types of blood specimens. Some specimens require a serum sample and need to be drawn in a tube that allows the blood to clot. Others require a whole-blood or plasma specimen and need to be drawn in a tube that does not allow the blood to clot. **Additives** are put into the tubes during manufacturing. The

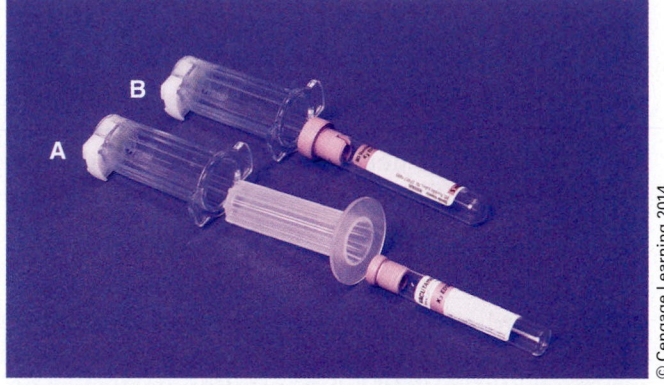

Figure 40-12 Holders for vacuum tube system. (A) Adult holder. (B) Pediatric tube using an adapter.

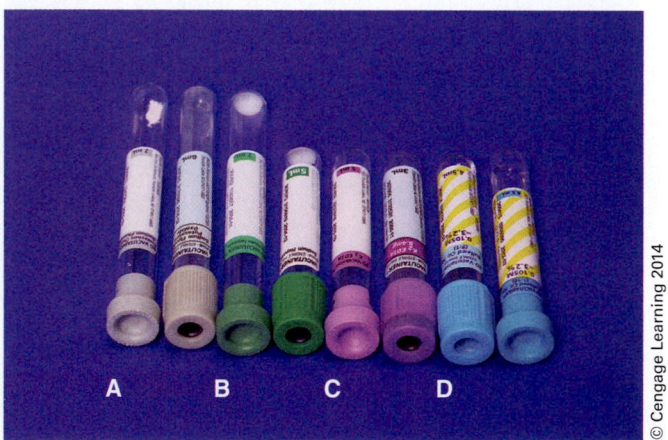

Figure 40-11 Standard anticoagulant tubes with conventional rubber stopper and Hemogard twist off closures. (A) Gray top, tube contains antiglycolytic agent; left tube with rubber stopper, right tube with twist off Hemogard top. (B) Green top, tube contains heparin anticoagulant; left tube with rubber stopper, right tube with twist off Hemogard top. (C) Lavender top, tube contains EDTA anticoagulant; left tube with rubber stopper, right tube with twist off Hemogard top. (D) Light blue top, tube contains sodium citrate; left tube with twist off Hemogard top, right tube with rubber stopper.

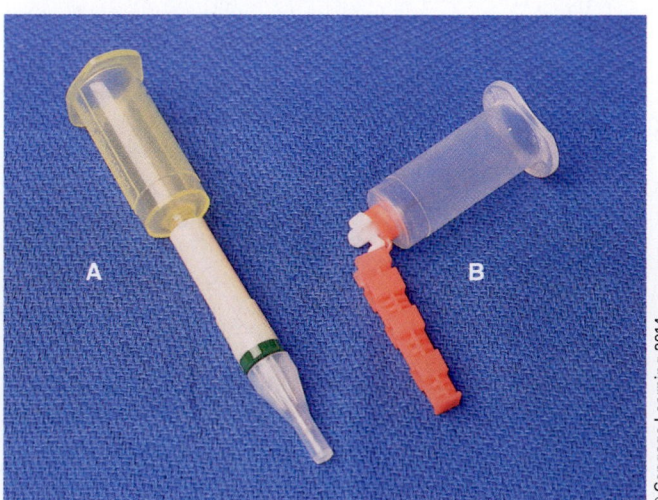

Figure 40-13 Safety tube holders. (A) Safety needle and holder. (B) Locking cover.

Table 40-3   Steps to Blood Clotting

1. Uncoagulated blood

2. Calcium utilized

3. Prothrombin converts to thrombin

4. Fibrinogen converts to fibrin

5. Clot forms

© Cengage Learning 2014

additive may be an anticoagulant to prevent clotting of the blood, a chemical to help preserve the blood, or a substance to accelerate the clotting process (called a clot activator). Some tubes also contain gel plugs, which act as separators between the blood cells/clot and the serum/plasma. An anticoagulant is a chemical substance that prevents the clotting by removing calcium in the form of calcium salts or by inhibiting the conversion of prothrombin to thrombin. Coagulation occurs naturally according to the steps in Table 40-3. If a step is prevented, the blood does not clot.

A tube containing an anticoagulant removes one of the steps in the process, preventing the blood from clotting. The step removed depends on the anticoagulant used. The basic anticoagulants used consist of oxalates, citrates, ethylenediaminetetraacetic acid (EDTA), or heparin (Figure 40-14). Anticoagulants are identified by tube color. It is important to use the correct anticoagulant for the test because the improper anticoagulant can alter test results.

Clot activators consist of silica (small glass) particles on the sides of the tubes that initiate the clotting process. The silica particles work as a catalyst for the clotting process by promoting the clotting process. The plastic vacuum tubes with the red tops have clot activators in them. The glass red top vacuum tubes do not.

Serum and plasma tubes can also be purchased with a thixotropic separator gel (Figure 40-15). The gel is an inert material that undergoes a temporary change in **viscosity** during centrifugation. When centrifuged, the gel changes to a liquid and moves up the sides of the tube to create a barrier between the blood cells or clot and the liquid portion of the blood. The gel then forms a solid plug and separates the cells/clot from the plasma/serum (Figure 40-16).

Red Top		
Contains:	None	
Effects on Specimen:	Blood clots, and the serum is separated by centrifugation	
Uses:	Chemistries, immunology and serology, blood bank (cross-match)	

Red-Gray Mottled Top ("Tiger top")		
Contains:	Serum separating tube (SST) with clot activator	
Effects on Specimen:	Forms clot quickly and separates the serum with SST gel at the bottom of the tube	
Uses:	Blood type screening and chemistries	

Gold Top		
Contains:	Separating gel and clot activator	
Effects on Specimen:	Serum separator tube (SST) contains a gel at the bottom to separate the blood from serum on centrifugation	
Uses:	Serology, endocrine, immunology, including HIV testing	

Light Green Top		
Contains:	Plasma separating tube (Na heparin)	
Effects on Specimen:	Anticoagulants with lithium heparin: plasma is separated with PST gel at the bottom of the tube	
Uses:	Chemistries	

Lavender/Purple Top		
Contains:	EDTA (liquid form)	
Effects on Specimen:	Forms calcium salts to remove calcium	
Uses:	Hematology (CBC) and blood bank (cross-match); requires a full draw—invert 8 times to prevent clotting and platelet clumping	

Light Blue Top		
Contains:	Sodium citrate (Na citrate)	
Effects on Specimen:	Forms calcium salts to remove calcium	
Uses:	Coagulation tests (PT, PTT, TCT, CMV), tube must be filled 100%	

Figure 40-14   Collection tubes and their additives for phlebotomy. (continues)

Dark Green Top

Contains:	Sodium heparin or lithium heparin
Effects on Specimen:	Inactivates thrombin and thromboplastin
Uses:	Ammonia, lactate, HLA typing For lithium level, use sodium heparin For ammonia level, use sodium or lithium heparin

Dark Blue/Royal Blue Top

Contains:	Sodium heparin or Na_2 EDTA
Effects on Specimen:	Forms calcium salts Tube is designed to contain no contaminating metals
Uses:	Toxicology and trace element testing (zinc, copper, lead, mercury) and drug level testing

Light Gray Top

Contains:	Sodium fluoride and potassium oxalate
Effects on Specimen:	Antiglycolytic agent preserves glucose up to 5 days
Uses:	For lithium level, use sodium heparin Glucose requires a full draw (may cause hemolysis if short draw)

Yellow Top

Contains:	ACD (acid-citrate-dextose)
Effects on Specimen:	Complement inactivation
Uses:	Paternity testing, DNA studies

Tan/Brown Top

Contains:	Sodium heparin
Effects on Specimen:	Inactivates thrombin and thromboplastin
Uses:	Serum lead determination

Black Top

Contains:	Sodium citrate (buffered)
Effects on Specimen:	Forms calcium salts to remove calcium
Uses:	Westergren sedimentation rate; requires a full draw

Orange Top

Contains:	Thrombin
Effects on Specimen:	Quickly clots blood
Uses:	STAT serum chemistries

© Cengage Learning 2014

Figure 40-14 (continued)

ACTIONS OF ADDITIVES

Additive	Action
Potassium oxalate	Binds calcium
Sodium fluoride	Inhibits glycolysis
Sodium citrate	Binds calcium
EDTA	Binds calcium
Lithium heparin	Inhibits prothrombin to thrombin
No additive	Clot naturally forms
Sodium polyanethol sulfonate (SPS)	Binds calcium
Glass particles/silica	Promotes clotting
Ammonium heparin	Inhibits prothrombin to thrombin

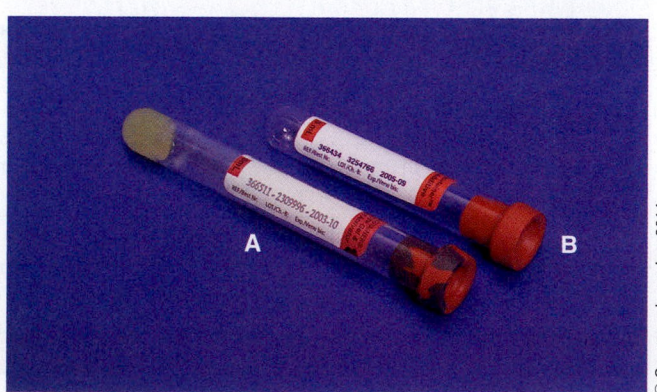

© Cengage Learning 2014

Figure 40-15 Standard vacuum tubes. (A) SST (red/gray or "speckled top") top tube contains clot activators and thixotropic gel. (B) Standard red top (glass) tube contains no anticoagulant but might contain glass particles/silica on the inside walls to irritate the thrombocytes to promote clotting.

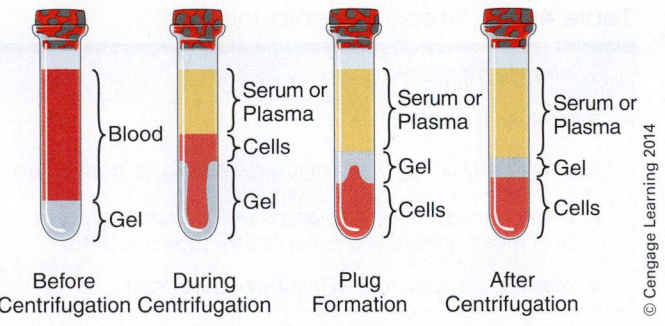

Figure 40-16 Separator thixotropic gel tube showing stages of the centrifugation process works.

Order of Draw

The order in which blood is drawn or mixed with the additives is important. A revised Order of Draw was published in 2003 by CLSI and is still the standard. See Table 40-4. Sterile collection bottles (for blood cultures) need to be filled first to prevent any contamination. After the sterile culture tubes are drawn, the order for the other tubes is related to the additives in them. The clot activator in the red and speckled-top tubes is now considered an additive, even though it is not a chemical anticoagulant. It does not matter whether the blood is drawn directly into a vacuum tube or into a syringe, then transferred to the vacuum tube. The order of the tubes remains the same for either method. Table 40-4 also lists the order of draw.

Table 40-4 Standard Order of Draw—CLSI Guidelines as of December 2008

Blood culture tubes or vials	Yellow top or culture bottles
Sodium citrate	Light blue top
Serum tubes	Red top and red/gray top (SST)
Heparin tubes	Green tops, light and dark
EDTA tubes	Lavender top, then pink, white, or royal blue
Glycolytic inhibitor	Gray top
Fibrin degradable products	Dark blue

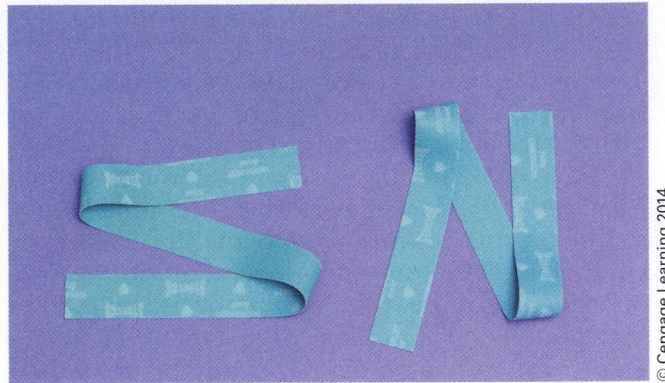

Figure 40-17 One kind of tourniquet.

Tourniquets

The **tourniquet**, when applied to the arm, constricts the flow of blood in the arm and makes the veins more prominent. The tourniquet is a soft, pliable, rubber or elastic strip approximately 1 inch wide by 15 to 18 inches long (Figure 40-17). The elastic strip serves as the best tourniquet for all conditions. The elastic strip can easily be released with one hand. Being about 1 inch wide, it does not cut into the patient's arm but distributes the pressure. The tourniquet can easily be disinfected but is inexpensive enough that it should be replaced often. If the tourniquet is obviously contaminated, it should be discarded into biohazard waste. If a patient has been identified as having a latex hypersensitivity, you must use a nonlatex tourniquet. Latex-free tourniquets are readily available and inexpensive, so they can be used for all patients regardless of latex allergy or hypersensitivity.

A blood pressure cuff can also be used as a tourniquet. Its use is primarily for veins that are difficult to locate using a standard tourniquet. The blood pressure should be taken first, and then the cuff should be maintained slightly below the diastolic pressure (average: 40 mm Hg).

CRITICAL THINKING

Which vacuum tube would you use to draw a serum specimen: lavender or red top? Why did you choose that tube? What differentiates the two tubes?

Specimen Collection Trays

The medical assistant may need a specimen collection tray to hold all the equipment necessary for proper specimen collection. The tray can be taken to the patient in the examination room so that whatever procedure is performed the phlebotomy can be conducted without searching for the proper equipment. The trays vary depending on the type of collections done. Because the tray is also used to transport blood specimens, the OSHA *Bloodborne Pathogen Standard* requires the tray be all red or prominently labeled with an approved biohazard symbol. The tray is usually preferred because it is more portable and can easily be taken to the patient. The trays come in a variety of sizes and shapes to better fit the preference and needs of the individual collecting the blood sample (Figure 40-18). Sometimes the equipment is stored in a special drawer for venipuncture equipment in each examination room or in a central laboratory area.

VENIPUNCTURE TECHNIQUE

Venipuncture is a detailed process that consists of many steps (Table 40-5).

Approaching the Patient

  The first step to a successful venipuncture is to put the patient at ease. The medical assistant uses many skills

Table 40-5 Steps in Venipuncture

1. Identify the patient.
2. Verify test ordered.
3. Verify diet/drug restrictions, e.g., fasting vs. nonfasting.
4. Wash hands. Put on gloves, as well as safety glasses and mask, if there is a potential for blood splatter.
5. Assemble supplies and inspect equipment.
6. Reassure the patient and explain the procedure.
7. Position the patient.
8. Verify paperwork and tubes.
9. Perform venipuncture.
10. Fill the tubes.
11. Bandage the patient's arm.
12. Dispose of sharps in the proper container.
13. Label the tubes.
14. Remove gloves and other PPE. Dispose of properly. Wash hands.
15. Chill specimen (only for certain tests).
16. Process paperwork. Complete laboratory requisition.
17. Send correctly labeled tubes to the office laboratory or prepare them to be sent to a reference laboratory.
18. Document procedure.

© Cengage Learning 2014

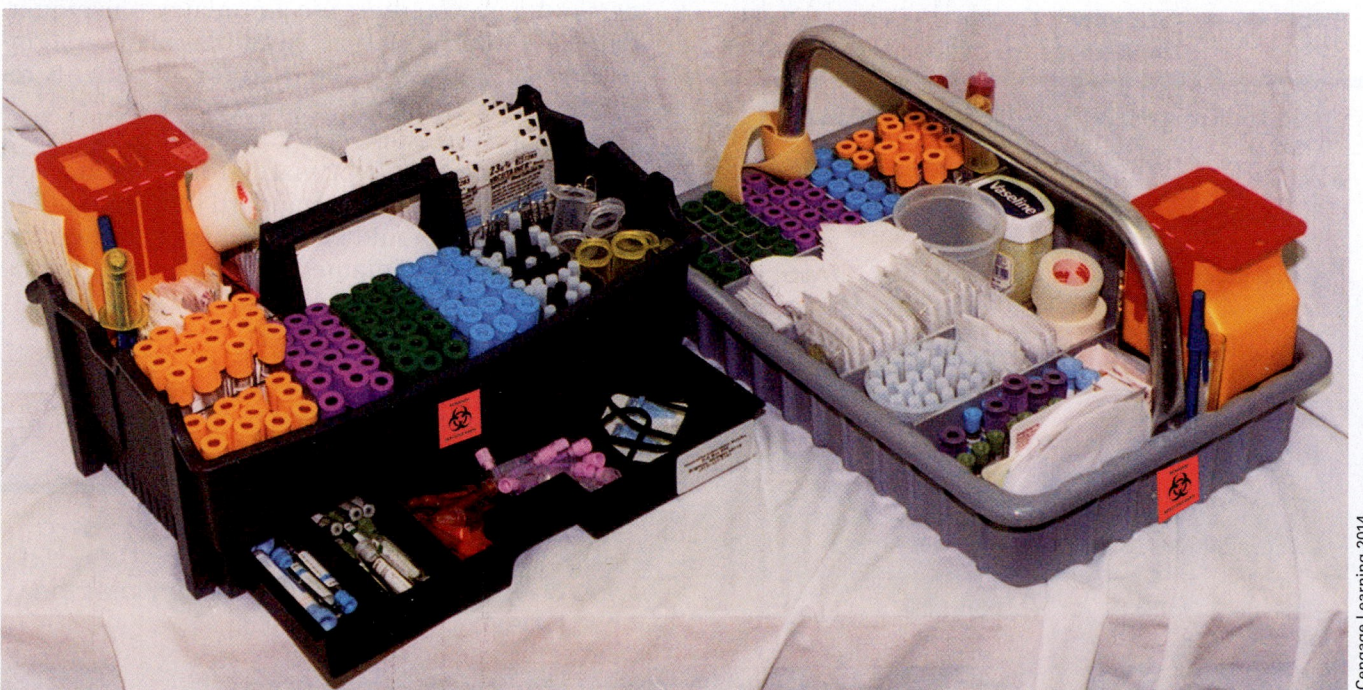

Figure 40-18 Two types of well-stocked phlebotomy trays.

© Cengage Learning 2014

when interacting with patients during phlebotomy. Three of the skills used are:

1. Social skills
2. Technical skills
3. Administrative skills

Social skills are used by the medical assistant to obtain cooperation from the patient. Some patients will be calm, whereas others may be extremely frightened. The nicest patient may be irritable and may even become physically or emotionally abusive when placed in the unfamiliar health care setting. The medical assistant uses social skills to put the patient at ease, allay the patient's fears, and persuade the patient to allow blood to be drawn.

After calming the patient and explaining the procedure, the medical assistant uses technical skills to perform the phlebotomy with a minimum of pain to the patient. As important as it is to obtain a good specimen, it is equally important to treat the patient with empathy. Using social and technical skills, the medical assistant can provide a positive experience for the patient. A patient who has had a positive experience will talk with friends and neighbors about that experience, which could result in new patients for the physician's office, the clinic, or the laboratory.

 For the medical assistant, administrative skills involve drawing the correct patient's blood and correctly labeling the specimen. Incorrect labeling constitutes the greatest number of errors in phlebotomy. All patient specimens must be positively identified on the primary container, the container that holds the specimen, to avoid any errors in reporting of results, thereby affecting patient diagnosis or treatment.

Preparing Supplies and Greeting the Patient

Prepare all supplies and equipment before the venipuncture. Place all tubes within easy reach to avoid crossing over the patient and possibly moving the needle after it is in the patient. Remember that occasionally a tube will not fill completely; therefore, it is best to keep a few spare tubes or have the phlebotomy tray within reach.

Patient and Specimen Identification

Proper patient and specimen identification is essential to accurate patient testing. The results of specimen testing will be incorrect if the specimen

GREETING THE PATIENT

1. Reassure the patient that the procedure is going to be simple and there will only be a slight inconvenience.

2. Be friendly and outgoing and talk to the patient, explaining the procedure. Polite conversation with all patients gives them the feeling someone cares about them.

3. Do not tell the patient that the procedure will not be painful. Explain that the procedure can be slightly uncomfortable but you will take care to cause the least discomfort possible. If the patient seems overly concerned about pain, check frequently with him or her to see how he or she is doing. If the patient seems extremely apprehensive, ask if he or she would prefer to lie down during the procedure. This may prevent further problems if the patient faints.

4. Exhibit concern for patients, because this will result in more satisfied patients who will return in the future for care from the same provider.

is not accurately identified. When entering the room, do not say "Mr. Jones, I'm here to draw your blood," assuming that if the patient says "Yes" he is Mr. Jones. The patient may not have been paying attention and may answer yes even if it is not his name. Ask the patient to state his or her full name. If the patient is unable to communicate with you, or if you are in an inpatient environment such as a hospital or extended care facility, always check the patient's identification wristband or check with the caretaker. In the ambulatory setting, a good policy is to ask for picture identification from non-English-speaking patients.

Once the medical assistant has identified the patient and the blood is drawn, the specimen needs proper identification. The patient's first and last name, middle initial, date of birth, any assigned identification number, the date, the time, and the initials of the person collecting the specimen must be written on the tube immediately after drawing the patient's blood. Label the tubes clearly, using a permanent marker, before leaving the patient's presence. By doing so, if the tubes are taken to the physician's office laboratory or an outside reference laboratory, the specimens will be properly identified. Any paperwork or forms accompanying the specimens must be checked with the blood tubes to verify that names and numbers match.

EHR Many offices are using various types of computer systems for test ordering and result reporting. The computer label has several advantages in that it lists the specific tests that are ordered and the required specimen and specimen requirements. The label can also be adhesive so it can be attached directly to the tube. Smaller labels can also be printed at the same time for smaller specimens. An **aliquot** specimen is a portion of a specimen that has been taken for use or storage. The computer has multiple advantages in timing the printing of orders, sorting lists of orders for one patient at one time, and speeding entry of draw times and test results. The computer labels print off in a roll with one label following the other. Two attached labels (Figure 40-19A and B) require special attention. One label must be checked carefully with the other to ensure that each label is for the same person, date, and time. Labels may also contain bar codes to assist in electronic patient and specimen identification. With computerized systems, the medical assistant will verify by entering information into the computer when the blood is drawn.

Positioning the Patient

The position of the patient is critical for proper patient blood collection. The best position is the position that is comfortable for the patient and the health care professional. Proper positioning of

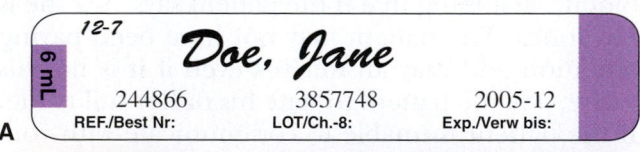

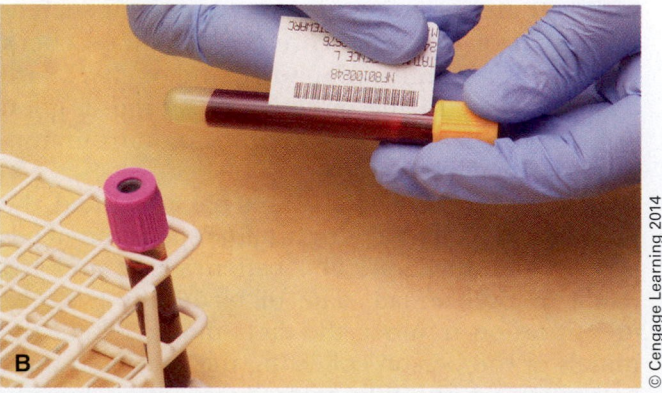

Figure 40-19 (A) Adhesive computer-generated labels for identifying specimen tubes from one patient. (B) The medical assistant applies a computer-generated label to the patient's specimen tube.

the patient will make the patient feel more at ease and facilitate the performance of the venipuncture.

Selecting the Appropriate Venipuncture Site

The appropriate venipuncture site can vary depending on the patient. The usual site that is first checked is the antecubital region of the arm.

The primary vein used in the antecubital region of the arm is the median cubital vein. This is usually the prominent vein in the middle of the bend of the arm (see Figure 40-4). The basilic or cephalic vein can be used as an alternative. These veins may not be accessible or may not be prominent enough to obtain a blood sample. The next step is to go to the back of the hand to determine other possibilities. The veins in the back of the hand have the tendency to "roll" more than the arm veins because they are not supported by as much tissue and are closer to the surface. To avoid

---

POSITIONING THE PATIENT

Before a patient's blood is drawn, discuss with the patient any previous problems with blood being taken. Usually one of two situations must be addressed:

1. Patients who do not have a problem with having blood drawn.
   a. The patient must be in a seated or reclining position before any attempt is made to draw blood.
   b. Do not allow the patient to sit on a tall stool or stand while drawing blood. There is always the possibility that the patient will faint (syncope) and be injured.
   c. The sitting position requires a chair with adequate arm supports that are adjustable for the best venipuncture position.

2. Patients who will faint (syncope).
   a. Apprehensive patients and patients who indicate they have fainted in the past when having blood drawn should be instructed to lie down.
   b. The reclining position is the ideal position from which to draw a blood sample from the patient.
   c. A pillow may be required to help support the patient's arm by keeping it straight for easier venous access.

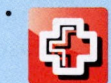
this, the vein will have to be held in place securely while a smaller gauge needle or a butterfly is used. The hand veins are ideal for a 3- to 5-mL syringe with a 22-gauge needle. Careful, slow pulling on the syringe will obtain the blood sample without collapsing the vein or hemolyzing the blood. The veins at the back of the wrist are also an alternative, but they are generally much more painful than the other sites. The foot and ankle veins may also be used if the patient's provider gives permission to use them and the medical assistant is properly trained to perform venipuncture on the lower extremities. The veins in the foot or ankle will also have the tendency to "roll." The medical assistant will in all likelihood never draw from the foot or ankle, but this is an area that will give an acceptable blood sample when all other attempts have failed.

The order for checking for the best available site is: (1) antecubital region of the arm, (2) back of hand, (3) back of wrist, and (4) ankle or foot. The next alternative is to have a more experienced medical assistant check. If venous access is not possible, draw the sample by capillary puncture if the test can be performed on a capillary specimen. Check the laboratory manual for criteria.

Applying the Tourniquet

A tourniquet must be used to assist the medical assistant in feeling a vein. The tourniquet is applied 3 to 4 inches above the intended puncture site. It is applied tightly enough to slow the flow of blood in the veins but not so tightly as to prevent the flow of blood in the arteries (Figures 40-20A–D). This is similar to damming a small stream. When a stream is dammed, the water forms a pond in front of the dam. With the tourniquet applied, the veins fill with blood, pooling in the veins below the tourniquet. This pooling of blood makes the veins more prominent. The veins can then be **palpated** (examined with the fingertips)

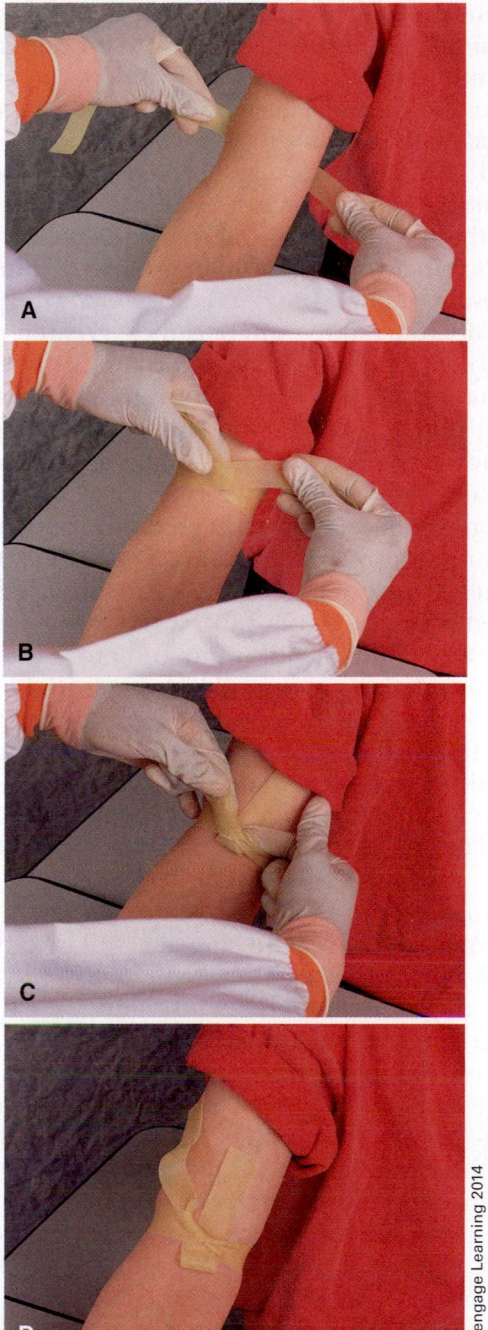

© Cengage Learning 2014

Figure 40-20   Applying a tourniquet. (A) Wrap the tourniquet around the arm 3 to 4 inches above the venipuncture site. Keeping the tourniquet flat to the skin will help minimize the discomfort felt by the patient. (B) Stretch the tourniquet tight and cross the ends. (C) While holding the ends tight, tuck one portion of the tourniquet under the other. (D) The tourniquet should not be loose and the ends should be secure. The ends of the tourniquet should be pointed upward and not hanging into the intended venipuncture site.

to determine their direction, depth, and size. The tourniquet should be on the arm no longer than 1 minute. A tourniquet that is left on too long will cause **hemoconcentration** of the blood, an increased concentration of constituents in the blood sample that may lead to inaccurate test results. If the patient has sensitive skin or a skin problem, the tourniquet should be applied over the patient's upper arm clothing or a piece of gauze pad. This will minimize the discomfort felt by the patient.

The tourniquet often causes greater discomfort for patients than the venipuncture itself. The tourniquet should ideally be removed as soon as blood flow is established. This is not practical for the novice medical assistant. The act of removing the tourniquet may move the needle or vein just enough so that no more blood can be obtained and a second venipuncture must be performed. It is recommended to wait until just before the needle is removed from the patient to remove the tourniquet. If the tourniquet is not removed before the needle is removed, the patient will bleed heavily. Blood will be forced out of the needle hole and into the surrounding tissue, resulting in a **hematoma** (an accumulation of blood around the venipuncture site).

Performing a Safe Venipuncture

The first step in actual collection of a venous blood specimen is to find the site that will give the best blood return. The vein must be palpated with the tip of the index finger. Feel for and trace the path of the vein several times. Avoid using the thumb because it has a pulse and is not as sensitive as the rest of the fingers. The vein will feel soft and bouncy to the touch. The roundness of the vein and the direction it follows may be determined. Palpate the path of the vein to determine the direction for needle insertion and feel the contour, across the vessel to find the 'bouncy' touch. Both actions will assure a better site selection for the blood draw. All veins are not straight up and down the arm. If no veins become prominent, retie the tourniquet tighter but not so tightly as to stop the

flow of arterial blood into the arm. If the tourniquet is tied tightly enough to stop arterial blood flow, the patient will no longer have a pulse in the wrist. If this occurs, immediately remove the tourniquet because this indicates that blood has ceased flowing below the tourniquet.

If the "vein" that is felt has a pulsing action to it, it is an artery, not a vein, and the vessel should not be punctured (see Safety Box). Tendons can be deceptive and give the appearance of veins. They do not have the soft, bouncy feel and will be hard to the touch. Puncturing a tendon will give no blood return and will be painful to the patient. Nerves also run the length of the arm. The nerves cannot be seen or felt, but by avoiding deep, probing venipunctures, the chance of puncturing a nerve will be diminished. If the patient complains that the venipuncture is extremely painful, it is best to stop and try another site.

Veins of **edematous** arms, which are swollen because of fluid in the tissue, will not be prominent and the tourniquet will not be effective because of the swelling. Using the tourniquet in this instance may cause tissue damage. Areas of scarring should also be avoided because of possible injury or excessive pain to the patient. Specimens collected from an area of a hematoma may cause erroneous test results. If another vein site is not available, the specimen is collected distal from the hematoma. Because of the potential for harm to the patient due to lymphostasis (the stoppage of the flow of lymph), the arm on the side of a mastectomy or any lymphatic compromise should be avoided. If the

CRITICAL THINKING

You are having a difficult time getting the needle to cooperate when putting together a butterfly system and you accidentally contaminate it. The patient has the tourniquet already on her arm. What do you do? Why? Is there something else you could have done?

SAFETY BOX

 If you accidentally puncture an artery, you will see that the blood is a brighter color. This is due to the oxygenation of arterial blood versus venous blood. Go ahead and calmly fill the tubes. Often the laboratory can run the blood tests on arterial blood just as with venous blood. After the needle is removed, pressure needs to be held for a full 3 minutes (longer if the patient is taking a blood thinner such as Coumadin). As with any phlebotomy procedure, make sure the bleeding has stopped before the patient leaves your care. While the patient is still there, check with the lab. If the test requires venous blood, you will need to repeat the procedure.

CORRECT HAND POSITION TO HOLD A SYRINGE

1. The needle is attached to the syringe.
2. Hold the syringe and needle system in your dominant hand, cradling it on your four fingers. A right-handed person would hold the syringe in the right hand, leaving the left hand to pull on the plunger. A left-handed person would do the opposite.
3. Place the thumb on top of the syringe (Figure 40-21).
4. With the syringe held in this position, turn it slightly so the bevel of the needle is facing up.
5. Hold the hand in such a position that by tilting the point of the needle down slightly the needle will enter the skin at a 15-degree angle and about 0.5 cm below the point where the vein was felt.

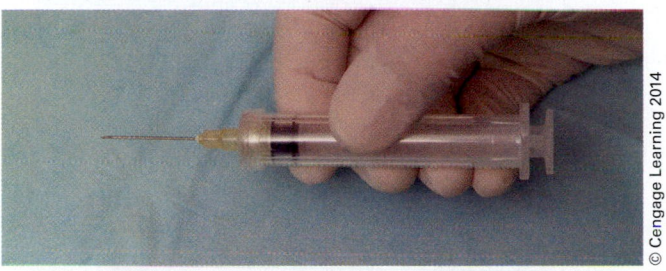

© Cengage Learning 2014

Figure 40-21   Proper hand position to hold a syringe for blood collection.

patient has had a double mastectomy, a physician should be consulted before drawing the blood.

SPECIMEN COLLECTION

The patient has been identified, requisition/orders and tubes have been verified, equipment has been assembled, and the patient is in a comfortable position. Hand washing is the most critical step to preventing the spread of infection. Before touching the patient, medical assistants should wash their hands. It is good practice to wash your hands in view of the patient to give the patient confidence in your technique. The next step is to tie the tourniquet. Have the patient close the hand, and then select a vein. If possible, place the patient's arm in a downward position. After locating an acceptable vein, mentally map the location. Set mental sites on the vein by visualizing the puncture site as the target for an accurate puncture. Cleanse the site with a gauze pad wet with 70% isopropyl alcohol

solution. A commercially prepared alcohol pad or one with 0.5% chlorhexidine in alcohol may also be used. Wipe the skin firmly with an alcohol pad. This removes any oil, sweat, perfume, lotions, and skin contaminations. This process is often referred to as "defatting" the skin. Allow the area to air dry, or you may dry it with a clean cotton ball or gauze pad. Puncturing the skin through wet alcohol can cause hemolysis of the specimen and give the patient a stinging sensation. Residual alcohol can also contaminate the specimen.

Some authorities suggest putting on gloves first and then palpating for the vein. This technique is required for the patient who is isolated because of a communicable disease and is good practice for all patients. Standard Precautions require that personal protective equipment be worn when there is a chance of coming in contact with blood and body fluid. If the patient has veins that are difficult to palpate, the gloves can be put on after the site has been palpated and before the cleansing. To avoid forgetting where the collection site is, palpate the vein 1 to 2 inches above and below the intended puncture site. It helps the medical assistant feel that the vein is located in a straight line and these points can be used to "reset" the mental crosshairs without contaminating the venipuncture site. Safety glasses and a mask must be worn if there is a potential for blood splatter.

The Syringe Technique

The syringe technique is used less often than the vacuum tube method. The syringe is ideal for collecting small volumes of blood from fragile, thin, or "rolling" veins or veins on the back of the hand or from the foot. Pulling on the plunger of the syringe creates suction; the larger the syringe, the greater the suction that can be obtained. Too great a suction might cause the vein to collapse. Vein collapse can be avoided by pulling the plunger slowly and by resting between pulls to allow the vein to refill. Because pediatric and geriatric patients often have thin and fragile veins, the syringe is the preferred method of venipuncture for them. The use of a syringe larger than 15 mL is not recommended. If more than 12 mL is needed, the butterfly collection method should be considered. Syringe draws are also ideal in special procedures when the blood must be transferred to a different container. Procedure 40-2 gives detailed instructions for venipuncture with syringe.

When a syringe is used, the blood obtained must be placed in appropriate containers. The order of filling the tubes is important.

CORRECT NEEDLE POSITION

The patient will experience the least amount of pain if the bevel of the needle is facing upward when the needle is inserted into the vein. The bevel of the needle is upward when the opening in the needle is visible when you look straight down on the needle as it is inserted. This position also helps prevent the suction from causing the inside wall of the vein to adhere to the needle bevel, thus occluding the needle.

The needle should be inserted at a 15-degree angle to the surface of the skin (Figure 40-22).

The skin should be held taut until the needle has been inserted. This technique allows the point of the needle to enter the skin with little drag or bunching of the skin, thereby reducing the discomfort of the puncture.

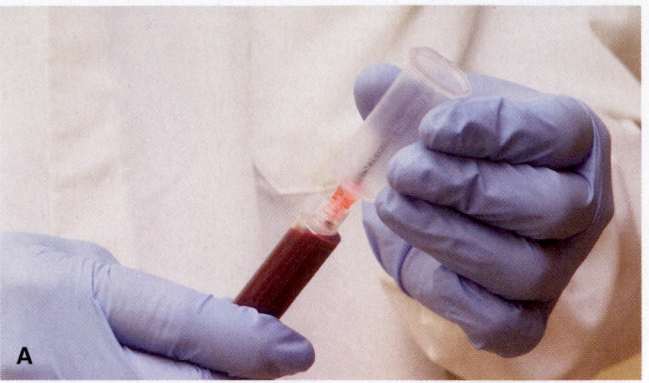

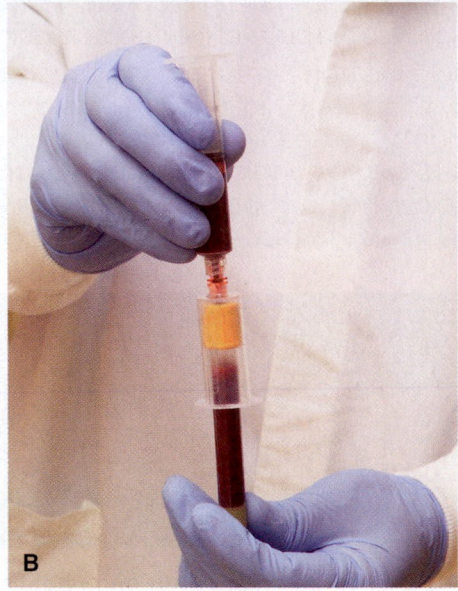

Figure 40-23 (A) The medical assistant attaches the BD Vacutainer Blood Transfer Device. (B) The device is used to safely transfer blood from a syringe to a vacuum tube.

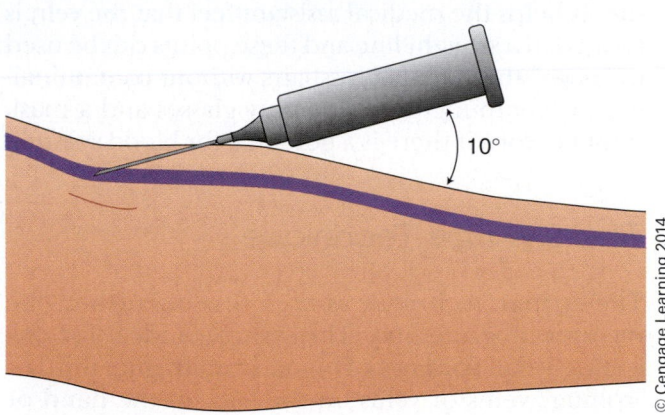

Figure 40-22 Proper angle of needle insertion for venipuncture.

 When transferring blood from a syringe to a vacuum tube, keep these safety features in mind:

- Never transfer to a vacuum tube using a needle. When transferring from a syringe to a vacuum tube, use a safety transfer device.
- Never push the blood into the vacuum tube. It will fill on its own.
- Always wear gloves, goggles, and face guard when performing this procedure.

The use of a needle to transfer blood from a syringe to a vacuum tube or culture bottle is unsafe and prohibited by OSHA. The use of a safety system such as the BD Vacutainer Blood Transfer Device is recommended (Figure 40-23). After drawing the blood into the syringe, activate the needle's safety mechanism, then remove the needle and dispose of it. Connect the needleless syringe to the transfer device. Insert a vacuum tube to the device and allow the blood to transfer from the syringe to the tube using the tube's vacuum. Never push on the syringe plunger or force the blood into the tube. This could cause the tube's stopper to pop off. When the appropriate tubes have been filled, dispose of the entire syringe and transfer assembly as one unit according to your clinic policies.

Immediately after filling, mix any tubes containing additives (Figure 40-24).

© Cengage Learning 2014

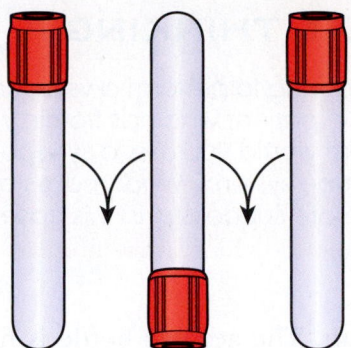

BD Vacutainer™ Tube Type	Closure Color	Number of Inversions
EDTA	Lavender	8–10
Sodium citrate	Light blue	3–4
SST with gel	Tiger (red gray) or gold	5
Serum	Red	5
Sodium fluoride	Gray	8–10
Heparin	Green	8–10

© Cengage Learning 2014

Figure 40-24 Vacuum tubes should be inverted several times (not shaken) to mix the additives well.

Vacuum Tube Specimen Collection

The vacuum tube system is an improvement over the syringe method yet maintains many similarities. When the syringe method is used, a vacuum is created as the medical assistant pulls on the syringe plunger. The vacuum tube method has the vacuum already in the tube. Another advantage of the vacuum tube system is that with multiple blood samples, syringes do not need to be changed; only the tubes need to be changed.

The similarity between the vacuum tube system and the syringe system is that the holder and needle are held in the same manner (Figure 40-25). The syringe is held in a manner that allows the medical assistant access to pull on the plunger. Access must be left in the vacuum tube system for one tube to be pulled out and another inserted. The hand that pulled on the plunger of the syringe is the hand that changes tubes with the vacuum tube system.

The procedure for venipuncture with the vacuum tube system follows the same steps as the syringe method with only slight variations.

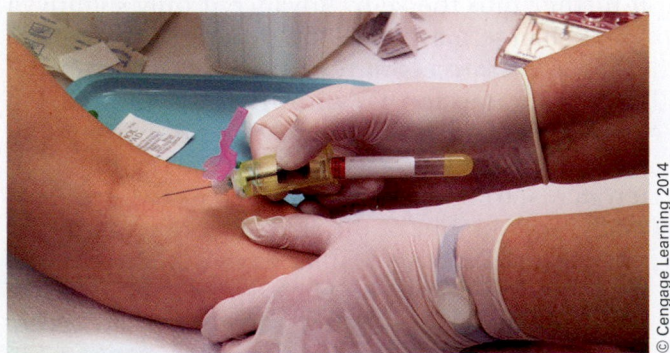

© Cengage Learning 2014

Figure 40-25 Proper hand position to hold a vacuum tube system.

Butterfly Needle Collection System

The butterfly collection system combines the benefits of the syringe system and the vacuum tube system. The butterfly collection system has on one end a 21- or 23-gauge needle with attached plastic wings. Six or twelve inches of tubing leads from the needle. On the other end of this tubing is a hub that can attach to a syringe. A needle covered by a rubber sleeve can also be attached to the tubing. The covered needle screws into an evacuated tube holder (Figure 40-26).

The butterfly system is used for small veins that are difficult to puncture with the vacuum tube system and standard vacuum tube system needle. The system also facilitates drawing from veins that have a tendency to collapse. The winged needle of the butterfly needle will slide into a small surface vein in the back of the hand, wrist, or foot. Instead of entering the vein at the usual 15-degree angle,

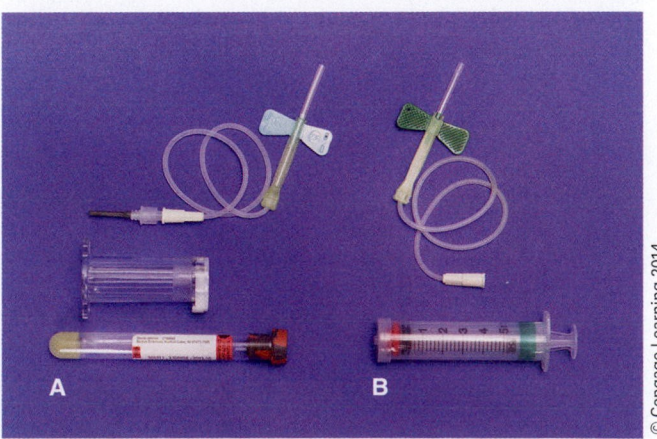

© Cengage Learning 2014

Figure 40-26 Butterfly needle sets with connections for either (A) a vacuum tube or (B) a Luer-Lok tipped syringe.

the winged needle is inserted at a 5- to 10-degree angle, and then threaded into the vein. This procedure anchors the needle in the center of a small vein that is inaccessible by other methods. If the patient moves, the tubing gives flexibility so the needle will stay anchored and not pull out of the vein. The butterfly collection set works well on children who have small veins and the tendency to move while blood is being collected.

The system also gives the adaptability of initiating a draw with a syringe and then finishing it with the evacuated tube system. A syringe can be filled for procedures that require a syringe sample. It can then be removed, and the vacuum tube system can be attached for multiple tube collection. Remember to draw into or transfer into the vacuum tubes in the proper order (see Table 40-4). Although the butterfly collection system has many benefits, it is not used for all collections. It is more expensive than the needle system. The additional expense is unnecessary for the majority of venipunctures.

Blood Cultures

Occasionally a patient will need to have blood collected for culture. The culture will determine if the patient has pathogens in the blood. Normally blood is sterile. When drawing blood for cultures, use a surgical solution (often Betadine) rather than alcohol and sterile rather than clean procedure. This means using sterile gloves; do not wipe away the surgical solution, touch the puncture site, or in any way compromise the sterile process. The blood is collected into special transport bottles, which are like vacuum tubes but shaped differently (Figure 40-27). The blood culture bottle contains transport media to preserve any microorganisms present while they are transported to the laboratory for culture. Because it is unknown whether the pathogen is anaerobic (living without oxygen) or aerobic (living with oxygen), blood is collected

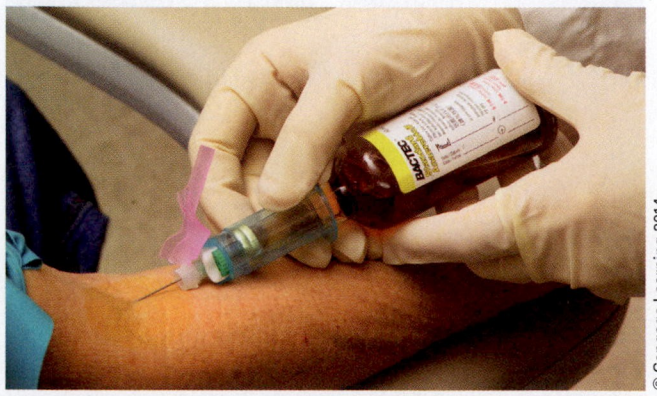

Figure 40-27 Blood being drawn for cultures.

© Cengage Learning 2014

CRITICAL THINKING

You are preparing to perform a venipuncture on a geriatric patient who has fragile veins. Which system would you use: a syringe or a vacuum tube system? What makes one technique more successful in this case?

to test for both. The aerobic bottle is filled first, then the anaerobic bottle is filled.

Patient Reactions

Patients can have a variety of reactions to having their blood drawn. The medical assistant must anticipate these reactions and respond appropriately as quickly as possible. The most common patient reaction is pain. The patient will indicate that the venipuncture is painful. Slightly reposition the needle, and then loosen the tourniquet. Loosening the tourniquet often helps because the tourniquet may be pinching the arm and causing discomfort rather than the needle. Avoid deep, probing venipunctures because they may go deeply into the arm and get too close to the nerves. If the pain is intolerable, discontinue the venipuncture.

Other possible patient reactions and the medical assistant's appropriate responses are listed in Table 40-6.

The Unsuccessful Venipuncture

Methods of vein stimulation are shown in Table 40-7. When a blood sample cannot be obtained, it may be necessary to change the position of the needle. Rotate the needle half a turn. The bevel of the needle may be against the wall of the vein. If the needle has not penetrated the vein far enough, advance it further into the vein. Advance it only slightly; a small change may mean the difference between a failed and a successful venipuncture. If the needle has penetrated too far into the vein, pull back a little. Always withdraw the needle slowly when the venipuncture has been unsuccessful. The blood often may start coming just as it seems the needle is ready to come out of the skin. The tube used may not have sufficient vacuum. Try another tube before withdrawing the needle.

Probing the site is not recommended. Probing is painful to the patient and may cause a hematoma. Never attempt a venipuncture more than two times. If a blood sample cannot be obtained after two attempts, have another person attempt the

Table 40-6 Patient Reactions to Blood Draws

Patient Reaction	Medical Assistant Response
Syncope (fainting)	Immediately remove the tourniquet, then the needle, and stop the patient from falling. Lower the patient's head and arms. Wipe the patient's forehead and back of the neck with a cold compress if necessary. If the patient does not respond, notify the provider, and place a pillow under the patient's legs.
Nausea	If a patient becomes nauseated, apply cold compresses to the patient's forehead. Give the patient an emesis basin, and have facial tissues ready if the nausea does not diminish. Advise the patient that deep slow breathing through the mouth may help lessen the nausea.
Insulin shock or hypoglycemia	The first signs of insulin shock are a cold sweat and pallor similar to the signs of syncope. The patient becomes weak and shaky, sudden mental confusion may follow, and it appears as though the patient's personality changes instantly. Call the provider if the patient loses consciousness. This can happen especially to patients having a fasting blood sugar test.
Convulsions	The patient loses consciousness and exhibits violent or mild convulsive motions. Do not try to restrain the patient. Move objects or furniture out of the way to prevent the patient from striking objects and being hurt. Help the patient to the floor and into a reclining position. The patient usually recovers within a few minutes. Notify the provider about the patient's reaction. The provider will determine when to release the patient.

© Cengage Learning 2014

draw. Notify the patient's provider if two medical assistants have been unsuccessful.

Criteria for Rejection of a Specimen

The primary goal of the medical assistant is to provide an acceptable specimen for laboratory testing as required by the provider. Certain general criteria must be met for a specimen to be acceptable. If the criteria are not met, the specimen is rejected and another venipuncture of the patient must be performed.

Table 40-8 lists quality-assurance controls for specimen collection and processing. The list is not all inclusive. The type of specimen that is acceptable and the volume required are determined by the procedure ordered. The quality-control checks done by the laboratory may indicate the results are valid. if the results do not agree with what the provider believes is the patient's diagnosis, the blood specimen may need to be redrawn to confirm the results. This is accomplished by either retesting the specimen or collecting another sample. This will either reconfirm that blood was drawn from the correct patient or that the patient's test results changed significantly.

Factors Affecting Laboratory Values

Numerous variables can affect laboratory test results. The specimens are tested by analytic instruments that give accurate and precise results. These results will accurately reflect what is wrong with the patient only if the specimen is collected correctly. The medical assistant is responsible for collecting and caring for the specimen properly. When in doubt of how to care for a specimen, refer to the manual supplied by the laboratory or contact the laboratory for specific instructions. It is always better to ask the question and perform the proper procedure than not to ask

Table 40-7 Methods of Vein Stimulation

1. Position the patient's arm lower than his or her heart.

2. Reapply the tourniquet; it may not be tight enough.

3. Massage the arm from the wrist to the elbow to encourage venous return.

4. Tap sharply at the venipuncture site with your fingertips. This can cause the veins to dilate.

5. Use a blood pressure cuff in place of the tourniquet. Pump it to about 40–60 mm Hg.

6. Warm the venipuncture site with a warming device or a warm washcloth (not hotter than 100°F).

7. Have the patient make a fist. Do not have the patient pump his or her fist; that can cause a false high level of potassium in the specimen.

© Cengage Learning 2014

Table 40-8 Quality Assurance for Specimen Collection and Processing

1. Each specimen must have its own label attached to the specimen's primary container.

2. Each specimen must have a laboratory requisition label.

3. Labels must have the patient's complete name and identification number, date of birth, date and time, and your signature.

4. Specimens in syringes with needles still attached are unacceptable.

5. Specimens must be in the appropriate anticoagulant.

6. Blood collection tubes with anticoagulant must be at least 75% full. All blood collection tubes for coagulation testing must be at least 90% full.

7. Uncoagulated blood specimens must be free of clots.

8. Certain tests require specimens to be free of hemolysis and **lipemia**, a milky appearance due to lipids.

9. The specimen may need to be recollected if the results do not agree with what the provider believes is the diagnosis of the patient.

10. Do not combine partially filled tubes.

11. Do not mix tubes of different additives.

12. As soon as possible, invert tubes 8 to 10 times to prevent microclots from forming (see Figure 40-24).

13. Mix tubes gently to prevent **hemolysis** of specimen.

© Cengage Learning 2014

Table 40-9 Factors Affecting Laboratory Results

Factor	Effect
Blood alcohol	When drawing a specimen for blood alcohol testing, a nonalcohol-based antiseptic should be used to clean the venipuncture site. The cleansing alcohol may falsely elevate the test result.
Diurnal rhythm	Some specimens must be drawn at timed intervals because of medication or diurnal (daily) rhythm. The exact time of collection must be noted on the specimen.
Exercise	Strenuous short-term exercise can make the heart work harder and increase the heart enzymes. Long-term exercise such as that performed by highly trained runners can cause erroneous results due to runner's anemia.
Fasting	If the patient is not in fasting state when fasting is required, the results of tests may not be accurate.
Hemolysis	Destruction of red blood cell membrane and release of intercellular contents into serum/plasma can be caused by not allowing alcohol to air-dry at venipuncture site, using a needle that is too small (less than 22-gauge), forcing the blood into a Vacutainer tube from a syringe, or shaking the Vacutainer tube instead of mixing by gentle inversion when mixing tubes with additives.
Heparin	Using incorrect heparin can interfere with the tests being run on the patient.
Stress	In children, violent crying before a specimen is collected can increase the white blood cell count.
Tourniquet on too long	Hemoconcentration can occur, causing a change in chemical concentration.
Volume	Not enough blood will cause a dilution factor, which can change the size of the cells and therefore produce a variation in test results.

© Cengage Learning 2014

and have to repeat the venipuncture. In addition, if you ever do need to repeat a venipuncture because of improper collection or handling of the specimen, the patient should not be billed for the second collection. Patient physiologic factors may also contribute to inaccurate results. Other factors that can alter results are listed in Table 40-9.

Occasionally, a specimen requires protection from light, incubation, refrigeration, or chilling immediately after collection. Any delay in these requirements will alter the results. The laboratory manual will direct you as to which specimens need to be chilled. See Table 40-10 for examples of special handling requirements.

The medical assistant is not the only person who can affect test results. The patient can knowingly or unknowingly alter the results by certain

Table 40-10 Common Laboratory Tests that Require Special Handling

Laboratory Test	Special Handling
A, vitamin	Protect from light by wrapping tube in foil
Acid phosphatase	Deliver to laboratory within 1 hour. Separate and freeze serum after clotting
Adrenocorticotropic hormone (ACTH)	Place in ice slurry
Alcohol, blood	Do NOT use alcohol pad to clean site
Ammonia	Place in ice slurry
B_6, vitamin	Protect from light by wrapping tube in foil
B_{12}, vitamin	Protect from light by wrapping tube in foil
Beta-carotene	Protect from light by wrapping tube in foil
Bilirubin, total or direct	Protect from light by wrapping tube in foil
Catecholamines	Place in ice slurry
Clot retraction	Incubate in 37°C until clotted
Cold agglutinins	Warm tube, incubate in 37°C
Complement C4	Separate and freeze serum after clotting
Complement, total (CH50)	Let clot in refrigerator, separate immediately and freeze immediately
Complement, total (CH100)	Let clot in refrigerator, separate immediately and freeze immediately
Cryofibrinogen	Warm tube, incubate in 37°C
Gastrin	Place in ice slurry
Gentamicin	Label peak or trough and time of last medication
Glucose tolerance	Label tubes with time intervals of draw specimens
Human leukocyte antigen (HLA-B27)	Do NOT refrigerate or freeze, record date and time collected
Lactic acid	Place in ice slurry
Parathyroid hormone (PTH)	Place in ice slurry
Partial thromboplastin time (PTT)	Refrigerate, test within 4 hours of drawing specimen
pH/blood gas	Place in ice slurry
Porphyrins	Protect from light by wrapping tube in foil
Prostate-specific antigen	Deliver to laboratory within 1 hour, separate, freeze serum after clotting
Prostatic acid phosphatase	Deliver to laboratory within 1 hour, separate, freeze serum after clotting
Prothrombin time (PT)	Refrigerate
Pyruvate	Place in ice slurry
Red blood cell folate	Protect from light by wrapping tube in foil
Renin	Place in ice slurry
Thioridazine (Mellaril)	Protect from light by wrapping tube in foil
Tobramycin	Label peak or trough and time of last medication

Source: Courtesy of Sheri R. Greimes, CMA (AAMA), PBT (ASCP), RMA, RPT (AMT).

actions. For example, a patient has consumed a cup of coffee but claims not to have had anything to eat or drink. The patient is often under the misconception that black coffee without sugar will not be a problem. Caffeine and smoking affect the metabolism and can affect the test results.

CAPILLARY PUNCTURE

Venipuncture is the most frequently performed phlebotomy procedure, but it is not the procedure of choice in all circumstances. An alternative to venipuncture is capillary puncture, also known as dermal puncture or skin puncture.

Capillary puncture is a method of obtaining one to several drops of blood for a variety of tests. With proper instruments, tests such as a complete blood count, RBC count, white blood cell (WBC) count, hemoglobin, and hematocrit can be run. One drop of blood can be used to test glucose blood levels, a few drops of blood can fill capillary tubes, and several drops can complete a phenylketonuria (PKU) test card. Tests that cannot be run on capillary blood specimens are sedimentation rates, blood cultures, coagulation studies, and any other tests requiring large amounts of serum or plasma.

Capillary puncture is the method of choice with two types of patients: when patient blood volume is a concern, such as with infants, and when vein access is difficult, such as with burned or scarred patients. Capillary puncture should not be used when a patient is edematous, dehydrated, or has poor peripheral circulation.

Composition of Capillary Blood

Blood obtained via capillary puncture is a mixture of blood from arterioles, venules, capillaries, and interstitial fluid. In most instances, a capillary puncture specimen most resembles arterial blood. There may be significant differences between specimens obtained by capillary puncture and those collected by venipuncture. For example, the glucose level may be increased in capillary blood, whereas the potassium, calcium, and total protein levels may be decreased. It is therefore important to always note on the specimen when capillary blood has been obtained.

Capillary Puncture Sites

The usual site for capillary puncture in adults and children is the fingertip (Figure 40-28). In adults, the ring finger is often selected because it usually is not callused. In infants, the lateral or medial

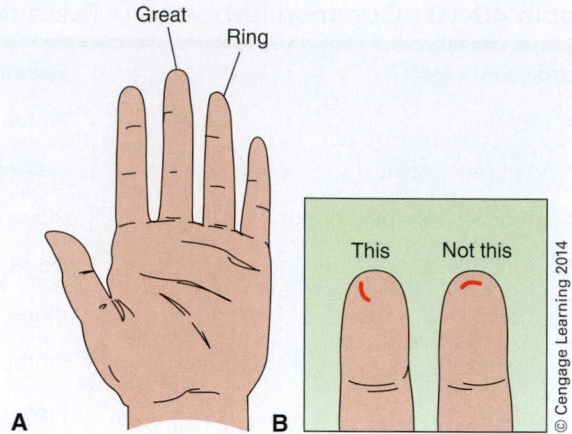

Figure 40-28 (A) Capillary blood collection sites. (B) Correct direction of capillary puncture.

plantar surface of the heel pad is usually used, and the procedure is often called a heelstick. The heelstick is most often performed when testing for PKU, which is covered in detail in Chapter 44.

Preparing the Capillary Puncture Site

The area selected for a capillary puncture must be carefully prepared. The puncture site will be warm if blood circulation is adequate. Coolness of the skin indicates decreased circulation. To increase circulation, the site can be gently massaged, or a warm, moist towel, face cloth, or warm pack (at a temperature not higher than 100°F) can be placed on the site for 3 to 5 minutes.

Alcohol-soaked gauze or cotton should be used to cleanse and disinfect the puncture site. The site should then be allowed to air-dry, or dry with a gauze pad. A cotton ball is not recommended because the tiny cotton fibers can stay on the puncture site, assisting in clotting, which is not desirable at this point. When the puncture is complete, a cotton ball can be used as a compress. Residual alcohol at the puncture site results in hemolysis of the specimen, which may affect test results, as well as cause a burning sensation to the patient. Betadine® (povidone-iodine) should not be used to clean the puncture site. Blood contaminated with iodine may falsely increase certain blood chemistries.

Performing the Puncture

Safety glasses, a mask, and gloves should be worn by the medical assistant while performing capillary puncture. Some patients bleed quite readily from the puncture, so be sure to have extra gauze on hand. The patient's hand and finger should be held so the puncture site is readily accessible. The puncture is made at the tip of the fleshy pad and slightly to the side (see Figure 40-28). The skin near the chosen site should be pulled taut. If the tips of the fingers are heavily callused or thickened, a lancet with a longer point may be used. Capillary punctures are performed using semiautomated devices such as the disposable Microtainer® Brand Safety Flow Lancet®.

The BD Microtainer® Genie Lancet is shown in Figure 40-29. After cleansing the puncture site, twist off the indicator as directed on the tab. Press the safety lancet firmly against the puncture site. Hold the lancet between your fingers and press the white button with your thumb. The lancet should not bounce off the skin. The puncture should be performed in one quick, steady movement. Once you have depressed the plunger, the button will lock into the housing and the needle will be permanently encapsulated. Practice working the lancets until you are comfortable with the action.

Collecting the Blood Sample

The first drop of blood is wiped away with dry, sterile gauze because it contains tissue fluid, which dilutes the blood drop and can also activate clotting. The second and following drops of blood are used for test samples. Depending on the tests to be performed, the blood may be collected in capillary tubes or other capillary collecting devices. Capillary tubes are small-diameter glass or plastic tubes that are open at both ends. Capillary tubes are extremely fragile and care should be taken to prevent breakage. The tubes have a colored line around

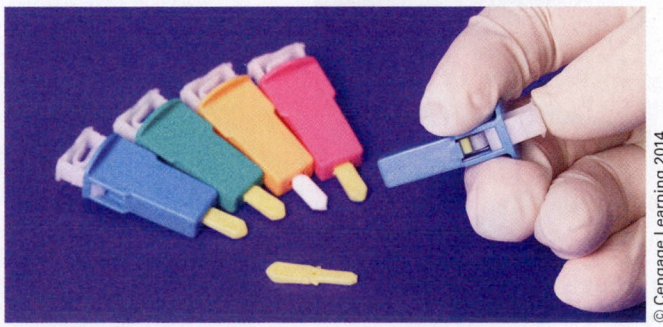

© Cengage Learning 2014

Figure 40-29   Microtainer brand lancets are available in different types for various purposes. They are color coded and have specific information on their packaging.

one end. A red or black line indicates that the tube contains heparin, an anticoagulant, and will yield a nonclotted specimen. A blue line indicates that the tube contains no anticoagulant and will yield a clotted specimen. When taking the blood sample directly from the puncture site, a capillary tube that contains anticoagulant would be used; when taking blood from a vacuum tube that already has anticoagulant in it, the plain capillary tube would be used. Capillary tubes are used for many tests, depending on the equipment available. Chapter 41 explains how to use capillary tubes to check hematocrit levels. When capillary tubes are used for hematocrit tests, they are called microhematocrit tubes.

It may be necessary to massage the finger to increase the blood flow. It is best to massage the whole hand, taking care not to apply direct pressure near the puncture site. Squeezing the fingertip should be avoided; this forces tissue fluid into the blood sample and dilutes it or may cause hemolysis. Do not use a scooping technique when collecting blood from the puncture site. Scooping can break the RBC membranes, leading to hemolysis.

Figure 40-30 shows the basic steps to follow when filling a capillary tube. Allow well-rounded drops of blood to form at the puncture site. Holding the capillary tube at a horizontal position, gently touch the tip of tube to the top of the blood drop. The blood will enter the tube through "capillary action" caused by surface tension. Take care to not tilt the tube downward, which can cause air to enter the tube, nor upward, which can cause blood to come out of the tube. Continue to fill the tube until it is two-thirds to three-quarters full. When the tube is sufficiently filled, remove it from the drop and, at the same time, place your gloved finger over the opposite end of the tube. This will prevent the blood from flowing out of the tube. Keep your gloved finger over the end of the tube and, using your other hand, wipe off any residue blood from the outside of the tube with a gauze pad. Gently place the end of the tube into the sealing clay. Sealing clay trays are specially made for this purpose. They have numbered sections to help identify the samples. Some capillary tubes have plastic caps. Carefully follow the manufacturer's instructions for the type of tube you are using.

During the filling of the tubes, if the flow of blood begins to slow, rewipe the puncture site firmly with dry gauze (not a cotton ball). This action will dislodge the platelet plug and allow the blood to flow freely. Be sure the patient is relaxed. Have the patient take a deep breath. After filling

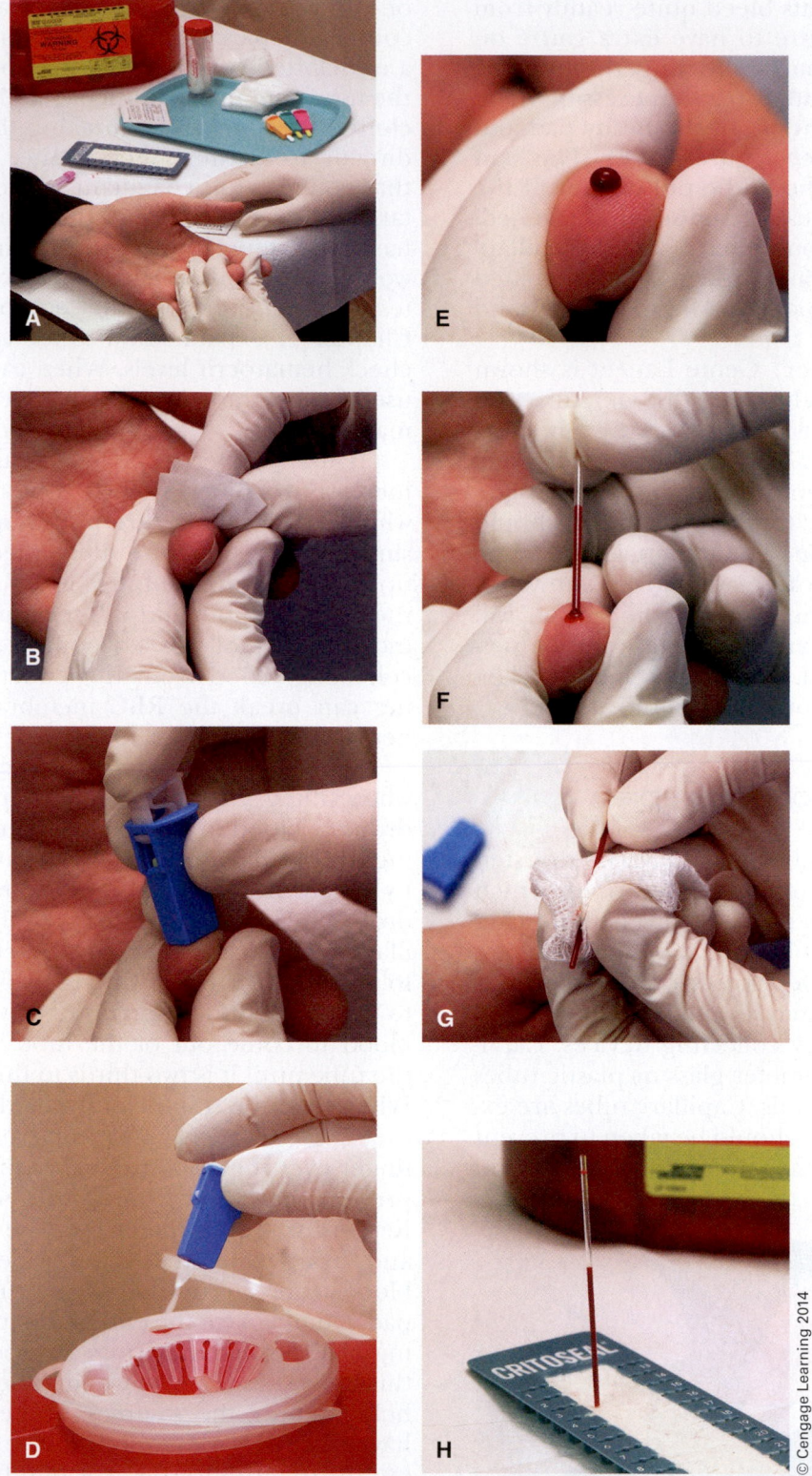

Figure 40-30 Collecting a specimen into a capillary tube through capillary puncture. (A) Assemble the necessary equipment and supplies and examine the finger for the best puncture site. (B) Clean the site with alcohol and allow the area to dry. (C) Perform the puncture. (D) Discard the lancet into a nearby sharps container. (E) Wipe off the first drop (not shown) and allow a well-rounded drop to form. (F) Holding the capillary tube horizontally, touch the end to the drop and allow the tube to fill. (G) Carefully wipe the residue blood off the tube. (H) Gently place the end of the tube into the sealing clay. Repeat to collect a second tube. Draw at least two tubes; some laboratories require three. Follow your laboratory manual instructions.

the required number of tubes, apply a cotton ball compress to the puncture site. The patient can usually help hold the compress. The compression should be held in place for 1 to 3 minutes, depending on the patient. If the patient is taking aspirin, Coumadin, or other anticoagulants, compression should be for at least 5 minutes.

 In many ways the procedure for capillary puncture is similar to the other collection procedures discussed in this chapter (e.g., patient identification, safety precautions, specimen labeling). Procedure 40-5 provides a detailed description of capillary puncture.

 ## PROCEDURE 40-1

Palpating a Vein and Preparing a Patient for Venipuncture

STANDARD PRECAUTIONS:

PURPOSE:
To palpate a vein and assess patient preparation prior to performing venipuncture.

EQUIPMENT/SUPPLIES:
Gloves
Tourniquet

PROCEDURE STEPS:

1. *Introduce yourself by name and credential. Identify the patient and explain the procedure.* Ask the patient's name and verify it with the computer label or identification number. If a fasting specimen is required, verify that the patient has not had anything to eat or drink except water for 12 hours. RATIONALE: Proper identification of the patient and specimen and ensuring that the patient has properly prepared for the blood tests are quality-control and quality-assurance measures.

2. Wash hands. Put on gloves.

3. Apply tourniquet 2 to 3 inches above the venipuncture site. Apply tightly enough to slow venous blood flow but not so tight that blood flow in arteries is stopped (see Figure 40-31A). RATIONALE: Applying the tourniquet too tightly can lead to excessive engorgement of the veins, causing blood to enter the tissues during puncture, further causing a hematoma.

4. Have the patient close the hand and place the patient's arm in a downward position. Do not allow the patient to pump his or her hand. RATIONALE: Having the patient close his or her hand and positioning the arm below the heart causes enlargement of the vein, allowing for an easier, more successful puncture. Pumping of the hand can lead to excessive engorgement of the vein, causing blood to leak into surrounding tissue during the puncture, which will cause a hematoma to occur.

5. Palpate the antecubital space of the arm, feeling for the basilic or cephalic vein with the tip of your middle or ring finger. Feel for a soft bounce and a roundness to the vein. RATIONALE: The tip of the middle or ring finger is less callused and more sensitive than the tip of the index finger. Veins will have a soft round feel.

6. After locating an acceptable vein, mentally map the location. Visualize the puncture site. Follow the direction of the vein with your finger tip, making a mental note of any turns, dips, and twists. RATIONALE: Mentally mapping the location and visualizing the puncture site will help in planning a successful direction.

7. If a vein cannot be found in the antecubital space of either arm, then the hand veins must be checked following the same procedure. The butterfly technique is more successful for hand venipuncture. RATIONALE: Butterfly is more successful because the hand veins have a greater tendency to roll and are smaller than the veins in the arm.

PROCEDURE 40-2
Venipuncture by Syringe

STANDARD PRECAUTIONS:

   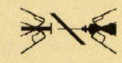

PURPOSE:
To obtain venous blood acceptable for laboratory testing as requested by the provider.

EQUIPMENT/SUPPLIES:

Gloves	Cotton balls
Goggles and mask	Adhesive bandage or tape
10 mL syringe, 21-gauge needle	Sharps container and biohazard red bag
Vacuum tube(s) or special collection tube(s)	Test tube rack
	Biohazard transport bag (optional)
Tourniquet	Lab requisition (optional)
70% isopropyl alcohol swab	

PROCEDURE STEPS:

1. Assemble the supplies. RATIONALE: Organizing supplies before the procedure ensures a more timely and professional process.

2. *Introduce yourself by name and credential.* Position and identify the patient. *Ask the patient's name and verify it* with the tests ordered and the computer label or identification number. If a fasting specimen is required, verify that the patient has not had anything to eat or drink except water for 12 hours. RATIONALE: Proper identification of the patient and the tests ordered and ensuring that the patient is properly prepared for the blood tests are all quality-control and quality-assurance measures.

3. *Explain the procedure and expectations to the patient. Allay the patient's fears regarding the procedure to help him feel safe and comfortable.* RATIONALE: Explaining the procedure and allaying the patient's fears will assure the patient that you are concerned about any apprehension he may have and that you are open to discussing his concerns.

4. Wash hands and apply gloves and goggles/mask. RATIONALE: Clean hands further protect the patient. Gloves protect you. Goggles/mask should be worn if there is a possibility of blood splatter.

5. Open the sterile needle and sterile syringe packages and assemble if necessary. Pull the plunger halfway out and push it all the way in again. RATIONALE: Preparing the equipment ahead of time ensures a smoother process. Syringes can stick when new, so pulling once on the plunger prevents it from sticking during the venipuncture.

6. Select the proper vacuum tubes for later transfer of the specimen; tap all tubes containing anticoagulants and check the expiration dates. Arrange them in a holding rack in proper order. RATIONALE: Having the supplies ready and in the rack saves confusion later. The rack is a safety item so you are not holding the tube while transferring the specimen. Tapping the tubes ensures that all the additive is dislodged from the stopper and wall of the tubes. Checking expiration dates is a quality-assurance measure.

7. Apply the tourniquet (Figure 40-31A) and select a site. See Procedure 40-1. RATIONALE: Applying the tourniquet causes the vein to enlarge for easier venipuncture.

8. Ask the patient to close the hand. The patient must not pump the hand. Place the hand in a downward position. RATIONALE: Closing the hand and placing the arm in a downward position further enlarges the vein, allowing for easier venipuncture. Pumping the hand can damage the quality of the specimen collected.

9. Select a vein, noting the location and direction of the vein. RATIONALE: This allows you to prepare mentally for the venipuncture.

10. Cleanse the site with an alcohol swab with one firm swipe (Figure 40-31B). Avoid touching the site after cleansing. RATIONALE: Alcohol removes body oils, sweat, and other contaminants. The site should stay as clean as possible.

11. Draw the skin taut with your thumb by placing it 1 to 2 inches below the puncture site. RATIONALE: This will anchor the vein.

12. With the bevel up, line up the needle with the direction of the vein and perform the puncture (Figure 40-31C). The point of the needle should enter the skin about ¼ inch below where the vein was palpated. With experience, a sensation of entering the vein can be felt. Once the vein has been entered, do not move the needle from

Procedure 40-2 (continued)

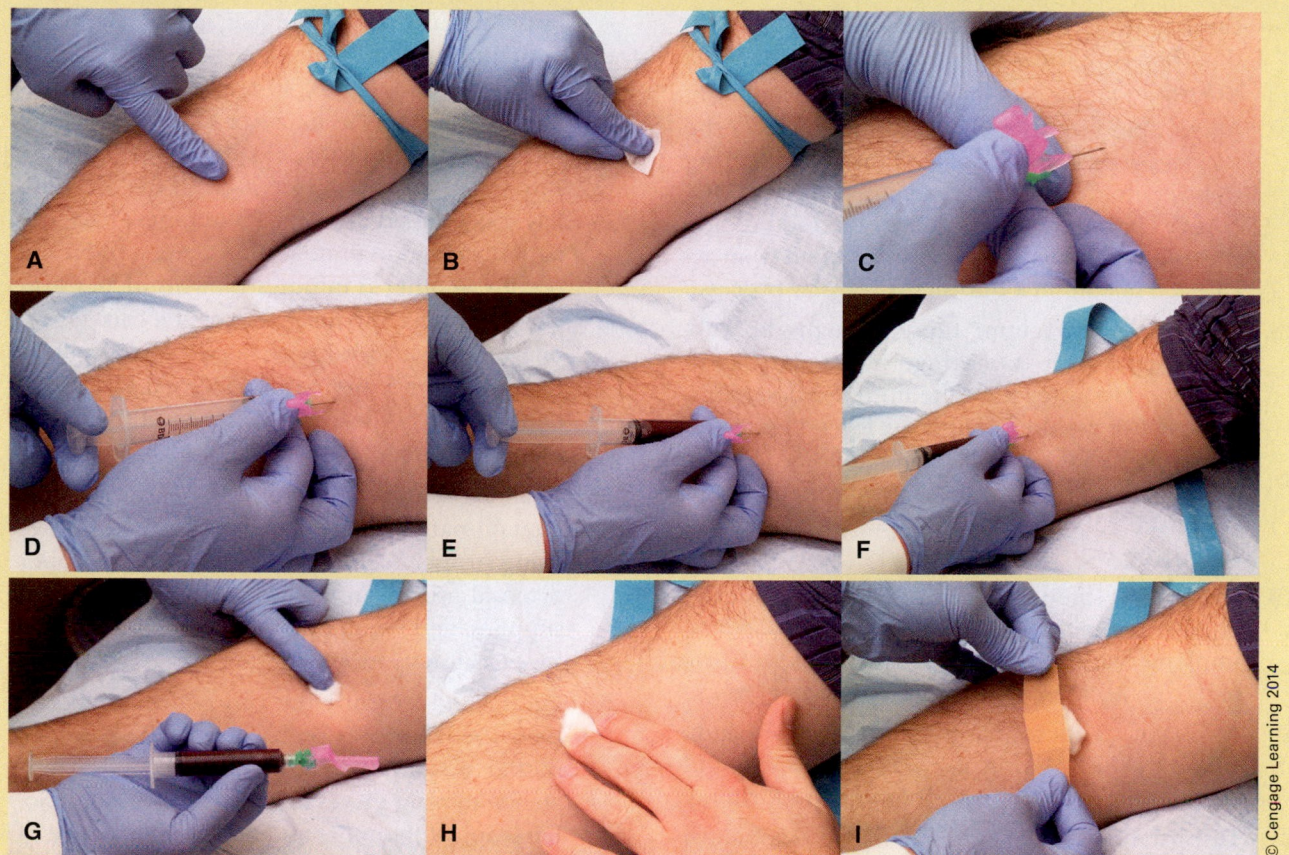

Figure 40-31 Performing a venipuncture with the syringe method. (A) Apply tourniquet and find vein. (B) Apply alcohol in one quick motion and allow to dry. Area can be wiped with a clean 2 × 2 gauze (do not use a cotton ball). (C) Draw skin taut (not shown) and insert needle. (D) Let go of skin and use that hand to pull back on the plunger. (E) Withdraw blood slowly, until the syringe is full. (F) Release tourniquet. (G) Apply a clean cotton ball immediately after withdrawing needle. (H) Have patient apply pressure to the site until a clot forms. (I) Apply a bandage over the site.

side to side. Do not push down or pull up the needle. The needle can be moved in or out gently if needed to locate the vein. RATIONALE: Lining up the needle with the vein is a mental exercise to help enter the vein in the proper direction. Entering the skin a fraction of an inch below the palpated site will aid in entering the vein at the correct site. This will align the needle so that it will enter the vein.

13. Let go of the skin and use that hand to pull back on the plunger (Figure 40-31D). Pull gently and only as fast as the syringe fills (Figure 40-31E). If the vein collapses, stop pulling on the plunger and let the vein refill. RATIONALE: Pulling too rapidly or too hard can cause the vein to collapse.

14. When the syringe is full, have the patient open the hand. Remove the tourniquet (Figure 40-31F). RATIONALE: Opening the hand and removing

the tourniquet releases the pressure so the needle can be removed.

15. Lightly place a cotton ball above the puncture site and remove the needle in the same direction as inserted (Figure 40-31G). RATIONALE: Holding the cotton ball above the site allows for immediate pressure to be applied once the needle is removed.

16. Apply pressure to the site for 2 to 3 minutes, or longer if the patient is taking prescribed anticoagulants (blood thinners) such as warfarin (Coumadin) or is taking aspirin or an herbal blood thinner such as ginkgo biloba. Let the patient assist by holding the pressure if desired (Figure 41-31H). The patient can elevate the arm but should be instructed not to bend the elbow. RATIONALE: Two to three minutes is usually enough time for the bleeding to stop. Elevating

continues

Procedure 40-2 (continued)

the arm while holding pressure aids in the clotting. Bending the elbow can cause a hematoma to form.

17. Aliquot blood into the appropriate tubes in the rack in the proper order (see Table 40-4). During transfer, hold each tube at the base only. RATIONALE: Having the tubes in the rack and holding the tubes at the base protects your hand from accidental needlestick during the transfer process.

18. Puncture the vacuum tube through the rubber stopper with the syringe needle and allow the blood to enter the tube until the flow stops. Never push on the plunger or force blood into the tube. RATIONALE: Pushing on the plunger and forcing blood into the vacuum tube can cause the rubber stopper to pop off, splashing blood.

19. Implement safety mechanism or devices on the needle immediately. RATIONALE: Immediate implementation of safety mechanisms will protect from accidental needlesticks.

20. Mix any anticoagulant tubes immediately. RATIONALE: Mixing the anticoagulants right away minimizes the chance of miniclots forming.

21. Discard the syringe and needle into a sharps container and the contaminated cotton ball and other contaminated waste into a red biohazard bag. RATIONALE: Proper disposal of sharps and biohazard waste protects all personnel.

22. Label all tubes before leaving the room. If any special treatment is required for the specimens, institute the handling protocol right away. RATIONALE: Labeling the tubes right away lessens the chances of a mix-up error. Proper handling of specimens ensures an accurate test result.

23. Check the patient. Observe him or her for signs of stress. RATIONALE: Venipuncture can be stressful for some patients.

24. When sufficient pressure has been applied to stop the bleeding, apply a small pressure bandage by pulling a cotton ball in half, applying it to the puncture site, and placing an adhesive bandage or tape over it (Figure 40-31I). Instruct the patient to remove the bandage in 20 minutes. If the patient is sensitive or allergic to latex, be sure to use nonlatex paper tape. If the bleeding has not stopped after 2 to 3 minutes, have the patient continue to hold direct pressure on the site for another 5 minutes with his or her arm elevated above the heart. He or she can do this by lying down with his or her arm on a pillow. Recheck after 5 minutes. RATIONALE: The patient should not leave your care until the bleeding has stopped.

25. Disinfect tray and supplies and dispose of all contaminated items properly. Remove gloves using proper technique. RATIONALE: Proper disposal and disinfection of all contaminated supplies and equipment protects from exposure to biohazardous substances.

26. Wash hands, record the procedure, and complete the laboratory requisition in the presence of the patient. RATIONALE: Washing hands after removing gloves further protects from biohazardous substances and lessens the chance of cross contamination to the patient's chart and the laboratory requisition. Completing the documentation and requisition as soon as possible after the procedure ensures the patient's sample is with the right requisition and improves accuracy.

27. Place specimen and requisition into biohazard transport bag and notify the laboratory that the specimen is ready for pickup.

DOCUMENTATION:

11/13/XX 2:54 PM   Venipuncture performed right arm for CBC and sed rate. Specimens sent to Inner City Lab. Identification. #987654321. Patient tolerated the procedure well and will call back tomorrow for the test results. Joe Guerrero, CMA (AAMA)

PROCEDURE 40-3

Venipuncture by Vacuum Tube System

STANDARD PRECAUTIONS:

   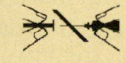

PURPOSE:

To obtain venous blood acceptable for laboratory testing as requested by a provider.

EQUIPMENT/SUPPLIES:

Gloves	21-gauge multidraw needle
Goggles and mask	Vacuum tube(s) or
Vacuum tube	special collection
adapter/holder	tube(s)
Lab requisition	Tourniquet
(optional)	Adhesive bandage or tape
70% isopropyl	Sharps container and
alcohol swab	biohazard red bag
Cotton balls	Biohazard transport bag
2 × 2 gauze	

PROCEDURE STEPS:

1. *Introduce yourself by name and credential.* RATIONALE: The patient has a right to know who is performing a procedure on him and what your credentials are. You will also be exhibiting professionalism.

2. *Explain the procedure and expectations to the patient. Allay the patient's fears regarding the procedure to help him feel safe and comfortable.* RATIONALE: Explaining the procedure and allaying the patient's fears will assure the patient that you are concerned about any apprehension he may have and that you are open to discussing his concerns.

3. Position and identify the patient. *Ask the patient's name and verify it* with the tests ordered and the computer label or identification number. If a fasting specimen is required, verify that the patient has not had anything to eat or drink except water for 12 hours. RATIONALE: Proper identification of the patient and the tests ordered and ensuring that the patient is properly prepared for the blood tests are all quality-control and quality-assurance measures.

4. Wash hands and apply gloves and goggles/mask. RATIONALE: Clean hands further protect the patient. Gloves protect you. Goggles/mask should be worn if there is a possibility of blood splatter.

5. Break the seal on the shorter needle; thread the shorter needle into the holder/adapter. Select the first tube and gently place it into the holder/adapter (do not puncture the tube yet). RATIONALE: Preparing the equipment ahead of time ensures a smoother process.

6. Tap all tubes containing anticoagulants and check the expiration dates. RATIONALE: Tapping the tubes ensures that all the additive is dislodged from the stopper and wall of the tubes. Checking expiration dates is a quality-assurance measure.

7. Select a site and apply the tourniquet (see Procedure 40-1). RATIONALE: Applying the tourniquet causes the vein to enlarge for easier venipuncture.

8. Ask the patient to close the hand. The patient must not pump the hand. Place the hand in a downward position. RATIONALE: Closing the hand and placing the arm in a downward position further enlarges the vein, allowing for easier venipuncture. Pumping the hand can damage the quality of the specimen collected.

9. Select a vein, noting the location and direction of the vein. RATIONALE: This allows you to prepare mentally for the venipuncture (Figure 40-32A).

10. Cleanse the site with an alcohol swab with one firm swipe. RATIONALE: Alcohol removes body oils and contamination (Figure 40-32B).

11. Avoid touching the site after cleansing. RATIONALE: The site should stay as clean as possible.

12. Draw the skin taut with your thumb by placing it 1 to 2 inches below the puncture site. RATIONALE: This will anchor the vein.

13. With the bevel up, line up the needle with the direction of the vein and perform the puncture. The point of the needle should enter the skin about ¼ inch below where the vein was palpated. With experience, a sensation of entering the vein can be felt. Once the vein has been entered, do not move the needle. RATIONALE: Lining up the needle with the vein is a mental exercise to help enter the vein in the proper direction. Entering the skin a fraction of an inch below the palpated site will aid in entering the vein at the palpated site (Figure 40-32C).

14. Let go of the skin and use that hand to grasp the flange of the vacuum tube holder and push the tube forward until the needle has completely entered the tube (Figure 40-32D). Do not change

continues

Procedure 40-3 (continued)

hands while performing venipuncture. The hand performing the venipuncture is the hand that is holding the vacuum tube holder. The other hand is free for tube insertion and removal. RATIONALE: Using the flange of the adapter helps you hold the needle steady while changing tubes. Changing hands while performing venipuncture could cause the needle to move.

15. Fill the tube until the vacuum is exhausted and the blood flow stops. Rotate tubes so the label is down. RATIONALE: Letting the tubes completely fill will ensure the right ratio of blood to additive. Positioning the label down enables you to see the tube filling.

16. When the blood ceases, gently remove the vacuum tube from the needle and holder. Do this by grasping the tube with the fingers and palm of your spare hand and using your thumb to push off from the flange of the holder (Figure 40-32E). RATIONALE: Using the flange will help steady the needle.

17. Immediately mix the blood in the anticoagulant tubes by gently inverting them several times. RATIONALE: Mixing the anticoagulant tubes right away minimizes the chance of miniclots forming.

18. Insert the second tube onto the needle by using the same motion as the first tube (Figure 40-32F). Let it fill; then remove it with

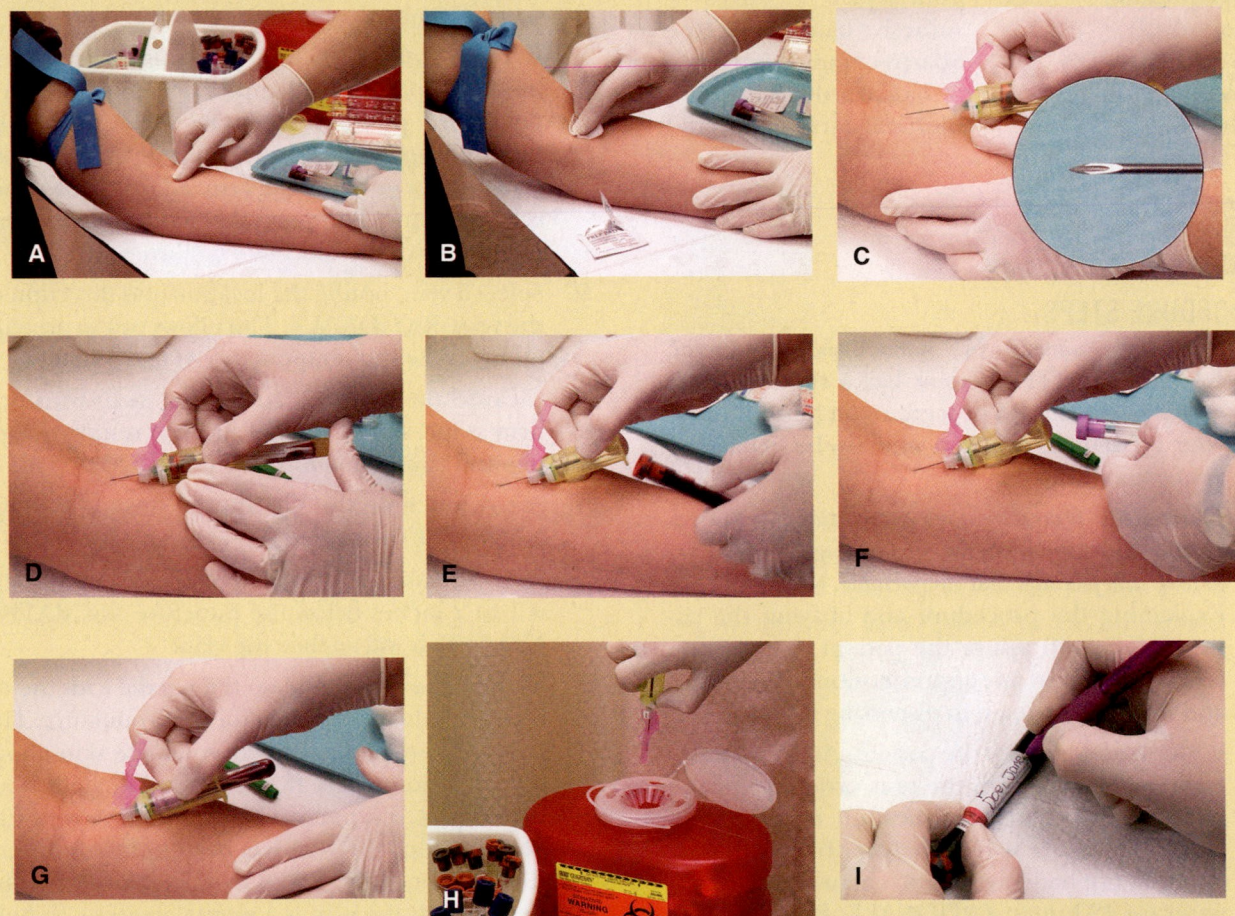

Figure 40-32   Performing a venipuncture with a vacuum tube assembly. (A) After tying the tourniquet, palpate the vein. (B) Cleanse the site with alcohol. Allow area to dry or wipe with a clean 2 × 2 gauze. (C) While holding the skin taut, hold needle with bevel up and penetrate the vein with a smooth rapid movement. (D) Grasp the flange of the vacuum tube holder to push the vacuum tube onto the needle. (E) When the tube has stopped filling, remove it gently from the needle and holder using the flange to push from. Invert it several times to mix the additives. (F) Place another tube onto the needle and let it fill. (G) When the last tube has filled, gently remove it from the holder. Release the tourniquet (not shown) and smoothly remove the needle from the vein, immediately applying pressure with the cotton ball. Mix well by inverting several times. (H) Dispose of the needle and holder into a nearby sharps container. (I) Properly label the tubes.

Procedure 40-3 (continued)

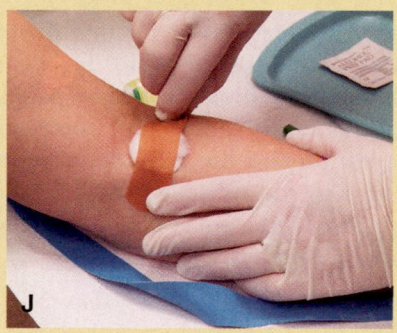

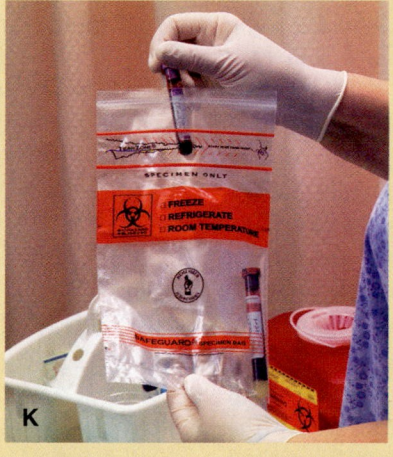

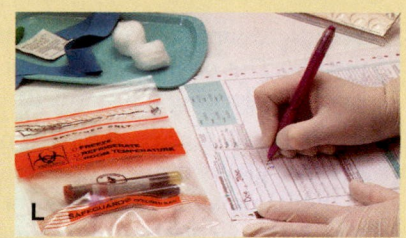

© Cengage Learning 2014

Figure 40-32   (Continued) (J) Check the patient, apply a bandage. (K) Package the specimens properly for transport (be aware of special storage or treatment needed, such as centrifugation or refrigeration). (L) Complete the laboratory requisition and document the procedure in the patient's chart or electronic medical record.

the same motion as the first tube. Invert it several times if it contains anticoagulants. RATIONALE: Mixing the additives prevents the blood from coagulating.

19. When the last tube has filled, remove it from the needle. Ask the patient to open his or her hand and release the tourniquet. RATIONALE: Removing the last tube from the needle prevents any residual suction from drawing blood through the tissues when needle is removed from the vein. Opening the hand and removing the tourniquet relieves pressure so the needle can be removed without causing excessive blood loss through the puncture site.

20. Lightly place the cotton ball above the puncture site and smoothly remove the needle from the arm in the same direction of insertion. RATIONALE: Holding the cotton ball above the site allows for immediate pressure to be applied once the needle is removed.

21. Immediately activate the safety device. RATIONALE: Activating the safety device protects you from accidental needlesticks (Figure 40-32H).

22. Apply pressure on the site for 2 to 3 minutes. Let the patient assist by holding the pressure. Ask him or her not the bend his or her arm, but he or she can elevate his or her arm while applying pressure. RATIONALE: Two to three minutes is usually enough time for bleeding to stop. Hold pressure for longer if the patient is taking prescribed anticoagulants (blood thinners) such as warfarin (Coumadin) or taking aspirin

or an herbal blood thinner such as ginkgo biloba. Elevating the arm while holding pressure aids in the clotting. Bending the elbow can cause a hematoma to form.

23. Dispose of the needle into a sharps container and the contaminated cotton ball and other contaminated waste into a biohazard red bag. RATIONALE: Proper disposal of sharps and biohazard waste protects all personnel.

24. Label all the tubes before leaving the patient (Figure 40-32I). If any special treatment is required for the specimens, institute the handling protocol right away. RATIONALE: Labeling the tubes right away lessens the chances of a mix-up error. Proper handling of the specimens ensures accurate test results.

25. Check the patient. Observe him or her for signs of stress. He or she should stop bleeding within 2 to 3 minutes. If the bleeding has stopped, apply a small pressure bandage by pulling a cotton ball in half, applying it to the site, and placing an adhesive bandage or tape over it (Figure 40-32J). The patient should be instructed to remove the bandage in about 20 minutes. If the patient is sensitive to latex, be sure to use a nonlatex paper tape. If the bleeding has not stopped, have the patient continue to hold direct pressure another 5 minutes with his or her arm elevated above his or her heart level. Have him or her lie down with his or her arm up on a pillow. Recheck the site after 5 minutes of additional direct pressure. RATIONALE: Check the patient for signs of distress

continues

Procedure 40-3 (continued)

because venipuncture can be stressful for some people. The patient should not leave your care until the bleeding has stopped.

26. Disinfect all surfaces and supplies/equipment. Remove gloves using proper technique. Dispose of contaminated items appropriately. RATIONALE: Proper disposal and disinfection of all contaminated supplies and equipment protects from exposure to dangerous biohazard substances.

27. Wash hands, record the procedure, and complete the laboratory requisition in the presence of the patient. Place specimen and requisition into biohazard transport bag and notify the laboratory that the specimen is ready for pickup (Figures 40-32K and L). RATIONALE: Washing

hands after removing gloves further protects you from biohazard substances and lessens the chance of cross contamination to the patient's chart and the laboratory requisition. Completing the documentation and the requisition as soon as possible and in the presence of the patient improves accuracy and assures that the patient's sample is the right requisition.

DOCUMENTATION:

4/27/XX 8:36 AM   Venipuncture performed on left arm for CBC, Hgb & Hct, and thyroid panel. Samples sent to Inner City Lab. Patient ID # 56776523. Patient tolerated the procedure well and will return on 4/30/XX for a recheck. Joe Guerrero, CMA (AAMA)

PROCEDURE 40-4

Venipuncture by Butterfly Needle System

STANDARD PRECAUTIONS:

   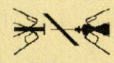

PURPOSE:
To obtain venous blood acceptable for laboratory testing as requested by a provider.

EQUIPMENT/SUPPLIES:
Gloves
Goggles and mask
Vacuum tube holder if using a vacuum tube connection
A 10- to 15-mL/cc syringe if using a syringe connection
Butterfly needle system with 21-gauge needle (use a multisample needle system with a Luer-Lok adapter for attaching to the vacuum tube and a hypodermic needle for syringe attachment)
Vacuum tubes if appropriate
Tourniquet
70% isopropyl alcohol swab
2 × 2 gauze
Adhesive bandage or tape
Sharps container and biohazard red bag
Lab transport bag and requisition (optional)

PROCEDURE STEPS:

1. Assemble the supplies. RATIONALE: Organizing supplies before the procedure ensures a more timely and professional process.

2. *Introduce yourself by name and credential.* RATIONALE: The patient has a right to know who is performing a procedure on him and what your credentials are. You will also be exhibiting professionalism.

3. Position and identify the patient. *Ask the patient's name and verify it* with the computer label or identification number. If a fasting specimen is required, verify that the patient has not had anything to eat or drink except water for 12 hours. RATIONALE: Proper identification of the patient and the tests ordered and verifying that the patient is properly prepared are quality-control and quality-assurance measures.

4. *Explain the procedure and expectations to the patient. Allay the patient's fears regarding the procedure to help him feel safe and comfortable.* RATIONALE: Explaining the procedure and allaying the

Procedure 40-4 (continued)

patient's fears will assure the patient that you are concerned about any apprehension he may have and that you are open to discussing his concerns.

5. Wash hands. Put on gloves, as well as goggles and mask if there is a potential for blood splatter. RATIONALE: Clean hands further protect the patient. Gloves and goggles/face shield protect you from any potential splatters.

6. Open the package of butterfly needle system. If using the multisample needle, connect the needle to the vacuum tube holder/adapter. If using the hypodermic needle and syringe, connect the needle to the syringe (Figure 40-33A). If using a syringe, set the vacuum tubes in a rack for later use. RATIONALE: The more organized you are before the venipuncture; the smoother the procedure will go.

7. Tap the vacuum tubes to be sure any additive is dislodged from the stopper and sides of the tube. Check the expiration dates. RATIONALE: Dislodging the additive will ensure proper ratio in the specimen. The tubes should not be older than their expiration date.

8. Apply the tourniquet. Select a vein. RATIONALE: Applying a tourniquet enlarges the vein, making it more accessible.

9. Ask the patient to close his or her hand (Figure 40-33B). The patient should not pump his or her hand. If possible, place the arm in a downward position. RATIONALE: Pumping of hand can lead to excessive engorgement of the vein, which can cause blood to enter the tissues during the puncture, causing a hematoma.

10. Select the vein, noting the direction and location of the vein. RATIONALE: You will want to enter the vein in the same direction it is going.

11. Cleanse the site with an alcohol swab using one swift firm swipe and allow to dry (Figure 40-33C). RATIONALE: Alcohol removes body oils and other contaminations. Puncturing the skin through wet alcohol can cause stinging and hemolysis of the specimen and will contaminate the specimen.

12. Avoid touching the site after cleansing. RATIONALE: Touching the skin will recontaminate it.

13. Draw the skin taut by placing your thumb 1 to 2 inches below the site and pulling down firmly. RATIONALE: This will anchor the vein.

14. Hold the wings of the butterfly together with the bevel up, line up the needle with the vein, and smoothly insert it into the vein at about a 5- to 10-degree angle (Figure 40-33D). RATIONALE: This process will cause the least amount of discomfort and provide the greatest success.

15. Remove your hand from holding the skin taut. RATIONALE: You will need one hand free to handle the other equipment.

16. If you are connected to a vacuum tube holder, grasp the flange of the vacuum tube holder and push the tube forward until the needle has completely entered the tube. RATIONALE: Using the flange when inserting and removing vacuum tubes will help the needle stay in position.

17. If you are connected to a syringe, pull gently on the syringe (Figure 40-33E). RATIONALE: Pulling too rapidly can cause the vein to collapse.

18. Do not change hands while performing venipuncture. The hand performing the venipuncture is the hand that is holding the vacuum tube holder. The other hand is for inserting and removing the vacuum tubes. RATIONALE: Changing hands can cause the needle to change position.

19. If you are collecting directly into vacuum tubes, remove and replace the vacuum tubes as explained in Procedure 40-3 until you have drawn the necessary amounts. If you are drawing into a syringe, you will be limited to the size of the syringe being used. RATIONALE: You do not have the option of removing and replacing the syringe during a draw.

20. When the syringe is filled, ask the patient to open his or her hand and release the tourniquet. RATIONALE: Opening of the hand and releasing the tourniquet takes the pressure off the vein and allows the blood to flow freely through the arm.

21. Lightly place a cotton ball above the puncture site and smoothly remove the needle from the arm in the same direction of insertion (Figure 40-33F). RATIONALE: You are getting the cotton ball ready so you can apply pressure on the puncture site immediately on removing the needle.

22. Activate the safety device of the butterfly needle immediately (Figure 40-33G). RATIONALE: The safety devices are better able to protect if activated immediately.

continues

Procedure 40-4 (continued)

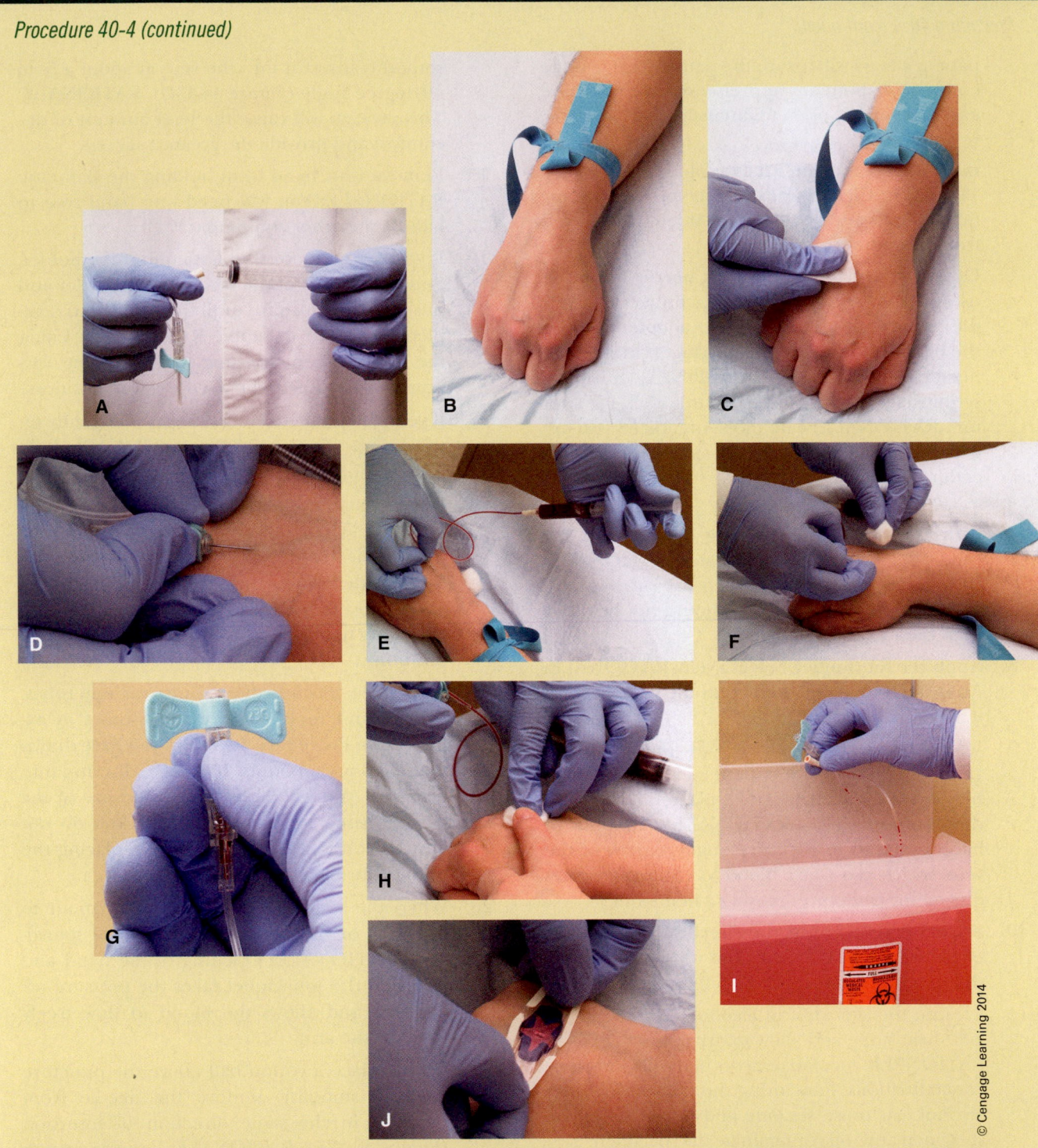

© Cengage Learning 2014

Figure 40-33   Performing a venipuncture with the butterfly needle system. (A) Open the package with the butterfly needle system and assemble the needle. In this case, the needle is connected to the syringe. (B) Apply the tourniquet and ask the patient to close his hand. (C) Cleanse the site using one swift wipe and allow to air dry. (D) Draw skin taut. While holding the wings of the butterfly together, line up the needle with the vein, and insert at a 5- to 10-degree angle. (E) Pull gently on the syringe, allowing it to fill. (F) When filled, have the patient relax his hand, and release the tourniquet. Place a cotton ball above the puncture site and remove the needle. (G) Activate the safety device of the butterfly needle. (H) Apply pressure on the site, and ask the patient to continue holding the pressure. (I) Dispose of the needle into a sharps container. (J) Apply a bandage to the site.

Procedure 40-4 (continued)

23. Apply pressure on the site. Let the patient assist by holding the pressure (Figure 40-33H). If drawing from the arm, ask him or her not the bend his or her arm. He or she can elevate his or her arm while applying pressure though. RATIONALE: Applying pressure and elevating the arm lessens the chance of bruising, whereas bending the elbow increases the chance of the patient forming a hematoma.

24. If using a syringe, aliquot blood into the appropriate tubes as outlined in Procedure 40-2. RATIONALE: Following proper procedure when transferring blood from the syringe into the vacuum tubes ensures the best specimens for testing.

25. Dispose of the needle into a sharps container (Figure 40-33I). RATIONALE: Immediate disposal of contaminated needles is the safest practice.

26. Label all the tubes. RATIONALE: Not labeling the tubes right away increases the likelihood of a mix-up error.

27. Check the patient. Observe him or her for signs of stress. RATIONALE: Patient safety is a primary concern. Venipuncture can be difficult for some patients.

28. The patient should stop bleeding within 2 to 3 minutes. If the bleeding has stopped, apply a small pressure bandage by pulling a cotton ball in half, applying it to the site, and placing an adhesive bandage or tape over it (Figure 40-33J). The patient should be instructed to remove the bandage in about 20 minutes. If the patient is sensitive to latex, be sure to use a nonlatex paper tape. If the bleeding has not stopped, have the patient continue to hold pressure another 5 minutes with his or her arm elevated above his or her heart level, then recheck. RATIONALE: The patient should not be released from your care until the bleeding has stopped.

29. Clean up tray and supplies; dispose of contaminated cotton ball. Remove gloves using proper technique. Discard gloves into biohazard container and disinfect goggles. RATIONALE: Proper disposal and disinfection of contaminated supplies and equipment protects from exposure to biohazard substances.

30. Wash hands, record the procedure, and complete the laboratory requisition. Place specimen and requisition into biohazard transfer bag in the presence of the patient and notify the laboratory that the specimen is ready for pickup. RATIONALE: Washing hands after removing the gloves further protects from biohazard substances and lessens the chance of cross contamination to the patient's chart and laboratory requisition. Completing the documentation and requisition as soon as possible after the procedure and in the presence of the patient improves accuracy and ensures the patient's sample is with the right requisition.

DOCUMENTATION:

11/13/XX 2:54 PM   Venipuncture performed on right hand for CBC and sed rate. Specimen sent to Inner City Lab. Identification #987654321. Patient tolerated the procedure well and will call back tomorrow for the test results. Joe Guerrero, CMA (AAMA)

PROCEDURE 40-5
Capillary Puncture

STANDARD PRECAUTIONS:

    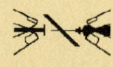

PURPOSE:
To obtain capillary blood acceptable for laboratory testing as requested by a provider.

EQUIPMENT/SUPPLIES:
Gloves
70% isopropyl alcohol swab
Microcollection tubes or capillary tubes
Safety lancet
Gauze 2 × 2
Adhesive bandage or tape
Sharps container
Cotton balls

continues

Procedure 40-5 (continued)

Biohazard red bag
Laboratory requisition (optional)
Biohazard transport bag (optional)

PROCEDURE STEPS:

1. Assemble the supplies. RATIONALE: Organizing the supplies before the procedure ensures a more timely and professional process.

2. *Identify the patient, introduce yourself by name and credential*, and recheck the provider's orders. RATIONALE: Introducing yourself and explaining the procedure will establish a professional relationship with the patient and might help put him or her at ease. Identifying the patient and rechecking the provider's orders will ensure the proper tests will be performed on the right patient.

3. *Explain the procedure and expectations to the patient. Allay the patient's fears regarding the procedure to help him feel safe and comfortable.* RATIONALE: Explaining the procedure and allaying the patient's fears will assure the patient that you are concerned about any apprehension he may have and that you are open to discussing his concerns.

4. Wash hands and apply gloves. RATIONALE: Washing your hands protects the patient, and applying gloves protects you.

5. Select the puncture site on the fleshy part of the ring or middle finger, avoiding the very tip and the extreme sides. RATIONALE: The ring and middle fingers generally will have fewer calluses and less scarring. The tip and sides are more sensitive than the fleshy part.

6. Have the patient wash his or her hands in very warm water; if necessary, apply a warming pack to the fingertip, encourage the patient to relax, and provide a comfortable, professional atmosphere. RATIONALE: The patient washing his or her hands in very warm water provides two benefits: his or her hands will be cleaner and warmer, which encourages blood flow to the area. Applying a warming pack to the fingertips will further encourage blood flow. A relaxed patient in a comfortable, professional atmosphere is more likely to provide a better sample.

7. Clean the selected puncture site with alcohol swab and allow it to air dry or dry it with a gauze pad. RATIONALE: Alcohol will remove any residue soap or debris. Allowing the alcohol to dry will prevent irritation and stinging. If the site is wiped dry, the irritation of the gauze pad will further encourage blood to the area.

8. Holding the distal phalange firmly, perform the puncture across the lines of the fingerprint rather than along the lines. RATIONALE: Holding the distal phalange firmly will add support to the finger and prevent the patient from pulling back on the finger during the puncture. Puncturing across the fingerprint will assist the blood to form a drop rather than flow across the fingertip.

9. Using a gauze pad, wipe away the first drop. RATIONALE: The first drop usually contains contamination from the alcohol and tissue fluid and would not be a good representation of the blood sample needed. Using gauze rather than cotton to wipe it away lessens the likelihood of it clotting too quickly.

10. Collect the specimen according to the test being performed (see Chapter 41 for hemoglobin and hematocrit; see Chapter 44 for PKU, glucose, and other specialty tests performed on capillary blood).

11. Have patient hold firm, direct pressure on the site with a cotton ball for at least 2 minutes. If the bleeding has stopped, an adhesive strip can be applied. If the bleeding has not stopped yet, hold firm, direct pressure on the site for another 5 minutes and then recheck. Adhesive strips are not recommended for patients younger than 2 years. RATIONALE: A cotton ball is used because the cotton fibers further encourage clotting at the puncture site. The bleeding should be stopped before the patient leaves your care. Adhesive strips for children younger than 2 years are not recommended because they are a choking hazard.

12. Disinfect the area and equipment, remove gloves, and dispose of them into a biohazard waste container/red bag. Wash hands. RATIONALE: Biohazard waste should be controlled for everyone's protection. Hand washing after removing gloves further protects you.

13. Record the procedure. If the test is being sent to an outside laboratory, complete the requisition in the presence of the patient, insert both

Procedure 40-5 (continued)

into the biohazard transport bag, and alert the laboratory to pick up the specimen. If the test is to be performed in your POL, proceed with the completion of the test immediately, record the results, and *notify the provider of the results.* RATIONALE: Documentation is critical for good patient records. Completing the laboratory requisition in the presence of the patient provides accurate insurance and personal information

if needed for the insurance forms and for your medical records.

DOCUMENTATION:

4/27/XX 8:15 AM   Capillary puncture performed left ring finger for Hgb A1c. Patient tolerated the procedure well. Dr. Lewis is scheduled to see the patient today to discuss progress. Joe Guerrero, CMA (AAMA)———————

PROCEDURE 40-6

Obtaining a Capillary Specimen for Transport Using a Microtainer Transport Unit

STANDARD PRECAUTIONS:

   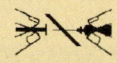

PURPOSE:

To obtain a specimen of capillary blood for transport to a laboratory for testing, using a Microtainer.

EQUIPMENT/SUPPLIES:

Capillary puncture supplies:
   Gloves
   70% isopropyl alcohol swab
   Gauze
   Safety lancet
   Cotton balls
   Gauze pads
   Adhesive bandage
   Sharps container and biohazard waste receptacle
Microtainer transport unit
Laboratory requisition
Small sturdy container with a tightly fitting lid (such as a urine specimen cup or red top vacuum tube)
Biohazard specimen transport bag

PROCEDURE STEPS:

1. Determine the appropriateness of submitting a capillary specimen for the specific test you are performing. RATIONALE: Not all tests can be performed on capillary specimens.

2. Assemble the supplies. RATIONALE: Organizing the supplies before the procedure ensures a more timely and professional process.

3. *Identify the patient, introduce yourself by name and credential*, and recheck the provider's orders. RATIONALE: Introducing yourself and explaining the procedure will establish a professional relationship with the patient and might help put him or her at ease. Identifying the patient and rechecking the provider's orders will ensure the proper tests will be performed on the right patient.

4. *Explain the procedure and expectations to the patient. Allay the patient's fears regarding the procedure to help him feel safe and comfortable.* RATIONALE: Explaining the procedure and allaying the patient's fears will assure the patient that you are concerned about any apprehension he may have and that you are open to discussing his concerns.

5. Wash hands, apply gloves, and perform the capillary puncture according to Procedure 40-5. RATIONALE: Washing your hands protects the patient, and applying gloves protects you.

6. Discard the first drop of blood. Wipe it away with a gauze square. RATIONALE: The first drop can contain mostly alcohol residue and tissue fluid and would not be a good representation of the blood sample needed. Using gauze rather than cotton to wipe it away lessens the likelihood of it clotting too quickly.

continues

Procedure 40-6 (continued)

7. Allow a good size drop to form. RATIONALE: Allowing a good size drop to form is a good idea with any capillary specimen; the blood is more likely to stay in a drop and not flow over the finger.

8. Scoop the drop into the Microtainer (Figure 40-34A). RATIONALE: This is the method used to get the specimen into the tip of the Microtainer.

9. Tip the Microtainer, allowing the drop to slide into the tube (Figure 40-34B). RATIONALE: As soon as a drop is obtained on the scoop it should be moved into the tube where it can mix with the additive.

10. Gently agitate the tube. RATIONALE: Agitating the tube allows the additive to mix with the blood.

11. Continue collection of blood until the tube is filled (Figure 40-34C). RATIONALE: The tube must be filled to the fill line to ensure the proper ratio of blood to additive.

12. Provide the patient with a cotton ball and ask him or her to hold pressure on the puncture site. RATIONALE: The pressure with a cotton ball will encourage the wound to clot.

13. Remove the scoop from the Microtainer and discard the scoop into the sharps container (Figure 40-34D). RATIONALE: The scoop is contaminated with blood and therefore is considered to be biohazard waste. Being hard plastic, it is capable of scratching someone, so the sharps container is safer than the red bag waste receptacle.

14. Remove the colored cap from the back of the Microtainer and place it securely onto the opening. RATIONALE: Placing the cap securely onto the Microtainer will ensure

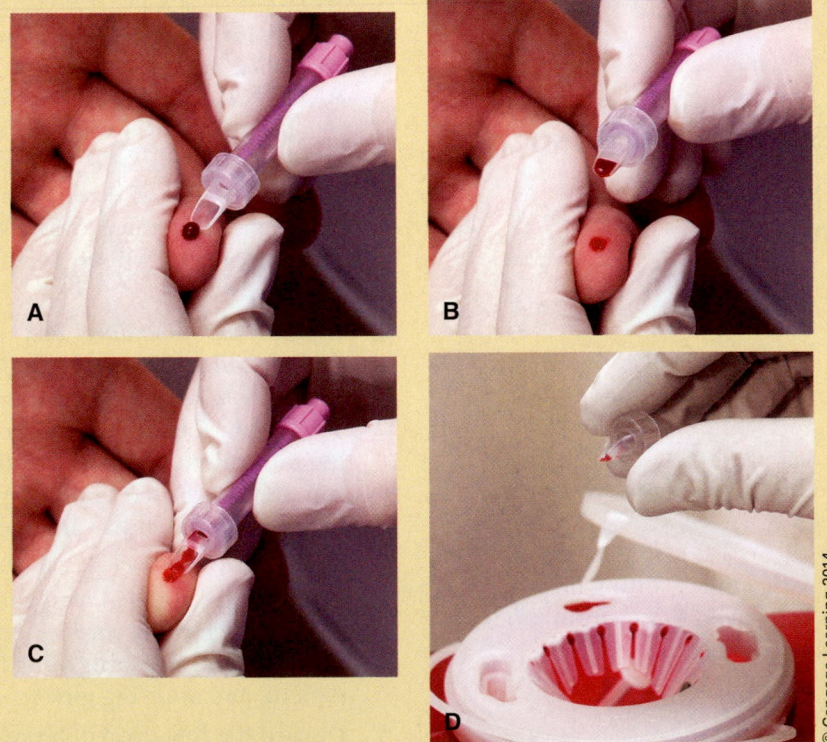

© Cengage Learning 2014

Figure 40-34 Collecting a capillary specimen for transport. (A) After wiping away the first drop (not shown), allow drop to form. Touch the scoop on the collection Microtainer tube to the blood droplet. (B) Tip the collection Microtainer tube up so that the blood flows into the tube. Agitate it gently to mix the anticoagulant with the blood. (C) Continue collecting the blood until the collection Microtainer tube is filled to the marked level. (D) Remove the scoop from the collection Microtainer tube and dispose of the scoop into a nearby sharps container.

Procedure 40-6 (continued)

the specimen will stay in the Microtainer during handling and transport.

15. Place the capped Microtainer into a small sturdy container with a tight-fitting lid. RATIONALE: Placing the Microtainer in another container protects it from being uncapped and (because of its small size) lost in transport. The Microtainer is also not large enough for adequate labeling.

16. Label the container. RATIONALE: Proper labeling ensures the proper tests on the right specimen.

17. Fill out the laboratory requisition while the patient is present. Place the specimen and the requisition into the biohazard transport bag in their separate compartments. RATIONALE: Any questions about the patient's address and insurance can be answered immediately if the patient is present while you complete the form.

18. Check the patient's puncture site. If bleeding has stopped, apply an adhesive strip, answer any questions the patient has, and release the patient. RATIONALE: Caring for the patient both physically and emotionally shows a professional dedication to your job.

19. Document procedure in patient's chart or electronic medical record and notify the laboratory that the specimen is ready for pickup. RATIONALE: Documentation ensures that the proper information is recorded into the patient's chart or electronic medical record.

DOCUMENTATION:

3/3/XX 4:15 PM   Capillary puncture was performed for a CBC. Specimen (Microtainer) sent to Inner City Laboratory. Patient tolerated the procedure well and will call in on Friday (3/6/XX) for the results. No return appointment scheduled.
W. Slawson, CMA (AAMA)

 ## PROCEDURE 40-7
Obtaining Blood for Blood Culture

STANDARD PRECAUTIONS:

   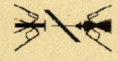

PURPOSE:
While performing venipuncture from two separate sites, prepare two culture bottles of blood from each site for culture (four total).

EQUIPMENT/SUPPLIES:
Nonsterile gloves for use with povidone-iodine solution
Sterile gloves
Laboratory requisition and transport bag
Blood culture bottles, anaerobic and aerobic (usually four: two bottles each for two sets of cultures)
70% isopropyl alcohol
Povidone-iodine solution swabs or towelettes
Venipuncture supplies (according to method used) for two separate sites
Biohazard red bag

Sharps container
Labeling pen
Biohazard transport bag

PROCEDURE STEPS:

1. *Identify the patient and introduce yourself by name and credential.* RATIONALE: Identifying the patient and rechecking the provider's orders will ensure the proper tests will be performed on the right patient. Introducing yourself and stating your credentials demonstrates professionalism and helps to reassure the patient.

2. *Explain the procedure and expectations to the patient. Allay the patient's fears regarding the procedure to help him feel safe and comfortable.* RATIONALE: Explaining the procedure and allaying the patient's fears will assure the patient that you are

continues

Procedure 40-7 (continued)

concerned about any apprehension he may have and that you are open to discussing his concerns.

3. Ensure that the patient has not initiated antimicrobial therapy. RATIONALE: Antibiotic therapy can interfere with the culture results. If the patient has started antibiotics, the name and strength of the antibiotic, dosage, duration, and last dose must be documented clearly on the laboratory report.

4. Wash hands and put on gloves. RATIONALE: Washing hands before any laboratory process prevents contamination of the specimen. Gloving provides personal protection.

5. Assemble equipment and supplies according to the venipuncture procedure being used and the laboratory requirements (Figure 40-35A). Check expiration dates on all collection and culture supplies. RATIONALE: Organizing your work area prevents confusion and error due to missing supplies. Usually two separate sites are used for collection, with two bottles (one aerobe and one anaerobe) from each site. Occasionally, three sites will be necessary. Expired supplies and culture bottles must not be used.

6. Place the culture bottles on a flat surface within reach during the procedure. Mark the correct fill line on both bottles at 10 mL per bottle (1–3 mL per bottle for pediatric patients). RATIONALE: Marking the fill line helps in viewing the proper amount during the procedure.

7. Prepare the venipuncture site with isopropyl alcohol and allow to dry, then apply povidone-iodine in progressively larger concentric circles from the inside outward (Figure 40-35B). The iodine must remain on the skin for 1 full minute and be allowed to dry naturally. The venipuncture site should not be touched after the skin is disinfected. RATIONALE: Alcohol removes oils and other debris, the povidone-iodine is a more thorough antiseptic. One full minute is required to ensure antisepsis. Touching the site may recontaminate it.

8. Cleanse the bottle tops with alcohol and povidone-iodine solution. RATIONALE: The bottle tops need to be disinfected to remove contamination. *NOTE:* Some laboratory guidelines state that iodine can disintegrate the rubber stopper and therefore should not be used. Follow your laboratory guidelines as stated in your laboratory manual.

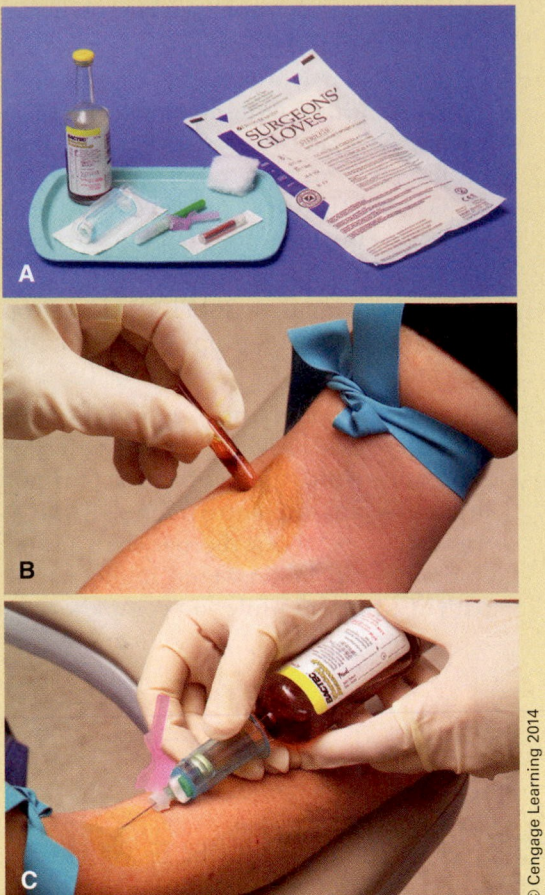

© Cengage Learning 2014

Figure 40-35 Obtaining blood for blood culture. (A) Assemble equipment and supplies (only one culture bottle shown). (B) Prepare the venipuncture site with alcohol and allow to dry, then apply povidone-iodine in concentric circles from the inside outward. Allow the iodine to dry naturally. (C) Perform venipuncture. Insert the aerobic culture bottle onto the needle and fill to the appropriate line.

9. Remove the preparation gloves and apply the sterile gloves using sterile procedure. RATIONALE: Sterile gloves will ensure the procedure will be as sterile as possible.

10. Perform venipuncture according to method used. Insert the aerobic culture bottle onto the needle (Figure 40-35C). Fill to the appropriate line, usually 10 mL per bottle (1–3 for pediatric patients). Remove the first bottle, invert 8 to 10 times, and apply the second (anaerobic) bottle. Fill. Remove the second bottle and invert 8 to 10 times. RATIONALE: Follow your laboratory manual guidelines. The aerobic bottle should be filled first because there will be some residual air in the needle. The anaerobic bottle will then collect only blood. Inverting the bottles ensures

Procedure 40-7 (continued)

the culture media will be well mixed with the blood.

11. Complete the venipuncture procedure as determined by the method used. Remove the remaining iodine from the skin with isopropyl alcohol. RATIONALE: The next two bottles will be filled from a different site. The iodine solution can irritate the skin and should be removed.

12. Perform venipuncture at the second site, repeating the process as stated above. The second and subsequent culture bottles must be collected within 30 minutes of the first. RATIONALE: The 30-minute time frame allows for an accurate assessment of the microorganisms present at that particular date and time.

13. The culture bottles should be stored at room temperature and not refrigerated. RATIONALE: Room temperature is ideal for the cultures so organisms are not destroyed.

14. Label the bottles with the patient's name, date, time, and other required information. RATIONALE: Labeling with the required information prevents mix-ups of specimens and ensures a quality timeline. Specimens will be rejected if not labeled properly.

15. Dispose of all contaminated supplies, disinfect all surfaces, remove gloves, and wash hands. RATIONALE: Using appropriate disposal techniques and disinfecting all surfaces according to Standard Precautions safely control biohazard substances.

16. Complete the laboratory requisition in the presence of the patient including the date and time of each specimen collected, any antibiotic

therapy the patient is on, the name and strength of the antibiotic, as well as the dosage, duration, and the last dose taken. Include the clinical diagnosis and any special organisms suspected or to rule out. The laboratory requisition must indicate if the culture is for *brucella* or *francisella*. The information on the laboratory requisition should match exactly the information given on the bottles. RATIONALE: Labeling with the required information prevents mix-ups of specimens, ensures a quality timeline, and ensures the laboratory will have the necessary information. Specimens will be rejected if there is a discrepancy between the information on the bottle and the information on the laboratory requisition.

17. Place the specimen and the requisition in the biohazard transport bag in their separate compartments and notify the laboratory that the specimen is ready for pickup. RATIONALE: The biohazard transport bag separates the specimen from the requisition and protects the laboratory personnel.

18. Document the procedure in the laboratory section of the patient's chart or electronic medical record. RATIONALE: Necessary information and the patient's chart or electronic medical record will be accurate and complete.

DOCUMENTATION:

08/06/20XX Venipuncture performed and specimens obtained from both right and left antecubital spaces for blood cultures. Specimens sent to Inner City Lab. Patient ID #56776533. Patient tolerated procedure well and instructed to call us on Wednesday for the results. Joe Guerrero, CMA (AAMA) ⎯⎯⎯⎯⎯⎯⎯⎯⎯⎯⎯

CASE STUDY 40-1

Refer to the scenario at the beginning of the chapter.

CASE STUDY REVIEW

1. What types of information will patients be able to share with Bruce about their previous venipuncture experiences?

2. How can Bruce use that information to better serve the patients?

3. Do you think patients are a good source of information about their bodies and their reactions to past experiences?

CASE STUDY 40-2

Inner City Health Care is short-staffed today, and medical assistant Liz Corbin is feeling pressed for time. She has many tasks to complete, but first she must perform a venipuncture. She greets the patient, Wayne Elder, in a perfunctory manner, discouraging time-wasting conversation. Although Wayne appears apprehensive, he is not resistant, so Liz quickly assembles the necessary supplies, applies the tourniquet, and inserts the needle. While she is drawing his blood, Wayne faints.

CASE STUDY REVIEW

1. What should Liz do now?
2. What could Liz have done to prevent this situation from occurring?
3. In the future, what are some steps Liz can take to provide a positive experience for venipuncture patients?

SUMMARY

With a little practice, the medical assistant will become an expert at phlebotomy. The skills of phlebotomy cannot be learned primarily from a textbook; continuous practice will develop the skill to perfection. It may take months before the medical assistant feels comfortable and is able to obtain a sample without difficulty.

In all procedures, safety is of the utmost consideration. Dispose of all sharps properly and separately from the noncontaminated trash. Proper hand cleansing between patients and wearing gloves, goggles, and masks with each phlebotomy will ensure safety for both the patient and the medical assistant.

Proper specimen collection and handling of the specimen after collection by the medical assistant will ensure that the patient obtains the most accurate result. The specimen must be treated in such a way that the integrity of the specimen is maintained. The quality of the sample must be the same when collected as when tested. Correct method of draw, order of draw, and the correct handling of the sample after collection will reduce the number of factors affecting the sample and give the most accurate result possible.

Good communication skills are critical in putting the patient at ease while drawing her blood. Medical assistants should always present a professional image and set the stage for professional interaction with the patient and her family. Active listening skills and the ability to respond appropriately, honestly, and diplomatically while being cognizant of professional boundaries will all help provide for a more positive experience.

Medical assistants should be aware of current laws and regulations regarding their scope of practice, credentials, and professional training requirements when performing clinical patient procedures.

STUDY FOR SUCCESS

To reinforce your knowledge and skills of information presented in this chapter:

- Review the *Key Terms*
- Role-play with other students to apply attributes of professionalism pertinent to this chapter.
- Consider the *Case Studies* and discuss your conclusions
- Answer the questions in the *Certification Review*
- Apply your knowledge by completing the *Activities* in the *Study Guide* and the *Games and Quizzes* in the StudyWARE **StudyWARE** software on the *Premium Website*
- Perform the *Procedures* using the *Competency Assessment Checklists* in the *Competency Manual*
- Practice your problem-solving skills with the *Critical Thinking Challenge 3.0* on the *Premium Website*

CERTIFICATION REVIEW

1. Drawing blood with a 25-gauge needle increases the chance for:
   a. vein collapse
   b. hematomas
   c. hemoconcentration
   d. hemolysis

2. An anticoagulant is an additive placed in vacuum tubes to:
   a. dilute the blood before testing
   b. ensure the sterility of the tube
   c. make the blood clot faster
   d. prevent the blood from clotting

3. When collecting a blood sample with a vacuum tube system, the last tube drawn is withdrawn from the holder before removing the needle from the patient to:
   a. avoid hematoma at the venipuncture site
   b. avoid dripping blood out the end of the needle
   c. prevent clotting of the blood
   d. cause the blood to clot

4. Leaving the tourniquet on a patient's arm for an extended length of time before drawing blood may cause:
   a. hemoconcentration
   b. specimen hemolysis
   c. stress
   d. bruising

5. The single most important way to prevent the spread of infection from patient to patient is:
   a. gowning and gloving
   b. hand washing
   c. always wearing masks
   d. avoid breathing on clients

6. Under Standard Precautions, all used needles are to be disposed of in the following manner:
   a. recapped
   b. discarded intact in a sharps container
   c. bent
   d. broken or cut off

7. When drawing multiple specimens in vacuum tubes, it is important to fill which of the following color-stoppered tubes first?
   a. Light blue
   b. Green
   c. Lavender
   d. Red

8. The anticoagulant of choice when drawing coagulation studies such as PT and APTT is:
   a. (red) no anticoagulant
   b. (light blue) sodium citrate
   c. (lavender) EDTA
   d. (green) heparin

9. When the medical assistant cannot perform a venipuncture successfully after two attempts, the medical assistant should:
   a. try at least two more times
   b. notify the provider
   c. ask another medical assistant to try
   d. request the test for the next day

10. If the blood is drawn too quickly from a small vein, the vein has a tendency to:
    a. collapse
    b. bruise
    c. disintegrate
    d. roll

11. What is OSHA's policy about choosing the safest needle systems to prevent accidental needlestick injuries?
    a. The clinic administrators can choose whatever is most cost effective.
    b. The clinic administrators should carefully choose the safest system for their staff.
    c. The clinic administrators must select the safest equipment based on feedback from the people who are using the needles.
    d. OSHA is not interfering with the clinics' rights to use any system they choose.

REFERENCES/BIBLIOGRAPHY

Walters, N. J., Estridge, B. H., & Reynold, A. P. (2011). *Basic Clinical Laboratory Techniques (6th ed.)* Clifton Park, NY: Delmar Cengage Learning.

CHAPTER 41

Hematology

OUTLINE

Hematologic Tests

Hemoglobin and Hematocrit Tests

  Hemoglobin

  Hematocrit

White and Red Blood Cell Counts

  White Blood Cells and Differential

Red Blood Cells

Platelets

Erythrocyte Indices

  Understanding RBC Indices

  Using Erythrocyte Indices to Diagnose

Erythrocyte Sedimentation Rates (ESR or SED Rate)

  Wintrobe Method

Westergren Method

Using the ESR to Screen

C-Reactive Proteins

Coagulation Studies

Automated Hematology

LEARNING OUTCOMES

1. Define, spell, and pronounce the key terms as presented in the glossary.
2. Describe the process of hematopoiesis.
3. List the five types of normal white blood cells and give the identifying characteristics and role of each.
4. Explain to a fellow student the role of the red blood cell and the platelets.
5. Discuss how the clinical science of hematology and the complete blood count (CBC) are used in the diagnosis and treatment of disease.
6. Discuss how the hemoglobin, hematocrit, erythrocyte to indices, and ESR are used to diagnose.
7. Apply mathematical computations to solve the equation of erythrocyte indices (using RBC count, hemoglobin and hematocrit).
8. Describe CRP and its uses as a screening test for general infection and inflammation.
9. Analyze the professionalism questions and apply them to this chapter's content.

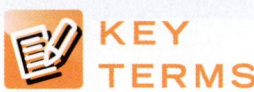

KEY TERMS

anisocytosis

basophil

C-reactive protein (CRP)

complete blood count (CBC)

eosinophil

erythrocyte (red blood cell or RBC)

erythrocyte indices

erythrocyte sedimentation rate (ESR or sed rate)

erythropoietin

hematocrit (Hct or crit)

hematopoiesis

hemoglobin (Hgb)

hemoglobinopathy

hypochromic

leukocyte (white blood cell or WBC)

lymphocyte

macrocytic

microcytic

monocyte

neutrophil

normochromic

normocytic

protime

reticulocyte (retic)

thrombocyte (platelet)

ATTRIBUTES OF PROFESSIONALISM

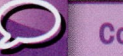 **Communication**

- Did you introduce yourself? Did you identify the patient through name and birth date or other identifying feature?
- Did you listen to and acknowledge the patient?
- Did you speak at the patient's level of understanding?
- Did you provide appropriate responses/feedback?
- Did you explain procedures and expectations to the patient?
- Did you allay patient's fears regarding the procedure being performed and help them feel safe and comfortable?
- Did you respond honestly and diplomatically to the patient's concerns?

 Presentation

- Were you dressed and groomed appropriately?
- Were you courteous, patient, and respectful to the patient?
- Did you display a positive attitude?
- Did you display a calm, professional, and caring manner?

 Competency

- Did you pay attention to detail?
- Did you ask questions if you were out of your comfort zone or did not have the experience to carry out tasks?
- Were you knowledgeable and accountable?
- Did you recognize the importance of local, state, and federal legislation and regulations in the practice setting?

 Integrity

- Did you work within your scope of practice?
- Did you immediately report any error you had made?

SCENARIO

The providers in the clinic of Drs. Lewis and King often order hematologic tests to assist them in diagnosing and treating patients. As she performs the tests in the providers' office laboratory, medical assistant Audrey Jones uses her knowledge of hematology every day. Audrey is comfortable performing waived lab tests because she understands the purposes and procedures of the tests. She always follows all safety and quality-control guidelines to protect herself and others and to ensure the accuracy of test results.

INTRODUCTION

Hematology is the study of the blood cells and coagulation in both normal and diseased states. The two main components of the blood are plasma (the liquid portion) and cells. Cells of the blood are also known as the formed elements of the blood. The study of hematology is usually limited to the cellular components of the blood and does not include the chemistry of the blood. See Chapter 44 for the chemistry of blood and tests related to blood chemistry.

*The cellular components of blood include **erythrocytes (red blood cells [RBCs])**, **leukocytes (white blood cells [WBCs])**, and **thrombocytes (platelets)**. Blood has many different functions. RBCs are responsible for supplying oxygen to all the cells of the body and removing the waste product of the cells: carbon dioxide. WBCs are involved in fighting infection, as well as producing antibodies for the immune system to defend against foreign antigens. There are five basic types of WBCs and they all have specific disease-fighting functions. Platelets are involved in hemostasis, the control of bleeding. Figure 40-2 shows the cellular elements of blood.*

*   **Hematopoiesis** *is defined as the formation of blood cells (Figure 41-1). The process of hematopoiesis, as well as the blood-forming tissues of the body, are included in the study of hematology. In the embryo, hematopoiesis occurs in the yolk sac, liver, and spleen. After we are born, the primary site for the production of erythrocytes, granulocytes, and platelets is the bone marrow. Lymphocytes are also produced in the bone marrow, as well as in the lymph nodes. At birth, most of the bone marrow in the body is capable of producing blood cells. This process is confined to the bone marrow of the ribs, vertebrae, sternum, and iliac crest by the age of 20 years. Bone marrow that is producing cells is known as red marrow. As the area for hematopoiesis is reduced, the red bone marrow is replaced by yellow marrow, which is stored fat. When a provider collects a bone marrow sample in an adult, the site chosen for sampling is the sternum or the iliac crest because this is where the blood cells are still being produced.*

HEMATOLOGIC TESTS

Hematologic tests are the second most common tests performed in the provider's office laboratory (POL). The most common test is the urinalysis. The cellular components of the blood may be affected by changes in either the blood-forming organs or in other tissues of the body. The study of these changes forms the basis of hematologic tests performed in the POL.

Hematologic tests performed in the clinical laboratory include:

- Hemoglobin
- Hematocrit

SPOTLIGHT ON CERTIFICATION

RMA Content Outline
- Asepsis
- Laboratory procedures

CMA (AAMA) Content Outline
- Principles of infection control
- Processing specimens
- Quality control
- Performing selected tests

CMAS Content Outline
- Asepsis in the medical office

CRITICAL THINKING

What do you think would happen if you did not have any leukocytes? What would your symptoms be?

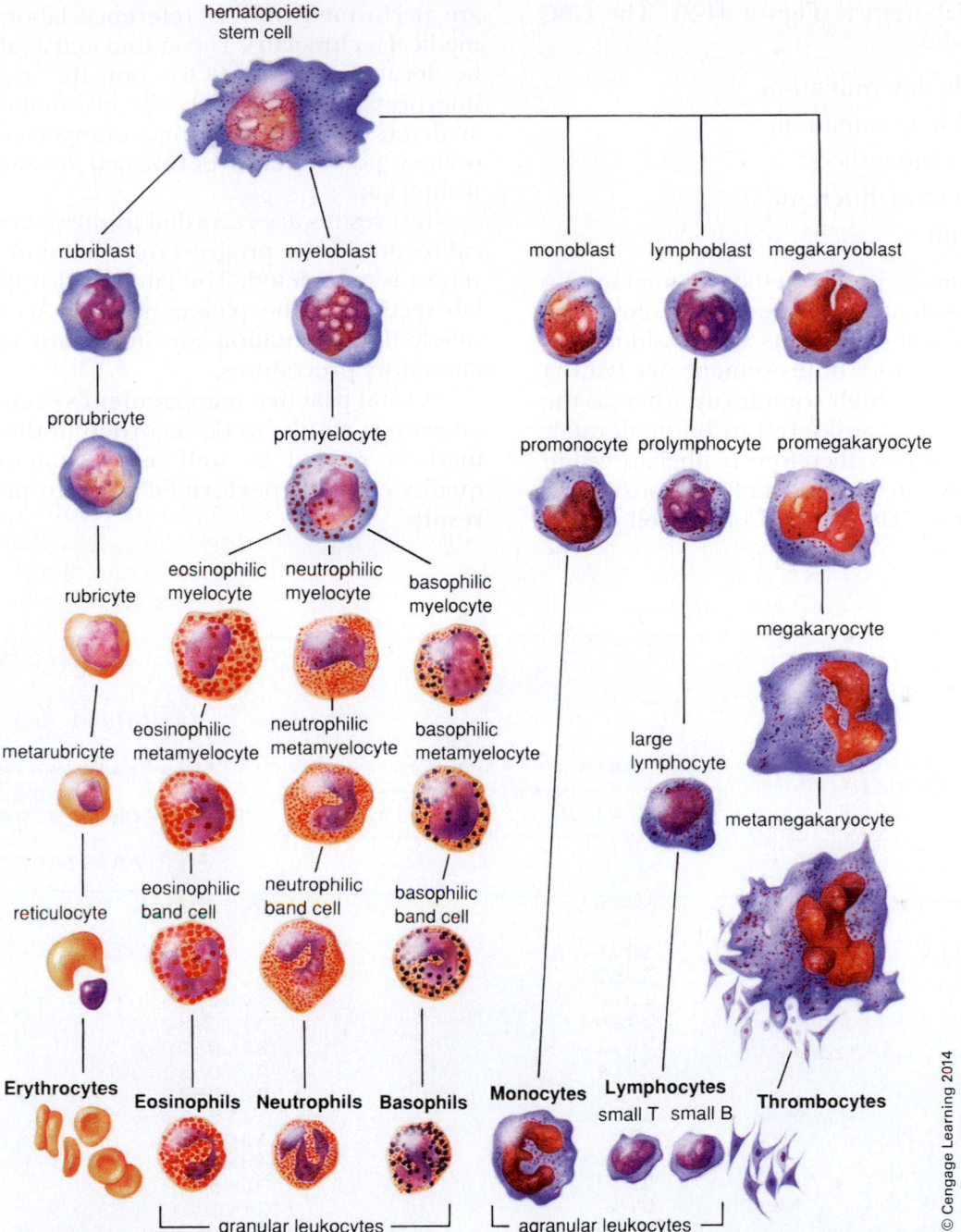

hematopoietic stem cell

rubriblast   myeloblast   monoblast   lymphoblast   megakaryoblast

prorubricyte   promyelocyte   promonocyte   prolymphocyte   promegakaryocyte

rubricyte   eosinophilic myelocyte   neutrophilic myelocyte   basophilic myelocyte

megakaryocyte

metarubricyte   eosinophilic metamyelocyte   neutrophilic metamyelocyte   basophilic metamyelocyte   large lymphocyte   metamegakaryocyte

reticulocyte   eosinophilic band cell   neutrophilic band cell   basophilic band cell

Erythrocytes   **Eosinophils**   **Neutrophils**   **Basophils**   **Monocytes**   **Lymphocytes** small T   small B   **Thrombocytes**

└─────── granular leukocytes ───────┘   └─── agranular leukocytes ───┘

© Cengage Learning 2014

Figure 41-1   Hematopoiesis showing blood cells and platelet formation starting with hematopoietic stem cell.

- WBC count
- Differential WBC count
- RBC count
- RBC indices
- Platelet count
- Erythrocyte sedimentation rate (ESR)
- Prothrombin time (PT)

The results of these hematologic tests provide valuable information used by the provider in making a diagnosis, evaluating a patient's progress, and regulating further treatment.

The laboratory test ordered most frequently on blood in the ambulatory care setting is the **complete blood count (CBC)**. The exact number of parameters included in the CBC will vary from laboratory to laboratory (Figure 41-2). The CBC generally includes:

- Hemoglobin determination
- Hematocrit determination
- RBC count (and indices)
- WBC count (and differential)
- Platelet count

All these tests can be performed by manual testing procedures or with an automated hematology analyzer. Manual blood cell counts are considered by the Clinical Laboratory Improvement Act (CLIA) to be of moderate to high complexity, whereas the automated tests are considered to be moderately complex; therefore, neither are within the medical assistant's scope of practice. The manual blood cell counts

are performed only at reference laboratories by medical technicians. The automated analyzers may be located in the POL, but the testing and interpretation of the tests, the maintenance of the analyzers, as well as training and supervision of laboratory personnel is performed by the medical technician.

Test results are recorded in the patient's medical record in the progress notes section and a lab report is completed. The lab report is filed in the lab section of the patient record. Accurate and timely documentation are important in medical laboratory procedures.

A total practice management system (TPMS) allows test results to be recorded in the patient's medical record as well as documentation of quality controls performed prior to patient test results.

```
Pat Name:                                                    Page:   1
Unit #/Acct #:
Loc:
Phys-Service:

***********************************************************************
In:   11/12/XX 0843     ---------------------              Spec: Blood
Out:  11/12/XX 1002     | CBC WITH DIFFERENTIAL |          Techs: V185 T180*
Coll Time: 11/12/XX 0840 ---------------------
Order Phys:                                           [A9331600017/4590]

Result Name                 Result                Reference Range

WBC(10*3/ul):               12.6  H               4.8-10.8
RBC(10*6/ul):               4.51                  4.2-5.4
Hgb(gm/dl):                 12.8                  12.0-16.0
Hct(%):                     37.9                  37.0-47.0
MCV(fl):                    84.1                  81.0-99.0
MCH(pg):                    28.4                  27.0-31.0
MCHC(gm/dl):                33.8                  32.0-36.0
RDW(%):                     13.6                  11.5-14.5
Plt Cnt(X(10)3):            303                   130-450
Neutrophil(%):              62.0                  43-75
Lymph(%):                   29.7                  20-51
Mono (%):                   5.9                   2-11
Eos(%):                     2.0                   0-7.5
Basos(%):                   0.4                   0-2
Neutrophil(X(10)3):         9.3   H               1.5-6.6
Lymph (X(10)3):             2     L               1.5-3.5
Mono(X(10)3):               0.4                   0-1.0
Eos (X(10)3):               0.1                   0-0.7
Baso(X(10)3):               0.0                   0-0.1


-----------------------------------------------------------------------
               End of Report - 03/09/XX 15:34




Single Test Report-HEMATOLOGY
```

Figure 41-2 Hematology report form.

HEMOGLOBIN AND HEMATOCRIT TESTS

Hemoglobin (Hgb) and **hematocrit (Hct or crit)** tests are part of the CBC, however they are frequently ordered separate from a CBC. They have a unique relationship with each other and are rarely ordered individually. Both the hemoglobin and the hematocrit are performed to obtain similar information about RBCs in relation to the rest of the blood sample, but they also give decidedly different information. In normal results, the hemoglobin often will be about one third the number of the hematocrit.

Hemoglobin

Hemoglobin is the major component of the RBC and serves to transport oxygen and carbon dioxide through the body. Hemoglobin, which is responsible for about 85% of the dry weight of the RBC, is a conjugated (combined) protein composed of heme and globin. A single hemoglobin molecule consists of four globin chains with a heme group attached to each globin (Figure 41-3). The central component of each heme group is an iron molecule. One oxygen molecule can be transported to each heme group; therefore, each RBC can carry four oxygen molecules.

Synthesis of the heme portion of the hemoglobin molecule requires iron, which is usually obtained through our diets. The daily iron requirement for an adult man is about 0.5 mg/day, whereas a menstruating woman requires about four times that much, or 2 mg/day.

Hemoglobin carries about 95% of the oxygen to the body cells and carries away about 27% of the carbon dioxide. The RBCs pick up the oxygen in the lungs from when we breathe in, and they drop off the carbon dioxide in the lungs to be expelled when we breathe out. The rest of the carbon dioxide is removed through other processes. Oxygenated hemoglobin is bright red, and hemoglobin unbound to oxygen is darker. This explains the bright red color of arterial blood (going from the lungs and to the cells) and the darker color of venous blood (going back to the lungs).

A second function of hemoglobin is as a blood buffer; that is, hemoglobin helps maintain the proper pH balance of the blood as it picks up and drops off oxygen and carbon dioxide.

The production of new RBCs and consequently the formation of new hemoglobin is triggered by a hormone called **erythropoietin**, which is produced in the kidney. The erythropoietin process is activated when the body cells sense a low oxygen level.

There are several forms of hemoglobin. Hemoglobin A (Hgb A) is the most common form found in adults. The other hemoglobin types are abnormal and are responsible for a group of diseases known as **hemoglobinopathies**. These abnormal forms of hemoglobin include hemoglobin S (Hgb S), hemoglobin C, and hemoglobin E. Hgb S is the most common abnormal form of hemoglobin observed in the laboratory. It is the form of hemoglobin that causes sickle cell anemia. When Hgb S molecules are subjected to certain conditions, they alter the physical structure of the RBCs. The RBCs assume a sickle shape, which makes it difficult, if not impossible, for the cell to pass through a capillary bed.

The most frequent hemoglobin disease seen in the ambulatory care setting is anemia, with iron deficiency anemia being the most common type. A decrease of available iron in the body is the most common cause of this type of anemia. Lack of available iron can be caused by insufficient intake through the diet (called nutritional anemia); losing iron because of a bleeding problem (called hemorrhagic anemia); or less commonly, congenital defects, industrial toxins, diseases of bone marrow (aplastic anemia), and a variety of other disorders. In nutritional anemia, the laboratory finding usually shows a normal or near-normal hematocrit (because these patients have the right percentage of RBCs) but a low hemoglobin. Their RBCs are hypochromic (pale) because they lack

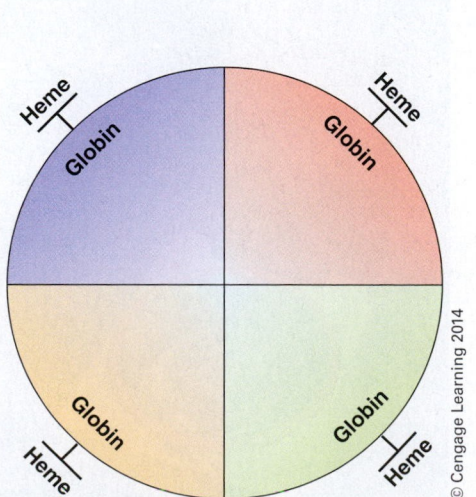

© Cengage Learning 2014

Figure 41-3   A normal hemoglobin molecule containing four globin chains with a heme group attached to each globin. One oxygen molecule can be transported by each heme group.

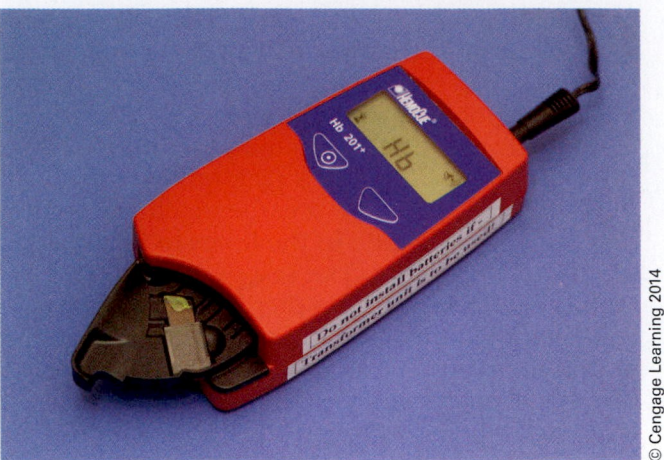

Figure 41-4 HemoCue instrument used for automated test.

Table 41-1 Normal Hemoglobin Values or Reference Ranges by Age and/or Sex

Newborn	15–20 g/dL
Age 3 months	9–14 g/dL
Age 10 months	12–14.5 g/dL
Adult female	12–16 g/dL
Adult male	13–18 g/dL

© Cengage Learning 2014

oxygen. The main symptom of anemia, fatigue, is also caused by lack of oxygen.

Hemoglobin is measured in the POL using an automated device called the HemoCue (Figure 41-4). The HemoCue is an infrared analyzer that measures the density of the hemoglobin pigment by light refraction. The more hemoglobin present in the sample, the more light is refracted. This is a quick method, uses only a small drop of blood, and gives immediate results (see Procedure 41-1).

CAUTION: The solution within the Hemo-Cue is poisonous. Precautions to observe when working with any reagents includes wearing gloves, working in a well-ventilated area, properly disposing of used reagents, wiping up all spills, and hand washing.

The normal reference values for hemoglobin vary according to both the age and sex of the individual (Table 41-1).

Hematocrit

Hematocrit (packed RBC volume) is the ratio of the volume of packed RBCs to that of the whole-blood specimen. Packed RBC volume is expressed as a percentage of the whole specimen. This is achieved manually or by automated methods. Most medical assistants working in ambulatory care settings use the manual microhematocrit method (see Procedure 41-2). It requires only a few drops of blood either directly into a microhematocrit tube obtained by capillary draw, or the sample can be taken from a vacuum tube containing ethylene-diaminetetraacetic acid

(EDTA) after a venipuncture. Chapter 40 explains both capillary draw and venipuncture.

The cellular components of the blood sample separate into layers when they are centrifuged at high speeds (Figure 41-5 and Figure 41-6). The cellular layers arrange themselves with the RBCs at the bottom of the tube. RBCs are the most numerous and the heaviest of the cellular components. WBCs and platelets form a thin layer called the buffy coat on top of the erythrocytes. The buffy coat has a whitish tan appearance. The plasma often is so clear it is difficult to see.

The WBC count of the sample can be estimated by measuring the buffy coat thickness. Each 0.1 mm of the buffy coat equals approximately 1,000 WBC/mm^3. Therefore, a buffy coat of 1 mm

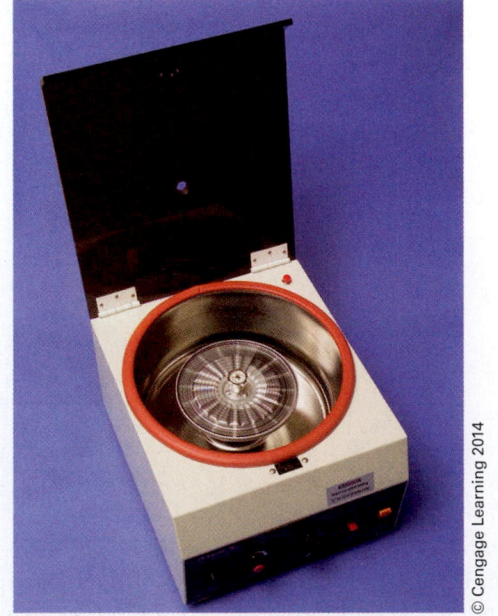

Figure 41-5 Microhematocrit centrifuge.

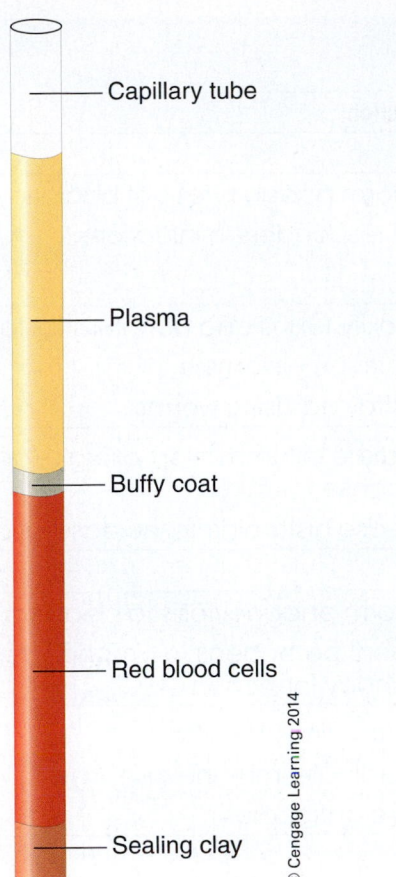

Figure 41-6 Diagram of packed cell column in the hematocrit tube showing separation of cellular components after centrifugation.

would equal a leukocyte count of approximately 10,000 WBCs/mm^3, and a 0.5 mm reading would equal 5,000 WBCs/mm^3. The cell counts may be reported in units of microliters (mcL), which are equivalent to cubic millimeters.

The normal values of hematocrit vary according to the age and sex of the individual (Table 41-2).

Sources of error associated with the microhematocrit method include improper centrifugation,

Table 41-2 Normal Hematocrit Values or Reference Ranges by Age and/ or Sex

Newborn	45–60%
1-year-old child	27–44%
Adult female	36–46%
Adult male	40–55%

resulting in increased trapped plasma, and improper reading of the packed RBC volume, such as including the buffy coat layer.

 Procedure 41-2 explains the microhematocrit method of determining blood hematocrit levels. Review the Chapter 40 sections on capillary tubes and capillary draw together with Procedure 40-5.

WHITE AND RED BLOOD CELL COUNTS

 WBC and RBC counts can be performed using either a manual or automated method. Because neither method is considered CLIA waived, neither is within the scope of practice for the medical assistant. The Introduction discusses the functions of blood cells, and you will learn much more in your anatomy and physiology course. The formation of blood cells was shown in Figure 41-1. Because blood cell counts are not performed by medical assistants, this section does not discuss the test process itself but rather the diagnostic implications of the leukocyte count with the differential.

White Blood Cells and Differential

WBCs do not necessarily remain within the blood vessels like RBCs do. They leave the blood vessels and travel to the tissues of the body to find and destroy pathogens. When a "bacterial battle" is fought in an area and many WBCs have died, the "battlefield" may be too large for the body to clean up. In these cases, pus can occur. A localized accumulation of pus is called an abscess and often must be incised (lanced) to aid in the removal of the pus. Chapter 31 discusses incision and drainage surgery for the purpose of incising and draining an abscess. Antibiotics are useful in some cases to help the leukocytes fight off the bacteria and remove the infection. When leukocytes travel into the tissues, most of them do not return to the bloodstream. The **lymphocyte** is the only type that does; it travels to the lymphatic system where it is specialized and matured (hence, its name), then returns to the bloodstream to await a mission. The normal values for white blood cells vary with age. Babies need more, because they have not yet built up antibody protections (Table 41-3).

WBCs or leukocytes can be divided into two basic groups: granulocytes, which contain granules within their cytoplasm, and agranulocytes, which do not contain granules. The presence of granules

LEUKOCYTE FUNCTION GUIDE

Cell Type	Function
Granulocytes	
Neutrophils • Mature neutrophils are called segs • Immature neutrophils are called bands or stabs	Perform phagocytosis of bacteria and fungi First responders in infections
Eosinophils	Detoxify toxins and harmful substances Neutralize histamine Destroy parasitic worms
Basophils	Mediate inflammation, allergic/antigen response Release histamine to increase inflammation
Agranulocytes	
Monocytes	Perform phagocytosis to clean up Present pathogens to lymphocytes for antibody formation
Lymphocytes B-cells T-cells	Destroy viruses Coordinate immune response Make antibodies

Table 41-3 Normal Leukocyte Counts

	Leukocyte Count (cells/mm³)	
Age	**Average**	**Reference Range**
Newborn	18,000	9,000–30,000
1-year-old toddler	11,000	6,000–14,000
6-year-old child	8,000	4,500–12,000
Adult	7,000	4,500–11,000

© Cengage Learning 2014

can be visualized by the trained eye after a staining process during the manual WBC count. Even during the automated method, the leukocyte is identified by the contents of the cytoplasm and the shape of their nuclei. The granulocytes are the **neutrophils, basophils**, and **eosinophils** (notice they all end in *-phil*, which will help you remember their cytoplasm is "filled" with granules). The agranulocytes are the lymphocytes and the monocytes.

The nuclei of the leukocytes differ from each other, as well as the cytoplasm. All three of the granulocytes contain nuclei that are multilobed or segmented (sometimes they are even called segs). They are described as being polymorphonuclear cells (*poly* means "many," *morpho* means "shape," and *nuclear* means "nucleus"). The immature neutrophil has a nucleus that has not yet formed lobes and is called a band cell (or stab cell) because its nucleus looks sort of like a comma. The agranulocytes do not form lobed nuclei; their nuclei are rounded in a single mass. Because of their single nuclei, the agranulocytes are sometimes called mononuclear (meaning one nucleus). Because so many different names can be confusing, this chapter provides an identification guide and pictures for you (see Table 41-4, Leukocyte Function Guide box, and Figure 41-7).

Each of the five types provide specialized protection. Some of their methods include phagocytosis, detoxification, inflammation, and immune response.

Phagocytosis is an engulfing process performed by all leukocytes, but especially the neutrophils and the monocytes. Once the bacteria or particles are engulfed, the material is destroyed by enzymes

Table 41-4　Normal Values for a Differential Leukocyte Count in Adults

Neutrophil Bands: 3–5%
Neutrophil bands increase in appendicitis and many other diseases.

Neutrophil Segs: 54–62%
Segmented neutrophils increase in appendicitis and many other diseases. An elevation in neutrophils usually is indicative of an infectious disease.

Lymphocytes: 25–33%
Lymphocytes increase with infectious mononucleosis, lymphocytic leukemia, and many diseases of viral origin.

Monocytes: 3–7%
Monocytes increase in tuberculosis and monocytic leukemia.

Eosinophils: 1–3%
Eosinophils increase with allergic reactions, hay fever, and parasitic infections.

Basophils: 0–1%
Basophils increase in polycythemia vera, chicken pox, and ulcerative colitis.

© Cengage Learning 2014

present in the leukocyte. Phagocytosis is so important as a means of protection, we would die if our leukocytes lost their ability to perform this process.

Detoxification is a neutralizing process that is effective against poisons and other harmful substances. Eosinophils use detoxification to control allergic reactions and histamine production.

Inflammation is a general process that occurs as a sequence of events. Chapter 22 explains the inflammatory process in more detail. The leukocyte most actively involved in inflammation is the basophil, which releases histamine into injured tissue to increase inflammation (antihistamines work to reduce inflammation). Basophils also contain the anticoagulant heparin. The basophil synchronizes the entire inflammatory process; thus, the poison is rendered harmless, the offending agents are eliminated, and the area is cleaned up of all the necrotic tissue and is ready for repair.

Immune response is a series of complicated and involved specific antigen–antibody reactions. Simply stated, when a harmful substance enters the human body, the adaptive immune response provided by the lymphocyte destroys the harmful substance. A "memory" is created so that the next time the body is exposed, it recognizes the intruder

and is better able to prevent the illness again. This is called immunity. Immunity can be permanent or temporary, passively acquired or actively acquired. Passively acquired immunity is gifted to us either in utero (congenital or natural) or through an injection (artificial). Actively acquired immunity requires us to actively fight off a disease, and because we actively take part in creating the immunity, it is usually permanent. Passively acquired immunities do not make us sick, but they usually do not last longer than 6 months.

Not only do the leukocytes fight off pathogens/toxins in a variety of ways, they also are fairly specific in the types of pathogens they do battle with (see Table 41-4). Neutrophils are the most numerous of all leukocytes and for good reason. They are there to destroy bacteria, which is our most common enemy. The second largest group is the lymphocytes, and they fight our second most common enemy: viruses. Lymphocytes are also involved in immune responses, which explains why we have immunity to viruses and not to other substances or microbes. Basophils release histamine to increase inflammation into injured tissues. Inflammation usually is our friend, but sometimes the inflammation is too severe.

This is what can happen in an allergic reaction. Eosinophils are especially well suited to battle the inflammation accompanying allergic-type reactions because they neutralize the histamines. **Monocytes** can be likened to the "cleanup crew" because these "big eaters" come in later to clean up the battlefield of the cellular debris and other substances.

Red Blood Cells

RBCs (erythrocytes) are very different from WBCs in composition, function, and numbers (Table 41-5). Remember from the Introduction that erythrocytes are responsible for carrying oxygen to the body's cells and bringing back the carbon dioxide. To have room to carry the oxygen and carbon dioxide molecules, the erythrocyte leaves its nucleus in the bone marrow where it is formed. The nucleus is used again and again to create other erythrocytes. Our bodies are efficient at recycling raw materials. If an erythrocyte is released from the bone marrow before it is mature, it may retain some of its nucleus material. It is then called a **reticulocyte (retic)**. About 1% of the circulating erythrocytes are reticulocytes, and an increase in the number of circulating reticulocytes is an indication that the body needs more erythrocytes. This can occur

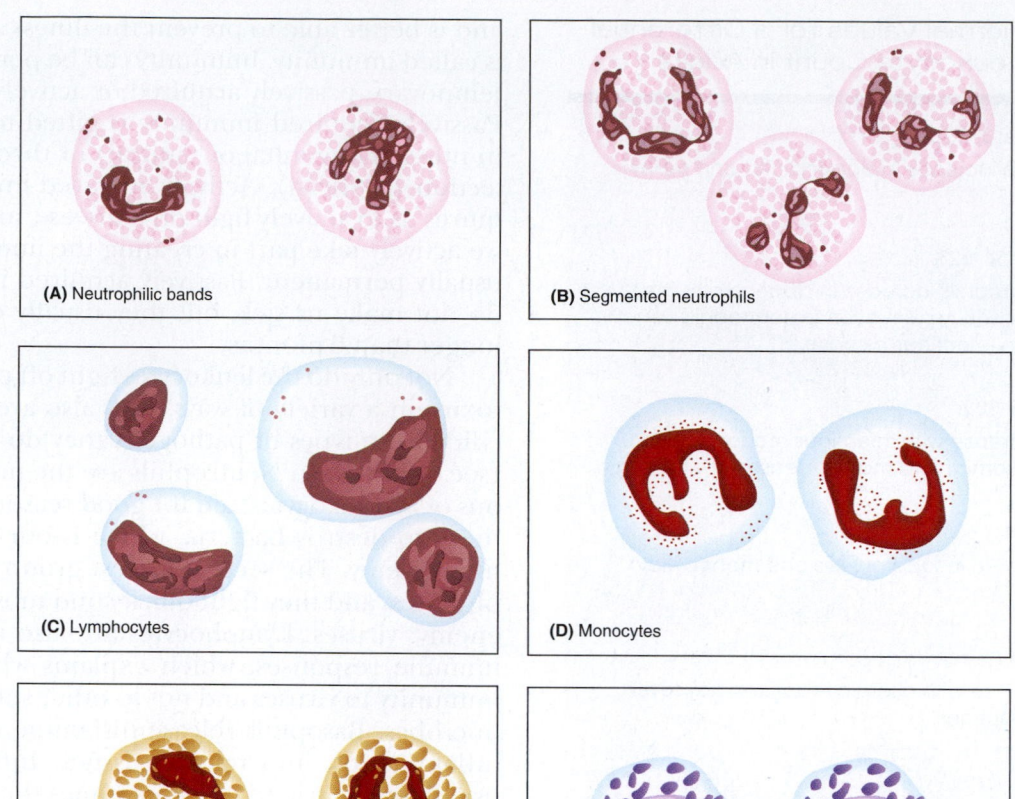

(A) Neutrophilic bands

(B) Segmented neutrophils

(C) Lymphocytes

(D) Monocytes

(E) Eosinophils

(F) Basophils

© Cengage Learning 2014

Figure 41-7   Various types of leukocytes from a stained blood smear.

Table 41-5   Normal Erythrocyte Counts

Age	Reference Range
Newborn	$5.0–6.5 \times 10^6/mm^3$
1-year-old child	$4.0–5.0 \times 10^6/mm^3$
Adult female	$4.0–5.5 \times 10^6/mm^3$
Adult male	$4.5–6.0 \times 10^6/mm^3$

© Cengage Learning 2014

in cases of hemorrhage and anemia. Erythrocytes can be of varying sizes. When erythrocytes are of normal size, they are called **normocytic**. Those that are larger are called **macrocytic**, and those that are smaller are called **microcytic**. When the erythrocytes show marked variation in size, the condition is called **anisocytosis**. The normal erythrocyte has a round or slightly oval shape. If the shape of the erythrocytes show marked variation, the condition is known as poikilocytosis.

The RBC should contain hemoglobin that fills about half of the cell. The RBC is biconcave, so most of the hemoglobin is seen around the outer part of the cell. The central area of the RBC is pale. RBCs with the proper amount of hemoglobin are called **normochromic**. Those that do not have enough hemoglobin, that demonstrate too large of a pale central area, are called **hypochromic**.

PLATELETS

The normal number of platelets (thrombocytes) is 140,000 to 400,000 per microliter of blood. Thrombocytes are actually fragments of cells. Like mature erythrocytes, thrombocytes have no nuclei. Thrombocytes are involved in the clotting of blood, or coagulation. Coagulation is a complex series of events that contains 13 distinct steps. A brief overview is provided

Examples of blood cell changes associated with disease states:

1. When a patient is experiencing an acute appendicitis, the white blood cell count increases rapidly with a high percentage of neutrophils. There is also an increase in the number of early or younger forms of these cells.
2. Patients who are suffering from a viral infection, especially adults, frequently experience a reduction in white blood cells and an increase in the percentage of lymphocytes. Patients with infectious mononucleosis have increased numbers of lymphocytes, many of which are atypical.
3. When patients have iron deficiency anemia, their indices demonstrate red blood cells that show marked reduction in hemoglobin content. Their erythrocytes appear hypochromic, lacking or low in color, because they lack the normal amount of hemoglobin in the red blood cells.

CLINICAL LABORATORY IMPROVEMENT AMENDMENT, 1988 (CLIA '88) REGULATION REGARDING WBC DIFFERENTIAL COUNTS

- Laboratories that are certified for waiver-level testing only are not permitted to perform manual WBC differential counts.
- Laboratories with a moderate-complexity certification can perform a manual differential WBC count but may only identify and report normal cells.
- Laboratories certified to perform tests of high complexity can perform a manual differential WBC count and are permitted to identify and report both abnormal and normal cells.
- Laboratories with moderate to complex certification can perform automated WBC counts including the reporting of abnormal results. Only qualified medical technicians and higher personnel may use and maintain the machines.

See Chapter 38 for details on CLIA '88 regulations.

here. When the body is physically injured, chemicals are released. Included in these chemicals are thromboplastin from injured tissues and plasma proteins and factors released from platelets. These chemicals form prothrombin activator. Prothrombin activator (with calcium) converts (activates) a blood protein called prothrombin into thrombin. Thrombin converts another blood protein called fibrinogen into fibrin. Fibrin is stringy and traps the sticky blood cells in a web at the site of injury, forming a plug of sorts. Eventually, the plug starts drying up, shrinks (pulling the edges of a wound together), and forms a scab.

What is really fascinating about the clotting of blood is why blood does not normally clot inside the blood vessels. Two chemicals made in the human body prevent that from happening. One is heparin, which is released from basophils and endothelial cells, and the other is antithrombin, which is released by the liver. The body needs blood to clot to stop bleeding, but it is important that blood not clot inside the body where it can cause problems and even death.

ERYTHROCYTE INDICES

The **erythrocyte indices** include the mean corpuscular (cell) volume (MCV), the mean corpuscular hemoglobin (MCH), and the mean corpuscular hemoglobin concentration (MCHC). These indices (plural for index) are calculations that provide information about the size of the RBCs and the hemoglobin content. The blood parameters needed to calculate all three indices are the RBC count, the hematocrit, and the hemoglobin. The erythrocyte indices values are important in the diagnosis or classification and treatment of different types of anemia. Table 41-6 shows normal values for the erythrocyte indices.

Before the automated hematology instrument became commonly used in the ambulatory care setting, the erythrocyte indices were not included as a part of the CBC because the RBC count was not an accurate measurement.

Table 41-6 Normal Values for the Erythrocyte Indices

MCV	80–100 fL
MCH	27–33 pg
MCHC	32–36 g/dL

© Cengage Learning 2014

The following formulas are used to calculate the erythrocyte indices:

$$MCV = \frac{Hematocrit}{RBC \text{ (in millions)}} \times 10$$

The result is reported in femtoliters (fL), a unit of volume 10^{-15} L, formerly reported in cubic microns (μm^3). This index gives the average volume of RBCs in the sample.

$$MCH = \frac{Hemoglobin \text{ (in grams)}}{RBC \text{ (in millions)}} \times 10$$

The result is expressed in picograms (pg), a micro microgram, or 1×10^{-12} g. This index estimates the weight of hemoglobin in RBCs of the sample.

$$MCHC = \frac{Hemoglobin \text{ (in grams)}}{Hematocrit} \times 10$$

This result is expressed in grams/deciliter (g/dL). The MCHC is the average concentration of hemoglobin in a given volume of packed RBCs (hematocrit).

Understanding RBC Indices

If we think of the red blood cells as water balloons filled with red-colored water, we might better understand the indices: The red-colored water signifies the hemoglobin inside the red blood cell. We have a basket of water balloons to signify our blood sample.

Because each water balloon is a different size (as are our red blood cells), we would need to measure the size of all of them to get the average volume or mass. We would add together the size/mass of all the balloons in our basket, then divide that number by the number of balloons in the basket. This gives us the average (mean) mass (volume), or MCV.

If we use MCH in the above example, we are measuring the average amount/concentration of water in the balloons. To measure this, we would pop each balloon, measure the total amount of water, and then divide by how many balloons there were. This would give us the average (mean) amount of red water (hemoglobin), or MCH.

CRITICAL THINKING

If the patient's hematocrit is 37 and the RBC count is 5 million, what would the MCV be?

Using the same water balloon comparison for explaining the MCHC, it would be the intensity of the red water within all the balloons. Some of the balloons might contain light red water, some might contain dark red water. The average of the intensity would give us the average (mean) intensity (concentration), or the MCHC.

All of these numbers together tell us about how many balloons (RBC) there are in the basket/sample, their average size (volume), how much they contain (amount hemoglobin/water), and the average concentration/intensity of the red water (hemoglobin) within all of them.

Understanding the relationship between the MCV, MCH, and MCHC helps to better understand what is happening when a patient is anemic due to low hemoglobin within each RBC versus a patient who is anemic due to low RBC count and so forth.

Using Erythrocyte Indices to Diagnose

The MCH and MCV are increased in megaloblastic anemias such as vitamin B_{12} and folate deficiency anemias. They also are increased in acute blood loss anemia, chronic hemolytic anemias, aplastic anemias, hypothyroidism, and liver disease. The MCH and MCV are decreased in hypochromic and microcytic anemias, including iron deficiency anemia, thalassemias, and occasionally in hyperthyroidism.

The MCHC is increased in hereditary spherocytosis. It is normal in macrocytosis. The MCHC is decreased in iron deficiency anemia. The stained blood smear of a person with iron deficiency anemia demonstrates RBCs that are both hypochromic and microcytic.

ERYTHROCYTE SEDIMENTATION RATES (ESR OR SED RATE)

The **erythrocyte sedimentation rate (ESR)**, as the name implies, is a measurement of the rate at which the RBCs in a well-mixed, anticoagulated blood sample will fall, or settle, toward the bottom when it is placed in a vertical tube. This test is commonly referred to in the laboratory as a "sed rate" (see Procedure 41-3). The ESR has been used for many years in the diagnosis and treatment of many disease states of the body, especially systemic inflammation. It is an inexpensive, accurate, and easy test to perform. Two factors that influence the sedimentation rate are the condition of the surface membrane of the RBC and changes in the level of fibrinogen in the plasma of the blood. During disease conditions in the body, the surface membrane of the RBC is altered, as well as the levels of fibrinogen, and this affects the rate at which the RBCs fall in the tube. RBCs will demonstrate this change even after the disease has subsided because RBCs have an average life of 120 days. For this reason, the ESR is a more accurate tool in diagnosing the onset of a disease than in checking the progress of treatment.

There is a commercial rapid ESR test available using centrifugation with results in 4 minutes. Two traditional methods of performing the ESR test are the Wintrobe method and the Westergren method. Both methods will provide the same information.

Wintrobe Method

An EDTA venous blood sample is thoroughly mixed. With the use of a Pasteur pipette, the blood is transferred to a Wintrobe tube. The blood is added to the left zero mark at the top of the tube. It is important that no air bubbles are present in the blood column. The tube is placed exactly vertical in a rack and allowed to stand for exactly 60 minutes. The test is read by determining the number of millimeters (mm) the red cells have settled. The tube has a total capacity of 100 mm. The test is reported in millimeters per hour (Figure 41-8). Table 41-7 lists normal values for the Wintrobe method of ESR.

Westergren Method

The Westergren method differs from the Wintrobe method in that the blood sample is mixed with 3.8% sodium citrate solution before the tube is filled. The blood and sodium citrate are mixed and the tube is filled to the zero mark and placed exactly vertical in a rack. The tube is read after exactly 60 minutes, and the test is reported in millimeters per hour. Table 41-8 gives normal values for the Westergren method of ESR.

The Polymedco company produces a Sediplast® system to perform a Westergren ESR that is self-filling. It is a completely closed system that protects laboratory personnel from the risks associated with blood handling. The Sediplast® ESR System is shown in Figure 41-9.

The following guidelines should be followed when performing Wintrobe and Westergren ESR procedures to ensure accurate test results:

1. The tube must remain exactly vertical during the 1-hour test time.

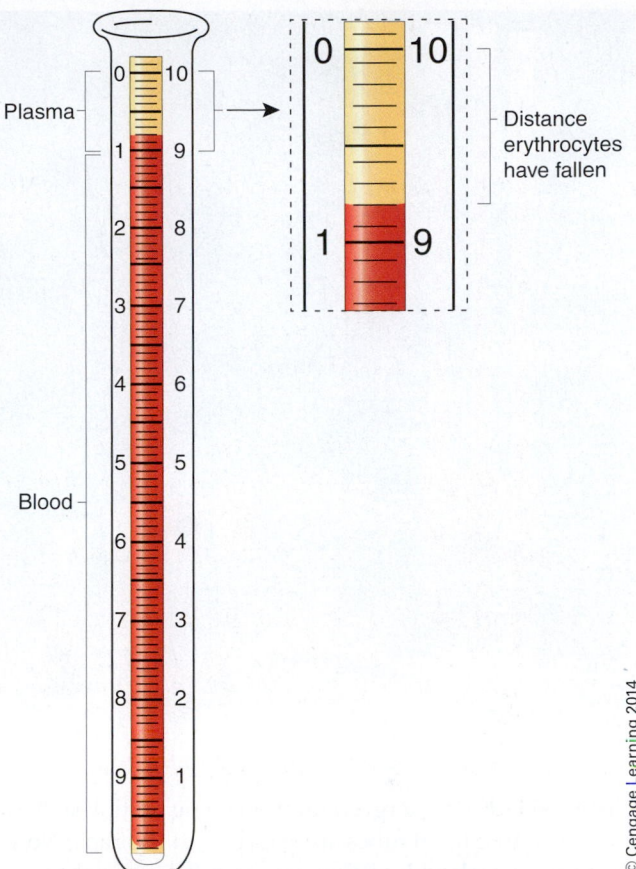

Figure 41-8 Wintrobe sedimentation tube showing settling of cells. The example shows a sedimentation of 8 mm.

© Cengage Learning 2014

Table 41-7 Normal Values for the Wintrobe Method of ESR

Male patients	0–9 mm/hr
Female patients	0–20 mm/hr

© Cengage Learning 2014

Table 41-8 Normal Values for the Westergren Method of ESR

Male patients younger than 50 years	0–15 mm/hr
Male patients older than 50 years	0–20 mm/hr
Female patients younger than 50 years	0–20 mm/hr
Female patients older than 50 years	0–30 mm/hr

© Cengage Learning 2014

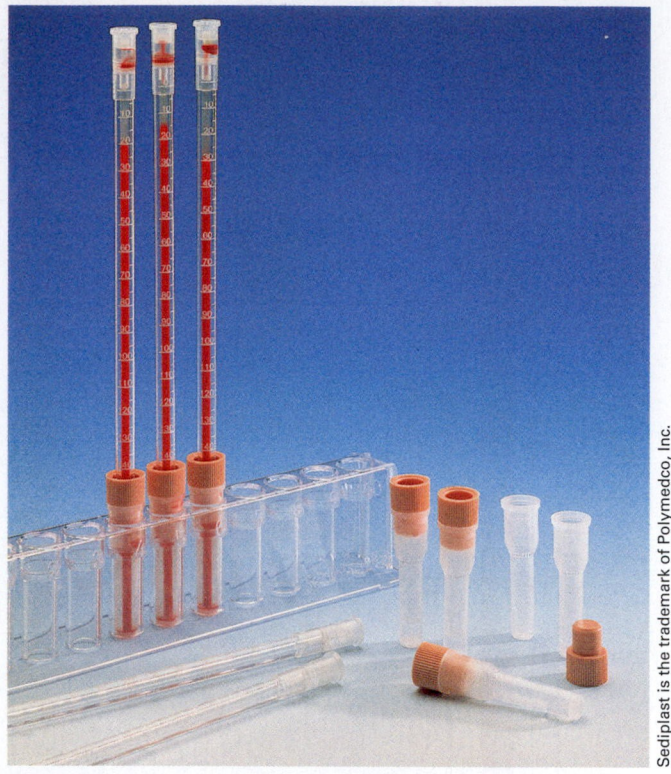

Sediplast is the trademark of Polymedco, Inc.

Figure 41-9 Westergren method using Sediplast® ESR System. Three filled tubes are standing in the rack. Note the diluting vials with sodium citrate solution (right).

2. The test must be read at exactly 60 minutes (1 hour).

3. The counter on which the rack is placed must be free of vibrations.

4. The test should be set up within 2 hours after the blood is drawn.

5. The test should be conducted at room temperature.

6. The tube should not be placed in a draft, and it should not be exposed to direct sunlight.

7. The column of blood must be free of bubbles.

The erythrocytes in normal, nondiseased blood tend to remain suspended in the plasma. They do not aggregate (clump) together to form rouleaux. Rouleaux are a phenomenon where RBCs form aggregates that look like rolls or stacks of coins (Figure 41-10).

This aggregate form causes the rate of sedimentation to increase. RBCs have membrane properties that tend to make them remain separated in the plasma. During certain diseased states, this repelling property is lost and the RBCs tend to aggregate.

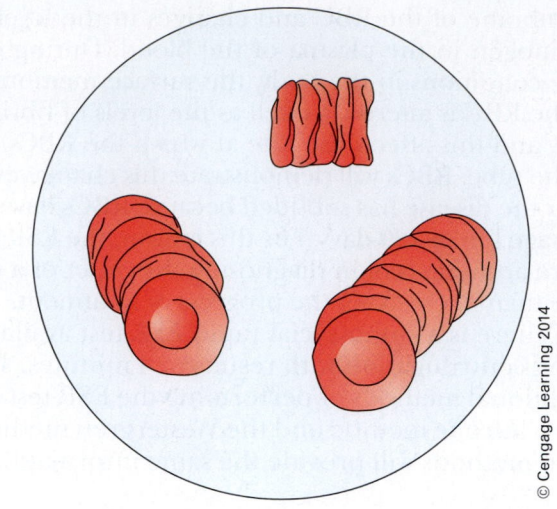

© Cengage Learning 2014

Figure 41-10 Erythrocytes forming rouleaux.

Using the ESR to Screen

ESRs are increased in infections, acute stress, inflammatory diseases, tissue destruction, and other conditions that lead to an increase in plasma fibrinogen. They are also increased with menstruation, pregnancy, lupus, malignant neoplasms, and multiple myeloma. With anemia, the ESR increases according to the severity of the condition.

The ESR may be normal in osteoarthritis and in some cases of cirrhosis and malaria. ESR values are decreased in polycythemia, spherocytosis, and sickle cell anemia.

C-REACTIVE PROTEINS

Another screening blood test for inflammation is **C-reactive protein** or **CRP**. The CRP level will rise and drop quicker than the ESR, giving the provider more timely information about the effectiveness of treatment. The CRP is not affected by as many other factors as the ESR, making it a better inflammation indicator than the ESR.

Like the ESR, CRP is helpful in determining systemic inflammatory conditions such as autoimmune diseases, inflammatory bowel conditions, and some forms of arthritis. While it is not specifically diagnostic for any one disease, it can serve as a marker for general infection and inflammation, and, once the disease or condition is diagnosed, it can help determine the effectiveness of treatment.

CRP is made by the liver and released into the bloodstream. It increases when infection and inflammation are present. It has been used for many years as an indicator of bacterial and viral infections.

Due to the more recent studies showing the correlation between vascular inflammation and heart disease, a more sensitive CRP-related test called hsCRP (highly sensitive C-reactive protein) has gained popularity in detecting vascular inflammation that can indicate coronary artery disease and cardiovascular disease. The hsCRP is used in conjunction with the traditional lipid profile and cardiac risk assessment.

COAGULATION STUDIES

Persons prone to forming blood clots often are medicated with anticoagulants (blood thinners) such as Coumadin or Pradaxa (diabigatran). Patients on Coumadin are monitored regularly to assure that their blood can clot within a reasonable amount of time, which ensures that the patient is taking the correct dosage of the blood thinning medication. The method of monitoring coagulation time is called the prothrombin time (PT) or, more commonly, the **protime**. The protime is reported in the time (seconds) it takes for the patient's blood to clot and in the international normalized ratio (INR). We still refer to both tests as protime. Currently the INR is more useful because it is standardized, that is, it can be universally applied, in contrast to the timing test, which can vary quite a bit from facility to facility. Normal blood will clot in about 11 to 13 seconds. The provider will want the patient taking anticoagulant medication to have a protime of approximately 16 to 18 seconds and INR of 2.0 to 2.6 (sometimes higher). If blood clots too soon, the anticoagulant medication is not at a therapeutic level. If the blood clotting takes too long (prolonged clotting), then the patient is taking too much medication. An INR of 1.0 is considered ineffective; 5.0 is considered dangerous.

Because activities of daily living, such as diet, can interfere with clotting factors, the protime usually is tested on a regular basis, weekly at the beginning of treatment, then monthly or less frequently as treatment progresses. If the patient experiences frequent unusual bruising or bleeding that might indicate an imbalance in clotting ability, then the protime test can be run "on demand". Some foods rich in vitamin K (e.g., dark leafy vegetables), alcohol, vitamins and supplements, aspirin, and many other medications can interfere with anticoagulant therapy. Health care professionals must interview the patient carefully about what is being taken. Patient education and patient compliance are both important components of effective treatment with anticoagulants.

The protime test is also used as a screening test for people who have liver disease or clotting factor disease or who are vitamin K deficient.

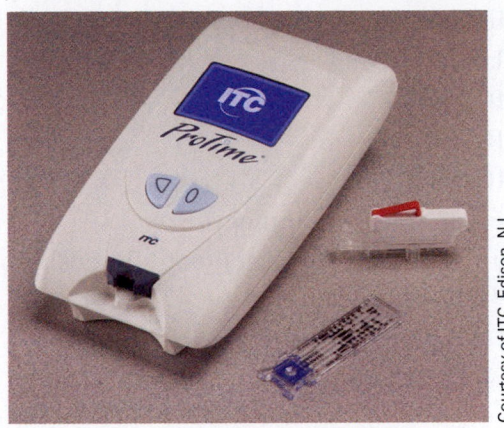

Figure 41-11 ProTime coagulation analyzer.

 The protime is a simple CLIA waived test that is performed on a drop of blood (Figure 41-11). Procedure 41-4 describes the step-by-step process.

AUTOMATED HEMATOLOGY

 Use of the automated or semiautomated hematology instruments is not categorized as waived testing under CLIA and therefore is not within the medical assistant's scope of practice without further education and training. CLIA has allowed many specific analyzers into the waived category, such as the hemoglobin and protime analyzers. All procedures performed with automated instrumentation are modifications of manual methods. Automated hematology procedures have many advantages over the manual methods. They are faster, less expensive, simple to operate, and accurate. The instruments can be calibrated and lend themselves to control testing. Most are equipped with printers that produce hard copy results. Many can store quality-control results and print out quality-control data summary sheets.

In addition to performing a wide variety of hematologic tests, many automated hematology instruments also calculate part or all of the RBC indices and print the results. Some automated hematology instruments can be connected to other computers in the medical facility.

The hematologic parameters that are available on different automated office hematology instruments are:

- RBC count
- WBC count
- Hemoglobin

- Hematocrit
- Platelet count
- MCV
- MCH
- MCHC
- Percentage of granulocytes
- Granulocyte count (neutrophils, eosinophils, basophils)
- Percentage of lymphocytes/monocytes

- Non granulocyte count (lymphocytes and monocytes)
- Mid-cell count (monocytes and band neutrophils)
- Percentage of mid-cells
- Lymphocyte count
- Percentage of lymphocytes
- RBC distribution width (RDW)

PROCEDURE 41-1

Hemoglobin Determination Using a CLIA Waived Hemoglobin Analyzer

STANDARD PRECAUTIONS:

  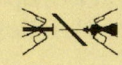

PURPOSE:
Properly and safely perform an automated hemoglobin determination to evaluate the oxygen-carrying capacity of the blood.

EQUIPMENT/SUPPLIES:
Gloves
Biohazard container
Sharps container
Capillary puncture equipment
   70% isopropyl alcohol
   Safety lancet
   Cotton ball
   Gauze 2 × 2
   Adhesive bandage
CLIA waived hemoglobin analyzer with test slides

PROCEDURE STEPS:

1. Assemble and organize equipment and supplies. RATIONALE: Being organized helps the process go more smoothly and professionally.

2. Wash hands and put on gloves. RATIONALE: Hand washing and gloving protects the patient and you.

3. Turn on the analyzer and calibrate or standardize according to the manufacturer's instructions (Figure 41-12A). RATIONALE: Turn on analyzer to warm machine up, calibrate to maintain quality controls.

4. *Introduce yourself by name and credential, identify the patient,* and recheck the provider's orders. RATIONALE: Introducing yourself and stating your credentials demonstrates professionalism and helps to reassure the patient. Identifying the patient and rechecking the provider's orders will ensure the proper tests will be performed on the right patient.

5. *Explain the procedure and expectations to the patient. Allay the patient's fears regarding the procedure to help him or her feel safe and comfortable.* RATIONALE: Explaining the procedure and allaying the patient's fears will assure the patient that you are concerned about any apprehension he or she may have and that you are open to discussing the patient's concerns.

6. Select the site, prepare the site, and perform the capillary puncture (see Chapter 40). Wipe away the first drop with gauze. RATIONALE: The first drop may be contaminated with tissue fluid. Using gauze rather than a cotton ball will discourage a clot from forming.

7. Apply the second drop of blood into the slide reservoir using the appropriate technique for the analyzer (Figure 41-12B). RATIONALE: Each machine has a slightly different applicator device and technique.

8. Apply a cotton ball to the puncture site and ask the patient to hold pressure for 2 minutes. RATIONALE: Cotton will assist the site to clot during the 2 minutes the pressure is held.

9. Place the slide into the analyzer and perform appropriate steps as required by the manufacturer's instructions. RATIONALE: Each manufacturer has specific processes for use with its analyzer.

Procedure 41-1 (continued)

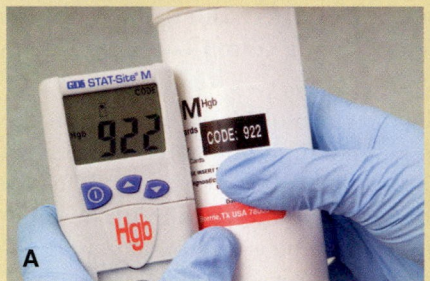 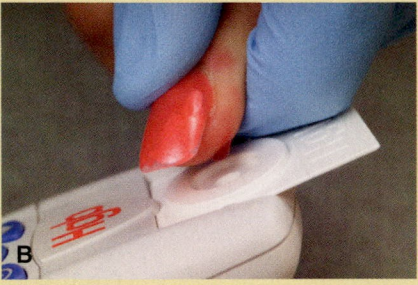 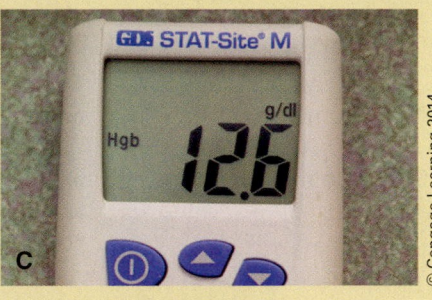

Figure 41-12 (A) Turn on the machine and perform control testing if necessary. Always follow the manufacturer's instructions. (B) Place the patient's drop of blood into the slide reservoir. (C) Read and record the hemoglobin value.

10. Read and make a note of the test results (Figure 41-12C). RATIONALE: Making a note helps you retain the results until they can be charted in the patient's medical record.

11. Assess the patient and apply a bandage strip to the puncture site. RATIONALE: The patient should not leave your care until the bleeding has stopped. Do not apply a fingertip bandage to an infant or young child because it could pose a choking hazard.

12. Disinfect analyzer according to manufacturer's instructions. Discard all contaminated equipment and supplies into appropriate biohazard waste receptacles. Disinfect counter space. RATIONALE: Using disinfectants not recommended by the manufacturer could harm the analyzer. Use sharps containers for sharp supplies and red bags for contaminated cotton ball and gloves.

13. Discard note, remove gloves and discard into biohazard container, and wash hands. RATIONALE: Washing hands removes residual contamination.

14. Document the procedure in the patient's medical record in the progress notes charting section and complete a lab report. File the lab report in the lab section of the patient record. RATIONALE: Accurate and timely documentation are important in medical laboratory procedures.

DOCUMENTATION:

08/06/20XX Capillary puncture performed for hemoglobin determination. Specimen tested in our lab. Dr. Rice notified of results and report filed in patient records. Patient tolerated the procedure well and Dr. Rice discussed results with her. Joe Guerrero, CMA (AAMA)——————————

Laboratory Report

Patient Name ___Diane Pankey___ Date ___08-06-20XX___

Hematocrit ___—___ % Hemoglobin ___14.5___ gm/dL

___Joe Guerrero, CMA (AAMA)___
MA signature

PROCEDURE 41-2

Microhematocrit Determination

STANDARD PRECAUTIONS:

  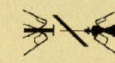

PURPOSE:
Properly and safely perform a microhematocrit determination.

EQUIPMENT/SUPPLIES:
Gloves
Biohazard container
Sharps container
Capillary puncture equipment
   70% isopropyl alcohol
   Safety lancet

continues

© Cengage Learning 2014

Procedure 41-2 (continued)

Cotton ball
Gauze 2 × 2
Adhesive bandage
Microhematocrit tubes (heparinized, plastic, self-sealing or use sealing clay)
Microhematocrit centrifuge and reader

PROCEDURE STEPS:

1. Assemble and organize equipment and supplies. RATIONALE: Being organized helps the process go more smoothly and professionally.

2. Wash hands and put on gloves. RATIONALE: Hand washing and gloving protects the patient, and you.

3. *Introduce yourself by name and credential, identify the patient,* and recheck the provider's orders. RATIONALE: Introducing yourself and stating your credentials demonstrates professionalism and helps to reassure the patient. Identifying the patient and rechecking the provider's orders will ensure the proper tests will be performed on the right patient.

4. *Explain the procedure and expectations to the patient. Allay the patient's fears regarding the procedure to help him or her feel safe and comfortable.* RATIONALE: Explaining the procedure and allaying the patient's fears will assure the patient that you are concerned about any apprehension he or she may have and that you are open to discussing the patient's concerns.

5. Select the site, prepare the site, and perform the capillary puncture (see Chapter 40). Wipe away the first drop with gauze. RATIONALE: The first drop may be contaminated with tissue fluid. Using gauze rather than a cotton ball will discourage a clot from forming.

6. Allow the second drop of blood to form on the patient's finger. Holding the microhematocrit tube horizontally, touch the end onto the top of the blood drop and let the tube fill by capillary action until the tube is approximately ¾ full (Figure 41-13A and Figure 41-13B).

7. With a 2 × 2 gauze, wipe off the end of the tube. Gently place the tube into clay until a plug is formed or use self-sealing tube (Figure 41-13C). RATIONALE: Wiping the end of the tube of blood lessens contamination to the clay holder. Sealing the tube prevents the specimen from being forced out during centrifugation.

8. Repeat the procedure with one more tube. RATIONALE: The two tubes balance one another in the centrifuge and the amounts are averaged to get the hematocrit results.

9. Apply a cotton ball to the puncture site and ask the patient to hold pressure for 2 minutes. RATIONALE: Cotton will assist the site to clot during the 2 minutes the pressure is held.

10. Place the tubes into the centrifuge with sealed ends outward against the gasket. Make certain the tubes balance each other across the centrifuge. Fasten the lid securely, lock into place, and turn the centrifuge on. Set the timer and spin for the appropriate amount of time as required by the manufacturer's instructions. RATIONALE: Centrifugal force requires that the outside ends of the tubes be plugged to prevent the specimen from

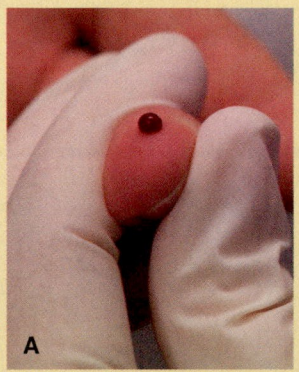
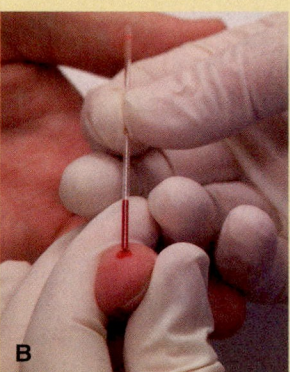
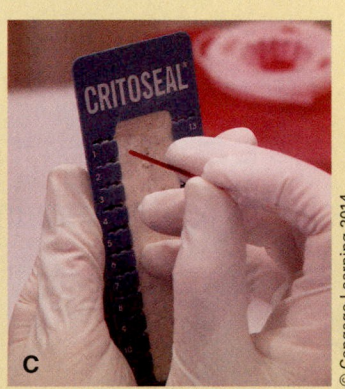

A   B   C

© Cengage Learning 2014

Figure 41-13 (A) Perform the capillary puncture, and wipe away the first drop with gauze. Allow the second drop of blood to form on the patient's finger. (B) Holding the microhematocrit tube horizontally, touch the end onto the top of the blood drop and let the tube fill by capillary action until it is approximately ¾ full. (C) Seal the microhematocrit tube with sealing clay.

Procedure 41-2 (continued)

leaking out. Balancing the tubes and locking the lid ensure laboratory safety and prevents breakage.

11. Assess the patient and apply a bandage strip to the puncture site. RATIONALE: The patient should not leave your care until the bleeding has stopped. Do not apply a fingertip bandage to an infant or young child because it could pose a choking hazard.

12. Allow the centrifuge to come to a complete stop before touching it. Remove the tubes. Using a reader or accompanying graph, determine the hematocrit level. Read and make a note of the test results. RATIONALE: A spinning centrifuge is very dangerous and can cause a friction burn if touched. Making a note helps you retain the results until they can be charted in the patient's medical record.

13. Discard all contaminated equipment and supplies into appropriate biohazard waste receptacles. Disinfect counter space and centrifuge according to manufacturer's instructions. RATIONALE: Using disinfectants not recommended by the manufacturer could harm the analyzer. Use sharps containers for sharp supplies and red bags for contaminated cotton ball and gloves.

14. Remove gloves and discard into biohazard container, and wash hands. RATIONALE: Washing hands removes residual contamination.

15. Document the procedure in the patient's medical record in the progress notes charting section and complete a lab report. *Notify the provider of the results* and file the lab report in the lab section of the patient record. RATIONALE: Accurate and timely documentation are important in medical laboratory procedures.

DOCUMENTATION:

08/06/20XX   Capillary puncture performed on patient's left middle finger for hematocrit determination. Specimen tested in our labs. Dr. notified of result and report filed. Patient tolerated the procedure well and Dr. Rice discussed results with her. Joe Guerrero, CMA (AAMA)

Laboratory Report

Patient Name ____*Diane Pankey*____ Date __*08-06-20XX*__

Hematocrit __*38*__ %   Hemoglobin ____—____ gm/dL

____*Joe Guerrero, CMA (AAMA)*____
MA signature

PROCEDURE 41-3
Erythrocyte Sedimentation Rate

STANDARD PRECAUTIONS:

     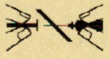

PURPOSE:
Properly and safely examine a blood sample by using either the Sediplast® (Westergren) or Wintrobe method to determine the ESR.

EQUIPMENT/SUPPLIES:
Gloves
Sample of venous blood collected in EDTA
Sediplast® kit (or other ESR kit):
  Sedivial and sedirack
  Sediplast® autozeroing pipette
  Pipette capable of delivering up to 1.0 mL
Wintrobe method:
  Wintrobe sedimentation tube (disposable or reusable)
  Wintrobe sedimentation rack
  Long-stem Pasteur-type pipette with rubber bulb
Timer
Disinfectant
Biohazard disposal container
Acrylic face shield or goggles and mask
Sharps container
NOTE: Consult the manufacturer's package insert for specific instructions for the ESR kit being used.

PROCEDURE STEPS:
1. Wash hands and put on gloves.
2. Assemble equipment and materials.
3. Gently mix blood sample for 2 minutes.
4. Perform either method a (Sediplast® ESR) or method b (Wintrobe):
   a. Sediplast® ESR (modified Westergren) method:
      (1) Remove stopper on sedivial and fill to the indicated mark with 0.8 mL blood.

continues

Procedure 41-3 (continued)

Replace stopper and invert vial several times to mix (or mix using pipette).

(2) Place sedivial in Sediplast® rack on a level surface.

(3) Gently insert the disposable Sediplast® pipette through the pierceable stopper with a twisting motion and push down until the pipette rests on the bottom of the vial. The pipette will autozero the blood and any excess will flow into the sealed reservoir compartment.

(4) Set timer for 1 hour.

(5) Return blood sample to proper storage. (If no laboratory work will be performed during the incubation, remove gloves, discard appropriately, and wash hands. Reglove before handling test materials.)

(6) Let the pipette stand undisturbed for exactly 1 hour, and then read the results of the ESR: Use the scale on the tube to measure the distance from the top of the plasma to the top of the RBCs.

(7) Record the sedimentation rate: ESR (Mod. Westergren, 1 hr) = _____ mm.

(8) Dispose of tube and vial in appropriate biohazard container.

b. Wintrobe method:

(1) Place tube in Wintrobe sedimentation rack.

(2) Check the leveling bubble to ensure that the Wintrobe rack is level.

(3) Fill Wintrobe tube to the zero mark with well-mixed blood using the Pasteur pipette and being careful not to over fill. *NOTE:* Tube must be filled from the bottom to avoid getting air bubbles in the tube.

(4) Set timer for 1 hour. Be certain the tube is vertical and left undisturbed for the entire hour.

(5) Return blood sample to proper storage. (If no other laboratory work is scheduled, remove gloves, discard appropriately, and wash hands. Reglove before handling test materials.)

(6) Measure the distance the erythrocytes have fallen (in mm): after exactly 1 hour, use the scale on the tube to measure the distance from the top of the plasma to the top of the RBCs.

(7) Record the sedimentation rate: ESR (Wintrobe, 1 hr) = _____ mm.

(8) Disinfect and clean equipment and return to storage.

NOTE: If disposable equipment is used, dispose of in biohazard container.

5. Clean work area with surface disinfectant.

6. Remove gloves and discard into biohazard container.

7. Wash hands.

8. Document the procedure in the patient's medical record in the progress notes charting section and complete a lab report. Notify the provider of the results file the lab report in the lab section of the patient record. RATIONALE: Accurate and timely documentation are important in medical laboratory procedures.

DOCUMENTATION:

08/06/20XX   ESR performed on venous sample. Results filed in patient's chart. Dr. Rice discussed results with him. Joe Guerrero, CMA (AAMA) ————————————————

Laboratory Report

Patient Name _____ *George Pankey* _____ Date _*08-06-20XX*_

Erythrocyte Sedimentation Rate _*17*_ mm/hr

*Joe Guerrero, CMA (AAMA)*
MA signature

PROCEDURE 41-4

Prothrombin Time (Using CLIA Waived ProTime Analyzer)

STANDARD PRECAUTIONS:

  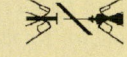

PURPOSE:

Properly and safely perform an automated prothrombin time determination to evaluate the clotting time of a drop of blood.

EQUIPMENT/SUPPLIES:

Gloves
Biohazard container
Sharps container
Capillary puncture equipment
  70% isopropyl alcohol
  Tenderlett lancet
  Cotton ball
  Gauze 2 × 2
  Adhesive bandage
CLIA Waived ProTime Analyzer (ITC ProTime-3)
  with accessories

PROCEDURE STEPS:

1. Assemble and organize equipment and supplies. Check expiration dates. RATIONALE: Being organized helps the process go more smoothly and professionally.

2. Wash hands and put on gloves. RATIONALE: Hand washing and gloving protects the patient and you.

3. Turn on the ProTime-3 and follow the prompts. Insert the test cuvette into the analyzer. RATIONALE: Turn on analyzer to warm up machine, calibrate to maintain quality controls.

4. *Introduce yourself by name and credential, identify the patient,* and recheck the provider's orders. RATIONALE: Introducing yourself and stating your credentials demonstrates professionalism and helps to reassure the patient. Identifying the patient and rechecking the provider's orders will ensure the proper tests will be performed on the right patient.

5. *Explain the procedure and expectations to the patient. Allay the patient's fears regarding the procedure to help him or her feel safe and comfortable.* RATIONALE: Explaining the procedure and allaying the patient's fears will assure the patient that you are concerned about any apprehension he or she may have and that you are open to discussing the patient's concerns.

6. Select the site, prepare the site, and perform the capillary puncture using the Tenderlett lancet. Remember to use gauze to wipe away the first drop. RATIONALE: The Tenderlett lancet contains the reservoir required for use with the ProTime-3.

7. Fill the Tenderlett lancet cup to the fill line and then place it onto the cuvette, which was placed into the machine in Step 3. Be sure it is snapped into place. Press the start button. RATIONALE: The Tenderlett cup is calibrated for the analyzer and must be properly placed for the test to run correctly.

8. Apply a cotton ball and ask the patient to hold pressure for 3 to 5 minutes. RATIONALE: A patient having this test performed usually has a delayed clotting time. Assess that the bleeding has stopped and apply bandage. RATIONALE: A patient should never leave your care until the bleeding has stopped.

9. Stay by the analyzer and await a prompt to remove the Tenderlett lancet device. When prompted, immediately remove the device and discard it into a nearby sharps container. RATIONALE: The device must be removed as soon as the clot has formed. This must be done very quickly, within seconds. The Tenderlett device contains a lancet and must be discarded into a sharps container.

10. Read the clotting time in seconds and the INR. Record the results. RATIONALE: Results should be recorded as soon as possible to decrease the chance of error.

11. *Notify the provider* immediately if the results fall within a critical range. RATIONALE: If the patient has a seriously delayed clotting time, the risk of a serious event occurring (such as a stroke) is greater. The provider must be notified immediately in order to adjust the anticoagulant dosage and/or prescribe other treatment.

continues

Procedure 41-4 (continued)

12. Disinfect analyzer according to manufacturer's instructions, discard all contaminated equipment and supplies into appropriate biohazard waste receptacles, and disinfect counter space. Remove gloves and wash hands. RATIONALE: Using disinfectants not recommended by the manufacturer could harm the analyzer. Use sharps containers for sharp supplies and red bags for contaminated cotton ball and gloves. Washing hands removes residual contamination.

13. Document the procedure in the patient's medical record in the progress notes charting section and complete a lab report. File the lab report in the lab section of the patient record. RATIONALE: Accurate and timely documentation are important in medical laboratory procedures.

DOCUMENTATION:

08/06/20XX   Capillary puncture performed on patient's right ring finger for protime determination. Specimen tested in our lab. Results given to Dr. Rice. Report filed in patient record. Patient tolerated the procedure well and Dr. Rice discussed results with her. Joe Guerrero, CMA (AAMA)—————————

Laboratory Report

Patient Name   Cynthia Januszewski   Date   08-06-20XX

Protime   16 seconds   INR   2.0

Joe Guerrero, CMA (AAMA)
MA signature

CASE STUDY 41-1

Refer to the scenario at the beginning of the chapter.

CASE STUDY REVIEW

1. What should Audrey do if the clinic buys a new machine for laboratory analysis that she is not familiar with?

2. How can Audrey be sure that she is using the laboratory analyzers properly and that the patient test results are accurate?

3. Who should Audrey consult if she has questions about how to perform a test using an analyzer?

CASE STUDY 41-2

Today is busier than usual at Drs. Lewis and King. While she is performing an ESR for Jim Marshal, a patient in his late 30s, medical assistant Audrey Jones is called on to help with another patient. She hurriedly places the sedimentation rack on top of an incubator in the sunlight by an open window and leaves to assist Dr. King.

CASE STUDY REVIEW

1. List two ways in which the test results may be affected.

2. What are the normal Westergren ESR values for male and female patients younger than 50 years?

3. What are the best conditions for an accurate test?

SUMMARY

Hematology tests are the second most frequently performed tests in the ambulatory care setting. Only urinalysis is performed more frequently. Medical assistants must have a knowledge of hematology to accurately and efficiently perform the tests. The study of hematology includes hematopoiesis, which is the formation of the blood elements, as well as the hematologic tests and their relation to the pathology of the body.

This chapter introduced the more common hematologic tests that are performed in the ambulatory care setting, including all the parts of the CBC, the ESR methods, and the erythrocyte indices. All of these tests are used by the provider in the diagnosis and treatment of disease.

Most of the hematology procedures performed in today's ambulatory care setting use some type of automated instrumentation. Some automated hematology instruments require a diluted blood sample, whereas others do not. Both methods of automated instrumentation are discussed in this chapter.

 Blood specimens used in the sampling of hematologic procedures are biohazardous material. Be sure to follow Universal and Standard Precautions when you work with these specimens (see Chapter 22).

STUDY FOR SUCCESS

To reinforce your knowledge and skills of information presented in this chapter:

- Review the *Key Terms*

- Role-play with other students to apply attributes of professionalism pertinent to this chapter.

- Consider the *Case Studies* and discuss your conclusions

- Answer the questions in the *Certification Review*

- Apply your knowledge by completing the *Activities* in the *Study Guide* and the *Games and Quizzes* in the StudyWARE (StudyWARE) software on the *Premium Website*

- Perform the *Procedures* using the *Competency Assessment Checklists* in the *Competency Manual*

- Practice your problem-solving skills with the *Critical Thinking Challenge 3.0* on the *Premium Website*

Additional resources for this chapter include:

- Module 22 of the *Medical Assisting Learning Lab*

- *CourseMate for Delmar's Comprehensive Medical Assisting*

- *WebTutor for Delmar's Comprehensive Medical Assisting*

CERTIFICATION REVIEW

1. Which of the following is *not* a cellular component of blood?
   a. Erythrocytes
   b. Leukocytes
   c. Thrombocytes
   d. Erythropoietin

2. The formation of blood cells is defined as:
   a. erythropoietin
   b. hematopoiesis
   c. mean corpuscular volume
   d. hemoglobinopathy

3. Sickle cell anemia, a hereditary disease, has which type of hemoglobin?
   a. Hemoglobin S
   b. Hemoglobin A
   c. Hemoglobin E
   d. Hemoglobin C

4. The volume of packed red cells compared with the total volume of the sample is calculated for which test?
   a. Hematocrit
   b. Hemoglobin
   c. MCH
   d. MCV

5. The most common white cell type found in the granulocytic series is the:
   a. lymphocyte
   b. monocyte
   c. neutrophil
   d. basophil

6. The erythrocyte indices are used for the diagnosis, classification, and treatment of different:
   a. infections
   b. anemias
   c. inflammatory diseases
   d. neoplasms

7. Which hematologic test result shows an increase with infections, inflammatory disease, acute stress, and tissue destruction?
   a. Hemoglobin
   b. MCV
   c. Hematocrit
   d. ESR

8. The most frequent hemoglobin disease seen in the ambulatory care setting is:
   a. iron deficiency anemia
   b. sickle cell anemia
   c. leukemia
   d. anisocytosis

9. Which test within a CBC is within the scope of practice of a medical assistant under CLIA's waived test category?
   a. Using a HemoCue® to determine a hemoglobin level
   b. Using a hemacytometer to count WBCs manually
   c. Using the Unopette system to count RBCs manually
   d. Using an automated blood analyzer that requires calculations and mixing of reagents

10. The highly sensitive C-reactive protein (hsCRP) test is used for detecting:
    a. any type of protein in the blood
    b. vascular inflammation
    c. very specific diseases such as lupus
    d. anemia and leukemia

REFERENCES/BIBLIOGRAPHY

Walters, N. J., Estridge, B. H., & Reynolds, A. P. (2011). *Basic Clinical Laboratory Techniques* (6th ed). Clifton Park, NY: Delmar Cengage Learning.

OUTLINE

Urine Formation
  Filtration
  Reabsorption
  Secretion
Urine Composition
Safety
Quality Control
Clinical Laboratory
  Improvement Amendments
  of 1988 (CLIA '88)

Urine Containers
Urine Collection
  Urine Specimen Types
  Collection Methods
Culture and Sensitivity of Urine
Examination of Urine
  Physical Examination
  of Urine

Chemical Examination
  of Urine
Microscopic Examination
  of Urine Sediment
Urinalysis Report
Drug Screening

LEARNING OUTCOMES

1. Define, spell, and pronounce the key terms as presented in the glossary.
2. Use language/verbal skills that enable the patient's understanding.
3. Display sensitivity to the patient's rights and feelings in collecting specimens.
4. Explain the rationale for performing a proper clean catch collection to a patient.
5. Explain the process of urine formation.
6. Discuss the importance of safety procedures and quality control when working with urine.
7. Describe the importance of proper collection and preservation of 24-hour urine specimens.

8. Identify the proper technique for examining the physical characteristics of a urine specimen.
9. Perform urinalysis (excluding microscopy).
10. Identify the proper method of preparing urine sediment for microscopic examination.
11. Identify normal and abnormal structures found during the microscopic examination of urine sediment.
12. Analyze the professionalism questions and apply them to this chapter's content.

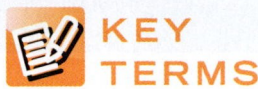

KEY TERMS

acid/base balance

amorphous

bilirubin

bilirubinuria

casts

chain of custody

circadian rhythm

creatinine

critical values

crystals

glucosuria

hematuria

hyaline

ketoacidosis

ketone

ketonuria

ketosis

leukocyte esterase

midstream collection

pH

reagent test strip

refractometer

sediment

specific gravity

supernatant

turbid

urea

urinary tract
  infection (UTI)

urobilinogen

ATTRIBUTES OF PROFESSIONALISM

Communication

- Did you introduce yourself? Did you identify the patient through name and birth date or other identifying feature?
- Did you listen to and acknowledge the patient?
- Did you speak at the patient's level of understanding?
- Did you provide appropriate responses/feedback?
- Did you explain procedures and expectations to the patient?
- Did you allay patients' fears regarding the procedure being performed and help them feel safe and comfortable?
- Did you respond honestly and diplomatically to the patient's concerns?

Presentation

- Were you dressed and groomed appropriately?
- Were you courteous, patient, and respectful to the patient?
- Did you display a positive attitude?
- Did you display a calm, professional, and caring manner?

Competency

- Did you pay attention to detail?
- Did you ask questions if you were out of your comfort zone or did not have the experience to carry out tasks?
- Were you knowledgeable and accountable?

Integrity

- Did you work within your scope of practice?
- Did you immediately report any error you had made?

SCENARIO

At Inner City Health Care, clinical medical assistant Wanda Slawson performs many urinalyses. Although urinalysis is a routine procedure, Wanda recognizes its importance as a diagnostic tool, and she performs each test carefully to ensure accurate results. Wanda takes time to instruct patients in the proper collection procedures. She encourages patients to ask questions before collecting the urine sample, and she provides written instructions for easy reference. When she performs the urinalysis, Wanda follows safety and quality control guidelines. By paying attention to the details of the procedure, Wanda does her best to ensure the quality of the urinalysis results.

INTRODUCTION

Examination of the urine (urinalysis) as a diagnostic tool for many diseases has been performed for centuries by medical practitioners. Urinalysis refers to the study of urine as an aid in patient diagnosis or to follow the course of disease. The urine examination is a routine part of most physical examinations.

The routine urinalysis is one of the most frequently performed procedures in the medical office laboratory. Many tests can be performed on one urine sample. This procedure is often ordered because urine is easily obtained, and much information about the body's metabolism may be gained from the results of this testing.

When providers order a "routine urinalysis," they expect timely and accurate results. Results can indicate a systemic disease process or renal (kidney) or urinary tract disease.

Practice, experience, and attention to detail are the most important tools in achieving quality results. Following Standard Precautions when working with any body fluid is mandatory.

URINE FORMATION

Before discussing the analysis of urine, it is helpful to understand how urine is formed in the human body. The formation and excretion of urine is the principal way the body excretes water and gets rid of waste. These waste products, if not removed, rapidly can become toxic.

The kidney is a highly specialized organ that eliminates soluble (dissolved in water) waste products of metabolism. Urine is formed in the kidney and is excreted from the body by way of the urinary tract system (Figure 42-1). The kidney also regulates the fluid outside the cells of the body by eliminating certain fluids and returning other fluids, maintaining a careful balance (homeostasis). In this manner, the body is protected from dramatic changes in fluid volume, acidity and alkalinity **(acid/base balance)**, composition, and pressure.

There are two kidneys, one on each side of the body. They are about 11 to 12 cm long and 5 to 6 cm wide. Kidneys are shaped like a lima bean with their concave border directed toward the midline of the body. The left kidney is slightly higher than the right.

Filtration

The kidney filters waste products, salts, and excess fluid from the blood. The filtering unit of the kidney is called the glomerulus. The part of the kidney that concentrates the filtered material is called the tubule. Together, the glomerulus

---

SPOTLIGHT ON CERTIFICATION

RMA Content Outline
- Anatomy and physiology
- Patient education
- Asepsis
- Laboratory procedures

CMA (AAMA) Content Outline
- Systems, including structure, function, related conditions, and diseases
- Patient instruction
- Legislation
- Principles of infection control
- Collecting and processing specimens; diagnostic testing

CMAS Content Outline
- Asepsis in the medical office
- Communication

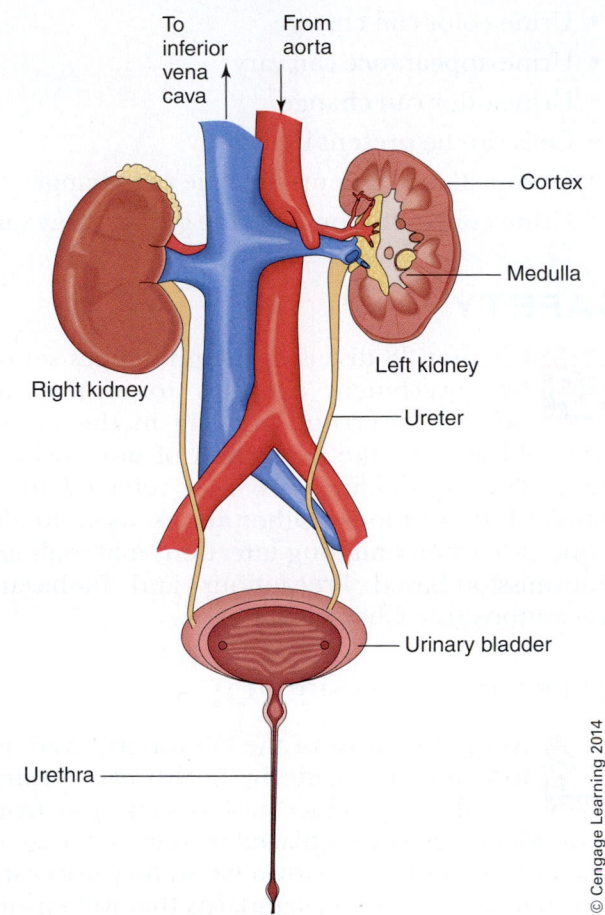

Figure 42-1 The urinary system.

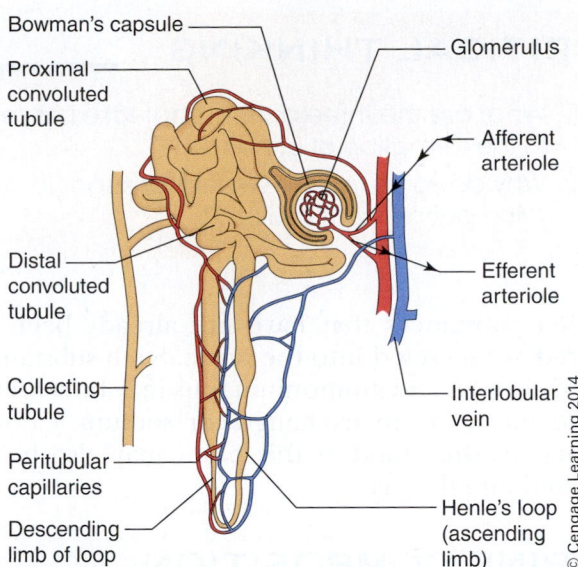

Figure 42-2 Parts of the nephron, including the glomerulus.

and the tubule combine to form the nephron (Figure 42-2).

Most of the work of the kidney is done by the nephrons. There are approximately one million nephrons in each kidney. Each minute, more than 1,000 mL of blood flows through the kidney to be cleansed. In the glomerulus, certain substances are filtered out of the blood. The remaining filtrate then passes into the tubule where various changes occur. Substances filtered out from the body can include water, ammonia, electrolytes, glucose, amino acids, **creatinine**, and **urea**. These wastes leave the body in the eliminated urine.

For example, when diabetics have excess sugar in their blood, the body attempts to eliminate the excess glucose through the urine. Routine urinalysis testing will reveal the excess glucose, alerting the provider to the presence of too much glucose. In this manner, diabetes can be investigated, and it can be an indication that a patient with diabetes is not taking enough insulin to control the glucose in the blood.

Reabsorption

While passing through the kidney, some substances may need to be reabsorbed by the blood. Approximately 180 L of filtrate is produced daily by the body, but only 1 to 2 L of urine is eliminated from the normally functioning human body. Therefore, much of the filtrate, including water, sodium, chloride, potassium, bicarbonate, glucose, calcium, and amino acids, is reabsorbed into the body.

Under normal conditions, blood cells and most proteins stay in the blood plasma because they are too large to pass through the walls of the capillaries of the glomerulus. If blood cells and excess protein are found in the urine, the provider is alerted that the kidney is not filtering properly due to an irregular condition affecting the urinary tract.

As long as the concentration of glucose in the blood is less than 180 mg/dL (milligrams per deciliter), the glucose will be completely reabsorbed. If the level increases to more than 180 mg/dL, the glucose is not reabsorbed. Substances such as glucose that are reabsorbed in relation to their concentration in the blood are known as threshold substances. Homeostasis usually requires sugar and protein to be almost completely reabsorbed, whereas other threshold substances such as creatinine, amino acids, potassium, sodium, and chloride are only partially reabsorbed.

Secretion

Near the end of the blood's journey through the kidney, specifically in the distal convoluted tubule, other substances that have not already been filtered are secreted into the urine. Such substances as hydrogen and ammonium ions may be secreted into the urine in exchange for sodium. Certain drugs in the blood at this point may also be secreted into the urine.

URINE COMPOSITION

After urine progresses through a healthy kidney, it is approximately 96% water and 4% dissolved substances, most of which come from either dietary intake or metabolic waste products. These substances are primarily urea, salt, sulfates, and phosphates. Abnormal constituents of urine include red and white blood cells, fat, glucose, casts, bile, acetone, and hemoglobin (Table 42-1).

When certain disease processes occur in the human body, the following changes in urine production and composition can occur:

- The amount of urine excreted can increase or decrease

Table 42-1 Normal and Abnormal Substances in Urine

Normal	Abnormal
Urea	Bile
Uric acid	Blood
Creatinine	Fat
Sodium	Glucose
Potassium	Protein
Ammonium	White blood cells
Sulfate	Urobilinogen
Chloride	Microorganisms (bacteria, parasites)

© Cengage Learning 2014

- Urine color can change
- Urine appearance can vary
- Urine odor can change
- Cells can be present in urine
- Chemical constituents in urine can change
- Urine concentration (specific gravity) may vary

SAFETY

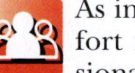 Chapter 38 discusses the guidelines set up by government agencies to ensure the safety of everyone working in the health care field and for the protection of our environment. These guidelines are now referred to as Standard Precautions. Other terms used to describe care when handling infectious materials are Transmission-Based Precautions and biohazard precautions (see Chapter 22).

QUALITY CONTROL

As in every area of the laboratory, every effort must be made by health care professionals to produce test results free from error. Much pressure is placed by regulatory agencies on facilities that perform laboratory tests such as urinalysis to maintain standards that will ensure reliable results. Quality control (QC) programs are an important part of urine testing to ensure accurate and reliable results for the patient. QC programs must be incorporated into every urine

PRECAUTIONS TO USE WHEN HANDLING URINE SPECIMENS

- Treat all specimens as if they were infectious, handling them with gloved hands.
- Avoid splashes or creation of aerosols when handling or disposing of urine specimens. Wearing face shields will prevent splashes from getting into the eyes, nose, or mouth.
- Process urine specimens as soon as possible.
- Store urine specimens appropriately in a designated refrigerator that contains no food or drink items.
- Dispose of urine appropriately, possibly in a designated sink (run water to wash the specimen into the drain) or toilet.

testing procedure. Because many of the tests are interpreted by visual examination, the QC procedures are dependent on the expertise of the person performing the examination.

Testing protocols must be written out and available to personnel. Records of testing must be maintained. Equipment and instruments used for urine testing must be maintained and checked daily for proper calibration. If the instrument should require recalibration, the manufacturer's instructions are provided with the instrument.

Always be careful to perform the QC procedures *exactly* as you perform the procedures on actual patient samples. Documentation of the performance of daily control testing must be kept for at least 3 years. With computer storage, the data can be stored indefinitely. Commercially available urine control samples can be purchased from a number of manufacturers. Positive and negative controls should be run each day on all tests to be performed. Control results should be recorded on a daily log for easy access. The control samples should be stored as directed by the manufacturer.

CLINICAL LABORATORY IMPROVEMENT AMENDMENTS OF 1988 (CLIA '88)

The regulations under the new CLIA are discussed in Chapter 38. Several CLIA '88 regulations apply to the medical assistant performing urine testing. They include:

- Appropriate training in the methodology of the test being performed

- Understanding of urine-testing QC procedures

- Proficiency in the use of instrumentation, being able to troubleshoot problems

- Knowledge of the stability and proper storage of reagents (substances involved in urine testing)

- Awareness of factors that influence test results

- Knowledge of how to verify test results

- The microscopic examination of urine is designated by CLIA to be a PPMP (provider-performed microscopy procedure) and therefore must be performed by a provider. The medical assistant is trained and able to prepare the slide for viewing and reading by the provider. The medical assistant should always take the opportunity to view the slide and discuss the finding with the provider as part of professional development and continued education.

URINE CONTAINERS

The first step toward achieving proper results during laboratory testing is proper collection of the specimen to be tested. There are a variety of containers (Figure 42-3) used for urine collection, including nonsterile containers for random specimens (urinalysis), sterile containers for cultures (testing specimens for growth of bacteria), and 24-hour collection containers with added preservatives.

Just before handing the urine specimen cup to the patient, label the cup with the patient's name, the date, and the time. Some facilities require more information, so follow the protocol of your facility. Always use a permanent marker so the information stays clear. Always label the cup, not the lid. This practice ensures that the specimen will not be separated from the label if the lid is removed. If the patient is unable to procure a specimen, discard the cup and then give the patient a new cup if the patient is later able to give a specimen.

EHR When using electronic medical records, computer-generated labels can be printed. One label can be applied to the cup and other labels used for additional tests ordered, if appropriate. An example of an additional lab test is a culture and sensitivity of the urine, as explained later in this chapter.

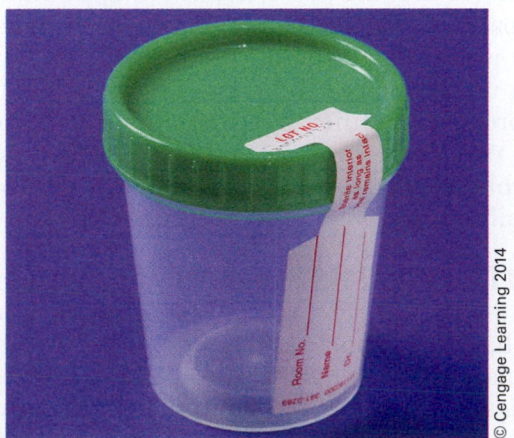

© Cengage Learning 2014

Figure 42-3 Urine collection containers should be calibrated, clear, and have a secure lid.

Occasionally, a patient will bring a sample with him or her in a generic container from home. General recommendations are to provide the patient with a new urine specimen cup and request a fresh sample. The exception to this rule would be if the patient has brought a "first morning void" specimen in an appropriate container.

URINE COLLECTION

Urine Specimen Types

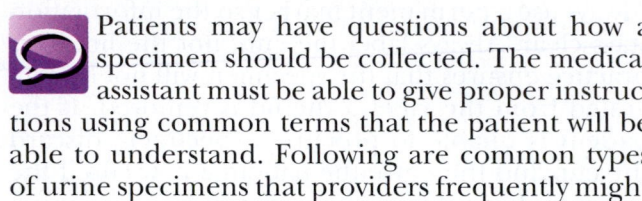 Patients may have questions about how a specimen should be collected. The medical assistant must be able to give proper instructions using common terms that the patient will be able to understand. Following are common types of urine specimens that providers frequently might order.

Random (Spot) Specimen. Random (spot) urine samples are specimens that can be obtained at any time and are the most common collection performed in the outpatient setting. Random simply means that there is no particular time placed on the collection. Patients are requested to give a specimen whenever they are present for their appointment. If the patient has already voided, not knowing a specimen would be required, the medical assistant may offer the patient several cups of water in an attempt to procure another specimen. Because the kidneys constantly produce urine, the patient should be able to provide another specimen within 15 to 20 minutes of drinking several cups of water.

First Morning Void Specimen. The first morning void is typically the most concentrated specimen and has a higher acid pH (which helps preserve the cellular components). It is preferred, but because it is less convenient, it is seldom ordered unless the patient is an inpatient or is in a controlled setting.

Fasting/Timed Specimens. A fasting (going without food and drink except water) urine specimen is ordered less often than a random specimen. The provider may want to measure a urinary substance without interference from food intake. Some providers may require an overnight fast. Others may ask the patient to have a meal and then urinate four hours later.

It is up to the medical assistant to give the patient proper instruction as to how to collect a fasting, or timed, specimen. Written directions given to the patient in addition to oral instructions are best. A regular urinalysis container can be used for a fasting specimen. It does not require a sterile container.

Twenty-Four-Hour Specimen. Urine varies in its concentration of certain substances at different times during any 24-hour period because of circadian rhythm and the intake of food and water. For instance, the amount of water excreted is greatest from 10 to noon and from 4 to 6 PM. Chloride is in its highest concentration from noon to 2 PM. Therefore, a 24-hour specimen is sometimes requested when quantitative tests (measuring the amount) for different substances are desired. The results of this type of collection then will be expressed in *units per 24 hours*. Some commonly tested substances include sodium, potassium, calcium, and creatinine.

The container used to collect this amount of urine should be of adequate size. Usually a one-gallon, dark-colored plastic bottle is used. For measuring urine constituents, preservatives need to be added to the bottle before the collection begins. Without the preservative, these substances may break down and be impossible to quantify. Preservatives include thymol, toluene, and certain acids.

Urine collected over a 24-hour period may be refrigerated between collections. After the collection is complete, it must be returned to the medical laboratory as soon as possible.

Many 24-hour urine bottles contain preservatives. Some preservatives are strong acids or bases. As with all laboratory chemicals, the medical assistant and the patient should avoid contact between the preservative and the skin. The urine specimen should be collected into a smaller container and then poured carefully into the main container. Vapors must not be inhaled when adding the specimen to the container. The patient's written instructions should contain a warning about avoiding contact with preservatives.

Providers sometimes choose to have a 2-hour or a 12-hour specimen instead of the usual 24-hour collection. All of the collection steps for a 24-hour specimen apply. Recording the time of day is important.

Collection Methods

In addition to ordering the type of urine specimen desired (random, fasting, 24-hour), the provider might also order a certain type of collection method to collect the specific sample. These methods include clean-catch midstream and catheterized collection.

Clean-Catch Midstream Collection.
To avoid as much contamination as possible when collecting a specimen, providers prefer that the patient cleanse the genital area before collection. The clean-catch order means that cleansing towelettes are provided in addition to a urine container. Male patients are directed to cleanse the urethral opening twice with cleansing towelettes, and female patients are directed to cleanse the urethral area with three swipes, using three separate towelettes. (See Patient Education box and Procedure 42-7 for complete instructions.) Female patients should also be instructed to notify the medical assistant if they are menstruating during the collection.

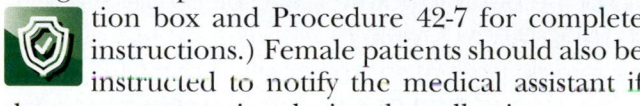

After cleansing, the patient should begin to urinate into the toilet. The patient begins urinating, pulls the cup into the urine stream and collects the sample, then removes the cup from the stream and voids the rest of the urine into the toilet. This is called a midstream specimen. The midstream urine should be as free of contamination as possible.

Catheterized Collection.
Urinary catheterization involves insertion of a sterile flexible tube into the urinary bladder through the urethra. Although urinary catheterization is performed for many reasons, this section discusses only the use of catheterization as a way to obtain a urinary sample (see Procedures 30-22 and 30-23).

Obtaining a urine specimen by catheterization is required when a completely sterile specimen is needed or when the patient is unable to follow cleansing instructions. The patient may not understand the language, may be mentally unable to comprehend the instructions, or may be physically unable to perform the process. It is the medical assistant's responsibility to determine if the patient understands the instructions for obtaining a clean-catch **midstream** urine sample and is able to perform the process.

Catheterization is a sterile procedure and is only performed under a provider's order and only by health care professionals who have been adequately trained. Because the urinary bladder is considered a sterile environment, if the catheterization is not performed properly, bacteria may be introduced into the patient's bladder, which can cause a bladder infection.

CULTURE AND SENSITIVITY OF URINE

Occasionally, the provider orders a culture and sensitivity (C&S) of a urine specimen. The medical assistant is responsible for preparing the sample for transport. A commonly used system is the urine culture and sensitivity transport kit (see Procedure 42-6).

EXAMINATION OF URINE

Urine should be examined in a fresh state, preferably while still warm if possible. However, on rare occasion the urine sample cannot be tested immediately. If immediate testing is not possible, the

---

PATIENT EDUCATION

24-Hour Urine Collection

1. When giving a patient any type of instructions, make sure that the patient understands the importance of each step. Always provide written instructions as well. Emphasize that failing to follow the instructions will cause the results to be invalid, requiring another collection.

2. The patient begins a 24-hour collection by emptying the bladder and not keeping the specimen. The container is then labeled with the time of bladder emptying. Patients generally start the collection between 6 and 8 PM, but any 24-hour period is acceptable.

3. Explain that each time the patient urinates within the 24-hour period, the urine is transferred into the collection container.

4. Instruct the patient to refrigerate the container between urinations if required.

5. Explain that at the end of the 24-hour period, the patient should urinate and transfer the urine into the container. The exact time should be written on the label as the "ended" or "completed" time.

6. The most common errors in the 24-hour urine specimen collection are the inclusion of the first voided specimen and the discarding of one or more of the voided specimens during the 24-hour period. Be sure the patient understands these steps.

PATIENT EDUCATION

Clean-Catch, Midstream Urine Specimen Collection Instructions

1. The patient should be provided with a clean or sterile covered urine cup, a pair of gloves, and adequate cleansing towelettes (three for female patients, two for male patients). The cup should be labeled with the patient's name and the date. Caution the patient not to contaminate the inside of the cup. A shelf near the toilet is extremely helpful for patients, allowing them to have the towelettes and cup within reach during collection of the specimen.

2. Instruct the patient in proper cleansing of the genital area. It is best to give the patient written instructions as well. Men and women should have separate instructions. The written instructions should be posted next to the toilet for reference by the patient during the procedure. Logically, the female instructions should be posted on the wall beside the toilet at reading level while she is sitting, and the male instructions should be posted on the wall behind the toilet at reading level while he is standing. Laminating the instruction documents protects the writing from any sprays or splashes.

   - *Men.* After thoroughly washing his hands, the male patient should retract the foreskin on the penis (if not circumcised). A cleansing towelette should be used to cleanse the urethral opening with a single stroke directed from the tip of the penis toward the ring of the glans. The cleansing procedure should be repeated again using a new towelette.

   - *Women.* After thoroughly washing her hands, the female patient should position herself comfortably on the toilet seat and spread her knees as far apart as she can. She should spread the outer vulval folds and hold them open with one hand. With the other hand, using the first towelette, the patient should cleanse on one side from front to back with one swipe, disposing of the towelette into the toilet. With the second towelette, she should wipe on the other side front to back with one swipe, disposing of that towelette into the toilet. While still holding the vulval folds open, she should use the third towelette to wipe the urethral opening front to back with one swipe. She may dispose of that towelette into the toilet, too. She should continue to hold the vulval folds open until she has completed the collection of the urine specimen.

3. Instruct the patient also about the midstream collection technique. Explain why it is necessary. These instructions should also be written and included with the clean-catch written directions.

   - After cleansing the area using the clean-catch directions, the patient should begin to void into the toilet. The specimen cup should then be held into the stream until it is about half full, then the cup should be removed from the stream. Assure the patient that urinalysis can be performed on a small amount of urine if they are unable to give half a cup. The patient may finish urinating into the toilet. Only the middle portion of the urine flow is included in the sample. After the specimen has been collected, the container should be capped. After securely capping the urine cup, the patient may cleanse the outside of the cup if desired. The patient should always avoid touching the inside of both the container and the lid.

4. The patient should be instructed on where/how to return the specimen to the medical assistant. Some providers' office laboratories (POLs) have a special shelf with a small door opening into the laboratory, whereas other offices prefer the patient actually hand the specimen to the medical assistant directly. Either way, the specimen should be taken immediately into the laboratory by the medical assistant.

5. All surface areas in the restroom should be immediately decontaminated in preparation for the next patient.

urine should be refrigerated at about 4°C (39°F) or stored on ice. The urinalysis should be performed as soon as possible, preferably within 2 hours. **Crystals** and **casts** begin to break down after 2 hours. Any time delay allows bacteria to multiply and can lead to inaccurate microbiology results.

The routine urinalysis procedure is composed of three parts:

- *Physical* examination of the urine
- *Chemical* examination of the urine
- *Microscopic* examination of urine sediment

 The medical assistant should wash hands, put on gloves, and follow all the safety guidelines when performing any of the following procedures. Some facilities require eye protection when pouring urine or performing any procedure where splashing of urine into the eye could occur. All surface areas in the restroom should be decontaminated immediately after procuring or testing urine specimens.

Physical Examination of Urine

When the medical assistant begins the process of performing a urinalysis, the first step is performing the physical examination. This examination consists of:

- Assessing the volume of the urine specimen, making sure that the amount is sufficient for testing
- Observing and recording the color, appearance, and transparency of the specimen
- Noting any unusual urine odor
- Measuring the specific gravity of the specimen

Procedure 42-1 describes how to assess the volume, color, appearance, transparency, and odor of urine. Procedure 42-2 describes testing for the specific gravity.

Specimen Volume. The first step in performing a urinalysis is to determine if the sample's volume is adequate for testing.

The medical assistant must have enough urine to fill a test tube with at least 10 mL (about two teaspoons) of urine with enough leftover in the specimen cup to completely insert and wet a chemical reagent strip and to culture if ordered.

The volume usually requested of the patient is a half cup, but patients should be assured that samples of much less volume can be tested. If the patient is only able to submit a small volume of urine, the provider will determine priority of which tests to perform according to the patient's suspected diagnosis. For example, if only a test for protein and glucose is requested, then only enough urine

to process the chemical reagent strip portion is needed. However, if a test for microscopic examination of the urine, such as to diagnose a bladder infection, is requested, then a full test tube is needed as well as some extra urine for a culture. These tests are thoroughly discussed later in this chapter.

The provider should be consulted for further direction if the amount of urine submitted is less than needed for the complete urinalysis. The urinalysis report should reflect that the quantity was not sufficient for complete testing. The medical assistant should write "QNS" (quantity not sufficient), where applicable, or follow clinic protocol.

If the patient is able to give less than 10 mL of urine for the test tube, the medical assistant should make a note of the amount of urine used. For example, if the patient provides 5 mL, the medical assistant may go ahead with the microscopic examination of urine but should note on the report that the specimen was only 5 mL. The rationale for this notation becomes clear when you understand that the amount of a substance found in 10 mL of urine will be less in a smaller sample. In other words, if the patient has five white blood cells in 10 mL of urine, he or she might only have two to three white blood cells in 5 mL of urine. Unless the notation is made that the sample was smaller, the provider may diagnose incorrectly.

Most clinics/POLs do not require that the urine volume be noted unless it is less than adequate for a complete urinalysis.

Urine Color. There is a wide range of color in normal urine, usually ranging from a pale yellow to a dark yellow or amber (Figure 42-4). The range of color usually is the result of the concentration of the urine. A darker color generally indicates

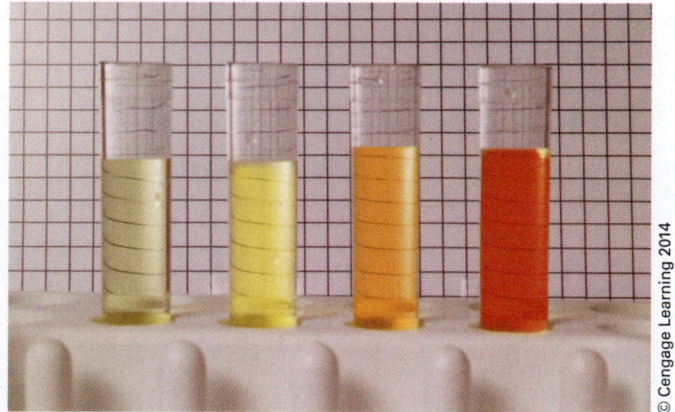

Figure 42-4 Normal urine can range in color from straw and yellow, to amber. Abnormal urine (depending on its constituents) can be red, brown, fluorescent orange, and more.

© Cengage Learning 2014

a more concentrated urine. The color of urine comes from normal metabolic processes, the end products of which are deposited in the urine.

After assessing the adequacy of the urine volume, the medical assistant then observes and records the color of the urine (see Procedure 42-1).

The diet and certain drugs can add substances to the urine that give it a specific color. The medical assistant should be familiar with common reasons for abnormally colored urine and whether they are pathologic (due to a disease process) or nonpathologic abnormalities. For example, the most common pathologic cause of red urine is the presence of red blood cells, known as **hematuria**. Red blood cells in urine may indicate bleeding in the urinary tract either because of a bladder infection or a kidney stone. A nonpathologic example of abnormally colored urine is the medication phenazopyridine (Pyridium), which can turn the urine bright orange. Table 42-2 lists several urine color variations and possible causes.

Urine Transparency. In order to assess transparency, the urine should be viewed through a clear cup or tube. Urine is considered clear if a line of print can be read through it. Urine transparency normally is not significant by itself. However, it may be helpful when included with the rest of the urinalysis information. Transparency

Table 42-2 Urine Colors and Possible Causes

Color	Possible Cause
Straw to yellow	Normal
Orange to amber	Concentrated urine
Colorless	Dilute urine
Deep yellow	Vitamin intake
Bright orange	Drugs, usually phenazopyridine (Pyridium)
Orange-brown	Urobilin
Greenish orange	Bilirubin
Smokey	Red blood cells
Wine red/reddish brown	Hemoglobin pigments
Green or blue	Methylene blue

© Cengage Learning 2014

of urine usually is recorded as clear, cloudy, hazy, or **turbid** (opaque) (Procedure 42-1). These descriptive terms may vary in different facilities.

There are many causes of cloudy urine, most of which are considered normal. Cloudiness could be attributed to contamination from vaginal discharges, white blood cells, bacteria, or yeast. As urine cools, sometimes crystals form that may give urine a cloudy appearance.

Urine Odor. With experience, the medical assistant will recognize certain odors in the urine that can indicate specific conditions. Odors, though not recorded on the final laboratory urinalysis report, should not be disregarded. For example, the urine of a diabetic patient who may have a condition known as **ketoacidosis** may have a sweet odor. Urine full of bacteria will have a foul odor that is easily recognized.

Urine Specific Gravity. **Specific gravity** is defined as the ratio of the weight of a given volume of a substance to the weight of the same volume of distilled water at the same temperature. Distilled water used as the reference point has been given the specific gravity value of 1.000. The specific gravity of urine indicates the concentrations of solids such as phosphates, chlorides, proteins, sugars, and urea that are dissolved in urine.

Variations in urine specific gravity can give the provider diagnostic information. In uncontrolled diabetes, glucose is released into the patient's urine. Glucose molecules are dense and may give the urine a high specific gravity. Another reason for high specific gravity readings is dehydration, because less fluid is being released by the body in relation to whatever chemicals are in the urine. The color of this urine will also probably be darker. In a well-hydrated patient, the specific gravity is low, meaning that the urine is mostly water. The normal range of specific gravity for urine is from 1.005 to 1.030. Specific gravity is highest in the first morning samples because the urine is more concentrated.

Specific gravity is often tested by using either a test strip, urinometer, or refractometer. A urinometer is a calibrated, floating device. A **refractometer** measures the amount of light that is bent by particles suspended in a liquid. A specific gravity reading is also available in conjunction with chemical testing on some reagent strips. The urinometer is the least accurate method and perhaps the most difficult; therefore, it is being replaced by either the refractometer or reagent test strips in most POLs.

Urinometer. A urinometer is made from a small glass tube weighted to float in a sample of urine (usually 15 mL). The glass tube has been calibrated, and the stem of the tube has been marked accordingly to read 1.000 at the bottom of the meniscus in distilled

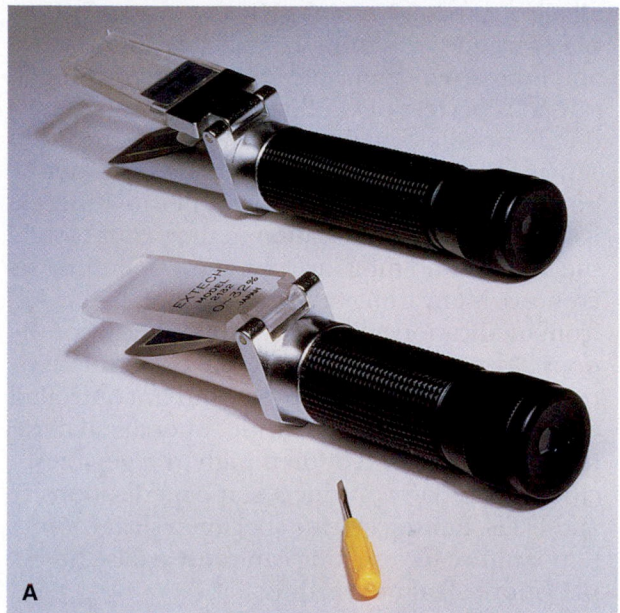

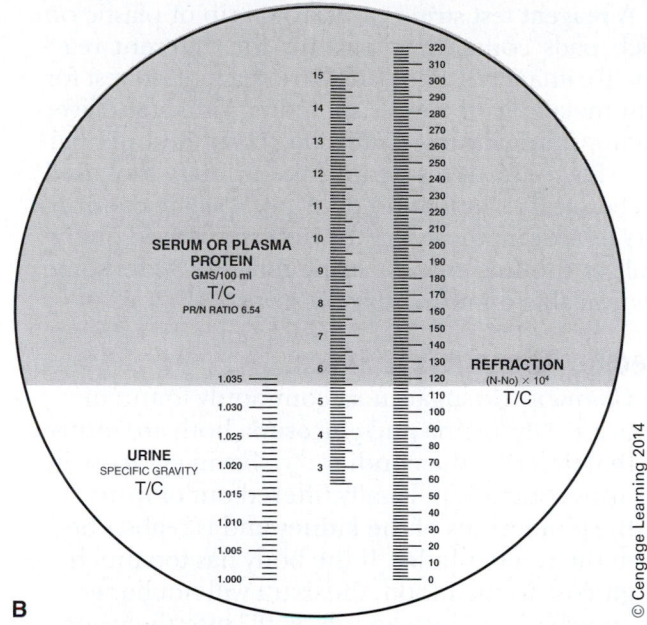

Figure 42-5   (A) Refractometers. (B) Specific gravity as viewed through a refractometer.

water at room temperature. The meniscus is the curvature that appears in a liquid's upper surface when the liquid is placed in a container. The medical assistant reads the specific gravity of the urine from the stem at the meniscus. However, the temperature of the urine must be taken into account if it differs from 70°F, which is normal room temperature. The buoyancy of a liquid changes with the temperature. If the urine is allowed to come to room temperature, the medical assistant risks the physical and chemical changes that can occur to urine when left for more than 20 minutes. It is because of these and other conflicting processes (such as human error) that the urinometer is not recommended as the best option for measuring the weight (specific gravity) of urine.

Refractometer. The most common tool for determining the specific gravity of liquids is the refractometer (Figures 42-5A and B). This instrument measures the refractive index of urine, which is the speed at which light travels through the air as compared with the speed at which it passes through urine. Light is slowed, and therefore bent, as it encounters particles—the more particles, the more bend. The bend can be used to determine the total number of particles and is not affected by the weight of the particles.

The refractometer reading is about 0.002 less than that of the true specific gravity. This slight difference is more than made up for by the ease of using the instrument and the instrument's reliability. This instrument only needs a drop or two of urine, and the result does not have to be adjusted for temperature as long as the temperature is between 60° and 100°F (see Procedure 42-2).

Reagent Test Strips. Reagent test strips that include specific gravity are available through many medical laboratory supply companies. Look for SG in the name, such as brands MultiStix 10 SG or Chemstrip 10 SG (the "10" designates there are 10 tests included on those particular test strips). Keep in mind that the more tests available on the reagent test strips, the more expensive the product will be.

Chemical Examination of Urine

After the physical testing of a urine specimen, the next step in urinalysis testing is chemical testing. This procedure once was complex, but today many manufacturers have made the task simple through a wide range of ready-to-use reagents and the reagent test strip (Figure 42-6).

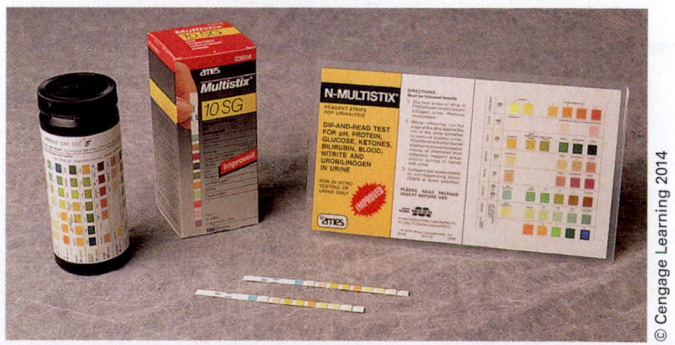

Figure 42-6   Chemical reagent test strips with color-coded chart.

A **reagent test strip** is a narrow strip of plastic on which pads containing reagents for different reactions are attached. The pads have reagents to test for many metabolic processes, including kidney and liver functions, **urinary tract infection (UTI)**, and **pH** balance. The reagent test strip is the primary tool used for chemical examination of urine. Specific confirmatory tests or methods may be necessary based on the result of the reagent test strip. Table 42-3 lists some tests available on urine reagent strips.

Specific Reagent Test Strips.

- *Glucose* is the sugar most commonly found in urine. Glycosuria and **glucosuria** both are terms that describe the condition of having glucose in urine. Sugar is normally filtered out of urine in the glomerulus of the kidney and is reabsorbed in the renal tubules. If the body has too much glucose in the blood, the extra will not be reabsorbed and instead will "spill" into the urine. Reagent test strips are embedded with an enzyme called glucose oxidase, which detects glucose. Of course the first pathological condition we think of for glucosuria is diabetes, but other nonpathological conditions can cause some glucose to spill into the urine. Glucose is stored by the liver and used for energy. Although unusual, conditions such as extreme physical or emotional stress can cause the liver to put a lot of glucose into the blood. Eating an unusual amount of sugar can also cause high amounts of glucose in the blood and either of these conditions can cause excess glucose to be lost in the urine. These nonpathological causes are some of the reasons further testing is required before a diagnosis of diabetes can be made.

- *pH* is the abbreviation for potential hydrogen ion concentration. The pH test determines if the urine is alkaline or acidic. The scale for pH runs from 0 for the most acidic to 14 for the most

alkaline or base. Neutral pH, of course, is 7. The pH of urine varies from 4.5 to 8. The kidneys and lungs are responsible for helping the blood stay at its perfect pH (7.35 to 7.45). The kidneys do this by adjusting the substances they secrete. A person can die if the blood is too acidic (acidosis) or too alkaline (alkalosis). Because there is so little room for deviation in the pH of blood, the kidneys and lungs are constantly adjusting secretions. Many things affect the pH of the urine, from medication and diet to pathological conditions. Diets high in protein, some medications, renal tuberculosis, high fevers, and uncontrolled diabetes can cause acidic urine, whereas alkaline urine can be caused by diets high in vegetables, citrus fruits, dairy products, some medications, and UTIs. Letting a urine specimen sit at room temperature for too long can cause a false high-pH (more alkaline) reading.

- *Protein* (albumin) may be secreted in very small (trace) amounts by the kidneys. The presence of protein in urine (proteinuria) occasionally has a nonpathological basis such as excessive exercise, exposure to extreme heat or cold, or acute emotional stress. Any substantial and/or consistent presence of protein in urine is of concern for renal disease. Proteins are large compounds and can only get through the filtering system (glomerulus) of the kidney if there has been damage to the glomeruli. Think of a volleyball net that a small golf ball could pass through but not a larger basketball, unless there are holes (damage) to the net. Damage can be caused by many things: diseases, toxins, or systemic conditions such as diabetes and uncontrolled hypertension. Any condition that causes the blood pressure to increase in the nephron can also cause damage to the glomeruli. A false high-protein reading can occur when large amounts of WBCs, RBCs, epithelial cells, or bacteria are present in the urine. When these four types of cells rupture in urine, they can release protein, causing a false-positive reading. It is important to note, too, that any protein reading in dilute urine is of concern because a normal SG in the same patient would show a much higher level of proteinuria. Thus, it is important to look at the SG of the specimen whenever protein is found in urine.

- **Ketones** are formed whenever the body uses fat/fatty acids for energy rather than carbohydrates/sugars. This can happen whenever there is a low intake of carbohydrates/sugars such as in dieting and in certain metabolic disorders such

Table 42-3 Chemical Testing Available on Urine Reagent Test Strips

pH	Blood
Protein	**Urobilinogen**
Glucose	Nitrite
Ketones	**Leukocyte esterase**
Bilirubin	Specific gravity

© Cengage Learning 2014

as diabetes. In diabetes, the body lacks insulin or is unable to use sugar properly for energy, so it uses fatty acids. Insulin is a chemical that helps the body use sugar for energy, so some diabetics replace their insulin. As fats are broken down, ketone bodies form and "spill" into the urine. The presence of ketones in urine is called **ketonuria**. The burning of fats for energy is called *ketosis* or sometimes *lipolysis*. Persons on carbohydrate-careful diets often use chemical reagent test strips to check if their urine contains ketones, thus indicating that their bodies are burning fats. **Ketosis** should not be confused with ketoacidosis, which is a dangerous condition for diabetics and alcoholics.

- **Bilirubin** is a yellow-orange substance that comes from the breakdown of hemoglobin. Hemoglobin is contained within the red blood cells. Because individual RBCs live for only 120 days, they are constantly breaking down and being replaced. When the RBCs "die," the "heme" part of the hemoglobin circulates in the blood until the liver filters it out. The liver is responsible for changing the heme into a water-soluble substance called bilirubin. Before it gets to the liver, it is called "indirect" or "free" bilirubin. After it leaves the liver, it is called direct or conjugated bilirubin. The liver sends the conjugated bilirubin to the gall bladder where it is released with bile into the small intestine. When there is a blockage in the liver or gall bladder ducts or when there is a disorder or disease of the liver, the bilirubin cannot get past the gall bladder to the small intestine, so it continues to circulate in the blood. This excess of bilirubin in the blood can lead to yellow-orange skin called *jaundice*. The body will try to get rid of extra bilirubin through the urine. Hence, any detection of bilirubin in the urine **(bilirubinuria)** can be indicative of a problem in the liver and/or gall bladder. Newborn babies can be jaundiced because their systems are not mature enough to rid the bile. Because bilirubin breaks down in sunlight, we treat jaundiced babies with special "bili-lights" to help them break down the bilirubin in their skin. Knowing that bilirubin is so unstable, we need to protect it from light in our urine samples, another good reason to test urine samples immediately. Keep in mind that further testing is required before a diagnosis can be made, because bilirubinuria is a symptom, not a disease.

- *Blood* in urine is called *hematuria*. If the blood in the urine is not from a nonpathogenic source, such as a contaminate from menstruation, it is indicative of a bladder infection (often called a *urinary tract infection* [UTI]), irritation of the urinary tract from a kidney stone, or, rarely, a neoplasm. Many chemical reagent test strips differentiate between hemoglobin and intact red blood cells. Hemoglobin in urine is called *hemoglobinuria* and can indicate pathogenic conditions such as severe infectious diseases, transfusion reactions, and hemolytic anemias. A nonpathogenic cause of hemoglobinuria occurs when the urine is allowed to sit too long, so any RBCs present start breaking down, thus releasing their hemoglobin. Sometimes the chemical reagent test strips indicate the presence of blood in the urine, but no blood cells are seen during the microscopic examination. This is an example of hemoglobin being present rather than the intact RBCs. The presence of blood in urine is combined with the patient symptoms and other tests to arrive at a diagnosis.

- *Urobilinogen* is a substance formed when bacteria in the digestive tract breaks down bilirubin. A very small percentage is excreted in the urine and is increased in liver disease. Urobilinogen gives color to feces.

- *Nitrite* forms in urine when certain pathogenic bacteria are present. These specific bacteria convert normal nitrate in urine to abnormal nitrite; thus, nitrite in urine is always indicative of the presence of these pathogenic bacteria in sufficient quantities to cause a bladder infection. Whenever nitrite is positive in a urine sample, white blood cells, bacteria, and often red blood cells also will be seen. The provider often orders a urine culture to determine the type of bacteria and the best medication to eradicate it.

- *Leukocytes* are white blood cells. They may be either granulocytes or agranulocytes. Either type can fight urinary tract infectious bacteria, and either type may be present in infected urine. You will learn more about specific WBCs in another chapter. The chemical reagent test strips will only detect esterase from granulocytes and will not detect the presence of agranulocytes, so a microscopic examination is still important as well as a urine culture and sensitivity. These results along with the patient's symptoms will help the provider diagnose and treat the UTI.

- *Specific gravity* (SG) has been discussed previously in this chapter and is available as a test option on many brands of chemical reagent test strips. The normal SG for urine is between 1.005 (very dilute urine) to 1.030 (concentrated urine).

Reagent Test Strip Quality Control.

Reagent test strips are easy to use, but the complexity of the chemical testing should not be overlooked. As with any chemical reaction, each test involves multiple steps that are sensitive to temperature, time, dilution, and other factors. Outdated strips or reagents should never be used, so be sure to check the expiration date every time. To get optimum results, a certain amount of care must be taken when handling and storing the reagent strips. They must not be exposed to moisture, volatile substances, direct sunlight, or excess heat. The strips should not be removed from their original container except at the time of use. Always follow the manufacturer's instructions for storage. Test results are represented by a color change. The test result is compared with a color chart on the label of the reagent test strip container. Employees performing this test should be tested for color blindness as many of the color changes are subtle.

Reagent test strips are ready to use directly from their container. Correct QC procedures should be followed as required by CLIA '88 and the facility where the testing is performed. This usually includes using a QC urine sample (with predetermined results). All that is needed for this testing are the strips, QC specimen, and patient specimens. Procedure 42-3 explains how to perform a urinalysis chemical examination.

Automated urine analyzers (Figure 42-7) capable of timing and reading the test strip are available.

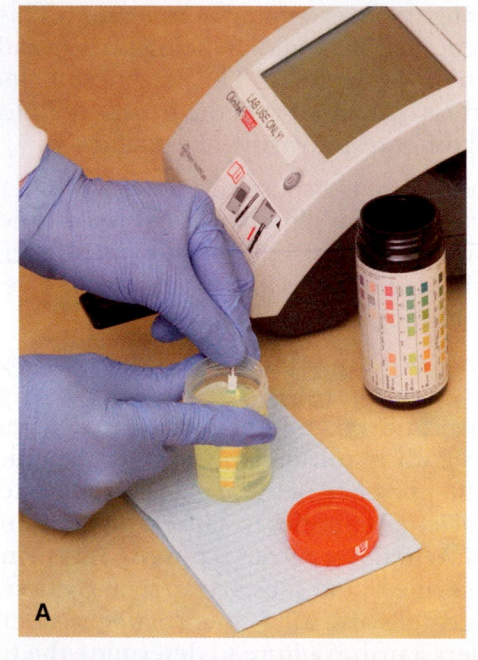

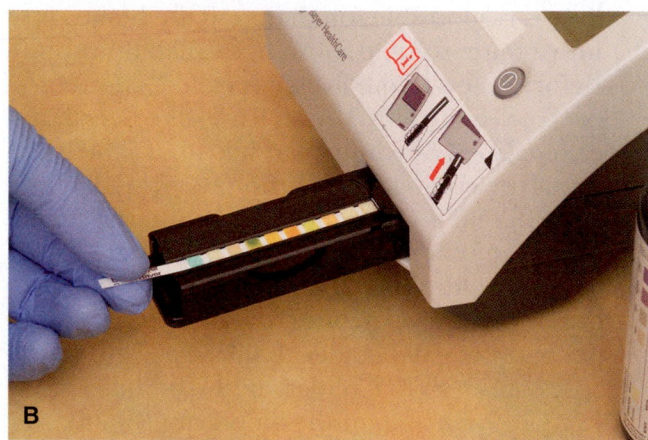

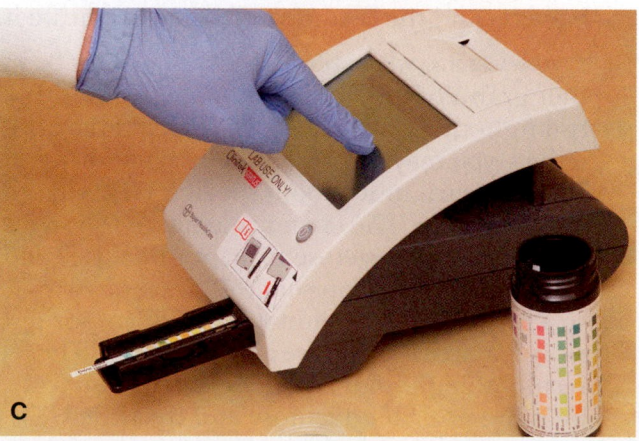

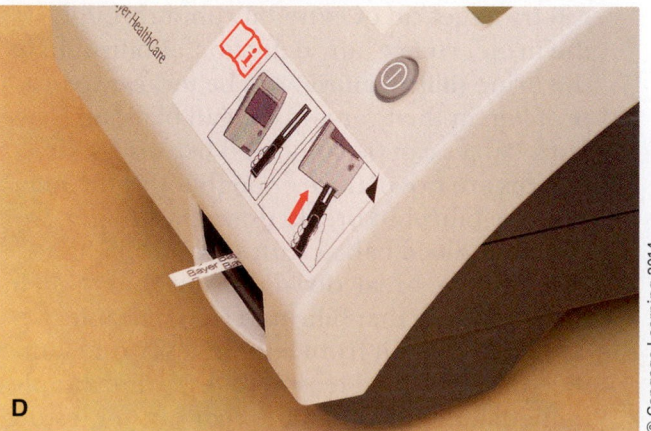

Figure 42-7 Automated urine analyzers are used frequently because of their accuracy. (A) The reagent strip is immersed in the urine specimen and then tapped lightly on a paper towel to remove excess urine. (B) The strip is placed into the machine. (C, D) The test is selected, and the machine pulls the strip into the machine to be analyzed.

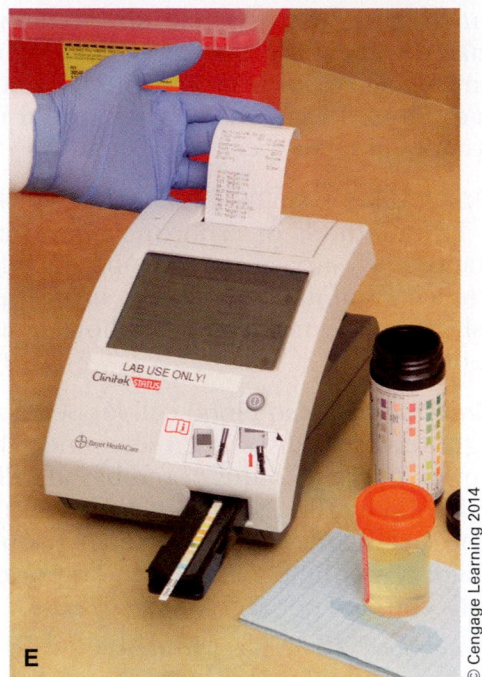

© Cengage Learning 2014

Figure 42-7 (*continued*) (E) Results are printed from the machine.

These instruments can be expensive and are not available in small laboratories. Currently, automated urine analyzers are used more frequently because they are more accurate and reduce human error.

When reporting results, it is important to use the proper units and terms as directed by your laboratory. An example of the sensitivity of the reagent strips is shown in Table 42-4 (there is variation in sensitivity among manufacturers).

Microscopic Examination of Urine Sediment

In addition to the physical and chemical examination of urine, the medical assistant should be familiar with the microscopic examination of urine. CLIA '88 considers the microscopic examination of urine to be a PPMP and not within the category of waived tests. Nevertheless, the medical assistant must be able to properly centrifuge the specimen

Table 42-4   Reagent Strip Sensitivity

Test	Range	Normal Value
pH	5–9	5–8
Protein	Negative to positive*	Negative
Glucose	Negative to >1,000 mg/dL	Negative
Ketone	Negative to >80 mg/dL	Negative
Bilirubin	Negative to large	Negative
Blood	Negative to large	Negative
Leukocyte esterase	Negative to large	Negative
Nitrites	Negative to positive	Negative
Urobilinogen	0.2–8.0 mg/dL	2.0 mg/dL
Specific gravity	1.000–1.035	Varies greatly

© Cengage Learning 2014

*Note that positive results in a newborn for glucose, ketone, and protein are considered **critical values** and should be reported to the provider immediately.

and set up a slide of the urine sediment for the provider to examine. It is recommended that the medical assistant have a working knowledge of all urine sediment, the pathologic significance of the components, and how to report the presence of sediment components. The **sediment** (insoluble material) at the bottom of the centrifuge tube is used for the microscopic examination (see Chapter 39 for proper use of the microscope). The microscopic examination is helpful in determining kidney disease, disorders of the urinary tract, and systemic disease. It is particularly important that urine be freshly voided and examined as soon as possible to prevent deterioration of sediment components.

One of the most important items to have on hand when performing a microscopic urine examination is a urine color atlas. It takes years to be able to correctly identify abnormal components of urine. A color atlas should always be available to the medical assistant to help with identification.

Some laboratories make use of urine stains to add color to certain structures in the urine sediment. Sedi-Stain® is an example of such a stain (Figure 42-8).

CRITICAL THINKING

If a medical assistant is color blind, does that mean she/he cannot perform the chemical testing of urine? What (if any) accommodations can be made for her/him?

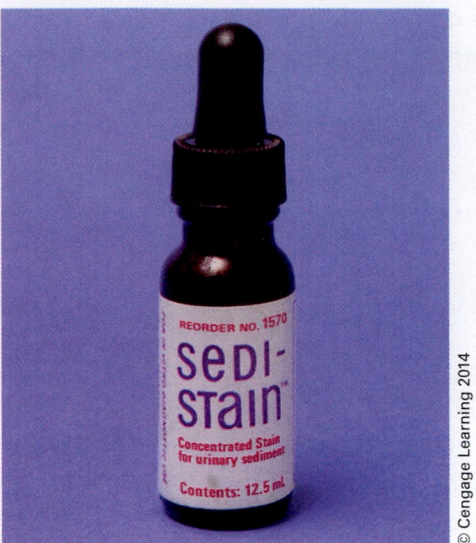

© Cengage Learning 2014

Figure 42-8 Sedi-Stain® is an example of a stain used in laboratories.

Sediment Components. Sediment is obtained by centrifugation of 10 to 15 mL of urine. The solid substances, such as cells and crystals, are forced to the bottom of the test tube, leaving clear fluid called supernatant on the top. The **supernatant** urine is carefully poured off. Most urine test tubes are specifically formed to assist in the process of pouring off all but 1 mL of the supernatant fluid. This is accomplished by quickly inverting the tube completely upside down (do not shake the tube in this position). When returned to the upright position, the 1 mL of fluid will be present in the bottom of the tube, together with the urine sediment. This is the perfect amount of supernatant fluid needed to resuspend the sediment. Try the inversion process first with plain water until you are able to perform it easily. After the supernatant has been poured off, the sediment needs to be resuspended or mixed back into the 1 mL of fluid. This mixing can be accomplished by gently tapping the tube on the counter or flicking it with your finger until the sediment and cellular components have all been mixed and resuspended in the fluid. A drop of sediment is then placed on a slide and examined microscopically.

When viewing a normal urine specimen, the medical assistant may see very little under the microscope. Squamous epithelial cells (Figure 42-9A) may be seen, especially in women. These cells have no medical significance because they are skin cells continuously sloughed off into the urine. They are generally reported as few, moderate, or many. If the provider sees many epithelial cells in the urine

specimen, it is indicative that the specimen is contaminated with skin cells. Better education of the patient of the reasons for and the technique of a clean-catch midstream collection should result in a less contaminated specimen.

Abnormal Urine Sediment Cells and Microorganisms. The methods of reporting abnormal urine sediment may vary among health facilities. Microscopic examination of the urine sediment may show one or more of the following cells and microorganisms:

- *Red blood cells.* Red blood cells appear as pale, light-refractive disks when seen under high power. Large amounts of red blood cells in urine (hematuria) indicate disease or trauma. These cells are counted in a microscopic field (high-power field, or HPF) and reported as cells counted per HPF (e.g., 10/HPF).

- *White blood cells.* A few white blood cells can appear in normal urine. More than four white blood cells in urine often indicate a UTI. White blood cells are slightly larger than red blood cells, may appear granular, and have a visible nucleus (the red blood cell has no nucleus). Figure 42-9B shows white blood cells in urine. White blood cells are reported in the same manner as red blood cells.

- *Renal tubular epithelial cells.* Renal tubular epithelial cells (Figure 42-9C) can indicate kidney disease if they are present in large numbers. They can be confused with both white blood cells and other epithelial cells. Renal and vaginal epithelial cells are smaller than squamous epithelial cells. Renal epithelia are rounder and vaginal epithelia are more oblong with pointed ends. They are also reported in the same manner as white and red blood cells.

- *Bacteria.* Bacteria can appear as tiny round or rod-shaped objects (Figure 42-9D). Rod-shaped bacteria are generally easier to see because round bacteria may appear as **amorphous**, or shapeless, material. Bacteria often seem to be shaking or vibrating. This is called Brownian movement and is caused by the molecules of water bumping against the bacteria. Bacteria can be very active, actually moving across the microscopic field. If many bacteria are seen and the specimen is not an obviously contaminated specimen, the indication is usually a UTI. The provider will consider the patient's symptoms in addition to the results of the urinalysis to make a diagnosis and will often order a C&S of the urine. Bacteria can be reported

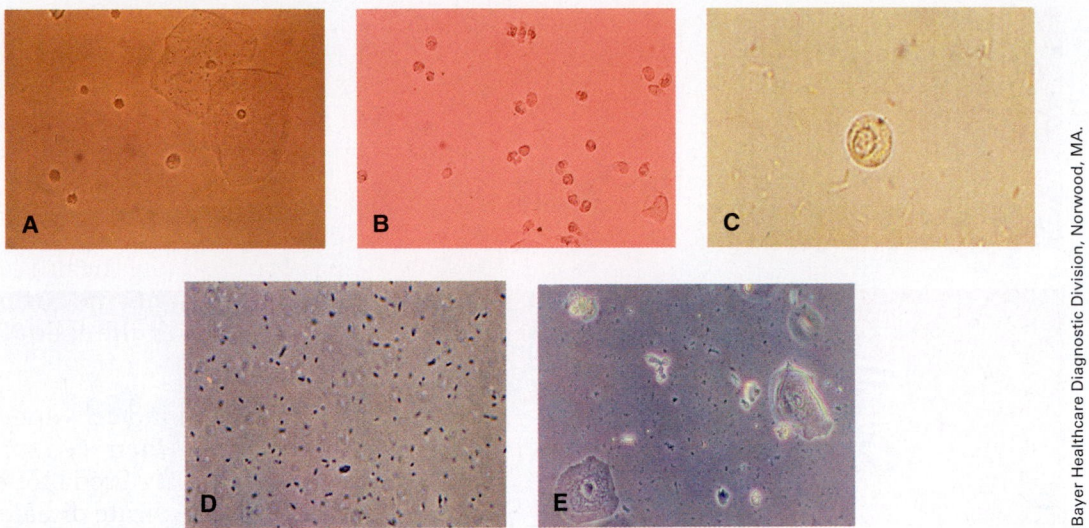

Bayer Healthcare Diagnostic Division, Norwood, MA.

Figure 42-9 (A) Squamous epithelial cells. (B) White blood cells. (C) Renal epithelial cells. (D) Bacteria in urine sediment. (E) Yeasts and squamous epithelial cells.

as few, moderate, or many. If both rod-shaped and round bacteria are seen in the same specimen, they may be reported as mixed bacteria. Mixed bacteria more often indicate a contaminated specimen rather than an infection.

- *Yeast.* Yeast cells (Figure 42-9E) may be present in urine, possibly indicating a yeast infection in the urinary tract. Yeast cells are smaller than red blood cells but may appear similar to them. Yeasts are round and can be observed to be budding. To distinguish between yeast and red blood cells, a drop of dilute acetic acid is added to the urine sediment. The acetic acid will cause the red blood cells to hemolyze, making the yeast more easily viewed. The most common yeast found is *Candida albicans.* Yeasts are reported as the amount per HPF.

- *Parasites.* The most frequently seen parasite in urine is *Trichomonas vaginalis* (Figure 42-10). *Trichomonas* is a parasite that can infect the urinary tract. It is often recognized by the movement of its tail (flagella). Always check with a provider or someone more familiar with these organisms before reporting this organism.

- *Sperm.* Sperm is reported when seen in male and female urine. Sperm have oval bodies with one long, thin flagella (Figure 42-11A).

- *Artifacts.* Hair, fibers, powder, and oil are among the substances that may appear in urine sediment as a result of contamination during collection or later. If a structure cannot be identified using a good urine atlas, it probably is an artifact. A urine atlas will show

illustrations of artifacts. If in doubt, get an expert opinion (Figure 42-11B and C).

Crystals in Urinary Sediment. Crystals make up unorganized urine sediment. Because crystals are interesting, the tendency of the novice examiner is to pay attention to them. However, they are the

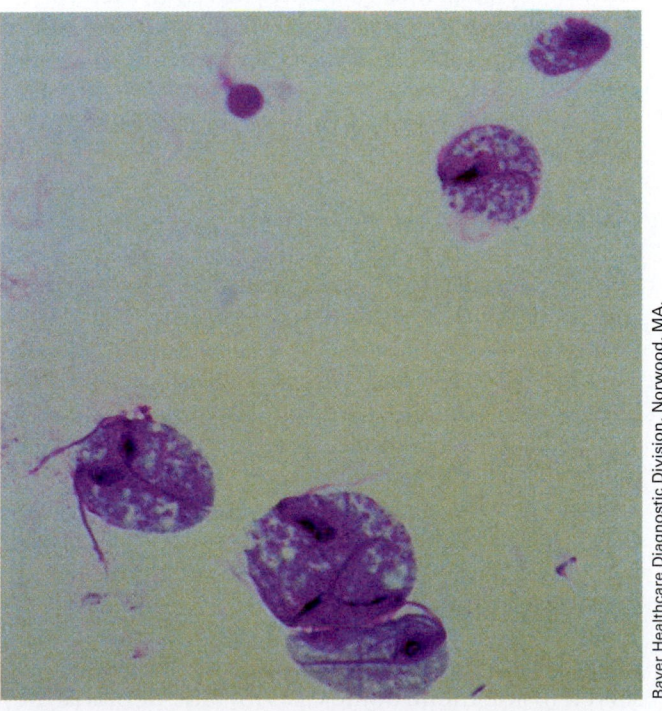

Bayer Healthcare Diagnostic Division, Norwood, MA.

Figure 42-10 *Trichomonas* in stained urine sediment.

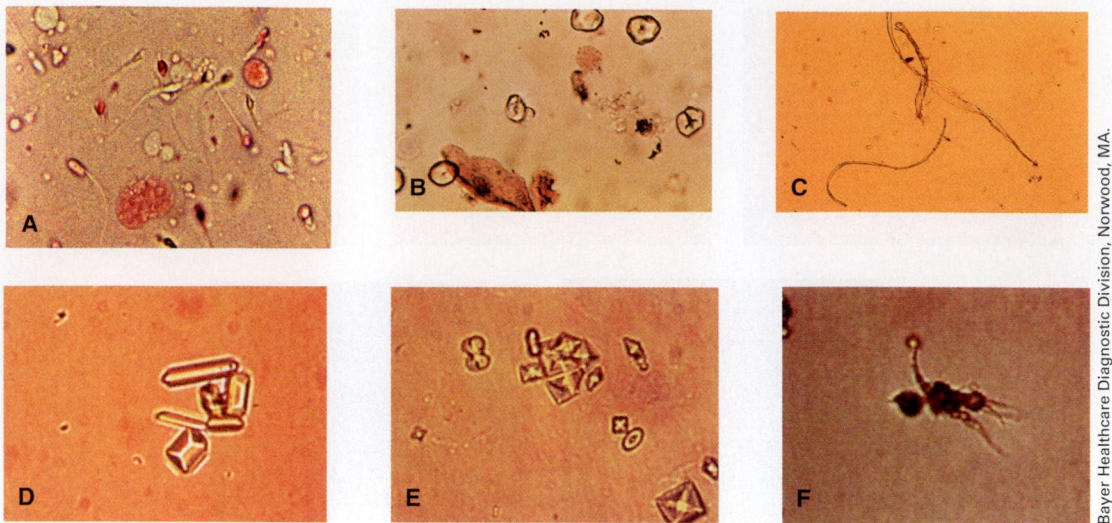

Bayer Healthcare Diagnostic Division, Norwood, MA.

Figure 42-11 Crystals and miscellaneous structures that can appear in urine. (A) Spermatozoa. (B) Starch granules. (C) Cotton fibers. (D) Triple phosphate. (E) Calcium oxalate. (F) Ammonium biurate.

most insignificant part of the urinary sediment. These crystals include calcium phosphate, triple phosphate, calcium oxalate, amorphous phosphates and urates, and calcium carbonate. These crystals generally form as urine specimens stand, especially when refrigerated. Many laboratories do report these crystals. Refer to a urine color atlas to identify crystals. Figures 42-11D–F illustrate several kinds of crystals that can be found in urine.

Some specific crystals in urine that should be particularly noted if seen because they may indicate disease states are uric acid, cystine, and sulfa drug crystals. Refer to a urine atlas for the shape of these crystals.

Casts in Urinary Sediment. Casts are important to see and identify in urine sediment. It takes a great deal of experience and expertise to recognize the many different kinds of casts that can be in sediment.

Casts are formed when protein accumulates and precipitates in the kidney tubules. The casts are then washed into the urine. Most casts are made from a particular type of protein called Tamm-Horsfall mucoprotein. Other proteins can also form casts. Serum proteins can form waxy casts. The presence of casts in the urine may indicate kidney disease.

Casts are cylindrical with rounded or flat ends. They are classified according to the substances observed inside them. Some casts include debris as they are forming and may appear cellular or granular.

The most common cast seen in urine sediment is the **hyaline** cast. Rare hyaline casts can be seen in normal urine but increase with any kidney disease. They can also be seen as a result of fever, emotional stress, or strenuous exercise. Hyaline casts are nearly transparent and can be difficult to see under the microscope without some light adjustment.

Other types of casts include granular casts, containing remnants of disintegrated cells that appear as fine or coarse granules. Cellular casts may contain epithelial cells, red blood cells, or white blood cells. Figure 42-12 illustrates hyaline, granular, and cellular casts.

Identification of casts in urine requires an experienced eye (see Procedures 42-4 and 42-5).

Urinalysis Report

When reporting the results of a urinalysis, you may use a ready-made form, or your clinic may create a form specifically for your practice. When using electronic medical records, test results are entered directly into the patient's medical record on the computer (Figure 42-13). No printed report is needed unless the patient requires a hard copy (printed document). The report should contain the patient's name, the type of urine specimen (voided or catheterized and whether it was a clean-catch midstream specimen), the provider who ordered the urinalysis, the medical assistant performing the physical and chemical portions of

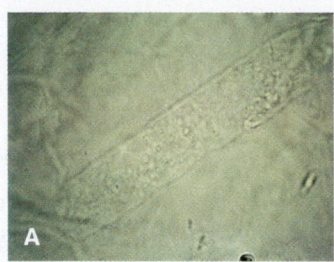 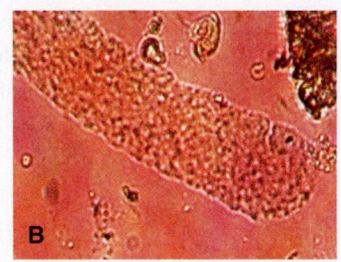 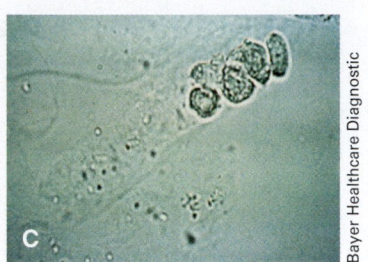

Bayer Healthcare Diagnostic Division, Norwood, MA.

Figure 42-12 Casts in urine sediment. (A) Hyaline. (B) Granular. (C) Cellular.

Patient: Noni Moody						Chart # 684-23				MA: W. Slawson, CMA (AAMA)				URINALYSIS	
Req. by: Dr. Rice							Date/Time Spec. Rec'd: 01-12-XX 10 AM				Date Test Completed: 01-12-XX 10:15 AM				
	TEST	NORM	RESULT	TEST	NORM	RESULT		TEST	NORM	RESULT	TEST	NORM	RESULT		
☒ VOID	Color	Yellow	Dk yellow	Protein	Neg	neg.	MICRO	WBC	0–2	few	Bact.	Trace	tr.		
☒ CC	Glucose	Neg	neg.	Nitrite	Neg	neg.		RBC	0–2	10	Mucus	None	─o─		
☐ CATH	Ketone	Neg	neg.	Leuk	Neg	tr.		Epith.	Few	─o─	Casts	Occ	─o─		
☐ TURBID	Sp. Gr.	1.005-1.030	1.024					Cryst.	None	─o─					
☐ HAZY	Blood	Neg	tr.				OTHER:								
☒ CLEAR	Ph	5 – 8	6.5												

Inner City Health Care

Patient: Maggie Radliff						Chart # 376-42				MA: W. Slawson, CMA (AAMA)				URINALYSIS	
Req. by: Dr. Rice							Date/Time Spec. Rec'd: 02-14-XX 3 PM				Date Test Completed: 02-14-XX 3:10 PM				
	TEST	NORM	RESULT	TEST	NORM	RESULT		TEST	NORM	RESULT	TEST	NORM	RESULT		
☒ VOID	Color	Yellow	Amber	Protein	Neg	neg.	MICRO	WBC	0–2	20 – 30	Bact.	Trace	many		
☒ CC	Glucose	Neg	neg.	Nitrite	Neg	+2		RBC	0–2	TNTC	Mucus	None	─o─		
☐ CATH	Ketone	Neg	neg.	Leuk	Neg	+3		Epith.	Few	few	Casts	Occ	─o─		
☐ TURBID	Sp. Gr.	1.005-1.030	1.024					Cryst.	None	─o─					
☒ HAZY	Blood	Neg	+3				OTHER:								
☒ CLEAR	Ph	5 – 8	8												

Inner City Health Care

Patient: Elaine Hardin						Chart # 1036-02				MA: W. Slawson, CMA (AAMA)				URINALYSIS	
Req. by: Dr.							Date/Time Spec. Rec'd: 04-27-XX 11:00 AM				Date Test Completed: 04-27-XX 11:15 AM				
	TEST	NORM	RESULT	TEST	NORM	RESULT		TEST	NORM	RESULT	TEST	NORM	RESULT		
☒ VOID	Color	Yellow	yellow	Protein	Neg	neg.	MICRO	WBC	0–2	─o─	Bact.	Trace	mixed		
☒ CC	Glucose	Neg	neg.	Nitrite	Neg	neg.		RBC	0–2	occas	Mucus	None	─o─		
☐ CATH	Ketone	Neg	neg.	Leuk	Neg	neg.		Epith.	Few	few	Casts	Occ	─o─		
☐ TURBID	Sp. Gr.	1.005-1.030	1.015					Cryst.	None	─o─					
☒ HAZY	Blood	Neg	neg.				OTHER:								
☒ CLEAR	Ph	5 – 8	5.0												

Inner City Health Care

Patient: Gwen Black						Chart # 986-08				MA: W. Slawson, CMA (AAMA)				URINALYSIS	
Req. by: Dr.							Date/Time Spec. Rec'd: 08-31-XX 2:30 PM				Date Test Completed: 08-31-XX 2:45 PM				
	TEST	NORM	RESULT	TEST	NORM	RESULT		TEST	NORM	RESULT	TEST	NORM	RESULT		
☒ VOID	Color	Yellow	Lt yellow	Protein	Neg	neg.	MICRO	WBC	0–2	─o─	Bact.	Trace	tr.		
☒ CC	Glucose	Neg	2+	Nitrite	Neg	neg.		RBC	0–2	─o─	Mucus	None	─o─		
☐ CATH	Ketone	Neg	─o─	Leuk	Neg	neg.		Epith.	Few	few	Casts	Occ	─o─		
☐ TURBID	Sp. Gr.	1.005-1.030	1.010					Cryst.	None	─o─					
☐ HAZY	Blood	Neg	neg.				OTHER:								
☒ CLEAR	Ph	5 – 8	5.5												

Inner City Health Care

© Cengage Learning 2014

Figure 42-13 Examples of handwritten urinalysis reports.

the urinalysis, the date and time the specimen was obtained and the date and time it was tested, and the findings (see Figure 42-13 and Figure 42-14 for examples of handwritten and automated urinalysis reports).

DRUG SCREENING

Testing for drugs is becoming more common during the job interview process. Some clinics specialize in occupational health, offering pre-employment physicals including drug screening.

A Brenda Stoaks   03-18-20XX

```
GLU     Negative
BIL     Negative
KET     Negative
SG      <=1.005
*BLO    Trace-intact*
PH      5.5
PRO     Negative
URO     0.2 E.U./dL
NIT     Negative
LEU     Negative
```

B Katie Oberleitner   06-18-20XX

```
GLU     Negative
BIL     Negative
KET     Negative
SG      >=1.030
*BLO    Trace-intact*
PH      5.5
*PRO    100 mg/dL    *
URO     0.2 E.U./dL
NIT     Negative
LEU     Negative
```

C Janie Carter   12-02-20XX

```
GLU     Negative
BIL     Negative
KET     Negative
SG      1.015
*BLO    Large        *
PH      5.5
*PRO    100 mg/dL    *
URO     0.2 E.U./dL
*NIT    Positive     *
*LEU    Moderate     *
```

© Cengage Learning 2014

Figure 42-14 Examples of urinalysis reports from automated urine analyzer.

The actual test is simple and is CLIA waived, but there are detailed protocols and legal documentations that need to be strictly adhered to. The POL should be certified to perform drug testing, and all clinical personnel should receive special training. A **chain of custody** must take place so that the specimen is guarded against tampering and to guarantee the integrity of the specimen.

Some basic criteria in the process are as follows:

- When the patient arrives, he or she must show photo ID, which is copied. The copy is signed.
- The patient signs a consent form for the testing and completes a questionnaire.
- The urine collection cup has a built in thermometer to ensure the urine is fresh and is at body temperature.
- The patient is asked to leave coats and bags with the clinic personnel, and these items should be secured.
- The bathroom and patient are inspected for chemicals and/or urine samples that do not belong to the patient.
- In the case of a legal court-ordered drug test, the collection of the urine is monitored. Monitoring may occur in all drug testing, depending on clinic policy.
- After the sample is collected, the temperature is recorded and the sample is sealed and secured for transport to a testing facility. The patient signs to verify that the sample is his or hers.
- If a CLIA-waived test kit is used in the POL, a test strip is dipped into the urine, and the reagent will react qualitatively (positive, negative, or sometimes inconclusive) for various substances during a specific amount of time. Inconclusive samples must be tested further.

PROCEDURE 42-1

Assessing Urine Volume, Color, and Clarity (Physical Urinalysis)

STANDARD PRECAUTIONS:

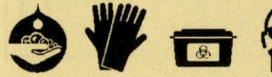

PURPOSE:
Determine and document the volume, color, and clarity of a urine sample.

NOTE: This procedure is separated from the complete urinalysis for instructional purposes only. The physical examination of urine is always performed along with the chemical analysis and usually includes the microscopic examination as well. For a complete urinalysis, see Procedure 42-5.

EQUIPMENT/SUPPLIES:
Gloves
Urine container
Laboratory report form
Biohazard container
Disinfectant cleaner

Procedure 42-1 (continued)

PROCEDURE STEPS:

1. Wash hands and put on gloves. RATIONALE: Washing hands before any laboratory process prevents contamination of the specimen. Gloving provides personal protection.

2. Assemble equipment and supplies. RATIONALE: Organizing your work area prevents confusion and error caused by missing supplies.

3. Follow all safety guidelines, being careful not to splash the urine specimen. Wipe up all spills immediately with disinfectant cleaner. RATIONALE: Preventing splashes and spills will prevent exposure to biohazardous substances. Cleaning any spill immediately prevents further contamination and risk for exposure.

4. Examine the specimen for proper labeling, *paying attention to detail*. Any unlabeled specimen is not to be tested. If the missing, unlabeled specimen cannot be identified, the patient should be notified to submit a new specimen. The provider ordering the test should be notified of the delay. The specimen should be labeled on the cup, not the lid. RATIONALE: An unlabeled specimen cannot be proven to come from any particular patient and we should never guess or assume whose specimen it is. The provider should be notified so that he or she is kept informed about the processing of laboratory tests he or she orders. The specimen should be labeled on the cup rather than the lid, because the lid can be removed from the specimen and mixed up with other lids.

5. Ensure the lid is securely tightened and mix the urine thoroughly. RATIONALE: Securing the lid will prevent leaking of urine while mixing. Mixing the specimen will suspend all particles and cellular components in the specimen so that the urine that is poured into the centrifuge tube contains a good sampling of the specimen.

6. Measure and note the amount of urine in the specimen if it is less than 10 mL. The amount of the specimen does not have to be noted if it is more than 10 mL. RATIONALE: If the sample is less than 10 mL, the sample is considered an inadequate amount. If unable to obtain an adequate amount, the testing may still be run on the sample, but the exact amount of the specimen should be well noted on the laboratory report form, and the test should be run according to the priority set by the provider. For example, he or she may request only a C&S be performed or only chemical testing using chemical reagent test strips rather than a complete urinalysis. Samples that are not of adequate quantity to perform the test ordered should be marked as QNS (quantity not sufficient).

7. Note and assess the urine color. Many medical assistants find it helpful to assess the color against a white background. Be sure to have good lighting. In the practice setting, comparing a variety of urine specimens with each other will help with learning about color assessment (see Table 42-2 for appropriate urine color descriptors). RATIONALE: The color of urine is helpful in predicting the concentration of the specimen. The white background helps with assessment of the color; good lighting also is helpful. Urine color names should come only from accepted color descriptors, not from arbitrary names.

8. After the volume and color have been assessed and recorded, assess the clarity of the urine. Holding the urine against a white background with good lighting, observe it for cloudiness. If you can clearly see print through the urine, it is said to be clear. If the urine appears cloudy, it is said to be slightly cloudy, cloudy, or very cloudy/turbid. Record the description on the report form. RATIONALE: The clarity of the urine is useful in predicting the presence of contaminants such as skin cells, mucus, and other debris.

9. At this point you would proceed to the chemical analysis of urine. RATIONALE: Urinalysis always includes both the physical and the chemical examination of the urine specimen and usually the microscopic as well. (For complete urinalysis, see Procedure 42-5).

10. Dispose of the specimen into the toilet or designated sink and all supplies into appropriate biohazard containers. Disinfect all reusable equipment and all surfaces. RATIONALE: Using appropriate disposal techniques and disinfecting all surfaces according to Standard Precautions safely controls all biohazard substances.

11. Remove gloves. Wash hands.

12. Document procedure in patient's chart or electronic medical record.

PROCEDURE 42-2

Using the Refractometer to Measure Specific Gravity (Physical Urinalysis, Continued)

STANDARD PRECAUTIONS:

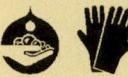

PURPOSE:

Measure and record the specific gravity of a urine specimen.

NOTE: This procedure is separated from the complete urinalysis for instructional purposes only. The physical examination of urine is always performed along with the chemical analysis and usually includes the microscopic examination as well. For a complete urinalysis, see Procedure 42-5.

EQUIPMENT/SUPPLIES:

Refractometer	Lint-free tissues
Urine sample	Biohazard container
Gloves	Disinfectant cleaners
Pipettes	Laboratory report form
Distilled water	

PROCEDURE STEPS:

1. Wash hands and put on gloves. RATIONALE: Washing hands before any laboratory process prevents contamination of the specimen. Gloving provides personal protection.

2. Assemble equipment and supplies. RATIONALE: Organizing your work area prevents confusion and error caused by missing supplies.

3. Follow all safety guidelines, being careful not to splash the urine specimen. Wipe up all spills immediately with disinfectant cleaner. RATIONALE: Preventing splashes and spills will prevent exposure to biohazardous substances. Cleaning any spill immediately prevents further contamination and risk for exposure.

4. QC must be performed on the refractometer before every use. This is accomplished by checking the specific gravity of a drop of distilled water:

   a. Clean the surface of the prism and the cover with lint-free tissue and distilled water. Wipe dry.

   b. Depending on the type of refractometer used, you may either apply the drop and then close the cover, or close the cover and apply the drop of distilled water to the notched portion of the cover so it flows over the prism. (Figure 42-15A).

   c. With the instrument tilted to allow light to enter, view the scale and read the specific gravity number (Figure 42-15B). It should be exactly 1.000.

   d. If the QC test shows the refractometer to be calibrated properly, you may record the results on your QC sheet and proceed to test the urine specimen (Step 5). If the QC test shows the refractometer to be inaccurate (the refractometer does not measure the second sample of distilled water accurately), the instrument is not calibrated properly. Use the small screwdriver to adjust the calibration. Do this adjustment using distilled water until the gauge reads 1.000.

5. Test the urine specimen exactly as the distilled water was tested and record the specific gravity on the urinalysis report form (Figure 42-15C).

6. At this point you would proceed to the chemical analysis of urine. RATIONALE: Urinalysis always includes both the physical and the chemical examination of the urine specimen and usually the microscopic as well. For a complete urinalysis, see Procedure 42-5.

7. Dispose of the specimen into the toilet or designated sink and all supplies into appropriate biohazard containers. Disinfect all reusable equipment and all surfaces. RATIONALE: Using appropriate disposal techniques and disinfecting all surfaces according to Standard Precautions safely controls all biohazard substances.

8. Remove gloves. Wash hands.

9. Document procedure in patient's chart or electronic medical record.

Procedure 42-2 (continued)

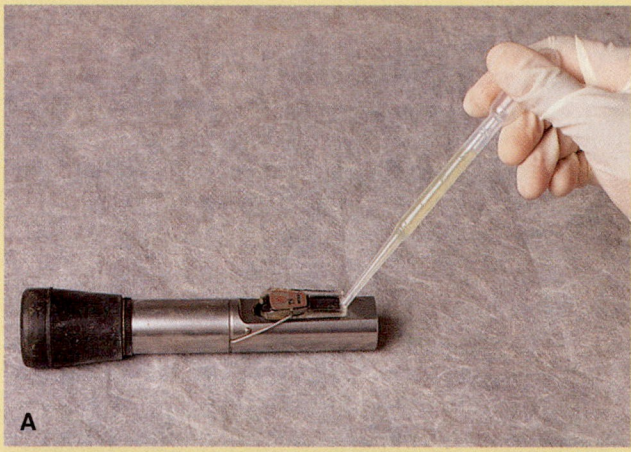

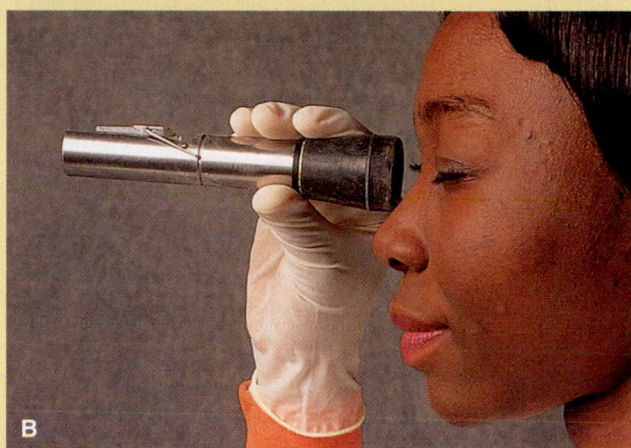

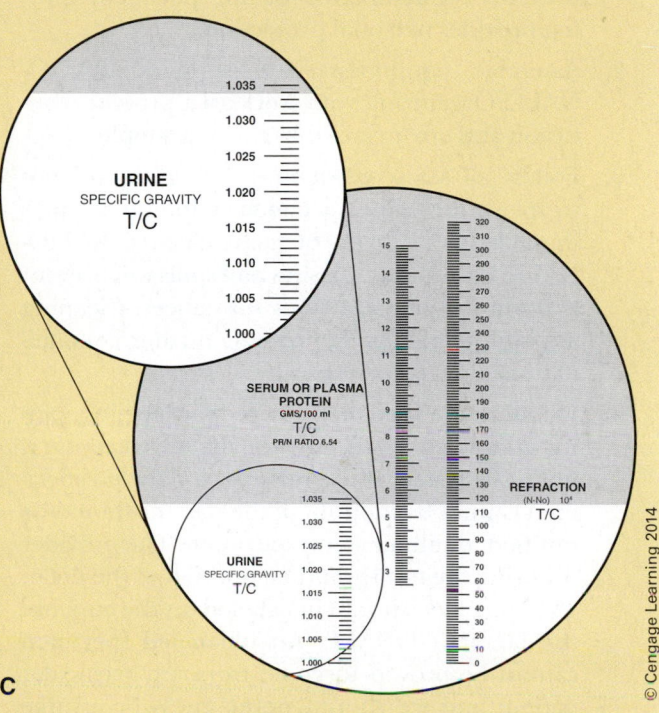

Figure 42-15   (A) A pipette or dropper may be used to fill the refractometer with urine. (B) The medical assistant looks through the refractometer. The instrument is held toward a light source. (C) The specific gravity readout.

PROCEDURE 42-3
Performing a Chemical Urinalysis

STANDARD PRECAUTIONS:

PURPOSE:

Detect any abnormal chemical constituents of a urine specimen.

NOTE: This procedure is separated from the complete urinalysis for instructional purposes only. The chemical analysis of urine is always performed along with the physical examination and usually includes the microscopic examination as well. For a complete urinalysis, see Procedure 42-5.

EQUIPMENT/SUPPLIES:

Gloves
Urine test strips
Urine specimen
Biohazard container
Disinfectant cleaner
Laboratory report form

continues

Procedure 42-3 (continued)

PROCEDURE STEPS:

1. Wash hands and put on gloves. RATIONALE: Washing hands before any laboratory process prevents contamination of the specimen. Gloving provides personal protection.

2. Assemble equipment and supplies. RATIONALE: Organizing your work area prevents confusion and error caused by missing supplies.

3. Follow all safety guidelines, being careful not to splash the urine specimen. Wipe up all spills immediately with disinfectant cleaner. RATIONALE: Preventing splashes and spills will prevent exposure to biohazardous substances. Cleaning any spill immediately prevents further contamination and risk for exposure.

4. Examine the specimen for proper labeling, *paying attention to detail*. Any unlabeled specimen is not to be tested. If the missing, unlabeled specimen cannot be identified, the patient should be notified to submit a new specimen. The provider ordering the test should be notified of the delay. The specimen should be labeled on the cup, not the lid. RATIONALE: An unlabeled specimen cannot be proven to come from any particular patient and we should never guess or assume whose specimen it is. The provider should be notified so that he or she is kept informed about the processing of laboratory tests he or she orders. The specimen should be labeled on the cup rather than the lid, because the lid can be removed from the specimen and mixed up with other lids.

5. Ensure the lid is securely tightened and mix the urine thoroughly. RATIONALE: Securing the lid will prevent leaking of urine while mixing. Mixing the specimen will suspend all particles and cellular components in the specimen so that the urine that is poured into the centrifuge tube contains a good sampling of the specimen.

6. If you are planning to perform a complete urinalysis, label a urine centrifuge tube with the patient's name and pour 10 mL into the tube for the microscopic examination. Set aside in the centrifuge. RATIONALE: Setting this portion of the sample aside ensures that it is not contaminated by the chemicals of the test strips or the process of the chemical examination.

7. Read and follow the manufacturer's instructions, *paying attention to detail*. The following procedure is a basic guideline. RATIONALE: Each manufacturer will provide specific instructions related to their product. Even manufacturers whose test strips you are already familiar with could change their instructions. The package insert should be read carefully every time a new package is used.

8. Remove a test strip from the container and replace the cap tightly. RATIONALE: Strips are adversely affected by light and moisture and should always be kept sterile in the original container with the lid securely on.

9. Immerse the test strip completely in the well-mixed urine and remove it immediately (Figure 42-16A). While removing the test strip from the cup, tap it gently onto a paper towel to remove excess urine (Figure 42-16B). RATIONALE: Removing the excess urine prevents the specimen from cross contamination of adjacent chemical pads on the strip, which can cause inaccurate results.

10. Properly time the test for each test pad. RATIONALE: Proper timing is essential for accurate results. The manufacturer's instructions will clearly list the proper time for each test.

11. Holding the test strip close to the container (or chart) but not touching it, compare the color of the pads on the test strip with the color guides on the container (or chart) (Figure 42-16C). RATIONALE: Touching the chart or container with the wet test strip will contaminate the chart/container with urine. If this accidentally happens, be sure to disinfect the surface well.

12. Record the results on the laboratory report form.

13. At this point you would proceed to setting up for the microscopic examination, if ordered. RATIONALE: Urinalysis always includes both the physical and the chemical examination of the urine specimen and usually the microscopic as well. For a complete urinalysis, see Procedure 42-5.

14. Dispose of the specimen into the toilet or designated sink and all supplies into appropriate biohazard containers. Disinfect all reusable equipment and all surfaces. RATIONALE: Using appropriate disposal techniques and disinfecting all surfaces according to Standard Precautions safely controls all biohazard substances.

15. Remove gloves. Wash hands.

16. Document procedure in patient's chart or electronic medical record.

Procedure 42-3 (continued)

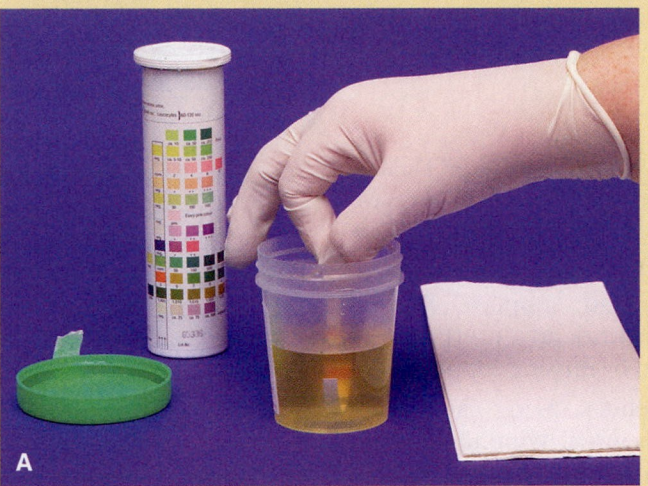

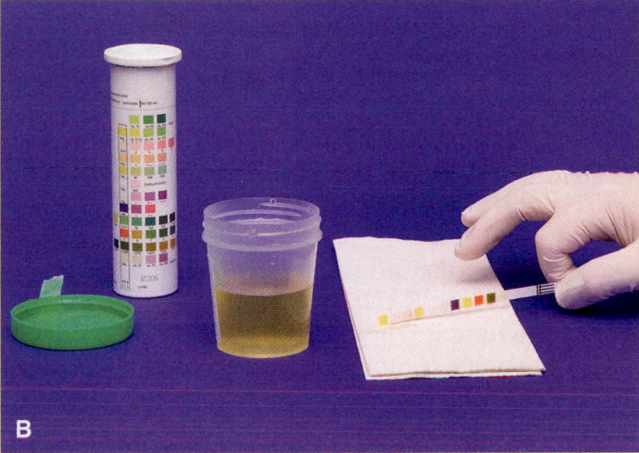

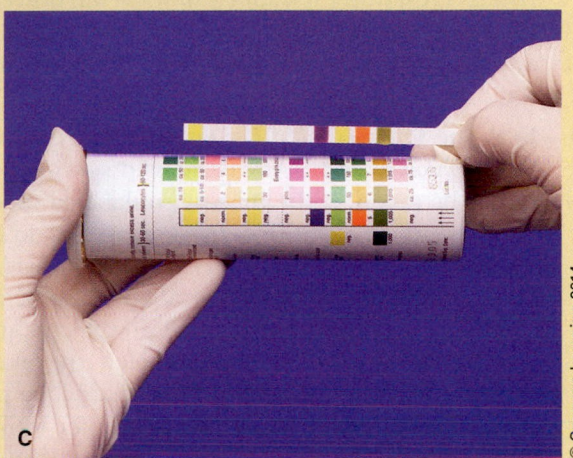

© Cengage Learning 2014

Figure 42-16 Performing a chemical examination of urine. (A) Immerse the reagent strip into the urine. (B) Remove the strip and tap it lightly on a paper towel to remove excess urine. (C) Read the strip by matching the color on the strip to the color chart. Take care not to touch the strip onto the color chart.

PROCEDURE 42-4

Preparing Slide for Microscopic Examination of Urine Sediment

STANDARD PRECAUTIONS:

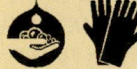

PURPOSE:

Prepare slide for a microscopic examination of urine sediment

NOTE: This procedure is separated from the physical and chemical urinalysis for instructional purposes only. The physical and chemical analyses of urine are always performed prior to the microscopic examination. (For a complete urinalysis, see Procedure 42-5).

EQUIPMENT/SUPPLIES:

Gloves	Centrifuge tubes
Microscope	and holder
Centrifuge	Urine atlas guide
Microscope slides	Disinfectant cleaner
Coverslips	Biohazard container
Disposable pipettes	Sedi-Stain® (optional)
Sharps container	

continues

Procedure 42-4 (continued)

PROCEDURE STEPS:

1. Wash hands and put on gloves. RATIONALE: Washing hands before any laboratory process prevents contamination of the specimen. Gloving provides personal protection.

2. Assemble equipment and supplies. RATIONALE: Organizing your work area prevents confusion and error caused by missing supplies.

3. Follow all safety guidelines, being careful not to splash the urine specimen. Wipe up all spills immediately with disinfectant cleaner. RATIONALE: Preventing splashes and spills will prevent exposure to biohazardous substances. Cleaning any spill immediately prevents further contamination and risk for exposure.

4. Examine the specimen for proper labeling, *paying attention to detail*. Any unlabeled specimen is not to be tested. If the missing, unlabeled specimen cannot be identified, the patient should be notified to submit a new specimen. The provider ordering the test should be notified of the delay. The specimen should be labeled on the cup, not the lid. RATIONALE: An unlabeled specimen cannot be proven to come from any particular patient and we should never guess or assume whose specimen it is. The provider should be notified so that he or she is kept informed about the processing of laboratory tests she or he orders. The specimen should be labeled on the cup rather than the lid, because the lid can be removed from the specimen and mixed up with other lids.

5. Ensure the lid is securely tightened and mix the urine thoroughly. RATIONALE: Securing the lid will prevent leaking of urine while mixing. Mixing the specimen will suspend all particles and cellular components in the specimen so that the urine poured into the centrifuge tube contains a good sampling of the specimen.

6. Label a urine centrifuge tube with the patient's name and pour 10 mL into the tube. Set into the centrifuge. Balance the centrifuge, securely close and lock the lid, and spin at 1,500 *g* (revolutions per minute) for 5 minutes. RATIONALE: The urine sediment will be forced to the bottom of the test tube and then will be placed on a slide for microscopic examination.

7. After centrifugation, pour off the supernatant, leaving about 1 mL in the bottom of the tube. Add two drops of Sedi-Stain® if desired. Remix the sediment by tapping gently on the counter or with your fingernail. RATIONALE: The test will be performed on the sediment only so the excess supernatant is not needed. Sedi-Stain® colors the cells and other elements for easier viewing.

8. Place a drop of the well-mixed sediment onto a clean microscope slide. Cover with a coverslip by holding the coverslip at an angle to the drop, bringing the edge close to the drop until the urine spreads along the edge of the coverslip, and then gently lower the coverslip onto the drop. Keep the tube. RATIONALE: Using this technique to place the coverslip onto the specimen will prevent air pockets from forming. Keep the tube in the event that a fresh slide needs to be prepared.

9. Place the slide onto the microscope stage but do not leave the light on. RATIONALE: Do not leave the light on because this will heat the slide and destroy the specimen.

10. Alert the provider that the slide is ready for viewing. RATIONALE: The microscopic examination is considered by CLIA to be in the moderately complex test category of PPMP. *Working within your scope of practice*, you are encouraged to view and discuss the microscopic examination with the provider as part of your professional development and continuing education. If you do view the slide before the provider views it, do not leave the light on. If the slide dries before the provider can view it, prepare a fresh slide.

11. *NOTE*: The following steps are included so the medical assistant can learn to examine urine microscopically even though the provider must perform the actual assessment.

    a. When examining urine sediment, it is important to keep the light subdued by lowering the condenser and to constantly vary the fine focus adjustment to view the structures that are faint. Proper lighting and focus adjustments take a great deal of practice.

    b. Scan the sediment using a 100× (low-power) magnification. A 100× magnification is achieved by using the 10× objective lens (The eyepiece lens (10×) multiplied

Procedure 42-4 (continued)

by the objective lens (10×) equals a 100× magnification).

c. View 10 to 15 fields and around the edges of the slide for casts. Casts are often forced to the edges. It may be necessary to use the 40× objective (400× magnification) to identify the casts.

d. Scan the slide using the 40× objective The eyepiece lens (10×) multiplied by the objective lens (40×) equals a magnification of 400× for other cells and formed elements. The count is obtained by averaging the number of each formed element or cell in 10 to 15 visualized fields.

12. After the provider is finished with the specimen and the patient has left the clinic, dispose of the specimen into the toilet or designated sink and all used supplies into appropriate biohazard containers. Disinfect all reusable equipment and all surfaces. Remove gloves and wash hands. RATIONALE: Using appropriate disposal techniques and disinfecting all surfaces according to Standard Precautions safely controls all biohazard substances. Remember that microscopic slides and coverslips are glass and should be placed into an appropriate biohazard sharps container.

PROCEDURE 42-5
Performing a Complete Urinalysis

STANDARD PRECAUTIONS:

PURPOSE:
Perform a complete urinalysis, including the physical, chemical, and microscopic examination within 30 minutes of obtaining the specimen.

EQUIPMENT/SUPPLIES:

Gloves	Reagent test strips
Urine specimen	Urine atlas
Pipettes	Refractometer
Centrifuge tube	Distilled water
Centrifuge	Lint-free tissues
Microscope	Biohazard container
Microscope slides	Sharps container
Coverslip	Disinfectant cleaner
Permanent marker	Laboratory report form
Sedi-Stain® (optional)	

PROCEDURE STEPS:
NOTE: The following procedure is a compilation and summary of the physical, chemical, and microscopic examination of urine (see Procedures 42-1, 42-2, 42-3, and 42-4). For details within each step, refer to the specific procedure as referenced.

1. Wash hands and put on gloves.

2. Assemble equipment and supplies.

3. Follow all safety guidelines.

4. Examine the specimen for proper labeling, ***paying attention to detail***.

5. Ensure the lid is securely tightened and mix the urine thoroughly.

6. Label a urine centrifuge tube with the patient's name, pour 10 mL into the tube and set it into the centrifuge. Balance the centrifuge, securely close and lock the lid, and spin at 1,500 *g* (revolutions per minute) for 5 minutes.

7. While the sample is being centrifuged, assess and record the color and clarity.

8. Perform the specific gravity test using a refractometer if specific gravity is not included in the chemical test strip.

9. Perform the chemical examination following the manufacturer's instructions. Record the results.

10. After centrifugation, pour off the supernatant, leaving about 1 mL in the bottom of the tube. Add two drops of Sedi-Stain® if desired. Remix the sediment by tapping gently on the counter or with your fingernail.

continues

Procedure 42-5 (continued)

11. Place a drop of the well-mixed sediment onto a clean microscope slide. Cover with a coverslip.

12. Place the slide onto the microscope stage and alert the provider that the slide is ready for viewing.

13. Dispose of the specimen into the toilet or designated sink and all supplies into appropriate biohazard containers. Disinfect all reusable equipment and all surfaces. Remember that microscopic slides and coverslips are glass and should be placed into an appropriate

biohazard sharps container. Remove gloves and wash hands.

14. File the completed laboratory report form into the laboratory section of the patient's chart or electronic medical record and document the procedure.

DOCUMENTATION:

11/13/XX 4:15 PM   Complete urinalysis performed on random voided specimen. Report filed. Joe Guerrero, CMA (AAMA)——————————

PROCEDURE 42-6

Utilizing a Urine Transport System for C&S

STANDARD PRECAUTIONS:

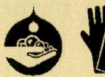

PURPOSE:

Prepare a urine specimen for transport using a culture and sensitivity transport kit.

EQUIPMENT/SUPPLIES:

Gloves
Sterile urine cup and specimen
Urine culture and sensitivity transport kit
Laboratory requisition
Paper towel

PROCEDURE STEPS:

1. Wash hands and put on gloves. RATIONALE: Washing hands before any laboratory process prevents contamination of the specimen. Gloving provides personal protection.

2. Assemble equipment and supplies (Figure 42-17A shows one type of system). RATIONALE: Organizing your work area prevents confusion and error caused by missing supplies.

3. Follow all safety guidelines, being careful not to splash the urine specimen. Wipe up all spills immediately with disinfectant cleaner. RATIONALE: Preventing splashes and spills will prevent exposure to biohazardous substances. Cleaning any spill immediately prevents further contamination and risk for exposure.

4. Examine the specimen for proper labeling, *paying attention to detail*. RATIONALE: The specimen cup must be properly labeled to ensure QC.

5. Check the urine C&S Transport kit expiration date. RATIONALE: If the kit has expired, the contents cannot be guaranteed sterile.

6. Open the urine C&S transport kit package (Figure 42-17B). Remove the cap from the specimen cup, placing the lid upside down on the paper towel. RATIONALE: The cap must be placed upside down to maintain the sterile inner surface.

7. Follow the manufacturer's instructions exactly:

   a. Place the urine tube in the tube adapter (Figure 42-17C) and the specimen straw into the urine within the specimen cup (Figure 42-17D).

   b. Advance urine tube into the adapter, pushing the tube onto the needle while keeping the specimen straw submerged in the urine.

Procedure 42-6 (continued)

c. Allow the vacuum in the urine tube to draw up the urine. Fill to the exhaustion of the vacuum within the tube (Figure 42-17E).

d. Remove the tube and the specimen straw/adapter unit and dispose of it into a biohazard container.

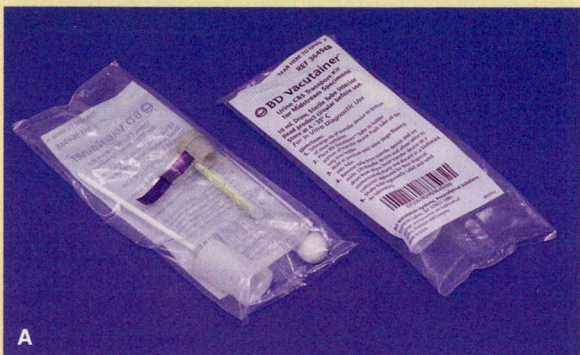

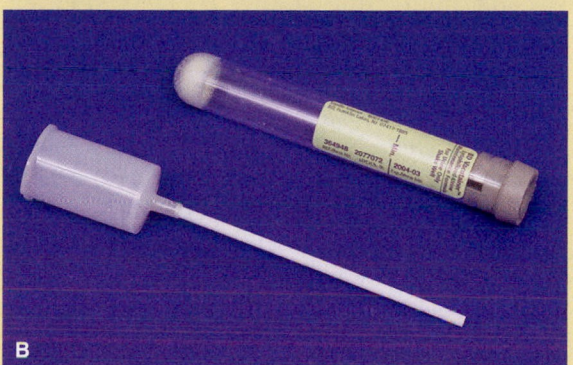

e. Gently invert the tube 8 to 10 times to mix the preservative within the tube.

8. Label the tube with patient's name, date, time, and other required information. RATIONALE: Labeling with the required information prevents mix-ups of specimens and ensures a quality timeline.

9. Dispose of all contaminated supplies, disinfect all surfaces, remove gloves, and wash hands. RATIONALE: Using appropriate disposal techniques and disinfecting all surfaces according to Standard Precautions safely controls biohazard substances.

10. Complete the laboratory requisition and document procedure in patient's chart or electronic medical record. RATIONALE: Proper documentation ensures the laboratory will have the necessary information and the patient's medical record will be accurate and complete.

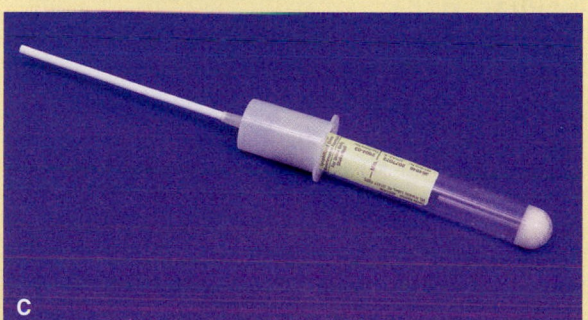

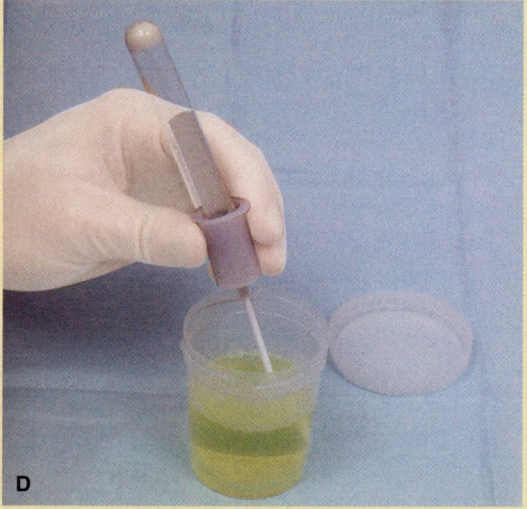

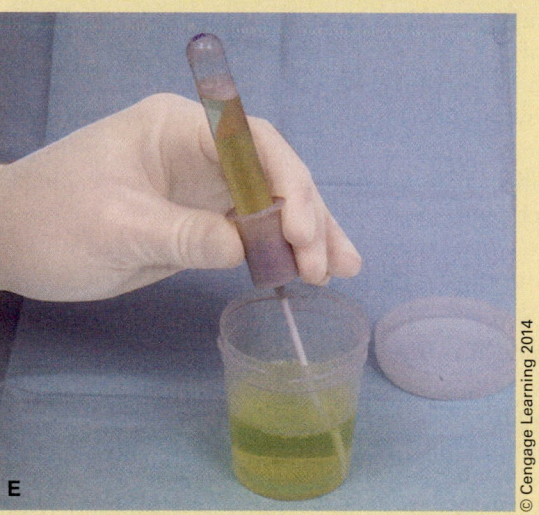

© Cengage Learning 2014

Figure 42-17 The urine transport kit for culture and sensitivity. (A) Packaged as a kit. (B) The components of the kit. (C) The tube is connected to the straw and adapter. (D) The end of the straw is placed in the urine (the vacuum tube is not pushed completely onto the adapter until the straw is submerged in the urine). (E) The vacuum in the tube draws up the urine.

PROCEDURE 42-7

Instructing a Patient in the Collection of a Clean-Catch, Midstream Urine Specimen

PURPOSE:

To instruct a patient on the proper technique of collecting a urine specimen suitable for urinalysis testing.

EQUIPMENT/SUPPLIES:

Gloves
Urine cup with a secure lid
Cleansing towelettes (two for males, three for females)
Marking pen
Written instructions posted in restroom

PROCEDURE STEPS:

1. Wash hands and assemble the supplies. RATIONALE: Always wash hands before working with each patient as a means of preventing disease transmission. Being organized ensures that the procedure will be performed in a professional manner.

2. *Introduce yourself by name and credential. Identify the patient*, and provide for a private area free from distractions. RATIONALE: Identifying the patient ensures that the right patient will have the right procedure. Introducing yourself and stating your credentials provides for a professional rapport with the patient. Providing for a private area ensures that the patient will have the freedom to ask questions and that confidentiality will be maintained. Being in an area that is free from distractions allows you to use a moderate voice volume and still be heard and understood by the patient.

3. Provide the patient with a capped urine cup labeled with his/her name, a pair of gloves, and the cleansing towelettes. RATIONALE: The cup should be labeled (not the cap) prior to giving it to the patient so there is not a chance of a mixup. Gloves will protect the patient's hand from contamination from the urine and from the genital area. The towelettes will be used for cleansing the area prior to obtaining the sample.

4. Show the patient the written instructions posted in the bathroom. RATIONALE: The patient should always have written instructions in case he or she forgets a step. The instructions should be posted at a level that can be read by the female patient while sitting and by the male patient while standing.

5. *Speaking to the patient's level of understanding*, explain why the urine sample should be a clean-catch midstream sample and what that means. RATIONALE: When the patient understands the reasons behind the instructions, he or she is much more likely to follow the steps completely.

6. Ask the patient to first wash his or her hands and apply the gloves. RATIONALE: Gloves are worn to protect the patient's hands from contamination.

7. *Demonstrate professionalism and courtesy to the patient* while you explain the cleansing process for a clean-catch: For the male patient, explain that he is to cleanse the urethral opening twice, using two separate towelettes before he begins to urinate. For the female patient, explain that she will need to spread her labia and cleanse from front to back first on one side, then the other, and lastly, in the middle. Explain that she is to hold her labia apart until the urine sample is obtained. RATIONALE: Demonstrating professionalism and courtesy will maintain a professional atmosphere and help put the patient at ease as some patients may become embarrassed with these instructions. Cleansing the urethral opening ensures that the sample will have no or few epithelial cells from the skin. Epithelial cells are quite large and can make the urine difficult to evaluate microscopically because the bacteria and other cells can be hidden behind them.

8. Explain the process of obtaining the midstream specimen: For both the male and the female patient, he or she is to bring the cup into the stream and obtain about half a cup before removing the cup from the stream. RATIONALE: The mid-stream catch is used to further prevent epithelial cells from entering the sample. If the

Procedure 42-7 (continued)

patient were to stop and start the urine flow, the chances of epithelial contamination increases.

9. Explain to the patient that he or she should secure the cap onto the cup. RATIONALE: The secure lid will prevent spillage.

10. The patient may rinse the outside of the capped cup if needed and towel dry it. RATIONALE: Rinsing and drying the outside of the cup will remove any urine that may be present.

11. The patient is to then remove the gloves, dispose of them into the red bag waste receptacle, and wash his or her hands. RATIONALE: Contaminated waste should always go into red bag receptacles. Hands should be washed to remove any residual powder from the gloves and/or contamination that may have touched the hands.

12. *Ask the patient if he or she has any questions and provide appropriate responses.* RATIONALE: Soliciting questions will encourage the patient to ask if there is something he or she does not understand. Providing appropriate responses will further the patient's understanding and ensure a cleaner specimen.

13. Using a paper towel as a barrier, the cup may be returned to the medical assistant or placed in the lab receptacle as directed. RATIONALE: The POL often has a shelf or designated area for the patient to place the urine sample onto. If not, the sample may be handed to the medical assistant. The paper towel creates a barrier between the specimen and the hand.

CASE STUDY 42-1

Refer to the scenario at the beginning of the chapter. Wanda is careful to prepare her patient properly so she gets a good sample, she pays attention to the details so that the test is run properly, and she cares about the quality of the results.

CASE STUDY REVIEW

1. What is the worst that can happen if the patient does not give a good clean-catch midstream urine sample?
2. What might happen if the reagents Wanda uses are outdated or have not been stored properly?
3. If Wanda does not care about the quality of the urine tests, how does that reflect on the rest of Wanda's work?

CASE STUDY 42-2

Linda Sterns came to Inner City Health Care today because she is experiencing frequent urination, itching, and burning when urinating. Dr. Rice ordered a urinalysis, which clinical medical assistant Wanda Slawson is performing. Wanda notes that the urine has a cloudy appearance and the chemical reagent test strip tests positive for nitrites. Wanda confers with Dr. Rice, who instructs her to prepare a slide for a microscopic examination of the specimen.

CASE STUDY REVIEW

1. Why might Dr. Rice want to examine this specimen microscopically?
2. How would the findings be reported?

SUMMARY

This chapter summarizes the basics of the urinalysis. Providers order a variety of tests on urine to help them determine or rule out certain abnormalities to make a correct diagnosis and prescribe treatment.

Urine is formed as blood is filtered through the kidney. Substances such as by-products of metabolism, mineral excesses, cells, bacteria, parasites, crystals, and casts can be found in the urine during examination.

It is important for the medical assistant to:

- Understand the proper collection techniques for urine specimens. Medical assistants often are called on to instruct patients on the proper collection procedures.
- Understand the safety guidelines involved with collecting and handling specimens, preservatives, and reagents. These guidelines must *always* be observed.
- Understand the importance of and the procedures for maintaining a consistent quality-control program.
- Understand how to properly perform the urinalysis, following up with proper confirmatory tests when necessary.
- Understand and be constantly aware of factors that may interfere with the accuracy of a urinalysis.
- Project a professional image and be able to use appropriate communication and active listening skills when providing care to patients.

STUDY FOR SUCCESS

To reinforce your knowledge and skills of information presented in this chapter:

- Review the *Key Terms*
- Role-play with other students to apply attributes of professionalism pertinent to this chapter.
- Consider the *Case Studies* and discuss your conclusions
- Answer the questions in the *Certification Review*
- Apply your knowledge by completing the Activities in the Study Guide and the *Games and Quizzes* in the StudyWARE **StudyWARE** software on the *Premium Website*
- Perform the *Procedures* using the *Competency Assessment Checklists* in the *Competency Manual*
- Practice your problem-solving skills with the Critical Thinking Challenge 3.0 on the *Premium Website*

Additional resources for this chapter include:

- Module 22 of the Medical Assisting Learning Lab
- *CourseMate for Delmar's Comprehensive Medical Assisting*
- *WebTutor for Delmar's Comprehensive Medical Assisting*

CERTIFICATION REVIEW

1. What safety guideline is important to follow during a routine urinalysis?
   a. Use the same pipette for all patients' urine samples
   b. Allow urine to sit at room temperature to ferment the urine properties
   c. Once tested, urine can be disposed of by the janitorial service
   d. Treat all specimens as if they were infectious

2. What are the three basic parts of a typical urine examination?
   a. Volumetric, chemical, and macroscopic
   b. Pathologic, chemical, and confirmatory
   c. Physical, chemical, and microscopic
   d. Random, 24-hour, and catheterized

3. What is the specimen of choice for routine urinalysis?
   a. Sterile
   b. Clean-catch
   c. Catheterized
   d. Timed

4. A diabetic patient will normally have an excess of what substance in the urine?
   a. Hemoglobin
   b. Glucose
   c. Insulin
   d. Sodium

5. What is the most common way of doing a chemical analysis of urine in a provider's office?
   a. Reagent test strip
   b. Microscopic examination
   c. Culture test
   d. Urinometer

6. Which substance or structure is automatically considered abnormal when found in urine?
   a. Phosphates
   b. Urea
   c. Blood
   d. Salt

7. What are three symptoms a patient might have that would indicate a need for a urinalysis?
   a. Nausea, vomiting, and fever
   b. Anorexia, diarrhea, and fever
   c. Abdominal pain, dysuria, and frequency
   d. Back pain, headache, and fever

8. Which casts are considered fairly normal in urine?
   a. Hyaline
   b. Red blood cell
   c. White blood cell
   d. Bacterial

9. Specific gravity of urine can be measured using which of the following?
   a. Urinometer
   b. Refractometer
   c. Chemical reagent strip
   d. All of the above

10. If a urine specimen is labeled as "QNS," what does it refer to?
    a. Quality not sufficient
    b. Quality not specific
    c. Quantity not sufficient
    d. Quantity not specific

REFERENCES/BIBLIOGRAPHY

Walters, N. J., Estridge, B. H., & Reynold, A. P. (2011). *Basic Clinical Laboratory Techniques* (6th ed.). Clifton Park, NY: Delmar Cengage Learning.

OUTLINE

The Medical Assistant's
  Role in the Microbiology
  Laboratory
Microbiology
  Classification
  Nomenclature
  Cell Structure
Equipment
  Autoclave
  Microscope
  Safety Hood
  Incubator
  Anaerobic Equipment
  Inoculating Equipment
  Incinerator
  Media
  Refrigerator

Safety When Handling
  Microbiology Specimens
  Personal Protective Equipment
  Work Area
  Specimen Handling
  Disposal of Waste and Spills
Quality Control
Collection Procedures
  Specific Collection
    Requirements for Cultures
Foodborne Illnesses
Microscopic Examination
  of Bacteria
  Bacterial Shapes
  Dyes (Stains)
  Simple Stain
  Differential Stain
  Acid-Fast Stain
  Special Techniques

Potassium Hydroxide
  Preparation
Culture Media
  Media Classification
Microbiology Culture
  Inoculating the Media
  Other Types of Streaking
  Primary Culture
  Subculture
Rapid Identification Systems
  Streptococcus Screening (Rapid
    Strep Testing)
Sensitivity Testing
Parasitology
  Examination Methods
  Specimen Collection
  Common Parasites
Mycology

LEARNING OUTCOMES

1. Define, spell, and pronounce the key terms as presented in the glossary.
2. Use language/verbal skills that enable a patient's understanding.
3. Describe basic bacterial cell structure.
4. Discuss quality control issues related to handling microbiology specimens.
5. Explain the types of microbiology specimens collected in the POL and how they are collected.
6. List different types of stains used to microscopically observe microorganisms.
7. Describe the significance of sensitivity testing.
8. List two parasites and two fungi that can be observed in the POL.
9. Obtain specimens for microbiological testing.
10. Perform CLIA waived immunology tests on serum.
11. Distinguish between normal and abnormal test results.
12. Analyze the professionalism questions and apply them to this chapter's content.

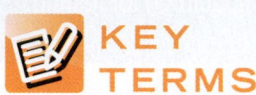

KEY TERMS

aerobic
agar
anaerobic
broth tubes
culture
dermatophytes
expectorate
genus
Gram stain
inoculate
mordant
morphology
mycology
nematode
normal flora
nosocomial
ova
parasitology
pathogen
potassium hydroxide (KOH)
protozoa
species
spores
stab culture
taxonomy
virology
wet mount
Wood's lamp

ATTRIBUTES OF PROFESSIONALISM

Communication

- Did you introduce yourself? Did you identify the patient through name and birth date or other identifying feature?
- Did you listen to and acknowledge the patient?
- Did you speak at the patient's level of understanding?
- Did you provide appropriate responses/feedback?
- Did you explain procedures and expectations to the patient?
- Did you allay patients' fears regarding the procedure being performed and help them feel safe and comfortable?
- Did you respond honestly and diplomatically to the patient's concerns?

Presentation

- Were you dressed and groomed appropriately?
- Were you courteous, patient, and respectful to the patient?
- Did you display a positive attitude?
- Did you display a calm, professional, and caring manner?

Competency

- Did you pay attention to detail?
- Did you ask questions if you were out of your comfort zone or did not have the experience to carry out tasks?
- Were you knowledgeable and accountable?

Integrity

- Did you work within your scope of practice?
- Did you immediately report any error you had made?

SCENARIO

To aid in diagnosing and treating patients, the providers at Drs. Lewis and King's office order tests to identify disease-causing bacteria, fungi, viruses, and parasites. Some of these tests, such as the quick tests for group A *Streptococcus,* are performed in the office laboratory, whereas other tests are sent to a reference laboratory. Regardless of where the test will be performed, medical assistant Joe Guerrero follows all Safety Precautions when handling specimens. He checks the test manufacturer's or laboratory's procedures and carefully completes each step. By following all safety guidelines and test procedures, Joe ensures his and others' safety. He also obtains a high-quality specimen for testing.

INTRODUCTION

The field of microbiology encompasses the study of all microorganisms, living structures that can be seen only with the powerful magnification of a microscope. The word microbiology comes from the Greek words micro ("small") and bios ("living"). The field of microbiology includes the study of such organisms as bacteria, fungi, viruses, parasites, and algae (Table 43-1).

Many medical textbooks in microbiology include extensive study of all of the preceding organisms, including lesser known species in each category. It is the goal of this chapter to introduce the student to the field of microbiology with emphasis on bacteria, fungi, and parasites. Safety while working with microorganisms in the laboratory is emphasized. The relation of bacteria to diseases also is explored.

THE MEDICAL ASSISTANT'S ROLE IN THE MICROBIOLOGY LABORATORY

The role of the medical assistant in microbiology within the physicians' office laboratory (POL) is to obtain specimens, test specimens within the Clinical Laboratory Improvement Act (CLIA) waived categories, and prepare slides and **cultures** for microscopic examination by the provider or for transport to an outside laboratory.

This chapter discusses cultures in detail. Simply put, a culture is a sample of a body secretion that is placed on special media to allow the bacteria to grow. Some samples of cultures discussed in this chapter are throat, sputum, urine, blood, vaginal and penile, and wound cultures. Cultures are usually allowed to grow in optimum temperatures and environments for at least 12 hours before they are examined for identification.

In certain test situations, a provider may request a sensitivity in addition to the culture. This test will identify which antibiotic(s) will effectively kill the microorganism identified as causing the infection.

In healthy individuals, several types of bacteria are found naturally in various parts of the body. These natural bacteria are called **normal flora**. These organisms are always present and help with the body's immune system. In disease, the causative microorganism is called a **pathogen** because it causes harm to the body.

 The medical assistant's technique must be exact to avoid laboratory error. The medical assistant also must ensure that the specimen for culture was taken with sterile supplies and delivered to the laboratory in a reasonable amount of time. Delivery time of the specimen or culture may vary depending on the type of specimen collected for culture. Some specimens may

SPOTLIGHT ON CERTIFICATION

RMA Content Outline
- Medical law
- Asepsis
- Laboratory procedures

CMA (AAMA) Content Outline
- Principles of equipment operation
- Principles of infection control
- Collecting and processing specimens and diagnostic testing

CMAS Content Outline
- Legal considerations
- Asepsis in the medical office

Table 43-1   Biologic Sciences

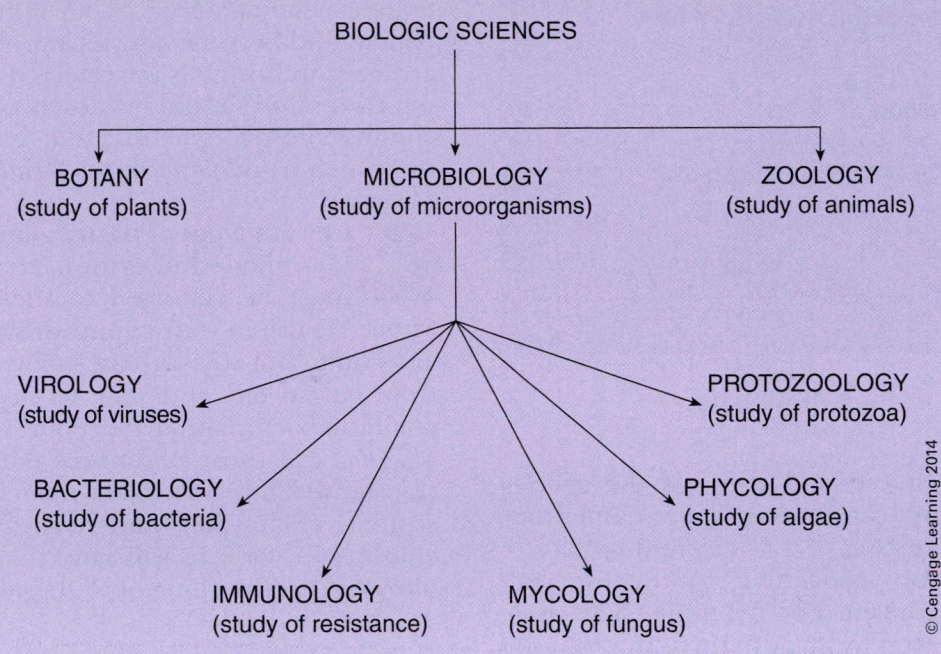

© Cengage Learning 2014

be refrigerated without harm. Some may be kept in holding media—media that will keep a specimen on a swab moist until it is cultured. These variations are discussed later in specimen processing.

By doing the smear, culture, and identification through biochemical tests, the microbiologist can identify the organism and aid the provider in diagnosing and treating the patient. Most identification of organisms can be done successfully within 12 to 24 hours. Some organisms may take longer to grow.

Many test kits are currently available to test for microbiologic pathogens; these kits are quick and fairly simple to perform. CLIA has identified which test kits are within their waived category and therefore appropriate for the medical assistant and other nonlaboratory medical personnel to perform. What used to take days and required the expertise of a laboratory technologist now takes minutes and can be performed within the POL and sometimes even within patients' homes. The at-home pregnancy tests were probably the first test kits available over the counter, but now there are literally hundreds. The test kits range from urine testing for cocaine and other drugs to cholesterol and cancer screening tests.

MICROBIOLOGY

Classification

Taxonomy deals with the classification of living organisms.

A common system divides living organisms into kingdoms. Before the discovery of the microscope in the sixteenth century, there were two known kingdoms, animal and plant. A new kingdom of microscopic organisms, the *Protista*, was developed because most microbes are neither plant nor animal. The members of this kingdom are called *protists* and are one-celled organisms (Table 43-2).

The microorganisms of importance in medical microbiology are divided into two groups: the lower protists, or *prokaryotes* (including blue-green algae and bacteria), and the higher protists, or *eukaryotes* (including **protozoa**, algae, and fungi).

Nomenclature

The system used for naming bacteria is a two-part system of names. Two Greek or Latin names are used, the first name being a **genus**, which

Table 43-2   Kingdom Protista

I. Lower protists: Prokaryotic— nuclear material not organized
   A. Bacteria
   B. Blue-green algae

II. Higher protists: Eukaryotic—true nucleus
   A. Algae
   B. Slime molds
   C. Fungus
   D. Protozoa

© Cengage Learning 2014

is capitalized. The second name is the **species** name, which is not capitalized. These names may reflect a characteristic of a bacterium or names of places or persons associated with the discovery of the microorganism. For example, *Salmonella typhi* was discovered by an American microbiologist named Salmon. The bacterium causes typhoid fever.

Individuals who study bacteria are referred to as bacteriologists or microbiologists. These individuals have taken extensive courses in the field of microbiology. In most laboratories, clinical laboratory scientists or assistants help perform microbiology procedures. The job of these individuals is to quickly and efficiently identify the organism in a given culture that has been properly obtained and brought to the laboratory within a reasonable time frame.

Together with routine bacteriologic cultures, many microbiology departments, especially in larger health care facilities, perform **parasitology** procedures for the identification of parasites; **virology** procedures for the identification of viruses; and **mycology** procedures for the identification of fungi. If an institution such as a clinic or POL is too small to properly identify many microorganisms, cultures often are sent to a reference laboratory. These laboratories are specialized laboratories with up-to-date equipment to handle large amounts of complex tests. In today's health care environment, it is cost-effective to centralize expensive and complex procedures. Instead of 10 small laboratories each having their own specialized equipment, one laboratory buys the equipment and runs the specialized test for all 10 laboratories.

The microbiology department works closely with the infection control department of a hospital to determine if certain organisms are causing infections throughout the hospital. These infections can be acquired by an immunosuppressed patient and become a serious problem. Infections acquired in hospitals are referred to as **nosocomial** infections and should be closely monitored. Some common nosocomial infections are caused by bacteria such as *Staphylococcus, Serratia,* and *Candida* (a yeast).

Certain types of bacteria and yeasts that are identified and grown in the laboratory must be reported to the Department of Public Health in your county or state because they are communicable diseases. These diseases vary from city to city and state to state. Some of the common bacteria that are reported are *Salmonella; Shigella;* and those organisms that cause sexually transmitted diseases (STDs), such as gonorrhea, syphilis, chlamydial, and herpes. The state and county you work in will have a list of reportable diseases that the clinic or POL will have posted.

Cell Structure

All living forms are alike in that their cells contain a nuclear material referred to as DNA (deoxyribonucleic acid), which carries special genetic information. The main structural difference of eukaryotes and prokaryotes is the arrangement of the nucleus. A eukaryote has a well-defined or true nucleus and is a higher form of microorganism. The prokaryote is a lower form of microorganism and has a simple nucleus that is not well defined.

The bacterial cell, classified as a lower protist, is a single-celled organism with a cytoplasmic cell membrane, cell wall, and nucleus. The nucleus is not well defined. The cell grows by taking in materials from the environment. After a certain amount of growth, the bacteria reproduce by division of the cell. Certain conditions are required for this reproduction to take place.

Figure 43-1 illustrates a basic bacterial cell. Not all bacteria possess flagella for motility, as some are not motile. Some bacteria can encapsulate themselves in protein, providing protection from antibiotic penetration and white blood cell attack. Once encapsulated they are called **spores**, an inactive state that can help bacteria resist chemicals, freezing, drying, radiation, and heating. Bacterial spores are so resistant they can live 150,000 years and can survive in dust. Tetanus is an example of a disease caused by bacteria that create spores.

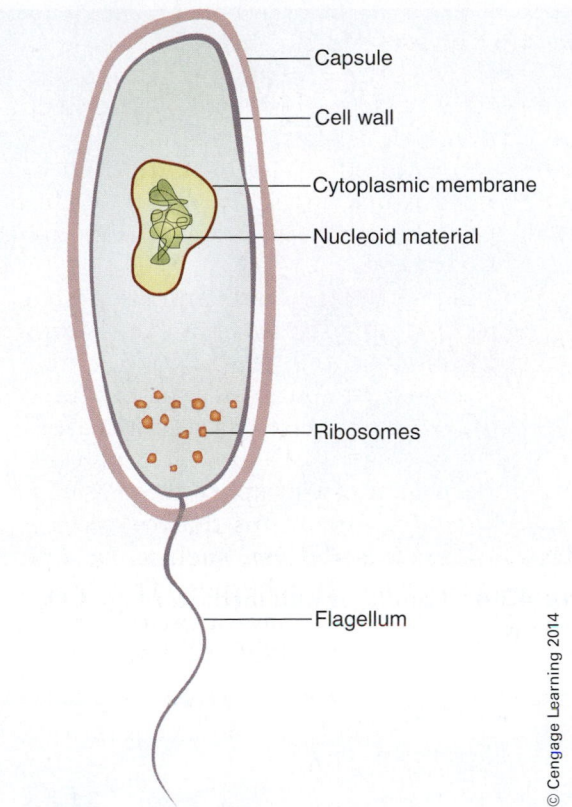

Figure 43-1 Basic bacterial cell.

EQUIPMENT

Basic equipment needed in a microbiology department of a clinic or a POL varies depending on the size of the facility. Most laboratories have some of the following equipment.

Autoclave

An autoclave (Figure 43-2) is used in the laboratory to sterilize equipment that may have been contaminated while processing specimens. It can be used to sterilize contaminated materials as well. The setting of 15 pounds per square inch and a temperature of 121°C for 15 to 20 minutes is sufficient to kill infectious agents, spores, viruses, and contaminants. Many laboratories no longer use autoclaves because of the use of presterilized and disposable equipment. (See Chapter 22 for more information on the autoclave.)

Microscope

An important piece of equipment for the POL or clinic is the microscope. This instrument is

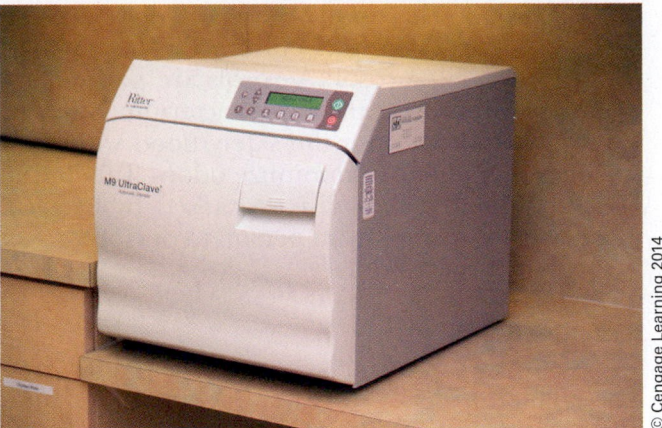

Figure 43-2 Small laboratory autoclave.

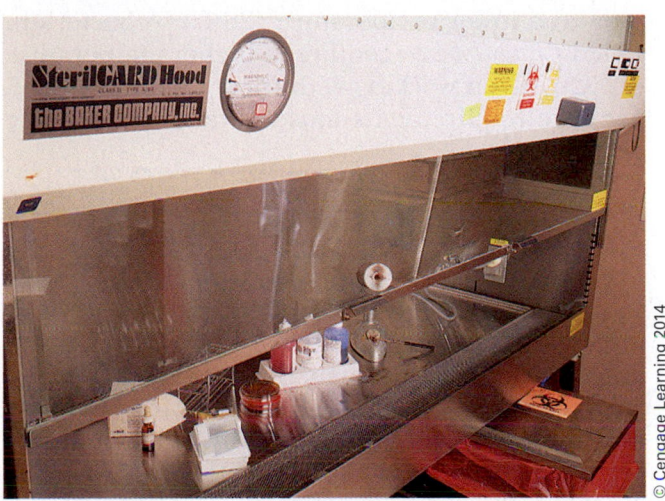

Figure 43-3 Laboratory safety hood.

used to view organisms that cannot be seen with the naked eye on a prepared slide. Skill in using the microscope is necessary to gain information from studying the slide. The microscope is a delicate instrument and should be cared for properly as stated by the manufacturer (see Chapter 39 for more information on the microscope).

Safety Hood

Some laboratories, especially if they are culturing specimens with aerosols, will have a safety hood (Figure 43-3). Aerosols are airborne particles that can be released into the air when culturing. They are potentially dangerous if inhaled. By using the safety hood, the health care worker is separated from the specimen by a glass in front of the face, with fumes and aerosols suctioned into the hood. The use of a safety hood is mandatory when performing a culture on a specimen with a potential aerosol. Aerosols are particularly dangerous in fungus and mycobacterium cultures. It is a good idea to use the safety hood with foul-smelling specimens to minimize odors. Tuberculosis is an example of a disease caused by bacteria that travel by aerosol from person to person.

Incubator

The incubator is a cabinet that has a constant temperature of 35 to 37°C. Most organisms, whether **aerobic** (grow well in oxygen) or **anaerobic** (will not grow well or at all in oxygen), grow at these temperatures. Some bacteria, such as *Yersinia*, grow at a lower temperature (26°C). A bacterium called *Campylobacter* requires a higher temperature (42°C). When working with these organisms, temperature requirements must be met for adequate growth.

Anaerobic Equipment

Certain types of cultures, such as deep-wound cultures, could contain anaerobic pathogens. At the time of culturing, the medical assistant sets up some cultures in an oxygenated environment, as well as an oxygen-reduced environment. Most laboratories post lists of cultures that need an anaerobic setup.

To grow anaerobic bacteria, the absence of oxygen is achieved by using something as simple as a candle jar (Figure 43-4) containing a lighted candle into which the inoculated petri dish is placed. When the cover is put on the jar, the burning of the candle will use up the available oxygen and generate carbon dioxide. Organisms such as *Neisseria gonorrhoeae*, which causes gonorrhea, need a high carbon dioxide atmosphere to survive. The use of a candle jar allows an easy collection and transport system that maximizes the recovery rate of certain microorganisms.

Another method of maintaining an anaerobic condition is a specialized jar called a gas pack jar (Figure 43-5). This jar contains a foil pack that, when activated, gives off carbon dioxide, decreasing the oxygen in the jar. Extensive culturing of anaerobes often is not performed by smaller laboratories. Anaerobic specimens are sent to reference laboratories better equipped to process them. Some small laboratories will perform a Gram stain on the suspected anaerobic cultures.

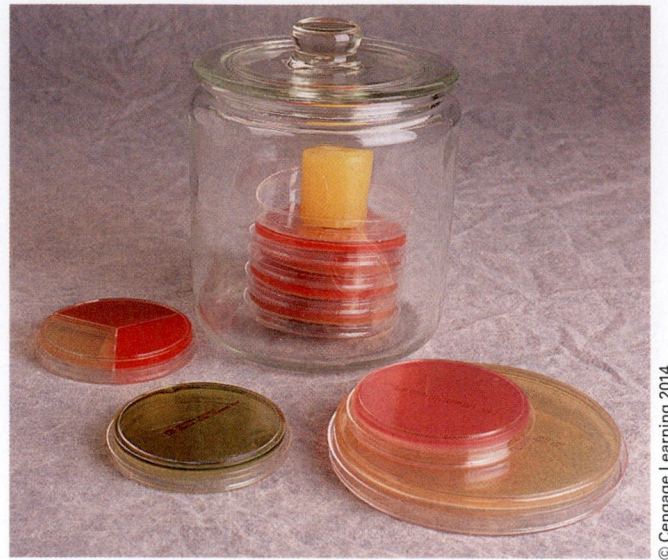

© Cengage Learning 2014

Figure 43-4 Candle jar with media for high CO_2 conditions.

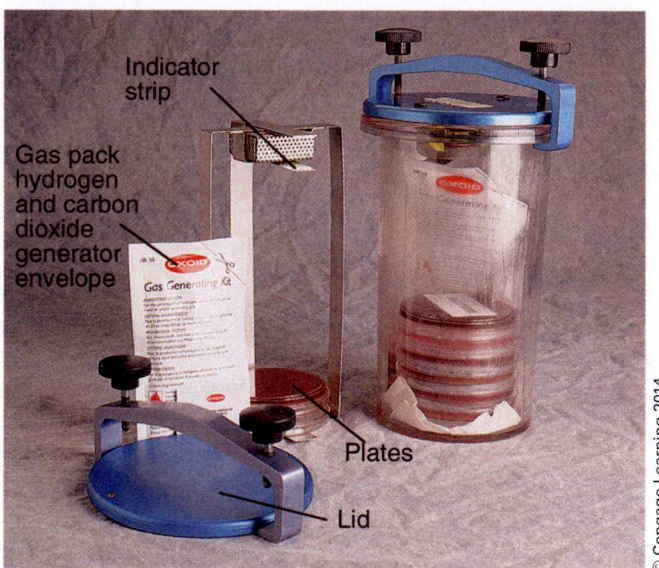

Indicator strip

Gas pack hydrogen and carbon dioxide generator envelope

Plates

Lid

© Cengage Learning 2014

Figure 43-5 Gas pack anaerobic system.

The **Gram stain** is the most common stain used to observe the gross morphologic features of bacteria and is discussed later in this chapter.

Inoculating Equipment

An *inoculating loop* (Figure 43-6) is a piece of wire with a rounded end and a handle at the other end. The loop is used to **inoculate** organisms onto a culture medium in a plate or broth. If it is made of wire, the loop can be flamed to sterilize it before and after use. As an alternative, sterile plastic

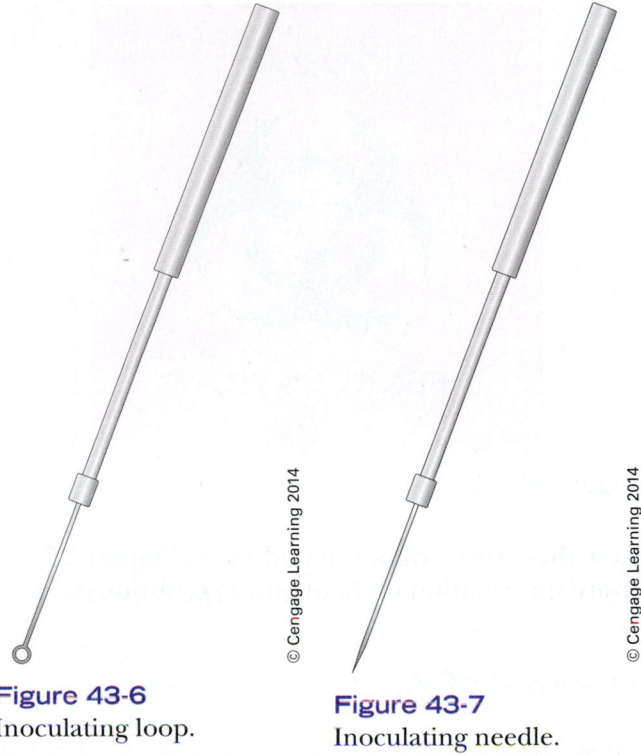

Figure 43-6
Inoculating loop.

Figure 43-7
Inoculating needle.

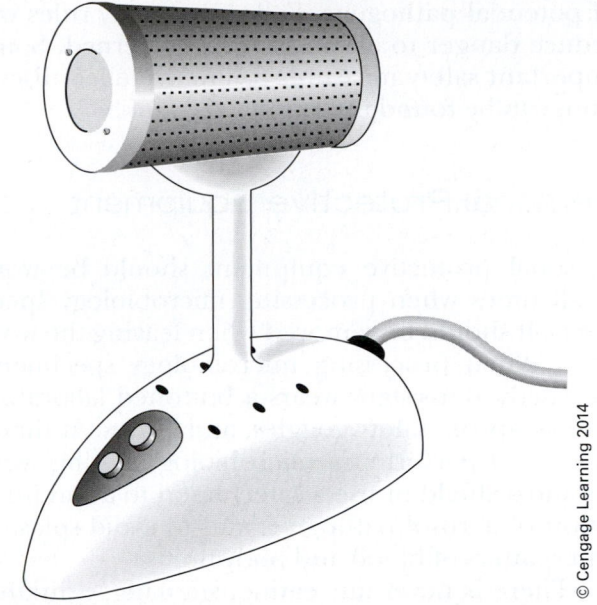

Figure 43-8   Electrical incinerator.

disposable loops can be used. These are one-time use and are disposed of in the biohazardous waste.

An *inoculating needle* (Figure 43-7) is similar to the loop but has a straight end. The needle is used when performing a **stab culture**, also known as "deep" inoculation. The needle is flamed, and the culture material is "stabbed" on the needle into medium in a tube.

Incinerator

Incineration is the quickest method of sterilizing the inoculating loop and needle. This can be accomplished by using an electrical incinerator (Figure 43-8) or a Bunsen burner (less popular today because of the open flame danger). When doing cultures, the inoculating needle or loop must be sterilized before and after it is used. This is done by placing the loop in the incinerator or passing through the flame of the Bunsen burner.

Media

In the microbiology laboratory the term media refers to a host of substances used to foster the growth of bacteria. It is listed in this section of basic equipment (Figure 43-9) but its use explained in detail later in the chapter under Culture Media.

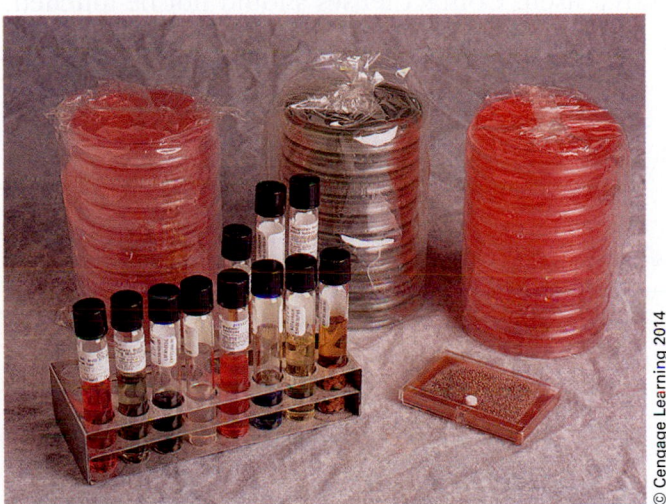

Figure 43-9   Various types of media tubes and plates.

Refrigerator

A refrigerator is needed to store certain materials, such as media and testing kits that need a temperature of 2 to 8°C. Food and drink should never be stored in the refrigerator with any specimens, kits, or media.

SAFETY WHEN HANDLING MICROBIOLOGY SPECIMENS

 Safety should be practiced in every area of the clinical laboratory at all times. Microbiology specimens can be dangerous because of potential pathogens. Following safety rules will reduce danger to all personnel concerned. Some important safety measures follow. Detailed discussions can be found in Chapters 22 and 38.

Personal Protective Equipment

Personal protective equipment should be worn at all times when processing microbiology specimens. It should be removed when leaving the work area. When processing microbiology specimens, the medical assistant wears a buttoned laboratory coat or apron, safety goggles, and gloves. At times, personnel performing microbiology testing work behind a shield or use a safety hood to avoid inhalation of aerosol pathogens and to avoid splashes and spatters of blood and body fluids.

There is never any eating, smoking, drinking, or putting objects into the mouth while working with microbiology specimens or in the laboratory area itself. Contact lenses should not be touched, nor should makeup be applied. The practice of washing hands several times should be a habit. Washing hands after glove removal is important.

Work Area

The counters where specimens are processed and set up should be cleaned with a strong germicide before and after daily use or immediately after a spill. Pathogens could be present where microbiology specimens are cultivated. This area should be dust-free and clean at all times.

Care should be taken not to have a cluttered work area. If using burners or incinerators, caution should be practiced to avoid body burns or fires.

Specimen Handling

Some microbiology specimens will be brought to the POL or clinic to be processed, so the medical assistant should look for leaks and contamination on the outside of the transporting containers. It is a good practice always to wear gloves when receiving specimens. Most specimens will arrive in an "outside" plastic bag to avoid danger to laboratory personnel. When sending specimens to an outside laboratory to be cultured, it is important to use the appropriate container to avoid contamination of others. Remember, if there is a possibility of an aerosol specimen, the specimen must be cultured under a safety hood. All specimens should be handled

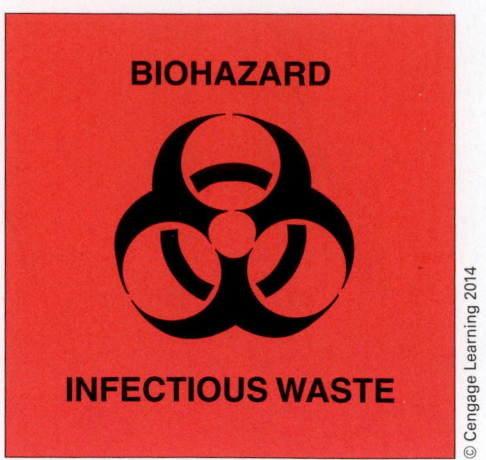

Figure 43-10 Biohazard symbol.

as if they were contaminated (see Chapter 22 for more information on Standard Precautions).

Disposal of Waste and Spills

Most facilities have a plan for disposal of dangerous biohazardous waste that should be strictly followed. Biohazardous waste generally is placed in red bags marked with the universal biohazard symbol (Figure 43-10). Most clinics or POLs employ an outside agency to dispose of waste. It is extremely important that biohazardous waste is not placed with the regular waste and disposal guidelines are followed.

If a spill should occur, follow the agency's or employer's rules. Remember to disinfect with a 5% phenol or a 10% bleach solution.

QUALITY CONTROL

Although quality control is practiced in all areas of the clinical laboratory, the microbiology department has equipment, media, and reagents that need quality-control checks with almost every test. The following list details some measures that are a part of a quality-control program in microbiology:

- All equipment with temperature controls should be monitored daily.
- The microscopes should be cleaned and kept dust-free.
- Testing for microorganism identification is often accomplished with the use of a special kit. When using kits for different tests, the positive and negative controls must be run at all times. Before use, the expiration date should be checked.

- Media of all types should not be used past the shelf life and should be stored at the proper temperatures. Your POL should have a specific list of bacteria to use on various media to test for growth. This list can be found in your laboratory manual.

- The laboratory manual should be updated periodically.

- All chemicals or reagents with Material Safety Data Sheets (MSDSs) should be available to reference when working with a chemical that is not familiar to you.

- Document all quality control testing in proper laboratory logs.

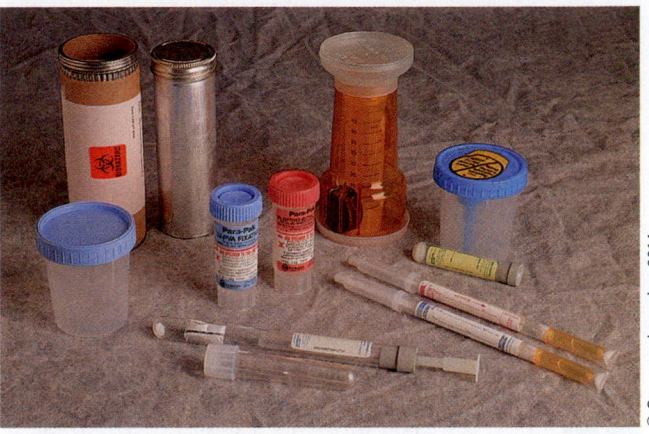

Figure 43-11 Various collection and transport containers for bacteriologic specimens.

COLLECTION PROCEDURES

When a provider needs identification of an organism that is causing infection, he or she orders a culture from that site. The culture specimen should be collected properly, delivered within a reasonable period, and collected in sufficient quantity. The results of the culture will depend on the quality of the original specimen. All specimens obtained for identification of infectious organisms must be taken from the site of the infection, not the surrounding area.

Once the specimen is collected correctly, it should be placed in the appropriate container and delivered to the laboratory soon after collection. Many organisms will die if not kept moist. Transport media can have a moistening agent to keep the specimen from drying out.

If a specimen comes into the laboratory in an improper container or has not been delivered within a reasonable period soon after collection, it must be rejected and another specimen obtained. The container in which the specimen has been placed should be sterile, and the right type should be used for a specific culture (Figure 43-11). Sterile containers are used for most collections, with the exception of stool collection containers, which do not have to be sterile. Culturette cultures are from swabs and should be kept moist. This system is a plastic tube that has a sterile swab used to collect the specimen and then is placed back into the tube. The tube contains a medium which keeps the swab moist and preserves the specimen.

The laboratory's success in isolating the causative pathogens depends on the following factors:

1. Proper collection from infection site
2. Collection of specimen during infectious period
3. Sufficient amount of specimen
4. Appropriate specimen container
5. Appropriate transport medium
6. Specimen labeled properly
7. Specimen delivered to the laboratory in a minimal amount of time
8. Specimen collected before the administration of antibiotics
9. Specimen inoculated onto proper media and placed in correct atmosphere to ensure growth

✓ When collecting specimens, it is important that the medical assistant carefully follow the instructions as designated in the laboratory manual. Standard Precautions must be strictly adhered to while obtaining and processing specimens and everyone (including couriers, receptionists, and laboratory assistants) handling specimens should wear gloves to protect themselves from leakage of the container and contamination with a pathogenic organism.

Specific Collection Requirements for Cultures

Urine. Patients should be instructed to obtain a clean-catch urine specimen in a sterile container. A clean-catch midstream specimen is obtained by first cleaning the genital area and then urinating midstream into a specimen container. Details of this procedure are found in Chapter 42. Patients should be given strict instructions so that a quality specimen for culturing can be obtained.

Sometimes a catheterization is done to collect a sterile urine specimen for culture. The urine must be collected into a sterile container.

© Cengage Learning 2014

Throat. When taking a throat specimen for culture, explain to the patient that a throat culture is necessary to identify certain organisms. Be sure to tell the patient that there may be some momentary discomfort in obtaining the specimen, especially if his or her throat is sore. Answer all questions about the process of obtaining the specimen. Throat culture specimens are taken using the culturette. As mentioned in the previous section, the culturette contains a sterile swab and growth medium for moisture to keep the bacteria viable.

 Once you have gathered all the necessary supplies (see Procedure 43-1) and put on gloves and a face shield, have the patient open his or her mouth and say "ah." This will lower the back of the tongue for better viewing (Figure 43-12A). Be sure to have a good light source available. Use a sterile tongue depressor to help hold the tongue down. While avoiding the tongue and inside of the cheeks, take the specimen directly from the affected area with the sterile swab. Once the specimen is obtained on the swab, place the swab back into the culturette (Figure 43-12B). The culturette is now ready for labeling and transport to the laboratory for testing (Figure 43-12C). As with any culture test ordered, a requisition stating the site from which the specimen was obtained is required.

  Throat swabs for the detection of group A *Streptococcus* infection (strep throat) usually are tested in the POL using a self-contained kit that produces quick results (see Procedure 43-3). Performing the rapid strep tests are well within the medical assistant's scope under CLIA's waived test category. More information about performing rapid strep tests is provided later in this chapter in the section on *Streptococcus* Screening.

Nose. A nasopharyngeal swab may be requested with a throat culture. This is collected with a swab on a thin wire. A separate swab may be used for each nostril. The patient tilts back the head, and each swab is gently inserted into each of the nostrils. The swab is then placed into a sterile tube and kept at room temperature for transport to the laboratory.

Wound. When culturing a wound, a sterile needle might be used to aspirate pus-filled fluid from the wound, or a swab is used. It is important to get the swab deep into the wound without touching the surrounding skin. Specimens for wound cultures often are placed in anaerobic transport medium, especially if the wound is not superficial.

Sputum. To collect this specimen correctly, the patient should cough deeply and **expectorate** into the sterile container (Figure 43-13). The specimen should be a first morning specimen and placed into a sterile container designed to protect all who handle the specimen from contamination.

Stool. Stool specimens are brought to the laboratory for various tests. If the stool is to be examined for **ova** (eggs) or parasites, the specimen should be as fresh as possible. Special containers often are used for ova and parasites. Stool specimens must

PATIENT EDUCATION

As you obtain throat cultures from patients, you may want to give them some helpful advice concerning their condition. Generally when a person has a sore throat, it is associated with other respiratory symptoms as well. The following suggestions may provide some relief from discomfort and help patients toward better health.

1. Advise patients to drink plenty of liquids, especially water, and to eat sensibly from the basic food groups.

2. Urge patients to get extra rest and dress comfortably (according to the weather/temperature outside).

3. Suggest use of gargles or throat lozenges (or both) to relieve painful sore throat.

4. Remind patients to avoid tobacco/smoking.

5. Instruct patients to cough/sneeze into tissue and discard into proper waste container wherever they are to prevent the spread of microorganisms. Because sewer waste is treated and disinfected, flushing a contaminated tissue is an effective method of disposal.

6. Remind patients to refrain from sharing drinking glasses and tableware and from intimate contact such as kissing while they are infected and still contagious. All eating utensils should be sanitized in hot water after use to avoid the spread of contagious diseases. Perhaps the most important educational advice is reminding patients to wash their hands frequently.

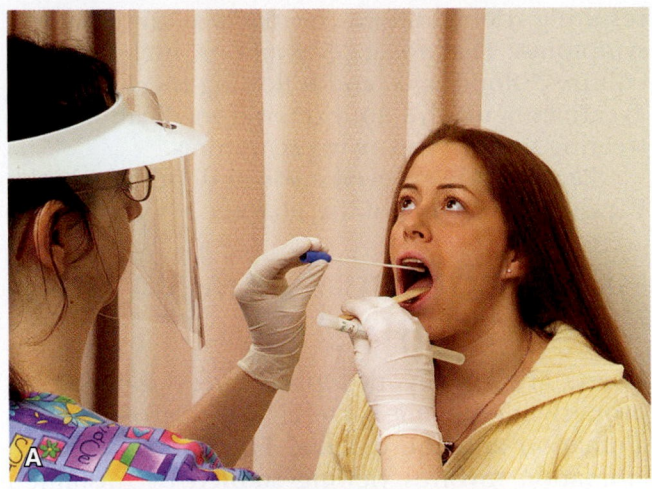

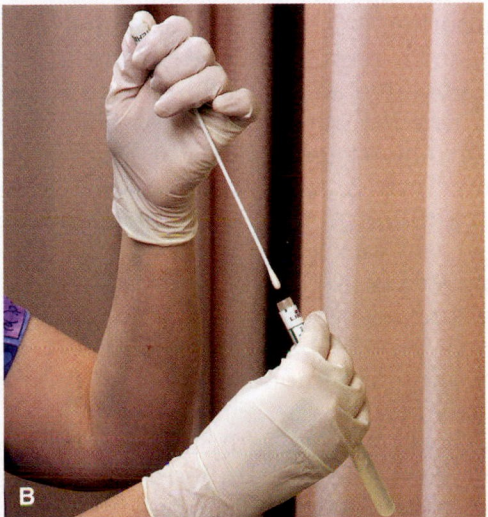

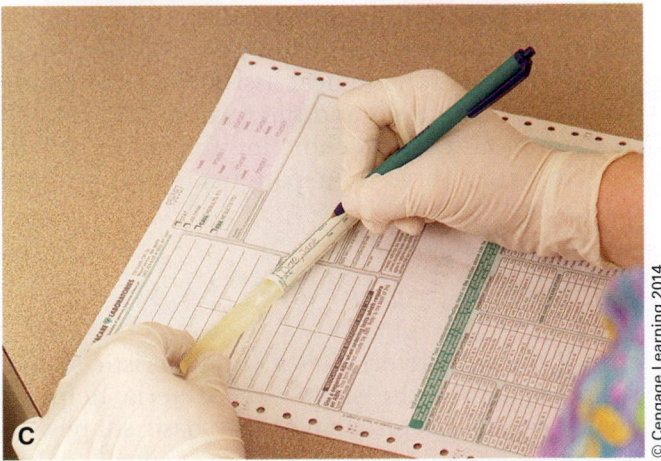

Figure 43-12   (A) The medical assistant obtains a throat culture using a culturette, taking care not to touch the cheeks or tongue. (B) After swabbing the patient's throat, the medical assistant returns the swab to the culturette, which contains the moist medium. (C) The culturette is labeled, and a requisition is completed in preparation for transport to the regional laboratory for testing.

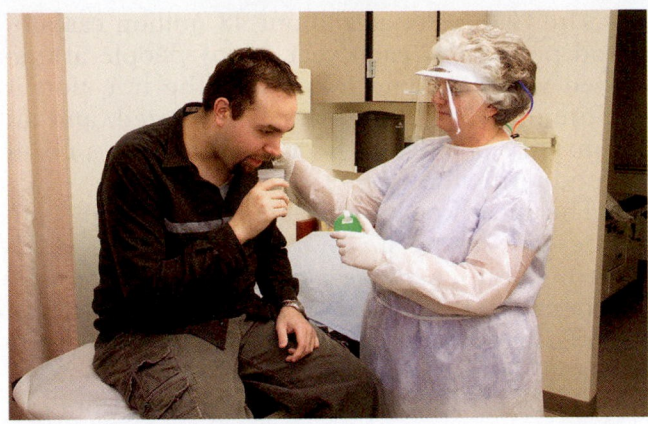

Figure 43-13   A patient gives a sputum sample.

be kept at between room temperature and body temperature. Refrigeration may destroy the parasites within the specimen.

For bacterial cultures of stool (as well as for ova and parasites), several different specimens may be sent for testing at different times. The collection containers for stool cultures do not have to be sterile, but they must be clean and have a tightfitting lid (see Procedure 43-4).

Cerebrospinal Fluid (CSF). The provider obtains CSF by doing a lumbar puncture (see Procedure 30-22). The fluid generally is dispersed in several departments of the clinical laboratory. Generally, the fluid goes first to the microbiology laboratory for a culture before it becomes contaminated by doing other tests. Before the culture set up, the tube should be placed in an incubator or left at room temperature. Refrigeration of spinal fluid can kill two common meningitis-causing bacteria, *Haemophilus influenzae* and *Neisseria meningitidis*. CSF culture is a STAT order for processing, and the medical assistant is responsible for calling the laboratory for immediate pickup.

Blood. Human blood is free from bacteria in a healthy human. If blood does become contaminated with bacteria, septicemia (septic blood infection) can result. Blood cultures are collected by the same means as regular blood collection, with special considerations to avoid any contamination of the blood. A variety of collection devices are available for collecting blood cultures, all requiring careful sterile techniques see Procedure 40-7 (blood culture collection).

FOODBORNE ILLNESSES

Foodborne illnesses from bacterial infections and parasites are a huge health care concern in the United States, becoming even more prevalent with the increase of international travel.

The CDC estimates about 48 million cases of "food poisoning" each year. Many people are afflicted without being aware and the infection is self-limiting. Still others are hospitalized, and an estimated 3,000 deaths occur each year as a result of foodborne illnesses.

The most well-known agents that cause foodborne illnesses are *Campylobacter, Clostridium botulinum* (botulism), *Cryptosporidium, Cyclospora, Escherichia coli,* hepatitis A virus, *Listeria,* norovirus, *Salmonella, Shigella, Staphylococcus aureus, Vibrio parahaemolyticus,* and *Vibrio vulnificus* (Figure 43-14). Some of these foodborne illnesses are contracted from raw or undercooked meats and seafood, some from contaminated food handlers, and some from unwashed produce.

Symptoms range from mild to severe diarrhea, nausea, vomiting, abdominal pain, fever, and the resulting dehydration, headaches, and flu-like symptoms. Diagnostic evaluations include stool cultures, blood tests, and following the symptoms. Treatments involve antibacterial medications and treating the accompanying symptoms.

Parasites are covered more in depth within the Parasitology section of this chapter.

MICROSCOPIC EXAMINATION OF BACTERIA

There are usually two procedures involved in properly identifying bacteria: the microscopic examination and the culture. The microscopic examination involves viewing stained or unstained bacteria through the microscope.

Culturing is a means of isolating a disease-causing microorganism for identification. A specimen is obtained and placed in a culture medium, which contains nutrients comparable to human tissue to encourage growth of microorganisms. The medium is **agar**, a gelatin-like substance, mixed with nutrients. The nutrients mixed in the agar will vary according to what each particular bacterium prefers. The section on Culture Media later discusses in detail the types of nutrients each type of bacterium prefers. Table 43-4 lists the more common bacteria and their growth requirements.

Microscopically identifying bacteria is not in CLIA's waived categories; therefore, although the medical assistant will not actually perform these tests, the staining information is included here to aid in understanding the staining and examination processes that culture specimens go through. It is important for medical assistants to be familiar with the processes and the terminology related to staining and microscopic identification of bacteria to better serve their patients, employer, and colleagues.

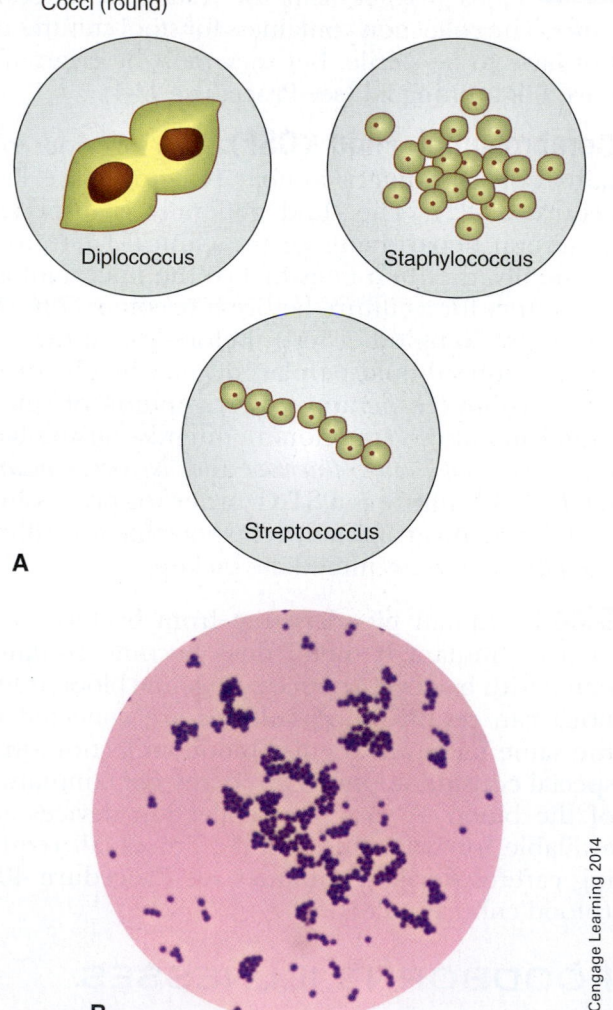

Cocci (round)

Diplococcus

Staphylococcus

Streptococcus

A

B

© Cengage Learning 2014

Figure 43-14 (A) Cocci (round). (B) Cocci, as seen through a microscope.

Bacterial Shapes

Each genus of bacteria has a characteristic shape. A knowledge of the shapes of bacteria helps in identification. Bacteria have three basic shapes:

1. *Cocci.* Cocci (Figure 43-14) are round, occurring in clusters, pairs, singles, and tetrads (groups of three). They are nonmotile microorganisms. (They do not move on their own accord.)

2. *Bacilli.* Bacilli are rod-shaped and can have rounded, straight, or pointed ends

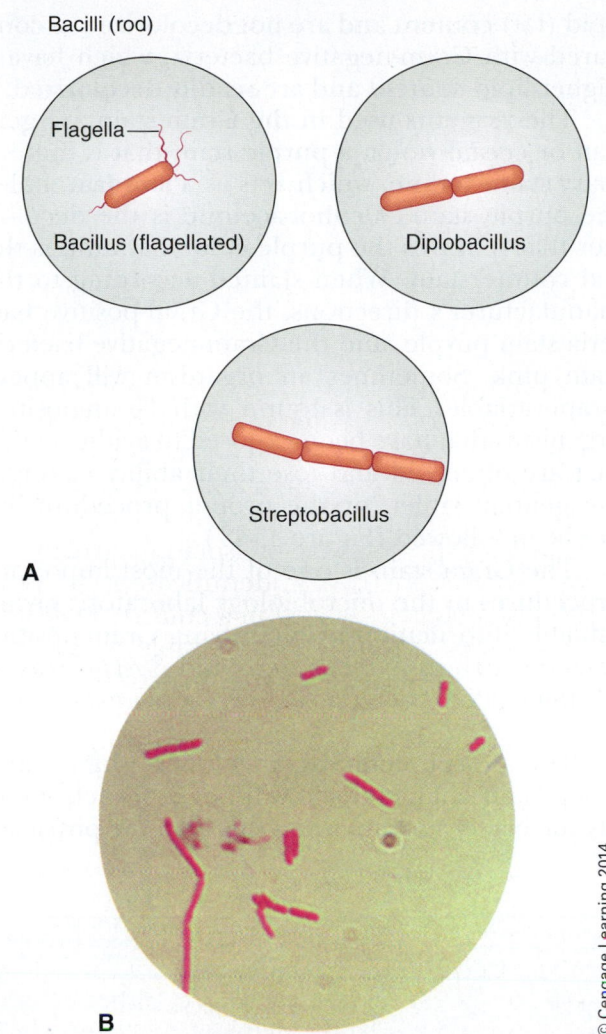

Bacilli (rod)

Flagella

Bacillus (flagellated)

Diplobacillus

Streptobacillus

A

B

Figure 43-15 (A) Bacilli (rod-shaped). (B) Bacilli, as seen through a microscope.

© Cengage Learning 2014

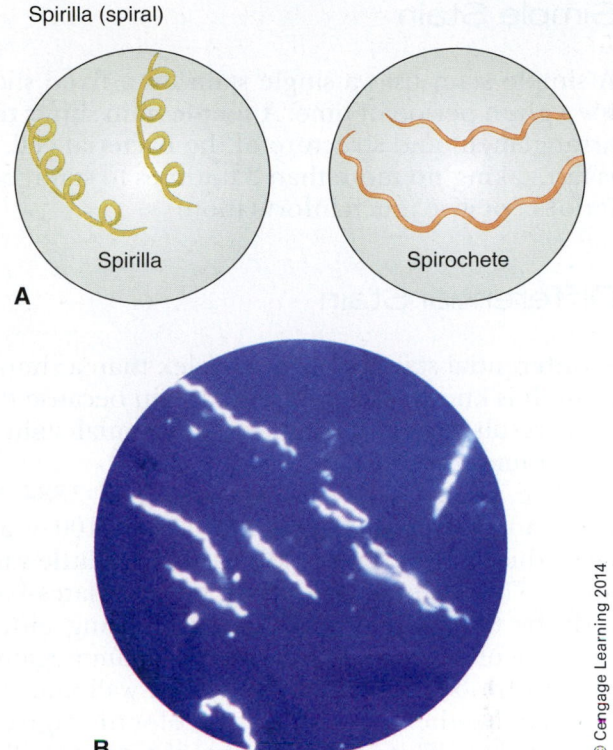

Spirilla (spiral)

Spirilla

Spirochete

A

B

Figure 43-16 (A) Spirilla (spiral). (B) Spirilla, as seen through a microscope.

© Cengage Learning 2014

(Figure 43-15). Some bacilli have flagella that give bacteria motility (movement). Most bacteria are the shape of bacilli.

3. *Spirilla.* Spirilla are spiral-shaped bacteria that have one too many turns (Figure 43-16). Most spirilla are motile.

The microscopic examination produces information that is often needed to identify bacteria. However, biochemical reactions and the sensitivity pattern (how the organisms respond to antibiotics) are also needed to make the full identification.

Dyes (Stains)

The dyes used in microbiology are derived from coal tar. These dyes are acidic or basic and impart a

color to the microorganism. Basic dyes carry a positive ion and stain structures that are acidic in nature. An acid dye carries a negative ion and stains structures that are basic (alkaline) in nature such as cytoplasmic structures. Several different types of stains are used depending on what test is ordered. (Table 43-3 lists stains and their uses.)

Table 43-3 Stains and Their Uses

Stain	Example
Simple	Carbolfuchsin Gentian violet Methylene blue Safranin
Differential	Gram Acid-fast (Ziehl-Neelsen, Kinyoun)
Special	Capsule (Welch negative) Flagella (Leifson) Nuclei (Feulgen) Spore (Doerner)

© Cengage Learning 2014

Simple Stain

A simple stain uses a single stain on a fixed slide for a given period of time. A simple stain shows the arrangement and structure of the bacterial cell. It is fast, taking no more than 3 minutes to stain, but it does not give much information.

Differential Stain

A differential stain is more complex than a simple stain. It is known as a differential stain because the stain result varies. A common differential stain is the Gram stain.

The Gram stain was developed in 1884 by Dr. Hans Christian Gram. More than 100 years later, this famous stain is still in use with little variation. This staining procedure differentiates bacteria by their Gram stain ability of being either negative or positive. A bacterium is Gram negative or positive by the nature of the cell wall and the ability of it either to retain or lose color through decolorization. This identification of Gram-positive or Gram-negative bacteria aids in identification of an organism. Gram-positive bacteria have a lower lipid (fat) content and are not decolorized as compared with Gram-negative bacteria, which have a higher lipid content and are readily decolorized.

The reagents used in the Gram stain are gentian or crystal violet, a purple stain that is the primary stain. Iodine, which acts as a **mordant**, holds the purple stain. Alcohol-acetone is the decolorizer that removes the purple color. Safranin is the red counterstain. When stained according to the manufacturer's directions, the Gram-positive bacteria stain purple, and the Gram-negative bacteria stain pink. Sometimes an organism will appear Gram-variable. This is found with Gram-positive organisms that have been exposed to acidic media, that are often old and lose their ability to retain the gentian violet, or the proper procedure has not been followed (Figure 43-17).

The Gram stain is one of the most important procedures in the microbiology laboratory, giving valuable information by identifying Gram-positive bacteria such as *Staphylococcus* and *Streptococcus* or Gram-negative bacteria such as *Escherichia coli* and *Proteus*.

The morphologic arrangement, shape, and Gram stain characteristic will begin to help identify the bacteria. Sometimes this is all the physician

Step	Time	Procedure	Result
1	1 minute	Primary stain: Apply crystal violet stain (purple) ↓ Rinse slide	All bacteria stain purple 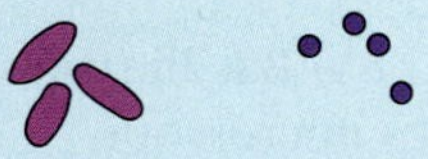
2	1 minute	Mordant: Apply Gram's iodine ↓ Rinse slide	All bacteria remain purple 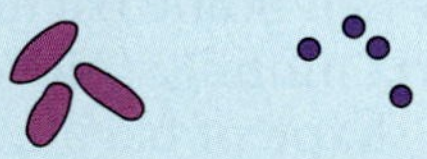
3	3 to 5 seconds	Decolorize: Apply alcohol ↓ Rinse slide	Purple stain is removed from Gram-negative cells 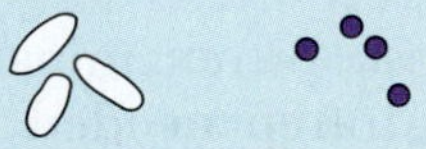
4	1 minute	Counterstain: Apply safranin stain (red) ↓ Rinse slide	Gram-negative cells appear pink-red; Gram-positive cells appear purple 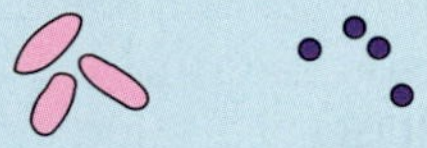

© Cengage Learning 2014

Figure 43-17 Steps in the Gram stain procedure.

needs to know to start treatment for a pathogenic organism. For example, the bacteria causing gonorrhea *(Neisseria gonorrhoeae)* is a distinctive organism, having a characteristic diplococci shape that resembles a coffee or kidney bean. Kidney or coffee bean is more readily identified through Gram staining.

Acid-Fast Stain

Another differential stain, which is often referred to as a specific stain, is the acid-fast stain. This stain is either differential or specific in that it allows microscopic examination of acid-fast organisms. This group of organisms does not respond well to the Gram stain and is difficult to stain under ordinary circumstances because of a waxy capsule cell wall that resists staining.

To stain these organisms, heat or a powerful dye is used in the procedure to stain the bacteria. The bacteria, once stained, resist decolorization with an acid alcohol, giving them the acid-fast name. The bacterium that causes tuberculosis is an acid-fast organism.

Two methods commonly used to stain acid-fast organisms are the Ziehl-Neelsen stain, which uses heat, and the Kinyoun stain, a cold method that does not include a heating process. Either of these stains is satisfactory.

Special Techniques

There are several special situations when more than the Gram stain or the shape and arrangement of an organism is needed to aid in the identification. Such situations would be the demonstration of the presence of flagella, spore, capsule, or nuclei of cells.

There also are microscopic examinations of organisms in a living state, without staining. Characteristics that can be studied by this method include motility, shape, and arrangement of organisms. This technique requires the microorganisms to be in a liquid suspension. The medical assistant often is responsible for setting up the slide for microscopic examination by the provider. Although microscopy is not a CLIA waived test, the medical assistant can certainly view the slides microscopically and discuss the finding with the provider as a learning exercise.

 For vaginal secretions, a swab of the vaginal discharge is placed in a sterile tube containing 1 mL normal saline and mixed. Then the suspension is viewed under a microscope. For stool or other bacterial specimens, a small amount of specimen is mixed with a drop of normal saline, then viewed under a microscope. These methods are known as the **wet-mount** preparation and the hanging drop preparation (see Procedure 43-2).

The wet-mount preparation is a valuable diagnostic tool in determining the cause of vaginosis. Bacterial vaginosis is identified by the presence of "clue cells," epithelial cells covered by coccobacillary bacteria. Motile trichomonads are seen with *Trichomonas vaginalis*. The presence of pseudohyphae indicates a yeast infection. In many cases, an accurate diagnosis can be made from the wet mount preparation, thus making more complex techniques unnecessary.

Potassium Hydroxide Preparation

Another type of wet preparation uses 10% solution of **potassium hydroxide (KOH)** in a wet preparation for the study of fungi and spores. The slide is prepared by using fragments of human hair, skin, or nails that could have fungus. KOH wet mounts are also useful for examining other body fluids such as vaginal swabs. These specimens are placed on a slide with a drop of 10% KOH and a cover-slip on top. The KOH will clear debris. The slide should sit at room temperature for about a half hour before examination for debris settlement.

The direct examination of specimens is best viewed with a phase or dark-field microscope rather than a bright-field microscope because of reduced illumination. If using a bright-field microscope, lower the condenser to reduce transmitted light. Proper disposal of these specimens is important because the organisms are alive and possibly pathogenic.

CULTURE MEDIA

After the proper collection of the specimen, the material collected must be inoculated on a proper culture medium. This is necessary for growth and eventual identification of an organism.

The results of culture, the growing of an organism on special media in the laboratory, are only as reliable as the method used in collecting the specimen. In addition, growth requirements of different organisms must be considered, such as moisture, temperature, oxygen, carbon dioxide, and essential nutrients. Organisms that are sensitive to drying must be put into transport medium immediately after collection to prevent loss of

Table 43-4   Common Bacteria and Their Growth Requirements

Organism	Disease	Medium	Oxygen Requirements
Streptococcus	Strep throat	Blood agar	$\downarrow O_2$, $\uparrow CO_2$
Neisseria gonorrhoeae	Gonorrhea	Chocolate agar, modified Thayer-Martin (MTM)	$\downarrow O_2$, $\uparrow CO_2$
Staphylococcus	Infections, boils	Blood agar	O_2
Escherichia coli	Urinary tract infection	Blood agar, eosin methylene blue (EMB), MacConkey	O_2

© Cengage Learning 2014

viability. Some bacteria require a specialized medium to grow and multiply. Aerobic bacteria grow only in the presence of oxygen. Anaerobic bacteria live and grow in the absence of oxygen. Examples of common bacteria and their growth requirements are listed in Table 43-4.

When specimens are collected for the laboratory, the microorganism's growth requirements must be considered. No matter how good the specimen, if an anaerobic organism is kept in an aerobic atmosphere while being transported to the reference laboratory, it will probably not survive. Special anaerobic transport systems must be used.

Neisseria gonorrhoeae, the causative agent of the STD gonorrhea, requires special media and an atmosphere of reduced oxygen and increased carbon dioxide. Therefore, the specimen must be collected from the patient and immediately placed on a special medium in a reduced oxygen atmosphere.

Medical assistants who send bacterial specimens to a reference laboratory must be familiar with the transport media the reference laboratory provides. Your laboratory manual explains how and when to use the various microbiology transport systems.

Media can be a solid, liquid, or semisolid substance that has the required nutrients to support the growth of bacteria. Such ingredients include vitamins, sugar, salt, minerals, and amino acids. Some media have the addition of special products such as egg, potato, meat, milk, blood, and dyes.

The solid form of media is called agar. Agar has an appearance similar to gelatin and is made of seaweed. When heated, agar is a liquid; when cooled, it solidifies. Agar is poured into a petri dish (a plastic dish used to grow bacteria) so the bacteria can be studied for gross **morphology** (form and structure). Agar can also be placed in tubes.

Semisolid medium is made by adding less agar. Medium in a liquid broth form is stored in tubes called **broth tubes** and allows for the observation of gas production, change in pH, and odor. Figure 43-9 shows many different types of media that can be used to identify bacteria. Medium can be purchased already prepared, or it can be produced from ingredients in the laboratory. Charts listing the proper media to set up for specific types of cultures generally are prominently displayed in the setup area of most microbiology laboratories.

Media Classification

There are several classifications of media, including:

- *Basic.* Basic media are used for general purposes and do not contain added nutrients. They will support the growth of many Gram-negative and Gram-positive organisms.

- *Differential.* Differential media contain substances that alter the appearance of some types of organisms and not other types. An eosin methylene blue (EMB) plate for lactose and nonlactose fermenters is an example of differential medium. The lactose fermenter can use lactose and looks different on the agar.

- *Selective.* Selective media support the growth of one type of organism while inhibiting the growth of another. This is done by the addition of a salt, dye, chemical, or antibiotic. A hektoen enteric (HE) plate for the growth of *Salmonella* and *Shigella* is a selective type of medium.

- *Enriched.* This type of medium contains substances that inhibit certain bacteria from growing. These media work well with cultures from sites that possess normal flora, such as the throat. The normal flora is inhibited and

Table 43-5 Common Microbiology Media by Classification and Use

Type	Name	Use
Basic	Trypticase agar Trypticase broth	Supports the growth of most organisms
Differential	Blood agar MacConkey Eosin methylene blue (EMB)	Supports the growth of *Streptococcus* and *Staphylococcus*; demonstrates hemolysis Certain Gram-negative organisms Escherichia coli
Selective	*Salmonella* and *Shigella* (SS) Hektoen Phenylethyl alcohol Mannitol salt Selenite (GN) broth Thayer-Martin Thioglycollate broth	Gram-negative *Salmonella* and *Shigella* Enteric organisms Inhibits Gram-negative growth Promotes growth of *Staphylococcus* Promotes growth of enteric organisms Promotes growth of *Neisseria* species Promotes growth of anaerobes
Enriched	Loefflers Chocolate Lowenstein-Jensen	Promotes growth of *Corynebacterium* Promotes growth of *Haemophilus* species Promotes growth of mycobacteria

© Cengage Learning 2014

pathogenic bacteria are encouraged to grow. Blood agar and chocolate agar are examples of enriched media.

All media that are used should first be checked with known organisms for quality control and for contaminants. The manufacturer will usually suggest a list of organisms for a quality-control check. A check for contaminants involves a thorough visual check of the plate before using it. It is also important to store media according to the manufacturer's direction. *Never use outdated media.*

Table 43-5 lists common media by classification and use. Table 43-6 lists media that might be selected for specific sources. All laboratories vary slightly in their recommendations of media to set up on specimens.

MICROBIOLOGY CULTURE
Inoculating the Media

After selecting the correct medium for the culture and observing the specimen to make sure it is properly collected, the specimen is inoculated onto the medium. If the specimen is on a swab, the swab is rolled directly onto the upper quadrant of the agar plate. If the specimen is a sputum or liquid, it is inoculated onto the plate with a loop.

The inoculum is spread back and forth in a sweeping motion with a flamed loop or needle.

After the agar plate has been inoculated and properly labeled, it should be turned upside down and placed in the proper environment for growth. By turning the agar upside down, any condensation that forms from bacterial growth will be on the inside lid.

Liquid broths and agar slant tubes have screw caps. These caps must not be screwed on too tightly because of gas production by some organisms that can break the tube.

Other Types of Streaking

Other types of streaking include the lawn streak. This streaking technique is used to place an organism over an entire area of an agar plate for sensitivity testing. The bacteria are spread over the entire plate using a swab (Figure 43-18), streaking over the entire area several times from different angles. After the streaking has been completed, discs saturated with different antibiotics are placed equidistant throughout the streaked area (Figure 43-19B).

The colony count is a streaking technique much like the lawn technique. This technique is used to plate urine cultures. A special calibrated urine loop is used to make the first streak, followed by a second streak that goes across the entire length of the initial streak. Then another

Table 43-6 Common Specimens, Suspected Pathogens, and Media Recommendations

Specimen Source	Potential Pathogens	Blood agar	Chocolate	Eosin Methylene Blue	MacConkey	Salmonella and Shigella Hektoen Enteric	Selenite	Thayer-Martin	Thioglycollate	CO₂
Eye/Ear	Neisseria gonorrhoeae Haemophilus species Staphylococcus aureus Streptococcus pyogenes Pseudomonas aeruginosa Moraxella species	x	x	x	x			x	x	x
Cerebrospinal fluid	Neisseria meningitidis Streptococcus pneumoniae Haemophilus influenzae	x	x						x	x
Throat	Streptococcus pyogenes	x								x
Sputum	Streptococcus pneumoniae	x								
Urine	Escherichia coli Klebsiella Proteus Pseudomonas aeruginosa Enterococcus	x		x	x					
Wounds	Staphylococcus Streptococcus Enterobacteriaceae Anaerobic bacteria	x	x	x	x				x	x
Stool	Salmonella Shigella			x	x	x	x			
Stool	Pathogenic E. coli Yersinia species									
Vaginal	Neisseria gonorrhoeae	x	x					x		x

© Cengage Learning 2014

complete streaking is placed over the original streaks after rotating the plate (Figure 43-19A). This method of using a calibrated loop to get a more accurate inoculation gives the provider an idea of how many colonies of bacteria are present.

Every laboratory will use slightly different ways of performing the basic streaks. The important factor is to use good aseptic techniques so there is no contamination from outside organisms, and all organisms that are streaked out are isolated enough to test further if necessary.

Primary Culture

After the medium has been incubated for 24 to 48 hours, the initial or primary culture is read.

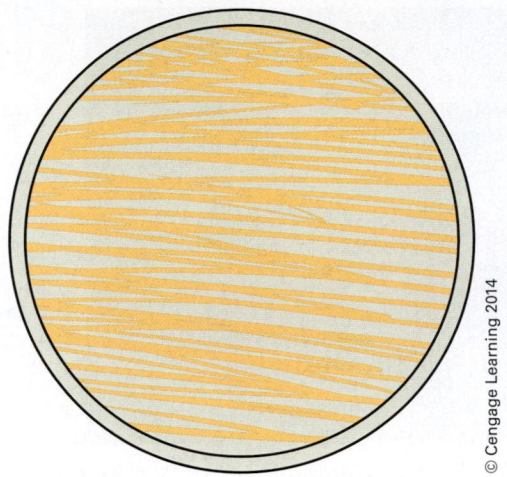

Figure 43-18   Lawn or spread streak.

Subculture

When working with bacterial cultures, there can be more than one pathogen growing in the culture. For instance, a wound culture may have both Gram-positive and Gram-negative organisms growing. To identify each organism, you must separate these bacteria to other media (Figure 43-20). It is also necessary at times to separate the pathogenic bacteria from the normal flora, as in the throat and sputum cultures. Some initial cultures do achieve excellent isolation without having to subculture.

RAPID IDENTIFICATION SYSTEMS

The age of high technology and computerized equipment has also made inroads into microbiology laboratories, clinics, and POLs. Many traditional methods of identifying bacteria have been replaced by rapid identification test kits.

Rapid test systems, which are CLIA waived, give a quick identification, are economical, and allow the provider to start treatment sooner. Rapid tests allow the provider to receive results while the patient is still in the office.

Streptococcus Screening (Rapid Strep Testing)

A number of instant or rapid test kits identify group A *Streptococcus* (also known as beta-hemolytic *Streptococcus* group A), the causative agent of a seriourjore (strep) throat. It is important to identify this Gram-positive *Streptococcus* as soon as possible because the bacteria can cause serious damage (i.e., kidney and heart valve damage) if not treated immediately with antibiotics.

This test is sensitive and eliminates false-positive results. The directions should be followed strictly to produce an accurate test result. The results are based on color development of a spot on the test filter. Test results are available in minutes.

A latex agglutination test for group A *Streptococcus* is based on an antigen and antibody agglutination. A throat swab is placed directly on the antibody-coated slide, and the presence of a positive test is seen by the appearance of agglutination (clumping). Although these tests are quick and convenient, the following rules should be followed strictly:

- Read and understand the manufacturer's instructions and directions before starting the test.
- Never use outdated materials.
- Observe all safety guidelines and precautions.

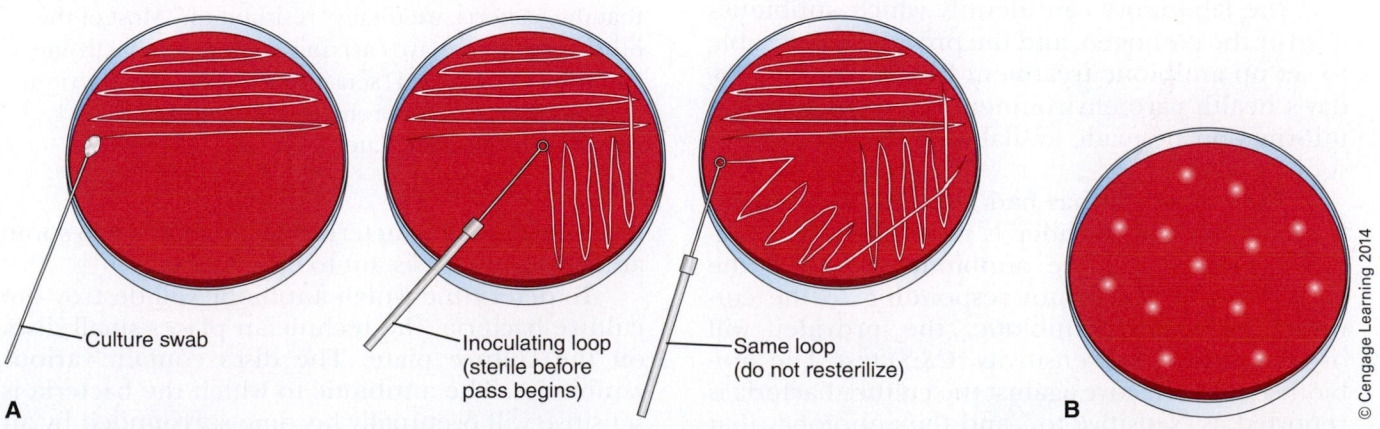

Culture swab

Inoculating loop (sterile before pass begins)

Same loop (do not resterilize)

A

B

Figure 43-19   Colony count streak.

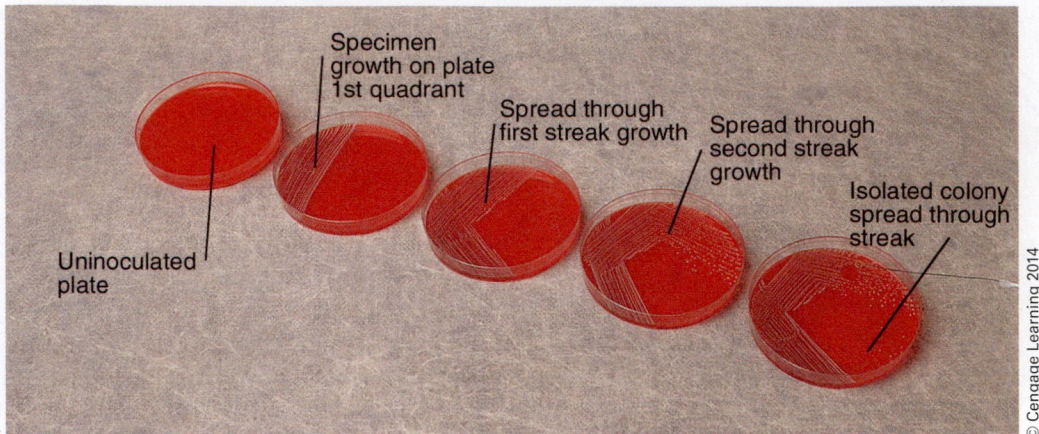

Figure 43-20 Stages of spreading out the bacteria to isolate colonies.

- Use the correct swab in taking the throat culture. Some cottons and chemicals on swab will interfere with the test reagents. If possible, use the swabs provided with the kit.

- Always run the positive and negative control together with the patient's actual test.

If a patient has symptoms of an infected throat and the slide test is negative, the provider will also order a regular throat culture to make sure there is no infection present. Latex agglutination kits can give false readings, and it is best to follow up with the throat culture. A list of all the CLIA waived rapid tests is available at the CDC website (http://www.cdc.gov) using the search words Waived Tests.

SENSITIVITY TESTING

Antibiotic sensitivity testing often is ordered on the pathogenic organisms recovered from the culturing process. By setting up an antibiotic sensitivity test, the laboratory can identify which antibiotics destroy the pathogen, and the provider will be able to set up antibiotic treatment for the patient. Today's health care environment demands that this information be made available to the provider as soon as possible.

When a patient has had multiple bacterial infections and the provider is concerned with prescribing an ineffective antibiotic, or when the bacterial infection is not responding to the currently prescribed antibiotic, the provider will order a culture and sensitivity (C&S) test. The antibiotic that is effective against the culture bacteria is reported as "sensitive to," and the antibiotics that are not effective will be reported as "resistant to,"

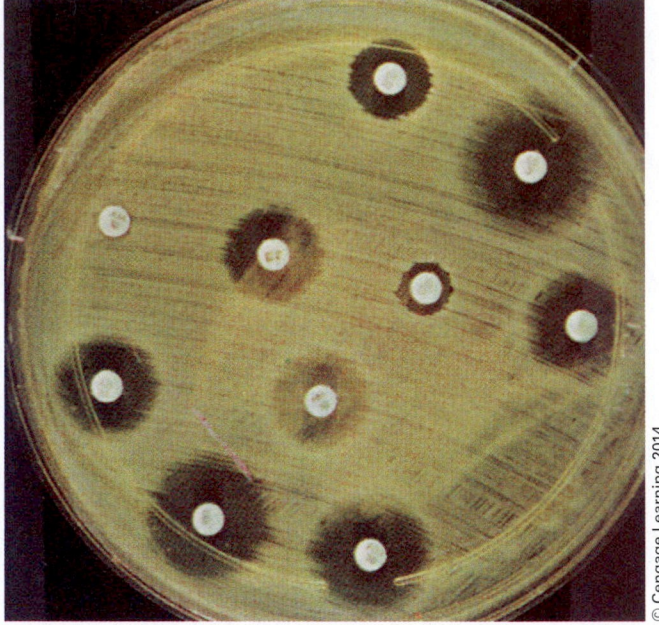

Figure 43-21 Culture plate showing antibiotic discs on bacteria. Note the one antibiotic disc in the left area that the bacteria are totally "resistant to." Most of the other antibiotics have carrying degrees of effectiveness and would be labeled "sensitive to." The one just right of the center area is barely effective and would be reported as "intermediate."

meaning that the bacteria will be sensitive to some antibiotics and resistant to others.

To determine which antibiotic will destroy the culture bacteria, the technician places small discs on the culture plate. The discs contain various antibiotics. The antibiotic to which the bacteria is sensitive will eventually become surrounded by an area of no growth (Figure 43-21).

Giardiasis
(Giardia intestinalis)

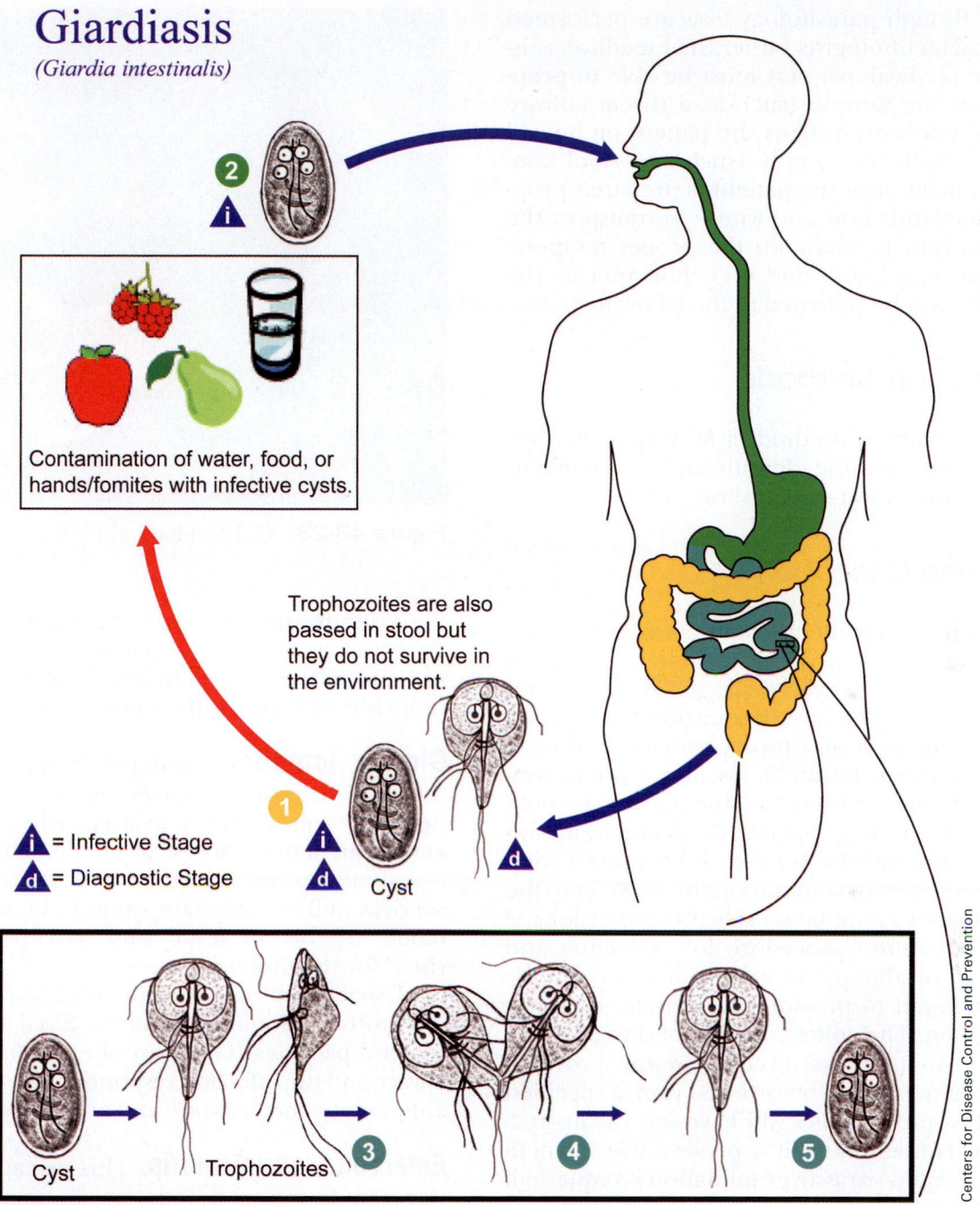

Contamination of water, food, or hands/fomites with infective cysts.

Trophozoites are also passed in stool but they do not survive in the environment.

i = Infective Stage

d = Diagnostic Stage

Cyst

Cyst   Trophozoites

Centers for Disease Control and Prevention

Figure 43-22 Giardia life cycle.

PARASITOLOGY

With the age of travel and more public awareness, we are beginning to see more parasitic infections. The field of parasitology is a vast one with many different types of parasites. They range from extremely small microscopic ones to those that are large and macroscopic. Parasites have varying life cycles. The degree of severity of illness depends on which parasite enters the human body and infects it. Parasites can be found in the blood, urine, or feces. The more common ones are found in the feces.

Different geographic areas have different types of parasites. Resettled immigrant populations may be infected with a parasite previously unseen in a geographic area. World travelers can also bring back rare parasitic infections from their adventures.

Even though parasitology tests are performed by medical technologists rather than medical assistants, the medical assistant must be able to properly obtain the sample (such as a throat culture or wound culture), instruct the patient on how to properly obtain the sample (such as a stool sample), and make sure the patient is prepared properly, understands how and where to transport the specimen, how to maintain the proper temperature of the specimen, and even how quickly the specimen must be returned to the laboratory.

Examination Methods

The most common method of fecal specimen examination for parasitic identification in a clinic or POL is the direct wet-mount slide.

Specimen Collection

Fecal specimens for identification of ova and parasites should be collected in wide-mouth containers with a tight lid to prevent leakage. The container should be put in a biohazard transport bag to avoid contamination and sent for examination immediately. The patient should be instructed not to contaminate the specimen with urine because it could interfere with testing. Special vials containing formalin are also available for ova and parasite testing that are preferred by some laboratories. Refer to the laboratory user's manual for specific instructions.

The laboratory procedure for collection and processing of the parasite specimen should be strictly followed to provide an accurate testing of the specimen. The collection time of the specimen should be followed as directed by the provider. Three specimens may be ordered over a specified period. Provider's clinics will have specific instructions and containers with a preservative in them when an ova and parasite examination is requested. When the specimen is sent for testing, it should be labeled correctly with the patient's name, date, and time of the specimen. It is important to know if the patient has been traveling, to what area of the world, and what is suspected by the provider to help aid in identification (see Procedure 43-4).

Common Parasites

Some of the more common parasites identified in the POL are *Giardia lamblia,* a type of intestinal Parasite (Figure 43-23), *Enterobius vermicularis,*

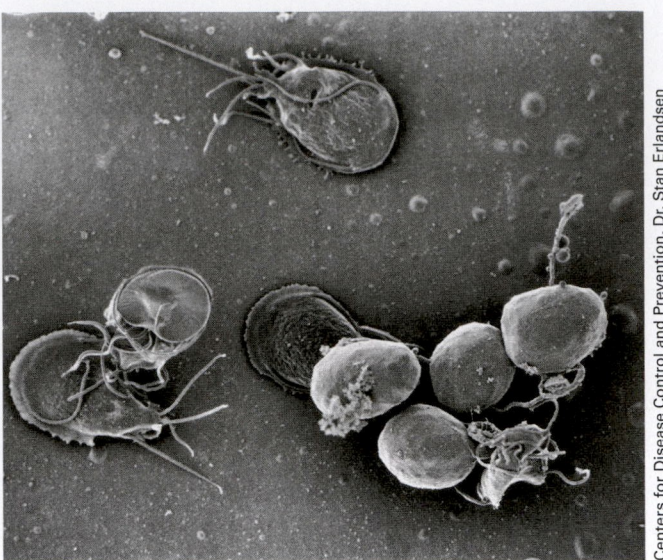

Figure 43-23   G. Lamblia.

the causative organism of pinworm infection, and *Trichomonas vaginalis,* a parasite that infects the urogenital tracts of men and women. Less common, but still seen, is the hookworm.

Giardia lamblia. Giardiasis is spread through the fecal to oral route (see Figure 43-22). Infection is certainly higher in areas where sanitation and clean water are less available. The organism is resistant to the chlorine levels in tap water and survives well in mountain streams, hence the nicknames of "beaver fever" and "backpacker's diarrhea" for the illness it causes.

Usual symptoms include diarrhea and multiple gastrointestinal complaints. Stool cultures for ova and parasites (O&P) are the diagnostic tests of choice and the infection responds well to antibiotics, antiparasitic medications, and antiprotozoal agents.

Enterobius vermicularis. This **nematode** (round worm) is found worldwide, predominantly in children. The adult worm is shaped like a pin, wide at one end and pointed at the other end. The female worm is larger than the male. Infection with pin worm can cause severe itching, irritability, and insomnia, depending on the severity of the infection. The adult female worm migrates to the anus at night, depositing ova (eggs) that cause itching during hatching. At times, the adult worm can be found around the anus and on the stool. The adult worm measures approximately 7 to 12 mm long. The egg is the infectious stage of the parasite (Figure 43-24).

To diagnose the presence of the parasite, either the adult worm or the ova have to be located

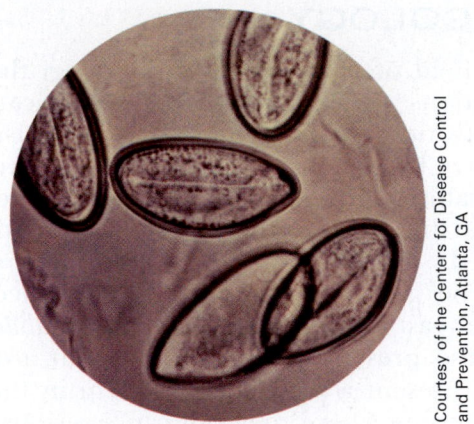

Figure 43-24   Pinworm ova, as seen through a microscope.

Courtesy of the Centers for Disease Control and Prevention, Atlanta, GA

in the specimen. A negative test should be confirmed by as many as six negative tests performed. The test is performed by taking a cellophane tape swab and placing the sticky side down to the skin around the anal area. The tape is placed on a slide and brought to the laboratory for examination (Figure 43-25).

Trichomonas vaginalis. This parasite is found in both men and women, but its presence is five times higher in women (men can harbor the organism for years without symptoms). Because men can harbor this parasite and have no symptoms, it is recommended that both partners be treated. This will prevent the ongoing reinfection of the female patient. The organism belongs to the flagellate (possesses flagella) class and is extremely motile. Infection with this flagellate causes a purulent yellowish green discharge and dysuria. The organism is recovered from the discharge or urine and is transmitted sexually.

ONLINE IMAGES AND INFORMATION ABOUT PARASITES

The Centers for Disease Control and Prevention (CDC) has an extensive website with a wealth of information about many health issues. Of particular interest to medical assistants and other health care professionals interested in parasites is the DPDx, a website that is maintained by the CDC's Division of Parasitic Diseases. Go to http://www.dpd.cdc.gov/dpdx and click on Image Library for a great college-level epidemiology image library.

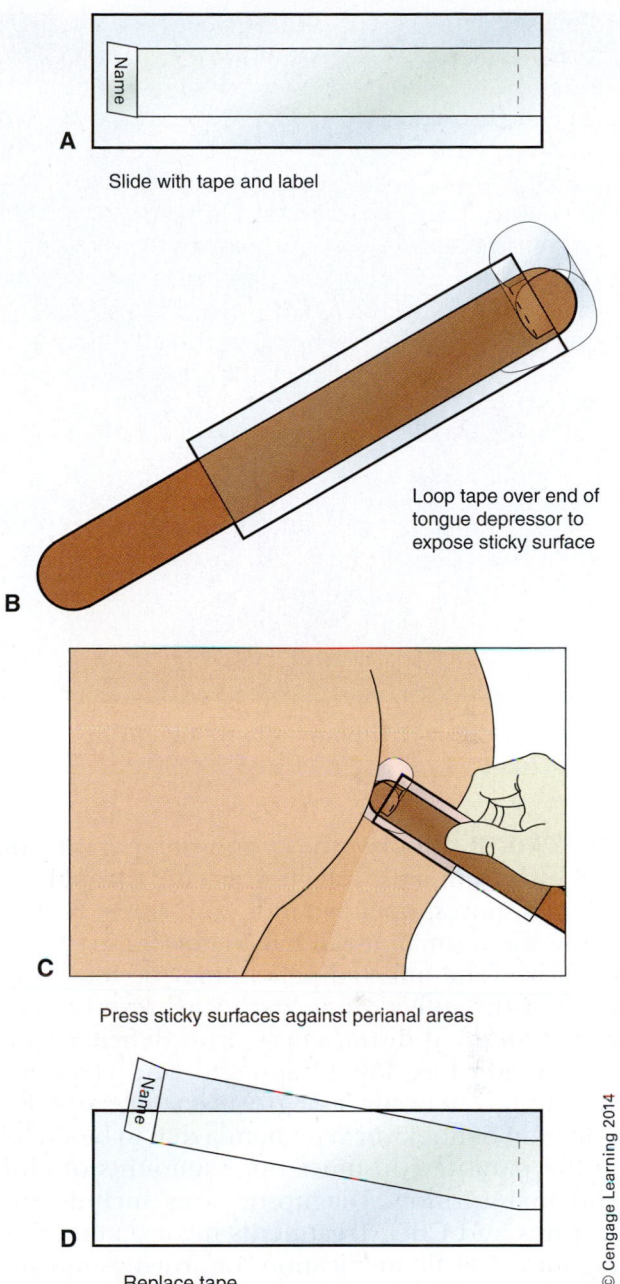

A   Slide with tape and label

B   Loop tape over end of tongue depressor to expose sticky surface

C   Press sticky surfaces against perianal areas

D   Replace tape

© Cengage Learning 2014

Figure 43-25   Technique for preparing and using a cellophane tape swab.

 The trichomonad is recovered in a wet preparation slide of spun urine or vaginal secretion mixed with a drop of saline (see Procedure 43-2). The specimen should not be contaminated with fecal material, which could contain *Trichomonas hominis,* another flagellate. The prepared slide is examined under the low and high objectives of the microscope to observe the motility and morphology of the parasite (Figure 43-26). There are also test kits and fluorescent stains used to diagnose this parasite.

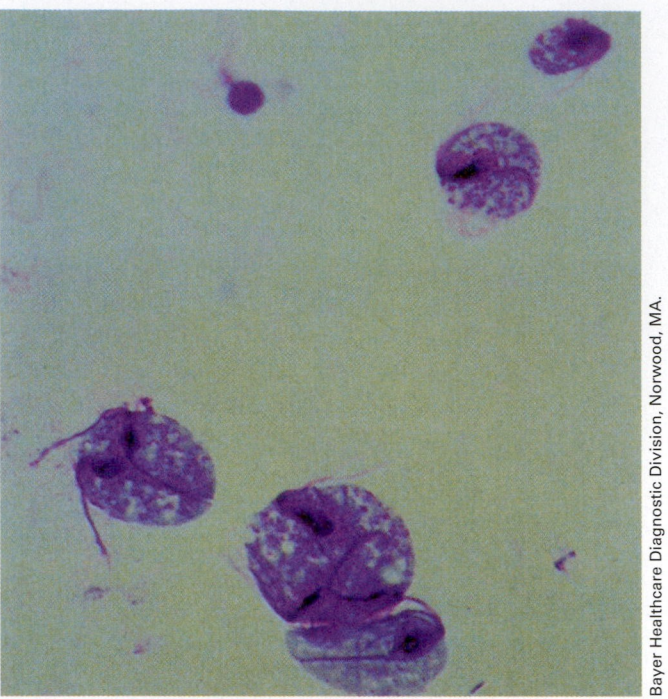

Bayer Healthcare Diagnostic Division, Norwood, MA.

Figure 43-26 Trichomonas in stained urine sediment.

Hookworm. Hookworm is another parasite that can infect humans. Infection occurs through hair follicles, pores, open wounds, and sores. Poor hygiene and warm moist climates allow these parasites to thrive. The infected person may be totally unaware of the infection at first. After several weeks, gastrointestinal disturbances, iron deficiency anemia, weight loss, loss of appetite, and respiratory symptoms will occur. The greatest concern with an infection of hookworm is anemia due to blood loss, as the parasite consumes huge amounts of blood and malnutrition. Diagnostic tests include stool cultures and CBC. Treatments involve administering antiparasitic medication, improving nutrition, and treating the complications of anemia.

MYCOLOGY

The field of mycology and the fungi that cause infections are extensive. Most identification and sensitivities testing for fungal organisms take place in larger laboratories and specific reference laboratories. Identification of two of the common fungal infections can be made quickly in the clinic or POL.

The genus *Candida* has several species that cause yeast infections in the body. *Candida* species are also present in the environment around us. They present a particular problem in the health care setting where they can cause serious nosocomial infections. Equipment can be easily contaminated with *Candida* organisms.

 Yeast infections commonly are found on the moist areas of the body and in the subcutaneous tissue. An infection with yeast can range from mild to serious. *Candida albicans* is the causative agent of vaginal yeast infections. The specimen is examined microscopically for the characteristic budding yeast forms (see Procedure 43-2). If the specimen is fluid and clear, it is placed on a slide with a drop of saline. If the specimen is thick, it should be mixed with 10% KOH (one drop) on the slide to clear away debris. Once the specimen is prepared, it is examined microscopically.

Another group of significant fungi that sometimes can be generally identified are the **dermatophytes**. These fungi cause infections on the hair, skin, and nails. The microscopic structure of these fungi is detailed. Some of the fungi that cause dermatophytic infections can be diagnosed using a **Wood's lamp**. This is a lamp with an ultraviolet light. Some dermatophytes will fluoresce (glow brightly) under this light.

Mycotic infections can also be identified through culture and kit identification systems. Fungi can produce heavy aerosols and should be processed and observed under a safety hood.

 PROCEDURE 43-1
Obtaining a Throat Specimen for Culture

STANDARD PRECAUTIONS:

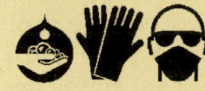

PURPOSE:
To obtain secretions from the nasopharnyx and tonsillar area for means of identifying a pathogenic microorganism.

Procedure 43-1 (continued)

EQUIPMENT/SUPPLIES:

Tongue depressor
Culture tube with applicator stick or commercially prepared culture collection system (culturette)
Label and requisition form
Gloves and face shield
Good light source
Biohazard transport bag

PROCEDURE STEPS:

1. *Introduce yourself by name and credential and identify the patient.* RATIONALE: Identifying yourself helps establish professional trust and rapport with the patient.

2. *Explain the procedure and expectations to the patient. Allay the patient's fears regarding the procedure to help him feel safe and comfortable.* RATIONALE: Explaining the procedure and allaying the patient's fears will assure the patient that you are concerned about any apprehension he may have and that you are open to discussing his concerns.

3. Have an emesis basin and tissues ready. RATIONALE: You will want to be prepared in case the patient spits up or vomits.

4. Have the patient in a sitting position. RATIONALE: The patient in a sitting position will facilitate better visualization of the throat area.

5. Wash hands, gather supplies, and apply gloves and face shield. RATIONALE: Washing hands before any patient contact will eliminate contamination. Gathering equipment before beginning the procedure ensures less chance of errors caused by missing supplies. Gloves and a face shield will offer personal protection in case the patient coughs, spits up, or vomits.

6. Ask the patient to open his or her mouth wide and then adjust the light source. RATIONALE: A widely opened mouth and properly adjusted light source will facilitate better visualization of the throat area.

7. Remove the swab from the culturette using sterile technique. RATIONALE: Using sterile technique maintains the sterility of the swab, which results in a quality specimen for culture.

8. Ask the patient to say "ah." Depress the tongue with the tongue depressor and swab the back of the throat and tonsillar area. Concentrate primarily on any red, raw areas and pustules. Take care to not touch the swab on the inside of the cheeks or on the tongue. RATIONALE: Having the patient say "ah" lowers the back of the tongue. Depressing the tongue reminds the patient to keep the mouth opened and assists in keeping the back of the tongue down. Swabbing only the tonsillar area and the back of the throat without touching the inside of the cheeks or the tongue ensures that the specimen will contain mostly the bacterial infectious agent (streptococci), if present, and not normal mouth flora or other contaminants. The red, raw areas and pustules will most likely contain the greatest concentration of streptococci.

9. Place the swab back into the culturette using sterile technique and crush the glass capsule containing the culture media. (*NOTE:* Some culturettes require a puncturing action to release the media. Follow the manufacturer's instructions.) RATIONALE: Using sterile technique avoids contaminating the specimen and having the specimen contaminate any other area. Crushing the glass capsule (or piercing the culture membrane) releases the culture medium, which will maintain the optimum environment for the specimen until it is tested at the regional laboratory.

10. *Paying attention to detail,* label the culturette according to the POL policy and requirements. RATIONALE: Proper and timely labeling of all specimens ensures that samples will not be mixed up with other patient samples.

11. Ensure patient comfort and answer any questions related to the testing. *Provide appropriate responses and feedback.* RATIONALE: Ensuring patient comfort and answering questions will establish professional *rapport.*

12. Discard contaminated supplies into a biohazard waste container. Disinfect all work surfaces. Remove gloves and face shield and discard appropriately. RATIONALE: Following Standard Precautions when disposing of contaminated supplies and disinfecting work surfaces will eliminate biohazard contaminations.

13. Wash hands. RATIONALE: Gloves protect hands from most but not all infectious microorganisms. Washing hands will remove residual powders and latex.

continues

Procedure 43-1 (continued)

14. Complete the laboratory requisition in the presence of the patient, then record procedure in patient's chart or electronic medical record. RATIONALE: Completing the laboratory requisition properly and in the presence of the patient will give the regional laboratory accurate information regarding the patient and the specimen. Charting the procedure will establish a timeline and document the procedure.

15. Place the specimen and the requisition in the biohazard transport bag in their separate compartments and notify the laboratory that the specimen is ready for pick up. RATIONALE: Any questions about the patient's contact information or insurance can be answered immediately if the patient is present. Completing the requisition in the presence of patient also ensures the right form accompanies the patient's sample.

DOCUMENTATION:

1/12/20XX 10:11 AM   Throat culture specimen obtained and sent to Inner City Laboratory for C&S. Patient tolerated the procedure well and will return for a follow-up visit and meditation, reevaluation in 2 days per Dr. King's request.
Appt scheduled 1/14 at 3:30 PM. Joe Guerrero, CMA (AAMA)

PROCEDURE 43-2
Wet-Mount and Hanging Drop Slide Preparations

STANDARD PRECAUTIONS:

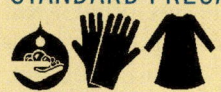

PURPOSE:
Prepare a slide for viewing live organisms for motility and identifying characteristics.

EQUIPMENT/SUPPLIES:
Gloves
Coverslips
Laboratory coat
Petroleum jelly
Clean glass slide
Dropper
Glass slide with concave well
Bacterial suspension

PROCEDURE STEPS:
1. Wash hands and apply gloves. RATIONALE: Washing hands before any procedure helps to eliminate contamination. Gloves will offer personal protection.

2. Assemble equipment and supplies. RATIONALE: Gathering equipment before beginning the procedure ensures less chance of errors caused by missing supplies.

3. For wet-mount slide preparation:

a. Place a drop of the bacterial suspension onto a clean glass slide (Figure 43-27A).

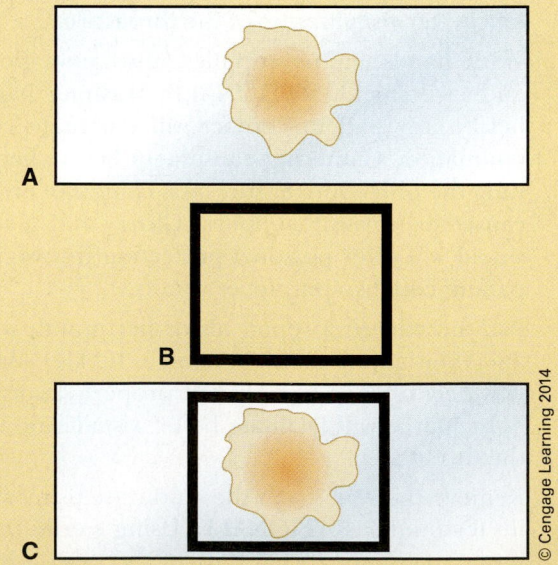

Figure 43-27 Wet-mount slide. (A) Specimen placed on a glass slide. (B) Coverslip with petroleum jelly on edges. (C) Coverslip placed directly on top of slide with specimen.

Procedure 43-2 (continued)

RATIONALE: The suspension of bacteria in a drop facilitates viewing.

b. Place petroleum jelly around the edges of the coverslip (Figure 40-27B) and place the coverslip on top of the bacterial suspension (Figure 40-27C). RATIONALE: The petroleum jelly cuts down on air currents and keeps the slide from drying out.

4. For hanging drop slide preparation:

a. Place the bacterial specimen (in suspension) in the center of the coverslip with petroleum jelly around the edges (Figure 40-28A). RATIONALE: For the suspended drop to be formed properly, this technique is used.

b. Invert the slide and place the concave well of the slide over the specimen drop on the coverslip (Figure 43-28B). RATIONALE: This method allows the slide well to protect the drop.

c. The slide is then carefully turned right side up for microscopic examination (Figure 43-28C). RATIONALE: The slide must be handled carefully to avoid slippage and disruption of the drop.

NOTE: After the smear is prepared properly, it can be observed microscopically at any power. Viewing the slide is considered by CLIA to be a provider-performed microscopy procedure. ***Working within your scope of practice assures a dedication to professional integrity.***

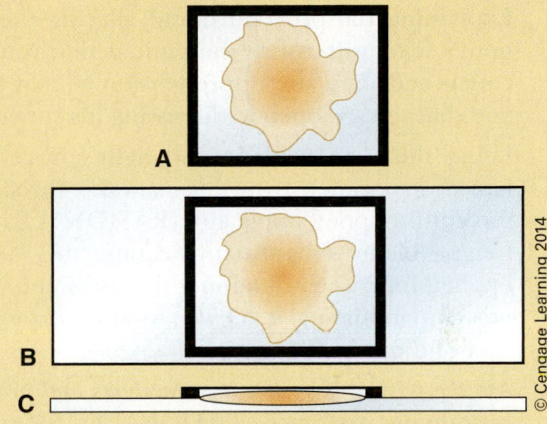

© Cengage Learning 2014

Figure 43-28 Hanging drop slide. (A) Specimen placed on coverslip. (B) Slide placed over coverslip. (C) Slide turned right side up for examination.

PROCEDURE 43-3

Performing Strep Throat Testing

STANDARD PRECAUTIONS:

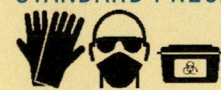

PURPOSE:

To test for streptococcus infection of the throat for diagnostic purposes. The following steps are intentionally general, so a variety of kits can be used.

EQUIPMENT/SUPPLIES:

Gloves
Commercial (CLIA waived) strep throat testing kit:
    Controls and reagents
    Sterile cotton-tipped swabs
    Test tubes and holder or receptacles (depending
       on the kit used)

Tongue blade
Adjustable light source
Laboratory report form

PROCEDURE STEPS:

1. Wash hands and apply personal protective equipment (PPE). RATIONALE: Hands should always be washed prior to working with patients to avoid transferring pathogens. PPE protects you from the patient in case he or she coughs or vomits during the procedure.

2. Assemble and organize equipment and supplies. RATIONALE: Organization presents a more professional image.

continues

Procedure 43-3 (continued)

3. ***Introduce yourself by name and credential, identify the patient.*** RATIONALE: Introducing yourself to the patient will gain his or her cooperation and establish a good rapport. Identifying the patient ensures that the right patient will receive the test.

4. ***Explain the procedure and expectations to the patient. Allay the patient's fears regarding the procedure to help him feel safe and comfortable.*** RATIONALE: Explaining the procedure and allaying the patient's fears will assure the patient that you are concerned about any apprehension he may have and that you are open to discussing his concerns.

5. Using the tongue blade and light source, obtain the specimen from the patient's throat on the cotton-tipped applicator. RATIONALE: The tongue blade will assist in keeping the mouth opened for ease in obtaining the specimen without contaminating it on the tongue, cheek, or roof of the mouth.

6. ***Ask the patient if he has any questions and provide appropriate responses.*** RATIONALE: Soliciting questions will encourage the patient to ask questions if she needs information. Providing appropriate feedback will enhance your professional relationship and help the patient understand better.

7. ***Paying attention to detail,*** follow the manufacturer's instructions exactly to perform the strep throat test. Be sure to also run the controls tests.

RATIONALE: Each manufacturer's kit varies slightly in the method used. The controls are to ensure quality results.

8. Properly dispose of all waste in biohazard container. Disinfect the equipment and the area. RATIONALE: Standard precautions are used to prevent disease transmission.

9. Complete the laboratory report form and notify the provider of the results. RATIONALE: The provider will treat the disease as soon as it is confirmed.

10. Document procedure in patient's chart or electronic medical record. RATIONALE: Proper documentation ensures good recordkeeping.

DOCUMENTATION:

04/27/20XX   Strep throat test performed in office. Patient tolerated procedure well, Dr. Lewis notified of results. Initialed report on file. Joe Guerrero, CMA (AAMA)———————

Laboratory Report

Patient Name   Lisa Carter   Date   04-27-20XX

Strep Throat Test _____negative_____

——————— Joe Guerrero, CMA (AAMA)
MA signature

PROCEDURE 43-4
Instructing a Patient on Obtaining a Fecal Specimen

STANDARD PRECAUTIONS:

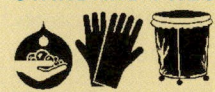

PURPOSE:
To instruct a patient in the correct collection of a fecal sample.

EQUIPMENT/SUPPLIES:
Gloves
Biohazard container
Sturdy, opaque, waterproof specimen container with a securely fitting lid
Special laboratory manual instructions if needed (depending on the test being performed)
Laboratory requisition form

Procedure 43-4 (continued)

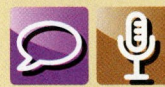

PROCEDURE STEPS:

1. Assemble and organize equipment and supplies. RATIONALE: Being organized helps the process go more smoothly and professionally.

2. *Introduce yourself by name and credential and identify the patient.* RATIONALE: Identifying the patient ensures that you have the right patient.

3. *Speaking to the patient's level of understanding, explain the procedure.* Provide written instructions as well. *Demonstrate professionalism and courtesy while you explain.* RATIONALE: Explaining the procedure in a manner the patient understands reassures him and helps ensure his cooperation. Demonstrating professionalism will help maintain a professional atmosphere and may help put the patient at ease, as some patient's may become embarrassed with these instructions. The written instructions will assist him in following the proper procedure.

4. Hand the patient the labeled specimen container, instructing him or her to deposit a sample of stool into the cup then securely set the lid onto it. RATIONALE: Labeling the container rather than the lid will ensure that the specimen will not be mixed up with another patient's sample in the laboratory. The sturdy lid will prevent leakage of the specimen during transport.

5. Caution the patient to avoid contaminating the stool specimen with urine. RATIONALE: Urine may interfere with the test.

6. Give the patient a biohazard transport bag and instructions on which pocket to put the specimen into and how to secure the bag. The medical assistant can place the laboratory requisition into the other pocket. RATIONALE: Using a bio-hazard transport bag and properly sealing it will prevent contamination during transport to the laboratory. Keeping the requisition in a separate pocket from the specimen further prevents contamination of the paperwork.

7. The patient should be prepared to transport the specimen to the laboratory as soon as possible while keeping the specimen at or just below body temperature. RATIONALE: If the stool is being tested for parasites and their eggs (ova and parasite, commonly called O&P), the laboratory will want to test the parasites while they are still viable.

8. *Ask the patient if he has any questions and provide appropriate responses. Demonstrate professionalism and courtesy while answering questions.* RATIONALE: Soliciting questions will encourage the patient to ask if there is something he doesn't understand. Providing appropriate responses will further the patient's understanding and ensure a cleaner specimen.

9. Document that the instructions were given to the patient, both orally and written. RATIONALE: Proper documentation serves as a record for future reference.

DOCUMENTATION:

5/10/20XX 3:30 PM   Patient instructed to provide a stool sample for O&P. Verbal and written instructions were given and understood well. Patient will take the sample to Inner City Laboratory for testing as soon as possible after procurement. Specimen Container Biohazard transport bag and lab requisition given. Patient will call for results in 48 hours, if he doesn't hear from us first. Barbara Dahl, CMA (AAMA), CPC—————

CASE STUDY 43-1

Refer to the scenario at the beginning of the chapter. You can see that Joe is very careful with all safety precautions when handling specimens.

CASE STUDY REVIEW

1. Name a few diseases Joe could contract from the specimens he handles.

2. Discuss the methods of transfer those diseases would take during transmission.

CASE STUDY 43-2

Mary O'Keefe has brought her 3-year-old son Chris to the clinic of Drs. Lewis and King with a temperature of 102°F and an extremely sore and red throat. He is irritable and crying. After examining Chris, Dr. King orders a quick test for group A *Streptococcus*. Medical assistant Joe Guerrero has a difficult time acquiring the throat swab for the test because of Chris's condition. The test is run, and the results are negative.

CASE STUDY REVIEW

1. What could be some reasons the test result is negative?
2. What other procedure can be done to diagnose strep throat?
3. How would the test in question 2 be set up?

SUMMARY

The field of microbiology is vast. Many microorganisms are pathogenic and can cause serious infection in patients. The successful culturing and identification of such organisms is an important aspect of the successful treatment of patients. All specimens that are processed in the POL should be handled carefully, and all safety guidelines should be followed.

For the pathogen to be identified correctly, the utmost care must be taken in obtaining the culture. Sterile equipment must be used. When the culture is processed, the correct microscopic examination, media, incubation, and confirmatory tests must be used correctly to identify the pathogen.

Often a sensitivity test will be requested together with the culture. The information from this test will guide the provider in selecting the appropriate treatment for the patient.

POLs vary in the type and number of cultures that are performed on the premises and those that are sent out to be performed in a reference laboratory. It is important to provide the best care for the patient by doing only those tests that a POL can reasonably handle given equipment, personnel limitations, and CLIA regulations.

In addition to performing bacterial identification, some POLs perform parasitology and mycology tests on a limited basis. When performing parasitology tests, it is important to obtain the proper specimen in the correct manner. When performing mycology tests, it is important to work under a safety hood to minimize the risk for exposure to spores from the fungal specimens.

Of utmost importance is the careful adherence to quality-control guidelines. These procedures ensure the integrity of test results.

STUDY FOR SUCCESS

To reinforce your knowledge and skills of information presented in this chapter:

- Review the *Key Terms*
- Role play with other students to apply attributes of professionalism pertinent to this chapter.
- Consider the *Case Studies* and discuss your conclusions
- Answer the questions in the *Certification Review*
- Apply your knowledge by completing the *Activities* in the *Study Guide* and the *Games and Quizzes* in the StudyWARE StudyWARE software on the *Premium Website*
- Perform the *Procedures* using the *Competency Assessment Checklists* in the *Competency Manual*
- Practice your problem-solving skills with the *Critical Thinking Challenge 3.0* on the *Premium Website*

Additional resources for this chapter include:

- Module 19 of the *Medical Assisting Learning Lab*
- *CourseMate for Delmar's Comprehensive Medical Assisting*
- *WebTutor for Delmar's Comprehensive Medical Assisting*

CERTIFICATION REVIEW

1. A structure that is *not* part of all bacterial cells is the:
   a. nucleus
   b. ribosome
   c. spore
   d. cell wall
2. An example of nonselective media would be media that:
   a. contain a substance that alters the appearance of some organisms
   b. will support the growth of all organisms and does not alter their appearance
   c. support the growth of one type of organism and inhibit the growth of other types of organisms
   d. identify the biochemical activity of some organisms
3. When a CSF culture cannot be set up immediately, it should be placed in the incubator or remain at room temperature as opposed to being placed in the refrigerator because some organisms are affected by a low temperature. An example of this type of organism would be:
   a. *Beta streptococci*
   b. *Neisseria meningitidis*
   c. *Streptococcus pneumoniae*
   d. *Staphylococcus aureus*
4. The best method of taking a specimen for the recovery of anaerobic organisms is to:
   a. swab deep and place into an anaerobic container
   b. aspirate purulent fluid and place into a test tube
   c. swab around the wound and place into an anaerobic container
   d. take as any other specimen for culture
5. Which of the following statements best describes the parasitic infections?
   a. In the USA we have access to clean drinking water and sanitary conditions so parasitic infections are rare.
   b. Parasitic infections are always immediately evident with gastrointestinal symptoms such as diarrhea, nausea, and fatigue.
   c. Parasitic infections do not affect wealthy and/or educated individuals.
   d. Parasitic infections can infect anyone in the United States through water, food, skin, and body openings.

6. The best treatment for a parasitic infection is:
   a. total and complete isolation of the infected person
   b. hospitalization and IV antibiotics
   c. antibiotics, antiparasitics, and/or antiprotozoal medications and treating other symptoms as appropriate
   d. let the infection run its course, the diarrhea and vomiting will rid the body of the parasite
7. When studying the form and structure of an organism, you are studying the:
   a. bacteriology
   b. morphology
   c. microbiology
   d. parasitology
8. An autoclave must be operated at 121°C and 15 #PSI for how long to be effective?
   a. 15 to 20 minutes
   b. 20 to 30 minutes
   c. 30 to 45 minutes
   d. 60 minutes
9. Which organism requires a high level of carbon dioxide to survive and grow?
   a. *Escherichia coli*
   b. *Nesseria gonorrhoeae*
   c. *Staphylococcus*
   d. All of the above
10. Which parasitic infection is also called "Pin Worm"?
    a. *Pseudomonas aeruginosa*
    b. *Candida albicans*
    c. *Enterobius vermicularis*
    d. *Trichomonas vaginalis*

REFERENCES/BIBLIOGRAPHY

Department of Health and Human Services, Centers for Disease Control and Prevention. Retrieved February 2012, from http://www.cdc.gov

U.S. Food and Drug Administration. Databases on the FDA Website. Retrieved February 2012, from http://www.fda.gov/search/databases.html

Walters, N. J., Estridge, B. H., & Reynold, A. P. (2011), *Basic Clinical Laboratory Techniques* (6th ed.) Clifton Park, NY: Delmar Cengage Learning.

CHAPTER 44

Specialty Laboratory Tests

OUTLINE

Urine Pregnancy Tests
 Commercial/Home Urine
  Pregnancy Tests
 False/Positive Pregnancy Test
  Results

Infectious Mononucleosis
 Transmission of EBV
 Symptoms of IM
 Treatment of IM
 Diagnosis of IM
 CLIA Waived IM Tests

Prothrombin Time

Blood Typing
 ABO Blood Typing
 Rh Blood Typing

Semen Analysis
 Semen Composition
 Altering Factors in Semen
  Analysis

Phenylketonuria Test
 Blood Testing for PKU

Tuberculosis
 Cause of TB

Resistance in Mycobacteria
Transmission of Infectious TB
Diagnosis of TB
Screening for TB: Skin
 Testing
The Mantoux Test

Blood Glucose
 Fasting Blood Glucose
 Two-Hour Postprandial Blood
  Glucose
 Glucose Tolerance Test
 Automated Methods of
  Glucose Analysis
 Testing Panels
 Glycosylated Hemoglobin

**Cholesterol, Lipids, and
Systemic Inflammation**
 The Chemistry of Cholesterol
 Functions of Cholesterol
 Lipoproteins and Cholesterol
  Transport
 Triglycerides
 Inflammation

Blood Chemistry Tests
 Alanine Aminotransferase
  (ALT)
 Albumin
 Alkaline Phosphatase (ALP)
 Aspartate Aminotransferase
  (AST)
 Bilirubin, Total and Direct
 Blood Urea Nitrogen Test
 Calcium
 Chloride
 Carbon Dioxide (CO_2)
 Creatinine
 Gamma Glutamyltransferase
  (GGT)
 Lactate Dehydrogenase
  (LDH)
 Phosphorus (Phosphate)
 Potassium (K)
 Sodium
 Total Protein
 Uric Acid

LEARNING OUTCOMES

1. Define, spell, and pronounce the key terms as presented in the glossary.
2. Use language/verbal skills that enable a patient's understanding.
3. Demonstrate respect for diversity in approaching patients and families.
4. Discuss quality-control issues related to handling laboratory specimens.
5. Explain the types of waived specialty tests performed in the POL and how specimens are collected.
6. Obtain specimens for specialty tests as covered in this chapter.
7. Select appropriate PPE for potentially infectious situations.
8. Perform CLIA waived chemistry tests covered in this chapter.
9. Distinguish between normal and abnormal test results.
10. Analyze the professionalism questions and apply them to this chapter's content.

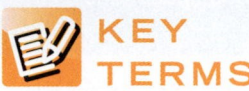

KEY TERMS

ABO blood group

bilirubin

blood urea nitrogen (BUN)

cholesterol

Guthrie screening test

high-density lipoprotein (HDL)

human chorionic gonadotropin (hCG)

low-density lipoprotein (LDL)

Mantoux test

phenylketonuria (PKU)

purified protein derivative (PPD)

Rh factor

triglycerides

ATTRIBUTES OF PROFESSIONALISM

Communication
- Did you introduce yourself? Did you identify the patient through name and birth date or other identifying feature?
- Did you speak at the patient's level of understanding?
- Did you provide appropriate responses/feedback?
- Did you explain procedures and expectations to the patient?
- Did you respond honestly and diplomatically to the patient's concerns?
- Did you demonstrate empathy in communicating with patients, family, and staff?

Presentation
- Were you dressed and groomed appropriately?
- Were you courteous, patient, and respectful to the patient?
- Did you display a positive attitude?
- Did you display a calm, professional, and caring manner?

Competency
- Did you pay attention to detail?
- Did you ask questions if you were out of your comfort zone or did not have the experience to carry out tasks?
- Did you recognize the importance of local, state, and federal legislation and regulations in the practice setting?
- Were you knowledgeable and accountable?

Initiative
- Did you direct the patient to other resources when necessary or helpful, with the approval of the provider?

Integrity
- Did you work within your scope of practice?
- Did you immediately report any error you had made?

SCENARIO

Audrey Jones, CMA (AAMA), has worked at Drs. Lewis and King's office for more than 5 years. In that time, Audrey has become proficient in obtaining specimens from patients for various laboratory tests. Audrey enjoys the work and finds it extremely challenging. She also realizes that communicating with patients to help them understand why their specimens are necessary for testing is just as important as being skillful in collecting and testing the specimens. Audrey has found that when she explains the reason the specimen is needed in terms patients can understand, they are often less fearful, which helps them relax. This can be especially helpful when collecting blood specimens.

INTRODUCTION

An increasing number of tests are performed in the ambulatory care setting, many of them by the medical assistant. To meet these new demands, the medical assistant must have a strong background in a variety of areas including medical terminology, Clinical Laboratory Improvement Amendments (CLIA) regulations, laboratory safety procedures, and specimen collection. Because many procedures require collection of a blood specimen, the medical assistant must also be an excellent phlebotomist. Good recordkeeping and communications skills round out the requirements. A quality-control program is necessary to ensure that the results are accurate and reliable. This will require a commitment on the part of the medical assistant to maintain the highest standards throughout the process.

A variety of specialty tests are covered in this chapter, including testing for pregnancy, infectious mononucleosis, tuberculosis (TB), and phenylketonuria (PKU), as well as blood types, hemoglobin A1c, and prothrombin time. This chapter also discusses the chemistry of blood, including chemistry panels, blood glucose, cholesterol, triglycerides, and other specialty laboratory tests such as semen analysis.

URINE PREGNANCY TESTS

Pregnancy tests are used when pregnancy is suspected. Pregnancy tests may also be used to rule out pregnancy before prescribing birth control pills, radiograph studies, certain antibiotics or other drugs, and for female patients who are to undergo surgery.

Pregnancy testing is based on detection of **human chorionic gonadotropin (hCG)**, a hormone secreted by the placenta that can be detected in the serum or urine of pregnant women as early as 5 days after conception. During pregnancy, hCG levels peak at about 8 weeks, then decrease to lower but detectable levels for the remainder of the pregnancy.

Commercial/Home Urine Pregnancy Tests

A variety of accurate and easy-to-use commercial tests are available for use in the medical office. Manufacturers of pregnancy test kits have designed them to be sensitive, to be easy to perform and interpret, and to give rapid results. Pregnancy tests are one of many tests available for purchase as an over-the-counter product. However, results of tests performed at home should be confirmed by a laboratory test using appropriate quality-control measures and properly trained personnel. CLIA has granted waived status to all urine pregnancy tests that use visual color comparison and specifically to the Bayer Corporations Clinitek 50 Urine

SPOTLIGHT ON CERTIFICATION

RMA Content Outline
- Medical law
- Patient education
- Laboratory procedures

CMA (AAMA) Content Outline
- Patient instruction
- Medicolegal guidelines and requirements
- Collecting and processing specimens; diagnostic testing

CMAS Content Outline
- Legal and ethical considerations
- Communication

Chemistry Analyzer for hCG in urine. Medical assistants qualify for the waived test category (COW) within the physicians' office laboratory (POL).

False/Positive Pregnancy Test Results

A positive reaction to any pregnancy test does not necessarily indicate a normal pregnancy; this is referred to as a 'false/positive' result. Detection of hCG can also indicate such abnormal conditions as an ectopic pregnancy, a developing hydatidiform mole of the uterus, choriocarcinoma, or cancer of the lung, stomach, uterus, pancreas, colon, or breast.

Quality Control. Kits must be stored and used at the temperature directed by the manufacturer. Most kits contain a built-in control; however, appropriate positive and negative urine controls must always be run with patient specimens. Kits and reagents must not be used after the expiration date. Manufacturer's instructions must be followed precisely for the particular test used.

PRECAUTIONS FOR PREGNANCY TESTING

1. Use a clean container for collection of the urine specimen. Disposable containers are preferred. Detergent residue on nondisposable containers may interfere with test results.

2. The first-voided morning urine has the highest concentration of hCG and is the preferred specimen. If this is not available, a urine specimen with a specific gravity of at least 1.010 is acceptable.

3. Although it is always best to run tests on fresh specimens, if the urine specimen cannot be tested immediately, it may be stored at 39° F for up to 24 hours. Both urine and serum specimens may be used with some test kits; other kits use only one or the other.

4. Allow refrigerated urine specimens and test reagents to come to room temperature before starting test procedures.

5. If using the slide test procedure:
   a. Avoid cross contamination with other urine specimens.
   b. Use a new stirrer for each test.

INFECTIOUS MONONUCLEOSIS

Infectious mononucleosi (IM) is a contagious disease that may have vague clinical symptoms and can mimic other diseases. Serologic tests are often the basis for an early diagnosis of the disease and may also be used to follow the course of the disease.

IM is commonly called "mono" or "kissing disease." The disease is a result of infection of the lymphocytes by the Epstein-Barr virus (EBV). EBV is common in our population. By 5 years of age, approximately 50% of the population is infected, increasing to 90% to 95% in adults. After the primary infection, the virus establishes a lifelong latency. The infectious virus may be isolated from saliva for several months, whereas antigens may be detected for life. In addition to causing IM, EBV has been implicated in other diseases such as nasopharyngeal carcinoma (NPC) and chronic fatigue syndrome.

Transmission of EBV

Transmission of EBV IM is primarily by saliva, which is why it is often referred to as "the kissing disease." EBV may also be spread by the sharing of drinking glasses and less often by blood transfusion. The disease is moderately contagious and is transmitted approximately 10% to 38% of the time in close social groups. In the home or in the hospital, careful hand washing will help prevent transmission of the virus.

Symptoms of IM

Mononucleosis is seen most often in children and young adults. Incubation may vary from 4 to 50 days; however, 7 to 14 days is the average. Infection in younger children is usually asymptomatic or manifests minor symptoms such as pharyngitis, otitis media, bronchitis, and other upper respiratory discomforts.

Classic symptoms usually occur when the primary infection is delayed until the second decade of life. IM is most often observed in the 15- to 25-year-old age group. Symptoms usually begin with a fever and swollen glands lasting for 3 to 5 days. Over the next 7 to 20 days, the patient may develop a headache; malaise; chest pain; a cough; tonsillitis; a rash; soft, swollen lymph nodes; and a swollen spleen. While the spleen is enlarged, the patient is advised to curtail activity, especially contact sports and rough activities, to prevent the rare, but serious, rupture of the spleen. Symptoms usually persist for 1 to 2 weeks and in more serious cases may last for more than 1 month.

Treatment of IM

Because there are currently no effective drugs available for EBV IM, treatment is primarily palliative, or supportive. Although a vaccine is not yet available, some important work in that direction is ongoing.

Diagnosis of IM

To properly diagnose IM, the provider must consider blood and serology test results together with the patient's symptoms.

Blood Test for IM. The hematologic tests for IM include white blood cell count and evaluation of the patient's lymphocytes. In IM, lymphocytosis, or increase in lymphocytes, usually occurs, and large numbers of lymphocytes (greater than 20%) have an unusual or atypical appearance.

Serologic Test for IM. Persons with IM produce antibodies called heterophile antibodies by the sixth to tenth day of the illness. Heterophile antibodies are antibodies that react with similar antigens in more than one species. They are usually of the IgM class.

Detection of heterophile antibodies combined with the blood tests and patient symptoms provide the basis for the diagnosis of IM. The serologic test is usually positive after the first week of illness. However, if test results are negative, the test should be repeated after 1 week if clinical symptoms are still present.

CLIA Waived IM Tests

Several manufacturers have produced CLIA waived test kits suitable for use by the medical assistant in the POL.

Kits for IM usually provide all the necessary reagents, materials, and controls. The laboratory must obtain only the specimen to be tested, which is usually a small sample of the patient's plasma or serum or a drop of capillary blood.

PROTHROMBIN TIME

Prothrombin time, which is also called protime, PT, and international normalized ratio (INR), is a test for blood's clotting ability. It is used often for people who are taking anticoagulant medications such as Coumadin (warfarin).

Coumadin targets Vitamin K molecules and is influenced by dietary intake of Vitamin K. This influence makes it an unstable treatment and regular monitoring is needed to make sure it is effective but not overly thinning the blood.

The desired levels of INR are 2.0 to 3.0. Refer to Chapter 41 for more information on coagulation tests and Procedure 41-4 for the process of running a prothrombin time test.

BLOOD TYPING

Blood types are based on the presence or absence of certain antigens on the surface of red blood cells (RBCs). Antibodies are protein molecules that are found in serum; they are also referred to as immunoglobulins (Ig). When RBC antigens and antibodies react, they cause the RBCs to agglutinate (clump). This process is called hemagglutination. Hemagglutination reactions are used in the typing of blood. The two major categories of blood typing are for the **ABO blood group** and the **Rh factor.** The ABO blood group consists of type A, type B, type AB, and type O. Within each of these types are the Rh factors, either Rh-positive (factor present) or Rh-negative (no factor).

The ABO and Rh systems place certain restrictions on how blood can be transfused from one individual to another. Depending on their blood type, individuals with a particular RBC antigen may have antibodies against the other types (Table 44-1). An incompatible blood transfusion results when the antigens of the donor RBCs react with the antibodies of the recipient RBCs. This is a potentially life-threatening situation that varies in severity from mild fever to anaphylaxis with severe intravascular hemolysis. Although ABO and Rh typing does not completely rule out the possibility of reaction, it greatly reduces the chances.

ABO Blood Typing

ABO blood typing is determined by the presence or absence of two major antigens, A and B. All

Table 44-1   Antigens and Antibodies in ABO and Rh Blood Systems

Blood Group/Type	Antigen on RBC	Serum Antibodies
O (universal donor)	None	Anti-A and anti-B
A	A	Anti-B
B	B	Anti-A
AB	A and B	None
Rh+	D	No anti-D*
Rh−	None	No anti-D*

© Cengage Learning 2014

*There are no naturally occurring antibodies to the Rh system.

people have one of the four blood group categories: A, B, AB, or O. People with group A RBCs have A antigens, group B RBCs have B antigens, group AB RBCs have antigens for both A and B, and group O RBCs lack both A and B antigens. Naturally occurring antibodies to the other antigen types are found in the serum.

Figure 44-1 illustrates how RBCs are tested for blood type. In the example, type O blood would have no reaction to either anti-A or anti-B, whereas type AB blood would have a reaction to both. By process of elimination, one can determine which type the specimen is. Because type O blood has neither antigens nor Rh factor, it is considered to be the "universal donor." Type AB+ blood has both antigens and an Rh factor so it is considered to be the universal recipient.

ABO type can be determined by the slide or tube method. The tube method is now most often used for blood typing. Because neither method is considered in the waived category by CLIA, they usually are not performed in the POL. Even if the patient carries a card listing his or her blood type, the patient's blood will be retested as a precaution. This is called a "blood cross and match" test. Nevertheless, it is a good idea to know your individual blood type and Rh factor.

Rh Blood Typing

Rh typing is routinely performed together with ABO typing. The Rh system is named for the rhesus monkey used in experiments that led to its discovery. The Rh factor is found on the surface of

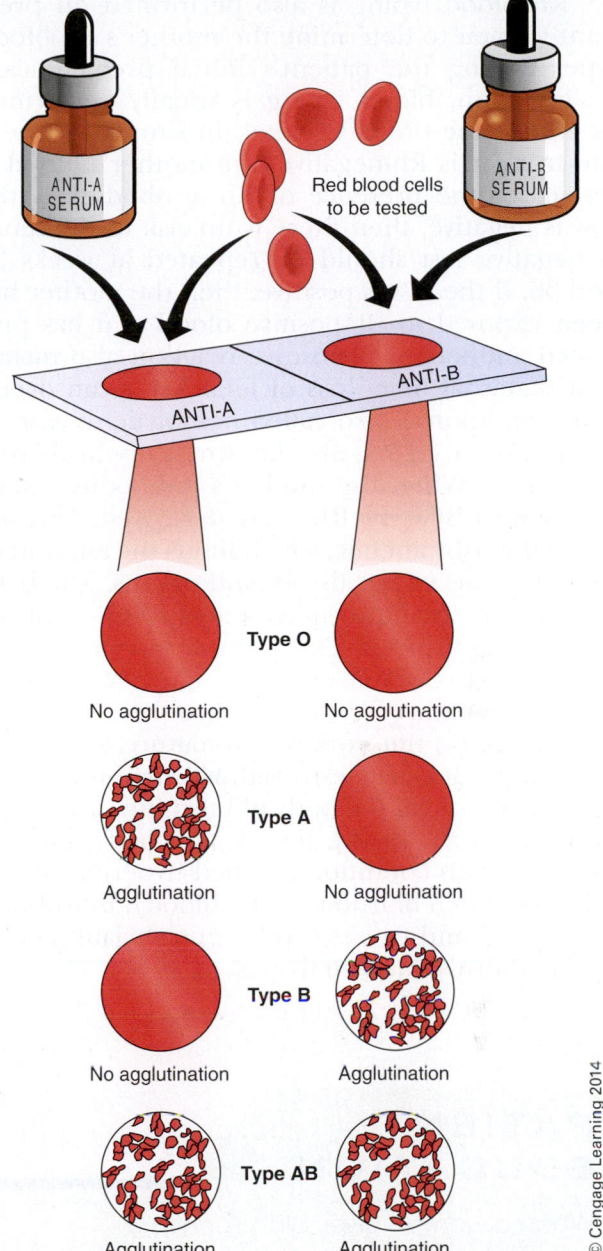

Figure 44-1   Blood typing the ABO groups.

© Cengage Learning 2014

RBCs. People possessing the Rh factor are said to have Rh-positive (Rh+) blood. Those without the Rh factor have Rh-negative (Rh−) blood.

About 85% of North Americans are Rh-positive; 15% are Rh-negative. Neither Rh-negative nor Rh-positive people have naturally occurring Rh antibodies in their blood. However, if an Rh-negative individual receives a transfusion of Rh-positive blood, he or she will develop antibodies to it. The antibodies take 2 weeks to develop. Both blood type and Rh factor must be taken into account for safe and successful transfusions.

Rh blood typing is also performed on pregnant women to determine the mother's Rh blood type. During the patient's initial prenatal care examination, blood typing is usually performed as part of the prenatal panel. In situations where the mother is Rh-negative, the mother's blood is tested for the presence of Rh antibodies. If the test is negative, then there is no risk to the fetus. A negative test should be repeated at weeks 30 and 36. If the test is positive, then the mother has been exposed to Rh-positive blood and has produced antibodies. A positive reaction also means that maternal hemolysis of fetal RBCs can occur. This condition is also called hemolytic disease of the newborn (HDN, also known as erythroblastosis fetalis). When the mother's antibodies attack the baby's RBCs, the RBCs are destroyed. This will make the baby anemic, which limits the amount of oxygen to his or her tissues and organs. The baby responds by trying to make more RBCs in his or her liver and spleen. This overuse can cause these two organs to become enlarged. The new RBCs are usually immature (called erythroblasts) and are not able to do the work of the mature RBC. Also, when the RBCs are destroyed, **bilirubin** is formed. Babies cannot rid the body of bilirubin, which can build up in the blood, tissues, and body fluids of the baby. This condition is called hyperbilirubinemia (too much bilirubin in the blood). Bilirubin is pigmented and causes a yellowing or jaundice of the newborn's skin and tissues.

This jaundice is not to be confused with the jaundice many newborns have, which is caused by a similar process but to a much less degree and with milder consequences. Hemolytic disease of the newborn (HDN) can be determined by evaluating the quantity of bilirubin in the amniotic fluid and in the newborn's blood.

HDN can cause severe complications for the newborn, ranging from the enlarged liver and anemia to seizures, brain damage, and even death.

Treatment before the baby is born can include intrauterine blood transfusions and early delivery if the baby is mature enough to survive. After the baby is born, blood transfusions, intravenous fluids, and help with respiration and oxygen intake may be necessary.

Fortunately, most cases of HDN can be prevented by administering RhoGAM to the Rh-negative mother. When injected into the mother, RhoGAM will prevent her from producing the RhD antibody. The injection must be administered at the 28th week of pregnancy and within 72 hours after delivery of an Rh-positive baby, miscarriage, or termination of pregnancy.

SEMEN ANALYSIS

With the progression of managed health care, more primary care providers are performing semen analysis in their offices to determine sperm cell counts before referring patients to fertility specialists. Examination of semen is also performed as part of a complete fertility work-up, to evaluate the effectiveness of a vasectomy, to determine paternity, and to substantiate rape cases.

When semen analysis is performed as part of a fertility work-up, the procedure involves macroscopic and microscopic analysis of seminal fluid for determination of total sperm count, percentage of motility, amount of semen, liquefaction time, the pH, the presence of white blood cells, fructose level, and percentage of normally formed sperm cells (Table 44-2). All male individuals will have variable sperm counts; therefore, a single analysis is insufficient. To achieve a reasonable estimate of these factors, the seminal analysis should be repeated at least three times over a 2-month period. A complete analysis will also include an evaluation of the partner's cervical secretions and sperm survival. This involves determining the ability of sperm to penetrate the mucus and maintain motility.

Postvasectomy semen analysis (PVSA) is evaluated a few weeks after surgery. If sperm are present at that time, then follow-up analysis is required.

PATIENT EDUCATION

When a woman gives birth (or has a miscarriage or abortion), some of the fetal blood can mix with the mother's as the placenta tears away from the uterus. When the Rh-negative woman is exposed to the baby's Rh-positive blood (there is an 85% chance that the baby is Rh-positive), she builds antibodies against the Rh factor. Consequently, during the next pregnancy, her antibodies (which cross the placental barrier) would attack the next Rh-positive baby's RBCs. Giving the woman an injection of RhoGAM after each exposure to the Rh antigens prevents her from building the antibodies. Rh-negative women will need RhoGAM each time they are exposed to the Rh factor.

Table 44-2 Reference Values for Semen Analysis

Parameter	Normal Range
Appearance	White, viscid, opaque
Volume	1.5–5 mL
pH	7.12–8.00
Total count	50–200 million
% normal sperm	At least 80%
% motility	At least 60%

© Cengage Learning 2014

Waived PVSA kits are now available for home use or use in the POL. The patient is not considered sterile until he has returned *two* samples, at least 1 week apart, that demonstrate no sperm, viable or dead. This typically will take several weeks. Until that time, an alternative method of birth control must be used.

Semen Composition

Semen is a composite solution produced by the testes and the accessory male reproductive organs. It consists primarily of spermatozoa suspended in seminal plasma. Because there is considerable variation in composition between different portions of the fluid as ejaculated, it is important to collect the entire sample. Refer to the Patient Education box for instructions to give to the male patient before semen analysis.

Altering Factors in Semen Analysis

Many factors can alter the results of semen analysis. Several drugs such as cyclophosphamide (Cytoxan) and nitrogen mustard reduce sperm count, as do certain conditions such as orchitis (inflammation of the testes), testicular atrophy, testicular failure, and obstruction of the vas deferens. Cigarette smoking is associated with a decrease in the volume of semen, whereas coffee drinking results in increased sperm density and an increase in the percentage of cells with abnormal morphology. Fever may temporarily suppress the count. Although research suggests that consumption of alcohol does not affect sperm function as measured by semen analysis, the patient is instructed to avoid alcohol for several days before testing as a precaution.

Although research suggests that fertility is most closely correlated with motility and morphology, men with very high (>200 million/mL) or very low (≤20 million/mL) counts are likely to be infertile. Patients with aspermia (no sperm) or oligospermia (low sperm count, ≤20 million/mL) should be endocrinologically evaluated for pituitary, testicular, adrenal, or thyroid abnormalities.

PATIENT EDUCATION

The following instructions should be given to male patients when a semen sample is required for analysis:

1. Advise the patient to avoid consumption of alcohol for several days before the test. He should also avoid ejaculation for 3 days before collection of the semen sample.

2. Provide the patient with instructions and a container. The entire sample should be collected in a clean, dry, glass bottle that has been labeled, including the date and time. The sample is collected by masturbation or interrupted coitus at home, or it may be collected at the medical office of the laboratory. A condom should never be used to collect a semen specimen due to the spermide content.

3. Specimens for complete fertility analysis collected outside the laboratory must be brought to the laboratory within 30 minutes. Postvasectomy specimens should be brought to the laboratory within 1 hour of collection.

4. The sample must be transported to the laboratory at 37°C (98.6°F). Low temperature during transport will decrease the motility of sperm. Temperature that is too warm could destroy the sperm. Keeping the sample close to his body during transport might be the best advice.

PHENYLKETONURIA TEST

Phenylketonuria (PKU) is an inherited condition in which the baby cannot metabolize protein properly. Phenylalanine is present in milk and other dairy proteins. If the baby has PKU, phenylalanine can build up in his or her brain and other organs and cause irreversible mental retardation, loss of muscle coordination, and other serious disorders. Diagnosis should be made early so that the baby can be put on a diet low in proteins. The baby should be tested at about 2 days old and again at 7 to 14 days old. Although a phenylalanine-restricted diet will prevent mental retardation, it will not cure the underlying condition. Routine screening of newborns for PKU is mandatory in all states and may be performed in the hospital or the medical office. The medical assistant's role is to properly explain the procedure to the infant's parents and to collect the blood specimen for analysis.

Many other tests can be performed using the blood sample sent on the PKU card, including tests for congenital hypothyroidism (CH), congenital adrenal hyperplasia (CAH), galactosemia, sickle cell disease, and others. The tests that are performed depend on individual state requirements.

Blood Testing for PKU

Excess phenylalanine can be detected in blood or in urine. Normal levels of phenylalanine are less than 2 mg/deciliter (dL); more than 4 mg/dL is considered elevated. The **Guthrie screening test** is used to evaluate blood and is considered more accurate than urine tests. Phenylalanine can be detected in the blood of infants with PKU after 3 to 4 days on a breast milk or formula milk diet. Testing of breast-fed infants is delayed a few days because of the lack of phenylalanine in colostrum, the first breast milk. Colostrum is produced for the first 2 to 3 days after birth and is rich in antibodies, protein, and calories. True breast milk production begins after this time. Positive results from blood testing are confirmed by measuring serum phenylalanine and tyrosine levels. Infants with PKU have increasing phenylalanine levels (>4 mg/dL) and decreasing tyrosine levels (<0.6 mg/dL).

The Guthrie test was developed to screen for phenylalanine in the blood, and the first test is usually performed before the discharge of infants from the hospital. However, with managed care and the trend toward very short hospital stays for newborns, many pediatrician offices are now performing this first test. Even though it may seem that testing for PKU right after birth wouldn't be

needed because the newborn hasn't had time to digest phenylalanine, some babies will show positive PKU and other abnormalities. Unfortunately some babies do not get their 2-week checkup, making this first PKU in the hospital all the more important. Capillary blood is collected from a heel stick onto a "filter paper" test card and sent to the laboratory for testing. Patient, provider, and test information, together with the blood samples, are placed directly on the laboratory test card, which is typically provided by most state Departments of Health (Figure 44-2). (See Procedure 44-3 and Chapter 40 for proper capillary puncture technique.)

Factors That May Influence the Guthrie Test. The following factors may influence the Guthrie test:

- Feeding problems such as vomiting may result in a false-negative reaction.
- Failure to ingest sufficient phenylalanine—testing before 3 to 4 days of the beginning of a milk diet—will result in a false-negative reaction.
- Premature infants may give false-positive test results because of a delay in the development of certain liver enzymes.
- Drugs such as salicylates, aspirin, or antibiotics taken by the mother (if breast-feeding) or the child may interfere with test results.

TUBERCULOSIS

Despite efforts to control its spread, tuberculosis (TB) infections are on the increase in the United States and around the world. Because tuberculosis morbidity is on the rise, increasing 14% from

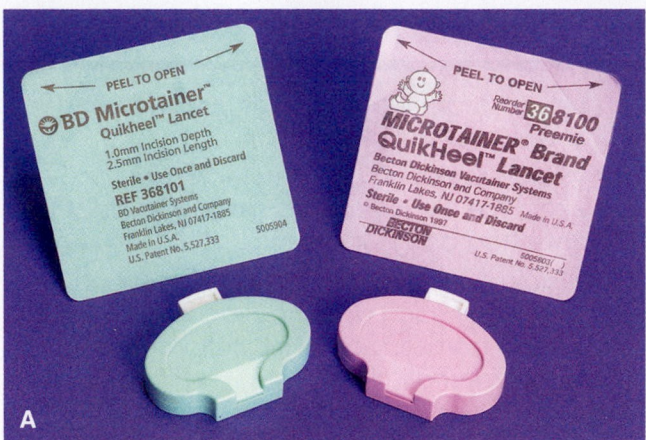

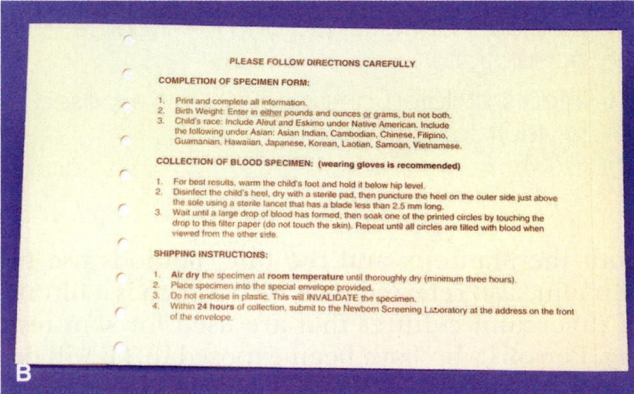

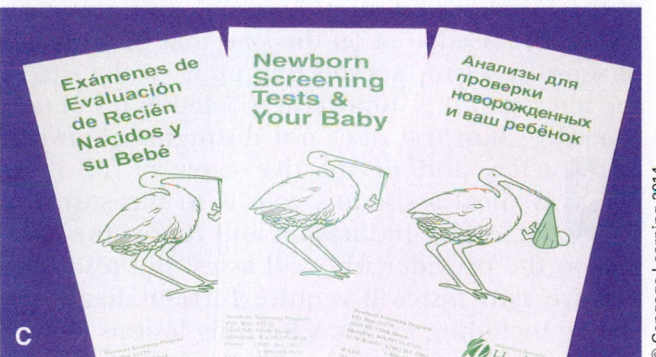

© Cengage Learning 2014

Figure 44-2 (A) Pediatric-sized safety lancets are available to vary the depth of the puncture. (B) The back of the PKU test card provides detailed instructions on performing the test and completing the card correctly. (C) Patient information and permission forms are available in a variety of languages.

1985 to 1997, more patients are screened now for the disease than ever before. The Advisory Council for Elimination of Tuberculosis, an independent group of TB-control experts, recommends screening all patients who fall into high-risk groups, or those who associate with high-risk groups, such as health care workers, including medical assistants. See the Current Family Practice Recommendations for TB Testing for a more complete list.

Cause of TB

Infectious TB is caused by the small, rod-shaped bacterium *Mycobacterium tuberculosis*. This aerobic bacterium is nonmotile and has a high content of lipid in its cell wall, making it difficult to stain using basic aniline dyes. For this reason, the Ziehl-Neelsen method was developed and is used as a tool for identification of mycobacteria. Mycobacteria will retain the red stain in the presence of acid alcohol and are therefore referred to as acid-fast. Other bacterial species stain blue.

Resistance in Mycobacteria

Mycobacteria exhibit an unusual degree of resistance on many fronts. They are able to tolerate drying and the effects of many disinfectants. Mycobacteria also show resistance to most antibiotics, making these infections difficult to treat. To help overcome bacterial resistance to antimicrobial agents, patients take two or three drugs for a period of 6 to 9 months. The most common drug used to fight TB is isoniazid (INH). Other drugs used are rifampin, pyrazinamide, ethambutol, and streptomycin.

Transmission of Infectious TB

Infectious TB is highly contagious, but is not spread by casual contact or even sharing drinks or kissing. Seventy-five percent of new cases occur by inhalation of cough-produced airborne droplets from symptomatic or asymptomatic persons. Crowded conditions contribute to this transmission. TB often is associated with poverty, poor nutrition, and crowded conditions such as what is often seen in prisons and mental health hospitals. A recent increase in TB is related to the increase in AIDS cases.

Diagnosis of TB

TB diagnosis differentiates between active and inactive TB, and the treatments differ. Active TB is a serious and contagious condition that requires isolation of the patient and aggressive treatment with several drugs over several months. TB can live in the body without causing illness and is referred to as latent or inactive TB. If the person becomes weakened through another illness or injury, the latent TB can become active, taking advantage of the person's weakened state.

Patients exhibiting a positive or questionable **purified protein derivative (PPD)** reaction should have a chest X-ray, tuberculin skin test (TST), or a sputum sample might be indicated. Reasons for a positive reaction to PPD are varied. First and most obvious is that the patient has been exposed to TB or has an active case of TB. Persons with an old, inactive case will also give a positive skin test, as will persons who have been vaccinated with BCG. BCG (bacille Calmette-Guerin) is a vaccine used in Europe and South America to help prevent childhood cases of TB. Persons who receive BCG may give a positive skin reaction for a minimum of 4 years and much longer in many cases. Many immigrants will show positive PPD because of a BCG vaccination. The chest X-ray is an important second step for those individuals, and a tuberculin blood test is less likely to give a false-positive result because it is not affected by the BCG vaccine.

Screening for TB: Skin Testing

Screening for TB may be performed as part of a routine medical examination or as a prerequisite for school or employment. In states where medical assistants can legally perform injections, they may be responsible for administration and interpretation of the skin test. The most accurate method used is the **Mantoux test**. The tine test, which is a multiple-puncture test, may still be used in some areas but is no longer recommended by the American Academy of Pediatrics.

Both the Mantoux and the tine methods use tuberculin, also referred to as PPD, which is a filtrate of tuberculin cultures that are used for skin testing. Persons who have been exposed to TB will develop a hypersensitive response to PPD resulting in the formation of an induration. An induration is a hard, raised area on the skin that is the result of sensitized lymphocytes migrating to the site of the injection. It is important to keep in mind that a positive skin test does not distinguish between active and or inactive cases of TB. The medical assistant's role is to measure the size of the induration and report the findings to the provider who will assess the results. A positive skin test will require further diagnostic testing including an X-ray for lung lesions and an acid-fast stain of sputum to examine for the presence of *Mycobacterium tuberculosis*. Because of the severity of the reaction, do not administer the skin test to persons who have had a positive reaction in the past.

The Mantoux Test

In the Mantoux test, 0.1 mL of 5 TU (toxin unit) strength PPD is injected intradermally using a 1-mL tuberculin syringe. A short (⅜–½ inch), 26 or 27 gauge needle is used. Care must be taken to inject the PPD so that a wheal forms (Figure 44-3). If the injection is too deep, it will be impossible to form the wheal. If the injection is too shallow, the PPD may leak onto the skin. Either of these two errors would invalidate the test results. It is also

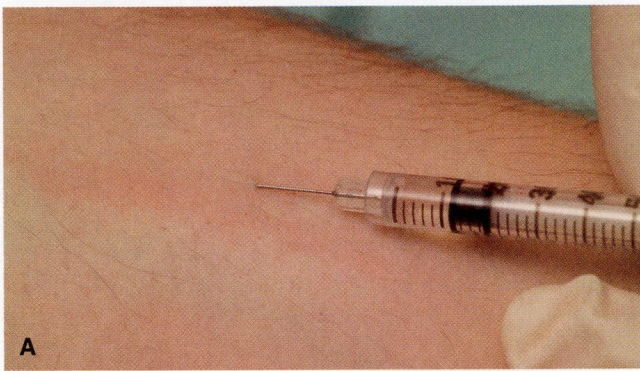

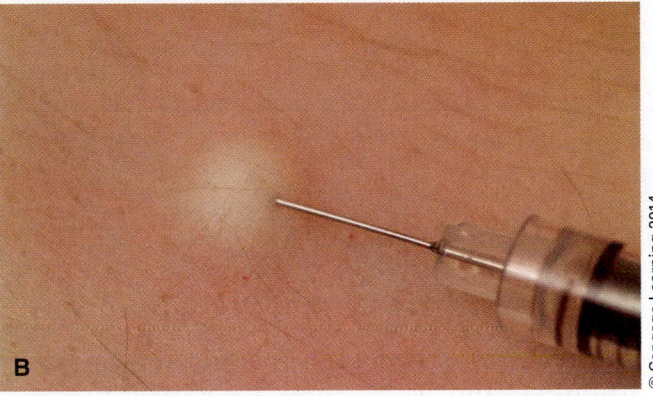

Figure 44-3 (A) Gently insert the needle just under the skin surface at about a 5-degree angle with the bevel up. Imbed the entire bevel. Slowly and carefully inject the medication. (B) A wheal should appear as a whitish raised bump.

important to draw exactly 0.1 mL of the PPD, because too much or too little will lead to erroneous test results. Refer to Procedure 36-7 for the complete injection procedure for the Mantoux test.

Reading the Results of the Mantoux TB Test.
The patient will have been instructed to return within 48 to 72 hours for an examination of the Mantoux injection site. If the patient delays the return visit more than 72 hours, the test cannot be properly assessed.

Gently feel and measure the induration (the hard raised area) (Figure 44-4). Do not include the area of redness or erythema in the measurement. Some patients will show swelling or localized raised hives and complain of itching at the injection site. These responses are not true indurations but rather are localized allergic reactions to the protein derivative and should not be misinterpreted as a positive response to the Mantoux test. Alert the physician to any unusual reactions. Do not repeat the Mantoux test if an allergic reaction has occurred.

The size of the induration is recorded for the provider to assess and determine further testing (Figure 44-5).

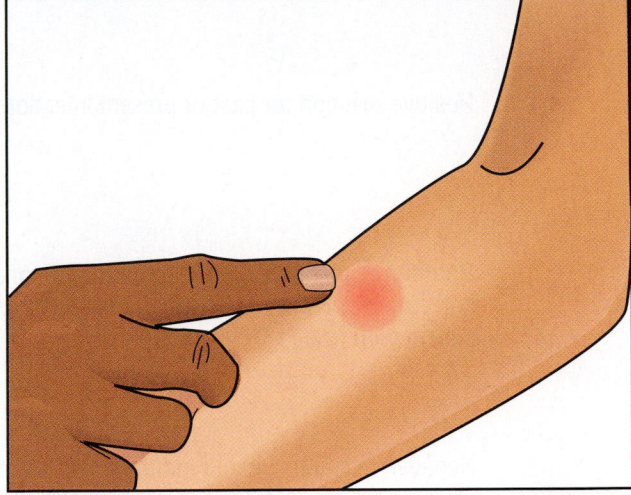

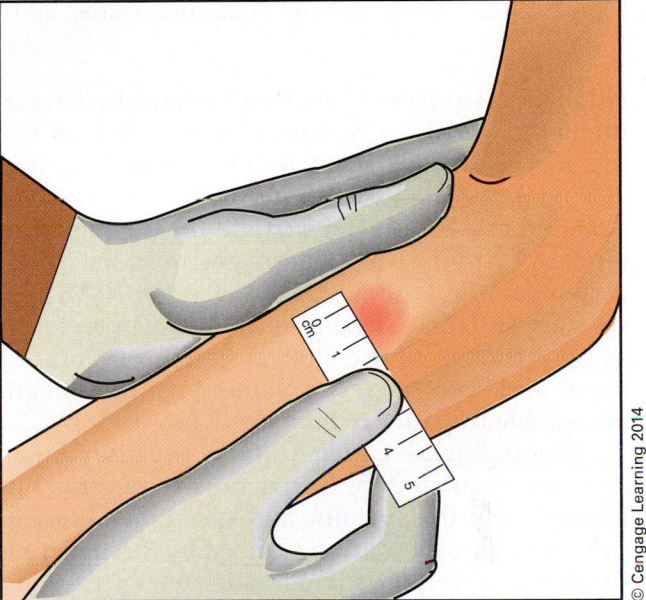

Figure 44-4 Gently inspect and measure the induration (the elevated firm area, not the area of redness or erythema) in response to the tuberculin test within 48 to 72 hours after administration. Some patients will have no induration.

BLOOD GLUCOSE

Glucose is the principal and almost exclusive carbohydrate found circulating in blood. It may also be detected in urine, cerebrospinal fluid, and semen. Glucose serves as an energy source for the body. Excess glucose is converted into glycogen for short-term storage in the liver and muscle cells, and as adipose tissue for long-term storage. Tests for blood glucose levels are commonly performed in the medical office. The results are used to screen for carbohydrate disorders such as hypoglycemia (low blood glucose level), hyperglycemia

© Cengage Learning 2014

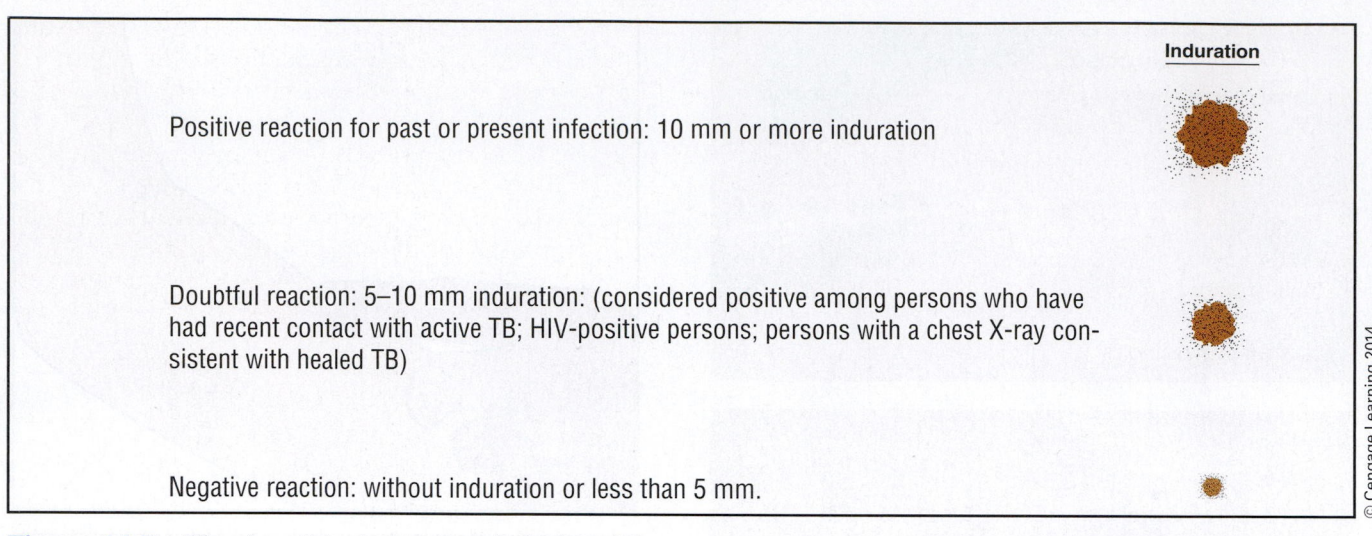

Induration

Positive reaction for past or present infection: 10 mm or more induration

Doubtful reaction: 5–10 mm induration: (considered positive among persons who have had recent contact with active TB; HIV-positive persons; persons with a chest X-ray consistent with healed TB)

Negative reaction: without induration or less than 5 mm.

© Cengage Learning 2014

Figure 44-5 The size of the induration (raised and firm area, not the redness) is measured and recorded as shown.

(high blood glucose level, which occurs in diabetes mellitus), and liver dysfunction. A variety of testing methods have been developed to diagnose, evaluate, and monitor abnormalities in carbohydrate metabolism. They include the fasting blood glucose (FBG), the 2-hour postprandial blood glucose, and the glucose tolerance test (GTT). All tests are discussed here, but the FBG is preferred as the first step in the clinical setting because it is easier and faster to perform, more convenient and acceptable to patients, and less expensive.

Blood glucose concentrations rise after a meal and are regulated by the action of several hormones including insulin and glucagon. Both insulin and glucagon are produced by the pancreas. Insulin is secreted by pancreatic cells in response to increased glucose levels and aids with the entry of glucose into cells for conversion into energy. Insulin is also required for proper storage of glucose (which is first converted into glycogen) in the liver and in muscle cells. Glucagon is secreted by the pancreas when blood sugar levels decrease and triggers the breakdown of glycogen to help increase and regulate blood sugar levels.

Fasting Blood Glucose

Evaluation of FBG levels is commonly used to screen for diabetes mellitus. Diabetes mellitus is a type of carbohydrate disorder characterized by insulin deficiency (or no insulin) and a state of hyperglycemia (*hyper* means "too much," *glyc* means "sugar," and *emia* means "blood").

The normal fasting value of glucose ranges from 70 to 110 mg/100 mL (mg/dL). Table 44-3

lists reference glucose values. A value of 120 mg/dL glucose is the dividing point between healthy and hyperglycemic individuals. Generally, truly increased glucose levels indicate diabetes mellitus. Other causes of hyperglycemia include Cushing's syndrome and acute stress response. Increased blood glucose levels should be further evaluated using the glucose tolerance test.

Two-Hour Postprandial Blood Glucose

The 2-hour postprandial (after eating) evaluation of blood glucose levels is used to screen for diabetes and to monitor insulin dosage. After fasting from midnight the night before, the patient eats a prescribed meal containing 75 to 100 g carbohydrate or consumes a 75 to 100 g glucose test load

PATIENT EDUCATION

In preparation for the test, the patient should be instructed to fast for 12 hours (except for water). A fasting blood sample is usually collected in the morning to minimize inconvenience to the patient. Certain drugs such as oral contraceptives, salicylates, diuretics, and steroids may alter the results, so the provider may restrict their use for 2 to 3 days before the test. The patient should receive both verbal and written instructions for the testing requirements and preparation.

Table 44-3 Reference Values For Blood Glucose Level

Test	Glucose Concentration (mg/dL)
Fasting	
Serum	70–110
Whole blood	60–100
Two-hour postprandial	≤110
Glucose tolerance (oral, serum)	
Fasting	70–110
1 hour	20–50 above fasting
2 hour	5–15 above fasting
3 hour	Fasting level or below

© Cengage Learning 2014

Values vary slightly between laboratories depending on testing method used.

solution such as Glucola®. Two hours later, a blood specimen is collected and tested for glucose concentration. Glucose levels will return to or fall below the fasting level within 2 hours in individuals without diabetes. Increased glucose levels should be further examined using the GTT.

According to the standards of the American Diabetes Association, a normal blood glucose is defined as less than 100 mg/dL in a fasting plasma glucose test and a 2-hour postload (75 g glucose load solution) value of less than 140 mg/dL.

A fasting plasma glucose test of 126 mg/dL or greater indicates a need for further testing, and a 2-hour postload value of 140 mg/dL or greater is a diagnosis of having "prediabetes" indicating a relatively high risk for development of diabetes.

A 2-hour postload value of 200 mg/dL or greater is a positive test for diabetes and should be confirmed on another day.

Glucose Tolerance Test

The GTT provides more detailed information used to assess insulin response to glucose and to diagnose diabetes.

When the patient arrives, he or she should be fasting (nothing but water) for at least 10 hours. A capillary specimen is drawn to determine the fasting blood sugar (FBS) level. If the FBS level is less than 200 mg/dL, then a venous specimen and urine specimen are obtained. These are labeled as fasting specimens with the date and time noted. If the results of the capillary test shows the FBS level greater than 200 mg/dL, the provider should be notified immediately. Hyperglycemia after fasting is abnormal and not an appropriate condition for

PATIENT EDUCATION

Let your patient know there are glucose meters available for them to choose from. All of them use the typical process of a drop of blood applied to a disposable "test strip" and inserted into the meter. The unit measures how much glucose is in the sample. All the meters display the result. Some meters allow a much smaller sample to be used and allow the sample to be taken from sites other than the fingertip (alternate site testing). Some meters record and store a number of test results, and some meters can connect to a personal computer to store results and print them out. Some new models have automatic timing, error codes and signals, or barcode readers to help with calibration. Some meters have a large display screen or spoken instructions for people with visual impairments. In choosing a meter, the patient should consider the following:

- Cost per strip
- Number of tests required per day
- Amount of blood needed for testing
- Testing speed
- Overall size and portability
- Cost of the meter
- Ability to store test results in memory
- Ability to test sites other than fingertip
- Other personal preferences

Many manufacturers offer free meters with the purchase of the test strips. Your clinic may be given free meters to give to patients together with a few sample strips in hopes the patient will continue to use that meter and purchase the strips. Unfortunately, the meters given to patients might not be the best choice for them, but they will continue to use it because their doctor gave it to them. Be sure to let patients know that there are many choices, and that the free meter you are giving them is not necessarily an endorsement of one meter over another.

further loading with additional glucose and may be dangerous to the patient.

After providing the fasting urine and blood specimens, the patient consumes a glucose test solution containing 1.75 g glucose/kilogram of body weight, or the standard adult dose of 75 to 100 g. The patient must consume the entire glucose solution within a 5-minute time frame. The test timing starts immediately after the patient has finished drinking the solution. If the patient should vomit within the first 30 minutes after drinking the solution, the test will be stopped and rescheduled on a different day. It is probably best not to mention this to the patient, though, because it is a rare occurrence and it is best not to have the patient worried about the possibility of vomiting. Blood and urine specimens are typically collected at 30 minutes, 1 hour, 2 hours, and 3 hours (and sometimes 6 hours) after ingestion of the glucose solution and are tested for glucose level. These measurements help determine the patient's ability to deal with increased glucose. During the test, the patient must not ingest anything (other than the solution) except water. The patient must also abstain from smoking, because smoking acts as a stimulant and increases blood glucose levels. The patient must also refrain from chewing gum, which stimulates the digestive process and also may add sugar to his or her system. Physical activity should be strongly discouraged because activity can activate sugar utilization in the body and affect the test results. Sedentary activity level is suggested.

During the second and third hours of the test, the patient may experience weakness, slight faintness, and perspire. These are all normal symptoms. If, however, the patient develops a headache, faints, or displays irrational speech or behavior, he or she may be experiencing hypoglycemic shock and the provider should be notified immediately.

The blood glucose level of patients without diabetes usually peaks 30 to 60 minutes after consumption of the test load at 160 to 180 mg/dL and returns to the fasting level after 2 to 3 hours. Patients with diabetes will still have increased glucose levels at the end of the test.

Automated Methods of Glucose Analysis

Several types of glucose analyzers are available that are suitable for POLs or small clinical laboratories. Many of these operate on the principle of reflectance photometry and use adaptations of the enzymatic methods of glucose analysis. One example of an instrument suitable for small laboratories is the HemoCue® blood glucose analyzer.

Dozens of small, inexpensive, handheld glucose meters are also made and are designed for home use by patients with diabetes. See the Patient Education box for some criteria for patients to consider when purchasing an at-home testing method. Most of these are suitable for use in point-of-care (POC) testing or in the provider's office (Figure 44-6).

Glucose controls can be purchased to check instrument performance. It is always necessary to use test materials that are made for a particular instrument only with that instrument.

All of these analyzers are designed to be easy to use and to give rapid results. With all instruments, it is necessary to use consistent proper specimen collection and testing technique to avoid variations in results.

The medical assistant often is responsible for providing education to patients on how to use glucometers, including maintenance and calibration of the meter. It is important that the medical assistant who works with patients with diabetes become familiar with a variety of meters and their differences and similarities.

Photometry Analyzers. The HemoCue® blood glucose system is a compact glucose analyzer based on the principle of photometry. The system consists of a compact photometer and disposable microcuvettes. The self-filling microcuvette automatically draws up 5 μL blood from a capillary puncture into its reaction chamber. The microcuvette is then placed into the holder and pushed into the photometer. The glucose concentration in milligrams per deciliter (mg/dL) is displayed within 45 to 240 seconds (Figure 44-7). This system is ideal for POLs and POC testing because of the stability of calibration and the minimum operator training required.

Reflectance Photometry Analyzers. Several glucose analyzers are available that are based on

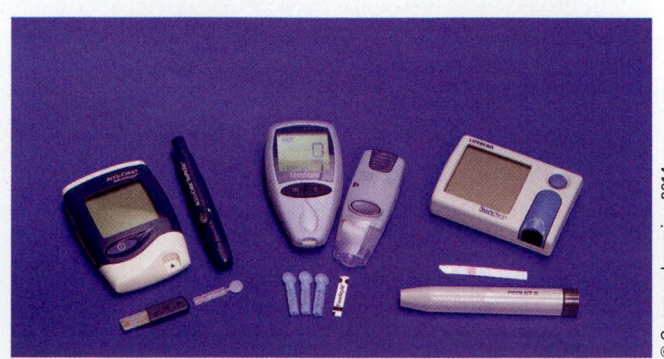

© Cengage Learning 2014

Figure 44-6 A variety of handheld glucose analyzers (commonly called glucometers) are available for home or clinic use.

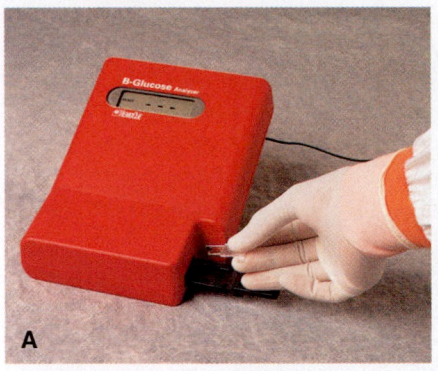
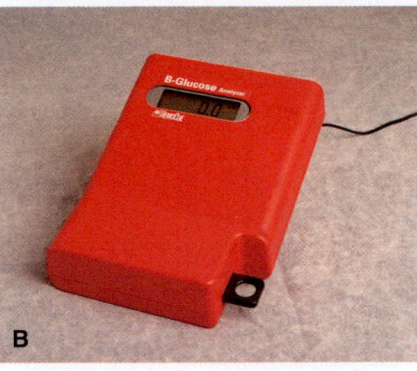
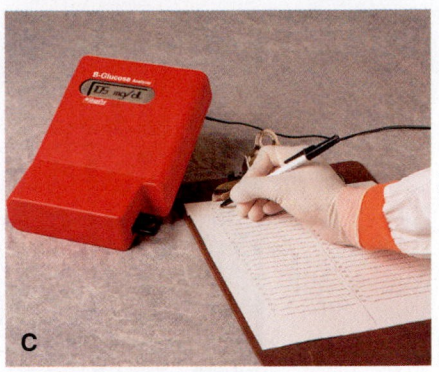

© Cengage Learning 2014

Figure 44-7   The HemoCue Blood Glucose System. (A) The patient's blood specimen is placed on the microcuvette. The microcuvette is inserted into its holder and pushed into the photometer. (B) Specimen is allowed to remain in the analyzer until test is completed. (C) When the analyzer has completed the testing, the results are displayed and recorded.

reflectance photometry. Blood from a fingerstick, serum, or plasma is applied to the reagent area of a test strip. The glucose in the sample reacts with the reagents in the pad(s), causing a color to form. The more glucose present in the sample, the darker or more intense the color. At the appropriate time, the strip is inserted into the test chamber and light is directed onto the test area. The amount of light reflected from the colored test area is measured by the photometer and converted to a digital readout showing the glucose concentration in milligrams per deciliter (or mg/dL). Most instruments give results in 1 to 3 minutes. Instructions included with the test strips must be followed carefully for reliable test results (see Procedure 44-4).

Testing Panels

Glucose testing may be part of a general chemistry panel test that can be useful in giving an overall view of an individual's state of health, especially when used in conjunction with other tests. Glucose testing may also be performed as part of a specific chemistry panel such as a glucose panel. Glucose serum levels are included in both the Basic Metabolic Panel (BMP) and the Comprehensive Metabolic Panel (CMP).

Glycosylated Hemoglobin

Glycosylated hemoglobin or hemoglobin A1c (HbA1c) determination is a blood test that measures how well the glucose level has been controlled over the past 2 to 3 months versus the conventional blood test that shows only current day status. Providers can use this test to determine

if patients with diabetes are consistently adhering to their diet and health guidelines or are adhering to their diet only for a day before their office visit.

Glycosylated hemoglobin is a stable molecule formed when sugar and hemoglobin bind together on the RBC. An increased finding of glycosylated hemoglobin indicates poor glucose control in the assessment of the diabetic patient.

When the RBC is first formed, it contains no glucose. If glucose is present at increased levels in the blood, the excess enters the RBC and attaches (glycates) to the hemoglobin. The more glucose is present, the more hemoglobin becomes glycated.

The A1c measures the percentage of the glycated hemoglobin. This offers us an average of the glucose in the blood over about 3 months. Most RBCs live about 120 days and maintain the glycated state.

What hemoglobin A1c does not do is indicate whether the patient has experienced hyperglycemia or hypoglycemia over that time frame because day-to-day readings of glucose levels are not provided; thus, it is not useful in adjusting insulin. Having the patient monitor his or her blood glucose level with a meter and keep a daily diary is a good way to look at his or her day-to-day blood glucose levels. Both tests are useful tools in helping manage diabetes.

The advantage of hemoglobin A1c not being affected by day-to-day variations in blood glucose levels is that the patient does not need to be fasting for this test.

CHOLESTEROL, LIPIDS AND SYSTEMIC INFLAMMATION

Cholesterol is a fatty compound that is essential for many vital life functions and is a normal constituent of blood. Although it is required for life, excess

ORGAN OR DISEASE PANELS — See reverse for components

Code	Test		Color
322744	Acute Hepatitis Panel	@ 80074	SST
322758	Basic Metabolic Panel (8)	80048	SST
322000	Comp Metabolic Panel (14)	80053	SST
303754	Electrolyte Panel	80051	SST
322755	Hepatic Function Panel (7)	@ 80076	SST
303756	Lipid Panel	% @ 80061	SST
322777	Renal Function Panel	80069	SST

HEMATOLOGY

Code	Test		Color
005009	CBC w Diff w Plt	@ 85025	LAV
115907	CBC w Diff w/o Plt	~	LAV
028142	CBC w/o Diff w Plt	@ 85027	LAV
005017	CBC w/o Diff w/o Plt	@ ~	LAV
005058	Hematocrit	85014	LAV
005041	Hemoglobin	@ 85018	LAV
005249	Platelet Count	@ 85049	LAV
005033	RBC Count	85041	LAV
005025	WBC Count	@ 85048	LAV
005090	WBC Differential	@ 85004	LAV

ALPHABETICAL/COMBINATION TESTS

Code	Test		Color
006049	ABO and Rh	86900 / 86901	LAV
001081	Albumin	82040	SST
001107	Alkaline Phosphatase	84075	SST
001545	ALT (SGPT)	84460	SST
001396	Amylase	82150	SST
006254	Antinuclear Antibodies	86038	SST
001123	AST (SGOT)	84450	SST
000810	B$_{12}$ and Folate	@ 82607 / 82746	SST
001099	Bilirubin, Total	82247	SST
001040	BUN	84520	SST

ALPHABETICAL TESTS CON'T

Code	Test		Color
001016	Calcium	82310	SST
007419	Carbamazepine (Tegretol®)	80156	SER
002139	CEA	@ 82378	SST
001065	Cholesterol, Total	% @ 82465	SST
001370	Creatinine	82565	SST
007385	Digoxin (Lanoxin®)	% @ 80162	SER
004515	Estradiol	82670	SST
004309	FSH	83001	SST
001958	GGTP	% @ 82977	SST
001818	Glucose, Plasma	% @ 82947	GRY
001032	Glucose, Serum	% @ 82947	SER
004556	hCG, Beta Subunit, Qual	% @ 84703	SST
004416	hCG, Beta Subunit, Quant	% @ 84702	SST
004036	hCG, Qualitative, Urine	81025	URN
001925	HDL Cholesterol	% @ 83718	SST
162289	Helicobacter pylori, IgG	86677	SST
006395	Hep B Surface Antibody	86706	SST
006510	Hep B Surface Antigen	87340	SST
140608	Hep C Antibody	86803	SST
001453	Hemoglobin A$_{1c}$	% @ 83036	LAV
083824	HIV-1 Antibodies *	% @ 86701	SST
001321	Iron and IBC	83540 / 83550	SST
001115	LDH	83615	SST
004283	LH	83002	SST
001404	Lipase	83690	SER
007708	Lithium (Eskalith®)	% @ 80178	SER
001537	Magnesium	83735	SST
007401	Phenytoin (Dilantin®)	% @ 80185	RED
001180	Potassium	84132	SST

ALPHABETICAL TESTS CON'T

Code	Test		Color
512094	PreGen-Plus™		
202945	Prenatal Profile 1	@	
004465	Prolactin	84146	SST
010322	PSA	% @ 84153 / G0103	SST
001073	Protein, Total	84155	SST
005199	Prothrombin Time (PT)	% @ 85610	BLU
020321	PT and PTT Activated	% @ 85610 / 85730	BLU
005207	PTT Activated	@ 85730	BLU
006502	Rheumatoid Arthritis Factor	@ 86431	SST
006072	RPR	@ 86592	SST
006197	Rubella Antibodies, IgG	86762	SST
005215	Sed Rate, Westergren	@ 85651	LAV
004226	Testosterone	84403	SST
001156	T3 Uptake	% @ 84479	SST
330015	Thyroid Cascade Profile	% @	SST
001149	Thyroxine (T$_4$)	@ 84436	SST
001974	Thyroxine (T$_4$) Free	% @ 84439	SST
001172	Triglycerides	% @ 84478	SST
002188	Triiodothyronine (T$_3$)	84480	SST
004259	TSH, 3rd generation	% @ 84443	SST
001057	Uric Acid	84550	SST
003038	Urinalysis Microscopic on Positives with	@ 81003	URN
003772	Urinalysis Microscopic	@ 81001	URN

MICROBIOLOGY – See Reverse Side

☐ ENDOCERVICAL ☐ THROAT ☐ URINE
☐ STOOL ☐ URETHRAL INDICATE SOURCE

OTHER

Code	Test		Source
008847	Urine Culture, Routine†	@ 87086	UriCul/Insrt
008169	Throat, Beta-Hemolytic Strep Cult, Group A	87081	Bact/Insrt
008342	Upper Respiratory Culture, Routine	† 87070	Bact/Insrt
180810	Lower Respiratory Culture	† 87070	Spec/Insrt
008334	Genital Culture, Routine	† 87070	Bact/Insrt
188128	Group B Strep Colonization Detection Cult/DNA Probe	87081 / 87149	Bact/Insrt
008144	Stool Culture †	87045 / 87046 X 2	Fecal/Insrt
008649	Aerobic	† 87070	Bact/Insrt
008623	Ova and Parasites	87177 / 88312	O&P Kit
164202	Chlamydia DNA Probe *	87490	Probe/Insrt
164210	N. gonorrhoeae DNA Probe *	87590	Probe/Insrt
164160	Chlamydia/GC DNA Probe w/Confirmation on positives *	PENDING	Probe/Insrt
096479	Chlamydia/GC DNA Probe without Confirmation	PENDING	Probe/Insrt
008904	Anaerobic Culture	87075	Aner/Insrt

† = ID / Susceptibility at Additional Charge
* = Confirmation at Additional Charge

OTHER TESTS / INDIVIDUAL PROFILE COMPONENTS
TEST # TEST NAMES

MATERNAL SERUM TESTING

017319 AFP Tetra @ % 017335 AFP X-tra @ %
017319 ... 017335 AFP X-tra @ %
GA: ___ wks ___ days on ___ by: LMP US EDD
DOB: ___ Maternal Wt: ___
Insulin Dependent: Yes No Repeat Test: Yes No
Type: Single Twins Other Race: Cau Blk Other
NTD History: ___
Other Indications: ___

© Cengage Learning 2014

Figure 44-8 Laboratory panels are combinations of tests related to a specific function, body organ, or organ system.

cholesterol is not a necessary part of the diet, except in babies and children. Sufficient quantities are manufactured by the body from carbohydrates and other fats. Cholesterol has been linked to coronary artery disease. According to the American Heart Association and the National Institutes of Health, cholesterol should not be restricted in babies and toddlers. Fats and cholesterol are important for normal growth and development. Babies and very young children should be on healthy diets, though, containing unsaturated and polyunsaturated oils and fats. From about 4 or 5 years old, they can be transitioned to heart-healthy foods such as nonfat milk. To help reduce the risk for coronary artery disease, nutritionists and agencies such as the American Heart Association and the National Cholesterol Education Program advise that fats make up no more than 30% of the total intake of calories daily, and that the concentration of cholesterol in blood not exceed 200 mg/dL. Cholesterol of 240 mg/dL or greater is considered to present a high risk for heart disease. Cholesterol levels between 200 and 239 mg/dL are considered borderline (see Procedure 44-5).

The Chemistry of Cholesterol

The cholesterol molecule consists of carbon, hydrogen, and oxygen. Cholesterol is a saturated, fatty acid. Saturated refers to the number of hydrogen atoms attached to the molecule. The more saturated the fat, the harder it is at room temperature. Fats of animal origin, for example, butter and animal fat, are saturated and are solid at room temperature. Monounsaturated and polyunsaturated fats are liquid at room temperature. Research into coronary artery disease has shown that saturated fats tend to increase levels of blood cholesterol. Monounsaturated fats (olive and peanut oils) do not change blood cholesterol levels, and polyunsaturated fats (corn, safflower, sunflower, and many fish oils) tend to reduce those levels.

Functions of Cholesterol

The human body is efficient at manufacturing cholesterol. Most cells are capable of doing so, especially the liver, the adrenal cortex, the testes, and the ovaries. All of the preceding cells, with the exception of the liver, use cholesterol to manufacture steroid hormones. In addition, cholesterol is an important component of bile and cellular

membranes. Although the body is efficient at making cholesterol, it is not as easily degraded and may accumulate in the body and reach dangerous levels.

In addition to what the body produces, humans take in additional cholesterol through the ingestion of meat, eggs, and dairy products (Figure 44-9). The liver metabolizes cholesterol to its free form, which is then bound to lipoprotein (fat + protein) and transported through the blood. Over time, excess cholesterol in the diet can result in a gradual increase of cholesterol concentration in the plasma. Increased

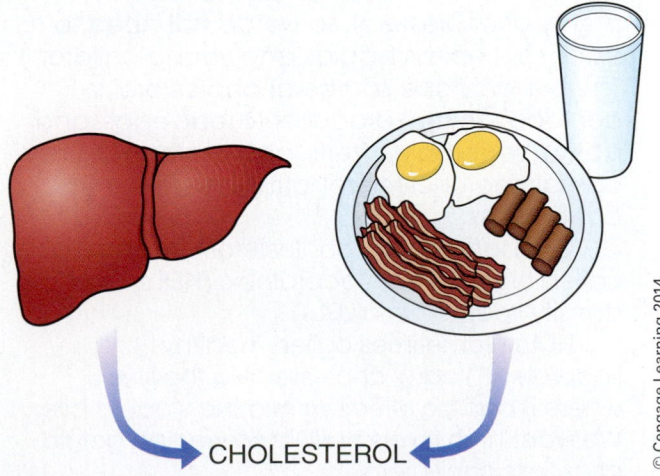

CHOLESTEROL

Figure 44-9 Cholesterol is created by the liver or obtained through animal sources of food such as meat, eggs, and dairy products.

© Cengage Learning 2014

concentrations of cholesterol in the plasma can increase to pathogenic levels. Some of the excess is stored in the liver, whereas some is deposited on the walls of blood vessels (atherosclerosis). Atherosclerosis of the coronary arteries is the most common cause of acute myocardial infarction (heart attack).

Lipoproteins and Cholesterol Transport

Two kinds of lipoprotein are involved in the transport of cholesterol through the body: **high-density lipoprotein (HDL)** and **low-density lipoprotein (LDL)**, Cholesterol bound to HDL is transported to the liver where it is excreted in the form of bile. HDL is sometimes referred to as good cholesterol. LDL cholesterol is deposited in the tissues as fat and inside the walls of blood vessels, and it is referred to as bad cholesterol. High levels of LDL are associated with an increased risk for coronary artery disease. Persons with coronary artery disease should have levels of less than 100 mg/dL LDL, whereas those without the disease should have levels of less than 160 mg/dL. Desirable values

for HDL and LDL are shown in Table 44-4. Levels of HDL and LDL are influenced by many factors, both genetic and environmental. It is possible to increase HDL levels through a combination of weight loss, a diet low in saturated fats, exercise, and cessation of smoking.

Blood cholesterol may be reported as total cholesterol or as total cholesterol and the HDL and LDL fractions. Cholesterol screening is used to help identify patients who are at a high risk for heart disease.

Cholesterol testing is part of a lipid profile that also evaluates lipoproteins and triglycerides to help identify patients at a high risk for heart disease. Figure 44-8 shows tests performed for lipid profiles on the laboratory form.

Triglycerides

Triglycerides are a type of lipid found in the blood that serve as a source of energy. Fatty acids and glycerol from the diet are converted into triglycerides by the liver. When triglyceride levels in the blood are excessive, they are deposited throughout the body as adipose tissue (commonly known

PATIENT EDUCATION

The Simple Scoop on Cholesterol

Cholesterol can be a confusing subject to try to explain to patients. Here is a very basic explanation that may help them:

Our bodies need cholesterol and we get it in two ways. We eat it and our liver manufactures it. Our liver manufactures plenty of cholesterol, so we do not need to eat it (except as babies and young children). There is only one source of cholesterol in our food: animal products (meat, eggs, and dairy). Vegetables, fruits, and grains naturally contain no cholesterol, although they may contain oils.

Our bodies have cholesterol transporters called high-density lipoproteins (HDLs) and low-density lipoproteins (LDLs).

HDLs (sometimes called "healthy lipoprotein") carry cholesterol to the liver where it can be released into the stool as bile. We want high levels of HDLs so we can get rid of excess cholesterol.

LDLs (sometimes referred to as the "lousy lipoprotein") carry cholesterol to our tissues

and blood vessels where it is stored and can cause problems such as blocked arteries, fatty liver, and obesity. We want low levels of the LDLs so we can have less risk for heart disease and arterial disease.

Fats and oils can also be confusing. Saturated fats are solid at room temperature and come from animal fats and butter and from manufactured products such as hydrogenated fats. These are the worst fats. Unsaturated fats, which are liquid at room temperature, may be in two forms: monounsaturated fats (*mono* means "single") and polyunsaturated fats (*poly* means "many"). Monounsaturated fats such as olive and peanut oils do not affect blood cholesterol levels, whereas polyunsaturated fats such as corn, safflower, sunflower, and fish oils will actually reduce blood cholesterol levels.

Triglycerides are a type of lipid found in our blood that provides energy. If we have too much in our blood, it is also stored in our tissues as fat. The liver converts some of our foods (fatty acids and glycerol) into triglycerides.

Table 44-4   Values for Cholesterol, HDL, LDL, and Triglycerides

Measurement	Values
Triglycerides	
desirable	<150
borderline high	150–199
high	200–499
very high	>500
Total Cholesterol (with no other risk factors such as hypertension and/or diabetes)	
Desirable	<200
Less desirable	200–239
At risk	>240
HDL (good cholesterol)	
Desirable	>60
At risk for women	<50
At risk for men	<40
LDL (bad cholesterol)	
Optimal	<100
Borderline risk	130–160
High risk	>190

All values are measured in milligrams per deciliter (mg/dL).

© Cengage Learning 2014

as fat). Triglycerides are transported within the bloodstream by LDL and very low-density lipoproteins (VLDLs).

Many factors influence serum triglyceride levels. Serum triglyceride concentration will increase moderately after ingesting a meal containing fat, peaking 4 to 5 hours later. Increased concentrations of triglycerides are associated with an increased risk for coronary and vascular disease.

Inflammation

With the escalating rates of heart disease in the United States, and the seemingly ineffective treatments of dietary changes and medications, there has been a shifted focus on systemic inflammation as being the predominant cause of heart disease. It has long been determined that inflammation is what causes cholesterol to accumulate in the arteries. The simple causes of systemic inflammation are said to be due to bacteria, viruses, toxins, and certain types of foods, namely, overprocessed,

prepackaged foods and foods high in sugars and omega-6 fatty acids.

Overly processed foods use omega-6 oils to sustain shelf life. The consumption of so many omega-6 oils causes an imbalance with the healthier omega-3 oils. The ratio should be a 3:1, rather than the more commonly found ratio of 15:1 or higher. Overeating overly processed, prepackaged foods loaded with omega-6 oils and sugars often leads to obesity, which leads to the inflammation, high blood pressure, heart disease, diabetes, and even Alzheimer's disease. Simply put, we were never meant to consume overly processed, prepackaged food products and should return to eating foods in their natural state.

C-reactive protein (CRP) and the more sensitive hs-CRP are blood tests to determine systemic inflammation and are currently being used in conjunction with traditional cholesterol blood tests and patient assessment to determine cardiac risk. Because CRP is an inflammation indicator, it can also be elevated as a result of acute arthritis and infections (see Chapter 41 for more information on CRP).

BLOOD CHEMISTRY TESTS

There are many natural chemicals in blood. The amounts of those chemicals are controlled by the efficiency of the body's organs and organ systems and certainly by environmental factors such as diet, smoking, drugs, and activity, as well as genetic composition.

The provider can order a general chemistry panel (BMP or CMP) or specific panels. A panel is a series of tests related to a body system, organ, or function. In interpreting a chemistry panel, the provider can determine pathology within the organ or malfunctions.

This chapter discusses each of the components briefly and explains some of the conditions and diseases that can cause these chemical tests to be abnormal. Keep in mind that all laboratory chemistry tests can vary slightly from laboratory to laboratory. Also remember that no one test, just like no one symptom, will make a diagnosis independent of other clues. The provider is considering laboratory tests together with the clinical picture, patient symptoms, and many other data in finalizing a diagnosis or diagnoses.

Alanine Aminotransferase (ALT)

ALT is an enzyme found in liver tissue. A high level indicates liver damage. A normal ALT level is less than 45 units/L.

Albumin

Most of the protein in plasma is albumin. It is responsible for transporting many small molecules (such as calcium, drugs, and bilirubin). It is synthesized in the liver; thus, low levels of albumin may indicate liver disease. It may also result from kidney disease, because the kidney is allowing too much albumin to spill into the urine. Low albumin may also be caused by malnutrition or a low-protein diet. A normal albumin level is 3.4 to 5.4 mg/dL.

Alkaline Phosphatase (ALP)

ALP is an enzyme. It is present in all our body tissues but mostly in the liver and bone. When levels are high in the blood, liver or bone disease must be suspected. A normal ALP level is 44 to 147 IU/L.

Aspartate Aminotransferase (AST)

AST is found in the muscle cells (heart and skeletal muscles) and in the liver. High levels cannot indicate specifically liver disease, but it is considered together with other liver enzymes. It is also used to monitor patients who have had heart muscle damage (such as heart attacks), but it is not the best or only enzyme tested for that purpose. A normal AST level is 10 to 34 International Units/L.

Bilirubin, Total and Direct

Bilirubin is a yellow-orange substance that comes from the breakdown of hemoglobin. Hemoglobin is contained within the RBCs. Because individual RBCs live for only 120 days, they are constantly breaking down and being replaced. When the RBCs "die," the "heme" part of the hemoglobin circulates in the blood until the liver filters it out. The liver is responsible for changing the "heme" into a water-soluble substance called bilirubin. Before it reaches the liver, it is called "indirect" or "free" bilirubin. After it leaves the liver, it is called "direct" or "conjugated" bilirubin. The liver sends the conjugated bilirubin to the gallbladder where it is released with bile into the small intestine. When there is a blockage in the liver/gallbladder ducts or a disorder/disease of the liver, the bilirubin cannot get past the gallbladder to the small intestine, so it continues to circulate in the blood. This excess of bilirubin in the blood can lead to a yellow-orange coloring of the skin called jaundice. The body will try to get rid of extra bilirubin through the urine. Hence, any detection of bilirubin in the urine (bilirubinuria) can be indicative of a problem in the liver or gallbladder. When the bilirubin level increases, it causes the skin and whites of the eyes to become yellow. This change to yellow is called jaundice. Newborn babies can be jaundiced because their systems are not sophisticated enough to get rid of the bile. Because bilirubin breaks down in sunlight, babies with jaundice are treated with special "bili-lights" to help them break down the bilirubin in their skin. The total bilirubin test will indicate problems in the liver and the hepatic system. Notice the total bilirubin test is in the general panel and the direct bilirubin test is part of the hepatic panel. Some types of general blood problems can cause high levels of bilirubin because more blood cells are breaking down than usual. Normal bilirubin ranges are as follows:

Total bilirubin	0.1–0.2 mg/dL
Indirect bilirubin	0.1–0.7 mg/dL
Direct bilirubin	0.1–0.3 mg/dL
Newborn total bilirubin	1–12 mg/dL

Blood Urea Nitrogen Test

The **blood urea nitrogen (BUN)** test measures the concentration of urea in blood. The amount of urea in blood reflects the metabolic function of the liver and the excretory function of the kidneys. Most renal diseases result in inadequate excretion of urea from the body; therefore, increased concentrations of urea appear in the blood. BUN is one of several tests, including creatinine, that are used to screen for renal disease and is especially useful for evaluating glomerular function.

Excess protein in the diet is not stored in the body but is metabolized (catalyzed) for energy production. Urea is the nitrogenous end product of protein catabolism and is produced in the liver. It is deposited in the blood and carried to the kidneys for excretion. Surplus urea is measured as BUN. Normal values of urea vary but in adults range between 8 and 25 mg/dL; concentrations greater than 100 mg/dL indicate serious impairment of renal function. A slightly elevated BUN can indicate dehydration.

Calcium

All the cells in the human body need calcium for many functions. It is a critical element for bones, muscles, and the nervous system. Too much calcium can cause the muscles and nerves to become hyperactive, whereas too little calcium can cause the muscles and nerves not to function at all.

Muscle cramps (charlie horses) are often caused by low calcium. Calcium needs to be maintained within certain levels in the blood. If we eat more calcium than we need, the excess is stored in the bones. If our diets are low in calcium, the needed amount is pulled from the bones. The storage of excess calcium becomes less efficient as women lose estrogen, hence the need to take in adequate daily calcium to prevent osteoporosis as we age. A normal calcium level is 8.5 to 10.2 mg/dL.

Chloride

Chloride is an electrolyte. Its main function is to help with the electrical impulses of the cells. Chloride works closely with sodium. Changes in either sodium or chloride levels usually affect each other. A normal chloride level is 96 to 106 mEq/L.

Carbon Dioxide (CO$_2$)

Measuring CO$_2$ actually is measuring bicarbonate. This test is part of an arterial blood gas analysis. The kidneys are the main organs responsible for balancing CO$_2$. Anything that throws off the body's metabolic balance (excessive vomiting and diarrhea) can affect the CO$_2$ levels. The CO$_2$ levels in the blood are influenced by kidney and lung function. Normal CO$_2$ is 20 to 29 mEq/L.

Creatinine

Creatinine forms when muscle (creatine) breaks down. Logically, these levels will vary depending on the patient's size and muscularity. This test is used to determine kidney function, and is especially important for patients on diabetic or hypertension medications. A normal creatinine level is 0.8 to 1.4 mg/dL.

Gamma Glutamyltransferase (GGT)

The highest concentrations of GGT are in the liver and kidney. Abnormal levels usually indicate diseases of the liver, kidney, or bone. It is used in conjunction with other enzymes, especially ALP, to diagnose diseases. A normal GGT level is 0 to 51 International Units/L.

Lactate Dehydrogenase (LDH)

LDH is an enzyme found in many organs, especially the liver, heart, kidneys, brain, skeletal muscles, and lungs. Abnormal levels indicate tissue damage but are not specific by themselves. Like all enzymes, LDH is examined in conjunction with other tests. A normal LDH level is 105 to 133 International Units/L.

Phosphorus (Phosphate)

Phosphorus works closely with calcium, another electrolyte. It is used to assist in the proper assessment of calcium levels and to detect endocrine and kidney disorders. Phosphorus levels are related to uncontrolled diabetes and malnourished conditions. A normal phosphorus level is 2.4 to 4.1 mg/dL.

Potassium (K)

Potassium is an electrolyte and is critical to muscle and nerve function and for the transportation of nutrients and cellular wastes across cellular membranes. Abnormal levels of potassium can cause heart muscle irregularities and, if severe, can lead to cardiac arrest. Potassium is controlled by aldosterone, a hormone. Uncontrolled diabetes or excessive vomiting/diarrhea can cause abnormal potassium levels. Patients taking certain diuretics (such as Lasix) should be observed for low potassium. A normal potassium level is 3.7 to 5.2 mEq/L.

Sodium

Sodium is an electrolyte and works closely with chloride. Dietary intake of sodium is usually sufficient, and the kidney can excrete the excess. Sodium is closely related to fluid balance and retention. Normal sodium level is 135 to 145 mEq/L.

Total Protein

Total protein is a measurement of protein in the blood serum and can reflect the nutritional state of the body, liver, kidneys, and many other conditions. If the total protein is abnormal, then further, more specific tests will need to be performed to find out exactly the source of the problem. Of course, if the total protein is abnormal, other tests might show some abnormal levels, too. A normal total protein level is 6.0 to 8.3 mg/dL.

Uric Acid

Uric acid is created when purine is metabolized. It is usually secreted by the kidneys, but too much can build up as crystals in the body and seem to settle in the largest dependent joint, the great toe. This is known as gout. A normal uric acid level is 3.0 to 7.0 mg/dL.

PROCEDURE 44-1
Pregnancy Test

STANDARD PRECAUTIONS:

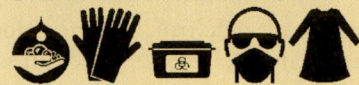

PURPOSE:
To perform the waived category visual determination test to detect hCG in urine to determine positive or negative pregnancy results.

EQUIPMENT/SUPPLIES:
Gloves
Urine specimen
Stopwatch
Disinfectant
Biohazard container
hCG negative and positive urine controls
Pregnancy test kit

PROCEDURE STEPS:

1. Wash hands and put on gloves. RATIONALE: While working with body fluids, such as urine, gloves should be worn as personal protection.

2. Assemble all equipment and supplies. RATIONALE: Organizing all equipment and supplies before running the test will eliminate errors caused by missing supplies.

3. *Paying attention to detail,* perform the test following the manufacturer's instructions. The following steps are intentionally general so a variety of kits can be used. RATIONALE: The manufacturer's instructions will differ from kit to kit. It is important, as a quality-assurance measure, for the instructions to be read and understood thoroughly. Any questions must be directed to the manufacturer.

   a. Determine materials are at room temperature.

   b. Apply urine to the test unit using dispenser provided (Figure 44-10A).

   c. Wait appropriate time interval (use stopwatch to time test).

   d. Apply first reagent/antibody to test unit using dispenser provided.

   e. Observe color development after appropriate time interval.

   f. Stop reaction.

   g. Consult manufacturer's package insert to interpret test results (Figure 44-10B).

4. Record the results of the test on a laboratory report form following laboratory policy. RATIONALE: Interpretation of results may differ from kit to kit according to the manufacturer's design, and even though laboratory processes are the same, policies and forms will differ from laboratory to laboratory.

5. Repeat steps with both positive and negative urine controls (Figures 44-10C). RATIONALE: Controls are performed to ensure the quality of the reagents and testing supplies. If a positive

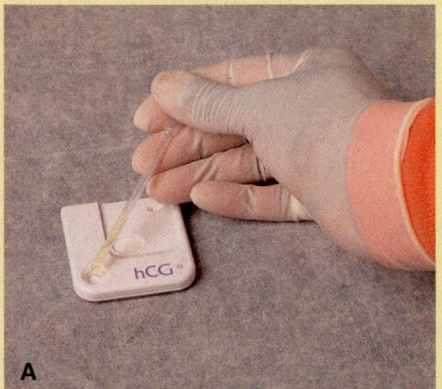

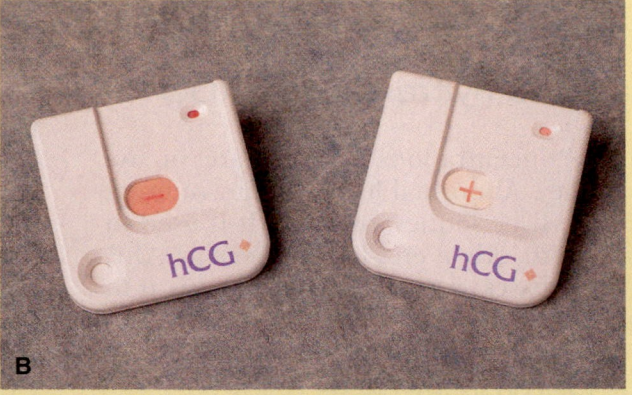

Figure 44-10 (A) Urine is placed in the test unit according to the manufacturer's instructions. (B) The package instructions specify how the test is to be interpreted. A common interpretation is with a negative sign (left) and a positive sign (right).

Procedure 44-1 (continued)

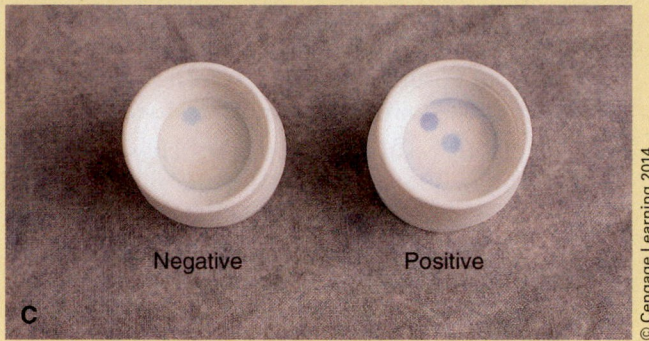
Negative   Positive

C

© Cengage Learning 2014

Figure 44-10 (*continued*) (C) Control tests must be performed according to the manufacturer's instructions. The results of the positive and negative controls test are shown.

control test does not show a positive result, then something is wrong with the reagent or the testing supplies. If the control test is not accurate, the patient's test will not be accurate either.

6. Disinfect reusable equipment. Discard disposable supplies into biohazard container. Dispose of specimen per laboratory policy. Clean work area with disinfectant. RATIONALE: Follow Standard Precautions and laboratory policies for disposal of biohazard substances and disinfection of supplies/equipment.

7. Remove gloves and discard into biohazard container. Wash hands. RATIONALE: Gloves protect hands from most but not all microorganisms. Hands should always be washed after removal of gloves to ensure complete protection and to remove glove powders and latex residue.

8. Document procedure in patient's chart or EHR. Complete a lab report. After the provider has initialed the report, it should be filled in the lab section of the patient's chart. RATIONALE: Documentation should refer the reader to the test result in the laboratory section of patient's chart.

DOCUMENTATION:

08/06/20XX Urine hCG test performed for pregnancy determination. Specimen tested in our lab. Results filed in lab section. Audrey Jones, CMA (AAMA) ————————

Laboratory Report

Patient Name ___Lynn Engle___ Date ___08-06-20XX___

Urine Pregnancy Test ___negative___

___Audrey Jones, CMA (AAMA)___
MA signature

PROCEDURE 44-2
Performing Infectious Mononucleosis Test

STANDARD PRECAUTIONS:

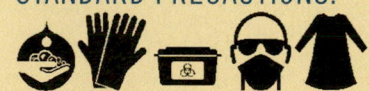

PURPOSE:
To perform an accurate test of serum or plasma to detect the presence or absence of antibodies of infectious mononucleosis (IM).

EQUIPMENT/SUPPLIES:
Gloves
Serum or plasma specimen
Stopwatch or lab timer
Surface disinfectant
CLIA waived test kit for IM
Biohazard container

PROCEDURE STEPS:
NOTE: These instructions are intentionally general so a variety of test kits may be used. The manufacturer's instructions will differ from kit to kit. It is important, as a quality-assurance measure, for the instructions to be thoroughly read and understood before performing the test. Any instructions not clearly understood should be clarified with the manufacturer.

1. Wash hands and put on gloves. RATIONALE: While working with body fluids, such as urine, gloves should be worn as personal protection.

continues

Procedure 44-2 (continued)

2. Assemble all equipment and supplies. RATIO-NALE: Organizing all equipment and supplies before running the test will eliminate errors caused by missing supplies.

3. *Paying attention to detail,* perform the test according to the manufacturer's instructions exactly. RATIONALE: The manufacturer's instructions will vary with each specific kit. Quality results are assured only when instructions are followed precisely.

4. Record the results on a laboratory report form following laboratory policy. RATIONALE: Even though laboratory processes are the same, policies and forms will differ from laboratory to laboratory.

5. Repeat the test procedure using positive and negative controls. RATIONALE: Controls are performed to ensure the quality of the reagents and testing supplies. If a positive control test does not show a positive result, then something is wrong with the reagent or the testing supplies. If the control test is not accurate, the patient's test will not be accurate either.

6. Discard contaminated materials into biohazard container. Dispose of specimen appropriately and disinfect reusable materials. Clean work area with disinfectant. RATIONALE: Follow Standard Precautions and laboratory policies for disposal of biohazard substances and disinfection of supplies/equipment.

7. Remove gloves and discard into biohazard container. Wash hands. RATIONALE: Gloves protect hands from most but not all microorganisms. Hands should always be washed after removal of gloves to ensure complete protection and to remove glove powders and latex residue.

8. Document results in the patient chart or EHR. Complete a lab report. After the provider has initialed the report, it should be filed in the lab section of patient's chart. RATIONALE: Documentation should refer the reader to the test result in the laboratory section of patient's chart.

DOCUMENTATION:

4/27/20XX 2:54 PM   Mononucleosis serum test performed. Results forwarded to provider and initialed. Report filed in laboratory section of the medical record. Joe Guerrero, CMA (AAMA)

DOCUMENTATION:

08/06/20XX   Venipuncture performed for infectious mononucleosis test. Specimen tested in our lab. Results filed in lab section of patient record. Patient tolerated the procedure well and Dr. Rice discussed results with her. Audrey Jones, CMA (AAMA)

Laboratory Report

Patient Name ____Noni Moo____   *Date* _08-06-20XX_

Infectious Mononucleosis Test ___negative___

___Audrey Jones, CMA (AAMA)___
MA signature

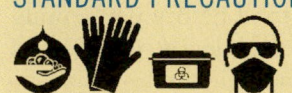

PROCEDURE 44-3
Obtaining Blood Specimen for Phenylketonuria (PKU) Test

STANDARD PRECAUTIONS:

PURPOSE:
To obtain a blood specimen using a PKU test card or "filter paper" to determine phenylalanine levels in newborns who are at least 3 days old.

EQUIPMENT/SUPPLIES:
Gloves
PKU filter paper test card and mailing envelope
Alcohol swabs
Cotton balls/gauze pads
Sterile pediatric-sized lancet
Biohazard waste container
Official Information Pamphlet

Procedure 44-3 (continued)

PROCEDURE STEPS:

1. Wash hands and put on gloves. RATIONALE: While working with body fluids, gloves should be worn as personal protection.

2. Identify the infant. ***Introduce yourself by name and credential and identify the patient and the parent(s).*** RATIONALE: Introducing yourself and stating your credentials will demonstrate professionalism and will help ensure the parent's cooperation. Identifying the patient and his parents will assure that you have the right patient.

3. ***Speaking to the parent's level of understanding, explain the procedure.*** Provide written information as well. ***Demonstrate professionalism and courtesy while you explain.*** RATIONALE: Explaining the

procedure in a manner the parent understands reassures him and helps ensure his cooperation. Demonstrating professionalism will help maintain a professional atmosphere and may help put the parent at ease as some parents may become apprehensive with this procedure. The written information is helpful to the parents and required by law.

4. Select and clean an appropriate puncture site (Figure 44-11A). Allow the alcohol to dry before the puncture. RATIONALE: Cleaning the site before puncture will remove any powders, oils, lotions, and contaminates. Allowing the alcohol to dry prevents the stick from stinging.

5. Grasp the infant's foot, taking care not to touch the cleansed area. Make a puncture approximately 1 to 2 mm deep in the infant's heel, making sure the infant's lateral, or side, portion of the heel pad is used. A pediatric-sized lancet, which limits the depth of puncture, should be used (Figure 44-11B). If possible, recent puncture sites should always be avoided (see Procedure 40-5, Capillary Puncture).

6. Wipe away the first drop of blood with a gauze pad. RATIONALE: The first drop is diluted with

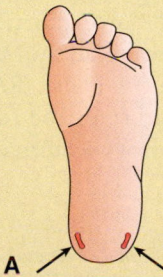

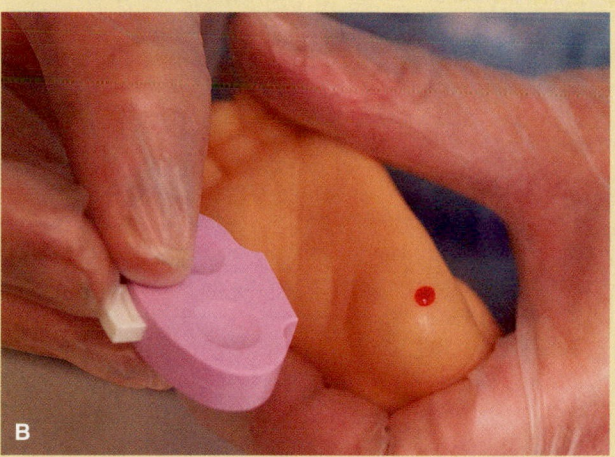

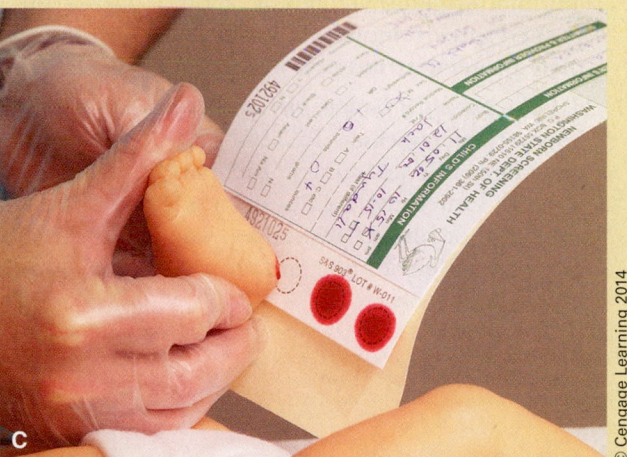

© Cengage Learning 2014

Figure 44-11   (A) Capillary blood collections sites on an infant's heel. (B) The infant's foot should be held securely with the nondominant hand while the dominant hand uses the pediatric lancet to perform the capillary heelstick. (C) Drops of blood are transferred from the capillary heelstick puncture site to the PKU filter card, completely filling all the circles.

continues

Procedure 44-3 (continued)

alcohol and should not be collected for the test. Using a gauze pad rather than a cotton ball is preferred because the cotton ball may leave tiny fibers on the puncture site. The fibers may encourage clotting, which will interfere with obtaining sufficient specimen for the test.

7. To collect blood for the test, press the back side of the filter paper test card against the infant's heel while exerting gentle pressure on the heel (Figure 44-11C). The drop of blood should be large enough to completely fill and soak through the circle. *Do not* layer the multiple blood drops within a single circle. Completely fill all of the circles on the test card. RATIONALE: Failure to do so will require a retest.

8. Hold a cotton ball over the puncture and apply gentle pressure until the bleeding stops. Do not apply a bandage. RATIONALE: The bleeding should be stopped before the patient is released from your care. Bandages are discouraged because they can be a choking hazard for infants and toddlers.

9. Properly dispose of all waste in biohazard container. RATIONALE: Follow Standard Precautions and laboratory policies for disposal of biohazard substances and disinfection of supplies/equipment.

10. Remove the gloves and wash hands. RATIONALE: Gloves protect hands from most but not all microorganisms. Hands should always be washed after removal of gloves to ensure complete protection and to remove glove powders.

11. ***Ask the parent if he has any questions and provide appropriate responses.*** RATIONALE: Soliciting questions will encourage the parent to ask if there is something he doesn't understand. Providing appropriate responses will further the parent's understanding and ensure a more cooperative follow-up.

12. Allow the PKU test card to completely dry on a nonabsorbent surface at room temperature. This will take about 2 hours. If collecting more than one card, *do not* lay one card on another when drying. RATIONALE: This could cause cross contamination of blood between the cards.

13. After the test card is dry, complete the PKU test card with all patient and provider information. RATIONALE: Allowing the blood to dry thoroughly before further handling lessens the chances of contaminating other parts of the form.

14. Place the test card in the mailer envelope and send it to the laboratory within 2 days. RATIONALE: It is important that the completed card be mailed as soon as possible to eliminate the breakdown of the contents within the specimen and to obtain the results as soon as possible to begin treatment if necessary.

15. Document the procedure in patient's chart. When test results are returned, they should be initialed by the provider and be placed in the lab section of patient's chart. RATIONALE: Documentation should refer the reader to the test result in the laboratory section of patient's chart.

DOCUMENTATION:

6/27/20XX 10:54 AM Capillary puncture performed on lateral aspect of left heel for PKU testing. Patient is 12 days old, currently taking no medication, and is not ill. Patient tolerated the procedure well and adequate specimen was obtained. PKU card completed and mailed. Audrey Jones, CMA (AAMA) —————————————————

7/10/20XX PKU test results received and initialed by Dr. King and filed in the laboratory section of the patient's medical record. The patient's parents were notified of the negative results per Dr. King's instructions. Audrey Jones, CMA (AAMA) —————————————————

PROCEDURE 44-4

Measurement of Blood Glucose Using an Automated Analyzer

STANDARD PRECAUTIONS:

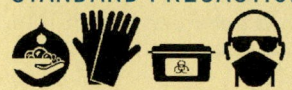

PURPOSE:
To measure blood glucose.

EQUIPMENT/SUPPLIES:
Gloves
Goggles
Safety lancet
Alcohol swabs
Glucose analyzer
Adhesive strip
Gauze 2 × 2
Control solutions for glucose analyzer
Test strips for glucose analyzer
Laboratory tissue
Cotton balls

PROCEDURE STEPS:

1. *Paying attention to detail,* review the manufacturer's manual for the specific glucose analyzer being used. Turn on the analyzer. RATIONALE: Always read and follow the manufacturer's instructions exactly for your particular analyzer to ensure accurate results.

2. Clean the work area and assemble all materials and supplies. RATIONALE: Organizing all equipment and supplies before running the test will eliminate errors caused by missing supplies.

3. Wash hands. Put on gloves and goggles. RATIONALE: Washing your hands ensures that your skin is clean before gloving and decreases contaminants. Applying personal protection equipment when working with body fluids will lessen the chances of exposure to dangerous biohazard substances.

4. Record the control ranges, control lot number, and test strip lot number. RATIONALE: Recording the lot numbers and control ranges is another type of quality-assurance measure and is required by CLIA for many automated tests.

5. Perform the check test and the control test according to the manufacturer's instructions. If both tests are within range, proceed to the glucose test. Repeat both tests if either is out of acceptable range. RATIONALE: Controls are performed to ensure the quality of the reagents and testing supplies. If a positive control test does not show a positive result, then something is wrong with the reagent or the testing supplies. If the control test is not accurate, the patient's test will not be accurate either.

To perform the glucose test:

1. Remove a test strip from the bottle and replace the lid. RATIONALE: Replacing the lid securely ensures that the reagents are protected from light and moisture.

2. Insert the test strip into the test chamber. RATIONALE: Follow the manufacturer's instructions for proper use of test kits.

3. Perform a capillary puncture (see Procedure 40-5). Wipe first drop with gauze. RATIONALE: Wiping the first drop away lessens the amount of tissue fluid in the specimen.

4. Apply a large drop of blood to the test strip. RATIONALE: The test requires a large drop of blood for accurate results. Let a large drop form before applying it to the test device.

5. While the test is running, check the puncture site. If the bleeding has stopped, apply an adhesive strip. RATIONALE: The test will take time to compute, allowing you time to treat the patient.

6. After the appropriate time interval has passed, read the glucose concentration. RATIONALE: The test requires an appropriate amount of time for accurate results.

7. Properly dispose of all waste in a biohazard waste container. RATIONALE: Follow Standard Precautions and laboratory policies for disposal of biohazard substances and disinfection of supplies/equipment.

continues

Procedure 44-4 (continued)

8. Remove gloves and wash hands. RATIONALE: Gloves protect hands from most but not all microorganisms. Hands should always be washed after removal of gloves to ensure complete protection and to remove glove powders.

9. Document the procedure in the progress notes. Complete a lab report. After the provider has initialed the report, it should be filed in the lab section of patient's chart. RATIONALE: The documentation should refer the reader to the laboratory section of patient's chart.

DOCUMENTATION:

08/06/20XX   Finger stick performed for blood glucose. Specimen tested in our lab. Results filed in lab section. Patient tolerated the procedure well and Dr. Rice discussed results with her. Audrey Jones, CMA (AAMA)

Laboratory Report

*Patient Name ___Maggie Radliff___   Date _08-06-20XX_*

Blood Glucose ___108___ mg/dL

___Audrey Jones, CMA (AAMA)___

MA signature

PROCEDURE 44-5
Cholesterol Testing

STANDARD PRECAUTIONS:

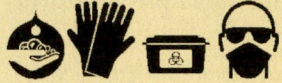

PURPOSE:

To measure cholesterol and triglyceride for monitoring purposes. For cholesterol, HDL, LDL, or triglyceride monitoring. *NOTE:* The following steps are intentionally general so a variety of kits can be used. The manufacturer's instructions will differ from kit to kit. It is important, as a quality-assurance measure, for the instructions to be read and understood thoroughly. Any questions must be directed to the manufacturer.

EQUIPMENT/SUPPLIES:

Gloves
Blood collecting equipment
Pipettes with disposable tips
Chlorine bleach
CLIA waived commercial kit for manual
   determination of cholesterol
Controls and standards
Marking pen
Biohazard container

PROCEDURE STEPS:

1. Assemble all necessary equipment and materials. RATIONALE: Organizing all equipment and supplies before running the test will eliminate errors caused by missing supplies and will show the patient a more professional process.

2. Wash hands; apply gloves. RATIONALE: Washing your hands ensures that your skin is clean before gloving and decreases contaminants. Applying personal protection equipment when working with body fluids will lessen the chances of exposure to dangerous biohazard substances.

3. Obtain a blood sample from the patient, either by fingerstick or venipuncture, depending on the manufacturer's instructions (see Chapter 40). RATIONALE: Always read and follow the manufacturer's instructions to ensure accurate results.

4. ***Paying attention to detail,*** follow the manufacturer's instructions to perform the cholesterol test. Be sure to run the controls also. RATIONALE: Following all manufacturer's instructions will

Procedure 44-5 (continued)

assure accurate test results. Controls are performed to ensure the quality of the reagents and testing supplies. If the control test is not accurate, the patient's test will not be accurate either.

5. Properly dispose of all waste in biohazard container. RATIONALE: Follow Standard Precautions when disposing of sharps and biohazard and contaminated waste.

6. Record the results of the test on a laboratory report form and document the procedure in the patient's chart. After the provider has initialed the report, file it in the patient's chart. RATIONALE: The chart note should refer the reader to the laboratory section of the patient's chart.

DOCUMENTATION:

08/06/20XX   Finger stick performed for serum cholesterol Specimen tested in our lab. Initialed results filed in the lab section of the chart. Dr. Rice discussed the results with the patient. Audrey Jones, CMA (AAMA)——————————

Laboratory Report

Patient Name ____Terri Smith____   Date _08-06-20XX_

Serum Cholesterol ___150___ mg/dL

_____Audrey Jones, CMA (AAMA)_____
MA signature

CASE STUDY 44-1

Refer to the scenario at the beginning of the chapter.

Audrey takes pride in paying attention to every detail when performing lab tests. She is also committed to explaining processes to her patients and increasing their comfort level.

CASE STUDY REVIEW

1. What are some key points to adhere to when performing testing using a CLIA waived test kit to ensure accuracy?
2. What are some specific ways you can reassure a patient to have confidence in your ability?

CASE STUDY 44-2

Anna Preciado, CMA (AAMA), a clinical medical assistant with Drs. Lewis and King, has performed many venipunctures during her training at college, throughout her practicum, and since her employment with Drs. Lewis and King. She has not, however, performed a heelstick capillary draw since she was in college and even then she practiced on a doll. Until now another medical assistant in the clinic was doing all the heelstick capillary draws for PKU testing, but Anna is ready to start performing them herself. She is concerned and understandably nervous about performing this procedure on an infant.

CASE STUDY REVIEW

1. What course of action should Anna take to prepare herself for performing a procedure that she has not done in several years?
2. Once Anna feels she is technically ready to perform the PKU blood test, what should she do to ensure that the procedure goes well?

SUMMARY

CLIA has identified many rapid test kits and automated methods for use in the ambulatory care setting in the waived category. For all of the tests discussed in this chapter, it is important for the medical assistant to have a basic understanding of the principles involved and the proper sampling procedures required. Safety procedures and Standard Precautions must be observed at all times and include the proper disposal of infectious materials and reagents. Gloves and goggles are always used when obtaining samples and while performing the actual test. Careful documentation by the medical assistant will help the provider in the diagnosis of the patient.

STUDY FOR SUCCESS

To reinforce your knowledge and skills of information presented in this chapter:

- Review the *Key Terms*
- Role-play with other students to apply attributes of professionalism pertinent to this chapter.
- Consider the *Case Studies* and discuss your conclusions
- Answer the questions in the *Certification Review*
- Apply your knowledge by completing the *Activities* in the *Study Guide* and the *Games and Quizzes* in the StudyWARE (StudyWARE) software on the *Premium Website*
- Perform the *Procedures* using the *Competency Assessment Checklists* in the *Competency Manual*
- Practice your problem-solving skills with the *Critical Thinking Challenge 3.0* on the *Premium Website*

Additional resources for this chapter include:

- *CourseMate for Delmar's Comprehensive Medical Assisting*
- *WebTutor for Delmar's Comprehensive Medical Assisting*

CERTIFICATION REVIEW

1. In addition to pregnancy, a positive hCG test can be found in the following pathologic conditions *except:*
   a. ectopic pregnancy
   b. hydatidiform mole of the uterus
   c. pelvic inflammatory disease
   d. cancer of the lung
2. If a urine sample for a pregnancy test cannot be tested immediately, it may be stored in the following way for 24 hours:
   a. room temperature, 25°C
   b. body temperature, 37°C
   c. frozen
   d. refrigerated at 4°C
3. The kissing disease is synonymous with the disease:
   a. tuberculosis
   b. infectious mononucleosis
   c. hemolytic anemia
   d. hypoglycemia
4. Serum or blood would be the specimen for all but the following test:
   a. ABO typing
   b. testing for EBV
   c. cholesterol
   d. hCG hormone
   e. all of the above

5. Which of the following statements is incorrect regarding blood type:
   a. type A RBCs have A antigens on the cell
   b. type B RBCs have B antigens on the cell
   c. type O RBCs have A and B antigens on the cell
   d. type AB RBCs have both A and B antigens on the cell
6. Which of the following is a *true* statement about the Rh factor?
   a. Rh factor is a rare blood type.
   b. Rh factor is present on all RBCs.
   c. Rh factor was discovered by experiments on rhesus monkeys.
   d. People without the Rh factor on their RBCs have naturally occurring antibodies called anti-D in their plasma.
7. When instructing a patient in the correct collection of a specimen for semen analysis, all of the following should be considered *except:*
   a. avoid the consumption of alcohol several days before the test
   b. collection of semen into a condom is unacceptable
   c. specimen should be transported to the laboratory at 37°C within 30 minutes of collection
   d. avoid the consumption of fats several days before the test

8. Testing for PKU is done on:
   a. newborns
   b. children 1 to 3 years of age
   c. teenagers
   d. adults older than 40 years
9. The best site location for a tuberculin Mantoux test is:
   a. back of the hand
   b. forearm 3 to 4 inches from bend of arm
   c. ½ inch above the back of the knee
   d. upper part of the arm in the deltoid muscle

10. A patient with hypoglycemia would have a blood glucose level of:
    a. 50–70 mg/dL
    b. 70–110 mg/dL
    c. 110–150 mg/dL
    d. 150–200 mg/dL

REFERENCES/BIBLIOGRAPHY

Department of Health and Human Services, Centers for Disease Control and Prevention. Retrieved February 2012, from http://www.cdc.gov

U.S. Food and Drug Administration. *Databases on the FDA Website.* Retrieved February 2012, from http://www.fda.gov/search/databases.html

Walters, N. J., Estridge, B. H., & Reynold, A. P. (2011). *Basic clinical laboratory techniques* (5th ed.). Clifton Park, NY: Delmar Cengage Learning.

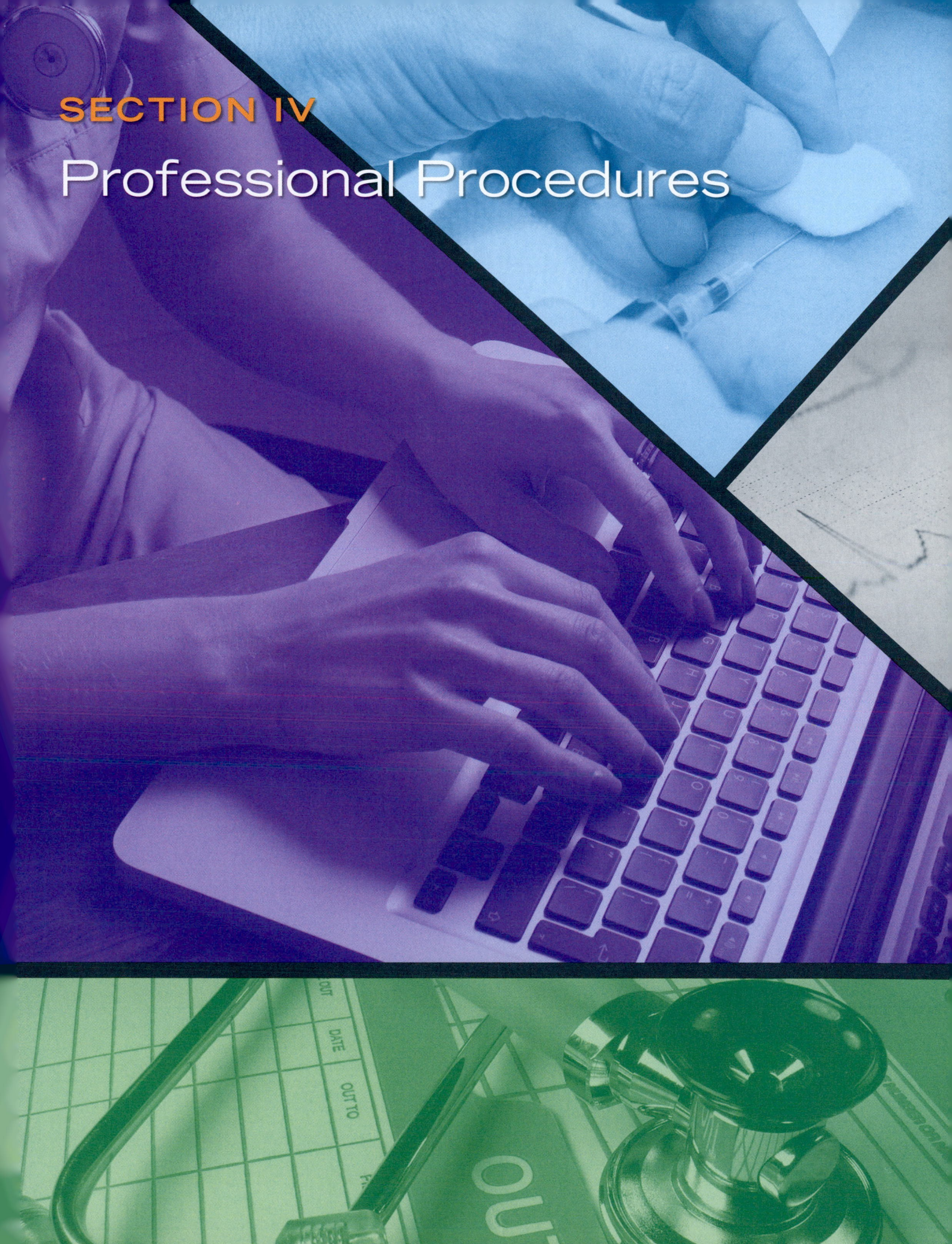

SECTION IV

Professional Procedures

UNIT X

Clinic and Human Resources Management

CHAPTER 45
The Medical Assistant as Clinic Manager 1394

CHAPTER 46
The Medical Assistant as Human Resources Manager .. 1434

OUTLINE

The Medical Assistant as Clinic Manager

Qualities of a Manager
  Clinic Manager Attitude
  Professionalism

Management Styles
  Authoritarian Style
  Participatory Style
  Management by Walking Around

Risk Management

Importance of Teamwork
  Getting the Team Started
  Using a Team to Solve a Problem
  Planning and Implementing a Solution
  Recognition

Supervising Personnel
  Staff and Team Meetings
  Conflict Resolution

Harassment in the Workplace
  Assimilating New Personnel
  Employees with Chemical Dependencies or Emotional Problems
  Evaluating Employees and Planning Salary Review
  Dismissing Employees

Procedure Manual
  Organization of the Procedure Manual
  Updating and Reviewing the Procedure Manual

HIPAA Implications

Travel Arrangements
  Itinerary

Time Management

Marketing Functions
  Seminars
  Brochures
  Newsletters

Press Releases
Special Events

Social Media in the Medical Clinic

Records and Financial Management
  Electronic Health Records and the Clinic Manager
  Payroll Processing

Facility and Equipment Management
  Administrative and Clinical Inventory of Supplies and Equipment
  Administrative and Clinical Equipment Calibration and Maintenance

Liability Coverage and Bonding
Legal Issues

LEARNING OUTCOMES

1. Define, spell, and pronounce the key terms as presented in the glossary.
2. Describe the qualities of a manager.
3. Discuss characteristics of managers and leaders.
4. Differentiate between authoritarian and participatory management styles.
5. Describe management by walking around and its usefulness in ambulatory care settings.
6. Recall a minimum of four common risks and risk-control measures.
7. List three benefits of a teamwork approach.
8. Discuss the importance of a meeting agenda.
9. Describe appropriate evaluation tools for employees.
10. Recall effective methods of resolving conflict.
11. Identify the steps required to make travel arrangements.
12. Define the term itinerary and list important information the itinerary should contain.
13. List three methods of increasing productivity and efficient time management.
14. Describe the purpose of a procedure manual.
15. Discuss the impact of HIPAA's privacy policy in ambulatory care settings.
16. Describe the general concept of marketing and recall at least three marketing tools.
17. Discuss the role of social media in the medical clinic.
18. Describe the purpose and benefit of marketing.
19. Discuss the steps involved in the inventory of administrative and clinical supplies and equipment.
20. Discuss the steps involved in administrative and clinical equipment calibration and maintenance.
21. Analyze the professionalism questions and apply them to this chapter's content.

KEY TERMS

agenda
ancillary services
authoritarian manager
benchmark
benefit
bond
brainstorming
conflict resolution
embezzle
fringe benefit
"going bare"
itinerary
liability
malpractice
management by
    walking around
    (MBWA)
marketing
mentor
minutes
negligence
participatory manager
practicum
procedure manual
professional liability
    insurance
profit sharing
risk management
salary review
self-actualization
shadow
social media
subordinate
teamwork
work statement

ATTRIBUTES OF PROFESSIONALISM

Communication

- Did you display appropriate body language?
- Did you demonstrate empathy in communicating with patients, family, and staff?
- Did you apply active listening skills?
- Did you demonstrate awareness of how an individual's personal appearance affects anticipated responses?
- Does your knowledge allow you to speak easily with all members of the health care team?
- Did you follow up with collateral allied health professionals to optimize the patient's plan of care?

Presentation

- Were you dressed and groomed appropriately?
- Did you display a positive attitude?
- Did you display a calm, professional, and caring manner?

Competency

- Did you pay attention to detail?
- Did you ask questions if you were out of your comfort zone or did not have the experience to carry out tasks?
- Did you display sound judgment?
- Were you knowledgeable and accountable?
- Did you recognize the importance of local, state, and federal legislation and regulations in the practice setting?

Initiative

- Did you show initiative?
- Did you develop a strategic plan to achieve your goals? Was your plan realistic?
- Did you seek out opportunities to expand your knowledge base?
- Were you flexible and dependable?
- Did you implement time management principles to maintain effective office function?
- Did you assist coworkers when appropriate?
- Did you seek ways to improve the morale of your work place?

Integrity

- Did you work within your scope of practice?
- Did you acknowledge the scope of practice of other health care professionals?
- Did you protect personal boundaries?
- Did you demonstrate respect for individual diversity?
- Did you immediately report any error you had made?
- Did you report situations that were harmful or illegal?
- Did you maintain your moral and ethical standards?
- Did you do "the right thing" even when no one was observing?

SCENARIO

Marilyn Johnson, CMA (AAMA), has been employed by Drs. Lewis and King's clinic for the past 8 years. Three years ago, she was promoted to the position of clinic manager when the facility added the second clinic for its associates in a nearby suburb. Marilyn has a baccalaureate degree in business administration. Her responsibilities at Drs. Lewis and King's clinic include various duties involving personnel, finances, and efficiency.

INTRODUCTION

The drive to improve the productivity of the medical clinic, precipitated by managed care, Medicare, and insurance limits placed on fees, has broadened the scope of employment options and job marketability for medical assistants. This has created an opportunity for medical assistants to advance to the position of clinic manager.

In small clinics, the position of clinic manager may include the duties of the human resources (HR) representative; in larger clinics, these positions will be independent. This book treats them as separate positions (see Chapter 46). In the larger facilities, the clinic manager and HR representative must coordinate their personnel-related functions into a seamless organization.

THE MEDICAL ASSISTANT AS CLINIC MANAGER

The manager of a medical clinic or ambulatory care facility can have vast and diverse responsibilities. This chapter covers the following clinic manager duties:

1. Make travel arrangements and prepare an itinerary
2. Arrange and maintain practice insurance and develop risk management strategies
3. Supervise clinic personnel
4. Approve financial transactions and account disposition; generate financial reports as needed
5. Supervise the purchase and storage of clinic supplies
6. Prepare staff meeting agenda, conduct the meeting, and record minutes
7. Supervise the purchase, repair, and maintenance of clinic equipment
8. Assist in improving work flow and clinic efficiencies (time management)
9. Create and update the clinic procedure manual, Material Safety Data Sheets (MSDSs), and Health Insurance Portability and Accountability Act (HIPAA) manual
10. Prepare patient education materials and arrange patient/community education workshops as needed

SPOTLIGHT ON CERTIFICATION

RMA Content Outline
- Medical law
- Medical ethics
- Human relations

CMA (AAMA) Content Outline
- Basic principles (psychology)
- Working as a team member to achieve goals
- Medicolegal guidelines & requirements
- Computer concepts
- Records management
- Resource information and community services
- Maintaining the office environment
- Office policies and procedures
- Practice finances

CMAS Content Outline
- Legal and ethical considerations
- Professionalism
- Patient information and community resources
- Medical records management
- Medical office financial management
- Medical office management

> ## TREAT OTHERS AS YOU WOULD LIKE TO BE TREATED!

Figure 45-1   The Golden Rule.

QUALITIES OF A MANAGER

A clinic manager should not feel the need to be superior to employees but should strive to develop a synergistic organization. The best manager is like an orchestra conductor. He or she constructively blends together the skills and abilities of diverse people to produce a smooth and efficient team. The result is an organization having greater capability than would be achievable by the individuals acting independently.

The clinic manager should have two overarching goals:

- Get the job done.
- Make the process enjoyable.

This does not mean work should be one big party. It means developing ownership for the work, pride in doing the job well, and a sense of teamwork. There will be times when employees will not like having to stay late to meet important deadlines, but through developed self-actualization, they will take enjoyment from even the most undesirable task.

A good clinic manager needs to be two persons in one body: leader and manager. The two functions are different, and the good manager will use some of each characteristic in meeting objectives. Table 45-1 lists the differences between an authoritarian-style manager and a leader/manager.

Table 45-1   Differences Between an Authoritarian-style Manager and a Leader/Manager

Authoritarian	Leader
• Establishes and adheres to written procedures	• Empowers people
• Focused on short-range goals	• Inspires by example
• Authoritarian style of management	• Vision and long-range goals
• Bottom line all important	• Consensus or team style of management
• Does things right	• Does the right thing
• Annual raises	• Pay for performance
• Reluctant to change	• Not afraid of change

Good managers are leaders, providing their coworkers with vision, guidance, and a feeling of ownership in the process. They do these things without threats, usually through the power of their personal charisma. It is also important that managers clearly convey their expectations to their employees. Possibly nothing leads to ill feeling between the manager and an employee more than failure to let the employee know what is expected of him or her. Furthermore, a lack of expectations stifles career growth and organizational vitality. Good leaders need to blend many admirable personality traits of leadership to be successful and still control the resources entrusted to them.

Before proceeding with a listing of qualities of a leader/manager, a rule that defines almost all of the ethical qualities needs to be mentioned (Figure 45-1). Some texts call it the Golden Rule; this rule will make the difference between a manager who is successful and one who fails miserably. The rule needs no explanation and will serve any manager well in any circumstance.

Qualities needed by a leader/manager include the following:

- *Effective communication skills.* Communication skills include written and oral methods. The manager must communicate clearly, diplomatically, tactfully, and with respect for the feelings of others.
- *Fair-mindedness.* It is important to always be fair with coworkers. Decisions that impact one fellow employee create a ripple effect. That is, you may have to make the same decision for another employee at another time. Decisions should be based, as much as possible, on the assumption that what is granted to one employee will be granted to others in similar situations. This approach will decrease the risk for being accused of playing favorites or being unfair.
- *Objectivity.* The clinic manager must be able to view challenges without bias or prejudice. For example, when promotions are made, the clinic manager must be able to focus on the job description criteria and individual qualifications without introducing personal preference.

- *Organizational skills.* Being organized includes being able to prioritize tasks, working efficiently and methodically. Know when and be willing to delegate tasks when others have the expertise and time to complete the task within the time lines.

- *People skills.* The clinic manager must like people in general and enjoy working with them. Building confidence and self-esteem in others and being interested in promoting constructive relationships are essential qualities of the clinic manager. The ability to function as an effective team leader provides a role model for other staff members to emulate.

- *Problem-solving skills.* The clinic manager must be a problem solver. This may include being creative and doing away with old paradigms and traditional approaches to solving a problem. When difficult issues arise, focus on the situation, issue, or behavior, not on the person. A discussion about solving the problem without laying blame is much more productive. Positive solutions may be more readily attained when discussing what was observed rather than what was told by someone else.

- *Technical expertise.* Have a working knowledge of each procedure performed in the clinic, although it is not necessary to be the acknowledged technical expert. A good clinic manager is continually learning and encourages **subordinates** to seek opportunities to continue their education and advance their technical skills.

- *Truthfulness.* Lead by example! If an honest mistake is made, be the first to admit to the error and seek the best solution for preventing it from happening again. Respond honestly to requests. For example, two staff members ask for the same day off. The clinic manager will make the decision that only one member may have the day off and will review the policy manual to determine the appropriate criteria for designating who will have the request granted.

Clinic Manager Attitude

 Many managers share a common enemy—themselves. The part of ourselves that is our enemy is our mind and the outlook we have on the world. People who succeed attribute positive results to their own actions. People who underachieve or fail usually attribute negative results to

someone else or to chance, over which they have no control. Because underachievers feel helpless to affect results, psychologists conclude that their motivation to succeed is diminished. A low achiever would be unlikely to have a personal risk management system in place. They would feel they could not affect events. The more positive person could easily take steps to avoid these problems.

The effect of a negative mindset does not stop with failure to accept responsibility for the things that happen to each of us, it continues on. Unless we change our outlook, we lower our expectations and begin accepting the mediocre. Individuals who feel they are helpless to affect events become afraid of success as well as failure, and they subconsciously find a way to fail to avoid the challenges success will bring.

How do you change your mindset? The following are a few suggestions considered helpful:

- Come to terms with what you would have to change if you are to be successful, and be ready for the change.
- Identify what you really want to achieve.
- Put your goals in writing using positive terms (say "I will," not "I'll try").
- Begin with small, achievable goals.
- Eliminate poor habits such as procrastination.
- Tune out negative thoughts and focus on positive thoughts.

We are what we think we are. Be careful of your mindset, it can derail you and your job as a manager.

Professionalism

 The medical assistant as clinic manager must exhibit professional behavior at all times. He or she must be courteous and diplomatic and demonstrate a

CRITICAL THINKING

How does the clinic manager begin to develop good working relationships with other community service organizations to better serve and provide for the patient's health care needs? How would this improve the quality of public relations?

responsible and positive attitude. All verbal and written communications should be accurate and correct and should follow appropriate guidelines. The clinic manager should demonstrate knowledge of federal and state health care legislation and regulations and must perform within legal and ethical boundaries. All documentation must be performed appropriately.

The clinic manager serves as a liaison between the provider, patient, and other professionals. Therefore, professional demeanor in all respects must be followed. It is not uncommon to be called on to locate community resources and information for patients and employers. A good working relationship with other community service organizations fosters the sharing of information vital to your patient's health care needs and 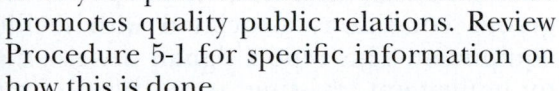 promotes quality public relations. Review Procedure 5-1 for specific information on how this is done.

MANAGEMENT STYLES

There are many books written on management styles; however, it is possible to break all of them down into only two basic styles, each with an infinite number of variations. Because this is not a management text, we take a straightforward view and look at only the fundamental styles: authoritarian and participatory. We also examine a third management style, managing by walking around, which, although not a people interaction style, is an effective management technique for keeping abreast of what is going on in an organization.

Authoritarian Style

Authoritarian managers operate on the premise that most workers cannot make a contribution without being directed, sometimes in the minutest detail, and even if they could, they would not be inclined to do so. This type of manager believes in the carrot and stick approach to motivate people to work. The carrot is monetary reward, and the stick is docked pay or being reprimanded or fired. The personality of the manager tends to influence natural tendencies of style. Individuals who are task or procedure oriented tend to be authoritarian. Authority control is easily accomplished in the case of simple tasks that can readily be structured and defined. Authoritarian managers try to control work to the maximum extent possible, for example, micro-management. Complex jobs, however, are difficult for the authoritarian manager to control.

Sometimes a manager needs to use the authoritarian style. It should be used quite sparingly because it may destroy morale and personal incentive. An assumption regarding the character of an employee frequently becomes a self-fulfilling prophecy. Workers with an authoritarian manager either give up and quit, or they become mindless robots. As a manager, you use the authoritarian style in the case of new employees until you have a chance to determine their capabilities, in the case of a worker who has proved to be without self-motivation, or in supervising short-term temporary labor.

Can an authoritarian manager style work in the twenty-first century? Yes. It has worked for a few well-respected, large companies in the United States, but this occurred only because management had unlimited resources to use as a carrot for rewarding employees. Most managers will not have these resources.

Participatory Style

The **participatory management** style is based on the premise that the worker is capable and wants to do a good job. The best known form of participatory management is the use of teams to do work tasks. This type of management is well suited to complex tasks where each member can contribute his specialty to the job at hand. The manager's function in this type of system is communicating direction and vision to the team and selling the team on the importance of the task. Providing the team with the necessary resources required is an important managerial function. Managers using this type of style need to be comfortable teaching, coaching, communicating, inspiring, and motivating. Workers engaged in a participatory management style are motivated by much more than monetary reward and develop an ownership for the work in which they are involved. Although the carrot is still important, their reward comes from teamwork, peer recognition, and self-actualization, that is, the pleasure derived from doing a job well and being recognized for it. Competition between teams is sometimes used as a motivation technique.

Management by Walking Around

Management by walking around (MBWA) is not really a management style but rather a technique for keeping the manager informed about the health of his or her organization. This style consists of just what the title says, the manager walks around looking at what is going on in the organization and talks with employees to get their opinion on how things could be done better. The manager collects data on new ideas; in a participatory system, a team is assigned to study and come up with a better way of doing the work. The manager must be careful to make sure his or her motives are not to micromanage and to convey this to the workers.

RISK MANAGEMENT

 The clinic manager should formulate a **risk management** procedure that assesses risks to which he or she and the organization is exposed and take steps to develop contingencies that minimize probable risks. Some common risks and risk-control measures are:

- *Loss of a critical employee.* Have cross training of employees to permit them to assume the duties of an employee who is ill or terminates his or her employment.

- *Failure of a supplier or contractor.* Maintain sufficient inventory to permit contracting with a secondary supplier before critical shortages occur. Monitor the status of orders so that you are aware of any failures in delivery before they have a negative impact and so that supplies can be obtained from a second source. Have a list of secondary sources.

- *Accidental disclosure of confidential information through error or unauthorized entry.* Have protocols in place regarding breach of confidentiality and defining steps to be taken in the event information is compromised. Define protocols to patients alerting them to the unlikely but potential possibility of accidental disclosure. Notify patients immediately if confidential information is compromised and work with them for resolution.

- *Computer failure.* Back up the system regularly. Have a secondary system that permits the clinic to operate until repairs are effected. Have a maintenance contract in place with a reputable firm permitting overnight repair.

- *Injury to a staff member or nonemployee.* Continually review safety procedures and conduct safety surveys. Have adequate liability insurance for the medical clinic.

- *Managerial position change.* Continuously network with friends and associates to permit you to rapidly seek a new position before experiencing a job loss. It's always easier to get a job while you still have a job.

Incident reports are required to notify managers of events involving injuries to patients, visitors, or staff; medical errors or omissions; breech of confidential information; and potentially dangerous conditions associated with facilities or equipment. This report signals the risk manager to implement existing protocols to minimize risk. Medical incident reports are confidential and cannot be released to anyone without a signed release of information agreement. The medical incident report form is an administrative document and is not considered part of the medical record. Procedure 45-1 provides steps for completing a medical incident report.

IMPORTANCE OF TEAMWORK

The use of **teamwork** to improve the efficiency of the clinic at first may seem incongruent to your desire to improve clinic efficiency, because it seems that several people are now involved in solving a problem that you as the manager should solve and explain. Teamwork builds morale and actually results in getting more accomplished with the resources you have because the team members develop ownership of the solution to a problem and want to make it work. When it works, it flatters them and builds their esteem.

The efficiency of a team results from collectively working together to plan how to "work smarter" and how to dovetail tasks and support each other so that wasted effort is avoided. To achieve all of these things, a team not only must be given the responsibility and the authority to plan and execute their plan to solve a problem, but they must know your expectations for them. Sometimes this means that you, the clinic manager, must stick your neck out for them. They will reward you handsomely for doing so.

Getting the Team Started

A successful teamwork approach is not a mysterious event that just happens; it is the result of a clear vision, specific goals, and a well-planned strategy on the part of the team leader. For teamwork to be successful, individual team members must understand and support the specifics of the problem they are being asked to solve. This is probably the most significant task of the team leader or the clinic manager. It is helpful in taking this important step to let the team develop its own **work statement**, for in this way they assume ownership of the goals and objectives you want them to achieve. The work statement frequently outlines specific tasks and their sequential order of accomplishment. Its purpose is to ensure that everyone is working toward the team goals and objectives.

A major pitfall at this stage may be diverse opinions that can lead to a work statement that does not meet the manager's goals and objectives for the team. It is your job as clinic manager to try to direct the team back to what you want them to work on without undermining their team spirit. Take care at this stage not to begin making assignments or to let team members start solving the problem until the work statement is complete. Under some circumstances, it may be necessary for you, the clinic manager, to exercise your authority in defining the work statement, but be careful, because this approach could harm the team's collective spirit.

The next step in team development is to establish a timetable for achieving results and identifying the standards that must be maintained. Without a timetable, a team feels no sense of urgency and tends to lose direction. You also have to paint a clear picture of the standards that must be maintained as you attempt to solve the problem. You should let the team develop both the standards and the timetable, but with your leadership and support.

Using a Team to Solve a Problem

Problem solution is the next step in team development. Some people call this stage **brainstorming** a solution. Brainstorming is fun, but unless it is controlled by the leader, it will bog down into needless arguments and hurt feelings. In a successful brainstorming session, everyone feels free to contribute solutions to the problem without any consideration for practicality or flaws in the proposal. Only after everyone has had a chance to speak are the solutions looked at in terms of practicality and for technical correctness. At this point the team should not look at what is wrong with the solution, but what needs to be done to make it a workable solution.

Prioritization of the solutions comes next. To do this, it is helpful to assign scores for impact on solving the problem and for changeability, or the difficulty in implementing a particular solution in your clinic environment. The result is a list of solutions to the problem in descending order from the greatest impact on the problem with the least cost or difficulty in implementation. Do a needs assessment, remove yourself from the issue, and look at it from a different perspective. **Benchmark** (compare) your facility to other facilities and organizations to see how they accomplish tasks, compensate employees, and so on.

Planning and Implementing a Solution

The team should work out a detailed plan for implementation of the selected solution, including a schedule. Assignments should be made, resources of equipment and funds available to the team should be defined, and any remaining problems should be assigned to subteams that will function just as the primary team did in solving them. The team should continue to meet to discuss progress and to resolve additional problems that may occur.

Recognition

A successful team should not be disbanded until it is acknowledged for its efforts and physical recognition is given in the case of an important problem that was solved. In some cases, a dinner or luncheon is in order. This is the most important phase of team development, because it is responsible for developing a team spirit or sense of **self-actualization** within the organization. Once this spirit is implanted into an organization, it becomes infectious.

SUPERVISING PERSONNEL

Creating an atmosphere in which open and honest communication can take place is critical to supervising personnel. This type of communication may be encouraged through the establishment of regular staff meetings, with each staff member sharing ideas for improvement and areas of concern. Eliciting the help of others in problem-solving strategies promotes harmony (Figure 45-2).

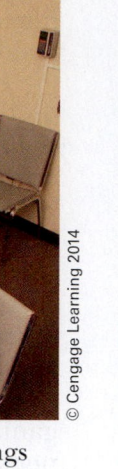

Figure 45-2 Consistently scheduled staff meetings promote communication and harmony among the health care team.

Staff and Team Meetings

The clinic manager usually initiates the staff and team meeting idea and should officiate at such meetings. Failure of the clinic manager to be present may convey a message that the meeting is an event not worthy of attention. It is important that the clinic manager be familiar with basic parliamentary procedures. The purchase of books such as *Robert's Rules of Order* or *Parliamentary Procedure at a Glance* is an excellent investment.

Successful staff and team meetings are announced well in advance or on established time lines to enable the majority of clinic personnel to attend. An **agenda** identifying the subjects to be covered during a given meeting should be issued before the meeting so that each attendee arrives prepared with input or questions relevant to the topics. Procedure 45-2 outlines the procedural steps for creating a meeting agenda. Figure 45-3 shows a sample agenda. Each meeting should end with opportunity for nonagenda items to be discussed or suggested for inclusion in the next meeting. The meeting should have a fixed time to end.

A written record in the form of **minutes** should be maintained and sent to all team members regardless of whether they attended the meeting. This policy keeps all members informed about policy changes and decisions that impact the clinic operations. The minutes also trigger a reminder for any new procedures or revisions to be made in the procedure manual. See Chapter 15 for additional information related to agendas and minutes.

The minutes for a staff and team meeting should record action plans under each agenda

AGENDA

STAFF MEETING Wednesday, February 16, 20XX
2:00 PM — Conference Room

1. Read and approve minutes of last meeting

2. Reports

   A. Satellite facility — Marilyn Johnson

   B. Patient flow — Joe Guerrero

   C.

3. Discussion of new telephone system

4. Unfinished Business

   A. Review new procedure manual pages

   B.

5. New Business

   A. Appoint committee for design of new marketing brochure

   B.

6. Open discussion and/or topics for next meeting's agenda

7. Set next meeting time

8. Adjourn

Figure 45-3 Sample meeting agenda.

topic. Summarize all action items agreed to in the meeting in one section of the minutes. This facilitates easy access to information at a later date should it be required.

The date, time, and place of the next meeting should be included. The person preparing the minutes should always sign them. A copy of the minutes should always be maintained in a book for easy reference.

Conflict Resolution

A good clinic/human resource manager is a master at **conflict resolution**, solving problems between any two parties. The most difficult task is to prevent or solve conflicts that occur between employees and supervisors or providers. Most conflict occurs because of poor communication or a misunderstanding; thus effective communication is a goal for any manager.

Volumes of materials have been written about successful conflict management. One can probably never get enough material on the subject. Some guidelines that may be helpful in preventing conflicts include the following:

- Listen to your employees. What do they say? What do they communicate nonverbally?
- Manage by walking around and talking to your employees.
- Do not tolerate negative comments or actions among employees.
- Encourage an open-door policy for concerns and complaints.
- Be a role model for all employees.
- Keep confidences.

A clinic/human resource manager who cares about each employee, who "carries water for the workers in the trenches," and who administers fairly and honestly creates an environment where conflict is at a minimum.

When conflicts arise, do not avoid taking immediate action to resolve the issue even if it appears to be superficially resolved. It will resurface at the first instance of stress between the individuals. Conflicts usually are the result of misunderstanding. In some cases the manager can mediate the issue and resolve the contentious behavior, but this places you in the role of judge and jury, and one party will feel injured or abused regardless of the outcome. Mediation is the only approach when the conflict is between a provider or supervisor and an employee. In all other instances the best approach is to use a confrontational approach. The two persons having a conflict are brought together and asked to express their conflicting opinions without interruption. The purpose is to communicate what each perceives to be the problem. If an obvious solution that is acceptable to both parties does not appear, the manager must insist that the parties come up with an acceptable solution to the conflict. (This latter step is not appropriate for conflicts between an employee and a superior in the organization.) In doing so both parties have ownership of the resolution.

HARASSMENT IN THE WORKPLACE

Harassment consists of verbal or physical behavior/conduct that is (a) unwelcome; (b) based on a protected class (e.g., race, sex, age, national origin, veteran status, or sexual orientation); (c) severe or pervasive; and (d) has a negative impact or creates a hostile environment. As a manager, you are legally responsible for ensuring nondiscrimination and preventing harassment. You, as a manager, may be innocent of any kind of sexual harassment yourself, but if the workplace you manage is construed as hostile by any one of your employees and you do not take appropriate action, you and your clinic can be held liable in a court of law.

 When an employee contacts you or you become aware of harassment, you should immediately contact your Human Resources Equal Opportunity Office (EOO). If your facility does not have an EOO, you should collect facts and confront the offending individuals or group, clearly notifying them that the offensive behavior must stop immediately. A report of the incident should be placed in the file of the offending individuals, with a written warning that a future incident will result in termination.

The manager must carefully evaluate the facts surrounding an incident. It is not uncommon for innocent events to be perceived as harassment. When there is conflict between people who are in some way different from each other, simple misunderstandings can be perceived as harassment. Blatant harassment is far less common than this kind of muddled interaction. Although some situations do involve malicious intent, many are largely the result of poor communication, and it is the manager's responsibility to differentiate between the two.

Every employer needs a comprehensive policy that prohibits all types of harassment. The policy needs to include a definition of what could constitute harassment or create a hostile work environment, information on who to report to, and a nonretaliation provision. This policy must be made available to all employees.

Assimilating New Personnel

The goal in the assimilation of new personnel into the workplace is to make it happen as seamlessly as possible. The clinic manager and HR representative usually assume this task jointly, with the clinic manager being responsible for orientation in medical protocols and procedures, and the HR representative handling orientation regarding medical practice rules and regulations and any legal implications.

New Personnel Orientation. The new personnel orientation process consists of orienting and training new employees in the medical protocols and procedures unique to the practice. If the procedure manual is detailed and accurate, this manual now becomes a guide for new employees.

It is important to introduce new employees to other staff members and to assign a **mentor** who can respond to questions that new employees may raise. Sometimes the individual leaving a position still is present and is asked to assist in the orientation process. This is especially beneficial if there is a good working relationship between the employee who is leaving and the management of the practice. Depending on the responsibilities of the new employee, a supervisor may be asked to monitor all procedures for a period for accuracy, safety, and patient protection.

The orientation should clearly present what is expected of new employees and explain that, at the end of their probationary period, their performance will be evaluated to determine if full-time employment will be offered. The same procedures followed for new employees should be followed for student practicums, with the exception that expectations and the evaluation process may vary.

Probation and Evaluation. It is common for a new employee to be placed on probation for 60 to 90 days. During this period, both the employee and supervisory personnel determine if the position is a suitable match for both employer and employee. Near the end of the probation period, the employee should be officially evaluated to determine how competently he or she is performing the assigned tasks/duties. The employee should also be given an opportunity to express their personal thoughts relative to job satisfaction. Figure 45-4 shows a sample probationary employee evaluation form. The evaluation becomes part of the employee's personnel record at the end of the probation period.

Supervising Student Practicums. The student **practicum** is a transitional stage that provides opportunity for the student to apply theory learned in the classroom to a health care setting through practical, hands-on experience. Some institutions use the term *externship* or *internship,* and still others operate through a cooperative education program. The number of hours for the practicum are predetermined together with criteria for site selection and tasks to be performed by the student.

The clinic manager should schedule an information interview with the student before the practicum begins. During this time, the expectations of the clinic manager and the student may be established. A tour of the facility and introductions

---

PROBATIONARY EMPLOYEE EVALUATION FORM

Name _____

Hire Date _____

Job Title _____

Pay Rate_____ Supervisor _____

Do you recommend the employee continue in employment?

_____ Yes _____ No

Please state your reasons for whatever action you recommend. Use the guidelines below to make your decision.

1. Has the employee required more training than is normally needed for the job?

2. Has the employee grasped this job with very little training?

3. Is the employee performing at, above, or below (circle one) the standard for this job?

4. If below, when do you expect the employee to reach the standard?

5. Does the employee get along well with all staff members?

6. Has the employee maintained a good attendance record and a good work attitude?

7. Has the employee expressed any dissatisfactions?

_____ _____
Supervisor's Signature   Date

© Cengage Learning 2014

Figure 45-4 Sample probationary employee evaluation.

to key personnel aid the student in feeling more comfortable the first day of "work."

Because the student will be writing in medical records where correct spelling is mandatory or may be scheduling appointments and must write telephone numbers without transposition, some pretesting may be offered. By giving a spelling test of 10 commonly used medical terms or verbally stating five telephone numbers for the student to write down, an immediate evaluation is attained.

The clinic manager should directly supervise or identify someone else to supervise the student. During the first few days of the practicum, the student may simply **shadow** the supervisor, learning the routine, provider preferences, and protocols for that particular clinic. As the student begins to feel comfortable in the new environment, minimal tasks should be assigned. Based on the student's ability to follow directions and perform tasks, increased skill–level tasks may be added.

The supervisor will direct and evaluate the student's progress; schedule activities that will provide experience in all aspects of medical assisting, including administrative, clinical, and laboratory procedures; maintain accurate records of attendance and hours "worked"; and communicate the student's progress to the medical assisting supervisor from the educational institution. Procedure 45-3 provides steps for supervising a student practicum.

When working with students, it is important to remember that they still have much to learn and will need lots of reassuring guidance. When you take time to explain each step and to provide the rationale for each, students will learn more quickly. Demonstrating new or different techniques and approaches helps students by providing them with options that they may find more comfortable.

Remember that this type of learning is stressful. The student is not yet accustomed to communication with a "real" patient, let alone working with a provider. Your role as clinic manager is to reduce as much stress as possible for everyone concerned. Introduce the student to the patient and ask the patient's permission to allow the student to perform a procedure. Many patients will be tolerant when they realize the circumstances and will be quite cooperative.

Employees with Chemical Dependencies or Emotional Problems

Employees with chemical dependencies or emotional problems are ill and are to be treated as such. Approach the situation constructively rather than punitively. Make a commitment to the employee, to the rest of the staff, and to the patients that at no time will patient care be put at risk. Help an employee with a problem to find the support and counseling necessary. No staff member should be permitted to remain on the premise with impaired judgment while under the influence of alcohol or controlled substances. If chemical dependency treatment is necessary, make accommodation as seems appropriate or is warranted. Everyone occasionally feels discouraged and distressed. Hopefully, the provider–employer and the manager are able to recognize problems before they become too serious.

It has been said that one in four individuals will experience some form of a mental health problem during the course of a year. Work-related stress is the base cause of a significant degree of mental ill health. Plan for and create a work environment that reduces as much stress as possible. Actions to consider may include the following:

1. Properly educate and train all employees for their positions.
2. Encourage teamwork and reward those who help each other.
3. Mandate "break periods" in the day for each employee.
4. Create a pleasant work environment (plants, water, music, and so on).
5. Establish a blowing off steam place for when employees are especially frustrated.
6. Take everyone out for lunch at least once a quarter.
7. Have regular staff meetings to discuss employee concerns and clinic improvements.
8. Celebrate birthdays and special occasions (i.e., length of service).

Keep in mind that a happy employee who feels valued in his or her position will stay much longer than someone who is unhappy and does not feel valued.

Evaluating Employees and Planning Salary Review

It is important that all employees know whether they are performing their job as expected and know how they can improve their performance if necessary.

Performance Evaluation. Not only is evaluation of employees necessary during the probation period, but it is necessary for current employees as well. Evaluations should be performed no less than once a year on the anniversary of the hire date. Some clinic managers may wish to evaluate an employee more often, especially if a problem has surfaced in an evaluation.

The evaluation may take many forms; it can be formal or informal; it may involve more than one person. The results of the evaluation, however, must be a part of the employee's personnel record. For that reason, a formal evaluation is preferred. Many practices use a written evaluation that requires that the employee evaluate himself before meeting with the clinic manager (Figure 45-5). The clinic manager uses the same form for evaluation.

PERFORMANCE REVIEW FORM

_____   _____
Employee Name   Title

_____   _____
Supervisor   Department

TYPE OF REVIEW (Check One)

_____ Quarterly

_____ Annual

_____ Probation

_____ Other _____

Review Period Covered _____ to _____

PERFORMANCE DEFINITIONS (To be used for general performance rating and job specific criteria rating.)

5 = Outstanding	Performance that is clearly superior, beyond the call of duty, or substantially above standard level. Seldom attained level of performance but achievable.
4 = Above Standard	Very commendable performance; exceeds the norm for the job.
3 = Standard	Competent and consistent performance; expected level of activity and performance for the job. Most often rating received.
2 = Below Standard	Performance needs improvement. This level of performance is unacceptable; needs improvement to meet the standards for the job. **Employee new to the job:** Performance might receive below standard rating due to lack of job knowledge and is expected to improve with experience. **Experienced Employee:** Performance is below acceptable level and requires direction and/or counsel.
1 = Unsatisfactory	Performance is unacceptable. Job activity is clearly and substantially lacking in quality, quantity, or timeliness. May also not be meeting cost or budget constraints. Needs much improvement to meet the standards for the job.

| (office use only)
EVALUATION SUMMARY

Total I _____

Total II _____ | FINAL RATING: CHECK ONE (clinic use only)

_____ Merit Increase Recommended

_____ No Merit Increase—Satisfactory Performance/No Growth

_____ No Merit Increase (Probationary/Special Evaluation)

_____ No Merit Increase (Performance Probation)

_____ Re-evaluate in 90 Days for Unsatisfactory or in 180 Days for Needed Improvement |

GENERAL PERFORMANCE RATING (PART I)

General Criteria	Rating	Comments Supporting Rating
1. **Patient Relations:** How well does the employee communicate a "we care" image to the patients, visitors, providers, and fellow employees?		
2. **Work Responsibilities:** What is the quality of the employee's work relative to quality, quantity, and timeliness?		
3. **Teamwork:** Does the employee have a team spirit? Does the employee interact well with coworkers/supervisor/manager?		(continues)

Figure 45-5 Sample performance review form.

General Criteria	Rating	Comments Supporting Rating
4. **Adaptability:** Is the employee open to change and new ideas? Does the employee remain flexible to changes in routine, workload, and assignments?		
5. **Personal Appearance:** How well does the employee maintain appropriate personal appearance, including proper attire, hygiene?		
6. **Communication:** Does the employee communicate well? Is information given and received clearly? Does he/she have good verbal and written skills?		
7. **Dependability:** Can the employee be relied upon for good attendance? Does the employee perform and follow through on work without supervisory intervention or assistance?		

Subtotal I _____ ÷ 7 General Criteria = _____

JOB-SPECIFIC CRITERIA RATING (PART II) (To be used with Job Description attached)

Responsibility and Standard	Rating	Comments Supporting Rating
Complete a section for each responsibility listed on the employee's job description.		

Subtotal II _____ ÷ _____ = _____
job duties

Contributions made since last review:

_____

_____

Education or training received since last review:

_____

_____

Action to be taken based on performance:

_____

_____

Comments:

_____

_____

_____

_____   _____
Employee Signature   Date

_____   _____
Supervisor Signature   Date

_____   _____
Provider Signature   Date

Figure 45-5   (continued)

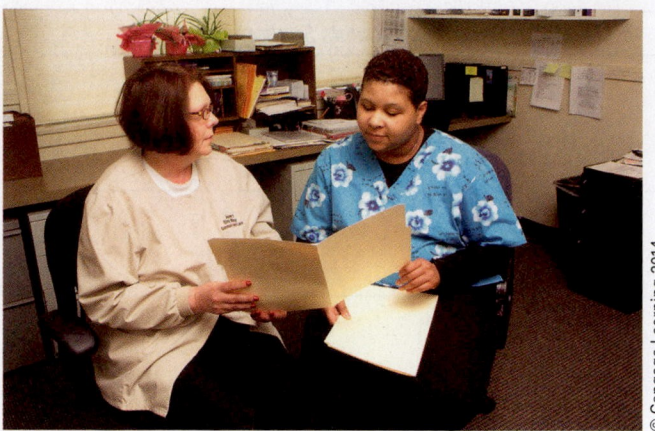

© Cengage Learning 2014

Figure 45-6 A comfortable, private setting encourages discussions during an employee performance review.

During the meeting, notes are compared as the evaluation is conducted.

The climate of the performance evaluation should be comfortable and provide privacy (Figure 45-6). The meeting should be friendly, but the employee must sense the importance of the evaluation. Do not allow any disagreements to escalate into arguments during the evaluation. Without reading the employee's self-evaluation, ask the employee to tell about the self-assessment. Acknowledge the employee's point of view and identify where you agree or differ from the self-assessment. Be prepared to describe specific examples of positive performance and negative performance.

When negative performance is identified, ask the employee for possible solutions. Then a plan can be determined to alter the negative performance. In this way, a trusting atmosphere is established in that both of you are working together for a solution that will benefit the medical practice. Always look for and seek a win-win situation whenever possible. The action plan determined should then be evaluated at the next performance evaluation.

At the close of the evaluation, always express your confidence in the individual to make any changes necessary, offer assistance where needed, and thank the employee for participating. End any evaluation with a positive statement about some portion of the employee's performance.

There are occasions when reviews are performed more frequently than annually. A review would occur 2 to 3 months after a significant promotion to measure how things are progressing. Reviews occur more often when general performance falls well short of past efforts or a serious error in judgment has been made. This type of review may end with a reprimand, a warning to correct the problem by a given date, or possibly, immediate dismissal. Document any steps to be taken to correct a problem and any reason that is cause for dismissal.

Salary Review. Although the practice is common in some areas, it may be better not to tie salary increases or bonuses with the annual performance evaluation. Conduct the **salary review** at the beginning of the new year separate from performance evaluations.

Salary review is important. Unfortunately, in smaller medical clinic and ambulatory care settings, the review of salary may have to be raised by the employee. Provider-employers tend to forget that their employees have been with them for over a year without a raise or a discussion of financial reimbursement. If this is the case, it is perfectly acceptable for the employee to raise the issue on a yearly basis. However, the best approach is for the clinic manager to conduct salary reviews at the beginning or end of each calendar year.

Data should be collected before a salary review. The clinic manager should network with other clinic managers in the local area to determine wages and salaries for comparable individuals with comparable skills. Remember, also, that it is far more cost-effective to reward good employees with a salary increase than it is to train a new employee who commands a lesser salary than current employees. Reward employees well and provide benefits that encourage them to stay with the practice. Employees who stay with the practice for a long time not only fully understand how best to serve their provider-employers, they have established a relationship with patients that is beneficial.

How much of a raise is to be awarded at the time of salary review is difficult to determine and depends on many factors that might include the profits of the year, the patient load, the workload, and the current cost of living.

The critical shortage of health care employees today is reflected in the shortage of medical assistants across the country. Newspapers advertising for individuals to work in the ambulatory care setting tell the story. A consideration worth mentioning is that often the salary does not match the education, experience, and special training required of someone working in the health care field. Educators often hear, "Why would I spend a year or more in education to be paid what I would make working in a fast food restaurant?" Because it is costly in time and resources to replace employees, it is best to invest that cost into a fair and just salary increase for valued employees.

Dismissing Employees

Most clinic/human resource managers do not enjoy rating the performance of other employees, particularly when difficult topics are involved and it may be necessary to dismiss an employee. However, the written performance evaluation actually establishes the format for such a dismissal when necessary and is more likely to remove the emotion from the situation. Involuntary dismissal is still difficult when it is necessary.

Involuntary Dismissal. Involuntary dismissal results from two primary causes: poor performance or serious violation of clinic policies or job descriptions. When it becomes apparent to the clinic manager that the effectiveness of an employee is dropping well below expectations, it will be known in the review or a performance review may be called. The review allows the employee to be informed of the shortcomings, to explain any reasons for the present situation, and to determine a plan to alleviate the problem. If the problem is a serious one, probation is usually invoked and any lack of significant improvement in the time provided results in immediate dismissal.

When the problem is a violation of either clinic policy or procedures, both a verbal and a written warning are given to the employee. Involuntary dismissal follows if the situation persists. Dismissal may be immediate if the action is a serious violation of policy. Serious violations depend on the clinic practice, but some causes for immediate dismissal include theft, making fraudulent claims against insurance, placing the patient in jeopardy by not practicing safe techniques, and breach of patient confidentiality.

Some key points to keep in mind when dismissal is necessary are:

1. The dismissal should be made in privacy.
2. Take no longer than 10 minutes for the dismissal.
3. Be direct, firm, and to the point in identifying reasons.
4. Do not engage in an in-depth discussion of performance.
5. Explain terms of dismissal (keys, clearing out area of personal items, final paperwork).
6. Listen to employee's opinion and emotions; it is not necessary to agree.
7. Accompany the employee to his or her desk to pack his or her belongings.
8. Escort the employee out of the facility; do not allow him or her to finish the work of the day.

Voluntary Dismissal. Other reasons for dismissal may be more pleasant. Changes in personnel occur for many good reasons, and people voluntarily leave their jobs. They may relocate, seek advancement in another facility, or simply have personal reasons for leaving. These employees will give their manager proper notice and will be able to turn their current projects and duties over to their replacements. They have time to say good-bye to their friends and leave with a good feeling about their employment.

PROCEDURE MANUAL

The **procedure manual** provides detailed information relative to the performance of tasks within the facility in which one is employed. Each procedure manual should be designed for that specific clinic setting and should satisfy its requirements.

The procedure manual serves as a guide to the employee assigned a specific task and may also be useful in evaluating the employee's performance. If a temporary employee is assigned the task, the procedure manual will be invaluable in assuring that each procedure is completed as outlined.

The provider(s) and the clinic manager should have copies of the procedure manual, and all employees should have access to the procedure manual. Copies of individual sections may be given to the employee responsible for the task; the employee should be instructed to follow these guidelines and told that they may be used as employee evaluation tools. If all employees have access to the clinic computer system, the procedures manual can be made available in electronic format.

Organization of the Procedure Manual

It is best to use a loose-leaf binder with separator pages denoting each procedure. Many clinic managers find it helpful to divide the binder into administrative and clinical sections with subdivisions for each primary task performed (Figure 45-7).

To facilitate using the procedure manual, a consistent format should be developed and used

Administrative Section	Clinical Section	Administrative/Clinical Sections
Personnel Management	Physical Examinations	HIPAA and ADA compliance
Communication	Infection Control	Creating a Safe Environment
(oral and written)	Collecting Specimens	Evacuation Procedures
Patient Scheduling	Laboratory Procedures	Emergency Codes
Records Management	Surgical Asepsis	Fire Safety
Financial Management	Emergencies	Fire Extinguisher Safety
Facility and Equipment	Material Safety Data Sheets	Response to National
Management	(MSDS)	Disaster or Emergency
	OSHA	Medical Assistant Response to
	CLIA '88	Disaster Preparedness

© Cengage Learning 2014

Figure 45-7 Many clinics find that dividing the procedure manual into tabular sections helps organize the material. A table of contents with page numbers helps locate information easily.

throughout the manual. Each procedure should be a step-by-step outline or list of steps to be taken to complete a task as desired in that facility. Providing the rationale for a step, when appropriate, enhances the learning process, especially for new staff members. Material Safety Data Sheets (MSDSs) are required to be maintained in the clinic and available for personnel to reference at any time. MSDS must be compiled for all chemicals considered hazardous and maintained in an appropriate manual. Some clinics opt to maintain these records in a separate tabbed section of the procedure manual. Others choose to maintain a separate MSDS manual. The information must be reviewed and updated on a regular basis. See Chapter 38 for detailed information regarding MSDS. Procedure 45-4 provides steps for developing and maintaining a procedure manual.

Updating and Reviewing the Procedure Manual

When new procedures are added to the clinic routine, a new procedure page should be developed immediately. The new page is useful as an educational tool or job aid while team members are learning new techniques.

An annual page-by-page review should be done to ascertain if each procedure is still being used and to ensure that each page is correct in each detail and satisfies all criteria established by the staff personnel. This contributes to an efficient clinic and gives all employees a sense of pride and satisfaction that they are performing within the scope of their training and to their greatest potential.

The procedure manual should be reviewed by personnel performing the various tasks, and their suggestions should be evaluated and incorporated into the revisions when appropriate. All new procedure pages and revisions should be dated (e.g., Rev. 02/15/XX).

HIPAA IMPLICATIONS

HIPAA regulations require each clinic to develop a separate HIPAA manual that is in either an electronic form or a paper manual. The manual spells out all policies and procedures of the practice and security management measures; identifies the security officer; addresses workforce security issues, information access concerns, security awareness and training, security incidents, and contingency plans; evaluates security effectiveness; and contains copies of all business associate contracts.

The HIPAA manual must be available to all employees and updated on a regular basis. During an audit, the clinic manager will be asked to produce the HIPAA manual for review and to establish compliance with all regulations. All documentation of policies and procedures are to be kept for 6 years even though the wording has changed or been eliminated. If an incident is under investigation, this allows an investigator to go back to what a policy said 6 years ago.

TRAVEL ARRANGEMENTS

The clinic manager may be asked to make travel arrangements for providers going on vacation or to conventions, symposiums, or out-of-town seminars and continuing medical education (CME) courses. If the providers do a fair amount of travel or if they live in a metropolitan area, they may use the services of a travel agent. Attention to detail is extremely important in preventing travel disruptions.

Read carefully the instructions for completing registration forms, complete them, and mail them as quickly as possible to secure reservations to conventions and so forth. Next make hotel and travel arrangements. General information regarding the provider's travel preferences should be maintained in a file and referred to when making travel arrangements. Helpful information to maintain in this file includes:

- Name of travel agents used in the past (ranked by reputation an clinic recommendation)
- Provider's or clinic credit card numbers
- Car rental preference
- Preferred airline, class of travel, seating choice
- Hotel/motel accommodations (bed size, suite, studio, connecting rooms, price range, amenities)
- Shuttle service

Next, contact the travel agent and identify the destination, date and time for departure and return, number traveling in party, and seating preference. A travel agent can assist with rental car and hotel accommodations, if needed. Take your time and pay attention to details. When tickets are received, always check to see that all departure and arrival times match what is needed and that a confirmation number has been provided for car rentals and hotel arrangements. Procedure 45-5 outlines the procedural steps involved in making travel arrangements through a travel agent.

The Internet can be used to search for the lowest-cost air, auto, and lodging reservations. The procedures do not require extensive knowledge of travel and airline reservation protocols. Searching for information on the Internet requires the use of a search engine if you do not already have a list of favorite travel Websites. A search engine is a special computer program available through your Internet service provider. With a search engine, you enter only the subject of your search, and the Web provides a list of Websites related to your subject. For example, if you are making travel arrangements, you might access a search engine such as Google.com and enter the key words "air fares." The engine returns either a list of Websites or asks you to further refine your subject, with suggestions

such as cheap air fares, international travel, and so on. Once you refine your search, you may have choices such as Travelocity.com, Expedia.com, or Priceline.com. Select the appropriate Websites and follow its instructions.

Priceline.com and similar Websites are services that allow you to name the price you want to pay; Priceline finds a major airline willing to release seats on flights where they have unsold space. You need to have a reasonable idea of the price of the service you are trying to purchase; unreasonably low bids will just waste your time and effort. Procedure 45-6 outlines the steps for making travel arrangements via the Internet.

Itinerary

If you have used a travel agent in making the travel arrangements, the agency most likely will provide several copies of the **itinerary**. An itinerary is a detailed plan for a proposed trip. The clinic should maintain one copy of the itinerary in case the provider must be reached for emergencies. The provider should have one copy to carry with him or her and a copy to leave with family members. You may need to develop the itinerary if you have made the travel arrangements via computer. Figure 45-8 shows a sample travel itinerary.

Important information to be included on any itinerary includes:

- *Air travel.* Departure and arrival date and time, meals, airline name and telephone number, airport
- *Car rental.* Name of provider, telephone number, confirmation number
- *Hotel/motel.* Name, confirmation number, dates, telephone number
- *Meeting location.* Name, address, room number, telephone number

TIME MANAGEMENT

Time management is an item of critical importance to the manager. You may have upward of 20 staff members putting demands on your time, and added to this are vendors, your superiors, business associates, and a host of others. A manager has not a moment to lose in the day, so managing time makes the difference between a normal 8- or 10-hour day and a

TRAVEL ITINERARY

James Whitney, MD
Inner City Health Care
400 Inner City Way
Seattle, WA 98400

15 Sept 20XX   INVOICE: 880133795

29 Sept Friday

USAIR	630	Coach Class	Equip-Boeing 757 Jet	
LV: Seattle		11:55P	Nonstop Miles-2125	Confirmed
AR: Pittsburgh		7:23A	Elapsed time-4:28	Arrival Date-30Sept
			Seat-31C	

30 Sept-Saturday

Alamo			1 Compact 2/4 DR Drop-101CT	Confirmed
Pickup-Pittsburgh			Pittsburgh Airport Chg-USD .00	
Rate-	59.98	Base rate	Guaranteed	Extra Hr 10.00-UN
Phone-412-472-5060				

Confirmation-1870649

01 Oct Sunday

USAIR	1419	Coach Class	Equip-Boeing 737 Jet	
LV: Pittsburgh		3:05P	Nonstop Miles-2125	Confirmed
AR: Seattle		5:27P	Elapsed time-5:22	
Lunch			Seat-20A	

Ticket Number/s:

Whitney/James	3570933		BA Card	$461.00
Air Transportation	$416.36	Tax 44.64	TOTAL	$461.00
		Sub Total		$461.00
		Credit Card Payment		$461.00-
		Amount Due		0.00

TICKET IS NON REFUNDABLE. TRIP INSURANCE IS AVAILABLE. RECONFIRM ALL FLTS 24 HRS PRIOR TO DEPARTURE

Figure 45-8 Sample travel itinerary.

15-hour or more day. The following suggestions are some proven means of managing your time whether in management or as a salaried employee.

- *Handle items once.* Once the mail is opened, sorted, and prioritized, try to handle it only once more, when action is taken with it. Picking it up, reading it, and setting it down again without taking action is a real waste of time.
- *Develop a to-do list.* At the end of each day prepare a list of things you plan to complete the next day and try to work down this list.

Prioritize the list by importance or by practical order.

- *Guard your time.* Schedule meetings with personnel and vendors so that they do not fragment your time, making you have to restart a task and get up to speed over and over again. Although modern management practice is to have an open-door policy with employees, this does not mean you should allow them to come into your office whenever they think about it. Have them schedule time with you. Make them think about what they want to discuss and do not let them monopolize your time. This is also true of meeting with vendors; require vendors to schedule ahead a time to meet with you.

- *Delegate work.* Assign others or a team to perform some of the functions discussed in this chapter. Having a team prepare weekly work schedules and vacation schedules results in less bickering and feelings of favoritism that you would have to spend time defusing if you made the schedules yourself. This does not mean that you do not have to approve them and, in some instances, make the hard decisions, but it results in your people having ownership in the decisions.

MARKETING FUNCTIONS

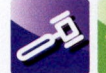 Effective communication skills are essential in the management of the ambulatory care setting. These skills are used by the clinic manager inside the ambulatory care setting to establish friendly, professional relationships with colleagues and patients. Communication is just as critical when relating to external audiences, such as other organizations, potential new patients, and community members. Developing relationships outside the clinic is often called marketing, a concept that clinic managers may use to enhance the image and visibility of an ambulatory care setting while also providing benefits to patients, potential patients, and the neighboring community.

In its broadest sense, **marketing** can be defined as the process by which the provider of services makes the consumer aware of the scope and quality of these services. Although marketing is a tool traditionally used by for-profit organizations to promote and sell products and services, it has become increasingly acceptable among health care organizations, whether they are for- or not-for-profit.

Marketing functions and materials are diverse and can include presence on social media sites, seminars and workshops, patient education brochures, brochures that describe the ambulatory care setting and its scope of services, HIPAA policies, newsletters, press releases, and special events such as open houses or participation in community health care events. Depending on the size and resources of the medical clinic, the manager may choose to use all or some of these tools (Figure 45-9).

 When producing written material and organizing events, it is essential that ethical guidelines be respected at all times. Marketing tools should be appropriate,

in good taste, and designed to quietly enhance the reputation of the clinic. Cultural issues should always be considered. For example, patient education brochures for a practice with many Spanish-speaking patients should be produced in bilingual editions, with English on one side and Spanish on the other. Legal issues are important as well; when presenting material of a medical nature, it is extremely important that information be accurate and up to date.

Effective marketing is a valuable tool for the clinic manager, especially as managed care calls on all health care professionals to become more competitive to survive. Marketing can increase visibility and credibility. The effective manager enlists the talents and skills of the entire team in developing a marketing plan.

Seminars

As consumers become increasingly aware of lifestyle choices, they look to health care professionals for information and guidance. Seminars and workshops are useful vehicles for presenting health-related information; while expert advice can be given, there is also the opportunity for patients and health care professionals to interact.

Seminars can be organized to meet patient and community needs. Some popular seminar topics include hypertension, diabetes, eating disorders, and exercise and weight management programs.

No matter what the topic area, the content should be oriented to the lay person's level of understanding, with a focused message and a delivery designed to maintain attention. Interactive seminars, which encourage audience participation, can be productive and enjoyable. Audiovisuals, such as PowerPoint™ slides, provide visual reinforcement. Handouts, either from professional organizations or those produced by clinic staff, can elaborate on seminar content and help the participant review and remember what was said.

Brochures

Despite the promise of a paperless society, brochures continue to be valuable sources of information. In the health care setting, patients welcome a rack of brochures as a source of current, accurate background on medical issues. New patients also find that a brochure on clinic services answers many questions about the practice, its philosophy, and its scope of services and gives provider profiles.

Marketing Tool	Potential Uses and Value	Marketing Tool	Potential Uses and Value
Seminars	Can educate patients and provide good will in the community. All staff—administrative and clinical—can work as a team to organize, publicize, and deliver the seminars.	Special Events	Special events are an effective way to join with other community organizations to promote wellness. They can include participation in health fairs, cosponsorship of a charity event, or an open house on the premises to acquaint the community with new services or equipment.
Brochures	Brochures are typically of two types: patient education brochures and brochures on clinic services. Can be simple 8-1/2" x 11" fact sheets, with text only, or more elaborate brochures folded to 4" x 9" that incorporate both text and graphics or photos. Both types of brochures are informative for patients and present a professional image of the ambulatory care setting.	Social Media	As lifestyles become more oriented to electronic forms of communication, social media (i.e., social networking, tweeting, and blogging) are being exploited as sources of information by consumers. These social media platforms must be added to the traditional vehicles used by health care institutions to provide health care–related information. Social media can be used to make your organization a looked-to source of medical information as well as a respected source of health care. Blogging can be employed to convey health management information and can be linked to a Facebook page for the medical facility, and tweeting can be used to present medical reminders and timely notices of needs for immunizations or steps to be taken as flu season arrives. Photo and video sharing sites can be used to convey medical information that can better be transmitted visually. All of these social media forms are new tools available for educating customers as well as for providing an online presence for the twenty-first century medical facility.
Practice Website and E-zines	The practice Website is an excellent means of promoting the practice. Personnel can be introduced, and procedures and technologies can be discussed. The E-zine approach is rapidly catching on as a promotional tool. It can be e-mailed to patients so it saves time and money. The patient may choose to view, delete, or save to read at a later time.		
Newsletters	Newsletters can be produced on a biannual or quarterly basis and can form the nucleus of a marketing program. Because they are versatile tools, they can include a wide range of information from health-related articles to staff introductions to insurance updates. They should be sent to individuals on the clinic's mailing list and be available in the reception area.		
Press Releases	Periodic press releases on new equipment, new staff, and expanded or remodeled clinic space can be a vital link to the local community.		

Figure 45-9   Marketing tools and their use in a medical environment.

Today, it is possible to produce a professional-looking brochure in the clinic using a computer program that integrates text and graphics. If a brochure is produced in-house, it is important to consider writing, design, and production. Writing should be clear, to the point, and grammatically correct. Always proofread carefully before printing. Design should be kept simple. Avoid the use of too many typefaces; choose a typeface and size for readability, and, if using artwork or photography, consider its reproduction qualities. Black or another dark ink against a light background is best for readability.

Often, a local printer can advise the clinic manager on how to prepare a brochure or handout for printing. The simplest handouts can be quick-copied (a high-speed photocopy) on a white or lightly colored or textured stock. After printing, brochures should be made accessible to patients and other visitors in a rack or neatly arranged in

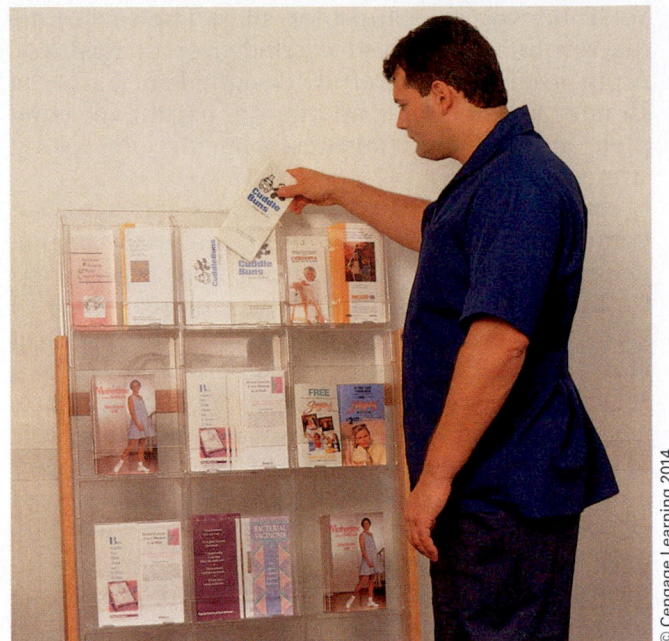

Figure 45-10   Brochures and handouts should be accessible and inviting to patients and clinic visitors.

piles (Figure 45-10). Occasionally, a brochure is mailed; one that folds to 4 × 9 inches fits into a standard #10 business envelope.

Patient Education Brochures. Like seminars, patient education brochures can address a variety of topics, including hypertension, diabetes, eating disorders, and exercise and weight management programs. When writing these brochures, always research material carefully, request permission for copyrighted materials, and present the information in a manner that is accessible to your patient population.

Clinic Brochures. A brochure on the practice can provide a wide range of information and orient the new patient to the practice. One way to determine what information to include is to develop a list of frequently asked patient questions. Once this list is compiled, it can serve as the beginning of the brochure outline. Issues to consider might include:

- Brief history of the practice
- Brief résumés or credentials of providers
- Philosophy of the practice
- Scope of services
- How to reach the practice in case of emergency
- Insurances accepted

- Rights of patients
- Policies regarding the release of information
- Scheduling information: how to schedule an appointment, cancellation policies
- Amenities on the premises, such as parking, pharmacy, laboratory
- Location, map if necessary, and location of satellite clinics

Newsletters

Newsletters are effective communication tools because they encourage regular contact with patients and other readers. Newsletters are a versatile medium; they can contain patient education articles, updates on staff changes, awards, information on insurance carriers, calendars of events, and even recipes that are consistent with a healthful lifestyle.

Most newsletters can be written and produced in the clinic. Like brochures, they should be simple in design and format. An additional factor in newsletter production is mailing; an up-to-date database must be maintained, postal regulations followed, and costs of mailing considered.

Press Releases

Press releases are simple, inexpensive marketing tools. Use them to announce new staff, promote a new service, or publicize a series of seminars. If a professional, courteous relationship is developed with the local press, most will be happy to receive and publish releases. When writing releases, always follow proper format, which includes a date of release, a contact person's name and telephone number, and a short headline. Releases are best kept to one double-spaced typed page. At the end of the release, type "30" or a number sign (#). Maintain an active list of local newspapers and editors' names so that you can mail or fax the release to the appropriate editor.

Special Events

Although they can be time-consuming to organize and participate in, special events are rewarding because they present an opportunity to interact with the community. They have high visibility; often a group of community organizations collaborate to cosponsor an event such as a walk-a-thon, blood pressure clinic, health fair for seniors, or wellness day for children and families. Sponsorship can be as simple as a donation to the cause; other times, staffing a booth or offering a service such as blood pressure checks is appropriate.

Like all marketing efforts, special events require organizational skills and teamwork, but they often result in heightened communication with the community and provide an educational service to patients and their families.

SOCIAL MEDIA IN THE MEDICAL CLINIC

Social media is an instrument of communication enabling communication in both directions. The telephone was an early means of social communication, but its reach to a mass audience was limited. Social media can take on many different forms. Definitions of some of these social media forms are:

- *Webinar.* A seminar or lecture delivered over the Internet. It can be one-way (webcast) or with audience interaction.

- *Social networking.* Interact by adding friends, commenting on profiles, and joining groups and having discussions. Facebook, MySpace, and LinkedIn are examples of this form of social media, as is Twitter on a micro scale.

- *Blogs.* A Website on which an individual or group of users record opinions and information.

- *Social photo and video sharing.* Interact by sharing photos or videos and commenting on user submissions. YouTube in an example of this form.

- *Wikis.* Interact by adding articles and editing existing articles. Wikipedia is an example of this form.

Social media in all its forms is a powerful new tool unleashed on the world only in the twenty-first century. The social media revolution became part of political campaigns in the 2008 U.S. elections, and it may rival armies and nuclear weapons in its ability to change world events. The Arab uprisings of 2010–2011 in Egypt, Yemen, Syria, and Libya were all spurred on by the power of social media. In these events the call to arms went out on Facebook-type sites, coordination was achieved on Twitter sites, and the world was informed using YouTube-type sites and blog sites. The social media revolution has also carried over to business. A purposeful and carefully designed social media strategy must become an integral part of any complete and directed business plan or job-seeking strategy.

Social media gives you a voice and a way to communicate with patients and potential consumers, to find qualified employees, and to verify the background of persons seeking employment with your organization. It personalizes the medical clinic and helps you to spread your message in a relaxed and conversational way. Social media projects your clinic as a personality. You want the clinic to become a respected source of information to the patient. This is the type of business plan observed in the highly successful "Oprah Winfrey" show. She became a respected and interactive source of information that sold both products and herself as a brand in the process.

A business plan is just another name for a marketing plan. The product can be your organization as a place of employment, something you manufacture, or a service such as a medical practice. A marketer can generally not expect prospective customers or clients to be receptive to a blatant marketing message in and of itself. A majority of persons hearing your message prefer their information to come from industry experts and academics or personal associates. A marketing plan must be designed using "authority building" techniques to establish you and your site as the premier authority that your prospective client will trust or that a prospective employee will be interested in. Consumers, and prospective patients in the case of a medical clinic, are very likely to make buying decisions based on what they read and see in social networking platforms only if presented by someone in whom they have developed trust.

The first question you must ask yourself in order to pick out the right social network is "What do you want out of a social network?" Are you looking into social networks to attract new patients, or to make contacts to locate prospective employees? Large general interest social networks such as MySpace or Facebook would be good advertising platforms, while a business-oriented social network such as LinkedIn would be better for making contacts helpful in searching for prospective employees. Beyond the business community, there are plenty of social networks that cater to different interests, and where there is not a specific network devoted to every interest, most social networks contain user-created groups that help people with similar interests connect. Many networks allow you to search for people or organizations having your interests, such as graduating from a specific school, or having the same hometown, or being interested in a given occupation.

When selecting and joining a social network, the first thing you want to do is establish a public profile. You want to take care in designing this, as it is what you show to the world. It is not a diary, so no secrets or trashing the competition. You want to make your company attractive and interesting to your audience. Persons seeking employment list their Professional Headline and Current Position. When they are unemployed they should be truthful and discuss the last position held. Most sites have a blog. You can establish yourself as knowledgeable on a subject or product. By establishing credibility (authority building) on the blog you will draw contacts to your profile and hopefully potential patients.

The power of social networking as a marketing tool is illustrated by a feature of Facebook called the "Like" button. This button, which looks like a pointing finger, links your website to the visitor's Facebook profile if he or she likes your site and clicks on the "Like" button. Your site, through his or her profile, becomes visible to all his or her friends and his or her Facebook page becomes a living testimonial to your product or organization. In other words, the "Like" button instantly adds social functionality to your site. In addition, you have the ability to publish updates to the user. One contact now becomes hundreds.

Many clinic managers are perplexed over whether social networking should be allowed by employees while at work. Many managers have a perception of employees hanging out on cyberspace wasting time. Experts on the subject do not support this perception. They feel that social networking can contribute to team building and can motivate employees, especially in small companies where the staff may be isolated from each other. The result has been increased productivity in most instances. Prohibition of social networking can result in the loss of valued employees. The answer to the question probably lies between total prohibition and uncontrolled use resulting in abuse. If social networking is allowed on the job, protocols should be in place to prevent HIPAA violations, to define where and when social networking is acceptable, and to prohibit bullying of colleagues. A manager must use caution in monitoring employee actions online to avoid overstepping legal boundaries.

RECORDS AND FINANCIAL MANAGEMENT

Providers entrust a great deal of responsibility to their medical clinic managers. The daily payments received through the mail and clinic visits must be processed and prepared for banking. Clinic expenses must be processed and paid in a timely fashion to capitalize on any discounts available. Employee requirements and records such as Social Security records; Withholding Allowance Certificates (W-4 forms) indicating the number of exemptions claimed (Figure 45-11); and Employment Eligibility Verification Forms (Form I-9) ensuring that all persons employed are either United States citizens, lawfully admitted aliens, or aliens authorized to work in the United States must be completed and filed with the appropriate federal agencies. Also, state and local tax records must be maintained for each employee.

Electronic Health Records and the Clinic Manager

The Total Practice Management System (TPMS) discussed in Chapter 11 is the nerve center for the clinic manager as he or she orchestrates a smooth-running organization. It provides all of the data needed by the clinic manager at the click of a mouse or a few keystrokes. Table 45-2 lists sample data types and the resulting actions by the manager.

Payroll Processing

In some cases, it is the client manager's responsibility to prepare payroll checks for each employee and record all deductions withheld. A W-2 form (Figure 45-12) summarizing all earnings and deductions for the year must be prepared for each employee by January 31 of each year. The Social Security Administration must receive a summary report of W-2 forms each year.

To comply with all federal, state, and local governmental regulations, it is important that the clinic manager who processes payroll maintain complete, up-to-date records on every employee. This information should be gathered from new employees and updated every year and with any change in employee status. For more specific information regarding printed and electronic filing

Form W-4 (2012)

Purpose. Complete Form W-4 so that your employer can withhold the correct federal income tax from your pay. Consider completing a new Form W-4 each year and when your personal or financial situation changes.

Exemption from withholding. If you are exempt, complete **only** lines 1, 2, 3, 4, and 7 and sign the form to validate it. Your exemption for 2012 expires February 18, 2013. See Pub. 505, Tax Withholding and Estimated Tax.

Note. If another person can claim you as a dependent on his or her tax return, you cannot claim exemption from withholding if your income exceeds $950 and includes more than $300 of unearned income (for example, interest and dividends).

Basic instructions. If you are not exempt, complete the **Personal Allowances Worksheet** below. The worksheets on page 2 further adjust your withholding allowances based on itemized deductions, certain credits, adjustments to income, or two-earners/multiple jobs situations.

Complete all worksheets that apply. However, you may claim fewer (or zero) allowances. For regular wages, withholding must be based on allowances you claimed and may not be a flat amount or percentage of wages.

Head of household. Generally, you can claim head of household filing status on your tax return only if you are unmarried and pay more than 50% of the costs of keeping up a home for yourself and your dependent(s) or other qualifying individuals. See Pub. 501, Exemptions, Standard Deduction, and Filing Information, for information.

Tax credits. You can take projected tax credits into account in figuring your allowable number of withholding allowances. Credits for child or dependent care expenses and the child tax credit may be claimed using the **Personal Allowances Worksheet** below. See Pub. 505 for information on converting your other credits into withholding allowances.

Nonwage income. If you have a large amount of nonwage income, such as interest or dividends, consider making estimated tax payments using Form 1040-ES, Estimated Tax for Individuals. Otherwise, you may owe additional tax. If you have pension or annuity income, see Pub. 505 to find out if you should adjust your withholding on Form W-4 or W-4P.

Two earners or multiple jobs. If you have a working spouse or more than one job, figure the total number of allowances you are entitled to claim on all jobs using worksheets from only one Form W-4. Your withholding usually will be most accurate when all allowances are claimed on the Form W-4 for the highest paying job and zero allowances are claimed on the others. See Pub. 505 for details.

Nonresident alien. If you are a nonresident alien, see Notice 1392, Supplemental Form W-4 Instructions for Nonresident Aliens, before completing this form.

Check your withholding. After your Form W-4 takes effect, use Pub. 505 to see how the amount you are having withheld compares to your projected total tax for 2012. See Pub. 505, especially if your earnings exceed $130,000 (Single) or $180,000 (Married).

Future developments. The IRS has created a page on IRS.gov for information about Form W-4, at *www.irs.gov/w4.* Information about any future developments affecting Form W-4 (such as legislation enacted after we release it) will be posted on that page.

Personal Allowances Worksheet (Keep for your records.)

A	Enter "1" for **yourself** if no one else can claim you as a dependent	A _____
B	Enter "1" if: { • You are single and have only one job; or • You are married, have only one job, and your spouse does not work; or • Your wages from a second job or your spouse's wages (or the total of both) are $1,500 or less. } . . .	B _____
C	Enter "1" for your **spouse**. But, you may choose to enter "-0-" if you are married and have either a working spouse or more than one job. (Entering "-0-" may help you avoid having too little tax withheld.)	C _____
D	Enter number of **dependents** (other than your spouse or yourself) you will claim on your tax return	D _____
E	Enter "1" if you will file as **head of household** on your tax return (see conditions under **Head of household** above) . .	E _____
F	Enter "1" if you have at least $1,900 of **child or dependent care expenses** for which you plan to claim a credit	F _____
	(**Note.** Do **not** include child support payments. See Pub. 503, Child and Dependent Care Expenses, for details.)	
G	**Child Tax Credit** (including additional child tax credit). See Pub. 972, Child Tax Credit, for more information.	
	• If your total income will be less than $61,000 ($90,000 if married), enter "2" for each eligible child; then **less** "1" if you have three to seven eligible children or **less** "2" if you have eight or more eligible children.	
	• If your total income will be between $61,000 and $84,000 ($90,000 and $119,000 if married), enter "1" for each eligible child . . .	G _____
H	Add lines A through G and enter total here. (**Note.** This may be different from the number of exemptions you claim on your tax return.) ▶ H _____	

For accuracy, complete all worksheets that apply.	{ • If you plan to **itemize** or **claim adjustments to income** and want to reduce your withholding, see the **Deductions and Adjustments Worksheet** on page 2. • If you are **single and have more than one job** or are **married and you and your spouse both work** and the combined earnings from all jobs exceed $40,000 ($10,000 if married), see the **Two-Earners/Multiple Jobs Worksheet** on page 2 to avoid having too little tax withheld. • If **neither** of the above situations applies, **stop here** and enter the number from line H on line 5 of Form W-4 below. }

- **Separate here and give Form W-4 to your employer. Keep the top part for your records.** -

Form **W-4** Department of the Treasury Internal Revenue Service	**Employee's Withholding Allowance Certificate** ▶ Whether you are entitled to claim a certain number of allowances or exemption from withholding is subject to review by the IRS. Your employer may be required to send a copy of this form to the IRS.	OMB No. 1545-0074 20**12**

1 Your first name and middle initial	Last name	2 **Your social security number**

Home address (number and street or rural route)

3 ☐ Single   ☐ Married   ☐ Married, but withhold at higher Single rate.
Note. If married, but legally separated, or spouse is a nonresident alien, check the "Single" box.

City or town, state, and ZIP code

4 If your last name differs from that shown on your social security card, check here. You must call 1-800-772-1213 for a replacement card. ▶ ☐

5	Total number of allowances you are claiming (from line **H** above **or** from the applicable worksheet on page 2)	5	
6	Additional amount, if any, you want withheld from each paycheck	6	$
7	I claim exemption from withholding for 2012, and I certify that I meet **both** of the following conditions for exemption.		
	• Last year I had a right to a refund of **all** federal income tax withheld because I had **no** tax liability, **and**		
	• This year I expect a refund of **all** federal income tax withheld because I expect to have **no** tax liability.		
	If you meet both conditions, write "Exempt" here . . . . ▶	7	

Under penalties of perjury, I declare that I have examined this certificate and, to the best of my knowledge and belief, it is true, correct, and complete.

Employee's signature
(This form is not valid unless you sign it.) ▶   Date ▶

8 Employer's name and address (Employer: Complete lines 8 and 10 only if sending to the IRS.)	9 Office code (optional)	10 Employer identification number (EIN)

For Privacy Act and Paperwork Reduction Act Notice, see page 2.   Cat. No. 10220Q   Form **W-4** (2012)

Figure 45-11 Form W-4 indicates the number of exemptions claimed by the employee for income tax purposes.

Form W-4 (2012) Page **2**

Deductions and Adjustments Worksheet

Note. Use this worksheet *only* if you plan to itemize deductions or claim certain credits or adjustments to income.

1	Enter an estimate of your 2012 itemized deductions. These include qualifying home mortgage interest, charitable contributions, state and local taxes, medical expenses in excess of 7.5% of your income, and miscellaneous deductions	**1**	$
2	Enter: { $11,900 if married filing jointly or qualifying widow(er) $8,700 if head of household $5,950 if single or married filing separately }	**2**	$
3	**Subtract** line 2 from line 1. If zero or less, enter "-0-"	**3**	$
4	Enter an estimate of your 2012 adjustments to income and any additional standard deduction (see Pub. 505)	**4**	$
5	**Add** lines 3 and 4 and enter the total. (Include any amount for credits from the *Converting Credits to Withholding Allowances for 2012 Form W-4* worksheet in Pub. 505.)	**5**	$
6	Enter an estimate of your 2012 nonwage income (such as dividends or interest) . . .	**6**	$
7	**Subtract** line 6 from line 5. If zero or less, enter "-0-"	**7**	$
8	**Divide** the amount on line 7 by $3,800 and enter the result here. Drop any fraction	**8**	
9	Enter the number from the **Personal Allowances Worksheet**, line H, page 1	**9**	
10	**Add** lines 8 and 9 and enter the total here. If you plan to use the **Two-Earners/Multiple Jobs Worksheet**, also enter this total on line 1 below. Otherwise, **stop here** and enter this total on Form W-4, line 5, page 1	**10**	

Two-Earners/Multiple Jobs Worksheet (See *Two earners or multiple jobs* on page 1.)

Note. Use this worksheet *only* if the instructions under line H on page 1 direct you here.

1	Enter the number from line H, page 1 (or from line 10 above if you used the **Deductions and Adjustments Worksheet**)	**1**	
2	Find the number in **Table 1** below that applies to the **LOWEST** paying job and enter it here. **However,** if you are married filing jointly and wages from the highest paying job are $65,000 or less, do not enter more than "3"	**2**	
3	If line 1 is **more than or equal to** line 2, subtract line 2 from line 1. Enter the result here (if zero, enter "-0-") and on Form W-4, line 5, page 1. **Do not** use the rest of this worksheet	**3**	
Note.	If line 1 is **less than** line 2, enter "-0-" on Form W-4, line 5, page 1. Complete lines 4 through 9 below to figure the additional withholding amount necessary to avoid a year-end tax bill.		
4	Enter the number from line 2 of this worksheet **4**		
5	Enter the number from line 1 of this worksheet **5**		
6	**Subtract** line 5 from line 4	**6**	
7	Find the amount in **Table 2** below that applies to the **HIGHEST** paying job and enter it here	**7**	$
8	**Multiply** line 7 by line 6 and enter the result here. This is the additional annual withholding needed . .	**8**	$
9	Divide line 8 by the number of pay periods remaining in 2012. For example, divide by 26 if you are paid every two weeks and you complete this form in December 2011. Enter the result here and on Form W-4, line 6, page 1. This is the additional amount to be withheld from each paycheck	**9**	$

Table 1				Table 2			
Married Filing Jointly		**All Others**		**Married Filing Jointly**		**All Others**	
If wages from **LOWEST** paying job are—	Enter on line 2 above	If wages from **LOWEST** paying job are—	Enter on line 2 above	If wages from **HIGHEST** paying job are—	Enter on line 7 above	If wages from **HIGHEST** paying job are—	Enter on line 7 above
$0 - $5,000	0	$0 - $8,000	0	$0 - $70,000	$570	$0 - $35,000	$570
5,001 - 12,000	1	8,001 - 15,000	1	70,001 - 125,000	950	35,001 - 90,000	950
12,001 - 22,000	2	15,001 - 25,000	2	125,001 - 190,000	1,060	90,001 - 170,000	1,060
22,001 - 25,000	3	25,001 - 30,000	3	190,001 - 340,000	1,250	170,001 - 375,000	1,250
25,001 - 30,000	4	30,001 - 40,000	4	340,001 and over	1,330	375,001 and over	1,330
30,001 - 40,000	5	40,001 - 50,000	5				
40,001 - 48,000	6	50,001 - 65,000	6				
48,001 - 55,000	7	65,001 - 80,000	7				
55,001 - 65,000	8	80,001 - 95,000	8				
65,001 - 72,000	9	95,001 - 120,000	9				
72,001 - 85,000	10	120,001 and over	10				
85,001 - 97,000	11						
97,001 - 110,000	12						
110,001 - 120,000	13						
120,001 - 135,000	14						
135,001 and over	15						

U.S. Internal Revenue Service

Figure 45-11 (continued)

Table 45-2 Clinic Manager Actions in Response to TPMS Data

Data	Action by Clinic Manager
Staffing requirements and appointment schedules	Hire or terminate employees, obtain additional clinic space and equipment, adjust vacation schedules
Equipment and supplies requests, and inventory data	Issue purchase orders, authorize payment of invoices, secure vendors and suppliers, negotiate maintenance contracts
Financial and billing reports	Practice financial status reports, instructions for coding and billing on past due accounts, actions on billing denied due to coding errors
Employee time sheets	Payroll authorization, corrective actions for missed work
Medical records	Review if patient demographics and HIPAA requirements are current
Personnel data	Progress reviews, salary reviews, W-4 forms, corrective actions, licenses, malpractice insurance contracts

© Cengage Learning 2014

Preparing Payroll Checks.

When preparing payroll checks, it is important to keep a record of all tax and insurance amounts deducted from an employee's earnings. Many ambulatory care settings that operate on a manual bookkeeping system find that the write-it-once system is the most efficient way to accurately maintain these records. Payroll records should include:

- Employee name, address, and telephone number
- Social Security number
- Date of employment

Each paycheck stub should contain:

- Number of hours worked, including regular and overtime (if hourly)
- Dates of pay period
- Date of check
- Gross salary
- Itemized deductions for federal income tax, Social Security (FICA) tax, state tax, and city or local tax
- Itemized deductions for health insurance and disability insurance
- Other deductions such as uniforms, loan payments, and so on
- Net salary (gross earnings minus taxes and deductions)

 Procedure 45-7 provides steps for processing payroll.

forms, go to the Internal Revenue Service Websites (http://www.irs.gov) for detailed instructions. It is a good idea to have employees update their W-4 form each year in case they want to adjust their deductions or make any other change. To accomplish this, many payroll managers include a new W-4 form with the first paycheck at the beginning of each year. Every employee file should contain the employee's Social Security number; number of exemptions claimed on the W-4 Form; employee's gross salary; and all deductions withheld for all taxes, including Social Security, federal, state, local, and unemployment tax (where applicable), and disability insurance (where applicable).

To process payroll, the provider's clinic must have a federal tax reporting number, obtained from the Internal Revenue Service. In some states, a state employer number also is needed.

Figuring Employee Taxes.

When figuring federal income taxes and Social Security taxes, use the "Circular E" tables provided by the Internal Revenue Service. Federal tax is based on amount earned, marital status, number of exemptions claimed, and length of pay period. State and city or local taxes are typically a percentage of the gross earnings.

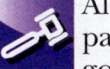 All federal and state taxes withheld must be paid on a quarterly basis to the appropriate government offices. These monies should be accompanied by the required reporting forms. It is important to observe deposit requirements for withheld income tax and Social Security and Medicare taxes. These requirements, which change frequently, are listed in the Federal Employer's Tax Guide, available from the U.S. Government Printing Office, Internal Revenue Service (or online at http://www.irs.gov).

22222	Void ☐	**a** Employee's social security number	For Official Use Only ▶ OMB No. 1545-0008	

b Employer identification number (EIN)	**1** Wages, tips, other compensation	**2** Federal income tax withheld
c Employer's name, address, and ZIP code	**3** Social security wages	**4** Social security tax withheld
	5 Medicare wages and tips	**6** Medicare tax withheld
	7 Social security tips	**8** Allocated tips
d Control number	**9**	**10** Dependent care benefits
e Employee's first name and initial Last name Suff.	**11** Nonqualified plans	**12a** See instructions for box 12
	13 Statutory employee ☐ Retirement plan ☐ Third-party sick pay ☐	**12b**
	14 Other	**12c**
		12d
f Employee's address and ZIP code		

15 State Employer's state ID number	**16** State wages, tips, etc.	**17** State income tax	**18** Local wages, tips, etc.	**19** Local income tax	**20** Locality name

Form **W-2** **Wage and Tax Statement**   **2012**   Department of the Treasury—Internal Revenue Service

Copy A For Social Security Administration — Send this entire page with Form W-3 to the Social Security Administration; photocopies are **not** acceptable.

For Privacy Act and Paperwork Reduction Act Notice, see the separate instructions.

Cat. No. 10134D

Do Not Cut, Fold, or Staple Forms on This Page

U.S. Internal Revenue Service.

Figure 45-12   Form W-2 summarizes all earnings and deductions for the year and must be prepared for each employee by January 31.

Managing Benefits and Other Responsibilities.

Benefits, or additional remuneration to the salary earned by full-time employees, must be managed and records maintained for each employee. Examples of benefits include paid vacation, paid holidays, health/dental insurance, disability, insurance **profit-sharing** options, and complimentary health care. Some ambulatory care settings may refer to all or some of these benefits as **fringe benefits**.

Other responsibilities of the clinic manager include maintaining a personnel file for each employee providing his or her history with the facility, application for the current position, evaluations, promotions, problems, awards, entitlements, legal forms required by state and federal agencies, and so on. All Occupational Safety and Health Administration (OSHA) data, hazard material training and documentation, HIPAA training documentation, cardiopulmonary resuscitation (CPR) certifications, immunization records, AIDS education, and confidentiality agreement must be recorded and maintained.

FACILITY AND EQUIPMENT MANAGEMENT

The physical plant or building must be observed and maintained with safety being a key ingredient. It should be the responsibility of each staff member to report to the clinic manager any facility repairs that require attention and suggest replacement or recommend new pieces of equipment as required by the practice to support the health care needs of its population.

The clinic manager usually is responsible for maintenance of the clinic and may hire **ancillary services** to provide janitorial and laundry services, dispose of hazardous materials, and maintain aquariums or plants that may enhance the environment of the facility. The clinic manager must be cognitive of the importance of patient confidentiality when ancillary services are present. Ancillary services must not view confidential material. A signed Business Associate agreement must be on file for each ancillary service contracted.

Magazine subscriptions and health-related literature for the reception area are the responsibility of the clinic manager. Selections should be made carefully, keeping in mind the interests of the patients and their cultures. These materials should not be kept once they become dog-eared, torn, or outdated. The use of plastic protectors and appropriate storage shelving aid in keeping the area and materials tidy.

The clinic manager, together with the provider, is responsible for facility improvements, including any necessary repairs, decorating and color scheme, and floor plan suggestions. The wise clinic manager does not make these decisions independently but asks for suggestions from staff members. Remember, the team-building approach adds a cohesive element to any clinic environment.

Administrative and Clinical Inventory of Supplies and Equipment

All administrative and clinical supplies and equipment in the facility must be inventoried. Maintaining a sufficient inventory of administrative and medical supplies requires implementation of a system for taking inventory of supplies frequently enough to permit placing and receiving an order before a shortage occurs. Large facilities frequently use the TPMS to inventory items that normally would be billed as part of a procedure, but this will not identify routinely used medical and administrative supplies.

Medical clinics operate on a budget, so comparison shopping is prudent. Many companies have online catalogs with full descriptions and prices of their products. The cost of an item is not the only consideration when purchasing inventory. Consider the following:

- Warranties
- Bulk orders
- Maintenance agreements
- Quality and durability
- Personal preferences
- Cost factors

Online ordering via the Internet can save time and money. When placing orders, select those suppliers with secure Websites; it is generally safe to use credit cards with these vendors. Supplies also can be ordered through hardcopy catalogs. Review Chapter 19 for specifics in completing a purchase order. Benchmarking with other medical clinics nets valuable information in determining reputable vendors.

When an order is received, it must be opened and checked properly. Look first for the packing slip, which lists the items ordered and the items shipped. Verify that no items have been substituted or back-ordered. Each item unpacked must be checked against the packing slip to be sure there are no discrepancies. Write the date the shipment was received, who verified it, and any follow-up information. The new stock should be stored appropriately.

Some items purchased come with a warranty. A warranty usually is activated online at the vendor's Websites or by using a warranty card packaged with the purchased item. Warranty cards are similar to postcards and establish the purchase date and name and address of the purchaser. The returned warranty information provides the vendor with information should it be necessary to notify the buyer of recalls or defective parts. It is also proof of purchase and gives the length of time the warranty is in effect.

It is important to create a file for each piece of equipment in the medical clinic. Information in this file should include:

- Date of purchase and original receipt
- Manufacturer name, address, and telephone number
- Model number and owner's manual
- Technical support information and telephone number
- Warranty information
- Service agreement
- Date last serviced
- Routine maintenance or calibration information

 The steps for inventorying supplies and equipment for administrative and clinical needs are given in Procedure 45-8.

Administrative and Clinical Equipment Calibration and Maintenance

Administrative and clinical equipment must be cleaned, calibrated, and maintained on a regular basis. Most clinics use a computer spreadsheet or relational-type database, depending on the size of the facility. The database identifies the equipment by name or type, its assigned facility identification number, location in the facility, warranty expiration date, service period, dates when service and calibration were last performed, and when the next service or calibration will be required. The database also may identify service contracts for equipment not maintained or calibrated by facility personnel and information on equipment service contractors such as contacts, phone numbers, and addresses. The database is backed up by a paper file containing operation manuals, warranty information, and service contracts.

Administrative equipment such as the computer should be cleaned and maintained regularly. Review Chapter 11 for suggestions on routine maintenance. Telephones as well as any other pieces of equipment should be cleaned and working order checked.

Laboratory and clinical equipment must be maintained and quality-control measures utilized. Calibration checks are required for a number of pieces of equipment: sphygmomanometers and centrifuges, to name two. Microscopes and various types of scopes used during physical examinations and specialty procedures contain light sources that must be checked before each use. A replacement supply of bulbs should be available. See Chapter 38 for more information on quality control and safety in the medical laboratory. Assigning a clinical laboratory manager to oversee the equipment is a good idea. Procedure 45-9 provides steps for routine maintenance and calibration of clinical equipment.

The clinic storage areas should be well maintained, and each item should always be put back in its place with lids replaced properly to prevent any accidents. Medication storage requires special attention. Many medications must be stored at certain temperatures, kept dry, or stored in dark, airtight containers. All medications, including samples, must be kept out of patient access areas. Narcotics should always be stored in a separate locked cabinet. Dispensing requires two individuals to sign off when narcotic supplies are used. A daily inventory should be maintained.

LIABILITY COVERAGE AND BONDING

Negligence is performing an act that a reasonable and prudent provider would not perform or failure to perform an act that a reasonable and prudent provider would perform. The common term used to describe professional **liability** or legal responsibility today is **malpractice**. It is much easier to prevent malpractice than to defend it in litigation; therefore every effort should be taken to prevent negligence. Events that could result in a malpractice litigation invariably will occur from time to time in even the best of medical clinics. When such an incident occurs, complete honesty with the patient and insurance carrier is the best policy. Protocols should be implemented or existing ones revised to prevent any future occurrences, and all steps necessary to minimize risk to the patient should be taken.

Insurance policies specifically designed to protect the provider's assets in the event a liability claim is filed and awarded in the patient's favor are available. Any provider not carrying such insurance is said to be "**going bare**" and would personally be responsible for any court costs, damages, and attorney fees if a malpractice suit were lost.

Practicing medical assistants should carry **professional liability insurance** for protection. Medical assistants who are members of the American Association of Medical Assistants (AAMA) have the option of purchasing personal and professional insurance through the organization at corporate rates.

Some providers carry the names of their employees on their policies. If this is the case, always ask to see the policy and verify that your name is printed on the policy—no name indicates no coverage. The manager may need to see that professional liability insurance has been purchased, all appropriate names are listed, and the premiums are paid in a timely fashion.

Professional liability insurance is important if the provider–employer is sued. In this event, the provider and the medical assistant could be named in the suit. If the case were lost, both the provider and the medical assistant could be liable.

Individuals who are responsible for handling financial records and money in the medical clinic may be bonded. A **bond** is purchased for a cash value in an employee's name that ensures that the provider will recover the amount of loss in the event that an employee **embezzles** funds. It is the clinic manager or the HR manager's responsibility to ask prospective employees if they are bondable. Individuals who are not bondable may not be the best candidates for the position.

LEGAL ISSUES

The clinic manager must be aware of and follow all state and federal regulations impacting the practice. Information related to the Clinical Laboratory Improvement Amendments of 1988 (CLIA '88) and the Occupational Safety and Health Administration (OSHA) can be found in Chapter 38. Federal regulations related to provider clinic laboratories (POLs) are discussed in Chapter 38. The Centers for Medicare and Medicaid Services Website also is helpful (http://www.cms.gov).

PROCEDURE 45-1
Completing a Medical Incident Report

PURPOSE:
To complete an accurate medical incident report providing all legally required information and to submit it in a timely manner.

EQUIPMENT/SUPPLIES:
Appropriate medical incident report form
Computer with Incident Report Software
Notes taken regarding incident

PROCEDURE STEPS:

1. *Report situations that were harmful* by discussing the incident with the employee(s) involved and read notes of pertinent information. Ask those who witnessed the incident to log when, where, and what they saw in their own words. RATIONALE: Provides an understanding of what happened and ensures all the information needed is documented.

2. *Paying attention to detail*, when complete the clinic-approved Medical Incident Report form. A single-sheet, multiple-copy form is best. The form should contain basic patient identification data, a checklist of different incidents, and a space for written comments. RATIONALE: Ensures that all information needed is documented.

3. The person completing the incident report form should be the individual who witnessed the incident, first discovered the incident, or is most familiar with the incident. RATIONALE: This ensures the most accurate recording of the incident.

4. Each section of the form must be completed. The incident description should be a brief narrative consisting of an objective description of the facts but should not draw any conclusions. Quotes should be used when appropriate with any unwitnessed incidents (e.g., "Patient states . . ."). The name(s) of any witnesses should be included on the report as well as employees directly involved in the incident. RATIONALE: To provide unbiased information without making judgments.

5. *Implement time management principles.* Incident reports must be submitted in a timely manner to the appropriate administrator or office following protocol identified in the Procedure Manual for the clinic. *Did you display sound judgment?* RATIONALE: Ensures that appropriate documentation and action is taken for follow-up.

PROCEDURE 45-2
Preparing a Meeting Agenda

PURPOSE:
To prepare a meeting agenda, a list of specific items to be discussed or acted on, to maintain the focus of the group and allow business to be transacted in a timely fashion.

EQUIPMENT/SUPPLIES:
List of participants
Order of business
Names of individuals giving reports
Names of any guest speakers
Computer and paper to print agendas

PROCEDURE STEPS:

1. *Pay attention to detail.* Reserve proposed date, time, and place of meeting. RATIONALE: Ensures that the facilities are available for the meeting.

2. *Pay attention to detail.* Collect information for meeting agenda by previewing the previous meeting's minutes for old business items, checking with others for report items, and determining any new business items. RATIONALE: Ensures that all old and new business items have been identified.

3. Prepare a hard copy of the agenda and have it approved by the chair of the meeting. RATIONALE: Confirmation by the chair of the agenda content ensures that agenda is correct and complete.

4. *Implement time management principles.* Send agenda to meeting participants a few days in advance of the meeting. RATIONALE: Permits participants to prepare for the meeting by completing any tasks required and preparing any necessary documentation.

PROCEDURE 45-3

Supervising a Student Practicum

PURPOSE:

To prepare a training path for a student being assigned to the clinic. To make the involved clinic personnel aware of their responsibilities. To preplan which tasks the student performs and in what sequence they will be assigned. To make the practicum successful by providing as much supervision and assistance as necessary.

EQUIPMENT/SUPPLIES:

None needed

PROCEDURE STEPS:

1. *Pay attention to detail.* Review the clinical practicum contract or agreement between your agency and the educational institution. RATIONALE: Guidelines and procedures are reviewed and refreshed in your mind.

2. Determine the amount of supervision the student will require. RATIONALE: Prepares you to speak with the student and site supervisor regarding supervision.

3. Identify the supervisor who will be immediately responsible for the student. RATIONALE: Establishes a person who knows he or she is to supervise the student and be responsible for the practicum procedures.

4. *Working within your scope of practice,* plan what tasks the student will be allowed or encouraged to perform. RATIONALE: The clinic may or may not permit the student to perform invasive procedures. Determining tasks the student can and cannot perform beforehand promotes a better relationship.

5. Create a schedule outlining the time the student will be assigned to each unit. RATIONALE:

Establishing a schedule keeps everyone appraised of what is happening and when.

6. *Develop a strategic, realistic plan to achieve your goals* by orientating the student as soon as he or she arrives at the clinic. Include a tour of the clinic and introduction to the staff. RATIONALE: Orients student and staff to each other and establishes guidelines for procedures.

7. Give the student work a copy of the clinic Policy Manual and the "work" schedule for the entire practicum. Answer any questions the student might have. RATIONALE: Orients student and staff to each other and establishes guidelines for procedures.

8. *Pay attention to detail* by maintaining an accurate record of the hours the student works. Also log the date and reason for any missed days, late arrivals, or early dismissals. RATIONALE: Provides necessary documentation for the hours completed by the student.

9. Check with the student frequently to be sure the student is receiving meaningful training from the work experience. RATIONALE: Verifies that necessary training is being provided.

10. Consult providers and staff members with whom the student has worked for their opinion of the student's capabilities. Follow up on any problems that might be identified. RATIONALE: Verifies that necessary training is being provided.

11. Report the student's progress to the medical assisting supervisor from the educational institution. This person usually visits once or twice each rotation. RATIONALE: Verifies that necessary training is being provided.

12. Prepare the student evaluation report from comments provided by the supervisor assigned and each employee who worked with the student. RATIONALE: Provides necessary documentation for the practicum experience.

PROCEDURE 45-4

Developing and Maintaining a Procedure Manual

PURPOSE:
To develop and maintain a comprehensive, up-to-date procedure manual covering each clinical, technical, and administrative procedure in the clinic, with step-by-step directions and rationales for performing each task.

EQUIPMENT/SUPPLIES:
Computer (electronic storage allows changes and revisions to be made easily)
Binder, such as a three-ring binder
Paper
Standard procedure manual format

PROCEDURE STEPS:

1. *Pay attention to detail* by writing step-by-step procedures and rationales for each clinical, technical, and administrative function. Each procedure is written by experienced employees close to the function and then reviewed by a supervisor and clinic manager. Rationales help employees understand *why* something is done. RATIONALE: Establishes consistent guidelines to be followed.

2. Include regular maintenance instructions and flow sheets for cleaning, servicing, and calibrating of all clinic equipment, both in the clinical and in the administrative areas. RATIONALE: Equipment needs to be cleaned and maintained on a regular basis to ensure it is working properly and that it lasts as long as needed. Some manufacturer guarantees and service contracts require regular cleaning and maintenance, especially on new and leased equipment. Instructions are necessary so that the task can be performed properly. The flow sheets provide documentation of dates the equipment was cleaned, serviced, and/or calibrated and the person who performed the task.

3. Include step-by-step instructions on how to accomplish each task in the clinic in both the clinical and administrative areas. RATIONALE: Clear and concise instructions ensure that each task is consistently performed to the clinic standards.

4. Include local and out-of-the-area resources for clinical and administrative staff, providers, and patients. Provide a listing in each area with contact information and services provided. RATIONALE: The procedures and instructions listed in the Procedure Manual should provide supporting documentation needed for accomplishing each task. For example, if the clinic requires that local public transportation resources be given to each patient who needs transportation, the Procedure Manual has a listing of all transportation available in the area with telephone numbers and schedules. This document could either be printed from the computer or photocopied from the manual and provided to the patient.

5. *Recognize the importance of local, state, and federal legislation and regulations* that are related to processes performed in both clinical and administrative areas. RATIONALE: Having a listing of the rules and regulations assists in performing those regulated duties correctly and legally.

6. Include the clinic procedures and flow sheets for taking inventory in each of the areas and instructions on ordering procedures. RATIONALE: When a clinic has processes clearly written for managing inventory and ordering of equipment and supplies, the clinic is less likely to run out of needed items and may even be able to take advantage of discounts offered by manufacturers.

7. Collect the procedures into the Clinic Procedure Manual. RATIONALE: Provides a reference guide with step-by-step instructions and examples where appropriate.

8. Store one complete manual in a common library area. Provide a completed copy to the provider-employer and the clinic manager. Distribute appropriate sections to the various departments. RATIONALE: Provides a reference guide with step-by-step instructions and examples where appropriate.

9. Review the procedure manual annually and add any new procedures, delete or modify as necessary, and indicate the revision date (e.g., Rev. 10/12/XX). RATIONALE: Maintains current clinic protocols.

PROCEDURE 45-5

Making Travel Arrangements with a Travel Agent

PURPOSE:
To make travel arrangements for the provider.

EQUIPMENT/SUPPLIES:
Travel plan
Telephone and telephone directory
Computer
Provider's or clinic credit card to pay for reservations

PROCEDURE STEPS:

1. ***Pay attention to detail*** by confirming the trip dates, time, and place for departure and arrival; preferred mode of transportation (plane, train, bus, car); number of travelers; preferred lodging type and price range; and whether travelers' checks are required. RATIONALE: Confirming pertinent travel details ensures that correct arrangements will be made.

2. Make travel and lodging reservations by calling travel agent or using the computer for online ticket services. RATIONALE: Ensures that space for provider is reserved at desired times.

3. Pick up tickets or arrange for their delivery.

4. Check to see that ticket arrangements are accurate (dates, times, places).

5. Check to see that car rental and lodging accommodations are accurate and confirmed. RATIONALE: Avoids inaccuracies and confusion with schedule.

6. Make additional copies of the itinerary or create the itinerary if making arrangements via computer. The itinerary should list date and time of departures and arrivals, including flight numbers and seat assignments. Note mode of transportation to lodging (shuttle, bus, car, taxi). Include name, address, and telephone number of lodgings and meeting places.

7. Maintain one copy of the itinerary in the clinic file.

8. Give several copies of the itinerary to the provider. RATIONALE: Ensures that a copy is on file with the clinic and that there are sufficient copies for the traveler(s) and their families.

PROCEDURE 45-6

Making Travel Arrangements via the Internet

PURPOSE:
To make travel arrangements for the provider using the Internet.

EQUIPMENT/SUPPLIES:
Travel plan
Computer
Provider's or clinic credit card to pay for reservations.

PROCEDURE STEPS:

1. ***Pay attention to detail*** by confirming the planned trip: dates, time, and place for departure and arrival; preferred mode of transportation (plane, train, bus, car); number of travelers; preferred lodging type and price range; and whether travelers' checks are required. RATIONALE: Confirming pertinent travel details ensures that correct arrangements will be made.

2. Go to the computer and access the Internet.

3. ***Show initiative*** by selecting a search engine to locate Web pages using the key term "air fares." Web pages may provide links to air fares, auto reservations, and hotel/motel reservations. Follow Web page instructions for making arrangements. Review and copy confirmation of your transaction. RATIONALE: The Internet can be a time saver and a cost effective way of securing travel arrangements.

continues

Procedure 45-6 (continued)

4. Pick up tickets or arrange for their delivery, if necessary. Tickets purchased on the Internet can be mailed or picked up at an airport, or they can be electronic tickets.

5. Make additional copies of the itinerary or create the itinerary. The itinerary should list date and time of departures and arrivals, including flight numbers and seat assignments. Note the mode of transportation to lodging (shuttle, bus, car, taxi). Include name, address, and telephone number of lodgings and meeting places.

6. Maintain one copy of the itinerary in the clinic file.

7. Give several copies of the itinerary to the provider. RATIONALE: Ensures that a copy is on file with the clinic and that there are sufficient copies for the traveler(s) and their families.

PROCEDURE 45-7
Processing Employee Payroll

PURPOSE:
To process payroll compensating employees, calculating all deductions accurately.

EQUIPMENT/SUPPLIES:
Computer and payroll software or checkbook
Tax withholding tables
Federal Employers Tax Guide

PROCEDURE STEPS:

1. Verify that copies of the employee's Social Security card and current I-9 and W-4 forms are in each employee file. RATIONALE: Provides verification that employee is eligible to work in the United States and to calculate withholding amounts that should be deducted from paychecks.

2. Review time cards looking for any tardiness, early dismissals, or absences. RATIONALE: To access any problems that could lead to termination. Be sure to document any that may be found and action taken.

3. Calculate the salary or hourly wages due to the employee for the work period. RATIONALE: To determine the amount owed each employee.

4. *Pay attention to detail* by calculating any deductions that must be withheld from the paycheck. These may include federal, state, and local taxes; Social Security withholdings; Medicare withholdings; insurance; savings; or donations. RATIONALE: To ensure compliance with all federal, state, and local laws and satisfy that all proper deductions are made.

5. Use computer and payroll software or hand write the payroll check and explanation of deductions.

6. Distribute individual payroll checks in envelopes according to clinic protocol. RATIONALE: Ensures compliance and confidentiality issues are maintained.

PROCEDURE 45-8

Perform an Inventory of Equipment and Supplies

PURPOSE:
To develop an inventory of expendable administrative and clinical supplies in a medical clinic.

EQUIPMENT/SUPPLIES:
Computer
Printout of most recent inventory spreadsheet, listing items by storage location, name and identification code, number of items, minimum quantity requiring reorder, date and quantity of last reorder, and expiration dates of items, if any.
Clipboard, pad of reorder forms, pen or pencil.

PROCEDURE STEPS:

1. *Pay attention to detail.* Compare number of items on hand corresponding to each name or code identification number with the printout, and write in the new inventory number on the printout. RATIONALE: To determine what is on hand and what needs to be ordered.

2. If the number of any item is less than the minimum quantity, fill out a reorder form listing completely the name, identification number, and quantity required.

3. Repeat the previous step for each storage location on the inventory printout sheet.

4. After completing the inventory, enter the new inventory information, including date of inventory, quantity, and date of reorder request, into the computer database. RATIONALE: To determine what needs to be ordered.

5. Forward the reorder forms to the person responsible for purchasing. RATIONALE: To forward information to the person responsible for reordering supplies and equipment.

NOTE: If the clinic uses handheld computers on a wireless network, all of the printouts and reorder forms can be entered directly into the computer record while doing the inventory, making unnecessary the reentry and preparation of reorder forms. If the handheld computer is not networked, it will be necessary to download or sync the data after completing the inventory.

PROCEDURE 45-9

Perform Routine Maintenance and Calibration of Clinical Equipment

PURPOSE:
To ensure the operability and calibration of clinical equipment.

EQUIPMENT/SUPPLIES:
Equipment list with maintenance or calibration requirements
Clipboard, pen with black ink, maintenance log and service calendar log forms, and deficiency tags
Access to operation and service manuals of equipment to be serviced
Access to any necessary maintenance tools and supplies

PROCEDURE STEPS:

1. Locate the number assigned by the clinic manager to identify the equipment being serviced, and verify serial number, manufacturer/maker, technical support phone number, warranty information, and last date of service. RATIONALE: Provides medical assistant with all information needed for maintenance and servicing of equipment.

continues

Procedure 45-9 (continued)

2. *Pay attention to detail* by visually inspecting each piece of equipment associated with the clinical area.
   - *Practice risk management principles* by checking for any frayed electrical cords, loose connections, or safety issues such as tripping hazards associated with electrical cords.
   - Clean each item according to manufacturer specifications, and replace light bulbs and batteries if necessary.

   RATIONALE: Equipment works more efficiently when clean and all parts are working properly.
3. Check to ensure the equipment meets operational/calibration standards as defined in the operation and service manual. Recalibrate the equipment following the instructions in the manual if required. RATIONALE: Calibration standards must be maintained for correct results.

4. *Follow necessary safety precautions* and tag any equipment not meeting operational standards and report the deficiency. RATIONALE: Equipment must be either replaced or repaired to ensure proper results.
5. Fill out and sign the maintenance record sheet if the equipment meets operations standards. RATIONALE: Documents routine maintenance was performed.
6. *Pay attention to detail.* Complete documentation form by verifying information for each piece of equipment serviced and/or calibrated. Complete the appropriate information for service using the Service Calendar Log form. RATIONALE: Documents what has been done and the date completed.

NOTE: The equipment list, maintenance records, and deficiency reports may be included in the TPMS of many practices.

DOCUMENTATION EXAMPLE:
Maintenance Log

Name of Equipment	Serial Number	Mfg/ Maker	Technical Support Phone Number	Purchase Date	Service Plan	Last Serviced	Completed By
EKG #8	80462	HP	xxx-xxx-xxxx	1/20/xx	On file	6/12/xx	bql
Centrifuge #3	79031	HP	xxx-xxx-xxxx	7/20/xx	On file	6/12/xx	bql

Service Calendar Log Form

January	February	March	April	May	June	July	August	September	October	November	December

CASE STUDY 45-1

Refer to the scenario at the beginning of the chapter.

Drs. Lewis and King have requested sigmoidoscopy procedures to be scheduled for two different patients. The patients are scheduled. Both patients are put on a strict diet and pretest protocol for several days to prepare for the procedures. The day of the appointments, Marilyn Johnson, CMA (AAMA) and clinic manager, discovers that the two sigmoidoscopy procedures have been scheduled at the same time. The problem is that the clinic has only one sigmoidoscope available.

CASE STUDY REVIEW

1. Divide the class into two groups to discuss problem-solving solutions. Assume that rescheduling a patient is not an acceptable solution because of the patient's pretest protocol. The patients would be upset if the procedure could not be performed due to a scheduling problem.
2. How could this problem have been avoided?
3. Both patients have been told about the scheduling problem and one is upset and argumentative. What role should the clinic manager assume in this predicament?

CASE STUDY 45-2

Anita Juarez, the clinic administrative medical assistant, speaks privately with Jane O'Hara, the clinic manager and the person responsible for personnel. Anita has a suspicious lump in her breast. She has seen both her internist and a surgeon for evaluation. Next week, she will have the lump removed, perhaps even a complete mastectomy. Anita is concerned about the time she will need to be away from the clinic.

CASE STUDY REVIEW

1. Identify the first and immediate concerns to be addressed.
2. What action might be taken to help both Anita and the clinic manager address these concerns?
3. Is it helpful to plan for the best results, the worst results, or both?

SUMMARY

The clinic manager is the glue that holds the clinic together and keeps it running smoothly. When the manager sets a positive example for others and is considerate and aware of the diversity of others, a positive environment is created for teamwork. A teamwork approach enables the entire clinic to be more productive, provide the best health care, and foster an enjoyable work relationship.

The role of clinic manager varies greatly depending on the size of the medical practice, the provider's trust in the manager's competency level, and the provider's comfort in delegating authority to others. An effective clinic manager is a tremendous asset to providers. The personal and financial rewards are worthwhile to the medical assistant who desires a new dimension to explore and enjoys a challenge.

STUDY FOR SUCCESS

To reinforce your knowledge and skills of information presented in this chapter:

- Review the *Key Terms*
- Role-play with other students to apply attributes of professionalism pertinent to this chapter.
- Consider the *Case Studies* and discuss your conclusions
- Answer the questions in the *Certification Review*
- Apply your knowledge by completing the *Activities* in the *Study Guide* and the *Games and Quizzes* in the StudyWARE **StudyWARE** software on the *Premium Website*

continues

STUDY FOR SUCCESS (CONTINUED)

- Perform the *Procedures* using the *Competency Assessment Checklists* in the *Competency Manual*
- Practice your problem-solving skills with the *Critical Thinking Challenge 3.0* on the *Premium Website*

Additional resources for this chapter include:

- Module 12 of the *Medical Assisting Learning Lab*
- *CourseMate for Delmar's Comprehensive Medical Assisting*
- *WebTutor for Delmar's Comprehensive Medical Assisting*

CERTIFICATION REVIEW

1. For teamwork to be successful, individual team members must:
   a. do as they are told by the clinic manager
   b. not ask why they are doing something a certain way
   c. understand and support the task
   d. think independently and solve the problem on their own

2. Meeting minutes:
   a. should address each agenda topic and include a brief summary of discussions, actions taken, name of each person making a motion, the exact wording of motions, and motion approval or defeat
   b. are a detailed plan for a proposed trip
   c. include information regarding mode of transportation and lodging reservations
   d. must follow parliamentary procedures

3. When working with practicum students, it is important to remember that:
   a. they should have expert knowledge about their field
   b. they do not need supervision when working with a patient
   c. they are experienced with working on real patients
   d. they have much to learn

4. Which of the following statements is *not* correct regarding a student practicum?
   a. It is a transitional stage that provides opportunity for students to apply theory learned in the classroom to a health care setting through hands-on experience.
   b. It assumes that the student is an employee who does not need to be introduced to patients.
   c. It may require the student to shadow another medical assistant for a few days.
   d. It involves an evaluation of the student's progress.

5. The procedure manual:
   a. is a detailed plan for a proposed trip
   b. provides detailed information regarding mode of transportation and lodging reservations
   c. provides detailed information relative to the performance of tasks within the health care facility
   d. summarizes action details of staff meetings

6. Developing relationships outside the clinic is often called:
   a. marketing
   b. benchmarking
   c. advertising
   d. sales

7. Record and financial management involves all of the following *except:*
   a. payroll processing
   b. preparing payroll checks
   c. figuring taxes
   d. equipment and supplies maintenance

8. Controlled substances must:
   a. be kept separate from other drugs
   b. be stored in a separate locked cabinet
   c. be recorded in a book that is maintained daily
   d. all of the above

9. Social media may be used by the medical clinic for all of the following *except:*
   a. to make your organization a looked-to source of medical information
   b. to promote personal tweeting
   c. to convey health management information
   d. to link to the organization's Facebook page

10. The procedure manual:
    a. serves as a guide to the employee assigned a specific task
    b. may be used in evaluating the employee's performance
    c. is invaluable in assuring that each procedure is completed as outlined
    d. should be generic so that any clinic could follow the procedures
11. The authoritarian style of management:
    a. operates on the premise that most workers cannot make a contribution without being directed
    b. is based on the premise that the worker is capable and wants to do a good job
    c. often uses teams to do work tasks
    d. is also known as MBWA

12. Benefits of social media in the medical clinic:
    a. provides another way to communicate with patients and potential consumers
    b. provides a way to find employees and to verify the background of persons seeking employment
    c. projects your clinic's personality
    d. all of the above

REFERENCES/BIBLIOGRAPHY

Colbert, B. J. (2000). *Workplace readiness for health occupations.* Clifton Park, NY: Delmar Cengage Learning.

ingenix. (2003). *HIPAA tool kit.* Salt Lake City, UT: St. Anthony Publishing/Medicode.

Krager, D., & Krager, C. (2005). *HIPAA for medical office personnel.* Clifton Park, NY: Delmar Cengage Learning.

"Like" Button (n.d.). Retrieved from http://developers.facebook.com/docs/opengraph/

Nations, D. (n.d.). What Is Social Media? What Are Social Media Sites? About.com Web Trends, retrieved from http://webtrends.about.com/od/web20/a/social-media.htm

Sobell, S. (2011, June). Social Networking @ Work, *The Costro Connection.*

CHAPTER 46

The Medical Assistant as Human Resources Manager

OUTLINE

Tasks Performed by the Human Resources Manager

The Clinic Policy Manual

Recruiting and Hiring Clinic Personnel
- Job Descriptions
- Recruiting
- Preparing to Interview Applicants

The Employment Interview

Selecting the Finalists

Orienting New Personnel

Dismissing Employees
- Exit Interview

Maintaining Personnel Records

Complying with Personnel Laws

Special Policy Considerations
- Temporary Employees
- Smoking Policy
- Discrimination

Providing/Planning Employee Instruction and Education

LEARNING OUTCOMES

1. Define, spell, and pronounce the key terms as presented in the glossary.
2. Interpret the role of the human resources manager.
3. Explain the function of the clinic policy manual.
4. Analyze methods of recruiting employees for a medical practice.
5. Conduct an employment interview.
6. Categorize items to keep in an employee's personnel record.
7. List and define a minimum of four laws related to personnel management.
8. Compare and contrast voluntary and involuntary separations.
9. Recall continuing education possibilities for employees.
10. Analyze the professionalism questions and apply them to this chapter's content.

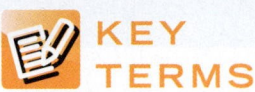 KEY TERMS

exit interview
involuntary dismissal
job description
letter of reference
letter of resignation
overtime
probation

ATTRIBUTES OF PROFESSIONALISM

 Communication
- Does your knowledge allow you to speak easily with all members of the health care team?

 Presentation
- Were you dressed appropriately?
- Did you display a positive attitude?

 Competency
- Did you pay attention to detail?
- Did you display sound judgment?
- Did you remain calm in a crisis?
- Were you knowledgeable and accountable?
- Did you recognize the importance of local, state, and federal legislation and regulations in the practice setting?

 Initiative
- Were you proactive?
- Did you show initiative?
- Did you develop a strategic plan to achieve your goals? Was your plan realistic?
- Did you seek opportunities to expand your knowledge base?
- Were your respectful of others?

 Integrity
- Did you work within your scope of practice?
- Did you demonstrate respect for individual diversity?
- Did you protect and maintain confidentiality?
- Did you maintain your moral and ethical standards?

INTRODUCTION

As you near the end of your studies and preparations to enter the field of health care, it is helpful for you to know how human resource managers are likely to function in the hiring process.

The medical assistant's employment responsibilities are many and varied. As you learned in Chapter 45, often they become clinic managers and assume a quite different function in the medical setting once they have been employed in the field and gained sufficient experience. The size of the ambulatory care setting and the number of employees likely determines if a human resources (HR) manager is a part of the practice. Whether the HR manager heads an HR department in a large, corporate medical setting with the title Human Resources Manager, or is a medical assistant/clinic manager who has HR responsibilities, there are some common tasks assigned as specific HR duties.

TASKS PERFORMED BY THE HUMAN RESOURCES MANAGER

A search for employment is likely to involve interactions with individuals with the title of human resources manager. It can be helpful to understand that position and their responsibilities when applying for a position. Tasks usually assigned to the HR manager include determining job descriptions for, hiring, and orienting employees; maintaining employee personnel records that include credentials and continuing education units (CEUs); and managing employee separations. With today's quest for greater clinic efficiency and the tremendous increase in federal and state regulatory requirements, the skills required of an HR manager have greatly broadened. Former responsibilities have been expanded to include preparing the policy manual, scheduling employee evaluations, preventing and investigating discrimination and harassment claims, and complying with regulatory agencies. The HR manager also assists in providing training and educational opportunities for employees so they are current in all aspects of quality patient care.

Increasingly, HR managers are expected to be able to support the organization's efforts that focus on productivity, service, and quality. In a climate in which there are too few persons for the positions to be filled and the delivery methods for health care are changing almost daily, productivity, service, and quality are essential to a successful practice. It becomes the responsibility of the HR manager to see that every employee's productivity level is high, that the service is A+, and that quality is at the highest level. Today's customers, the patients, often choose their health care provider, even within their health insurance limitations, on the basis of service and quality.

  The position of HR manager now requires a higher level of education and experience to better grasp the legal and regulatory aspects of personnel management. The HR manager also must have excellent people skills, a strong sense of fairness, and the ability to resolve conflicts. None of this is accomplished in a vacuum. It requires working in close cooperation with the clinic manager and the employer(s).

This chapter discusses these responsibilities in the following separate but overlapping functions:

1. Creating and updating the clinic policy manual
2. Recruiting and hiring clinic personnel
3. Orienting new personnel
4. Scheduling salary reviews
5. Conducting exit interviews
6. Maintaining personnel records
7. Complying with all state and federal regulations regarding personnel
8. Planning/providing employee training and education
9. Maintaining records of credentials, licensure, certifications, and CEUs, such as cardiopulmonary resuscitation (CPR)

THE CLINIC POLICY MANUAL

The procedure manual described in Chapter 45 identifies specific methods and steps in performing tasks. The policy manual provides more general guidelines for clinic practices and will be introduced to new employees very quickly following the hiring process (Table 46-1).

The policy manual identifies clear guidelines and directions required of all employees. It also defines appropriate expectations and boundaries of the employment relationship. Having written policies means not having to determine a policy on a case-by-case basis. Policy manuals will vary by the size of the practice or problems to be addressed, but some topics include the mission statement of the practice, biographic data on each provider, employment policies, wage and salary policies, benefits to be awarded, and employee conduct expectations.

Table 46-1   Possible Content of Policy and Procedure Manuals

Policy Manual	Procedure Manual
Mission statement	Details of procedures performed
Employer(s) biographic data	Administrative procedures
Employment issues	Clinical procedures
Wages, salaries, and benefits	Safety issues
Employee conduct	Asepsis
Confidentiality guidelines	Material Safety Data Sheets
HIPAA compliance	Emergency protocol

© Cengage Learning 2014

Establishing and stating the mission of the practice clearly identifies the goals and objectives to be sought by each employee. Having biographic data of each provider helps employees to respond to queries from patients about a provider's experience, education, and interests.

Employment policies might include statements on equal employment opportunity, job requirements for particular positions and to whom the person reports, recruitment and selection procedures, orientation of new employees, probation, and dismissal. Wage and salary policies should be in writing. How are employees classified? What are the working hours, how is overtime compensated, and how are salary increases determined? What benefits (medical, retirement, vacation, holidays, sick leave, and profit sharing) does the practice have? The answers to such questions are part of the policy manual.

A discussion of employee conduct is another component of the policy manual. A statement regarding the strict confidentiality of all information received in the practice is essential in this area of the policy manual and often includes a form requiring a signature from the new hire assuring they fully understand the consequences of any breach in confidentiality. Guidelines should be established about uniforms, dress codes, appearance, and personal hygiene. Can an employee hold a second job outside the practice? Are staff members responsible for housekeeping duties? Is updated certification required? If so, what accommodations are made for continuing education requirements?

When the policy manual is computerized, changes and updates are easily made. Any changes made are to be shared with employees so that everyone is up to date on policies. Having a policy manual with clearly written directives helps employees understand the expectations and boundaries of the employment relationship. The policy manual is reviewed with each new employee and updated on a regular basis. Procedure 46-1 provides details on developing and maintaining a policy manual.

RECRUITING AND HIRING CLINIC PERSONNEL

The majority of employees in the ambulatory or primary care center are full-time, part-time, or occasionally independent contractor employees. Full-time employees generally work 30 hours or more per week; part-time employees work less than 30 hours per week. Either may be paid by the hour. Full-time employees may be salaried and are exempt from overtime regulations. Most part-time employees are paid by the hour. Benefits are often different between full- and part-time employees. Independent contractors who are employed usually work with the facility to perform specific predetermined tasks at a predetermined rate of pay for the services provided and are not eligible for benefits from the clinic.

Before recruiting and hiring personnel to fill positions within the medical facility, the HR manager and employers must understand exactly what the role and responsibilities of the position are by having a current job description for the position. They must follow a recruiting policy that is effective and fair and that observes all appropriate laws and regulations.

Job Descriptions

Before any position is filled, a **job description** must be in place. This usually is created cooperatively by the clinic manager and the employer(s). Once the job qualifications are defined, the lead personnel and HR manager can begin efforts to fill the position.

In daily operations most job descriptions are on file, but if the situation involves a new or greatly expanded clinic, a complete set of job descriptions is needed before recruiting can begin. Even

when a written description is on file, it should be reviewed when a new employee is to be hired. The person who is leaving the position is often an excellent resource for the accuracy of the current job description and any changes that should be made.

The job description must include basic qualifications necessary for the position and have enough information to provide both the supervisor and the employee with a clear outline of what the position entails (Figure 46-1). Necessary work

---

JOB DESCRIPTION

POSITION TITLE:
Administrative Medical Assistant

REPORTS TO:
Clinic Manager and Provider–Employer(s)

RESPONSIBILITIES AND DUTIES:
- Being a therapeutic and helpful receptionist
  1. Answer telephone as quickly as possible, hopefully by the second ring
  2. Greet all patients warmly and with a helpful attitude
- Manage time efficiently with appropriate scheduling for patients and professional staff
  1. Schedule patients according to their needs, scheduling guidelines, staff availability, and equipment readiness
  2. Call to remind patients of their visit the day before appointment
- Responding to patient requests on the telephone and in person
  1. Ascertain reason for request
  2. Satisfy patient request or refer patient to one who can
- Preparing patient charts for professional staff
  1. Print schedules and encounter forms
  2. Pull patient charts late afternoon the day before appointment; print as necessary
  3. Check charts for completeness
  4. Attach encounter form when patient arrives to check in

AUTHORITY BOUNDARIES:
The Clinic manager will assist in answering questions. Remember that it is better to ask than to make an error. Screening concerns not identified in a policy/procedure manual also can be directed to the clinical medical assisting staff.

POSITION REQUIREMENTS:
Two years' experience and/or graduate of a medical assistant program. CMA (AAMA), RMA, or CMAS preferred.

© Cengage Learning 2014

Figure 46-1 Sample job description for administrative medical assistant.

experience, skills, education, and any special certification or licensure that is expected is to be identified in the job description. Procedure 46-2 provides details on preparing job descriptions.

Another important point with respect to the job description is that a review and update of the description should be done every year. Most positions change constantly, whether from a minor shifting of duties or the addition of some new technical procedure or device. Without updating a job description, a person with the wrong qualifications may be recruited to fill a vacancy.

When seeking employment it is most helpful to understand the job description for the position being sought and to make certain that your qualifications fit that description.

Recruiting

A major challenge facing the HR manager today is recruitment. Medical assistants are listed among the top 10 occupations, with expected employment growth much faster than average through 2018, according to the U.S. Department of Labor, Bureau of Labor Statistics. One reason for this demand is the aging of the U.S. population and the demands made upon primary or ambulatory care. Medical assistants with formal education, instruction, and appropriate certification will be in high demand. When employers have been unsuccessful in recruiting qualified medical assistants, they have turned to contracting for some work, such as transcription and billing.

 Once the hiring need is determined, the HR manager begins the recruitment process. Often a process called networking is a highly effective method of finding employees. Networking is a process in which people of similar interests exchange information in social, business, or professional relationships. A survey conducted by Jobvite in 2010 indicated that nearly 75 percent of companies

use social media networks to recruit employees. LinkedIn was the most popular, followed by Facebook and Twitter. The HR manager may network with members of the American Association of Medical Assistants (AAMA) and express an interest in a new employee for an open position. Current employees are often an excellent resource because they may know of a qualified person who is looking for a position.

The medical assistant departments of nearby colleges are another good resource. Medical assisting students may find employment through their practicum experience near the end of their coursework. Individuals who volunteer to shadow, follow, or work in a facility are often seen as potential employees. Although newspaper advertisements or Craigslist may generate many résumés, they are only marginally effective as search tools. It is often far too time consuming to review the large volume of applications generated by this approach. There are a number of medical employment Internet sites that identify positions for medical assistant personnel, often in specific locales.

Preparing to Interview Applicants

Once several applicants have expressed interest in the position, preparation for the interview begins. The HR manager should have a number of résumés to consider. Some applicants may have already completed a job application if they dropped off a résumé. The résumés and applications can be reviewed together. Some important points to remember in reading these documents follow.

When considering education, look beyond the degree earned. Look for a good performance record at school and the kinds of supplemental education achieved. Does attendance at seminars and short-course training programs relate to your position needs? When reading a person's work history, make note of any unexplained gaps in employment. You may want to ask specific questions in the interview. Has advancement been gained in each new position? Are the responsibilities and duties of the applicant's positions explained, or

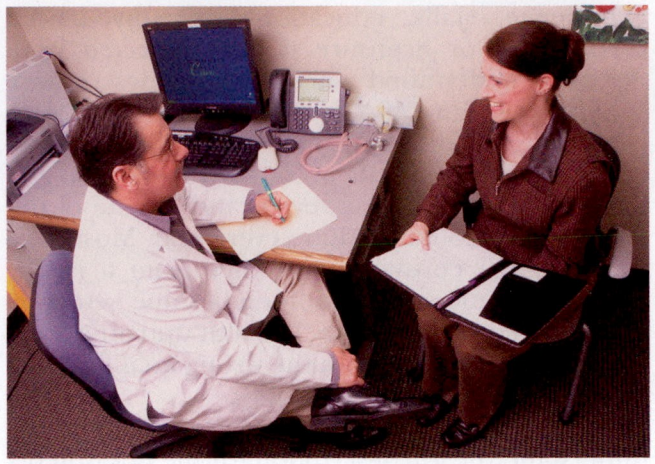

© Cengage Learning 2014

Figure 46-2 The interview can be conducted on a one-on-one basis with only the applicant and one staff member or with several staff members meeting with the applicant at once.

will questions need to be asked of the prospective employee?

Look for information that indicates if this candidate really enjoys the kind of work setting you have. Is the applicant comfortable serving the infirm? Can you truly identify the level of skill from the descriptions, or are the applicant's skills descriptions vague? The cover letter, if one is included, should address the specifics required of your position. Does the person display a negative or a positive attitude? Do not excuse any errors or unprofessional appearance in the job application or the résumé. Each should be perfect in all aspects. An individual who is careless in this respect is likely to be careless in the position.

Some applications will be discarded when compared to the preceding guidelines. With the remaining candidates, determine who is to be interviewed and make telephone calls to establish interviews. You may make note of the quality of speaking skills, especially if this person will be using the telephone in the position. Make an interview appointment date with only those who seem truly interested in the position during your telephone conversation.

The Employment Interview

The employment interview is usually conducted by only one person if second interviews are anticipated. The provider-employer, clinic manager, or

another employee may be present in either the first or the second interview, however (Figure 46-2). The interviewer(s) will want to review the application and résumé before the interview for particular points to ask the candidate. Before the interview, those doing the interviewing should establish a set of questions for all of the applicants. These predetermined questions will help avoid one applicant being given advantages over another and will help ensure continuity throughout all the interviews. An interview worksheet is an excellent tool to use to make certain that the interview process is fair and equitable with each candidate. The worksheet should provide enough room for notes taken during the interview.

Suggested items for the interview worksheet are:

- Applicant's name
- Telephone number
- Education and experience
- Work experience
- Special skills
- Professional demeanor
- Voice and mannerisms specific to position
- Questions and responses
- Ability to problem solve when given a scenario
- Any health-related or work-related problems applicant discloses
- Interviewer's personal impressions and recommendations

Conduct interviews in a quiet and private setting. Do not schedule interviews back to back

General Questions

- What are your strengths and weaknesses?
- Why did you leave your last position?
- Identify what is most important to you in a position.

Questions Related to Work Relationships

- Describe an individual you have enjoyed working with.
- Explain how a conflict with a coworker was resolved.
- How would a coworker describe you?

Questions Related to Problem Solving

- Describe a work-related decision that made you very proud.
- Identify a task/procedure/assignment you could not do, and explain why.
- How do you approach a task when it seems mundane or boring?

Questions Related to Integrity

- If asked to do something you believe is illegal or unethical, what would you do?
- Tell us about a time when you broke a confidence.
- If you saw a coworker put a patient at risk, what would you do?

© Cengage Learning 2014

Figure 46-3   Common interview questions.

without time to collect your thoughts or to allow you to compare notes with others participating in the interview. Ask job-related questions. For example, describe your last position. What did you like best about it? What did you like least? What is most important to you about a position? Describe your administrative and clinical skills. Figure 46-3 shows some sample questions. Let the applicant do the most of the talking.

Any questions related to age, sex, race, religion, or national origin are inappropriate. Inquiries about medical history, drug use, or arrest records may not be made (see Chapter 7). Keep your questions related to performance on the job. If you may want to bond this employee, you may ask candidates if they have been bonded before or are willing to be bonded. It may be best to leave salary discussions for a second interview, but it can also be helpful to determine if applicants' salary expectations are in line with what you can offer. A question such as "What salary are you expecting?" is appropriate. Do not make a job offer until all the candidates selected for interview have been interviewed, and do not prejudge someone on any factor other than the person's qualifications during or after the interview.

At the close of the interview, let the applicant know when a decision will be made or whether a second interview will be conducted and how notification will be made. A tour of the facility and introduction to key staff members may be offered but are not necessary at the time of the first interview. Finally, thank the applicant for participating in the interview and being interested in the position.

Selecting the Finalists

Shortly after the final interview is completed, the HR manager should compare notes with all the others involved in the interviews to select the top candidates. This is done by comparing notes and impressions from the interviews and by taking into consideration the ability of a candidate to work with patients and colleagues who might have a variety of problems and cultural backgrounds. The next step is to check references from former employers, supervisors, coworkers, and instructors. A large corporate medical practice may even have a consent form each candidate is asked to sign that gives permission to check references and call former employers and instructors. You may need to recognize, however, that even with a signed release from a potential new employee, many organizations and businesses restrict the release of reference information to only name, dates of employment, and title of position served. Telephone checks for references are an excellent strategy because you receive an immediate response. If you stress confidentiality when you make the contact, it will be easier for the person to respond to your questions. When possible, always check with more than one reference and former employer to get an accurate assessment of the candidate. All reference information is to be kept confidential. A sample telephone reference check form is shown in Figure 46-4.

A checklist of questions to ask might include:

1. What were the dates of employment of (name of applicant) in your firm?
2. Describe the position held.
3. Reason for leaving the position?
4. Strong points of the employee?
5. Limitations of the employee?
6. Can you comment on attendance and dependability?
7. Would you rehire?
8. Anything else we should know about this candidate?

TELEPHONE REFERENCE

Name of Applicant _____

Person Contacted _____

Position and Name of Business _____

_____

Telephone Number _____

Relationship to Applicant _____

- May I verify the employment history of (applicant's name) who is applying for a position with our medical clinic?

  _____, 20_____ to _____, 20_____

- Describe the responsibilities held by this individual.

- Identify the salary _____

- What are this individual's strong points?

- What are this individual's weak points?

- Describe this individual's overall attitude toward the position and toward patients.

- Please comment on dependability and attendance.

- Given the opportunity, would you rehire? Why or why not?

- Why did this individual leave the position?

- Describe personal and professional growth this individual made while in your firm.

- Is there anything else you would like to tell us?

Reference call made by _____

Date _____

© Cengage Learning 2014

Figure 46-4 Sample form to use for telephone references.

Offer the position when a first-choice candidate has been determined and indicate when a response is needed. Be prepared with a second-choice candidate should the preferred candidate respond negatively. At the time of the offer, the candidate should understand the salary offered, the starting date, the practice policies, and the benefits. When a candidate has accepted the position, a confirmation letter should be written that clearly spells out details discussed earlier. Give specific instructions on when and where the new employee should report the first day on the job. If practical, the employee should be given the policy and procedure manuals to read. Employers are required by federal law to verify that all employees are authorized to work. This is done by having the candidate complete an Eligibility Verification (I-9) form (see Case Study 46-2).

For the unsuccessful applicants, send a letter explaining that "we have selected another candidate whose qualifications and experience more closely meet our needs at this time. We would like to keep your résumé on file should another suitable position become available." Copies of these letters, as well as the interview checklists, should be kept for a minimum of 6 months should any questions arise regarding your choice of candidates. Procedure 46-3 provides details on interviewing.

ORIENTING NEW PERSONNEL

Orienting new employees is usually the responsibility of both the clinic manager and lead personnel who are most likely to work the closest with the new employee. It is common for a new employee to be placed on **probation** for 30 to 60 days, during which time both the employee and supervisory personnel may determine if the environment and the position are satisfactory for the employee. Procedure 46-4 outlines how to orient personnel.

Elements important to orientation include the introduction of the new employee to other staff members, assigning a mentor who can respond to questions, and making the employee aware of the procedures to be performed in this new position. If the procedure manual is detailed and accurate, this manual now becomes the daily guide for the new employee. Sometimes the individual leaving a position may still be present and is asked to assist in the orientation process. This is especially beneficial if there is a good working relationship between the employee who is leaving and the management of the practice. Depending on the responsibilities of the new employee, a supervisor may be asked to monitor for a period all the new employee's procedures for accuracy, safety, and patient protection. During the probation period, the employee should be officially evaluated by the clinic manager.

DISMISSING EMPLOYEES

The function of employee dismissal or separation falls mostly to the clinic manager; however, in a large facility with an HR representative, discussing dismissal or separation with that individual can be quite beneficial. Such a discussion ensures that all the information necessary is in place before a separation. There are voluntary and involuntary separations or dismissals.

Voluntary separations usually occur when an employee is relocating, advancing to another position elsewhere, retiring, or leaving for personal reasons. A letter of resignation is usually submitted to both the clinic manager and the HR representative. These employees will give their manager proper notice and may be able to turn current projects and duties over to their replacement. There is also time to say good-bye to their colleagues and have a good feeling about their employment.

Involuntary dismissals or separations usually occur when an employee's performance is poor or there has been a serious violation of the clinic policies or job description. The clinic manager is aware of poor performance through the probationary reviews. Verbal and written warnings must be given to the employee and are to be well documented. Dismissal can be immediate if there is a serious breach of clinic policy. The HR director can provide necessary detail to the clinic manager and/or provider(s) regarding when and if immediate dismissal is recommended. If a clinic manager expects any serious difficulties with an employee during an immediate dismissal, the HR director or another person appointed to assist should be present when the employee is notified (see Chapter 45 for a more detailed discussion).

Exit Interview

An **exit interview** is an excellent opportunity for the employee who voluntarily leaves a practice and the HR manager to discuss the positive and negative aspects of the job and what changes might be made for a new person coming into the facility. A sample exit interview form is shown in Figure 46-5. It also allows the opportunity for the employee to ask for a **letter of reference** or to view the personnel file before leaving. In a voluntary separation, a **letter of resignation** for the personnel file is necessary.

Any separation process, voluntary or involuntary, must include a statement in the personnel file. For involuntary separation, be certain that the reasons for the dismissal are well documented in

EXIT INTERVIEW FORM

1. What did you like and dislike about the work you have been doing?
   (Including: support on the job; opportunity for personal growth; recognition and rewards)

2. What kind of people have you found the providers, your immediate supervisor, and co-workers to be?
   (Including: attitude; fairness; scheduling and assignment of work; work expectations; technical competence; assistance and guidance available; team spirit)

3. What is your view of our management practices and policies?
   (Including: clarity and fairness of practice policies; communications; management and staff)

4. How have you felt about performance appraisals, your salary and benefits?
   (Including: adequacy of salary; regularity and fairness of appraisals)

5. What are your principal reasons for leaving the practice?
   (Including: primary dissatisfactions; job or personal changes)

6. In what areas do you feel we need to improve?

Interviewer signature: _____   Date _____

Employee signature: _____   Date _____

From Ricardo, M. (1992). Personnel management handbook (2nd ed.). New York: The McGraw-Hill Companies, Inc. Copyright 1992. Reprinted with permission.

Figure 46-5   Sample exit interview form.

an honest, nonjudgmental statement. State only the facts in the personnel file; do not state opinion. Remember that employees have the right to view their personnel file at any time.

Employers are always to be informed of any dismissal as quickly as possible. As indicated above, some may be involved in the actual dismissal process.

MAINTAINING PERSONNEL RECORDS

An important aspect of the responsibilities of the HR manager is maintaining personnel records. All documentation and correspondence related to each employee from application to dismissal, ranging from awards to reprimands and including the formal reviews, must be kept in the confidential personnel file. Access to this file is limited to certain management personnel and the employee. Not all of these people are allowed to see the entire file. These files are usually kept for a period of 3 to 5 years after employees leave the practice. Some of the personnel files may be maintained electronically on the computer. However, access to those files must be protected so that only those with authorized access are able to open the files or make changes to them.

This file also includes the kind of information normally maintained for payroll and business practices. That information includes the name, address, telephone number, and Social Security number of employee. The position title, date of beginning employment, rate of pay (hourly or otherwise), total overtime pay, deductions or additions to wages, wages paid each pay period, and the date the employee leaves the practice also are included.

COMPLYING WITH PERSONNEL LAWS

Only a brief introduction to the laws related to the ambulatory care setting are given in this section; therefore, this text is not meant to be a legal guide for an HR manager. The practice attorney should always be contacted if there is any question regarding personnel laws, which may vary in some states depending on the size of the practice.

Overtime must be addressed in each practice. Who is reimbursed for overtime and how is that reimbursement determined? Typically, administrative medical assistants, insurance billers, medical transcriptionists, and clinical medical assistants are likely to be paid overtime. Overtime pay at a rate of not less than one and one-half times the regular rate of pay after a 40-hour work week is standard. Each week stands alone and one week cannot compensate for another. If the practice does not want to be involved in overtime situations, require that any overtime be preauthorized in advance.

The Equal Pay Act of 1963 prevents wage discrimination for jobs that require equal skill, effort, and responsibility. The Civil Rights Act of 1964 prevents employers from discriminating against individuals on the basis of race, color, religion, sex, age, or national origin (see Chapter 7).

Sexual harassment violates Title VII of the Civil Rights Act. Steps must be taken to ensure that all employees are working in an atmosphere that is not hostile, where sexual gestures, the presence of pornographic or offensive materials, or obscene language are not allowed (see Chapter 7).

Employees have a right to expect safe working conditions. The Occupational Safety and Health Act (OSH Act) was established to prevent injuries and illnesses resulting from unsafe or unhealthy working conditions (see Chapter 22 for a detailed discussion of the standards and requirements, especially in the section on bloodborne pathogens, that went into effect in 1992). Compliance with this law requires that each employee be aware of possible risks associated with chemical hazards and how to protect themselves. Because there are many of these hazards in a medical practice, compliance and protection for employees are extremely important, and training sessions should be held in this area.

The Immigration Reform Act requires employers to verify the right of employees to work in the United States. Documentation acceptable for verification is a Social Security card or birth certificate. The U.S. Department of Justice Immigration and Naturalization Service will provide instructions and a form for employees and employers to complete, commonly referred to as the I-9 or Employment Eligibility Verification form.

Employers cannot discriminate against or condemn any full-time employee for jury duty. Although the employer does not have to continue pay during jury duty, the employee cannot lose seniority, insurance, or other benefits. Many employers continue an employee's full pay during the time of service on a jury because the reimbursement for jury service is minimal. This is a way to benefit employees and encourage good citizenship.

This list is by no means comprehensive but does include personnel regulations most likely to affect the medical practice. Any concerns should be directed to the practice's attorney.

SPECIAL POLICY CONSIDERATIONS

Several other managerial issues may arise in a medical setting for which the clinic manager and the HR manager will have to plan. These can include policies for temporary employees, rules of conduct, avoiding discrimination, and having a support system in place for employees who need physical or emotional help.

Temporary Employees

Temporary employees who may be employed for 90 days or less include students who are serving an internship or practicum from a local college and are practicing their skills for when they will be on the job. They should be reviewed on a regular basis in cooperation with their college supervisor. Give them as much actual hands-on experience as possible; they are future employees. Accommodating students in the practice is a two-way benefit. Students learn what reality is in the ambulatory care setting and are able to practice newly developed skills. Current staff members in the facility are "sharpened" by the students' presence. Teaching and monitoring someone's actions always results in sharpening and rethinking the skills of the current staff. Many HR directors and managers depend on these programs for future job applicants.

Smoking Policy

Smoking on the premises, especially at a health care facility, is a concern. The majority of health care facilities do not allow smoking at all. Additionally, some states and cities have laws that restrict smoking. When a policy is established, it should cover everyone—employers, employees, *and* patients. The objective is to have a policy that is workable and enforceable, promotes health, encourages employee morale and productivity, and sets examples for patients.

Discrimination

The Americans with Disabilities Act (ADA) prohibits discrimination by all private employers with 15 or more employees. Some states may further prohibit discrimination in facilities based on a much smaller size of their workforce. *All* public entities are prohibited from discrimination against qualified individuals with disabilities. The ADA establishes guidelines prohibiting discrimination against a "qualified individual with a disability" in regard to employment. Someone with a disability who satisfies the skills necessary for the job; has the experience, education, and any other job requirements; and who, with reasonable accommodation, can perform the job cannot be discriminated against. Employers often find that persons with disabilities are their finest employees.

Persons who are HIV-positive or have AIDS are included in the guidelines set forth by the ADA. Persons with HIV/AIDS cannot be discriminated against. It can be assumed that if a safe working environment is provided when all employees follow the rules for Standard Precautions, then reasonable accommodation has been made for the person with HIV or AIDS.

An employer cannot refuse the job to a qualified person based on the belief that in the future the employee may become too ill to work. The hiring decision must be based on the individual's ability to perform the functions of the position at the present time. If a current employee reveals to the manager that he or she is HIV positive or has AIDS, that information must be kept confidential and must be kept apart from the general personnel file. The manager may choose to hold a discussion at that time of what accommodations might be needed in the future.

PROVIDING/PLANNING EMPLOYEE INSTRUCTION AND EDUCATION

Health care changes daily—new procedures are established; a better technique is discovered for performing a particular task. Major changes regularly occur in medical insurance. Computer systems are updated or new software is added. A more sophisticated telephone system is installed to make certain patients are responded to promptly. New state or federal regulations mandate additional education or compliance in safety. New medications become available that providers may prescribe and employees must understand. All this demands that employees receive a continuing and constant update in their area of employment.

Instruction and education may be accomplished within the practice or outside the practice. When an employee is a member of a professional organization such as the American Association of Medical Assistants, many monthly meetings include continuing education opportunities. Numerous seminars and conferences held throughout the country may be beneficial to employees. Local hospitals often have continuing education opportunities that may be beneficial. Managers will keep abreast of these opportunities and encourage employees to attend. Any continuing education opportunity that may benefit the employee on the job and the medical practice itself should ideally be paid for by the employer(s). Credentialed employees will always need to update skills and earn CEUs to maintain their credentials in active status. An important function of HR is to make CEU opportunities available to employees.

It is often best to provide employee instruction and education within the facility when the necessary instruction is specific to the medical practice. For instance, instruction on new computer software is apt to be specific to the particular setting.

When sophisticated new equipment is purchased, companies often provide in-house instruction for the individuals who will be using the equipment. Take advantage of as many of those opportunities as are available and for as many of your employees as possible. When the instruction is quite expensive or time consuming, make certain at least person receives the instruction. Then have that individual teach others. Whenever possible, provide instruction outside of regular hours when patients are not being seen—before the clinic opens or after the clinic closes or during a lunch period. Always pay employees for any time served over their regular working hours. Offer certificates for any in-services.

Careful attention to continuing education and instruction for employees will pay for itself many times over again. The more confident and secure employees feel in the skills they are expected to perform, the more satisfied the practice's patients will be.

PROCEDURE 46-1

Develop and Maintain a Policy Manual

PURPOSE:
To develop and maintain a comprehensive, up-to-date policy manual of all clinic policies relating to employee practices, benefits, clinic conduct, and so on.

EQUIPMENT/SUPPLIES:
Computer
Binder, such as a three-ring
Paper
Standard policy manual format

PROCEDURE STEPS:

1. *Paying attention to detail,* develop precise, written clinic policies detailing all necessary information pertaining to the staff and their positions. The information should include benefits, vacation, sick leave, hours, dress codes, evaluations, rules of conduct, and grounds for dismissal. RATIONALE: Well-defined policies clearly outlined for each employee are necessary for efficient and effective staff operations.

2. Identify procedures for reimbursing overtime, preventing discrimination and harassment, creating a safe working environment, and allowing for jury duty.

3. Include a policy statement related to rules of conduct.

4. Identify steps to follow should an employee become disabled during employment.

5. Determine what employee opportunities for continuing education, if any, will be reimbursed; include requirements for recertification or licensure.

6. Provide a copy of the policy manual for each employee. RATIONALE: Each employee is made aware of facility policies.

7. Review and update the policy manual regularly. Add or delete items as necessary, dating each revised page. RATIONALE: Policy manual will always be current.

PROCEDURE 46-2

Prepare a Job Description

PURPOSE:
To provide a precise definition of the tasks assigned to a job; to determine the expectations and level of competency required; and to specify the experience, training, and education needed to perform the job for purposes of recruiting and performance evaluation.

EQUIPMENT/SUPPLIES:
Computer
Paper
Standard job description format

Procedure 46-2 (continued)

PROCEDURE STEPS:

1. *Paying attention to detail,* describe each task that creates the job. RATIONALE: A detailed job description identifies clear expectations for each employee.

2. List special medical, technical, or clerical skills required.

3. Determine the level of education, instruction, and experience required for the position.

4. Determine where the job fits in the overall structure of the practice.

5. Specify any unusual working conditions (hours, locations, and so on) that may apply.

6. Describe career path opportunities.

PROCEDURE 46-3
Conduct Interviews

PURPOSE:
To screen applicants for training, experience, and characteristics to select the best candidate to fill the position vacancy.

PROCEDURE STEPS:

1. *Paying attention to detail,* review résumés and applications received.

2. Select candidates who most closely match the education and experience being sought.

3. *Develop a strategic plan* for conducting the interviews by creating an interview worksheet for each candidate listing points to cover.

4. Select an interview team; this team should always include the HR or clinic manager and the immediate supervisor to whom the candidate will report.

5. Call personally to schedule interviews. RATIONALE: This allows you to judge the applicant's telephone manners and voice.

6. *Maintain ethical standards* by reminding the interviewers of various legal restrictions concerning questions to be asked.

7. Conduct interviews in a private, quiet setting. RATIONALE: Careful interviewing of potential employees is an important step in hiring the best candidate for the position.

8. Put the applicant at ease by beginning with an overview about the practice and staff, briefly describing the job, and answering preliminary questions.

9. Ask questions about the applicant's work experience and educational background using the résumé and interview worksheet as a guide.

10. Provide the most promising applicants additional information on benefits and a tour of the clinic, if practical.

11. Applicant's general salary requirements may be discussed, but avoid discussion of a specific salary until a formal offer is tendered.

12. Inform the applicants when a decision will be made and thank each for participating in the interview.

13. Do not make a job offer until all the candidates have been interviewed.

14. Check references of all prospective employees.

15. Establish a second interview between the provider-employer(s) and the qualified candidate if necessary.

16. Confirm accepted job offers in writing, specifying details of the offer and acceptance. RATIONALE: A written document provides proof of hiring and employment details.

17. *Show respect* by notifying all unsuccessful applicants by letter when the position has been filled. RATIONALE: Makes a positive statement to those not hired and keeps the doors open for future employment possibilities.

PROCEDURE 46-4
Orient Personnel

PURPOSE:

To acquaint new employees with clinic policies, staff, what the job encompasses, procedures to be performed, and job performance expectations.

PROCEDURE STEPS:

1. Tour the facilities and introduce the clinic staff.
2. Complete employee-related documents and explain their purpose.
3. Explain the benefits program.
4. Present the clinic policy manual and discuss its key elements.
5. *Review federal and state regulatory precautions for medical facilities.*
6. Review the job description.
7. Explain and demonstrate procedures to be performed and the use of procedure manuals supporting these procedures.
8. Demonstrate the use of any specialized equipment.
9. Assign a mentor from the staff to help with the orientation. RATIONALE: Without proper orientation and training, even the best new employee can fail.

CASE STUDY 46-1

Refer to the scenario at the beginning of the chapter.

It is sometimes difficult for Jane O'Hara, CMA (AAMA), to complete her responsibilities as both the clinic manager and the human resources manager.

CASE STUDY REVIEW

1. What steps might Jane take to manage her many and time-consuming tasks comfortably?
2. What responsibilities, if any, that normally fall to the human resources manager could be assigned to other staff members?

CASE STUDY 46-2

Daly Jacobsen, RMA (AMT), is an administrative medical assistant at Inner City Health Care. The HR manager has suggested that she might expand her skills and learn some of the procedures in the hiring process. A new medical assistant who specializes in nutrition is coming on board. Daly has been asked to make certain the I-9 form is completed appropriately. The HR manager tells Daly that she will need to download the latest form before completion.

CASE STUDY REVIEW

1. Daly knows that the I-9 is a government form verifying employment eligibility. What keywords might she use in her Internet search to find the form?
2. Once the form has been located, identify the specific rules necessary in completion of the form. What document in List A would a number of prospective employees most likely have?
3. In what area of the clinic might you post the lists of acceptable documents for the I-9 form?
4. With what agency is the form filed on successful completion?

CASE STUDY 46-3

Charles Kensington has just been hired as the HR manager in a large metropolitan clinic. In studying the policy manual, he notes that there is no defined policy for sick leave or bereavement leave. Describe the steps he might take to write such a policy.

CASE STUDY REVIEW

1. To whom should he speak regarding what currently occurs when an employee is ill or when there is a death in the family?
2. What might Charles consider in writing this policy?
3. How should a policy be approved once it is written?
4. What parameters would you suggest for the policy?

SUMMARY

As shown in this discussion, HR management is a challenge. It is, however, a rewarding one. While provider-employers are responsible for patients' physical care, the management team is responsible for hiring and maintaining the employees in the organization. The HR manager who is successful will hire the right people for the open positions and monitor employees in a way that enables and encourages them to give the best patient care possible. The medical assistant who has good communication skills and acquires additional education and experience in HR management will always have variety on the job and will have the satisfaction of watching a health care team run smoothly and efficiently.

STUDY FOR SUCCESS

To reinforce your knowledge and skills of information presented in this chapter:

- Review the *Key Terms*
- Role-play with other students to apply attributes of professionalism pertinent to this chapter.
- Consider the *Case Studies* and discuss your conclusions
- Answer the questions in the *Certification Review*
- Apply your knowledge by completing the *Activities* in the *Study Guide* and the *Games and Quizzes* in the StudyWARE (StudyWARE) software on the *Premium Website*
- Perform the *Procedures* using the *Competency Assessment Checklists* in the *Competency Manual*
- Practice your problem-solving skills with the *Critical Thinking Challenge 3.0* on the *Premium Website*

Additional resources for this chapter include:

- *CourseMate for Delmar's Comprehensive Medical Assisting*
- *WebTutor for Delmar's Comprehensive Medical Assisting*

CERTIFICATION REVIEW

1. HR managers:
   a. need no special education for the position
   b. are responsible for hiring and orienting personnel
   c. often work longer hours than other employees
   d. both b and c

2. Which of the following questions may be asked in an interview?
   a. How old are you?
   b. Have you ever been arrested?
   c. Can you supply a birth certificate or a Social Security card?
   d. Do you plan to start a family soon?

3. When a candidate has been accepted for a position, the HR manager should:
   a. call the candidate to determine what salary is preferred
   b. write a letter defining the position details
   c. check references listed by the candidate
   d. notify patients of a staff change

4. Overtime hours in the medical facility:
   a. are to be expected as part of the position
   b. do not require prior authorization
   c. are usually paid at no less than one and one-half times the regular pay rate
   d. are paid only to managers

5. The HR manager will work closely with:
   a. the provider-employer(s)
   b. the clinic manager
   c. all employees
   d. all of the above

6. OSHA:
   a. requires employers to verify an employee's right to work in the United States
   b. protects employees who have disabilities from employment discrimination
   c. protects employees with chemical dependencies or emotional problems
   d. protects employees from unsafe or unhealthy working conditions

7. The best area for hiring medical employees comes from:
   a. students in a business college
   b. newspaper advertisements
   c. networking sources
   d. the state's unemployment office

8. Employees receiving instruction or education necessary to the position:
   a. will seek that instruction after hours and not expect reimbursement
   b. will be current and up-to-date in the health care field
   c. should always be paid for any time served over regular working hours
   d. both b and c

9. Personnel records:
   a. are usually kept for 3 to 5 years after employment ends and may include payroll data
   b. are not available for everyone to view and must be kept confidential
   c. include all papers related to employment and personal data
   d. all of the above

10. Dismissal or separation:
    a. may be voluntary or involuntary
    b. should always be documented
    c. is a good time for an exit interview
    d. all of the above

REFERENCES/BIBLIOGRAPHY

Fallon, Jr., F. L. (2007). *Human resource management in health care: Principles and practice.* Bowling Green, OH: Bowling Green State University.

Mathis, R. L., & Jackson, J. H. (2004). *Healthcare human resource management* (10th ed.). Cincinnati, OH: South-Western College Publishing.

McWay, D. C. (2008). *Today's health information management.* Clifton Park, NY: Delmar Cengage Learning.

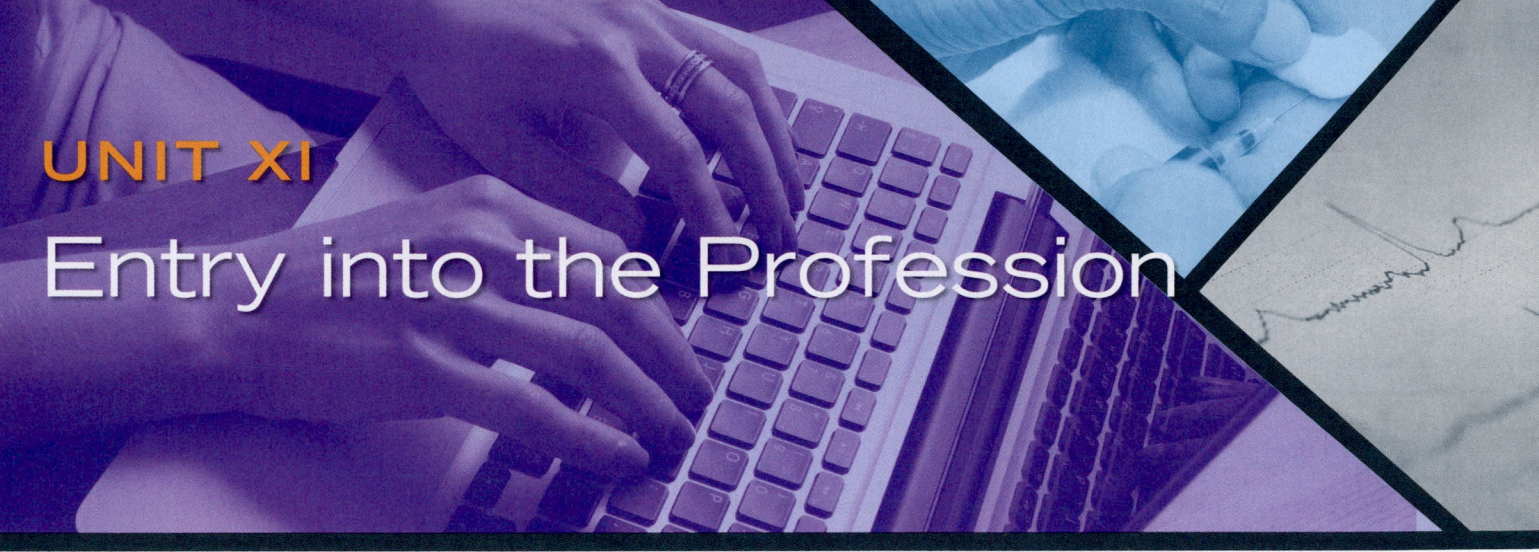

UNIT XI
Entry into the Profession

CHAPTER 47
Preparing for Medical Assisting Credentials 1452

CHAPTER 48
Employment Strategies 1466

Preparing for Medical Assisting Credentials

OUTLINE

Purpose of Certification
  Certification Agencies
Preparing for Certification
  Examinations
American Association
  of Medical Assistants (AAMA)
  Certified Medical
    Assistant (AAMA)
    Examination Format
    and Content
  Certified Medical Assistant
    (AAMA) Application
    Process
  Certified Medical Assistant
    (AAMA) Examination
    Scheduling and
    Administration
  Certified Medical Assistant
    (AAMA) Recertification

American Medical
  Technologists (AMT)
  Registered Medical
    Assistant (AMT)
    Examination Format
    and Content
  Registered Medical Assistant
    (AMT) Application Process
  Registered Medical Assistant
    (AMT) Examination
    Scheduling and
    Administration
  Registered Medical Assistant
    (AMT) Recertification
National Healthcareer
  Association (NHA)
  Certified Clinical Medical
    Assistant and Certified
    Medical Administrative
    Assistant Examination
    Format and Content

Certified Clinical Medical
  Assistant and Certified
  Medical Administrative
  Assistant Application
  Process
Certified Clinical Medical
  Assistant and Certified
  Medical Administrative
  Assistant Examination
  Scheduling and
  Administration
Certified Clinical Medical
  Assistant and Certified
  Medical Administrative
  Assistant Recertification
Professional Organizations
  American Association of
    Medical Assistants (AAMA)
  American Medical
    Technologists (AMT)
  National Healthcareer
    Association (NHA)

LEARNING OUTCOMES

1. Define, spell, and pronounce all of the key terms as presented in this chapter.

2. List the necessary qualifications to sit for the certified medical assistant (AAMA) certification examination.

3. State when the certified medical assistant (AAMA) certification examination is offered and state the registration deadlines.

4. List the necessary qualifications to sit for the registered medical assistant examination.

5. State when the registered medical assistant examination is offered and state the registration protocols.

6. Differentiate between being certified and being registered.

7. Discuss the National Healthcareer Association and its options for medical assisting certification.

8. Identify the benefits of certification and registration.

9. Describe several methods for pursuing continuing education opportunities.

10. Explain when recertification must take place for the CMA (AAMA).

11. Describe the procedure for recertification for the registered medical assistant.

12. Analyze the professionalism questions and apply them to this chapter's content.

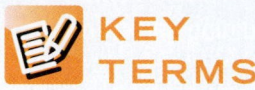

KEY TERMS

Accrediting Bureau of Health Education Schools (ABHES)

American Association of Medical Assistants (AAMA)

American Medical Technologists (AMT)

certification examination

Certified Clinical Medical Assistant (CCMA)

Certified Medical Administrative Assistant (CMAA)

Certified Medical Administrative Specialist (CMAS)

Certified Medical Assistant (CMA [AAMA])

Commission on Accreditation of Allied Health Education Programs (CAAHEP)

continuing education units (CEUs)

National Healthcareer Association (NHA)

recertification

Registered Medical Assistant (RMA [AMT])

Task Force for Test Construction (TFTC)

ATTRIBUTES OF PROFESSIONALISM

Presentation
- Were you dressed and groomed appropriately?
- Did you display a positive attitude?
- Did you display a calm, professional, and caring manner?

Competency
- Did you pay attention to detail?
- Did you display sound judgment?
- Did you remain calm in a crisis?
- Were you knowledgeable and accountable?
- Did you recognize the importance of local, state, and federal legislation and regulations in the practice setting?

Initiative
- Did you show initiative?
- Did you develop a strategic plan to achieve your goals? Was your plan realistic?
- Did you seek out opportunities to expand your knowledge base?
- Were you flexible and dependable?

Integrity
- Did you maintain your moral and ethical standards?
- Did you do the "right thing" even when no one was observing?

SCENARIO

Dr. Ray Reynolds currently is the senior provider at Inner City Health Care, a multiprovider urgent care center. When he began his practice 32 years ago, however, he had a private practice and employed one full-time and two part-time medical assistants. Dr. Reynolds felt the practice ran smoothly, except when an assistant had to be replaced. Retraining a new person consumed a great deal of valuable time. Even if the new employee came with experience from another medical practice, the procedures still required retraining.

Dr. Reynolds now finds that when he needs to replace a medical assistant, he looks at the applicants' résumés and interviews only those candidates who are Certified Medical Assistants or Registered Medical Assistants. The practice is too busy to spend time training and retraining new people.

INTRODUCTION

Forty years ago, medical assistants were trained on the job by the practitioner with whom they were employed. Quality control of training varied because there were no established criteria for evaluating such training. This chapter will present the purpose of certification, certifying agencies, and preparation for certification examinations.

PURPOSE OF CERTIFICATION

Certification is intended to set a consistent minimum standard for evaluating an individual's professional competence as a medical assistant. The medical assisting profession continues to be one of the fastest growing in the U.S. economy. Because of the demand for skilled medical assistants, increasing numbers of career-oriented candidates enter this profession annually. Certification acknowledges the professional has standard entry-level knowledge and skills. Successfully passing a **certification examination** builds personal self-esteem, confidence, and a positive attitude in performing the responsibilities assigned.

Other reasons for certification include help in your career advancement and compensation. Hiring providers view these credentials as professional and an indication of proficiency in entry-level skills. Individuals who are competent and interested in continued learning experiences are more apt to be rewarded with promotions and salary increases. Maintaining the credential demonstrates a lifelong commitment to professional development. The graduate medical assistant has a goal and challenge to which to aspire, first by earning the credential and second by maintaining the credential through continued education and recertification.

Some certifying agencies offer student membership into their organizations. This avenue provides excellent opportunities to network and be mentored by fellow professionals, to enroll in continuing education programs, and to receive many other membership perks.

CRITICAL THINKING

Take time to think through your personal medical assisting career goals. Will credentialing be an important consideration? Why or why not?

SPOTLIGHT ON CERTIFICATION

RMA Content Outline
- Medical law
- Oral and written communication

CMA (AAMA) Content Outline
- Professionalism
- Communication
- Medicolegal guidelines and requirements

CMAS Content Outline
- Legal and ethical considerations
- Professionalism
- Communication

Certification Agencies

The **American Association of Medical Assistants (AAMA)** offers examinations to certify the **Certified Medical Assistant (CMA [AAMA])**. The **American Medical Technologists (AMT)** offers examinations to certify the **Registered Medical Assistant (RMA [AMT])** and the **Certified Medical Administrative Specialist (CMAS [AMT])**. The **National Healthcareer Association (NHA)** is another agency offering certification to health care professionals. These professionals include the **Certified Clinical Medical Assistant (CCMA)** and the **Certified Medical Administrative Assistant (CMAA)**. Figure 47-1 illustrates a comparison of agencies providing certification for medical assistants.

Since January 1, 2008, medical assistants certified through AAMA have used the title "Certified Medical Assistant" or the abbreviation "CMA (AAMA)." This title indicates that a person whose services are competent—having graduated from a program accredited by the **Commission on Accreditation of Allied Health Education Programs (CAAHEP)** or the **Accrediting Bureau of Health Education Schools (ABHES)**, and having successfully passed the AAMA certification examination—will perform medical assisting services.

It has become common practice for American Medical Technologist certificants to use "RMA (AMT)" to indicate their competency and graduation from an ABHES accredited program. When responding to advertisements or during the interview process, "certified medical assistants" are responsible to make clear to prospective employers which credential they have been awarded.

PREPARING FOR CERTIFICATION EXAMINATIONS

Preparation for the examination requires planning, scheduling, and discipline. It is important to plan well in advance to ensure confidence and a passing score to earn your credential. If you are sitting for the examination immediately on graduation, your preparation time for the examination may only allow 2 to 3 months. If you have been out of school for some time or your work experience has been very specialized, you may need longer to prepare for the examination.

During the planning stage, determine the date you want to sit for the examination. Check with the appropriate Web site or call the appropriate examination department to obtain the current application form. The application form contains information such as dates, times, and locations of test sites; policies regarding deadlines; incomplete applications; examination verification information; and information regarding study guides.

It is important to consider having a study group or partner. The right study environment can be invaluable to your success for several reasons. First, it is important to select a study partner or group

Certification Details

Certifying Agency	American Association of Medical Assistants (AAMA)	American Medical Technologists (AMT)	National Healthcareer Association (NHA)
Credential	CMA (AAMA)	RMA (AMT) or CMAS (AMT)	CCMA or CMAA
Certification Exam	Computer-based national exam, offered at Prometric testing centers (www.prometric.com)	Computer-based national exam offered at Pearson Vue testing centers (www.pearsonvue.com), or paper exam by appointment	National exam taken by online or paper exam
Number of Questions and Make-up of Exam	200 multiple choice questions Topics from the Content Outline for the CMA (AAMA). (Only 180 of the questions will be scored, the other 20 are trial questions for future exams.)	200–210 multiple choice questions Clinical, Administrative, and General questions	200 multiple choice questions Separate tests for CCMA and CMAA (exam completion time approximately 90 minutes)
Continuing Education	AAMA-approved CEUs: 60 points every 5 years 10 Clinical 10 Administrative 10 General 30 Discretionary	Certification Continuation Program (CCP): 30 points every 3 years AMT and AMTIE* offer several CE options for credits	Continuing education (CE) program: 5 credits per year Home study program taken online, downloaded, or using printed copies

*American Technologists Institute For Education

© Cengage Learning 2014

Figure 47-1   Comparison of agencies providing certification.

who shares your commitment to a successful outcome and who plans to sit for the examination on or near the same date you have selected. A study partner can also give you some accountability for keeping to the planned schedule.

Once it has been determined when and where you will sit for the examination and who your study partner(s), if any, will be, a meeting should be scheduled to discuss the review/study approach. It may be that your group will decide to review/study each subject provided in the Curriculum Content Outline accompanying the application. Other groups review/study only those areas in which they feel less confident. A plan that meets the needs of each group member and that all can agree to works best.

Meeting once or twice a week helps the group stay focused and on task. Independent study should be done throughout the week. During the independent study time, each group member may be asked to write 10 multiple choice questions relevant to the weeks' study topic. Answers to these questions should be on a separate page. Some find it helpful to also provide the rationale or textbook page number that supports their answer. When the group meets, a discussion of the study topic could take place and copies of the questions could be distributed for answering. The questions could then be corrected and discussion of any questionable or missed answers could take place.

Once a schedule has been established and agreed on, discipline is required. It is critical that each group member spend time individually preparing for the next group meeting. Someone should be put in charge of each group meeting to keep the event from turning into a social event. To help with this, it is a good idea to set a specific time limit for the study/review session. If individuals want to visit after the session, they are free to do that without disrupting the purpose of the session. All members should be committed to being prepared and attending each scheduled review/study session.

AMERICAN ASSOCIATION OF MEDICAL ASSISTANTS (AAMA)

The AAMA is an organization whose objective is to promote skills and professionalism, protect the medical assistants' right to practice, and encourage consistent health care delivery through professional certification. The AAMA is a sponsoring member of the Commission on Accreditation of Allied Health Education Programs (CAAHEP). CAAHEP establishes the standards for medical assisting programs and is the issuing body of the accreditation for AAMA.

Only graduates of CAAHEP- and Accrediting Bureau of Health Education Schools (ABHES)-accredited medical assistant programs may sit for the Certified Medical Assistant exam. To locate either CAAHEP or ABHES medical assisting programs, go to http://www.aama-ntl.org and click on *About AAMA*. Follow the drop-down menu for specific information.

Eligibility categories and documentation requirements to sit for the Certified Medical Assistant exam include the following:

- *Category 1.* The candidate must be a CAAHEP or ABHES graduating student or recent graduate. Verification of graduation date is required as documentation.

- *Category 2.* The candidate may be a CAAHEP or ABHES nonrecent graduate. A nonrecent graduate is one with a graduation date more than 12 months prior to the examination date. An official transcript and verification of graduation date are required documentation.

- *Category 3.* The candidate may be a recertificant, a Certified Medical Assistant® applying for the CMA Examination to recertify his or her credential.

The AAMA Endowment is a not-for-profit corporation that provides funding for two purposes:

- Awarding of scholarships to students in CAAHEP-accredited medical assisting education programs

- Accreditation of medical assisting education programs through CAAHEP

The Medical Assisting Education Review Board (MAERB) operates under the authority of the endowment and evaluates medical assisting programs according to standards adopted by the endowment and the CAAHEP. The MAERB recommends programs to CAAHEP for accreditation. The MAERB also reviews standards for medical assisting curricula, conducts accreditation workshops for educators, and provides medical assisting educators with current information about CAAHEP, accreditation laws, policies, and practices. CAAHEP's purpose is to accredit entry-level, allied health education programs.

Certified Medical Assistant (AAMA) Examination Format and Content

The AAMA certification examination is a comprehensive test of the knowledge actually used in today's medical clinic. The content is drawn from an in-depth analysis of the numerous tasks medical assistants perform on a daily basis.

Examination questions are formulated by the Certifying Board's **Task Force for Test Construction (TFTC)**. This group is composed of practicing medical assistants, providers, and medical assisting educators from across the United States. The TFTC updates the examination annually to reflect changes in medical assistants' day-to-day responsibilities, as well as the latest developments in medical knowledge and technology.

The three major areas tested include:

1. *General.* Medical Terminology, Anatomy and Physiology, Psychology, Professionalism, Communication, and Medicolegal Guidelines and Requirements
2. *Administrative.* Data Entry, Equipment, Records Management, Screening and Processing Mail, Scheduling and Monitoring Appointments, Resource Information and Community Services, Managing the Office, Office Policies and Procedures, and Practice Finances
3. *Clinical.* Principles of Infection Control, Treatment Area, Patient Preparation and Assisting the Provider, Patient History Interview, Collecting and Processing Specimens; Diagnostic Testing, Preparing and Administering Medications, Emergencies, First Aid, and Nutrition

Students must enroll as an AAMA member before their graduation date to be eligible for the reduced student rate. Once they are a student member they may stay at the student rate for 1 year after graduation if they do not choose to be an active or associate member and pay the higher dues amount. The additional year of membership at the reduced rate helps the recent graduate maintain membership while finding a job and becoming established in a career.

Certified Medical Assistant (AAMA) Application Process

 Candidates should read all instructions carefully before completing the application form. Incomplete or incorrect applications will not be processed and will be returned to the candidate. Postmark deadlines for applications, cancellations, and examination location changes are strictly enforced.

Applications are available from the AAMA Certification Department, 7999 Eagle Way, Chicago, IL 60678-1079. The application may also be downloaded from the AAMA Web site (http://www.aama-ntl.org).

It is recommended that the application be sent by certified mail, return receipt requested to verify delivery. The application must be typewritten or printed using black ink only. Be sure the application is signed and dated properly and the eligibility category section is completed appropriately. Applications take up to 45 days after the postmark date to process.

Tear off the application page from the instruction pamphlet. Do not mail the instructions back with the application. Keep this information for future reference together with a copy of everything submitted, including a copy of your completed payment check or money order. If you are paying by VISA or MasterCard, provide the requested information at the top of the application.

The CMA (AAMA) content outline identifies the subject matter that will be covered on the examination. It is available on the AAMA Web site. A sample 120-question examination is available to help assess your knowledge of the categories tested and the format used to formulate the questions. The Content Outline for the CMA (AAMA) Certification/Recertification Examination is also included.

Certified Medical Assistant (AAMA) Examination Scheduling and Administration

The AAMA certification examination is made up of 200 multiple choice questions, covering topics listed on the Content Outline for the CMA (AAMA) Certification/Recertification Examination. The CMA (AAMA) certification examination is offered via computer-based testing (CBT). Candidates whose applications are accepted will receive a Scheduling Permit containing instructions for making a testing appointment, and will be able to select locations and flexible testing times at Prometric test centers throughout the United States. To schedule examination appointments, candidates go to www.prometric.com and select a test center and appointment test time. Centers are open 9:00 am to 5:00 pm Monday through Saturday. An email confirming your appointment will be sent to you.

Photo identification is required for admission to the examination. Candidates are not permitted to bring any items except identification in the examination area. Candidates are allowed 3 hours and 15 minutes to complete the exam, which includes a 15 minute tutorial.

All exam candidates will receive an unofficial pass/fail result immediately upon completion of the exam. An official report of your scores will be mailed within 6 to 10 weeks after the exam date.

Certified Medical Assistant (AAMA) Recertification

All newly certified and recertifying CMAs (AAMA) will be current through the end of the calendar month of initial certification or most recent recertification for 60 months after initial certification or most recent recertification.

Recertification can be achieved either by reexamination or by the continuing education method. Recertification credits are evaluated on supportive documentation and on their relevancy to medical assisting as defined by the AAMA Medical Assistant Role Delineation Study or the Content Outline for the Certification/Recertification Examination.

A total of 60 points is necessary to recertify the CMA (AAMA) credential. A minimum of 10 points is required in each category: general, administrative, and clinical. The remaining 30 points can be accumulated in any of the three content areas or from any combination of the three categories. At least 30 of the required 60 recertification points must be accumulated from AAMA-approved **continuing education units (CEUs)**. If desired, all 60 points may be AAMA CEUs.

CMAs (AAMA) applying for recertification must also provide documentation of current cardiopulmonary resuscitation (CPR) certification for health care professionals or providers. Acceptable courses of CPR include the American Red Cross and the American Heart Association. The components of certification must include adult and pediatric CPR and obstructed airway training and Automated External Defibrillator (AED) instruction.

Applicants who accumulate all 60 points through AAMA CEUs, and in the correct content areas, can order a recertification over the telephone. Application fees still apply; however, an application form is not required. All CMAs employed or seeking employment must have current certified status to use the CMA (AAMA) credential.

Continuing education courses are offered by local, state, and national AAMA groups. Guided study programs are also available through AAMA's "Quest for Excellence" program. *CMA Today,* the official bimonthly publication of AAMA, provides articles designated for CEUs.

A CMA (AAMA) need not be a member of the AAMA nor currently employed to recertify. The entire recertification by continuing education instructions and application can be downloaded from AAMA's Web site (http://www.aama-ntl.org). Review of recertification applications can take up to 90 days. If all criteria are met, recertification is granted. The date that the application is postmarked to the AAMA Executive Office will be the date of recertification.

CRITICAL THINKING

You will graduate from a CAAHEP-accredited program in June and want to sit for the CMA examination the last Saturday of June (the same month in which you graduate). Go to the AAMA web site and determine when your application must be postmarked for acceptance for this test date.

On successfully passing the Certification Examination and earning the CMA (AAMA) credential, one should begin to document all CEUs earned. It is important to have the following information for CEU documentation:

- Complete date of the activity
- Sponsor (group or organization issuing the credit for the continuing education activity)
- Program title
- Amount and type of credit earned (e.g., CEU, CME, contact hour or college credit)
- Recertification points (AAMA CEUs or other credit)
- Points per content area (general, administrative, clinical)

On meeting recertification requirements, the applicants receives an identification card, which indicates the year of recertification and the expiration date.

AMERICAN MEDICAL TECHNOLOGISTS (AMT)

The American Medical Technologists (AMT) awards the registered medical assistant RMA (AMT) credential to individuals graduating from ABHES-accredited medical assisting programs who successfully pass their examination. ABHES is recognized by the U.S. Department of Education for accreditation of postsecondary schools offering traditional instruction as well as instruction by distance delivery.

The AMT also offers certification for the certified medical administrative specialist (CMAS). The CMAS (AMT) is employed primarily in the "administrative area" of provider clinics, or hospitals. They must understand and use medical terminology properly and be skilled in all administrative tasks performed in health care settings. Each individual state decides the scope of practice for the CMAS (AMT), with most states not requiring licensure.

Additional information regarding CMAS (AMT) education requirements, duties performed, working conditions, employment outlook, and estimated earnings can be found online at http://www.americanmedtech.org. Simply click on Certified Medical Administrative Specialist to access the information.

Registered Medical Assistant (AMT) Examination Format and Content

AMT certification examinations are intended to evaluate the competence of entry-level practitioners. The Education, Qualifications, and Standards Committee of American Medical Technologists develops registered medical assistant RMA (AMT) examinations. The medical assistant committee writes test questions and reviews questions submitted from other sources (e.g., instructors, experts, practitioners, and other individuals associated with the medical assistant profession). The medical assistant committee also determines certification requirements and addresses standard-setting issues related to the credential. Once test construction has been completed, the examination is reviewed and approved by the AMT Board of Directors.

The AMT registration examination consists of 200 to 210 four-option multiple-choice questions. Examinees are required to select the single best answer; multiple answers for a single item are scored as incorrect. Test questions may require examinees to recall facts, interpret graphic illustrations, interpret information presented in case studies, analyze situations, or solve problems. The approximate percentages of questions in content areas are as follows:

1. General Medical Assisting Knowledge—41.0%
   - Anatomy and physiology
   - Medical terminology
   - Medical law
   - Medical ethics
   - Human relations
   - Patient education
2. Administrative Medical Assisting—24.0%
   - Insurance
   - Financial bookkeeping
   - Medical secretarial-administrative medical assistant
3. Clinical Medical Assisting—35.0%
   - Asepsis
   - Sterilization
   - Instruments
   - Vital signs
   - Physical examinations
   - Clinical pharmacology
   - Minor surgery
   - Therapeutic modalities
   - Laboratory procedures
   - Electrocardiography
   - First aid

Registered Medical Assistant (AMT) Application Process

The following criteria have been established for applicants sitting for the RMA (AMT) examination:

1. Applicant shall be of good moral character and at least 18 years of age.
2. Applicant shall be a graduate of an accredited high school or acceptable equivalent.
3. Applicant must meet one of the following requirements:
   a. Applicant shall be a graduate of a(n):
      - Medical assisting program that holds programmatic accreditation by (or is in a postsecondary school or college that holds institutional accreditation by) the ABHES or the CAAHEP.

- Medical assisting program in a post-secondary school or college that has institutional accreditation by a Regional Accrediting Commission or by a national accrediting organization approved by the U.S. Department of Education. That program must include a minimum of 720 clock hours (or equivalent) of training in medical assisting skills (including a clinical practicum of no less than 160 hours).
- Formal medical services training program of the U.S. Armed Forces.

b. Applicant shall have been employed in the profession of medical assisting for a minimum of five years, no more than two years of which may have been as an instructor in a postsecondary medical assisting program.

4. Applicants applying under criteria 3 a or b *must* take and pass the AMT certification examination for RMA.

5. The AMT Board of Directors has further determined that applicants who have passed a generalist medical assistant certification examination offered by another medical assisting certification body (provided that examination has been approved for this purpose by the AMT Board of Directors), who have been working in the medical assisting field for the past 3 of 5 years, and who meet all other AMT training and experience requirements may be considered for RMA (AMT) certification without further examination.

Applications can be downloaded from AMT's Web site (http://www.americanmedtech.com) either in print and fill-in format or as online fill-in format. A useful handbook for the AMT candidate is available at http://www.americanmedtech.org/files/rma%20handbook.pdf.

Registered Medical Assistant (AMT) Examination Scheduling and Administration

All applications must be completed online or printed clearly except for the signatures required. All ancillary documentation must also be submitted (e.g., application fee; proof of high school graduation or equivalent; official final transcripts stating graduation from medical assistant school, college, or training program [with school seal affixed or notarized]).

When the AMT Registrar has received the application and all required information, an authorization letter containing a toll-free number is mailed to you. You can then contact Pearson Vue locations at http://www.pearsonvue.com/amt to schedule a date and time to take the examination. Two forms of valid identification are required, both bearing your signature and at least one bearing your photo. Photo identification is limited to a driver's license, state-issued identification card, military identification, or passport.

All AMT registration examination tests are available in paper-and-pencil format or in computerized formats at over 200 locations in the United States, its territories, and Canada. Tests can be scheduled daily except Sundays and holidays. Both formats are identical in length; however, experience has shown the computerized test takes less time to complete. Your computerized test score is displayed moments after you complete your test. A paper copy of your result letter is provided to you before you leave the testing center.

Registered Medical Assistant (AMT) Recertification

The AMT has established the Certification Continuation Program (CCP) for continuing education points. Certification will be suspended following a 30-day grace period if proper documentation is not submitted.

Each RMA (AMT) is required to accumulate 30 points, which must be turned in every 3 years for recertification. A Compliance Evaluation Worksheet and Attestation will be mailed close to the 3-year mark. This worksheet must be completed, signed, and returned to AMT by the due date. Retaking the RMA examination is not an option for reinstatement or recertification.

NATIONAL HEALTHCAREER ASSOCIATION (NHA)

The National Healthcareer Association (NHA) also offers national certification examinations for health care professionals. NHA works with educational institutions throughout the country on curriculum development, competency testing, and preparation and administration of their examination and offers a continuing education (CE) program. The NHA is dedicated to the following:

- Set guidelines for national certification competencies/standards
- Ensure a high level of performance among health care professionals
- Establish educational/continuing education requirements
- Adhere to the highest ethical standards

Certified Clinical Medical Assistant and Certified Medical Administrative Assistant Examination Format and Content

The NHA certifies the Certified Clinical Medical Assistant (CCMA) and the Certified Medical Administrative Assistant (CMAA) among other health career professions. Criteria for taking the NHA certification examinations include one of the following: The applicant must have a high school diploma and have recently successfully completed an NHA-approved training program, or the applicant must have either a high school diploma or equivalency and have recently worked in the field of certification for a minimum of 1 year as a full-time employee. Work experience must be documented in writing and signed by the director or employer.

The NHA offers several methods to help prepare candidates for their national certification examination. All students applying for NHA certification examination receive NHA Study Guides. Separate tests are taken for each healthcareer certification. The CCMA and the CMAA test is composed of multiple choice questions and takes approximately one and one-half hours to complete. The CMAA exam contains 100 questions and the CCMA contains 200 questions to complete.

The examination is offered in traditional pencil-and-paper formats or can be taken online at any of the specified approved locations. For details regarding testing, contact the NHA by telephone at 1-800-499-9092 or email them at info@nhanow.com or visit the Web site at http://www.nhanow.com. You will receive a confirmation notice of your seating including the date and location of the examination.

Certified Clinical Medical Assistant and Certified Medical Administrative Assistant Application Process

There are four ways to apply or register for the NHA national certification examination:

- Online using http://www.nhanow.com. Go directly to the secured registration page and submit the registration form using Visa, MasterCard, Discover, American Express, or school voucher.
- The registration form can be downloaded and printed. Once it is filled out completely, it can be mailed along with payment. Address and mail to:

  National Healthcareer Association

  7 Ridgedale Ave, Suite 203

  Cedar Knolls, NJ 07927
- The completed registration form can be faxed to NHA with credit card information or school voucher. The fax number is 1-973-644-4797.
- Telephone the Customer Service Department at 1-800-449-9092. You can then complete the registration over the phone. You will need your credit card number and expiration date or school voucher accessible for payment information.

Certified Clinical Medical Assistant and Certified Medical Administrative Assistant Examination Scheduling and Administration

The NHA examination can be scheduled at any of the specified approved locations:

- Training Schools/Colleges—Check with your school for details
- Testing Sites—Over 550 PSI/LaserGrade testing sites nationwide
- Experienced individuals can take examinations at their place of employment

NOTE: All examinations are required to have an exam proctor present.

Certified Clinical Medical Assistant and Certified Medical Administrative Assistant Recertification

NHA offers a Continuing Education (CE) Program to make the process of continuing education more convenient for the health care professional. Courses in this program can be taken at your convenience at home.

New industry standards require that each NHA-certified health care professional complete 10 CE credits every two years.

Currently there are thirty CE credits available online with two options for completing NHA CE credits:

Option 1: complete 5 online CE credits each year.

Option 2: complete 10 online CE credits every two years.

In the event that certification expires, reinstatement is permitted within one year of the expiration date. If reinstatement is initiated within one year of the expiration date, the individual must submit evidence of 15 completed CE credits, and pay a renewal and reinstatement fee. After one year from the expiration date, reinstatement is not permitted and the individual must apply and take the Certification Examination again to become recertified.

Applicants who pass the examination will be nationally certified as recognized by the NHA. They will receive a certification certificate suitable for framing and a wallet-size ID certification card containing their national certification number. CE credits will be reviewed by NHA, and a sticker to apply to the certification ID card will be mailed if the credits are accepted.

PROFESSIONAL ORGANIZATIONS

 Professional organizations have evolved to establish standards by which medical assistants and medical assisting programs are evaluated. Programs accredited by agencies must meet certain criteria, and students must pass national examinations to become certified. Medical assistants are not licensed and need not be certified to meet employment requirements; however, those certified are viewed as professionals with entry-level skills and a commitment to continued education.

American Association of Medical Assistants (AAMA)

 The AAMA was instrumental in defining the scope of training required for the profession and developed standards and guidelines by which programs could become accredited and the medical assistant credentialed. Membership in the AAMA offers many benefits, which include, but are not limited to, the following:

- Medical assisting news and health care information through the bimonthly magazine *CMA Today*
- CEUs for AAMA activities entered in the Continuing Education Registry and access to your transcript online
- Educational events provided by local chapters, state societies, and national meetings
- Answers to legal questions regarding job-related issues
- If eligible, application for the prestigious CMA examination at a reduced fee
- Discounts on car rentals, conventions, workshop and seminar fees, and self-study courses
- Opportunity to network with other practicing medical assistants

American Medical Technologists (AMT)

 The AMT is another nonprofit certification agency and professional membership association representing allied health care individuals. It certifies medical assistants by awarding the RMA (AMT) national credential to those candidates successfully satisfying requirements. AMT has many local chapters, 38 state societies, and a Uniform Services Committee. Each of these societies meets regularly and annually for a national convention.

AMT benefits and services include:

- Continuing education through the *Journal of Continuing Education Topics & Issues* published three times a year
- AMT's Institute for Education (AMTIE), which monitors continued education credits and sends a "report card" each year
- Four scholarships available to members who want to return to school and five scholarships for current students enrolled in allied health care programs
- State societies that offer opportunities for continued education, activities, and networking
- Peer recognition through AMT's prestigious RMA (AMT) credential
- Personal discount programs

National Healthcareer Association (NHA)

 The NHA serves as a reliable resource for up-to-date information on health career opportunities, training programs, education opportunities, and industry forecasts. The NHA newsletter *The NHA Today* is well respected and provides current trends, articles, and information regarding the health care field.

NHA benefits and services include:

- National certification
- Continuing education opportunities
- Collaboration with educational institutions in curriculum development and competency testing
- Annual Continuing Education Program
- Elite Membership Program that puts you in touch with a team of placement specialists to expand job opportunities

CASE STUDY 47-1

Refer to the scenario at the beginning of the chapter.

CASE STUDY REVIEW

1. Discuss the advantages of certification to the medical assistant.

2. Discuss the advantages of certification to the provider.

3. How does certification set a consistent minimum standard for evaluating professional competence as a medical assistant?

CASE STUDY 47-2

It is May, and Nancy McFarland, who graduated from an ABHES-accredited program 4.5 years ago, is beginning to research the procedures and requirements for taking the RMA examination. Nancy completed her internship at Inner City Health Care and was hired to work there full time (35 hours per week) when she graduated.

CASE STUDY REVIEW

1. If Nancy wants to take the examination in January, what is the procedure for applying?

2. Nancy is setting up a study schedule. She plans to review course textbooks and tests, purchase a study guide, and set up a study group. Develop a simple study schedule.

3. What criteria should Nancy use when asking people to join her study group?

SUMMARY

Many advantages for certification/recertification and registration have been discussed in this chapter. Although certification examinations are not legally required for practicing medical assistants, it is the goal of CAAHEP- and ABHES-accredited institutions to encourage graduates to sit for and maintain their credentials. Membership in the AAMA or in the AMT is also encouraged.

With nearly 400 local AAMA chapters and 51 affiliate state societies, there is the benefit of networking with others in the profession. As an information source for both professional and association issues, the executive staff at the AAMA's national headquarters is available to answer questions at a toll-free number (1-800-228-2262).

AMT currently has 38 chapters that meet regularly and allow networking with other RMA (AMT) practitioners plus other allied health professionals registered through the AMT, including phlebotomists, medical laboratory technicians, and dental assistants.

The NHA offers national certification examinations for CMAAs and CCMAs among other health care professionals. NHA offers CE programs and encourages recertification.

STUDY FOR SUCCESS

To reinforce your knowledge and skills of information presented in this chapter:

- Review the *Key Terms*
- Role-play with other students to apply attributes of professionalism pertinent to this chapter.
- Consider the *Case Studies* and discuss your conclusions
- Answer the questions in the *Certification Review*
- Apply your knowledge by completing the *Activities* in the *Study Guide* and the *Games and Quizzes* in the StudyWARE **StudyWARE** software on the *Premium Website*

Additional resources for this chapter include:

- Module 1 of the *Medical Assisting Learning Lab*
- *CourseMate for Delmar's Comprehensive Medical Assisting*
- *WebTutor for Delmar's Comprehensive Medical Assisting*

CERTIFICATION REVIEW

1. The goal and challenge of each graduating medical assistant should be to:
   a. find employment
   b. have a good benefit package
   c. possess entry-level skills
   d. earn the CMA/RMA credential and maintain it

2. The certification examination is:
   a. a comprehensive test based on tasks medical assistants perform daily
   b. all true/false questions
   c. developed by the AMTIE
   d. developed by the NBME

3. Benefits of membership in a professional organization such as AAMA or AMT include all of the following *except:*
   a. discounted rates on legal representation
   b. legal advice
   c. nationwide networking opportunities
   d. professional journal publications

4. Recertification of the CMA (AAMA) credential options include:
   a. submit work experience
   b. reexamination or CEU method
   c. submit on-the-job training
   d. submit military training

5. To keep the RMA (AMT) credential current, an individual must earn:
   a. 10 credits every two years
   b. 30 points every three years
   c. 30 points every five years
   d. 60 points every five years

6. The RMA was established by the:
   a. ABHES
   b. CAAHEP
   c. AMT
   d. AAMA

7. The NHA offers medical assisting certification for which of the following?
   a. CMA
   b. RMA
   c. CCMA and CMAA
   d. CMAS

8. RMA examinations:
   a. are offered at Pearson Vue locations
   b. are offered twice a year
   c. are offered three times a year
   d. are offered six times a year

9. Only graduates of CAAHEP- and ABHES-accredited medical assisting programs may sit for which credential(s):
   a. CCMA
   b. CMAS
   c. CMA (AAMA)
   d. CMAA

10. To retain certification, industry standards require that each NHA-certified health care professional complete:
    a. 10 credits every two years
    b. 30 points every three years
    c. 30 points every five years
    d. 10 credits every five years

REFERENCES/BIBLIOGRAPHY

American Association of Medical Assistants. (2013). *AAMA certification/recertification examination for medical assistants.* Retrieved January 7, 2013, from http://www.aama-ntl.org

American Association of Medical Assistants. (n.d.). FAQs *on* CMA (AAMA) *certification.* Retrieved January 7, 2013, from http://www.aama-ntl.org

American Medical Technologists. (n.d.). Certifying Excellence in Allied Health, retrieved January 7, 2013, from http://www.americanmedtech.org

National Healthcareer Association. (n.d.). NHA *national certification examination.* Retrieved January 7, 2013, from http://www.NHAnow.com

Simmers, L. (2004). *Diversified health occupations* (6th ed.). Clifton Park: NY: Delmar Cengage Learning.

OUTLINE

Developing a Strategy
  Attitude and Mindset
  Self-Assessment
Job Search Analysis and
  Research
Social Media in Your Job
  Search
Résumé Preparation
  Résumé Specifications
  Clear and Concise Résumés
  Accomplishments

References
  Accuracy
  Résumé Styles
  Vital Résumé Information
Application/Cover Letters
Completing the Application
  Form
The Interview Process
  The Look of Success
  Preparing for the Interview
  The Actual Interview

Interviewing the Employer
  Closing the Interview
Interview Follow-Up
  Follow-Up Letter
  Follow Up by Telephone
After You Are Employed
  Dealing with Difficult People
  Getting a Raise
Professionalism

LEARNING OUTCOMES

1. Define, spell, and pronounce the key terms as presented in the glossary.
2. List the steps involved in job analysis and research.
3. Describe a contact tracker and its usefulness.
4. Give three examples of accomplishment statements.
5. Differentiate chronologic, functional, targeted, and online résumés.

6. Identify the purpose and content of a cover letter.
7. Demonstrate effective ways to anticipate and respond to an interviewer's questions.
8. Describe appropriate overall appearance and dress for an interview.
9. Identify the benefits of writing a follow-up letter.
10. Analyze the professionalism questions and apply them to this chapter's content.

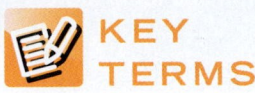

KEY TERMS

accomplishment statements

application/ cover letter

application form

benefits

bullet point

career objective

chronologic résumé

contact tracker

direct skills

e-résumé

functional résumé

internet blogs

interview

keywords

power verbs

references

résumé

targeted résumé

transferable skills

ATTRIBUTES OF PROFESSIONALISM

Communication
- Did you introduce yourself?
- Did you provide appropriate responses/feedback?
- Did you display appropriate body language?
- Did you respond honestly and diplomatically?
- Did you apply active listening skills?
- Did you demonstrate awareness of how an individual's personal appearance affects anticipated responses?
- Does your knowledge allow you to speak easily with all members of the health care team?
- Did you maintain eye contact during the communication?
- Did you refrain from sharing your personal experiences?

Presentation
- Were you dressed and groomed appropriately?
- Were you courteous, patient, and respectful?
- Did you display a positive attitude?
- Did you display a calm, professional, and caring manner?

Competency
- Did you pay attention to detail?
- Did you ask questions if you were out of your comfort zone or did not have the experience to carry out tasks?
- Did you display sound judgment?
- Were you knowledgeable and accountable?

Initiative
- Did you show initiative?
- Did you develop a strategic plan to achieve your goals? Was your plan realistic?
- Did you seek out opportunities to expand your knowledge base?
- Were you flexible and dependable?
- Were you respectful of others?

Integrity
- Did you demonstrate respect for individual diversity?
- Did you maintain your moral and ethical standards?
- Did you do the "right thing" even when no one was observing?

SCENARIO

Eun Mee Soo, RMA (AMT), is a graduate of an accredited medical assisting program and recently passed the certification examination. While attending school, Eun Mee was employed part-time as a sales representative in one of the city's prestigious clothing stores. She has no medical work experience except her practicum at Inner City Health Care. She is now preparing her résumé

and beginning her job search. Eun Mee plans to move out of state (she always dreamed of moving north), so she will also be looking for a new apartment. All of these changes are a bit unsettling for Eun Mee. She is beginning to wonder if she should defer relocating at this time and stay close to home until she feels more secure.

INTRODUCTION

So you are about to graduate from the medical assistant program! This time is often unsettling because many changes are occurring. The loss of security the classroom environment provided, the loss of contact with fellow classmates, and the loss of a structured schedule are just a few changes. Questions such as: Am I ready for my first job? How do I find a job? What do I say at the interview? begin to surface.

The focus on employment may represent apprehension and doubt or be sparked with anticipation and a sense of fulfillment. This chapter provides direction and answers some of the questions related to the job search.

DEVELOPING A STRATEGY

 It is best to begin developing your job search strategy early in your training as a medical assistant. If you have not started this phase, determine to begin today.

The first step in developing a strategy is to look at reality. You and maybe a hundred other medical assistants may be applying for the same job position. How are *you* different from every other person applying for this job? The following sections will help make *you* stand out, be different, and hopefully be successful in your job search.

Attitude and Mindset

One important quality an employer looks for in employees is their attitude. Your attitude is not something you turn on and off or learn in school. It is the result of your innate personality combined with the events that mold you during your life. Your instructors and acquaintances have a significant impact over who you are. Your attitude is reflected by how you react to:

1. Taking direction
2. Seeking excellence or doing just enough to get by
3. Meeting your employer's needs, not just looking forward to payday

4. Assuming responsibility for your actions versus considering your problems to be someone else's fault

If you find yourself having a negative attitude in any of the ways mentioned in the preceding list, you need to make an effort to change while you are still in training. An employer will zero in on a negative attitude and eliminate you as a candidate almost immediately. While your formal training is important and you can be retrained to do things the way a new employer desires, your attitude takes time to change and requires a willingness to make the change. Develop a strategy to evolve a positive attitude while you are still in school because this is a time when you will have professional guidance and resources, as well as excellent role models.

SPOTLIGHT ON CERTIFICATION

RMA Content Outline
- Medical law
- Human relations
- Oral and written communications

CMA (AAMA) Content Outline
- Displaying professional attitude
- Job readiness and seeking employment
- Professional communication and behavior
- Medicolegal guidelines and requirements

CMAS Content Outline
- Legal and ethical considerations
- Professionalism
- Communication

Beyond a positive attitude, being successful in your search for a job requires positive thinking on your part. There is a good position out there for you. Finding it is your first job. Those individuals who are successful at finding that first job devote many hours per week at job strategy tactics. You should not become discouraged by rejection but learn from it and apply what you have learned to the next interview opportunity.

Self-Assessment

As you begin your job search campaign, you should identify what you want in a job. It is always better to do work you enjoy in the type of practice you find most interesting. Take a moment now to complete the self-evaluation work sheet shown in Figure 48-1. When you have finished, you will have some idea of the type of practice you would like

---

SELF-EVALUATION WORK SHEET

Respond to the following questions honestly and sincerely. They are meant to assist you in self-assessment.

1. List your three strongest attributes as related to people, data, or things.

    i.e., Interpersonal skills related to people

    Accuracy related to data

    Mechanical ability related to things

    _____ related to _____

    _____ related to _____

    _____ related to _____

2. List your three weakest attributes as related to people, data, or things.

    _____ related to _____

    _____ related to _____

    _____ related to _____

3. How do you express yourself? Excellent, Good, Fair, Poor

    Orally _____ In writing _____

4. Do you work well as a leader of a group or team? Yes _____ No _____

5. Do you prefer to work alone? Yes _____ No _____

6. Can you work under stress/pressure? Yes _____ No _____

7. Do you enjoy new ideas and situations? Yes _____ No _____

8. Are you comfortable with routines/schedules? Yes _____ No _____

9. Which work environment do you prefer?

    Single-provider setting _____   Multiple-provider setting _____

    Small clinic setting _____   Large clinic setting _____

10. Which type of practice do you prefer?

    Pediatrics _____   Obstetrics/Gynecology _____

    Geriatrics _____   General Medicine _____

    Internal Medicine _____   Other _____

11. Which work setting do you prefer?

    Front office (reception) _____   Back office (assisting provider) _____

    Laboratory (phlebotomy) _____   Administrative (coding/billing) _____

© Cengage Learning 2014

Figure 48-1 Self-evaluation work sheets can help determine a person's strengths, weaknesses, and preferences before a job search begins.

to work in and what position you would find most satisfying.

Before you begin a self-assessment, review what a medical assistant does, determine what level pay can be expected, and compare that with your personal skills and financial requirements. In some practices you may specialize in administrative or clinical duties; in others you may be expected to function in both specialties.

A medical assistant is salaried, with yearly earnings varying between $20,810 and $40,190, inflation adjusted to 2010. Entry-level salaries will be closer to the lower figure but will vary depending on credentials, practicum performance, and geographic location. Medical assistants who can show proficiency in both administrative and clinical capability command higher salaries in some medical settings.

As part of the self-assessment you should evaluate what direct and transferable skills you have that will make you a contributing member of the medical team. **Direct skills** are the medical procedures you have acquired in school and in which you are proficient. **Transferable skills** are those skills that would be useful in a wide variety of professions and may have been perfected during the education process or learned in other employment settings. Leadership, communication, writing, computer literacy, keyboarding, linguistics, and spelling are some examples of transferable skills. List your personal direct and transferable skills on paper now.

When you have completed this portion of the self-assessment, you will be in a better position to determine what type of job to seek. You will also have identified the skills that you can highlight as you prepare your application/cover letter and résumé.

The final part of your self-assessment is conducting a budgetary needs analysis to determine how much income you need to make per month to meet your living expenses.

The budgetary analysis should include a list of the **benefits** you find necessary, such as medical, dental, and vision insurance; a 401k program; and stock options. You also might need to consider work schedule, location/travel, and child care leave policies.

To accomplish this, begin to keep a diary of all purchases and payments. By reviewing your checkbook register and credit card statements, you should be able to itemize basic expenditures, such as rent, utilities, payments (car, credit card), food, clothing, insurance, and taxes. Once a monthly expenditure record is established, the amount of money needed to meet living expenses can be calculated.

JOB SEARCH ANALYSIS AND RESEARCH

The job analysis and research phase of your job search should start before graduation. Telephoning or visiting various clinics and asking questions to determine what the duties of a medical assistant are in different types of practices will help to further clarify where you would like to work and will help you become acquainted with a potential employer or identify a possible site for practicum experience. If you visit the facility, dress appropriately, just as you would for an interview. You want to impress the clinic personnel just as if it were a formal interview. Remember to send a letter thanking the person taking time on the telephone or authorizing the visit.

Based on the self-assessment you completed and the preliminary job analysis, you know what type of clinic or practice you want to work in, so now is the time to compile a list of potential employers in the geographic area where you want to work. Begin your job search by networking with students who have graduated before you and are successfully employed. Networking via social media is becoming another important job search resource and should be investigated thoroughly. Statistics tell us that 80% of positions are filled through networking contacts. Next compile a list from the Yellow Pages, Job Expositions, the Internet, Want Ads, for your specialty in the local papers, American Association of Medical Assistants (AAMA) or American Medical Technologists (AMT) publications, and contacts acquired through attending state and local meetings. Other sources are your program director and instructors and the network of contacts at the site where you did your practicum. A practicum site is frequently your best prospect for employment because they will know your capabilities and your attitude and have expended time and resources in your training. If the site is hiring and you performed well, experience has shown that most sites will frequently hire the intern.

Candidate job sites can also be found through employment agencies. These agencies usually charge a fee, although sometimes the employer pays the fee. Extreme caution should be exercised in dealing with agencies because fees are sometimes excessive. Fees should only be paid after successfully obtaining a job and never for getting an interview.

Prioritize the list based on your assessment of chances of employment. Sites where you have personal contacts or where you have done your practicum should be at the top of the list, with sites

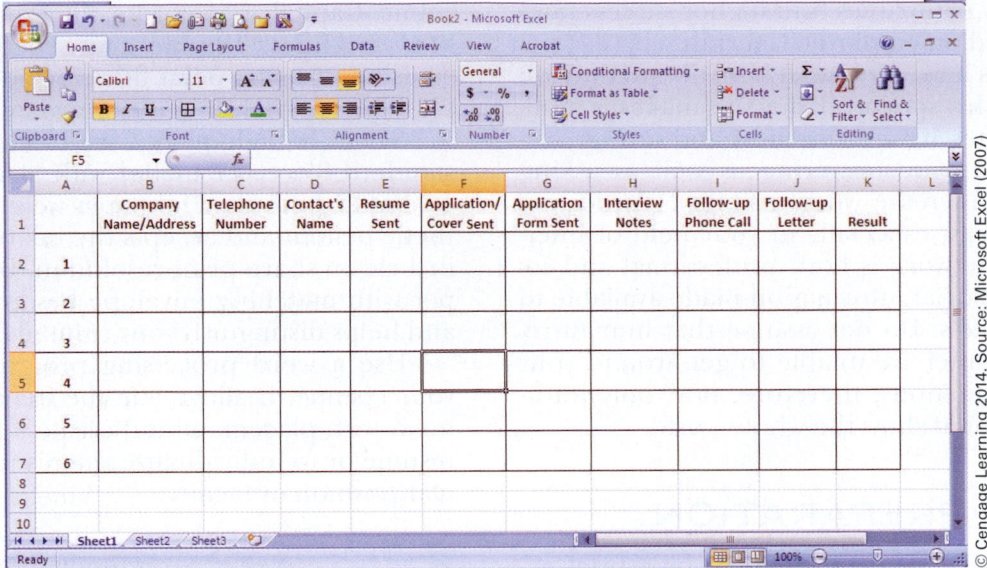

Figure 48-2 A simple contact tracker such as this can help organize all communication you have with potential employers.

advertising for help wanted next. Further down the list should be sites that, in sales parlance, would be called cold prospecting. You can further prioritize the list by putting your personal choices at the top each category.

Now is the time to complete detailed homework or research on each prospective employer. Start collecting information on each prospective site, identifying their services, policies, fees and insurance protocol, hours of service, number of providers, and very importantly their mission statement and philosophy of practice criteria. Brochures may be available in their clinics, on the Internet, and in wellness publications for patients. Pamphlets on new procedures are other sources of this information. You can use this information to prepare the cover letter for your résumé and to brief yourself should you be invited for an interview.

As part of a serious job search, you should contact many individuals and will need some means of recording the contacts, their responses, and your actions. Figure 48-2 shows a helpful sample **contact tracker**. It should be used to prevent confusion and to keep track of valuable information and action items.

SOCIAL MEDIA IN YOUR JOB SEARCH

Social networking is a powerful tool in searching for employment because it permits networking, the most effective means of finding a job today. The most effective strategy is to go to one of the social and professional sites listed in Table 48-1 and prepare your profile. Following this you will search for jobs in your field and persons in your field of interest and then narrow the search to the target geographic area. You will build a network of contacts, but attempt to limit them to people you know or have something in common with such as school or other outside interests. In doing this you present your credentials while developing contacts to help locate openings which may never be advertised,

Table 48-1 Top Social Media Sites for Job Search

- LinkedIn—a directory of professionals and companies
- Facebook—more of a social network, but includes professional data as well
- KODA—a hybrid between LinkedIn and Facebook
- Twitter—a social network and microblogging site using instant messaging
- MySpace—a social networking site similar to Facebook
- Ning—a social network created to customize networks on any subject

© Cengage Learning 2014

because many companies find higher success rates in hiring based on employee referrals.

Some sites have a job search section to find job listings. Use this section if the site makes it available. Some sites have a question and answer section. Participate in answering as well as asking questions to increase your visibility. Participate in **Internet blogs**, especially in your field of interest. When a network is both professional and social, limit the social information made available to business contacts. Do not assume that human resources personnel are unable to get around your site access limitations; therefore, post only information you would show the whole world.

RÉSUMÉ PREPARATION

A **résumé** is a summary data sheet or a brief account of your qualifications and progress in the career you have chosen and should include both direct and transferable skills. The purpose of your résumé is to sell you. It provides an opportunity to describe your education, what you have done, and what you can do, and it lists those who can vouch for your integrity and experience. A résumé that is well thought out and written in such a way as to create interest in what you have to contribute to the employer may reward you with many interviews. During the interview your résumé serves as a reference from which the interviewer may be prompted to ask questions.

Résumé Specifications

The résumé should be limited to one page in length whenever possible. One-page résumés work well if you have less than ten years of experience, or when pursuing a radical change in your career and your experience is not related to your new goal. However, today's trend finds the two-page résumé just as acceptable. Experienced job seekers may discover the one-page résumé limits their ability to share valuable skills and work experience with a prospective employer.

Each page should contain your name and the page number. Keep a 1- to 1½-inch margin on all four sides of the page to create a picture-like

Copy or design your own contact tracker form and document all pertinent information regarding your job search contacts.

frame. Capitalize major headings and single space between lines. Double space between sections. The use of **bullet point** lists instead of paragraphs aids the interviewer in gleaning key points quickly.

Select a high-quality bond stationery that is standard 8½ × 11 inches with a weight between 16 and 25 pounds. This paper weight provides aesthetic benefit and accepts the ink better, resulting in a clean, sharp print resolution. Buff or ivory paper with matching envelope has great eye appeal and helps distinguish your résumé from others.

Use a word processing program to produce your résumé. It allows you the freedom to experiment with placement and create a picture-perfect résumé or to individualize the résumé for a particular position or facility.

Clear and Concise Résumés

Your résumé must be concise and easy to read and understand. Use statements that are positive, reflect confidence, and portray you as a problem solver. Be sure that any information given within your résumé or application form is not misleading or exaggerated. Leave out the word *I* when writing your résumé. This is your personal résumé, and it is understood that you are referring to yourself.

Accomplishments

Use **accomplishment statements** if you have them from your practicum or work experience. Accomplishment statements begin with power verbs and give a brief description of what you did and the demonstrable results that were produced. Figure 48-3 provides a list of sample **power verbs**. Some accomplishment statement examples are "Utilized computer skills to schedule and reschedule patient appointments" and "Demonstrated skills in setting up sterile trays and assisting with sterile procedures."

References

Select a variety of **references** to be included with your résumé. References should be listed on a separate sheet of paper that matches your résumé. Remember to include the same letterhead as on your résumé on the references page. An individual who knows you or has worked with you long enough to make an honest assessment and recommendation regarding your background history is an excellent reference person. Use only nonrelated persons as

Accompanied	Composed	Engineered	Integrated	Overcame	Relayed
Accumulated	Computed	Entertained	Interpreted	Packaged	Renewed
Achieved	Conducted	Enumerated	Interviewed	Packed	Reorganized
Acquired	Conferred	Established	Introduced	Paid	Repaired
Administered	Constructed	Estimated	Inspected	Participated	Replaced
Admitted	Consulted	Evaluated	Inventoried	Patrolled	Reported
Advised	Contacted	Examined	Investigated	Perfected	Requested
Allowed	Contracted	Exchanged	Invoiced	Piloted	Researched
Analyzed	Contrasted	Exhibited	Issued	Placed	Responsible for
Answered	Contributed	Expanded	Judged	Planned	Retrieved
Applied	Controlled	Expedited	Justified	Posted	Revised
Appointed	Converted	Experienced	Kept	Prepared	Routed
Appraised	Convinced	Fabricated	Learned	Prescribed	Scheduled
Arranged	Coordinated	Facilitated	Lectured	Presented	Secured
Assembled	Copied	Figured	Led	Priced	Selected
Assessed	Corrected	Filled	Licensed	Printed	Sent
Assigned	Corresponded	Financed	Listed	Processed	Separated
Attached	Counseled	Finished	Listened	Procured	Served as
Attained	Created	Fitted	Loaded	Produced	Serviced
Attended	Debated	Fixed	Located	Programmed	Set up
Authorized	Decided	Formalized	Logged	Promoted	Showed
Balanced	Delegated	Formulated	Mailed	Prompted	Sold
Billed	Delivered	Fulfilled	Maintained	Proofread	Solicited
Bought	Demonstrated	Generated	Managed	Proposed	Sorted
Budgeted	Deposited	Graded	Manufactured	Proved	Stocked
Built	Described	Graphed	Marked	Provided	Stored
Calculated	Detailed	Greeted	Marketed	Published	Straightened
Cashed	Determined	Headed	Measured	Purchased	Summarized
Catalogued	Developed	Hired	Met	Ran	Supervised
Changed	Devised	Identified	Modified	Rated	Supplied
Charged	Diagnosed	Implemented	Monitored	Read	Taught
Charted	Directed	Improved	Motivated	Rearranged	Telephoned
Classified	Discovered	Improvised	Negotiated	Rebuilt	Tested
Cleaned	Dismantled	Increased	Nominated	Recalled	Trained
Cleared	Dispatched	Indexed	Noted	Received	Transferred
Closed	Distributed	Indicated	Notified	Recommended	Transported
Coded	Documented	Influenced	Observed	Reconciled	Typed
Collated	Drew	Informed	Obtained	Recorded	Verified
Collected	Drove	Initiated	Opened	Reduced	
Commanded	Earned	Inspected	Operated	Referred	
Communicated	Educated	Installed	Ordered	Registered	
Compiled	Employed	Instructed	Organized	Regulated	
Completed	Encouraged	Insured	Outlined	Related	

Figure 48-3   These sample power verbs may help you define your previous job responsibilities.

references unless the work relationship has been formalized.

Choose references who are well respected and are clear speakers and writers. No matter how much someone likes you and your work, they may not be helpful to you if they cannot convey the information in a business-like manner. Professional references such as a former instructor, provider, practicum supervisor, or fellow coworker are excellent choices.

Always ask permission to use someone as a reference *before* the name is printed on the reference list. Verify the correct spelling of the reference's name, title, place of employment and position, and telephone number for prospective employers.

Help your references aid you in obtaining an interview and employment. A personal visit or telephone call to discuss your career objectives and how you plan to conduct your job search will be helpful. Ask for any suggestions they may have to offer. Provide them with a copy of your résumé and cover letter. This helps them visualize the position for which you are applying and picture how you may benefit that employer.

Keep in touch with references. Check back to see who has called and how things went. Knowing what employers ask may produce some valuable pointers for your next letter, résumé, or interview.

Finally, thank your references. They will appreciate knowing how you are doing and that you value their assistance.

Leave out "References Upon Request" if necessary to shorten your résumé to save space. Employers know they can ask for references at a later date.

Accuracy

Proofread, proofread, and proofread your résumé. Ask someone who is a good speller or one of your references to edit your résumé. Then proofread it again yourself. Do not rely on your computer spell check; it does not differentiate between words such as *to, too,* and *two* or *here* and *hear.* Eliminate repetition of information such as task descriptions. Summarize employment before 10 years ago or leave it off entirely if not relevant to the position you are seeking.

Résumé Styles

Various résumé styles have been developed, each having specific advantages and disadvantages. Choose the style or combination of styles that best describes your strengths and ability to do the job. It may be advantageous to check with the human resources department of the facility to which you are applying to determine if they have a résumé style preference.

Chronologic Résumé. Your **chronologic résumé** should be organized so that the most important information you want to share is the first thing the reader sees. If your job experience is your greatest asset and may set you apart from other applicants, put your work history and job skills first. If your education and training is your best professional feature, put your education and training first. Some medical managers and human resources directors take only 10 seconds to scan a résumé. You want them to see clearly and quickly what you have to offer.

The chronologic résumé is advantageous when:

- The position is in a highly traditional field, such as teaching, law, or health care, where specific employers are of paramount interest
- You are staying in the same field as prior jobs
- Job history shows real growth and development
- Prior titles are impressive

The chronologic résumé is *not* advantageous when:

- Your work history is spotty
- You are changing career goals
- You have been in the same job for many years
- You are looking for your first job

Figure 48-4 illustrates a chronologic résumé.

Functional Résumé. The **functional résumé** highlights specialty areas of accomplishment and strengths. It allows you to organize them in an order that supports your work objective.

The functional résumé is advantageous when:

- Your experience can be sorted into areas of function, i.e., administrative, clinical, supervisory
- You are changing careers
- You are reentering the job market after an absence
- Your career path or growth is not clear from a chronologic listing
- You have had a variety of different, apparently unconnected work experiences
- Much of your work has been volunteer, freelance, or temporary
- You want to eliminate repetition of descriptions of job duties
- You have extensive specialized experience

The functional résumé is *not* advantageous when:

- You want to emphasize a management growth pattern

ASHLEY JACKSON, CMA (AAMA)
2031 Craig Street ~ Renton, Washington 98055

Work: 206-878-1545   Cell: 206-835-9879
Home: 253-838-6690   email: asjack@pinetree.com

WORK EXPERIENCE

September, 20XX–Present   GROUP HEALTH COOPERATIVE
Directed support for a dermatology/surgery practice.
Patient preparation.
Medical and surgical asepsis.
Assist with sterile procedures.
Patient follow-up.

June, 20XX–August, 20XX   VALLEY INTERNAL MEDICINE
Clinical responsibilities.
Assisted with surgeries in ambulatory care setting.
Patient preparation.
Medical and surgical asepsis.
Assisted with sterile procedures.

March, 20XX–June, 20XX   VALLEY INTERNAL MEDICINE
Medical Assistant Practicum
Administrative duties and clinical responsibilities utilizing all medical assisting skills, including patient induction, chief complaint, vital
signs, patient preparation, EKGs, medical and surgical asepsis, and
sterile procedures.

EDUCATION/CERTIFICATION

Associate in Applied Science degree, June, 20XX, Highline Community College,
Des Moines, Washington, 98198-9800.

Certified Medical Assistant (AAMA), June, 20XX.

© Cengage Learning 2014

Figure 48-4 Sample chronologic résumé.

- Your most recent employers are highly prestigious and the specific employers are of paramount interest

A sample of a functional résumé for a person
reentering the job market is shown in Figure 48-5.

Targeted Résumé. The **targeted résumé** is best
for focusing on a clear, specific job target. It
should contain a **career objective** and list your
skills, capabilities, and any supporting accomplishments related to that objective. This résumé
style enables graduating students to list classes
related to their career objective, grade point average, student awards, and achievements. This information adds substance to a résumé when work

experience is minimal and should be at the beginning of the résumé because it is your most significant asset.

The targeted résumé is advantageous when:

- You are very clear about your job target.

- You have had a variety of experiences that appear unrelated to each other but that include
skills that you can use in a skills list related to
your job target.

- You can go in several directions and want a different résumé for each.

- You are just starting your career and have little
experience but know what you want, and are
clear about your capabilities.

JOAN BISHOP, RMA (AMT)
4320 Sprig Street
Renton, Washington 98055

Work: 206-878-1545   Cell: 206-835-9879
Home: 253-838-6690   email: jbishop@abc.net

TEACHING:

Instructed community groups on issues related to child abuse.

Taught volunteers how to set up community program for victims of domestic violence.

Conducted workshops for parents of abused children.

Instructed public school teachers on signs and symptoms of potential and actual child abuse.

COUNSELING:

Consulted with parents for probable child abuse and suggested courses of action.

Worked with social workers on individual cases, in both urban and suburban settings.

Counseled single parents on appropriate coping behaviors.

Handled pre-take interviewing of many individual abused children.

ORGANIZATION/COORDINATION:

Coordinated transition of children between original home and foster home.

Served as liaison between community health agencies and schools.

Wrote proposal to state for county funds to educate single parents and teachers.

WORK HISTORY:

20XX–20XX   Community Mental Health Center, Tacoma, Washington
Volunteer Coordinator—Child Abuse Program

20XX–20XX   C.A.R.E.—Child-Abuse Rescue-Education, Trenton, New Jersey
County Representative

EDUCATION:

20XX   B.S. Sociology, Douglass College, New Brunswick, New Jersey

© Cengage Learning 2014

Figure 48-5   Sample functional résumé. This style is useful for a person reentering the job market.

- You are able to keep your résumé on a flash drive.

  The targeted résumé is *not* advantageous when:

- You want to use one résumé for several different applications.

- You are not clear about your abilities and accomplishments.

Figure 48-6 and Figure 48-7 show samples of targeted résumés.

Online Résumé. Job searches more frequently will be conducted online using applications (e-applications) from the Web site of the organization selected by the applicant, or on a social networking site in the form of a personal profile. All of the admonishments in the previous paragraphs regarding content, spelling, accuracy, and clarity apply online. The items that are most important with an online application are the need to develop an exciting presentation and brevity. If you do not catch the eye of the reviewer within the first few

ASHLEY JACKSON, CMA (AAMA)
2031 Craig Street ~ Renton, Washington 98055

Work: 206-878-1545   Cell: 206-835-9879
Home: 253-838-6690   email: asjack@pinetree.com

CAREER OBJECTIVES: To obtain a position as a medical assistant in an ambulatory care/surgery facility that allows use and development of clinical skills.

ACHIEVEMENTS:
Certified Medical Assistant.
Graduate of an Accredited Medical Assistant Program accredited by the Commission on Accreditation of Allied Health Education Programs (CAAHEP).
Experienced in providing assistance with surgeries in an ambulatory care setting.
Excellent communication and interpersonal skills.

SKILLS AND CAPABILITIES:
Post-surgery patient follow-up.
Patient induction.
Vital signs.
Patient preparation.
EKGs.
Medical and surgical asepsis.
Sterile procedures.

WORK HISTORY:

September, 20XX to present	Group Health Cooperative, Seattle, WA Surgical Medical Assistant.
June, 20XX–August, 20XX	Valley Internal Medicine, Renton, WA Clinical Medical Assistant.
March 20XX–June, 20XX	Valley Internal Medicine, Renton, WA Practicum Student/Trainee.

EDUCATION/CERTIFICATION:
Associate in Applied Science Degree, Highline Community College.
Certified Medical Assistant (AAMA).

AFFILIATIONS:
American Association of Medical Assistants.

© Cengage Learning 2014

Figure 48-6 Sample targeted résumé. This style is useful when focusing on a specific job target.

sentences, the submission or posting is likely to be a waste of time; therefore, careful selection of words in your self-description is critical.

E-Résumé. An electronic résumé, also known as an **e-résumé**, is electronically delivered via email, submitted to Internet job boards, or placed on Web pages. When employers post jobs on their own Web sites, they generally expect job seekers to respond electronically.

Special care must be taken when preparing the e-résumé because many employers place résumés directly into searchable databases. The following points should be considered:

- Formatting must be removed before the résumé can be placed in a database. Submitting a formatted résumé may cause it to be eliminated.
- Submit a text résumé, also known as a text-based résumé, plain-text résumé, or ASCII text résumé. These variations are preferred when submitting résumés electronically.

Ashley Jackson, CMA (AAMA)
1321 Craig Street
Renton, Washington 98055
(253) 838-6690
Cell (206) 835-9879
Asjackson@pinetree.com

Professional Profile

Eager to utilize my medical assisting knowledge and skills in an ambulatory/surgery facility that allows further development of clinical skills.
- Dedicated to meeting the needs of individual patients at their level of need.
- Committed team member approach to care delivered to patients.

What People Say:

"Ashley's positive attitude is a strong asset as it helps guide her actions, thoughts, and words. Ashley uses her strong knowledge base to make critical thinking choices."
   Stephanie Young, CMA (AAMA)
   Group Health Cooperative

"Ashley builds strong relationships with her co-workers, supervisors, providers, and patients. She shows interest in their lives and models respect, kindness, and empathy. She truly cares about people."
   Martha Marshall, RN
   Valley Internal Medicine

"Ashley's clinical critical thinking skills are excellent. She is competent and works well with others to see that quality care is provided to each patient in an efficient and timely manner."
   Donald Blackburn, PA
   Valley Internal Medicine

Education, Honors, and Certification

Associate in Applied Science
Highline Community College, Des Moines, Washington
Overall GPA: 3.9
Dean's List
Current Red Cross First Aid and CPR cards
Certified Medical Assistant, (AAMA)
President SeaTac Chapter of AAMA

Work Experience

Group Health Cooperative Seattle, Washington
September, 20XX to present
- Post-surgery patient follow-up
- Patient induction
- Vital signs
- Patient preparation
- EKGs
- Medical and surgical asepsis
- Sterile procedures

Valley Internal Medical, Renton, Washington
June, 20XX to August, 2011
- EKGs
- Patient preparation
- Medical and surgical asepsis
- Surgical Procedures

© Cengage Learning 2014

Figure 48-7 Sample targeted résumé. This style is useful when focusing on a specific job target.

- The e-résumé is not visually appealing. Eye appeal is not required because its main purpose is to be placed into one of the keyword-searchable databases.
- The text résumé is not vulnerable to viruses and is compatible across computer programs and platforms.

- The text résumé is versatile and can be used for:
  - Posting on job boards
  - Pasting piece-by-piece into the profile forms of job boards, such as Monster.com
  - Pasting into the body of an email to be sent to prospective employers

- Converting to a Web-based HTML résumé
- Sending as an attachment to prospective employers
- Conversion to a scannable résumé

Employers are often inundated with résumés from job seekers each time they advertise a position opening. Therefore, in an effort to save time and to determine the best-qualified candidates for the position, employers digitize the résumés to create an electronic résumé. Using software to search for specific **keywords** that relate to the position, the numbers of candidates can quickly be narrowed. If you apply for a job with a company that searches databases for keywords and your résumé does not conform, you may not be considered for the position.

How do you determine keywords? Begin scrutinizing employment ads and list keywords repeatedly mentioned in association with jobs that interest you. Nouns that relate to the skills and experience the employer is looking for will quickly surface. Keywords may include:

- Job-specific skills/profession-specific words (e.g., specialty experience, bilingual, scheduling, data entry, insurance verification, telephone and communication skills, laboratory/X-ray experience)
- Technologic terms and descriptions of technical expertise (including hardware and software in which you are proficient, e.g., PRISM, DEXA experience)
- Job titles, certifications (e.g., RMA, CMA [AAMA], RMA [AMT], CMAS)
- Types of degrees, names of colleges (e.g., AAS, BA)
- Awards received, professional organization memberships (e.g., Dean's list, scholarships, certificates, AAMA or AMT member)

Keywords should be used throughout the résumé, but they should be front loaded. Front loaded means to use as many keywords as possible in the first 100 words of the résumé. A good goal is to aim for 25 to 35 keywords. This may be achieved by using synonyms, various forms of the keyword, and using both the spelled-out and acronym versions of common terms. If a person reviews the résumé, he or she will see enough keywords to process it through the software search.

Social Network Personal Profile.

The first thing you will do after selecting a social media site is to prepare a personal profile. It is the key to being found by a potential employer. LinkedIn and some other sites allow you to have a professional headline that is an eye-catching way of drawing attention to you up front. As an example, "Medical Assistant" is common and does not separate you from the other job seekers. A more exciting and enticing headline might be "Patient Friendly & Proactive Paraprofessional." The headline should draw a favorable picture in the mind of the reviewer. Truthful creativity is an important factor in preparing a headline for your profile. Caution—some sites automatically list your job title. Edit the line to something more exciting and eye-catching.

The personal profile will contain a tabulation of information on past employment, education, and the type of employment sought. The list of educational institutions should be complete, as should the list of past employers. The employer list should be more extensive than you would use in all other résumés. Recruiters frequently search for people who have worked at a particular company or attended a given school in the past, and if you do not include them in your list they will not find you. LinkedIn allows people to search for former colleagues by looking for employer names. If you do not list all your employers, you are missing the chance to identify people who are possible references.

Online references are very important. Your connections (friends and persons you follow online working in the facilities you are targeting) who give a positive recommendation are valuable in getting you to the top of the list of applicants. Be sure to list all professional associations and certifications because employers frequently choose to search for these rather than previous employers.

In preparing your personal profile, here are some key words that paint a favorable picture of you and are frequently "hot buttons" for reviewers:

- Accepts Responsibility
- Open
- Positive Attitude
- Integrity
- Committed
- People Skills
- Organized
- Dependable
- Proactive

Do not limit your choice keywords to these terms only. Use words taken from the facility Web site, from contacts you might have with employees, and from using the suggestions in the previous

E-Résumé section. Online résumés often allow you to add a photo to your profile. A headshot is recommended (size < 100 × 100 pixels).

Detail out the "Specialties" section of your profile. Emphasize your accomplishments and experience, not just your skills. This section should be results oriented and should use as many keywords as are truthful and applicable. Create a personal URL if you are using LinkedIn. Other search engines such as Google will list your LinkedIn profile first when a search is made for your name.

Vital Résumé Information

All résumé styles must contain certain vital information about the job applicant. Essential information includes:

- Your full name and credential, address including street number, city, state, and zip code.
- Your telephone number or a number where a message can be left. The telephone selected should be one you are confident will be answered in a professional manner. Always include the area code with the number.
- Your email address.
- Your education. Begin with the most recent school attended and include the name, address, and graduation date with the diploma, certificate, or degree earned.
- Work experience. List company name and address. Do not underestimate the value of any job; relate transferable skills to your career objective.
- Skills that are necessary for the job. The list can be completed from your program curriculum. Be careful not to list course titles that have no meaning to the reader. It is much better to list the skills obtained in courses.

The following are the top errors found in résumés:

- Typographical and grammatical errors
- Lack of specifics on work training or history
- Use of same résumé for all job applications (résumé should be tailored to specific job)
- Emphasizing what you did instead of highlighting your accomplishments
- Stating objectives that do not focus on the needs of the employer
- Lack of power verbs and keywords

- Not mentioning jobs that gave you transferable skills
- Lying or exaggerating about skills and experience
- Eliminating key accomplishments in order to meet a one-page goal

APPLICATION/COVER LETTERS

The **application/cover letter** is a means of introducing yourself and submitting your résumé to a potential employer with the goal of obtaining an interview. A well-written cover letter highlights your qualifications and experience for employment and enhances the information contained within your résumé. It should reflect how your skills satisfy the employer's needs. The letter should follow a standard business style and should not be more than one page in length. It should be printed on the same paper as the résumé.

Because this may be your first contact with a potential employer, the letter should sell you and describe your intentions regarding employment, display your personality, and create an interest in reading your enclosed résumé.

Some guidelines to follow in writing the application/cover letter include:

1. Address your letter to a specific individual whenever possible. You may need to make a telephone call to obtain the name, title, and correct spelling.
2. Keep the letter concise, use correct grammar and spelling, and follow standard business letter format (formality is key).
3. The first paragraph should state your reason for writing and focus the reader's attention. It should not give as a reason "in response to a help wanted ad."
4. The second paragraph should identify how your education, experience, and qualifications relate to the job and refer to the enclosed résumé.
5. The last paragraph should close with a request for an interview.
6. Have someone with management experience review your cover letter. This could be your practicum supervisor, an instructor, a friend, or an acquaintance who is in a supervisory position.
7. Do not reproduce cover letters. An original letter should be sent to each individual.

8. The cover letter should be placed on top of the résumé and mailed in a business-size envelope that matches its contents or in an 8½ × 11 manila envelope containing your return address.

9. Do not staple the cover letter to the résumé.

A sample of an application/cover letter is shown in Figure 48-8A.

An alternate example of an application/cover letter using Information Mapping® to highlight and draw attention to specific information in your letter is shown in Figure 48-8B. This format is considered easier to read because the focus is on specific blocks of information. In addition, its uniqueness draws attention to your letter and may result in your being selected when competition is keen.

COMPLETING THE APPLICATION FORM

Sooner or later during the job search you will be asked to complete an **application form**. How well you complete this task may be a key factor in obtaining an interview and that first job.

Reading through the application form questions, you may be tempted to write in "See résumé" rather than repeat pertinent information already contained within your résumé. Do not fall into this pitfall. Answer every item completely. The application is organized in the manner that suits the clinic, whereas individual résumés are organized in a variety of ways. Finding specific information on a résumé is more

---

2031 Craig Street
Renton, Washington 98055
August 22, 20XX

Sarah Molles, Manager
Seattle Group Health Cooperative
304 Fourth Avenue
Seattle, Washington 98124-1716

Dear Ms. Molles:

I am interested in the medical assistant position to assist in a dermatology surgery practice. I meet the qualifications and would like to be considered for the position.

I am currently a certified clinical medical assistant certified through the National Healthcareer Association (NHA). I have experience as a clinical assistant in an internal medicine clinic and have excellent communication and interpersonal skills.

I will be available Tuesday and Thursday afternoons from 1:00 p.m. to 4:00 p.m. I will call you next Thursday to set up an appointment for an interview.

Yours truly,

Porscha Dolan, CCMA

Enclosure, Résumé

© Cengage Learning 2014

Figure 48-8A Sample application/cover letter.

2031 Craig Street
Renton, Washington 98055
August 22, 20XX

Sarah Molles, Manager
Seattle Group Health Cooperative
304 Fourth Avenue
Seattle, Washington 98124-1716

SUBJECT: SURGICAL MEDICAL ASSISTANT POSITION

Background	I am interested in the medical assistant position to assist in a dermatology surgery practice. I meet the qualifications and would like to be considered for the position.
Qualifications	I am currently a certified medical assistant graduated from a 2-year program accredited by the Commission on Accreditation of Allied Health Education Programs (CAAHEP). I have experience as a clinical assistant in an internal medicine clinic and have excellent communication and interpersonal skills.
Requested Action	I will be available Tuesday and Thursday afternoons from 1:00 p.m. to 4:00 p.m. I will call you next Thursday to set up an appointment for an interview.

Yours truly,

Ashley Jackson, CMA (AAMA)

Enclosure, Résumé

© Cengage Learning 2014

Figure 48-8B   Sample information mapped letter.

time consuming for the clinic, whereas finding the same information on the job application is easy and quick because they know where to look for it. Read all the directions carefully. Look for seemingly insignificant directions placed at the top or bottom of the page that state "Print Carefully," "Complete in Your Own Hand-writing," or "Please Type." Employers may use this to assess your ability to read and follow directions and pay attention to detail.

If the application is to be handwritten, use black ink to complete the form. Black ink is considered legal and often is an indelible (permanent) ink and is more legible if the form must be duplicated. Concentrate when completing the form and be sure to print clearly and make no errors. When

possible, copy the application before beginning in case an error is made.

The current trend is toward online application forms. These forms are prepared by keying information into the appropriate spaces or blocks by using a computer. The completed forms are printed and mailed to the prospective employer or sent electronically. Sending electronically is increasingly the preferred method. All of the concerns relative to care in following instructions, providing complete and accurate information, and proofreading the application for any errors before sending are applicable.

If you are asked to list experience but the application does not specify "paid experience," be sure to list any volunteer or practicum experience that relates to the position you are seeking. Volunteer work can be important as an indicator of your willingness to work, your ability to serve the public, and your organizational skills.

You may be asked to complete the application form "on the spot." Plan ahead for this event and carry a completed copy of your résumé, reference list, and application/cover letter with you. Also carry with you information not included in your résumé, such as which years you attended high school and your salary history. A pocket spelling wordbook or dictionary may be a useful tool to carry for those who find spelling challenging. These documents should provide all the information needed to complete the application form and may be submitted with the application form. This demonstrates to the potential employer your seriousness and preparedness for finding a job.

THE INTERVIEW PROCESS

If your application/cover letter, résumé, and application form have made a favorable impression with the organization, you may be invited for an interview. An **interview** is a meeting in which you and the interviewer discuss the employment opportunities within that particular organization. It is the interviewer's responsibility to determine if you have the personality, education, and skills to perform the job.

 The interviewer uses the interview process to *assess* appearance, attitude, and dependability. The interviewer also tries to verify that you have been honest in the skills you claim to have mastered. You, on the other hand, are selling your qualifications and assessing if this is an organization in which you want to be employed.

Being well prepared for the interview will increase your self-confidence and ability to focus during the actual interview. Knowing that your application/cover letter, résumé, and references all support your career goal and objectives allows you time to concentrate on interview preparation and presentation.

The Look of Success

The look of success begins with the outward appearance. First impressions are lasting, so strive for a favorable, professional look from head to toe. Appropriate conservative attire is important. Remember, your goal is to sell your professional abilities.

Hair should be clean and healthy looking, and worn in an appropriate style for the ambulatory care setting. Long hair should be worn off the collar in perhaps a French braid or twist. Strive for a neat, professional style.

The skin should have a healthy glow. Consultation with a cosmetician may prove helpful in solving skin problems or may provide an opportunity for trying new products. A basic understanding of your personal skin type and selection of cosmetics that complement your skin tone aid in the presentation of a professional appearance. The natural look is most appropriate for the medical clinic.

A daily shower and use of personal hygiene products is advised. Remember to use caution where perfumes and scents are concerned because many magnify when the body is under stress and the scent may be offensive or cause allergic reactions in others. Smokers should be aware that smoke odor carries in their hair, skin, and clothing. This odor may not be acceptable in health care settings.

Fingernails should be short and oval shaped or have rounded corners. Only clear nail polish should be worn in the ambulatory care setting if you are not working in the clinical area. Nail polish that is chipped or cracked must be removed or replaced immediately because it creates crevices in which pathogens may hide, multiply, and spread.

First impressions are lasting, so make yours professional in all respects. Conservative business attire is appropriate. Smart casual attire is appropriate for both men and women. This consists of a skirt and blouse or a tailored pantsuit for women and slacks and dress shirt with or without a tie for men. Pay attention to details such as your accessories and shoe selection. Accessories should be small and tasteful. Shoes should be clean, polished, and in good repair. They should fit properly and be comfortable and easy to walk in (Figure 48-9).

Women may carry a small purse if necessary. A portfolio is recommended in which to keep an extra copy of your résumé, reference list, application, and cover letter. A pen should be handy. Do not plan to search in either a purse or a portfolio for a pen or papers, keys, and so forth. Be sure that your cell phone is turned off before entering the clinic.

When you feel well and know that you look good, you project a confident and professional appearance. In other words, you are professionally poised. *Webster's Dictionary* defines *poise* as balance and stability; ease and dignity of manner. Personal poise combines all of the previously mentioned body appearances plus smoothness of movement and physical flexibility.

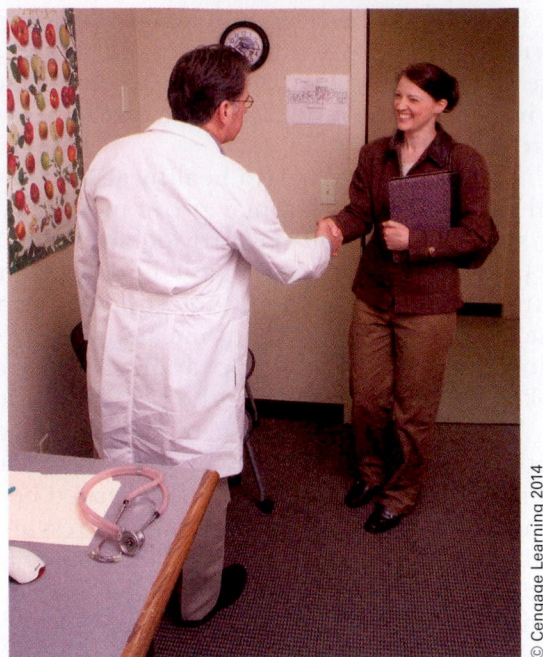

© Cengage Learning 2014

Figure 48-9 Medical assistant appropriately dressed and prepared for the interview.

Preparing for the Interview

Before the interview takes place, carefully research the organization offering the position. Study the organization's mission statement, financial reports, future projections, and any other information available. Be prepared to relate your skills and interests to the needs of this organization. In other words, what can you contribute and why should they hire you? The interview is your opportunity to sell yourself and identify ways in which you can benefit the employer.

Bring a copy of your résumé and cover letter to the interview just in case the interviewer cannot locate the original or wants another copy. You should also have copies of letters of recommendation, a list of references, a copy of your transcript from the schools you attended, and copies of any

CRITICAL THINKING

If you are a smoker, how can you minimize the smoke odor carried on your person before you go on a job interview? Make a list and prioritize each suggestion into a plan of action.

certificates such as AIDS training, First Aid, and CPR. These items should not be presented unless dictated by events that take place during the interview. You might also have with you the name of the interviewer and a copy of any questions you plan to ask the interviewer. A last-minute review will refocus your thoughts before you go into the interview. Keep your list available for quick reference in the event your mind goes blank when you are asked if you have questions.

To arrive 5 to 10 minutes early, check a map for directions or make a trip the day before your interview. Try to travel about the same time as you would for the interview so you have an idea of the time it takes, traffic flow, construction areas encountered, and parking availability. Plan for inclement weather (raincoat, umbrella, shoes). It is a good idea to make a quick trip to the restroom on arrival to change shoes or recheck your appearance.

Introduce yourself confidently to the administrative medical assistant and identify by name the person you wish to see and the time of your appointment. Always arrive alone. The employer wants to see you and sense your self-reliance and responsibility. While you wait, try to relax and observe the clinic setting, other employees, what they are wearing, and their manner of conducting business. This may be helpful to you during the interview and in making a decision to work there.

Figure 48-10 lists reasons why employers do not hire applicants.

The Actual Interview

When you enter an interviewer's office, think of yourself as a guest and take your cues from him or her. Most interviewers will introduce themselves and extend a hand. A firm handshake, responding by introducing yourself, and smiling confidently convey a positive professional image. Remain standing until you are invited to be seated. Keep your personal items on your lap or place them on the floor near your chair. Do not invade the interviewer's territory by placing your things on the desk.

Sit erect in the chair with your feet flat on the on the floor or cross only your ankles. Avoid nervous mannerisms while you speak and maintain good eye contact, but do not stare the interviewer down. Be natural and positive about the position, organization, and yourself. Present a professional image by using medical terminology when

REASONS FOR EMPLOYERS NOT HIRING

Employers in business were asked to list reasons for not hiring a job seeker. Given in rank order (from most unwanted to least unwanted), the 15 biggest gripes are as follows:

1. Poor appearance (not dressed properly, poorly groomed).
2. Acting like a know-it-all.
3. Cannot express self clearly; poor voice, diction, grammar.
4. Lack of planning for work—no purpose or goals.
5. Lack of confidence or poise.
6. No interest in or enthusiasm for the job.
7. Not active in school extracurricular programs.
8. Interested only in the best dollar offer.
9. Poor school record (academic, attendance).
10. Unwilling to start at the bottom.
11. Making excuses, hedges on unfavorable record.
12. No tact.
13. Not mature.
14. No curiosity about the job.
15. Critical of past employers.

Courtesy of Highline Community College, Counseling/Career Center, Des Moines, WA.

Figure 48-10 Reasons for employers not hiring.

responding to questions or providing information. Observe the interviewer carefully for cues. Respond to questions completely, trying not to repeat yourself or give more information than was requested.

Be prepared for the kinds of questions that may be asked during the interview process. Ask yourself, "If I were the employer, what would I want to know about the applicant?" Figure 48-11 gives examples of standard questions asked by most employers. Consider how you would respond to each question.

Remember that the interviewer is asking questions to determine if you are qualified for the position and if you are the kind of person who will fit into the organization. *Think* before answering questions; try to provide the information requested in a positive and professional manner. Do not respond with slang terms. *Listen* carefully so that you understand what information the question is requesting. *Ask* for clarification if you are uncertain. This demonstrates your ability to be open enough to ask questions when in doubt.

TYPICAL QUESTIONS ASKED DURING AN INTERVIEW

1. I see from your résumé you graduated from _____ college. What did that college have to offer that others didn't?
2. What subjects did you enjoy the most and why?
3. What do you see yourself doing 5 years from now?
4. What salary do you expect and what do you think it will be in 5 or 10 years?
5. What do you consider to be your greatest strengths and weaknesses?
6. How do you think a friend or professor who knows you well would describe you?
7. What qualifications do you have that make you think you would be successful in this position?
8. In what ways do you think you can make a contribution to our organization?
9. What two or three accomplishments have given you the most satisfaction?
10. What didn't you like about your last employer?
11. How well do you work under pressure?
12. Will you be able to work overtime occasionally?
13. How do you respond to criticism?
14. How would you respond if a patient or coworker made advances toward you?
15. How would you handle following procedures with which you do not agree?
16. Describe a specific medical procedure.
17. Do you have any questions you would like to ask?
18. How would you establish credibility quickly with our team?
19. What attracted you to this clinic?
20. What is the last book you read?
21. Why should we hire you?
22. What is your personal mission statement?

© Cengage Learning 2014

Figure 48-11 Knowing how you would answer some of these typical questions can prepare you for your interview.

Interviewing the Employer

The worst thing that can happen to an entry-level employee is to be hired and then have to quit or be fired because of a conflict with the employer. The interview process is a two-way street. You, the interviewee, should also interview the potential employer. The following are danger signs of an employer who could make your work life very difficult:

- Disrespectful behavior during the interview toward other staff members or to you

- Signs of insecurity by the manager
- Lack of enthusiasm toward the organization
- Shows signs of being highly stressed
- Negative attitude in statements
- Arrogance or answers own questions
- Uses the pronoun "I" excessively

You have to read the interviewer because some of the signs listed could be attributed to a "bad day". If too many signals are showing or, after prudent questioning on your part, you still have concerns, perhaps you should look for employment elsewhere to avoid the possibility of damaging your future career.

Following are a few questions you might ask the interviewer to resolve some of these concerns raised by observations:

- How would you describe the clinic culture?
- How do you handle differing opinions on how best to accomplish tasks?
- How are employee accomplishments recognized?
- What is the leadership style at the clinic?
- What is the attitude toward professional growth and educational opportunities?

Answers to these questions will help you determine if the clinic culture is one you can embrace.

Closing the Interview

By observing the interviewer and listening carefully, you will be able to determine when the interviewer feels he or she has enough information about you to make a decision. Usually during the closing the interviewer asks if you have any additional questions. This is your opportunity to collect information helpful in making a decision to accept or decline an offer. Your questions provide another opportunity to sell yourself, show that you have done your homework about the organization, and have listened carefully during the interview. Select three or four questions that will help you the most.

Questions about the organization are excellent choices. Examples are:

- "What are the opportunities for advancement with this organization?"
- "I read that your organization has educational benefits. Could you explain briefly how that program works?"
- "You mentioned in-house training programs for employees. Could you give one or two examples?"

You may also have some questions about the job itself. Examples of these types of questions are:

- "Is this a newly created position? If so, what results are you hoping to see?"
- "Was the last person in this position promoted? What contributed to their advancement?"
- "What do you consider the most difficult task on this job?"
- "What are the lines of authority for this position?"

Do not use this question time to ask about salary, sick leave, vacations, or retirement benefits. At this point, your focus should be on the value and skills you can contribute to the organization. These questions may be asked during a second interview or when a position is offered.

Before you leave, thank the interviewer for taking time to discuss the position with you. If you definitely are interested in the position, ask to be considered as a candidate for the position. If follow-up procedures have not been explained, now is the time to ask when the final selection will be made and how you will be notified. A firm handshake as you leave, a pleasant smile, and confidence as you exit will leave a professional picture in the interviewer's mind.

INTERVIEW FOLLOW-UP

Following up after the interview is essential. This is the time to telephone your references to let them know the name of the organization and the person's name with whom you interviewed, something about the position, and your qualifications. Share any information that will help your references support you in obtaining the position.

Follow-Up Letter

Take time to write a follow-up letter or handwritten note to the interviewer a day or two after your interview to thank him or her for the time spent interviewing you. The letter should be written in standard business format and printed on the same paper as your application/cover letter and résumé. Be sure that all spelling and grammar are correct.

The follow-up letter provides another opportunity to express your interest in the organization and the position. You can briefly emphasize the experience and skills you have to offer and again request being considered a candidate for the position.

Record the mailing date on your contact tracker and keep a copy of the letter in a file

2031 Craig Street
Renton, Washington 98055
August 28, 20XX

Sarah Molles, Manager
Seattle Group Health Cooperative
304 Fourth Avenue
Seattle, Washington 98124-1716

Dear Ms. Molles,

Thank you for scheduling a personal interview with me last Wednesday, August 26, at 9:45AM. I enjoyed discussing the medical assistant position open in one of your dermatology surgery practices. I would like to be considered for the position.

After talking with you, I feel my qualifications match closely with those you requested. My communication and interpersonal skills are excellent and a necessary ingredient for any medical assistant.

I look forward to hearing from you September 5 as you mentioned during the interview. If there are any questions I may answer, please telephone me.

Sincerely,

Ashley Jackson

Ashley Jackson, CMA (AAMA)
(206) 255-1365

Figure 48-12   Sample follow-up letter.

with other information about the organization. Figure 48-12 shows a sample follow-up letter.

Follow Up By Telephone

Allow a few days for your follow-up letter to reach the interviewer. If you do not hear from the interviewer within a week or by the designated time established during the interview, you may call to ask if you are still being considered for the position or if a decision has been made.

Speak directly into the mouthpiece of the telephone using good diction and voice volume. Identify yourself and provide some information to aid the interviewer in recalling who you are. Perhaps mentioning the date you interviewed will suffice. Be polite and professional, and remember to thank the individual for speaking with you. At the end of the conversation say good-bye and wait until the other person hangs up before you break the connection. Log the telephone call and its response on your contact tracker for future reference.

AFTER YOU ARE EMPLOYED

You are now a newly employed medical assistant. What do you do now to advance your career? Following are some suggestions:

- Make sure your workstation is set up and you have what you need to do the job
- Practice good time management skills
- Try to allow time for emergencies, which will occur
- Do not be a know-it-all; ask other employees how they do things around here
- Get to know colleagues and be part of the team
- Seek feedback on how you are doing your job
- Create a professional image

Dealing with Difficult People

Sooner or later you will encounter coworkers who could be described as just plain "jerks." Jerks may be defined as persons who use power to belittle and ridicule people who work under them. These people may be foul-mouthed, power hungry, bullies, uncouth, or unethical. There are several ways to free yourself from jerks.

- Check out emotionally (attempt to ignore the comments); indifference is an underrated virtue
- Try to move to a different position within the organization
- If all else fails, change jobs

Getting a Raise

One of the main reasons people do not get a raise is because they do not ask. This is particularly true of professional women. It has been reported that less than half ask for a raise or promotion within a 12-month period. Of those that did ask, almost three quarters received a raise or promotion. After taking into consideration the wages of persons with similar job descriptions and experience, if your salary appears to be lagging you should not feel uncomfortable asking for a raise at your next favorable performance review.

CRITICAL THINKING

As you begin to prepare for a job interview, how can you prepare yourself to reflect a professional image, attitude, and demeanor, and verbal and nonverbal communication skills, as well as articulately describe your skills and abilities to fit the position to which you are applying? Develop a complete written checklist and review it before each interview.

PROFESSIONALISM

   Areas of professionalism directly related to the medical clinic may include:

- Display a professional manner and image. The chapter content stresses the importance of having a positive attitude, taking pride in doing the best you can, being prepared, and dressing appropriately for job interviews.
- Promote your CMA (AAMA), RMA (AMT), CMAS, or other credential. On graduation from an accredited school, you will be ready to sit for the national certification examination. On notification of passing the examination, you will be awarded the appropriate credential. When signing your name, include your credential and educate others regarding its significance.

CASE STUDY 48-1

Refer to the scenario at the beginning of the chapter.

CASE STUDY REVIEW

1. Which résumé style represents Eun Mee best and why?

2. List transferable skills that Eun Mee may want to include in her résumé.

3. What is the purpose of an accomplishment statement? Provide examples Eun Mee might use.

CASE STUDY 48-2

Drs. Lewis and King maintain a two-provider family practitioner clinic. They are in need of a new medical assistant to take the place of one who will be leaving at the end of the month. They have scheduled interviews with five applicants. Eun Mee Soo is the first candidate to be interviewed.

CASE STUDY REVIEW

1. Eun Mee wants to bring some papers to the interview. What is the best way to do this? What paperwork should she bring with her?

2. Why should Eun Mee arrive 5 to 10 minutes early for the interview?

3. How should Eun Mee enter the room?

SUMMARY

Finding your first job is your first job. How well you research, plan, prepare, and implement your tasks will make the difference between being hired and not being hired. Learn from each interview session. Recall the questions that were asked and formulate answers that you feel would be appropriate for your next interview. Tell everyone you are looking for a job and solicit their help. Follow up on all leads and do not become discouraged.

Once you have been hired at that first job, continue your learning experience. Ask appropriate questions and try not to ask the same question a second or third time. Pay attention to details and learn individual preferences. Become a team player and look for ways you can help others. Carry your share of responsibility and do not be afraid to admit you are unfamiliar with certain aspects of the clinic. Employers need to know you can be trusted to work within the scope of your education and not beyond. Practice being an asset to your employer.

STUDY FOR SUCCESS

To reinforce your knowledge and skills of information presented in this chapter:

- Review the *Key Terms*
- Role-play with other students to apply attributes of professionalism pertinent to this chapter.
- Consider the *Case Studies* and discuss your conclusions
- Answer the questions in the *Certification Review*
- Apply your knowledge by completing the *Activities* in the *Study Guide* and the *Games and Quizzes* in the StudyWARE **StudyWARE** software on the *Premium Website*
- Practice your problem-solving skills with the *Critical Thinking Challenge 3.0* on the *Premium Website*

Additional resources for this chapter include:

- Module 28 of the *Medical Assisting Learning Lab*
- *CourseMate for Delmar's Comprehensive Medical Assisting*
- *WebTutor for Delmar's Comprehensive Medical Assisting*

CERTIFICATION REVIEW

1. The résumé:
   a. is a summary data sheet or brief account of your qualifications and progress in your career
   b. is also known as a contact tracker
   c. always includes references
   d. is used to introduce yourself and identify qualifications

2. References:
   a. must always be listed on the résumé
   b. should be a relative
   c. should be someone who likes you and your work but may not be a good communicator
   d. should be someone who knows you or has worked with you long enough to make an honest assessment of your capabilities and integrity

3. The targeted résumé is advantageous:
   a. when prior titles are impressive
   b. when reentering the job market after an absence
   c. when you are just starting your career and have little experience
   d. when you have extensive specialized experience

4. The application/cover letter:
   a. is a detailed data sheet describing your vital information, education, and experience
   b. introduces you to a prospective employer and captures their interest in you as a candidate for the position
   c. lists individuals who can vouch for you
   d. should be lengthy and detailed

5. The interview:
   a. does not require much thought or preparation
   b. requires you to think before answering questions, listen carefully, and ask for clarification if uncertain of the question
   c. provides time to ask questions about salary, vacation, and benefits
   d. does not require any follow-up
6. Preparing for the interview:
   a. bathe yourself, groom your hair and fingernails, and wear clean and pressed conservative business attire
   b. allow adequate time to get to the interview
   c. prepare a packet to give the interviewer containing certificates, letters of recommendation, a list of references, and your list of questions
   d. all of the above
7. Job analysis should include:
   a. compiling a list of potential employers
   b. gathering information about employers in whom you have interest
   c. preparing a budgetary needs analysis
   d. all of the above
8. The best source for job search data is:
   a. the Internet
   b. friends and acquaintances
   c. the Yellow Pages and classified ads
   d. all of the above

9. The purpose of a résumé is:
   a. to sell yourself
   b. to provide references
   c. to assist in maintaining your contact tracker
   d. to provide an opportunity to use social media
10. Accomplishment statements:
    a. are power verbs that give a brief description of what you did and the results produced
    b. a list of contacts and their responses and your actions
    c. a list of who you know or have worked with
    d. a brief account of your qualifications and progress in your career
11. Follow-up after the interview includes all of the following *except:*
    a. telephoning references to update them
    b. sending a follow-up letter
    c. asking references to call interviewer and put in a good word for you
    d. following up with a telephone call
12. Online résumés:
    a. use social media sites
    b. require a personal profile
    c. use key words or hot buttons for reviewers
    d. never allow photos

REFERENCES/BIBLIOGRAPHY

Farr, M. (n.d.). Making your résumé-friendly: 10 steps. Retrieved from http://www.careerbuilder.com/Article/CB-403-Cover-Letters-Resumes-Making-Your-R%C3%A9sum%C3%A9-E-Friendly-10-Steps/ http://www.grovo.com/browse/product/linkedin-personal-profile

Farr, M. (2000). *Quick resume & cover letter book.* Indianapolis, IN: JIST Works, Inc.

Fletcher, L. (n.d.). How to write a LinkedIn profile. Retrieved from http://www.blueskyresumes.com/free-resume-help/article/how-to-write-a-linkedin-profile/

Keir, L., Wise, B. A., Krebs, C., Kelley-Arney, C. (2008). *Medical assisting: Administrative and clinical competencies (6th ed.).* Clifton Park, NY: Delmar Cengage Learning.

Levy, R. (n.d.). How to use social media in your job search. Retrieved from http://jobsearch.about.com/od/networking/a/socialmedia.htm

LinkedIn defined (2009, January). Retrieved from http://www.socialmediadefined.com/2009/01/30/linkedin-defined/

Nobel, D. F. (2000). *Gallery of best resumes for people without a four-year degree.* Indianapolis, IN: JIST Works, Inc.

Schawbel, D. (2009, January). 7 secrets to getting your next job using social media. Retrieved from http://mashable.com/2009/01/05/job-search-secrets/

Sindell, M., & Sindell, T. (2006). *Sink or swim.* Avon, MA: Adams Media Publishing.

Washington, T. (2000). *Resume power selling yourself on paper in the new millennium.* Indianapolis, IN: JIST Works, Inc.

Zedlitz, R. H. (2003). *How to get a job in health care.* Clifton Park, NY: Delmar Cengage Learning.

ā	before			auscultation and palpation
āā	of each			auscultation and percussion
AAMA	American Association of Medical Assistants		APC	ambulatory payment classifications
AAP	American Academy of Pediatrics		apps	applications
AAPC	American Academy of Professional Coders		aq	water
ab	abortion		A/R	accounts receivable
abd	abdomen		ARDS	acute (or adult) respiratory distress syndrome
ABE	acute bacterial endocarditis			
ABG	arterial blood gases		ARRA	American Recovery and Reinvestment Act
ABHES	Accrediting Bureau of Health Education Schools		ARU	automated routing unit
			ASA	acetylsalicylic acid
ABO	blood groups		ASAP	as soon as possible
ac	before meals (ante cibum)		ASC	atypical squamous cell
	acute		ASCAD	arteriosclerotic coronary artery disease
ACAP	Alliance of Claims Assistance Professionals			athrosclerotic coronary artery disease
ACIP	Advisory Committee on Immunization Practices		ASC US	atypical squamous cell of uncertain significance
ACOG	American Congress of Obstetricians and Gynecologists		ASCVD	arteriosclerotic cardiovascular disease
				atherosclerotic cardiovascular disease
ACTH	adrenocorticotropic hormone		A&W	alive and well
ADA	Americans with Disabilities Act			
ADHD	attention deficit hyperactivity disorder		Ba	barium
ADL	activities of daily living		BaE	barium enema
ad lib	as desired		BBB	bundle branch block
adm	admission		BC	birth control
AED	automated external defibrillator		BCP	birth control pills
AES	Advanced Encryption Standard		BC/BS	Blue Cross/Blue Shield
AFP	alpha-fetoprotein		BE	bacterial endocarditis
AHD	arteriosclerotic heart disease		bid	twice a day
	atherosclerotic heart disease		bil	bilateral
AHDI	Association for Healthcare Documentation Integrity		BM	basal metabolism
				bowel movement
AHIMA	American Health Information Management Association		BMI	body mass index
			BMR	basal metabolism rate
AIDS	acquired immunodeficiency syndrome		BNA	budget neutrality adjuster
alb	albumin		BP	blood pressure
AM	before noon (ante meridiem)		BPH	benign prostatic hypertrophy
AMA	against medical advice		BS	blood sugar
	American Medical Association			bowel sounds
AMBA	American Medical Billing Association			breath sounds
AMI	acute myocardial infarction		BSA	body surface area
amt	amount		BSL	blood sugar level
AMT	American Medical Technologists		BSN	bowel sounds normal
AMTIE	American Medical Technologists Institute for Excellence		BSO	bilateral salpingo-oophorectomy
			BSR	blood sedimentation rate
ant	anterior		BUN	blood urea nitrogen
ante	before		BW	below waist
A&P	anatomy and physiology			birth weight
	anterior and posterior			body weight
			Bx	biopsy

C	Celsius
	centigrade
c̄	with
C1	first cervical vertebra
CA	cancer
	carcinoma
Ca	calcium
CAAHEP	Commission on Accreditation of Allied Health Education Programs
CAD	coronary artery disease
CAHD	coronary arteriosclerotic heart disease
	coronary athersclerotic heart disease
caps	capsules
CAM	complementary and alternative medicine
CAT	computerized axial tomography
CBC	complete blood count
CBT	computer-based testing
CC	chief complaint
CCA	Certified Coding Associate
CCHIT	Certification Commission for Health Information Technology
CCMA	Certified Clinical Medical Assistant
CCP	Certification Continuation Program
CCR	continuity of care record
CCS	Certified Coding Specialist
CCS-P	Certified Coding Specialist–Physician-Based
CCT	cardiac computerized tomography
CCU	coronary care unit
C&D	cystoscopy and dilation
CDC	U.S. Centers for Disease Control and Prevention
CE	continuing education
cerv	cervical
	cervix
CEU	continuing education unit
CF	conversion factor
CHAMPVA	Civilian Health and Medical Program of the Department of Veterans Administration
CHD	childhood disease
	congenital heart disease
	congestive heart disease
	coronary heart disease
CHEDDAR	chief complaint, history, examination, details of problems, drugs and dosages, assessment, return visit if applicable
CHF	congestive heart failure
CHO	carbohydrate
CIN	cervical intraepithelial neoplasia
ck	check
Cl	chlorine
cldy	cloudy
CLIA	Clinical Laboratory Improvement Amendments
cm	centimeter
CMA (AAMA)	Certified Medical Assistant through the American Association of Medical Assistants
CMAA	Certified Medical Administrative Assistant
CMAS	Certified Medical Administrative Specialist
CME	continuing medical education
CMR	cardiac magnetic resonance
CMS	Centers for Medicare and Medicaid Services
CMT	Certified Medical Transcriptionist
CNS	central nervous system

C/O	complains of
CO$_2$	carbon dioxide
COB	coordination of benefits
COPD	chronic obstructive pulmonary disease
CPC	Certified Professional Coder
CPC-A	Certified Professional Coder–Apprentice
CPC-H	Certified Professional Coder–Hospital
CPC-HA	Certified Professional Coder–Hospital Apprentice
CPR	cardiopulmonary resuscitation
CPT	Current Procedural Terminology
CPU	central processing unit
CRB	Curriculum Review Board
crit	hematocrit
CS	cerebrospinal
	cesarean section
C&S	culture and sensitivity
CSF	cerebrospinal fluid
CT	computerized tomography
CVA	cerebrovascular accident
CVE	capsule video endoscopy
CVP	central venous pressure
CVS	chorionic villus sampling
cx	cervix
CXR	chest X-ray
cysto	cystoscopic examination
	cystoscopy
DACUM	developing a curriculum
DC	doctor of chiropractic
D&C	dilation and curettage
d/c	discontinue and discharge
DDS	doctor of dentistry
DEA	U.S. Drug Enforcement Agency
dec	decrease
DEERS	Defense Enrollment Eligibility Reporting System
del	delivery
DES	diethylstilbestrol
DHHS	U.S. Department of Health and Human Services
diab	diabetic
	diabetes
diag	diagnosis
diff	differential white blood cell count
dil	dilute
disc	discontinue
disp	dispense
DM	diabetes mellitus
DNA	deoxyribonucleic acid
	does not apply
DNR	do not resuscitate
DO	doctor of osteopathy
DOA	dead on arrival
DOB	date of birth
DOD	date of death
DOE	dyspnea on exertion
dos	dosage
DPI	dry powder inhaler
DPM	doctor of podiatric medicine
DPT	diphtheria, pertussis, and tetanus
DR	delivery room

Dr	doctor		fl	fluid
DRGs	diagnosis-related groups		fl oz	fluid ounce
DS	discharge summary		FMP	first menstrual period
DSD	dry sterile dressing		FP	family practice
dsg	dressing		freq	frequent
DT	delirium tremens		FSH	follicle-stimulating hormone
DTR	deep tendon reflex		ft	foot
D&V	diarrhea and vomiting		FTA	fluorescent treponemal antibody
DW	distilled water		FTP	file transfer protocol
D/W	dextrose in water		fx	fracture
dx	diagnosis			
			G	gravida
ea	each		g	gram
EAP	extensible authentication protocol		GB	gallbladder
EBV	Epstein–Barr virus		GC	gonococcus
ECG	electrocardiogram			gonorrhea
echo	echocardiogram		GERD	gastroesophageal reflux disease
	echoencephalogram		GI	gastrointestinal
E. coli	*Escherichia coli*		gm	gram
ECT	electroconvulsive therapy		GP	general practice
	electronic claims transmission		GPCI	Geographic Practice Cost Index
EDC	estimated date of confinement or expected date of confinement		gr	grain
			grav	pregnancy
EDD	estimated date of delivery or expected date of delivery		GTH	gonadotropic hormone
			GTT	glucose tolerance test
EEG	electroencephalogram		gtt(s)	drop (drops)
EENT	eyes, ears, nose, and throat		GU	genitourinary
e.g.	for example		GYN	gynecology
EHR	electronic health record			
EKG	electrocardiogram		h	hour
elix	elixir		HAI	healthcare–associated infection
email	electronic mail		HBP	high blood pressure
EMG	electromyography		HCFA	U.S. Health Care Financing Administration
EMR	electronic medical record		hCG	human chorionic gonadotropin
EMS	emergency medical service		HCl	hydrochloric acid
ENT	ear, nose, and throat		HCPCS	Healthcare Common Procedure Coding System
EOB	explanation of benefits			
eos	eosinophil		Hct	hematocrit
EPA	Environmental Protection Agency		HCVD	hypertensive cardiovascular disease
EPCA-2	early prostate cancer antigen-2		HEENT	head, eyes, ears, nose, and throat
EPO	exclusive provider organization		HEPA	high-efficiency particulate air
eq	equivalent		Hgb	hemoglobin
ER	emergency room		H&H	hemoglobin and hematocrit
ERT	estrogen replacement therapy		HIPAA	Health Insurance Portability and Accountability Act
ESR	erythrocyte sedimentation rate			
EST	electroshock therapy		HMO	health maintenance organization
exam	examination		H/O	history of
ext	extract		H₂O	water
			H&P	history and physical
F	Fahrenheit		HPI	history of present illness
	female		HPV	human papillomavirus
FAS	fetal alcohol syndrome		HR	human resources
fax	facsimile		HRS	Healthcare Reimbursement Specialist
FBS	fasting blood sugar		HRT	hormone replacement therapy
FDA	U.S. Food and Drug Administration		HSV1	herpes simplex virus 1
FECA	Federal Employees Compensation Act Program		HSV2	herpes simplex virus 2
			HT	hormone therapy
FH	family history		ht	height
FHR	fetal heart rate		hx	history
FHS	fetal heart sound		Hz	hertz

ICCU	intensive coronary care unit		M	male
ICD-9-CM	International Classification of Diseases, 9th revision, Clinical Modification		m	meter
			MA	medical allowable
ICU	intensive care unit		MBCD	management by coaching and development
ID	intradermal		MBCE	management by competitive edge
I&D	incision and drainage		MBDM	management by decision models
IDS	integrated delivery system		MBP	management by performance
IM	internal medicine		MBS	management by styles
	intramuscular		MBWA	management by wandering around
imp	impression		MBWS	management by work simplification
inf	infusion		MCHC	mean corpuscular hemoglobin and red cell indices
inj	injection			
I&O	intake and output		MCO	managed care organization
IOM	Institute of Medicine		MCV	mean corpuscular volume and red cell indices
IPA	independent physician association		MD	doctor of medicine
IPV	intimate partner violence			muscular dystrophy
IPPB	intermittent positive pressure breathing		MDI	metered dose inhaler
IPPS	inpatient prospective payment systems		MDR	minimum daily requirement
ISP	Internet service provider		med	medicine
IT	information technology		mEq/L	milliequivalents per liter
IUD	intrauterine device		MFS	Medicare fee schedule
IV	intravenous		mg	milligram
IVF	in vitro fertilization		MH	marital history
IVP	intravenous pyelogram			medical history
				menstrual history
JAAMT	*Journal of the American Association for Medical Transcription*		MHx	medical history
			MI	maturation index
JAMA	*Journal of the American Medical Association*			myocardial infarction
			mL	milliliter
K	potassium		mm	millimeter
kg	kilogram		mm³	cubic millimeter
KOH	potassium hydroxide		mm Hg	millimeters of mercury
KUB	kidney, ureter, and bladder		MMR	measles, mumps, and rubella
kV	kilovolt		MOM	milk of magnesia
			mono	mononucleosis
Ⓛ	left		MP	menstrual period
	liter		MRC	Medical Reserve Corps
l	length		MRI	magnetic resonance imaging
LA	left atrium		MRIA	magnetic resonance imaging angiography
	lactic acid		MRSA	methicillin resistant *Staphylococcus aureus*
L&A	light and accommodation		MS	mitral stenosis
lab	laboratory			multiple sclerosis
lac	laceration		MSDS	material safety data sheets
LAN	local area network		MSHA	Mine Safety and Health Administration
lap	laparotomy		MT	medical technologist
LASIK	laser-assisted in-situ keratomileusis			medical transcriptionist
lat	lateral		multip	multipara
lb	pound		MVP	mitral valve prolapse
LBBB	left bundle branch block			
LDL	low-density lipoprotein		NA	not applicable
LE	lupus erythematosus		NaCl	sodium chloride
LEEP	loop electrosurgical excision procedure		NACP	National Association of Claims Assistance Professionals
liq	liquid			
LLQ	lower left quadrant		narc	narcotic
LMP	last menstrual period		NB	newborn
LP	lumbar puncture		NCAI	National Coalition for Adult Immunization
LRQ	lower right quadrant		N/C	no complaints
LUQ	left upper quadrant		ND	doctor of naturopathy
L&W	living and well		NEBA	National Electronic Billers Alliance
lymphs	lymphocytes		NEC	not elsewhere classified
			neg	negative

NG	nasogastric		posteroanterior
NGU	nongonococcal urethritis	PAC	phenacetin, aspirin, and codeine
NHA	National Healthcareer Association		premature atrial contraction
NIDDM	noninsulin-dependent diabetes mellitus	PACS	picture archiving and communications systems
NL	normal limits	Pap	Papanicolaou (smear, test)
NMP	normal menstrual period	PAR	participating provider
noct	at night	para	number of pregnancies
Non-PAR	nonparticipating provider	para I	primipara
non rep	do not repeat	PAT	paroxysmal atrial tachycardia
NOS	not otherwise specified	path	pathology
NPI	national provider identification	PBI	protein-bound iodine
NPO	nothing by mouth	pc	after meals
NR	no refill	PC	personal computer
	nonreactive	PCA	patient-controlled analgesic
	normal range	PCC	Poison Control Center
	nonspecific	PCN	penicillin
NS	normal saline	PCP	primary care provider
	not significant	PCR	polymerase chain reaction
	not sufficient	PCV	packed cell volume
N&T	nose and throat	PDA	personal digital assistant
N&V	nausea and vomiting	PDR	*Physician's Desk Reference*
NVD	nausea, vomiting, and diarrhea	PE	physical examination
		peds	pediatrics
O	oral	PEG	pneumoencephalography
	oxygen	PERRLA	pupils equal, round, regular, react to light, and accommodation
O$_2$	oxygen		
OB	obstetrics	PET	positron emission transmission or tomography
OB-GYN	obstetrics-gynecology	PH	past history
OC	office call		personal history
	on call		public health
	oral contraceptive	pH	hydrogen in concentration
occ	occasionally	PHI	protected health information
OCR	Office of Civil Rights	PHO	physician-hospital organization
	optical character reader	PI	present illness
OGTT	oral glucose tolerance test		pulmonary infarction
OM	office manager	PID	pelvic inflammatory disease
OOB	out of bed	PKU	phenylketonuria
OP	outpatient	PM	after noon (post meridiem)
O&P	ova and parasites		post mortem (after death)
OPIM	other potentially infectious material	PMN	polymorphonuclear neutrophils
OPPS	outpatient prospective payment systems	PMP	past menstrual period
OPV	oral polio vaccine	PMS	premenstrual syndrome
OR	operating room	PNC	penicillin
	operative report	PO	postoperative
ortho	orthopedics	po	by mouth
os	mouth	POB	place of birth
OSHA	U.S. Occupational Safety and Health Administration	POLST	physician orders for life-sustaining treatment
OT	occupational therapist	POMR	problem-oriented medical record
	occupational therapy	POS	point-of-service plan
OTC	over the counter	pos	positive
OURQ	outer upper right quadrant	poss	possible
OV	office visit	postop	postoperative
OWCP	Office Workers' Compensation Programs	PP	present problem
oz	ounce		postprandial
		PPB	positive pressure breathing
p̄	after	PPBS	postprandial blood sugar
P	phosphorus	PPD	purified protein derivative
	pulse	PPO	preferred provider organization
P&A	percussion and auscultation	preop	preoperative
PA	physician's assistant	primip	woman bearing first child

prn	as the occasion arises, as necessary
procto	proctoscopy
prog	prognosis
PROM	premature rupture of membranes
pro-time	prothrombin time
PRSP	penicillin-resistant *Streptococcus* pneumonia
PSA	prostate-specific antigen
PSRO	Professional Standards Review Organization
PT	physical therapy
	prothrombin time
pt	patient
PTA	prior to admission
PTT	partial thromboplastin time
pulv	powder
PVC	premature ventricular contraction
px	physical examination
	prognosis
$\bar{q}$	each; every
q AM	every morning
QA	quality assurance
qh	every hour
q (2, 3, 4)h	every 2, 3, or 4 hours
qid	four times a day
QISMC	Quality Improvement System for Managed Care
qns	quantity not sufficient
qs	of sufficient quantity
qt	quart
®	registration
	right
RAM	random access memory
RBC	red blood cell
RBC/hpf	red blood cells per high power field
RBCM	red blood cell mass
RBCV	red blood cell volume
RBRVS	Resource-Based Relative Value Scale
REM	rapid eye movement
resp	respiration
Rh	rhesus (factor)
Rh−	rhesus negative
Rh+	rhesus positive
RHD	rheumatic heart disease
RLQ	right lower quadrant
RMA (AMT)	Registered Medical Assistant
RNA	ribonucleic acid
R/O	rule out
ROA	received on account
ROM	range of motion
	read-only memory
ROS	review of systems
ROTA	rotavirus
RT	radiation therapy
RUQ	right upper quadrant
RVUs	relative value units
Rx	prescription

S	subjective data (POMR)
$\bar{s}$	without
S&A	sugar and acetone (urine)
SA	sinoatrial
SARS	severe acute respiratory syndrome
SBE	shortness of breath on exertion
	subacute bacterial endocarditis
SE	standard error
sed rate	sedimentation rate
segs	segmented neutrophils
seq	sequela
SF	scarlet fever
	spinal fluid
SG	specific gravity
SH	social history
SIDS	sudden infant death syndrome
sig	instructions, directions
sigmoid	sigmoidoscopy
SIL	squamous interepithelial lesion
SMA 12/60	Sequential Multiple Analyzer (12-test serum profile)
SOAP	subjective data, objective data, assessment, and plan
SOAPER	subjective, objective, assessment, plan, education, response
SOB	shortness of breath
SOF	signature on file
sol	solution
solv	solvent
SOMR	source-oriented medical record
SOP	standard operating procedure
SOS	if necessary
spec	specimen
sp gr	specific gravity
spont ab	spontaneous abortion
SR	sedimentation rate
SS	signs and symptoms
$\bar{s}\bar{s}$	one-half
SSI	Supplemental Security Income
SSL	service sockets layer
Staph	Staphylococcus
stat	immediately
STD	sexually transmitted disease
Strep	Streptococcus
subq	subcutaneous
supp	suppository
surg	surgery
sx	signs
	symptoms
sym	symptoms
syr	syrup
T	temperature
T_3	tri-iodothyronine
T_4	thyroxine
T&A	tonsillectomy and adenoidectomy
tab	tablet
TAT	temporal artery thermometer
TB	tuberculin
	tuberculosis

TBS	The Bethesda System
tbs	tablespoon
TC	throat culture
	tissue culture
	total capacity
	total cholesterol
TDD	telecommunication device for the deaf
temp	temperature
TENS	transcutaneous electrical nerve stimulator
TFTC	Task Force for Test Construction
ther	therapy
therap	therapeutic
TIA	transient ischemic attack
tid	three times a day
tinct	tincture
TLC	tender loving care
TLS	transport layer security
TMJ	temporomandibular joint
top	topically
TOPV	trivalent oral poliovirus vaccine
TP	total protein
TPI	treponema pallidum immobilization test
TPMS	Total Practice Management System
TPN	total parenteral nutrition
TPR	temperature, pulse, and respiration
tr	tincture
trig	triglycerides
TSH	thyroid-stimulating hormone
tsp	teaspoon
TSS	toxic shock syndrome
TTY	teletype communications
TUR	transurethral resection
tus	cough
Tx or tx	treatment
T&X	type and cross match
UA	urinalysis
UB04	Uniform Bill 04
UCG	urinary chorionic gonadotropin
UCHD	usual childhood diseases
UCR	usual, customary, reasonable
ULQ	upper left quadrant
ung	ointment
UNICEF	United Nations International Children's Emergency Fund
UR	utilization review
urg	urgent
URI	upper respiratory infection
URL	Uniform Resource Locator
urol	urology
URQ	upper right quadrant
URT	upper respiratory tract
URTI	upper respiratory tract infection
USB	universal system bus port
USMLE	United States Medical Licensing Examination
USP	United States Pharmacopoeia
UT	urinary tract
UTI	urinary tract infection
UV	ultraviolet

vac	vaccine
vag	vagina
	vaginal
VD	venereal disease
VDRL	Venereal Disease Research Laboratory
VIS	vaccine information statement
vit	vitamin
vit cap	vital capacity
vol	volume
VoIP	voice over Internet protocol
VRE	vancomycin-resistant enterococcus
VRS	voice recognition software
VS	vital signs
WAN	wide area network
WBC	white blood cell
WDWN	well developed, well nourished
WHO	World Health Organization
WN	well nourished
WNF	well-nourished female
WNL	within normal limits
WNM	well-nourished male
WO	written order
w/o	without
wt	weight
WVE	wireless video endoscopy
$\bar{x}$	except
x	multiply by
XDR TB	extensively drug-resistant tuberculosis
XR	X-ray
YOB	year of birth
yr	year

Symbols

*	birth
†	death
♂	male
♀	female
+	positive
−	negative
±	positive or negative, indefinite
÷	divide by
=	equal to
>	greater than
<	less than
×	multiply by
#	number, pound
'	foot, minute
"	inch, second

Top 200 Brand-Name Drugs in the U.S. Market by Dispensed Prescriptions, 2010

1. Hydrocodone/APAP (Watson)
2. Amoxicillin (Teva)
3. Hydrocodone/APAP (Mallinckrodt)
4. Lipitor (Pfizer)
5. Levothyroxine Sodium (Mylan)
6. Lisinopril (Lupin)
7. Simvastatin (Lupin)
8. Plavix (Bristol-Myers Squibb/Sanofi-Aventis)
9. Nexium (AstraZeneca)
10. Singulair (Merck)
11. Metoprolol Tartate (Mylan)
12. Simvastatin (Teva)
13. Lexapro (Forest)
14. Synthroid (Abbot)
15. Azithromycin (Teva)
16. Crestor (AstraZeneca)
17. Levothyroxine Sodium (Lannett)
18. Proair HFA (Teva)
19. Metformin HCL (Teva)
20. Sertraline HCL (Greenstone)
21. Ibuprofen (Rx) (Amneal)
22. Metroprolol Succinate (Par)
23. Azithromycin (Greenstone)
24. Zolpidem Tartrate (Teva)
25. Advair Diskus (GlaxoSmithKline)
26. Furosemide (Mylan)
27. Hydrochlorothiazide (Teva)
28. Omeprazole (Rx) (Mylan)
29. Trazodone HCL (Teva)
30. Lisinopril (Teva)
31. Simvastatin (Dr. Reddy's)
32. Diovan (Novartis)
33. Tramadol (Amneal)
34. Hydrocodone/APAP (Qualitest)
35. Cymbalta (Lilly)
36. Warfarin Sodium (Teva)
37. Amlodipine Besylate (Mylan)
38. Omeprazole (Sandoz)
39. Oxycodone/APAP (Mallinckrodt)
40. Amlodipine Besylate (Greenstone)
41. Sulfamethoxazole/Trimethoprim (Amneal)
42. Seroquel (AstraZeneca)
43. Promethazine HCL (Sandoz)
44. Ventolin HFA (GlaxoSmithKline)
45. Fluticasone Propionate (Roxane)
46. Alprazolam (Actavis)
47. Clonazepam (Teva)
48. Amoxicillin Trihydrate/Potassium Clavulanate (Sandoz)
49. Hydrochlorothiazide (Qualitest)
50. Warfarin Sodium (Taro)
51. Diovan HCT (Novartis)
52. Actos (Takeda)
53. Pravastatin Sodium (Teva)
54. Oxycodone/APAP (Watson)
55. Vitamin D (Teva)
56. Fluoxetine HCL (Teva)
57. Alprazolam (Greenstone)
58. Lantus (Sanofi-Aventis)
59. Atenolol (Mylan)
60. Fluconazole (Teva)
61. Lisinopril/Hydrochlorothiazide (Lupin)
62. Metoprolol Succinate (Watson)
63. Levaquin (Ortho-McNeil-Janssen)
64. Aricept (Eisai)
65. Celebrex (Pfizer)
66. APAP/Codeine (Teva)
67. Nasonex (Schering)
68. Metformin HCL (Zydus)
69. Amoxicillin (Sandoz)
70. Ciprofloxacin HCL (Watson)
71. Triamterene/Hydrochlorothiazide (Sandoz)
72. Omeprazole (Rx) (Kremers Urban)
73. Prednisone (West-Ward)
74. Lyrica (Pfizer)
75. Alendronate Sodium (Teva)

76. Tricor (Abbott)
77. Effexor XR (Pfizer)
78. Lorazepam (Activis)
79. Viagra (Pfizer)
80. Zetia (Merck/Schering-Plough)
81. Lisinopril (Sandoz)
82. Meloxicam (Lupin)
83. Citalopram Hydrobromide (Torrent)
84. Cephalexin (Lupin)
85. Vytorin (Merck/Schering-Plough)
86. Spiriva Handihaler (Boehringer Ingelheim)
87. Gabapentin (Amneal)
88. Alprazolam (Sandoz)
89. Abilify (Otsuka)
90. Lisinopril (Mylan)
91. Amoxicillin Trihydrate/Potassium Clavulanate (Teva)
92. Potassium Chloride (Watson)
93. Cyclobenzaprin HCL (Cadista)
94. Methylprednisolone (Cadista)
95. Concerta (Ortho-McNeil-Janssen)
96. Fexofenadine HCL (Teva)
97. Carvedilol (Teva)
98. Propoxyphen-N/APAP (Qualitest)
99. Furosemide (Teva)
100. Carisoprodol (Qualitest)
101. Digoxin (Lannett)
102. Cyclobenzaprine HCL (Mylan)
103. Citalopram Hydrobromide (Aurobindo)
104. Namenda (Forest)
105. Atenolol (Sandoz)
106. Diazepam (Mylan)
107. Amlodipine Besylate (Lupin)
108. Atenolol (Teva)
109. Loestrin 24 Fe (Warner-Chilcott)
110. Premarin (Pfizer)
111. Benicar (Daiichi Sankyo)
112. Gabapentin (Greenstone)
113. Ibuprofen (Rx) (Dr. Reddy's)
114. Allopurinal (Mylan)
115. Penicillin VK (Teva)
116. Clonazepam (Mylan)
117. Simvastatin (Aurobindo)
118. Januvia (Merck)
119. Alprazolam (Mylan)
120. Amitriptyline HCL (Mylan)
121. Clonidine HCL (Mylan)
122. Tramadol HCL (Teva)

123. Cialis (Lilly)
124. Xalatan (Pfizer)
125. Vyvanse (Shire)
126. Niaspan (Abbott)
127. Amlodipine Besylate (Camber)
128. Oxycontin (Purdue)
129. Atenolol (Zydus)
130. Levoxyl (King)
131. Azithromycin (Sandoz)
132. Naproxen (Teva)
133. Fluticasone Propionate (Apotex)
134. Zolpidem Tartate (Torrent)
135. Lisonopril (Watson)
136. Amlodipine Besylate/Benazepril (Teva)
137. Atenolol (Ranbaxy)
138. Fluoxetine HCL (Sandoz)
139. Prednisone (Watson)
140. Gabapentin (Actavis)
141. Oxycodone HCL (Mallinckrodt)
142. Actonel (Warner-Chilcott)
143. Folic Acid (West-Ward)
144. Potassium Chloride (Sandoz)
145. Klor-Con M20 (Upsher-Smith)
146. Benicar HCT (Daiichi Sankyo)
147. Hydrocodone/APAP (Amneal)
148. Flovent HFA (GlaxoSmithKline)
149. Prednisone (Qualitest)
150. Doxycycline Hyclate (West-Ward)
151. Alendronate Sodium (Watson)
152. Pantoprazole Sodium (Pfizer)
153. Albuterol (Mylan)
154. Furosemide (Sandoz)
155. Yaz-28 (Bayer)
156. Simvastatin (Zydus)
157. Flomax (Boehringer Ingelheim)
158. Metformin HCL ER (Teva)
159. Triamterene/Hydrocholorthiazide (Mylan)
160. Fenofexadine HCL (Prasco)
161. Paroxetine HCL (Zydus)
162. Nuvaring (Organon)
163. Suboxone (Reckitt Benckiser)
164. Furosemide (Ranbaxy)
165. Enalapril Maleate (Mylan)
166. Lovastatin (Lupin)
167. Omeprazole (Rx) (Dr. Reddy's)
168. Lovaza (GlaxoSmithKline)
169. Propoxyphen-N/APAP (Teva)
170. Cephalexin (Teva)

171. Glyburide (Teva)
172. Ciprofloxacin HCL (Dr. Reddy's)
173. Trinessa-28 (Watson)
174. Benazepril HCL (Teva)
175. Zyprexa (Lilly)
176. Prednisone (Roxane)
177. Amoxicillin (Greenstone)
178. Ocella (Teva)
179. Detrol LA (Pfizer)
180. Isosorbide Mononitrate (Kremers Urban)
181. Cheratussin AC (Qualitest)
182. Hydrochlorothiazide (Cadista Pharm)
183. Amphetamine Salts (Teva)
184. Sertraline HCL (Camber)
185. Proventil HFA (Schering)

186. Ambien CR (Sanofi-Aventis)
187. Naproxen (Glenmark)
188. Ranitidine HCL (Glenmark)
189. Amoxicillin (Aurobindo)
190. Famotidine (Teva)
191. Diltiazem 24Hr (Teva)
192. Toprol-XL (AstraZeneca)
193. Cefdinir (Sandoz)
194. Carvedilol (Mylan)
195. Klor-Con 10 (Upsher-Smith)
196. Mupirocin (Teva)
197. Verapamil SR (Teva)
198. Sertraline HCL (Lupin)
199. Combivent (Boehringer Ingelheim)
200. Lorazepam (Watson)

AAMA 2007–2008
Occupational Analysis of the CMA (AAMA)*

In furtherance of its leadership role in the profession, the American Association of Medical Assistants (AAMA) has completed the following *2007–2008 Occupational Analysis of the CMA (AAMA)*. In previous years, this document was titled *AAMA Role Delineation Study: Occupational Analysis of the Medical Assisting Profession.*

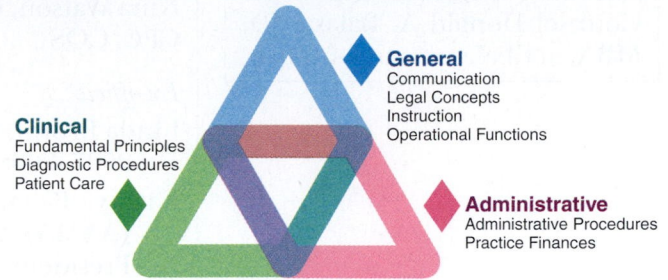

Clinical
Fundamental Principles
Diagnostic Procedures
Patient Care

General
Communication
Legal Concepts
Instruction
Operational Functions

Administrative
Administrative Procedures
Practice Finances

A Necessary Distinction

A professional's skills are largely determined by professional education. The CMA (AAMA) is the only credential that requires candidates to be graduates of a programmatically accredited medical assisting program. Therefore, it is appropriate and necessary that the qualifying language "of the CMA (AAMA)" be incorporated into this document's title.

About the Survey

A survey was sent to a random sample of CMAs (AAMA)—AAMA members and non-members. The CMA (AAMA) represents a medical assistant who has been certified by the Certifying Board of the AAMA. Of the 15,500 surveys distributed, 3,658 were collected and analyzed, resulting in a 95 percent confidence level. The results obtained from the sample are within ±1.6 percent of the results if all 15,500 individuals had responded.

Analysis Highlights

Today's CMA (AAMA) is expected not only to master the body of knowledge of the profession, but also to apply this knowledge in the complex and fast-paced world of ambulatory health care. Thus, critical thinking is emphasized in this *Occupational Analysis.*

Another dimension in the *Occupational Analysis* reflects the growing awareness that the CMA (AAMA) is uniquely qualified to "speak the patient's language" and serve as a "communication liaison" between the busy physician and patients. The roles of the CMA (AAMA) as "patient advocate" and "health coach," as well as "communication liaison," are given appropriate prominence in this document.

All health professionals have been expected to refine their knowledge and skills in responding to natural and manmade emergencies, and the vital roles of CMAs (AAMA) have come into increasing focus in recent years. In keeping with this priority, the *Occupational Analysis* includes emergency-related functions under Communication, Instruction, and Patient Care.

Uses of the Study

This document provides valuable data to the Certifying Board (CB) and the Continuing Education Board (CEB) of the AAMA, as well as to the Medical Assistant Education Review Board (MAERB). However, the *Occupational Analysis* should not be confused with the following documents:

- *Content Outline of the CMA (AAMA) Certification/Recertification Examination,* published by the CB
- *Advanced Practice of Medical Assisting,* published by the CEB
- *Standards and Guidelines for Medical Assisting Educational Programs,* published by CAAHEP
- *Curriculum Content and Competencies,* published by the CRB

*Permission is granted from the American Association of Medical Assistants.

Legal Scope of Practice

This *Occupational Analysis* does not delineate the legal scope of medical assisting practice. Legally delegable responsibilities vary from state to state. Scope of practice questions should be directed to AAMA Executive Director and Legal Counsel Donald A. Balasa, JD, MBA, at dbalasa@aama-ntl.org.

Occupational Analysis Committee

Chair: Charlene Couch, CMA (AAMA)

Karen Minchella, CMA (AAMA), PhD

Rebecca Walker, CMA (AAMA), CP

Nina Watson, CMA (AAMA), CPC, COS

Ex officio

Linda Brown, CMA (AAMA), 2007–2008 President

Kathryn Panagiotacos, CMA (AAMA), 2007–2008 Vice President

Donald A. Balasa, JD, MBA, Executive Director

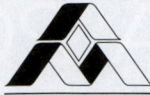

AMERICAN ASSOCIATION OF MEDICAL ASSISTANTS
20 N. WACKER DR., STE. 1575
CHICAGO, ILLINOIS 60606
website: www.aama-ntl.org   800/228-2262

General, Clinical, and Administrative Skills* of the CMA (AAMA)

General Skills

◆ Communication

- Recognize and respect cultural diversity
- Adapt communications to individual's understanding
- Employ professional telephone and interpersonal techniques
- Recognize and respond effectively to verbal, nonverbal, and written communications
- Utilize and apply medical terminology appropriately
- Receive, organize, prioritize, store, and maintain transmittable information utilizing electronic technology
- Serve as "communication liaison" between the physician and patient
- Serve as patient advocate professional and health coach in a team approach in health care
- Identify basics of office emergency preparedness

◆ Legal Concepts

- Perform within legal (including federal and state statutes, regulations, opinions, and rulings) and ethical boundaries
- Document patient communication and clinical treatments accurately and appropriately
- Maintain medical records
- Follow employer's established policies dealing with the health care contract
- Comply with established risk management and safety procedures
- Recognize professional credentialing criteria
- Identify and respond to issues of confidentiality

◆ Instruction

- Function as a health care advocate to meet individual's needs
- Educate individuals in office policies and procedures
- Educate the patient within the scope of practice and as directed by supervising physician in health maintenance, disease prevention, and compliance with patient's treatment plan
- Identify community resources for health maintenance and disease prevention to meet individual patient needs

◆ Operational Functions

- Perform inventory of supplies and equipment
- Perform routine maintenance of administrative and clinical equipment
- Apply computer and other electronic equipment techniques to support office operations
- Perform methods of quality control
- Maintain current list of community resources, including those for emergency preparedness and other patient care needs
- Collaborate with local community resources for emergency preparedness
- Educate patients in their responsibilities relating to third-party reimbursements

Clinical Skills

◆ Fundamental Principles

- Identify the roles and responsibilities of the medical assistant in the clinical setting
- Identify the roles and responsibilities of other team members in the medical office
- Apply principles of aseptic technique and infection control
- Practice Standard Precautions, including handwashing and disposal of biohazardous materials
- Perform sterilization techniques
- Comply with quality assurance practices

◆ Diagnostic Procedures

- Collect and process specimens
- Perform CLIA-waived tests
- Perform electrocardiography and respiratory testing
- Perform phlebotomy, including venipuncture and capillary puncture
- Utilize knowledge of principles of radiology

◆ Patient Care

- Perform initial-response screening following protocols approved by supervising physician
- Obtain, evaluate, and record patient history employing critical thinking skills
- Obtain vital signs
- Prepare and maintain examination and treatment areas
- Prepare patient for examinations, procedures and treatments
- Assist with examinations, procedures, and treatments
- Maintain examination/treatment rooms, including inventory of supplies and equipment
- Prepare and administer oral and parenteral (excluding IV) medications and immunizations *(as directed by supervising physician and as permitted by state law)*
- Utilize knowledge of principles of IV therapy
- Maintain medication and immunization records
- Screen and follow up test results
- Recognize and respond to emergencies

Administrative Skills

◆ Administrative Procedures

- Schedule, coordinate, and monitor appointments
- Schedule inpatient/outpatient admissions and procedures
- Apply third-party and managed care policies, procedures, and guidelines
- Establish, organize, and maintain patient medical record
- File medical records appropriately

◆ Practice Finances

- Perform procedural and diagnostic coding for reimbursement
- Perform billing and collection procedures
- Perform administrative functions, including book-keeping and financial procedures
- Prepare submittable ("clean") insurance forms

*All skills require decision making based on critical thinking concepts.

Medical Assisting Task List*

The various tasks that medical assistants perform include, but are not necessarily limited to, those on the following list.

The tasks presented in this inventory are considered by American Medical Technologists to be representative of the medical assisting job role. This document should be considered dynamic, to reflect the medical assistant's evolving role with respect to contemporary health care. Therefore, tasks may be added, removed, or modified on an on-going basis.

Medical Assistants that meet AMT's qualifications and pass a certification examination are certified as a Registered Medical Assistant (RMA).

I. GENERAL MEDICAL ASSISTING KNOWLEDGE

A. Anatomy and Physiology
1. Body systems
2. Disorders and diseases of the body

B. Medical Terminology
1. Word parts
2. Medical terms
3. Common abbreviations and symbols
4. Spelling

C. Medical Law
1. Medical law
2. Licensure, certification, and registration

D. Medical Ethics
1. Principles of medical ethics
2. Ethical conduct
3. Professional development

E. Human Relations
1. Patient relations
2. Interpersonal skills
3. Cultural diversity

F. Patient Education
1. Identify and apply proper communication methods in patient instruction
2. Develop, assemble, and maintain patient resource materials

II. ADMINISTRATIVE MEDICAL ASSISTING

A. Insurance
1. Medical insurance terminology
2. Various insurance plans
3. Claim forms
4. Electronic insurance claims
5. ICD-9CM/CPT Coding applications
6. HIPAA mandated coding systems
7. Financial applications of medical insurance

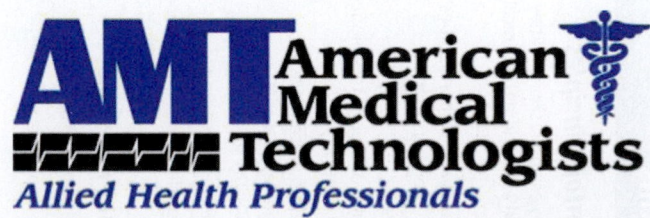

Allied Health Professionals

*Permission is granted from the American Medical Technologists.

B. Financial Bookkeeping
  1. Medical finance terminology
  2. Patient billing procedures
  3. Collection procedures
  4. Fundamental medical office accounting procedures
  5. Office banking procedures
  6. Employee payroll
  7. Financial calculations and accounting procedures

C. Medical Secretarial—Receptionist
  1. Medical terminology associated with receptionist duties
  2. General reception of patients and visitors
  3. Appointment scheduling systems
  4. Oral and written communications
  5. Medical records management
  6. Charting guidelines and regulations
  7. Protect, store, and retain medical records according to HIPAA regulations
  8. Release of protected health information adhering to HIPAA regulations
  9. Transcription of dictation
  10. Supplies and equipment management
  11. Medical office computer applications
  12. Compliance with OSHA guidelines and regulations of office safety

III. CLINICAL MEDICAL ASSISTING

A. Asepsis
  1. Medical terminology
  2. State/Federal universal bloodborne pathogen/body fluid precautions
  3. Medical/surgical asepsis procedure

B. Sterilization
  1. Medical terminology associated with sterilization
  2. Sanitization, disinfection, and sterilization procedures
  3. Record keeping procedures

C. Instruments
  1. Specialty instruments and parts
  2. Usage of common instruments
  3. Care and handling of disposable and reusable instruments

D. Vital Signs/Mensurations
  1. Blood pressure, pulse, respiration measurements
  2. Height, weight, circumference measurements
  3. Various temperature measurements
  4. Recognize normal and abnormal measurement results

E. Physical Examinations
  1. Patient history information
  2. Proper charting procedures
  3. Patient positions for examinations
  4. Methods of examinations
  5. Specialty examinations
  6. Visual acuity/Ishihara (color blindness) measurements
  7. Allergy testing procedures
  8. Normal/abnormal results

F. Clinical Pharmacology
  1. Medical terminology associated with pharmacology
  2. Commonly used drugs and their categories
  3. Various routes of medication administration
  4. Parenteral administration of medications (subcutaneous, intramuscular, intradermal, Z-Tract)
  5. Classes or drug schedules and legal prescriptions requirements for each
  6. Drug Enforcement Agency regulations for ordering, dispensing, storage, and documentation of medication use
  7. Drug Reference books (PDR, Pharmacopeia, Facts and Comparisons, Nurses Handbook)

G. Minor Surgery
  1. Surgical supplies and instruments
  2. Asepsis in surgical procedures
  3. Surgical tray preparation and sterile field respect
  4. Prevention of pathogen transmission
  5. Patient surgical preparation procedures
  6. Assisting physician with minor surgery including set-up
  7. Dressing and bandaging techniques
  8. Suture and staple removal
  9. Biohazard waste disposal procedures
  10. Instruct patient in pre- and postsurgical care

H. Therapeutic Modalities
  1. Various standard therapeutic modalities
  2. Alternative/complementary therapies
  3. Instruct patient in assistive devices, body mechanics, and home care
I. Laboratory Procedures
  1. Medical laboratory terminology
  2. OSHA safety guidelines
  3. Quality control and assessment regulations
  4. Operate and maintain laboratory equipment
  5. CLIA-waived laboratory testing procedures
  6. Capillary, dermal, and venipuncture procedures
  7. Office specimen collection such as: urine, throat, vaginal, wound cultures, stool, sputum, etc.
  8. Specimen handling and preparation

  9. Laboratory recording according to state and federal guidelines
  10. Adhere to the MA Scope of Practice in the laboratory
J. Electrocardiography
  1. Standard, 12 lead ECG testing
  2. Mounting techniques for permanent record
  3. Rhythm strip ECG monitoring on Lead II
K. First Aid
  1. Emergencies and first aid procedures
  2. Emergency crash cart supplies
  3. Legal responsibilities as a first responder

American Medical Technologists
10700 W. Higgins Road
Rosemont, Illinois 60018
Phone: (847) 823-5169 – Fax: (847) 823-0458
Website: www.amt1.com

Software Support:
The Critical Thinking Challenge and Medical Office Simulation Software

TECHNICAL SUPPORT INFORMATION

Technical Support at Delmar Cengage Learning is available from 8:30 AM to 9:00 PM, Eastern Standard Time.

- Telephone: 1-800-648-7450
- Email: delmar.help@cengage.com

ABOUT THE CRITICAL THINKING CHALLENGE 3.0

The new Critical Thinking Challenge (CTC) 3.0 is a game that simulates a 3-month practicum at Birch Hill Family Practice. In this game, you'll be confronted with a series of situations in which you have to use critical thinking skills to select the most correct action in response to the situation. Your actions will be evaluated by how the decision has affected the patient, the practice, and your career. You will also be awarded points for your overall decision making. The 3.0 version includes 12 all-new video-based scenarios that include more follow-on scenarios, depending on the decisions made. After successfully completing the program, you can print out a Certificate of Completion.

Setup and Time Requirements

The program can be accessed from the Premium Website. Completion of the game requires about 45–60 minutes of your time.

After watching the Overview video, you must **set up your character as male or female** by clicking the appropriate button. You can turn on Subtitles by clicking the buttons in the upper right corner of the game window. You can **turn Subtitles on or off** at any point in the game. Subtitles are available in both **English (EN)** and **Spanish (ES)**.

To **adjust the volume level**, click on the Volume button at the upper right side of the game window. Then, move the fader to the desired setting. Click outside of the volume window to return to the game.

To exit the Critical Thinking Challenge, close out of your browser window. Your score will be saved, and you can begin at the same point where you left off.

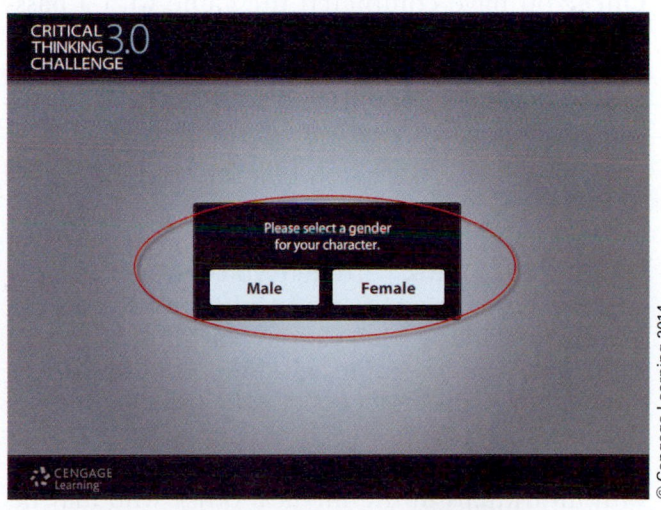

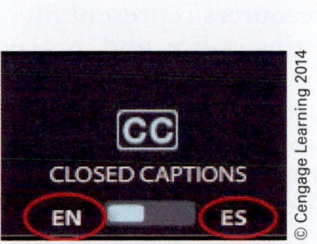

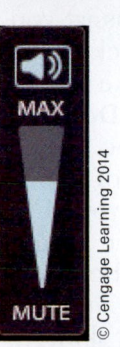

Playing the Game

You are a character in each situation in the game. Each situation is a video presented from your point of view. In most cases, you will be directly involved in the situation, interacting with other staff members or patients; in other instances, you will be a witness to the situation. However, in every situation presented, you must use your critical thinking skills to respond.

The object of the game is to receive an offer of employment from the medical practice.

The Situations. You will need to view each video situation **to determine the best action** to take. To control the pace of the narrative, use the video buttons at the bottom of the game window. These allow you to play and pause the narration. You can forward and reverse the narration by clicking ahead or behind in the progress bar at the bottom of the game window. After you view the video scenario, you are presented with three possible actions that you can take.

Your first time through the game, you will be required to finish the scenarios in order, beginning with the first scenario. Future scenarios will be locked until you finish each one in sequence. Once you have completed the game with a passing grade, you will be able to go back and view each scenario again in any order. Once you have passed, you are encouraged to go back through the scenarios and view the consequences of having chosen incorrect responses to the action questions.

Using Resources. To help you choose the most correct action, you may **consult your Resources Panel** by clicking the Resources button on the right side of the game window. The Resources Panel allows you to access People and Documents resources.

The **People resources** allow you to interact with individuals in the medical office who may be able to assist you in choosing the appropriate action. Click on the staff member with whom you would like to speak.

The **Documents resources** represent files that would be found in the policy and procedure manual of a medical office and that may be able to help you. Each resource may only be viewed once per action question. Keep in mind that not all the resources may be helpful to you, depending on the situation. Always use your critical thinking skills!

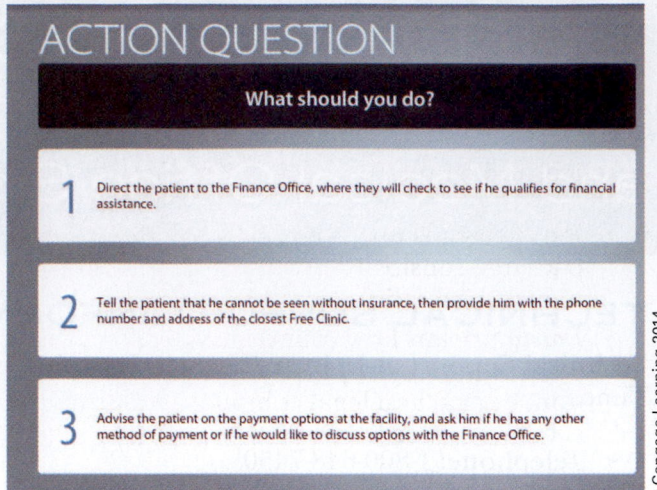

ACTION QUESTION

What should you do?

1 Direct the patient to the Finance Office, where they will check to see if he qualifies for financial assistance.

2 Tell the patient that he cannot be seen without insurance, then provide him with the phone number and address of the closest Free Clinic.

3 Advise the patient on the payment options at the facility, and ask him if he has any other method of payment or if he would like to discuss options with the Finance Office.

© Cengage Learning 2014

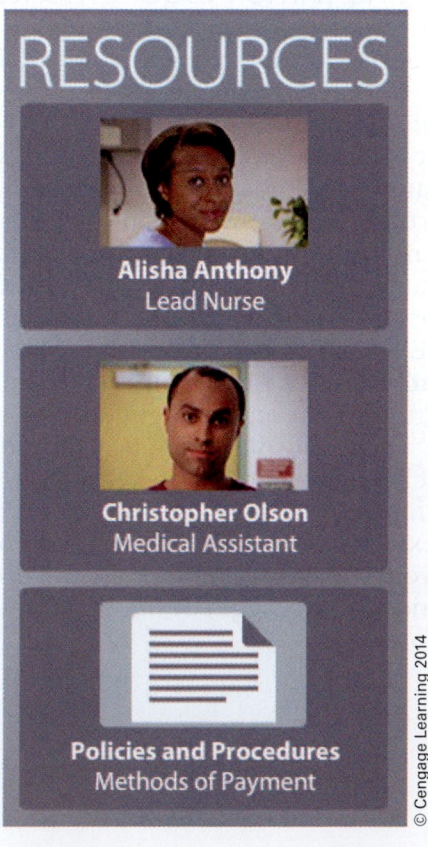

RESOURCES

Alisha Anthony
Lead Nurse

Christopher Olson
Medical Assistant

Policies and Procedures
Methods of Payment

© Cengage Learning 2014

Evaluation and Points Awarded

When you have finished consulting your resources, select one of the actions presented. Your decisions are then **evaluated in three categories**: patient, practice, and employee.

- *Patient* means how your decision affects the patient—sensitivity, privacy, health, convenience, and satisfaction.
- *Practice* means how your decisions affect the medical office—reputation, patient retention, ethical and legal compliance, or medical malpractice liability.
- *Employee* means how your decisions affect your career as a medical assistant—employability, professionalism, effectiveness, reputation, ethical and legal compliance, or medical malpractice liability.

When you have completed a scenario, you will receive video feedback from the office manager at Birch Hill Family Practice that discusses the merits of your decision and the outcome of the situation. You will then be given detailed written feedback addressing all three evaluation categories. You will also be awarded points for your overall decision-making skills.

You will **receive points according to the merits of the action** chosen:

- You will receive full credit for selecting the best action.
- You will receive partial credit for selecting a good action to take, but not the best action.
- You will not receive any credit for selecting the least desirable action.

At any time, you can print a score report. Click on the **report** icon at the upper right side of the main menu. The score report lists your overall score, as well as your individual scenario scores on both your first attempt at playing the game and your best attempt.

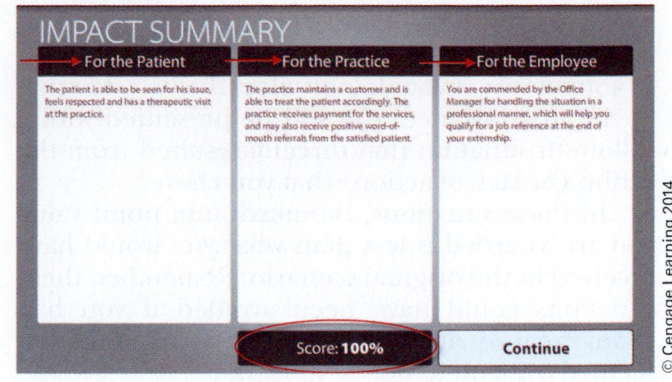

© Cengage Learning 2014

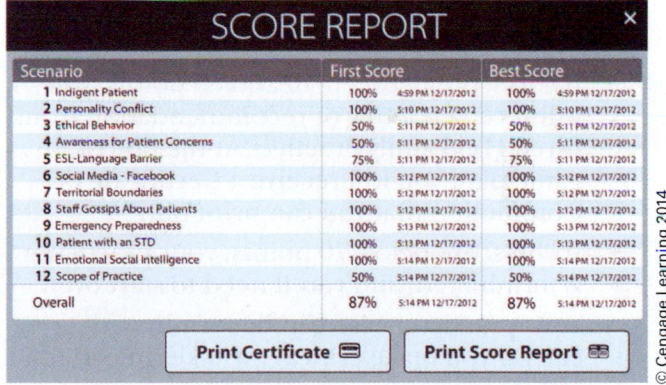

© Cengage Learning 2014

Follow-on Situations

In some cases, if you do not select the best decision in the first instance, you will be presented with a follow-on situation that directly resulted from the action (or lack of action) that you chose.

In these situations, the maximum point value you are awarded is less than what you would have received in the original scenario. Remember, these situations could have been avoided if you had taken the most appropriate action at first, even if it seemed difficult to do.

As the action questions become more challenging, the later scenarios contain more potential follow-on videos than earlier scenarios.

Scoring the Game

Your goal is to be hired by Birch Hill Family Practice as a full-time medical assistant. On the other hand, if you show a serious lack of critical thinking skills that threatens the well-being of the medical office or the patients, the office manager will terminate your practicum and you'll have to start over.

- You will receive a job offer to work in the office if you score above 85 points in the game. At the end of game play, you will receive a Certificate of Completion that you can print out.

- If you score between 70 and 85 points, you will receive a letter of recommendation from Birch Hill Family Practice. At the end of game play, you will receive a Certificate of Completion that you can print out.

- If you score below 70 points, your practicum is terminated, and you'll need to start over.

- Your practicum also can be terminated early if you make critical mistakes in certain scenarios.

As you continue throughout the game, a progress bar at the bottom of the main menu shows your cumulative score. This allows you to keep track of how many points you have received, and how close you are to receiving a passing grade.

Once you have completed the game, you will be able to improve upon your scores by choosing the most correct answer in those scenarios where you did not receive full marks. If you improve your scores, the score report will update your **best attempt** score. Your scores will not be negatively impacted by choosing incorrect answers after your first time through the game. In subsequent attempts, your score can only be improved upon.

© Cengage Learning 2014

ABOUT MEDICAL OFFICE SIMULATION SOFTWARE 2.0

In Medical Office Simulation Software (MOSS), the Main Menu screen orients you to the general functions of most practice management software programs. Basic components common to most practice management software include the following: Patient Registration, File Maintenance, Procedure Posting, Insurance Billing, Posting Payments, Patient Billing, Report Generation, and Appointment Scheduling.

What's new in MOSS 2.0:

- Uses Microsoft Access 2007 and is compatible with Windows Vista.
- Claims Tracking is a new area of the program that simulates receiving an electronic explanation of benefits (EOB) or remittance advice (RA) from an insurance carrier.
- CMS-1500 forms populate based on insurance type selected to meet the needs of medical billing programs.
- Each insurance carrier has a fee schedule.
- Date parameters have been expanded to a 5-year range.
- Search functionality has been improved.
- Reports functionality has been improved.
- New reports have been added: monthly report, aging patient balance report, and individual patient balance report.

- Adjustment functionality is corrected to the type of adjustment; additional adjustment types have been added.
- Patient ledger report has been added to track payment history.
- Prebilling report has been added prior to generating claims.
- Expanded seed data have been added to the program.

Installation and Setup Requirements

1. Take the MOSS 2.0 CD in the back of this book and place it into your CD-ROM drive.
2. MOSS 2.0 should begin setup automatically. Follow the on-screen prompts to install MOSS and Access Runtime.
3. If MOSS does not begin setup automatically, follow these instructions:
   - Double-click on My Computer.
   - Double-click the Control Panel icon.
   - Double-click Add/Remove Programs.
   - Click the Install button, and follow the on-screen prompts.
4. When MOSS is finished installing, it will be accessible through the Start menu:

Start > All Programs > Medical Office Simulation Software > MOSS

At the **logon screen**, click OK to enter MOSS. Your user name and password are already loaded for you. You can change your password after you have logged in by going to the File Maintenance area of the software.

MOSS 2.0 is a single-user program that is designed to be used with various procedures in the administrative section of this book. Procedures that use MOSS are clearly marked in the procedure title.

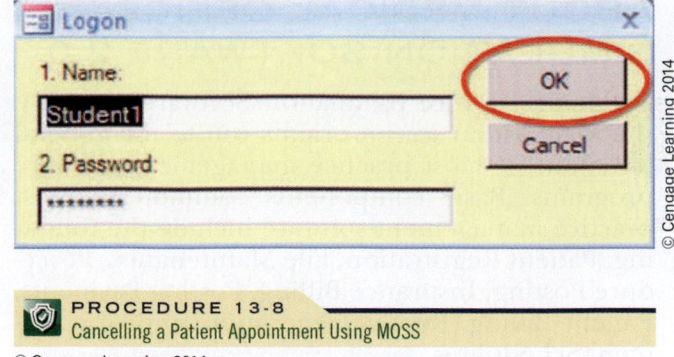

PROCEDURE 13-8
Cancelling a Patient Appointment Using MOSS

© Cengage Learning 2014

Changing Your Password.
Once in the program, **select File Maintenance** from the Main Menu screen.

Select the button next to **1. Change Password**.

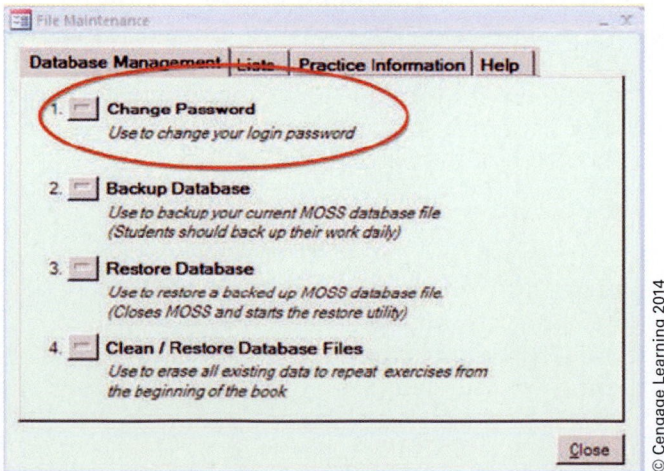

Enter the current password "Student1" and then your new password.

Click **Change Password** when you are finished. If you change your password, we recommend that you write down your new password and keep it in a secure place.

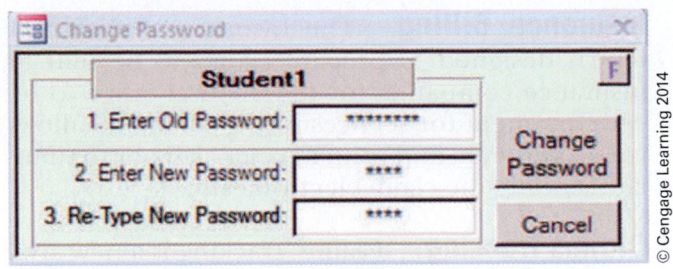

Sections of the Program

MOSS features a **Main Menu screen** consisting of buttons that provide access to specific areas.

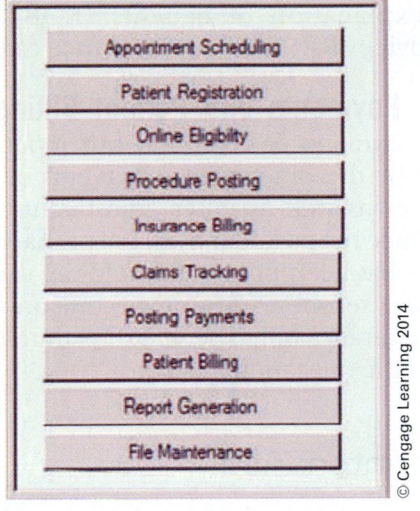

Alternatively, you can use **the icon bar** along the top left to quickly access the areas of the software, or you can navigate the software by using the **pull-down menus** below the software title bar.

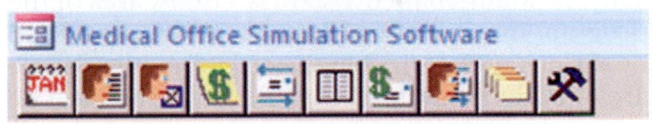

Patient Registration. The Patient Registration area allows you to input information about each patient in the practice, including demographic, Health Insurance Portability and Accountability Act (HIPAA), and medical insurance information. From the Main Menu screen, click on the Patient Registration button to search for a patient or to add a new patient, using the command buttons along the bottom of the patient selection dialog box.

Appointment Scheduling. The Appointment Scheduling System enables you to make appointments and to cancel, reschedule, and search for appointments. MOSS allows for block scheduling as well as several print features, including appointment cards and daily schedules.

Procedure Posting. In the Procedure Posting System, patient fees for services are applied, as well as relevant information such as service dates and place of service information. When procedures are input into the procedure posting system, the software assigns the fee to be charged according to the fee schedule for the patient's insurance.

Insurance Billing. The Insurance Billing System is designed to prepare claims to be sent to insurance companies for the medical office to receive payment for services provided. MOSS allows you to generate and print a paper claim or to simulate sending the claim electronically.

Claims Tracking. Claims Tracking is a new area of the program that simulates receiving an electronic explanation of benefits (EOB) or remittance advice (RA) from an insurance carrier.

Posting Payments and Patient Billing. In the Posting Payments System, you can input payments received by the practice from patients or insurance companies as well as enter adjustments to the account. Once the payment from the primary insurance company has been posted, the software can generate a claim to a secondary insurance company, if applicable, or generate a bill to be sent directly to the patient to collect the outstanding balance.

File Maintenance

The File Maintenance System is a utility area of the program that contains common information used by various systems within the software. It is also an area where the setup of the software system can be adjusted or customized.

Feedback Mode and Balloon Help. Under the Help tab in File Maintenance, you can **turn Feedback Mode and Balloon Help Mode on or off**. Feedback Mode will alert you when essential fields have not been completed before allowing data to be saved. Balloon Help offers explanations, clarification, and reminders for certain fields.

Creating Backup Files. You can create a backup file of the work you've completed in the program at any time. Click on File Maintenance, and then click the button next to **2. Backup Database**.

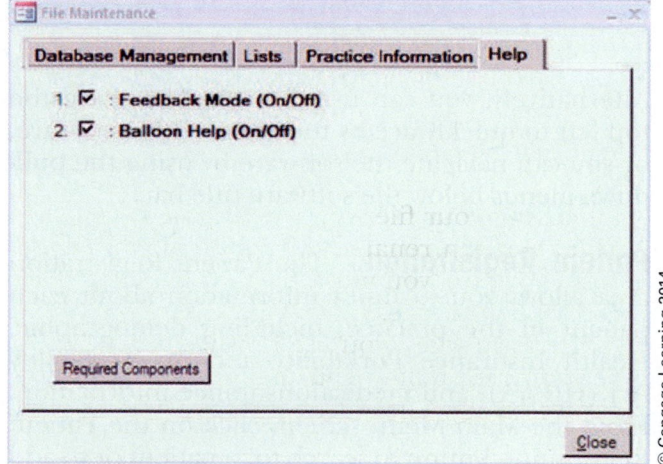

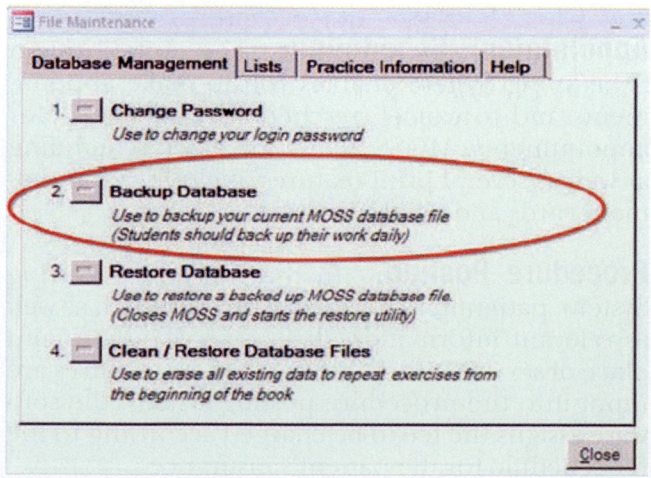

Click **Yes** at the prompt.

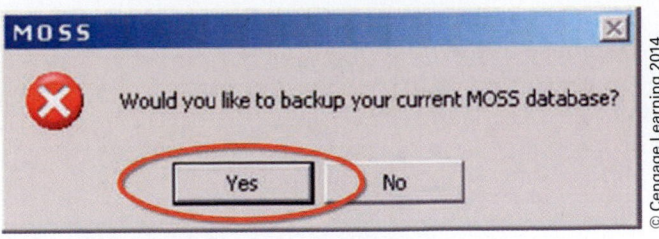

Now, select a location to **save your backup file**. We recommend that you save the database on a flash drive (in most computers, this is your E:/ or F:/ computer drive).

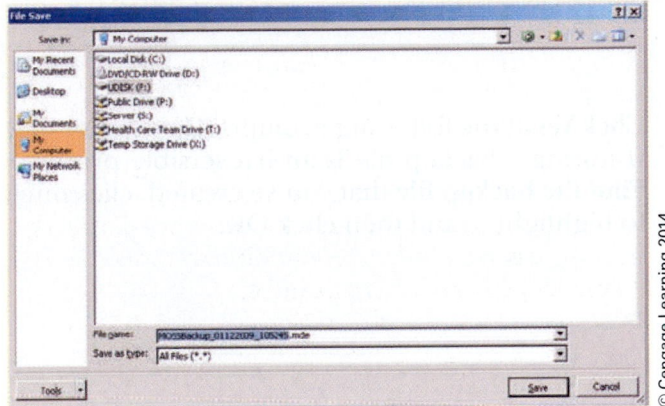

When saving your file, you can choose to rename the file. You can rename the file to anything you choose; however, you must **keep the file extension .mde in the file name**.

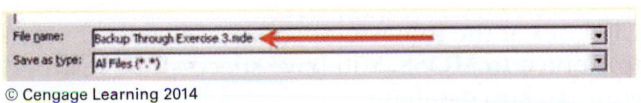

Click Save when you are finished. You will receive a prompt telling you that your file was created successfully. Click OK.

Restoring Backup Files. You can restore a backup file of the work you've saved in the program at any time. Click on File Maintenance, and then click the button next to **3. Restore Database**. Note that restoring a backup file is an irreversible process.

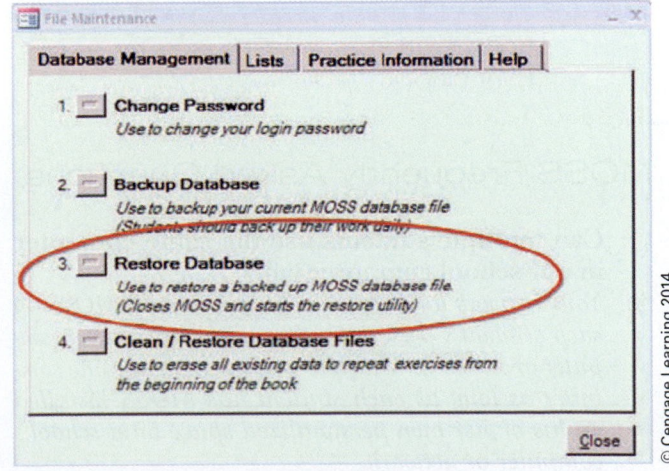

Click Yes at the prompt. Click **Restore MOSS from Database** at the next prompt.

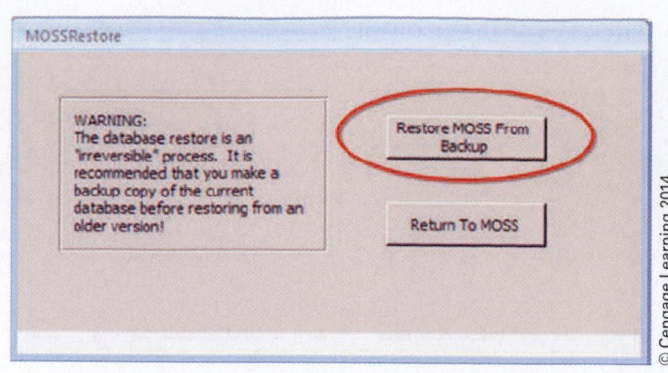

Click Yes at the following prompt. (Remember that restoring a backup file is an irreversible process.) **Find the backup file** that you've created, click once to highlight it, and then click OK.

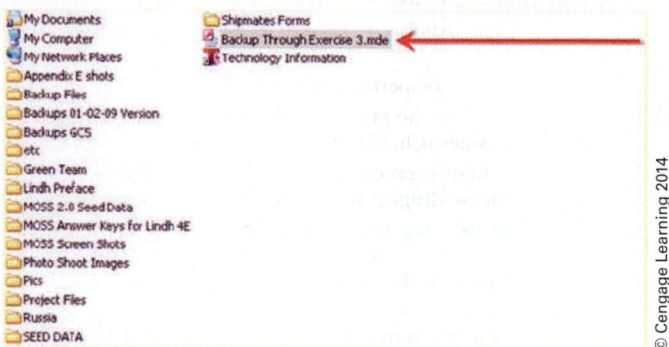

Click Yes at the following prompt. Click the button to **Return to MOSS**. You have successfully restored your backup database.

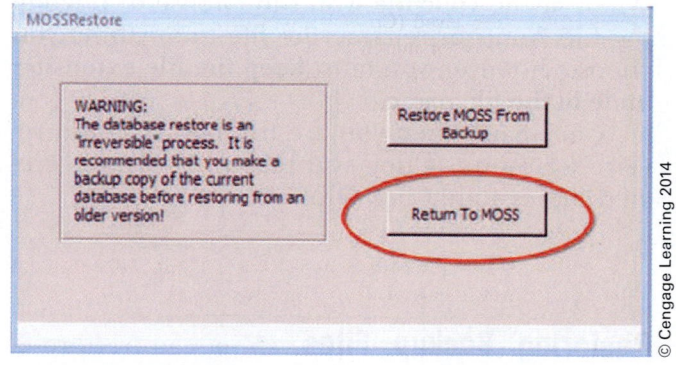

MOSS Frequently Asked Questions

Q: **Can multiple students use the same computer in our school computer lab?**

A: *Your network administrator should install MOSS on each student's personalized space on a school's computer or network. Multiple students can use one computer **as long as each student has MOSS installed on his or her own personalized space on a school's computer or network.***

For programs that do not have network privileges, students should use the backup/restore utility in MOSS, saving the MOSS.mde file to a flash drive.

Q: **I have Microsoft Access on my computer. Do I need to install Access Runtime on my computer?**

A: *Yes, you should install Access Runtime on your computer to go along with the program. It will not cause any problems to your system or otherwise interfere with the Microsoft Access program on your computer.*

Glossary of Terms

Note: The equivalent Spanish word follows in parentheses in green.

abduction (abducción) motion away from the midline of the body (Ch. 33).

ABO blood group (grupo sanguíneo ABO) genetically determined system of antigens found on the surface of erythrocytes. The population can be divided into four ABO blood groups: A, B, AB, and O (Ch. 44).

abortion (aborto) expulsion of the products of conception before viability (Ch. 26).

abrasion (abrasión) a superficial scraping of the epidermis (Ch. 9).

absorption (absorción) the process whereby the drug passes into the body fluids and tissues (Ch. 35).

abuse (abuso) misuse; excessive or improper use, especially of narcotics or psychoactive drugs (Ch. 17, 35).

accession record (numeric system) (registro de entrada [sistema de ordenación por número]) logbook used to assign numbers to correspondence or patients (Ch. 14).

accomplishment statements (declaraciones de logros) statements that begin with a power verb and give a brief description of what you did, and the demonstrable results that were produced (Ch. 48).

accounting (contabilidad) system of monitoring the financial status of a facility and the financial results of its activities, providing information for decision making (Ch. 21).

accounts payable (cuentas por pagar) sum owed by a business for services or goods received (Ch. 19); also unwritten promise to pay a supplier for property or merchandise purchased on credit or for a service rendered (Ch. 21).

accounts receivable (cuentas por cobrar) amount owed to a business for services or goods supplied (Ch. 19).

accounts receivable (A/R) ratio assets (relación de cuentas por cobrar a activos) outstanding accounts receivable divided by the average monthly gross income for the past 12 months (Ch. 20, 21).

accreditation (acreditación) process whereby recognition is granted to an educational program for maintaining standards that qualify its graduates for professional practice; to provide with credentials (Ch. 1).

Accrediting Bureau of Health Education Schools (ABHES) (Junta de Acreditación de Escuelas de Educación en Salud [ABHES]) entity accrediting private, postsecondary institutions in the U.S. which offer allied health education programs as well as programmatic accreditation of medical assistant, medical laboratory technician, and surgical technology programs (Ch. 47).

accrual basis accounting (contabilidad según el principio del devengo) reports income at the time charges are generated (Ch. 21).

acid/base balance (equilibrio ácido-básico) condition that occurs when the net rate at which the body produces acids or bases is equal to the net rate at which acids or bases are excreted (Ch. 42).

acquired immunodeficiency syndrome (AIDS) (síndrome de inmunodeficiencia adquirida [SIDA]) disorder of the immune system caused by a human immunodeficiency virus (HIV), a retrovirus that destroys the body's ability to fight infection. As the disease progresses, the individual becomes overcome by disorders, including cancers and opportunistic infections. There is no known cure for AIDS (Ch. 22).

active listening (escucha activa) received message is paraphrased back to the sender to verify the correct message was decoded (Ch. 5).

activities of daily living (ADL) (actividades de la vida diaria [AVD]) activities usually performed during a typical day that involve caring for oneself, such as eating and brushing teeth (Ch. 33).

acupuncture (acupuntura) treatment to relieve pain and disease by puncturing the skin with thin needles at specific points (Ch. 2).

acute or adult respiratory distress syndrome (ARDS) (Síndrome de dificultad respiratoria aguda o de adulto [ARDS]) a life-threatening condition that occurs when there is severe fluid buildup and hemorrhage in the lungs (Ch. 30).

additive (aditivo) any material placed in a tube that maintains or facilitates the integrity and function of the specimen (Ch. 40).

adduction (aducción) motion toward the midline of the body (Ch. 33).

adjustments (ajustes) increases or decreases to patient accounts not due to charges incurred or payments received (Ch. 17, 19).

administer (administrar) to give a medication (Ch. 7, 35, 36).

administrative law (derecho administrativo) establishes agencies that are given the power to make laws and enact regulations (Ch. 7).

aegis (auspicio) sponsorship or protection (Ch. 38).

aerobic (aerobio) organism that requires oxygen for growth (Ch. 43).

aerosolized (aerosolizado) dispensed by means of a mist (Ch. 27).

aerosols (aerosoles) particles from potentially infectious materials that may be released in the air (Ch. 43).

afebrile (afebril) without fever (Ch. 24).

agar (agar) a gelatin-like substance extracted from red algae that contains nutrients and moisture for bacteria growth (Ch. 43).

agenda (orden del día) printed list of topics to be discussed during a meeting, sometimes giving time allocation (Ch. 15, 45).

agent (agente) person representing another (Ch. 7).

airborne transmission (transmisión por aire) spread of disease-causing microorganisms over long distances through the air (Ch. 22).

aliquot (alícuota) part of the whole specimen that has been taken off for use or storage (Ch. 40).

allergen (alérgeno) any substance that causes signs of allergy; examples are inhalants such as dust and pollen, foods such as wheat and strawberries, drugs, penicillin, chemicals, heat, bacteria (Ch. 30).

allergy (alergia) acquired hypersensitivity to a substance (allergen) that does not normally cause a reaction (Ch. 23).

allopathic (alopático) method of treating disease with remedies that produce effects different from those caused by the disease itself. Most traditional practitioners today are considered allopathic practitioners (Ch. 3).

alternative dispute resolution (ADR) (resolución alternativa de conflictos [RAC]) an alternative to trial that encourages the parties to settle their differences out of court (Ch. 7).

ambulation (ambulación) ability to walk (Ch. 33).

ambulatory care setting (entorno de atención ambulatoria) health care environment where services are provided on an outpatient basis. *Ambulatory* is from the Latin and means "capable of walking." Examples include the solo-provider's office, the group practice, the urgent care center, and the health maintenance organization (Ch. 1, 2).

American Association of Medical Assistants (AAMA) (Asociación Estadounidense de Asistentes Médicos [AAMA]) professional organization dedicated to serving the interests of Certified Medical Assistants (Ch. 47).

American Medical Technologists (AMT) (Tecnólogos Médicos Estadounidenses [AMT]) national organization which credentials health care professionals, including Registered Medical Assistants (RMA) and Certified Medical Administrative Specialists (CMAS) (Ch. 47).

amino acid (aminoácido) basic structural unit of protein (Ch. 34).

amniocentesis (amniocentesis) surgical puncture of the amniotic sac to remove fluid for laboratory analysis (Ch. 22, 26).

amniotomy (amniotomía) artificial rupture of the amniotic sac (Ch. 26).

amoebic dysentery (disentería amébica) infectious intestinal disease caused by amoebas and characterized by inflammation of the mucous membrane of the colon (Ch. 22).

amorphous (amorfo) shapeless; possessing no definite form (Ch. 42).

amplified (amplificado) made larger or enlarged. The amplifier of the electrocardiograph enlarges the electrical impulse activity and the recording can be read more easily (Ch. 37).

amplitude (amplitud) amount, extent, size, abundance, or fullness (Ch. 37).

anaerobic (anaerobio) organism that needs little or no oxygen for growth (Ch. 43).

anaphylaxis (anafilaxia) hypersensitive state of the body to a foreign protein or drug (Ch. 9, 35).

ancillary services (servicios auxiliares) professional occupational companies hired to complete a specific job (Ch. 45).

andropause (andropausia) midlife changes in a male (Ch. 29).

anesthesia (anestesia) loss of feeling or sensation; an anesthetic is any mechanism that causes anesthesia (Ch. 31).

angiogram (angiograma) series of X-rays of a blood vessel(s) after injection of a radiopaque substance (Ch. 37).

anisocytosis (anisocitosis) marked variation in the size of cells (Ch. 41).

anorexia (anorexia) loss of appetite (Ch. 22, 30).

answering services (servicios de respuesta) services employed to answer the calls of an ambulatory care setting after hours; unlike an answering machine, a live operator answers the call and forwards it appropriately (Ch. 12).

antibacterial (antibacteriano) capable of destroying bacteria, often applied to a wound in the form of an ointment or cream (Ch. 31).

antibody (anticuerpo) specific chemical produced by B cells of the immune system in response to an antigen (Ch. 22).

anticoagulant (anticoagulante) chemical in a blood tube that prevents the clotting of the blood by removing the calcium from the blood or by stopping the formation of thrombin (Ch. 40).

antigen (antígeno) substance such as bacteria or other agents that the body recognizes as foreign; the stimulus for antibody production (Ch. 22, 44).

antioxidant (antioxidante) something that prevents oxidation (Ch. 34).

aphasia (afasia) the inability to speak (Ch. 30).

apical (apical) pertaining to the apex of the heart. A site for measuring heart rate with a stethoscope (Ch. 24).

apnea (apnea) cessation or absence of normal spontaneous breathing (Ch. 24, 36).

appendicular skeleton (esqueleto apendicular) skeleton that consists of the pectoral and pelvic girdles and the upper and lower extremities. The pelvic girdle attaches the upper extremities to the trunk (Ch. 30).

application/cover letter (solicitud/carta de presentación) letter used to introduce yourself and your résumé to a prospective employer with the goal of obtaining an interview (Ch. 48).

application form (formulario de solicitud) form devised by a prospective employer to collect information relative to qualifications, education, and experience in employment (Ch. 48).

application software (software de aplicación) software that performs a specific data-processing function (Ch. 11).

approximate (aproximar) to bring together the edges of a wound (Ch. 31).

apps (aplicaciones) generic term for any standalone bit of software. Computer programs purpose-built for a specific function. Software office suites are giving way to a new era of individual single function programs usually downloaded from the Internet (Ch. 11).

arbitration (arbitraje) a form of dispute resolution that allows a neutral party to settle the dispute (Ch. 7).

arrhythmia (arritmia) deviation from the normal pattern or rhythm of the heartbeat (Ch. 24, 37).

arteriosclerosis (arteriosclerosis) hardening of the arteries caused by buildup of plaque, a deposit of fatty substances on the artery lining (Ch. 29).

articulating (elocuente) expressing oneself clearly and distinctly (Ch. 12).

artifact (artefacto) anything artificially produced (Ch. 37).

ascorbic acid (ácido ascórbico) vitamin C (Ch. 34).

ascultation (auscultación) using a stethoscope, determines the blood pressure reading that is documented in a patient's chart (Ch. 25).

asepsis (asepsia) protecting against infection caused by pathogenic microorganisms (Ch. 3).

aseptic (aséptico) freedom from any infectious material; absence of microorganisms (Ch. 22).

assay (ensayo) analysis of a substance to determine constituents and relative proportion of each (Ch. 39).

assets (activos) properties of value that are owned by a business entity (Ch. 21).

assignment of benefits (asignación de beneficios) signing over of benefits by the beneficiary to another party (Ch. 17).

Association for Healthcare Documentation Integrity (AHDI) (Asociación para la Integridad de la Documentación del Cuidado de la Salud [AHDI]) professional organization in the field of medical transcription/editing (Ch. 16).

associate's degree (Título de técnico) a degree granted by a junior college at the end of a two-year course (Ch. 1).

ataxia (ataxia) defective muscular coordination, primarily seen when attempting voluntary muscular movements (Ch. 25).

atherosclerosis (aterosclerosis) a form of arteriosclerosis marked by calcium deposits in the arterial linings (Ch. 24).

attribute (atributo) inherent characteristic (Ch. 1).

auditor (auditor) a person responsible for determining the final content of a document and the document's correctness in every aspect (Ch. 16).

augment (aumentar) to add or increase (Ch. 37).

auricle (aurícula) the external ear, also called pinna (Ch. 30).

auscultatory gap (brecha auscultatoria) while measuring blood pressure, the tapping sounds heard may disappear between the Korotkoff phases of sound (Ch. 24).

authentication (autenticación) dictating provider signs or authenticates the document indicating that the information was accurate and complete at the time of signing (Ch. 16).

authoritarian manager (gerente autoritario) operates on the premise that most workers cannot make a contribution without being directed (Ch. 45).

autoclave (autoclave) used to achieve sterilization. The autoclave uses steam under pressure to obtain higher temperatures than can be achieved with boiling (Ch. 31).

automated external defibrillator (AED) (desfibrilador externo automatizado [DEA]) portable, self-contained, automatic device with voice instructions on use for individuals in cardiac arrest. It is used externally to electronically "shock" the myocardium into contracting again. Same as cardioversion (Ch. 9).

automated routing unit (ARU) (enrutador automático [ARU]) telephone system that answers a call and uses a recorded voice to identify departments or services (Ch. 12).

autopsy report (informe de autopsia) also called an autopsy protocol, a necropsy report, or a medical examiner report. Autopsies are performed to determine the cause of death or to ascertain and confirm disease presence (Ch. 16).

avulsion (avulsión) an open wound in which the skin is torn off and bleeding is profuse (Ch. 9).

axial skeleton (esqueleto axial) consists of bones that lie around the center of the body (Ch. 30).

bachelor's degree (licenciatura) four-year academic degree conferred by colleges and universities (Ch. 1).

bacilli (bacilo) one of the three classifications of bacteria; rod shaped (Ch. 22).

backup (hacer una copia de seguridad) copying or saving data to a secure location to prevent loss of data in the event of a disaster (Ch. 11).

balance (balancear) amount owed (N); to verify posting accuracy (V); records difference between debit and credit columns (Ch. 19).

balance sheet (balance general) itemized statement of assets, liabilities, and equity; a statement of financial condition (Ch. 21).

balanitis (balanitis) the swelling and/or inflammation of the glans penis (Ch. 28).

bandage (venda) nonsterile gauze or other material applied over a sterile dressing to protect and immobilize (Ch. 9, 31).

bariatrics (bariátrica) the branch of medicine that deals with prevention, control, and treatment of obesity (Ch. 30).

barrier (barrera) obstacle that exists to protect an individual from contact with blood or other potentially infected materials. Called personal protective equipment (PPE), barriers include gloves, masks, face shields, laboratory coats, protective eyewear, and gowns (Ch. 22).

Bartholin gland (glándula de Bartolino) one of two small mucous glands located at the vaginal opening at the base of the labia majora (Ch. 26).

basal metabolic rate (BMR) (índice metabólico basal [IMB]) level of energy required when the body is at rest (Ch. 34).

baseline (valor de referencia) known or initial measurement against which future measurements are compared (Ch. 24, 39); also, flat, horizontal line that separates the various waves of the ECG cycle (Ch. 37).

basophil (basófilo) granulocytic white blood cell with dark purple cytoplasmic granules. It is the least common of the white blood cells (Ch. 41).

benchmark (comparador de rendimiento) making a comparison among different organizations relative to how they accomplish tasks, such as office computerization, organizing file systems, and employee remuneration (Ch. 45).

beneficiary (beneficiario) person under a policy eligible to receive benefits (Ch. 17).

benefit (beneficio) remuneration that is in addition to the salary (Ch. 45, 48).

benefit period (período de beneficios) the specified time during which benefits will be paid under certain types of health insurance coverages (Ch. 17).

beriberi (beriberi) disease caused by a deficiency in vitamin B (thiamin), characterized by headaches, depression, anorexia, constipation, tachycardia, edema, and heart failure (Ch. 34).

Betadine® (Betadine®) brand of povidone-iodine solution used as a skin antiseptic. Betadine® is also available in a scrub (soap) solution (Ch. 31).

bias (sesgo) slant toward a particular belief (Ch. 5).

bilirubin (bilirrubina) orange–yellow pigment that forms from the breakdown of hemoglobin in damaged red blood cells. Bilirubin usually travels in the bloodstream to the liver, where it is converted to a water-soluble form and is excreted into the bile (Ch. 42, 44).

bilirubinuria (bilirrubinuria) the presence of bilirubin in urine (Ch. 42).

bimanual examination (examen bimanual) an examination performed by the provider using two hands to examine the internal pelvic organs. Two fingers of one hand are inserted into the vagina and the other hand presses on the outside of the abdominal wall. Shape, consistency, and position of the pelvic organs can be determined (Ch. 26).

bioethics (bioética) branch of medical ethics concerned with moral issues resulting from high technology and sophisticated medical research. Social issues such as genetic engineering, abortion, and fetal tissue research raise important bioethical questions (Ch. 8).

biohazard (riesgo biológico) material that has been in contact with body fluid and is capable of transmitting disease (Ch. 22).

biopsy (biopsia) removal of a small piece of living tissue from an organ or other part of the body for microscopic examination to confirm or establish a diagnosis (Ch. 30, 39).

biotransformation (biotransformación) the chemical alteration that a drug undergoes in the body, usually in the liver (Ch. 35).

bipolar (bipolar) having two poles or processes (Ch. 37).

birthday rule (regla del cumpleaños) method to determine which of two or more policies covering a dependent child will be primary; that parent with the birthday falling first in the calendar year has the primary policy (Ch. 17).

blind copy (copia oculta) protects the privacy of email. Other recipients cannot identify who else may have received the transmitted message (Ch. 15).

bloodborne (transmisión sanguínea) means of transmission of an infectious disease (such as HIV and HBV) via human blood (Ch. 22).

bloodborne pathogen (patógeno transmitido por la sangre) microorganism capable of causing disease found in blood or components of blood (Ch. 22).

blood urea nitrogen (BUN) (nitrógeno ureico en sangre [BUN]) nitrogen in the blood in the form of urea. The level of nitrogen in the blood is an indicator of kidney function (Ch. 44).

body fluid (líquido corporal) any secretion or excretion from the human body such as vaginal, cerebrospinal, synovial, pleural, pericardial, peritoneal, amniotic, sputum, and saliva (Ch. 38).

body language (lenguaje corporal) nonverbal communication that includes unconscious body movements, gestures, and facial expressions that accompany verbal messages (Ch. 5).

body mechanics (mecánica corporal) practice of using certain key muscle groups together with correct body alignment to avoid injury when lifting or moving heavy or awkward objects (Ch. 33).

body surface area (BSA) (área de superficie corporal [ASC]) a highly accurate method for calculating medication dosages for infants and children up to 12 years of age (Ch. 36).

bond (fianza) binding agreement with an employee ensuring recovery of financial loss should funds be stolen or embezzled (Ch. 45).

bond paper (papel bond) durable, strong paper usually used for correspondence (Ch. 15).

bradycardia (sinus) (bradicardia [sinusal]) slow (less than 60 beats per minute), but regular heartbeat (Ch. 24, 37).

bradypnea (bradipnea) abnormally slowed respiratory rate (Ch. 24).

brainstorming (tormenta de ideas) process of developing ideas through a synergistic interaction among participants in an environment free of criticism (Ch. 45).

Braxton–Hicks (Braxton–Hicks) irregular, intermittent, and painless uterine contractions; also known as false labor (Ch. 26).

bronchi (bronquios) bifurcates from the trachea into each lung that terminate in the bronchial tubes (Ch. 30).

bronchodilator (broncodilatador) a drug that expands the bronchial tubes (Ch. 30).

broth tubes (tubos de caldo) tubes filled with a broth substance that will support the growth of certain microorganisms (Ch. 43).

bruits (ruidos) sound of venous or arterial origin heard on auscultation (Ch. 25).

bubonic plague (peste bubónica) infectious disease with a high fatality rate transmitted to humans from infected rats and ground squirrels by the bite of the rat flea (Ch. 3).

buffer words (palabras de relleno) expendable words used while answering the telephone (Ch. 12).

buffy coat (capa leucocitaria) layer of white blood cells and platelets that forms at the interface between the plasma and red blood cells in a tube of blood containing an anticoagulant (Ch. 40).

bulbourethral glands (glándulas bulbouretrales) located internally at the base of the penis and are part of the male reproductive system. These glands are responsible for the manufacture and discharge of a clear viscous secretion known as pre-ejaculate. This fluid lubricates the urethra in preparation for ejaculation (Ch. 28).

bulimia (bulimia) a syndrome in which an individual binges on food and then purges by inducing vomiting (Ch. 30, 34).

bullet point (viñeta) asterisk or dot followed by a descriptive phrase; helps the reader identify important points easily (Ch. 48).

bundled codes (códigos agrupados) a grouping of several services that are directly related to a specific procedure and are paid as one (Ch. 18).

burnout (agotamiento profesional) a state of fatigue or frustration brought about by a devotion to a cause, a way of life, or a relationship that failed to produce the expected reward (Ch. 4).

c-reactive protein (CRP) (proteína C reactiva [CRP]) screening blood test for inflammation (Ch. 41).

cachectic (caquéctico) describes a state of ill health, malnutrition, and wasting (Ch. 34).

calibration (calibración) determination of the accuracy of an instrument by comparing the information provided with an accepted standard known to be accurate (Ch. 37, 38).

calorie (caloría) unit of heat. The large Calorie (which is always capitalized) is used in discussion of human nutrition. The large Calorie is also expressed as the kilogram calorie (kcal), equal to 1,000 small calories (Ch. 34).

candidiasis (candidiasis) infection of the skin or mucous membrane with any species of *Candida* (Ch. 26).

cannula (nasal) tubing (cánula) used to deliver oxygen (Ch. 36); also, the blunting member in a Bio-Plexus Puncture Guard® needle (Ch. 40).

capitation (capitación) use of the number of members enrolled in a plan to determine salary of the provider; the provider is paid a fixed fee for each member no matter how many times that member is seen by the provider (Ch. 17).

caption (leyenda) method of designation used on file guides (Ch. 14).

carbuncle (ántrax) necrotizing infection of skin and tissue composed of a cluster of boils (Ch. 30).

carcinoma in situ (carcinoma in situ) cancer that does not extend beyond the basement membrane (Ch. 26).

cardiac catheterization (cateterismo cardíaco) passage of a catheter into the heart through an arm or leg vein and blood vessels leading into the heart. The purpose is to obtain cardiac blood samples, detect abnormalities, and determine intracardiac pressure. Contrast medium can be injected and a coronary artery angiogram can be performed (Ch. 37).

cardiac cycle (ciclo cardíaco) period from the beginning of one heartbeat to the beginning of the next succeeding beat, including systole and diastole. One complete heartbeat (Ch. 37).

cardiogenic (cardiogénico) a type of shock in which the cardiac muscle is unable to contract and adequately provide blood to the body (Ch. 9).

cardiopulmonary resuscitation (CPR) (reanimación cardiopulmonar [RCP]) combination of rescue breathing and chest compressions performed by a trained individual on a patient experiencing cardiac arrest (Ch. 9).

cardioversion (cardioversión) conversion of a pathological cardiac rhythm (arrhythmia), such as ventricular fibrillation, to normal sinus rhythm (Ch. 9, 37).

career objective (objetivo profesional) expresses your career goal and the position for which you are applying (Ch. 48).

carotene (caroteno) vitamin A (Ch. 34).

carrier (portador) person who harbors a pathogenic organism and who is capable of transmitting the organism to others (Ch. 22).

cash basis accounting (contabilidad de caja) reports income at the time money is collected (Ch. 21).

cashier's check (cheque de caja) bank's own check drawn against the bank's account (Ch. 19).

casts (cilindros) tiny structures usually formed by deposits of protein or other substances on the walls of renal tubules; in urine, they can indicate kidney disease (Ch. 42).

catalyst (catalizador) substance that allows a chemical reaction to proceed at a much quicker rate and without as much energy input (Ch. 34).

cataract (catarata) opacity of the eye lens that usually occurs from aging, trauma, or disease (Ch. 10).

catheterization (cateterismo) insertion of a catheter tube into the body for evacuating fluids or injecting fluids into body cavities. In urinary catheterization, the tube is inserted through the urethra into the bladder for withdrawal of urine (Ch. 25).

cathode (cátodo) a negative electrode from which electrons are emitted (Ch. 32).

caustic (cáustico) corrosive and burning; destructive to living tissue (Ch. 22, 31).

cauterize (cauterizar) to destroy tissue through application of a caustic agent, a hot instrument, an electric current, or other agent (Ch. 9).

cautery (cauterio) destruction of tissue by burning (Ch. 31).

cell-mediated immunity (inmunidad mediada por células) the regulatory activities of T cells during the specific immune response (Ch. 22).

cellular telephones (teléfonos celulares) a short range portable device used for voice or data communication over a network of base stations known as cell sites. The cell sites are interconnected to the public switched telephone network (Ch. 12).

cellulose (celulosa) type of indigestible fiber made of carbohydrates found in plants (Ch. 34).

Centers for Medicare and Medicaid Services (CMS) (Centros de Servicios de Medicare y Medicaid [CMS]) formerly known as HCFA. CMS is a federal agency within the U.S. Department of Health and Human Services (DHHS). The agency administers Medicare, Medicaid, and the State Children's Health Insurance Program (SCHIP). CMS also administers the Health Insurance Portability and Accountability Act of 1996 (HIPAA) and Clinical Laboratory Improvement Act of 1988 (CLIA '88) (Ch. 17).

central processing unit (CPU) (unidad de procesamiento central [CPU]) brain of the computer that performs instructions defined by software (Ch. 11).

centrifuge (centrifugador) device that spins tubes using centrifugal force to separate the fluid portion of blood from the formed elements (Ch. 40).

cerebral vascular accident (CVA) (accidente cerebrovascular [ACV]) loss of blood supply to the brain (anoxia); also referred to as a stroke (Ch. 30).

certification (certificación) guarantees as being true or as represented by or as meeting a standard (Ch. 1).

certification examination (examen de certificación) standardized means of evaluating medical assistant competency (Ch. 47).

certified check (cheque certificado) depositor's own check that the bank has indicated with a date and signature to be good for the amount written (Ch. 19).

Certified Clinical Medical Assistant (CCMA) (Asistente Clínico Médico Certificado [CCMA]) an NHA certification for a clinical medical assistant. (Ch. 1, 47).

Certified Medical Administrative Assistant (CMAA) (Asistente Administrativo Médico Certificado [CMAA]) an NHA certification for a medical administrative assistant (Ch. 47).

Certified Medical Administrative Specialist (CMAS) (Especialista Administrativo Médico Certificado [CMAS]) an AMT certification for a medical administrative specialist (Ch. 47).

Certified Medical Assistant (CMA [AAMA]) (Asistente Médico Certificado [CMA (AAMA)]) a certified medical assistant who has successfully completed the AAMA's national certification examination (Ch. 1, 47).

Certified Medical Transcriptionist (CMT) (Transcriptor Médico Certificado [CMT]) completion of a two-part certification examination administered by the Association for Healthcare Documentation Integrity (AHDI) (Ch. 16).

cerumen (cerumen) a substance secreted by glands at the outer third of the ear canal (Ch. 30).

cervical punch biopsy (biopsia cervical en sacabocados) a biopsy of the uterine cervix using an instrument, the end of which is a punch (Ch. 26).

cesarean section (operación cesárea) delivery of fetus through surgical incision into the uterus (Ch. 26).

chart notes (notas clínicas) (also called progress notes) provider's formal or informal notes about presenting problem, physical findings, and plan for treatment for a patient examined in the office, clinic, acute care center, or emergency department (Ch. 16).

check register (registro de cheques)   record of checks written; categorized into separate and identified columns (Ch. 21).

cheilosis (queilosis)   caused by a deficiency of vitamin B₂ (riboflavin) and characterized by sores on the lips and cracks in the corners of the mouth (Ch. 34).

Cheyne–Stokes (Cheyne–Stoke)   regular pattern of irregular breathing rate often seen in children and that may be seen in brain dysfunction (Ch. 24).

chief complaint (CC) (queja principal [QP])   specific symptom or problem for which the patient is seeing the provider today (Ch. 16, 23).

chlamydia (clamidia)   a bacterium that causes one of the most prevalent sexually transmitted diseases (Ch. 26).

cholecalciferol (colecalciferol)   vitamin D (Ch. 34).

cholesterol (colesterol)   sterol lipid that is widely distributed in animal tissues. Cholesterol is produced in the liver and is a component of bile (Ch. 44).

chronologic résumé (curriculum vitae cronológico)   résumé format used when you have employment experience (Ch. 48).

circadian rhythm (ritmo circadiano)   pattern based on a 24-hour cycle emphasizing the repetition of certain physiologic phenomena such as eating and sleeping (Ch. 42).

circumcision (circuncisión)   the surgical removal of the foreskin (prepuce) of the penis (Ch. 27).

circumduction (circunducción)   circular motion of a body part (Ch. 33).

civil law (derecho civil)   law related to actions between individuals (Ch. 7).

clinical email (correo electrónico clínico)   type of email established using defined protocols as a means of communication between providers and established patients (Ch. 12).

claim register (registro de reclamaciones)   diary or register of claims submitted to each insurance carrier. When payment is received, the date and amount of payment is entered in the register (Ch. 18).

claustrophobia (claustrofobia)   fear of being confined in any space (Ch. 32).

clinical chemistry (química clínica)   analysis and study of blood, body fluids, excreta, and tissues in the diagnosis and treatment of disease (Ch. 39).

clinical diagnosis (diagnóstico clínico)   identification of a disease by history, laboratory studies, and symptoms (Ch. 23, 39).

closed questions (preguntas cerradas)   questions answered with a yes or no (Ch. 5).

clustering (agrupación)   a grouping together of nonverbal messages into statements or conclusions. Can also be used to describe a scheduling system where patients with similar complaint/conditions are scheduled consecutively (example is scheduling all the allergy injections for 3:00 PM to 4:00 PM every Tuesday and Thursday) (Ch. 5).

CMS 1500 (08/05) (CMS 1500 [08/05])   formerly known as the HCFA 1500 form that is the office health insurance claim form for Medicare and Medicaid (Ch. 18).

cobalamina (cobalamina)   vitamin B₁₂ (Ch. 34).

cochlear implantation (implante coclear)   an electrical device that receives sounds and transmits the resulting signal to electrodes implanted in the cochlea. The signal stimulates the cochlea and the individual is able to perceive sound (Ch. 27).

coenzyme (coenzima)   substance that enhances a catalyst (Ch. 34).

cognitive functioning (funcionamiento cognitivo)   awareness with perception, reasoning, judgment, intuition, and memory (Ch. 29).

coinsurance (coseguro)   that percentage paid by the company or that paid by the insured (Ch. 17).

collection ratio (relación de cobranza)   gross income divided by the amount that could have been collected less disallowances (Ch. 20, 21).

colonoscopy (colonoscopia)   visual examination of the colon with a lighted scope (Ch. 30).

colposcopy (colposcopia)   visual examination of vaginal and cervical tissues using a colposcope following abnormal Pap smear. A magnifying lens and powerful lights are used (Ch. 26).

comedone (comedón)   blackhead; usually the result of blocked sebaceous glands caused by acne (Ch. 30).

Commission on Accreditation of Allied Health Education Programs (CAAHEP) (Comisión de Acreditación de Programas Educativos Asociados a la Salud [CAAHEP])   entity accrediting over 2,000 educational programs in 20 health sciences professions (Ch. 47).

common law (derecho consuetudinario)   refers to laws developed in England and France and brought to the United States by the early settlers; sometimes referred to as judge-made law (Ch. 7).

communicable (transmisible)   contagious. Capable of being transmitted from one person to another either directly or indirectly (Ch. 22, 38).

compensation (compensación)   overemphasizing of characteristics to make up for a real or imagined failure or handicap (Ch. 5).

competency (competencia)   legally qualified or adequate (Ch. 1).

complete blood count (CBC) (recuento sanguíneo completo [RSC])   battery of hematologic tests consisting of hemoglobin, hematocrit, total white blood cell count including differential, total red blood cell count, including indices, and platelets (Ch. 41).

compliance (cumplimiento)   conformity in fulfilling official requirements (Ch. 1).

compounding (composición)   combining two or more substances in definite proportions (Ch. 36).

condenser (condensador)   in a microscope, directs a beam of light from the source to the specimen (Ch. 39).

condylomata (condiloma)   a wartlike lesion of viral origin found on external genitalia or perianal region (Ch. 26).

confidentiality (confidencialidad)   ethical and legal rules in regard to patient privacy (Ch. 16).

confidentiality agreement (acuerdo de confidencialidad)   when signed, the agreement signifies that the medical transcriptionist is committed to keep all patient information confidential (Ch. 16).

conflict resolution (resolución de conflictos)   solving problems between coworkers or any two parties (Ch. 45).

congenital anomalies (anomalías congénitas)   being born with; existing at time of birth (Ch. 26).

congruency (congruencia)   the verbal message and the nonverbal message must agree (Ch. 5).

constitutional law (derecho constitucional)   consists of laws that are made by constitutions of the United States or individual states (Ch. 7).

constriction band (banda de constricción)   term used to replace tourniquet (no longer used) in emergencies. A band of material used to control severe bleeding in an extremity that has been injured due to trauma. The band is applied above the source of bleeding, but not so tight that it restricts the flow of blood completely. Some slight trickling of blood should be evident. This action avoids loss of an extremity because of complete blood flow restriction. Complete blood flow restriction results in no blood flow to the extremity's cells and tissues; therefore, the cells, tissues, and body part receive no oxygen and die (Ch. 9).

consultation report (informe de consulta)   document that reports the findings and advice of another provider requested to see a patient by the attending provider (Ch. 16).

contact tracker (seguidor de contactos)   form used to keep track of employment contact information such as name of employer, name of contact person, address and telephone number, date of first contact, résumé sent, interview date, follow-up information, and dates (Ch. 48).

contact transmission (transmisión por contacto)   spread of disease-causing microorganisms by directly or indirectly touching the source of the infection or by touching an object or environmental surface (Ch. 22).

contaminate (contaminar)   to make something unclean; often used to describe a sterile area being made "unsterile" or exposing a clean area to a pathogenic substance (Ch. 22, 31).

continuing education units (CEU) (unidades de educación continua [UEC])   method for earning points toward recertification (Ch. 47).

contraception (anticoncepción)   voluntary prevention of pregnancy (Ch. 26).

contract law (derecho contractual) law that refers to agreements between individuals and entities that are binding (Ch. 7).

contracting (contraer) acquiring an infection from pathogens (Ch. 22).

contracture (contractura) occurs when the body is in a non-moving state. The usually flexible connective tissues become stiffened and are replaced with fiber-like tissues (Ch. 33).

contraindication (contraindicación) any symptom or circumstance indicating that the use of a particular drug is inappropriate when it would otherwise be advisable. For example, the use of alcoholic beverages is a contraindication when the drug Flagyl® is prescribed (Ch. 35).

control test (prueba de control) test of a sample of known results used to compare with the results of a patient's sample (Ch. 39).

coordination of benefits (COB) (coordinación de beneficios [COB]) the provision of an insurance contract that limits benefits to 100% of the cost (Ch. 17).

co-payment (copago) payment required when seen by the provider (Ch. 17).

cost accounting (Contabilidad de costos) helps to determine what it costs the ambulatory care setting to perform particular services and is an integral part of managerial accounting (Ch. 21).

cost analysis (análisis de costos) procedure that determines the costs of each service (Ch. 21).

cost ratio (relación de costos) formula that shows the cost of a procedure or service and helps determine the financial value of maintaining certain services (Ch. 21).

cough etiquette (protocolo de manejo de la tos) coughing/sneezing into a tissue to prevent microorganisms from spreading to others. Includes properly disposing of tissue into a waste receptacle and washing hands as soon as possible (Ch. 22).

countershock (contrachoque) application of an electric current to the heart directly or indirectly to alter a disturbance in cardiac rhythm (Ch. 37).

coupling agent (agente de acoplamiento) an agent used when ultrasonography is used; enhances penetration of sound waves through tissue (Ch. 26).

crash tray or cart (bandeja o carro de parada) tray or portable cart that contains medications and supplies needed for emergency and first aid procedures (Ch. 9).

creatinine (creatinina) waste product formed in muscle that is excreted by the kidneys; increased in blood and urine when kidney function is abnormal (Ch. 42).

credentialed (acreditado) testimonials showing that a person is entitled to credit or has a right to exercise official power (Ch. 1).

credit (crédito) decreases balance due; column used for entering payments (Ch. 19).

crepitation (crepitación) grating sound heard on movement of ends of a broken bone (Ch. 9).

criminal law (derecho penal) law related to wrongs committed against the welfare and safety of society as a whole (Ch. 7).

critical values (valores críticos) test results that indicate a potentially life-threatening or greatly debilitating situation that must be reported to the provider immediately (Ch. 42).

cross-reference (referencia cruzada) notation in a file to direct the reader to a specific record that may be filed under more than one name/subject (e.g., married name/maiden name or foreign names) where the surname is not easily recognizable (Ch. 14).

cryopreservation (crioconservación) storage of biologic materials (sperm, embryo, tissue, plasma) at extremely cold temperature for use at a later time (Ch. 8).

cryosurgery (criocirugía) the destruction of tissue by application of extreme cold, silver nitrate, and carbon dioxide (Ch. 26).

cryptorchidism (criptorquidia) undescended testicle (Ch. 28).

crystals (crystals) found in normal urine sediment having no particular significance; should be noted because they may indicate disease states (Ch. 42).

cultural brokering (intermediación cultural) the act of bridging, linking, or mediating between groups or persons through the process of reducing conflict or producing change (Ch. 5).

culture (cultura) the attitudes and behavior that are characteristic of a particular social group or organization (Ch. 5).

culture and sensitivity (cultivo y sensibilidad) often referred to as C&S. The sample is cultured for bacteria and then is exposed to various antibiotics to determine what the bacteria is sensitive (and resistant) to (Ch. 39, 42).

cultures (cultivos) microorganisms cultivated in a nutrient medium (Ch. 42, 43).

Current Procedural Terminology (CPT) (Terminología Actual sobre Procedimientos [TAP]) standard codes for procedures and services. Used by most ambulatory care settings in encoding the claim form and recognized by most insurance carriers (Ch. 18).

current reports (informes actuales) reports such as history and physical examinations that should be complete within 24 hours (Ch. 16).

cyanosis (cianosis) discoloration of the skin due to abnormal amounts of reduced hemoglobin in the blood caused by decreased oxygen and increased carbon dioxide in the blood (Ch. 25).

cystitis (cistitis) inflammation of the bladder (Ch. 29).

cytology (citología) science that deals with the formation, structure, and function of cells (Ch. 39).

data storage device (dispositivo de almacenamiento de datos) device capable of permanently or temporarily storing digital data (Ch. 11).

data storage memory (memoria de almacenamiento de datos) permanent memory not part of the motherboard. Uses any suitable data storage device. Can be read-only or read-write type of memory (Ch. 11).

day sheet (hoja diaria) form used with pegboard system to record daily patient transactions (Ch. 19).

debit (debe) used for entering charges and description of services; column is on the left (Ch. 19).

debris (detritos) remains of broken down or damaged cells or tissues (Ch. 22).

declination form (formulario de rechazo) written formal refusal (Ch. 22).

decode (decodificar) to translate into language that is easily understood; to interpret (Ch. 5).

deductible (deducible) that amount of incurred medical expenses that must be met before the insurance policy will begin to pay (Ch. 17).

defendant (demandado) person who defends action brought in litigation (Ch. 7).

Defense Enrollment Eligible Reporting System (DEERS) (Sistema de Informes de Elegibilidad para la Inscripción en Defensa [DEERS]) a system operated by the Department of Defense and used by TRICARE contractors to determine and confirm the eligibility of beneficiaries (Ch. 17).

defense mechanism (mecanismo de defensa) behavior that protects the psyche from guilt, anxiety, or shame (Ch. 5).

defibrillation (desfibrilación) stopping fibrillation of the heart by use of drugs or by physical means (Ch. 37).

defibrillator (desfibrilador) a machine that delivers an electric current to alter a disturbance in cardiac rhythm (Ch. 37).

defragmentation (desfragmentación) reorganization of information on a hard disk to store files as continuous units rather than as small packets. A computer with little fragmentation of files will operate at a higher speed (Ch. 11).

dementia (demencia) impairment of intellectual function that is progressive and interferes with normal activities (Ch. 29).

demyelination (desmielinización) destruction of the myelin sheath; often a factor in multiple sclerosis (Ch. 30).

denial (rechazo) rejection of or refusal to acknowledge (Ch. 5).

Denver Developmental Screening Test (Prueba de evaluación del desarrollo de Denver) used to determine motor skills development levels (Ch. 27).

deoxygenated (desoxigenada) blood that is high in carbon dioxide, low in oxygen, and pumped through the heart to the lungs where the carbon dioxide is exchanged for oxygen (Ch. 37).

depolarize (despolarizar) process of reducing to a nonpolarized condition. Generation of an electrical current is enhanced. Electrical activity generated when the atria or ventricles contract (Ch. 37).

deposition (declaración)   oral testimony given by an individual with a court reporter and attorneys for both sides present; often used as part of the discovery process (Ch. 7).

dermatophytes (dermatofitos)   category of fungi causing infections of hair, skin, and nails (Ch. 43).

dexterity (destreza)   skill and ease in using the hands (Ch. 1).

diabetes mellitus (diabetes mellitus)   chronic disorder of carbohydrate metabolism characterized by hyperglycemia and resulting from inadequate production or utilization of insulin (Ch. 44).

diagnosis (diagnóstico)   determination of disease or condition (Ch. 39).

diastole (diástole)   one component of blood pressure measurement representing the lowest amount of pressure exerted during the cardiac cycle; the force exerted on the arterial walls during cardiac relaxation (Ch. 24, 37).

diethylstilbestrol (DES) (dietilestilbestrol [DES])   a synthetic hormone used therapeutically in menopausal disturbances. It should not be given during pregnancy. It has been related to cervicovaginal malignances in daughters of mothers who had it prescribed for them to treat a threatened abortion. DES has been related to reproductive disorders in males whose mothers took it during pregnancy (Ch. 26).

differential diagnosis (diagnóstico diferencial)   diagnosis based on comparison of symptoms of similar diseases (Ch. 39).

digestion (digestión)   breaking down of food into smaller particles. It can be either physical or chemical (Ch. 34).

dilation (dilatación)   expansion of an orifice or organ (Ch. 26).

diploma (diploma)   a document bearing record of graduation from or of a degree conferred by an educational institution (Ch. 1).

direct skills (habilidades directas)   skills that are job specific. Skill in taking a blood pressure reading would be specific to the medical field (Ch. 18).

discharge summary (DS) (resumen de alta médica [DS])   medical reports that document the hospitalization history of a patient (Ch. 16).

discovery (exhibición de pruebas)   the time in which both parties are allowed access to all information and evidence related to a case; follows the subpoena process (Ch. 7).

disinfection (desinfección)   use of chemicals or boiling water to free an item from infectious materials but not its spores (Ch. 22).

dislocation (luxación)   displacement of a bone or joint from its normal position (Ch. 9, 30).

dispense (dosificar)   prepare and give out a medication to be taken at a later time (Ch. 7, 35, 36).

displacement (desplazamiento)   displacing negative feelings onto something or someone else with no significance to the situation (Ch. 5).

disposition (temperamento)   temperament, character, personality (Ch. 1).

distribution (distribución)   the process whereby the drug is transported from the blood to the intended site of action, site of biotransformation, site of storage, and site of elimination (Ch. 35).

diuretic (diurético)   substance that causes less water to be reabsorbed by the kidney and therefore causes water to be excreted from the body (Ch. 34).

DNA (ADN)   deoxyribonucleic acid; important nuclear material that carries genetic codes (Ch. 39).

doctrine (doctrina)   principle of law established through past decisions (Ch. 7).

documentation (documentación)   written material that accompanies purchased software containing the information necessary for using the software appropriately; sometimes known as the manual (Ch. 11, 22); also, providing factual support through written information (Ch. 22).

Doppler (doppler)   a noninvasive technique used with ultrasonography to evaluate blood flow through major arteries and veins of the arms, legs, and neck. It can reveal blood clots or blockages (Ch. 32).

dorsal recumbent (decúbito dorsal)   in this position, patients lie on their back (dorsal) face up, legs separated, knees flexed with feet flat on the table (Ch. 25).

dorsiflexion (dorsiflexión)   moving the foot upward at the ankle joint (Ch. 33).

dosimeter (dosímetro)   a device for measuring X-ray output (Ch. 32).

down-coding (baja de codificación)   insurance carriers down-code if documentation or codes are ambiguous and reimburse for the lowest possible fee (Ch. 18).

donut hole (período sin cobertura)   within the Medicare Part D prescription drug program, the donut hole is the phase of coverage in which all costs are covered by the enrollee rather than CMS (Ch. 17).

dressing (apósito)   sterile gauze or other material applied directly to a wound to absorb secretions and to protect (Ch. 9, 31).

driver (controlador)   computer program designed to convert data output from one device to a format compatible with another device (Ch. 11).

droplet transmission (transmisión por gotitas)   method of spreading disease from respiratory secretions through the air. Spread is usually confined to within 3 feet of the infected patient (Ch. 22).

durable power of attorney for health care (poder legal duradero para atención médica)   legal form that allows a designated person to act on another's behalf in regard to health care choices (Ch. 6, 7).

dysmenorrhea (dismenorrea)   painful menses (Ch. 26).

dyspareunia (dispareunia)   painful intercourse (Ch. 26).

dysplasia (displasia)   abnormal development of tissue (Ch. 26).

dyspnea (disnea)   shortness of breath or labored/difficult breathing (Ch. 24, 29).

dysuria (disuria)   painful or difficult urination (Ch. 30).

E codes (códigos E)   ICD-9-CM codes for the external causes of injury, poisoning, or other adverse reactions that explain how the injury occurred (Ch. 18).

echocardiogram (ecocardiograma)   noninvasive diagnostic method that uses ultrasound to visualize internal cardiac structure, including valves (Ch. 32).

eclampsia (eclampsia)   complication of pregnancy that includes general edema, hypertension, proteinuria, and convulsions (Ch. 26).

ectopic pregnancy (embarazo ectópico)   implementation of the fertilized ovum outside of the uterine cavity (Ch. 26).

edematous (edematoso)   abnormal accumulation of fluid in the tissues resulting in swelling (Ch. 40).

editor (corrector)   see auditor (Ch. 16).

effacement (borramiento)   thinning and shortening of the cervical canal during labor to permit passage of fetus (Ch. 26).

effleurage (effleurage)   deep or gentle stroking massage (Ch. 33).

EHR (RSE)   see **electronic health record** (Ch. 11).

electrocardiogram (electrocardiograma)   record of the electrical activity of the heart; showing P, QRS, and T waves (Ch. 37).

electrocardiograph (electrocardiografío)   instrument for recording the electrical activity of the heart (Ch. 37).

electrocardiography (electrocardiografía)   process of recording the electrical activity originating in the heart (Ch. 37).

electrode (electrodo)   also known as a sensor. Used to conduct electricity from the body to the electrocardiograph (Ch. 37).

electrolyte (electrolito)   substances that conduct electricity whose components are important in maintaining fluid and acid–base balance (Ch. 34, 37, 39).

electronic health record (EHR) (registro de salud electrónico [RSE])   a patients' electronic medical records from multiple sources combined into one master database (Ch. 11).

electronic mail (email)   the process of sending, receiving, storing, and forwarding messages in digital form over computer networks (Ch. 12).

electronic medical record (EMR) (registro médico electrónico [RME])   patient medical record from a single medical practice, hospital, or pharmacy (Ch. 11, 16).

electrosurgery (electrocirugía)   uses an electric current in a concentrated area to either cut or destroy tissue whenever pathologic examination is not required (Ch. 31).

elimination (eliminación)   the process whereby the drug is excreted from the body. Elimination occurs via the gastrointestinal tract, respiratory tract, skin, mucous membranes, and mammary glands (Ch. 35).

emancipated minor (menor emancipado) persons under age 18 years who are financially responsible for themselves and free of parental care (Ch. 7).

embezzle (malversar) to appropriate fraudulently to one's own use (Ch. 45).

Emergency Medical Services (EMS) (Servicios Médicos de Emergencia [SME]) a local network of police, fire, and medical personnel trained to respond to emergency situations. In many communities, the system is activated by calling 911 (Ch. 9).

empathy (empatía) ability to be objectively aware of and have insight into another's feelings, emotions, and behaviors, and to be aware of the significance and meaning of these to the other person (Ch. 1, 29).

emphysema (enfisema) chronic pulmonary disease characterized by dilated and damaged alveoli (Ch. 24).

EMR (RME) see **electronic medical record** (Ch. 11).

encode (encoding) (codificar [codificación]) creating a message to be sent (Ch. 5).

encounter form (formulario de visita) formerly known as a charge slip or superbill. A copy of the encounter form is given to the patient after seeing the provider. It identifies the procedures performed, diagnoses, charges, and when to return (Ch. 18, 19).

encrypted email (correo electrónico cifrado) the process of coding email to render the transmission essentially secure (Ch. 12).

encryption technology (tecnología de cifrado) converts information into code; used to protect privacy and confidentiality of individuals in computer software (Ch. 13).

endometriosis (endometriosis) tissue that resembles the endometrium invades various locations in the pelvic cavity and elsewhere (Ch. 26).

endoscopy (endoscopia) visual examination of body cavities with a lighted scope (Ch. 30).

engineering controls (controles de ingeniería) physical or mechanical devices that isolate or remove health hazards from the workplace (Ch. 22).

enunciation (dicción) speaking clearly; articulating (Ch. 12).

eosinophil (eosinófilos) granulocytic white blood cell with red eosin-stained granules in the cytoplasm. It is elevated in cases of allergies (Ch. 41).

epidemic (epidemia) an infectious disease that attacks many persons at the same time in the same location (Ch. 22).

epidemiology (epidemiología) field of science that studies the history, cause, and patterns of infectious diseases (Ch. 22).

epididymitis (epididimitis) inflammation of the tubes on the testis (Ch. 28).

epinephrine (epinefrina) used to treat allergic reactions (Ch. 9); also, hormone also known as adrenaline. Epinephrine is manufactured as a chemical (pharmaceutical preparation) and is often mixed with local anesthetics for use as a vasoconstrictor in minor surgery (Ch. 31).

e-résumé (curriculum vitae electrónico) electronic résumés may be delivered electronically via e-mail, submitted to Internet job boards, or placed on Web pages (Ch. 48).

erectile dysfunction (ED) (disfunción eréctil [DE]) impotence; occurs when a man is unable to achieve or to sustain an erection of the penis during sexual intercourse (Ch. 28).

ergonomics (ergonomía) scientific study of work and space, including factors that influence worker productivity and that affect workers' health (Ch. 11).

erythema (eritema) redness or inflammation of the skin or mucous membranes that is the result of dilatation and congestion of superficial capillaries (Ch. 30).

erythrocyte (eritrocito) red blood cell, one of the formed elements of the blood (Ch. 40, 41).

erythrocyte indices (índices de eritrocitos) three equations that provide information about the sizes and hemoglobin content of red blood cells. These include the mean corpuscular cell volume, mean corpuscular hemoglobin, and mean corpuscular hemoglobin volume (Ch. 41).

erythrocyte sedimentation rate (velocidad de eritrosedimentación) measurement of how far the red cells in a sample of blood settle in one hour (Ch. 41).

erythropoietin (eritropoyetina) hormone that causes production of new red blood cells (Ch. 41).

esophageal varices (várices esofágicas) tortuous dilation of the esophageal vein associated with any condition that causes obstruction of drainage from the esophageal veins into the portal vein of the liver. Seen in cirrhosis of the liver and alcoholism (Ch. 32).

Ethernet (Ethernet) references the networking of computers using metallic conductors or hard wires (Ch. 11).

ethics (ética) defined in terms of what is morally right and wrong; ethics will differ from person to person; often defined by a code or creed as in the Code of Ethics from the American Association of Medical Assistants (AAMA) (Ch. 8).

etiquette (etiqueta) manners, politeness, proper behavior (Ch. 12).

eupnea (eupnea) normal breathing (Ch. 24).

eversion (eversión) moving a body part outward (Ch. 33).

exclusion (exclusión) specific disease or condition listed in an insurance policy for which the policy will not pay (Ch. 17).

exclusive provider organization (EPO) (organización de proveedor exclusivo [EPO]) a closed-panel preferred organization (PPO) plan where enrollees receive no benefits if they opt to receive care from a provider who is not in the EPO (Ch. 17).

excretion (excreción) waste matter. The elimination of waste products from the body (Ch. 22, 38).

exit interview (entrevista de salida) opportunity for departing employees to provide their positive and negative opinions of the position and facility (Ch. 46).

expectorate (expectorar) act of coughing up material from airways that lead to the lungs (Ch. 43).

expert witness (testigo experto) individual with highly specialized knowledge and skills in a particular area who testifies to a standard of care (Ch. 7).

explanation of benefits (EOB) (explicación de beneficios [EDB]) insurance report that is sent with claim payments explaining the reimbursement of the insurance carrier (Ch. 18).

explicit (explícito) fully revealed or expressed without ambiguity or vagueness, leaving no question as to intent (Ch. 9).

expressed contract (contrato explícito) written or verbal contract that specifically describes what each party in the contract will do (Ch. 7).

extension (extensión) straightening of a body part (Ch. 33).

external respiration (respiración externa) ventilation of the lungs when the exchange of oxygen and carbon dioxide takes place (Ch. 30).

externship (práctica laboral) transition stage between the classroom and actual employment; may also be referred to as internship or practicum (Ch. 1, 45).

extracellular (extracelular) pertaining to the environment outside of a body cell (Ch. 34).

exudate (exudado) accumulated fluid in a cavity; an oozing of pus; matter that penetrates through vessel walls into adjoining tissue (Ch. 27, 31).

facilitate (facilitar) to make an action or process easier (Ch. 1).

Fair Debt Collection Practice Act (Ley sobre Prácticas Justas para el Cobro de Deudas) 1977 federal law that outlines collection practices (Ch. 20).

fat-soluble (soluble en lípidos) pertaining to substances that are hydrophobic and therefore dissolve better in fat (Ch. 34).

fax (facsimile) (fax [facsímilx]) machine that sends documents from one location to another by way of telephone lines (Ch. 12).

febrile (febril) having a fever (Ch. 24).

felony (delito mayor) a serious crime such as murder, larceny (thefts of large sums of money), assault, and rape (Ch. 7).

female genital mutilation (mutilación genital femenina) Partial or complete removal of the clitoris, partial or total removal of the labia minora and/or labia majoria, narrowing the vaginal opening by creating a covering seal, and the pricking, piercing, or cauterizing of genitals (Ch. 8).

fenestrated (fenestrado) having openings. A sterile, fenestrated drape is used in surgery. It has an opening (round) in it to expose only the operative site. The remainder of the drape covers the patient and is a sterile area (Ch. 31).

fenestrated drape (paño fenestrado) a type of drape with an opening, usually round, that can be placed with the opening over a particular body area; used in surgery and for proctologic examinations (Ch. 25).

financial accounting (contabilidad financiera) provides information primarily for entities external to the organization such as the government (Ch. 21).

firewall (cortafuegos) hardware device or software program designed to prevent unauthorized access to a computer system (Ch. 11).

first aid (primeros auxilios) immediate (or first) care provided to persons who are suddenly ill or injured; first aid is typically followed by more comprehensive care and treatment (Ch. 9).

fiscal intermediary (intermediario fiscal) local administrator for Medicare (Ch. 17).

fixed cost (costo fijo) cost that does not vary in total as the number of patients vary (Ch. 21).

flag (indicador de mensaje) method of identifying a blank space or a question regarding dictator's meaning by attaching a note or marker to indicate the question (Ch. 16).

flash drive (unidad flash) solid-state data storage device (Ch. 11).

flexion (flexión) bending of a body part (Ch. 33).

fluoroscope (fluoroscope) a device consisting of a screen; mounts separately or with an X-ray tube that shows the images of objects interposed between the table and the screen (Ch. 32).

folic acid (ácido fólico) one of the B-complex vitamins (Ch. 34).

fomite (fómite) substance that absorbs and transmits infectious material; for example, contaminated items such as equipment (Ch. 22).

fontanel (fontanela) soft spot lying between the cranial bones of the skull of a fetus, newborn, and infant (Ch. 27).

form letter (carta tipo) letter containing the same content in the body but sent to different individuals (Ch. 15).

formalin (formalina) an aqueous solution of 37% formaldehyde (Ch. 26).

Fowler's (Fowler) patients sit in a position with the back of the examination table raised to either 45 degrees (semi-Fowler's) or 90 degrees (high-fowler's). Legs rest flat on the table. A pillow may be placed under the knees. This position is used for patients having cardiovascular or respiratory problems to facilitate their breathing, and for examination of the upper body and head (Ch. 25).

fracture (fractura) break in a bone. There are several types of fractures, but all are classified as either open or closed fractures (Ch. 9).

fraud (fraude) deliberate misrepresentation of facts (Ch. 17).

frenulum (frenillo) of the tongue, a fold of mucous membrane located under the tongue attaching the tongue to the floor of the mouth (Ch. 24).

frequency (frecuencia) urinating frequently (Ch. 30).

friable (friable) easily broken (Ch. 31).

fringe benefit (beneficio complementario) benefit above and beyond salary to which an employee may be entitled. Examples include health and life insurance, paid vacation, sick days, personal days, and tuition reimbursement for courses related to employment (Ch. 2, 45).

fulgarated (fulgurado) destroyed by electric current (Ch. 26).

full block letter (carta de bloque completo) major letter style in which all lines begin flush with the left margin. This style is suggested for offices desiring a contemporary-looking, efficient letter (Ch. 15).

fume hood (campana de humo) type of hood or barrier used in the laboratory to capture chemical vapors and fumes and move them away from health care workers and into a building's exhaust fan system (Ch. 38).

functional résumé (curriculum vitae funcional) résumé format used to highlight specialty areas of accomplishment and strengths (Ch. 48).

furuncle (forúnculo) localized, suppurative staphylococcal skin infection originating in a gland or hair follicle (Ch. 30).

gait (marcha) manner or style of walking including rhythm and speed (Ch. 33).

gait belt (cinturón de marcha) safety belt worn by the patient around the waist that provides a firm handhold for the caregiver when transferring the patient or when assisting in ambulation (Ch. 33).

galvanometer (galvanómetro) mechanism in the electrocardiograph that changes the voltage into a mechanical motion for recording purposes (Ch. 37).

genetic engineering (ingeniería genética) alteration, manipulation, replacement, or repair of genetic material (Ch. 8).

genitalia (genitales) the reproductive organs, internal and external (Ch. 24).

genus (género) first Greek or Latin name given to a microorganism; always capitalized (Ch. 43).

geriatrics (geriatría) the branch of medicine concerned with the problems of aging (Ch. 29).

gerontology (gerontología) the scientific study of the problems associated with aging (Ch. 29).

gestation (gestación) period of development from fertilization to birth (Ch. 26).

gestational diabetes (diabetes gestacional) diabetes that first manifests clinically during pregnancy. It usually subsides after delivery (Ch. 26).

gestures/mannerisms (gestos/ademanes) movement of various body parts while communicating (Ch. 5).

glaucoma (glaucoma) condition caused by increased intraocular pressure due to a buildup of aqueous humor. This results in mild visual disturbances with little or no pain but can lead to severe visual impairment if untreated (Ch. 30).

glucose (glucosa) simple sugar that is a major source of energy in the human body; monitoring of blood glucose levels in urine and blood is a vital diagnostic test in diabetes and other disorders; also a test on a reagent strip (Ch. 39, 42).

glucosuria (glucosuria) the presence of glucose in urine (also correct is glycosuria) (Ch. 42).

glycogen (glicógeno) carbohydrate form used for storage of sugar in the body (Ch. 34).

goal (meta) result or achievement toward which effort is directed (Ch. 4).

"going bare" ("estar desprotegido") said of a provider who does not carry professional liability insurance (Ch. 45).

goniometer (goniómetro) instrument used to measure the angle of a joint's range of motion (Ch. 33).

goniometry (goniometría) measurement of joint motion (Ch. 33).

Good Samaritan laws (leyes del Buen Samaritano) laws designed to protect individuals from legal action when rendering emergency medical aid, without compensation, within the areas of their training and expertise (Ch. 12).

Gram stain (tinción de Gram) named for its inventor, Hans Christian Gram, and is, therefore, always capitalized; most common stain used in microbiology to observe gross morphologic features of bacteria; a differential stain, allowing differentiation between Gram-negative and Gram-positive organisms (Ch. 43).

gravidity (gravidez) total number of pregnancies a woman has had regardless of duration, including a present one (Ch. 26).

gross contamination (contaminación importante) highly infectious material present (Ch. 22).

gross examination (examen macroscópico) viewing specimens with the naked eye (Ch. 16).

guarantor (garante) the person identified as responsible for payment of the bill (Ch. 19).

Guthrie screening test (prueba de detección de Guthrie) also known as newborn screening test; diagnostic test for the detection of phenylketonuria (PKU) (Ch. 44).

hard drive (disco duro) a nonvolatile storage device that stores digitally encoded data on rapidly rotating rigid disks with magnetic surfaces.

The capacity is approximately 100 GB. The device is either permanently installed within the computer case or can be portable (Ch. 11).

hardware (hardware)   physical equipment used by the computer system to process data (Ch. 11).

hard-wired networks (redes con cableado físico)   networks connected by metallic conductors or cables; under some circumstances, optical cables could be used (Ch. 11).

health care proxy (poder para la atención médica)   a document that allows a patient to appoint an agent to make health care decisions in the event that the patient is unable to do so (Ch. 6).

Health Insurance Portability and Accountability Act (HIPAA) (Ley de Portabilidad y Responsabilidad de Seguros de Salud [HIPAA])   government rules, regulations, and procedures resulting from legislation designed to protect the confidentiality of patient information (Ch. 7, 16).

health maintenance organization (HMO) (organización de mantenimiento de la salud [HMO])   type of managed care operation that is typically set up as a for-profit corporation with salaried employees. HMOs "with walls" offer a range of medical services under one roof; HMOs "without walls" typically contract with providers in the community to provide patient services for an agreed-upon fee (Ch. 2, 17).

Healthcare Common Procedure Coding System (HCPCS) (Sistema de Códigos de Procedimientos Comunes de la Atención Médica [HCPCS])   a coding system consisting of the CPT, national codes (level II), and local codes (level III); previously known as HCFA Common Procedure Coding System (Ch. 18).

hematocrit (hematocrito)   percentage of red blood cells within a specimen of anticoagulated whole blood (Ch. 41).

hematology (hematología)   study of blood and the blood-forming tissues (Ch. 39, 40, 41).

hematoma (hematoma)   a large bruise, accumulation of blood around the venipuncture site during or after venipuncture caused by the leakage of blood from where the needle punctured the vein (Ch. 40).

hematopoiesis (hematopoyesis)   formation of blood cells (Ch. 41).

hematuria (hematuria)   abnormal presence of blood in urine, symptomatic of many disorders of the genitourinary system and renal diseases (Ch. 30, 42).

hemiplegia (hemiplejía)   paralysis of one side of the body (Ch. 33).

hemoconcentration (hemoconcentración)   pooling of blood at the location of the venipuncture caused by leaving the tourniquet on the arm longer than one minute, resulting in inaccurate blood samples (Ch. 40).

hemoglobin (hemoglobina)   molecule within the red blood cell that transports oxygen (Ch. 41).

hemoglobinopathy (hemoglobinopatía)   inherited disease resulting from the formation of an abnormal hemoglobin molecule (Ch. 41).

hemolysis (hemólisis)   rupturing of the red blood cells during the process of blood collection. The serum or plasma becomes contaminated and has a reddish color (Ch. 40).

hemoptysis (hemoptisis)   spitting up of blood arising from the mouth, larynx, trachea, bronchi, or lungs characterized by a sudden attack of coughing with production of bloody sputum (Ch. 30).

heterophile antibody (anticuerpo heterófilo)   antibody that reacts with other than the specific antigens as seen in infectious mononucleosis (Ch. 44).

Hibeclens® (Hibeclens®)   brand of antiseptic soap solution (Ch. 31).

hierarchy of needs (jerarquía de necesidades)   needs that are arranged in a specific order or rank; sequential arrangement. Associated with Abraham Maslow (Ch. 5).

high-context communication (comunicación de alto contexto)   communication style that involves great reliance on body language, reference to objects in the environment, and culturally relevant phraseology to convey an idea. Relies on the listener knowing related events through close association with the speaker or culture (Ch. 5).

high-density lipoprotein (HDL) (lipoproteína de alta densidad [HDL])   lipoprotein in the blood composed primarily of protein; removes cholesterol from peripheral tissues and transports them to the liver for excretion (Ch. 44).

histology (histología)   study of a tissue biopsy sample for the determination of disease (Ch. 39).

history and physical examination report (H&P) (informe de historia clínica y examen físico [H&P])   report of patient's history and physical examination to document reason for visit (Ch. 16).

history of present illness (HPI) (antecedentes de enfermedad actual [AEA])   the chronologic description of the development of the patient's illness (Ch. 16).

holding media (medios de sostén)   specific media used in the transport of microorganisms to support the life of the organisms until they can be put on nutrient medium in the laboratory (Ch. 43).

Holter monitor (monitor Holter)   a portable continuous recording of cardiac activity for a 24-hour period (Ch. 37).

homeopathy (homeopatía)   a healing modality that uses diluted doses of certain substances to create an "energy imprint" in the body to bring about a cure (Ch. 2).

homeostasis (homeostasia)   state of equilibrium of internal environment (Ch. 34).

hordeolum (hordéolo)   inflamed sebaceous gland of the eyelid caused by bacterial infection; stye (Ch. 30).

hormone replacement therapy (HRT) (terapia de reemplazo hormonal [TRH])   the replacement of hormones lacking from the patient's system. In this case, HRT refers to the replacement of varying levels of estrogen and progesterone in perimenopausal or postmenopausal women (Ch. 26).

hospital-based laboratories (laboratorios con base en el hospital)   hospital-owned laboratories that perform most tests required by the hospital and local communities (Ch. 39).

human chorionic gonadotropin (hCG) (gonadotropina coriónica humana [hCG])   hormone secreted by the trophoblast after fertilization of the ovum. It may be detected in the blood and urine of pregnant women (Ch. 26, 44).

human immunodeficiency virus (HIV) (virus de la inmunodeficiencia humana [VIH])   virus causing AIDS; it is a retrovirus that ultimately destroys immune system cells (Ch. 22).

humoral immunity (inmunidad humoral)   immunity mediated by antibodies in body fluids such as plasma and lymph (Ch. 22).

hyaline (hialino)   transparent, clear; hyaline casts consist of mucuprotein, they are transparent and often difficult to see in urine (Ch. 42).

hydrocollator pack (paquete de hidrocolator)   pack filled with gel that is warmed in a water bath (Ch. 33).

hydrogen peroxide (peróxido de hidrógeno)   antibacterial solution that has a mechanical cleansing action (Ch. 31).

hyperemesis gravidarum (hiperemesis gravídica)   severe nausea and vomiting during pregnancy with inability to eat; may lead to severe dehydration (Ch. 26).

hyperextension (hiperextensión)   position of maximum extension, or extending a body part beyond its normal limits (Ch. 33).

hyperglycemia (hiperglucemia)   increased levels of blood glucose. Hyperglycemia does not necessarily mean that the patient is diabetic but may be an indication of prediabetes (Ch. 44).

hyperpnea (hiperpnea)   increased respiratory rate and depth as seen in exercise, pain, fever, and hysteria (Ch. 24).

hypertension (hipertensión)   blood pressure that is consistently greater than 140/90 mm Hg (Ch. 24).

hyperthermia (hipertermia)   body temperature above normal range; an unusually high fever (Ch. 29).

hyperventilation (hiperventilación)   ventilation rate that is greater than metabolically necessary, potentially leading to alkalosis (Ch. 24).

hypochromic (hipocrómico)   less color than normal (Ch. 41).

hypoglycemia (hipoglucemia)   state of having a lower than normal blood glucose level (Ch. 40, 44).

hypogonadism (hipogonadismo)   when the testes produce little or no testosterone (Ch. 28).

hypotension (hipotensión)   abnormally low blood pressure resulting in inadequate tissue profusion and oxygenation (Ch. 24).

hypothermia (hipotermia)   extremely dangerous cold-related condition that can result in death if the individual does not receive care and if the progression of hypothermia is not reversed. Symptoms include shivering, cold skin, and confusion (Ch. 9, 29).

hypoventilation (hipoventilación)   decrease in respiration rate with shallow depth of respiration (Ch. 24).

hypovolemic (hipovolémico)   a type of shock in which the body has lost blood or fluid volumen to such an extent that there is not enough circulating volumen to fill the ventricles. The heart attempts to compensate by increasing the heart rate (Ch. 9).

hypoxemia (hipoxemia)   lack of oxygen in the blood (Ch. 36).

hypoxia (hypoxia)   oxygen deficiency (Ch. 26).

hysterosalpingogram (histerosalpingograma)   X-ray of uterus and fallopian tubes using a contrast medium (Ch. 26).

immune system (sistema inmunitario)   body's strong line of defense against invading microorganisms. The body recognizes foreign substances such as microorganisms and produces substances to fight them off. Antibodies, white blood cells, digestive enzymes, and resistance of the skin are some examples (Ch. 22).

immunity (inmunidad)   ability of the body to resist specific pathogens and their toxins (Ch. 22).

immunoglobulins (inmunoglobulinas)   family of proteins capable of acting as antibodies, thereby protecting individuals from pathogenic microorganisms; also, antibodies produced by the cells of the immune response system (Ch. 22).

immunohematology (inmunohematología)   study of blood group antigens and antibodies; blood banking (Ch. 39).

immunology (inmunología)   the study of the components of the immune system and their function (Ch. 39).

immunomodulator (inmunomodulador)   a substance that has the ability to change immune responses (Ch. 22).

immunosuppressed (inmunosuprimido)   referring to a patient whose immune system is unhealthy because of disease, medication, and genetics; these patients can be particularly susceptible to attack by microorganisms (Ch. 22).

implantable cardioverter/defibrillator (ICD) (cardioversor/desfibrilador)   an implantable device used for life-threatening arrhythmias. Its purpose is to shock the heart out of the arrhythmia and into a more normal sinus rhythm (Ch. 37).

implicit (implícito)   capable of being understood from something else though unexpressed; implied (Ch. 9).

implied consent (consentimiento implícito)   consent assumed by the health care provider, typically in an emergency that threatens the patient's life. Implied consent also occurs in more subtle ways in the health care environment; for example, when a patient willingly rolls up the sleeve to receive an injection (Ch. 7).

implied contract (contrato implícito)   contract indicated by actions rather than words (Ch. 7).

improvise (improvisar)   to make, invent, or arrange in an unplanned or spontaneous manner (Ch. 1).

in vitro fertilization (IVF) (fertilización in vitro [IVF])   the ovum is fertilized in a culture dish, allowed to grow, and then implanted into the uterus (Ch. 8).

income statement (estado de resultados)   financial statement showing net profit or loss (Ch. 21).

incompetence (incompetencia)   legally, a person who is insane, inadequate, or not an adult (Ch. 7).

incontinence (incontinencia)   uncontrollable loss of urine or feces (Ch. 29).

increment (incremento)   an increase or addition in number, size, or extent (Ch. 24).

independent provider association (IPA) (Asociación Independiente de Médicos [IPA])   independent network of physicians in private practice who contract with the association to treat patients for an agreed-upon fee (Ch. 2).

indexing (indexar)   selecting the name, subject, or number under which to file a record and determining the order in which the units should be considered (Ch. 14).

indirect statements (declaraciones indirectas)   means of eliciting a response from a patient by turning a question into a statement of interest (Ch. 5).

infection (infección)   invasion of pathogens into living tissue (Ch. 31).

infection control (control de infecciones)   methods to eliminate or reduce the transmission of infectious microorganisms (Ch. 22).

infectious agent (agente infeccioso)   pathogen responsible for a specific infectious disease (Ch. 22).

infectious mononucleosis (mononucleosis infecciosa)   acute infectious disease primarily affecting the lymphoid tissue, caused by the Epstein–Barr virus (Ch. 44).

infectious waste (residuos patógenos)   items that have come in contact with patient blood or body fluids. Contaminated items (Ch. 22).

infertility (infertilidad)   the inability or diminished ability to conceive is known (Ch. 28).

inflammation (inflamación)   the normal nonspecific immune response by the body to any type of injury (trauma, bacterial, viral, and temperature extremes) (Ch. 31).

inflammatory response (respuesta inflamatoria)   body's defense against the threat of infection or trauma. Characterized by redness, pain, heat, and swelling (Ch. 22).

informed consent (consentimiento informado)   consent given by the patient who is made aware of any procedure to be performed, its risks, expected outcomes, and alternatives (Ch. 7, 31).

inner-directed people (personas con autodeterminación)   people who decide for themselves what they want to do with their lives (Ch. 4).

inoculate (inocular)   to place colonies of microorganisms onto nutrient media (Ch. 43).

input device (dispositivo de entrada)   a device used to input data into a computer (Ch. 11).

instrument tray (bandeja de instrumentos)   see **Mayo stand** (Ch. 31).

insulin (insulina)   hormone secreted by beta cells of the islets of Langerhans of the pancreas essential for the proper metabolism of glucose (Ch. 44).

integrated delivery system (IDS) (sistema de prestación de servicios médicos integrado [IDS])   a health care organization of affiliated provider sites combined under a single ownership that offers the full spectrum of managed health care (Ch. 17).

integrative medicine (medicina integradora)   bringing together of two or more treatment modalities so they function as a harmonious whole, as seen in alternative forms of health care (Ch. 2).

internal respiration (respiración interna)   passage of oxygen from the blood into the cells (Ch. 30).

***International Classification of Diseases, 9th Revision, Clinical Modification* (ICD-9-CM) (Clasificación Internacional de Enfermedades, 9.ª Revisión, Modificación Clínica [CIE-9-MC])**   standard diagnosis codes used to identify a patient's medical problem. Used by most ambulatory care settings in encoding the claim form and recognized by most insurance carriers (Ch. 18).

internet blogs (blogs de Internet)   web site having commentary, description of events or other material maintained on a regular basis. The blog is usually interactive allowing visitors to leave comments (Ch. 48).

internship (pasantía)   transition stage between classroom and employment (Ch. 1).

interrogatory (interrogatorio)   a written set of questions that must be answered, under oath, within a specific time period; part of the discovery process (Ch. 7).

interview (entrevista)   meeting in which you and the interviewer discuss employment opportunities and strengths you can contribute to the organization (Ch. 48).

interview techniques (técnicas de entrevista)   methods of encouraging the best communication between the applicant and the interviewer (Ch. 5).

intimate partner violence (IPV) (violencia de pareja [IPV])   refers to violence or abuse between a spouse or former spouse; boyfriend, girlfriend or former boyfriend/girlfriend; and same-sex or heterosexual intimate partner or former same-sex or heterosexual intimate partner (Ch. 7, 8).

intraepithelium (intraepitelial)   within the epithelium (Ch. 26).

intravenous pyelogram (pielograma intravenoso)   radiographic studies of the kidneys, ureters, and bladder using a contrast medium (Ch. 28, 30).

invasive procedure (procedimiento invasivo) surgical technique or a procedure that requires penetration of the skin or a body opening. The potential for pathogenic microorganisms to enter the body exists (Ch. 22, 39).

inversion (inversión) moving a body part inward (Ch. 33).

involuntary dismissal (despido involuntario) termination of employment based on poor job performance or violation of office policies (Ch. 46).

involution (involución) return of the uterus to normal size and shape after childbirth (Ch. 26).

ionizing radiation (radiación ionizante) X-ray beams (Ch. 32).

ischemia (isquemia) local and temporary lack of blood to an organ or part caused by obstruction of circulation (Ch. 37).

isoelectric (isoeléctrico) having equal electrical potentials. It is represented on the ECG as the flat horizontal line, the baseline (Ch. 37).

isolation (aislamiento) separating a patient with certain infections or communicable diseases from other individuals (Ch. 22).

isolation categories (categorías de aislamiento) system of seven categories developed by the Centers for Disease Control (CDC) that isolates patients according to known infections. These categories have been condensed into three Transmission-Based Precautions based on air, contact, and droplet routes of transmission (Ch. 22).

isopropyl alcohol (alcohol isopropílico) commonly called rubbing alcohol; 70% alcohol solution commonly used as a cleaner (Ch. 31).

isotope (isótopo) a chemical element (Ch. 32).

itinerary (itinerario) detailed written plan of a proposed trip (Ch. 45).

jargon (jerga) words, phrases, or terminology specific to a profession (Ch. 12).

jaundice (ictericia) yellow discolorization of the skin and sclera caused by excess bilirubin in the blood (Ch. 22, 25).

jet injection (inyección a chorro) an injection given under the skin without a needle, using the force of the liquid under pressure to pierce the skin (Ch. 22).

job description (descripción del trabajo) outline of tasks, duties, and responsibilities for every position in the office (Ch. 46).

Joint Commission (Comisión Conjunta) formerly the Joint Commision on Accreditation of Healthcare Organizations, a commission established to improve the quality of care and services provided in organized health care setting, through a voluntary accreditation process (Ch. 16).

ketoacidosis (cetoacidosis) accumulation of ketones in the body, occurring primarily as a complication of diabetes mellitus; if left untreated, it could cause coma (Ch. 42).

ketone (cetona) chemical compound produced during an increased metabolism of fat; also, test on a reagent strip (Ch. 42).

ketonuria (cetonuria) having ketones in urine (Ch. 42).

ketosis (cetosis) a condition of the body burning fatty acids for energy in the absence of appropriate glucose/carbohydrates; may be referred to as lipolysis (Ch. 42).

key (keyed) (mecanografiar) to input data by keystrokes on a computer keyboard (Ch. 15).

key unit (unidad clave) first indexing unit of the filing segment (Ch. 14).

keywords (palabras clave) words that relate to a job-specific position. Keywords may be job-specific skills or profession-specific words (Ch. 48).

kinesics (cinésica) study of body language (Ch. 5).

labyrinthitis (laberintitis) inflammation of inner ear or labyrinth (Ch. 25).

lackluster (deslucido) dull, lacking in sheen (Ch. 9).

Lamaze (Lamaze) technique consisting of breathing exercises to facilitate delivery (Ch. 26).

laparoscopy (laparoscopía) a procedure in which a lighted instrument is used to view the inside of the pelvic cavity (Ch. 26).

LASIK (LASIK) abbreviation for laser-assisted in situ keratomileusis, a kind of eye surgery using lasers to change the shape of the cornea eliminating or reducing the need for corrective lenses in cases of severe myopia (nearsightedness) (Ch. 10).

lead wire (alambre guía) a conductor attached to an electrocardiograph. Consists of limb leads and chest leads (Ch. 37).

ledger (libro mayor) record of charges, payments, and adjustments for individual patient or family (Ch. 19).

lesion (lesión) injury or wound. A circumscribed area of tissue that has been altered pathologically (Ch. 22, 30).

letter of reference (carta de referencia) letter usually written by an employee's past employer describing the employee's performance, attitude, or qualifications. This letter is presented to a potential employer when applying for a new job (Ch. 46).

letter of resignation (carta de renuncia) letter informing the current employer of the employee's decision to resign from a current position (Ch. 46).

leukocyte (leucocito) white blood cell, one of the formed elements of blood (Ch. 40, 41).

leukocyte esterase (esterasa leucocitaria) test on a reagent strip that indicates the presence of white blood cells in the urinary tract (Ch. 42).

liability (pasivo) debts and financial obligations for which one is responsible (Ch. 21); legal responsibility (Ch. 45).

libel (calumnia) false and malicious writing about another constituting a defamation of character (Ch. 7).

libido (libido) sexual drive (Ch. 28).

license (licencia) permission by competent authority (the state) to engage in a profession; permission to act (Ch. 1); permission statement authorizing the use of copyrighted computer software (Ch. 11).

licensure (matrícula) granting of licenses to practice a profession (Ch. 1).

ligature (ligadura) length of suture thread without a needle, used for tying off vessels during surgery (Ch. 31).

lipemia (lipemia) excessive amount of fat (lipids) in the blood, resulting in a blood sample that has a milky appearance (Ch. 40).

liquid nitrogen (nitrógeno líquido) commonly and incorrectly referred to as dry ice, liquid nitrogen is a volatile freezing agent used to destroy unwanted tissue such as warts (Ch. 31).

lithotomy (litotomía) patients lie on their back similar to the dorsal recumbent position except the buttocks should be as close to the bottom edge of the table as possible, and feet are placed in stirrups attached to the foot of the table (Ch. 25).

litigation (litigio) court action (Ch. 7).

living will (testamento en vida) document allowing a person to make choices related to treatment in a life-threatening illness (Ch. 6).

local area network (LAN) (red de área local [LAN]) network of computers usually in one office or building (Ch. 11).

lochia (loquios) discharge from the uterus of blood, mucus, and tissue during the period after childbirth (Ch. 22, 26).

long-range goals (metas a largo plazo) achievements that may take three to five years to accomplish (Ch. 4).

low-context communication (comunicación de bajo contexto) communication style that uses few environmental or cultural idioms to convey an idea or concept. Ideas are spelled out explicitly (Ch. 5).

low-density lipoprotein (LDL) (lipoproteína de baja densidad [LDL]) lipoprotein in the blood composed primarily of cholesterol. The cholesterol carried by LDL may be deposited in peripheral tissues and is associated with an increased risk for heart disease (Ch. 44).

lumbar puncture (punción lumbar) surgical puncture of the lumbar area of the intervertebral spaces to aspirate cerebrospinal fluid for laboratory analysis (Ch. 22).

lumen (luz) the space within an artery, vein, intestine, needles, and catheter or tube (Ch. 24).

lymphocyte (linfocito) white blood cell with a dense nonsegmented nucleus and lacking granules in the cytoplasm (Ch. 41).

lyophilized (liofilizado) the process of rapidly freezing a substance at extremely low temperatures and then dehydrating the substance in a high vacuum (freeze drying) (Ch. 27).

M codes (morphology codes) (códigos M [códigos morfológicos]) found in the ICD-9-CM and used primarily with cancer registries. M codes further identify behavior and the cell type of a neoplasm (Ch. 18).

macroallocation (macroasignación) of scarce medical resources; decisions are made by Congress, health systems agencies, and insurance companies (Ch. 8).

macrocytic (macrocítico) term that describes a larger than normal cell (Ch. 41).

macular degeneration (degeneración macular) degeneration of the macula area of the retina caused by aging; a leading cause of visual impairment in people older than 50 years, making it difficult to do fine work (Ch. 29).

major mineral (mineral principal) mineral that is required in large amounts by the body (Ch. 34).

malabsorption (malabsorción) inadequate absorption of nutrients from the intestinal tract (Ch. 30).

malaise (malestar) discomfort, uneasiness, or indisposition, often indicative of infection (Ch. 22, 30).

malaria (paludismo) acute infectious disease caused by the presence of protozoan parasites within the red blood cells; usually comes from the bite of a female mosquito (Ch. 3, 22).

malfeasance (fechoría) conduct that is illegal or contrary to an official's obligations (Ch. 7).

malpractice (mala praxis) professional negligence (Ch. 7, 45).

man-in-the-middle attack (ataque de intermediario (man-in-the-middle) a form of attack where the hacker connects independently and transparently with two parties so that they each think they are communicating directly to each other. The hacker can then intercept all transmitted information (Ch. 11).

managed care operation (establecimiento de atención administrada) any health care setting or delivery system that is designed to reduce the cost of care while still providing access to care (Ch. 2).

managed care organization (MCO) (organización de atención administrada [MCO]) a health insurance organization that adheres to the principles of strong dependence on selective contracting with providers, the use of primary care physicians, prospective and retrospective utilization management, use of treatment guidelines for high cost chronic disorders, and an emphasis on preventive care, education, and patient compliance with treatment plans (Ch. 17).

management by walking around (MBWA) (gestión itinerante [MBWA]) a technique for keeping managers informed about the health of their organization (Ch. 45).

managerial accounting (contabilidad administrativa) generates financial information that can enable more efficient internal management (Ch. 21).

mandate (mandato) formal order to obey certain rules and regulations (Ch. 38).

manometer (manómetro) device for measuring a liquid or gaseous pressure. The measurement is expressed in millimeters of mercury or water (Ch. 24).

Mantoux test (prueba de Mantoux) test for tuberculosis involving the intracutaneous injection of purified protein derivative (see PPD) (Ch. 44).

marketing (comercialización) process by which the provider of services makes the consumer aware of the scope and quality of those services. Marketing tools might include public relations, brochures, patient education seminars, and newsletters (Ch. 45).

masking (ocultamiento) attempt to conceal or repress true feelings or the message (Ch. 5).

matrix (matriz) to establish an appointment matrix, a provider's unavailable time slots are marked with an X. Patients are not scheduled during those times (Ch. 13).

mature minor (menor maduro) a person, usually younger than 18 years, who is able to understand and appreciate the consequences of treatment despite their young age (Ch. 7).

Mayo stand (mesa de Mayo) portable metal tray table used for setting up small sterile fields for minor surgery and procedures (Ch. 31).

meconium (meconio) first feces of newborn (Ch. 26).

mediation (mediación) dispute resolution that allows a facilitator to help the two parties settle their differences and come to an acceptable solution (Ch. 7).

medical asepsis (asepsia médica) clean and free from infection (Ch. 22, 38).

medically indigent (médicamente indigente) refers to those individuals unable to pay for their own medical coverage (Ch. 7).

Medicare Part A (Medicare Parte A) benefits covering inpatient hospital and skilled nursing facilities, hospice care, and blood transfusion (Ch. 17).

Medicare Part B (Medicare Parte B) benefits covering outpatient hospital and health care provider services (Ch. 17).

Medicare Part C (Medicare Parte C) commonly referred to as Medicare advantage plans. These plans are approved by Medicare and are run by private companies (Ch. 17).

Medicare Part D (Medicare Parte D) prescription drug coverage by Medicare (Ch. 17).

Medigap policy (póliza de Medigap) an individual plan covering the patient's Medicare deductible and co-pay obligations that fulfills the federal government standards for Medicare supplemental insurance (Ch. 17).

memorandum (memorándum) interoffice correspondence, usually referred to as a memo (Ch. 15).

memory (memoria) refers to storage of computer data. Memory can be volatile (lost when computer is turned off) or nonvolatile (permanently written to storage device) (Ch. 11).

meniscus (menisco) curvature appearing in a liquid's upper surface when a liquid is placed in a container (Ch. 24, 36).

mensuration (medición) a method of examination using the process of measuring. The measurements of height and weight, the length of a limb, and the amount of flexion and extension of an extremity are all forms of mensuration (Ch. 25).

mentor (mentor) person assigned or requested to assist in training, guiding, or coaching another (Ch. 45).

metabolism (metabolismo) total of all changes, chemical and physical, that take place in the body (Ch. 34).

metastasis (metástasis) in cancer, malignant cells spread from the primary growth to a new location (Ch. 28).

metered dose inhaler (inhalador de dosis medida) a device used to deliver a prescribed amount of medication to the respiratory tract, especially the lungs (Ch. 30).

metrorrhagia (metrorragia) uterine bleeding at irregular intervals (Ch. 26).

microallocation (microasignación) of scarce medical resources; decisions are made by providers and individual members of the health care team (Ch. 8).

microbiology (microbiología) branch of biology dealing with the study of microscopic forms of life (Ch. 39, 43).

microcytic (microcítico) term describing a smaller than normal cell (Ch. 41).

microorganism (microorganismo) microscopic living creature capable of transmission and reproduction in specific circumstances (Ch. 22).

microscopic examination (examen microscópico) viewing a specimen with the aid of a microscope (Ch. 16).

midstream collection (recolección de mitad de micción) urine sample collected in the middle of a flow of urine (Ch. 42).

minor (menor) person who has not reached the age of majority, usually 18 years (Ch. 7).

minutes (actas) written record of topics discussed and actions taken during meeting sessions (Ch. 15, 45).

misdemeanor (contravención) a lesser crime; misdemeanors vary from state to state in their definition. Punishment is usually probation or a time of public service and a fine (Ch. 7).

misfeasance (irregularidad) a civil law term referring to a lawful act that is improperly or unlawfully executed (Ch. 7).

modalities (modalidades) physical agents such as heat, cold, light, water, and electricity used to treat muscular or joint malfunction (Ch. 33).

modified block letter, indented (carta estilo bloque modificado, con sangría) modified letter style with indented paragraphs. Paragraphs in this style of letter may be indented five spaces (Ch. 15).

modified block letter, standard (carta estilo bloque modificado, estándar) major letter style where all lines begin at the left margin with the exception of the date line, complimentary closure, and keyed signature. The exceptions usually begin at the center position or a few spaces to the right of center (Ch. 15).

modified wave scheduling (planificación en olas modificada) system where multiple patients are scheduled at the beginning of each hour, followed by single appointments every 10 to 20 minutes the rest of the hour (Ch. 13).

modifier (modificador) an additional code that may be added to a five-digit CPT code to further explain the service provided (Ch. 18).

modulated (modulado) speech that varies in pitch and intensity (Ch. 12).

money market savings accounts (cuentas de ahorro del mercado monetario) bank accounts that pay a higher interest rate (money market rate) than standard savings accounts and permit writing a limited number of checks (Ch. 19).

monocyte (monocito) white blood cell without cytoplasmic granules that has a large convoluted nonsegmented nucleus (Ch. 41).

morbid obesity (obesidad mórbida) obesity so severe that it can result in serious diseases (Ch. 30).

morbidity (morbilidad) number of cases of disease in a specific population (Ch. 22).

mordant (mordiente) substance that causes dye to adhere to an object; iodine is a mordant in Gram stain (Ch. 43).

morphology (morfología) form and structure of an organism (Ch. 22, 43).

mortality (mortalidad) the ratio of the number of deaths to a given population (Ch. 22).

mounting (montaje) process of applying in sequence a portion of each of the 12 leads of the ECG recording onto a commercially prepared mounting form or plain sheet of paper as part of the patient's permanent record (Ch. 37).

moxibustion (moxibustión) ancient Chinese method of treatment that uses a powdered plant substance on the skin to raise a blister (Ch. 3).

multigravida (multigrávida) a woman who has been pregnant more than once (Ch. 26).

mycology (micología) study of fungi (Ch. 39, 43).

myocardial infarction (infarto de miocardio) a heart attack; usually caused by a blockage of one or more of the coronary arteries (Ch. 9, 37).

myopia (miopía) nearsightedness; caused by an elongated (shaped) eyeball and the image is focused in the front of the retina resulting in the inability to focus on objects at a distance (Ch. 30).

myringotomy (miringotomía) incision into the tympanic membrane; part of the treatment for otitis media (Ch. 27).

Nägele's rule (regla de Nägele) usual method for calculating expected date of birth (Ch. 26).

National Healthcareer Association (NHA) (Asociación Nacional de Profesiones de Salud [NHA]) an association that offers national certification examinations for health care professionals. NHA works with educational institutions on curriculum development, competency testing, and preparation and administration of their examination for certification (Ch. 47).

negligence (negligencia) failure to exercise a certain standard of care (Ch. 7, 45).

nematode (nematodo) round worm (Ch. 43).

neonatal (neonatal) pertaining to newborn (Ch. 26).

neonate (neonato) newborn (Ch. 27).

network interface (interfaz de red) software, servers, and cable connections used to link computers (Ch. 11).

networking (conexión en red) connecting two or more computers together to share files and hardware. The system is called a network

(Ch. 11); process in which people of similar interests exchange information in social, business, or professional relationships (Ch. 46).

neurogenic (neurogénico) a type of shock in which there is injury or trauma to the nervous system causing the loss of tone in the vessels resulting in massive dilation of arterioles and venuoles. This results in a dramatic drop in blood pressure (Ch. 9).

neutrophil (neutrófilo) the most common type of granulocytic white blood cell (Ch. 41).

nevus (nevo) a mole (Ch. 29).

niacin (niacina) one of the B-complex vitamins (Ch. 34).

nocturia (nocturia) excessive urination during the night (Ch. 28, 30).

nomogram (nomograma) graph that shows the relation among numeric values. Body surface area (BSA) of a patient can be estimated by its use (Ch. 36).

noncompliant (inobservancia) failure to follow a required command or instruction (Ch. 7).

nonconsecutive filing (archivado no consecutivo) numeric filing method where numbers are considered in ascending order using subsets of figures within a number; for example, in the number 574 19 2863: 2863 is unit 1, 19 is unit 2, 574 is unit 3 (Ch. 14).

nonfeasance (omisión) a civil law term referring to the failure to perform an act, official duty, or legal requirement (Ch. 7).

noninvasive procedure (procedimiento no invasivo) a procedure that does require penetrating the skin or a body opening (Ch. 37).

normal flora (flora normal) microorganisms that are normally present in a specific site (Ch. 22, 43).

normal saline (solución salina normal) a solution of sodium chloride (salt) and distilled water. It has the same osmotic pressure as blood serum. It is also known as isotonic or physiologic saline (Ch. 9).

normal sinus rhythm (ritmo sinusal normal) term used to describe the heart's rhythm when it is within the normal range (Ch. 37).

normochromic (normocrómico) of normal color, in this case, when referring to red blood cells (Ch. 41).

normocytic (normocítico) term that describes a normal-sized cell (Ch. 41).

nosocomial (intrahospitalaria) infection acquired in a health care setting (hospital, clinic, nursing home) (Ch. 22, 43).

notary (notary public) (escribano público) someone with the legal capacity to witness and certify documents; can take depositions (Ch. 19).

nullipara (nulípara) a woman who has not carried a pregnancy to the stage of viability (Ch. 26).

nutrient (nutriente) ingested substance that helps the body stay in its homeostatic state (Ch. 34).

nutrition (nutrición) study of the bringing of nutrients into the body and how the body uses these nutrients (Ch. 34).

nystagmus (nistagmo) continuous involuntary movement of the eyes (Ch. 30).

objective (objetivo) a patient sign that is visible, palpable, or measurable by an observer (Ch. 23); also, magnifying lens that is closest to the object being viewed with a microscope (Ch. 39).

occluder (oclusor) instrument used to obstruct or close off vision or light (Ch. 30).

occlusion (oclusión) closure of a passage (Ch. 9).

old reports (informes anteriores) reports such as a discharge summary that should be completed within 71 hours (Ch. 16).

oliguria (oliguria) decrease in urine output (Ch. 30).

open-ended questions (preguntas abiertas) questions that encourage verbalization and response; questions that seek a response beyond a simple yes or no (Ch. 5).

operating system (OS) (sistema operativo [SO]) software used to control the computer and its peripheral equipment. Also referred to as system software (Ch. 11).

operative report (OR) (informe quirúrgico [OR]) medical report that chronicles the details of a surgical procedure (Ch. 16).

opportunistic infection (infección oportunista) an infection that results from a defective immune system that cannot defend itself from pathogens normally found in the environment (Ch. 22).

optical character reader (OCR) (lector óptico de caracteres [OCR]) U.S. Postal Service's computerized scanner that reads addresses printed on letter mail. If the information is properly formatted, then the OCR will find a match in its address files and print a bar code on the lower right edge of the envelope (Ch. 15).

orchidectomy (orquidectomía) surgical excision of a testicle (Ch. 28).

organomercurial (compuestos organomercuriales) any mercury-containing organic compound (Ch. 27).

orthopnea (ortopnea) difficulty breathing in any position other than an upright position (Ch. 24).

oscilloscope (osciloscopio) an electronic device used for recording electrical activity of the heart, brain, and muscular tissues (Ch. 32, 37).

osteoporosis (osteoporosis) a thinning of the long bones, pelvic bones, and vertebrae (Ch. 29).

otoscope (otoscopio) instrument used to examine the external ear canal and tympanic membrane (Ch. 30).

out guide or sheet (señalador o marcador) card, folder, or slip of paper inserted temporarily in the files to replace a record that has been retrieved from the files (Ch. 14).

outer-directed people (personas influenciables) people who let events, other people, or environmental factors dictate their behavior (Ch. 4).

output device (dispositivo de salida) a device used to output data from a computer. Includes printers, faxes, data storage drivers, screens, and plotters (Ch. 11).

outsourcing (subcontratación) the practice of contracting with a service outside of the clinic or hospital to a company where the task can be accomplished at a lower cost and with a faster turnaround time (Ch. 16).

ova (óvulos) eggs, in this case, eggs of a parasite (Ch. 43).

overtime (horas extra) money paid at a rate of not less than one and one-half times the regular rate of pay after a 40-hour work week is completed (Ch. 46).

owner's equity (patrimonio neto) amount by which business assets exceed business liabilities. Also called net worth, proprietorship, and capital (Ch. 21).

oxidation (oxidación) process of a substance combining with oxygen (Ch. 34).

oxytocin (oxitocina) a pituitary hormone that stimulates the muscles of the uterus to contract, thus inducing labor (Ch. 26).

palliative (paliativa) measures taken to relieve symptoms of disease (Ch. 6, 22, 32).

pallor (palidez) lack of color, paleness (Ch. 25).

palpate (palpar) to feel with fingertips, to search for a vein with a pressure and release touch (Ch. 25, 40).

panel (panel) a series of tests related to a particular organ or organ system of body function. For example, a liver panel would check many different functions of the liver. Previously called a "profile" (Ch. 39).

paracentesis (paracentesis) puncture of a cavity for removal of fluid (Ch. 22).

parasitology (parasitología) study of organisms (parasites and their eggs) that live within or on another organism and at the expense of that organism (Ch. 39, 43).

parasympathetic nervous system (sistema nervioso parasimpático) part of the autonomic nervous system that returns the body to its normal state after stress has subsided (Ch. 4).

parenteral (parenteral) injection of a liquid substance into the body via a route other than the alimentary canal (Ch. 22, 36).

parity (paridad) carrying a pregnancy to the point of viability regardless of the outcome (Ch. 26).

participatory manager (gerente participativo) operates on the premise that the worker is capable and wants to do a good job (Ch. 45).

parturition (parir) the process of giving birth (Ch. 26).

patch (parche) modification to software to fix deficiencies in the software. Frequently downloaded from the software supplier's Web site or from floppy disks provided by the supplier (Ch. 11).

patent (permeable) open, not blocked (Ch. 26).

pathogen (patógeno) disease-producing microorganism (Ch. 22, 43).

pathology report (informe de patología) medical reports generated to describe the gross and microscopic examinations performed during a surgical procedure (Ch. 16, 31).

Patient Self-Determination Act (PSDA) (Ley de Autodeterminación del Paciente [PSDA]) the Act that includes the Advance Directive giving patients the right to be involved in their health care decisions (Ch. 7).

patient service centers (centros de servicio al paciente) satellite laboratory facilities located in convenient areas for patients where specimens can be collected or dropped off (Ch. 39).

payee (beneficiario) person named on check who is to receive the amount indicated (Ch. 19).

peak (pico) the opposite of "trough," this is the point at which a drug is at its highest level in the body, usually about 30 minutes after administration. In lab tests, the peak would tell the provider the strongest influence the drug would have on the body at that particular dose (Ch. 39).

pegboard system (sistema de tablero de clavijas) most commonly used manual medical accounts receivable system (Ch. 19).

pellagra (pelagra) disease caused by a deficiency in vitamin B3 (nicotinic acid) characterized by sores on the skin, diarrhea, anxiety, confusion, and death if not treated (Ch. 34).

pelvic inflammatory disease (enfermedad inflamatoria pélvica) infection of uterus, fallopian tubes, and adjacent pelvic structures; most common causes are gonorrhea and chlamydia, spread as sexually transmitted diseases (Ch. 26).

percussion (percusión) the process of eliciting sounds from the body by tapping with either a percussion hammer or fingers. The vibrations and sounds from underlying organs and cavities can be felt and heard (Ch. 25).

percutaneous transluminal coronary angioplasty (PTCA) (angioplastía transluminal coronaria percutánea [PTCA]) a procedure that widens a narrowed or blocked coronary artery (Ch. 37).

peripheral (periférico) away from the center of the body (Ch. 24).

pernicious anemia (anemia perniciosa) chronic anemia caused by lack of hydrochloric acid in the stomach; weakness, fatigue, tingling of extremities, and even heart failure can result; vitamin B12 injections are the treatment for this condition (Ch. 29).

personal computer (PC) (computadora personal [PC]) any computer whose price, size, and capabilities make it useful for individuals to use with no intervening computer operator. Also known as a microcomputer (Ch. 11).

petri dish (placa de Petri) plastic dish into which agar is placed for the purpose of growing bacteria (Ch. 43).

petrissage (petrissage) a kneading movement in massage (Ch. 33).

petty cash (caja chica) small sum kept on hand for minor or unexpected expenses (Ch. 19).

Peyronie's Disease (enfermedad de Peyronie) curvature of the penis during erection (Ch. 28).

pH (pH) scale that indicates the relative alkalinity or acidity of a solution; measurement of hydrogen ion concentration (Ch. 42).

phacoemulsification (facoemulsificación) treatment for cataracts. An ultrasonic device is used to disintegrate the cataract of the lens of the eye, which is then aspirated and removed (Ch. 30).

pharmacogenomics (farmacogenómica) the study of the response of the body to various chemical compounds based on an individual's genetic inheritance (Ch. 35).

pharmacokinetics (farmacocinética) refers to the way a drug is handled by the body (Ch. 36).

pharmacology (farmacología) study of drugs; the science concerned with the history, origin, sources, physical and chemical properties, and uses of drugs and their effects on living organisms (Ch. 35).

pharmacopoeia (farmacopea) book describing drugs and their preparation or a collection or stock of drugs (Ch. 3).

pharmazooticals (Fármacos derivados de animales) drugs obtained from tissues such as the adrenal glands of animals (Ch. 35).

phenylketonuria (PKU) (fenilcetonuria [FCU]) a hereditary disease caused by the body's inability to oxidize the amino acid phenylalanine. If not discovered and treated early, brain damage can occur, causing severe mental retardation (Ch. 27, 44).

phishing (Suplantación de identidad) a practice where the recipient of email is directed to go to a website to provide information to his bank, the IRS, or other official organization. The website is actually a fake made to resemble the real thing, and when information is given, it goes to the consumer fraud criminal (Ch. 11).

phlebotomy (flebotomía) process of collecting blood (Ch. 22, 40).

physicians' office laboratories (POL) (laboratorios del consultorio de los médicos [POL]) laboratories within physicians' offices where common office laboratory tests are performed (Ch. 39).

phytomedicines (fitomedicinas) herbs used as medicinal plants. They contain plant material as their active ingredient (Ch. 36).

placenta abruptio (desprendimiento de la placenta) sudden and abrupt separation of the placenta from uterine wall (Ch. 26).

placenta previa (placenta previa) placenta lies low in uterus and can partially or completely cover the cervical os (Ch. 26).

plaintiff (demandante) person bringing charges in litigation (Ch. 7).

plantar flexion (flexión plantar) moving the foot downward at the ankle (Ch. 33).

plasma (plasma) fluid portion of blood from a tube containing anticoagulant. This fluid contains fibrinogen (Ch. 40).

pluralistic (pluralism) (pluralista [pluralismo]) society where there are several distinct ethnic, religious, or cultural groups that coexist with one another (Ch. 3).

point-of-service (POS) device (dispositivo de punto de servicio [POS]) device allowing direct communication between a medical office and the health care plan's computer (Ch. 18).

point-of-service (POS) plan (plan de punto de servicio [POS]) a plan that allows direct communication between a medical office and the health insurance company (Ch. 17).

polyp (pólipo) tumor with a stem found in nose, uterus, bladder, colon, or rectum (Ch. 30).

port (puerto) shortened term for portal—an entry way. When related to intravenous therapy, it is a type of adapter that can serve as additional means for infusing fluids or medications. The port can be attached to the primary tubing. The port has a needleless entry site (Ch. 36).

portfolio (cartera) notebook or file containing examples of materials commonly used (Ch. 15).

Positron Emission Tomography (PET) (tomografía por emisión de positrones [PET]) a radiographic procedure that uses a computer and a radioactive substance. The radioactive substance is injected into the patient's body and gives off charged particles. They combine with particles in the patient's body to produce color images that reveal the amount of metabolic activity in an organ or structure (Ch. 31).

postcoital (poscoital) period of time following (after) intercourse (Ch. 26).

posting (asiento) recording financial transactions into a bookkeeping or accounting system (Ch. 19).

potassium hydroxide (KOH) (hidróxido de potasio [KOH]) 10% solution placed on vaginal smears, as well as skin scrapings, hair, and other dry substances, to dissolve excess debris. This clears the vision field for better viewing of fungi and spores (Ch. 43).

power verbs (verbos de acción) action words used to describe your attributes and strengths (Ch. 48).

practicum (práctica) transitional stage providing opportunity to apply theory learned in the classroom to a health care setting through practical, hands-on experience (Ch. 1, 45).

preauthorization (autorización previa) obtaining an insurance carrier's consent to proceed with patient care and treatment. Unless authorization is obtained, insurance carriers may not pay benefits for specific problems (Ch. 17).

precedents (precedentes) refers to rulings made at an earlier time and include decisions made in a court, interpretations of a constitution, and statutory law decisions (Ch. 7).

precipitate (precipitado) substance in the form of fine particles that separates from a solution if allowed to stand for a time (Ch. 36).

precordial (precordial) pertaining to the area on the anterior surface of the body overlying the heart (Ch. 37).

preeclampsia (preeclampsia) a complication of pregnancy characterized by generalized edema, hypertension, and proteinuria (Ch. 26).

preferred provider organization (PPO) (organización de proveedor preferido [PPO]) organization of providers who network together to offer discounts to purchasers of heath care insurance (Ch. 2, 17).

prejudice (prejuicio) opinion or judgment that is formed before all the facts are known (Ch. 5).

prenatal (prenatal) time period between fertilization and birth (Ch. 26).

presbycusis (presbiacusia) progressive loss of hearing caused by the normal aging process (Ch. 29).

present problem (PP) (problema presente [PP]) see **chief complaint (CC)** (Ch. 16).

prescribe (recetar) to order or recommend the use of a drug, diet, or other form of therapy (Ch. 7, 35).

preservative (conservante) chemical added to food to keep it fresh longer or added to urine to preserve it for testing (Ch. 34, 42).

priapism (priapismo) defined as an erection lasting more than four hours and can occur with or without sexual stimulation (Ch. 28).

primary care provider (PCP) (médico de atención primaria [PCP]) primary care provider for a patient; all care is coordinated through the PCP (Ch. 17).

primary container (recipiente principal) container that directly contains the specimen (Ch. 40).

primigravida (primigrávida) a woman pregnant for the first time (Ch. 26).

privileged (privilegiada) confidential information that may only be communicated with the patient's permission or by court order (Ch. 16).

probate court (tribunal sucesorio) court that administers estates and validates wills (Ch. 20).

probation (período de prueba) period during which the employee and supervisory personnel may determine if both the environment and the position are satisfactory for the employee (Ch. 46).

problem-oriented medical record (POMR) (historia clínica orientada al problema [POMR]) a type of patient chart recordkeeping that uses a sheet at a prominent location in the chart to list vital identification data. Patient medical problems are identified by a number that corresponds to the charting; for example, bronchitis is #1, a broken wrist is #2, and so forth (Ch. 14, 23).

procedure manual (manual de procedimientos) manual providing detailed information relative to the performance of tasks within the job description (Ch. 45).

processed food (alimentos procesados) food that is no longer in a whole, natural state; cooked or packaged with parts removed or ingredients added (Ch. 34).

professional liability insurance (seguro de responsabilidad profesional) insurance policy designed to protect assets in the event a claim for damages resulting from negligence is filed and awarded (Ch. 45).

professionalism (profesionalismo) the qualities that characterize or distinguish a professional person who conforms to the technical and ethical standards of the profession (Ch. 1).

proficiency testing (prueba de aptitud) sample tests performed in a clinical laboratory to determine with what degree of accuracy tests are being performed. Testing samples are checked in the same manner as patient specimens (Ch. 38).

profit sharing (participación en las ganancias) sharing in the financial profits, gains, and benefits of an organization (Ch. 45).

progress notes (notas de evolución) also called chart notes. Provider's formal or informal notes about presenting problem, physical findings, and plan for treatment for a patient examined in the office, clinic, acute care center, or emergency department (Ch. 16).

projection (proyección)   act of placing one's own feelings on another (Ch. 5).

pronation (pronación)   moving the arm so the palm is down (Ch. 33).

prone (prono)   in this postion, the patient is instructed to lie face down on the table with head turned to side; arms may be placed above the head or along the side of the body. The drape must cover from the mid-chest area to the legs (Ch. 25).

pronunciation (pronunciación)   saying words correctly (Ch. 12).

proofread (revisar)   to read a document to verify the accuracy of content and that correct grammar, spelling, punctuation, and capitalization were used (Ch. 15, 16).

proprietary (empresa de propiedad privada)   privately owned and managed facility, a profit-making organization (Ch. 1).

prostaglandin (prostaglandina)   modulator of biochemical activity in tissues (Ch. 26).

prostatitis (prostatitis)   an inflammation of the prostate gland (Ch. 28).

proteinuria (proteinuria)   protein in the urine (Ch. 30).

protime (tiempo de protrombina)   method of monitoring coagulation time (Ch. 41).

protozoa (protozoos)   one-celled animals divided into four groups: amoebae, flagellates, ciliates, and coccidia (Ch. 43).

provider performed microscopy procedure (PPMP) (procedimiento de microscopia realizada por el proveedor [PPM])   a CLIA term for those microscopic examinations that require the expertise of a physician or mid-level provider qualified in microscopic examinations. The PPMP is part of the CLIA's moderately complex category of tests (Ch. 38).

pruritus (prurito)   itchiness (Ch. 35).

psychomotor retardation (retraso psicomotor)   slowing of physical and mental responses; may be seen in depression (Ch. 6).

puerperium (puerperio)   the period from the end of the third stage of labor until involution of uterus is complete, usually three to six weeks (Ch. 26).

pulmonary edema (edema pulmonar)   accumulation of serous fluid in the air vesicles and interstitial tissues of the lungs (Ch. 38).

pulse oximeter (oxímetro de pulso)   a device (similar to a clip) that can be attached to a finger or bridge of the nose. It measures oxygen concentration in the blood (Ch. 24).

purging (purga)   method of maintaining order in the files by separating active from inactive and closed files (Ch. 14).

purified protein derivative (PPD) (derivado proteico purificado [DPP])   filtrate obtained from *Mycobacterium* cultures used for intradermal testing for tuberculosis (Ch. 44).

purulent (purulento)   forming or containing pus (Ch. 22).

pyorrhea (piorrea)   discharge of pus from the gums, around the teeth (Ch. 25).

pyrexia (pirexia)   fever (Ch. 24).

pyridoxine (piridoxina)   vitamin B_6 (Ch. 34).

pyuria (piuria)   pus in the urine (Ch. 30).

qualitative test (prueba cualitativa)   analysis to identify quality or characteristics of components, such as size, shape, and maturity of cells (Ch. 39).

quality assurance (QA) (aseguramiento de calidad [QA])   process to provide accurate, complete, consistent health care documentation in a timely manner while making every reasonable effort to resolve inconsistencies, inaccuracies, risk management issues, and other problems (Ch. 16, 38).

quality control (control de calidad)   measures used to monitor the processing of laboratory specimens. Includes proper use, storage, handling, stability, expiration dates, and indications for measuring precision and accuracy of analytic processes (Ch. 38, 42, 43).

quantitative test (prueba cuantitativa)   analysis that can identify quantity or actual number counts such as counting the number of blood cells (Ch. 39).

radioactive (radioactivo)   emits rays or particles from nucleus (Ch. 32).

radiograph (radiografía)   the film on which an image is produced through exposure to X-rays (Ch. 32).

radiology and imaging reports (informes de radiología y de diagnóstico por imágenes)   medical reports that describe the findings and interpretations of the radiologist (Ch. 16).

radiolucent (radiolúcido)   allowing X-rays to pass through. A dark area appears on the radiograph (Ch. 32).

radionuclides (radionúclidos)   atoms that disintegrate by emitting electromagnetic radiation (Ch. 32).

radiopaque (radiopaco)   impenetrable to X-rays. A light area appears on the radiograph (Ch. 32).

radiopharmaceuticals (sustancias radiofarmacéuticas)   radioactive chemicals used in testing the location, size, outline, or function of tissue, organs, vessels, or body fluids (Ch. 32).

rales (estertores)   abnormal bubbling or crackling sound heard by auscultation during the inspiratory phase of respiration (Ch. 24).

random access memory (RAM) (memoria de acceso aleatorio [RAM])   a type of computer memory that can be written to and read from. The word *random* means that any one location can be read at any time. RAM commonly refers to the internal memory of a computer. RAM is usually a fast, temporary memory area where data and programs reside until saved or until the power is turned off (Ch. 11).

range of motion (ROM) (amplitud de movimiento [ROM])   amount of movement that is present in a joint (Ch. 33).

ratchets (trinquetes)   locking mechanisms on the handles of many surgical instruments (Ch. 31).

rationalization (racionalización)   act of justification, usually illogically, that one uses to keep from facing the truth of the situation (Ch. 5).

read-only memory (ROM) (memoria de sólo lectura [ROM])   permanently stored computer data that cannot be overwritten without special devices. Stores instructions required to start up the computer. Located on the motherboard (Ch. 11).

reagent (reactivo)   chemical substance that detects or synthesizes other substances in a chemical reaction; used in laboratory analyses because it is known to react in a specific way (Ch. 39, 42, 43).

reagent test strip (tira de prueba reactiva)   narrow strip of plastic on which pads containing reagents are attached; used in the urinalysis chemical examination to detect glucose, bilirubin, ketones, specific gravity, blood, pH, urobilinogen, nitrites, and leukocyte esterase (Ch. 42).

recertification (nueva certificación)   documentation admitted to support continued education for maintaining a professional credential (Ch. 47).

redundant array of independent disk (RAID) (matriz redundante de discos independientes [RAID])   a data storage scheme that uses multiple hard drives to share or replicate data among the drives (Ch. 11).

reference laboratories (laboratorios de referencia)   independent, regionally located laboratories used by hospitals for complex, expensive, or specialized tests (Ch. 39).

reference values (valores de referencia)   also referred to as normal value, normal range, or reference range; range of values that includes 95% of test results for a normal healthy population (Ch. 39).

references (referencias)   individuals who have known or worked with a person long enough to make an honest assessment and recommendation regarding the person's background history (Ch. 48).

referral (remisión)   term used by managed care facilities for authorization for someone other than the patient's primary care provider to treat the patient (Ch. 17).

refractometer (refractómetro)   instrument that measures the refractive index of a substance or solution; used in the urinalysis physical examination to measure the urine specimen's specific gravity (Ch. 42).

Registered Medical Assistant (RMA) (Asistente Médico Matriculado [RMA])   credential awarded for successfully passing the AMT examination (Ch. 1, 47).

registered medical transcriptionist (RMT) (transcriptor médico registrado [RMT])   completion of a two-part certification examination administered by the Association for Healthcare Documentation Integrity (AHDI) (Ch. 16).

regression (regresión)   moving back to a former stage to escape conflict or fear (Ch. 5).

regulated waste (residuos regulados) any waste that contains infectious material that would pose a threat due to possible transmission of pathogenic microorganisms (Ch. 22).

rehabilitation medicine (medicina de rehabilitación) field of medical disciplines that seeks to restore an individual or body part to normal or near-normal function after an illness or injury using physical and mechanical agents (Ch. 33).

reimbursement (reembolso) payment (Ch. 38).

remittance advice (aviso de pago) summarizes all of the benefits paid to a provider within a particular period of time; includes all of the patients covered by a specific insurance company for the time period (Ch. 17).

repolarization (repolarización) reestablishment of a polarized state in a muscle after contraction (Ch. 37).

repression (represión) coping with an overwhelming situation by temporarily forgetting it; temporary amnesia (Ch. 5).

requisition (solicitud) request form sent with a specimen specifying tests to be performed on the specimen; most common tests are separated into logical categories with additional space for writing special requests (Ch. 38, 39).

rescue breathing (respiración de rescate) performed on individuals in respiratory arrest, rescue breathing is a mouth-to-mouth (using appropriate protective equipment) or mouth-to-nose procedure that provides oxygen to the patient until emergency personnel arrive (Ch. 9).

residual urine (orina residual) amount of urine remaining in bladder immediately after voiding; seen with hyperplasia of prostate (Ch. 29).

resistance (resistencia) ability of the immune system to resist or withstand an infectious disease (Ch. 22).

resource-based relative value scale (RBRVS) (escala de valores relativos basada en recursos [RBRVS]) basis for the Medicare fee schedule (Ch. 17).

résumé (curriculum vitae) written summary data sheet or brief account of qualifications and progress in your chosen career (Ch. 48).

retention (retención) urine held in the bladder; inability to empty the bladder (Ch. 28).

reticulocyte (reticulocito) an erythrocyte that is released from the bone marrow before it is mature and retains some of its nucleus material (Ch. 41).

retrolental fibroplasia (fibroplasia retrolenticular) disease of blood vessels of retina in newborns (Ch. 36).

review of systems (ROS) (revisión de sistemas [ROS]) inquires about the system directly related to the problems identified in the history of the present illness (Ch. 16).

Rh factor (factor Rh) blood factor indicating the presence or absence of the Rh antigen on the surface of human erythrocytes (Ch. 44).

rhythm strip (tira de ritmo) ECG recording of a single lead, usually lead II, that is used to determine the rhythm of the heart beat. An arrhythmia can more easily be seen in a rhythm strip because it is run longer per provider's request (Ch. 37).

riboflavin (riboflavina) vitamin B_2 (Ch. 34).

rickettsiae (rickettsiae) intracellular parasitic, small nonmotive bacteria (Ch. 22).

risk management (gestión de riesgos) techniques adhered to in the ambulatory care setting that keep the practice, its environment, and its procedures as safe for the patient as possible. Proper risk management also reduces the possibility of negligence that leads to torts and malpractice suits (Ch. 7, 9, 16, 45).

roadblocks (obstáculos) verbal or nonverbal messages that block communication (Ch. 5).

rosacea (rosácea) a chronic skin condition characterized by pustules, papules, erythema, and hyperplasia. Its cause is unknown (Ch. 30).

rotation (rotación) turning a body part around its axis (Ch. 33).

salary review (revisión de salario) informing the employee of his or her revised base pay rate (Ch. 45).

salicylates (salicilatos) aspirin-type drugs that can cause ulcers because of their irritation to the gastrointestinal tract (Ch. 30).

sanitization (higienización) cleaning or scrubbing contaminated instruments or fomites to remove tissue, debris, or other contaminants (Ch. 22).

saturated fat (grasa saturada) fats that are typically solid at room temperature, most commonly found in animal products, such as butter, milk, cream, and eggs as well as coconut and palm oils (Ch. 34).

scabies (sarna) infectious skin disease caused by the itch mite (*Sarcoptes scabiei*), which is transmitted by direct contact with infected persons (Ch. 22).

scleroderma (esclerodermia) slowly progressing disease characterized by deposition of fibrous connective tissue in the skin and in internal organs (Ch. 25).

scoop technique (técnica de una sola mano) a one-handed technique used to "scoop" up and cover a used needle only if a sharp's container is not immediately available, the covering (cap) over the needle is not manipulated in any way; it is then disposed of in the nearest sharps container (Ch. 22).

scope of practice (ámbito de práctica) the range of clinical procedures and activities that are allowed by law for a profession (Ch. 1).

screening (prueba de detección) evaluating patient symptoms to determine emergent needs. Sometimes used to determine the next best course of action when assisting a provider in giving appropriate patient care (Ch. 42).

scrotum (escroto) a soft tissue structure that holds the testes (Ch. 28).

scurvy (escorbuto) a deficiency in vitamin C characterized by the abnormal formation of bones and teeth. Signs of hemorrhage can appear, such as bruising (Ch. 34).

secretion (secreción) substance produced by the cells of glandular organs from materials in the blood (Ch. 22, 38).

sediment (sedimento) insoluble material that settles to the bottom of a liquid; material examined in the urinalysis microscopic examination (Ch. 42).

self-actualization (autorealización) being all that you can be; developing your full potential and experiencing fulfillment (Ch. 4, 45).

self-insurance (autoseguro) insurance carried by large companies, nonprofit organizations, and government to reduce costs and gain more control of their finances. Each plan differs in coverage and claim filing requirements (Ch. 17).

semen (semen) thick, viscid secretion discharged from the urethra of males at orgasm. It is a mixed product containing various fluids and spermatozoa. In postvasectomy males, spermatozoa is absent in semen (Ch. 44).

senile (senil) mental and physical weakness sometimes associated with aging (Ch. 29).

sensitivity (sensibilidad) test in which an organism is placed with antibiotics to determine which antibiotic will effectively kill the organism with the smallest dose (see also culture and sensitivity) (Ch. 43).

sensor (sensor) term used to describe a metallic-coated paper tab that is applied to the patient's body in preparation for an ECG (also known as electrode). Sensors are placed on specific locations on the skin, then attached to the ECG with wires. The sensors conduct electricity from the patient to the ECG machine (Ch. 37).

sensorineural (neurosensorial) permanent hearing loss that results from damage or malformation of the middle ear and auditory nerve (Ch. 27).

septic (sepsis) Overwhelming infection that usually occurs in critically ill patients. Chemicals are released into the blood stream that cause vasodilatation and other organic products that are harmful to the organs and tissues. The vasodilation and decreased ability of the cells and tissues to utilize oxygen is the basis for this type of shock (Ch. 9).

septicemia (septicemia) invasion of pathogenic bacteria into the bloodstream (Ch. 3).

serum (suero) liquid portion of blood obtained after blood has been allowed to clot (Ch. 39, 40).

server (servidor) computer with massive hard drive capacity that is used to link other computers together so that data can be shared by multiple users. A computer system in an ambulatory care facility is likely to be linked or networked with a central server (Ch. 11).

service sockets layer (SSL) (servicio sockets layer [SSL])   A protocol designed to allow secure Web-based transfer of data using encryption (Ch. 11).

severe acute respiratory syndrome (SARS) (síndrome respiratorio agudo y grave [SARS])   a viral outbreak of a respiratory illness first reported in Asia in 2003; spread by close person-to-person contact and characterized by fever and respiratory symptoms (Ch. 22).

shadow (aprendizaje por observación)   follow a supervisor or delegated subordinate to learn facility protocol (Ch. 45).

sharps (objetos filosos)   needles or scalpels or other sharp instruments that are capable of causing a penetrating or puncture wound of the skin (Ch. 22).

shock (shock)   potentially serious condition in which the circulatory system is not providing enough blood to all parts of the body, causing the body's organs to fail to function properly (Ch. 9).

short-range goals (metas a corto plazo)   long-range goals are dissected and reassembled into smaller, more manageable time segments (Ch. 4).

sickle cell anemia (anemia drepanocítica)   an inherited blood disorder that may shorten life span (Ch. 26).

sigmoidoscopy (sigmoidoscopiá)   a diagnostic examination of the interior of the sigmoid colon (Ch. 30).

silver nitrate (nitrato de plata)   caustic astringent antiseptic. As a weak liquid, it is applied to the eyes of newborns to prevent infections at birth. In the medical office, it is most often seen as a solid substance impregnated onto the end of a wooden applicator. Silver nitrate applicator sticks contain hydrochloric acid and other chemicals and are commonly used to cauterize small blood vessels in the nose or other mucous membranes (Ch. 31).

sim's (sims)   in this position, the patient is instructed to lie on the left side; the left arm and shoulder may be drawn back behind the body. The left knee is slightly flexed to support the body, and the right knee is flexed sharply (Ch. 25).

simplified letter (carta simplificada)   major letter style recommended by the Administrative Management Society that omits the salutation and complimentary closure. All lines are keyed flush with the left margin. In medical offices, this style is most often used when sending a form letter (Ch. 15).

sitz bath (baño de asiento)   a warm water bath, in which only the hips and buttocks are immersed (Ch. 31).

slander (calumnia)   false and malicious words about another constituting a defamation of character (Ch. 7).

smartphone (teléfono inteligente)   a device that lets you make telephone calls, but also adds in features that you might find on a personal digital assistant or a small personal computer. Some examples are the ability to take pictures, send and receive e-mail, and edit office documents and a host of other functions frequently called apps (Ch. 12).

Snellen chart (Gráfica de Snellen)   consists of the alphabet letters in various combinations starting at the top with a large E, and letters of descending size by line toward the bottom. Each line is labeled with the visual acuity measurement (Ch. 30).

SOAP (SOAP)   acronym for patient progress notes based on subjective impressions (S), objective clinical evidence (O), assessment or diagnosis (A), and plans for further studies (P) (Ch. 14, 23).

social media (medios sociales)   web-based media for social interaction (Ch. 45).

sodium hydroxide (hidróxido de sodio)   chemical used to chemically burn and destroy tissue; usually in a liquid state when used in minor surgery (Ch. 31).

sodium hypochlorite (hipoclorito de sodio)   household bleach (Ch. 22).

software (software)   equivalent of a computer program or programs (Ch. 11).

solvent (solvente)   producing a solution, dissolving (Ch. 22).

sonographer (ecografista)   professionally trained individual capable of performing the ultrasound examination (Ch. 37).

source-oriented medical record (SOMR) (historia clínica orientada a la fuente [SOMR])   a type of patient chart record keeping that includes separate sections for different sources of patient information, such as laboratory reports, pathology reports, and progress notes (Ch. 14, 23).

species (especie)   second Greek or Latin name given to microorganisms; the species name is not capitalized (Ch. 43).

specific gravity (densidad específica)   ratio of weight of a given volume of a substance to the weight of the same volume of distilled water at the same temperature; test often performed during the urinalysis physical examination (can also appear on the reagent strip) (Ch. 42).

spermatogenesis (espermatogénesis)   the formation of mature sperm (Ch. 28).

spill kit (kit para derrames)   commercially packaged materials containing supplies and equipment needed to clean up a spill of a biohazardous substance (Ch. 22).

spirometry (espirometría)   test to measure the air capacity of the lungs (Ch. 30).

splint (férula)   any device used to immobilize a body part. Often used by EMS personnel (Ch. 9).

spores (esporas)   an inactive state of some bacteria in which they are capsulated in protein. The encapsulation protects them from heat, chemicals, freezing, desiccation, and radiation. Spores can live for tens of thousands of years with no nutrient. When they are placed onto fertile soil (such as human tissue), they can become activated and grow. Tetanus is one type of bacteria that creates spores (Ch. 43).

sprain (esguince)   injury to a joint, often an ankle, knee, or wrist, that involves a tearing of the ligaments. Most sprains are minor and heal quickly; others are more severe, include swelling, and may not heal properly if the patient continues to put stress on the sprained joint (Ch. 9).

sputum (esputo)   substance from the respiratory tract expelled by coughing (Ch. 22).

stab culture (cultivo por punción)   culture where the microorganism is stabbed for deep penetration into tubed solid media (Ch. 43).

standard (patrón)   rules established to measure quality, weight, extent, or value (Ch. 22, 38).

Standard Precautions (Precauciones Estándar)   precautions developed in 1996 by the Centers for Disease Control and Prevention (CDC) that augment universal precautions and body substance isolation practices. They provide a wider range of protection and are used any time there is contact with blood, moist body fluid (except perspiration), mucous membranes, or nonintact skin. They are designed to protect all health care providers, patients, and visitors (Ch. 9, 22).

status asthmaticus (estado asmático)   severe episode of asthma that does not respond to ordinary treatment (Ch. 36).

statute of limitations (ley de prescripción)   statute that defines the period in which legal action can take place (Ch. 20).

statutory law (derecho estatutario)   refers to the body of laws established by states (Ch. 7).

steam sterilization (esterilización por vapor)   the most widely used method of sterilization used in the medical office. An autoclave, basically a pressure cooker, is used to achieve sterilization (Ch. 31).

sterile field (campo estéril)   an area that is considered sterile, usually designated by a sterile drape. The area contains sterile supplies and instruments needed for a particular sterile procedure or surgery (Ch. 31).

stertorous (estertoroso)   snoring sound heard with labored breathing (Ch. 24).

stomatitis (estomatitis)   inflammation of the mouth associated with chemotherapy. Can include swelling, redness, halitosis, ulcerations (Ch. 32).

strabismus (estrabismo)   disorder of the eye in which optic axes cannot be directed to the same object (cross-eye) (Ch. 30).

strain (distensión)   injury to the soft tissue between joints that involves the tearing of muscles or tendons. Strains often occur in the neck, back, or thigh muscles (Ch. 9).

stream scheduling (programación ininterrumpida)   system where patients are seen on a continuous basis throughout the day; for example, at 15-, 30-, or 60-minute intervals, each patient having a distinct appointment time (Ch. 13).

stress (estrés) body's response to change; can be manifested in a variety of ways, including changes in blood pressure, heart rate, and onset of headache (Ch. 4).

stressors (factores estresantes) demands to change that cause stress (Ch. 4).

strictures (estenosis) narrowing of a tubelike structure such as the esophagus or urethra (Ch. 31).

stridor (estridor) crowing sound heard on inspiration, the result of an upper airway obstruction (Ch. 24).

stylus (estilete) heated slender wire of the electrocardiograph that melts the wax off of the ECG paper during the recording (Ch. 37).

subjective (subjetivo) symptom that is felt by the patient but not observable by others (Ch. 23).

sublimation (sublimación) redirecting a socially unacceptable impulse into one that is socially acceptable (Ch. 5).

subordinate (subordinado) in an organization, a person under the direction of (reporting to) a person of greater authority (Ch. 45).

subpoena (citación) written command designating a person to appear in court under penalty for failure to appear (Ch. 7).

supercomputer (supercomputadora) fastest, largest, and most expensive of the four classes of computers currently being manufactured (Ch. 11).

supernatant (sobrenadante) urine that appears above the sediment when centrifuged; poured off before sediment is examined in the urinalysis microscopic examination (Ch. 42).

supination (supinación) moving the arm so the palm is up (Ch. 33).

supine (supina) this position is assumed when lying flat facing up. It is used for examination of the anterior surface of the body from head to toe (Ch. 25).

supine hypotension (hipotensión supina) a condition that may occur when the woman is lying in supine position; the heavy, large uterus presses on the inferior vena cava and aorta, reducing blood flow back to the heart (Ch. 26).

suppressed immune system (sistema inmunitario con inmunosupresión) term used to describe an immune system unable to function normally due to the presence of a disease such as AIDS (Ch. 38).

suppurant (supurante) an agent causing pus formation (Ch. 31).

suppurative (supurativo) producing or associated with the generation of pus (Ch. 27).

surge protection (protección contra sobretensiones) protection of the fragile electronics from spikes in electrical voltage that occur on electric distribution lines (Ch. 11).

surgery cards (tarjetas de cirugía) written reference for surgeries and procedures (Ch. 31).

surgical asepsis (asepsia quirúrgica) procedures that render objects sterile; techniques to maintain sterile conditions during invasive procedures (Ch. 22, 31).

surrogate (sustituto) substitute; someone who substitutes for another (Ch. 8).

suture (sutura) surgical material or thread; may describe the act of sewing with the surgical thread and needle (Ch. 31).

swaged (estampada) a surgical needle attached, during manufacturing, to a length of suture material (Ch. 31).

symmetry (simetría) correspondence in shape, size, and position of body parts on opposite sides of the body (Ch. 25).

sympathetic nervous system (sistema nervioso simpático) large part of the autonomic nervous system that prepares the body for fight-or-flight (Ch. 4).

syncope (síncope) fainting (Ch. 9, 37).

system software (software de sistema) see **operating system** (Ch. 11).

systole (sístole) one component of blood pressure measure-ment representing the highest amount of pressure exerted during the cardiac cycle; the force exerted on the arterial walls during cardiac contraction (Ch. 24, 37).

tachycardia, sinus (taquicardia sinusal) abnormally rapid heartbeat greater than 100 beats/minute. A type of cardiac arrhythmia (Ch. 24, 37).

tachypnea (taquipnea) abnormal increased rate of breathing (Ch. 24).

tape drive (unidad de cinta) data storage device that uses magnetic tape as the storage media (Ch. 11).

targeted résumé (curriculum vitae dirigido al objetivo) résumé format utilized when focusing on a clear, specific job target (Ch. 48).

Task Force for Test Construction (TFTC) (Fuerza de Tareas para la Elaboración de Exámenes [TFTC]) committee of professionals whose responsibility is to update the CMA examination annually to reflect changes in medical assistants' responsibilities and to include new developments in medical knowledge and technology (Ch. 47).

taut (tirante) to pull or draw tight a surface, such as skin (Ch. 36).

taxonomy (taxonomía) classification of organisms into appropriate categories (Ch. 43).

Tay–Sachs (Tay–Sachs) an inherited disease that is usually fatal (Ch. 26).

teamwork (trabajo en equipo) persons synergistically working together (Ch. 45).

test cable (cable de prueba) accessory device that attaches between the Holter monitor and the electrocardiograph to check for correct waveform and lack of artifact (Ch. 37).

testicular torsion (torsión testicular) a twisting of the spermatic cord (Ch. 28).

thalassemia (talasemia) a hereditary anemia that may be fatal (Ch. 26).

thallium scan (gammagrafía con talio) chemical element given intravenously and used in cardiac stress tests. The radioisotope localizes in the myocardium, and a scanning device picks up the distribution of the thallium and can identify blockages in the coronary arteries. An accurate test for coronary artery disease (Ch. 37).

therapeutic communication (comunicación terapéutica) use of specific and well-defined professional communication skills to create a feeling of comfort for patients even when difficult or unpleasant information must be exchanged (Ch. 5).

therapeutic drug monitoring (TDM) (monitoreo de fármacos terapéuticos [TDM]) periodic blood tests to determine the effectiveness of a particular drug. Drugs will have a therapeutic level that must be attained in order for the drug to be therapeutic or effective. If the blood level of the drug is below the range of therapeutic effectiveness, the provider will probably increase the dosage. Likewise, if the drug is above the therapeutic range, the provider will probably lower it (Ch. 39).

thermolabile (termolábil) easily affected by heat (Ch. 31).

thermophile (termófilo) resistant to destruction by heat. Characteristic of some bacteria (Ch. 31).

thermotherapy (termoterapia) use of heat to treat a physical condition (Ch. 33).

thiamin (tiamina) vitamin B_1 (Ch. 34).

thixotropic separator gel (gel separador tixotrópico) gel material capable of forming an interface between the cells and fluid portion of the blood as a result of centrifugation (Ch. 40).

thoracentesis (toracentesis) surgical puncture of the thoracic cavity to aspirate fluid (Ch. 22).

thrombocyte (trombocito) (platelet) cellular fragment of megataryocyte; plays an important role in blood coagulation, hemostasis, and clot formation (Ch. 40, 41).

tickler file (archivo de recordatorios) system to remind of action to be taken on a certain date (Ch. 14).

time focus (enfoque en el tiempo) defines the period of time that is important and to which an individual's actions are directed or oriented (Ch. 5).

tinnitus (tinnitus) ringing or buzzing sound in the ear (Ch. 25).

titer (título) measurement of amount of antibody present against a particular antigen (Ch. 26).

tocopherol (tocoferol) vitamin E (Ch. 34).

tonometer (tonometría) used to measure the intraocular eye pressure of patients older than 35 years (Ch. 25).

tort (agravio)   wrongful act that results in injury to one person by another (Ch. 7).

tort law (derecho de responsabilidad civil)   laws that stem from torts, or wrongful acts that cause harm to one person, by another (Ch. 7).

Total Practice Management System (TPMS) (Sistema de Gestión de Prácticas Total [TPMS])   a category of software that deals with all the day-to-day operations of a medical practice (Ch. 11).

tourniquet (torniquete)   device used to facilitate vein prominence (Ch. 40).

toxicity (toxicidad)   the level at which a drug or chemical becomes poisonous or toxic. Some substances, such as certain metals, are considered toxic at any level of accidental exposure (Ch. 39).

trace mineral (oligomineral)   mineral required by the body in small amounts (Ch. 34).

tracing (trazado)   graphic record usually of an event that changes with time, as with the electrical activity of the heart (Ch. 37).

transcriber (transcriptor)   device that makes it possible to transform voice recordings into a transcript or printed documents (Ch. 16).

transdermal (transdérmico)   system of medication delivery that consists of a small adhesive patch that may be applied to intact skin near the treatment site (Ch. 35).

transducer (transductor)   device that converts one form of energy to another. During an ultrasound procedure, the transducer picks up echoes and converts them to electrical energy. The energy is transformed into digitalized images that can be viewed and printed. Photographs of the image can be taken (Ch. 32, 37).

transferable skills (habilidades transferibles)   skills that would be used in a host of different and unrelated occupations. Keyboarding skill is an example of a transferable skill. It could be used by a secretary, data entry clerk, medical assistant, or clothing manufacturer (Ch. 48).

transient ischemic attack (ataque isquémico transitorio)   temporary interference with blood flow to brain; may last only a few moments or several hours; neurologic symptoms occur (Ch. 29).

transmission (transmisión)   spread of infectious disease by direct contact, indirect contact, inhalation, ingestion, or blood-borne contact (Ch. 22).

Transmission-Based Precautions (Precauciones Basadas en la Transmisión)   second tier of Centers for Disease Control and Prevention (CDC) guidelines that applies to specific categories of patients and that include air, contact, and droplet precautions. Transmission-Based Precautions are always used in addition to Standard Precautions (Ch. 22).

transurethral resection (resección transuretral)   removal of prostate tissue using a device inserted through the urethra (Ch. 28).

traveler's check (cheque de viajero)   often used in place of cash when traveling; available in denominations of $20 to $100; requires a signature at place of purchase as well as signature at the time the check is used (Ch. 19).

trephination (trepanación)   cutting out a circular section (Ch. 3).

triage (triage)   screening to determine which patient is treated first when two or more patients present with emergencies simultaneously (Ch. 9).

trial balance (saldo de comprobación)   created by totaling debit balances and credit balances to confirm that total debits equal total credits (Ch. 21).

TRICARE (TRICARE)   formerly the Civilian Health and Medical Program for Uniformed Services (CHAMPUS). TRICARE offers HMO, PPO, and fee-for-service medical insurance for dependents of active duty and retired military personnel and dependents of personnel who died while on active duty (Ch. 17).

trichomoniasis (tricomoniasis)   infestation with a *Trichomonas* parasite, which may be transmitted through sexual intercourse (Ch. 22, 26).

triglycerides (triglicéridos)   form of fat in the bloodstream that functions to store energy (Ch. 44).

trimester (trimestre)   three months; one third of the gestational period of pregnancy (Ch. 26).

triple option plan (plan de opción triple)   a managed care model allowing enrollees the option of traditional, HMO, or PPO health plans (Ch. 17).

trough (valle)   the opposite of "peak," this is the point at which the drug is at its lowest level in the body. Usually this occurs just before the next dose is administered. In lab tests, the trough will tell the physician the weakest influence the drug would have on the body at that particular dose (Ch. 39).

Truth-in-Lending Act (Ley de Veracidad en los Préstamos)   also known as the Consumer Credit Protection Act of 1968; an act requiring providers of installment credit to state the charges in writing and to express the interest as an annual rate (Ch. 20).

tuberculosis (TB) (tuberculosis [TB])   infectious disease caused by the bacterium *Mycobacterium tuberculosis* (Ch. 44).

turbid (turbio)   opaque, not clear. Used to describe urine that is cloudy (Ch. 42).

turnaround time (plazo de entrega)   specific time limits established for completion of medical reports (Ch. 16).

tympanostomy (timpanostomía)   placement of a tube through the tympanic membrane to allow ventilation of the middle ear; part of the treatment for otitis media (Ch. 27, 30).

typhus (typhoid) (tifus [tifoide])   acute infectious disease that causes severe headache, rash, high fever, and progressive neurologic involvement. Prevalent where conditions are unsanitary and congested (Ch. 3).

ultrasonic cleaner (limpiador ultrasónico)   machine that uses the energy of high-frequency sound waves that agitate to sanitize instruments before sterilization (Ch. 22).

ultrasonography (ecografía)   process of placing a handheld transducer against a body area to be tested. The transducer sends sound waves through the skin and the various internal organs. When echoes are formed and sent back the transducer converts them into electrical energy. This energy is transformed into a picture on a monitor or printed on paper. Photographs of the images can be taken and become part of the patient's permanent record (Ch. 26, 37).

ultrasound (ultrasonido)   use of high-frequency sound waves for therapeutic reasons to generate heat in deep tissue (Ch. 33).

unbundling codes (códigos de desagregación)   refers to separating the components of a procedure and reporting them as billable codes with charges to increase reimbursement rates (Ch. 18).

undifferentiated (no diferenciada)   a change in the character of a cell(s) toward a malignant state (Ch. 22).

undoing (reparación)   actions designed to make amends to cancel out inappropriate behavior (Ch. 5).

Uniform Bill 04 (UB04) (Factura Uniforme 04 [UB04])   unique billing form used extensively by acute care facilities for processing inpatient and outpatient claims (Ch. 18).

uniform resource locater (URL) (localizador uniforme de recursos [URL])   the address that defines the route to a file on the Web or any other Internet facility (Ch. 12).

unipolar (unipolar)   having or pertaining to one pole process (Ch. 37).

unit (unidad)   each part of a name (business or person), words, or numbers that will be indexed and coded for filing (Ch. 14).

unit dose (dosis unitaria)   premeasured amount of medication, individually packaged on a per-dose basis (Ch. 36).

universal emergency medical identification symbol (símbolo universal de identificación médica para emergencias)   identification sometimes carried by individuals to identify health problems they may have (Ch. 9).

Universal Precautions (Precauciones Universales)   guidelines established by the Centers for Disease Control and Prevention (CDC) for the protection of health care workers from infectious diseases (Ch. 22).

universal serial bus (USB) port (puerto de bus universal en serie [USB])   a type of data entry portal or bus for computer data (Ch. 11).

unsterile field (campo no estéril)   area that is adjacent to the sterile field where items needed can be accessed, opened, and supplied by an individual who does not wear sterile garb (Ch. 31).

up-coding (sobrecodificación) also known as code creep, overcoding, and overbilling. Up-coding occurs when the insurance carrier deliberately bills a higher rate service than what was performed to obtain greater reimbursements (Ch. 18).

urea (urea) principal end product of protein metabolism (Ch. 42).

urgency (urgencia) the need to urinate immediately (Ch. 30).

urinalysis (análisis de orina) examination of the physical, chemical, and microscopic properties of urine (Ch. 39, 42).

urinary tract infection (UTI) (infección del tracto urinario [ITU]) also referred to as a bladder infection (Ch. 42).

urobilinogen (urobilinógeno) colorless compound produced in the intestine after the breakdown by bacteria of bilirubin (Ch. 42).

urticaria (urticaria) hives (Ch. 30, 35).

usual, customary, and reasonable (UCR) (usual, acostumbrado y razonable [UCR]) fee schedule often used by Medicare and some insurance carriers. *Usual* refers to the fee typically charged by a provider for certain procedures; *customary* is based on the average charge for a specific procedure by all provider practicing the same specialty in a defined geographic region; and *reasonable* refers to the midrange of fees charged for this procedure (Ch. 17).

utilization review (UR) (revisión de utilización [RU]) review of medical services before they can be performed (Ch. 21).

V codes (códigos V) ICD-9-CM codes representing either factors that influence a person's health status or legitimate reasons for contacting the health facility when the patient has no definitive diagnosis or active symptom of any disorder (Ch. 17, 18).

vaccine (vacuna) pharmacologic agent capable of producing artificial active immunity (Ch. 22).

variable cost (costo variable) cost that varies in direct proportion to volume (Ch. 21).

vas deferens (conducto deferente) a muscular tube that connects the testes with the urethra (Ch. 28).

vasoconstriction (vasoconstricción) narrowing or constricting of blood vessels (Ch. 33).

vasovagal syncope (síncope vasovagal) sudden faint due to hypotension induced by response of the autonomic nervous system to abrupt emotional stress, pain, or trauma (Ch. 9).

vector (vector) a carrier of disease, usually an insect, that is the causative organism of disease from infected to noninfected individuals (Ch. 22).

venipuncture (venopunción) puncturing into a vein with a needle to obtain a blood sample (Ch. 40).

vertigo (vértigo) the sensation of moving around in space; dizziness, lightheadedness (Ch. 25).

vesicular (vesicular) characterized by the presence of vesicles. Vesicles are blisters or other elevations on the skin (Ch. 22, 26).

viable (viable) able to live, grow, and develop after birth; usually 24 weeks or greater than 1 pound (Ch. 26).

virology (virología) study of viruses (Ch. 39, 43).

virtual local area network (VLAN) (red de área local virtual [VLAN]) A VLAN is a subset of a network that connects only authorized computers together excluding all others. By separating sensitive data from the rest of the network it decreases the chance that unauthorized persons can access the data (Ch. 11).

virulence (virulencia) an organism's relative power and degree of pathogenicity (Ch. 22).

viscosity (viscosidad) degree of thickness of a liquid (Ch. 40).

vitiligo (vitíligo) skin disorder characterized by smooth white spots on various areas of the body (Ch. 25).

voice over Internet protocol (VoIP) (protocolo de voz por Internet [VoIP]) the real-time transmission of voice signals over the Internet or Internet Protocol (IP) network (Ch. 12).

voice recognition software (VRS) (software de reconocimiento de voz) software that translates voice commands and is used in place of a mouse and keyboard (Ch. 16).

volatile (volátil) easily evaporated (Ch. 31).

voucher check (cheque con comprobante) check with detachable form used to detail reason check is drawn; commonly used in payroll checks (Ch. 19).

waived (prueba de baja complejidad) used to describe a category of clinical laboratory tests that are simple, unvarying, and require a minimum of judgment and interpretation (Ch. 38).

watermark (sello de agua) design incorporated in paper during the papermaking process that is visible when the paper is held up to the light (Ch. 15).

water-soluble (soluble en agua) pertaining to substances that are hydrophilic and therefore dissolve better in water (Ch. 34).

wave scheduling (planificación en olas) system where patients are scheduled for the first half hour of every hour and then are seen throughout the hour (Ch. 13).

wet mount (preparación en fresco) a method of adding liquid, usually saline or potassium hydrochloride, to a specimen on a slide for examination and preservation. The specimen is placed on a slide and one drop of saline (for diagnosis of trichomonas vaginalis) or potassium hydroxide (for diagnosis of vaginal yeast infections) is applied and mixes with the specimen. It is then covered with a coverslip and examined microscopically (Ch. 26, 43).

wheal (roncha) slight elevation of skin that can be produced as a result of an intradermal injection such as the Mantoux/PPD test for TB (Ch. 44).

wheezes (sibilancia) high-pitched musical sound heard on expiration, often the result of an obstruction or narrowing of respiratory passages (Ch. 24).

wide area network (WAN) (red de área amplia [WAN]) connecting together of computers on a large area for the purpose of sharing data (Ch. 11).

WiFi connection (conexión WiFi) connection via a universal wireless network standard that uses radio waves (Ch. 11).

WiMAX (WiMAX) Telecommunications technology that uses radio spectrum to transmit between digital devices. Sometimes referred to as WiFi on steroids; WiMAX has the ability to transmit over far greater distances and to handle much more data at higher transmission rates. Third generation (3G) and fourth generation (4G) systems are in use (Ch. 11).

wireless local area network (WLAN) (red de área local inalámbrica [WLAN]) a type of local area network that uses high-frequency radio waves rather than wires to communicate between nodes (Ch. 11).

Wood's lamp (lámpara de Wood) special lights used to detect organisms that fluoresce such as certain fungi, bacteria, and parasites. Scabies and ringworm are two examples. Scratches in the eye may be detected using a Woods lamp after the eye has been stained with a fluorescent dye. Also used in determining margin dissection of melanoma (Ch. 43).

work practice controls (controles de prácticas laborales) measures used in the workplace that consist of physical equipment and mechanical devices to control employee exposure to bloodborne pathogens and other potentially infectious materials. Examples are sharps disposal containers, handwashing facilities, personal protective equipment, and eyewash stations (Ch. 22).

work statement (declaración de trabajo) concise description of the work you plan to accomplish (Ch. 45).

Workers' Compensation insurance (seguro de indemnización por accidentes de trabajo) medical and paycheck insurance for workers who sustain injuries associated with their employment (Ch. 17).

wound (herida) a break in the continuity of soft parts of body structures caused by violence or trauma to tissues. In an open wound, skin is broken as in a laceration, abrasion, avulsion, or incision. In a closed wound, skin is not broken as in contusion, ecchymosis, or hematoma (Ch. 9).

xerophthalmia (xeroftalmía) dry, lusterless mucous membranes of the eyes (Ch. 34).

yellow fever (fiebre amarilla) acute infectious disease where a person develops jaundice, vomits, hemorrhages, and has a fever; caused mostly by mosquitoes (Ch. 3).

ZIP+4 (ZIP+4) standard zip code including four additional digits that identify a postal delivery area. Mail will be processed more efficiently and effectively with the use of the ZIP+4 code in the address (Ch. 15).

Glosario de términos

abducción (abduction) movimiento que consiste en alejarse de la línea media del cuerpo (Ch. 33).

aborto (abortion) expulsión de los productos de la concepción antes de llegar a la viabilidad (Ch. 26).

abrasión (abrasion) raspado superficial de la epidermis (Ch. 9).

absorción (absorption) proceso mediante el cual el fármaco pasa a los fluidos y tejidos del organismo (Ch. 35).

abuso (abuse) mal uso, uso excesivo o inadecuado, especialmente de fármacos narcóticos o psicofármacos (Ch. 17, 35).

accidente cerebrovascular (ACV) (cerebral vascular accident [CVA]) pérdida de suministro de sangre al cerebro (anoxia); también denominado apoplejía (Ch. 30).

ácido ascórbico (ascorbic acid) vitamina C (Ch. 34).

ácido fólico (folic acid) una de las vitaminas del complejo B (Ch. 34).

acreditación (accreditation) proceso por el cual se otorga reconocimiento a un programa educativo por cumplir las normas que califican a sus graduados para el ejercicio de la profesión; proporcionar credenciales (Ch. 1).

acreditado (credentialed) pruebas que demuestran que una persona tiene derecho a un crédito o a ejercer su facultad oficial (Ch. 1).

actas (minutes) registro escrito de los temas tratados y las medidas adoptadas durante las sesiones de reuniones (Ch. 15, 45).

actividades de la vida diaria (AVD) (activities of daily living [ADL]) actividades que generalmente se realizan durante un día típico que incluyen el cuidado propio, por ejemplo, comer y cepillarse los dientes (Ch. 33).

activos (assets) bienes de valor que posee una entidad comercial (Ch. 21).

acuerdo de confidencialidad (confidentiality agreement) cuando se firma este acuerdo, significa que el transcriptor médico se compromete a mantener la confidencialidad de toda la información de los pacientes (Ch. 16).

acupuntura (acupuncture) tratamiento para aliviar el dolor y las enfermedades mediante la inserción en la piel de agujas finas en puntos específicos (Ch. 2).

aditivo (additive) cualquier material que se coloca en un tubo que mantiene o facilita la integridad y la función de la muestra para análisis (Ch. 40).

administrar (administer) dar un medicamento (Ch. 7, 35, 36).

ADN (DNA) ácido desoxirribonucleico; material nuclear importante que contiene códigos genéticos (Ch. 39, 43).

aducción (adduction) movimiento que consiste en acercarse a la línea media del cuerpo (Ch. 33).

aerobio (aerobic) organismo que requiere oxígeno para crecer (Ch. 43).

aerosoles (aerosols) partículas de materiales potencialmente infecciosos que puedan liberarse a la atmósfera (Ch. 22, 43).

aerosolizado (aerosolized) aplicado por medio de un atomizador (Ch. 27).

afasia (aphasia) la incapacidad de hablar (Ch. 30).

afebril (afebrile) sin fiebre (Ch. 24).

agar (agar) sustancia gelatinosa extraída de algas rojas que contiene nutrientes y humedad para el crecimiento de bacterias (Ch. 43).

agente (agent) persona que representa a otra (Ch. 7).

agente de acoplamiento (coupling agent) agente usado en una ecografía que mejora la penetración de ondas sonoras a través de los tejidos (Ch. 26).

agente infeccioso (infectious agent) patógeno responsable de una enfermedad infecciosa específica (Ch. 22).

agotamiento profesional (burnout) estado de cansancio o frustración ocasionado por la dedicación a una causa, forma de vida o a una relación que no produjo el resultado esperado (Ch. 5).

agravio (tort) acto ilegítimo en el que una persona provoca una lesión a otra persona (Ch. 7).

agrupación (clustering) unión de mensajes no verbales para formar oraciones o conclusiones. También se puede usar para describir un sistema de programación en el cual los pacientes con quejas o afecciones similares se programan consecutivamente (por ejemplo, la programación de todas las infecciones alérgicas entre las 3:00 p. m. y las 4:00 p. m. todos los martes y los jueves) (Ch. 4).

aislamiento (isolation) separar a un paciente con ciertas infecciones o enfermedades transmisibles de otras personas (Ch. 22).

ajustes (adjustments) aumento o disminución en las cuentas de pacientes que no se deben a los cargos incurridos o a los pagos recibidos (Ch. 17, 19).

alambre guía (lead wire) conductor conectado a un electrocardiógrafo. Tiene derivaciones para las extremidades y para el tórax (Ch. 37).

alcohol isopropílico (isopropyl alcohol) comúnmente llamado alcohol de botiquín; solución de alcohol al 70% que se usa comúnmente como limpiador (Ch. 31).

alérgeno (allergen) cualquier sustancia que produce signos de alergia, por ejemplo, inhalantes como polvo y polen, alimentos como trigo y fresas, fármacos, penicilina, sustancias químicas, calor, bacterias (Ch. 30).

alergia (allergy) hipersensibilidad adquirida a una sustancia (alérgeno) que normalmente no causa una reacción (Ch. 23, 31).

alícuota (aliquot) parte de la muestra completa que se ha retirado para usarla o almacenarla (Ch. 40).

alimentos procesados (processed food) alimentos que ya no están en su estado íntegro y natural; cocinados o envasados sin algunas partes o con ingredientes agregados (Ch. 34).

alopático (allopathic) método para tratar enfermedades con remedios que producen efectos diferentes a los provocados por la propia enfermedad. La mayoría de los profesionales de la salud tradicionales hoy son considerados profesionales alopáticos (Ch. 3).

ámbito de práctica (scope of practice) campo de aplicación de los procedimientos y las actividades clínicas que se permiten por ley para una profesión (Ch. 1).

ambulación (ambulation) capacidad para caminar (Ch. 33).

aminoácido (amino acid) unidad estructural básica de la proteína (Ch. 34).

amniocentesis (amniocentesis) punción quirúrgica del saco amniótico para extraer líquido para análisis de laboratorio (Ch. 22, 26).

amniotomía (amniotomy) ruptura artificial del saco amniótico (Ch. 26).

amorfo (amorphous) sin forma; que no posee forma definida (Ch. 42).

amplificado (amplified) agrandado o aumentado. El amplificador del electrocardiógrafo agranda la actividad del impulso cardíaco, por lo que el registro se puede leer más fácilmente (Ch. 37).

amplitud (amplitude) cantidad, extensión, tamaño, abundancia o plenitud (Ch. 37).

amplitud de movimiento (ROM) (range of motion [ROM]) grado de movimiento presente en una articulación (Ch. 33).

anaerobio (anaerobic) organismo que requiere poco oxígeno o que no necesita oxígeno para crecer (Ch. 43).

anafilaxia (anaphylaxis) hipersensibilidad del cuerpo ante una proteína o fármaco extraño (Ch. 9, 35).

análisis de costos (cost analysis) procedimiento que determina los costos de cada servicio (Ch. 21).

análisis de orina (urinalysis) examen de las propiedades físicas, químicas y microscópicas de la orina (Ch. 39, 42).

andropausia (andropause) cambios que se producen en hombres de mediana edad (Ch. 29).

anemia drepanocítica (sickle cell anemia) trastorno sanguíneo congénito que puede acortar la vida (Ch. 26).

anemia perniciosa (pernicious anemia) anemia crónica causada por la falta de ácido clorhídrico en el estómago; puede provocar debilidad, cansancio, hormigueo en las extremidades y hasta insuficiencia cardíaca; las inyecciones con vitamina B₁₂ son el tratamiento usado para esta enfermedad (Ch. 29).

angiograma (angiogram) serie radiográfica de un vaso sanguíneo después de la inyección de una sustancia radiopaca (Ch. 37).

angioplastía transluminal coronaria percutánea (PTCA) (percutaneous transluminal coronary angioplasty [PTCA]) procedimiento que ensancha una arteria coronada estrecha o bloqueada (Ch. 37).

anisocitosis (anisocytosis) variación marcada del tamaño de las células (Ch. 41).

anomalías congénitas (congenital anomalies) anomalías de nacimiento, que existen en el momento del nacimiento (Ch. 26).

anorexia (anorexia) pérdida del apetito (Ch. 22).

antecedentes de enfermedad actual (AEA) (history of present illness [HPI]) descripción cronológica del desarrollo de la enfermedad del paciente (Ch. 16).

antibacteriano (antibacterial) que puede destruir bacterias; a menudo se aplica en una herida en forma de ungüento o crema (Ch. 31).

anticoagulante (anticoagulant) sustancia química en tubos de sangre que impide la coagulación de la sangre al quitar el calcio de la sangre o al detener la formación de trombina (Ch. 40).

anticoncepción (contraception) prevención voluntaria del embarazo (Ch. 26).

anticuerpo (antibody) sustancia química específica producida por las células B del sistema inmunitario como respuesta a un antígeno (Ch. 22, 44).

anticuerpo heterófilo (heterophile antibody) anticuerpo que reacciona con otros que no son los antígenos específicos, como se observa en la mononucleosis infecciosa (Ch. 44).

antígeno (antigen) sustancias, tales como bacterias u otro agentes, que el cuerpo reconoce como extrañas; estímulo para la producción de anticuerpos (Ch. 22, 44).

antioxidante (antioxidant) algo que impide la oxidación (Ch. 34).

ántrax (carbuncle) infección necrosante de la piel y del tejido formada por un agrupamiento de forúnculos (Ch. 30).

apical (apical) perteneciente al vértice o punta del corazón. Lugar para medir la frecuencia cardíaca con un estetoscopio (Ch. 24).

aplicaciones (apps) término genérico para cualquier software independiente. Programas informáticos diseñados especialmente para una función específica. Los paquetes de software para oficina están dando paso a una nueva era de programas de funciones individuales generalmente descargados de Internet (Ch. 11).

apnea (apnea) cese o ausencia de respiración espontánea normal (Ch. 24, 36).

apósito (dressing) gasa estéril u otro material que se aplica directamente en una herida para absorber secreciones y como protección (Ch. 9, 31).

aprendizaje por observación (shadow) seguir de cerca a un supervisor o a un subordinado delegado para aprender el protocolo del establecimiento (Ch. 45).

aproximar (approximate) juntar los bordes de una herida (Ch. 31).

arbitraje (arbitration) forma de resolución de conflictos que permite a una parte neutral resolver una disputa (Ch. 7).

archivado no consecutivo (nonconsecutive filing) método de archivado numérico en el cual los números se consideran en orden ascendente usando subconjuntos de cifras dentro de un número; por ejemplo, en el número 574 19 2863: 2863 es la unidad 1, 19 es la unidad 2, 574 es la unidad 3 (Ch. 14).

archivo de recordatorios (tickler file) sistema para recordar que se debe ejecutar una acción en una fecha determinada (Ch. 14).

área de superficie corporal (ASC) (body surface area [BSA]) método sumamente exacto para calcular las dosis de medicamentos para bebés y niños de hasta 12 años (Ch. 36).

arritmia (arrhythmia) desviación del patrón o ritmo normal del latido cardíaco (Ch. 24, 37).

artefacto (artifact) cualquier cosa que se produce artificialmente (Ch. 37).

arteriosclerosis (arteriosclerosis) endurecimiento de las arterias causado por la acumulación de placa, un depósito de sustancias grasas en las paredes de las arterias (Ch. 29).

aseguramiento de calidad (QA) (quality assurance [QA]) proceso para proporcionar documentación de atención médica exacta, completa y uniforme en forma oportuna a la vez que se toman todas las medidas razonables para resolver incoherencias, imprecisiones, cuestiones de gestión de riesgos y otros problemas (Ch. 16, 38).

asepsia (asepsis) protección contra las infecciones causadas por microorganismos patógenos (Ch. 3).

asepsia médica (medical asepsis) limpio y libre de infecciones (Ch. 22, 38).

asepsia quirúrgica (surgical asepsis) procedimientos para esterilizar los objetos; técnicas para mantener las condiciones estériles durante los procedimientos invasivos (Ch. 22, 31).

aséptico (aseptic) libre de cualquier material infeccioso; ausencia de microorganismos (Ch. 22, 30).

asiento (posting) registro de transacciones financieras en un sistema contable o de teneduría de libros (Ch. 19).

asignación de beneficios (assignment of benefits) cesión de beneficios por parte del beneficiario a un tercero (Ch. 17).

Asistente Administrativo Médico Certificado (CMAA) (Certified Medical Administrative Assistant [CMAA]) certificación de la NHA para asistente administrativo médico (Ch. 47).

Asistente Clínico Médico Certificado (CCMA) (Certified Clinical Medical Assistant [CCMA]) certificación de la NHA para asistente clínico médico (Ch. 47).

Asistente Médico Certificado (CMA [AAMA]) (Certified Medical Assistant [CMA (AAMA)]) asistente médico certificado que ha completado con éxito el examen de certificación nacional de la Asociación Estadounidense de Asistentes Médicos (AAMA, por sus siglas en inglés) (Ch. 1, 47).

Asistente Médico Matriculado (RMA) (Registered Medical Assistant [RMA]) credencial otorgada por aprobar con éxito el examen de los Tecnólogos Médicos Estadounidenses (AMT, por sus siglas en inglés) (Ch. 1, 47).

Asociación Estadounidense de Asistentes Médicos (AAMA) (American Association of Medical Assistants [AAMA]) organización profesional dedicada a atender los intereses de los Asistentes Médicos Certificados (Ch. 47).

Asociación Independiente de Médicos (IPA) (independent provider association [IPA]) red independiente de médicos en la práctica privada que tienen contrato con la asociación para tratar pacientes a cambio de una tarifa convenida (Ch. 2).

Asociación Nacional de Profesiones de Salud (NHA) (National Healthcareer Association [NHA]) asociación que ofrece exámenes de certificación nacional para profesionales de la atención médica. La NHA trabaja con instituciones educativas en el desarrollo de planes de estudio, pruebas de competencias y preparación y administración de su examen de certificación (Ch. 47).

Asociación para la Integridad de la Documentación del Cuidado de la Salud (AHDI) (Association for Healthcare Documentation Integrity [AHDI]) organización sin fines de lucro fundada por los transcriptores médicos para promover la profesión (Ch. 16).

aspirar (aspirate) eliminar mediante succión (Ch. 22).

ataque de intermediario (man-in-the-middle) (man-in-the-middle attack) una forma de ataque en la que el pirata informático se conecta de manera independiente y transparente con dos partes de modo que cada una de ellas piensa que se está comunicando directamente con la otra. El pirata informático puede interceptar toda la información transmitida (Ch. 11).

ataque isquémico transitorio (transient ischemic attack) interferencia temporal en el flujo sanguíneo que va al cerebro; puede durar sólo unos momentos o varias horas; puede haber síntomas neurológicos (Ch. 29).

ataxia (ataxia) trastorno caracterizado por la alteración de la coordinación muscular que se observa principalmente cuando se intenta hacer movimientos musculares voluntarios (Ch. 25).

aterosclerosis (atherosclerosis) forma de arteriosclerosis marcada por depósitos de calcio en las paredes arteriales (Ch. 24).

atributo (attribute) característica inherente (Ch. 1).

auditor (auditor) persona responsable de determinar el contenido final de un documento y la exactitud en cada aspecto informado (Ch. 16).

aumentar (augment) agregar o incrementar (Ch. 37).

aurícula (auricle) el oído externo, también llamado pabellón auricular (Ch. 30).

auscultación (ascultation) mediante el uso de un estetoscopio, determina la lectura de la presión sanguínea que se documenta en el expediente del paciente (Ch. 25).

auspicio (aegis) patrocinio o protección (Ch. 38).

autenticación (authentication) la persona que dicta la información firma o autentica el documento para indicar que la información era exacta y completa en el momento de firmar (Ch. 16).

autoclave (autoclave) se utiliza para realizar la esterilización. La autoclave utiliza vapor bajo presión para obtener temperaturas más altas que las alcanzadas con ebullición (Ch. 31).

autorealización (self-actualization) ser todo lo que se puede ser; desarrollar todo el potencial y experimentar la sensación de logro (Ch. 5, 45).

autorización previa (preauthorization) proceso por el cual se obtiene el consentimiento de la compañía de seguros antes de proceder con la atención y el tratamiento de un paciente. Si no se obtiene la autorización, quizás las compañías de seguros no paguen los beneficios para problemas específicos (Ch. 17).

autoseguro (self-insurance) seguro contratado por las grandes empresas, organizaciones sin fines de lucro y por los gobiernos para reducir los costos y obtener más control de sus finanzas. Cada plan difiere en cuanto a su cobertura y a los requisitos para presentar reclamaciones (Ch. 17).

aviso de pago (remittance advice) resume todos los beneficios pagados a un proveedor dentro de un periodo de tiempo particular; incluye a todos los pacientes cubiertos por una compañía aseguradora específica para el período de tiempo (Ch. 17).

avulsión (avulsion) herida abierta en la que la piel se desgarra y el sangrado es profuso (Ch. 9).

bacilo (bacilli) una de las tres clasificaciones de la bacteria; tiene forma de bastoncillo (Ch. 22).

baja de codificación (down-coding) las compañías de seguros bajan de codificación si la documentación o los códigos son ambiguos y reembolsan la tarifa más baja posible (Ch. 18).

balance general (balance sheet) estado detallado de los activos, los pasivos y el patrimonio; estado de situación patrimonial (Ch. 21).

balancear (balance) verificar la exactitud de un asiento; registra la diferencia entre las columnas del debe y el haber (Ch. 19).

balanitis (balanitis) la hinchazón y/o la inflamación del glande peniano (Ch. 28).

banda de constricción (constriction band) término usado para reemplazar a torniquete (que ya no se usa) en emergencias. Se usa una banda de material para controlar una hemorragia importante de una extremidad que ha sufrido una lesión por un traumatismo. La banda se aplica por encima del origen de la hemorragia pero no tan ajustada de modo que no restrinja el flujo de sangre completamente. Habrá un ligero goteo de sangre. Esta acción evita la pérdida de una extremidad debido a la restricción completa del flujo sanguíneo. Si esto sucede, no hay flujo sanguíneo hacia las células y los tejidos de la extremidad, por lo que las células, los tejidos y esa parte del cuerpo no reciben oxígeno y se mueren (Ch. 9).

bandeja de instrumentos (instrument tray) ver mesa de Mayo (Ch. 31).

bandeja o carro de parada (crash tray or cart) bandeja o carro portátil que contiene medicamentos y suministros necesarios para urgencias y procedimientos de primeros auxilios (Ch. 9).

baño de asiento (sitz bath) baño con agua tibia, en el que sólo se sumergen las caderas y las nalgas (Ch. 31).

bariátrica (bariatrics) rama de la medicina que se ocupa de la prevención, el control y el tratamiento de la obesidad (Ch. 30).

barrera (barrier) obstáculo que existe para proteger a una persona del contacto con la sangre o con otros materiales posiblemente infectados. Llamado equipo de protección personal (EPP), las barreras incluyen guantes, máscaras, protectores faciales, guardapolvos de laboratorio, gafas de protección y batas (Ch. 22).

basófilo (basophil) glóbulo blanco granulocítico con gránulos citoplásmicos de color púrpura oscuro. Es el menos común de los glóbulos blancos (Ch. 41).

beneficiario (beneficiary) persona que reúne los requisitos para recibir beneficios en virtud de una póliza (Ch. 17).

beneficiario (payee) persona nombrada en el cheque y que recibirá el importe indicado (Ch. 19).

beneficio (benefit) remuneración que se agrega al sueldo (Ch. 45, 48).

beneficio complementario (fringe benefit) beneficio que supera el sueldo que tiene derecho a cobrar un empleado. Los ejemplos incluyen seguro de salud y de vida, vacaciones pagas, licencia por enfermedad, días de licencia por razones particulares y reembolso de matrícula para cursos relacionados con el trabajo (Ch. 2, 45).

beriberi (beriberi) enfermedad causada por una deficiencia de vitamina B (tiamina) y caracterizada por dolor de cabeza, depresión, anorexia, estreñimiento, taquicardia, edema e insuficiencia cardíaca (Ch. 34).

Betadine® (Betadine®) marca de una solución de povidona yodada usada como antiséptico para la piel. Betadine® también está disponible como solución jabonosa (en forma de jabón) (Ch. 31).

bilirrubina (bilirubin) pigmento de color entre amarillento y anaranjado que se forma a partir de la descomposición de la hemoglobina en glóbulos rojos dañados. La bilirrubina generalmente se transporta en el torrente sanguíneo hacia el hígado, donde se convierte en una forma soluble al agua y se excreta en la bilis (Ch. 42, 44).

bilirrubinuria (bilirubinuria) presencia de bilirrubina en la orina (Ch. 42).

bioética (bioethics) rama de la ética médica que se ocupa de las cuestiones morales que surgen de la investigación médica sofisticada y del uso de tecnología avanzada. Las cuestiones sociales como ingeniería genética, aborto e investigación en tejido fetal plantean importantes preguntas bioéticas (Ch. 8).

biopsia (biopsy) extracción de una pequeña parte de tejido vivo de un órgano o de otra parte del cuerpo para examinarla microscópicamente y confirmar o establecer un diagnóstico (Ch. 30, 39).

biopsia cervical en sacabocados (cervical punch biopsy) biopsia del cuello uterino usando un instrumento cuyo extremo es un sacabocados (Ch. 26).

biotransformación (biotransformation) la alteración química que experimenta un fármaco en el organismo, usualmente en el hígado (Ch. 35).

bipolar (bipolar) que tiene dos polos o procesos (Ch. 37).

blogs de Internet (internet blogs) sitio web que publica comentarios, descripción de eventos u otro material periódicamente. El blog habitualmente es interactivo y permite que los visitantes dejen comentarios (Ch. 48).

borramiento (effacement) adelgazamiento y acortamiento del conducto cervical durante el parto para permitir el paso de feto (Ch. 26).

bradicardia sinusal (bradycardia [sinus]) frecuencia cardíaca lenta (menos de 60 latidos por minuto) pero regular (Ch. 24, 37).

bradipnea (bradypnea) frecuencia respiratoria anormalmente baja (Ch. 24).

Braxton–Hicks (Braxton–Hicks) contracciones irregulares, intermitentes e indoloras delútero; también conocidas como contracciones falsas (Ch. 26).

brecha auscultatoria (ausculatatory gap) mientras se mide la presión arterial, los sonidos de golpeteo que se oyen pueden desaparecer entre las fases de los ruidos de Korotkoff (Ch. 24).

broncodilatador (bronchodilator) fármaco que expande los tubos bronquiales (Ch. 30).

bronquios (bronchi) bifurcaciones de la tráquea que se ramifican hacia cada pulmón y terminan en los tubos bronquiales (Ch. 30).

bulimia (bulimia) es un síndrome durante el cual la persona come en exceso y luego se purga induciendo el vómito (Ch. 30, 34).

cable de prueba (test cable) dispositivo accesorio que se conecta entre el monitor Holter y el electrocardiógrafo para verificar que la forma de onda sea correcta y que no haya artefactos (Ch. 37).

caja chica (petty cash) pequeña suma que se tiene a mano para gastos menores o imprevistos (Ch. 19).

calibración (calibration) determinación de la exactitud de un instrumento comparando la información suministrada con un patrón aceptado del cual se conoce su exactitud (Ch. 37, 38).

caloría (calorie) unidad de calor. La Caloría grande (que a menudo se escribe con mayúscula) se usa para hablar de la alimentación en seres humanos. La Caloría grande también se expresa como kilocaloría (kcal) y equivale a 1,000 calorías pequeñas (Ch. 34).

calumnia (libel) escrito falso y malicioso sobre otra persona que constituye una difamación de la persona (Ch. 7).

calumnia (slander) dichos falsos y maliciosos sobre otra persona que constituyen una difamación del carácter de una persona (Ch. 7).

campana de humo (fume hood) tipo de campana o barrera que se usa en el laboratorio para atrapar los vapores y los humos químicos y desviarlos lejos de los profesionales de la atención médica por el sistema de extracción de aire del edificio (Ch. 38).

campo estéril (sterile field) área que se considera estéril, usualmente designada por un paño estéril. El área contiene insumos e instrumentos estériles que se usarán en un procedimiento particular o cirugía estériles (Ch. 31).

campo no estéril (unsterile field) área adyacente al campo estéril en la que una persona que no usa vestimenta estéril puede entrar, abrir y suministrar elementos necesarios (Ch. 31).

candidiasis (candidiasis) infección de la piel o de la membrana mucosa con alguna especie de *Candida* (Ch. 26).

capa leucocitaria (buffy coat) capa de glóbulos blancos y plaquetas que se forma en la interfaz entre el plasma y los glóbulos rojos en un tubo de sangre que contiene anticoagulante (Ch. 40).

capitación (capitation) uso de la cantidad de miembros inscritos en un plan para determinar el sueldo del proveedor; el proveedor recibe un pago fijo por cada miembro, independientemente de cuántas veces ese miembro consulte al proveedor (Ch. 17).

caquéctico (cachectic) describe un estado de mala salud, desnutrición y consunción (Ch. 34).

carcinoma in situ (carcinoma in situ) cáncer que no se extiende más allá de la membrana basal (Ch. 26).

cardiogénico (cardiogenic) tipo de choque en el que el músculo cardíaco no puede contraerse y proporcionar sangre al cuerpo adecuadamente (Ch. 9).

cardioversión (cardioversion) conversión de un ritmo cardíaco patológico (arritmia), como fibrilación ventricular, al ritmo sinusal normal (Ch. 9, 37).

cardioversor/desfibrilador (cardioverter/defibrillator) dispositivo implantable usado para arritmias que ponen en riesgo la vida. Su objetivo es aplicar descargas eléctricas para eliminar la arritmia y lograr un ritmo sinusal más normal (Ch. 37).

caroteno (carotene) vitamina A (Ch. 34).

carta de bloque completo (full block letter) estilo de carta principal en el cual todos los renglones de los párrafos comienzan alineados en el margen izquierdo. Este estilo se sugiere para oficinas que desean una carta eficiente y de aspecto contemporáneo (Ch. 15).

carta de referencia (letter of reference) carta generalmente escrita por el ex empleador de un empleado en el que se describe el desempeño, la actitud o las aptitudes del empleado. Esta carta se presenta a un posible empleador cuando el candidato se postula para un nuevo empleo (Ch. 46).

carta de renuncia (letter of resignation) carta en la que se informa al empleador actual sobre la decisión del empleado de renunciar al puesto actual (Ch. 46).

carta estilo bloque modificado, con sangría (modified block letter, indented) estilo de carta modificado con párrafos con sangría. Los párrafos de este estilo de carta pueden tener sangría de cinco espacios (Ch. 15).

carta estilo bloque modificado, estándar (modified block letter, standard) estilo de carta principal en el que todos los renglones comienzan en el margen izquierdo excepto el renglón de la fecha, el cierre de cortesía y la firma mecanografiada. Las excepciones generalmente comienzan en la posición central o a una distancia de unos espacios a la derecha del centro (Ch. 15).

carta simplificada (simplified letter) estilo de carta principal recomendado por la Sociedad de Gestión Administrativa (Administrative Management Society) que omite el saludo y el cierre de cortesía. Todos los renglones se escriben alineados en el margen izquierdo. En los consultorios médicos, este estilo es el más usado para enviar una carta tipo (Ch. 15).

carta tipo (form letter) carta que tiene el mismo contenido en el cuerpo pero que se envía a diferentes personas (Ch. 15).

cartera (portfolio) cuaderno o dossier que contiene ejemplos de materiales que se usan comúnmente (Ch. 15).

catalizador (catalyst) sustancia que permite que una reacción química se desarrolle a un ritmo mucho mayor y sin demasiado ingreso de energía (Ch. 34).

catarata (cataract) opacidad de la lente del ojo que usualmente se produce por envejecimiento, trauma o enfermedad (Ch. 10).

categorías de aislamiento (isolation categories) sistema de siete categorías desarrollado por los Centros para el Control de Enfermedades (CDC, por sus siglas en inglés) que aísla a los pacientes de acuerdo con las infecciones conocidas. Estas categorías se han condensado en tres Precauciones basadas en la transmisión, según si la vía de transmisión es por aire, por contacto o por gotitas (Ch. 22).

cateterismo (catheterization) inserción de un catéter en el cuerpo para evacuar líquidos o inyectarlos en las cavidades corporales. En el cateterismo urinario, el tubo se introduce a través de la uretra hacia la vejiga para extraer orina (Ch. 25).

cateterismo cardíaco (cardiac catheterization) pasaje de un catéter hacia el corazón a través de una vena del brazo o de la pierna y de los vasos sanguíneos que van al corazón. El objetivo es obtener muestras de sangre cardíaca, detectar anormalidades y determinar la presión intracardíaca. Se puede inyectar un medio de contraste y se puede realizar una angiografía coronaria (Ch. 37).

cátodo (cathode) electrodo negativo que emite electrones (Ch. 32).

cáustico (caustic) que quema y corroe, que destruye el tejido humano (Ch. 22, 31).

cauterio (cautery) destrucción de tejido al quemarlo (Ch. 31).

cauterizar (cauterize) destruir tejido a través de la aplicación de un agente cáustico, un instrumento caliente, una corriente eléctrica u otro agente (Ch. 9).

celulosa (cellulose) tipo de fibra no digerible compuesta por los hidratos de carbono que se encuentran en las plantas (Ch. 34).

centrifugador (centrifuge) dispositivo que hace girar tubos usando la fuerza centrífuga para separar la parte líquida de la sangre de los elementos más densos (Ch. 40).

centros de servicio al paciente (patient service centres) instalaciones de laboratorio satélite ubicadas en áreas convenientes para pacientes donde se pueden recolectar y dejar las muestras para análisis (Ch. 39).

Centros de Servicios de Medicare y Medicaid (CMS) (Centers for Medicare and Medicaid Services [CMS]) Antes conocido como Administración para el Financiamiento de la Atención Médica (HCFA, por sus siglas en inglés). CMS es una agencia federal dentro del Departamento de Salud y Servicios Humanos (DHHS, por sus siglas en inglés) de los EE. UU. La agencia administra Medicare, Medicaid y el Programa Estatal de Seguro Médico para Niños (SCHIP, por sus siglas en inglés). CMS también administra la Ley de Portabilidad y Responsabilidad de Seguros de Salud (HIPAA, por sus siglas en inglés) de 1996 y la Ley de Mejoras de Laboratorios Clínicos (CLIA, por sus siglas en inglés) de 1988 (Ch. 17).

certificación (certification) garantía que indica que es verdadero o que se rige por un estándar o que lo cumple (Ch. 1).

cerumen (cerumen) sustancia segregada por las glándulas ubicadas en el tercio exterior del canal auditivo (Ch. 30).

cetoacidosis (ketoacidosis) acumulación de cetonas en el cuerpo, que se produce principalmente como complicación de la diabetes mellitus; si no se trata puede provocar coma (Ch. 42).

cetona (ketone) compuesto químico producido durante un aumento del metabolismo de los lípidos; también, prueba con una tira reactiva (Ch. 42).

cetonuria (ketonuria) presencia de cetonas en la orina (Ch. 42).

cetosis (ketosis) afección en la que el cuerpo quema los ácidos grasos para obtener energía en la ausencia de la glucosa o los carbohidratos correspondientes; se puede llamar también lipólisis (Ch. 42).

cheque certificado (certified check) cheque propio del depositante que, según lo indica el banco con fecha y firma, tiene los fondos de respaldo del importe escrito (Ch. 19).

cheque con comprobante (voucher check) cheque con un formulario recortable que se usa para detallar el motivo por el que se libra el cheque; generalmente se usa en los cheques de nómina (Ch. 19).

cheque de caja (cashier's check) cheque propio del banco librado a cargo de la cuenta del banco (Ch. 19).

cheque de viajero (traveler's check) a menudo se usa en lugar de efectivo en los viajes; disponible en denominaciones de $20 a $100; requiere la firma en el lugar de compra y la firma en el momento de usar el cheque (Ch. 19).

Cheyne–Stoke (Cheyne–stroke) patrón regular de frecuencia respiratoria irregular que a menudo se observa en niños y que puede verse en la disfunción cerebral (Ch. 24).

cianosis (cyanosis) decoloración de la piel debido a cantidades anormales de hemoglobina reducida en la sangre, provocada por la disminución del oxígeno y el aumento del dióxido de carbono en la sangre (Ch. 25).

ciclo cardíaco (cardiac cycle) período desde el inicio de un latido cardíaco hasta el comienzo del siguiente latido, que incluye la sístole y la diástole. Un latido completo del corazón (Ch. 37).

cilindros (casts) estructuras diminutas que generalmente se forman por depósitos de proteína u otras sustancias en las paredes de los túbulos renales; en la orina, pueden indicar enfermedad renal (Ch. 42).

cinésica (kinesics) estudio de lenguaje corporal (Ch. 4).

cinturón de marcha (gait belt) cinturón de seguridad que usa el paciente alrededor de la cintura y que permite un asimiento firme a la persona que está a cargo de su cuidado al transferir al paciente o al ayudarlo en la ambulación (Ch. 33).

circuncisión (circumcision) la extirpación quirúrgica de la piel móvil (prepucio) del pene (Ch. 27).

circunducción (circumduction) movimiento circular de una parte del cuerpo (Ch. 33).

cistitis (cystitis) inflamación de la vejiga (Ch. 29).

citación (subpoena) orden por escrito que designa a una persona para que comparezca ante un tribunal bajo pena de recibir penalización por rebeldía (Ch. 7).

citología (cytology) ciencia que trata sobre la formación, la estructura y la función de las células (Ch. 39).

clamidia (chlamydia) bacteria que causa una de las enfermedades de transmisión sexual más frecuente (Ch. 26).

Clasificación Internacional de Enfermedades, 9.ª Revisión, Modificación Clínica **(CIE-9-MC)** *(International Classification of Diseases, 9th Revision, Clinical Modification* **[ICD-9-CM])** códigos de diagnóstico estándar usados para identificar la enfermedad de un paciente. Se usa en la mayoría de los entornos de atención ambulatoria para codificar el formulario de reclamación y es reconocida por la mayoría de las compañías de seguros (Ch. 18).

claustrofobia (claustrophobia) miedo de estar confinado en algún espacio (Ch. 32).

CMS 1500 (08-05) (CMS 1500 [08-05]) antes conocido como el formulario HCFA 1500, que es el formulario de reclamación del seguro de salud para Medicare y Medicaid (Ch. 18).

cobalamina (cobalamina) vitamina B_{12} (Ch. 34).

codificar (codificación) (encode [encoding]) crear un mensaje para enviarlo (Ch. 4).

códigos agrupados (bundled codes) agrupamiento de varios servicios que están directamente relacionados con un procedimiento específico y se pagan como uno solo (Ch. 18).

códigos de desagregación (unbundling codes) se refiere a separar los componentes de un procedimiento e informarlos como códigos facturables con los cargos para aumentar las tasas de reembolso (Ch. 18).

códigos E (E codes) códigos ICD-9-CM para las causas externas de lesiones, intoxicación u otras reacciones adversas que explican cómo se produjo la lesión (Ch. 18).

códigos M (códigos morfológicos) (M codes [morphology codes]) se encuentran en el ICD-9-CM y se usan principalmente con registros de cáncer. Los códigos M identifican el comportamiento y el tipo celular de una neoplasia (Ch. 18).

códigos V (V codes) códigos de la Clasificación Internacional de Enfermedades, 9.ª Revisión, Modificación Clínica (ICD-9-CM, por sus siglas en inglés) que representan factores que influyen en el estado de salud de una persona o razones legítimas para comunicarse con el centro de salud cuando el paciente no tiene un diagnóstico definitivo o un síntoma activo de algún trastorno (Ch. 18).

coenzima (coenzyme) sustancia que potencia un catalizador (Ch. 34).

colecalciferol (cholecalciferol) vitamina D (Ch. 34).

colesterol (cholesterol) lípido esterol ampliamente distribuido en tejidos animales. El colesterol se produce en el hígado y es un componente de la bilis (Ch. 44).

colonoscopia (colonoscopy) examen visual del colon con una sonda con luz (Ch. 30).

colposcopia (colposcopy) examen visual de los tejidos vaginales y cervicales usando un colposcopio e indicado después de un Papanicolaou con resultado anormal. Se usa una lente con aumento y luces potentes (Ch. 26).

comedón (comedone) espinilla, generalmente resultado de glándulas sebáceas obstruidas por el acné (Ch. 30).

comercialización (marketing) proceso por el cual el proveedor de servicios comunica al consumidor el alcance y la calidad de los servicios. Las herramientas de comercialización incluyen relaciones públicas, folletos, seminarios de educación para pacientes y boletines (Ch. 45).

Comisión Conjunta (Joint Commission) anteriormente conocida como Comisión Conjunta para la Acreditación de Organizaciones de Cuidado de la Salud; comisión establecida para mejorar la calidad de la atención y de los servicios provistos en el entorno organizado de la atención médica a través de un proceso de acreditación voluntario (Ch. 16).

Comisión de Acreditación de Programas Educativos Asociados a la Salud (CAAHEP) (Commission on Accreditation of Allied Health Education Programs [CAAHEP]) entidad que acredita más de 2,000 programas educacionales en el campo de las profesiones de las ciencias de la salud (Ch. 1, 47).

comparador de rendimiento (benchmark) comparación entre diferentes organizaciones con respecto a la forma en que realizan las tareas, por ejemplo, informatización de oficinas, organización de sistemas de archivos y remuneración de empleados (Ch. 11, 45).

compensación (compensation) exageración de características para compensar una deficiencia o una desventaja real o imaginada (Ch. 4).

competencia (competency) legalmente apto o adecuado (Ch. 1).

composición (compounding) combinación de dos o más sustancias en proporciones definidas (Ch. 36).

compuestos organomercuriales (organomercurial) cualquier compuesto orgánico que contenga mercurio (Ch. 27).

computadora personal (PC) (personal computer [PC]) cualquier computadora que por su precio, tamaño y capacidad resultaútil para ser usada por un solo usuario, sin la intervención de operadores de computadora. También conocida como microcomputadora (Ch. 11).

comunicación de alto contexto (high-context communication) estilo de comunicación que depende en gran parte del lenguaje corporal, la referencia a los objetos del entorno y la fraseología culturalmente relevante para transmitir una idea. Depende de que el interlocutor conozca los acontecimientos relacionados a través de una asociación estrecha con el hablante o la cultura (Ch. 4).

comunicación de bajo contexto (low-context communication) estilo de comunicación que usa pocas expresiones idiomáticas del ambiente o cultura para trasmitir una idea o un concepto. Las ideas se explican explícitamente (Ch. 4).

comunicación terapéutica (therapeutic communication) uso de habilidades de comunicación profesionales específicas y bien definidas para crear una sensación de comodidad para los pacientes, aun cuando se debe dar información difícil o desagradable (Ch. 4).

condensador (condenser) en un microscopio, dirige un haz de luz desde la fuente hasta la muestra (Ch. 39).

condiloma (condylomata) lesión verrugosa de origen viral que se presenta en los genitales externos o en la región perianal (Ch. 26).

conducto deferente (vas deferens) tubo muscular que conecta los testículos con la uretra (Ch. 28).

conexión en red (networking) conectar dos o más computadoras para compartir archivos y hardware. El sistema se llama red (Ch. 11).

confidencialidad (confidentiality) reglas éticas y legales con respecto a la privacidad del paciente (Ch. 16).

congruencia (congruency) cuando deben coincidir el mensaje verbal y el no verbal (Ch. 4).

consentimiento implícito (implied consent) consentimiento sobreentendido por el proveedor de atención médica, generalmente en una emergencia que pone en riesgo la vida del paciente. También ocurre de formas más sutiles en el entorno de atención médica; por ejemplo, cuando un paciente levanta las mangas voluntariamente para recibir una inyección (Ch. 7).

consentimiento informado (informed consent) consentimiento dado por el paciente en el que se le explica el procedimiento que se realizará, sus riesgos, los resultados esperados y las alternativas (Ch. 7, 31).

conservante (preservative) sustancia química que se agrega a los alimentos para mantenerlos frescos durante más tiempo o que se agrega a la orina para conservala para el análisis (Ch. 34, 42).

constreñirse (constrict) achicarse en diámetro (Ch. 40).

contabilidad administrativa (managerial accounting) genera información financiera que puede dar lugar a una administración interna más eficaz (Ch. 21).

contabilidad (accounting) sistema de control de la situación financiera de un establecimiento y de los resultados económicos de sus actividades, que proporciona información para la toma de decisiones (Ch. 21).

contabilidad de caja (cash basis accounting) informa sobre los ingresos en el momento en que se cobra el dinero (Ch. 21).

Contabilidad de costos (cost accounting) ayuda a determinar cuánto le cuesta al entorno de atención ambulatoria prestar servicios particulares y es parte integral de la contabilidad administrativa (Ch. 21).

contabilidad financiera (financial accounting) proporciona información principalmente a entidades externas a la organización, como el gobierno (Ch. 21).

contabilidad según el principio del devengo (accrual basis accounting) informa sobre los ingresos en el momento en que se generan los cargos (Ch. 21).

contaminación importante (gross contamination) presencia de material marcadamente infeccioso (Ch. 22).

contaminar (contaminate) ensuciar algo; a menudo se usa para describir un área estéril que pasó a ser "no estéril" o la exposición de un área limpia a un agente patógeno (Ch. 22, 31).

contrachoque (countershock) aplicación de una corriente eléctrica en el corazón directa o indirectamente para modificar una alteración en el ritmo cardíaco (Ch. 37).

contractura (contracture) se produce cuando el cuerpo está en un estado sin movimiento. Los tejidos conectivos usualmente flexibles se vuelven rígidos y son reemplazados por tejidos similares a la fibra (Ch. 33).

contraer (contracting) adquirir una infección por patógenos (Ch. 22).

contraindicación (contraindication) cualquier síntoma o circunstancia que indica que el uso de un fármaco en particular es inapropiado cuando sí se recomendaría en otra situación. Por ejemplo, el uso de bebidas alcohólicas es una contraindicación cuando se receta el medicamento Flagyl® (Ch. 35).

contrato explícito (expressed contract) contrato escrito o verbal que describe específicamente lo que hará cada parte del contrato (Ch. 7).

contrato implícito (implied contract) contrato indicado por acciones en lugar de palabras (Ch. 7).

contravención (misdemeanor) delito menor; la definición de contravención varía según el estado. El castigo generalmente es libertad condicional o un tiempo de prestación de un servicio público y una multa (Ch. 7).

control de calidad (quality control) mediciones usadas para verificar el procesamiento de muestras de laboratorio. Incluye el uso correcto, el almacenamiento, la manipulación, la estabilidad, las fechas de vencimiento y las indicaciones para lograr precisión en las mediciones y exactitud en los procesos analíticos (Ch. 38, 42, 43).

control de infecciones (infection control) métodos para eliminar o reducir la transmisión de microorganismos infecciosos (Ch. 22).

controlador (driver) programa informático diseñado para convertir la salida de datos de un dispositivo a un formato compatible con otro dispositivo (Ch. 11).

controles de ingeniería (engineering controls) dispositivos físicos o mecánicos que aíslan o eliminan los riesgos para la salud del lugar de trabajo (Ch. 22).

controles de prácticas laborales (work practice controls) medidas usadas en el lugar de trabajo que constan de equipo físico y dispositivos mecánicos para controlar la exposición de los empleados a los patógenos transmitidos por la sangre y otros materiales potencialmente infecciosos. Algunos ejemplos son recipientes para desechar objetos filosos, instalaciones para lavarse las manos, equipo de protección personal y estaciones para lavarse los ojos (Ch. 22).

coordinación de beneficios (COB) (coordination of benefits [COB]) disposición de un contrato de seguro que limita los beneficios al 100% del costo (Ch. 17).

correo electrónico (email) el proceso de envío, recepción, almacenamiento y reenvío de mensajes en forma digital por redes informáticas (Ch. 12).

copago (co-payment) pago que se debe hacer cuando se consulta al proveedor (Ch. 17).

copia oculta (blind copy) protege la privacidad del correo electrónico. Los demás destinatarios no pueden identificar las otras personas que recibieron el mensaje transmitido (Ch. 15).

corrector (editor) ver auditor (Ch. 16).

correo electrónico cifrado (encrypted Email) proceso para codificar el correo electrónico de modo de lograr una transmisión esencialmente segura (Ch. 12).

correo electrónico clínico (clinical Email) tipo de correo electrónico establecido usando protocolos definidos como medio de comunicación entre proveedores y pacientes establecidos (Ch. 12).

cortafuegos (firewall) dispositivo de hardware o programa de software diseñado para impedir el acceso no autorizado a un sistema informático (Ch. 11).

coseguro (coinsurance) porcentaje pagado por la empresa o que paga el asegurado (Ch. 17).

costo fijo (fixed cost) costo que no varía en total a medida que varía la cantidad de pacientes (Ch. 21).

costo variable (variable cost) costo que varía en proporción directa al volumen (Ch. 21).

creatinina (creatinine) producto de desecho formado en el músculo que se excreta por los riñones; aumenta en la sangre y la orina cuando la función renal es anormal (Ch. 42).

crñdito (credit) reducción de un saldo deudor (Ch. 19).

crepitación (crepitation) sonido rechinante que se escucha al mover los extremos de un hueso fracturado (Ch. 9).

criocirugía (cryosurgery) destrucción de tejido mediante la aplicación de frío extremo, nitrato de plata y dióxido de carbono (Ch. 26).

crioconservación (cryopreservation) almacenamiento de materiales biológicos (esperma, embriones, tejido, plasma) a temperaturas sumamente frías para usarlos en otro momento (Ch. 8).

crioterapia (cryotherapy) uso del frío para tratar un problema físico (Ch. 33).

criptorquidia (cryptorchidism) testículo que no ha descendido (Ch. 28).

cristales (crystals) se encuentran en el sedimento normal de la orina y no tienen importancia en particular; se debe prestar atención a la presencia de cristales ya que pueden indicar estados de enfermedad (Ch. 42).

cuentas de ahorro del mercado monetario (money market savings accounts) cuentas bancarias que pagan una tasa de interés más alta (tasa del mercado monetario) que las cuentas de ahorros estándar y permiten librar una cantidad limitada de cheques (Ch. 19).

cuentas por cobrar (accounts receivable) importe adeudado a una empresa por servicios o productos suministrados (Ch. 19).

cuentas por pagar (accounts payable) suma adeudada por una empresa por servicios o productos recibidos (Ch. 19); también, compromiso no escrito de pagar a un proveedor por bienes o mercadería comprada a crédito o por un servicio prestado (Ch. 21).

cultivo por punción (stab culture) cultivo en el cual en el microorganismo es introducido para penetración profunda en medios sólidos en tubos (Ch. 43).

cultivo y sensibilidad (culture and sensitivity) a menudo se conoce por la sigla C&S del inglés. Se cultiva la muestra para que desarrolle bacterias y luego se la expone a diversos antibióticos para determinar a qué son sensibles (y resistentes) las bacterias (Ch. 39, 42).

cultivos (cultures) microorganismos cultivados en un medio de nutrientes (Ch. 42, 43).

cultura (culture) actitudes y comportamientos característicos de un grupo u organización social en particular (Ch. 4).

cumplimiento (compliance) observancia de los requisitos oficiales (Ch. 1).

curriculum vitae (résumé) hoja de datos resumidos escritos o recuento breve de aptitudes y de avance en la profesión elegida (Ch. 48).

curriculum vitae cronológico (chronologic résumé) formato de currículum vitae cuando se tiene experiencia laboral (Ch. 48).

curriculum vitae dirigido al objetivo (targeted résumé) formato de currículum vitae que se usa al concentrarse en un objetivo laboral específico y claro (Ch. 48).

curriculum vitae electrónico (e-résumé) el currículum vitae electrónico se puede enviar electrónicamente por correo electrónico, enviarse a las bolsas de trabajo en Internet o publicarse en páginas web (Ch. 48).

curriculum vitae funcional (functional résumé) formato de currículum vitae usado para destacar áreas de especialidad con sus logros y fortalezas (Ch. 48).

debe (debit) columna de la izquierda (Ch. 19).

débito (debit) se usa para asentar los gastos y la descripción de los servicios (Ch. 19).

declaración (deposition) testimonio oral dado por una persona en presencia de un taquígrafo judicial y abogados de ambas partes; a menudo se usa como parte del proceso de exhibición de pruebas (Ch. 7).

declaración de trabajo (work statement) descripción concisa del trabajo que planea realizar (Ch. 45).

declaraciones de logros (accomplishment statements) declaraciones que comienzan con un verbo de acción y describen brevemente lo que usted hizo y los resultados demostrables que se obtuvieron (Ch. 48).

declaraciones indirectas (indirect statements) medio de provocar una respuesta de un paciente transformando una pregunta en una declaración de interés (Ch. 4).

decodificar (decode) traducir a un idioma que sea fácil de entender; interpretar (Ch. 4).

decúbito dorsal (dorsal recumbent) es esta posición, los pacientes se recuestan boca arriba (dorsal), con las piernas separadas, las piernas flexionadas con los pies apoyados en la mesa (Ch. 25).

deducible (deductible) importe de gastos medicos incurridos al que se debe llegar antes de que la póliza de seguro comience a pagar (Ch. 17).

degeneración macular (macular degeneration) degeneración de la mácula de la retina debido al envejecimiento; causa principal del deterioro visual en personas mayores de 50 años que dificulta las tareas minuciosas (Ch. 29).

delito mayor (felony) delito grave, como homicidio, hurto (robo de grandes sumas de dinero), agresión violenta y violación (Ch. 7).

demandado (defendant) persona que contesta una demanda presentada en un litigio (Ch. 7).

demandante (plaintiff) persona que presenta cargos en un litigio (Ch. 7).

demencia (dementia) deterioro de la función intelectual que es progresivo e interfiere en las actividades normales (Ch. 29).

densidad específica (specific gravity) relación entre el peso de un volumen dado de una sustancia con el peso del mismo volumen de agua destilada a la misma temperatura; prueba que a menudo se realiza durante el examen físico del análisis de orina (también puede aparecer en la prueba de tira reactiva) (Ch. 42).

derecho administrativo (administrative law) establece los organismos que tienen la facultad de dictar leyes y promulgar reglamentaciones (Ch. 7).

derecho civil (civil law) leyes relacionadas con actos entre personas (Ch. 7).

derecho constitucional (constitutional law) consiste en leyes establecidas por las constituciones de los Estados Unidos o de los estados individuales (Ch. 7).

derecho consuetudinario (common law) referente a las leyes desarrolladas en Inglaterra y Francia e introducidas en los Estados Unidos por los primeros colonos; a veces llamada derecho de creación judicial (Ch. 7).

derecho contractual (contract law) leyes que se refieren a los contratos vinculantes entre personas y entidades (Ch. 7).

derecho de responsabilidad civil (tort law) leyes que se originan en los agravios o en los actos ilegítimos en los que una persona provoca daños a otra persona (Ch. 7).

derecho estatutario (statutory law) se refiere al cuerpo de leyes establecidas por los estados (Ch. 7).

derecho penal (criminal law) leyes relacionadas con los delitos cometidos contra el bienestar y la seguridad de la sociedad en su conjunto (Ch. 7).

derivado proteico purificado (DPP) (purified protein derivative [PPD]) filtrado obtenido de los cultivos de *Mycobacterium* usados para pruebas intradérmicas de tuberculosis (Ch. 44).

dermatofitos (dermatophytes) categoría de hongos que provocan infecciones en el cabello, la piel y las uñas (Ch. 43).

descripción del trabajo (job description) descripción de tareas, obligaciones y responsabilidades para cada cargo en la oficina (Ch. 46).

desfibrilación (defibrillation) detener la fibrilación del corazón usando fármacos o por medios físicos (Ch. 37).

desfibrilador (defibrillator) equipo que aplica una corriente eléctrica para modificar una alteración del ritmo cardíaco (Ch. 37).

desfibrilador externo automatizado (DEA) (automated external defibrillator [AED]) dispositivo automático, portátil y autónomo con instrucciones de voz sobre el uso para personas con paro cardíaco. Se utiliza externamente para aplicar electrónicamente una "descarga eléctrica"al miocardio y hacer que se contraiga nuevamente. Igual que la cardioversión (Ch. 9).

desfragmentación (defragmentation) reorganización de la información en un disco duro para guardar archivos como unidades continuas en vez de paquetes pequeños. Una computadora con poca fragmentación de archivos funcionará a mayor velocidad (Ch. 11).

desinfección (disinfection) uso de productos químicos o agua hirviendo para liberar a un objeto de materiales infecciosos pero no de sus esporas (Ch. 22).

deslucido (lackluster) opaco, que le falta brillo (Ch. 9).

desmielinización (demyelination) destrucción de la vaina de mielina, a menudo un factor observado en la esclerosis múltiple (Ch. 30).

desoxigenada (deoxygenated) sangre con alto contenido de dióxido de carbono y bajo contenido de oxígeno que se bombea del corazón a los pulmones, donde el dióxido de carbono se intercambia por oxígeno (Ch. 37).

despido involuntario (involuntary dismissal) desvinculación del empleo debido a un desempeño laboral deficiente o a la violación de las políticas de la oficina (Ch. 46).

desplazamiento (displacement) trasladar sentimientos negativos a algo o alguien sin tener en cuenta la situación (Ch. 4).

despolarizar (depolarize) proceso para reducir hasta un estado no polarizado. Así, se mejora la generación de una corriente eléctrica. La actividad eléctrica generada cuando se contraen las aurículas o los ventrículos (Ch. 37).

desprendimiento de la placenta (placenta abruptio) separación repentina y abrupta de la placenta de la pared uterina (Ch. 26).

destreza (dexterity) habilidad y facilidad para usar las manos (Ch. 1).

detritos (debris) restos de células o tejidos descompuestos o dañados (Ch. 22).

diabetes gestacional (gestational diabetes) diabetes que se manifiesta clínicamente por primera vez durante el embarazo. Por lo general, desaparece despuñs del parto (Ch. 26).

diabetes mellitus (diabetes mellitus) trastorno crónico del metabolismo de los carbohidratos que se caracteriza por hiperglucemia y que es resultado de la producción o el uso inadecuado de la insulina (Ch. 44).

diafragma (diaphragm) lente u otro objeto que se abre y se cierra para aumentar o disminuir la cantidad de luz sobre el objeto que se ilumina. Se refiere a un diafragma óptico como en un microscopio (el diafragma se usa para el control de natalidad y también es el músculo respiratorio principal) (Ch. 39).

diagnóstico (diagnosis) determinación de una enfermedad o afección (Ch. 39).

diagnóstico clínico (clinical diagnosis) identificación de una enfermedad por antecedentes, estudios de laboratorio y síntomas (Ch. 23, 39).

diagnóstico diferencial (differential diagnosis) diagnóstico basado en la comparación de síntomas de enfermedades similares (Ch. 39).

diástole (diastole) un componente de la medición de la presión arterial que representa la presión más baja durante el ciclo cardíaco; fuerza ejercida sobre las paredes arteriales durante la relajación cardíaca (Ch. 24, 37).

dicción (enunciation) hablar con claridad y buena expresión (Ch. 12).

dietilestilbestrol (DES) (diethylstilbestrol [DES]) hormona sintñtica usada terapéuticamente en trastornos menopáusicos. No se debe administrar durante el embarazo. Se la ha relacionado con tumores malignos cérvicovaginales en hijas de madres que tomaron la hormona para tratar una amenaza de aborto. DES ha sido relacionado con enfermedades reproductivas en hombres cuyas madres tomaron la hormona durante el embarazo (Ch. 26).

digestión (digestion) descomposición de los alimentos en partículas más pequeñas. Puede ser física o química (Ch. 34).

dilatación (dilation) expansión de un orificio u órgano (Ch. 26).

dilatarse (dilate) agrandarse en diámetro (Ch. 40).

diploma (diploma) documento en el consta la graduación de una institución educativa o el título que ésta otorga (Ch. 1).

disco duro (hard drive) dispositivo de almacenamiento no volátil que conserva la información almacenada por medio de un sistema de grabación magnetica digital en discos metálicos que giran a gran velocidad. La capacidad es de aproximadamente 100GB. El dispositivo puede estar instalado permanentemente dentro de la carcasa de la computadora o ser portátil (Ch. 11).

disentería amébica (amoebic dysentery) enfermedad intestinal infecciosa provocada por amebas y caracterizada por inflamación de la membrana mucosa del colon (Ch. 22).

disfunción eréctil (DE) (erectile dysfunction [ED]) impotencia; ocurre cuando un hombre no puede alcanzar o mantener una erección del pene durante la relación sexual (Ch. 28).

dismenorrea (dysmenorrhea) menstruaciones dolorosas (Ch. 26).

disnea (dyspnea) falta de aire o dificultad para respirar (Ch. 24).

dispareunia (dyspareunia) coito doloroso (Ch. 26).

displasia (dysplasia) desarrollo anormal de tejido (Ch. 26).

dispositivo de almacenamiento de datos (data storage device) dispositivo que puede guardar datos digitales en forma permanente o temporal (Ch. 11).

dispositivo de entrada (input device) dispositivo usado para ingresar datos en una computadora (Ch. 11).

dispositivo de punto de servicio (POS) (point-of-service [POS] device) dispositivo que permite la comunicación directa entre un consultorio médico y la computadora del plan de atención médica (Ch. 18).

dispositivo de salida (output device) dispositivo usado para sacar información de una computadora. Incluye impresoras, faxes, unidades de almacenamiento de datos, pantallas y trazadores (Ch. 11).

distensión (strain) lesión en el tejido blando entre las articulaciones que consiste en el desgarro de músculos o tendones. Las distensiones a menudo se presentan en el cuello, la espalda o los músculos de los muslos (Ch. 9).

distribución (distribution) el proceso mediante el cual el fármaco es transportado desde la sangre al sitio de acción previsto, el sitio de biotransformación, el sitio de almacenamiento y el sitio de eliminación (Ch. 35).

disuria (dysuria) dolor o dificultad al orinar (Ch. 30).

diurético (diuretic) sustancia por cuya acción el riñón reabsorbe menos agua y, por lo tanto, el agua se excreta del cuerpo (Ch. 34).

doctrina (doctrine) principio de ley establecido a través de decisiones pasadas (Ch. 7).

documentación (documentation) material escrito que acompaña la compra de software y que incluye la información necesaria para usar el software correctamente; a veces se conoce como manual (Ch. 11, 22); también, que proporciona apoyo exacto a través de información escrita (Ch. 22).

doppler (doppler) técnica no invasiva usada junto con la ecografía para evaluar el flujo sanguíneo a través de las venas y arterias principales de los brazos, las piernas y el cuello. Puede revelar coágulos de sangre u obstrucciones en el flujo sanguíneo (Ch. 32).

dorsiflexión (dorsiflexion) movimiento del pie hacia arriba a la altura de la articulación del tobillo (Ch. 33).

dosificar (dispense) preparar y dar un medicamento para que se tome posteriormente (Ch. 7, 36, 36).

dosímetro (dosimeter) dispositivo para medir la radiación generada (Ch. 32).

dosis unitaria (unit dose) cantidad medida previamente de medicamento, envasada individualmente para cada dosis (Ch. 36).

eclampsia (eclampsia) complicación del embarazo que incluye edema general, hipertensión, proteinuria y convulsiones (Ch. 26).

ecocardiograma (echocardiogram) método de diagnóstico no invasivo que usa el ultrasonido para visualizar la estructura cardíaca interna, incluidas las válvulas (Ch. 32).

ecografía (ultrasonography) proceso de colocar un transductor manual contra una parte del cuerpo que se desea examinar. El transductor envía ondas de sonido a través de la piel y de los diversos órganos internos. Cuando se forman los ecos y regresan, el transductor los convierte en energía eléctrica. Esta energía se transforma en una imagen en un monitor o se imprime en papel. Se pueden tomar fotografías de las imágenes que pueden ser parte del registro permanente del paciente (Ch. 26, 37).

ecografista (sonographer) persona capacitada profesionalmente para realizar un examen de ecografía (Ch. 37).

edema pulmonar (pulmonary edema) acumulación de líquido seroso en las vesículas aéreas y los tejidos intersticiales de los pulmones (Ch. 38).

edematoso (edematous) acumulación anormal de líquidos en los tejidos que produce inflamación (Ch. 40).

effleurage (effleurage) masaje que emplea golpes prolongados o suaves (Ch. 33).

electrocardiografía (electrocardiography) proceso para registrar la actividad eléctrica que se origina en el corazón (Ch. 37).

electrocardiógrafo (electrocardiograph) instrumento para registrar la actividad eléctrica del corazón (Ch. 37).

electrocardiograma (electrocardiogram) registro de la actividad cardíaca del corazón que muestra ondas P, QRS y T (Ch. 37).

electrocirugía (electrosurgery) utiliza una corriente eléctrica en un área concentrada para cortar o destruir tejido siempre que no se requiera examen patológico (Ch. 31).

electrodo (electrode) también conocido como sensor. Se usa para conducir electricidad del cuerpo al electrocardiógrafo (Ch. 37).

electrolito (electrolyte) sustancias que conducen electricidad cuyos componentes son importantes para mantener el equilibrio acidobásico y de líquidos (Ch. 34, 37, 39).

eliminación (elimination) el proceso mediante el cual el fármaco se excreta del organismo. La eliminación se produce por medio del tracto intestinal, el tracto respiratorio, la piel, las membranas mucosas y las glándulas mamarias (Ch. 35).

elocuente (articulating) que se expresa con claridad y con fluidez (Ch. 12).

embarazo ectópico (ectopic pregnancy) implementación del óvulo fecundado fuera de la cavidad uterina (Ch. 26, 44).

empatía (empathy) capacidad de percibir y entender los sentimientos, las emociones y los comportamientos de otra persona, y de percibir la importancia y el significado que tienen para la otra persona (Ch. 1, 29).

empresa de propiedad privada (proprietary) establecimiento de propiedad y administración privada; organización con fines de lucro (Ch. 1).

endometriosis (endometriosis) invasión por parte de tejido similar al endometrio en diversas zonas de la cavidad pélvica y en otras partes (Ch. 26).

endoscopia (endoscopy) examen visual de las cavidades corporales con una sonda con luz (Ch. 22).

enfermedad de Peyronie (Peyronie's Disease) curvatura del pene durante la erección (Ch. 28).

enfermedad endémica (endemic) enfermedad que se presenta continuamente o en ciclos con una cierta cantidad de casos previstos durante un período determinado (Ch. 22).

enfermedad inflamatoria pélvica (pelvic inflammatory disease) infección del útero, las trompas de Falopio y las estructuras pélvicas adyacentes; las causas más comunes son gonorrea y clamidia; se propaga como las enfermedades de transmisión sexual (Ch. 26).

enfisema (emphysema) enfermedad pulmonar crónica que se caracteriza por dilatación y daño alveolar (Ch. 24).

enfoque en el tiempo (time focus) define el período de tiempo que es importante para una persona y hacia el cual se dirigen y se orientan las acciones de una persona (Ch. 4).

enrutador automático (ARU) (automated routing unit [ARU]) sistema telefónico que responde a una llamada y usa una voz grabada para identificar departamentos o servicios (Ch. 12).

ensayo (assay) análisis de una sustancia para determinar sus componentes y la proporción relativa de cada uno (Ch. 39).

entorno de atención ambulatoria (ambulatory care setting) entorno de atención de la salud en la que se brindan servicios a personas que no están hospitalizadas. *Ambulatorio* proviene del latín y significa "que puede caminar". Los ejemplos incluyen el consultorio de un proveedor único, el ejercicio profesional grupal, el centro de atención de urgencias y la organización de mantenimiento de la salud (Ch. 1, 2).

entrevista (interview) reunión en la que usted y el entrevistador hablan sobre las oportunidades laborales y las fortalezas que puede aportar a la organización (Ch. 48).

entrevista de salida (exit interview) oportunidad para que los empleados que abandonan la empresa den sus opiniones positivas y negativas del puesto de trabajo y del establecimiento (Ch. 46).

eosinófilos (eosinophil) glóbulo blanco granulocítico con gránulos que se tiñen de rojo con eosina en el citoplasma. Su número es elevado en casos de alergias (Ch. 41).

epidemia (epidemic) enfermedad infecciosa que ataca a muchas personas al mismo tiempo en el mismo lugar geográfico (Ch. 22).

epidemiología (epidemiology) campo de la ciencia que estudia los antecedentes, las causas y los patrones de enfermedades infecciosas (Ch. 22).

epididimitis (epididymitis) inflamación de los conductos en el testículo (Ch. 28).

epinefrina (epinephrine) usada para tratar reacciones alérgicas (Ch. 9); también, hormona llamada también adrenalina. La epinefrina se fabrica como sustancia química (preparado farmacéutico) y a menudo se mezcla con anestésicos locales para usar como vasoconstrictor en cirugías menores (Ch. 31).

equilibrio ácido-básico (acid/base balance) estado que se presenta cuando la tasa neta a la cual el cuerpo produce ácidos o bases es igual a la tasa neta a la cual se excretan los ácidos o las bases (Ch. 42).

ergonomía (ergonomics) estudio científico del trabajo y del espacio, incluidos los factores que afectan la productividad de los empleados y su salud (Ch. 11).

eritema (erythema) enrojecimiento o inflamación de la piel o de las membranas mucosas producto de la dilatación y de la congestión de los capilares superficiales (Ch. 30).

eritrocito (erythrocyte) glóbulo rojo, uno de los componentes de la sangre (Ch. 40, 41).

eritropoyetina (erythropoietin) hormona causante de la producción de nuevos glóbulos rojos (Ch. 41).

escala de valores relativos basada en recursos (RBRVS) (resource-based relative value scale [RBRVS]) base para el esquema de tarifas de Medicare (Ch. 17).

esclerodermia (scleroderma) enfermedad que avanza lentamente y que se caracteriza por el depósito de tejido conectivo fibroso en la piel y los órganos internos (Ch. 25).

escorbuto (scurvy) deficiencia de vitamina C caracterizada por la formación anormal de huesos y dientes. Pueden aparecer signos de hemorragia como hematomas (Ch. 34).

escribano público (notary public) persona con la capacidad legal para dar fe y certificar documentos; puede tomar declaraciones juradas (Ch. 19).

escroto (scrotum) estructura de tejido blando que sostiene los testículos (Ch. 28).

escucha activa (active listening) mensaje recibido que se vuelve a parafrasear al remitente para verificar que se ha decodificado el mensaje correcto (Ch. 4).

esguince (sprain) lesión en una articulación, a menudo el tobillo, la rodilla o la muñeca, en la que se desgarran los ligamentos. La mayoría de los esguinces son menores y se curan rápidamente, pero otros pueden ser más graves, con inflamación, y no curarse adecuadamente si el paciente sigue aplicando presión sobre la articulación desgarrada (Ch. 9).

especie (species) segundo nombre griego o latino dado a los microorganismos; el nombre de la especie no va con mayúscula (Ch. 43).

Especialista Administrativo Médico Certificado (CMAS) **(Certified Medical Administrative Specialist [CMAS])** certificación de la AMT para especialista administrativo médico (Ch. 47).

espermatogénesis (spermatogenesis) la formación de esperma maduro (Ch. 28).

espirometría (spirometry) prueba para medir la capacidad respiratoria de los pulmones (Ch. 30).

esporas (spores) estado inactivo de algunas bacterias en el cual se encapsulan en proteínas. El encapsulamiento las protege del calor, de las sustancias químicas, del congelamiento, de la desecación y de la radiación. Las esporas pueden vivir decenas de miles de años sin nutrientes. Cuando se colocan en suelo fértil (como el tejido humano), pueden activarse y crecer. El tétanos es un tipo de bacteria que crea esporas (Ch. 43).

esputo (sputum) sustancia de las vías respiratorias que se expulsa con la tos (Ch. 22).

esqueleto apendicular (appendicular skeleton) esqueleto formado por los cinturones pectoral y pélvico y las extremidades superiores e inferiores. El cinturón pélvico conecta las extremidades superiores con el tronco (Ch. 30).

esqueleto axial (axial skeleton) formado por huesos que se encuentran alrededor del centro del cuerpo (Ch. 30).

establecimiento de atención administrada (managed care operation) cualquier entorno o sistema de prestación de atención médica diseñado para reducir el costo de la atención y, al mismo tiempo, proveer acceso a ella (Ch. 2).

estado asmático (status asthmaticus) episodio severo de asma que no responde al tratamiento común (Ch. 36).

estado de resultados (income statement) estado contable que muestra las ganancias o las pérdidas netas (Ch. 21).

estampada (swaged) aguja quirúrgica adherida a un tramo de material de sutura durante la costura (Ch. 31).

"estar desprotegido" ("going bare") se dice del proveedor que no contrata seguro por responsabilidad profesional (Ch. 45).

estenosis (strictures) estrechamiento de una estructura de forma tubular, como el esófago o la uretra (Ch. 31).

esterasa leucocitaria (leukocyte esterase) prueba sobre una tira reactiva que indica la presencia de glóbulos blancos en las vías urinarias (Ch. 42).

esterilización por vapor (steam sterilization) el método más utilizado de esterilización en el consultorio médico. Para lograr la esterilización, se utiliza una autoclave, que básicamente es una olla a presión (Ch. 31).

estertores (rales) ruido anormal burbujeante o crujiente que se escucha en la auscultación durante la inspiración (Ch. 24).

estertoroso (stertorous) ruido de ronquido que se escucha cuando la persona tiene dificultad para respirar (Ch. 24).

estilete (stylus) cable delgado caliente del electrocardiógrafo que derrite la cera del papel del ECG durante el registro (Ch. 37).

estomatitis (stomatitis) inflamación de la boca relacionada con la quimioterapia. Puede incluir hinchazón, enrojecimiento, halitosis y ulceraciones (Ch. 32).

estrabismo (strabismus) trastorno de la vista en el cual los ejes ópticos no se pueden dirigir al mismo objeto (bizquera) (Ch. 30).

estrés (stress) respuesta del cuerpo a los cambios; se puede manifestar en una variedad de formas, incluidos los cambios en la presión arterial, la frecuencia cardíaca y la aparición de dolores de cabeza (Ch. 5).

estridor (stridor) ruido como de graznido que se escucha en la inspiración, resultado de una obstrucción en las vías aéreas superiores (Ch. 24).

Ethernet (Ethernet) se refiere a la conexión en red de computadoras usando conductores metálicos o cables físicos (Ch. 11).

ética (ethics) se define en términos de lo que se considera moralmente bien o mal; la ética varía según la persona y a menudo se define mediante un código o credo como el Código de Ética de la AAMA (Ch. 8).

etiqueta (etiquette) modales, cortesía, comportamiento apropiado (Ch. 12).

eupnea (eupnea) respiración normal (Ch. 24).

eversión (eversion) rotación de una parte del cuerpo hacia afuera (Ch. 33).

examen bimanual (bimanual examination) examen realizado por el proveedor usando ambas manos para examinar los órganos pélvicos internos. Se introducen dos dedos de una mano en la vagina y la otra mano presiona el exterior de la pared abdominal. De este modo, se puede determinar la forma, la consistencia y la posición de los órganos pélvicos (Ch. 26).

examen de certificación (certification examination) medio estandarizado de evaluar la competencia del asistente médico (Ch. 47).

examen macroscópico (gross examination) ver muestras a simple vista (Ch. 16).

examen microscópico (microscopic examination) visualizar una muestra con la ayuda del microscopio (Ch. 16).

exclusión (exclusion) enfermedad o afección específica enumerada en una póliza de seguro que no cubre dicha póliza (Ch. 17).

excoriación (excoriated) abrasión de la epidermis por traumatismo, sustancias químicas, quemaduras u otras causas (Ch. 22).

excreción (excretion) sustancia de desecho. La eliminación de los productos de desecho del cuerpo (Ch. 22, 38).

exhibición de pruebas (discovery) momento en que ambas partes tienen acceso a toda la información y la evidencia relacionada con un caso; después del proceso de citación (Ch. 7).

expectorar (expectorate) acto de toser material y expulsarlo desde las vías aéreas que conducen a los pulmones (Ch. 22, 43).

explicación de beneficios (EDB) (explanation of benefits [EOB]) informe del seguro que se envía con los pagos de reclamaciones para explicar el reembolso de la compañía de seguros (Ch. 19).

explícito (explicit) totalmente revelado o expresado sin ser ambiguo o equívoco, que no deja dudas sobre su intención (Ch. 9).

extensión (extension) enderezamiento de una parte del cuerpo (Ch. 33).

extracelular (extracellular) relacionado con el entorno fuera de una célula del cuerpo (Ch. 34).

exudado (exudate) líquido acumulado en una cavidad; supuración de pus; sustancia que atraviesa las paredes de los vasos hacia el tejido contiguo (Ch. 22, 27, 31).

facilitar (facilitate) hacer que una acción o un proceso sean más fáciles (Ch. 1).

facoemulsificación (phacoemulsification) tratamiento para las cataratas. Se usa un dispositivo ultrasónico para desintegrar la catarata del cristalino del ojo, que luego se aspira y se retira (Ch. 30).

factor Rh (Rh factor) factor sanguíneo que indica la presencia o la ausencia del antígeno Rh en la superficie de los eritrocitos humanos (Ch. 44).

factores estresantes (stressors) exigencias de cambio que producen estrés (Ch. 5).

Factura Uniforme 04 (UB04) (Uniform Bill 04 [UB04]) formulario de facturación único que usan ampliamente los centros de cuidados agudos para procesar los reclamos de hospitalización y atención ambulatoria (Ch. 18).

farmacología (pharmacology) estudio de los fármacos; ciencia que se ocupa de la historia, el origen, las fuentes, las propiedades físicas y químicas, y los usos de los fármacos y sus efectos en los organismos vivos (Ch. 35).

farmacopea (pharmacopoeia) libro que describe los fármacos y su preparación, o una recopilación o inventario de fármacos (Ch. 3).

farmacocinética (pharmacokinetics) se refiere a la manera en la que el organismo maneja un fármaco (Ch. 36).

farmacogenómica (pharmacogenomics) el estudio de la respuesta del cuerpo a diferentes compuestos químicos según la herencia genética de un individuo (Ch. 35).

Fármacos derivados de animales (pharmazooticals) fármacos obtenidos a partir de tejidos como las glándulas suprarrenales de los animales (Ch. 35).

fax (facsímil) (fax [facsimile]) máquina que envía documentos de un lugar a otro a través de líneas telefónicas (Ch. 12).

febril (febrile) que tiene fiebre (Ch. 24).

fechoría (malfeasance) conducta ilegal o contraria a las obligaciones de un funcionario (Ch. 7).

fenestrado (fenestrated) que tiene orificios. Paño fenestrado y estéril que se usa en cirugía. Tiene un orificio (redondo) para exponer solamente la zona quirúrgica. El resto del paño cubre al paciente y es una zona estéril (Ch. 31).

fenilcetonuria (FCU) (phenylketonuria [PKU]) enfermedad hereditaria causada por la incapacidad del cuerpo de oxidar el aminoácido fenilalanina. Si no se descubre y se trata a tiempo, puede producirse daño cerebral y un consecuente retraso mental grave (Ch. 27, 44).

fertilización in vitro (IVF) (in vitro fertilization [IVF]) el ovario es fertilizado en una placa de cultivo, se lo deja crecer y luego se implanta en el útero (Ch. 8).

férula (splint) cualquier dispositivo para inmovilizar una parte del cuerpo. Usado con frecuencia por el personal del Servicio de Emergencias Médicas (EMS, por sus siglas en inglés) (Ch. 9).

fianza (bond) acuerdo vinculante con un empleado por el cual se garantiza la recuperación de una pérdida financiera en el caso de que se roben o se malversen fondos (Ch. 45).

fibroplasia retrolenticular (retrolental fibroplasia) enfermedad de los vasos sanguíneos de la retina en el recién nacido (Ch. 36).

fiebre amarilla (yellow fever) enfermedad infecciosa aguda en la que una persona presenta ictericia, vómitos, hemorragias y fiebre; provocada principalmente por los mosquitos (Ch. 3).

fitomedicinas (phytomedicines) hierbas usadas como plantas medicinales. Contienen material derivado de plantas como su principio activo (Ch. 36).

flebotomía (phlebotomy) proceso para recolectar sangre (Ch. 22, 40).

flexión (flexion) acción de doblar una parte del cuerpo (Ch. 33).

flexión plantar (plantar flexion) movimiento descendente del pie a la altura del tobillo (Ch. 33).

flora normal (normal flora) microorganismos que normalmente están presentes en un lugar específico (Ch. 22, 43).

fluoroscopio (fluoroscope) dispositivo que consiste en una pantalla; se monta en forma separada o con un tubo de rayos X que muestra imágenes de objetos interpuestos entre la mesa y la pantalla (Ch. 32).

fómite (fomite) sustancia que absorbe y transmite material infeccioso; por ejemplo, elementos contaminados como los equipos (Ch. 22).

fontanela (fontanel) espacio blando que se encuentra entre los huesos del cráneo del feto, del recién nacido y del bebé (Ch. 27).

forense (forensic) aplicar conocimiento cinetífico a asuntos legales (Ch. 38).

formalina (formalin) solución acuosa de formaldehído al 37% (Ch. 26).

formar redes de contactos (networking) proceso por el cual personas de intereses similares intercambian información en relaciones sociales, comerciales o profesionales (Ch. 46).

formulario de rechazo (declination form) negativa formal por escrito (Ch. 22).

formulario de solicitud (application form) formulario diseñado por un posible empleador para recabar información relacionada con las aptitudes, la educación y la experiencia en el empleo (Ch. 48).

formulario de visita (encounter form) antes conocido como comprobante de servicio o superfactura. Se entrega una copia del formulario de visita al paciente después de consultar al proveedor. Este formulario identifica los procedimientos realizados, los diagnósticos, las tarifas y cuándo debe regresar (Ch. 18, 19).

forúnculo (furuncle) infección cutánea, estafilocócica, supurante y localizada que se origina en una glándula o folículo piloso (Ch. 30).

Fowler (Fowler's) los pacientes se sientan en una posición con la espalda en la mesa de examen elevada a 45 grados (semi-Fowler) o 90 grados (Fowler alta) Las piernas reposan apoyadas en la mesa. Puede colocarse una almohada debajo de las rodillas. Esta posición se utiliza en pacientes que tienen problemas cardiovasculares o respiratorios para facilitar su respiración y para el examen de la parte superior del cuerpo y la cabeza (Ch. 25).

fractura (fracture) rotura de un hueso. Hay varios tipos de fracturas, pero todas se clasifican como fractura abierta o cerrada (Ch. 9).

fractura cerrada (closed fracture) fractura sin complicaciones en la cual el hueso no atraviesa la piel (Ch. 30).

fraude (fraud) tergiversación deliberada de los hechos (Ch. 17).

frecuencia (frequency) que orina a menudo (Ch. 30).

frenillo (frenulum) de la lengua, pliegue de membrana mucosa ubicado debajo de la lengua y que une la lengua a la base de la boca (Ch. 24).

friable (friable) que se quiebra fácilmente (Ch. 31).

Fuerza de Tareas para la Elaboración de Exámenes (TFTC) (Task Force for Test Construction [TFTC]) comisión de profesionales cuya responsabilidad es actualizar el examen de los Asistentes Médicos Certificados (CMA, por sus siglas en inglés) anualmente para reflejar los cambios en las responsabilidades de asistentes médicos y para incluir nuevos desarrollos en la tecnología y los conocimientos médicos (Ch. 47).

fulgurado (fulgarated) destruido por la corriente eléctrica (Ch. 26).

funcionamiento cognitivo (cognitive functioning) conocimiento con percepción, razonamiento, juicio, intuición y memoria (Ch. 29).

galvanómetro (galvanometer) mecanismo del electrocardiógrafo que transforma el voltaje en un movimiento mecánico para poder registrarlo (Ch. 37).

gammagrafía con talio (thallium scan) elemento químico que se administra en forma intravenosa y se usa en las pruebas de esfuerzo cardíaco. El radioisótopo se ubica en el miocardio y un escáner capta la distribución del talio y puede identificar obstrucciones en las arterias coronarias. Prueba exacta para enfermedades de las arterias coronarias (Ch. 37).

garante (guarantor) persona identificada como responsable del pago de la factura (Ch. 19).

gel separador tixotrópico (thixotropic separator gel) gel que puede formar una interfaz entre las células y la parte líquida de la sangre como resultado de la centrifugación (Ch. 40).

género (genus) primer nombre griego o latino dado a un microorganismo; siempre se escribe la primera letra con mayúscula (Ch. 43).

genitales (genitalia) órganos reproductivos, internos y externos (Ch. 26).

gerente autoritario (authoritarian manager) opera bajo la premisa de que la mayoría de los empleados no pueden hacer su aporte sin que se les ordene hacerlo (Ch. 45).

gerente participativo (participatory manager) opera bajo la premisa de que el empleado puede y quiere hacer un buen trabajo (Ch. 45).

geriatría (geriatrics) rama de la medicina que se ocupa de los problemas del envejecimiento (Ch. 29).

gerontología (gerontology) estudio científico de los problemas relacionados con el envejecimiento (Ch. 29).

gestación (gestation) período de desarrollo desde la fertilización al nacimiento (Ch. 26).

gestión de riesgos (risk management) técnicas respetadas en el entorno de atención ambulatoria que mantienen en la mayor medida posible la seguridad para el paciente de la práctica, de su entorno y de los procedimientos. Una gestión de riesgos adecuada también reduce la posibilidad de negligencia y los resultantes juicios por agravios y mala praxis (Ch. 7, 9, 16, 45).

gestión itinerante (MBWA) (management by walking around [MBWA]) técnica para mantener a los gerentes informados sobre el estado de su organización (Ch. 45).

gestos/ademanes (gestures/mannerisms) movimiento de diversas partes del cuerpo durante la comunicación (Ch. 4).

glándula de Bartolino (Bartholin gland) una de dos glándulas mucosas pequeñas ubicadas en el vestíbulo de la vagina en la base de los labios mayores (Ch. 26).

glándulas bulbouretrales (bulbourethral glands) están ubicadas internamente en la base del pene y son parte del sistema reproductivo masculino. Estas glándulas son responsables de la producción y la descarga de una secreción viscosa transparente conocida como líquido preseminal. Este fluido lubrica la uretra para preparar la eyaculación (Ch. 28).

glaucoma (glaucoma) trastorno causado por aumento de la presión intraocular debido a la acumulación de humor acuoso. Esto produce molestias visuales con poco o ningún dolor, pero puede ocasionar discapacidad visual grave en caso de no recibir tratamiento (Ch. 30).

glicógeno (glycogen) forma de hidrato de carbono que se usa para almacenar azúcar en el cuerpo (Ch. 34).

glucosa (glucose) azúcar simple que es la fuente principal de energía del cuerpo humano; el control de los niveles de glucosa en sangre en la orina y la sangre es una prueba de diagnóstico fundamental para la diabetes y otros trastornos; también es una prueba con una tira reactiva (Ch. 39, 42).

glucosuria (glucosuria) presencia de glucosa en la orina (también es correcto decir glicosuria) (Ch. 42).

gonadotropina coriónica humana (hCG) (human chorionic gonadotropin [hCG]) hormona secretada por el trofoblasto después de la fertilización del óvulo. Se puede detectar en la sangre y en la orina de mujeres embarazadas (Ch. 26, 44).

goniometría (goniometry) medición del movimiento articular (Ch. 33).

goniómetro (goniometer) instrumento usado para medir el ángulo de la amplitud de movimiento que tiene una articulación (Ch. 33).

Gráfica de Snellen (Snellen chart) las letras del abecedario conformadas en diferentes combinaciones, comenzando en la parte superior con una gran E y letras en tamaño descendente por línea hacia la parte inferior. Cada línea tiene una etiqueta con la medición de agudeza visual (Ch. 30).

grasa saturada (saturated fat) grasas que se caracterizan por ser sólidas a temperatura ambiente, se encuentran por lo general en productos de origen animal, como la mantequilla, leche, crema y huevos, como también en los aceites de palma y coco (Ch. 34).

gravidez (gravidity) cantidad total de embarazos que ha tenido una mujer, independientemente de la duración, incluido el actual (Ch. 26).

grupo sanguíneo ABO (ABO blood group) sistema de antígenos genéticamente determinados que se encuentra en la superficie de los eritrocitos. La población puede dividirse en cuatro grupos sanguíneos ABO: A, B, AB y O (Ch. 44).

haber (credit) columna usada para asentar pagos (Ch. 19).

habilidades directas (direct skills) habilidades específicas del trabajo. La habilidad para tomar una lectura de presión arterial sería específica del campo médico (Ch. 48).

habilidades transferibles (transferable skills) habilidades que se usarían en una serie de ocupaciones diferentes y no relacionadas. Saber mecanografía es un ejemplo de habilidad transferible. Pueden emplearla una secretaria, el empleado que ingresa datos, el asistente médico o el fabricante de ropa (Ch. 48).

hacer una copia de seguridad (backup) copiar o guardar datos en un lugar seguro para evitar perderlos en el caso de un desastre (Ch. 11).

hardware (hardware) equipo físico que usa el sistema informático para procesar los datos (Ch. 11).

hematocrito (hematocrit) porcentaje de glóbulos rojos dentro de una muestra de sangre entera anticoagulada (Ch. 41).

hematología (hematology) estudio de la sangre y de los tejidos que forman la sangre (Ch. 39, 41).

hematoma (hematoma) un moretón de tamaño considerable, acumulación de sangre alrededor de la zona de venopunción, durante o despuñs de ésta, provocada por el derrame de sangre del lugar en donde la aguja penetró la vena (Ch. 31, 40).

hematopoyesis (hematopoiesis) formación de células sanguíneas (Ch. 41).

hematuria (hematuria) presencia anormal de sangre en la orina, síntoma de muchos trastornos del sistema genitourinario y de enfermedades renales (Ch. 30, 42).

hemiplejía (hemiplegia) parálisis de un lado del cuerpo (Ch. 33).

hemoconcentración (hemoconcentration) acumulación de sangre en el lugar de la venopunción provocada al dejar el torniquete del brazo más de un minuto, lo que produce muestras sanguíneas inexactas (Ch. 40).

hemoglobina (hemoglobin) molécula dentro de los glóbulos rojos que transporta oxígeno (Ch. 41).

hemoglobinopatía (hemoglobinopathy) enfermedad heredada producto de la formación de una molécula de hemoglobina anormal (Ch. 41).

hemólisis (hemolysis) ruptura de los glóbulos rojos durante el proceso de recolección de sangre. El suero o el plasma se contaminan y tienen color rojizo (Ch. 40).

hemoptisis (hemoptysis) expectoración de sangre que proviene de la boca, de la laringe, de la tráquea, de los bronquios o de los pulmones, caracterizada por un repentino ataque de tos con producción de esputo sanguinolento (Ch. 30).

herida (wound) ruptura en la continuidad de las partes blandas de las estructuras corporales por violencia o traumatismo en los tejidos. En el caso de una herida abierta, la piel está abierta como en el caso de una laceración, abrasión, avulsión o incisión. En una herida cerrada, la piel no se rompe como en el caso de contusión, equimosis o hematoma (Ch. 9).

hialino (hyaline) transparente, cristalino; los cilindros hialinos están compuestos por mucoproteína, son transparentes y a menudo difíciles de ver en la orina (Ch. 42).

Hibeclens® (Hibeclens®) marca de solución de jabón antiséptico (Ch. 31).

hidróxido de potasio (KOH) (potassium hydroxide [KOH]) la solución al 10% colocada en los frotis vaginales, asícomo también en las raspaduras de piel, el cabello y otras sustancias secas para disolver el exceso de detritos. Esto despeja el campo visual para visualizar mejor los hongos y las esporas (Ch. 26, 43).

hidróxido de sodio (sodium hydroxide) sustancia química usada para quemar químicamente y destruir el tejido, generalmente en estado líquido cuando se usa en cirugía menor (Ch. 31).

higienización (sanitization) limpieza o fregado de instrumentos o fómites contaminados para eliminar tejidos, detritos u otros contaminantes (Ch. 22).

hiperemesis gravídica (hyperemesis gravidarum) náuseas y vómitos intensos durante el embarazo con imposibilidad de comer; puede provocar deshidratación grave (Ch. 26).

hiperextensión (hyperextension) posición de máxima extensión o extensión de una parte del cuerpo más allá de sus límites normales (Ch. 33).

hiperglucemia (hyperglycemia) aumento de los niveles de glucosa en sangre. La hiperglucemia no significa necesariamente que el paciente sea diabético sino que puede ser indicación de prediabetes (Ch. 44).

hiperpnea (hyperpnea) aumento de la frecuencia y la profundidad respiratoria, como se observa al hacer ejercicio, con el dolor, la fiebre y la histeria (Ch. 24).

hipertensión (hypertension) presión arterial que es regularmente superior a 140/90 mm Hg (Ch. 24).

hipertermia (hyperthermia) temperatura corporal superior al rango normal, fiebre inusualmente alta (Ch. 29).

hiperventilación (hyperventilation) frecuencia de ventilación superior a lo metabólicamente necesario que puede provocar alcalosis (Ch. 24).

hipoclorito de sodio (sodium hypochlorite) lejía de uso doméstico (Ch. 22).

hipocrómico (hypochromic) menos color de lo normal (Ch. 41).

hipoglucemia (hypoglycemia) estado en el cual el nivel de glucosa en sangre es inferior a lo normal (Ch. 40, 44).

hipogonadismo (hypogonadism) se presenta cuando los testículos producen poca o ninguna testosterona (Ch. 28).

hipotensión (hypotension) presión arterial anormalmente baja que produce profusión y oxigenación inadecuada de los tejidos (Ch. 24).

hipotensión supina (supine hypotension) afección que puede producirse cuando una mujer está recostada en posición supina; el útero grande y pesado presiona la vena cava inferior y la aorta, reduciendo el flujo de regreso al corazón (Ch. 26).

hipotermia (hypothermia) afección sumamente peligrosa relacionada con el frío que puede provocar la muerte si la persona no recibe atención y si no se revierte su avance. Los síntomas incluyen escalofríos, piel fría y confusión (Ch. 9, 29).

hipoventilación (hypoventilation) disminución de la frecuencia respiratoria con respiración superficial o poco profunda (Ch. 24).

hipovolémico (hypovolemic) es un tipo de choque en el cual el cuerpo ha perdido volumen de sangre o fluido a tal punto que no hay suficiente volumen circulante para llenar los ventrículos. El corazón intenta compensar amentando la frecuencia cardíaca (Ch. 9).

hipoxemia (hypoxemia) falta de oxígeno en la sangre (Ch. 36).

hipoxia (hypoxia) deficiencia de oxígeno (Ch. 26).

histerosalpingograma (hysterosalpingogram) radiografía delútero y de las trompas de Falopio usando un medio de contraste (Ch. 26).

histología (histology) estudio de la biopsia de la muestra de tejido para determinar una enfermedad (Ch. 39).

historia clínica orientada a la fuente (SOMR) (source-oriented medical record [SOMR]) tipo de registro de las fichas clínicas que incluye secciones separadas para diferentes fuentes de información de pacientes, como informes de laboratorio, informes de patología y notas de evolución (Ch. 14, 23).

historia clínica orientada al problema (POMR) (problem-oriented medical record [POMR]) forma de documentación de las fichas clínicas que usa una hoja en un lugar visible de la ficha para enumerar los datos de identificación vitales. Los problemas médicos de los pacientes se identifican por un número que corresponde a la ficha; por ejemplo, bronquitis es el N.° 1, fractura de muñeca es el N.° 2 y así sucesivamente (Ch. 14, 23).

hoja diaria (day sheet) formulario usado con el sistema de tablero de clavijas para registrar las transacciones diarias de pacientes (Ch. 19).

homeopatía (homeopathy) modalidad de curación que usa dosis diluidas de ciertas sustancias para crear una "huella de energía" en el cuerpo y dar lugar a la cura (Ch. 2).

homeostasia (homeostasis) estado de equilibrio del entorno interno (Ch. 34).

horas extra (overtime) dinero pagado a una tarifa no inferior a una hora y media de la tarifa habitual de pago después de completar una semana de trabajo de 40 horas (Ch. 46).

hordéolo (hordeolum) inflamación de la glándula sebácea en el párpado ocasionada por infección bacteriana; orzuelo (Ch. 30).

ictericia (jaundice) coloración amarillenta de la piel y de la esclerótica provocada por el exceso de bilirrubina en la sangre (Ch. 22, 25).

infarto de miocardio (myocardial infarction) ataque cardíaco; usualmente causado por un bloqueo de una o más arterias coronarias (Ch. 9, 37).

infertilidad (infertility) la incapacidad o capacidad disminuida de concebir (Ch. 28).

implante coclear (cochlear implantation) dispositivo eléctrico que recibe sonidos y transmite la señal resultante a los electrodos implantados en la cóclea. La señal estimula la cóclea y así la persona puede percibir sonidos (Ch. 27).

implícito (implicit) capaz de ser entendido aunque no esté expresado; tácito (Ch. 9).

improvisar (improvise) hacer, inventar u organizar en forma no planificada o espontánea (Ch. 1).

incompetencia (incompetence) legalmente, persona que es demente, inepta o no adulta (Ch. 7).

incontinencia (incontinence) incapacidad para controlar la orina o las heces (Ch. 29).

incremento (increment) aumento o suma en cuanto al número, tamaño o medida (Ch. 24).

indexar (indexing) seleccionar el nombre, el sujeto o el número conforme al cual se archiva un registro y determinar el orden en el cual se deben considerar las unidades (Ch. 14).

indicador de mensaje (flag) método para identificar un espacio en blanco o una pregunta sobre el significado de la persona que dicta; para ello, se agrega una nota o un marcador que indica la pregunta (Ch. 16).

índice metabólico basal (IMB) (basal metabolic rate [BMR]) nivel de energía necesario cuando el cuerpo está en reposo (Ch. 34).

índices de eritrocitos (erythrocyte indices) tres ecuaciones que proporcionan información sobre los tamaños y el contenido de hemoglobina de los glóbulos rojos. Éstos incluyen el volumen celular corpuscular medio, la hemoglobina corpuscular media y el volumen de hemoglobina corpuscular media (Ch. 41).

infarto (infarction) área de tejido de un órgano o de una parte del cuerpo que se necrosa (se muere) después de que se detiene el suministro sanguíneo (Ch. 37).

infección (infection) invasión de patógenos en el tejido vivo (Ch. 31).

infección del tracto urinario (ITU) (urinary tract infection [UTI]) también conocida como infección de la vejiga (Ch. 42).

infección oportunista (opportunistic infection) infección producto de un defecto en el sistema inmunitario que no se puede defender de los patógenos que normalmente se encuentran en el medio ambiente (Ch. 22).

inflamación (inflammation) respuesta inmunitaria no específica normal que tiene el cuerpo ante cualquier tipo de lesión (traumatismo, bacteriana, viral y por temperaturas extremas) (Ch. 31).

informe de autopsia (autopsy report) también llamado protocolo de autopsia, informe de necropsia o informe del médico forense. Las autopsias se realizan para determinar la causa de la muerte o para establecer y confirmar la presencia de enfermedad (Ch. 16).

informe de consulta (consultation report) documento que informa las conclusiones y el consejo de otro proveedor que revisó a un paciente a pedido del proveedor principal que lo atiende (Ch. 16).

informe de historia clínica y examen físico (H&P) (history and physical examination report [H&P]) informe de la historia clínica y examen físico de un paciente para documentar el motivo de la consulta (Ch. 16).

informe de patología (pathology report) informes médicos generados para describir los exámenes macro y microscópicos realizados durante un procedimiento quirúrgico (Ch. 16, 31).

informe quirúrgico (OR) (operative report [OR]) informe médico que documenta los detalles de un procedimiento quirúrgico (Ch. 16).

informes actuales (current reports) informes como antecedentes y exámenes físicos que se deben realizar en el plazo de 24 horas (Ch. 16).

informes anteriores (old reports) informes como el resumen del alta que se deben completar en el plazo de 71 horas (Ch. 16).

informes de radiología y de diagnóstico por imágenes (radiology and imaging reports) informes médicos que describen los resultados y las interpretaciones del radiólogo (Ch. 16).

ingeniería genética (genetic engineering) alteración, manipulación, sustitución o reparación de material genético (Ch. 8).

inhalador de dosis medida (metered dose inhaler) dispositivo usado para aplicar una cantidad recetada de medicamento en las vías respiratorias, especialmente los pulmones (Ch. 30).

inmunidad (immunity) capacidad del cuerpo de resistir patógenos específicos y sus toxinas (Ch. 22).

inmunidad humoral (humoral immunity) inmunidad mediada por anticuerpos en los líquidos corporales, como por ejemplo, el plasma y la linfa (Ch. 22).

inmunidad mediada por células (cell-mediated immunity) actividades reguladoras de las células T durante la respuesta inmunitaria específica (Ch. 22).

inmunoglobulinas (immunoglobulins) familia de proteínas capaces de actuar como anticuerpos que, de este modo, protegen a las personas de los microorganismos patógenos; también, anticuerpos producidos por las células del sistema de respuesta inmunitaria (Ch. 30).

inmunohematología (immunohematology) estudio de los antígenos y los anticuerpos del grupo sanguíneo; banco de sangre (Ch. 39).

inmunología (immunology) estudio de los componentes del sistema inmunitario y su función (Ch. 39).

inmunomodulador (immunomodulator) sustancia que tiene la capacidad de modificar las respuestas inmunitarias (Ch. 22, 43).

inmunosuprimido (immunosuppressed) paciente cuyo sistema inmunitario no está sano debido a enfermedad, medicamentos y genética. Estos pacientes pueden ser especialmente susceptibles al ataque de microorganismos (Ch. 22, 43).

inobservancia (noncompliant) no seguir una orden o una instrucción exigida (Ch. 7).

inoculación (inoculation) inyección (Ch. 22).

inocular (inoculate) colocar colonias de microorganismos en medios nutrientes (Ch. 43).

insulina (insulin) hormona segregada por células beta de los islotes de Langerhans del páncreas esencial para el metabolismo correcto de la glucosa (Ch. 44).

interfaz de red (network interface) software, servidores y conexiones de cable usadas para conectar computadoras (Ch. 11).

intermediación cultural (cultural brokering) acto de comunicar, vincular o mediar entre grupos o personas reduciendo los conflictos o produciendo cambios (Ch. 4).

intermediario fiscal (fiscal intermediary) administrador local de Medicare (Ch. 17).

interrogatorio (interrogatory) conjunto de preguntas escritas que se deben responder, bajo juramento, dentro de un período específico de tiempo; parte de un proceso de exhibición de pruebas (Ch. 7).

intraepitelial (intraepithelium) dentro del epitelio (Ch. 26).

intrahospitalaria (nosocomial) infección adquirida en un entorno de atención médica (hospital, clínica, hogar de ancianos) (Ch. 22).

inversión (inversion) movimiento de una parte del cuerpo hacia adentro (Ch. 33).

involución (involution) regreso del útero a su tamaño y forma normales después del parto (Ch. 26).

inyección a chorro (jet injection) inyección administrada debajo de la piel sin aguja, usando la fuerza del líquido bajo presión para atravesar la piel (Ch. 22).

irregularidad (misfeasance) término del derecho civil que se refiere a un acto legal que se ejecuta en forma incorrecta o ilegítima (Ch. 7).

isoeléctrico (isoelectric) que tiene potenciales eléctricos iguales. Se representa en el ECG como la línea horizontal plana de base (Ch. 37).

isótopo (isotope) un elemento químico (Ch. 32).

isquemia (ischemia) falta temporal y local de sangre en un órgano o parte provocada por la obstrucción de la circulación (Ch. 37).

itinerario (itinerary) plan por escrito detallado de un viaje propuesto (Ch. 45).

jerarquía de necesidades (hierarchy of needs) necesidades que se organizan en un orden o posicionamiento específico, disposición secuencial. Relacionado con Abraham Maslow (Ch. 4).

jerga (jargon) palabras, frases o terminología específica de una profesión (Ch. 12).

Junta de Acreditación de Escuelas de Educación en Salud (ABHES) (Accrediting Bureau of Health Education Schools [ABHES]) entidad que acredita a las empresas privadas, instituciones de educación superior en los EE.UU. que ofrecen programas de educación de salud auxiliares, como también acreditación programática de asistencia médica, asociado en tecnología médica y programas de enfermería quirúrgica (Ch. 1, 47).

kit para derrames (spill kit) materiales envasados comercialmente que contienen insumos y equipos necesarios para limpiar un derrame de una sustancia biológica peligrosa (Ch. 22).

laberintitis (labyrinthitis) inflamación del oído interno o laberinto (Ch. 25).

laboratorios con base en el hospital (hospital-based laboratories) laboratorios de propiedad del hospital que realizan la mayoría de las pruebas que requiere el hospital y las comunidades locales (Ch. 39).

laboratorios de referencia (reference laboratories) laboratorios independientes, ubicados por región, que usan los hospitales para pruebas complejas, caras o especializadas (Ch. 39).

laboratorios del consultorio de los médicos (POL) (physicians' office laboratories [POL]) laboratorios dentro de los consultorios de los médicos donde se realizan análisis de laboratorio comunes en el consultorio (Ch. 39).

Lamaze (Lamaze) técnica que consiste en ejercicios de respiración para facilitar el parto (Ch. 26).

lámpara de Wood (Wood's lamp) fuente de iluminación especial usada para detectar organismos que brillan con la luz, como ciertos hongos, bacteria y parásitos. Dos ejemplos son la sarna y la tiña. Con la lámpara de Wood es posible detectar rasguños en el ojo después de que éste ha sido impregnado con colorante fluorescente. También usada para determinar el margen de disección de un melanoma (Ch. 43).

laparoscopía (laparoscopy) procedimiento en el que se utiliza un instrumento con luz para ver el interior de la cavidad pélvica (Ch. 26).

LASIK (LASIK) abreviatura de "laser-assisted in situ keratomileusis" (queratomileusis in situ asistida con láser), un tipo de cirugía ocular de la córnea que elimina o reduce la necesidad de usar lentes correctivas en casos de miopía grave (Ch. 10).

lector óptico de caracteres (OCR) (optical character reader [OCR]) escáner computarizado del Servicio Postal de los EE. UU. que lee las direcciones impresas en la correspondencia. Si la información está correctamente formateada, entonces el OCR encontrará una coincidencia en los archivos de direcciones e imprimirá un código de barra en el margen inferior derecho del sobre (Ch. 15).

lenguaje corporal (body language) comunicación no verbal que incluye movimientos corporales inconscientes, gestos y expresiones faciales que acompañan los mensajes verbales (Ch. 4).

lesión (lesion) lastimadura o herida. Zona limitada de tejido que se ha alterado patológicamente (Ch. 22, 30).

leucocito (leukocyte) glóbulo blanco, uno de los componentes de la sangre (Ch. 40, 41).

Ley de Autodeterminación del Paciente (PSDA) (Patient Self-Determination Act [PSDA]) ley que incluye la Directiva Avanzada que les otorga a los pacientes el derecho a participar en las decisiones sobre su atención médica (Ch. 7).

Ley de Portabilidad y Responsabilidad de Seguros de Salud (HIPAA) (Health Insurance Portability and Accountability Act [HIPAA]) normas, reglamentaciones y procedimientos gubernamentales producto de la legislación destinada a proteger la confidencialidad de la información de los pacientes (Ch. 16).

ley de prescripción (statute of limitations) ley que define el período durante el cual puede tener lugar la acción legal (Ch. 20).

Ley de Veracidad en los Préstamos (Truth-in-Lending Act) también conocida como Ley de Protección de Créditos del Consumidor de 1968; ley que exige a los proveedores de créditos en cuotas que declaren los cargos por escrito y que expresen el interés en forma de tasa anual (Ch. 20).

Ley sobre Prácticas Justas para el Cobro de Deudas (Fair Debt Collection Practice Act) ley federal de 1977 que establece las prácticas de cobro de deudas (Ch. 20).

leyenda (caption) método de designación usado en guías de archivos (Ch. 14).

leyes del Buen Samaritano (Good Samaritan laws) leyes diseñadas para proteger a las personas contra acciones legales cuando prestan asistencia médica de emergencia, sin retribución, dentro de las áreas de su formación y pericia (Ch. 12).

libido (libido) impulso sexual (Ch. 28).

libro mayor (ledger) registro de gastos, pagos y ajustes relacionados con el paciente o la familia (Ch. 19).

licencia (license) declaración de permiso que autoriza el uso de software informático con derecho de autor (Ch. 11).

licenciatura (bachelor's degree)   título académico de cuatro años de estudio conferido por universidades e instituciones de enseñanza superior (Ch. 1).

ligadura (ligature)   longitud del hilo de sutura sin aguja, usada para cerrar vasos durante la cirugía (Ch. 31).

limpiador ultrasónico (ultrasonic cleaner)   máquina que usa la energía de ondas de sonido de alta frecuencia que se agitan para desinfectar instrumentos antes de la esterilización (Ch. 22).

linfocito (lymphocyte)   glóbulo blanco con un núcleo no segmentado denso y que carece de gránulos en el citoplasma (Ch. 41).

liofilizado (lyophilized)   proceso por el cual se congela rápidamente una sustancia a temperaturas sumamente bajas y luego se deshidrata la sustancia en alto vacío (secado por congelación) (Ch. 27).

lipemia (lipemia)   cantidad excesiva de grasas (lípidos) en la sangre, lo que produce una muestra sanguínea que tiene aspecto lechoso (Ch. 40).

lipoproteína de alta densidad (HDL) (high-density lipoprotein [HDL])   lipoproteína de la sangre compuesta principalmente de proteína; elimina el colesterol de los tejidos periféricos y los transporta al hígado para la excreción (Ch. 44).

lipoproteína de baja densidad (LDL) (low-density lipoprotein [LDL])   lipoproteína de la sangre compuesta principalmente de colesterol. El colesterol que transporta la LDL se puede depositar en los tejidos periféricos y se asocia con un mayor riesgo de enfermedad cardíaca (Ch. 44).

líquido corporal (body fluid)   toda secreción o excreción del cuerpo humano, por ejemplo, vaginal, cefalorraquídeo, sinovial, pleural, pericárdico, peritoneal, amniótico, esputo y saliva (Ch. 38).

litigio (litigation)   acción judicial (Ch. 7).

litotomía (lithotomy)   los pacientes se recuestan de espalda en posición decúbito dorsal, excepto por las nalgas que deben estar lo más cerca posible del borde inferior de la mesa y los pies colocados en estribos fijados al pie de la mesa (Ch. 25).

localizador uniforme de recursos (URL) (uniform resource locater [URL])   dirección que define la ruta para llegar a un archivo en la Web o en cualquier otra instalación de Internet (Ch. 12).

loquios (lochia)   secreción uterina de sangre, moco y tejido presente durante el período posterior al parto (Ch. 22, 26).

luxación (dislocation)   desplazamiento de un hueso o de una articulación de su posición normal (Ch. 30).

luz (lumen)   espacio dentro de una arteria, vena, intestino, agujas y catéter o tubo (Ch. 24).

macroasignación (macroallocation)   de recursos médicos escasos; decisiones que toma el Congreso, las agencias de sistemas de salud y las compañías de seguro (Ch. 8).

macrocítico (macrocytic)   término que describe una célula más grande de lo normal (Ch. 41).

mala praxis (malpractice)   negligencia profesional (Ch. 7, 45).

malabsorción (malabsorption)   absorción inadecuada de los nutrientes del tracto intestinal (Ch. 30).

malestar (malaise)   molestia, incomodidad o indisposición, a menudo indicador de infección (Ch. 22, 30).

malversar (embezzle)   apropiarse fraudulentamente para uso propio (Ch. 45).

mandato (mandate)   orden formal de obedecer ciertas normas y reglamentaciones (Ch. 38).

manómetro (manometer)   dispositivo para medir la presión líquida o gaseosa. La medición se expresa en milímetros de mercurio o agua (Ch. 24).

manual de procedimientos (procedure manual)   manual que proporciona información detallada relacionada con el desempeño de tareas dentro de la descripción del cargo (Ch. 45).

marcha (gait)   manera o estilo de caminar, incluidos el ritmo y la velocidad (Ch. 33).

matrícula (license)   permiso expedido por la autoridad competente (el estado) para ejercer una profesión; permiso de actuar (Ch. 1).

matriculación (licensure)   otorgamiento de matrículas para ejercer una profesión (Ch. 1).

matriz (matrix)   para establecer una matriz de citas, los espacios de tiempo no disponibles del proveedor se marcan con una X. Los pacientes no se programan durante esos horarios (Ch. 13).

matriz redundante de discos independientes (RAID) (redundant array independent disk [RAID])   esquema de almacenamiento de datos que usa múltiples discos duros para compartir o replicar datos entre las unidades (Ch. 11).

mecánica corporal (body mechanics)   práctica de uso de ciertos grupos musculares clave junto con una alineación corporal correcta para evitar lesiones al levantar o trasladar objetos pesados o difíciles de trasladar (Ch. 33).

mecanismo de defensa (defense mechanism)   comportamiento que protege la psiquis de culpa, ansiedad o vergüenza (Ch. 4).

meconio (meconium)   primeras heces del recién nacido (Ch. 26).

mediación (mediation)   resolución de conflictos que permite al mediador ayudar a ambas partes a conciliar las diferencias y a llegar a una solución aceptable (Ch. 7).

médicamente indigente (medically indigent)   se refiere a las personas que no pueden pagar su propia cobertura médica (Ch. 7).

Medicare Parte A (Medicare Part A)   beneficios que cubren la hospitalización en hospitales y en centros de enfermería especializada, la atención en hospicios y transfusiones de sangre (Ch. 17).

Medicare Parte B (Medicare Part B)   beneficios que cubren la atención ambulatoria en hospitales y los servicios de proveedores de atención médica (Ch. 17).

Medicare Parte C (Medicare Part C)   comúnmente se los llama planes de Medicare Advantage. Estos planes están aprobados por Medicare y son administrados por empresas privadas (Ch. 17).

Medicare Parte D (Medicare Part D)   cobertura de medicamentos recetados por parte de Medicare (Ch. 17).

medicina de rehabilitación (rehabilitation medicine)   campo de las disciplinas médicas que procura restablecer la función normal, o casi normal, de una persona o de una parte del cuerpo después de una enfermedad o lesión usando agentes físicos y mecánicos (Ch. 33).

medicina integradora (integrative medicine)   conjunción de dos o más modalidades de tratamiento para que funcionen como un todo armonioso, como se observa en las formas alternativas de la atención médica (Ch. 2).

médico de atención primaria (PCP) (primary care physician [PCP])   médico de atención primaria de un paciente a través del cual se coordina toda la atención (Ch. 17).

medición (mensuration)   método de examen mediante el uso del proceso de medición. Las medidas de altura y peso, la longitud de un miembro y la cantidad de flexión y extensión de una extremidad son todas formas de medición (Ch. 25).

medios de sostén (holding media)   medios específicos en el transporte de microorganismos para sustentar la vida de los organismos hasta que se coloquen en un medio nutriente en el laboratorio (Ch. 43).

medios sociales (social media)   medios basados en la red para la interacción social (Ch. 45).

memorándum (memorandum)   correspondencia que se usa dentro de la oficina, comúnmente llamada memorando (Ch. 15).

memoria (memory)   se refiere al almacenamiento de datos en la computadora. La memoria puede ser volátil (se pierde cuando se apaga la computadora) o no volátil (escrita permanentemente en un dispositivo de almacenamiento) (Ch. 11).

memoria de acceso aleatorio (RAM) (random access memory [RAM])   tipo de memoria de computadora que se puede escribir y leer. La palabra *aleatorio* significa que se puede leer en cualquier ubicación en cualquier momento. RAM comúnmente se refiere a la memoria interna de una computadora. RAM generalmente es un área de memoria temporal rápida donde residen los datos y los programas hasta que se guardan o hasta que se desconecta la energía (Ch. 11).

memoria de almacenamiento de datos (data storage memory)   memoria permanente que no forma parte de la placa madre. Usa cualquier dispositivo de almacenamiento de datos adecuado. Puede ser memoria de sólo lectura o de lectura/escritura (Ch. 11).

memoria de sólo lectura (ROM) (read-only memory [ROM]) datos almacenados permanentemente en la computadora que no se pueden sobrescribir sin dispositivos especiales. Se requieren instrucciones de almacenamiento para iniciar la computadora. Se encuentra en la placa madre (Ch. 11).

menisco (meniscus) curvatura en la superficie de arriba de un líquido cuando se lo coloca en un recipiente (Ch. 24, 36).

menor (minor) persona que no ha alcanzado la mayoría de edad, generalmente 18 años (Ch. 7).

menor emancipado (emancipated minor) personas menores de 18 años que son financieramente responsables de sí mismas y libres del cuidado paterno (Ch. 7).

menor maduro (mature minor) persona, generalmente menor de 18 años, que puede entender y medir las consecuencias del tratamiento a pesar de su corta edad (Ch. 7).

mentor (mentor) persona asignada o solicitada para ayudar en la capacitación, la orientación o la instrucción de otra (Ch. 45).

mesa de Mayo (Mayo stand) mesa con bandeja metálica portátil para establecer pequeños campos estériles para cirugías y procedimientos menores (Ch. 31).

meta (goal) resultado o logro hacia el cual se dirigen todos los esfuerzos (Ch. 5).

metabolismo (metabolism) totalidad de todos los cambios, químicos y físicos, que se producen en el cuerpo (Ch. 34).

metas a corto plazo (short-range goals) las metas a largo plazo se dividen y se reacomodan en segmentos de tiempo más cortos y más manejables (Ch. 5).

metas a largo plazo (long-range goals) logros que pueden tardar de tres a cinco años en concretarse (Ch. 5).

metástasis (metastasis) en cáncer, diseminación de células malignas a partir de un tumor primario a una nueva ubicación (Ch. 28).

metrorragia (metrorrhagia) hemorragia uterina en intervalos irregulares (Ch. 26).

micología (mycology) estudio de los hongos (Ch. 39, 43).

microasignación (microallocation) de recursos médicos escasos; decisiones que toman los proveedores y los miembros individuales del equipo de atención médica (Ch. 8).

microbiología (microbiology) rama de la biología que trata del estudio de formas microscópicas de vida (Ch. 39, 43).

microcítico (microcytic) término que describe una célula más pequeña de lo normal (Ch. 41).

microorganismo (microorganism) ser vivo microscópico capaz de transmitirse y reproducirse en circunstancias específicas (Ch. 22).

mineral principal (major mineral) mineral que el cuerpo requiere en grandes cantidades (Ch. 34).

miopía (myopia) visión corta; es ocasionada por un globo ocular alargado; la imagen se enfoca en la parte delantera de la retina, lo que produce la imposibilidad de enfocar objetos a distancia (Ch. 30).

miringotomía (myringotomy) incisión en la membrana timpánica; parte del tratamiento para la otitis media (Ch. 27).

modalidades (modalities) agentes físicos como calor, frío, luz, agua y electricidad usados para tratar disfunciones musculares o articulares (Ch. 33).

modificador (modifier) código adicional que se puede agregar a un código CPT de cinco dígitos para explicar el servicio provisto (Ch. 18).

modulado (modulated) habla que varía en tono e intensidad (Ch. 12).

monitor Holter (Holter monitor) un registro continuo portátil de actividad cardíaca para un período de 24 horas (Ch. 37).

monitoreo de fármacos terapéuticos (TDM) (therapeutic drug monitoring [TDM]) análisis de sangre periódicos para determinar la eficacia de un fármaco en particular. Los fármacos deberán alcanzar un nivel terapéutico para que sean terapéuticos o eficaces. Si el nivel en sangre del fármaco está por debajo del espectro de eficacia terapéutica, el proveedor probablemente aumentará la dosis. Del mismo

modo, si el fármaco supera el espectro terapéutico, el proveedor probablemente la reducirá (Ch. 39).

monocito (monocyte) glóbulo blanco sin gránulos citoplasmáticos que tiene un núcleo grande no segmentado y arriñonado (Ch. 41).

mononucleosis infecciosa (infectious mononucleosis) enfermedad infecciosa aguda que afecta principalmente el tejido linfoide, provocada por el virus de Epstein-Barr (Ch. 44).

montaje (mounting) proceso que aplica de manera secuencial una parte de cada una de las 12 derivaciones del registro del ECG en un formulario o planilla de montaje de papel preparada comercialmente, como parte del registro permanente del paciente (Ch. 37).

morbilidad (morbidity) cantidad de casos de enfermedad en una población específica (Ch. 22).

mordiente (mordant) sustancia que fija el colorante a un objeto; el yodo es un mordiente en la tinción de Gram (Ch. 43).

morfología (morphology) forma y estructura de un organismo (Ch. 22, 43).

mortalidad (mortality) la proporción del número de muertes en una población dada (Ch. 22).

moxibustión (moxibustion) antiguo método chino de tratamiento que usa una sustancia de una planta en polvo sobre la piel para provocar una ampolla (Ch. 3).

multigrávida (multigravida) mujer que ha estado embarazada más de una vez (Ch. 26).

mutilación genital femenina (female genital mutilation) eliminación parcial o completa del clítoris, eliminación parcial o total de los labios menores y/o los labios mayores, estrechamiento del orificio vaginal mediante la creación de un sello recubridor y la pinchadura, la perforación o la cauterización de los genitales (Ch. 8).

negligencia (negligence) falta de cumplimiento de un determinado estándar de atención (Ch. 7, 45).

nematodo (nematode) gusano redondo (Ch. 43).

neonatal (neonatal) relativo al recién nacido (Ch. 26).

neonato (neonate) recién nacido (Ch. 27).

neurogénico (neurogenic) tipo de choque en el que hay una lesión o un trauma en el sistema nervioso que ocasiona la pérdida del tono en los vasos sanguíneos, ocasionando dilatación masiva de las arteriolas y las vénulas. Esto produce una caída drástica de la presión sanguínea (Ch. 9).

neurosensorial (sensorineural) pérdida permanente de la audición producto del daño o una malformación del oído medio y el nervio auditivo (Ch. 27).

neutrófilo (neutrophil) el tipo más común de glóbulo blanco granulocítico (Ch. 41).

nevo (nevus) lunar (Ch. 29).

niacina (niacin) una de las vitaminas del complejo B (Ch. 34).

nistagmo (nystagmus) movimiento involuntario continuo de los ojos (Ch. 30).

nitrato de plata (silver nitrate) antiséptico astringente cáustico. En su forma de líquido débil, se aplica en los ojos de los recién nacidos para prevenir infecciones en el nacimiento. En el consultorio médico, a menudo se usa como sustancia sólida impregnada en el extremo de un aplicador de madera. Las varillas del aplicador de nitrato de plata contienen ácido clorhídrico y otras sustancias químicas y comúnmente se usan para cauterizar pequeños vasos sanguíneos en la nariz o en otras membranas mucosas (Ch. 31).

nitrógeno líquido (liquid nitrogen) llamado comúnmente, y erróneamente, hielo seco; el nitrógeno líquido es un agente congelante volátil usado para destruir tejido no deseado como las verrugas (Ch. 31).

nitrógeno ureico en sangre (BUN) (blood urea nitrogen [BUN]) nitrógeno en la sangre en forma de urea. El nivel de nitrógeno en la sangre es un indicador de la función renal (Ch. 44).

no diferenciada (undifferentiated) degeneración maligna de una célula (Ch. 22).

nocturia (nocturia) micción excesiva durante la noche (Ch. 28, 30).

nomograma (nomogram) gráfico que muestra la relación entre valores numéricos. Con él se puede calcular el área de superficie corporal (ASC) de un paciente (Ch. 36).

normocítico (normocytic) término que describe una célula de tamaño normal (Ch. 41).

normocrómico (normochromic) de color normal, en este caso, cuando se refiere a glóbulos rojos (Ch. 41).

notas clínicas (chart notes) (también llamadas notas de evolución) observaciones formales o informales del proveedor sobre la presentación de un problema, los resultados físicos y el plan de tratamiento para un paciente examinado en el consultorio, la clínica, el centro de cuidados agudos o el departamento de emergencias (Ch. 16).

notas de evolución (progress notes) también llamadas notas clínicas. Observaciones formales o informales del proveedor sobre la presentación de un problema, los resultados físicos y el plan de tratamiento de un paciente examinado en el consultorio, la clínica, un centro de cuidados agudos o el departamento de emergencias (Ch. 16).

nueva certificación (recertification) documentación admitida como prueba de educación continua para mantener una credencial profesional (Ch. 47).

nulípara (nullipara) mujer que no ha llevado un embarazo hasta el estadio de viabilidad (Ch. 26).

nutrición (nutrition) estudio de cómo se incorporan los nutrientes al cuerpo y cómo éste los usa (Ch. 34).

nutriente (nutrient) sustancia ingerida que ayuda al cuerpo a mantenerse en estado homeostático (Ch. 34).

obesidad mórbida (morbid obesity) obesidad tan grave que puede provocar una enfermedad grave (Ch. 30).

objetivo (objective) signo del paciente que es visible, palpable o mensurable para el observador (Ch. 23); también; lente con aumento que es el que está más cerca del objeto cuando se lo observa con un microscopio (Ch. 39).

objetivo profesional (career objective) expresa su objetivo en su profesión y el cargo para el que se postula (Ch. 48).

objetos filosos (sharps) agujas o escalpelos u otros instrumentos con punta que pueden penetrar o perforar una herida en la piel (Ch. 22).

obstáculos (roadblocks) mensajes verbales o no verbales que obstaculizan la comunicación (Ch. 4).

oclusión (occlusion) cierre de una vía (Ch. 9).

oclusor (occluder) instrumento usado para obstruir o cerrar la visión o la luz (Ch. 30).

ocultamiento (masking) intento de ocultar o reprimir los sentimientos o el mensaje verdaderos (Ch. 4).

ofuscación (obfuscation) enredar o confundir las cosas (Ch. 12).

oligomineral (trace mineral) mineral que el cuerpo necesita en pequeñas cantidades (Ch. 34).

oliguria (oliguria) disminución en la producción de orina (Ch. 30).

omisión (nonfeasance) término del derecho civil que se refiere a la falta de cumplimiento de un acto, una obligación oficial o un requisito legal (Ch. 7).

operación cesárea (cesarean section) nacimiento del feto a través de una incisión quirúrgica en elútero (Ch. 26).

orden del día (agenda) lista impresa de temas que se tratarán durante una reunión, que a veces establece el tiempo asignado (Ch. 15, 45).

organización de atención administrada (MCO) (managed care organization [MCO]) organización de seguros de salud que se rige según los principios de fuerte dependencia en la contratación selectiva de los proveedores, el uso de médicos de atención primaria, gestión de utilización prospectiva y retrospectiva, uso de pautas de tratamiento para trastornos crónicos de alto costo y énfasis en la atención preventiva, la educación y el cumplimiento de los planes de tratamiento por parte del paciente (Ch. 17).

organización de mantenimiento de la salud (HMO) (health maintenance organization [HMO]) tipo de actividad de atención administrada que generalmente se constituye como una empresa con fines de lucro con empleados remunerados. Las HMO "con paredes" ofrecen una variedad de servicios médicos bajo un solo techo; las HMO "sin paredes" por lo general contratan a proveedores de la comunidad para brindar servicios a los pacientes a cambio de una tarifa acordada (Ch. 2, 17).

organización de proveedor exclusivo (EPO) (exclusive provider organization [EPO]) plan de organización de proveedor preferido (PPO, por sus siglas en inglés) de conjunto cerrado en la cual los afiliados no reciben ningún beneficio si optan por recibir atención de un proveedor que no está en la EPO (Ch. 17).

organización de proveedor preferido (PPO) (preferred provider organization [PPO]) organización de proveedores que forman una red para ofrecer descuentos a los compradores de seguros de salud (Ch. 17).

orina residual (residual urine) cantidad de orina que queda en la vejiga inmediatamente después de vaciarla; se observa con la hiperplasia de próstata (Ch. 28, 29).

orquidectomía (orchidectomy) extirpación quirúrgica de un testículo (Ch. 28).

ortopnea (orthopnea) dificultad para respirar en cualquier posición que no sea en posición vertical (Ch. 24).

osciloscopio (oscilloscope) dispositivo electrónico usado para registrar la actividad eléctrica del corazón, el cerebro y los tejidos musculares (Ch. 32, 37).

osteoporosis (osteoporosis) disminución de la densidad de los huesos largos, los huesos pélvicos y las vértebras (Ch. 29).

otoscopio (otoscope) instrumento usado para examinar el conducto auditivo externo y la membrana timpánica (Ch. 30).

óvulos (ova) huevos, en este caso, huevos de parásitos (Ch. 43).

oxidación (oxidation) proceso en el cual una sustancia se combina con el oxígeno (Ch. 34).

oxímetro de pulso (pulse oximeter) dispositivo (similar a un clip) que se puede sujetar al dedo o al puente de la nariz. Mide la concentración de oxígeno en la sangre (Ch. 24).

oxitocina (oxytocin) hormona hipofisaria que estimula la contracción de los músculos delútero y así induce el parto (Ch. 26).

palabras clave (keywords) palabras relacionadas con un puesto específico en un trabajo. Las palabras clave pueden ser habilidades específicas de un trabajo o palabras específicas de la profesión (Ch. 48).

palabras de relleno (buffer words) palabras prescindibles que se usan mientras se atiende el teléfono (Ch. 12).

paliativa (palliative) medida adoptada para aliviar los síntomas de la enfermedad (Ch. 22, 32).

palidez (pallor) falta de color, lividez (Ch. 25).

palpar (palpate) sentir con la yema de los dedos, buscar la vena con el tacto presionando y soltando (Ch. 40).

paludismo (malaria) enfermedad infecciosa aguda provocada por la presencia de parásitos protozoarios dentro de los glóbulos rojos; generalmente es consecuencia de la picadura de un mosquito hembra (Ch. 3, 22).

panel (panel) serie de pruebas relacionadas con un órgano o sistema de órganos en particular del funcionamiento corporal. Por ejemplo, un panel hepático controla muchas funciones diferentes del hígado. Antes llamado "perfil" (Ch. 39).

pantalla antirreflejo (antiglare screen) filtro que se coloca sobre la pantalla del monitor de un equipo de computación para reducir el reflejo (Ch. 11).

paño fenestrado (fenestrated drape) tipo de paño con un orificio, generalmente redondo, que se puede colocar con el orificio sobre un área particular del cuerpo; se usa en cirugía y para exámenes proctológicos (Ch. 25).

papel bond (bond paper) papel duradero y más resistente que generalmente se usa para correspondencia (Ch. 15).

paquete de hidrocolator (hydrocollator pack) paquete lleno con gel que se calienta a baño María (Ch. 33).

paracentesis (paracentesis) punción de una cavidad para extraer líquido (Ch. 22).

parasitología (parasitology) estudio de organismos (parásitos y los huevos) que viven en o dentro de otro organismo y a costa de él (Ch. 39, 43).

parche (patch) modificación en el software para arreglar deficiencias en él. A menudo se descarga del sitio web del proveedor del software o de disquetes suministrados por el proveedor (Ch. 11).

parenteral (parenteral) inyección de una sustancia líquida en el cuerpo mediante una vía alternativa al canal alimentario (Ch. 22, 36).

paridad (parity) llevar un embarazo hasta el punto de viabilidad independientemente del resultado (Ch. 26).

parir (parturition) proceso de dar a luz (Ch. 26).

participación en las ganancias (profit sharing) compartir las utilidades, las ganancias y los beneficios de una organización (Ch. 45).

pasantía (internship) etapa de transición entre las clases y el empleo (Ch. 1).

pasivo (liability) deudas y obligaciones financieras de las cuales uno es responsable (Ch. 21).

patógeno (pathogen) microorganismo que produce enfermedades (Ch. 22, 43).

patógeno transmitido por la sangre (bloodborne pathogen) microorganismo capaz de producir una enfermedad y que se encuentra en la sangre o en los hemoderivados (Ch. 22).

patrimonio neto (owner's equity) monto en que los activos de la empresa superan los pasivos. También llamado activo neto, patrimonio y capital contable (Ch. 21).

patrón (standard) normas establecidas para medir la calidad, el peso, el alcance o el valor (Ch. 22, 38).

pelagra (pellagra) enfermedad producida por una deficiencia de vitamina B$_3$ (ácido nicotínico) caracterizada por llagas en la piel, diarrea, ansiedad, confusión y muerte, si no se trata (Ch. 34).

percepción (perception) comprensión consciente de los sentimientos propios y de los demás (Ch. 4).

percusión (percussion) el proceso de provocación de sonidos del cuerpo mediante golpes suaves con un martillo de percusión o con los dedos. Las vibraciones y los sonidos de los órganos y las cavidades subyacentes pueden sentirse y oírse (Ch. 25).

periférico (peripheral) alejado del centro del cuerpo (Ch. 24).

período de beneficios (benefit period) tiempo especificado durante el cual los beneficios se pagarán en virtud de ciertos tipos de coberturas de seguro médico (Ch. 17).

período de prueba (probation) período durante el cual el empleado y el personal de supervisión pueden determinar si el entorno y el cargo son satisfactorios para el empleado (Ch. 46).

período sin cobertura (donut hole) dentro del programa de medicamentos recetados de la Parte D de Medicare, el período sin cobertura es la etapa en la cual todos los costos son cubiertos por el afiliado en lugar de los CMS (Ch. 17).

permeable (patent) abierto, no obstruido (Ch. 26).

peróxido de hidrógeno (hydrogen peroxide) solución antibacteriana que tiene una acción de limpieza mecánica (Ch. 31).

personas con autodeterminación (inner-directed people) personas que deciden por sí mismas lo que quieren hacer con su vida (Ch. 5).

personas influenciables (outer-directed people) personas que permiten que los acontecimientos, que otras personas o que los factores ambientales determinen su comportamiento (Ch. 5).

peste bubónica (bubonic plague) enfermedad infecciosa con alta tasa de mortalidad que es transmitida a los seres humanos a través de ratas y ardillas terrestres infectadas que fueron mordidas por la pulga de las ratas (Ch. 3).

petrissage (petrissage) movimiento de amasamiento en masaje (Ch. 33).

pH (pH) escala que indica la alcalinidad o la acidez relativa de la solución; medición de la concentración de iones de hidrógeno (Ch. 42).

pico (peak) lo opuesto de "valle", es el punto en el cual el fármaco alcanza su mayor nivel en el cuerpo, generalmente tiene lugar aproximadamente a los 30 minutos después de la administración. En las pruebas de laboratorio, el pico indica al proveedor la mayor influencia que tendría el fármaco en el cuerpo con esa dosis en particular (Ch. 38).

pielograma intravenoso (intravenous pyelogram) estudios radiográficos de los riñones, uréter y vejiga usando un medio de contraste (Ch. 28).

piorrea (pyorrhea) secreción de pus de las encías, alrededor de los dientes (Ch. 25).

pirexia (pyrexia) fiebre (Ch. 24).

piridoxina (pyridoxine) vitamina B$_6$ (Ch. 34).

piuria (pyuria) pus en la orina (Ch. 30).

placa de Petri (petri dish) placa plástica en la que se coloca el agar para el crecimiento de bacterias (Ch. 43).

placenta previa (placenta previa) la placenta se implanta en la parte inferior delútero y puede cubrir parcial o completamente el orificio cervical (Ch. 26).

plan de opción triple (triple option plan) modelo de atención administrada que permite a los afiliados la opción de elegir planes de salud tradicionales, HMO o PPO (Ch. 17).

plan de punto de servicio (POS) (point-of-service [POS] plan) plan que permite la comunicación directa entre un consultorio médico y la compañía de seguros de salud (Ch. 17).

planificación en olas (wave scheduling) sistema en el que los pacientes se programan para la primera media hora de cada hora y luego se atienden durante toda la hora (Ch. 13).

planificación en olas modificada (modified wave scheduling) sistema en el que se programan varios pacientes al comienzo de cada hora, seguidos de citas individuales cada 10 a 20 minutos el resto de la hora (Ch. 13).

plasma (plasma) parte líquida de la sangre de un tubo que contiene anticoagulante. Este líquido contiene fibrinógeno (Ch. 40).

plazo de entrega (turnaround time) límite de tiempo específico establecido para terminar los informes médicos (Ch. 16).

pleiteador (litigious) propenso a involucrarse en demandas judiciales (Ch. 1).

pluralista (pluralismo) (pluralistic [pluralism]) sociedad en la que coexisten distintos grupos étnicos, religiosos o culturales diferentes (Ch. 3).

poder legal duradero para atención médica (durable power of attorney for health care) formulario legal que permite a una persona designada actuar en nombre de otra con respecto a las opciones de atención médica (Ch. 6, 7).

poder para la atención médica (health care proxy) documento que permite que un paciente designe a un representante para tomar decisiones sobre la atención médica en caso que el paciente no pueda hacerlo (Ch. 6).

pólipo (polyp) tumor pediculado que se presenta en la nariz, elútero, la vejiga, el colon o el recto (Ch. 30).

póliza de Medigap (Medigap policy) plan individual que cubre el deducible de Medicare del paciente y las obligaciones de copago que cumple con las normas del gobierno federal en cuanto al seguro complementario de Medicare (Ch. 17).

portador (carrier) persona que aloja un agente patógeno y que puede transmitirlo a otras personas (Ch. 22).

poscoital (postcoital) período de tiempo que le sigue al (después) coito (Ch. 26).

práctica (practicum) etapa de transición que brinda la oportunidad de aplicar la teoría aprendida en el aula en un entorno de atención médica a través de experiencia práctica y activa (Ch. 1, 45).

práctica laboral (externship) etapa de transición entre los estudios y el empleo real; también se conoce como pasantía o práctica (Ch. 1, 24, 45).

Precauciones Basadas en la Transmisión (Transmission-Based Precautions) segundo nivel de las pautas de los Centros para el Control y la Prevención de Enfermedades (CDC, por sus siglas en inglés) que se aplica a categorías específicas de pacientes y que incluyen precauciones para transmisión por aire, por contacto y por gotitas. Se usan siempre en conjunto con las Precauciones Estándar (Ch. 22).

Precauciones Estándar (Standard Precautions) precauciones desarrolladas en 1996 por los Centros para el Control y la Prevención de

Enfermedades (CDC, por sus siglas en inglés) que amplían las precauciones universales y las prácticas de aislamiento de sustancias corporales. Proporcionan una variedad más amplia de protección y se usan en cualquier momento que exista contacto con la sangre, los líquidos corporales húmedos (excepto la sudoración), las membranas mucosas o la piel no intacta. Tienen como objetivo proteger a todos los proveedores de atención médica, los pacientes y los visitantes (Ch. 9, 22).

Precauciones Universales (Universal Precautions)   pautas establecidas por los Centros para el Control y la Prevención de Enfermedades (CDC, por sus siglas en inglés) para proteger a los profesionales de la atención médica de las enfermedades infecciosas (Ch. 22).

precedentes (precedents)   se refiere a los fallos dictados anteriormente e incluyen decisiones tomadas en el tribunal, interpretaciones de una constitución y decisiones del derecho estatutario (Ch. 7).

precipitado (precipitate)   sustancia en forma de partículas finas que se separa de una solución si se deja reposar durante un tiempo (Ch. 36).

precordial (precordial)   perteneciente al área de la superficie anterior del cuerpo situada sobre el corazón (Ch. 37).

preeclampsia (preeclampsia)   complicación del embarazo que se caracteriza por edema generalizado, hipertensión y proteinuria (Ch. 26).

preexistente (preexisting)   lesión o enfermedad que se presenta antes de una fecha determinada (Ch. 22).

preguntas abiertas (open-ended questions)   preguntas que incentivan la verbalización y la respuesta; preguntas que buscan obtener una respuesta que va más allá del simple sí o no (Ch. 4).

preguntas cerradas (closed questions)   preguntas cuya respuesta es sí o no (Ch. 4).

prejuicio (prejudice)   opinión o juicio que se forma antes de conocer los hechos (Ch. 4).

prenatal (prenatal)   período de tiempo entre la fertilización y el nacimiento (Ch. 26).

preparación en fresco (wet mount)   método para agregar líquido, generalmente solución salina o hidrocloruro de potasio a una muestra en un portaobjetos para examinarla y conservarla. La muestra se coloca en un portaobjetos y se aplica una gota de solución salina (para diagnóstico de *Trichomonas vaginalis*) o hidróxido de potasio (para diagnóstico de infecciones vaginales por hongos) y se mezcla con la muestra. Luego se tapa con un cubreobjeto y se examina microscópicamente (Ch. 26, 43).

presbiacusia (presbycusis)   pérdida progresiva de la audición provocada por el proceso normal de envejecimiento (Ch. 29).

priapismo (priapism)   definido como una erección que dura más de cuatro horas y puede producirse con o sin estimulación sexual (Ch. 28).

primeros auxilios (first aid)   cuidados inmediatos (o primeros cuidados) que se brindan a personas que se enferman o se lesionan repentinamente; en general, después de los primeros auxilios se brinda atención y tratamiento integrales (Ch. 9).

primigrávida (primigravida)   mujer embarazada por primera vez (Ch. 26).

privilegiada (privileged)   información confidencial sobre la cual sólo se puede informar con el permiso del paciente o por orden judicial (Ch. 16).

problema presente (PP) (present problem [PP])   ver queja principal (QP) (Ch. 16).

procedimiento de microscopia realizada por el proveedor (PPMP) (provider performed microscopy procedure [PPMP])   término de la Ley de Mejoras de Laboratorios Clínicos (CLIA, por sus siglas en inglés) para aquellos exámenes microscópicos que requieren la pericia de un médico o de un proveedor de nivel medio calificado en exámenes microscópicos. El PPMP es parte de la categoría de pruebas moderadamente complejas de la ley CLIA (Ch. 38).

procedimiento invasivo (invasive procedure)   procedimiento que requiere atravesar la piel o hacer una incisión en el cuerpo (Ch. 22, 39).

procedimiento no invasivo (noninvasive procedure)   procedimiento que no requiere atravesar la piel o hacer una incisión en el cuerpo (Ch. 37).

profesionalismo (professionalism)   cualidades que caracterizan o distinguen a un profesional que cumple con las normas técnicas y éticas de la profesión (Ch. 1).

programación ininterrumpida (stream scheduling)   sistema en el que se atiende a los pacientes en forma continua durante el día; por ejemplo, a intervalos de 15, 30 ó 60 minutos, en el cual cada paciente tiene un horario de cita definido (Ch. 13).

pronación (pronation)   movimiento del brazo de modo que la palma quede hacia abajo (Ch. 33).

prono (prone)   en esta posición, se indica al paciente que se recueste boca abajo en la mesa con la cabeza volteada a un lado; los brazos pueden colocarse por encima de la cabeza o a lo largo del costado del cuerpo. El paño debe cubrir desde el área media del pecho hasta las piernas (Ch. 25).

pronunciación (pronunciation)   decir las palabras correctamente (Ch. 12).

prostaglandina (prostaglandin)   modulador de la actividad bioquímica en los tejidos (Ch. 26).

prostatitis (prostatitis)   inflamación de la glándula de la próstata (Ch. 28).

protección contra sobretensiones (surge protection)   protección de los componentes electrónicos frágiles contra las corrientes de fuga en el voltaje eléctrico que se producen en las líneas de distribución de energía (Ch. 11).

proteína C reactiva (CRP) (c-reactive protein [CRP])   análisis sanguíneo para detectar la inflamación (Ch. 41).

proteinuria (proteinuria)   proteína en la orina (Ch. 30).

protocolo de manejo de la tos (cough etiquette)   toser/estornudar en un pañuelo de papel tisú para impedir que los microorganismos se transmitan a otras personas. Incluye saber cómo desechar correctamente el pañuelo en un recipiente de residuos y lavarse las manos lo antes posible (Ch. 22).

protocolo de voz por Internet (VoIP) (voice over Internet protocol [VoIP])   transmisión en tiempo real de señales de voz a través de Internet o de la red del protocolo de Internet (IP) (Ch. 12).

protozoos (protozoa)   animales unicelulares que se dividen en cuatro grupos: amebas, flagelados, ciliados y coccidios (Ch. 43).

proyección (projection)   acto de atribuir sentimientos propios a otra persona (Ch. 4).

prueba cualitativa (qualitative test)   análisis para identificar las cualidades o las características de los componentes, como tamaño, forma y madurez de las células (Ch. 39).

prueba cuantitativa (quantitative test)   análisis que puede identificar la cantidad o el recuento de cantidades reales como el recuento de la cantidad de células sanguíneas (Ch. 39).

prueba de aptitud (proficiency testing)   pruebas de muestras realizadas en un laboratorio clínico para determinar con qué grado de exactitud se realizan las pruebas. Las muestras de prueba se verifican del mismo modo que las muestras de los pacientes (Ch. 38).

prueba de baja complejidad (waived)   se usa para describir una categoría de pruebas de laboratorio clínico que son simples, invariables y que requieren un mínimo de criterio e interpretación (Ch. 38).

prueba de control (control test)   prueba de una muestra de resultados conocidos usados para compararlos con los resultados de la muestra de un paciente (Ch. 39).

prueba de detección (screening)   evaluación de los síntomas del paciente para detectar necesidades emergentes. Algunas veces se realizan como ayuda al proveedor de salud para determinar las mejores medidas a tomar en cuanto al cuidado más apropiado para el paciente (Ch. 42).

prueba de detección de Guthrie (Guthrie screening test)   también conocida como prueba del talón; prueba de diagnóstico para la detección de fenilcetonuria (FCU) (Ch. 44).

Prueba de evaluación del desarrollo de Denver (Denver Developmental Screening Test) utilizada para determinar los niveles de desarrollo de las habilidades motrices (Ch. 27).

prueba de Mantoux (Mantoux test) prueba para determinar la presencia de tuberculosis que consiste en la inyección intradérmica de derivado proteico purificado (ver DPP) (Ch. 44).

prurito (pruritus) picazón (Ch. 22, 35).

puerperio (puerperium) período desde el final de la tercera etapa del parto hasta que se completa la involución delútero, generalmente de tres a seis semanas (Ch. 26).

puerto (port) término abreviado de portal, vía de ingreso. Cuando se refiere a la terapia intravenosa, es un tipo de adaptador que puede servir como medio adicional para infundir líquidos o medicamentos. El puerto se puede conectar al tubo principal. Tiene un lugar de entrada sin aguja (Ch. 36).

puerto de bus universal en serie (USB) (universal serial bus [USB] port) tipo de portal o bus de entrada de datos para datos informáticos (Ch. 11).

punción lumbar (lumbar puncture) punción quirúrgica del área lumbar de los espacios intervertebrales para aspirar el líquido cefalorraquídeo para análisis de laboratorio (Ch. 22, 43).

purga (purging) método para mantener ordenados los archivos separando los archivos activos de los inactivos y cerrados (Ch. 14).

purulento (purulent) que produce o contiene pus (Ch. 22).

queilosis (cheilosis) trastorno provocado por una deficiencia de vitamina B2 (riboflavina) y caracterizado por llagas en los labios y grietas en las comisuras de la boca (Ch. 34).

queja principal (QP) (chief complaint [CC]) síntoma o problema específico por el cual el paciente consulta al proveedor hoy (Ch. 16, 23).

química clínica (clinical chemistry) análisis y estudio de la sangre, los líquidos corporales, los excrementos y los tejidos en el diagnóstico y el tratamiento de enfermedades (Ch. 39).

racionalización (rationalization) acto de justificación, generalmente ilógico, que se usa para no enfrentar la verdad de la situación (Ch. 4).

radiación ionizante (ionizing radiation) haces de rayos X (Ch. 32).

radioactivo (radioactive) emite rayos o partículas desde el núcleo (Ch. 32).

radiografía (radiograph) placa en la cual se produce una imagen a través de la exposición a los rayos X (Ch. 32).

radiolúcido (radiolucent) que permite que lo atraviesen los rayos X. Aparece un área oscura en la radiografía (Ch. 32).

radionúclidos (radionuclides) átomos que se desintegran emitiendo radiación electromagnética (Ch. 32).

radiopaco (radiopaque) impenetrable para los rayos X. Aparece un área clara en la radiografía (Ch. 32).

reactivo (reagent) sustancia química que detecta o sintetiza otras sustancias en una reacción química; se usa en los análisis de laboratorio porque se conoce su reacción de una forma específica (Ch. 39, 42, 43).

reanimación cardiopulmonar (RCP) (cardiopulmonary resuscitation [CPR]) combinación de respiración artificial de rescate y compresiones torácicas realizada por una persona capacitada a un paciente que presenta paro cardíaco (Ch. 9).

recetar (prescribe) indicar o recomendar el uso de un fármaco, una dieta u otra forma de terapia (Ch. 7, 35).

rechazo (denial) renuencia o negativa a aceptar algo (Ch. 4).

recipiente principal (primary container) recipiente que contiene directamente a la muestra (Ch. 40).

recolección de mitad de micción (midstream Collection) muestra de orina recogida a la mitad de la micción (Ch. 42).

recuento sanguíneo completo (RSC) (complete blood count [CBC]) batería de análisis hematológicos que consisten en hemoglobina, hematocrito, recuento total de glóbulos blancos que incluye diferencial, recuento total de glóbulos rojos, que incluyeíndices y plaquetas (Ch. 41).

red de área amplia (WAN) (wide area network [WAN]) conexión de múltiples computadoras juntas en un área grande con el fin de compartir datos (Ch. 11).

red de área local (LAN) (local area network [LAN]) red de computadoras generalmente en una oficina o edificio (Ch. 11).

red de área local inalámbrica (WLAN) (wireless local area network [WLAN]) un tipo de red de área local que utiliza ondas de alta frecuencia en lugar de cables para comunicar entre nodos (Ch. 11).

red de área local virtual (VLAN) virtual local area network [VLAN]) Una Vlan es un subconjunto de una red que conecta solo computadoras autorizadas entre sí excluyendo a todas las demás. Al separar los datos delicados del resto de la red, disminuye la posibilidad de que personas no autorizadas puedan acceder a los datos (Ch. 11).

redes con cableado físico (hard-wired networks) redes conectadas por conductores metálicos o cables; en algunas circunstancias, se pueden usar cables ópticos (Ch. 11).

reembolso (reimbursement) pago (Ch. 38).

referencia cruzada (cross-reference) anotación en un expediente para guiar al lector hacia un registro específico que puede estar archivado bajo más de un nombre/sujeto (p. ej., nombre de casado/nombre de soltera o nombres extranjeros) cuando el apellido no es fácilmente reconocible (Ch. 14).

referencias (references) personas que conocen a otra persona o han trabajado con ella el tiempo suficiente para hacer una evaluación sincera y una recomendación con respecto a los antecedentes de la persona (Ch. 48).

refractómetro (refractometer) instrumento que mide elíndice de refracción de una sustancia o solución; se usa en el examen físico del análisis de orina para medir la densidad urinaria de una muestra de orina (Ch. 42).

registro de cheques (check register) registro de los cheques emitidos, categorizados en columnas separadas e identificadas (Ch. 21).

registro de entrada (sistema de ordenación por número) (accession record [numeric system]) libro de registro usado para asignar números a la correspondencia o a los pacientes (Ch. 14).

registro de reclamaciones (claim register) diario o registro de reclamaciones presentado a cada aseguradora. Cuando se recibe el pago, se escribe la fecha y el importe del pago en el registro (Ch. 18).

registro de salud electrónico (RSE) (electronic health record [EHR]) registros médicos electrónicos de un paciente de varias fuentes combinados en una base de datos principal (Ch. 11).

registro médico electrónico (RME) (electronic medical record [EMR]) registro médico del paciente de unaúnica práctica médica, hospital o farmacia (Ch. 11, 16).

regla de Nägele (Nägele's rule) método habitual para calcular la fecha prevista del parto (Ch. 26).

regla del cumpleaños (birthday rule) método para determinar cuál de dos o más pólizas que cubren a un niño dependiente será la principal, es decir, la póliza del padre o de la madre que cumpla años primero en el año calendario será la póliza principal (Ch. 17).

regresión (regression) movimiento hacia atrás hasta una etapa anterior para escapar del conflicto o de los miedos (Ch. 4).

relación de cobranza (collection ratio) ingresos brutos divididos por el importe que se podría haber cobrado menos los rechazos (Ch. 20, 21).

relación de costos (cost ratio) fórmula que muestra el costo de un procedimiento o servicio y ayuda a determinar el valor financiero de mantener determinados servicio (Ch. 21).

relación de cuentas por cobrar a activos (accounts receivable [A/R] ratio assets) cuentas por cobrar pendientes de pago divididas por los ingresos brutos mensuales promedio durante losúltimos 12 meses (Ch. 20, 21).

remisión (referral) término usado por los centros de atención administrada para autorizar a otro proveedor, que no sea el proveedor de atención primaria, para que atienda al paciente (Ch. 17).

reparación (undoing) acciones destinadas a subsanar y anular un comportamiento inapropiado (Ch. 4).

repolarización (repolarization) restitución de un estado polarizado en un músculo después de una contracción (Ch. 37).

represión (repression) forma de sobrellevar una situación abrumadora olvidándola temporalmente; amnesia temporal (Ch. 4).

resección transuretral (transurethral resection) extirpación de tejido de la próstata usando un dispositivo que se introduce a través de la uretra (Ch. 28).

residuos patógenos (infectious waste) elementos que han estado en contacto con la sangre o los líquidos corporales del paciente. Elementos contaminados (Ch. 22).

residuos regulados (regulated waste) residuos que contienen material infeccioso que representaría una amenaza debido a la posible transmisión de microorganismos patógenos (Ch. 22).

resistencia (resistance) capacidad del sistema inmunitario para resistir o enfrentar las enfermedades infecciosas (Ch. 22).

resolución alternativa de conflictos (RAC) (alternative dispute resolution [ADR]) una alternativa al juicio que alienta a las partes a resolver sus diferencias fuera de un tribunal (Ch. 7).

resolución de conflictos (conflict resolution) solución de problemas entre compañeros de trabajo o entre dos partes dadas (Ch. 45).

respiración de rescate (rescue breathing) realizada en personas con paro respiratorio, la respiración de rescate es un procedimiento boca a boca (usando equipo de protección apropiado) o boca a nariz que proporciona oxígeno al paciente hasta que llegue el personal de emergencia (Ch. 9).

respiración externa (external respiration) ventilación de los pulmones cuando se produce el intercambio de oxígeno y dióxido de carbono (Ch. 30).

respiración interna (internal respiration) paso de oxígeno de la sangre a las células (Ch. 30).

responsabilidad (liability) responsabilidad legal (Ch. 45).

respuesta inflamatoria (inflammatory response) defensa del cuerpo contra la amenaza de infección o traumatismo. Se caracteriza por enrojecimiento, dolor, calor e hinchazón (Ch. 22).

resumen de alta médica (DS) (discharge summary [DS]) informes médicos que documentan el historial de hospitalización de un paciente (Ch. 16).

retención (retention) orina que se retiene en la vejiga; incapacidad de vaciar la vejiga (Ch. 28).

reticulocito (reticulocyte) eritrocito que es liberado de la médula ósea antes de que esté maduro y que retiene parte de su material nuclear (Ch. 41).

retraso psicomotor (psychomotor retardation) disminución de las respuestas físicas y mentales; se puede observar en la depresión (Ch. 6).

revisar (proofread) leer un documento para verificar que el contenido sea exacto y que se hayan usado correctamente las normas de gramática, ortografía, puntuación y uso de mayúsculas (Ch. 15, 16).

revisión de salario (salary review) informar al empleado sobre su sueldo base por hora revisado (Ch. 45).

revisión de sistemas (ROS) (review of systems [ROS]) consultas sobre el sistema directamente relacionadas con problemas identificados en la historia de la enfermedad presente (Ch. 16).

revisión de utilización (RU) (utilization review [UR]) revisión de los servicios médicos antes de que se brinden (Ch. 21).

riboflavina (riboflavin) vitamina B_2 (Ch. 34).

rickettsiae (rickettsiae) pequeña bacteria inmóvil parasítica intracelular (Ch. 22).

riesgo biológico (biohazard) material que ha estado en contacto con líquidos corporales y puede transmitir enfermedades (Ch. 22).

ritmo circadiano (circadian rhythm) patrón que se basa en un ciclo de 24 horas y que remarca la repetición de ciertos fenómenos fisiológicos como comer y dormir (Ch. 42).

ritmo sinusal normal (normal sinus rhythm) término usado para describir el ritmo cardíaco cuando está dentro del intervalo normal (Ch. 37).

RME (EMR) ver registros médicos electrónicos (Ch. 11).

roncha (wheal) ligera elevación de la piel que se puede producir al aplicar una inyección intradérmica, como la prueba de Mantoux para la tuberculosis (Ch. 44).

rosácea (rosacea) enfermedad crónica de la piel caracterizada por pústulas, pápulas, eritema e hiperplasia. Se desconoce su causa (Ch. 30).

rotación (rotation) giro de una parte del cuerpo alrededor de su eje (Ch. 33); también, oportunidad para pasar 2 o 3 semanas en una variedad de entornos de atención médica (Ch. 40).

RSE (HER) ver registros de salud electrónicos (Ch. 11).

ruidos (bruits) sonido de origen venoso o arterial que se escucha en la auscultación (Ch. 25).

saldo (balance) monto adeudado (Ch. 19).

saldo de comprobación (trial balance) creado sumando los saldos deudores y los saldos acreedores para confirmar que el total de débitos sea igual al total de créditos (Ch. 21).

salicilatos (salicylates) fármacos similares a las aspirinas que pueden producirúlceras porque irritan el tracto gastrointestinal (Ch. 30).

sarna (scabies) enfermedad infecciosa de la piel provocada por ácaros *(Sarcoptes scabiei),* que se transmite por contacto directo con las personas infectadas (Ch. 22).

secreción (secretion) sustancia producida por las células de los órganos glandulares a partir de materiales en la sangre (Ch. 22, 38).

sedimento (sediment) material insoluble que se deposita en el fondo de un líquido; material examinado en el examen microscópico de análisis de orina (Ch. 42).

seguidor de contactos (contact tracker) formulario usado para realizar el seguimiento de la información de contacto laboral, como nombre del empleador, nombre de la persona de contacto, dirección y número telefónico, fecha del primer contacto, currículum vitae enviado, fecha de la entrevista, información de seguimiento y fechas (Ch. 48).

seguro de indemnización por accidentes de trabajo (Workers' Compensation insurance) seguro médico y salarial para los trabajadores que sufren lesiones relacionadas con el empleo (Ch. 17).

seguro de responsabilidad profesional (professional liability insurance) póliza de seguro cuyo objetivo es proteger los activos en el caso en que se presente o se dé lugar a una reclamación por daños y perjuicios producto de la negligencia (Ch. 45).

sello de agua (watermark) diseño incorporado al papel durante el proceso de fabricación del papel que es visible cuando se sostiene el papel ante la luz (Ch. 15).

semen (semen) secreción espesa y viscosa segregada por la uretra de los hombres en el orgasmo. Es un producto mixto que contiene distintos líquidos y espermatozoides. El esperma está ausente en el semen de los hombres que se han practicado la vasectomía (Ch. 44).

senil (senile) debilidad mental y física a veces relacionada con el envejecimiento (Ch. 29).

sensibilidad (sensitivity) prueba en la cual se coloca un antibiótico en un organismo para determinar cuál antibiótico eliminará eficazmente el organismo con la menor dosis (ver también cultivo y sensibilidad) (Ch. 43).

sensor (sensor) término usado para describir una lengüeta de papel recubierta en metal que se aplica en el cuerpo del paciente como preparación para un ECG (también conocido como electrodo). Los sensores se colocan en lugares específicos de la piel y luego se conectan al ECG con cables. Los sensores conducen la electricidad desde el paciente hasta el equipo de electrocardiografía (Ch. 37).

señalador o marcador (out guide or sheet) tarjeta, carpeta o tira de papel insertada provisoriamente en los archivos para reemplazar un registro que fue retirado de allí (Ch. 14).

sepsis (septic) infección generalizada que habitualmente se produce en pacientes gravemente enfermos. Se liberan químicos en el torrente sanguíneo que causan vasodilatación y otros productos orgánicos que son nocivos para los órganos y los tejidos. La vasodilatación y la disminución de la capacidad de las células y los tejidos para utilizar el oxígeno son la base para este tipo de choque (Ch. 9).

septicemia (septicemia) invasión de bacterias patógenas en el torrente sanguíneo (Ch. 3).

servicio sockets layer (SSL) (service sockets layer [SSL]) protocolo diseñado para permitir la transferencia segura de datos basados en la red usando la encriptación (Ch. 11).

servidor (server) computadora con capacidad de disco duro masiva que se usa para conectar otras computadoras entre sí de modo que múltiples usuarios puedan compartir los datos. Probablemente un sistema informático de un centro de atención ambulatoria estará vinculado o conectado en red con un servidor central (Ch. 11).

servicios auxiliares (ancillary services) empresas ocupacionales profesionales contratadas para completar un trabajo específico (Ch. 45).

servicios de respuesta (answering services) servicios empleados para responder a las llamadas de entornos de atención ambulatoria después del horario de atención; a diferencia de un contestador automático, un operador en vivo responde a la llamada y la deriva según corresponda (Ch. 12).

Servicios Médicos de Emergencia (SME) (Emergency Medical Services [EMS]) red local de policía, bomberos y personal médico capacitado para responder a situaciones de emergencia. En muchas comunidades, el sistema se activa llamando al 911 (Ch. 9).

sesgo (bias) tendencia hacia una creencia en particular (Ch. 4).

shock (shock) afección potencialmente grave en la que el sistema circulatorio no suministra sangre suficiente a todas las partes del cuerpo y que provoca que los órganos del cuerpo no funcionen correctamente (Ch. 9).

sibilancia (wheezes) ruido de tono alto que se escucha en la expiración, a menudo resultado de una obstrucción o estrechamiento de las vías respiratorias (Ch. 24).

sigmoidoscopía (sigmoidoscopy) examen de diagnóstico del interior del colon sigmoide (Ch. 30).

símbolo universal de identificación médica para emergencias (universal emergency medical identification symbol) identificación que a veces llevan puesta las personas para identificar los problemas de salud que tienen (Ch. 9).

simetría (symmetry) correspondencia de forma, tamaño y posición de las partes del cuerpo en lados contrarios del cuerpo (Ch. 25).

sims (sim's) en esta posición, se indica al paciente recostarse sobre el lado izquierdo; el brazo izquierdo y el hombro deben llevarse detrás del cuerpo. La rodilla izquierda se flexiona ligeramente para apoyar el cuerpo y la rodilla derecha se flexiona de forma definida. (Ch. 25).

síncope (syncope) desmayo (Ch. 9, 37).

síncope vasovagal (vasovagal syncope) desmayo repentino debido a la hipotensión inducida por la respuesta del sistema nervioso autónomo al estrés emocional, al dolor o a un traumatismo abrupto (Ch. 9).

Síndrome de dificultad respiratoria aguda o de adulto (ARDS) (acute or adult respiratory distress syndrome [ARDS]) trastorno potencialmente letal que se produce cuando hay acumulación grave de líquido y hemorragia en los pulmones (Ch. 30).

síndrome de inmunodeficiencia adquirida (SIDA) (acquired immunodeficiency syndrome [AIDS]) trastorno del sistema inmunitario causado por el virus de inmunodeficiencia humana (VIH), un retrovirus que destruye la capacidad del cuerpo para combatir las infecciones. A medida que la enfermedad avanza, los trastornos, que incluyen cáncer e infecciones oportunistas, van doblegando a la persona. No existe cura conocida para el SIDA (Ch. 22).

síndrome respiratorio agudo y grave (SARS) (severe acute respiratory syndrome [SARS]) brote viral de una enfermedad respiratoria que se informó en Asia por primera vez en 2003; se contagia por contacto estrecho de persona a persona y se caracteriza por fiebre y síntomas respiratorios (Ch. 22).

Sistema de Códigos de Procedimientos Comunes de la Atención Médica (HCPCS) (Healthcare Common Procedure Coding System [HCPCS]) sistema de códigos que consta de la Terminología Actual de Procedimientos (CPT, por sus siglas en inglés), códigos nacionales (nivel II) y códigos locales (nivel III); antes conocido como Sistema de Códigos de Procedimientos Comunes HCFA (Ch. 18).

Sistema de Gestión de Prácticas Total (TPMS) (Total Practice Management System [TPMS]) categoría de software que maneja todas las operaciones diarias de la práctica médica (Ch. 11).

Sistema de Informes de Elegibilidad para la Inscripción en Defensa (DEERS) (Defense Enrollment Eligible Reporting System [DEERS]) sistema operado por el Departamento de Defensa y usado por los contratistas de TRICARE para determinar y confirmar la elegibilidad de los beneficiarios (Ch. 17).

sistema de prestación de servicios médicos integrado (IDS) (integrated delivery system [IDS]) organización de atención médica de centros de proveedores afiliados combinados bajo una única propiedad que ofrece el espectro completo de atención médica administrada (Ch. 17).

sistema de tablero de clavijas (pegboard system) sistema manual de cuentas médicas por cobrar que se usa con más frecuencia (Ch. 19).

sistema inmunitario (immune system) mecanismo de defensa del cuerpo contra los microorganismos invasores. El cuerpo reconoce las sustancias extrañas, como los microorganismos, y produce sustancias para combatirlos. Algunos ejemplos son los anticuerpos, los glóbulos blancos, las enzimas digestivas y la resistencia de la piel (Ch. 22).

sistema inmunitario con inmunosupresión (suppressed immune system) término usado para describir un sistema inmunitario que no puede funcionar normalmente debido a la presencia de una enfermedad como el SIDA (Ch. 38).

sistema nervioso parasimpático (parasympathetic nervous system) parte del sistema nervioso autónomo que hace que el cuerpo vuelva a su estado normal después de que disminuye el estrés (Ch. 5).

sistema nervioso simpático (sympathetic nervous system) gran parte del sistema nervioso autónomo que prepara el cuerpo para la reacción de lucha o huída (Ch. 5).

sistema operativo (SO) (operating system [OS]) software usado para controlar la computadora y su equipo periférico. También se lo conoce como software de sistema (Ch. 11).

sístole (systole) un componente de la medición de presión arterial que representa la presión más alta durante el ciclo cardíaco; fuerza ejercida sobre las paredes arteriales durante la contracción cardíaca (Ch. 24, 37).

SOAP (SOAP) sigla de las notas de evolución del paciente basadas en las impresiones subjetivas (S), la evidencia clínica objetiva (O), análisis o diagnóstico (A) y planes para estudios adicionales (P) (Ch. 14, 23).

sobrecodificación (up-coding) también conocido como incremento de códigos y sobrefacturación. La sobrecodificación ocurre cuando la compañía de seguros intencionalmente factura un servicio que tiene una tarifa mayor del que se prestó para obtener mayores reembolsos (Ch. 19).

sobrenadante (supernatant) orina que aparece encima del sedimento cuando se centrifuga; lo drenado antes de que el sedimento sea examinado en el examen microscópico del análisis de orina (Ch. 42).

software (software) equivalente de programa informático (Ch. 11).

software de aplicación (application software) software que realiza una función específica de procesamiento de datos (Ch. 11).

software de reconocimiento de voz (voice recognition software [VRS]) software que traduce comandos de voz y se usa en lugar del mouse y del teclado (Ch. 16).

software de sistema (system software) ver sistema operativo (Ch. 11).

solicitud (requisition) formulario de pedido que se envía con una muestra y que especifica las pruebas que se deben realizar; las pruebas más comunes se separan en categorías lógicas con espacio adicional para escribir pedidos especiales (Ch. 38, 39).

solicitud/carta de presentación (application/cover letter) carta que se usa para presentarse y para enviar el curriculum vitae a un posible empleador a fin de obtener una entrevista (Ch. 48).

soluble en agua (water-soluble) relativo a sustancias que son hidrofílicas y, por lo tanto, se disuelven mejor en agua (Ch. 34).

soluble en lípidos (fat-soluble) relativo a sustancias que son hidrofóbicas y, por lo tanto, se disuelven mejor en los lípidos (Ch. 34).

solución salina normal (normal saline) solución de cloruro de sodio (sal) y agua destilada. Tiene la misma presión osmótica que el suero sanguíneo. También se la conoce como solución salina isotónica o fisiológica (Ch. 9).

solvente (solvent) que produce una solución, que se disuelve (Ch. 22).

subcontratación (outsourcing) la práctica de la contratación de un servicio externo a la clínica o al hospital de una empresa en la que se realiza la tarea a un costo menor y con un tiempo de respuesta más rápido (Ch. 16).

subjetivo (subjective) síntoma que siente el paciente pero que los demás no pueden observar (Ch. 23).

sublimación (sublimation) redirigir un impulso socialmente inaceptable hacia uno que sea socialmente aceptable (Ch. 4).

subordinado (subordinate) en una organización, persona bajo la dirección (o el mando) de una persona de mayor autoridad (Ch. 45).

suero (serum) parte líquida de la sangre que se obtiene después de que se ha dejado coagular la sangre (Ch. 39, 40).

supercomputadora (supercomputer) la más veloz, grande y cara de las cuatro clases de computadoras que se fabrican actualmente (Ch. 11).

supina (supine) esta posición se asume en reposo boca arriba. Se utiliza para el examen de la superficie anterior del cuerpo desde la cabeza hasta los pies (Ch. 25).

supinación (supination) movimiento del brazo de modo que la palma quede hacia arriba (Ch. 33).

Suplantación de identidad (phishing) práctica en la que el receptor de un correo electrónico es dirigido a un sitio web para proporcionar información a su banco, Hacienda u otra organización oficial. El sitio web es en realidad una farsa preparada para parecerse a algo auténtico y, cuando se suministra la información, esta pasa al delincuente que comete fraude al consumidor (Ch. 11).

supurante (suppurant) agente que produce formación de pus (Ch. 31).

supurativo (suppurative) que produce la generación de pus o relacionado con ello (Ch. 27).

sustancias radiofarmacéuticas (radiopharmaceuticals) sustancias químicas radioactivas usadas en pruebas de ubicación, tamaño, contorno o función de tejidos, órganos, vasos o líquidos corporales (Ch. 32).

sustituto (surrogate) suplente; alguien que reemplaza a otro (Ch. 8).

sutura (suture) material o hilo quirúrgico; puede describir el acto de coser con hilo y aguja quirúrgicos (Ch. 31).

talasemia (thalassemia) anemia hereditaria que puede ser mortal (Ch. 26).

taquicardia sinusal (tachycardia, sinus) latido cardíaco anormalmente rápido superior a 100 latidos/minuto. Tipo de arritmia cardíaca (Ch. 24, 37).

taquipnea (tachypnea) aumento anormal en la frecuencia de la respiración (Ch. 24).

tarjetas de cirugía (surgery cards) referencia escrita para cirugías y procedimientos (Ch. 31).

taxonomía (taxonomy) clasificación de organismos en categorías apropiadas (Ch. 43).

Tay–Sachs (Tay–Sachs) enfermedad congénita que generalmente es mortal (Ch. 26).

teclear (key) ingresar datos mediante teclas en el teclado de la computadora (Ch. 15).

técnica de una sola mano (scoop technique) técnica que usa una sola mano para recoger y tapar una aguja usadaúnicamente si no hay disponible de manera inmediata un recipiente para objetos filosos; no se manipula la cubierta (tapa) de la aguja de ningún modo; luego se la desecha en el recipiente de objetos filosos más próximo (Ch. 22).

técnicas de entrevista (interview techniques) métodos para promover una mejor comunicación entre el postulante y el entrevistador (Ch. 4).

tecnología de cifrado (encryption technology) convierte la información en un código; se usa para proteger la privacidad y la confidencialidad de las personas en el software informático (Ch. 13).

Tecnólogos Médicos Estadounidenses (AMT) (American Medical Technologists [AMT]) organización médica que acredita a los profesionales de atención médica, incluidos los Asistentes Médicos Matriculados (RMA, por sus siglas en inglés) y los Especialistas Administrativos Médicos Certificados (CMAS, por sus siglas en inglés) (Ch. 1, 47).

teléfonos celulares (cellular telephones) dispositivo portátil de corto alcance usado para comunicación de voz o datos en una red de estaciones base llamadas sitio de celda. El sitio de celda está interconectado a la red telefónica conmutada (Ch. 12).

teléfono inteligente (smartphone) dispositivo que permite hacer llamadas telefónicas, pero además cuenta con funciones que podrían encontrarse en un asistente digital personal o una pequeña computadora personal. Algunos ejemplos son la capacidad para tomar fotografías, enviar y recibir correos electrónicos, editar documentos de Office y muchas otras funciones frecuentemente llamadas aplicaciones (Ch. 12).

temperamento (disposition) modo de ser, carácter, personalidad (Ch. 1).

terapia de reemplazo hormonal (TRH) (hormone replacement therapy [HRT]) reemplazo de las hormonas faltantes en el sistema del paciente. En este caso, la TRH se refiere al reemplazo de diferentes niveles de estrógeno y progesterona en mujeres perimenopáusicas y posmenopáusicas (Ch. 26, 39).

Terminología Actual sobre Procedimientos (TAP) (Current Procedural Terminology [CPT]) códigos estándar para procedimientos y servicios. Se usa en la mayoría de los entornos de atención ambulatoria para codificar el formulario de reclamación y es reconocida por la mayoría de las compañías de seguros (Ch. 19).

termófilo (thermophile) resistente a la destrucción por el calor. Característico de algunas bacterias (Ch. 31).

termolábil (thermolabile) afectado fácilmente por el calor (Ch. 22).

termoterapia (thermotherapy) uso del calor para tratar una afección física (Ch. 33).

testamento en vida (living will) documento que permite que una persona tome decisiones relacionadas con el tratamiento de una enfermedad con riesgo de muerte (Ch. 6).

testigo experto (expert witness) persona con conocimientos y habilidades sumamente especializadas en un área en particular que atestigua con respecto a un estándar de atención (Ch. 7).

tiamina (thiamin) vitamina B_1 (Ch. 34).

tiempo de protrombina (protime) método de control del tiempo de coagulación (Ch. 41).

tifus (tifoide) (typhus [typhoid]) enfermedad infecciosa aguda que produce dolor de cabeza intenso, sarpullido, fiebre alta y compromiso neurológico progresivo. Es frecuente en lugares donde las condiciones son insalubres y de hacinamiento (Ch. 3).

timpanostomía (tympanostomy) colocación de un tubo por la membrana timpánica para permitir la ventilación del oído medio; parte del tratamiento de la otitis media (Ch. 27).

tinción de Gram (Gram stain) su nombre proviene de su inventor, Hans Christian Gram, y por lo tanto "Gram" se escribe siempre con mayúscula; tinción más común usada en microbiología para observar las características morfológicas de las bacterias; tinción diferencial que permite la diferenciación entre organismos gramnegativos y grampositivos (Ch. 43).

tinnitus (tinnitus) repiqueteo o zumbido en el oído (Ch. 25).

tira de prueba reactiva (reagent test strip) tira estrecha de plástico en la cual se pegan almohadillas que contienen reactivos; se usa en el examen químico de análisis de orina para detectar, glucosa, bilirrubina, cetonas, densidad urinaria, sangre, pH, urobilinógeno, nitritos y esterasa leucocitaria (Ch. 42).

tira de ritmo (rhythm strip) registro del ECG de unaúnica derivación, generalmente la derivación II, que se usa para determinar el ritmo del latido cardíaco. La arritmia se puede observar más fácilmente en una tira de ritmo porque se prolonga más tiempo, de acuerdo con el pedido del proveedor (Ch. 37).

tirante (taut) estirar o tensar una superficie, como la piel (Ch. 36).

título (titer) medición de la cantidad de anticuerpos presentes contra un antígeno en particular (Ch. 26).

Título de técnico (associate's degree) título otorgado por un colegio universitario al final de un curso de dos años (Ch. 1).

tocoferol (tocopherol) vitamina E (Ch. 34).

tomografía por emisión de positrones (PET) (Positron Emission Tomography [PET]) procedimiento radiográfico que utiliza una computadora y una sustancia radiactiva. La sustancia radiactiva se inyecta en el cuerpo del paciente y emite partículas cargadas. Estas se combinan con partículas en el organismo del paciente para producir imágenes en color que revelan la cantidad de actividad metabólica en un órgano o una estructura (Ch. 31).

tonometría (tonometer) utilizada para medir la presión intraocular de los pacientes mayores de 35 años (Ch. 25).

toracentesis (thoracentesis) punción quirúrgica de la cavidad torácica para aspirar líquido (Ch. 22).

tormenta de ideas (brainstorming) proceso para desarrollar ideas a través de la interacción sinérgica entre los participantes en un entorno libre de críticas (Ch. 45).

torniquete (tourniquet) dispositivo usado para facilitar la prominencia de la vena (Ch. 40).

torsión testicular (testicular torsion) retorcimiento del cordón espermático (Ch. 28).

toxicidad (toxicity) nivel a partir del cual un fármaco o sustancia química es tóxico o nocivo. Algunas sustancias, como algunos metales, son consideradas tóxicas en cualquier nivel de exposición accidental (Ch. 39).

trabajo en equipo (teamwork) personas que trabajan juntas en forma sinérgica (Ch. 45).

transcriptor (transcriber) dispositivo que permite transformar las grabaciones de voz en documentos transcritos o impresos (Ch. 16).

Transcriptor Médico Certificado (CMT) (Certified Medical Transcriptionist [CMT]) terminación de las dos partes del examen de certificación administrado por la Asociación para la Integridad de la Documentación del Cuidado de la Salud (AHDI, por sus siglas en inglés) (Ch. 16).

transcriptor médico registrado (RMT) (registered medical transcriptionist [RMT]) finalización de un examen de certificación de dos partes administrado por la Association for Healthcare Documentation Integrity (AHDI, Asociación para la Integridad de la Documentación sobre Atención de la Salud) (Ch. 16).

transdérmico (transdermal) sistema de administración de medicamentos que consiste en un pequeño parche adhesivo que puede aplicarse sobre la piel intacta cerca del sitio del tratamiento (Ch. 35).

transductor (transducer) dispositivo que convierte una forma de energía en otra. Durante un procedimiento de ecografía, el transductor registra los ecos y los convierte en energía eléctrica. La energía se transforma en imágenes digitalizadas que se pueden ver o imprimir. Se pueden tomar fotografías de la imagen (Ch. 32, 37).

transiluminador (transilluminator) instrumento usado para inspeccionar una cavidad o un órgano pasando una luz a través de las paredes (Ch. 28).

transmisible (communicable) contagioso; que puede transmitirse de una persona a otra directa o indirectamente (Ch. 22, 38).

transmisión (transmission) propagación de una enfermedad infecciosa por contacto directo, contacto indirecto, inhalación, ingestión o por transmisión sanguínea (Ch. 22).

transmisión por aire (airborne transmission) propagación de microorganismos causantes de enfermedades por el aire a través de largas distancias (Ch. 22).

transmisión por contacto (contact transmission) diseminación de microorganismos causantes de enfermedades al tocar directa o indirectamente la fuente de la infección o al tocar un objeto o una superficie del ambiente (Ch. 22).

transmisión por gotitas (droplet transmission) método de diseminación de las enfermedades por secreciones respiratorias a través del aire. La diseminación por lo general se limita a 3 pies del paciente infectado (Ch. 22).

transmisión sanguínea (bloodborne) medio de transmisión de una enfermedad infecciosa (como VIH y VHB) a través de la sangre humana (Ch. 22).

trazado (tracing) registro gráfico por lo general de un episodio que cambia con el tiempo y con la actividad eléctrica del corazón (Ch. 37).

trepanación (trephination) corte de una sección circular (Ch. 3).

triage selección para determinar cuáles pacientes son tratados en primer lugar cuando dos o más pacientes se presentan con emergencias simultáneamente (Ch. 9).

tribunal sucesorio (probate court) tribunal que administra sucesiones y valida los testamentos (Ch. 20).

TRICARE (TRICARE) antes llamado Programa Médico y de Salud Civil de los Servicios Uniformados (CHAMPUS, por sus siglas en inglés). TRICARE ofrece HMO, PPO y seguro médico con pago por servicio para dependientes de personal militar en servicio activo y retirado y para dependientes del personal que falleció mientras prestaban servicio (Ch. 17).

tricomoniasis (trichomoniasis) infestación con el parásito *Trichomonas*, que se puede transmitir a través de las relaciones sexuales (Ch. 22, 26).

triglicéridos (triglycerides) forma de lípido del torrente sanguíneo que sirve para almacenar energía (Ch. 44).

trimestre (trimester) tres meses; un tercio del período de gestación del embarazo (Ch. 26).

trinquetes (ratchets) mecanismos de trabado en los mangos de muchos instrumentos quirúrgicos (Ch. 31).

trombocito (thrombocyte) (plaqueta) fragmento celular del megacariocito; cumple un papel importante en la coagulación de la sangre, la hemostasia y la formación de coágulos (Ch. 40, 41).

tuberculosis (TB) (tuberculosis [TB]) enfermedad infecciosa causada por la bacteria *Mycobacterium tuberculosis* (Ch. 44).

tubo de cánula (nasal) (cannula [nasal] tubing) usado para administrar oxígeno (Ch. 36); también, la parte con punta roma de una aguja Bio-Plexus Punctur-Guard® (Ch. 40).

tubos de caldo (broth tubes) tubos llenados con un medio de cultivo líquido llamado caldo que permitirá el crecimiento de determinados microorganismos (Ch. 43).

turbio (turbid) opaco, no claro. Utilizado para describir la orina que es opaca (Ch. 42).

ultrasonido (ultrasound) uso de ondas de sonido de alta frecuencia por motivos terapéuticos para generar calor en tejidos profundos (Ch. 33).

unidad (unit) cada parte del nombre (empresa o persona), palabras o números que se indexarán y se codificarán para archivado (Ch. 14).

unidad clave (key unit) primera unidad de indexación del segmento de archivado (Ch. 14).

unidad de cinta (tape drive) dispositivo de almacenamiento de datos que usa cinta magnética como medio de almacenamiento (Ch. 11).

unidad de procesamiento central (CPU) (central processing unit [CPU]) cerebro de la computadora que ejecuta las instrucciones definidas por el software (Ch. 11).

unidad flash (flash drive) dispositivo de almacenamiento de datos en estado sólido (Ch. 11).

unidades de educación continua (UEC) (continuing education units [CEU]) método para obtener puntos a través de una nueva certificación (Ch. 47).

unipolar (unipolar) que tiene o se relaciona con un proceso de un polo (Ch. 37).

urea (urea) producto final principal del metabolismo de las proteínas (Ch. 42).

urgencia (urgency) necesidad de orinar de inmediato (Ch. 30).

urobilinógeno (urobilinogen) compuesto incoloro producido en el intestino después de que las bacterias descomponen la bilirrubina (Ch. 42).

urticaria (urticaria) roncha (Ch. 35).

usual, acostumbrado y razonable (UCR) (usual, customary, and reasonable [UCR]) programa de tarifas que generalmente usan

Medicare y algunas compañías aseguradoras. *Usual* se refiere a la tarifa que generalmente cobra un proveedor por determinados procedimientos; *acostumbrado* se basa en la tarifa promedio para un procedimiento específico que cobran todos los proveedores que ejercen la misma especialidad en una región geográfica determinada; *y razonable* se refiere al nivel medio de tarifas que se cobran por ese procedimiento (Ch. 17).

vacuna (vaccine) agente farmacológico que puede producir inmunidad activa artificial (Ch. 22).

valle (trough) lo opuesto de "pico", es el punto en el cual el fármaco alcanza su nivel más bajo en el cuerpo. Generalmente ocurre justo antes de administrar la dosis siguiente. En las pruebas de laboratorio, el valle indica al proveedor la influencia más débil que tendría el fármaco en el cuerpo con esa dosis en particular (Ch. 38).

valor de referencia (baseline) medición inicial o conocida con la que se comparan mediciones futuras (Ch. 24, 39); también, línea plana y horizontal que separa las distintas ondas del ciclo del electrocardiograma (ECG) (Ch. 37).

valores críticos (critical values) resultados de una prueba que indican la existencia de una situación con posible riesgo para la vida o sumamente debilitante que se debe informar al proveedor de inmediato (Ch. 42).

valores de referencia (reference values) también llamado valor normal, intervalo normal o intervalo de referencia; intervalo de valores que incluye el 95% de los resultados de pruebas de una población normal sana (Ch. 39).

várices esofágicas (esophageal varices) dilatación tortuosa de la vena esofágica relacionada con cualquier afección que produce la obstrucción del drenaje de las venas esofágicas hacia la vena portal del hígado. Ver cirrosis hepática y alcoholismo (Ch. 32).

vasoconstricción (vasoconstriction) estrechamiento o constricción de los vasos sanguíneos (Ch. 33).

vector (vector) un portador de enfermedad, generalmente un insecto, que es el organismo causante de la enfermedad de personas infectadas a no infectadas (Ch. 22).

velocidad de eritrosedimentación (erythrocyte sedimentation rate) medición de cuánto se asientan los glóbulos rojos en una muestra de sangre en una hora (Ch. 41).

venda (bandage) gasa no estéril u otro material que se aplica sobre un apósito estéril para proteger e inmovilizar un área (Ch. 9, 31).

venopunción (venipuncture) punción en la vena con una aguja para obtener una muestra de sangre (Ch. 40).

verbos de acción (power verbs) palabras indicadoras de acción que se usan para describir sus atributos y sus fortalezas (Ch. 48).

vértigo (vertigo) sensación de pérdida de equilibrio o desvanecimiento; mareos (Ch. 25).

vesicular (vesicular) caracterizado por la presencia de vesículas. Las vesículas son ampollas u otras elevaciones de la piel (Ch. 22, 26).

viable (viable) que puede vivir, crecer y desarrollarse después del nacimiento; generalmente de 24 semanas o más de 1 libra (Ch. 26).

viñeta (bullet point) asterisco o punto seguido de una frase descriptiva que ayuda al lector a identificar puntos importantes con facilidad (Ch. 48).

violencia de pareja (IPV) (intimate partner violence [IPV]) se refiere a la violencia o el abuso entre un cónyuge o ex cónyuge, novio o novia, ex novio o ex novia y pareja del mismo sexo o heterosexual o ex pareja del mismo sexo o heterosexual (Ch. 7, 8).

virología (virology) estudio de los virus (Ch. 39, 43).

virulencia (virulence) potencia relativa de un organismo y grado de patogenicidad (Ch. 22).

virus de Epstein-Barr (VEB) (Epstein–Barr virus [EBV]) se cree que este virus es la causa de la mononucleosis infecciosa y que está involucrado en afecciones como el linfoma de Burkitt africano y el carcinoma nasofaríngeo (Ch. 44).

virus de la inmunodeficiencia humana (VIH) (human immunodeficiency virus [HIV]) virus del SIDA; es un retrovirus que con el tiempo destruye las células del sistema inmunitario (Ch. 22).

viscosidad (viscosity) grado de espesor de un líquido (Ch. 40).

vitíligo (vitiligo) trastorno de la piel caracterizado por manchas blancas claras en diversas áreas del cuerpo (Ch. 25).

volátil (volatile) que se evapora fácilmente (Ch. 31).

WiMAX (WiMAX) Tecnología de las comunicaciones que utiliza el espectro radioeléctrico para transmitir entre dispositivos digitales. WiMAX, a veces denominada WiFi con esteroides, tiene la capacidad de transmitir a distancias superiores y manejar muchos más datos a frecuencias de transmisión más altas. Se utilizan los sistemas de tercera generación (3G) y cuarta generación (4G) (Ch. 11).

xeroftalmía (xerophthalmia) membranas mucosas secas y opacas de los ojos (Ch. 34).

ZIP+4 (ZIP+4) código postal estándar que incluye cuatro dígitos adicionales que identifican el área de envío postal. El correo se procesará en forma más eficaz y eficiente con el uso del código ZIP+4 en la dirección (Ch. 15).

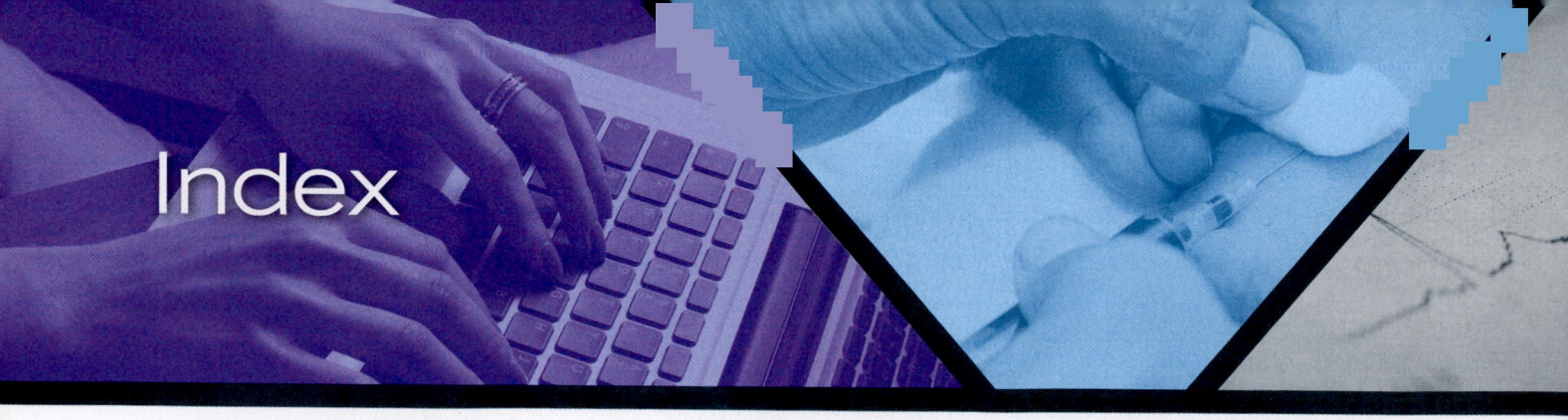

Index

Note: Page references in **bold type** refer to boxes, procedures, figures, and tables.

A

AAMA. *See* American Association of Medical Assistants (AAMA)
Abbreviations
    common medical, 1491–1497
    for patient charts, 585–587, **586**
    for prescriptions, 1082–1084, **1083, 1084**
    of states, **341**
    of street suffixes, **341**
Abdominal aortic aneurysm, **816**
Abdominal examination, **641,** 643
ABO blood typing, 1362–1363, **1363**
Abortion, 149–150, 662–663
Abscess, **788, 790**
Abuse
    child, 124, 144, **145,** 145–146, 738–739
    elder, 125, 144–145, **145**
    ethical issues related to, 144–145
    intimate partner, 125, 143, **145**
Acceptance, as grief stage, 100
Accidents, in older adults, 775
Accountability, 15
Accounting practices
    accounts payable, 490
    accounts receivable trial balance,
      489–490, **496**
    cost analysis and, 491
    day-end summary, 489
    disbursement records, 490
    double-entry system, 487
    financial records and, 491
    function of, 490–491
    income earned reporting, 491–494, **492, 493**
    legal and ethical guidelines for, 494–495
    pegboard system and, 435, **436,** 439, 487
    single-entry system, 486–487
    TPMS, 487–488, **488**
    use of computer service bureau for, 488–489
Accounts payable, 490
Accounts receivable ratio, 469, 470, 494
Accounts receivable trial balance, 489–490, **496**
Accreditation
    ABHES, 9
    CAAHEP, 9, 181
Accrediting Bureau of Health Education Schools
    (ABHES), 9, 33, 1455
Accrual basis, 491
Acid-fast stain, 1341
Acme stage, of infectious disease, 519
Acne, **788, 790**
Activated charcoal, **1067**
Active files, 314
Active listening, 72, 84
Acupressure, **32**
Acupuncture, 31, 43

Acute respiratory distress syndrome
    (ARDS), **810, 812**
Acute stage, of infectious disease, 519
Acute stress, 58
Acute viral hepatitis diseases, 526, **528–529**
Additives, 1228–1229, **1229, 1230**
Adenocarcinomas, 683
Administrative law, 110
    examples of, 110–114
Administrative Simplification Compliance Act
    (ASCA) (2005), 417
Adolescents
    ethical issues related to, **147**
    growth and development in, 726–727
    nutrition for, 1027
Adrenaline, **1067**
Adson, 903
Adults, ethical issues related to, **147**
Advanced Beneficiary Notification (ABN), 433, 915
Advanced Encryption Standard (AES), 218
Advance directives
    examples of, **126–128**
    explanation of, 125, 129
Advanced Registered Nurse Practitioners
    (ARNPs), 36
Advertising, 143
Aerosols, 738
Afebrile, 595
Agar, 1342
Age
    communication and, 76, **77**
    cultural diversity in calculation of, **574**
Aged reports, 365
Agenda. *See* Meeting agenda
Aging. *See also* Gerontology; Older adults
    facts about, 770–771, **771**
    health in, 779–780
    memory impairment and, 776–777
AIDS, 98, 526. *See also* HIV/AIDS
Airborne precautions, **533**
Airborne transmission, 513, 531
Alanine aminotransferase (ALT), 1377
Albumin, 1378
Albuterol, **1067**
Alcohol-based hand rubs (ABHR), **554–555**
Alcohol use
    effects of, **1072–1073**
    during pregnancy, 666
Alkaline phosphatase (ALP), 1378
Allergenic extracts, 1115–1116
Allergy skin testing, 787, 790–791
Allied Bureau of Health Education Schools
    (ABHES), 1456
Allied health professionals
    health unit coordinators as, 33
    job descriptions for various, **34**
    medical assistants as, 32–33
    medical laboratory technologists as, 33
    nurses as, 35–36
    pharmacists as, 35

    pharmacy technicians as, 35
    phlebotomists as, 35
    physical therapists as, 35, **36**
    physical therapy assistants as, 35
    physicians assistants as, 36
    registered dietitians as, 33, 35
Allopathic, 43
Alphabetic filing system, 308, **319–320**
Alpha-fetoprotein test, 660
Alpha-Z filing system, 306–307, **307**
Alternative dispute resolution (ADR), 122
Alternative medicine, 32, **32**
Alzheimer's disease, **793**
Amblyopia, **799**
Ambulation, 978, **996–1001**
Ambulatory care settings. *See also* Computerized
    medical clinics
    boutique or concierge practices as, 26–27
    design and environment in, 192, **192,**
      196–198, **197**
    educational materials in, 195–196
    emergencies in, 158–159
    explanation of, 24
    individual and group practices as, 24–26
    legal compliance in, 198–199
    managed care operations as, 26
    medical assistants in, 7
    overview of, 192
    predictions for future, 203
    procedure to close, 202–203
    procedure to open, 202
    reception area in, **193–195,** 193–196
    safety issues for, 199–202, **201, 204–205**
    urgent care centers as, 26
    welcoming environment in, 193
American Association of Medical Assistants (AAMA)
    background of, **15,** 15–16, 1462
    certification offered by, 16, 19, 1455, 1456–1458
    code of ethics of, 138, **139,** 142
    continuing education and, 16
    educational and certification standards of, 19
    liability insurance offered by, 121
    medical assistant definition of, 6, 7
    2007–2008 Occupational Analysis of the CMA,
      1501–1503
American Chiropractic Association, code of ethics, 142
American Heart Association, 179, **180**
American Medical Association (AMA)
    code of ethics, 138, **139,** 142
    confidentiality policy of, 227–228, **230**
    physician's office laboratories and, 1183
American Medical Technologists (AMT)
    certification offered by, 16, **17,** 1455, 1459–1460
    function of, 16–17, 1462
    on scope of practice, 19
American Recovery and Reinvestment Act (2009)
    (ARRA), 222–223
American Reinvestment and Recovery Act (2009), 298
American Society of Radiologic Technologists
    (ASRT), 19

Americans with Disabilities Act (1990) (ADA)
  explanation of, 111
  facility design and, **192, 193,** 198–199
  telephone communications and, 254
Amniocentesis, 660, 662
Amniotic fluid, 535
Amoebic dysentery, 510
Amorphous, 1308
Amphetamine, **1070**
Amplified DNA probe test, 692, **700–701**
Ampules, **1123–1125**
Amyl nitrite, **1072**
Amyotropic lateral sclerosis (ALS), **793, 796**
Anabolic steroids, **1072**
Anaerobic equipment, 1332, **1332**
Analgesic, **1055**
Anaphylaxis, 1063
Ancillary services, 1421
Anderson, Elizabeth G., **49**
Andropause, 775
Anemias, 775, **819, 820,** 1271
Aneroid manometers, 606
Aneroid sphygmomanometer, 606–607
Anesthesia, 404, 912
Anesthesiologist assistants (AAs), **34**
Anesthetics, 912–914, **914, 1055**
Anger, 99–100
Angina pectoris, **816, 818,** 1156
Angiography, 798, **959, 960**
Anorexia nervosa, 59, **828, 833,** 1027
Answering machines, 255
Answering services, 255
Antacids, **1055**
Anthrax, 552, **552,** 1066
Antianemic, **1055**
Antianxiety medications, **1055**
Antiarrythmic medication, **1055**
Antibacterial creams, 912
Antibiotic-resistant bacteria, 47, **514,** 515
Antibiotics, **1055**
Antibodies, 516, 517
Anticholesterol medication, **1056**
Anticholinergic medication, **1056**
Anticoagulants, **1056,** 1222, **1228–1229**
Anticonvulsants, **1056**
Antidepressants, **1056**
Antidiarrheals, **1057**
Antidote, **1057**
Antiemetics, **1057**
Antihistamines, **1057**
Antihyperlipidemic medication, **1057**
Antihypertensives, **1057**
Antiinflammatories, **1058**
Antimanic medication, **1058**
Antineoplastic medication, **1058**
Antioxidants, 1016, **1019–1020,** 1022
Antipsychotics, **1058**
Antipyretic medication, **1058**
Antitussive medication, **1059**
Antiulcer medication, **1059**
Antiviral medication, **1059**
Antivirus protection programs (computer), 219–220
APGAR Score, **666,** 709
Aphasia, 792
Apical pulse, 603, **620–621, 746–747**
Apnea, 603, 604
Appearance. *See* Personal appearance
Appendicitis, **828, 833**
Appendicular skeleton, 821
Application/cover letters, 1480–1481, **1481, 1482**
Application forms, 1481–1483
Application software, 216–217
Appointment matrix, 279, **284–285**

Appointments. *See* Patient scheduling
Apps, 221, 223, 328
Aquamatic K-Pad, 990–991
Arbitration, 122
Archival storage, medical record, 317
Arms, examination of, **640**
Arm splints, **183–184**
Aromatherapy, **32**
Arrhythmias, 602, 1164–1165
Arteriosclerosis, **816,** 1030
Articulation, 241
Artifacts
  AC interference, 1154–1156, **1155**
  in urine, 1309
Artificial insemination, 149
Ascorbic acid, 1016, **1019**
Asepsis, 45
  medical, 45, 547–551, **549, 550, 553–555,**
    889, 890
  surgical, 888–890, **889**
Aspartate aminotransferase (AST), 1378
Aspiration, of joint fluid, **944–945**
Assisted reproductive technology (ART), 149, 666
Assisted suicide, 96, 151
Assistive devices
  canes as, 984, **984**
  crutches as, 980–983, **981–983**
  explanation of, 978–979
  types of, **979**
  walkers as, 980, **980**
  wheelchairs as, 984–985, **985**
Associate's degree, 8–9
Association for Healthcare Documentation Integrity
  (AHDI), 356, 359
Asthma, 737–738, **810, 812**
Astigmatism, **799, 802**
Atherosclerosis, 605, 1030
Athlete's foot, **788, 790**
Athletic trainers (ATs), **34**
Atrial fibrillation, 1157
Atropine, **1067**
Attention deficit hyperactivity disorder (ADHD), 738
Attitude, 13–14, **1468–1469**
Atypical squamous cells (ASCs), 683
Audiometry, **861–862**
Augmented leads, 1150–1151
Aural temperature, 600, **615,** 733
Auscultation, 632
Auscultatory gap, 608–609
Authoritarian managers, 1399
Authorization for Release of Health Care
  Information Form, 568, **570**
Autoclave, 892–896, **893–895, 925–929,** 1331, **1331**
Automated external defibrillator (AED), 179,
  179, 1160
Automated hematology, 1281–1282
Automated routing units (ARUs), 254–255
Automated urine analyzers, **1306,** 1306–1307, **1307**
Automatic electrocardiograph machines, 1146, 1148
Autopsy reports, 363, **366**
Avascular necrosis, **822**
Avian influenza, 504
Avulsion, **917**
Axial skeleton, 821
Axillary crutches, 980, **981, 982**
Axillary temperature, 600, **617–618,** 733

B

Bachelor's degree, 8–9
Bacilli, 1338–1339, **1339**
Back pain, **824, 825**

Bacteria
  cell structure for, 1330, **1331**
  drug-resistant, 47, **514,** 515
  explanation of, 506–507, 510
  growth requirements for, 1342, **1342**
  media to identify, 1342, **1343**
  microscopic examination of, 1338–1341,
    1339, 1340
  natural, 1328
  shapes of, 1338–1339
  in urine, 1302, 1308–1309
Bacterial diseases, common, **511**
Bacteriologists, 1330
Balance sheets, 491
Balanitis, 758
Bandages, 166–167, **167,** 912, **913, 914**
Banking procedures
  for checking accounts, 441–445, **444–446**
  for online banking, 440
  for savings accounts, 443
Bankruptcy, patient, 475
Bank statements, 445–446, **446, 456**
Banting, Frederick G., 45, **49**
Bargaining, 100
Bariatrics, 841–842
Bariatric surgery, 842
Barium enema, **843, 960**
Barium swallow test, 841, **841, 843, 959, 960**
Barnard, Christian, 45, **50**
Bartholin glands, 678, **689**
Barton, Clara, **49**
Basophils, 1274
Batanitis, **755**
Battery, 117–118
Bell's palsy, **793, 796**
Benadryl, **1067**
Benign prostatic hyperplasia, 761
Benign prostatic hypertrophy, **755**
Benzodiazepines, **1068–1069**
Best, Charles, 45
Betadine, 912
Bethesda system, 683
Bias, communication and, 78
Bilirubin, 1305, 1364, 1378
Bilirubinuria, 1305
Billing. *See also* Collections; Daily financial practices
  cycle system of, 469, **469**
  identifying accounts receivable for, **477**
  for insurance carriers, 471
  monthly, 468–469, **469**
  non-sufficient funds checks and, **479**
  for past-due accounts, 469
  patient statements and, 466–468, **477, 478**
  payment at time of service policy and,
    465–466
  policies for, 465
  Truth-in-Lending Act and, 466, **466**
Bill of Rights, 108
Bimanual pelvic examination, 678, **681**
Bioethics, 146, 150
Biofeedback, **32**
Biohazard labels, 543, **543**
Biohazardous waste, 1333, **1334**
Bioidentical hormone replacement therapy
  (BHRT), 685
Biopsies
  explanation of, 1203
  of kidney, 848
  of skin, 787
Bioterrorism, 551–552, **552,** 1066
Biotin, **1019**
Bipolar leads, 1149, 1150
Birth control, 148–149

Birth control pills, 668, **671**
Blackwell, Elizabeth, 48, **49**
Blanchard, Kenneth, 141
Bleeding
    control of, **182–183**
    external, 177
    internal, 178
Blogs, 1416, 1472
Blood
    from capillary puncture, 1244
    cellular components of, 1221–1222, **1222**
    hazard communication for, 543, **543**
    infection control and, 533
    in urine, 1305
Blood and lymph system
    diagnostic procedures for, 820
    disorders of, **819, 820**
    function of, 818
Bloodborne pathogens, 505, **530,** 539–540, 542
Bloodborne Pathogen Standard (Occupational
    Safety and Health Administration), 539–540,
    544–546, 1232
Blood chemistry tests, 1377–1379
Blood clotting, 1228–1229, **1229**
Blood collection, 1223–1224, **1224, 1225.** See also
    Phlebotomy
Blood culture, 1240, **1240,** 1261–1263, 1337
Blood glucose, 1369
Blood glucose tests, 1369–1373, **1371–1373,**
    1385–1386
Blood incompatibility, 667
Blood pressure
    abnormalities in, 609–611, **610**
    in children, 734, **734**
    equipment to measure, 605–608, **605–608**
    explanation of, 604–605
    normal, 609, **609**
    during pregnancy, **661**
    procedure to measure, 608–609, **609, 622–623**
Blood typing tests, 1362–1364, **1363**
Blood urea nitrogen (BUN), 844, 847, 1378
Blue Cross/Blue Shield (BC/BS), 382
Bluetooth, 218
Body fluids, 534–536
Body language, 73. See also Nonverbal
    communication
Body mass index (BMI), **844**
Body mechanics, 975–976, **976**
Body movements, 638
Body surface area (BSA), 1085, 1096, **1097**
Body temperature. See also Thermometers
    aural, 600
    in children, 733
    explanation of, 594–595
    measurement of, 599, **614–619**
    method to record, 600–601
    oral, 500, 599–600, **618–619**
    rectal and axillary, 600, **616–618**
    terms used to describe, 595, **596**
Bonding, 495
Bonds, 1423
Bone cancer, **822**
Bone densitometry, 962–963
Bookkeeping, 434–435, **436,** 486. See also Accounting
    practices
Botulism, **552,** 1066
Boutique medical practices, 26–27
Bradycardia, 602
Bradypnea, 603
Braille, 198, **199**
Brainstorming, 1401
Brand-name drugs, 1043–1044
Braxton-Hicks contractions, 667

Breast cancer, **689**
Breast examinations, 641, 643, **676,** 676–678, **677**
Breast-feeding, 1026
Breast milk, 536
Breast self-examination (BSE), **677,** 677–678
Breathing emergencies, 178–179, 181
Breath odors, 638–639
Breath sounds, 604
Brochures, 1413–1415, **1415**
Bronchitis, **810,** 812
Bronchodilators, **1059**
Broth tubes, 1342
Bruits, 632
Bubonic plague, 45, 1066
Buffy coat, 1222
Building. See Facility environment
Bulbourethral glands, 757
Bulimia, 59, **828, 833,** 1027
Bundled codes, 408
Burnout, 61–62. See also Stress
Burns
    classification of, 168, **169–171**
    explanation of, 168
    first-aid for, 168–169, **170–171**
    types of, 169, 171
Bursitis, **824, 825**
Bush, George W., 150, 298
Business letters. See also Written communication
    for collection purposes, 472, **473, 474, 478**
    components of, 328–329, **330, 331,** 331–332
    misused words in, 327, **328**
    proofreading of, 327–328, **329**
    spelling in, 327, **327**
    styles for, 332–334, **334, 335**
    supplies for, 334–337
    writing tips for, 326
Butryl nitrite, **1072**
Butterfly needle collection system, **1239,** 1239–1240,
    1254–1257

C

Calcium, **1021,** 1022, 1378–1379
Callus, **788, 790**
Calories, 1013
Cancer
    of blood, **819, 820**
    bone, **822**
    breast, **689**
    cervical, **689**
    colon, **829, 833, 840,** 1031
    endometrial, **689**
    lung, **811, 812**
    ovarian, 686
    overview of, 46–47
    pancreatic, **832, 834**
    penile, 757–758
    prostate, **755,** 762
    rectal, **832, 834**
    skin, **789–791**
    stomach, **832, 834**
    testicular, **755,** 759–760
    therapeutic diets for, 1031–1032
    therapeutic response to patients with, 98–99
    urinary bladder, **845,** 847
Candida, 1350
Candida albicans, 1350
Candidiasis, **689**
Canes, **978, 984, 984, 1001**
Cannabis, **1072**
Cannon, Walter, 58
Cannula, 1227

Capillary puncture, **1244–1246,** 1244–1247,
    1257–1259
Capillary specimen, **1259–1261**
Capitation, 392
Capsule video endoscopy (CVE), 835, **837**
Carbohydrates, 1010, **1010,** 1013, **1014, 1024**
Carbon dioxide (CO$_2$), 1379
Cardiac ablation, 1164
Cardiac arrhythmias, 1156–1157
Cardiac computerized tomography (CCT), 1165
Cardiac cycle, **1145,** 1145–1146
Cardiac electricity, **1150**
Cardiac magnetic resonance (CMR), 1165
Cardiomyopathy, **816**
Cardiopulmonary resuscitation (CPR), 125, 178,
    179, **179, 180,** 181
Cardiovascular disease, 1030–1031
Cardiovascular system, in older adults, 774
Cardioversion, 1159
CARE bill (March 30, 2007), 19, 957
Caregiving, cultural diversity and, 80, **81**
Carpal tunnel syndrome, 226, **793, 822, 825**
Cash
    on hand, 443–444
    petty, 448
Cash basis, 491
Cashier's checks, 443
Casts, 821, **826, 872–873,** 1310, **1311**
Catalyst, 1016
Cataract, **799, 802**
Catheterization. See Urinary catheterization
Catheterized urine collection, 1299
Cautery, 897
Celiac disease, **828, 833**
Cell-mediated immunity, 516
Cell structure, 1330, **1331**
Cellular phones, 261
Cellulose, 1023
Centers for Disease Control and Prevention (CDC)
    immunization guidelines of, 709
    infection control and, 538–539, 549, 551, 1176
Centers for Medicare and Medicaid Services (CMS),
    384, 491, 1087, **1204**
Central European diet, **1033**
Central processing unit (CPU), 212, 215, 225
Cerebral vascular accident (CVA), 178, **793, 796**
Cerebrospinal fluid aspiration, **850–852**
Cerebrospinal fluid (CSF), 534, 1337
Certificate of Training, **1190**
Certificate of Waver (COW) laboratories, **1183**
Certification
    AAMA, 16, 19, 1455, 1456–1458
    agencies granting, 1455, **1455**
    AMT, 16, **17,** 1459–1460
    CCMA, 17, 1461–1462
    CMA, **7,** 16, **16**
    CMAA, 17
    CMAS, **7,** 17
    examinations for, 1454–1456
    function of, 16, 18, **18**
    NCCT, 17–18, **18**
    NCMA, 18
    NHA, 17, 1460–1462
    purpose of, 1454
    RMA, **7,** 17
Certified clinical medical assistant (CCMA),
    1461–1462
Certified medical administrative assistant (CMAA),
    1455, 1461–1462
Certified medical administrative specialist (CMAS), 17
Certified medical assistants (CMAs), 7, 16, **16,** 1455,
    1457–1458
Cerumen, 807

Cervical cancer, **689**
Cervical cap, 668, **669, 670**
Cervical cone biopsy, 691
Cervical intraepithelial neoplasia (CIN), 681
Cervical punch biopsy, 691
Chain, Ernst, 45
Chalazion, **799**
Changu Chung-ching, **49**
Charts. *See* Patient charts
Checking accounts, 441–442
Checkout system, file, 313
Check register, 490
Checks
  acceptance of, 444–445
  lost or stolen, 445
  method to deposit, 443, **444, 454**
  nonsufficient funds, **454–455, 479**
  types of, 443
  writing and recording, 445, **445, 455–456**
CHEDDAR charting approach, 574, 575, 583
Chemical burns, 169
Chemical "cold" sterilization, 910, **924–925**
Chemical Hygiene Plan (CHP), 1184–1185,
  1185–1187, 1188–1189
Chemical Inventory Form, **1185**
Chemicals, avoiding exposure to, 1190–1191
Chemical sterilization, 891–892, 910
Chemical tissue destruction, 897
Chemical urinalysis, **1303,** 1303–1310, **1304,
  1306–1310, 1315–1317**
Chemotherapy, 47
Chest, examination of, **641,** 643
Chest circumference, 613, 732, **744–745**
Cheyne-Stokes, 603
Chicken pox, **525**
Chief complaint (CC), 360, 575
Child abuse
  ethical issues related to, 145–146
  explanation of, 124, 144, **145**
  guidelines to handle, 738–739
  signs of, 739
Children. *See also* Pediatrics
  apical pulse in, **746–747**
  calculation of medication dosages for, 1085,
    1096–1098, **1097**
  chest circumference and, **743–745**
  common disorders and diseases in, 736–739
  ethical issues related to, **147**
  failure to thrive in, 733
  growth and development stages of, 723–727, **724**
  growth patterns in, 727, **728–732, 743–745**
  length and weight measurements in, 727,
    743–745
  nutrition for, 1026–1027
  in reception areas, 195, **195**
  rectal temperature in, **745–746**
  respiratory rate in, **747**
  urine specimen collection in, 734–735, **747–748**
  vital signs in, 723, 725, 733–734, **734**
  weight and length measurement in, **743–745**
Chinese diet, **1033**
Chlamydia, **690,** 692, **700–701, 755, 762**
Chloride, **1021,** 1022, 1379
Cholangiography, **960**
Cholecystitis, **828, 833**
Cholecystogram, **843**
Cholecystography, **961**
Cholelithiasis, **829**
Cholesterol, 1024, 1030–1031, 1373–1376, **1375, 1376**
Cholesterol tests, 1375–1377, **1377, 1386–1387**
Chorionic villus sampling (CVS), 662
Chromium, 1022
Chronic obstructive pulmonary disease (COPD), **810**

Chronic stress, 59
Chronologic résumé, **1465,** 1474
Churchill, Winston, 141
Circadian rhythm, 1298
Circulatory system
  anatomy and physiology of, **1221,** 1221–1222,
    1222
  disorders of, **816–818**
  function of, 815
Circumcision, 676, 739
Civilian Health and Medical Program of the Veterans
  Administration (CHAMPVA), 387
Civil law, 110
Civil litigation. *See* Litigation process
Civil Rights Act (1964), Title VII, 110
Claim registry, 418
Clean-catch midstream collection, 1299, **1300,
  1322–1323**
Cleft palate, **825**
Clinical chemistry department, 1200
Clinical chemistry tests, **1201**
Clinical diagnosis, 1197
Clinical email, 259–260
Clinical Laboratory Improvement Amendments
  (1988) (CLIA), 681, 1176, 1177–1184, **1178,
  1179,** 1205, 1270, **1277**
Clinical laboratory technicians (CLTs), **34**
Clinic brochures, 1415
Clinic management
  employee dismissal and, 1409
  employee evaluation and, 1405, **1406–1408,**
    1408–1409
  of employees with chemical dependencies or
    emotional problems, 1405
  facility and equipment management and,
    1421–1423, **1429–1430**
  harassment and, 1403
  HIPAA implications and, 1410
  legal issues related to, 1423
  liability coverage and bonding and, 1423
  managerial qualities for, **1397,** 1397–1399
  managerial styles and, 1399–1400
  marketing aspect of, 1413–1416, **1414, 1415**
  medical assistants and, 1396
  medical incident reports and, **1424**
  meeting agenda and, **1424**
  personnel assimilation and, 1403–1405
  procedure manual for, 1409–1410,
    1410, 1426
  records and financial management aspects of,
    1417, **1418–1421,** 1420–1421, **1428**
  risk management procedures for, 1400
  social media and, 1416–1417
  supervising student practicum and, **1425**
  teamwork in, 1400–1401
  time management as aspect of, 1411–1413, **1412**
  travel arrangements and, 1410–1411, **1412,
    1427–1428**
Clinic policy manuals, 1437–1438, **1446**
Closed files, 314
Closed questions, 85
Closed wounds, 165, **918**
Clot activators, 1229
Cloud computing, 221, 328
Clustering scheduling, 275
CMS-1500 Form, 380, **381, 409, 411,** 412–413, **414,**
  415, **422–427**
Coagulation, 1229
Coagulation studies, 1281, **1281**
Cobalamin, **1018**
Cobalt, 1022
Cocaine, **1070**
Cocci, 1338

Codeine, **1068**
Codes of ethics
  American Association of Medical Assistants,
    138, **139,** 142
  American Chiropractic Association, 142
  American Medical Association, 138, 142
  American Osteopathic Association, 142
  explanation of, 15, 138–139
Coding. *See* Medical insurance coding
Coenzyme, 1016
Coinsurance, 377, 378
Cold-related illness, 173–174
Colds, 737
Cold therapy, 988–989, 991, **991**
Collection agencies, 472, 474
Collection letters, 472, **473, 474, 478**
Collection ratio, 469–470, 494
Collections. *See also* Billing
  accounts receivable ratio and, 470
  for aging accounts, 470
  insurance claims and, 471
  non-sufficient funds checks and, **479**
  outside agencies for, 472, 474
  policy schedule for, 471, **471**
  post/record collection adjustments and,
    479, 480
  professional attitude for, 476
  small claims court for, 474–475
  special situations related to, 475
  statute of limitations and, 475–476
  techniques for, 470–471
  telephone, 472, **476**
Collections ratio, 469–470
Colon cancer, **829, 833, 840,** 1031
Colonoscopy, 836, **837,** 839
Color, 197–198
Color blindness, **799, 802**
Color-coded filing systems, 306–308, **307**
Color vision, 804–805, **855–856**
Colposcopy, 686, 690, **690**
Comminuted fracture, **826**
Commission on Accreditation for Allied Health
  Education Programs (CAAHEP), 9, 33, 181,
  1146, 1455
Common cold, 737
Common law, 109
Common torts, 117–118
Communication. *See also* Therapeutic
  communication; Written communication
  about sensitive topics, 573
  across the life span, 574
  five Cs of, 72–73
  high-context, 80
  listening skills and, 72
  low-context, 80
  for medical assistants, **10,** 12, **12**
  multicultural, 84–85
  nonverbal, 73–76
  verbal, 72–73
Communication barriers
  age, 76, **77**
  bias and prejudice, 78
  cultural and religious, 80, **81–82,** 82
  defense mechanisms as, 78–80
  economic, 76
  education and life-experience, 76, 78
  environmental, 83–84
  human needs as, 82–83
  patients with special needs as, 83
  time-factor, 84
  verbal, 78, **79**
Communication cycle, 70–72, **71**
Compact disk (CD), 216

Compazine, **1067**
Compendium of Drug Therapy, 1052
Compensation, 80
Competency, **11,** 14
Complete blood count (CBC), 1269–1270
Complex carbohydrates, 1010, **1010**
Compliance programs, 419
Complimentary closing, 331
Computer-aided detection (CAD), 967
Computerized medical clinics. *See also* Computer
　systems
　　clinical and laboratory applications in, 223
　　confidentiality issues in, 221, 227–229, **230**
　　design considerations for, 223, 225
　　ergonomics and, 226–227, **227, 228**
　　general purpose applications for, 222
　　hardware for, 225–226, **234**
　　health records and, 222–223, **224**
　　installation of, 226
　　portable computers and, 223, **225**
　　professionalism in, 229–230
　　routine maintenance of, **231–232**
　　software for, 225, **232–233**
Computerized tomography (CT), 798, 964,
　964, 965, 1164
Computer monitors, 226, **226**
Computer networks, 217–218
Computer service bureaus, 488–489
Computer systems. *See also* Computerized medical
　clinics
　　backup devices for, 220
　　basic information for, 212–213, **213, 214**
　　cloud computing and, 221, 328
　　compatibility issues for, 217
　　documentation for, 217
　　hardware for, 215–216
　　maintenance of, 221–222, **231–232**
　　power and surge protection for, 220
　　security issues related to, 218–220, **220**
　　software for, 216–217
　　types of, 212–213
Computer tomography (CT), 798
Concierge medical practices, 26–27
Condoms, 668, **669, 670**
Condylomata, **690**
Confidentiality. *See also* Privacy
　　in computerized medical clinics, 221,
　　　227–229, **230**
　　in emergency situations, 159–160
　　ethical issues related to, 146
　　HIPAA and, 121, 143, 198, 227–229, 256,
　　　260, 310
　　legal issues related to, 121, 143, 198
　　of medical records, 316–317
　　in obstetrical history, 654
　　protocols for, 358–359
Confidential patient sign-in system, 273, **274**
Conflict resolution, 1402–1403
Congenital anomalies, 662
Congestive heart failure, **816, 818**
Conjunctivitis, **799, 802, 803**
Constitution, U.S., 108
Constitutions, state, 109
Consultation reports, 363, **364**
Consumer Protection Act (1967), Regulation Z, 113
Contact transmission, 513, 531
Continuation page heading, 332
Continuing education
　　AAMA promotion of, 16
　　AMT promotion of, 17
　　of employees, 1445–1446
　　importance of, 14
Continuity of care record (CCR), 580–581

Contraception
　　ethical issues related to, 148–149
　　explanation of, 668, **669**
　　sterilization as, 668, 672, **673**
　　types of, 668, **670–672,** 672–673
Contraceptives, **1059**
Contract law, 114–115
Contracts
　　explanation of, 114–115
　　termination of, 115, **115, 116**
Contract trackers, 1471, **1471**
Contrast media, 958, **959**
Controlled substances
　　classification of, 1046–1047
　　disposal of, 1047
　　e-prescribing of, 1049
　　explanation of, 112–113, 1049
　　medical assistants and, 1047
　　prescriptions for, 1082, **1082**
　　storage of, 1047
Controlled Substances Act (1970), 112–113, 1046
Control tests, 1205
Convalescent stage, of infectious disease, 519
Coordination of benefits (COB), 378–379
Co-payment, 378
Coping skills
　　burnout and, 61–63
　　goal setting and, 63–64
　　importance of, 58
　　stress and, 58–61
Copper, 1022
Copy notation, 332
Corneal abrasion, **799, 802**
Corns, **788, 790**
Coronary artery disease, **817, 818**
Corporations, **25**
Correspondence. *See* Written communication
Cost accounting, 490
Cost analysis, 491
Cost ratio, 494
Coumadin, 1362
Countershocks, 1159
Coupling agent, 662
Covey, Stephen R., 140–141
COX-2 inhibitor, **1060**
CPR. *See* Cardiopulmonary resuscitation (CPR)
Crash cart, 162–164, **163**
C-reactive protein (CRP), 1280–1281, 1377
Creams, **914**
Creatinine, 1295, 1379
Credit arrangements, 434
Criminal law, 109–110
Critical Thinking Challenge (CTC), 1507–1511
Crohn's disease, **829, 833**
Cross-referencing filing system, 311
Croup, 738
Crutches, **979,** 980–983, **981–983, 1000**
Cryosurgery, **691,** 691–692, 897
Crystals, in urine, 1309–1310, **1310**
Cultural brokering, 84–85
Cultural diversity
　　caregiving and, 80, **81–82**
　　communication guidelines for, 84–85
　　diet and, 1032, **1032–1035**
　　ethical issues related to, 144
　　life-threatening illness and, 94–95
　　nonverbal communication and, 74–76, 80
　　patient interviews and, 567–568, 572–573
　　pregnancy and, 654
　　reception area considerations related to, 195
Culture and sensitivity (C&S) urine specimen, 1299
Cultures, 1328
Cumulative trauma disorder, 226, 1191

Current Procedural Terminology (CPT),
　402, 404–406
Current reports, 365
Cyanosis, 639
Cycle billing, 469, **469**
Cystic fibrosis, **810, 812**
Cystitis, **845, 847**
Cystocele, **689**
Cystography, **961**
Cystoscopy, 847
Cytology department, 1203
Cytology tests, **1202**

D

Daily financial practices. *See also* Billing; Collections
　　banking procedures as, 440–446, **444–446,**
　　　454–456
　　bookkeeping as, 434–435, **436, 437**
　　credit arrangements as, 434
　　day sheet balancing as, **450–451**
　　insurance transactions as, **452–453**
　　patient fees as, 432–434, **451**
　　patient transactions records as, 436–440, **438,**
　　　441, 448–449, 453–454
　　petty cash as, **457**
　　supply and equipment purchases as,
　　　446–448, **447**
Data input devices, 215
Data output devices, 215
Data storage devices, 215–216
Data storage memory, 215–216
Date line, 328
Day-end summaries, 489
Day sheets, 439, **450–451**
Death and dying
　　cultural perspective on, 94, **577**
　　ethical issues related to, 151
Declining stage, of infectious disease, 519
Decoding, 71
Decongestants, **1060**
Decubitus ulcers, **788, 790**
Deductible, 378
Deep tendon reflexes (DTRs), 798
Defamation of character, 118
Defense Enrollment Eligible Reporting System
　　(DEERS), 387
Defense mechanisms, 78–79
Defibrillation, 1159–1160
Deltoid muscle, 720, 1111, 1113, **1113**
Dementia, 83, 776
Demographic data form, 568, **569**
Denial, 79, 99
Denver Developmental Screening Test, 725
Dependability, 14
Depolarization, 1144
Depressants, **1068–1070**
Depression, 97, 100
Dermatitis, **790**
Dermatophytes, 1350
Dermatophytosis, **789, 790**
Design considerations
　　for ambulatory care settings, 192, **192**
　　for computerized medical clinics, 223, 225
　　legal compliance and, 198–199
　　for lighting, 196–197
　　music and color and, 197–198
　　for noise reduction, 198
　　safety issues and, 199–202, **201**
　　for ventilation and infection control, 196
Desk Reference for Nonprescription Drugs, 1052
Detoxification, 1066, 1275

Dextrose, **1067**
Diabetes
    explanation of, 176–177
    therapeutic diets for, 1029–1030
    types of, 1091–1092
Diabetic coma, **177**
Diabetic retinopathy, **799, 802**
Diagnosis-related groups (DRGs), 391
Diagnostic imaging
    contrast media and, 958
    filing films and reports and, 967, **968**
    fluoroscopy as, 962–963
    nuclear medicine as, 968
    patient positioning for, 961–962
    patient preparation for, 958
    radiation equipment and, 957–958,
      958, 959
    radiation safety and, 956–957
    radiation therapy and, 967–968
    types of, **960–961, 963–966**, 963–967
Diagnostic medical sonographers (DMSs), **34**
Diagnostic tests. *See also specific tests*
    for digestive system, 827, 834
    for respiratory system, 813
    for sensory system, **799–801**
    for urinary system, 844, 847–848
Dialysis, 99
Diaphragms, 668, **669, 670**
Diarrhea, 827
Diastole, 605, 1145
Diazepam, **1067**
Dietary Supplement Health and Education Act
    (DSHEA), 1045
Diethylstilbestrol (DES), 681
Diets. *See also* Nutrition
    for cancer, 1031–1032
    culture and, 1032, **1032–1035**
    for diabetics, 1029–1030
    for individuals with cardiovascular disease,
      1030–1031
    for weight control, 1028–1029
Differential diagnosis, 1197
Differential stain, 1340–1341
Digestive system
    bariatrics and, 841–842
    conditions and disorders of, 827, **828–834**
    diagnostic tests for, 827, 834
    endoscopic procedures for, **834**, 834–837, **837**
    explanation of, 1009, **1009**
    fecal blood test for, 840, **840, 841**
    function of, 827, **834**
    in older adults, 774–775
    patient education on, **835**
    radiographic studies of, 840–841, **843**
    sigmoidoscopy and, 837–839
Digitalis, 1044
Digital thermometers, 598, **745–746**
Digital video/versatile disk (DVD), 216
Digoxin, **1067**
Dilation and curettage (D&C), 692–693
Dilators, 904, 907, **910**
Diplopia, **799**
Direct skills, 1470
Disaster response, 144, 200–202, **204**
Disbursement records, 490
Discharge summaries, 363, **365**
Discovery process, 122
Discrimination
    based on sexual orientation, 110
    employee, 110, 1445
    against individuals with disabilities, 111
Diseases. *See* Infectious diseases
Disinfection, 550–551

Dislocations, 162, **822, 825**
Displacement, 80
Disposable sensors, 1149
Disposable syringes, 1104
Disposable thermometers, 597–598, **618–619**
Disposition, 122
Diuretics, **1060**
Diuril, **1067**
Diverticulitis, **829, 833**
Diverticulosis, **833**
DNA tests, **1202**, 1203
Doctor of Chiropractic (DC), 27, 28, 30
Doctor of Medicine (MD)
    explanation of, 27–28
    specialists, **29–30**, 43
Doctor of Naturopathic Medicine (NMD), 30
Doctor of Naturopathy (ND), 27, 30–31
Doctor of Optometry (OD), 27
Doctor of Osteopathy (DO), 27, 28
"Doctor" title, 27
Documentation. *See* Patient history and
    documentation
Documents. *See* Medical documents
Doppler ultrasonography, 966
Dorsal recumbent position, 633, **634**
Dorsogluteal site, 1111, **1112**
Dosages. *See* Medication dosages
Dosimeters, 957
Double booking, 273, 275
Double-entry system, 487
Down-code, 408
Down Syndrome, 662
Drapes, **914**
Draping, 633
Drawing techniques, 913–914
Dressing change, **935–936**
Dressings, 166–167, 912, **914**
Drivers, 217
Droplet transmission, 513, 531
Drug abuse, 1066, **1068–1073**
Drug Abuse Prevention and Control Act, 1046
Drug administration. *See* Medication administration
Drug dosage. *See* Medication dosage
Drug-induced ulcers, **829, 833**
Drug-resistant bacteria, 47, **514**, 515
Drugs. *See* Medications
Drug screening, 1311–1312
Dry cold therapies, 991
Dry heat sterilization, 891
Dry heat therapy, 990–991
Dry sterile transfer forceps, 921, **921**
Duodenal ulcers, **830, 833**
Durable power of attorney for health care, 96, 129,
    130–131
Dying. *See* Death and dying
Dysmenorrhea, 675
Dyspareunia, 675
Dyspnea, 604, 809

E

Ear instillation, **862–863**
Ears. *See also* Sensory system
    description of, 805–806, **806**
    disorders of, **806**
    examination of, **640**, 642
    hearing measurement and, 806–808, **807, 808**
Eastern Orthodox diet, **1034**
Eating disorders, 59, **828, 833**, 1027
ECG. *See* Electrocardiography
Echocardiograms, 966
Echocardiography, 1163–1164

Eclampsia, 664
E codes, 407
Ectopic pregnancy, **659**, 663–664
Edematous arms, 1236
Education. *See also* Continuing education
    medical, 43–44
    for medical assistants, 7–9, **8**
    patient, 30, 74, 87, 129
EHR Incentive Program, 1087
The 8th Habit: From Effectiveness to Greatness (Covey), 139
Elder abuse, 125, 144–145, **145**, 777–779
Elderly patients. *See* Gerontology; Older adults
Electrical burns, 169, 171
Electrocardiograph machine, 1149
Electrocardiograph paper, **1145**, 1145–1146, 1149, **1149**
Electrocardiograph telephone transmissions, 1148
Electrocardiography
    artifact interference and, 1154
    basic procedures, 1154–1156, **1155**
    cardiac arrhythmias as, 1156–1159, **1157–1159**
    defibrillation and, 1159–1160, **1160**
    equipment for, 1149, **1149**
    heart rate calculation and, 1146
    holter monitor, **1167–1169**
    lead coding and, 1150
    mounting and, 1154
    myocardial infarctions and, 1156
    overview of, 1142
    sensor placement and, 1150–1151, **1151, 1152**
    standardization and adjustment of, 1153, **1153**
    standard resting, 1153–1154
    types of, 1146, **1147, 1148**, 1148–1149,
      1160–1164, **1161, 1162, 1165–1167**
Electrodes, 1149, 1150
Electroencephalography (EEG), 798
Electrolyte, 1149
Electromyography (EMG), 798, 988
Electroneurodiagnostic technologists (EEG-Ts), **34**
Electronic checks, 443
Electronic claims transmission (ECT), 471
Electronic health records (EHRs), 222–223, 229,
    240, 283. *See also* Electronic medical records
    (EMRs); Medical records
Electronic mail. *See* Email
Electronic medical records (EMRs). *See also* Medical
    records
    archival storage of, 317
    claim forms and, 412, **413**
    confidentiality issues for, 316–317
    function of, 222–223, 316–317, 354, 579–580,
      583, 1417
    health histories on, 571
    laboratory requisitions and, 571, 1208–1210, **1209**
    manual vs., **297**, 297–299
    physical examination in, 636, **637**
    prescriptions and, 1087
    transfer of data to, 317, 354–355
    use of, 298–299, **582**
Electronic thermometers, 598, **598**, 614
Electrostimulation of muscle, 988
Electrosurgery, 896–897, **897**
Email
    clinical, 259–260
    encryption of, 258–259
    etiquette for, **258**
    guidelines for, 257–258
    legal and ethical issues related to, 260
Emancipated minors, 120
Embezzlement, 494–495, 1423
Emergencies
    categories of, **160**
    EMS system for, 161
    Good Samaritan laws and, 161–162

Emergencies (*Continued*)
 medical crash cart for, 162–164, **163**
 911 calls for, 161
 preparing for, 162–164
 primary survey to assess, **160**, 160–161, **161**
 recognition of, 158–159
 responding to, 159–160
 safety practices for dealing with, 181
 universal precautions for, 162
Emergency Cardiovascular Care (ECC), 179
Emergency codes, 200
Emergency contraception, **672**
Emergency medical services (EMS), 161
Emergency medical technicians–paramedics
 (EMTs-Ps), **34**
Emergency medications, 1066, **1067**
Emergency preparedness, 144
Emergency procedures
 for arm splints, **183–184**
 for burns, 168–169, **169–171**, 171
 for cardiac arrest, 178
 cardiopulmonary resuscitation as, 179, **179**,
 180, 181
 for cold-related illness, 173–174
 to control bleeding, **182–183**
 for diabetes, 176–177, **177**
 for fainting, 175–176
 for heart attack, 178
 for heat-related illness, 173
 for hemorrhage, 177–178
 for insect stings, 175, **176**
 for musculoskeletal injuries, 171–173, **173**
 for poisoning, 174
 for respiratory emergencies, 178
 for seizures, 176
 for shock, 164–165, **165**
 for stroke, 178
 for wounds, 165–167, **167**
Emergency/urgent phone calls, 248–249
Emotional/psychological abuse, **145**
Empathy, 13, **13**, 84
Emphysema, **810, 812**
Employee discrimination, 110, 1445
Employees
 assimilation of new, 1403–1405
 with chemical dependencies or emotional
 problems, 1405
 dismissal of, 1409, 1443, **1443**
 education and training of, 1445–1446
 evaluation and salary review for, 1405,
 1406–1408, 1408–1409
 figuring taxes for, 1420
 managing benefits for, 1421
 orienting new, 1442, **1448**
 payroll checks for, 1420
 supervision of, 1401–1403, **1402**
 temporary, 1444–1445
Employment interviews, 1439–1441, **1441, 1447**,
 1483–1486, **1484, 1485**
Employment strategies
 application forms and, 1481–1483
 development of, 1468–1470, **1469**
 interview follow-up and, 1486–1487, **1487**
 job search analysis and research and, 1470–1471
 résumés and, 1472–1480, **1473, 1475–1478**
 social media as, **1471**, 1471–1472
Enclosure notation, 331–332
Encoding, 70–71
Encounter forms, 409, **410**, 436–437
Encryption, email, 258–259
Endometrial biopsy/sampling, 690–691
Endometrial cancer, **689**
Endometriosis, 666, 685, **685, 689**

Endoscopes, sterilization of, **924–925**
Endoscopic procedures, 834–837, **837**
Endoscopic retrograde cholangiopancreatography
 (ERCP), **837**
End-stage renal disease (ESRD), 99
Enema, 839
Energy balance, 1013–1014
Energy nutrients, **1009, 1010–1012**, 1010–1014.
 See also Nutrition
English-as-a-second-language patients,
 communication with, 83
Enterobiasis, **830, 833**
Enterobius vermicularis, 1348–1349, **1349**
Enunciation, 241
Envelopes, 336–337, **343–346**
Environmental factors, communication
 and, 83–84
Eosinophils, 1274
Ephedra, 1045, 1046
Epinephrine, 913, **1067**
Epidemics, 46–47, 518
Epidemiology, 505
Epididymitis, **755**, 756, 760
Epilepsy, **793, 796**
Episodic stress, 59
Epistaxis, 177, **799, 810, 812, 864–865**
Epstein-Barr virus (EBV), 1361
Equal Employment Opportunity Commission
 (EEOC), 110–111
Equal Opportunity Office (EOO), 1403
Equal Pay Act (1963), 111
Equipment/supplies. *See also* Instruments;
 specific supplies
 anesthetics as, 912–914
 calibration and maintenance of, 1422–1423
 drapes as, 911
 dressings and bandages as, 912, **913**
 guidelines to purchase, 446–448, **447**
 inventory of, 1422
 for medical records, 301–303, **302, 303**
 overview of, 910
 for physical examinations, 636, **636**
 solutions/creams/ointments as, 911–912
 sponges and wicks as, 911, **911, 912**
 types of, **914**
 for venipuncture, 1224–1229, **1226–1232**,
 1231–1232
Erectile dysfunction (ED), **755**, 757
E-résumé, 1477–1479
Ergonomics, 226–227, **227, 228**, 1191
Erikson, Erik, 76
Erythrocyte indices, **1277**, 1277–1278
Erythrocytes, 1221, 1268. *See also* Red blood cells
 (RBCs)
Erythrocyte sedimentation rate (ESR), 1278–1280,
 1279, 1280, 1285–1286
Erythropoietin, 1271
Escherichia coli, **512**
Esophagogastroduodenoscopy (EGD), **837, 838**
Essential hypertension, **817, 818**
Estates, 475
Estrogen, 684, 1022
Estrogen and progestin therapy (HT), 684, 685
Ethernet, 218
Ethical considerations
 for abortion and fetal tissue research,
 149–150
 for abuse, 144–145, **145**
 for accounting, 494–495
 for advertising, 143
 for allocation of scarce resources, 146
 for bioethical issues, 146
 for care of poor, 144

 for confidentiality, 143
 for culturally diverse clients, 142
 for death and dying, 151
 for disaster response and emergency
 preparedness, 144
 for email, 260
 five Ps of ethical power and, 141
 for genetic engineering, 150–151
 for health care providers, 142–146
 for HIV/AIDS, 148
 for hospice care, 151–152
 for life-cycle stages, **147**
 for medical assistants, 15, 138–140
 for medical insurance, 392–393
 for medical insurance coding, 419
 for medical records, 143
 overview of, 138
 for principle-centered leadership, 140–141
 for professional fees and charges, 143
 for professional rights and responsibilities, 144
 questions to check, 141–142
 for reproductive issues, 148–149
 for telephone communications, 252–253, **253**
 for written communication, 341
Ethics
 codes of, 15, 138–139, **139**, 142
 explanation of, 138
Eukaryotes, 1329, 1330
Evaluation procedures, 199–200
Examination
 basic components of, 636, **637, 638–639**
 of blood and lymph system, 818,
 819–820, 820
 of circulatory system, 815, **816–818**
 components of, 639, **640–642**, 642–644
 of digestive system, 827, **828–838**, 834–842,
 840–844, 844
 draping for, 633
 equipment and supplies for, 636, **636, 637**
 of integumentary system, 786–787, **787–791**,
 790–791
 of male reproductive system, 763, **764**
 methods of, 630–633
 of musculoskeletal system, 820–821, **821–826**
 of neurologic system, 791–792, 796–798
 positioning for, 633–635, **634, 635**
 procedure following, 644
 procedure to assist with, **645–647**
 of respiratory system, 809, **809–815**, 813–815
 role of medical assistant in, 630
 of sensory system, 798, 802–808
 of urinary system, 844, **845–850**, 847–850
Exclusions, 378
Exclusive provider organizations (EPOs), 382
Excretions, 1178
Excretory urography, **961**
Executive branch of government, 108
Exercise tolerance ECG, **1162**, 1162–1163
Exit interviews, 1443, **1443**
Expectorants, **1060**
Expectorate, 1336
Expert witnesses, 122
Explanation of benefits (EOB), 379, **379**, 419
Expressed contracts, 114
Extensible Authentication Protocol (EAP), 218
External bleeding, 177
External cause codes (E codes), 407
External otitis, **800, 806**
Exudates, 736, 918
Eye-curing lens, 1065
Eye instillation, **856–857**
Eye irrigation, **858–861**
Eye patch, **858**

Eyes. *See also* Sensory system
  description of, 798, 802–803, **803**
  disorders of, **802**
  examination of, **640,** 642
Eyestrain, 226

F

Facebook, 1416
Facial expressions, 74
Facility and equipment management, 1421–1423
Facsimile electrocardiograph, 1148
Failure to thrive, 733
Fair Debt Collection Practices Act (FDCPA), 472
Family and Medical Leave Act (1993)
    (FMLA), 111
Family history, 577
Family planning, **672**
Farsightedness, 802
Fast foods, 1026
Fasting blood glucose (FBG), 1370, **1371**
Fasting urine specimen, 1298
Fats, 1010–1011, **1011, 1012,** 1024, 1030–1031
Fat-soluble vitamins, 1016
Fax machines, 256–257, **257, 265–266**
Febrile, 595
Fecal occult blood test, 840, **840, 841,**
    874–875
Fecal specimens, **1354–1355**
Federal Age Discrimination Act (1967), 111
Federal government, branches of, 108
Feedback, 71–72, 86
Fees. *See* Patient fees
Fee schedules, 390–392, **391**
Feet, examination of, **642**
Female circumcision, 676
Female genital mutilation (FGM), 148
Female genitals. *See also* Gynecological
    examination
      anatomy of, **849**
      examination of, **641,** 644
Fertility, impaired, 665–667
Fertility awareness methods (FAM), 148
Fetal alcohol syndrome (FAS), **666**
Fetal heart rate, 662
Fetal tissue research, 150
Fever, 595, **596.** *See also* Body temperature
Fiber, 1023
Fibrocystic breasts, **689**
Fibromyalgia, **824, 825**
File folders, 302, **302,** 307–308
Files
      movable, 302
      open-shelf lateral, 301–302, **302**
      supplies for, **302,** 302–303, **303**
      vertical, 301, **302**
Filing procedures. *See also* Medical records
      for chart data, 313–314
      checkout, 313
      for correspondence, 315–316
      for cross-referencing, 311–312
      for locating missing files, 313
      for release marks, 312
      for retention and purging, 314, **314**
      for tickler files, 312
Filing systems. *See also* Medical records
      alphabetic, 308, **319–320**
      basic rules for, 303–305
      color-coded, 306–308, **307**
      criteria to choose, 310
      for medical documents in patient files,
        305–306, **306**

numeric, 308–309, **309, 310,** 320
subject, 309–310, **321**
Financial abuse, 145, **145**
Financial accounting, 490, 491
Financial issues, 96–97
Financial records, 491
Fire extinguishers, 200, **201, 204–205**
Fire safety, 200
Firewalls, 220
First-aid. *See* Emergency procedures
First-degree burns, 168, **169, 170**
First morning void specimen, 1298
Fixed costs, 491
Flash drives, 216
Fleming, Alexander, 45, **49**
Flexibility, 14
Florey, Howard, 45
Flu. *See* Influenza
Fluorine, 1022
Fluoroscopy, 962, **962**
Folate, **1018**
Follow-up letters, 1486–1487, **1487**
Fontanels, 724
Foodborne illnesses, 520, 1337–1338, **1338**
Food labels, 1023–1025, **1023–1025**
Forceps, 902–903, **905, 906**
Forearm crutches, 980–981, **981**
Fomites, 513
Formula method, to calculate medication
    dosage, 1091, 1094–1096
Form W-2, **1421**
Form W-4, **1418–1419,** 1420
Fowler's position, 634, **634**
Fractures, 172, **173,** 821, **825, 826**
Free radicals, 1016, 1019
Fringe benefits, 25
Frostbite, 173–174
Full block letters, 333
Fume hoods, 1184
Functional résumé, 1474–1475, **1476**
Fungi, 510, 1350

G

Gait, 638, 798, 981–983
Gait belt, 977
Galvanometer, 1149
Gamete intrafallopian transfer (GIFT), 666
Gamma glutamyltransferase (GGT), 1379
Gamma hydroxybutyric acid, **1068**
Gardasil, 675
Gas sterilization, 891
Gastric bypass, **842**
Gastric ulcers, 827, **830, 833**
Gastritis, **830, 833**
Gastroduodenoscopy, **837**
Gastroenteritis, 827, **830, 833**
Gastroesophageal reflux disease (GERD),
    830, 833
Gastrointestinal (GI) system. *See* Digestive system
General adaptation syndrome (GAS), 58, **59**
Generic drugs, 1043–1044
Genetically engineered pharmaceuticals, 1046
Genetic engineering, 150–151
Geniometer, 821, **821**
Genital examination, **641,** 643–644, 678
Genital herpes, **755, 762**
Genuineness, 84
Genus, 1329–1330
Geographic practice cost index (GPCI), 391
GERD. *See* Gastroesophageal reflux disease (GERD)
German measles, **523**

Gerontology. *See also* Older adults
  aging process and, 770–771, **771**
  explanation of, 770
  medical assistants role and, 776–779, **778**
  physiologic changes in, 771–775, **772–774**
  prevention of complications and, 775–776
  psychological changes and, 776
Gestational diabetes, 655, 664
Gestures, 75
Giardia lamblia, **1347,** 1348, **1348**
Giardiasis, 1348
Gibbon, John, **50**
Glaucoma, **800**
Gleason, Donald, 762
Gleason score, 762
Glomerulonephritis, **845, 847**
Glomerulus, 1294–1295, **1295**
Gloves, **555–558,** 718, **923–924**
Glucagon, 1370
Glucose, 1198, 1304
Glucose meters, **1371**
Glucose tests, 1369–1373, **1371–1373, 1385–1386**
Glucose tolerance test (GTT), 1371–1372
Glycosylated hemoglobin, 1373
Goals, 63–64
Goal setting, value of, 63–64
Goggles, 549
Going bare, 1423
Gonorrhea, **690, 700–701, 755, 762**
Good Samaritan laws, 125, 161–162
Gout, **822, 825**
Gowns, **557–558**
Gram stain, 1332, **1340,** 1340–1341
Gravida, 659
Gravidity, 658–659
Greenstick fracture, **826**
Grief, stages of, 99–100
Gross contamination, 547
Group medical practices, 24–25, **25**
Guarantor, 437
Guided imagery, **32**
Guides (file), 302–303, **303**
Guthrie screening test, 1366
Gynecological examination
      assisting with, 678–679
      breast examination and, **676,** 676–678, **677**
      female circumcision and, 676
      HPV and, 675, 681
      laboratory requisition for, 680, **682**
      Pap tests and, 674–676, 679–681, **679–681,** 683,
        683, 694–696
      recommendations for, 674–675
Gynecological issues
      complementary therapy for, 693
      contraception as, 668, **669–673,** 672–673
      endometriosis as, 666, 685, **685**
      infertility as, 665–667, 684
      list of common, **689–690**
      menopause as, 684–685
      ovarian cancer as, 686
      ovarian cysts as, 686, **686**
      pelvic inflammatory disease as, 665, 686
      sexually transmitted, **690**
Gynecological tests/treatments
      amplified DNA probe test as, 692, **692,**
        700–701
      cervical cone biopsy as, 691
      cervical punch biopsy as, 691
      colposcopy as, 686, 690
      cryosurgery as, 691–692
      dilation and curettage as, 692–693
      endometrial biopsy/sampling as, 690–691
      hormonal contraceptive insertion as, **698**

Gynecological tests/treatments (*Continued*)
   intrauterine device insertion as, **671–673,**
      696–697
   laparoscopy as, 666, 692, **693**
   list of common, **687–688**
   potassium hydroxide prep as, 692, **699–700**
   wet prep/wet mount as, 692, **699–700**
Gynecology, 654, 673–674

H

Haemophilus pertussis, **512**
Hahnemann, Samuel, **49**
Hallucinogens, **1070–1072**
Hands, examination of, **640**
Handwashing, 196, 538, 548, **549, 553–555,** 718.
   See also Asepsis
Harassment, 110–111, 1403
Hard drives, 215–216
Hardware (computer)
   compatibility issues for, 217
   for computerized medical clinics, 225–226, **234**
   description of, 215–216
   installation of, **234**
Hashish, **1072**
HCPCS. *See* Healthcare Common Procedure Coding
   System (HCPCS)
Head, examination of, 639, 641
Headaches, **796**
Head circumference, 731–732, **732, 744**
Head lag, 724
Health care
   availability of, 146
   explanation of, 376
   as right or privilege, 148
Healthcare-associated infection (HAI), 515
Healthcare Common Procedure Coding System
   (HCPCS), 402, 406
Health care directive form, **126.** *See also* Advance
   directives
Health care providers
   ethical guidelines for, 142–146
   regulation of, 18–19
Health Care Reform Act (2010), 146
Health care team
   allied health professionals on, 32–36
   chiropractors on, 28
   "doctor" title and, 27
   explanation of, 27
   integrative medicine and alternative health
      care practitioners on, 28, 30–31, **32**
   medical assistants on, 36
   medical doctors in, 27–28, **29–30**
   naturopathic practitioners on, 30–31
   oriental medicine practitioners and
      acupuncturists on, 31
   osteopaths in, 28
Health Information Technology Plan, 298
Health insurance. *See* Medical insurance
Health Insurance Portability and Accountability Act
   (1996) (HIPAA)
   clinic protocol and, **192,** 193, 358
   confidentiality and, 121, 143, 198, 227–229,
      256, 260, 310, 358, 568
   HIPAA manual and, 1410
   patient scheduling and, 273
   provisions of, 112
   scheduling and, 273
   telephone communications and, 253–254
Health insurance specialists, 393
Health maintenance organizations (HMOs), 24,
   378, 383

Health unit coordinators (HUCs), 33
Hearing. *See also* Ears
   in infants, 735
   measurement of, **807, 808**
   in older adults, 772, 777
Heart
   anatomy of, 1142–1143, **1143**
   electrical conduction system of,
      1143–1145, **1144**
   examination of, **641**
Heart attacks, 178, 1156
Heart disease, 1164
Heart rate
   in children, 733, **734**
   fetal, 662
Heat cramp, 173
Heating pads, 990–991
Heat-related illness, 173
Heat stroke, 173
Heat therapy, 988–991, **990**
Hegar dilators, 907
Height, 611, **612–613,** 624, **624,** 730–731
Hematocrit, 1272–1273
Hematocrit tests, 1271, 1272
Hematologic tests
   procedures for, 1270
   types of, **1201,** 1268–1270
Hematology
   automated, 1281–1282
   coagulation studies and, 1281
   C-reaction protein and, 1280–1281
   erythrocyte indices and, **1277,** 1277–1278
   erythrocyte sedimentation rates and, 1278–1280,
      1279, 1280, 1285–1286
   explanation of, 1220, 1268
   hematocrit and, **1272,** 1272–1273, **1273**
   hemoglobin and, **1271,** 1271–1272, **1282–1283**
   microhematocrit determination and, **1283–1285**
   platelets and, 1276–1277, **1277**
   prothrombin time and, **1287–1288**
   red blood cells and, 1275–1276, **1276**
   white blood cells and, 1273–1275, **1274, 1275**
Hematology department, 1200
Hematology Report Form, **1270**
Hematopoiesis, 1268, **1269**
Hematuria, 1305
Hemoconcentration, 1236
HemoCue, **1262,** 1272
Hemoglobinopathies, 1271
Hemoglobin tests, 1271, 1272, **1272, 1282–1283**
Hemoglobinuria, 1305
Hemoglobin, **1271,** 1271–1272
Hemolytic disease of the newborn (HDN), 1364
Hemophilia, **819**
Hemoptysis, 809
Hemorrhage, 177–178
Hemorrhoids, **831**
Hemorrhoid thrombectomy, **945–947**
Hemostatic forceps, 902–903
Hemostatics, **1060**
Hepatitis, **831, 833**
Hepatitis A virus (HAV), 526, **528–529**
Hepatitis B vaccination, 540, 542, **542, 545**
Hepatitis B virus (HBV), 526, **528–530, 762**
Hepatitis C virus (HCV), 504, 526, **528–529, 762**
Hepatitis D (HDV), 526
Hepatitis E (HEV), 526
Herbal supplements, 1020, 1044–1046, **1045**
Herniated disk, **822, 825**
Heroin, **1068**
Herpes simplex, **690**
Herpes zoster, **790, 794, 796**
Hiatal hernia, **831, 833**

Hibeclens, 912
Hierarchy of needs, 60, **82,** 82–83
High-context communication, 80
High-density lipoprotein (HDL), 1376, **1376**
Hindu diet, **1034**
HIPAA. *See* Health Insurance Portability and
   Accountability Act (HIPAA)
Hippocrates, 46, 48, **49**
Hippocratic Oath, 48, **48**
Hiring. *See* Recruiting/hiring
Histology department, 1203
Histology tests, **1202**
History and physical examination reports,
   360, **361**
History of present illness (HPI), 360
HIV/AIDS
   background of, 47, 504
   ethical issues related to, 148
   facts about, **520,** 526, **527–528,** 690, **762**
   patients with, 98
HMOs. *See* Health maintenance organizations
   (HMOs)
Hodgkin's disease, **819, 820**
Holter monitor, 1160–1162, **1161, 1162, 1167–1169**
Homeopathy, **32**
Hookworm, 1350
Hospice, 151–152
Hospital-based laboratories, 1198
Hospital inpatient prospective payment system
   (IPPS), 391
Hospital outpatient prospective payment system
   (OPPS), 391–392
Household measures, **1089,** 1089–1090, **1090**
Human chorionic gonadotropin (hCG), 1360
Human cloning, 151
Human Genome Project, 1043
Human growth and development, stages of, 76, **77**
Human papillomavirus (HPV), 675, 681
Human resources management
   clinic policy manual and, 1437–1438, **1446**
   compliance with personnel laws as function
      of, 1444
   discrimination and, 1445
   dismissing employees as function of, 1443, **1443**
   employee training/education as function
      of, 1445–1446
   maintaining personnel records as function
      of, 1443–1444
   orienting new personnel as function of,
      1442, **1448**
   recruiting and hiring as function of, **1438,**
      1438–1442, **1440, 1441, 1446–1447**
   smoking policy and, 1445
   tasks for, 1436–1437
   temporary employees and, 1444–1445
Humoral immunity, 516–517
Hunter, John, **49**
Hyaline casts, 1310
Hydrocodone, **1068**
Hydrocortisone, **1067**
Hydrogen peroxide, 912
Hydromorphone, **1068**
Hydrotherapy, **32**
Hyperemesis gravidarum, 664
Hyperopia, **800**
Hyperpnea, 604
Hypertension, 605, 610, **610,** 667, 1030
Hyperventilation, 604
Hypnotic agents, **1061**
Hypoglycemic agents, **1061**
Hypogonadism, 760
Hypotension, 611
Hypothermia, 174

Hypoventilation, 604
Hypoxia, 665
Hysterosalpingography, 665–666, **961**

I

ICD-9-CD. *See* International Classification of Diseases, 9th Revision, Clinical Modification (ICD-9-CM)
ICD-10-CD. *See* International Classification of Diseases, 10th Revision, Clinical Modification (ICD-10-CM)
Ice packs, 991, **991**
Identification labels, 302
Illness. *See also* Infectious diseases; Life-threatening illness
    attitudes toward, 44
    history of present, 576
    sudden, 175
Imaging techniques. *See* Diagnostic imaging
Immune responses, 516–518
Immune system, 516–518
Immunity, 516, 517
Immunizations
    administration guidelines for, **713–716,** 718–723, **719–722, 740–741**
    booster, 726
    classifications of, 518
    function of, 506, 518
    preparation of, 709, 713, 716
    recommended adult, **508–509**
    recordkeeping for, 716, **717, 741–742**
    schedules for, **710–712,** 717–718
Immunoglobins, 517
Immunohematology, 1200
Immunosuppressed populations, 505
Impacted cerumen, **800, 806**
Impacted fracture, **826**
Impetigo, **520, 789, 790**
Implanon, **698**
Implantable cardioverter defibrillator (ICD), 1165
Implantable devices, 1065
Implied consent, 120
Implied contracts, 114–115
Inactive files, 314
Incinerators, 1333, **1333**
Incisions, **917, 939–940, 942–944**
Income statements, 491, **492–493**
Incoming calls, **242,** 242–245, **261–262**
Incompetence, legal, 120
Incubation stage, of infectious disease, 518–519
Incubators, 1332
Indexing units, 303–304
Indirect statements, 85–86
Individual medical practices, 24–25, **25**
Individuals with disabilities, discrimination against, 111
Infants. *See also* Children; Newborns; Pediatrics
    ethical issues related to, **147**
    failure to thrive in, 733
    growth and development in, 723–725
    guidelines to lift and carry, 727–730
    hearing impairment screening in, 735
    injection guide for, 720
    length in, **729**
    measurement of, **743–745**
    nutrition for, 1026
    respiratory rate in, **747**
    taking rectal temperature in, **745–746**
    urine specimen collection from, 734–735, **735, 747–748**
    visual acuity in, 735, **736**

Infection control
    bioterrorism and, 551–552, **552**
    blood and body fluids and, 533–536
    bloodborne pathogen standard and, 539–540, **544–546**
    design principles and, 196
    during emergencies, 162
    federal agencies and, 538–539
    immunizations and, 718
    infectious waste disposal and, 537–538
    maximum process for, **551**
    medical asepsis and, 45, 547–551, **549, 550, 553–555**
    needlesticks and, 536–537
    OSHA regulations and, 539–540, **541,** 542–543, 546–547
    overview of, 504
    personal protective equipment for, 536, **555–560**
    principles of, 547
    standard precautions and, 162, 513, **532**
Infection cycle
    explanation of, 506, **507**
    infectious agents and, 506–507, 510–511
    mode of transmission and, 513
    portal of entry and, 514
    portal of exit and, 511, 513
    reservoir and, 511
    susceptible host and, 514–515
Infections
    incision and drainage of, **942–944**
    nosocomial, 1330
Infectious diseases. *See also specific diseases*
    agents of, 506–507, 510–511
    body's defense mechanisms to fight, 515–518
    causes of, 505–506
    common bacterial, **511, 512**
    common viral, **510**
    examples of, **520–525**
    fungal, **512**
    immunizations for, 506, **508–509**
    impact of, 505
    overview of, 504
    reporting requirements for, 529, **531**
    stages of, 518–519
    standard precautions for, 529, 531, **532–538,** 533, 539 (*See also* Infection control)
    transmission of, **507,** 513–515, 519, **520–525,** 526, 531
Infectious mononucleosis, **819,** 1361
Infectious mononucleosis tests, 1361–1362
Infectious waste, disposal of, 537–538, **538**
Infertility, 665–666, 684, 763
Inflammation, 516, **916,** 917, 1275, 1377
Inflammatory response, 516
Influenza, **520, 810, 812**
Informed consent
    explanation of, 118, 120, 915
    implied, 120
    legal incompetence and, 120
Informed consent forms, **119**
Inhalants, **1072**
Inhalation medications, 1065, 1116–1118, **1117, 1118**
Inhalers, 815, 1116
Initiative, **11,** 14
Injectable anesthetics, 913
Injections. *See also* Immunizations
    basic guidelines for, 1114–1115, **1125–1127**
    intradermal, 1110, 1111
    intramuscular, 719, **720, 721,** 1110–1114
    subcutaneous, **720, 722,** 1110, 1111
Inner-directed people, 63
Inoculating equipment, 1332–1333, **1333**

Inoculating needle, 1333, **1333**
Insect stings, 175
Inside address, 328
Inspection, 630–631
Institute of Medicine (IOM), 1086, 1087
Instruments. *See also* Equipment/supplies
    care of, 907–910
    categories of, 900, **901–910,** 902–907
    checking quality of, 1205
    explanation of, 900
    sterilization of, **925–929**
Insulin, **1067,** 1091–1093, **1092,** 1370
Insulin shock, **177**
Insurance. *See* Medical insurance
Insurance coding. *See* Medical insurance coding
Insurance fraud/abuse, 392–393
Integrated delivery systems (IDSs), 383
Integrative medicine, 28, 31–32
Integrity, **11,** 15
Integumentary system. *See also* Skin
    allergy skin testing and, 787, 790–791
    disorders of, **788–790**
    explanation of, 786–787, **787**
    in older adults, 772–773
    skin tests for, 790–791, **791**
Intentional torts, 117
Interactive videoconferencing, 260–261
Internal bleeding, 178
International Classification of Diseases
    9th Revision, Clinical Modification (ICD-9-CM), 402–403, 406–409, 412, **420**
    10th Revision, Clinical Modification (ICD-10-CM), 402–403
International direct distance dialing (IDDD), 251
International normalized ratio (INR), 1362
International Revenue Service, 110
Internet
    explanation of, 217
    secure sites on, 220, **220**
    security issues related to, 218–219
    travel arrangements using, 1411
    virus protection and, 219–220
Interpretive electrocardiograph, 1148–1149
Interrogatory, 122
Interviews
    cultural awareness during, 567–568, 572–573
    employment, 1439–1441, **1441, 1447,** 1483–1486, **1484, 1485**
    patient, 567–568, **571,** 571–573, **573**
    techniques for, 85–86
Intestinal protozoa, **512**
Intimate partner violence (IPV), 125, 145
Intradermal injections
    administration of, **1125–1127**
    of purified protein derivative, **1131–1132**
Intradermal test, 791
Intramuscular injections
    administration of, **1125–1127, 1129–1131**
    explanation of, 719, **720, 721**
    marking correct site for, 1111, **1112,** 1113–1114
    site selection for, 1110–1111
    Z-track method for, 1115, **1134–1136**
Intrauterine device (IUD)
    explanation of, **671–673**
    insertion of, **696–697**
Intravenous pyelogram (IVP), 761, 847, **848**
Intravenous therapy, 1108–1110, **1109**
Invasion of privacy, 118
Invasive, 1197
In vitro fertilization (IVF), 149, 666
Involuntary dismissal, 1409, 1443
Iron, 1022
Iron deficiency anemia, 1271

Irritable bowel syndrome (IBS), **831, 834**
Ischemia, **1156**
Islam, 43–44
Islamic diet, **1034**
Isoelectric line, 1145
Isolation categories (Centers for Disease Control), 538
Isopropyl alcohol, 912
Isuprel, **1067**
Italian diet, **1033**
Itinerary, 1411
Iyler, Patricia W., 72

J

Japanese diet, **1033**
Jaundice, 639, 1364, 1378
Jenner, Edward, **49**, 505
Jet injection, 537
Jewish diet, **1034**
Job application/cover letters, 1480–1481, **1481, 1482**
Job application forms, 1481–1483
Job descriptions, **1438,** 1438–1439, **1446–1447**
Job hunting. *See* Employment strategies
Job interviews, 1439–1441, **1441, 1447,** 1483–1486, **1484, 1485**
Job résumés, 1472–1480, **1473, 1475–1478**
Job search, 1470–1471
Joint fluid aspiration, **944–945**
Joint movement, 986, **986, 987**
Judicial branch of government, 108

K

Ketoacidosis, 1302
Ketones, 1304–1305
Ketonuria, 1305
Ketosis, 1305
Keyed signature, 331
Kidney biopsy, 848
Kidneys, function of, 1294–1295
Kidney transplants, 99
Kinesics, 73
Knee-chest position, 634–635
Koch, Robert, 45, **49,** 505
Kübler-Ross, Elisabeth, 99, 100
Kyphosis, **823**

L

Labor, **667,** 667–668
Laboratories
    departments in, **1120,** 1199–1200, 1202–1203
    microscopes in, 1211–1213, **1211–1214**
    panels of, 1203, **1204**
    personnel in, 1199, **1199**
    types of, 1198–1199
Laboratory procedures
    Clinical Laboratory Improvement Amendments and, 1177–1184, **1178, 1179**
    ergonomics and cumulative trauma disorders and, 1191
    OSHA regulations and, 1184–1185, **1184–1190,** 1188–1191
    quality control, 1205
    requisitions and reports as, 1205, **1206,** 1207–1209, **1208, 1209**
    safety and, 1176
    for specimens, **1209,** 1209–1210, **1210**
Laboratory Requisition Form, **1206**

Laboratory tests
    for adolescents, 726–727
    billing for, 1203
    blood chemistry, 1377–1379
    blood glucose, 1369–1373, **1371–1373**
    blood typing, 1362–1364, **1363**
    categories of, 1200, **1201–1202,** 1202–1203
    cholesterol and lipids, 1373, 1375–1377, **1375–1377**
    factors affecting results of, 1241–1242, **1242,** 1244
    infectious mononucleosis, 1361–1362
    overview of, 1196
    panels of, 1203, **1204**
    phenylketonuria, 1366, **1367, 1382–1384**
    pregnancy, 1360–1361, **1380–1381**
    prenatal, 657, **657**
    purpose of, 1197–1198
    quality controls for, 1205
    semen analysis, 1364–1365, **1365**
    systemic inflammation, 1377
    that require special handling, **1243**
    tuberculosis, 1366–1369, **1369**
Labyrinthitis, 642
Lacerations, **917, 939–940**
Lactate dehydrogenase (LDH), 1379
Lactation, nutrition and, 1025, 1026
Laennec, Rene, **49**
Lamaze method, 660
Laparoscopy, 666, 692, **693, 837**
Laryngitis, **810, 812**
Laser surgery, 897–898
Lasix, **1067**
Lateral position, 635, **635**
Latex sensitivity, **531**
Law. *See also* Legal issues; Legislation; Litigation process
    administrative, 110–114
    civil, 110
    common, 109
    contract, 114–115
    criminal, 109–110
    sources of, 108–109
    statutory, 109
    tort, 115–118
Laxatives, **1061**
Lead wires, 1150
Ledgers, patient, 437–439, **438**
Legal incompetence, 120
Legal issues. *See also* Law; Legislation; Litigation process
    for accounting, 494–495
    advance directives as, 125, **126–128,** 129, **130–131,** 132
    for clinic manager, 1423
    confidentiality as, 121, 143, 198 (*See also* Confidentiality)
    for email, 260
    informed consent as, 118, **119,** 120
    for medical insurance, 392–393
    for medical insurance coding, 419
    for patient scheduling, 277
    public duties as, 124–125
    related to human resource management, 1444
    risk management to avoid, 120–121
    statute of limitations as, 123
    for telephone communications, 252–253, **253**
    for written communication, 341
Legislation. *See also* Law; *specific laws*
    explanation of, 108–109
Legislative branch of government, 108
Legs, examination of, **642**
Leonardo da Vinci, 44
Lesions, 787

Letterhead, 335
Letter of reference, 1443
Letter of resignation, 1443
Letters. *See* Business letters; Written communication
Leukemia, **819, 820**
Leukocytes, 1221, 1268, 1273–1275, **1274–1276,** 1305. *See also* White blood cells
Liability insurance, 121, 1423
Licensed practical nurses (LPNs), 36
Licensure, 18, **18**
Lidocaine, **1067**
Life-threatening illness
    cancer as, 99–100
    challenges for medical assistants who have patients with, 100–101
    choices for patients that have, 95–97
    cultural perspective on, 94–95
    end-stage renal disease as, 99
    explanation of, 94
    grief and, 99–100
    HIV/AIDS as, 98
    psychological suffering in, 97–98
Lifting techniques, 976
Lighting, 196–197, **197**
Lignin, 1023
Lillehei, C. Walton, 45, **50**
Lipids. *See* Fats
Lipoproteins, 1376
Li Shih-chen, 44
Listening skills, function of, 72, 84
Lister, Joseph, 45, **49**
Lithium, 1044
Lithotomy position, 633–634, **634**
Litigation process. *See also* Law; Legal issues
    discovery period as, 122
    explanation of, 121, **123**
    pretrial conference in, 122
    subpoenas and, 121–122
    trial period in, 122–123
Living wills, 129
Local area network (LAN), 217
Long and short leg casts, 821
Long arm cast (LAC), 821
Long-distance telephone calls, 251–252
Long-range goals, 63
Loop ECG, 1162
Lordosis, **823**
Low-context communication, 80
Low-density lipoprotein (LDL), 1376, **1376**
LSD, **1070**
Lumbar puncture, 798, **850–852**
Lung cancer, **811, 812**
Lungs, examination of, **641**
Lybrel, **671**
Lyme disease, **521**
Lymph, 818
Lymphedema, **819, 820**
Lymphocytes, 1273
Lyophilized vaccination form, 718

M

Macroallocation, 146
Macular degeneration, **800**
Magnesium, 1022, **1021**
Magnetic disk drives, 215–216
Magnetic resonance imaging (MRI), 798, 964–965, **965, 966,** 1164
Mail
    incoming, 338–339, **340**
    outgoing, 339–341, **341, 343–348**
    postage rates for, 340, **340**

Mail merge, 337, **346–448**
Mainframe computers, 213
Malaria, 45, 47, 510
Male genitalia, **641,** 644
Male reproductive system
  anatomy of, 754, 756–757, **848**
  diseases and disorders of, **755**
  disorders of penis and, 757–758
  disorders of prostate and, 760–762, **761, 762**
  disorders of testes and, **758, 759,** 758–760
  infertility and, 763
  physical examination of, 763, **764**
  sexually transmitted diseases and, **755,**
    762, **762**
Malfeasance, 109
Malnutrition, in older adults, 775
Mammography, 674–675, **961,** 967
Managed care operations, 26
Managed care organizations (MCOs), 382
Managed care plans, 382–384, **393–394**
Management. *See* Clinic management
Management by walking around (MBWA),
  1399–1400
Managerial accounting, 490
Managers
  qualities of, 1397–1399
  styles of, 1399–1400
Mandates, 1180
Manganese, 1022
Manipulation, 633
Manometers, 606
Mantoux test, 1368–1369, **1369**
Manual medical records. *See* Medical records
Marijuana, **1072**
Marketing, 1413–1416, **1414, 1415**
Masks, **557–558**
Maslow, Abraham, 60, 61, 82
Massage, **32**
Massage therapy, 992, **992, 993**
Material Safety Data Sheet (MSDS), 1185,
  1186–1187, 1188
Mature minors, 120
M codes, 408
MDMA, **1070**
Mean corpuscular (cell) volume (MCV), 1277, 1278
Mean corpuscular hemoglobin concentration
  (MCHC), 1277, 1278
Mean corpuscular hemoglobin (MCH),
  1277, 1278
Measurement. *See also* Vital signs
  of chest circumference, 613, 732, **744–745**
  of head circumference, 731–732, **732, 744**
  of height, 611, **612, 613, 624,** 730–731
  of weight, 611–613, **613, 624–625, 743–745**
Media, in microbiology laboratory, 1333,
  1342–1343, **1343**
Mediation, 122
Medicaid
  administration of, 110
  explanation of, 386–387
  patient fees and, 433
Medical asepsis
  disinfection and, 550–551
  examples of, 548
  explanation of, 547, 1176
  hand washing and, 196, 548, **549, 553–555**
  sanitization and, 548–550, **549, 560**
  sterilization and, 551
  surgical vs., **889**
Medical assistants. *See also* Clinic management
  accreditation for, 9
  attributes of, 9, **10–11,** 12–15
  career opportunities for, 7

certification for, **7,** 16, 17, **18,** 58, 1454–1455,
  1455, 1457–1462
disaster preparedness for, 202, **204**
educational requirements for, 7–9, **8**
explanation of, 6, **34**
in health care team, 36
historical background of, 6–7
impact of Clinical Laboratory Improvement
  Amendments on, 1183–1184
importance of chemical standards to, 1189–1190
in microbiology laboratory, 1328–1329
national association for, 15–16
negligence and, 117
regulation of, 18–19
role in laboratory tests, 1205
role in phlebotomy, 1220–1221
role in rehabilitation, 974–975
role of, 32–33
role with controlled substances,
  1047, **1048,** 1049
role with geriatric patients, 776–779, **778**
scope of practice for, 18–19
strategies for newly employed, 1487–1488
supervision of, 6
task list for, 1504–1506
Medical Assisting Education Review Board
  (MAERB), 1456
Medical Bluetooth, 51
Medical crash cart, 162–164, **163**
Medical documents
  authentication of, 357–358
  autopsy reports as, 363, **366**
  chart notes and progress notes as, 360, **360**
  confidentiality and, 143, 358–359
  consultation reports as, 363, **364**
  discharge summaries as, 363, **365**
  filing procedure for, 305–306
  history and physical examination reports as,
    360, **361**
  medical correspondence as, 363, 365, **367**
  medical transcription and, 354–358, **357,**
    366, 368
  operative reports as, 361–362, **362**
  pathology reports as, 262–263, **363**
  radiology and imaging reports as, 360–361, **362**
  turnaround time for, 365
  types of, 359
Medical history, 576–577, **587.** *See also* Medical
  records; Patient history and documentation
Medical history form, 568, 570
Medical illustrators (MIs), **34**
Medical incident report, **1424**
Medical insurance
  CHAMPVA, 387
  fee schedules for, 390–392, **391**
  function of, 376–377
  legal and ethical issues related to, 392–393
  managed care, 382–384, **393–394**
  Medicaid, 386–387
  medical tourism, 388
  Medicare, 384–386, **384–386,** 391, **391, 396–397**
  posting payment and adjustments for, **452–453**
  referrals and, 389–390, **396**
  screening for, 388–389, **394–395**
  self-insurance, 388
  terminology for, 377–380
  traditional, 380, 382
  TRICARE, 387
  verifying eligibility for, **395**
  workers' compensation, 387–388
Medical insurance claims
  common errors in, 417
  electronic submission of, 417, **452**

forms for, 380, **381,** 409, **410, 411,** 412–413,
  414, 415, **416,** 417
insurance carrier's role in, 419
management of, 417–419, **418,** 471
Medical insurance coding
  accuracy of, 408–409
  for claim forms, 380, **381,** 409, **410, 411,**
    412–413, **414,** 415, **416,** 417, **422–427**
  clinical modification, **420–421**
  converting medical procedures to, **420**
  HCPCS, 402, 406
  ICD-10-CM and ICD-10-PCS, 402–403
  legal and ethical issues related to, 419
  for medical diagnoses, 406–409
  for medical procedures, 403–406
  overview of, 402
  third-party guidelines for, 412, **421**
Medical insurance specialists, 393
Medical laboratories. *See* Laboratories; Laboratory
  procedures; Laboratory tests
Medical laboratory technologists (MLTs), 33, **33**
Medical Office Simulation Software (MOSS), 222,
  223, 242, **244, 285–289,** 318, 319, 368–369, 395,
  451–454, 477–479, 496, **1511–1517**
Medical practice acts (state), 114, **114**
Medical records. *See also* Electronic health records
  (EHRs); Electronic medical records (EMRs);
  Patient history and documentation
  accuracy of, 299–300
  corrections to, 299–300, **319**
  correspondence in, 315–316
  equipment and supplies to maintain and
    access, 301–303, **302, 303**
  filing guidelines for, 303–314, **306, 307, 309,**
    310, 312, 319–321
  function of, 296, **297**
  manual vs. electronic, **297,** 297–299
  for new patients, **317–319**
  ownership of, 296–297
  releasing information for, 297
  retention of, 314, **314**
  types of, 300–301
Medical Reserve Corps (MRC), 181
Medical specialists, **29–30,** 43
Medical symbols, 1497
Medical tourism insurance, 388
Medical transcription
  authentication of, 357–358
  as career, 368
  changing role of, 354–358
  function of, 356–357, **357**
  outsourcing of, 355–356
  professionalism in, 368
  software for, **368–369**
Medicare
  administration of, 110
  coding for, 408
  explanation of, 384, **384**
  patient fees and, 433
  payment formula for, 391, **391, 396–397**
Medicare CMS-1500 Form, 380, **381,** 409, 411,
  412–413, **414,** 415, **422–427**
Medicare Part A, 384
Medicare Part B, 384–385, **385**
Medicare Part C, 385–386
Medicare Part D, 386
Medication administration
  of allergenic extracts, **1115,** 1115–1116
  from ampule, **1123–1125**
  errors in, 1101
  guidelines for, **1098,** 1098–1099
  for inhaled medication, 1116
  injection guidelines for, 1114–1115, **1125–1132**

Medication administration (*Continued*)
    intravenous, 1108–1111, **1109–1114**, 1113–1114
    legal and ethical issues related to, 1080–1082
    oral, 1102, **1102, 1119–1121**
    oxygen and, 1116–1118, **1117, 1118**
    parenteral, 1102–1108, **1103–1108**
    patient assessment prior to, 1101–1102
    from power, **1133–1134**
    "six rights" for, **1099**, 1099–1100
    from vial, **1121–1123**
    by Z-track intramuscular injection, 1115,
        1134–1136
Medication dosages
    for adults, 1093–1096
    age and, 1084–1085
    calculation of, 1086–1096, **1089, 1090**
    for children, 1085, 1096–1098, **1097**
    factors that determine, 1085
    gender and, 1085
    for medication measured in units, 1090–1093,
        1092, 1093
    weight and, 1085
Medication note, 1098, **1098**
Medications
    abuse of, 1066, **1068–1073**
    animal sources of, 1044
    classification of, 1054, **1055–1062**
    disposal of, 1050–1052
    emergency, 1066, **1067**
    forms of, 1064–1065
    genetically engineered, 1046
    herbal supplements as, 1044–1046, **1045**
    labels on, 1049, **1049**, 1050, **1051**, 1085–1086
    list of top 200 brand-name, 1498–1500
    methods to handle, 1052
    mineral sources of, 1044
    nonprescription, 1050
    patient education about, 1086
    plant sources of, 1044
    prescription, **263–264, 1049**, 1049–1050, **1050**
    principal actions of, 1054, **1055–1062**
    references and standards for,
        1052–1054, **1953**
    regulation of controlled, 1046–1049,
        1082, **1082**
    research and development of, 1043
    routes of administration for, 1063
    sound-alike, look-alike, 1084, **1085**
    storage and handling of, 1065
    synthetic, 1046
    types of names for, 1043–1044
    uses of, 1042–1043
Medicine
    attitude toward illness and, 44
    codes for, 405
    cultural heritage in, 42–43
    education for practice of, 43–44
    epidemics and, **46**, 46–47
    frontiers in, 48, 50–51
    historical background of, 44–45, **49–50**
    limitations of, 47
    Oriental, 31, 42–43
    significant contributors to, **49–50**
    women in, 48
Meeting agenda, 337–338, **338**, 1402,
    1402, 1424
Meeting minutes, 338, **339**
Melanoma, **789, 790**
Memoranda, 337, **338**
Memory impairment, in older adults, 776–777
Ménière's disease, **800, 806**
Meningitis, **521, 796**
Meniscus, 606

Menopause, 684–685, 775
Mensuration, 632, **632**
Mentors, 1404
Mercury sphygmomanometers, 605, **606**
Mercury thermometers, 597, **599**
Metered dose inhaler (MDI), **868–869**
Methamphetamine, **1070**
Methicillin-resistant *staphylococcus aureus*
    infections, **521**
Metric system, 1088–1090, **1089, 1099**
Metrorrhagia, 675
Mexican diet, **1033**
Michelangelo, 44
Microbiologists, 1330
Microbiology
    cell structure and, 1330, **1331**
    explanation of, 1328, **1329**
    nomenclature and, 1329–1330
Microbiology cultures
    classification of, 1341–1343, **1343**
    collection requirements for, 1335–1337, **1337**
    inoculating media for, 1343
    primary, 1344
    streaking and, 1343–1344, **1345**
    subcultures and, 1345, **1346**
    throat specimen for, **1350–1352**
Microbiology department, 1203
Microbiology laboratories
    dyes used in, **1339**, 1339–1341
    equipment in, 1331–1333, **1331–1333**
    examination of bacteria in, **1338–1340,**
        1338–1341
    fecal specimen for, **1354–1355**
    fungi and, 1350
    parasites and, 1347–1350, **1347–1350**
    quality control in, 1334–1335
    rapid identification systems in, 1345–1346
    role of medical assistant in, 1328–1329
    safety practices in, 1333–1334, **1334**
    sensitivity testing in, 1346, **1346**
    strep testing in, **1353–1354**
    wet-mount/hanging drop preparation, 692,
        699–700, 1352–1353
Microbiology tests, **1202**, 1203
Microcomputers, 213, **214**
Microhematocrit, **1272**
Microhematocrit determination, **1283–1285**
Microorganisms. *See also* Infection cycle
    classification of, 506–507, 510–511
    explanation of, 505
    growth requirements for, 506
Microscopes, 1211–1213, **1211–1214**
Middle Eastern diet, **1033**
Midstream specimen, 1299, **1300,**
    1322–1323
Minerals, 1020–1022, **1021**
Ming dynasty, 44
Minicomputers, 213
Minors, 120, 469
Misdemeanors, 109
Misused words, 327, **328**
Mitral valve stenosis, **817, 818**
Modified block style letters, 333, **333, 334**
Modified wave scheduling, 275
Modulated voice, 241
Moist cold therapy, 991, **991**
Moles, **788**
Molybdenum, 1022
Monosaccharide, 1010
Month-end sheets, 439–440
Monthly billing, 468–469
Morbidity, 504
Morbid obesity, 842

Mordant, 1340
Mormon diet, **1034**
Morphine, **1067, 1068**
Morphology codes (M codes), 408
Mortality, 504
Morton, W. T. G., 49
Moses, 49
Motion sickness, **800**
Mouth, examination of, **640**, 643
Movable file units, 302
Moxibustion, 43
Multichannel electrocardiograph, 1146, **1148,**
    1165–1167
Multiple sclerosis, **794, 796**
Multivitamin supplements, 1020
Murray, Joseph, **50**
Muscle relaxants, **1061**
Muscle testing, 987
Musculoskeletal system
    disorders of, **822–825**
    fractures of, 821, **828**
    function of, 820–821
    injuries to, 171–173, **173**
    in older adults, 773, **774**
Music therapy, 51
Myasthenia gravis, **823**
Mycobacterium tuberculosis, 1367, 1368
Mycology, 1330, 1350
Myocardial infarction (MI), 178, **817, 818**, 1156
Myopia, **800**
MyPlate Food Guidance System, 1014, **1014, 1015**
Myringotomy, 737, 807
MySpace, 1416

N

Nägele's Rule, 659
Narcan, **1067**
Narcolepsy, 604
Narcotics, **1068**
Nasal catheter, 1118
Nasal examination, **863–864**
Nasal instillation, **866**
Nasal irrigation, **865**
Nasal polyps, **801, 811, 812**
National Alliance for the Primary Prevention of
    sharps Injections (NAPPSI), 1108
National Center for Competency Testing (NCCT),
    17–18, **18**
National Center for Elder Abuse (NCEA), 779
National Certified Medical Assistant
    (NCMA), 18
National Fire Protection Association, color and
    number method, 1188, **1188, 1189**
National Healthcareer Association (NHA), 17, **17,**
    1460–1463
National Uniform Claim Committee (NUCC), 412,
    413, 415
Native American diet, **1032**
Native Americans, 44
Natural disasters, procedures for, 200–202, **204**
*NCAA Standards for the Accreditation of Certification
    Programs,* 16
Nearsightedness, **802**
Nebulizers, 815, **815**
Neck, **640**, 643
Needle-free injection, 718
Needle holders, 904, **907**
Needles
    for syringes, 1106–1108, **1107, 1108**
    for venipuncture, 1225–1227,
        1226, 1227

Needle selection, for immunizations, 718
Needlestick, 536–537, **537**
Needle-stick prevention devices, 1227, **1227**
Neglect, **145**
Negligence, 116–117, 1423
Negligent torts, 117
Neisseria gonorrhoeae, 1342
Nematode, 1348
Neonates, 708–709. *See also* Infants; Newborns
Nephron, 1295, **1295**
Nervous system, in older adults, 773
Networking, computer, 217–218
Network interfaces, 227
Neurologic system
    disorders of, **793–796**
    examination of, **642**, 792, **792**, 796–798, **852–853**
    explanation of, 791–792
Neutrophils, 1274
Newborns. *See also* Children; Infants; Pediatrics
    growth and development in, 723
    physical examination of, 708–709
Newsletters, 1415
Niacin, **1018**, 1020
Nightingale, Florence, **49**
Nitrite, 1305
Nitro-Dur, 1064, **1064**
Nitroglycerin, **1067**
Nitrous oxide, **1072**
Noise reduction, 198
Nomogram, 1096
Nondisposable syringes, 1104
Non-Hodgkin's lymphoma, **819, 820**
Noninsulin-dependent diabetes mellitus
    (NIDDM), 1093
Nonprescription drugs, 1050
Nonsocomial infection, 515
Nonspecific urethritis (NSU), **755**
Nonsteroidal antiinflammatory drugs
    (NSAIDs), **1061**
Nonsufficient funds checks, **454–455, 479**
Nonverbal communication
    congruency between verbal and, 76
    cultural diversity and, 74–76
    explanation of, 73–74
    facial expression and, 74
    gestures and mannerisms and, 75–76
    personal space and, 74–75
Normal flora, 507, 1328
Northern and Western European diet, **1033**
Nose, **640**, 642–643, 808. *See also* Sensory system
Nosebleeds, 177
Nose culture, 1336
Nosocomial infection, 1330
Nuclear medicine, 968
Nullipara, 659
Numeric filing system, 308–309, **309, 320**
Nurse practitioners (NPs), 36
Nurses, 35–36
Nurses' Health Study, 1031
Nutrition. *See also* Therapeutic diets
    for adolescents, 1027
    antioxidants and, 1016, 1019–1020
    breast-feeding and, 1026
    carbohydrates and, 1010, **1010**
    for children, 1026–1027
    culture and, 1032, **1032–1035**
    daily food plan for, **1015**
    energy balance and, 1013–1014
    fats and, 1010–1011, **1011, 1012**
    fiber and, 1023
    food labels and, 1023–1025, **1023–1025**
    herbal supplements and, 1020
    minerals and, 1020–1022, **1021**

for older adults, 1027
overview of, 1008–1010, **1009**
proteins and, 1011–1013
vitamins and, 1014, 1016, **1017–1019**
water and, 1022–1023
Nystagmus, **800**

O

Obama, Barack, 298, 377
Obesity, 841–842, 1013–1014, 1026, 1027, 1029, 1030
Oblique fracture, **826**
Observation, 630–631
Obstetrics. *See also* Pregnancy complications
    complementary therapy for, 693
    contraception and, 668, **669–673,** 672–673
    explanation of, 654, 655
    initial prenatal visit and, 655, **657,** 657–659,
        658, 693–694
    labor and, **667,** 667–668
    parturition and, **667,** 667–668
    postpartum period and, 668
    pregnancy disorders and, 662–667, **663, 665**
    return prenatal visits and, 659–660, **660, 661,**
        662, **693–694**
    tests and procedures for, 660, **660, 661,** 662
Occupational Analysis of the CMA (AAMA), 7
Occupational Safety and Health Act (1967)
    (OSH Act), 112
Occupational Safety and Health Administration
    (OSHA), 1098
    Bloodborne Pathogen Standard, 539–540,
        544–546, 1232
    ergonomics and, 1191
    health care regulation by, 1176, **1177**
    laboratory regulations of, 1184–1185,
        1184–1190, 1188–1191
    on safety needles, 1227
    sharps disposal and, 537
    student compliance with regulations of, **546,**
        546–547
Occupational therapists (OTs), **34, 975**
Office management. *See* Clinic management
Office policy manuals, 1437–1438, **1446**
Ointments, 912, **914**
Older adults. *See also* Gerontology
    abuse of, 125, 144–145, **145**
    aging process and, 770–771, **771**
    ambulatory care settings for, 203
    communication with, 574
    ethical issues related to, **147**
    health in, **779,** 779–780, **780**
    memory impairment in, 776–777
    nutrition for, 1027–1028
    physiologic changes in, 771–775, **772–774**
    prevention of complications in, 775–776
    psychological changes in, 776
    societal bias against, 770
Old reports, 365
Online résumé, 1476–1480
Open-ended questions, 85
Open hours scheduling, 273
Open-shelf lateral files, 301–302, **302**
Open wounds, 166, **917**
Operative reports, 361–362, **362**
Ophthalmic medical technicians (OMTs), **34**
Optical drives, 216
Oral hypoglycemic medication, 1093
Oral medication administration, 1102, **1102,**
    1119–1121
Oral temperature, 599–600, **614, 618–619**
Order of Draw (CLSI), 1231, **1231**

Organomercurial, 722
Oriental medicine, 31, 42–43
Orthopnea, 604
Oscilloscope, 966
OSHA. *See* Occupational Safety and Health Act
    (OSHA)
Osteoarthritis, **823, 825**
Osteoporosis, 773, **823, 825,** 1022
Otitis media, 736–737, **801, 806**
Otosclerosis, **801, 806**
Otoscopes, 905
Outer-directed people, 63
Out guides, 303, **303**
Outsourcing, 355–356
Ovarian cancer, 686
Ovarian cyst, 686, **686**
Over-the-counter (OTC) medications, 1050, 1086
Oxycodone, **1068**
Oxygen administration
    background of, 1116–1117
    dosage for, 1117
    methods for, **1117,** 1117–1118, **1118**
    by nasal cannula, **867–868**
Oxytocin, 667

P

Paget's disease, **825**
Pain, cultural perspective on, 95
Pain management, 96
Palliative agents, 506
Palliative care, 95, 967
Pallor, 639
Palmer, Daniel David, **49**
Palpation, 631, **631**
Pancreatic cancer, **832, 834**
Pancreatitis, **832, 834**
Pantothenic acid, **1019**
Papanicolaou, George, 45, **49**
Paper charts, 299, **317, 319.** *See also* Medical
    records
Pap tests, 674–676, 679–681, **679–681,** 683, **683,**
    694–696, 1177
Para, 659
Paraffin wax bath, 989–990, **990**
Paralytic poliomyelitis, 46, **46**
Parasites, 510, 737, 1309, 1348–1350,
    1348–1350
Parasitology
    explanation of, 1330, 1347–1348
    specimen collection for, 1348
Parasitology department, 1203
Parasitology tests, **1202**
Parasympathetic nervous system, 59
Parenteral medications
    administration of, 1102–1108, **1103–1108**
    equipment and supplies for, 1103–1108,
        1104–1108
    hazards associated with, 1103
    reasons for, 1103
    routes for, 1102–1103
Parkinson's disease, 51, 776, **794, 796**
Paroxysmal atrial tachycardia (PAT), 1157
Participatory management, 1399
Partnerships, **25**
Parturition, **667,** 667–668
Past-due accounts, 469
Pasteur, Louis, 45, **45, 49,** 505
Patch test, 791, **791**
Pathogens, 505, 1328
Pathology, codes for, 405
Pathology reports, 262–263, **363**

Patient accounts
    computerized, 440, **441**
    management of, 434–435, **448–449, 451–455**
    recording transactions in, 436–439, **438**
Patient Bill of Rights (American Hospital
    Association), 139
Patient care/preparation
    background of, 915
    for diagnostic imaging, 958–962
    informed consent and, 915
    medical assisting considerations for, 915–916
    postoperative instructions and, 916
    transfer methods for, 976–978, **978, 993–996**
    for wounds, 916–918, **917, 918**
Patient charts
    abbreviations for, 585–587, **586**
    CHEDDAR approach to, 574, 575, 583
    elements of, 313–314
    filing procedure for, 304–305
    methods for, 581, **581**, 582, 583, **583**
    notes on, 360, **360**
    organization of, 587
    rules for, 583, **584, 585**
    scanning of, 355
    SOAP/SOAPER approach to, 300, 301, 574,
        575, **575**, 583
Patient check-in, 280, **280**
Patient education, **30**, 74, 87, 129
    about medications, 1086
    on cholesterol, **1375**
    on digestive health, **835**
    on drug-resistant bacteria, **514**
    on health maintenance and disease
        prevention, **1035–1036**
    on hypertension, **610**
    on immunizations, **717**
    on inflammation, **916**
    for limited-English patients, 250
    on magnetic resonance imaging, **966**
    materials for, 195–196
    opportunities for, **644, 645**
    on pregnancy, 657–658, **658**
    in prescription medications, **1050**
    on prostate cancer, **762**
    on skin cancer, **791**
    on specimen collection, **1211**
    on throat cultures, **1336**
Patient education brochures, 1415
Patient fees
    adjustment of, 433–434
    discussion of, 433
    explanation of, 432
    method to determine, 432–433
    refund of, 434
Patient flow, analysis of, **276**, 276–277
Patient history and documentation. *See also* Medical
    records
    chief complaint and, 575–576
    communication across life span and, 574
    computerized health history for, 571
    cross-cultural model of, 567–568
    electronic, 583, **583**, 585
    family history in, 577
    HIPAA compliance and, 580
    medical history components and, 574–579,
        578–579, 587
    method of charting, 581, **581**, 582, 583, **584**,
        585, **585, 586**, 587
    patient information forms for, 568, **569,**
        570, **571**
    patient intake interview for, **571**, 571–573, **572**
    patient records and, 579–581
    preparation for, 567

purpose of, 566–567
    rules of charting, 583, **584–586**, 585–587
    social history in, 577
Patient information forms, 568, **569,** 570, **570**
Patient intake interview
    cultural diversity and, 572–573
    guidelines for, **571**, 571–572
    sensitivity when conducting, 573
Patient Protection and Affordable Care Act (2010),
    108, 377, 673
Patient records. *See* Medical records
Patients
    assistance for ambulation, 978
    blood draw reactions of, 1240, **1241**
    with life-threatening illness, 94–98
    medical charts for new, **317–319**
Patient scheduling
    appointment matrix in paper system and,
        284–285
    cancelling and rescheduling procedures for,
        280–281, **281, 288–289**
    function of, 272–273
    guidelines for, 278–282, **280, 281**
    for inpatient/outpatient admission procedures,
        283–284, **289–290**
    interpersonal skills for, 277
    legal issues related to, 277
    Medical Office Simulation Software for,
        285–289
    with paper scheduling, **285–286**
    patient flow and, **276**, 276–277
    reminder systems for, 281–282
    software for, 282–283
    for telephone appointments, 279–280
    types of, 273, **274**, 275–276
Patient Self-Determination Act (1990), 96, 129, 132
Patient service centers, 1198
Patients with special needs, communication and, 83
Payroll checks, 1420
Payroll processing, 1417, 1420
Peak, 1197
Peak expiratory flow rate (PEFR), 814, **814**
Peale, Norman Vincent, 141
Pediatric facilities, features of, 195, **195**
Pediatrics. *See also* Children
    adolescents and, 726–727
    chest circumference and, **743–745**
    common disorders and diseases in, 736–739
    explanation of, 708–709
    growth patterns and, 727, **728–732, 743–745**
    hearing screening and, 735
    immunizations and, 709, **710–717**, 713,
        716–723, **719–722, 740–742** (*See also*
        Immunizations)
    infants and, 723–725
    male circumcision and, 739
    measuring respiratory rate and, **747**
    newborns and, 723
    preschoolers and, 725–726
    school-aged children and, 726
    taking apical pulse and, 746–747
    taking rectal temperature and, 745–746
    toddlers and, 725
    urine specimen collection and, 734–735, **735,**
        747–748
    visual acuity screening and, 735, **736**
    vital signs and, 733–734, **734**
    weight and length measurement in, **743–745**
    well-baby visits and, 709
Pediculosis, 737
Pegboard system, 435, **436**, 439, 487. *See also*
    Accounting practices
Pelvic inflammatory disease (PID), 665, 686, **689**

Penicillin, 45
Penile cancer, 757–758
Penis
    disorders of, 757–758
    explanation of, 754
Percussion, 631–632, **632**
Percutaneous transluminal coronary angioplasty
    (PTCA), 1164
Percutaneous umbilical blood sampling (PUBS),
    662, 667
Pericardial fluid, 535
Pericarditis, **817, 818**
Peripheral arteries, 604
Peritoneal fluid, 535
Personal appearance
    of job applicants, 1483, **1484**
    of medical assistants, **12**, 12–13
    of patients, 638, **640**
Personal computers, 212, **214**
Personal digital assistants (PDAs), 218, 223
Personal fitness trainers (PFTs), **34**
Personal protective equipment (PPE)
    bloodborne pathogens and, 539, 540
    function of, 536, **536, 541**
    for handling microbiology specimens, 1334
    student use of, 546–547
    use of, **557–558**
Personal space, 74–75
Personnel. *See* Employees
Personnel records, 1443–1444
Pertussis, **521,** 738
Peter, Laurence, 63
Petty cash, 448, **457**
Peyronie's disease, 758
pH, 1304
Phagocytosis, 1274–1275
Pharmaceutical representatives, scheduling of, 282
Pharmacists (RPhs), 35
Pharmacogenomics, 1043
Pharmacology, 1042. *See also* Medication
    administration; Medication dosages; Medications
Pharmacopoeia, 42
Pharmacy technicians, 35
Pharmazooticals, 1044
Pharyngitis, **811, 812**
Phencyclidine, **1070**
Phenylketonuria (PKU), 709, 1366
Phenylketonuria tests, 1366, **1367, 1382–1384**
Phimosis, 758
Phlebotomists, 1220
Phlebotomy
    capillary puncture and, 1244–1245, **1244–1246,**
        1247, **1257–1259**
    capillary specimen for transport and, **1259–1261**
    circulatory system and, **1221**, 1221–1222, **1222**
    equipment for, 1224–1229, **1226–1232,**
        1231–1232
    explanation of, 1220
    obtaining blood for blood culture, **1261–1263**
    procedure for, 1223–1224, **1224, 1225**
    role of medical assistant in, 1220–1221
    specimen collection and, 1237–1242,
        1238–1243, 1244
    venipuncture technique for, **1232**, 1232–1237,
        1234, 1235, 1237, 1247–1257
Phosphorus, **1021**, 1022, 1379
Photometry analyzers, 1372, **1373**
Physical abuse, **145**
Physical activity, health benefits of, **1016**
Physical examination. *See* Examination
Physical therapists (PTs), 35, **36**, 975
Physical therapy assistants (PTAs), 35
Physician assistants (PAs), 36

Physician Orders for Life-Sustaining Treatment (POLST), 125, **127–128**
Physician's Desk Reference (PDR), 1050, 1052–1054, **1053**
Physician's office laboratories (POLs), 1179, 1183, 1184, 1198–1199, 1328
PillCam, 51, 835, 836, **837**
Placenta abruptio, 665
Placenta previa, 664–665, **665**
Plague, 552, **552**
Plasma, 1221–1223
Plaster casts, **872–873**. *See also* Casts
Platelets, **1222**, 1268, 1276–1277. *See also* Thrombocytes
Platform crutches, 981, **981**
Pleural fluid, 534
Pleurisy, **811, 812**
Pneumonia, **523, 811, 812**
Pneumonic plague, 1066
Pneumothorax, **811, 812**
Point of care techniques, 86–87
Point-of-care testing (POCT), 1198
Point-of-service (POS) device, 417–418, **418**
Point-of-service (POS) plans, 383
Poison Control Center, 174
Poisoning, 174
Policy manuals, 1437–1438, **1446**
Polio, 46, **46**
Polycystic kidneys, **845, 847**
Polysaccharides, 1010
Poor, care of, 144
Position, 75, **75**
Positioning, 633
Positron emission tomography (PET), 798, 963, **963**
Post-Exposure Management Record, 543
Post-lumbar puncture, **792**
Postoperative instructions, 916
Postpartum period, 668
Postscript, 332
Posture, 75, 226–227, 242, 638, 975–976, **976**
Postvasectomy semen analysis (PVSA), 1364–1365
Potassium, **1021**, 1022
Potassium hydroxide (KOH), 692, 1341
Power medication, reconstituting, **1133–1134**
The Power of Ethical Management (Blanchard/Peale), 141
Power verbs, 1472, **1473**
Practice-based scheduling, 276
Practicums, student, 8, 1404–1405, **1425**
Preauthorization, 389–390
Precertification, 389
Precipitate, 1099
Precordial leads, 1151
Preeclampsia, 655
Preexisting conditions, 378
Preferred provider organizations (PPOs), 24, 383
Pregnancy
    alcohol intake during, 666
    cultural difference in views of, 654
    initial prenatal visits during, 655, **657,** 657–659, **658, 693–694**
    normal uterine, 655, **656**
    nutrition and, 1025–1026
    patient education on, 657–658, **658**
    return prenatal visits during, 659–660, **660, 661,** 662, **693–694**
    x-rays and, 956–957
Pregnancy complications
    abortion/interruption of pregnancy as, 662–663
    blood incompatibility as, 667
    eclampsia as, 664
    ectopic pregnancy as, **659,** 663–664
    gestational diabetes as, 655, 664

hyperemesis gravidarum as, 664
    placenta previa as, 664–665, **665**
    preeclampsia as, 655
Pregnancy tests, 1360–1361, **1380–1381**
Prejudice, 78
Premature atrial contraction (PAC), 1156–1157
Premature ventricular contraction (PVC), 1157–1158
Premenstrual syndrome (PMS), **689**
Prenatal history, 658–659
Prenatal tests, 657, **657**
Prenatal visits
    initial, 655, **657,** 657–659, **658, 693–694**
    return, 659–660, **660, 661,** 662, **693–694**
Presbyopia, **802,** 804
Preschoolers, 725–726. *See also* Children
Prescriptions. *See also* Medications
    abbreviations and symbols used on, 1082–1084, **1083, 1084**
    for controlled substances, 1082, **1082**
    electronic, 1049
    explanation of, 1081–1082, **1082**
Presentation, 10, 12–14
Present problem (PP), 360
Press releases, 1415
Pretrial conference, 122
Preventive maintenance, 1205
Pridoxine, **1018**
Primary survey, for emergency assessment, **160,** 160–161, **161**
Principle-centered leadership, 140–141
Principle-Centered Leadership (Covey), 140
Prions, 511
Privacy. *See also* Confidentiality
    computer security and, 218–219
    invasion of, 118, 198
Probation, 1404, **1404,** 1442
Problem-oriented medical records (POMRs), 300–301, 581, 583
Procedure manual, 1409–1410, **1410, 1426**
Procedures. *See* Examinations
Proctologic table, 635, **635**
Proctosigmoidoscopy, **837,** 839
Prodromal stage, of infectious disease, 519
Professional fees, 143
Professionalism
    collections and, 476
    in computerized medical clinic, 229–230
    explanation of, 6, **10–11**
    in medical transcription, 368
    in telecommunications, 261
Professional liability insurance, 121, 1423
Professional organizations, 1462–1463
Proficiency tests, 1205
Progestin, 684
Progress notes, 360, **360**
Prokaryotes, 1329, 1330
Prone position, 635
Proofreader's marks, **329**
Proofreading, 327–328, **329**
Proportion, 1087–1088
Proportional method, to calculate medication dosage, 1091, 1094
Proprietary schools, 7
Prostaglandins, 667
Prostate
    disorders of, 760–762, **761**
    explanation of, 756
Prostate cancer, **755,** 762
Prostatitis, **755,** 760–761
Protected health information (PHI), 112, 256, 568
Protein, 1011–1013, **1014,** 1304, 1379
Prothrombin time, **1287–1288,** 1362

Protista, 1329, **1330**
Proton-pump inhibitor, **1062**
Protozoa, 1329
Provider-performed microscopy procedures (PPMPs), 1178, 1179, **1179,** 1181–1182, **1183**
Pruritus, **790,** 1063
Psoriasis, **789, 790**
Public duties, 124–125
Puerperium, 655. *See also* Postpartum period
Puerto Rican diet, **1033**
Pulmonary embolism (PE), **811, 812**
Pulse oximeters, 607–608, **608,** 814–815, **815, 871**
Pulse pressure, 609
Pulse/pulse rate
    abnormalities in, 602–603
    in children, 733
    explanation of, 601
    in infants, **746–747**
    measurement and evaluation of, 602, **619–621**
    method to record, 603
    normal, 602, **603**
Pulse sites, **601,** 601–602
Puncture, **917**
Purging, record, 314
Purified protein derivative (PPD), 1368
P wave, 1145
Pyelonephritis, **846, 847**
Pyridoxine, **1018,** 1020

Q

Qualitative tests, 1200
Quality assurance (QA), 356, 1178
Quality control, in microbiology laboratory, 1334–1335
Quantitative tests, 1200
Quinlan, Karen Ann, 151

R

Rabies, **795, 796**
Radial pulse, 603, **619–620**
Radiation therapy, 967–968
Radiographers, **34,** 956
Radiologic studies. *See also* Diagnostic imaging
    of digestive system, 840–841, **843**
    equipment for, 957–958, **958**
    patient preparation for, 958
    safety procedures for, 956–957
Radiology, 405, 956
Radiology reports, 360–361, **362**
Radiolucent, 958
Radiopaque, 958
Rales, 604
Random access memory (RAM), 215
Random (spot) urine sample, 1298
Range of motion exercises, 985–987, **986**
Rapid identification systems, 1345–1346
Ratio, 1087
Rationalization, 80
Read-only memory (ROM), 215
Reagents, 1205
Reagent test strips, **1303,** 1303–1307, **1304, 1306**
Receipts, 439
Reception area
    children in, 195, **195**
    cultural considerations for, 195
    design elements in, 197, **197**
    educational materials in, 195–196
    function of, **193,** 193–194

Receptionists, 194, **194**
Recognition, 86
Recruiting/hiring, **1438**, 1438–1442, **1440, 1441, 1446–1447**
Rectal cancer, **832, 834**
Rectal temperature, 600, **616–617, 733, 745–746**
Rectocele, **689**
Rectum, examination of, **641,** 644
Red blood cells (RBCs), 1222, **1222,** 1268, 1271–1272, 1275–1276, **1276,** 1278, 1308, 1362, 1364. *See also* Erythrocytes
Redundant array of independent disks (RAID) storage, 216
Reference initials, 331
Reference laboratories, 1198
References, for résumé, 1472–1474
Referral appointments, 278
Referrals, 389–390
Reflexes, 644
Refractometers, 1303, **1303, 1314–1315**
Refrigerators, 1333
Registered dietitians (RDs), 33–34
Registered health information administrators (RHIA), **34**
Registered health information technicians (RHITs), **34**
Registered medical assistants (RMAs), 17, **17,** 1455, 1460
Registered nurses (RNs), 35
Registration, 18, **18**
Regression, 79
Regulation Z of Consumer Protection Act (1967), 113
Rehabilitation procedures
  assisting patients to ambulate during, 978, **996–1001**
  assistive devices and, 978–985, **979–985**
  body mechanics and, 975–976, **976**
  for falling patients, **998–999**
  role of medical assistant during, 974–975
  safety considerations for, 976, **977**
  therapeutic exercises as, 985–988, **986, 987**
  therapeutic modalities as, 988–993, **990–993**
  transferring patients during, 976–978, **978**
Rehabilitative medicine, 974, **975**
Relaxation, 63
Release marks, filing, 312
Release of Information Form, 568, **570**
Reminder systems, 281–282
Remittance advice, 380, **380**
Renal calculi, **846, 847**
Renal tubular epithelial cells, 1308
Repolarization, 1145
Reportable diseases, 124
Repression, 79–80
Reproductive system. *See also* Contraception; Gynecological issues; Gynecological tests/ treatments; Male reproductive system; Pregnancy
  ethical concerns related to, 148–149
  in older adults, 775
Requisitions, laboratory, 1205, **1206,** 1207–1209, **1208, 1209**
Rescue breathing, 179
Res ipsa loquitur, 117
Resistance, 517
Resource-based relative value scale (RBRVS), 385, **386,** 390–391
Respect, 84
Respiration rate
  abnormalities in, 603–604
  explanation of, 603, **603**
  in infants, **747**
  measurement of, **622**
Respiratory emergencies, 178–179, 181
Respiratory syncytial virus (RVS), 738

Respiratory system
  conditions and disorders of, 809, **810–812**
  diagnostic tests for, 813
  function of, 809, **809**
  inhalers and, 815, **815**
  in older adults, 774
  peak expiratory flow rates and, 814, **814**
  pulse oximetry and, 814–815
  spirometry and, 813, **813–814**
Respiratory therapists (RRTs), **34**
Respondeat superior, 117
Résumés, 1472–1480, **1473, 1475–1478**
Retention, records, 314, **314**
Reticulocyte, 1275
Retinal detachment, **801–803**
Retinoblastoma, **801**
Retrograde pyelography, **961**
Review of systems (ROS), 577–579, **578–579**
Reye's syndrome, **795,** 796
Rh blood typing, **1363,** 1363–1364
Rheumatic fever, **817,** 818
Rheumatoid arthritis, **823,** 825
Rh factor, 667, 1363–1364, **1364**
RhoGAM, 667, **1364**
Rhythm strip, 1150
Riboflavin, **1018**
Rickets, **823,** 825
Rickettsiae, 510–511
Ringworm, **512**
Risk management, 120–121, 356, 1400
Roadblocks, 78, **79**
Roentgen, Wilhelm, **49,** 956
Roe v. Wade, 149, 150
Roman Catholic diet, **1034**
Roosevelt, Franklin D., 46
RU-486, 148–149, 672–673
Rubella, **523**

S

Saccharide, 1010
Safety
  facility design and, 199–202, **201**
  for oxygen administration, 1118
  during rehabilitation procedures, 976, **977,** 978
  venipuncture, **1236,** 1236–1237, **1237**
  when handling microbiology specimens, 1333–1334, **1334**
Safety hoods, **1331,** 1331–1332
Safety Training Form, **1190**
Saliva, 536
Salmonella typhi, 1330
Salutation, 329
Sanitization, 548–550, **549, 560**
SARS. *See* Severe acute respiratory syndrome (SARS)
Savings accounts, 443
Scabies, 510
Scales, 612, **612, 613**
Scalpels, 900, 902, **903**
Schatz, Albert, **49**
Scheduling. *See* Patient scheduling
Schiavo, Theresa, 151
Sciatica, **795,** 796
Scissors, 900, **902–904**
Scleroderma, **789**
Scoliosis, **823**
Scope of practice, 18
Scopes, 905, **907, 908**
Scratch test, 790–791
Screening
  for insurance, 388–389, **394–395**
  of phone calls, 248–249, **261–262,** 278

Scrotum, 756
Seasonique, **671**
Sebaceous cyst excision, **941–942**
Second-degree burns, 168, **169–171**
Secretions, 1178
Sedation, 95–96
Sedatives, **1062**
Seizures, 176
Selenium, 1022
Self-actualization, 1401
Self-assessment, **1469,** 1469–1470
Self-insurance, 388
Selye, Hans, 58, **59**
Semen, 535
Semen analysis, 1364–1365, **1365**
Seminars, 1413
Semmelweis, Ignaz, **49**
Sensitivity testing, 1328, 1346, **1346**
Sensors, 1149, 1150
Sensory system. *See also specific senses*
  disorders of, **799–801**
  ear and, 805–808, **805–808**
  explanation of, 698
  eyes and, 798, **802,** 802–805
  laboratory and diagnostic tests of, **799–801**
  nose and, 808, **864**
  in older adults, 771–772, **773**
Sequelae, 519
Serology (immunology) department, 1200, 1202
Serology (immunology) tests, **1201**
Serum, 1222
Servers, 216
Service Sockets Layer (SSL), 219
The 7 Habits of Highly Effective People (Covey), 140
Seventh Day Adventist diet, **1034**
Severe acute respiratory syndrome (SARS), 504, **811, 812**
Sexual abuse, **145**
Sexual exploitation, **145**
Sexual harassment, 110–111
Sexually transmitted diseases (STD), 668, **689, 690, 755,** 762, **762**
Sexual orientation, 110
Sharps containers, 536–537, **537,** 1108
Shock, 164–165, **165**
Short arm cast (SAC), 821
Short-range goals, 63–64
Sickle cell anemia, 662
Sighted guide techniques, **778**
Sigmoidoscopy, 837–839, **838, 840**
Silence, 86
Silvadene, 912
Simple stain, 1340
Simplified letter style, 334, **335**
Sim's position, 635, **635**
Single-channel electrocardiograph, **1145,** 1146, **1165–1167**
Single-entry system, 486–487
Sinusitis, **801, 811,** 812
Sitz bath, 989
"Six rights" of drug administration, 1099–1100, **1100**
Skin. *See also* Integumentary system
  appearance of, 639, **640**
  cross-section of, 787, **787**
  disorders of, **788–790**
  surgery preparations for, **938–939**
Skin cancer, **789–791**
Skin tests, 790–791
Skips, 475
Sleep apnea, 604
Small claims court, 474–475
Smallpox, **552**
Smallpox vaccine, 552

Smartphones, 223, **225, 261**
Smell, in older adults, 772
Smoking policy, 1445
Snake bites, **176**
Snellen chart, 804, **804, 853–854**
SOAP/SOAPER charting approach, 300, 301, 574, 575, **575**, 583
Social history, 577
Social media, 1416–1417, **1471**, 1471–1472
Social networking, 1416
Social Security Administration, 110
Social support, 62, 97
Sodium, **1021**, 1022, 1024, 1379
Software
    application, 216–217
    compatibility issues for, 217
    for computerized medical clinics, 225, **232–233**
    installation of, **232–233**
    system, 216
Solar radiation, 171
Sole proprietorships, **25**
Solutions, 911–912, **914**
Sonographer, 1164
Source-oriented medical records (SOMRs), 301, 581
Southeast Asian diet, **1033**
Spasm, **825**
Special events, 1415–1416
Special needs. *See* Patients with special needs
Species, 1330
Specific gravity
    explanation of, 1302
    of urine, 1302–1303, **1303**, 1305–1306
Specimen collection, 1209–1210, **1209–1211**, 1237–1242, **1238–1243**, 1244. *See also* Phlebotomy
Specimen collection trays, 1232, **1232**
Specula, 904–905, **907, 908**
Speech, 638
Speech therapy, **975**
Sperm, 1309
Spermatic cord, 756
Spermatogenesis, 756
Spermicides, 668, **670, 671**
Sphygmomanometers, 547, 605–607, **606, 607**
Spinal curvatures, **823, 825**
Spirilla, 1339, **1339**
Spirometry, **813**, 813–814, **870**
Splinter forceps, 903, **906**
Sponge forceps, 903–904, **906**
Sponges, 911, **911, 914**
Spores, 1330
Sports medicine, **975**
Sprains, 171–172, **824, 825**
Sputum specimen, 1336, **1337**
Squamous cell carcinoma, 683
Squamous interepithelial lesions (SILs), 683
St. Benedict of Nursia, 43
Staff meetings, 1402
Standard of care, 115–116
Standard Precautions, 162, 513, **532**, 1176, **1177**
Staphylococcus, 47
Staple removal, 899, **947–949**
Staples, 899, **899**
Static discharge protection, 220
Stat reports, 365
Stature, 638
Status asthmaticus, 1116
Statute of limitations, 123, 475–476
Statutory law, 109
Steam sterilization, 892–896, **893–895**
Stem cells, 51, 150, 151
Sterile fields, **929–933**
Sterile gloves, **923–924**. *See also* Gloves
Sterile trays, 918, **918**

Sterilization
    chemical "cold," 910, **924–925**
    methods of, 891–896, **893–895, 925–929**
    principles of, 890–891
Stertorous respiration, 604
Stethoscopes, 547
Stimulants, **1070**
Stomach cancer, **832, 834**
Stool specimens, 1336–1337
Strabismus, **801**
Strains, 172, **824, 825**
Streaking, 1343–1344, **1345**
Stream scheduling, 275–276
Strep throat testing, 1336, **1353–1354**
Streptococcus, 1345
Stress
    body's response to, 59, **59**
    categories of, 59
    causes of, 59–61
    effects of prolonged, 61–62
    explanation of, 58
Stress management
    goal setting for, 63–64
    techniques for, 62–63
Stressors, 58
Strictures, 907
Stridor, 604
Stroke, 178, **793**
Student practicums, 8, 1404–1405, **1425**
Stye, **801–803**
Subcutaneous injections, **720, 722, 1125–1129**
Subject filing system, 309–310, **321**
Sublimation, 80
Subpoenas, 121–122
Sudden illness, 175
Suicide, assisted, 96, 151
Sulfur, **1021**
Supercomputers, 213
Supine hypotension, 667
Supine position, 633, **633**
Supplementary health factor codes (V codes), 407
Supplies. *See* Equipment/supplies
Suppurant, 918
Suppurative otitis media, 736
Surge protection, 220
Surgery
    assisting with, **934–935**
    codes for, 404–405
    dry sterile transfer forceps for, 921, **921**
    preparation for, 918, **918–920**, 921, **938–939**
    tasks involved in, 918
Surgical asepsis, 888–890, **889**
Surgical procedures, types of office/ambulatory, 896
Surgical technologists (STs), **34**
Surrogacy, 149
Suture materials/supplies, **898**, 898–899, **899**
Suture needles, 899
Suture removal, **947–949**
Suturing, **939–940**
Swaged, 898
Symbols, medical, 1497
Sympathic nervous system, 59
Symptoms, review of, 577–579, **578–579**
Syncope, 1160
Synovial fluid, 534
Synthetic drugs, 1046
Syphilis, **690, 755, 762**
Syringes
    explanation of, 1103–1104
    frequently used, 1107
    method to prefill, 718

    parts of, 1104–1106, **1105**
    for venipuncture, 1225, **1226, 1237**, 1237–1238, **1248–1250**
System software, 216
Systole, 605, 1145

T

Tab-Alpha filing system, 306
Tablet PC, 223
Tachycardia, 602
Tachypnea, 603
Tape drives, 216
Targeted résumé, 1475–1476, **1477, 1478**
Task Force for Test Construction (TFTC), 1457
Taste, in older adults, 772
Taxonomy, 1329
Taylor, Andrew, **49**
Tay-Sachs disorder, 662
TB. *See* Tuberculosis (TB)
Team meetings, 1402
Teamwork, 1400–1401
TEAR, 100
Telecommunications. *See also* Telephone procedures
    ADA guidelines and, 254
    answering services and machines and, 255
    automated routing units and, 254–255
    cell phones and, 261
    in electronic health record environment, 240–241
    e-mail and, 257–260, **258**
    fax machines and, 256–257, **257, 265–266**
    HIPAA guidelines for, 253–254
    legal and ethical considerations for, 252–253, **253**, 260
    professionalism in, 261
    telephone directory use and, 250–251
    videoconferencing and, 260–261
    VoIP and, 255–256
Telephone directories, 250–251
Telephone procedures
    ADA requirements for, 254
    for angry callers, 249
    for answering services and machines, 255
    for automatic routing, 254–255
    for call transfers, 244–245
    for collections, 472, **476**
    for communicating with limited-English callers, 249–250
    for documentation, 250
    for emergency/urgent calls, 248–249
    for employment interview follow-up, 1487
    guidelines for, 241, **243**
    HIPAA guidelines for, 253–254
    for incoming calls, **242**, 242–245, **261–262**
    legal and ethical issues and, 252–253, **253**
    for long-distance calls, 251–252, **252**
    for message taking, 245, **245, 263**
    for older callers, 249
    for outgoing calls, 251–252
    personality and attitude and, 241–242, **243**
    for prescription refill calls, **263–264**
    for problem calls, **264–265**
    for referral calls, 248
    for routing calls, 245–250, **246**, 254–255
    for screening calls, 248–249, **261–263**, 278
    for telephone directory use, 250–251
Telephone references form, 1441, **1442**
Temperature. *See* Body temperature
Temporal artery temperature, 733
Temporal artery thermometers, 598–599, **599, 616**
Temporary employees, 1444–1445

Tendonitis, **824, 825**
Testes
    disorders of, **758,** 758–760, **759**
    explanation of, 756
Testicular cancer, **755,** 759–761
Testicular torsion, **755,** 758–759
Testicular trauma, 758
Testosterone, **1072**
Tetanus, 1330
Tetrahydrocannabinol, **1072**
Thalassemia, 662
Thallium stress test, 1163
Therapeutic communication. *See also*
Communication
    communication cycle and, 70–72, **71**
    community resources and, 87, **87–88**
    explanation of, 70
    interview techniques and, 85–86
    listening skills and, 72
    point of care techniques and, 86–87
Therapeutic communication barriers
    age, 76, **77**
    bias and prejudice, 78
    cultural and religious, 80, **81–82,** 82
    defense mechanisms as, 78–80
    economic, 76
    education and life-experience, 76, 78
    environmental, 83–84
    human needs as, 82–83
    patients with special needs as, 83
    time-factor, 84
    verbal, 78, **79**
Therapeutic diets. *See also* Nutrition
    for cancer, 1031–1032
    for diabetics, 1029–1030
    explanation of, 1028
    for individuals with cardiovascular disease, 1030–1031
    for weight control, 1028–1029
Therapeutic drug monitoring (TDM), 1197
Therapeutic exercises
    electromyography as, 988
    electrostimulation of muscle as, 988
    muscle testing, 987
    range of motion, 985–987, **986**
    types of, 987–988
Therapeutic modalities
    explanation of, 988
    heat and cold as, 988–989
    massage therapy as, 992, **992, 993**
    moist and dry cold as, 991, **991**
    moist and dry heat as, **989,** 989–991
    ultrasound as, 991–992
Thermometers. *See also* Body temperature
    cleaning and storing, 601
    disposable, 597–598, **618–619**
    electronic and digital, 598, **598, 614, 745–746**
    phaseout of mercury, 597, **599**
    temporal artery, 598–599, **599,** 616
    tympanic, 598
Thermotherapy, 988
Thiamin, **1017–1018**
Thimerosol, 722–723
ThinPrep Pap Test, 681
Third-degree burns, 168, **169, 171**
Third-party guidelines, 412, **421**
Third-party payers, 469
Thixotropic separator gel, 1229, **1231**
Throat, examination of, **640,** 643
Throat specimens, 1336, **1336, 1337, 1350–1352**
Thrombocytes, 1221, 1268. *See also* Platelets
Thrombophlebitis, **817, 818**
Tic douloureux, **795, 796**

Tickler files, 312, **312**
Time focus, 82
Time management, 1411–1413
Tine test, 1368
Title VII of Civil Rights Act (1964), 110
Toddlers. *See also* Children
    growth and development in, 725
Tonometer, 642
Tonsillitis, 737, **811, 812**
Topical spray anesthetics, 914
Torts
    common, 117–118
    explanation of, 115, 117
    negligence and, 116–117
    standard of care and scope of practice
        and, 115–116
Total practice management system (TPMS)
    for accounting, 487–488, **488**
    for billing and collections, 468
    explanation of, 222, **224**
    for medical records, **572**
    for telephone calls, 240, 247
    for test results, 1270
Total protein, 1379
Touch, 75–76, 195
Tourniquets, 166, 1231, **1231, 1235,** 1235–1236
Towel clamps, 904, **906**
Toxicology department, 1202–1203
Toxicology tests, **1202**
Toxic shock syndrome (TSS), **523**
TPMS. *See* Total practice management system (TPMS)
Trace minerals, 1022
Traditional insurance, 380, 382
Tranquilizers, **1062**
Transcription. *See* Medical transcription
Transcutaneous electric nerve stimulation
    (TENS), 988
Transdermal system of medication delivery, **1064,**
    1064–1065, **1065**
Transducer, 1163
Transferable skills, 1470
Transmission-Based Precautions, **1177**
Trans unsaturated fatty acids, **814,** 1011, **1011**
Transurethral resection of the prostate (TURP),
    761, **761**
Transverse fracture, **826**
Travel arrangements, 1410–1411, **1411, 1427–1428**
Traveler's checks, 443
Treadmill stress test, **1162,** 1162–1163
Trendelenburg position, 635
Trephination, 42
Trial, 122–123
TRICARE, 387
Trichomonas, **690,** 692
Trichomonas hominis, 1349
Trichomonas vaginalis, 1349, **1350**
Trichomoniasis, 510, **689**
Triglycerides, 1010, **1011,** 1376–1377
Trimester, 662
Triple option plans, 383
Trough, 1197
Trust, 84
Truth-in-Lending Act (1967), 466, **466**
Tubal ligation, 149, **672,** 673
Tuberculosis (TB), 45, 47, **524, 811–813,** 1366–1368
Tuberculosis tests, **1368,** 1368–1369, **1369**
Tularemia, 552, **552,** 1066
Turnaround time (TAT), 365
T wave, 1145
24-hour urine collection, 1298, **1299**
2007–2008 Occupational Analysis of the CMA (American
    Association of Medical Assistants), 1501–1503
Tympanic thermometers, 598, **615**

Tympanometry, 808
Tympanostomy, 807
Typhus, 45

U

Ultrasonic cleaning, 549, **550,** 909–910
Ultrasonography, 1163–1164
Ultrasound
    for diagnostic imaging, 662, 665, **966,** 966–967
    as therapeutic modality, 991–992
Unbundling, 408
Uniform Anatomical Gift Act (1968), 113
Uniform Bill 04 form, 415, **416**
Unipolar leads, 1150
United States Pharmacopeia/National Formulary, 1052
Universal Blood and Body Fluid Precautions, **1177**
Universal Precautions (Centers for Disease
    Control), 538
Universal Serial Bus (USB) port, 216
Urea, 1295
Urgent care centers, 26
Uric acid, 1379
Urinalysis
    chemical, **1303,** 1303–1310, **1304, 1306–1310,**
        1315–1317
    collection methods for, 1298–1299,
        1299–1300
    culture and sensitivity transport kit for,
        1320–1321
    drug screening and, 1311–1312
    explanation of, 844, 1198, 1294
    federal regulations and, 1297
    microscopic examination of urine sediment,
        1317–1319
    patient instructions for, **1299–1300,**
        1322–1323
    procedure for complete, **1319–1320**
    quality control for, 1296–1297
    reporting results of, 1310–1311, **1311**
    safety precautions for, 1296, **1296**
    specific gravity, **1314–1315**
    urine examination and, 1299, 1301–1303,
        1312–1313
Urinalysis department, 1200
Urinalysis tests, **1201**
Urinary bladder cancer, **845, 847**
Urinary catheterization
    explanation of, 633, 848–850, **849, 850**
    of females, **878–880**
    of males, **876–878**
Urinary system
    conditions and disorders of, 844, **845–847**
    description of, 844, 1294, **1295**
    diagnostic tests for, 844, 847–848
    diseases and disorders of, **846,** 847, 1304, 1308
    in older adults, 775
Urinary tract infection (UTI), 844, **846,** 1304, 1308
Urine
    chemical examination of, **1303,** 1303–1310,
        1304, 1306–1310, 1315–1317
    collection requirements for, 1335
    color of, **1301,** 1301–1302, **1302**
    composition of, 1296, **1296**
    containers for, **1297,** 1297–1298
    examination of, 1299, 1301–1303, **1312–1313**
    formation of, 1294–1296, **1295**
    microscopic examination of sediment in,
        1307–1310, **1308, 1309, 1317–1319**
    odor of, 1302
    precautions when handling, 1296, **1296,** 1297
    specific gravity of, 1302–1303, **1303**

specimen collection in children, 734–735, **747–748**
transparency of, 1302
Urine culture and sensitivity transport kit, **1320–1321**
Urine pregnancy tests, 1360–1361, **1380–1381**
Urine sediment
casts in, 1310, **1311**
crystals in, 1309–1310, **1310**
microscopic examination of, 1307–1310, **1308, 1309, 1317–1319**
Urinometers, 1302–1303
Urobilinogen, 1305
U.S. Southern diet, **1032**
Usual, customary, and reasonable (UCR) fees, 390
Uterine sound, 906, **908**
Utilization review (UR), **495**

V

Vaccinations. *See* Immunizations
Vaccine Adverse Event Reporting System (VAERS), 716
Vacutainer, 1228
Vacuum tubes, 1228, **1230**
Vacuum tube specimen collection, 1239, **1239, 1251–1254**
Vaginal ring, **671**
Vaginal secretions, 534
Vaginitis, **689**, 776
Valium, **1067**
Vancomycin resistant enterococcus (VRE), **524**
van Leeuwenhoek, Anton, **49**
Variable costs, 491
Varicella, **525**
Varicose veins, **817, 818**
Vas deferens, 756
Vasectomy, 668, **673**, 756, **756**
Vasoconstriction, 988
Vasodilators, **1062**
Vasopressors, **1062**
Vastibular neuritis, **801**
Vastus lateralis site, **1113**, 1113–1114
V codes, 407
Vector transmission, 513
Vegan diet, **1035**
Vegetarian diet, **1034**
Veins, method to palpate, **1247**
Venipuncture. *See also* Capillary puncture; Phlebotomy
equipment for, 1224–1229, **1226–1232,** 1231–1232
explanation of, 1220, 1223–1224
technique for, **1232**, 1232–1237, **1234, 1235, 1237, 1247–1257**
unsuccessful, 1240–1241
Ventricular arrhythmias, 1157–1159, **1158, 1159**
Ventricular fibrillation, 1159
Ventricular tachycardia, 1158–1159
Ventrogluteal site, 1111, **1112**
Verapamil, **1067**
Verbal communication, 72–73, 76. *See also* Communication; Therapeutic communication
Verruca, **790**
Vertical files, 301, **302**
Vertigo, 642
Vesalius, Andreas, **49**
Viability, age of, 659

Vials, **1121–1123**
Vibria cholerae, **512**
Videoconferencing, 260–261
Viral diseases, common, **510**
ViraPap, 681
Virology, 1330
Viruses, 506
Virus protection programs (computer), 219–220
Viscosity, 1229
Visual acuity, 735, **736**, 803–804, **853**
Visual impairment, in older adults, **771**, 771–772, **772**, 777, **778**
Vital signs. *See also* Measurement
accuracy in taking, 594
blood pressure as, 604–611, **605–610, 622–623**
body temperature as, 594–595, **596–600**, 597–601, **614–619**
in children, 723, 725, 733–734, **734**
explanation of, 594
pulse as, **601**, 601–603, **602, 619–621**
respiration as, **603**, 603–604, **622**
Vitamin A, 1016, **1017**
Vitamin B_1, **1017–1018**, 1019
Vitamin B_2, **1018**, 1019
Vitamin B_3, **1018**
Vitamin B_5, **1019**
Vitamin B_6, **1018**, 1020
Vitamin B_{12}, **1018**, 1020
Vitamin C, 1016, 1019, **1019**
Vitamin D, 1016, **1017**
Vitamin E, 1016, **1017**
Vitamin K, 1016, **1017**, 1362
Vitamins, 1014, 1016, **1017–1019**
Vitiligo, 639
Voice over Internet Protocol (VoIP), 218, 255–256
Voice recognition software (VRS), 356
Voluntary dismissal, 1409
Voucher checks, 443
VSED (voluntarily stop eating and drinking), 95

W

Waived tests, 1179
Walkers, **979**, 980, **980, 999–1000**
WAP2, 218
Warm soaks, 989
Warm wet compresses, 989
Warts, **788**
Water, as nutrient, 1022–1023
Waterfalls, 197, **197**
Water-soluble vitamins, 1016
Wave scheduling, 275
Webinars, 1416
Weight
in children, 727, 731, **743**
in infants, **729**, 731
measurement of, 611–613, **613, 624–625**, 639
during pregnancy, **661**
Weight control, therapeutic diets for, 1028–1029
Westergren method, **1279**, 1279–1280, **1280**
West Nile virus, 504, **525, 795, 796**
Wet-mount preparation, 692, **699–700, 1352–1353**
Wheelchairs, 984–985, **985**
Wheelchair transfers, **993–996**
Wheezes, 604
White blood cells, 1221, 1222, **1222**, 1268, 1273–1275, **1274, 1275**, 1308. *See also* Leukocytes
Whooping cough, **521**, 738

Wicks, **914**
Wide area network (WAN), 217
WiFi, 218
Wikis, 1416
Wilmut, Ian, **50**
WiMAX, 218
Windows, 197
Wintrobe method, 1279, **1279**
Wireless capsule endoscopy (WCE), 835, **837**
Wireless local area networks (WLANs), 218
Women, in medicine, 48
Wood's lamp, 1350
Workers' compensation insurance, 387–388
Workplace
harassment in, 110–111, 1403
stress in, 60–61
World Health Organization (WHO), 548
Would culture, 1336
Wounds
application of sterile adhesive skin closure strips to, **949–950**
care of, 916–918, **917, 918**
closed, 165, **918**
healing of, 165–167, **167**
irrigation of, **937–938**
open, 166, **917**
Written communication. *See also* Business letters
components of, 328–329, **330, 331**, 331–332
guidelines for, 326–328
legal and ethical issues related to, 341
as medical document, 363, 365, **367**
in medical records, 315–316
meeting agendas as, 337–338, **338**
meeting minutes as, 338, **339**
memoranda as, 337, **338**
preparing and composing, **342–343**
processing incoming, 338–339, **340**
processing outgoing, 339–341, **341, 343–348**
styles for, 332–334, **333–335**
supplies for, 334–337
types of, 337–338, **338, 339**

X

X-rays. *See also* Diagnostic imaging
contrast media and, 958, **959**
equipment for, 957–958, **958**
flat plate, 965
function of, 956
patient preparation for, 958
safety procedures for, 956–957

Y

Yeast cells, 1309
Yeast infections, 1350
Yellow fever, 45

Z

Zen macrobiotic diet, **1035**
Zinc, 1022
ZIP+4, 341
Zoll, Paul, **50**
Z-track intramuscular injection technique, 1115, **1134–1136**